Organic Psychiatry

LISHMAN'S

Organic Psychiatry
A Textbook of Neuropsychiatry

Anthony S. David

Simon Fleminger

Michael D. Kopelman

Simon Lovestone

John D.C. Mellers

FOREWORD BY
Marshal Folstein

FOURTH EDITION

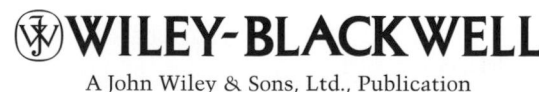

WILEY-BLACKWELL

A John Wiley & Sons, Ltd., Publication

Blackwell Publishing was acquired by John Wiley & Sons in February 2007. Blackwell's publishing program has been merged with Wiley's global Scientific, Technical and Medical business to form Wiley-Blackwell.

Registered office: John Wiley & Sons Ltd, The Atrium, Southern Gate, Chichester, West Sussex, PO19 8SQ, UK

Editorial offices: 9600 Garsington Road, Oxford, OX4 2DQ, UK
The Atrium, Southern Gate, Chichester, West Sussex, PO19 8SQ, UK
111 River Street, Hoboken, NJ 07030-5774, USA

For details of our global editorial offices, for customer services and for information about how to apply for permission to reuse the copyright material in this book please see our website at www.wiley.com/wiley-blackwell

Library of Congress Cataloging-in-Publication Data
Lishman's organic psychiatry : a textbook of neuropsychiatry / Anthony David . . . [et al.]. – 4th ed.
p. ; cm.
Rev. ed. of: Organic psychiatry / William Alwyn Lishman. 3rd. ed. 1998.
Includes bibliographical references and index.
ISBN: 978-1-4051-1860-6
1. Neuropsychiatry.   2. Neurobehavioral disorders–Etiology.
[DNLM: 1. Brain Diseases–complications.   2. Delirium, Dementia, Amnestic, Cognitive Disorders–etiology.   3. Neurobehavioral Manifestations. WM 220 L7692 2006]   I. Title: Organic psychiatry.   II. David, Anthony S.   III. Lishman, William Alwyn. Organic psychiatry.
RC386.L57 2006
616.89'071–dc22

2006005025

A catalogue record for this book is available from the British Library.

Set in 9.25/12 pt Palatino by SNP Best-set Typesetter Ltd., Hong Kong
Printed in Singapore by Fabulous Printers Pte Ltd.
1 2009

Contents

Contributor List, vi

Foreword, vii

Preface to the First Edition, ix

Preface to the Fourth Edition, xi

Part 1 | Principles

1 Basic Concepts in Neuropsychiatry, 3

2 Neuropsychology in Relation to Psychiatry, 29

3 Clinical Assessment, 103

Part 2 | Specific disorders

4 Head Injury, 167

5 Cerebral Tumours, 281

6 Epilepsy, 309

7 Intracranial Infections, 397

8 Cerebrovascular Disorders, 473

9 Alzheimer's Disease and Other Dementias (Including Pseudodementias), 543

10 Endocrine Diseases and Metabolic Disorders, 617

11 Addictive and Toxic Disorders, 689

12 Movement Disorders, 745

13 Sleep Disorders, 817

14 Other Disorders of the Nervous System, 845

Index, 907

Colour plates are found facing p. 468

Contributor List

Mayur Bodani, MRCP MRCPsych
Consultant Neuropsychiatrist
Department of Neuropsychiatry
West Kent Neurorehabilitation Unit
Sevenoaks Hospital
Sevenoaks
Kent

Meryl Dahlitz, MRCPsych
Honorary Research Fellow
Section of Cognitive Neuropsychiatry
Institute of Psychiatry
King's College
London

Anthony S. David, FRCP FRCPsych MSc MD FMedSci
Professor of Cognitive Neuropsychiatry
Institute of Psychiatry
King's College, London;
Honorary Consultant Psychiatrist
South London and Maudsley NHS Foundation Trust
London

Michael D. Dilley, BSc MB MRCPsych
Consultant & Honorary Senior Lecturer
Central & North West London NHS Foundation Trust
Soho Centre for Health and Care
London

Simon Fleminger, PhD FRCP FRCPsych
Consultant Neuropsychiatrist
South London and Maudsley NHS Foundation Trust
London

Marshal Folstein, MD
Professor of Psychiatry
Johns Hopkins Medical Institutions;
Professor of Psychiatry
Tufts School of Medicine
Boston, MA
USA

Neil A. Harrison, MBBS PhD MRCP MRCPsych
Clinical Research Fellow
Institute of Cognitive Neuroscience & Wellcome Trust
    Centre for Neuroimaging
University College;
Honorary SpR Neuropsychiatry
National Hospital for Neurology and Neurosurgery
London

Max Henderson, MBBS MSc MRCP MRCPsych
Locum Consultant and Lecturer in Liaison Psychiatry
Department of Psychological Medicine
Institute of Psychiatry
King's College
London

Michael D. Kopelman, PhD FBPsS FRCPsych
Professor of Neuropsychiatry
Institute of Psychiatry
King's College, London;
Consultant Neuropsychiatrist (St Thomas' Hospital)
South London and Maudsley NHS Foundation Trust
London

Simon Lovestone, PhD MRCPsych
Professor of Old Age Psychiatry
NIHR Biomedical Research Centre for Mental Health;
MRC Centre for Neurodegeneration Research;
Departments of Psychological Medicine and Neuroscience
Institute of Psychiatry
King's College
London

Nuria Mellado-Calvo, MSc MRCPsych
Locum Consultant Psychiatrist
South London and Maudsley NHS Foundation Trust
London

John D.C. Mellers, MBBS MRCPsych
Consultant Neuropsychiatrist
South London and Maudsley NHS Foundation Trust
London

Laurence J. Reed, PhD MRCPsych
Lecturer in Addiction Neurobiology
Institute of Psychiatry
King's College
London

Foreword

It is an honour to introduce to readers the fourth edition of Professor Alwyn Lishman's landmark book *Organic Psychiatry: The Psychological Consequences of Cerebral Disorder*, newly titled *Lishman's Organic Psychiatry: A Textbook of Neuropsychiatry*. Since its first publication in 1978, I have regularly referred to it in my clinical work and research on the psychiatric aspects of neurological disorders.

It was one of the first modern texts to compile knowledge of psychiatric aspects of neurological disorders, including cognition, mood, delusions, hallucinations, obsessions and phobia. Before its publication, patients who had neurological disorders were often deprived of expert psychiatric care, and clinical research workers could not take advantage of these experiments of nature to aid their search for brain–mind connections. *Organic Psychiatry* provided a basis for neuropsychiatric training, patient care and research.

Until early in the 20th century, neurology and psychiatry were, in a number of countries, considered to be a single discipline, but then neurologists such as Charcot and Freud postulated psychological and social roots for anxiety and abnormal behaviours, thus differentiating neurology from psychiatry. Soon, psychiatrists were receiving minimal neurological training and neurologists were receiving minimal psychiatric training. This separation had many consequences, not the least of which was the need for psychiatrists to be reintroduced to the psychiatric aspects of neurological disorders. Professor Lishman's historic text, in its several iterations, has filled this need and fostered the development of the subspecialty of neuropsychiatry.

Several psychiatrists who worked in the years prior to the publication of the first edition directly or indirectly influenced Lishman's work. Adolph Meyer, a psychiatrist and a neuroanatomist, invented a method for documenting the psychological and social context of mental states, now known as the 'case taking notes', which remains a framework for observations necessary for the formulation of individual cases and for research conjectures. At about the same time, Karl Jaspers published the monumental *General Psychopathology*. Jaspers was trained by Franz Nissl who was interested in cortical–subcortical connections and the correlation of psychological states with blood vessels, glia and cortical structures. Jaspers' book defined the methods of psychiatry and also compiled the elements of the mental state to be explained or understood in relation to neurological and social conditions.

Organic Psychiatry also reflects the thought of Jaspers' colleague in Heidelberg, Wilhelm (Willi) Mayer-Gross. Mayer-Gross came to London in 1934 to work with Mapother at the Bethlem and Maudsley hospitals. In 1939 he moved to Birmingham to teach and conduct research in psychiatry. Lishman was to become a medical student there a decade later. Mayer-Gross's major influence on Lishman most likely came through his textbook, *Clinical Psychiatry*, which he wrote with Eliot Slater and Martin Roth. As a neurology resident I was delighted to find a psychiatric text that presented the material in a straightforward descriptive manner, similar to a textbook of internal medicine. *Clinical Psychiatry* included chapters on Alzheimer's disease and other neurological disorders that cause psychiatric symptoms. It published Meyer's case taking notes and a brief, scored cognitive examination that influenced my formulation of the Mini Mental State examination. Lishman generally followed Mayer-Gross's approach, expanding the sections on neurological disorder and more importantly providing evidence for and against assertions that a particular disease caused specific symptoms.

Finally, Lishman was encouraged to undertake the writing of the book by Aubrey Lewis, the first Chairman of the Institute of Psychiatry in London who created what Jaspers called 'the genius of place' that produced Lishman and many other important 20th-century psychiatrists. Denis Hill, who succeeded Lewis as Chairman, continued this encouragement and wrote the foreword to the first edition of the book.

Each and every chapter of the fourth edition of *Organic Psychiatry* has been comprehensively revised and updated by a small group of experts, lead by Tony David, Lishman's successor at the Maudsley Hospital/Institute of Psychiatry, who have maintained the tradition set by Alwyn Lishman and invigorated it. The new textbook has expanded sections on neuropsychology and neuroimaging, both essential disciplines for neuropsychiatric practice and research. Neuropsychology developed from the localisationist ideas of Broca and Wernicke who discovered that discrete lesions of the brain were followed by disorders of language. This view has been replaced by the idea that dysfunction of cortical–subcortical networks has psychological effects. The modern field was initially based on the study of war injuries, and tried to localise psychological functions to discrete brain areas. Neuroimaging has in some ways supplanted or replaced the autopsy as a means for clinical pathological correlation. It has demonstrated the widespread cortical and subcortical networks involved in cognitive impairment and depression. Knowledge of the strengths and weaknesses of imaging technologies is critical for the work of neuropsychiatrists who should be able to evaluate scan results in relation to other clinical features. Interpretation must be cautious because, as the authors note, a lesion seen may or may not be causally related to the clinical features.

Also included is a separate chapter on sleep disorders, a common group of conditions at the interface between neurology and psychiatry, and the elevation of Alzheimer's disease to the chapter title covering this and related dementias. This reflects both its importance as a global health issue and the huge advances in the understanding of its genetic basis and underlying pathophysiology.

The authors' accurate and critical descriptions of the cognitive and non-cognitive features of neurological diseases bring some clarity to these complex interpretations, which reflect the brain–mind relationships. The new edition, like the earlier editions, will be an indispensable guide for the work of psychiatrists, neurologists and neuropsychologists and all students and practitioners working in neuropsychiatry, a growing clinical field.

Marshal Folstein MD, June 2009
Professor of Psychiatry, Johns Hopkins
Medical Institutions; Professor of Psychiatry,
Tufts School of Medicine, USA

Preface to the First Edition

The impetus for writing a book on organic psychiatry has come largely from clinical practice and teaching. Both reveal the lack of focused knowledge concerning the overlapping territories between psychiatry and neurology – a gap manifested in the paucity of textbook literature on the subject. Clearly, as with any borderland zone, there has been a risk of relative neglect as each separate discipline has proceeded on its specialised way, leaving, perhaps inevitably, an uneasy interface between.

Neurology deals directly with the apparatus of mind by investigating malfunction of the brain. Yet paradoxically it has often paid scant attention to mental disorder itself. Psychiatry on its part deals essentially with mental disorder, yet has had little in relative terms to do with the hardware upon which mind depends. The rich complexity of human behaviour, and the multitude of factors which can shape and distort it, have clearly demanded a multifaceted growth of clinical psychiatry; the subject had profited from psychodynamic, psychosocial and pharmacological approaches to mental disorder, but with the expert neurologist waiting in the wings the factor of brain malfunction has sometimes tended to be eclipsed. Sir Denis Hill, in his Foreword to the book, has touched on the dilemma and set it in much wider historical perspective.

It has therefore seemed worthwhile to attempt a comprehensive review of the cognitive, behavioural and emotional consequences of cerebral disorder, and the problems in this area which are encountered in clinical practice. The task proved greater than at first envisaged. In the first place neurology and psychiatry with their attendant disciplines have both proceeded apace, sometimes drawing closer together and sometimes further apart in their different approaches to disease. The literature on their common ground has correspondingly flourished, but in a scattered manner. Secondly it soon became obvious that a text devoted to psychiatric disorders associated with structural brain disease would be unduly restrictive, and that certain metabolic, toxic and other systemic disorders must also be considered if brain malfunction was to be the central theme.

Others could have argued for the inclusion of a good deal more than is here presented. Very little will be found on mental subnormality or child psychiatry since such fields are beyond the author's competence. And the temptation to speculate in detail on possible 'cerebral' contributions to the major functional psychoses has been resisted. Boundaries have in general been drawn short of hypothetical situations, and the work is mainly confined to disorders of cerebral function which are indubitable and well established.

Within the selected field coverage of different topics will no doubt be found inequitable. An avowed preoccupation with focal cerebral disorder, and the light which disease has thrown on regional brain function, will be apparent to the reader. But other considerations have also been at work. Some very rare disease processes are given considerable attention when their psychiatric components can on occasion be important or when important lessons have been learned from them. Similarly the selection of case reports will sometimes illustrate rare conditions or phenomena, if case presentation seems much better than lengthy description for communicating the essence of the matter. In the sections on treatment, physical approaches will often be described in more detail than psychotherapeutic or social interventions, without any necessary assumption that these have less important parts to play in overall management of the patient. Thus in many respects the emphases in the book must be construed, not as reflecting the absolute importance of a topic, but rather the particular slant indicated in a work devoted to organic aspects of psychiatry. Finally if scant attention seems to have been paid to purely psychological reactions to physical disorder this in no sense implies that such aspects are less intriguing or practically important. Matters of space and time, and the patience of the reader, have dictated that lines must be drawn, however arbitrarily and painfully.

Acknowledgements for the help of others are traditionally given, but the list would be long indeed if I were to pay tribute to all the teachers, colleagues and students who have fostered my interest and guided my thinking on the subjects dealt with herein. I will list instead those who have been directly concerned with the book and have often spent generous hours in detailed discussion and the reading of drafts. The late Sir Aubrey Lewis took a keen and encouraging interest in the earlier stages of the work. Sir Denis Hill has given both detailed criticism and constant helpful support. I am greatly indebted to him for generously providing a Foreword to the book. Special thanks must go to Dr Richard Pratt for reading large parts of the manuscript and allowing me to draw on his exceptional knowledge of the literature. Those who have criticized individual sections and chapters include Professor Frank Benson, Professor Robert Cawley, Dr Elaine Drewe, Dr Griffith Edwards, Professor George Fenton, Dr John Gunn, Dr Derek Hockaday, Dr Raymond Levy, Professor David Marsden, Dr David Parkes, Dr Felix Post and Dr Sabina Strich. Others who have helped in innumerable ways include Dr Christopher Colbourn, Mrs Isobel Colbourn, Dr John Cutting, Dr May Monro, Dr Maria Ron and Dr Brian Toone. Miss Helen Marshall put at my disposal her unrivalled expertise in guiding me to the rich store of information in the Institute of Psychiatry library. To all of these kind friends and colleagues I am very deeply grateful.

Finally I must record my gratitude to the two people who have been most intimately concerned of all. Mrs Dorothy Wiltshire has not only collaborated on an arduous task, but has positively welcomed the burden and done much to sustain my enthusiasm. Her expert secretarial skills and untiring patience have, in effect, made the venture possible. My wife, Marjorie, deserves the warmest thanks of all – meticulous help with the manuscripts and with problems of the English language have been but a tiny part; over several years she has paved the way, deflected obstacles and taken over numerous burdens in an ever-helpful manner which is most affectionately acknowledged.

Alwyn Lishman, June 1977

Preface to the Fourth Edition

When Alwyn Lishman suggested that I might edit the fourth edition of his famous tome my reaction was one of huge delight mixed with equal trepidation. It took five co-editors with the help of some young and energetic colleagues to finally complete the task, a fact that only goes to emphasise his monumental achievement in bringing about the previous three editions of *Organic Psychiatry*. It is clearly no longer tenable for a single person to maintain the level of detailed analysis and standard of exposition across the entire breadth of neuropsychiatry that Lishman set, given the explosion in neuroscientific and clinical insights over the last two decades.

The team of co-editors in many ways selected themselves, being firmly rooted in complementary aspects of neuropsychiatry, currently working as clinicians and academics at the Maudsley Hospital/Institute of Psychiatry and having various degrees of affiliation with Alwyn Lishman. I would like to take this opportunity to thank them for their undying enthusiasm, painstaking hard work and good humour.

This fourth edition has a new title that honours Lishman's original accomplishment but makes it clear that this is not a cosmetic makeover but a new textbook. The awesome task that was required of us was to somehow preserve the single authoritative authorial voice of Alwyn Lishman while at the same time bringing new perspectives and clinical research to bear on the topics of neuropsychiatry. The clinical descriptions are, of course, timeless and these have been left largely intact, but new classificatory systems, new understandings in biology and, to some extent, new treatment approaches have displaced much of the previous edition. Thanks to our sub-editors and publisher the format has been rendered more easy on the eye, with highlighted text and boxes of information. There are many more tables and illustrations. However, there has been no attempt to 'dumb down' the content. Readers seeking a quick and easy fix to ignorance in neuropsychiatry should look elsewhere.

The basic chapter structure remains although we begin with the principles of neuropsychiatry, which incorporates the previous small chapter on differential diagnosis. The next chapter is, as pointed out by Marshal Folstein, a new departure and brings in more neuropsychology which is of course a bedrock science for neuropsychiatry. The clinical assessment chapter includes illustrations, particularly of magnetic resonance brain images, as this is such a dominant diagnostic tool. The first chapter in the 'disorders' section is Head Injury, by Simon Fleminger, and brings in a raft of new material both in terms of pathophysiology and prognosis. The Cerebral Tumours chapter by Drs Fleminger and Mellado Calvo has also been extensively revised and it is pleasing to see more on treatment and effects of treatment in this chapter. John Mellers has carried out many fundamental revisions and additions to the Epilepsy chapter reflecting new approaches to classification, diagnosis and treatment in that field. In Intracranial Infections, Simon Fleminger, ably abetted by Mike Dilley, takes on infections of historic significance and very modern conditions, such as HIV-AIDS which Lishman introduced in the third edition, knowledge of which has now matured through the introduction of effective chemo- and immunotherapy. This is followed by the last of Simon Fleminger's contributions, Cerebrovascular Disorders, which contains information on new vascular syndromes of importance in neuropsychiatry. Simon Lovestone, a Professor of Old Age Psychiatry, has taken on Alzheimer's disease and other dementias. This chapter bears little resemblance to its equivalent in the previous edition, reflecting the massive strides in the understanding of Alzheimer's and related dementias from a molecular genetic point of view. The next two chapters, on endocrine/metabolic disorders and toxic disorders were both led by Mike Kopelman with the help of Neil Harrison, Lawrence Reed and Mayur Bodani. These chapters show considerable reworking from the previous edition but with toxic disorders, including effects of alcohol, continuing to exert its full weight. Indeed, in some respects the term 'organic psychiatry' more readily encompasses such issues, whereas neuropsychiatry can be interpreted in a very narrow sense as only applying to diseases of the brain. Clearly our preferred usage of neuropsychiatry includes the whole range of conditions that can affect brain and mind, directly and indirectly. In the movement disorders chapter John Mellers and Max Henderson bring recent discoveries in molecular genetics to the understanding of Parkinson's disease, dystonias and less common disorders of the basal ganglia. The next chapter is on sleep and related disorders and is ably managed by Mike Kopelman and Meryl Dahlitz. Sleep disorders were previously embedded within a 'ragbag' final chapter but such are the advances in the field that we felt that this cluster of very common as well as some esoteric disorders deserves a chapter in its own right. However, there remains the necessity for a final chapter bringing together other miscellaneous disorders and Simon Lovestone manfully took this on. It includes as before, psychiatric aspects of multiple sclerosis and neuromuscular conditions plus the paraneoplastic neuropsychiatric syndromes that in many ways constitute 'breaking news'; even now there are novel disorders to be discovered and described.

It has been a privilege to steer this effort to completion. It has been a wondrous, if sometimes tortuous, journey. Many people, too numerous to name, have helped along the way: clinicians, managers, neurophysiologists, neuropsychologists, etc. Special mention should go to the late Ginny Ng, consultant neuroradiologist who provided some of the MR images and helped educate all of us in their interpretation and, more recently, Naomi Sibtain, who has carried on this tradition. The publishers in their various incarnations have remained steadfastly behind the project. Finally, the greatest thanks must go to Alwyn Lishman himself for inspiring all of us to carry on his work and for providing a benign watchful presence as we do so.

Anthony S. David, January 2009

I am deeply grateful to my younger colleagues who have produced this new edition of 'Organic Psychiatry', and particularly to Professor Tony David who bravely undertook to coordinate their efforts. They have, at a stroke, liberated me from a somewhat daunting task, and at the same time brought the book forward into the new millennium.

When I look back on the preparation of previous editions I realise the extent of the debt I then owed to day-to-day clinical practice, coupled with the stimulation afforded by colleagues, students and research associates, not to mention the availability on site of a first-class library. In short, the unique atmosphere of the Institute of Psychiatry kept me, almost insensibly, abreast of progress. Now, well into my retirement, I have been forced to recognise that without this special environment it would be foolhardy to attempt to update the text once more myself.

The next important step was to free the new editors in turn, and leave them to proceed unfettered by any intrusions on my part. I could not have taken so bold a decision without close acquaintance with all of the editors and having the utmost confidence in them. They are clearly present-day leaders in the neuropsychiatric field and with special interests that bring added strengths to their capabilities for the task.

It has been a privilege to witness the extraordinary growth of interest and progress in this sub-specialty of psychiatry since the era when the first edition of the book was published in 1978. In part, this has derived from the astonishing advances in the neurosciences that have made brain structure and function increasingly relevant to mental, as well as neurological, disorder, also in part from the rapprochement between neurologists, psychiatrists and neuropsychologists as they pursue overlapping areas of research and clinical endeavour. The consequent burgeoning of knowledge and its attendant literature have gradually made it unrealistic for a single author to attempt to encompass the subject matter satisfactorily. My appreciation and my indebtedness towards the architects of this fourth edition are therefore great indeed.

Alwyn Lishman, January 2009

The distinction between symptoms and signs that is customary in general medicine is often difficult to make where psychological phenomena are concerned. To avoid repetition, 'symptoms' will often be used alone when both the patient's complaints and the psychological abnormalities detected by the examiner are being considered together. For similar reasons 'he' or 'his' will often be used when 'he/she' or 'his/her' would be more appropriate and correct.

PART 1

Principles

CHAPTER 1

Basic Concepts in Neuropsychiatry

Anthony S. David

Institute of Psychiatry, King's College, London

What is neuropsychiatry?

In most psychiatric illnesses the clinical picture is profoundly coloured and sometimes decisively shaped by factors specific to the individual and his environment. Hence the notorious difficulty in identifying separate disease processes in psychiatry. This is compounded still further, where most mental disorders are concerned, by the lack of collateral evidence by means of tissue pathology. Alwyn Lishman used the term 'organic psychiatry' to describe those disorders 'in which there is a high probability that appropriate examination and investigation will uncover some cerebral or systemic pathology responsible for, or contributing to, the mental condition'. He contrasted this with the term 'neuropsychiatry', which he took to be a more specific discipline at the interface between neurology and psychiatry, concerned with disorders that can be demonstrated to owe their origins 'to brain malfunction of a clearly identifiable nature' and thus not including endocrine, toxic and metabolic disorders. While these disorders operate via disturbances in brain function, they are, according to Lishman, the concern of general medicine rather than neurology. Despite the clarity and merits of this distinction, 'neuropsychiatry' has become the more widely used term and is generally not used in its more restrictive sense. It is used here synonymously with organic psychiatry but broader still to include those conditions that might appear at first sight to be caused by pathology of the nervous system with manifestations in the neurological domain, but which turn out not to be so; in fact psychological and social factors predominate in the clinical formulation – in other words, the so-called conversion disorders. Inclusion of such disorders may be justified on pragmatic grounds since they contribute to a sizeable proportion of the workload of the neuropsychiatrist and related health professional. Further, the differential diagnosis of conversion is, by definition, neurological; likewise, conversion disorders contribute to the differential diagnoses of most neuropsychiatric conditions.

Before leaving the issue of definitions, it is worth reiterating here two other aspects dealt with by Alwyn Lishman in his preface to the second and third editions of his textbook. First, we wholly subscribe to Lishman's injunction that neuropsychiatry 'must capitalise on all that psychiatry has to offer' including psychodynamic, social and cultural aspects, and that 'neuropsychiatric practice requires a widening not a narrowing of psychiatric skills and interests'. Second, neuropsychiatry does not claim to be the only branch of psychiatry where the brain and other biological systems are relevant, far from it. The term 'biological psychiatry' is rightly reserved for the approach (rather than the clinical discipline) concerned with 'pathophysiologies of a biological nature' which can be brought to bear on increasingly numerous if not all forms of psychiatric disorder to varying extents.

The psychological disturbances which result from brain pathology often share common ground that cuts across differences in background, personality and social situation. They are related to pathological processes within the brain, or acting on the brain, which can often be identified by the techniques of medical investigation. In these respects neuropsychiatry draws closer to the rest of medicine, and should at least in theory be amenable to a similar approach in leading towards useful clinicopathological correlations.

In large measure this is so. However, psychological symptoms are hard to identify objectively and can rarely be measured accurately. Difficulties of assessment increase abruptly as we ascend from basic motor and sensory processes to mental phenomena, and especially when we move from simple cognitive impairments to changes in emotion, personality and other complex aspects of behaviour. Moreover, when symptoms characteristic of the neuroses or major psychoses emerge in the brain-damaged person, it is necessary to consider the possibility that he may have been specially

Lishman's Organic Psychiatry: A Textbook of Neuropsychiatry, 4th edition.
© 2009 Blackwell Publishing.   ISBN 978-1-4051-1860-1

predisposed to their development. Ultimately, indeed, we are often forced back again to the problems of the main body of psychiatry, since the more complex effects of cerebral disorder can be properly assessed only when the whole individual is viewed in the context of his personal history and environment. The situation is therefore a good deal more complex than in most other branches of medicine, and the opportunities for relating abnormalities of behaviour to precise aspects of cerebral pathology are limited in several important respects.

Fortunately for the diagnostic process, neuropsychiatric disorders tend to have certain features in common that usually allow them to be distinguished from non-organic mental illnesses. Different varieties of pathological change are often associated with similar forms of impairment. Bonhoeffer (1909), who coined the term 'exogenous psychoses', deserves the credit for recognising this and discarding the Kraepelinian view that each noxious agent affecting the brain evokes a specific psychiatric picture. Impairment of consciousness, for example, may result from a number of toxic processes acting on the brain or from raised intracranial pressure; dementia may result from anoxia, from trauma or from primary degenerative disease. It is therefore possible to extract important symptoms and syndromes that indicate the possibility of cerebral disorder whatever the basic pathology and despite the colouring lent by pathoplastic features. Such symptoms form the cornerstone of diagnosis in neuropsychiatry and it is essential to recognise their earliest and most minor manifestations. Many disease processes affecting the brain will come to attention with psychological symptoms alone and well before the appearance of definite neurological signs, and it is often by the correct appreciation of these common forms of reaction that a mistaken diagnosis of non-organic (or so-called 'functional') psychiatric disorder will be avoided.

Other forms of presentation may indeed occur with change of personality, affective disturbance, neurotic symptoms or even pictures indicative of schizophrenia. The clinician must remain aware that occasionally a mental illness presenting in this way may be related to the early stages of cerebral disease. Such cases are not infrequent and their detection by judicious application of ever more sensitive and non-invasive investigations such as magnetic resonance imaging increasingly likely; however, as the condition progresses, organic mental symptoms will usually appear.

Basic concepts and terminology

This chapter describes various frameworks for grouping together the cardinal psychological symptoms and signs of cerebral disorder. The principal accent will be on the shared forms of reaction common to most individuals and to different pathological processes, though features particular to individuals are also briefly described where appropriate. The feature that distinguishes neuropsychiatric

disorders from the rest of psychiatry is cognitive impairment.

A main division is the temporal one, i.e. 'acute' and 'chronic' reactions. These terms are clinically useful for broad classification and for shorthand description of groups of clinical phenomena. A topographical distinction, namely 'focal' versus 'generalised' or 'diffuse', can be superimposed on this temporal division, so that both acute and chronic conditions can be focal or diffuse in nature.

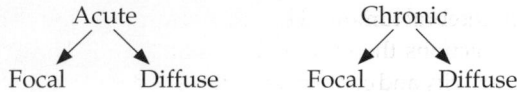

Acute versus chronic cerebral disorder

Acute organic reaction and *chronic organic reaction* are the terms best used for the first major division of organic psychiatric illnesses, each functioning as no more than a pointer to a class of problems, and serving only as starting points for further enquiries into aetiology. These terms carry implications for abruptness and onset and to some extent for the constellation of symptoms most in evidence. Each may show features not seen in the other, and requiring specific approaches for their identification. The terms also carry implications for likely duration, but not directly for ultimate prognosis. It is more usual for acute than for chronic organic reactions to recover, but the prognosis in each case will depend on the precise aetiology at work. A separate category of 'subacute organic reactions' is sometimes demarcated, and merely implies less sudden onset than the acute disorders, somewhat longer continuation, and an admixture of clinical symptoms characteristic of acute and chronic reactions. It must be accepted, however, that both acute and chronic reactions will vary in the degree of their acuteness or chronicity, and that in some cases the former will, with time, prove to merge into the latter.

The temporal dimension or time course is one of the most critical indicators in the evaluation of chronic neuropsychiatric conditions. The clinical course of the disorder reveals many clues as to its nature. These may be variously described as progressive, stepwise, relapsing and remitting, etc. A progressive course implies degeneration or the gradual expansion of a space-occupying lesion. A stepwise course classically describes the intermittent but accumulating deficit as a consequence of repeated vascular events. A relapsing and remitting course suggests an inflammatory processes, such as multiple sclerosis, especially where each relapse adds a residuum of impairment or disability. Acute disturbances followed by complete recovery suggest disorders of function such as physiological disruptions to cerebral or neural activity without the enduring stamp of tissue pathology, as occurs with electrical disturbances or transient metabolic upsets or indeed a 'non-organic' aetiology.

Generalised versus focal cerebral disorder

A great number of organic psychiatric disorders are due to widespread disturbance of brain function. This may be the result of diffuse disease processes within the brain, as in certain degenerative diseases, or of systemic disturbances, for example those leading to anoxia which impair brain function indirectly. Moreover, well-localised brain lesions may declare themselves only when secondary diffuse effects supervene, as with raised intracranial pressure in association with cerebral tumour. The majority of acute and chronic organic reactions therefore reflect widespread disorder of cerebral activity and contain symptoms of defective function in many spheres.

It has become customary to talk of 'generalised cerebral disorder' and to distinguish this from the effects of strictly focal pathology. However, it must be appreciated that both generalised and focal disturbances of brain function represent theoretical extremes that are rarely if ever encountered in practice. It is most unlikely that intrinsic brain disease is ever uniformly distributed throughout the brain, and some degree of focal emphasis can usually be discerned with careful observation. Extrinsic factors that impair brain function are likewise selective in their effects, sparing some neural or neurochemical systems while disrupting others. Impairment of consciousness, for example, represents interference with brainstem alerting functions while cardiovascular and respiratory functions are little affected. Similarly, disruption of cortical and subcortical functions very rarely occurs to an equivalent extent.

Strictly focal disorder, on the other hand, is also very rare except when purposely produced by surgical procedures. In naturally occurring disease we merely see a focal emphasis of pathology, which in greater or lesser degree is complicated by the additional effects of damage elsewhere.

Nevertheless it is of great importance in practical clinical terms to preserve the distinction between clinical pictures that result from widely disseminated or from relatively circumscribed brain dysfunction. The distinction is essential in the formulation of likely causes and thence in deciding the lines which investigation must follow. Each, in practice, contains different symptoms of fundamental importance.

The plan in this chapter will be first to describe in broad terms the characteristic clinical pictures seen in 'generalised' acute and chronic reactions, and then to summarise the salient features seen with focal damage or focal emphasis of pathology in specific brain regions. The focal significance of certain symptoms and symptom complexes is dealt with in more detail in Chapter 2.

Commonly used terms

The following are some commonly used terms of general clinical description.

Confusion refers to symptoms and signs which indicate that the patient is unable to think with his customary clarity and coherence. Cognitive impairment is often used nowadays as a portmanteau term in preference to confusion. It is seen in both organic and non-organic mental disturbances, and the term is useful merely as a shorthand clinical description of an important aspect of such mental states. In acute organic reactions, confusion is due largely to impairment of consciousness. In chronic organic reactions, it betrays the disruption of thought processes due to structural brain damage. In a whole range of psychiatric disorders, confusion of thinking may be much in evidence without any identifiable brain pathology whatever; similarly when powerful emotions from any cause interfere with the efficient ordering of cognitive processes. The term 'toxic confusional state' is widely used but can properly be applied only when toxic influences on the brain have been established.

Clouding of consciousness denotes the mildest stage of impairment of consciousness which is detectable clinically, on the continuum from full alertness and awareness to coma. As such it is manifest as slight impairment of thinking, attending, perceiving and remembering, in other words as mild global impairment of cognitive processes in association with reduced awareness of the environment. The patient will frequently, though not always, appear to be drowsy but this is not to be confused with the normal transition to sleep.

Twilight states. Among Bonhoeffer's 'forms of exogenous reaction' due to pathogenic factors acting on the brain, twilight states and delirium were separately demarcated. The essential features appear to include abrupt onset and ending, variable duration from hours to weeks, and the interruption of quiet periods of behaviour by unexpected and sometimes violent acts or outbursts of rage or fear. Other descriptions include dream-like 'oneiroid' states, vivid hallucinations and delusional ideas that dictate powerful affective disturbance. Clearly, therefore, the term is used to cover a variety of syndromes and can now have little useful meaning. It is, moreover, widely employed to describe hysterical manifestations in addition to acute organic reactions (particularly some types of complex partial seizure).

Coma represents the extreme of a graded continuum of impairment of consciousness, at the opposite pole of the spectrum from full alertness and awareness of the environment. The patient is incapable of sensing or responding adequately to external stimuli or inner needs, shows little or no spontaneous movement apart from respiration, and no evidence whatever of mental activity.

Coma is itself a graded phenomenon. At its deepest there is no reaction to stimuli of any intensity, and corneal, pupillary, pharyngeal, tendon and plantar reflexes are absent. Respiration is slow and sometimes periodic (Cheyne–Stokes respiration) and cardiovascular regulating processes may show signs of failure. Lighter degrees of coma (semicoma) allow partial response to stimulation, though this is incomplete, mostly non-purposive and usually consists of ineffectual movements or rubbing and scratching of the stimulated area. Bladder distension may call forth groaning or ill-coordinated motor stirring but the patient is still incontinent. Tendon reflexes may or may not be obtainable, and the plantars may be either flexor or extensor. The Glasgow Coma Scale, which has proved its usefulness for the grading of depth of coma, is described in Chapter 4, Measuring head injury severity.

Coma needs to be distinguished from deep sleep and from stupor. In deep sleep and in coma the pictures may be closely similar on superficial observation, but the sleeper can be roused again to normal consciousness by the efforts of the examiner. He may wake spontaneously to unaccustomed stimuli, or in response to inner sensations such as hunger or bladder distension. In sleep there is sporadic continuing mental activity in the form of dreams which leave traces in memory. Coma is more difficult to demarcate from stupor, which is described below. The distinguishing features usually accepted are that in coma the eyes remain shut even in response to strong arousal stimuli, do not resist passive opening, and do not appear to be watchful or follow moving objects; movements in response to stimulation are never purposeful, and there is no subsequent recall of events or inner fantasies from the time in question (see also persistent vegetative state, Chapter 4).

Stupor is an exceedingly difficult term to define, principally because it has been used widely in neurological and psychiatric practice to refer to conditions with markedly different causation. Sometimes it is used loosely and wrongly to refer to an intermediate stage on the continuum of impairment of consciousness that leads ultimately to coma; sometimes to refer to a syndrome characteristic of lesions in the neighbourhood of the diencephalon and upper brainstem and called akinetic mutism; and sometimes to clinical states superficially similar to this but due to hysterical, depressive or schizophrenic illness. Stupor is thus a term without definite nosological status, but valuable when properly used in referring, in essence, to a clinical syndrome of akinesis and mutism but with evidence of relative preservation of conscious awareness. There is a profound lack of responsiveness, and evidence of impairment, or at least putative or apparent impairment, of consciousness. Speech and spontaneous movement are absent or reduced to a minimum, and the patient is inaccessible to the great majority of external stimuli. Unlike coma and semicoma, however, the patient may at first sight appear to be conscious, since the eyes may be open and seem to be watchful. The patient may direct his gaze towards the examiner and the eyes may follow moving visual stimuli in a manner which appears to be purposeful rather than random. When the eyes are shut

they may resist passive opening. Relative preservation of consciousness is also betrayed by the response to stimulation: strong painful stimuli may induce blinking or purposeful coordinated efforts to dislodge the noxious agent. Moreover, in some cases there is subsequent recall of events or delusional fantasies occurring in the stuporose state.

Typically, spontaneous movements are absent but there may be tremors, coarse twitching or, in light stupor, restless stereotyped motor activity. The latter may seem to occur in response to hallucinatory experiences, or to display special meaning in stupors due to psychotic illness. Here also the resting posture may be awkward or bizarre, or it may be meaningful in the context of the patient's delusions. Reflexes are usually entirely normal. Complete mutism is the rule, but again there may sometimes be partially coherent muttering, or arousal may be possible to the extent of brief stereotyped exclamations. In light stupor there may be no sphincter disturbance, and even feeding may be possible with coaxing. Simple responses to commands may then be obtained, though these are slow, inaccurate and often ill-coordinated. The least severe examples may merge indefinably with severe psychomotor retardation in psychotic depression, or with severe blocking of thought and volition in catatonic schizophrenia. The causes of stupor and their differential diagnoses are considered later in this chapter.

Organic personality change. Brain damage often results in changes of temperament, or changed patterns of reaction to events and to other people. As a result, behavioural tendencies that have previously been enduring characteristics of the individual are found to be altered. Areas typically affected include the control of emotions and impulses and aspects of motivation and social judgement (Lipowski 1980). Such 'change of personality' is usually prominent in dementia, and is then seen along with cognitive defects. But sometimes brain damage may operate more directly by disruption of regional cerebral systems upon which the synthesis of the personality depends. This situation is compatible with excellent preservation of intellect to formal testing, yet the personality change is nonetheless organic in origin. Thus when disturbance of cognitive processes cannot be identified, the term 'organic personality change' is preferable to 'dementia'. Most examples occur with strictly focal brain damage, the best known being with lesions of the frontal lobes of the brain. A clear discontinuity between the current and premorbid personality is essential if this term is to retain its meaning.

Chronic amnesic syndrome. Disorder of memory, especially for recent events, is an integral part of dementia, but can also exist without global impairment of intellect. Such memory disturbance may emerge as the sole defect, as after bilateral hippocampal lesions, or more commonly may stand out as the obtrusive defect while other cognitive processes are but little affected. Such a syndrome may follow an acute organic reaction which clears to reveal a relatively isolated defect of memory, as when Wernicke's encephalopathy leads to Korsakoff's syndrome.

The term 'chronic amnesic syndrome' usefully describes the essential features of disorder in all its forms, and emphasises the distinction from dementia. It may be defined as an organic impairment of memory out of all proportion to other cognitive changes. A focal rather than a diffuse brain pathology can be confidently predicted as described. Unfortunately, the terms 'chronic amnesic syndrome' and 'Korsakoff's amnesic syndrome' are sometimes used interchangeably, the territory of the latter being allowed to expand considerably. Strictly speaking, the term 'Korsakoff's syndrome' should be restricted to those patients whose amnesia depends on lesions in the hypothalamus and diencephalon and is consequent upon thiamine deficiency.

Organic hallucinosis refers to a syndrome of recurrent or persistent hallucinations, occurring in a setting of full preservation of consciousness and awareness of the environment yet attributable to organic factors. The patient is not disorientated and proves capable of thinking with normal clarity throughout. The hallucinations occur mostly in the auditory or visual modalities but any sensory modality can be affected. Insight into the unreal nature of the phenomena may vary markedly in degree, but any delusions that occur are secondary to the hallucinatory experiences. Such a syndrome may be occasioned by circumscribed brain lesions, strategically placed to irritate cortical or subcortical areas, but is more commonly seen as a result of toxic processes. The hallucinations occurring during the early phase of alcohol withdrawal or after ingestion of hallucinogenic drugs are typical examples.

The prototypical acute and chronic organic reactions are delirium and dementia respectively. These have been operationally defined in the two current major classificatory systems, the Diagnostic and Statistical Manual of Mental Disorders (DSM)-IV and the International Classification of Diseases (ICD)-10 (Boxes 1.1 and 1.2).

Delirium. There are many meanings and definitions of this term, sometimes embracing all varieties of acute organic reaction, sometimes referring to the degree of overt disturbance, and sometimes confining its use to clinical pictures with certain specific features. Special characteristics have included wakefulness with ability to respond verbally, increased psychomotor activity, pronounced disturbance of affect, defective reality testing, or the appearance of productive symptoms in the form of illusions and hallucinations. Delirium tremens is often taken as a prototype for delirium, and contrasted with the 'simple confusion' of subdued cognitive impairment in other illnesses, although this is categorised separately in DSM and ICD. In the UK it was formerly

---

Box 1.1 DSM-IV and ICD-10 classifications of delirium

DSM-IV criteria

A Disturbance of consciousness (i.e. reduced clarity of the environment) with reduced ability to focus sustain or shift attention.

B A change in cognition (such as memory deficit, disorientation, language disturbance) or the development of a perceptual disturbance.

C The disturbance develops over a short period of time (usually hours to days) and tends to fluctuate during the course of the day.

D There is evidence from the history, physical examination or laboratory findings that the disturbance is caused by the direct physiological consequences of a general medical condition/ substance intoxication/withdrawal/multiple aetiologies. [Each subcategory has its own additional criteria including 'Delirium not otherwise specified'.]

ICD-10 criteria

(a) Impairment of consciousness and attention, with reduced ability to direct, focus, sustain, and shift attention.

(b) Global disturbance of cognition: perceptual distortions, illusions and hallucinations, mostly in the visual modality; impairment of abstract thinking and comprehension; impairment of immediate recall and recent memory; disorientation for time and sometimes place and person as well.

(c) Psychomotor disturbance which may consist of hypoactivity or hyperactivity or unpredictable shifts between the two.

(d) Disturbance of the sleep–wake cycle: insomnia, daytime drowsiness, sleep reversal; nocturnal worsening of symptoms; or disturbing dreams and nightmares which may continue as hallucinations on awakening.

(e) Emotional disturbances: depression, anxiety, fear, irritability, euphoria, apathy or perplexity.

---

traditional to reserve the term for patients whose acute cerebral disorder resulted in some degree of disturbed or disruptive behaviour, i.e. to emphasise the restless hyperactivity and emotional disturbance which is so commonly part of the picture. It is clear, however, that not all patients who meet current criteria for delirium present like this, some showing predominant listlessness, inertia and dulling of the senses. In a daily evaluation of 125 patients who met DSM-III criteria for delirium in a general hospital, Liptzin and Levkoff (1992) classified 15% as hyperactive, 19% as hypoactive, 52% as mixed and 14% as neither.

It is important to appreciate that consciousness is not merely quantitatively reduced in delirium, but also qualitatively changed. Typically the patient becomes preoccupied with his own inner world which is distorted by illusions, hallucinations and delusions, and sometimes by powerful

For an ICD-10 research diagnosis of dementia (World Health Organization 1993) there must be evidence of the following.

1 A decline in memory affecting both verbal and non-verbal material, sufficient at least to interfere with everyday activities.

2 A decline in other cognitive abilities, characterised by deterioration in judgement and thinking and in the general processing of information. Deterioration from a previously higher level of performance should be established. For a confident diagnosis both 1 and 2 must have been present for at least 6 months.

3 Preserved awareness of the environment during a period sufficiently long to allow the unequivocal demonstration of the symptoms in 1 and 2; when there are superimposed episodes of delirium, the diagnosis of dementia should be deferred.

4 Decline in emotional control or motivation, or a change in social behaviour manifest as at least one of emotional lability, irritability, apathy or coarsening of social behaviour.

DSM-IV specifies individual criteria for dementia of the Alzheimer-type, vascular dementia, etc., the common elements being as follows.

A The development of multiple cognitive deficits manifested by both:

1 memory impairment;

2 one or more of aphasia, apraxia, agnosia or disturbance of executive function (planning, organising, sequencing, abstracting).

B Such cognitive deficits cause significant impairment in social or occupational functioning, and represent a significant decline from a previous level of functioning.

C The course is characterised by gradual onset and continuing cognitive decline.

D The deficits do not occur exclusively during the course of a delirium.

Further inclusion and exclusion criteria then apply to the several varieties of dementia specified in DSM-IV.

affective changes derived therefrom or more directly from dysfunction of specific brain systems. Even though awareness of external events is impaired, arousal may be high, enabling these productive symptoms to occur. The fluctuations in severity are commonly accompanied by fluctuations in content, manifesting as a continuously changing clinical picture. Many different disturbances of cerebral function can lead to delirium, with little that can be regarded as specific in the clinical pictures that result. Toxic and metabolic disturbances are perhaps prone to be associated with listlessness and apathy, and infective processes and alcohol withdrawal syndromes with hyperactivity, fearfulness and prominent hallucinations.

DSM-IV divides the syndrome into delirium due to a general medical condition, substance-induced delirium, and delirium due to multiple aetiologies (American Psychiatric Association 1994). Fundamental to all is a disturbance of consciousness (i.e. reduced clarity of awareness of the environment) coupled with a reduced ability to focus, sustain or shift attention. Additional requirements are a change in cognition (such as memory deficit, disorientation or language disturbance) or the development of a perceptual disturbance (misinterpretations, illusions or hallucinations, mainly visual), with the proviso that these are not better accounted for by a pre-existing or evolving dementia. The disturbance develops over a short period of time (usually hours to days) and tends to fluctuate during the course of the day.

The ICD-10 classification (World Health Organization 1992) similarly stresses concurrent disturbances of consciousness and attention, along with changes in cognition, perception, psychomotor behaviour, sleep–wake cycle and emotion. The disorder is usually rapid in onset, with diurnal fluctuations, most cases recovering within 4 weeks or less but sometimes continuing for up to 6 months.

'*Dementia*' is used in two contexts which must be clearly distinguished: first to label a group of specific disease entities, and secondly to refer to a clinical syndrome that can have many other causes. The specific diseases for which the term is used are considered in Chapter 9. They are characterised by progressive and widespread and inexorable brain degeneration. When denoting a syndrome, however, the term may validly be used more widely, and can be defined very simply as an acquired global impairment of intellect, memory and personality, but without impairment of consciousness. As such it is almost always of long duration, usually progressive and often irreversible, but these features are not included as part of the definition.

The syndrome therefore consists of a constellation of symptoms that suggest chronic and widespread brain dysfunction. Global impairment of cognition or intellect is the central and essential feature, manifest as difficulty with memory, attention, thinking and comprehension. Other mental functions are usually affected concurrently, and changes of mood, personality and social behaviour may sometimes be the outstanding or even presenting features. Nevertheless 'dementia' should not be used to describe such changes unless intellectual deterioration can be identified.

Historically the term has acquired implications for inevitable decline and irreversibility. This remains true for the disease entities of dementia, but not for all the settings in which the syndrome may appear. The dementia accompanying general paresis can be arrested, and that due to head injury or normal-pressure hydrocephalus may improve with time or treatment. We are now in a new era of effective treatment for Alzheimer's and related dementias, at least in the short and medium terms. Thus when matters of prognosis are excluded from the definition, the term can be used whatever the cause of the syndrome and whatever future therapeutic discoveries may bring.

It is also important that the syndrome be defined in terms of global impairment of cognitive functions and not in terms of diffuse cerebral damage. Focal brain damage can sometimes lead to global impairment of intellect, memory and personality in addition to regional deficits. Frontal lobe tumours are notorious in this regard, and can produce a picture of dementia indistinguishable at first sight from other causes. In such cases it remains logical to use the term to describe the clinical picture which presents for attention, even though diffuse affection of brain tissue is not the immediate cause. Indeed some forms of dementia are best regarded as the end-result of multiple focal pathologies that coalesce and combine to impair functions globally, as in the vascular dementias. It is essential, therefore, to avoid defining the syndrome in terms of a pathology which has yet to be displayed.

The term is thus reserved for the description of a group of clinical symptoms, while all considerations of prognosis and aetiology are excluded from the definition. This has a certain practical importance, in that once the syndrome has been identified it must always dictate a search for ultimate causes. These may be focal or diffuse, within or without the brain, and may have possibilities for treatment.

Clinical picture in acute organic reactions (acute brain syndrome, acute confusional state, 'delirium')

The acute organic reactions are called forth by a great number of different pathological processes affecting the brain, including trauma, cerebral anoxia, epilepsy, metabolic derangements such as uraemia, or the toxic effects of drugs or alcohol. A list of causes is presented in Table 1.1. The onset is always fairly abrupt, though when slight in degree the disorder may not declare itself in an obvious fashion from the outset. The majority of acute organic reactions are reversible when the underlying pathology can be remedied, but some may progress directly to a chronic organic syndrome, as when an acute post-traumatic psychosis clears to reveal dementia or when Wernicke's encephalopathy results in an enduring amnesic syndrome.

The clinical pictures which result are essentially due to disruption of normal brain function by virtue of biochemical, electrical or mechanical disturbances. The symptomatology follows a surprisingly constant pattern despite these various causes. To some extent there are specific features depending on rate of development, the intensity and perhaps the nature of the noxious agent, but this variability is small in relative terms. The personality and background of the patient will also colour the picture, especially in minor affections and particularly where matters such as intensity of emotional

disturbance or content of delusional thinking are concerned. The main emphasis in what follows, however, will be on shared and common forms of reaction. There is a growing tendency to treat delirium as a problem in its own right with an epidemiology, collection of risk factors, prognosis and treatment strategies (see Burns *et al.* 2004 for review). This reverses years of neglect as a topic for clinical research. The settings in which delirium is most commonly seen, outside those in which acute infections of the central nervous system (CNS) are endemic, are services for the elderly, those undergoing palliative care and in the postoperative situation, especially following cardiothoracic procedures. Simple but comprehensive medical and nursing procedures to minimise and reduce the impact of delirium have now been the subject of clinical trials (Britton & Russell 2004). It is obvious that treatment of delirium should target the underlying cause, but managing a very disturbed patient in the mean time often requires judicious use of parenteral antipsychotic drugs or short-acting benzodiazepines.

Impairment of consciousness

Impairment of consciousness is the primary change in acute organic reactions, and in some degree is universal. It therefore holds a fundamentally important place in the detection of acute disturbances of brain function and in the assessment of their severity. Other features, such as disordered psychomotor activity, perception and emotion, may be more striking but are less constantly found and are also more variable in their manifestations.

Impairment of consciousness lies on a continuum that ranges from barely perceptible dulling of awareness to profound coma. Characteristically the impairment fluctuates when mild in degree, often worsening at night with fatigue and with decreased environmental stimulation. The fluctuations and the appearance of lucid intervals are observations of great clinical importance in the differential diagnosis of organic from non-organic psychiatric disorders, and also in distinguishing acute from chronic organic reactions. Daytime visits may find the patient at his best, and it is thus essential to pay attention to reports of changed behaviour as nightfall approaches.

Disorders of attention

In most conditions impairment of consciousness is accompanied by diminished arousal and alertness which become clinically apparent at some stage of the disorder. However, in others, such as delirium tremens, the patient may be hyperaroused and hyperalert. Arousal and alertness, in this context, refer to the readiness with which the patient responds to environmental stimuli, 'arousal' being best used to describe the physiological state of the organism and 'alertness' to describe the observational data from which this state is inferred.

However, preserved alertness is not the sole yardstick by which preservation of normal consciousness is assessed. To be useful alertness must be coupled with an ability to select discriminatingly between

Table 1.1 Causes of acute organic reactions.

Degenerative
Dementias complicated by infection, anoxia, etc.
Episode in Lewy body dementia

Space-occupying lesions
Cerebral tumour, subdural haematoma, cerebral abscess

Trauma
'Acute post-traumatic psychosis'

Infection/inflammation
Encephalitis, meningitis, HIV infection, subacute meningovascular syphilis, exanthemata, streptococcal infection, septicaemia, pneumonia, influenza, typhoid, typhus, cerebral malaria, trypanosomiasis, rheumatic chorea

Vascular
Acute cerebral thrombosis or embolism, episode in multi-infarct dementia, transient cerebral ischaemic attack, subarachnoid haemorrhage, hypertensive encephalopathy, systemic lupus erythematosus

Epileptic
Complex partial seizures, petit mal status, postictal states

Metabolic
Uraemia, liver disorder, electrolyte disturbances, alkalosis, acidosis, hypercapnia, remote effects of carcinoma, porphyria

Endocrine
Hyperthyroid crises, myxoedema, Addisonian crises, hypopituitarism, hypoparathyroidism and hyperparathyroidism, diabetic precoma, hypoglycaemia

Toxic
Alcohol: Wernicke's encephalopathy, delirium tremens
Drugs: benzodiazepines and other sedatives (including withdrawal), salicylate intoxication, cannabis, LSD, MDMA ('ecstasy'), prescribed medications (antiparkinsonian drugs, scopolamine, antidepressants, steroids, antiretrovirals, anticonvulsants, etc.)
Others: lead, arsenic, organic mercury compounds, carbon disulphide

Anoxic
Bronchopneumonia, congestive cardiac failure, cardiac dysrhythmias, silent coronary infarction, silent gastrointestinal bleeding, carbon monoxide poisoning, post anaesthesia

Vitamin lack
Thiamine (Wernicke's encephalopathy), nicotinic acid (pellagra, acute nicotinic acid deficiency encephalopathy), B_{12} and folic acid deficiency

LSD, lysergic acid diethylamide; MDMA, 3,4-methylenedioxymethamphetamine.

those stimuli which are important and meaningful and those which are not. Moreover, the relevant stimuli must gain access to conscious awareness where they can be related to past experience and present needs. For these purposes alertness must be accompanied by a capacity to attend. When consciousness is impaired, certain qualities of attention will invariably be found to be defective, qualities referred to as *phasic*, *modulated*, *selective* or *directed* attention.

These involve the capacity not merely to allow a stimulus to elicit a response, but to mobilise, focus, sustain and shift attention in a fluid and changing manner according to the needs of the moment. Whether the patient is hypoalert or hyperalert, it will often soon become apparent that such mechanisms are at fault. Failure to be selective can result in indiscriminate, often excessive, responses to stimuli with the result

that the patient is *distractible*; failure to mobilise and sustain attention is seen in *impaired concentration*; inability to shift attention can lead to *perseveration*. The examiner's difficulty in engaging with the patient may owe much to all these factors. A more pervasive change may also occur, whereby internal percepts, thoughts and images come to hold attention more readily than percepts from the environment, allowing them to become elaborated in an unrestrained manner. This would appear to be important in the genesis of the vivid affects, fantasies and hallucinations of 'delirium', as described earlier in this chapter.

A true appreciation of the patient's level of consciousness must therefore include assessment not only of alertness and responsivity, but also of capacity to attend in a discriminating manner to what is going on around.

A minor degree of impairment of consciousness may present merely with complaints of vague malaise and feelings of uncertainty. It may escape detection at the time and be revealed only in retrospect by the amnesic gap left for the period in question. Other sensitive indicators are minor difficulties in judging the passage of time, in focusing attention as described above, or in thinking coherently. The latter again may initially be more apparent subjectively than to external observation. Sometimes there may be neglect of appearance and of needs, or an episode of incontinence may be an early sign. The sleep–wakefulness cycle is almost universally disturbed in some degree, with various combinations of insomnia, vivid dreams and dream-like mentation (Lipowski 1980, 1990). The diurnal rhythm of activity is sometimes clearly disordered, with a tendency to somnolence by day and excitability at night.

With more severe degrees of impairment, the patient is observed to be slow in responding, loses the thread in conversation, and attention to outside events is hard to arouse and sustain. Responses to requests may betray inadequate understanding or lack of volition to carry them out. Later still the patient is clearly drowsy, sleeps excessively and, if rousable, shows only a torpid and muddled awareness.

Psychomotor behaviour

Motor behaviour usually diminishes progressively as impairment of consciousness increases. When left alone the patient shows little spontaneous activity and habitual acts such as eating are carried out in an automatic manner. The capacity for purposive action is diminished. When pressed to engage in activities the patient is slow, hesitant and often perseverative. He responds to external stimuli apathetically if at all, though highly charged subjective events such as hallucinatory experiences may still call forth abrupt and even excessive reactions. Speech is slow and sparse, answers stereotyped or incoherent, and difficult questions are usually ignored. There is often slurring, perseveration, or dysphasic difficulties. In severe cases there may be no more than incoherent muttering.

While the above is the rule with most acute affections of the brain, some show the reverse with restless hyperactivity and noisy disturbing behaviour. Delirium tremens and the deliria which accompany certain systemic infections are the well-known examples. Not surprisingly these florid cases figure disproportionately highly in most published accounts of acute organic reactions. Psychomotor activity is greatly increased, with an excessive tendency to startle reactions. Typically the overactivity consists of repetitive, purposeless behaviour, such as ceaseless groping or picking movements. Behaviour may be dictated by hallucinations and delusions, the patient turning for example to engage in imaginary conversation, or ransacking the bedclothes for objects thought to be hidden there. More rarely he may perform complex stereotyped movements, re-enacting the driving of a car or miming his usual work (occupational delirium). Sometimes there is dangerously belligerent behaviour. When purposive, the activities are usually misdirected, inappropriate or bizarre, and voluntary movements are often jerky and uneven. The overactivity is often accompanied by excitement with noisy shouting, laughing or crying. There may be pressure of speech with incoherent flight of ideas. Most of the behaviour is obviously dictated by the patient's own internal world, and alertness to external stimuli is seen to be impaired. Not uncommonly the clinical picture shows rapid changes from phases of overactivity to periods of apathy and aspontaneity.

Thinking and reasoning

Thought processes show characteristic changes when consciousness is impaired. In the early stages there is subjective slowing, with difficulty in focusing thoughts or formulating complex ideas. Mental fatigue may be obvious in the course of examination. Later, reasoning becomes less clear and coherent, logic is impaired and thinking is more concrete and literal. Even when speeded by high arousal, the thought content is seen to be banal and impoverished. Trains of thought become chaotic, showing in speech as fragmentation and incoherence.

An important change is in the relative importance of the internal and external worlds, and in the decreasing ability to preserve the distinction between the two. Thus perceptions and thoughts become inextricably interwoven (defective 'reality testing'). Comprehension of events is impaired, with inability to embrace the elements of experience and relate them meaningfully to one another (impaired 'grasp'). The patient may be unaware of the most obvious features of his situation, whether he is standing or lying, whether indoors or in the street. At the same time increased significance is attached to subjective experiences, ideas or false perceptions, which come to dominate the content of consciousness. Bizarre thoughts and fantasies intrude into awareness, and false significance is attached to external cues. Illusions and hallucinations readily arise, and vivid dream material may be carried over into waking life.

Ideas of reference and delusion formation may become prominent, depending to some extent on qualities in the premorbid personality. Delusions of persecution are especially common, and may well up suddenly with conviction. They usually betray their organic origin in being poorly elaborated, vague, transient and inconsistent. When consciousness is relatively clear, however, the delusions may be more coherently organised, with a picture more closely resembling schizophrenia. In rare cases delusions may persist when the patient has recovered from the acute illness, with an obstinate belief in the reality of the hallucinatory experiences that occurred.

Insight into cognitive difficulties is typically lost early, but may vary with fluctuations in the level of consciousness. Sometimes even in moderately severe affections the patient may be briefly roused to self-awareness and to a better appreciation of reality.

Memory

With impairment of consciousness there is disturbance of registration (encoding and learning), retention and recall. Registration of current experience is hampered by defects in attention, perception and comprehension. Accordingly, the immediate memory span for digits or similar material (working memory) is found to be reduced. Defective retention leads to difficulty with new learning and this is a sensitive clinical indicator in mild stages of disorder. Recent (episodic) memories prove to be faulty while long-term memories are reasonably intact, though with moderate impairment of consciousness both are found to suffer.

An early change is defective appreciation of the flow of time, and the jumbling of time sequences for recent events. This quickly leads to disorientation in time, which is sometimes regarded as the hallmark of acute organic reactions. However, disorientation may be transient in the early stages, and a normally orientated patient may prove later to be amnesic for all that passed during the interview in which he was examined.

Disorientation for place, and later still for person, follow with worsening of perceptual and cognitive disorganisation. Patients may maintain two incompatible attitudes towards their orientation without seeming aware of the inconsistency. This can emerge strikingly where orientation for place is concerned, the patient saying quite correctly, for example, that he is in hospital in one town yet interpreting his surroundings and behaving in every other way as though he were at home in another part of the country, a condition known as reduplicative paramnesia. Such correct and incorrect orientations may exist side by side in a vacillating and unrelated manner, or be reconciled by shallow rationalisations. The patient may insist that the two places are the same, or contiguous with each other, or confabulate a recent journey between the two. Reduplicative paramnesias may take a number of forms and are sometimes associated with misrecognition or reduplication of persons. They can be seen with chronic organic reactions as well, perhaps particularly in association with right hemisphere pathology (Ellis & Lewis 2001; see also Illusions of transformation, displacement or reduplication, later in this chapter). False memories and confabulation may occasionally be in evidence, and misidentifications, including pseudorecognition, are facilitated by the perceptual abnormalities described below.

On recovery there is typically a dense amnesic gap for the period of the acute illness, though where fluctuation has been marked islands of memory may remain. Sometimes sensory impressions, and especially vivid hallucinations, stand out clearly and are remembered in great detail when all else is forgotten, attesting again to the importance of subjective experience over external reality in severe stages of the disorder.

Perception

Quite commonly it is the more florid perceptual abnormalities that draw attention to the presence of an acute organic reaction in a patient suffering from some physical disease. However, these are not essential features in every case, and the diagnosis should be made by seeking out the subtle deficits in thinking, memory and attention which betray impairment of consciousness.

Early on the patient may be aware that perception requires unusual effort, particularly where vision is concerned. Sometimes, in contrast, perceptions appear subjectively to be hyperacute. Disturbances of vision include micropsia, macropsia or distortions of shape and position. Disordered auditory perception may hinder clear communication. There may be distortions of weight and size, or bizarre disorders of the body image in which body parts feel shrunken, enlarged, misplaced or even disconnected. The whole body may feel as though it is tilted or floating. Disordered perception of internal bodily sensations leads sometimes to bizarre complaints. Genuine physical symptoms such as vertigo, headache and paraesthesiae are likewise often reported in distorted fashion.

Depersonalisation and derealisation are common, though usually incompletely expressed. Dissolution of the perceptual boundaries between the self and the environment may give rise to terrifying feelings of imminent dissolution or loss of bodily and personal integrity.

Perceptual abnormalities readily lead to misinterpretations and illusions which are typically fleeting and changeable. The visual modality is affected most often. Difficulty with visual recognition combines with faulty thinking and memory to produce false recognitions and faulty orientation in place. The unfamiliar tends to be mistaken for the familiar, or may be interpreted as hostile or persecutory. Thus the patient may misidentify a nurse as a relative, or the doctor as an old friend or enemy. The hospital ward may be mistaken for home or prison. Chance noises may similarly be misinterpreted, contributing to delusion formation. The whole is often reinforced by disordered affects of fear and suspicion.

Hallucinations are also commonest in the visual modality, though tactile and auditory hallucinations occur as well. They probably derive partly from failure to distinguish inner images from outer percepts, and partly from vivid dreams carried over into the waking state as consciousness waxes and wanes. Simple visual hallucinations consist of flashes of light, geometrical patterns or colours. More complex phenomena, sometimes kaleidoscopic in nature, may occur, with fully formed hallucinations of scenes, people and animals. A bizarre fantastic quality is not uncommon. The hallucinated material may be grossly distorted, as with Lilliputian hallucinations where objects and people appear to be minute in size. The reality of the phenomena is fully accepted by the patient, who may react with fear and alarm but sometimes with interest or even amusement.

Hallucinations appear to be particularly characteristic of the acute organic reactions occasioned by certain pathological processes. Delirium tremens remains the classic example, with extremely florid hallucinations as described in Chapter 11. Along with hallucinogenic drugs, prescribed drugs with potent anticholinergic properties are also notorious for the wealth of formed and unformed hallucinations they may provoke. Animals are said to feature particularly frequently in the hallucinations of delirium tremens, and visual hallucinations of 'nets' were said to characterise the organic reactions seen in bromide intoxication when this was common. In the setting of delirium, sensory impairments appear to predispose to hallucinations in the corresponding modality and hence are common in the elderly.

Emotion

In early stages, mild depression, anxiety and irritability may be expected, though typically the affect is shallow. With deeper impairment, and further impoverishment of mental processes, apathy usually becomes the striking feature, and the whole course of the illness may pass with indifference and emotional withdrawal. More lively affects are seen in conjunction with increased psychomotor activity when affective disturbance may become intense. Anxiety and fear are especially common, increasing sometimes to terror and panic. A state of wondering perplexity forms a common background to other affective states. Depression is frequent, elation or anger less so. Paranoid attitudes may show in marked hostility and suspicion. The affective reactions are often fleeting and changeable with changing delusional ideas. Sudden displays of primitive and highly charged emotion are often called forth by hallucinatory experiences.

In part the emotional state is likely to be determined by the stress of the physical illness, and in part by a vague awareness of cognitive impairments. The individual's personality structure may contribute in considerable measure, some patients being predisposed to react by apathetic withdrawal and others by projection of fantasised dangers onto the environment. The extent of such influences has not been determined, nor the degree to which the picture is shaped by different pathogenic agents. There are strong clinical impressions that delirium tremens tends to be accompanied by intense fear, hepatic encephalopathy by euphoria or depression, and uraemia by apathy, but reliable and systematic comparisons have not been made. It is clear, moreover, that several factors are often operative together in leading to delirium in the individual patient, particularly in the elderly (Francis *et al.* 1990).

Other features

In the milder stages in particular, the definitive organic features may be less in evidence than those which depend on individual traits and characteristics. Psychological reactions to early cognitive impairment, or to the stress of the underlying physical disease, may dominate the picture and emerge in the form of neurotic symptoms. Similarly, vulnerable aspects of personality may be exaggerated, with the appearance of depressive, hypochondriacal or phobic features. Histrionic and importunate behaviour may sometimes be much in evidence. Hysterical conversion symptoms, usually transient but sometimes persistent, may lead to mistakes in diagnosis. Paranoid developments occur frequently, and can become the overriding feature at an early stage in susceptible individuals. A distinct schizophrenic colouring to the total clinical picture is likewise not uncommon. With progression of cognitive disorganisation the true situation usually becomes apparent, but mild self-limiting acute organic reactions can be misdiagnosed for some time as non-organic psychiatric illness.

Clinical picture in chronic organic reactions (chronic brain syndrome, chronic confusional state, 'dementia')

Chronic organic reactions, like acute organic reactions, result from many different pathological processes, yet the clinical picture shows a large measure of similarity from one condition to another. A focal emphasis of pathology may produce special patterns of impairment, but the purpose in what follows is to describe the general clinical picture and to emphasise the shared and common forms of reaction that occur.

While the majority of chronic organic reactions are due to diffuse and widespread affections of the brain, some owe their origins to focal pathology, so careful examination for signs of localising value must always be undertaken. The principal causes are listed in Table 1.2. Most of the illnesses concerned are slowly progressive with increasing disablement, but static pictures may be seen as with arrested general paresis, or gradual improvement may occur as after head injury. In a small but extremely important group, therapeutic intervention can decisively reverse the process, for example with myxoedema or normal-pressure hydrocephalus, or when a frontal meningioma is discovered to be the cause.

Mode of presentation

Some chronic organic reactions follow acute episodes such as trauma or anoxia, and are then revealed in full when the patient recovers consciousness, or else emerge by a process of transition from an acute organic reaction. The great majority, however, develop insidiously from the start.

Table 1.2 Causes of chronic organic reactions.

Degenerative
Alzheimer's disease, multi-infarct dementia, Lewy body dementia, frontal lobe dementia, Pick's, Huntington's and Creutzfeldt–Jakob diseases, normal-pressure hydrocephalus, multiple sclerosis, Parkinson's, Schilder's and Wilson's diseases, progressive supranuclear palsy, progressive multifocal leucoencephalopathy, progressive myoclonic epilepsy, metachromatic leucodystrophy, neuroacanthocytosis, Kufs' disease, mitochondrial myopathy, etc.

Space-occupying lesions
Cerebral tumour, subdural haematoma

Trauma
Post-traumatic dementia

Infection/inflammation
HIV-associated dementia, general paresis, chronic meningovascular syphilis, subacute and chronic encephalitis, multiple sclerosis

Vascular
Cerebral vascular disease, *état lacunaire*, cerebral autosomal-dominant arteriopathy with subcortical leucoencephalopathy (CADASIL)

Epileptic
'Epileptic dementia'

Metabolic
Uraemia, liver disorder, remote effects of carcinoma

Endocrine
Myxoedema, Addison's disease, hypopituitarism, hypoparathyroidism and hyperparathyroidism, hypoglycaemia

Toxic
Korsakoff's syndrome, 'alcoholic dementia', chronic intoxication with sedative drugs, manganese, carbon disulphide

Anoxic
Anaemia, congestive cardiac failure, chronic pulmonary disease, post anaesthesia, post carbon monoxide poisoning, post cardiac arrest

Vitamin lack
Lack of thiamine, nicotinic acid, B_{12}, folic acid

The commonest mode of onset is with evidence of impairment of memory or more general cognitive impairment with disorganisation of intellect. Failures of memory are usually noted earlier by relatives and workmates than by the patient himself. They show in missed appointments, apparent unawareness of recent happenings, a tendency to mix up times or to lose things. More general cognitive failure emerges in slipshod work and loss of overall efficiency. The patient may be noticed to think and speak less coherently than usual, to muddle money or to fail to grasp essentials.

Change in personality as the first manifestation is much less common, but when it occurs the patient is especially likely to come before the psychiatrist. Here intellectual deficits are mild or absent in the early stages, or pass unnoticed because of curtailment of activities and the use of props and evasions. Deterioration of manners may be the earliest sign,

or diminished awareness of the needs and feelings of others. Some social blunder may disclose the problem, such as stealing or disinhibited behaviour out of character for the individual. Sometimes the earliest change is merely the exaggeration of long-standing personality traits such as suspiciousness or egocentricity. Neurotic traits may be elaborated with the production of depressive, obsessional, hysterical or hypochondriacal symptoms. More rarely the illness presents with the picture of a psychotic illness of depressive, paranoid or schizophrenic type in especially predisposed individuals. It is then only by careful examination that the onset of cognitive impairment is revealed.

Whatever the form of presentation, the illness may declare itself abruptly even though its evolution has been insidious. Some episode of acute mental disturbance may bring the disease to attention. Or relatives may have adjusted to the slow decline until some dramatic instance forces their attention to the true situation. Not infrequently a tenuous adjustment is concealed until new demands must be met, for example on the death of a partner or a move to a new environment. Admission to hospital may be the step which reveals the disorder, and only careful retrospective enquiry then establishes that the onset has been gradual. Intercurrent illness may bring the situation to light by pushing the patient below the threshold at which the brain was previously coping, especially infection, anoxia or postoperative metabolic derangements.

General behaviour

Although cognitive impairment is the hallmark of chronic organic reactions, this may be manifest only indirectly by way of behavioural change. Typical early signs are loss of interest and initiative, inability to perform to the usual standard, or minor episodes of muddle and confusion. Episodes of bizarrely inappropriate behaviour may occur, as when a woman unloads her shopping in the oven or prepares a meal at an inappropriate time. As described above, some cases present with changes in the field of social behaviour well before impairment of cognitive processes is overt.

As the disorder progresses the same division is seen, some aspects of behaviour reflecting the intellectual disorganisation, and some the change in emotional control and social awareness. Intellectual impairment shows as incapacity for decisive action, loss of application and inability to persist in a consistent course of conduct. Despite full alertness and the preservation of normal levels of consciousness the patient fatigues readily on mental effort. He responds appropriately to stimuli within his limited range of comprehension and is capable of directed attention as the need arises, but powers of concentration are impaired. Various behavioural changes may come into play that reflect the attempts of the personality to cope with such defects. There is often restlessness, with purposeless overactivity or, alternatively, rigid adherence to routines and stereotyped behaviour. In this manner the patient may be enabled to cope for a while. When taxed beyond his ability, however, he may become evasive and sullen, or react abruptly with an explosion of primitive affect such as anger, anxiety or tears ('catastrophic reaction' after Kurt Goldstein). In the later stages hygiene and personal appearance are neglected and ritualistic hoarding may develop. Food is eaten sloppily, habits deteriorate and there is indifference to urinary or faecal incontinence. In contrast, however, some patients preserve superficial social competence until surprisingly late in the course of the disease.

Eventually, behaviour becomes futile and aimless, often with stereotypies and mannerisms. Impoverishment of thought is reflected in lack of purposive activity, and physical deterioration follows with increasing weakness and emaciation.

Thinking

Thinking is impaired both qualitatively and quantitatively. It becomes slowed with reduced powers of concentration and ready mental fatigue. The content of thought is impoverished, with fewer associations, inability to produce new ideas, and a tendency to dwell on set topics and memories from the past. Themes are banal and perseveration usually marked. The ability to reason logically and to manipulate concepts is impaired, likewise the ability to keep in mind various aspects of a situation simultaneously. Specific skills such as calculation are usually impaired from an early stage.

Intellectual flexibility is lost, leading to difficulty in shifting from one frame of reference to another. The lack of effective counter-ideas leads the patient to become tied to the immediate situations that arise, so that he is distracted by accidental impressions and events and becomes 'stimulus bound' to them. Such difficulties are compounded by inability to extract the essentials of a situation or experience. Abstract ideas present especial difficulty and concepts tend to be given their most literal interpretation (termed 'concretisation').

Judgement is impaired early. The patient's insight is poor and there may be little awareness of illness at all. The more the complexity of the domain of functioning, the greater the discrepancy between the individual's appraisal of his abilities and that of his carer. False ideas readily gain ground and paranoid ideation is particularly common. Ideas of reference may reflect an exaggeration of premorbid tendencies. Delusions are typically persecutory in nature and may owe much to limbic dysfunction (Cummings 1992). The complexity of their content tends to be inversely proportional to the severity of cognitive impairment, patients with severe dementia usually harbouring only simple and loosely structured false beliefs. Occasionally, however, they become entrenched and unshakeable. As Roth and Myers (1969) point out, they may be delusions in the technical sense, in that the beliefs are held in the face of evidence of their falsehood, but this is largely because the evidence fails to be understood not because it is rejected. Delusional themes are often crude and bizarre, typically of being robbed, poisoned, threatened or deprived. The exception is delusional misidentification, which appears to be particularly associated with organic brain changes. In the later stages thinking appears to be restricted to circumscribed reiterative themes, and becomes grossly fragmented, incoherent and disorganised.

Speech

The disturbances in thinking are mirrored in speech. The most characteristic disturbance is poverty of speech with excessive employment of clichés and set phrases. The pool of vocabulary is greatly reduced, and speech initiative is poor.

Sentences are often simple, incomplete and poorly constructed, with perseveration, stereotyped utterances and echolalia.

Paraphasic errors, and nominal dysphasia, are not uncommon. Barker and Lawson (1968) suggest that difficulty in word-finding is a general feature in dementia if care is taken to test with words of low frequency of usage. There may be little evidence of disability until the patient is pressed to name an object, whereupon he may show little awareness of his errors. This is in contrast to the situation in nominal dysphasia due to focal brain lesions. Sometimes he may improvise to produce new words, showing perseveration and 'clang' associations. Concretisation shows in the excessive use of words which refer to the self and the tendency for external stimuli to influence the words that are chosen.

Ultimately, speech becomes grossly disorganised and fragmented, and used exclusively in the service of bodily needs. The patient may become mute or capable only of a restricted range of semicoherent ejaculations.

Memory

Memory disturbance is frequently the earliest sign of a developing chronic organic reaction, and at first may be intermittent. Allison (1962) makes the important point that with diffuse as opposed to focal cerebral lesions the onset of memory disturbance can rarely be dated accurately because it has been of such gradual evolution. The onset may be marked by minor forgetfulness and 'absent-mindedness', or by more definite episodes in which new impressions fail to register and striking lapses of memory occur. Loss of topographical memory is often seen, with the patient losing his way when away from home. Disorientation in time is a frequent early sign; disorientation for place and person are found much later in development.

The memory defect is typically global, affecting all categories of material and remote as well as recent events, as described in Chapter 2. Failure at new learning is usually the most conspicuous sign, but rarely there is the sharp demarcation between remote and recent memory that characterises the purer amnesic syndromes. Recall is affected as well as registration and retention, as shown by increased success with prompting and better performance at recognition than at free recall. Memory for names is sometimes particularly affected. Temporal sequences are disorganised early, with faulty appreciation of the flow of time and mislocation of past events. Berlyne (1972) found that over one-third of an unselected group of demented patients showed unequivocal confabulation, sometimes representing a true memory displaced in time, but sometimes consisting of more sustained and elaborate productions.

Characteristically the patient's awareness of his memory difficulties is impaired, or there may even be an apparently motivated desire to hide the deficits with facile excuses and shallow confabulations. In the early stages the patient may show surprising ingenuity in covering up his failures, and may compensate by means of a rigid daily routine and the use of a notebook. Ultimately, however, memory for current events may fail completely and the patient may be able to produce only a few jumbled recollections from the past.

Emotion

Emotional changes form an integral part of the clinical picture in chronic organic reactions and deterioration of emotion and intellect frequently pursue a parallel course.

Early emotional changes probably reflect the struggle to cope with incipient intellectual deficits, and are coloured by premorbid personality characteristics. Anxiety is common, likewise depression with agitation and hypochondriacal features. Serious suicidal attempts may occur at this stage. Irritability leads to querulous morose behaviour, and sometimes to outbursts of anger and hostility. Perplexity and suspicion are other common early developments, leading to paranoid beliefs and attitudes.

Further deterioration produces emotional changes of a distinctive organic type. Affective blunting and shallowness may progress to states of apathy or empty euphoria. Emotions may take on a child-like aspect, with petulant importunate behaviour and short-lived excessive responses to trivial annoyances. Thus the death of a spouse may leave the patient unmoved, yet interference with some simple routine may provoke outbursts of anger.

Emotional control may show a characteristic threshold effect in which there is little response to mild stimulation but thereafter an excessive and prolonged disturbance. Emotional lability may be extreme, with episodes of pathological laughing and crying for little or no cause. The 'catastrophic reaction' may be observed when the patient is taxed beyond his ability to cope, as described in Chapter 2 (Psychiatric disturbance and aphasia) and Chapter 3 (Mood).

The ultimate picture in progressive disease represents a combination of these various emotional changes, but characterised above all by increasing emptiness of affect, shallowness, dullness and lack of emotional response.

Other features

The impact of chronic diffuse brain disease is not entirely unaffected by features specific to the individual. As already mentioned, neurotic manifestations may be conspicuous in mild stages of disorder. Hysterical conversion symptoms and obsessional disorders may figure prominently, the former perhaps by virtue of increased suggestibility and the latter as a mode of coping with reduced resources. A predisposition towards affective or schizophrenic psychosis may lend a distinctive colouring to the clinical picture and lead to mistaken diagnosis in the early stages. Hallucinations can occur in visual, auditory and tactile modalities, and are typically paranoid in content. With progressive disease all such manifestations are usually ultimately engulfed in the general pattern of intellectual and social decline.

The combination of acute and chronic organic reactions is of course much more common than would be predicted by their chance co-occurrence. Delirium superimposed on dementia is a common clinical problem and is recognised in international disease classificatory systems. Indeed, a dementing condition may be exposed for the first time by the superimposition of delirium following a relatively minor metabolic or toxic insult, due to the unnoticed loss of some theoretical cerebral 'reserve'. Other general psychiatric disorders when they occur in the setting of organic brain disease may be classified separately in the ICD and DSM schemes from their 'idiopathic', 'non-organic' counterparts.

Clinical picture in focal cerebral disorder

Strictly focal brain damage can be responsible for both acute and chronic organic reactions as well as rather characteristic 'neurobehavioural syndromes'. Symptoms and signs of localizing significance may then be much in evidence, and must be kept in mind in the clinical assessment of all patients who show organic psychiatric illnesses.

Epileptic phenomena, especially those of temporal lobe epilepsy, are clear examples of acute psychological disturbances due to focal brain dysfunction, also some of the disturbances seen after small acute cerebrovascular accidents. Wernicke's encephalopathy is another classic example, with its own distinctive chronic end-state in the chronic amnesic syndrome. For obvious reasons, however, focal brain disorder has been most comprehensively studied in slowly progressive or static lesions of long duration, which allow the focal components to be disentangled from any generalised deficits that coexist.

In Chapter 2, the complex problems of the focal significance of psychological symptoms are dealt with in detail. Here, those which emerge with fair consistency after lesions of different parts of the brain are described in summary form. Neurological defects are in general more reliable than psychological symptoms in pointing to the site of focal pathology, and these too will be included. In general focal signs and symptoms serve only to indicate the site of likely pathology, and are of relatively little value in themselves in suggesting the nature of the lesion.

Frontal lobes

Frontal lesions may confer distinctive changes of disposition and temperament subsumed under the term 'change of personality'. Most characteristic is disinhibition, with expansive over-familiarity, tactlessness, over-talkativeness, childish

excitement (moria) or prankish joking and punning (*Witzelsucht*). Social and ethical control may be diminished, with lack of concern for the future and for the consequence of actions. Sexual indiscretions and petty misdemeanours may occur, or gross errors of judgement with regard to financial and interpersonal matters. Sometimes there is marked indifference, even callous unconcern, for the feelings of others. Lack of insight into their social inappropriateness or the presence of any perturbation of health and functioning is characteristic. Elevation of mood is often seen, mainly as an empty and fatuous euphoria rather than as a true elation that communicates itself to the observer. In other cases the principal changes are lack of initiative, aspontaneity and profound slowing of psychomotor activity, particularly with frontal lobe tumours. This may progress to a state of extreme aspontaneity amounting virtually to stupor.

Concentration, attention and ability to carry out planned activity are impaired by these changes, but performance on tests of formal intelligence is often surprisingly well preserved once the patient's cooperation has been secured. Even with sharply circumscribed frontal lesions, however, the overall picture may at first sight strongly resemble a generalised dementing process. The hazards of misdiagnosis are increased by the 'silent' nature of frontal lobe lesions, which can allow them to grow large before declaring themselves with neurological signs.

When frontal lesions encroach upon the motor cortex or motor projections there will be contralateral spastic paresis, usually seen earliest in the face and more obvious on voluntary movement than emotional expression. Paresis may be extremely slight, and show only as slowness of repeated movements or falling away of the outstretched arm. A grasp reflex may be the only definite sign. Firmer evidence may be found in hyperactive tendon reflexes and a positive Babinski response. Characteristic decomposition of gait may be seen, with trunk ataxia or awkward postures.

Lesions affecting the orbital part of the frontal lobes may be associated with the 'forced utilisation' of objects presented to the patient, as described in Chapter 2 (Classical case reports). This appears to be an extension of the more commonly observed forced grasping. Posterior lesions of the dominant lobe may produce a primary motor dysphasia, a motor agraphia or an apraxia of the face and tongue. Ipsilateral optic atrophy or anosmia may result from orbital lesions of the lobe, the latter being commonly overlooked in clinical examination. Sphincteric incontinence may occur surprisingly early in view of the reasonable preservation of intellect, and is a valuable added indication.

Parietal lobes

Parietal lobe lesions are associated with a rather bewildering variety of complex cognitive disturbances, including defects of language and number sense, defective appreciation of external space, and disorders of the body image. Where some are concerned it is uncertain how far the lesions of the parietal lobe are alone responsible, or how far adjacent lesions in the temporal and occipital lobes contribute to the total picture. These matters are dealt with in Chapter 2, but the following is presented as a brief clinical guide.

Lesions of either parietal lobe may result in visuospatial difficulties and topographical disorientation. Visuospatial difficulties are most readily exposed by asking the patient to copy simple drawings or construct patterns from coloured blocks or matchsticks, tests which reveal the presence of visuospatial agnosia or constructional dyspraxia. Defective performance is seen more commonly with lesions of the non-dominant than dominant lobe but may occur with either. Difficulty in locating objects in space, or in describing the relationships between different objects by vision alone, may also be observed. Topographical disorientation is revealed by difficulty in learning or remembering the way about, with the result that the patient mislocates his bed in the ward, fails to find the bathroom or loses himself even in familiar surroundings.

Dominant parietal lobe lesions are associated with various forms of dysphasia, primary motor dysphasia being most in evidence with anterior lesions and primary sensory dysphasia with posterior lesions. The latter may include alexia in association with agraphia. Motor apraxia similarly accompanies dominant parietal lobe lesions, and usually affects the limbs of both sides of the body. Various components of Gerstmann's syndrome may be seen, namely finger agnosia, dyscalculia, right–left disorientation and agraphia. The syndrome is rarely seen in its entirety and individual components often occur along with other parietal lobe symptoms. Bilateral tactile agnosia is occasionally seen, as are various forms of visual agnosia when the lesion lies posteriorly in the parieto-occipital region.

Non-dominant parietal lobe lesions may produce disturbed appreciation of the body image and of external space, particularly involving the contralateral side. The left limbs may fail to be recognised or may be disowned by the patient. If paralysed or hemianaesthetic, the disability may be ignored or refuted (anosognosia), a part of the body may be felt to be absent (hemisomatognosia), or in rare cases there may be phantom reduplication of body parts. Neglect of the left half of external space may show in the omission of left-sided details when drawings are copied, or in the crowding of writing into the right-hand part of the paper. Left-hand turnings may be overlooked when finding the way about. 'Dressing dyspraxia' consists of muddle when inserting limbs into garments or putting garments over the head. In addition to visuospatial agnosia there may be a marked defect of the recognition of faces (prosopagnosia) when the lesion is posterior and involves the occipital lobe.

Neurological signs indicative of a parietal lobe lesion include cortical sensory loss and the phenomena of extinction and inattention. Cortical sensory loss consists not of analgesia but of a more complex impairment of sensation and difficulty with discrimination; objects cannot be identified by palpation (astereognosis), figures written on the hand cannot be named (agraphaesthesia), two-point discrimination is impaired, and the localisation of sensory stimuli is inaccurate. Sensory extinction (sensory inattention) is shown when two parts of the body are lightly touched simultaneously and that on the side contralateral to the lesion is not perceived. Visual inattention may be demonstrated by asking the patient to point to moving objects in both half-fields of vision; when two objects move simultaneously that in the contralateral half-field is ignored.

Sensory deficits are often accompanied by evidence of mild hemiparesis in the limbs contralateral to the lesion. Deep lesions affecting the optic radiation produce a contralateral homonymous hemianopia, usually more fully developed in the lower than the upper quadrants.

Temporal lobes

Lesions restricted to the poles of the temporal lobes can be entirely asymptomatic. More commonly, however, temporal lobe lesions are associated with disturbance of intellectual functioning, lesions of the dominant lobe more so than those of the non-dominant lobe.

Dominant temporal lesions may produce language difficulties alone. This is typically a sensory dysphasia, resulting in severe cases in jargon productions. More posterior lesions on the dominant side may also impair visual aspects of language in the form of alexia and agraphia. Parietal lobe symptomatology may then also appear by way of motor apraxia, constructional apraxia and aspects of Gerstmann's syndrome.

Non-dominant temporal lobe lesions often show a paucity of symptoms and signs. Sometimes, however, visuospatial difficulties are in evidence, also prosopagnosia and hemisomatognosia.

Bilateral lesions of the medial temporal lobe structures can produce amnesic syndromes of great severity and virtually uncontaminated by other intellectual disturbances (see Chapter 2, Medial temporal amnesia). Unilateral temporal lobe lesions lead to a more restricted disturbance of memory for certain classes of material along with related perceptual deficits, but this is rarely a spontaneous complaint and is usually revealed only by special testing. Lesions on the dominant side impair the learning and retention of verbal material even in the absence of overt dysphasia. Non-dominant lesions impair the learning and retention of non-verbal patterned stimuli, such as music, or faces and drawings to which a name cannot be attached.

Personality disturbances identical with those accompanying frontal lesions may occur, but will more commonly be associated with intellectual and neurological deficits.

Chronic temporal lobe lesions are notorious for their association with disturbance of personality, and particularly with emotional instability and aggression. Similarly lesions of the temporal lobe appear to carry an increased risk of psychotic disturbances akin to schizophrenia. Depersonalisation may be prominent, also disturbance of sexual function. Epileptic phenomena are common with temporal lobe lesions and give important evidence of localisation (Chapter 6).

The most reliable neurological sign of deep temporal lobe lesions is a contralateral homonymous upper quadrantic visual field defect, caused by interruption of the visual radiation in the central white matter. This sign alone may occasionally betray the presence of a temporal lobe lesion in a dementing process that has been attributed to diffuse brain damage. Deep lesions may also result in a mild contralateral hemiparesis or sensory loss due to encroachment upon fibres in the corona radiata. Equilibrium and hearing are not impaired, even by extensive unilateral lesions of the temporal neocortex.

Occipital lobes

Occipital lobe lesions lack well-established focal symptomatology except where vision is concerned. Complex disturbances of visual recognition characterise lesions of the parastriate areas. Agnosia for written or printed material (alexia without agraphia), colour agnosia and 'simultanagnosia' are characteristic of dominant occipital or occipitotemporal lesions, whereas bilateral pathology is usually present with visual object agnosia or prosopagnosia. Visuospatial agnosia occurs more commonly from non-dominant than from dominant occipitoparietal lesions, likewise metamorphopsia in which the appearance of objects is distorted. Complex visual hallucinations are said to occur more commonly from non-dominant than dominant occipital lesions.

Lesions of the striate cortex produce homonymous defects in the opposite half-field of vision and occasionally simple visual hallucinations of patterns, flashes of light, etc. Extensive bilateral lesions may produce cortical blindness, distinguished from peripheral blindness by the normal appearance of the optic fundi and the preservation of pupillary light reflexes.

Corpus callosum

Expanding corpus callosum lesions typically extend laterally into adjacent parts of the hemispheres, producing a picture of severe and rapid intellectual deterioration along with changes specific to the lobes involved. Anterior tumours produce marked frontal lobe disturbance, often with extreme psychomotor retardation and aspontaneity. Dysphasia, apraxia and asymmetrical pyramidal signs are common when the parietal lobes are affected. Involvement of diencephalic structures leads to somnolence, stupor and akinesis. Bizarre postural motor abnormalities may strongly resemble the pictures seen in catatonia. Disruption of communication between the two hemispheres may result in lack of access of the non-dominant hemisphere to the speech mechanisms in the dominant hemisphere; there will then be left-sided apraxia to verbal commands, with agraphia and astereognosis in the left hand (Geschwind 1965). Lesions restricted to the posterior part, in association with lesions of the left occipital lobe, may result in alexia without agraphia (or pure word blindness) for similar reasons.

Diencephalon and brainstem

The most characteristic symptoms of lesions in the deep midline structures of the brain are amnesia of the Korsakoff type and hypersomnia. These may stand out against a background of progressive intellectual deterioration or present initially as the sole disturbance. Amnesia that is strikingly more marked for recent than remote events, and is sometimes accompanied by confabulation, is characteristic of lesions in the neighbourhood of the third ventricle, aqueduct and posterior hypothalamus. Somnolence and hypersomnia suggest a lesion of the posterior diencephalon and upper midbrain. It may fluctuate in intensity, or occur in brief attacks suggestive of narcolepsy. Sometimes it may progress to states of profound stupor or coma. Akinetic mutism ('coma vigil') is a characteristic syndrome in which the patient lies immobile and mute, though the eyes may be open and follow moving objects (see Chapter 6, under Diencephalic tumours).

Intellectual deterioration may occur by virtue of raised intracranial pressure consequent upon obstruction of the cerebrospinal fluid circulation. Some focal lesions, however, produce rapidly progressive dementia without such generalised disturbance, particularly those originating within the thalamus. Features closely akin to the 'frontal lobe syndrome' may occur with diencephalic and brainstem lesions: disinhibition, indifference, carelessness and euphoria. Insight into the changes is said to be better preserved than with the equivalent pictures produced by frontal lobe lesions. Swings of mood and sudden outbursts of violent emotion are also held to be characteristic. Bilateral lesions within the upper brainstem and diencephalon, seen for example with pseudobulbar palsy, are associated with extreme emotional lability and 'emotional incontinence'. The patient laughs or cries excessively in response to trivial stimuli, yet if questioned he denies experiencing the degree of emotion he displays, and may well be distressed at his inability to control the response.

Focal neurological signs may be surprisingly absent in the early stages of progressive diencephalic lesions. Raised intracranial pressure with headache and papilloedema are found with the majority of obstructive lesions, though even here mental symptoms may be severe before this develops. Visual field defects will betray lesions such as craniopharyngiomas which grow upwards from the sella turcica and compress the optic chiasma. However, the patient who has considerable intellectual loss may make no complaint of the visual field disturbance, and testing can sometimes be impossible.

Disturbance of hypothalamic function can result in polydipsia, polyuria, hyperphagia and obesity or elevation of temperature. Amenorrhoea or impotence may occur in the adult, delayed or precocious sexual development in the child. Involvement of the pituitary gland will result in a wide variety of endocrine changes, which may, however, be overlooked for a time when psychiatric disturbance is prominent.

Thalamic lesions cause the sensory disturbances characteristic of parietal lobe lesions with, in addition, hypalgesia or analgesia to painful stimuli. Brainstem lesions cause characteristic cranial nerve palsies, along with evidence of dense long-tract motor and sensory disturbances.

Basal ganglia

Disorders of the basal ganglia are, in classical neurology, liable to present with one of the involuntary movements as their more visible manifestation. However, neuropsychiatric presentations of basal ganglia lesions are being increasingly recognised. Such lesions are commonly the result of degenerative conditions such as Parkinson's disease and Huntington's chorea and hence present with a gradually deteriorating course. By virtue of the strong reciprocal connections between the basal ganglia and the frontal lobes, many presentations have a strong 'frontal' flavour. These tend to be of the more 'negative' type, with slowing of thought, speech and movement and lack of spontaneity and motivation being most prominent. Indeed, depressive disorders are a common accompaniment as well as being a major part of the differential diagnosis. However, apathy may give way to irritability and diffuse cerebral dysfunctions. Rigid patterns of behaviour and repetitiveness may lead to frank obsessional–compulsive disorders. There is a particular constellation of cognitive deficits that has become known as the 'subcortical dementias' (see Table 1.3 and Chapter 12).

Differential diagnosis

The correct appraisal of patients with neuropsychiatric disorders is a test of both psychiatric and general medical skills. The detailed differential diagnosis of individual conditions will be considered in the appropriate sections elsewhere, but here certain general principles are outlined.

Of first importance is the ability to distinguish between organic and non-organic psychiatric illness, in other words to recognise when identifiable brain disorder is the root cause of the presenting clinical picture. The nature of the cerebral disorder must then be determined by a process of enquiry that proceeds logically in accordance with reasonable expectations. A distinction between acute and chronic organic reactions is often helpful in deciding on probabilities, as is the distinction between diffuse or focal cerebral disorder. Thereafter the range of possible causes remains wide, and will also be briefly discussed below.

Differentiation from non-organic conditions

There can be little difficulty in deciding on an organic aetiology when impairment of consciousness or of cognitive processes is marked, when there are epileptic fits, or when psychiatric symptoms are accompanied by obvious neurological symptoms and signs. But this is not always the case. Some organic disorders can present with hallucinations, affective change or schizophrenia-like symptomatology and lack clear organic accompaniments throughout their course. Others unfold very gradually, with indefinite organic features and with symptomatology suggestive of virtually any form of psychiatric illness. Special predisposition to neurotic forms of reaction, or to psychotic illness, may confer distinctive features which for some time obscure the true situation.

Table 1.3 Characteristics of the cortical and subcortical dementias.

Feature	Cortical (e.g. Alzheimer's disease)	Subcortical (e.g. Parkinson's and Huntington's diseases)
Language	Dysphasia early	Reduced output
Memory	Recall and recognition impaired	Some impairment in recall
Visuospatial	Impaired early	Impaired
Calculation	Impaired	Preserved until late
Executive function	Normal early	Reduced, especially spontaneity and flexibility
Psychomotor	Normal early	Slowed
Abnormal movements	None (myoclonus rare)	Chorea, tremor, stooped posture, etc.
Personality/behaviour	Preserved unless 'frontal lobe'	Apathetic, withdrawn
Mood	Euthymic; may lack awareness	Depression common

The converse is also true, since patients with non-organic psychiatric illness may show features that raise the possibility of cerebral disease. For example, disorientation and minor impairment of consciousness may be detected at the onset of acute schizophrenia, also sometimes in mania and agitated depression, yet without evidence of identifiable brain malfunction either at the time or subsequently. Similarly, cognitive impairment, including difficulty with recent memory, may accompany purely affective disorders particularly in later life, as discussed in Chapter 9. Features resembling delirium, including characteristic disturbances of thought processes and even hallucinations, can occur in mania (Hutchinson & David 1997) and follow psychological stress, as in sensory deprivation or sleep deprivation. It is probable that subtle perturbations of brain function underlie all such examples, though these are not yet identifiable by routine clinical investigation; moreover, the possibility of their presence has little practical implication for treatment.

Thus it is clear that the line of demarcation between organic and non-organic psychiatric disorders is not hard and fast, and in a substantial number of cases there can be continuing uncertainty. Some commentators use this to encourage an abandonment of the organic/non-organic distinction as if it were a primitive throwback to Cartesian dualism. However, while neuropsychiatry is the embodiment of an integrated approach to mind and body, it is not an excuse for woolly thinking or for ignoring the very real distinctions between classes of disorder. These distinctions remain valid and useful in practice for the great majority of cases. The margin for error is reduced when investigations are undertaken, but even so is not removed completely. Specialist investigations such as electroencephalography (EEG), psychometric testing, radiographic procedures and functional brain imaging techniques may all be helpful but can be equivocal and even misleading. It is important to remember that the more sensitive the technique, the more likely it is to yield false-positive results. Clinical examination therefore remains of the first importance, and is in any case the chief guideline that determines whether or not special investigations should be undertaken. Examples of patients in whom unusual problems in the differentiation between organic and non-organic disorder have arisen, often with surprising results, have been described by Lishman (1992).

Neurotic disorder may be simulated in the early stages of cerebral disease by virtue of diffuse complaints of anxiety, depression, irritability and insomnia. The patient may himself complain of forgetfulness and difficulty in concentration, but these tend to be discounted because of the multitude of other vague somatic symptoms. Involuntary movements, tremors and akathisia may be put down to simple anxiety. Phobic and obsessional symptomatology is not uncommon at the onset, and may remain a prominent feature for some considerable time. It is also well known that one must be wary of neurotic developments beginning only in middle life and when the previous mental constitution was good, also to seek for clear evidence of adequate immediate causes for their appearance.

Sometimes the clue may lie in the patient's attitude towards his symptoms. The organic patient will often tend to play down his deficits so that a graver picture is obtained from relatives than from the patient himself. The neurotic patient, by contrast, presses home his symptoms and actively seeks a remedy for them. The patient's evasiveness may raise suspicion, or when pressed he may display abrupt 'catastrophic' reactions of distress or anger. Typically also the organic patient's symptomatology lacks the richness and diversity seen in purely neurotic disorders.

Conversion ('hysterical') disorder may also be simulated by organic conditions. Acute organic reactions tend to fluctuate with periods of lucidity, and symptoms may thus be fleeting. A shallow affective quality and a tendency to make light of symptoms may suggest the *belle indifference* of hysteria. In mild delirium the cardinal features of impairment of consciousness and subtle deficits of attention may sometimes be hard to determine, and behaviour may be seemingly motivated for display. Thus it may be necessary to watch closely for signs of perseveration, slight dysarthria and other minimal features that betray the organic basis of the disorder.

Episodes of bizarre behaviour in hypoglycaemic attacks, or of paralysis in porphyria, provide well-known diagnostic hazards in which conversion disorders come to be suspected. Similar difficulty is sometimes found with periods of long-continued abnormal behaviour following encephalitis. Frank conversion symptoms may of course occur with chronic brain disease and be mistaken for the primary disorder. It is unclear how far these reflect in some way the direct effects of cerebral damage, or how far they merely represent a psychogenic response to the patient's partial awareness of his deficits. Again, it is axiomatic to view with grave suspicion 'hysterical' symptoms that make their first appearance only in middle life. The problem of the differential diagnosis of pseudodementia is discussed in Chapter 9.

Schizophrenic symptoms in association with cerebral disease can readily be misleading. A preponderance of visual over auditory hallucinations should raise suspicion of an organic disorder, similarly an empty or shallow affective colouring to delusional beliefs and passivity phenomena. Delusions in both acute and chronic organic reactions may take any of the forms seen in schizophrenia, but paranoid delusions are by far the most common. Certain qualities of the delusions strongly suggest an organic basis, namely those which are vague, poorly systematised, incoherent, fleeting and changeable, or restricted and stereotyped in content. Nevertheless, schizophrenic illnesses that are typical in every respect occasionally prove ultimately to be founded on identifiable cerebral disease. Disorders of the temporal lobes are the most likely to present with schizophrenia-like features.

Depressive symptoms can also give rise to difficulty. Ordinary affective disorder can be associated with marked slowness of thinking, difficulty with concentration and uncertainty with memory. There may be considerable doubt about the correct evaluation of such features, and psychometric testing may give equivocal results. The difficulties are increased when electroconvulsive treatments have already been given.

Features that may help in distinguishing primary depressive illness from organic psychiatric disorder include the careful appraisal of the setting in which disturbances of concentration and memory occur. In depressive illness it can often be observed that lack of interest or excessive anxiety prevent the focusing of attention on the matter in hand, rather than any pervasive difficulty with the organisation of thought and memory. Preoccupation with morbid thoughts may operate similarly. Typically the patient with uncomplicated depression is able to give a more coherent account of his discomforts and a more accurate chronology of his illness than would be possible in the presence of cerebral disease. These important aspects of differential diagnosis are considered more fully in the section on depressive pseudodementia (Chapter 9).

Personality disorder is especially liable to be suspected where frontal lobe dysfunction is concerned, for example following injury or in the early stages of a frontal dementia. Irresponsible behaviour or lapses of social conduct may be attributed to pre-existing personality factors, particularly when there has been some recent stress or problem in the patient's life. Here the essential clue will lie in a careful history from an informant which reveals the change that has occurred. Other avenues to the differential diagnosis are less reliable. Thus the patient may fail to display the classic features of frontal lobe disturbance at interview. And psychometric testing cannot always be relied upon in making the distinction; cognitive ability may be well preserved, and even tests specially devised to reveal frontal deficits can occasionally be misleading. Examples of frontal tumours or chronic infections presenting with change of disposition and behaviour are described in Chapter 2. Functional neuroimaging is increasingly being used to investigate the possibility of focal and generalised cerebral disorders presenting diagnostic difficulties. Frontal lobe dementia is described in Chapter 9. Special difficulty will of course arise in patients whose personality has always been abnormal.

Differentiation between acute and chronic organic reactions

In practice this distinction is most directly made from the history of the mode of onset of the disorder. A short history and firm knowledge of an acute onset will make a chronic organic reaction unlikely. Onset in association with a physical illness rather strongly suggests an acute organic reaction. However, when such leads are lacking close attention to phenomenology may be necessary.

Acute rather than chronic cerebral disorder is suggested when there are severe perceptual disturbances and distortions, with prominent illusions and hallucinations in the visual modality. Defective appreciation of reality may lead to rich and intrusive fantasies, in contrast to the emptiness and impoverishment of thought characteristic of chronic organic reactions. Similarly, in the presence of florid behaviour disturbance, this will be seen to be dictated by disturbed thought processes of a more sophisticated kind in acute than in chronic cerebral disorder. The affective state of the patient may also help with the distinction. In acute organic reactions the emotional disturbances are typically of a positive kind – fear or terror, perplexity and agitation – whereas the demented patient may be flat, apathetic and emotionally unresponsive. Emotional rapport can usually be established in patients showing clouding of consciousness, but tends to be poor in dementia.

This said, it must be recognised that in practice the differentiation between acute and chronic organic reactions can sometimes be very difficult. Despite careful observation, the distinction may come to be revealed only by the time course that is followed. For example, a prolonged subacute delirious state due to anoxia, uraemia or hepatic disorder can simulate dementia very closely. Or the patient may be admitted to hospital without a history to point to the acute and recent onset of the disorder. Perhaps most difficulty is encountered with elderly patients who show postoperative disturbances, due to metabolic derangements or anoxia, and in whom the mental state was incompletely evaluated beforehand. The electroencephalogram may provide some guidance in such examples (see Chapter 3, under Electroencephalography). The distinction between delirium and dementia may be aided by a simple list of contrasting features compiled by Butler and Zeman (2005) (Table 1.4).

Differentiation between diffuse and focal lesions

Symptoms and signs of localising significance must be carefully sought in all organic psychiatric disorders, and when discovered must not be ignored. Local disturbances of cerebral function can, of course, occur with progressive cortical disease before it is sufficiently extensive to produce a global dementia; well-known examples are a circumscribed amnesic syndrome in the early stages of Alzheimer's disease or a frontal lobe syndrome in Pick's disease (see Chapter 9). Evidence of focal brain damage may also emerge later in the course of such disorders when the pathological changes become especially advanced in certain regions of the brain. Signs of focal damage must therefore be carefully assessed in relation to the clinical picture as a whole, but will usually dictate that further investigations should be under-

Table 1.4 Delirium versus dementia. (From Butler & Zeman 2005.)

Feature	Delirium	Dementia
Onset	Abrupt/subacute	Insidious
Course	Fluctuating	Slow progression
Duration	Hours to weeks	Months to years
Alertness	Abnormally high or low	Typically normal
Sleep–wake cycle	Disrupted	Typically normal
Attention	Impaired	Relatively normal
Orientation	Impaired	Intact in early dementia
Working memory	Impaired	Intact in early dementia
Episodic memory	Impaired	Intact in early dementia
Thought	Disorganised, delusions	Impoverished
Speech	Slow/rapid, incoherent	Word finding difficulty
Perception	Illusions/hallucinations common	Usually intact in early dementia
Behaviour	Withdrawn/agitated	Varies: often intact early

taken. The important problem is to distinguish the essentially focal lesion from diffuse brain damage, because a remediable cause may then come to light. Finally, the neurological examination should always be supplemented by careful enquiry and observation for epileptic disturbances of focal origin.

Psychological symptoms of possible localising value include amnesia out of proportion to other cognitive deficits, dysphasia, somnolence, and the several aspects of parietal lobe symptomatology that have been discussed above. Mild dysphasia due to focal cerebral disease may be mistaken for early dementia when the patient's account is hesitant and incoherent, or when he is anxious and depressed as a result of his disability. However, careful observation usually shows that behaviour not involving language remains substantially intact. Dysphasic difficulties, and especially nominal dysphasia, may be seen with diffuse cerebral disorder, but then insight into the defect is less likely to be well preserved. Agnosic and apraxic deficits, and disturbances of the body image and of spatial orientation, likewise raise suspicion of focal cerebral disorder when severe and out of all proportion to other cognitive difficulties. Such deficits are, however, relatively common in acute organic reactions or when consciousness is impaired to a significant extent, and when chronic diffuse brain disease has progressed beyond the early stages.

Special investigatory procedures, as outlined in Chapter 3, are the most reliable arbiters in the distinction between focal and diffuse brain damage, and will often need to be undertaken before a firm differentiation is achieved.

Causes of acute and chronic organic reactions

The specific cause in the majority of cases will readily become apparent in the course of history-taking and examination. In many it is self-evident from the outset. Sometimes, however, the cause may be elusive and it is then essential to consider systematically a wide range of possibilities. These are shown in Tables 1.1 and 1.2.

It is helpful in approaching a given case to consider first the possible causes arising within the CNS itself, then derangements of cerebral function consequent upon disorders in other systems of the body. This division is reflected approximately in the ordering of causes in Tables 1.1 and 1.2. Even some of the very rare conditions are remediable, and enquiry must therefore be extensive when the solution is not soon forthcoming.

The antecedent history will give important clues, and it is essential that a relative or close acquaintance should be seen. The time and mode of onset must always be carefully established. The classic presenile and senile dementias usually begin insidiously and their history commonly extends over several months, whereas remediable illnesses often have an abrupt and relatively recent onset. Careful enquiry should always be made for a history of head injury, fits, alcoholism, drug abuse, recent illness or anaesthesia. Even in the absence of known head injury the possibility of subdural haematoma should be kept in mind, since this may follow trivial injury in arteriosclerotic subjects or be forgotten in alcoholics. It may be followed by a latent interval, and be accompanied by minimal neurological signs. A known epileptic tendency may suggest that the present disturbance is an unusually prolonged complex partial seizure or postictal state. Fits of recent onset may indicate a space-occupying lesion, or some acute cerebrovascular accident or injury that has left a residual focus of brain damage. A history of alcoholism or drug abuse may be long concealed in some cases, even on occasion by relatives as well as by the patient. Suspicion may only be raised by indirect evidence from the patient's attitude to enquiry or unwillingness for hospitalisation. A history of repeated episodes over a considerable period of time may strongly suggest that drug abuse is responsible.

Apart from self-administered drugs, it is always important to enquire about medication recently prescribed. This may have contributed by way of toxic effects, idiosyncratic reactions or the lowering of blood pressure. Diuretics given without proper supervision may have led to electrolyte depletion. If the patient is a known diabetic, enquiry must be made about previous hypoglycaemic reactions, the current dose of insulin and the current diet. The list of drugs that can affect cognitive functions is almost limitless and idiosyncratic reactions are always possible. Hence a high index of suspicion is required. A useful update on medications with propensity to cause neuropsychiatric effects is provided by Turjanski and Lloyd (2005).

A history of recent illness and operation should be noted, and also the quality of recovery from any recent anaesthetic. Previous episodes of dysphasia, paralysis or other neurological deficit will be suggestive of cerebral arterial disease. Any indications that the patient may be at risk of HIV infection should be noted, also a family history of illness such as Huntington's disease.

In patients with acute organic reactions it is still important to enquire for an antecedent history of failing memory or intellect over some period of time, since an incipient chronic dementia may be being aggravated by intercurrent disease. The adequacy of diet should be assessed in elderly patients, especially when living alone, or in patients of low intelligence and low economic means. Vitamin depletion is certainly not excluded in patients suffering from presenile or senile dementing illnesses and may be adding to the disability. Finally, in the more immediate history, specific enquiry should always be made for headache, vomiting or visual disturbance indicative of raised intracranial pressure, and in Elderly patients for breathlessness, ankle swelling or substernal pain which may indicate recent cardiac decompensation.

On examination one must pay attention to any appearance of physical ill health which may be token metabolic disorder, carcinoma or an infective process. The general appearance of the patient may indicate anaemia, or an endocrine disorder such as myxoedema that is otherwise easily missed. Dehydration may suggest uraemia or diabetic precoma. Muscular twitching suggests uraemia, electrolyte disturbance or hypoglycaemia. There may be skin lesions diagnostic of exanthemata or indicative of vitamin deficiency. It may be necessary to search closely, by 4-hourly temperature recording, for evidence of low-grade intermittent pyrexia indicating, for example, encephalitis or cerebral abscess. Finally, very careful general observation may sometimes reveal the choreiform movements diagnostic of early Huntington's chorea.

Examination of the CNS must pay careful attention to the optic fundi for signs of raised intracranial pressure, to abnormalities of pupil size or reactions indicative of syphilis, or nystagmus which may suggest drug intoxication. Transient disorders of external ocular movement may be the essential sign for confirming a diagnosis of Wernicke's encephalopathy. Evidence of focal neurological defects in motor or sensory systems (including unsuspected visual field defects) will suggest a space-occupying lesion or cerebrovascular disease. Neck stiffness may indicate subarachnoid haemorrhage or meningitis, and evidence of recent ear infection will raise the possibility of cerebral abscess.

Signs of arteriosclerosis should be noted both at the periphery and in the optic fundi. The patency of the carotid arteries should be tested by palpation and auscultation in the neck. Hypertension must be assessed, likewise evidence of cardiac failure, heart block or recent coronary infarction. Respiratory infection or inadequacy must also be noted as possible causes of cerebral anoxia. Even in the absence of hepatic or splenic enlargement it may be necessary to examine for liver flap, spider naevi or fetor hepaticus. It can be important to examine for prostatic enlargement. Carcinoma with secondary cerebral deposits, or secondary 'remote' effects upon the CNS, may need to be excluded by palpation of breasts, neck, axillae, and rectal and vaginal examinations. A chest X-ray will be obligatory for exclusion of carcinoma of the lung.

Investigations in every case should include haematology, erythrocyte sedimentation rate, blood urea, serum electrolytes and proteins, liver function tests, serum thyroxine, estimation of blood sugar, serological tests for syphilis, urine examination and chest radiography, no matter what may appear to be the cause. Skull radiography and EEG may be required, and computerised tomography (CT) or magnetic resonance imaging (MRI) will quite often be undertaken. It may be necessary to proceed with estimation of serum B_{12} and folate, or urinary examination for drugs or evidence of porphyria. An electrocardiogram may be indicated if silent myocardial infarction or Stokes–Adams attacks are suspected, along with other cardiovascular specialist investigations such as echocardiography, Doppler studies of the carotid arteries and coagulation screens. Immunological tests for autoantibodies and paraneoplastic markers may be valuable. The problems surrounding HIV testing and the need to obtain informed consent beforehand are discussed in Chapter 7. Lumbar puncture will sometimes be required when the diagnosis remains in doubt, in particular to confirm suspicions of intracranial infection. Further investigations such as a radioisotope scan or angiography will sometimes be indicated, though CT and MRI have greatly reduced the need for these.

Causes of stupor

Mention may be made of the differential diagnosis of stupor. The causes may be organic or non-organic, and the differential diagnosis must embrace schizophrenia, depression and hysteria in addition to organic brain dysfunction.

Joyston-Bechal (1966) examined the records of 100 cases of stupor diagnosed at the Bethlem Royal and Maudsley Hospitals in order to obtain an indication of the frequency of different causes. In this setting organic causes are seen in one-fifth. The essential features of the stupor were closely similar in the organic and non-organic cases. In 14 cases, the cause remained uncertain. Sometimes the true situation was unclear at the time of the patient's presentation, but was revealed in retrospect when the stupor had resolved. A more recent series (Johnson 1984) had twice the prevalence of 'organic' cases. This may reflect advances in diagnostic techniques, especially non-invasive neuroimaging. In Joyston-Bechal's (1966) series almost half of the stupors resolved within a week, and only one-fifth lasted more than a month. The six patients who remained in stupor for more than 6 months were all severely brain damaged.

Knowledge of the antecedent psychiatric history is often invaluable in suggesting the cause, and a careful neurological examination is always essential with special attention to signs that may indicate a diencephalic or upper brainstem lesion (see Diencephalon and brainstem, earlier in chapter). Patients with stupor due to non-organic psychiatric illness are more likely to show some partial preservation of ability to help with feeding or eliminative functions, though this is by no means invariable. The facial expression and posture is also more likely to be meaningful or show some emotional reaction to what is said or done. On recovery, patients with non-organic stupors often prove to have retained awareness of what transpired during the episode, whereas in organic stupor the level of awareness as well as the level of responsiveness is usually severely diminished.

Schizophrenic stupor is mainly a catatonic phenomenon, and is usually seen along with other catatonic features such as negativism, echopraxia, posturing or flexibilitas cerea. It tends to carry a poor prognosis in the long term. The patient's posture is often fixed and bizarre, and may have symbolic meaning in connection with his delusions. When disturbed the special posture is often resumed. The facial expression may be secretive or withdrawn, and may betray attention to hallucinatory experiences. Some schizophrenic stupors appear to represent withdrawal into a world of delusional fantasies, whereas in others it seems that nothing at all is experienced by the patient. The latter may represent a prolongation in severe form of schizophrenic blocking of thought and of willed action. After acute treatment with, for example, lorazepam or electroconvulsive therapy (ECT), some patients may dramatically recover and may then be able to explain that their immobile state was a response to beliefs or hallucinatory injunctions. In other cases the patient apparently has no recollection of the episode. An important diagnosis to consider is neuroleptic malignant syndrome, an idiosyncratic response to many antipsychotic drugs (see Chapter 11); regardless of cause, some authorities advocate ECT as an effective treatment (Fink & Taylor 2001).

Depressive stupor may occasionally be just as profound as the above, and the differentiation can be difficult if the antecedent psychiatric history is unknown. Usually it can be seen to develop out of severe psychomotor retardation, which increases until there is universal motor inhibition. The posture and expression are sometimes indicative of sadness and hopelessness, and silent tears may be shed. Sometimes, however, the expression is apathetic and vacant. Conscious awareness is usually fully retained and the patient can later relate most of what was said and done to him.

Manic stupor is usually described as uncommon. The expression may be of elation or ecstasy, and the patient may later report that his mind was filled with teeming ideas to the extent that he was unable to react to anything around him. Surprisingly, in Abrams and Taylor's (1976) prospective study of catatonic patients, mania emerged as the commonest diagnosis, applying also to the subgroup who had shown stupor.

Hysterical and psychogenic stupors usually occur in a situation of stress, and manifest superficial motives can often be discerned. Signs of conversion hysteria are commonly in evidence. The condition is more likely than others to wax and wane, and there may be a marked emotional reaction when sensitive subjects are discussed. Completely passive dependence on others for feeding and toilet functions is rare, and the patient may show signs of irritability and annoyance when moved against his wishes.

Organic stupor has many causes, the most urgent of which is raised intracranial pressure producing a medullary or midbrain pressure cone. Focal pathologies in the region of the posterior diencephalon or upper midbrain include tumours (especially craniopharyngiomas), infarctions, meningitis (especially tuberculous meningitis), neurosyphilis and formerly encephalitis lethargica. Senile or presenile dementias may lead to stupor late in their course, likewise HIV-associated dementia. Complex partial seizures may take this form, or alternatively stupor may follow briefly in the wake of an epileptic seizure.

When a brain lesion is responsible for stupor, the site will commonly lie in the upper brainstem or mesencephalon. Sometimes, however, it is due to involvement of the anteromedial frontal lobes and adjacent septal area (Segarra 1970). With stupors of brainstem origin the patient tends to be apathetic and somnolent most of the time and will frequently show pareses of external ocular movement. Patients with frontal stupor are more likely to appear alert, ready to be roused and with seeming vigilant gaze (hyperpathic akinetic mutism). Lesions of the anterior congulate and its subcortical connections seem to be implicated (Mega & Cohenour 1997).

Extracerebral causes that must be considered include a number of the conditions listed in Table 1.1. Pictures typical of stupor may occasionally be seen with uraemia, hypoglycaemia or liver disorder, or postoperatively with electrolyte disturbance or water intoxication. Endocrine disorders include myxoedema, Cushing's disease, Addison's disease, hypopituitarism and hyperparathyroidism. Stupor may also emerge with severe alcoholic intoxication, other intoxications, nicotinic acid deficiency encephalopathy, or terminally with certain infections such as typhus fever. It is important to remember that it can occasionally be seen as an adverse reaction to psychotropic medication; in Johnson's (1982) series of 25 cases, two were due to intoxication with lithium and one to excessive medication with flupenthixol. The neuroleptic malignant syndrome in either its full-blown or partial form should also be considered in any person exposed to antipsychotic drugs presenting with stupor and abnormally increased muscle tone. The presence of pyrexia and a raised creatine phosphokinase level form part of the diagnostic criteria.

Fortunately, with the great majority of organic causes there will be evidence of neurological dysfunction or systemic disturbance. In equivocal cases the EEG is often helpful in deciding between a psychiatric or a neurological aetiology. The absence of alpha rhythm and reduced reactivity is expected while faster rhythms may indicate a toxic or drug-induced state. Triphasic waves may be seen in hepatic and renal insufficiency in young adults and spindle coma patterns are believed to indicate brainstem dysfunction; the EEG may reveal previously unsuspected non-convulsive status epilepticus (Kaplan 2004). When psychogenic causes are suspected, an interview under Sodium amytal or a benzodiazepine may confirm the situation, while in schizophrenic and depressive stupors the response to ECT can be dramatic.

Causes of mutism

Mutism is rarely an isolated phenomenon, often occurring along with catatonic signs such as negativism, stereotypy, posturing or stupor. It may therefore be associated with the several psychiatric conditions discussed above. Important organic causes include head injury, posterior fossa surgery, encephalitis, frontal lobe lesions, the postictal phase of epilepsy, and endocrine disorders including hyperparathyroidism, myxoedema, diabetic ketoacidosis and Addison's disease (Gordon 2001). Complete speechlessless is rare in aphasic disorders since there is frequently some attempt to communicate or vocalise. The exception is the end stage of frontotemporal dementia.

Mutism without catatonic features may also be due to organic or non-organic causes. Dissociative states are among the commoner associated conditions, though here it is essential that severe dysphasia is excluded, as outlined in Chapter 2, Conversion disorders. In younger people, elective mutism is a relatively common reaction to a range of emotional disturbances and social anxiety.

Altshuler et al. (1986) drew together collected series of patients presenting with mutism and attempted to assess the

Table 1.5 Causes of mutism. (After Altshuler et al. 1986.)

All causes		Organic causes	
Schizophrenia	6	Stroke	4
Schizoaffective disorder	2	Postencephalitic disturbance	2
Other psychosis	1	Organic affective disorder	2
Affective disorder	3	Organic delusion syndrome	1
Organic disease	10	Phencyclidine psychosis	1
Total	22	Total	10

frequency of various causes. The pooled results showed that some 40% were likely to have affective disorder, 30% schizophrenia, 9% personality disorder and 17% an organic cerebral cause. In the remainder the responsible factors were uncertain. The diagnoses in these authors' own series of 22 patients presenting over a 2-year period are shown in Table 1.5; 14 of these had shown additional catatonic signs but eight had presented with mutism alone. Not uncommonly organic causes had been overlooked initially, for example in a patient with stroke who was first diagnosed as having hysterical aphonia, and in a patient with herpes encephalitis who was first thought to have catatonic schizophrenia. This emphasises the importance of careful neurological examination in every case.

Features stressed by Altshuler et al. as important in pointing to a neurological cause include irregular respiration, abnormal pupil responses, roving eye movements, facial weakness and an exaggerated jaw jerk. A psychiatric cause is suggested in patients who resist eye opening. Occasionally patients with a primary psychiatric disorder may be induced to whisper or communicate in writing, though the latter may also occur with infarctions leading to pure word-dumbness as described in Chapter 2 (Pure word-dumbness). The presence of accompanying catatonic phenomena cannot be relied upon as aiding the distinction between organic and non-organic causes. Again, however, an abreactive interview can often be informative.

References

Abrams, R. & Taylor, M.A. (1976) Catatonia: a prospective clinical study. *Archives of General Psychiatry* **33**, 579–581.

Allison, R.S. (1962) *The Senile Brain: A Clinical Study*. Edward Arnold, London.

Altshuler, L.L., Cummings, J.L. & Mills, M.J. (1986) Mutism: review, differential diagnosis, and report of 22 cases. *American Journal of Psychiatry* **143**, 1409–1414.

American Psychiatric Association (1994) *Diagnostic and Statistical Manual of Mental Disorders*, 4th edn. American Psychiatric Association, Washington, DC.

Barker, M.G. & Lawson, J.S. (1968) Nominal aphasia in dementia. *British Journal of Psychiatry* **114**, 1351–1356.

Berlyne, N. (1972) Confabulation. *British Journal of Psychiatry* **120**, 31–39.

Bonhoeffer, K. (1909) Exogenous psychoses. *Zentralblatt für Nervenheilkunde* **32**, 499–505. Translated by H. Marshall, in Hirsch, S.R. & Shepherd, M. (eds) *Themes and Variations in European Psychiatry*. John Wright, Bristol, 1974.

Britton, A. & Russell, R. (2004) Multidisciplinary team interventions for delirium in patients with chronic impairment. Cochrane Database of Systematic Reviews, CD000395.

Burns, A., Gallagley, A. & Byrne, J. (2004) Delirium. *Journal of Neurology, Neurosurgery and Psychiatry* **75**, 362–367.

Butler, C. & Zeman, A.Z.J. (2005) Neurological syndromes which can be mistaken for psychiatric conditions. *Journal of Neurology, Neurosurgery and Psychiatry* **76** (suppl. 1), 31–38.

Cummings, J.L. (1992) Psychosis in neurologic disease. Neurobiology and pathogenesis. *Neuropsychiatry, Neuropsychology and Behavioral Neurology* **5**, 144–150.

Ellis, H.D. & Lewis, M.B. (2001) Capgras delusion: a window on face recognition. *Trends in Cognitive Science* **5**, 149–156.

Fink, M. & Taylor, M.A. (2001) The many varieties of catatonia. *European Archives of Psychiatry and Clinical Neuroscience* **251** (suppl. 1), I8–I13.

Francis, J., Martin, D. & Kapoor, W.N. (1990) A prospective study of delirium in hospitalized elderly. *JAMA* **263**, 1097–1101.

Geschwind, N. (1965) Disconnexion syndromes in animals and man. *Brain* **88**, 237–294, 585–644.

Gordon, N. (2001) Mutism: elective or selective, and acquired. *Brain and Development* **23**, 83–87.

Hutchinson, G. & David, A. (1997) Manic pseudo-delirium: 2 case reports. *Behavioural Neurology* **10**, 21–23.

Johnson, J. (1982) Stupor: its diagnosis and management. *British Journal of Hospital Medicine* **27**, 530–532.

Johnson, J. (1984) Stupor: a review of 25 cases. *Acta Psychiatrica Scandinavica* **70**, 370–377.

Joyston-Bechal, M.P. (1966) The clinical features and outcome of stupor. *British Journal of Psychiatry* **117**, 967–981.

Kaplan, P.W. (2004) The EEG in metabolic encephalopathy and coma. *Journal of Clinical Neurophysiology* **21**, 307–318.

Lipowski, Z.J. (1980) *Delirium: Acute Brain Failure in Man*. Charles C. Thomas, Springfield, IL.

Lipowski, Z.J. (1990) *Delirium: Acute Confusional States*, 2nd edn. Oxford University Press, Oxford.

Liptzin, B. & Levkoff, S.E. (1992) An empirical study of delirium subtypes. *British Journal of Psychiatry* **161**, 843–845.

Lishman, W.A. (1992) Neuropsychiatry. A delicate balance. *Psychosomatics* **33**, 4–9.

Mega, M.S. & Cohenour, R.C. (1997) Akinetic mutism: disconnection of frontal–subcortical circuits. *Neuropsychiatry, Neuropsychology and Behavioral Neurology* **10**, 254–259.

Roth, M. & Myers, D.H. (1969) The diagnosis of dementia. *British Journal of Hospital Medicine* **2**, 705–717.

Segarra, J.M. (1970) Cerebral vascular disease and behavior. 1 The syndrome of the mesencephalic artery (basilar artery bifurcation). *Archives of Neurology* **22**, 408–418.

Turjanski, N. & Lloyd, G.G. (2005) Psychiatric side-effects of medications: recent developments. *Advances in Psychiatric Treatment* **11**, 58–70.

World Health Organization (1992) *The ICD-10 Classification of Mental and Behavioural Disorders: Clinical Descriptions and Diagnostic Guidelines*. World Health Organization, Geneva.

CHAPTER 2

Neuropsychology in Relation to Psychiatry

Anthony S. David and Michael D. Kopelman

Institute of Psychiatry, King's College, London

Historical and conceptual background

Neuropsychology is the branch of psychology concerned with the relationship between the brain, behaviour and thinking (cognition). The relationship is reciprocal in the sense that we understand the brain through its manifestations in psychology, including behaviour and cognition, and we gain an understanding of behaviour and cognition through the actions of the brain. The twin observations that perturbations to the brain may lead to predictable effects on its output and that the path from disturbed cognition and behaviour leads back to the brain and its functions form the cornerstone of neuropsychology. Such observations also serve to highlight the clinical underpinnings of the field even at its most academic. Indeed the founding fathers of neuropsychology were invariably clinicians whose area of practice approximated that of the modern neuropsychiatrist.

Certain psychological manifestations deserve particular attention because they are sometimes found in association with relatively circumscribed brain lesions. In every case they can also be seen with pathology which involves the brain diffusely or disturbs its functions widely, so their presence is by no means a certain indication of a single localised lesion. Nevertheless, when they emerge as isolated defects or stand out prominently against a background of mild impairment of other cerebral functions, they command especial care in the search for focal pathology.

What we ask of psychological symptoms as guides to focal pathology must be considerably less than we expect of neurological signs. The latter will often point with fair precision to the site of the lesion, but psychological symptoms can often tell us little more than that the pathology is unlikely to be diffuse. The careful analysis of dysphasia or of visual perceptual deficits may take us some way towards assessing the site of the lesion, but even here we must usually be content with rather broad indications of the areas of brain that fail to function. Thus with rare exceptions there remains uncertainty about the 'regional' as opposed to the 'focal' implications of most of the syndromes considered in this chapter. Some of them will be found to owe their origin, in different patients, to focal lesions in a variety of sites.

The majority of focal psychological symptoms represent defects of cognitive functioning. Less can be said with certainty about the focal significance of emotional, motivational or 'personality' abnormalities. 'Psychotic' symptoms, with a few exceptions, elude clear ties to focal brain pathology, and here other determinants are known to be more important. Nevertheless, certain non-cognitive disorders and even some psychotic manifestations do show interesting regional affiliations, and these will also be briefly reviewed.

Strictly focal brain damage or dysfunction is rare, except when produced by operations on the brain. In naturally occurring disease we see merely a focal emphasis in pathology, with effects that are then compounded by the effects of damage elsewhere. Focal head injury, for example, is usually accompanied by brain damage remote from the site of principal destruction; epileptic disturbances which originate focally disrupt other cerebral systems more or less widely; and circumscribed tumours produce distant effects by distortion of brain tissue, vascular complications or raised intracranial pressure. It is not surprising therefore that knowledge of regional cerebral disorder has been slow to accumulate and raises many areas of controversy. Brain imaging by computerised tomography (CT) or magnetic resonance imaging (MRI), and the more recent development of sophisticated functional imaging techniques, now hold promise of clarifying some of the problems in this area. Converging evidence from work with animals, experimental studies on healthy volunteers, simulations using mathematical and computer models and so forth have elevated research in neuropsychology to a key position in relation to medicine

Lishman's Organic Psychiatry: A Textbook of Neuropsychiatry, 4th edition.
© 2009 Blackwell Publishing.   ISBN 978-1-4051-1860-1

and psychiatry, rivalling in importance and excitement the unravelling of the genetic code.

While neuropsychology is a relatively young discipline, beginning in earnest around the mid-nineteenth century, its conceptual basis dates back to Hippocrates (*c*.425 BCE) and the doctrine that:

the source of our pleasure, merriment, laughter, and amusement, as of our grief, pain, anxiety and tears is none other than the brain. It is specially the organ which enables us to think, see, hear and to distinguish the ugly and the beautiful, the bad and the good, the pleasant and unpleasant.

And as for neuropsychiatry, he goes on:

It is the brain too which is the seat of madness and delirium, of the fears and frights which assail us . . . it is there where lies the cause of insomnia and sleep-walking, of thoughts that will not come, forgotten duties and eccentricities (quoted in Marshall and Gurd 2003).

Cerebral localisation

The paradigm shift came with the assertion that a particular part of the brain was the 'seat' of a particular psychic function, in this case articulate language. This is usually attributed to French neurologist Paul Broca in 1861, although some claim precedence for Marc Dax nearly 30 years earlier. A constant battle has run through neuropsychology ever since between those pursuing the 'localisationist' view and those with a more holistic view of brain functions, later termed 'equipotentiality' by Karl Lashley in the early part of the twentieth century. Such battles continue to the present day. Holistic views of brain function fitted well with early humoral theories of the mind and appeared to be upheld by the early experiments on pigeons by Flourens (1824) in the first part of the nineteenth century. Strict localisationist views gained impetus during this period from the widespread credibility accorded to Franz Joseph Gall and his followers. Gall initially proffered a sophisticated view of the modular nature of brain functions but lost credibility through the doctrines of phrenology, which ultimately reached the fantastic lengths of claiming cerebral centres for such functions as 'hope', 'patriotism' and 'attraction to wine'. Lashley's work specifically addressed acquisition of knowledge. In tests of maze learning in rats, it was shown that the size but not the location of the lesion was related to impairment of learning. Lashley's law of mass action expressed the view that learning ability is determined by the total mass of normally functioning cortex.

Since the end of the nineteenth century, there has been a steady though far from smooth accumulation of evidence concerning the cerebral representation of language and of other symbolic 'gnostic' functions. Unfortunately, much of this initially depended on uncritical compilations of case material, and at the turn of the century the 'diagram makers' were frequently in confusion. Hughlings Jackson's (1869) theory of *levels* of functional organisation within the nervous system, and the emergence of symptoms by a process of dissolution of such levels, received little attention at the time but has a strikingly contemporary ring, for instance in the classification of psychiatric symptoms as positive versus negative (or deficit) and the discussion of 'release' phenomena such as hallucinations. One of the issues is that strictly focal damage is rarely seen, and usually the lesion touches on several zones and damages several overlapping systems together. Moreover, the plasticity of organisation is such that the structure of a psychological function may vary with the particular mental task involved; for example the recall of one series may utilise a mnemonic logical path, and the recall of another series a path based on visual images. Finally, a clear distinction must always be maintained between the localisation of the pathology accounting for symptoms, and the localisation of the functions whose disturbance the symptoms represent.

Despite these necessary warnings, the careful description and experimental exploration of cases with discrete damage or highly specific deficits has led to genuine leaps in conceptual knowledge. This approach – with its emphasis on dissociations of function (i.e. the presence of a pattern of intact abilities and surprisingly marked impairments in an individual) or, even more informative, the contrasting patterns of intact abilities and marked impairments across individuals (the double dissociation) – has proved decisive in neuropsychology (Shallice 1988; McCarthy & Warrington 1990). For example, discrete lesions in the hypothalamic–diencephalic region, or damage restricted to the hippocampal areas as in the case of the patient H.M. (see Medial temporal amnesia, later), may virtually abolish new learning in any modality. Thus, contra Lashley, we now have clear evidence that the proper organisation of memory functions involves to some considerable degree discrete systems within the human brain. Finally, the search for focal deficits has also been extended into matters other than cognitive function. In animals, focal brain lesions can lead to dramatic changes of temperament (rage reactions or placidity) depending on the site of the lesion. The amygdala has been the focus of much research in this regard. And what of higher functions still such as 'personality' and social behaviour? Certainly in monkeys interesting results can follow focal extirpations of brain tissue. Such demonstrations continue to influence our understanding of emotional disorders in neuropsychiatry but with the advent of *in vivo* techniques of neuroimaging, less reliance need be placed on this type of animal experimentation.

An alternative to strict localisationism emerged in the early part of the twentieth century: the postulation of brain *systems* rather than discrete regions dedicated to functions. An early influential example is the 'circuit' described by Papez (1937) of the limbic system, which he thought constituted an essential mechanism for the elaboration of emotional experience and emotional expression. More recently, Alexander *et al.* (1990) have mapped another system or rather series of circuits that links the basal ganglia and thalamus to the frontal cortex, from which may be derived the basic architecture for motor control, initiation and inhibition of action and which is believed to be affected in tic disorders, obsessive–compulsive phenomena and regulation of affect. The implication is that lesions interrupting the anatomically distributed circuit at any point may result in a rather similar clinical picture.

Other groupings or organising principles that are supra-local include the division between the left and right cerebral hemispheres. As noted the close affiliation between the left hemisphere and language was part of Broca's original insight and attempts have been made to characterise the left and right hemispheres broadly in terms of a verbal/non-verbal processing. This dichotomy had to broaden to take account of accumulating evidence for, in particular, a greater range of specialised functions localised in the right hemisphere (including language related) and non-linguistic functions of the left, giving rise to other contrasting pairings, for example analytic–holistic, serial–parallel, general impersonal–specific personal, but none has achieved universal acceptance. A boost to the notion of lateralisation of cerebral functions came with the description of the disconnection syndromes, both naturally occurring and induced by surgical transection of the corpus callosum and cerebral commissures (Geschwind 1965; Bogen 1985). These syndromes accentuate functional specialisation but also, by definition, show how patterns of deficits and preserved abilities can arise through the disruption of pathways that convey information between specialised areas of the brain rather than disruption to the areas themselves.

Despite these fascinating debates regarding the basis of neuropsychological deficits, it is disturbed social behaviour and awareness that are at the root of the presenting complaints that dominate neuropsychiatric clinical practice. A recurring question is whether these can be localised to a part of the brain. If the favoured answer is 'yes', then the candidate region is usually the frontal lobes, as discussed briefly in Chapter 1 (and see Executive (frontal lobe) syndromes, later in this chapter). From a contemporary cognitive neuroscience point of view, the frontal lobes represent the greatest challenge. The current notion is that the frontal lobes subserve (with other parts of a network) a collection of executive functions, for example willed intentional action, inhibition of pre-potent responses, selective attention, set-shifting, working memory (holding and manipulating information online), reasoning and self-awareness and possibly 'general intelligence'. The 'executive' metaphor is intended to convey the idea that such higher-level functions arise through the coordinated and controlled activity of subsidiary functions rather than the higher functions themselves being localisable within the frontal cortex or other region (see Neuropsy-

chology of executive function, later for discussion). This would explain the myriad disparate manifestations of neuropsychiatric disorders found to be associated with disease or dysfunction of the frontal lobes. Finally, the unthinking tendency to attribute all that is interesting and unique about human behaviour to the frontal lobes in the misguided belief that this is in some way an explanation must be resisted (David 1992).

Modern neuropsychology

Many contemporary neuropsychological theories were anticipated by the so-called 'diagram-makers' of the late nineteenth century (Shallice 1988), but the inevitable limitations of their clinical data meant that their views came to be dismissed. The term 'neuropsychology' is often attributed to Hebb (1949) whose classic *The Organization of Behaviour* was subtitled *A Neuropsychological Theory*. However, Bruce (1985) pointed out that the word had a much earlier currency. Bruce attributed the word to Osler (1913) in an address at the Johns Hopkins Hospital, subsequently published. Bruce speculated that Lashley may have attended this address; Lashley's own first use of the term appears to have been in 1936, and he was appointed Research Professor of Neuropsychology at Harvard in 1937.

The huge growth of neuropsychology after the Second World War had, perhaps, three main sources. The first was the influence of Hebb's classic book, which drew ideas from many disciplines into a unified theory and anticipated many contemporary notions. The second was the excellent series of investigations of soldiers injured by penetrating missile wounds in the Second World War, which considerably advanced our knowledge of functional localisation (and its limitations); parallel studies occurred in the UK (Newcombe 1969), the former USSR (Luria 1964) and the USA (Semmes *et al.* 1963; Teuber 1962). Thirdly, Milner's pioneering studies of H.M. (Scoville & Milner 1957; Milner 1966) demonstrated in a dramatic fashion the devastating effects of circumscribed brain pathology, and the ways in which these could be investigated by detailed experimental techniques.

A very important consequence of this burgeoning interest was the founding of the journals *Neuropsychologia* and *Cortex*, both in 1963. The International Neuropsychological Society was formed in 1967. But there were limitations to empiricism across large patient groups, and the more theoretical approach of Elizabeth Warrington, her collaborators and successors in the UK produced important advances in our knowledge of topics such as amnesia, the acquired dyslexias, semantic memory and executive function. The intensive investigation of single cases to develop or refute cognitive models that were not that dissimilar from those of the 'diagram-makers' culminated in the foundation of the journal *Cognitive Neuropsychology* in 1984, exemplifying this approach. However, despite the enormous advances made in theoretical knowledge, there were always limitations to this approach, principally a tendency to over-generalise from the particular case and a failure to take account of other factors ('associations') that might be just as important in understanding cognitive performance as the identification of 'dissociations' in single cases. However, what seems most to have undermined the predominance of the 'single case' approach has been the requirements imposed by functional neuroimaging studies.

Current debates concern the relationship of findings from functional neuroimaging, which identify circuits recruited in association with cognitive performance, and lesion studies, which identify sites critical to a cognitive function. Debate continues about whether functional imaging studies can truly contribute to cognitive neuropsychological theory, as opposed to a different level of behavioural (neurophysiological) analysis (Coltheart 2006; Shallice 2003).

Disorders of memory

Memory disorder is a symptom of the utmost importance in psychiatric practice, in that it is one of the most sensitive indicators of brain damage or dysfunction, regardless of underlying pathology.

Neurological amnesias can be transient or persistent. Moreover, the persistent forms can be divided into two broad categories: those resulting from focal and those arising from diffuse cerebral disorder. In the former, amnesic defects can result from lesions in highly discrete parts of the brain and stand out against the relative preservation of other cognitive functions. In the latter, amnesic defects form an integral part of more widespread cortical and subcortical disease, as in dementia, or part of acute or subacute cerebral dysfunction, as in delirium. Moreover, memory loss can result from psychogenic disturbance, where there may be brain dysfunction but brain damage is not causative. Therefore, after a general background introduction, memory disorder is considered below in terms of (i) transient amnesias, (ii) the brain systems mainly involved in memory disorders, (iii) the clinical picture and pattern of neuropsychological deficits in common amnesic states, (iv) confabulation, (v) amnesia in diffuse cerebral disease, and (vi) psychogenic and psychiatric forms of memory loss.

General background introduction

The relationship between disorder of memory and cerebral pathology has repaid detailed study, and clinicopathological correlations have here reached firmer ground than where many other psychological symptoms are concerned. This is largely because many aspects of memory are amenable to objective testing and because relatively discrete lesions give rise to memory deficits and these lesions can be mimicked in animal investigations. These are both features that are rarely encountered in other psychiatric syndromes. However, many controversies remain.

Theories of memory exist at many levels. Physiological theories postulate changes in electrical activity of neurones and their interconnections; such theories serve to explain very short-term storage, but for the establishment of durable memories there must be the ability to withstand profound derangement of electrical activity as in anaesthesia, hypothermia or convulsions. Biochemical theories suggest changes in the synthesis of neurotransmitters and intracellular proteins, or changes in gene expression within the neurone, but fail to take account of how brain systems operate and interact. Connectionist theories follow Hebb (1949) in postulating anatomical changes in synaptic relationships between cells (e.g. Meeter & Murre 2004) but some of their postulates are not directly testable.

Squire (1987), Kandel and Hawkins (1992) and Tranel and Damasio (1995) have discussed findings in this area. Studies of the mollusc *Aplysia*, for example, have shown unequivocal evidence both of changes in transmitter release and morphological alterations in synapses during learning. The discovery that brief high-frequency stimulation can alter the excitability of postsynaptic cells in the hippocampus for several hours or even weeks (long-term potentiation, LTP) has also been shown to have relevance to learning. The initiation of LTP is subserved by the binding of glutamate to receptors on target cells, whereas its maintenance appears to depend on some factor, possibly nitric oxide, which acts in a retrograde manner on presynaptic terminals to enhance transmitter release. Both electrical and biochemical theories are brought together by the discovery that the N-methyl-D-aspartate (NMDA) glutamate receptor has a channel that opens to extracellular ions only when the cell is depolarised. This dual requirement for both receptor binding and electrical depolarisation suggests that NMDA receptors may act as conjunction detectors in the hippocampus with a role in associative learning. Nevertheless, the findings from biochemistry have been disappointing, both in terms of improving our understanding of human memory disorders and in terms of producing potent pharmacological agents for their treatment.

Two main regions of the brain that have emerged as especially significant in relation to anterograde amnesia are the diencephalon and the medial temporal lobes. They lie within circuitry that also encompasses the mamillary bodies, fornix and retrosplenium. Damage within this circuitry can selectively impair the capacity to form durable records of experience. It is associated also with a variable retrograde gap for memories laid down before the damage occurred (Rempel-Clower et al. 1996). It used to be thought that earlier memories remained substantially intact, and that these sites did not themselves represent the 'repositories' or storehouses of memories but were concerned with adding to the store and perhaps with retrieval from the store (Squire & Alvarez 1995).

However, a more recent view is that the hippocampus (perhaps together with other medial temporal structures) is indeed a component in the memory engram, acting as a pointer or index of memories for episodes, whatever their age (Nadel & Moscovitch 1997). According to this view, every time a memory is retrieved or reactivated a new trace is laid down, resulting in the accumulation of 'multiple traces'.

Besides these parts of the brain, other neural systems must be implicated in the processes of remembering. We preserve in memory mainly those things towards which attention is directed, and alerting and 'executive' mechanisms must therefore be involved. The emotional connotations of material can also influence memory recall (Lishman 1972, 1974; Master *et al.* 1983; Rubin & Schulkind 1997; Buchanan *et al.* 2005), and the amygdalae and frontal systems are implicated in this. Other variables affect the content of what is encoded and retrieved, such as interest and motivation, relevance, importance, and consistency with existing frames of reference (Bartlett 1932; Schacter 2001). Hence, memory provides fertile ground for the influence of psychosocial factors and, in extreme instances, for the occurrence of psychogenic impairment. In short, the clinicopathological correlations obtained in neurological amnesias may reveal only a part of the total mechanisms involved in remembering.

Transient amneslas

Transient amnesias can be particularly informative because they are dense and then, by definition, they recover.

Transient global amnesia (TGA) most commonly occurs in the middle-aged or elderly, more frequently in men. It encompasses a period of anterograde amnesia lasting several hours. It is characterised by repetitive questioning, and there may be some confusion, but unlike psychogenic forms of amnesia, patients do not report any loss of personal identity. It is sometimes preceded by a headache or nausea, a stressful life event, a medical procedure, intense emotion or vigorous exercise. Hodges and Ward (1989) found that the mean duration of amnesia was 4 hours and the maximum 12 hours. In 25% of their sample, there was a past history of migraine, which was considered likely to have had an aetiological role. In 7% of cases, the patient subsequently developed epilepsy, in the absence of any previous history of seizures. There was no association with a past history of, or risk factors for, vascular disorder or transient ischaemic attacks. In 60–70% of the sample, the aetiology was unknown. Similar findings were obtained by Miller *et al.* (1987) in a sample of 150 men and 127 women. Again, the incidence of cerebral vascular events was no higher than would be expected in this age group.

Neuropsychological testing during the episode confirms a profound anterograde amnesia on tests of both verbal and non-verbal memory, but retrograde amnesia is variable, usually being relatively brief but occasionally more exten-sive. Although the clinical impression is of complete recovery following the attack, both Miller *et al.* (1987) and Hodges and Oxbury (1990) found evidence of subtle but statistically significant residual impairments on some neuropsychological tests. There is now evidence from a number of sources that medial temporal lobe, vasospasm, hypoperfusion, and spreading depression within white matter is the underlying basis of TGA. Evidence supporting this hypothesis comes from investigations using single-photon emission computed tomography (SPECT), positron emission tomography (PET) and diffusion-weighted MRI.

Transient epileptic amnesia (TEA) is a term coined by Kapur (1990). It refers to that subgroup of TGA cases in which epilepsy appears to be the underlying cause. The main differences from other cases of TGA are that where seizure activity underlies the dysfunction, the episodes of memory loss are brief (1 hour or less), and that patients are more likely to experience multiple attacks (Hodges & Warlow 1990). It is important to note that standard electroencephalography (EEG) and CT or MRI findings are often normal; however, an epileptic basis to the disorder may be revealed on sleep-deprived EEG. Although 'transient epileptic amnesia' is a useful term, there may be variants within it, notably between cases in which the amnesic episodes are ictal and those in which they are postictal in nature. As will be mentioned below, it appears that many patients who report TEA attacks also describe 'gaps' in their past autobiographical memory. There is controversy about the nature of these autobiographical memory gaps, but the most parsimonious explanation would be that there have been clinically undetected brief runs of seizure activity in the past, which resulted in faulty (anterograde) encoding of very specific items in autobiographical memory. Hence the patients complain of 'gaps' in autobiographical memory rather than more global impairment.

Brain systems involved in memory disorder

Diencephalic amnesia

Lesions in the posterior hypothalamus and nearby midline structures were the first to be firmly linked with amnesia. They constitute the principal pathological basis of Korsakoff's syndrome, and involve areas around the third ventricle, the periaqueductal grey matter, the upper brainstem, certain thalamic nuclei and the posterior hypothalamus. The mamillary bodies along with the terminal portions of the fornices are nearly always affected, and publications reviewed by Brierley (1966) suggested that damage confined almost exclusively to the mamillary bodies can account for the Korsakoff memory defect. However, in a detailed neuropathological study Victor *et al.* (1971) argued that lesions in the medial dorsal nuclei of the thalamus were of more critical importance, and may in fact be crucial for the development of amnesic symptoms in Korsakoff's syndrome.

Debate has continued over the relative importance of the mamillary bodies and the thalamic nuclei in Korsakoff patients, or indeed whether both must be involved together (Mair *et al.* 1979). Kopelman (1995) has reviewed evidence suggesting that a circuit involving the mamillary bodies, the mamillothalamic tracts and the *anterior* (rather than the medial dorsal) nuclei of the thalamus may be particularly critical for memory formation. Investigations by Mayes *et al.* (1988) and Harding *et al.* (2000) have supported the importance of this circuitry, and of lesions to the anterior rather than medial dorsal thalamic nuclei.

The common cause for lesions in this situation is thiamine deficiency, the amnesic difficulties developing as a sequel to Wernicke's encephalopathy (Chapter 11, Wernicke's encephalopathy). Chronic alcoholism is nowadays by far the commonest cause of a Wernicke episode, but other established causes include carcinoma of the stomach, pregnancy, severe malnutrition, or persistent vomiting from any cause.

The term 'Korsakoff's syndrome' is probably best reserved for such cases where thiamine depletion is the underlying aetiology, and 'amnesic syndrome' can be used more generally to describe those disorders which follow other forms of damage to the same brain regions. Tumours in the neighbourhood of the hypothalamus and third ventricle may produce a closely similar picture (Guinan *et al.* 1998). Subarachnoid haemorrhage may occasionally be followed by a pronounced amnesic syndrome due to local haemorrhage or organisation of the clot in the basal regions of the brain. In the severe stages of tuberculous meningitis, a picture closely similar to Korsakoff's syndrome may be witnessed over many weeks; following recovery normal memory function gradually returns, leaving only an amnesic gap for the acute phase of the illness and a retrograde amnesia for a variable period before it (Williams & Smith 1954). The characteristic pathology of tuberculous meningitis in the amnesic phase is an inflammatory process with organisation of exudate, largely limited to the anterior basal cisterns of the brain and involving the mamillary region and the floor of the third ventricle. There is evidence to suggest that these regions have escaped the main impact of the infective process in those few cases where memory difficulties do not appear.

While the importance of diencephalic and hypothalamic lesions in relation to amnesia cannot be doubted, it is important to remember that the pathology of Korsakoff's syndrome involves additional brain regions, and that these may include structures which contain important neurochemical nuclei. There is usually concomitant frontal lobe atrophy, which may give rise to behavioural features such as apathy, and, when severe, can be the basis of confabulation (Kopelman 2002). Adrenergic, serotonergic and cholinergic depletions have all been reported in Korsakoff's syndrome with accompanying claims of aetiological importance. None of these has produced any major therapeutic advance to date, although this may be partly because there has been a dearth of adequate therapeutic trials in this disorder.

Medial temporal amnesia

Long after the description of Korsakoff's syndrome, an amnesic syndrome was described that was closely similar in phenomenology to that of the Korsakovian defect. This was first fully recognised after surgical extirpation of brain tissue for the relief of psychotic disorders and epilepsy (Scoville 1954; Scoville & Milner 1957). It results from bilateral lesions of the hippocampus and hippocampal gyrus, with variable involvement of structures within the parahippocampal gyri including the entorhinal, perirhinal and parahippocampal cortices (Corkin *et al.* 1997). In the surgical cases, the extent of their resection appeared to be roughly proportional to the severity of the memory disorder (Milner 1966), and bilateral lesions were required before a severe and global amnesia appeared. When amnesic symptoms have followed unilateral temporal lobe resection there has usually been evidence that the remaining hippocampal zone was also dysfunctional (Warrington & Duchen 1992). Unilateral resections generally give rise to a material-specific, more moderate memory impairment. Serafetinides and Falconer (1962) found that mild subjective forgetfulness sometimes followed unilateral right lobectomy, but in all such cases there was also evidence of a postoperative spike-discharging focus at the opposite temporal lobe, indicating dysfunction if not a lesion there.

Other aetiologies can also give rise to medial temporal amnesia. Cerebrovascular accidents may sometimes be followed by the acute onset of amnesic difficulties, as in the patient described by Victor *et al.* (1961) who suffered occlusion of each posterior cerebral artery in turn, and at autopsy was found to have lesions in the inferomedial portions of each temporal lobe. Two years intervened between the two strokes and it was only after the second episode that the amnesic syndrome appeared. The severe memory impairments that follow herpes encephalitis also result from pathology in this distribution, since the herpes simplex virus has a predilection for the medial temporal lobe structures Including the hippocampi (Brierley *et al.* 1960; Cermak & O'Connor 1983; Wilson *et al.* 1995; Stefanacci *et al.* 2000). Evidence from epilepsy similarly points to the importance of the hippocampal areas for memory, since these are the regions implicated in complex partial seizures where amnesia constitutes an essential feature of the attacks, and interictal memory complaints are common. Cerebral hypoxia or hypoxia/ischaemia is another cause of hippocampal amnesia as in the patient reported by Zola-Morgan *et al.* (1986) who developed a marked and persistent anterograde amnesia after ischaemic damage restricted to the CA1 fields of the hippocampi bilaterally.

High-resolution MRI has proved capable of visualising hippocampal damage during life in amnesic patients. Press *et al.* (1989) reported three patients with circumscribed amnesic states, one due to respiratory arrest and the others of unknown aetiology, all of whom showed bilateral hippocampal abnormalities on coronal T1-weighted images taken perpendicularly to the long axis of the hippocampus. Quantified measurements of the hippocampi on three-dimensional MRI have now been carried out in many investigations of amnesia and dementia (Chan *et al.* 2001; Colchester *et al.* 2001), and good correlations with measures of anterograde memory can be obtained (Kopelman *et al.* 2001).

Other brain structures implicated in memory processes

Early reports suggested that the fornix bundles, which provide the main connection between the hippocampi and the hypothalamic structures, could be cut bilaterally without disturbing memory (Dott 1938; Cairns & Mosberg 1951). Such patients, however, were not subjected to formal neuropsychological evaluation. More recently, memory deficits have been documented after lesions of the fornix, even in the absence of CT or MRI evidence of damage to other key memory structures (Grafman *et al.* 1985; Hodges & Carpenter 1991). The patient reported by Tucker *et al.* (1988) was particularly interesting in that a small focal astrocytoma of the left fornix led to a memory deficit confined to verbal material, much as would be expected from a left hippocampal lesion. Aggleton *et al.* (2000) reported memory disorder, particularly affecting recall memory, in a series of patients with choroid cysts implicating the fornix.

Disruption of the memory circuitry and resulting memory disorder also occurs in retrosplenial lesions arising from vascular accidents or with tumours of the splenium of the corpus callosum (Valenstein *et al.* 1987; Rudge & Warrington 1991). The retrosplenial cortex is situated in the cingulate gyrus just above and posterior to the splenium, and contains relays between the anterior nucleus of the thalamus and the medial temporal lobe. Retrosplenial hypometabolism is commonly found in amnesic disorders in fluorodeoxyglucose (FDG)-PET investigations, whatever the underlying aetiology (Reed *et al.* 1999, 2003, 2005; Nestor *et al.* 2003).

The role of the frontal lobes in memory has been increasingly highlighted, especially since the advent of functional neuroimaging. Operations on the frontal lobes rarely produce persistently severe memory disorders, though in the early postoperative period there may be a striking deficit of retention of current experience together with patchy retrograde amnesia (Klein 1952; Kral & Durost 1953). Whitty and Lewin (1960) described a transient memory disorder involving especially the temporal sequence of events following limited ablations of the anterior cingulate cortex. The early amnesic patient recorded by Mabille and Pitres (1913) was found to have symmetrical areas of infarction in the frontal white matter, strategically placed to interrupt long association fibres from the frontal lobes to other parts of the brain. More recently, Wheeler *et al.* (1995) reviewed the evidence on frontal lesions and memory, finding impairments in both

recall and recognition memory in the vast majority of studies.

It remains a matter of controversy whether the frontal lobes play a primary role in memory *per se* or merely influence memory processes by virtue of their involvement in attention and other executive functions. There are numerous pathways between the prefrontal cortex and the medial temporal lobe structures, and their interaction is a current topic of active research. It is now well established that there is frontal involvement in relation to special aspects of memory processes, for example in the suppression of irrelevant associations, in memory for temporal order and spatiotemporal context (source memory), and in the efficient retrieval of memories from the past (Mayes *et al.* 1985; Schacter 1987; Mayes 1988; Kopelman 1991). The role of superadded frontal lobe damage in Korsakoff's syndrome has been especially closely studied (see Chapter 11). There is hemispheric and subcortical (basal ganglia) specialisation for experience as displayed in verbal, visuospatial or motor learning. A temporal lobe (hippocampal) lesion in the hemisphere dominant for speech impairs the learning and retention of verbal material, resulting for example in forgetfulness for names, material read in newspapers or material heard in lectures. Conversely, patients with non-dominant temporal lobe lesions are impaired in memorising that which cannot be categorised in words, such as tunes, faces and meaningless drawings. There is now a considerable body of experimental data available on such distinctions between left and right hemisphere lesions.

There is now a vast literature on functional brain activation techniques (PET, fMRI) in memory, which it is beyond the scope of this chapter to review. However, early investigations suggested that the left frontal region was particularly involved in the encoding of episodic memories, whereas the right frontal region, together with the precuneus, was of particular importance in episodic memory retrieval (Shallice *et al.* 1994; Tulving *et al.* 1994; Fletcher *et al.* 1995). In contrast, other investigations have produced evidence of more traditional left–right material-specific asymmetries during memory encoding in both the medial temporal lobes and the prefrontal cortex (Golby *et al.* 2001). Many investigations have reported activations in the hippocampi and medial temporal lobe structures. Lepage *et al.* (1998) argued, on the basis of a matter-analysis, that anterior medial temporal activations were associated with memory encoding and posterior activations with retrieval, whereas Schacter and Wagner (1999) found that encoding activations were associated with both anterior and posterior activations. Some studies have examined the relationship between frontal and hippocampal activation in consolidation (Kopelman *et al.* 1997), whereas others have reported differential patterns of hippocampal and parahippocampal activation during more recollective or familiarity-based memory processes (Davachi *et al.* 2003; Ranganath *et al.* 2004).

There are also functional imaging studies that have examined the retrieval of more remote, episodic memories. Some investigations have reported greater hippocampal activation in the retrieval of recent, as opposed to remote, episodic memories (Haist *et al.* 2001; Mayes *et al.* 2004a), whereas other studies have found that medial temporal lobe structures (the hippocampi in particular) are significantly activated in retrieving both recent and remote autobiographical memories (Ryan *et al.* 2001; Maguire *et al.* 2001). More recently, Gilboa *et al.* (2004) reported that the pattern of activations within the hippocampi may vary between remote and recent memory retrieval, the latter tending to show more anteriorally positioned hippocampal activations.

Clinical picture and pattern of neuropsychological deficits in amnesia

Definitions

The clinical and neuropsychological pattern of deficits seen in amnesic states has been extensively studied in patients who are relatively free from other intellectual impairments, usually in patients with focal lesions in the diencephalon or medial temporal lobes. In clinical practice, there is often some degree of concomitant cortical atrophy and/or confounding psychological problems such as depression or post-traumatic stress disorder.

For purposes of clinical description, a somewhat arbitrary division can be made into immediate, recent and remote memory. The *immediate memory span* is reflected in the reproduction of material such as brief digit sequences which fall within the span of attention. This memory span appears to represent the functioning of short-term memory mechanisms, which need not, even in normal circumstances, lead to an enduring record. (Clinically, this is often interpreted as evidence that 'registration' is intact.) *Recent memory* is reflected in the ability to acquire and retain new knowledge (termed 'current memorising' or 'new learning') and is assumed to require a process of consolidation in addition to initial encoding or registration. Clinically, it is assessed by testing the ability to recall simple information (exceeding the memory span) after at least a minute has elapsed. *Remote memory* is reflected in the ability to recall events or facts acquired at a considerable distance in time, and certainly before the onset of the memory difficulties, i.e. an impairment in remote memory indicates retrograde amnesia.

In everyday clinical practice, it is convenient to employ the terms 'immediate', 'recent' and 'remote' as outlined above. Unfortunately, however, considerable confusion has arisen over some of the terms commonly used in referring to memory mechanisms. For example, 'short-term memory' is used by experimental psychologists as synonymous with the immediate memory span, whereas in medical practice it is usually taken as congruent with recent memory. The term

is best avoided or, if used, employed in a strictly experimentally defined (research) sense.

An important division is recognised between primary and secondary memory mechanisms both in animal and human experimental work. Each has certain characteristics not shared by the other. Primary memory has a strictly limited capacity, being able to hold only a small number of unrelated items of information at a time. Decay from it is rapid when rehearsal is prevented. This is the aspect of memory tested by the digit span. The material held in primary memory is retained in a form closely tied to the qualities of the initial percepts (timbre, visual detail, precise verbal content, etc.); it is largely non-selective, and material can be reproduced from it with minimal comprehension of the meaning. Subsequent entries to the system displace what is already there. Primary memory thus acts as a short-term back-up to perceptual experience, giving time for selective attention to focus on what is meaningful and valuable for processing into secondary memory.

Working memory (Baddeley 1976; Hitch 1984) is an elaboration of the concept of primary memory described above. It emphasises those components that can hold information in short-term storage and manipulate it while performing ongoing cognitive tasks, and it recognises the existence of different subsystems dealing with specialised forms of material. The 'articulatory loop', for example, deals with phonological information, the 'visuospatial scratch pad' with visual images. Suitable experimental paradigms, and studies in patients with brain lesions, can show the relative independence of the one from the other (Vallar & Papagno 1995).

Secondary memory has very different properties. Material held in secondary memory is encoded more commonly in semantic terms, i.e. in the form of meaningful schema or concepts, and the primary qualities of the percepts may become somewhat obscured. The result is a far more durable record. There is no known limit to the amount that can be stored. Secondary memory (also known as 'long-term memory' in experimental psychology) thus encompasses all material retained beyond a period of several seconds, and includes both recent and remote memories.

Studies carried out in both normal subjects and patients with amnesia have generally upheld these broad divisions, though complex interrelationships clearly exist between these memory storage systems. Valuable reviews of experimental work are to be found in Squire (1987) and Parkin (1987).

The *episodic–semantic* distinction was introduced by Tulving (1972) and relates to events and facts held within secondary memory. Episodic memory refers to memory for specific, personally experienced events or episodes from the individual's past and to the ability to travel back mentally in time. Semantic memory deals essentially with organised knowledge about the world which does not have a specific location in time or place – knowledge of objects, labels, vocabulary, principles and concepts. As such, it is a shared form of knowledge, much of which is acquired early in life. Both the episodic and semantic aspects of memory can be affected (or spared) in memory disorders. Hence, episodic memory is particularly (although not usually exclusively) affected in the amnesic syndrome, whereas semantic memory is particularly damaged in semantic dementia, involving focal temporal lobe atrophy.

A further distinction is made between *explicit* or *declarative* and *implicit* or *procedural* memory. Explicit or declarative memory refers to conscious awareness of past events or facts (Squire 1987). It embraces both episodic and semantic memory as defined above. Implicit memory refers to the facilitation of particular responses or to perceptuomotor skill acquisition and retention, which does not require (and may be inhibited by) conscious awareness of the learning episode. This 'knowing how' to do it is expressed in performance, not in conscious recollection. The phenomenon of 'priming' involves the facilitation of responses to cues such as previously perceived, partially completed or semantically related words. The various forms of procedural memory include motor skills (e.g. how to ride a bicycle or tie shoe laces) and the capacity to perform certain cognitive operations (e.g. how to solve certain types of puzzle). Implicit memory is characteristically preserved when explicit memory is severely disrupted in the amnesic syndrome.

Thus there appear to be several independent memory systems, and these are related to different neural networks within the brain. Explicit episodic memory is damaged by medial temporal and diencephalic lesions. There is some evidence that impairments in skill learning may be related to damage in the striatum, and priming effects to neocortical pathology (Squire 1986; Kopelman 2002). Semantic memory is particularly affected by atrophy or pathology in the inferior and lateral temporal lobes, more commonly on the left.

Clinical picture

In the amnesic syndrome, perception is unimpaired, the immediate memory span is well preserved, and there is severe impairment of new learning (anterograde amnesia) and a variable retrograde amnesia usually with a so-called 'temporal gradient', i.e. relative sparing of early memories.

Preservation of the immediate memory span is a point of importance clinically. Performance on a test of digit span is usually normal, and therefore will fail to reveal the existence even of a severe amnesic syndrome. Patients with bilateral temporal lobe resection, in whom good ability to cooperate is well preserved, have shown that in the absence of distraction such brief information can be retained for as long as several minutes by dint of constant verbal rehearsal. However, forgetting occurs as soon as new activity demands a shift away from the task in hand. Moreover, the learning of a list which only slightly exceeds the normal digit span is markedly impaired, revealing the essential difficulty in getting new material into longer term store (Drachman & Arbit 1966).

Current and recent memory (i.e. new learning) is severely impaired, and disorientation in time is almost universal. In the most extreme cases, new learning may be reduced to virtually nil, so that as time goes by there is a continuing and extending anterograde amnesia. If recovery subsequently occurs (e.g. following head injury), a dense and permanent gap will be left for the period of the illness. In less severe examples the problem shows as uncertainty about events that occurred minutes, days or weeks before, some being vaguely recalled and others having made no lasting impression at all. The retelling of simple stories is marked by gross omissions, incorrect juxtapositions and condensations of material. Testing reveals that the problem affects all types of material, both verbal and non-verbal, such as word associations, drawings and numbers.

It seems clear also that these defects of memory are to a large extent independent of the significance of the material involved. Events of high emotional significance may sometimes appear to be remembered especially well (Hamman *et al.* 1997) but this is not always the case. Milner (1966) reported of H.M.:

His initial emotional reaction may be intense, but it will be short-lived, since the incident provoking it will soon be forgotten. Thus, when informed of the death of his uncle, of whom he was very fond, he became extremely upset, but then appeared to forget the whole matter and from time to time thereafter would ask when his uncle was coming to visit them; each time, on hearing anew of his uncle's death, he would show the same intense dismay, with no sign of habituation.

Victor (1964), in a group of alcoholic Korsakoff patients, was unable to discern any factors that governed what was remembered and what was forgotten. A patient might fail to retain news of a bereavement which shocked him profoundly at the time, yet retain other matters of no significance whatever. More recently, evidence has been reported that a number of severe amnesic patients show very slow acquisition of semantic memories, possibly by cortical mechanisms, in the absence of discernible episodic memory acquisition (McCarthy *et al.* 2005).

Despite such pervasive deficits, procedural memory is well preserved, even in the most severely affected patients. Milner's (1966) patient, for example, showed a normal learning curve for a task of mirror drawing, even though on each test occasion he was completely unaware that he had tried the task before. Other motor and perceptual skills, such as on pursuit-rotor tasks or (more importantly) musical skills, are well preserved even if the patients lacks awareness of still having these skills (Corkin 1968; Starr & Phillips 1970; Wilson *et al.* 2008). 'Priming effects' are largely preserved, as when prior presentation of a word increases the tendency to produce that word when its initial letters are shown some minutes later (Squire *et al*. 1987). Thus the forms of memory that are accessible only in performance, and not as acts of conscious recollection or recognition, appear to be spared in the classic amnesic syndrome.

The retrograde amnesia often covers a period of months, years or even decades before the onset of the illness. This is usually dense for events just prior to the onset, but may be incomplete, patchy and lacking in detail for the earliest memories. Time sense is characteristically disordered within the retrograde gap, with jumbling of the sequential ordering of those events which are recalled. In patients with Korsakoff's syndrome of alcoholic origin, the retrograde amnesia characteristically extends back 20–25 years, sometimes longer, and shows a clear-cut temporal gradient (Kopelman 1989). In discrete amnesic syndromes of other aetiologies the retrograde amnesia is very variable according to case reports and experimental investigations. Some studies report a short retrograde loss of 2–4 years in hippocampal lesions (Reed & Squire 1998; Kapur & Brooks 1999), others a much more extensive retrograde loss (Viskontas *et al*. 2000; Cipolotti *et al*. 2001).

According to Ribot's (1882) 'law', early memories are always relatively preserved, but there is now considerable controversy about whether this always occurs or whether it reflects a clinical impression based on oft-repeated stories. The issue relates to the various theories which purport to explain the occurrence of retrograde amnesia (see below).

Disturbance of time sense and of the ordering of events is an outstanding characteristic, particularly in Korsakoff's syndrome. The patient may allocate some recent remembered event to the distant past, or (much more commonly) bring up a past event as a recent happening. He may condense long periods of time or telescope repeated happenings into one (Korsakoff 1889; Victor *et al*. 1971). This affects recent memory and the period of the retrograde gap particularly, but may be observed for more remote happenings as well. Talland (1965) suggested that the problem is due not to a loss of appreciation of the flow of time, but rather to 'contextual isolation'; that is to say, events within the memory store appear to lose relationship with the totality of experience which surrounds them, sometimes referred to as a loss of 'temporal tagging'.

Other cognitive functions are relatively well preserved, and the above amnesic deficits are out of all proportion to other disturbances of intellect or behaviour (Victor *et al*. 1971). In particular the patients are alert, responsive to their environments and without any evidence of clouding of consciousness. However, where pathology is more widespread, as can occur in Korsakoff's syndrome, cerebral hypoxia, vascular pathology or herpes encephalitis, the situation is less straightforward. Other cognitive functions may be disordered when carefully examined (Talland 1965; Zangwill 1966; Victor *et al*. 1971). Where there is concomitant frontal lobe involvement, there is often difficulty in sustaining mental activity, coupled with inflexibility of set and reduced capacity to shift attention from one task or train of thought to another. Thinking is usually stereotyped, perseverative and facile, with inadequate concept formation and defective ability to categorise. Butters and Cermak (1980) found visuo-perceptual impairments in Korsakoff patients when sought by special tests, for example the digit–symbol substitution test, hidden figures test, or tests requiring the sorting and discrimination of complex visual stimuli. However, all these impairments are nonetheless overshadowed by the prominence of the memory disorder. It is this disproportion between severe memory deficits and other (subtle) cognitive deficits that defines the amnesic syndrome. However, there are undoubtedly transitional forms between the classic picture and patients with variable degrees of more global cognitive impairment.

In Korsakoff's syndrome, and some other amnesic patients (e.g. following herpes encephalitis), there may be certain marked disturbances of personality. There is often a pronounced degree of apathy and loss of initiative, a bland or even fatuous disposition, and a tendency towards self-neglect. Left alone, the patient occupies himself poorly, makes few demands or enquiries from those around, and obeys instructions in a passive and indifferent manner. A virtual disinterest in alcohol may represent a particularly striking change. Lack of insight is also almost universal; few severely amnesic patients are overtly aware of their deficits, and in those who do the gravity of these defects is minimised or explained away by facile rationalisations.

The neuropsychological deficit

The amnesic syndrome was for many years regarded as reflecting a failure of consolidation of new experience. Thus while the immediate memory span is normal, and early memories may remain substantially intact, current experience cannot gain proper access to the secondary memory (Milner 1966). However, a simple consolidation hypothesis is hard pressed to explain why some forms of cueing can improve performance, or why patients can achieve better results on recognition tests than when tested by free recall. Moreover, if consolidation were the explanation of an extensive retrograde amnesia, where it occurs, this would imply that the process of physiological consolidation lasts for years, even decades.

Butters and colleagues stressed the role of deficient semantic encoding of information in leading to the poor performance of amnesic subjects (Butters & Cermak 1980). This, it was argued, might account in considerable degree for their failure to store material adequately. Thus, patients with Korsakoff's syndrome were found to rely unduly on simple acoustic encoding of the information they receive, rather than analysing it more deeply in terms of semantic meaning. Moreover, they use inappropriate strategies for the rehearsal and 'chunking' of information, all rendering information more susceptible to interference and rapid decay. When specifically instructed to attend to the semantic features of pre-sented stimuli, for example in terms of categories, attributes or meaning, patients with Korsakoff's syndrome are found to achieve a somewhat improved performance on memory tasks, although considerable impairment remains (Meudell et al. 1979; McDowell 1981).

Another theory is that there is a specific deficit in the amnesic patient's acquisition of contextual (e.g. temporal and spatial) information, resulting in disproportionate impairments in contextual memory (Huppert & Piercy 1976, 1978a; Mayes et al. 1985). More recently, this theory has evolved into a more generalised notion of a deficit in binding complex associations (Mayes & Downes 1997) or in binding the relations between items (Cohen et al. 1997). This specific deficit in combining complex associations or relations between items is usually attributed to hippocampal pathol-ogy, or dysfunction, and results in various related distinc-tions being postulated in amnesia, including those between recollection and familiarity memory, recall and recognition memory, remembering and knowing, as well as that between 'explicit' and 'implicit' memory.

Another possibility is that there is a specific deficit in 'storage' (retention) rather than in learning processes, at least in some amnesic patients. It was found that, after learning has been acquired, many amnesic patients show a normal rate of forgetting, at least on recognition memory tests (Huppert & Piercy 1978b; Kopelman & Stanhope 1997), but there is some evidence that patients with medial temporal lobe pathology might forget at an accelerated rate, even after learning has been acquired (Huppert & Piercy 1979; Parkin & Leng 1988). However, various studies have failed to demon-strate this (Kopelman 1985a; McKee & Squire 1992), although there is some evidence that, over and above their initial acquisition or learning deficit, amnesic patients show accel-erated forgetting when tested on recall (as opposed to recog-nition) memory tasks over a period of minutes (Kopelman & Stanhope 1997; Green & Kopelman 2002).

A further possibility is that the deficit occurs at retrieval. Warrington and Weiskrantz (1968) postulated that amnesic patients were unable to suppress inappropriate responses during recall and recognition memory tasks. They noted that such patients sometimes respond erroneously with what had been the correct responses to previous test items, and that the provision of retrieval cues can improve their per-formance. On the other hand, it was later found that healthy subjects exhibited these phenomena when given memory tests at relatively long delay intervals, suggesting that they were a consequence of poor memory rather than its cause (Mayes & Meudell 1981). Subsequently, Warrington and Wisekrantz (1982) retracted this view, arguing instead that lesions in diencephalic or medial temporal structures might 'disconnect' a critical memory circuit running between frontal cortex, subserving 'cognitive mediation', and a semantic memory system in the temporal lobes.

Amnesic syndrome or syndromes

In the past, there was an extensive debate concerning whether there was a differential pattern of amnesic deficit in compar-ing patients with diencephalic and those with medial tempo-ral lobe pathologies. On the one hand, Warrington and Weiskrantz (1982) argued that these structures were all part of the same memory circuitry, damage in which 'discon-nected' a frontal cognitive mediation system from a tempo-ral lobe semantic or conceptual memory system. In contrast, others argued for differential patterns of memory deficits on the basis of findings with respect to measures of forgetting rates or contextual (temporal and spatial) memory (Huppert & Piercy 1979; Parkin 1987). In general, although there may be subtle differences in contextual memory, these differential patterns have not been corroborated (Kopelman 2002). Moreover, although a broad distinction between executive processes and encoding/retrieval mechanisms remains valid, there is also considerable overlap with the effects of large (particularly bilateral) frontal lesions, and a review of the latter showed that virtually all studies have reported impairments in recall (and often recognition) memory (Wheeler et al. 1995).

More recently, differences have been sought between the effects of damage to hippocampal and parahippocampal (particularly perirhinal) structures. Aggleton and Shaw (1996) argued that patients with pathology confined to the hippocampi showed impairments on verbal and visual recall but not recognition memory, whereas damage to parahip-pocampal structures was required to produce an impairment in familiarity-based or recognition memory. There were problems with the meta-analysis on which this hypothesis was based, but supportive evidence has been obtained in a number of investigations, notably by Holdstock et al. (2002) and Mayes et al. (2004b). On the other hand, others have argued that when appropriate experimental controls are introduced, patients with pathology confined to the hippoc-ampi (as well as other amnesic patients) showed proportion-ate impairments on both recall and recognition memory procedures (Reed & Squire 1997; Manns et al. 2003; Kopelman et al. 2005). This issue remains hotly debated.

Lengthy retrograde amnesia

The short retrograde amnesia of several minutes' duration, such as commonly occurs after head injury, can plausibly be explained on the view that new learning requires a period of consolidation for stable long-term memory to be established. It is difficult, in contrast, to provide an explanation for the very long retrograde amnesias that may extend for years or decades before the onset of an amnesic syndrome. A number of authors have previously made this distinction between the different characteristics of short- and long-term retro-grade amnesia (Symonds 1966; Kapur 1999). These lengthy retrograde amnesias are often patchy, and the patient may show a so-called 'temporal gradient', i.e. relative sparing of early memories. Moreover, this lengthy retrograde amnesia may shrink with time (e.g. in head injury or tuberculous meningitis) but it can persist (e.g. in herpes encephalitis or Alzheimer dementia).

Neuropsychological studies have attempted to map the pattern of retrograde amnesia in amnesic disorders of various aetiologies. In a pioneering study, Sanders and Warrington (1971) employed a test requiring the recall and recognition of famous faces and a standardised questionnaire about public events from different time periods, finding a retrograde amnesia extending back many decades in a small group of amnesic patients. There was no evidence of a temporal gradient or sparing of early memories. In contrast, Albert *et al.* (1979, 1981), using closely similar tests, found striking evidence of a temporal gradient in patients with Korsakoff's syndrome, but not in patients with Huntington's dementia.

Subsequently, measures of personal or autobiographical memory were introduced (Zola-Morgan *et al.* 1983; Kopelman *et al.* 1989), and the debate has continued. For example, some authors have reported striking temporal gradients in amnesic patients (Kopelman 1989; Squire & Haist 1989; Kapur & Brooks 1999), whereas others have found 'flat' gradients in autobiographical memory and in the recall of public information, consistent with the original Sanders and Warrington finding (Viskontas *et al.* 2000; Cipolotti *et al.* 2001). Differential patterns across distinct diagnostic groups have been reported and, in general, there is a more 'gentle' temporal gradient in dementia patients, i.e. a lesser degree of sparing of early memories (Kopelman 1989; Kopelman *et al.* 1999).

Interesting hemispheric differences have been reported in memory-disordered patients. For example, De Renzi *et al.* (1987) reported a patient who was severely impaired after herpes encephalitis on a wide range of general or semantic information, but who appeared intact in retrieving autobiographical memories. This patient had extensive left temporal lobe damage. In contrast, others have reported disproportionate impairments in autobiographical memory with relative sparing of semantic knowledge in patients with predominantly right temporal lobe damage (O'Connor *et al.* 1992; Ogden 1993; Kopelman *et al.* 1999). This latter pattern has usually been attributed to the problems in retrieving the visual imagery associated with autobiographical memories.

These observations have implications for the interpretation of a lengthy retrograde amnesia. *Consolidation theory* assumes that a time-dependent physiological process is required to 'fix' memories in the brain, and to make them less vulnerable to the effects of brain pathology. This process has commonly been interpreted in terms of 'structural reallocation', which postulates that memories are initially dependent on (or stored in) medial temporal (or diencephalic) structures, particularly the hippocampi, but are later stored in the neocortex and are no longer dependent on the medial temporal/diencephalic system (Squire & Alvarez 1995;

Meeter & Murre 2004). This view predicts a temporal gradient in retrograde amnesia, as obtained in various studies cited above (Zola-Morgan *et al.* 1986; Kapur & Brooks 1999; Bayley *et al.* 2005). It is also supported by some fMRI investigations of remote memory, but is refuted by others. However, the theory cannot explain patients whose retrograde amnesia failed to show an unequivocal or any temporal gradient (Viskontas *et al.* 2000; Cipolotti *et al.* 2001). Moreover, a very extensive temporal gradient going back 20–30 years would imply that physiological consolidation must continue for a remarkably long time (Nadel & Moscovitch 1997).

The *semanticisation hypothesis* argues that, as memories for episodes are rehearsed, they adopt a more semantic form, losing their contextual immediacy or vividness, but protecting them from the effect of brain damage (Cermak 1984). In other words, the contextual components of these memories become attenuated or lost, making the memories feel much less immediate and vivid, but they are better preserved and protected against any subsequent retrieval deficit. One possibility is that this process involves the transfer of memories from the hippocampal system to the neocortex, in which case this theory overlaps with consolidation theory in postulating structural reallocation. A second possibility is that both episodic and semantic memories are stored in the neocortex, but only episodic memories require the hippocampus for their retrieval. A major problem for this theory is the finding that memories which are semantic virtually from the outset, such as knowledge of the meaning of new words, can also show a temporal gradient (Verfaellie *et al.* 1995).

Multiple trace theory, as mentioned briefly above, postulates that the hippocampi are continuously involved in the storage and retrieval (reactivation) of autobiographical memories, and that every time the reactivation of a memory trace occurs a new trace is laid down, resulting in 'multiple traces' (Nadel & Moscovitch 1997). In this theory, the memory trace for a specific episode is represented by a combination of 'binding codes' in the hippocampi and by fragments of information in neocortical association areas. The theory predicts that the extent of retrograde amnesia and the slope of the temporal gradient for autobiographical memories will depend on the size of hippocampal lesions or atrophy, and that a complete hippocampal transection would result in a 'flat' gradient for autobiographical memories. However, factual information is postulated as being stored in the neocortex independently of the episode in which it was acquired, and a steeper gradient for semantic than episodic memories is also predicted. Some functional activation investigations have provided findings consistent with this theory (Maguire *et al.* 2001; Ryan *et al.* 2001). On the other hand, many amnesic patients do indeed show a steep temporal gradient, as reported above, and Kopelman *et al.* (2003) failed to find the predicted significant correlations between hippocampal volumes and the extent or severity of retrograde amnesia in patients with primarily medial temporal lobe pathology.

Furthermore, retrograde amnesia gradients across autobiographical and semantic remote memory do not always fit the predicted pattern.

An alternative view, little discussed to date, is that the relative sparing of early memories in neurological amnesia reflects differences in the way that such early memories were originally encoded, making them more likely to be retrieved by healthy volunteers at a later date and also protecting them from the effects of subsequent brain damage. Kopelman *et al.* (1989) postulated such a hypothesis on the basis of age differences in the slope of temporal gradients in memory-disordered patients, and some recent observations would be consistent with such a hypothesis (Rubin & Schulkind 1997; Buchanan *et al.* 2005).

Disproportionate retrograde amnesia

Highly contentious is the nature of disproportionate retrograde amnesia, sometimes known as 'focal' or even 'isolated' retrograde amnesia. Many such cases have been reported in the literature, but they differ considerably in the circumstances and features of their onset, underlying clinical diagnosis, findings on neuroimaging, and the postulated site or sites of pathology, as well as in the adequacy of the clinical descriptions given. For example, Kapur *et al.* (1992) described a 26-year-old woman who had fallen from a horse, sustaining left and right frontal contusions, evident on CT, with subsequent signal alteration in the left and right temporal poles on MRI. This patient was severely impaired across all the remote memory tests with which she was investigated, but showed normal performance or only moderate impairment at various anterograde memory tests. However, the interpretation of her deficit was confounded by her subsequent development of various hysterical symptoms in the context of depression (Kapur 2000).

The underlying nature of such cases has been debated elsewhere (Kopelman 2000; Kapur 2000). Many of the cases described as 'focal retrograde amnesia' in fact showed evidence of anterograde memory impairment, especially for visuospatial material. Other cases showed poor anterograde memory in more moderate or subtle form across a number of tests, particularly story recall, face recognition memory, and delayed recall, begging the question of whether their failure reflects, in some sense, task demands and task difficulties. Some of the most convincing cases in this literature initially showed a severe anterograde amnesia as well as a severe retrograde amnesia. By the time of their assessment, the retrograde amnesia remained profound, whereas the anterograde amnesia had become only moderate, mild or minimal; in such cases, the real issue concerns differential patterns of recovery, and the way in which physiological or psychological factors can contribute to this. A further group of patients reported in the literature are those with TEA (see above), who commonly report 'gaps' in their autobiographical memories. However, it is not clear whether this has resulted from brief 'subclinical' runs of seizure activity in the past compromising encoding over short periods, or from current ictal activity inhibiting retrieval processes, or even causing an acceleration in the forgetting of 'old' memories; each of these views has been advocated. Finally, psychogenic factors may make an important contribution to the presence of a residual, disproportionately severe retrograde amnesia, and the reversed temporal gradient in psychogenic amnesia is identical to that seen in many cases of 'focal retrograde amnesia'. Psychogenic mechanisms may be important in those cases which follow a mild concussion, but also in some cases where there has been more severe brain pathology.

Confabulation

Confabulation can be a striking feature in amnesias, but in its 'spontaneous' form (see below) probably reflects concomitant ventromedial frontal pathology (Kopelman 1987a 2002). In the past, it has often (erroneously) been thought of as pathognomonic of diencephalic amnesia, but the relationship between diencephalic amnesia and confabulation has been greatly overstressed. When present, confabulation is commoner in the acute (Wernicke) stages than in the chronic phases of Korsakoff's syndrome but it is usually absent (Victor *et al.* 1971). It can also occur in temporal lobe amnesia (Wilson *et al.* 1995), but again it probably reflects concomitant frontal pathology. In general, it may appear as an evanescent phenomenon, or in rare cases it may last for many years.

Typically, the patient gives a reasonably coherent but false account of some recent event or experience, either in relation to his own activities or in response to suggestion by the examiner. Berlyne (1972) defined confabulation as 'a falsification of memory occurring in clear consciousness in association with an organically derived amnesia'. He upheld Bonhoeffer's early distinction between two varieties. The common 'momentary type' is brief in content, has reference to the recent past and has to be provoked. The content can sometimes be traced to a true memory that has become displaced in time or context. Much rarer is the 'fantastic type' in which a sustained and grandiose theme is elaborated, usually describing far-fetched adventures and experiences which clearly could not have taken place at any time. This form tends to occur spontaneously even without a provoking stimulus, and the content is often related to wish fulfillment and the seeking of prestige. Kopelman (1987a) preferred a classification simply into 'provoked' and 'spontaneous' confabulation, and has shown that the former appears in the context of efforts at recall by amnesic or dementia patients, whereas it is the latter that reflects specific (ventromedial) frontal pathology. Schnider *et al.* (1996) have provided important empirical evidence which supports this distinction.

Kopelman (1987a) was able to demonstrate examples of 'provoked' confabulation in healthy subjects when asked to recall prose passages after a considerable interval of time;

these were similar in nature to those sometimes observed in Korsakoff and Alzheimer patients when tested shortly after exposure, consisting mainly of additions of inaccurate or irrelevant material or changes in the sense of the passage. This type can thus be regarded as a 'normal' response to a faulty memory.

The evidence linking spontaneous confabulation to the presence of frontal lobe dysfunction includes the finding by Stuss et al. (1978) of five patients in whom frontal deficits, superadded to their memory problems, appeared to account for their persistent and extraordinary confabulation. Kapur and Coughlan (1980) were able to chart the change from fantastic to momentary confabulations in a patient with left frontal damage following subarachnoid haemorrhage, and to show that this change was paralleled by improvement in performance on frontal lobe or executive tests. Moscovitch and Melo (1997) reported that ventromedial pathology seemed to be the common factor in their patients, but others have disputed its critical importance (Dalla Barba 1993, 2002).

Sometimes confabulation may represent the residue of abnormal and confused experiences, including misidentifications and misinterpretations that occurred in the delirium of the initial Wernicke's encephalopathy. Thus, it commonly sets in as clouding of consciousness is receding and persists thereafter while insight into the unreal nature of the delirious experiences is lacking. As in delusions, the content of confabulation may appear 'motivated' or meaningful (Conway & Tacchi 1996).

Recent theories of spontaneous confabulation fall into three main groups. The first group of theories emphasises faulty specification and verification of memory retrieval. For example, Burgess and Shallice (1996) postulated deficits in a descriptor process, an editor process and a mediator process, which make differential contributions to the clinical phenomena of confabulation. Moscovitch and Melo (1997) put forward a somewhat similar argument, identifying a number of putative deficits in cue-retrieval, strategic search or faulty monitoring, the last resulting in erroneous memories not being edited out or suppressed. Likewise, Schacter et al. (1998) argued that an insufficiently 'focused' retrieval description, or an impairment in post-retrieval monitoring and verification, would give rise to confabulation. Moreover, encoding impairments would make subjects more liable to confabulatory errors at retrieval.

The second group of theories emphasises so-called source memory deficits, either with respect to confusion about the temporal context or sequence of memories, or in distinguishing between real and imagined memories. The belief that many confabulations may, in fact, be 'real' memories jumbled up and recalled inappropriately out of temporal sequence has a long history going back to Korsakoff (1889). In an empirical test of this hypothesis, Schnider et al. (1996) found that a small group of spontaneous confabulators were differentiated from other amnesic patients and healthy controls on the basis of errors at an 'implicit' temporal context memory test (see also below). In a variant of this hypothesis, Dalla Barba (1993) and Dalla Barba et al. (1999) have proposed that 'temporal consciousness' is intact but malfunctioning in confabulating patients, who are aware of a past, present and future (unlike amnesic patients) but, in making temporal judgements, they employ only the most stable elements from their long-term memory stores. Asked what they did yesterday or what they will do tomorrow, the patients reply with the well-established routines or habits of a lifetime, irrelevant to their present situation. Johnson et al. (1993) postulated a wider range of context, source or reality monitoring deficits, in which a confabulating patient is unable to distinguish 'real' from imagined experience. Schnider et al. (2001) have more recently interpreted their experimental findings in these terms, arguing that deficits in a filter mechanism within the ventromedial frontal cortex results in the confabulating patient being unable to distinguish real memories from irrelevant thoughts and information.

A third group of theories emphasises that multiple deficits may contribute to confabulation. For example, Shapiro et al. (1981) postulated that confabulation results from (i) impaired self-monitoring, (ii) a failure to inhibit memory errors and (iii) frequent perseverations, each of these deficits being related to a different aspect of frontal/executive function. Johnson et al. (1997) concluded that confabulation may reflect an interaction between (i) a vivid imagination, (ii) an inability to retrieve autobiographical memories systematically and (iii) impaired source monitoring. Kopelman et al. (1997) found that (i) many confabulations in episodic memory were associated with temporal context errors, (ii) confabulations particularly in semantic memory were associated with perseverative errors and (iii) other confabulations appear to be unchecked, instantaneous, ill-considered responses to immediate environmental and social cues.

Amnesia in diffuse cerebral disease

When associated with diffuse cerebral disorder, memory disorder is often subsumed among more widespread impairments of intellectual function, making precise analysis of the memory deficits more difficult. In delirium, the memory difficulties can be traced to the combination of an impairment of consciousness and to problems in attention and perception. In dementias, memory complaints are often the earliest manifestation, in part perhaps because memory difficulties tend to be more readily identified than other aspects of intellectual loss. However, studies of Alzheimer patients show that some patients initially manifest an amnesic picture, whereas other initially show a dysexecutive syndrome (Becker et al. 1992; Hodges et al. 2003). The general picture of the memory difficulties in acute and chronic neurological disorders has been discussed earlier in this chapter (see Clinical picture and pattern of neuropsychological deficits in amnesia). Certain distinctive features are summarised here for comparison with the picture in focal amnesic states.

The memory deficits in diffuse brain disease, such as Alzheimer's dementia, are extensive, affecting both recent and remote events to an obvious degree. Only rarely is there a clear-cut disturbance of anterograde memory with only a brief retrograde gap. However, recent events may be the most obviously affected, in part because of a lack of interest and involvement in current experiences. Remote memories may appear to be relatively intact, but their recall is often in fact banal, stereotyped and lacking in detail. There are now a large number of investigations reporting only a very gentle temporal gradient (relative sparing of early memories) in Alzheimer patients (Sagar *et al.* 1988; Kopelman 1989; Greene *et al.* 1995). Performance may be variable from one occasion to another, and capricious in that some events are easily recalled while others, apparently equally trivial or unimportant, are not. Indeed, part of the difficulty may lie in a failure to sustain attention and concentration on the general task of memory retrieval.

Evidence such as this suggests that the memory disorder in Alzheimer's dementia reflects diffuse cortical pathology as well as the characteristic atrophy and histopathological changes in the medial temporal lobes. Thus, the pattern of deficits is more extensive than that seen in the amnesic syndrome, and can be attributed to reduced neuronal interconnections, disrupted associations, impaired retrieval processes, and damage to the memory stores themselves. The immediate memory span is impaired (Miller 1973; Kaszniak *et al.* 1979), unlike the situation in patients with circumscribed amnesic syndromes, and forgetting occurs more rapidly within primary or working memory (Corkin 1982; Kopelman 1985a). However, once material has been acquired in secondary memory, forgetting rates on recognition memory tasks are surprisingly normal, suggesting that the main problem is in memory formation (Corkin *et al.* 1984; Kopelman 1985a), although faster forgetting can be found on recall memory tasks (Christensen *et al.* 1998). Kopelman and Corn (1988) reviewed and presented evidence that depletion within the cholinergic system in dementia can account only partially for the memory disorder encountered in such patients.

Findings in implicit memory in Alzheimer's dementia have been conflicting, and are closely tied to the specific test paradigms employed. The general picture that emerges in Alzheimer's disease is of preserved motor skill learning, as on pursuit-rotor tasks (Eslinger & Damasio 1986) and mirror reading (Deweer *et al.* 1993). On priming tasks, the findings are variable, depending on the precise experimental design (Shimamura *et al.* 1987; Brandt *et al.* 1988; Downes *et al.* 1996).

In Alzheimer's disease, the earliest and most intense pathological change is often in the hippocampal regions and this is correlated with the severity of the memory deficits (Brier-ley 1961; Corsellis 1970; Braak & Braak 1991). Conversely, in the *frontotemporal dementias*, the pathological process may initially spare the hippocampal regions, and here episodic memory problems are rarely an early manifestation.

Semantic dementia is a temporal lobe variant of frontotemporal dementia. Many of its features were described by Pick (1892), but the first neuropsychological description was by Warrington (1975) and the term was coined by Snowden *et al.* (1989) and further employed by Hodges *et al.* (1992). In this syndrome, there is severe impairment in semantic memory (especially involving naming, word-finding, and comprehension) with relatively preserved episodic memory (for events) in the context of intact visuospatial abilities, number skills, reasoning and problem-solving, with good orientation in time and place. It most commonly involves unilateral atrophy of the left temporal lobe or bilateral temporal lobe atrophy with relative sparing of medial temporal lobe structures, although MRI studies clearly show that severe atrophy of medial temporal structures also emerges. Cases of relatively isolated right temporal lobe atrophy have also been described (Evans *et al.* 1995). Remote memory for early autobiographical events may also appear affected (Snowden *et al.* 1996; Graham & Hodges 1997), but this is almost certainly a consequence of the patients' deficits in semantic memory interfering with autobiographical memory retrieval, rather than a deficit in autobiographical memory storage *per se* (Westmacott *et al.* 2001; Moss & Kopelman 2003). Survival from onset of symptoms is approximately 5–10 years (Hodges *et al.* 2003), and the underlying histopathology is very varied (Pick cells, motor neurone inclusions, non-specific changes) (Hodges *et al.* 2004).

In *normal ageing*, there are commonly memory impairments and the relationship between these and dementia has long been controversial. Huppert (1994) reviewed the attempts made to specify those aspects of memory most vulnerable to the ageing process, and the difficulty in generalising about the pathological substrates that might be responsible. In normal ageing, the impairments involve working memory or a lack of 'processing resources', so that performing a concurrent task while memorising is particularly difficult, and there are also particular problems in prospective memory (remembering to do something) and in remembering the contextual aspects of information (Huppert 1994; Parkin 1987). Dementia may represent accelerated ageing (Drachman *et al.* 1990) or it may represent a qualitatively distinct neuropsychological and neuropathological process superimposed on normal ageing (Huppert & Kopelman 1989). In recent years, the term 'mild cognitive impairment' has been used to describe elderly people with mild memory complaints associated with a moderate degree of hippocampal atrophy. If cases of mild vascular change, alcohol abuse, head injury or depression are rigorously excluded, there is now evidence that many of these cases 'convert' eventually to dementia (Lambon *et al.* 2003).

The pathological changes characteristic of ageing commonly involve the frontal and temporal lobes, but they are usually diffuse so that attribution of all the changes of normal ageing to, for example, frontal lobe or hippocampal atrophy is somewhat simplistic.

Psychogenic amnesia

Psychogenic amnesia is commonly either dense and global or restricted to circumscribed ('situation-specific') themes or events. When global it involves the blotting out of long periods or the whole of a person's past life, or even loss of personal identity. Amnesias of this severity do not occur in organic states unless at the same time there is abundant evidence of disturbance of consciousness or of severe disruption of cognitive functions generally. Interestingly, even with dense psychogenic amnesias there may sometimes be 'islands' of preserved memories that can be uncovered by careful questioning (Schacter et al. 1982). Inconsistencies in the account may also be noted. The subject with hysterical amnesia, for example, may insist that certain events could not have occurred during the period covered by the amnesic gap, while at the same time he is in no position to refute the proposition. More restricted (situation-specific) psychogenic amnesias will usually be found to centre on a traumatic event or circumscribed areas such as sexual abuse in childhood. Repeated episodes of psychogenic amnesia will frequently betray stereotyped themes or settings.

Psychogenic amnesia should be suspected when from the outset profound difficulty with retrieval of past events is coupled with normal ability to retain new information, and when there is an acute onset of memory loss for the entirety of a person's past. A delayed onset of the forgetting, e.g. following a minor head injury, is likewise sometimes seen in psychogenic but not in neurological amnesias. The focal retrograde amnesia syndrome has often been reported to arise in such circumstances, but its aetiology remains controversial (Kopelman 2000; Kapur 2000).

Kopelman (2002) discussed factors that appear to predispose to psychogenic amnesia, notably a severe precipitating stress, depressed mood or the experience of an earlier neurological amnesia in disorders such as head injury, epilepsy or alcoholism. In medicolegal practice, amnesia is often reported by offenders particularly in cases of homicide, occurring in 30–40% of cases, but is sometimes described in connection with other violent and non-violent offences. The amnesic episodes are typically fairly brief and knowledge of personal identity usually remains intact (Pyszora et al. 2003). Victims of offences such as rape (Mechanic et al. 1998) report similar amnesic gaps, and eyewitnesses of crime frequently make memory errors.

Special difficulties arise when neurological and psychological predisposing factors occur together. Psychogenic factors may sometimes be obtrusive in amnesias which are clearly due primarily to brain damage, or a neurological deficit may come to be selectively reinforced or perpetuated on a psychogenic basis. Such difficulties are well illustrated by the celebrated dispute, reviewed by Zangwill (1967), that surrounded the Grünthal–Störring case for more than 30 years. Kopelman et al. (1994) described a patient with transient epileptic amnesia who had previously been diagnosed as having a psychogenic fugue. In focal retrograde amnesia, however, the faulty attribution may be to neurological causation, and psychological factors have sometimes been neglected or ignored.

Possible mechanisms in psychogenic amnesia

The mechanisms may vary from case to case. Faulty encoding of information may explain some examples, as discussed below, while others may represent 'motivated forgetting', 'dissociation' or 'repression'. Another possibility is of a primary retrieval deficit reflecting mood-dependent phenomena. Sometimes there may indeed be a substrate in transient neurological memory dysfunction which dictates the form the psychogenic reaction takes, as in the alcoholic patient reported by Gudjonsson and Taylor (1985).

Certain cases of psychogenic amnesia may depend, at least in part, on failure in the initial processing of experience rather than on a process of forgetting or repression (Kopelman 1985b, 1987b). Thus Taylor and Kopelman (1984) found that inability to recall a criminal offence was frequent when this had been committed in a state of very high emotional arousal, in the context of florid psychotic delusions, or under heavy alcoholic intoxication. All such factors would be liable to impair normal registration of what was happening at the time. On the other hand, Pyszora et al. (2003) found that in a sizeable proportion of offenders amnesic for their crime, the amnesic gap diminishes substantially through time, leaving only a brief (1 minute or less) permanent amnesia for the actual killing. In such cases, there was evidence that dissociative mechanisms may have been important in the aetiology of the amnesia.

The neuropsychology of psychogenic amnesia can resemble, in certain respects, that seen following head trauma. As already mentioned, there may be 'islands' or fragments of preserved memory within the amnesic gap, which are often described as strange and unfamiliar. Performance at verbal learning tests is variable: it has been reported as unaffected, mildly affected or more severely impaired in different studies. Memory for procedural skills is often preserved, and this may also be true of other aspects of implicit memory, such as tests of priming, although there are again conflicting reports. Deliberate cueing of memories is seldom successful, but memory recovery is often facilitated by chance cues in the environment. For example, a patient, on seeing an author's name on the spine of a book, recalled that he had a friend of that name who was dying of cancer. On transfer to a psychiatric ward, he recollected the details of another psychiatric hospital admission years earlier.

Some functional imaging studies have produced evidence of changes in brain regions analogous to those purported to be implicated in neurological retrograde amnesia (Markowitsch *et al.* 1997; Glisky *et al.* 2004), although in general these studies find decreased frontal activations. Anderson and Green (2001) reported evidence that executive mechanisms can be recruited to prevent unwanted memories from entering awareness, and that repeated use of such strategies inhibits the subsequent recall of the suppressed memories. More particularly, Anderson *et al.* (2004) showed that this memory suppression is associated with *increased* activations in dorsolateral frontal cortex bilaterally, and with *diminished* bilateral activation in the hippocampi and the frontal poles. Hence, there is evidence that frontal executive mechanisms are implicated in psychogenic amnesia, but there are conflicting reports about whether this is correlated with increased or decreased frontal activation.

Memory disorder in the psychoses

While it used to be held that memory disorder was the hallmark of neurological brain damage, there are now indications that memory may also be defective in the psychoses. At an anecdotal level it is commonly noted that patients lack detailed knowledge of key features of their abnormal beliefs and experiences on recovery from schizophrenia or severe affective disorder. Moreover, depression has been shown to have a marked effect on the selective processes normally operative in memory, leading to readier recall and more accurate recognition of unpleasant compared with pleasant material (Lloyd & Lishman 1975; Dunbar & Lishman 1984; Teasdale & Spencer 1984). Among normal subjects such selectivity operates in the reverse direction.

However, there is also evidence that overall memory efficiency is impaired in patients with depression or schizophrenia. Cutting (1979) examined groups of patients with acute schizophrenia, chronic schizophrenia or major depression, and compared their memory test performance with normal subjects and with patients who had 'organic psychosyndromes'. The most prominent finding was that patients with chronic schizophrenia were impaired on verbal learning and pattern recognition tasks, their performance sometimes being comparable to patients with confusional states, dementia or Korsakoff's syndrome. The depressives were also impaired on both tasks but to a less marked degree. Acute schizophrenic patients performed poorly on verbal memory alone. It seemed unlikely that coincidental brain damage could be the explanation, but the possible effects of medication were harder to discount.

McKenna *et al.* (1990) evaluated a large group of acute and chronic schizophrenic patients on the Rivermead Behavioural Memory Test battery (Wilson *et al.* 1985) and found that poor performance was common and sometimes substantial. The level of memory impairment appeared occasionally to approach that of patients with overt brain damage. Tamlyn *et al.* (1992) confirmed such deficits in a more detailed

neuropsychological study of the same sample, finding that the pattern of impairment was similar to that of the classic amnesic syndrome. However, virtually all the patients were receiving neuroleptic medication and many were also taking anticholinergic drugs, which might have contributed to their poor performance. Saykin *et al.* (1991) demonstrated a disproportionate and apparently selective deficit on memory and learning tasks in 36 non-medicated acute schizophrenic patients.

Duffy and O'Carroll (1994) have reported a detailed study of 40 schizophrenic patients using the Rivermead Behavioural Memory Test battery, paired associate learning, and other memory tests. This was a heterogeneous sample of acute and chronic patients, all screened to exclude those with a history of alcohol or drug abuse, head injury or other brain disease. Poor performance was demonstrated on several tests: on the Rivermead battery the group was as likely to show significant memory impairment as the brain-damaged sample on which the battery was originally validated. The severity of impairment was related to age and to the chronicity of illness, but not to measures of motivation, severity of psychotic symptoms or amount of neuroleptic medication. Of particular interest were comparisons with a group of chronic Korsakoff patients. On tests of episodic memory the schizophrenics were considerably less impaired than the Korsakoff patients, only 50% of the schizophrenics scoring within the severely impaired range, but on a test of semantic memory (judgements of whether a series of factual sentences were true or false) they were significantly worse. McKenna *et al.* (1995) provided a detailed review of research into this and other aspects of memory in the disorder, including impaired episodic memory and spared procedural memory, analogous to findings in neurological amnesia (see Clinical picture and pattern of neuropsychological deficits in amnesia, earlier).

Disorders of language and the aphasias

Disturbance of language is an important source of evidence of focal brain disorder and, indeed, historically provided the chief impetus for attempts at correlating focal psychological deficits with regional brain pathology. Aphasic symptoms probably remain more useful clinically than any other cognitive defect in indicating the approximate site of brain pathology. (The term 'aphasia' and its derivatives is used in preference to dysphasia in line with growing convention in neuropsychological and linguistic circles but encompasses all varieties and severities of language disturbance.) Yet despite over 100 years of careful enquiry and observation the analysis of aphasia remains a controversial area, and beyond certain broad limits its relationship to regional cerebral disorder remains in many respects uncertain. This should not be surprising in view of the complex interrelationships that exist between different aspects of language processes, and the intimate way in which language must enter into many other cognitive functions and vice versa. The parts of the brain concerned with language are extensive, and necessarily diffused over a considerable territory so that auditory, visual and motor mechanisms can be subserved. Consequently cerebral lesions that produce aphasia can lead to many forms of deficit, and at the same time to other defects which render the appraisal of clinicopathological correlations difficult. Moreover, it is likely that there is individual variation in the anatomical substrate for language.

Cerebral dominance for language

The earliest observation of a relationship between anatomy and psychology to gain universal acceptance was that aphasia was overwhelmingly more common after lesions of the left hemisphere than the right. Later, right hemisphere lesions were reported to produce aphasia in left-handed subjects, and the general rule was proposed that the hemisphere contralateral to handedness governed speech. This has been upheld in large measure where right-handed subjects are concerned; the vast majority of cases of aphasia in right-handed subjects arise following lesions in the left hemisphere whereas the incidence is only about 1% when the lesion is right sided. However, it is now known from large unselected series of patients with brain lesions that left-handers also suffer aphasia more often from left than from right hemisphere lesions ('crossed aphasia'), in fact in a ratio of approximately 2:1. Bilateral speech representation appears to be more common in left-handers than right-handers, though remaining rare in both.

The most direct confirmation of these relationships has come from observing the transient effect on speech of injecting amobarbital into the carotid arteries of the left and right sides separately by the Wada technique (Wada & Rasmussen 1960; Rasmussen & Milner 1977). Amobarbital, 175 mg as a 10% solution, is injected over 2–3 seconds into the internal carotid artery. This results in a contralateral flaccid paralysis lasting several minutes during which the preservation or disruption of language can be briefly assessed. Rasmussen and Milner (1977) have reported 396 epileptic patients examined under such conditions. Among the right-handers 92% were found to have left hemisphere speech, 6% to have right hemisphere speech and in 2% there was bilateral representation. Among left-handers and ambidextrous patients (without early brain damage) 70% had left hemisphere speech, 15% right hemisphere speech and 15% had bilateral speech representation. In subjects with evidence of bilateral speech representation the speech defects were mild, from both the right- and left-sided injections. Functional MRI has begun to be used as a non-invasive method for determining cerebral dominance prior to surgery.

An alternative method for assessing language laterality applicable to clinical and non-clinical groups involves the use of dichotic listening. Verbal information in the form of, for example, consonant–vowel syllables is fed through earphones to the two ears, but in such a way that different information arrives at each ear simultaneously. The subject must report whatever he hears, and is found to report more accurately and comprehensively from the ear contralateral to the hemisphere subserving language, the so-called right ear advantage in right-handed subjects. The results are less clear-cut than with the Wada technique, but dichotic listening has the advantage of safety and lack of adverse effects.

The prevalence of handedness in the normal population varies according to how it is defined and measured. Nevertheless if asked which hand an individual habitually writes with, about 90% of people will say the right. Dominance for other skilled tasks, footedness and eyedness yield lower percentages. The proportion of left-handers is slightly but consistently higher in males than females. Cultural factors exert some influence over these figures: the performance of certain tasks with the left hand is taboo in some societies and pressure from educationalists, particularly in the first half of the twentieth century, forced many children to write with their right hands regardless of their preference. While it is generally agreed that genetic factors are the major determinant of handedness, there remains controversy regarding the precise mode of transmission and genetic model. Of neuropsychiatric interest is the issue of 'pathological left-handedness'. It has been suggested that a proportion of people become left-handed because of early damage to their left hemispheres that brings about a shift in cerebral dominance. The age of 10–12 years is generally accepted as the upper limit beyond which brain damage will not alter handedness and beyond which the second hemisphere will not develop fully adequate language skills by way of compensation. That shifts in cerebral dominance do occur in relation to early left hemisphere damage is strongly upheld by Rasmussen and Milner's (1977) results of intracarotid amobarbital injection already mentioned above. Where left-handedness or ambidexterity was accompanied by a history of early left hemisphere damage there was, in contrast to all other groups, a large percentage of cases with language representation in the right hemisphere (28% left hemisphere speech, 53% right hemisphere speech, 19% bilateral speech representation). From a population perspective it has been estimated that only about 1 in 20 left-handers is 'pathological'. Furthermore, a variety of non-specific developmental disorders and insults may increase the incidence of non-right-handedness, suggesting that this may be due to the failure of left hemisphere dominance for language to become established in the first place rather than it shifting.

Handedness, or more broadly laterality, has been investigated in relation to many psychiatric disorders but most particularly schizophrenia (see Structural brain imaging, and also Associations with regional brain pathology, later) where it has been shown that non-right-handedness is indeed more common. This appears to be due to an increase in left-handedness as well as mixed or 'ambiguous' handedness. Again, the finding is open to interpretation but is consistent with theories which postulate an abnormality in left hemisphere specialisation during development (Dragovic & Hammond 2005).

Yakovlev and Rakic (1966) reported that in fetal and newborn brains the corticospinal tract from the left hemisphere usually begins to decussate higher in the medulla than that coming from the right, and the corticospinal tract is usually larger on the right side of the cord than the left. Right hand preference, therefore, probably develops on the basis of the increased motor innervation available to the right side of the body. More directly, Geschwind and Levitsky (1968) examined 100 adult human brains at post-mortem and reported marked differences between the two hemispheres in the size of the planum temporale, which lies on the superior surface of the temporal lobe immediately behind Heschl's gyrus. This is the region that contains the auditory association cortex, and represents the classic Wernicke's area known to be important for language. Other related anatomical differences have been noted, for example the occipital lobe is usually wider on the left than the right, whereas the frontal lobe is wider on the right than the left; these asymmetries may be less striking or even reversed in left-handers. MRI has superseded post-mortem studies of laterality. A meta-analysis of all such anatomical data including MRI confirmed the left greater than right surface area and volume of the planum and different configuration of the left versus the right sylvian fissure in neurologically intact participants totalling several hundreds (Shapleske *et al.* 1999).

Evidence with regard to cerebral dominance for language has also come from observations after section of the corpus callosum for the relief of intractable epilepsy (Sperry 1966; Gazzaniga & Sperry 1967; Sperry & Gazzaniga 1967). As a result of the operation the two hemispheres are virtually isolated from each other and information can be fed tachistoscopically to either hemisphere alone by brief exposures in the opposite half-field of vision. When a picture of an object is exposed to the dominant hemisphere it can be named promptly or recorded in writing, but similar exposures to the non-dominant hemisphere meet with no such response. If pressed to answer after information has been fed to the non-dominant hemisphere, the patient may deny seeing anything, or alternatively the speaking hemisphere may resort to pure guesswork and produce a random response. Nonetheless, the patient can select the appropriate matching object, by means of palpation with the left hand, from among a group of objects concealed behind a screen, indicating that the non-dominant hemisphere has correctly perceived the picture despite the patient's inability to name it. In a similar way an object concealed from view can be named when palpated by the right hand but not when palpated by the left

hand. The non-dominant hemisphere is therefore mute as would have been expected.

In some of these patients, however, it seems certain that limited comprehension of language can take place in the non-dominant hemisphere. The left hand can correctly select or point to an object which corresponds to a name exposed briefly to the non-dominant hemisphere alone. That the dominant hemisphere can have played no part is shown by the failure of the right hand to perform accurately in this situation; moreover the subject cannot name the matching object if this has been selected by the left hand but remains concealed from view. Auditory comprehension can be demonstrated by flashing a picture to the non-dominant hemisphere and then asking the patient to signal when the matching word is read aloud to him; this he can do by signalling with the left hand but not with the right. Alternatively, a word can be spoken out loud and the patient asked to signal when the corresponding printed word is exposed visually to the non-dominant hemisphere. Ingenious research techniques that overcome the limitations of brief tachistoscopic presentations have allowed further exploration of the language capacities of the non-dominant hemisphere (Zaidel 1977, 1978; Gazzaniga 1983). It has become apparent that such capacities are present in a small proportion of patients. The degree of sophistication varies widely, from primitive levels of comprehension to the ability to detect semantic incongruities in sentences and to understand syntactic rules. It is *expressive* speech that appears to be most outside the capabilities of the normal right hemisphere as does normal inferential reasoning (Gazzaniga 1985).

Some exceedingly rare observations have been made on patients after total surgical removal of the dominant hemisphere. One such patient was investigated by Smith (1966) after left hemispherectomy for recurrence of a glioblastoma. The patient had previously been strongly right-handed. In the immediate postoperative period there was, as expected, a severe sensory and motor dysphasia along with right hemiplegia and hemianopia. Even then, however, he could follow some simple commands, indicating some preservation of comprehension of speech. He could also utter emotional expletives such as 'Goddamit' with good articulation, at a time when single words could not be repeated and when there was no ability at all to communicate in propositional speech. Suddenly in the tenth postoperative week he asked his nurse 'What does "B.M." mean?' in response to her enquiry about his bowel movements. Thereafter the occasional use of fragments of propositional speech increased, along with ability to repeat progressively longer sentences on command, though most of the time the patient remained incapable of speaking voluntarily. Comprehension of speech, in contrast, appeared to reach approximately normal levels at 1 year postoperatively before the tumour recurred (Smith 1972). Of particular interest in view of the evidence linking musical functions with the minor hemisphere (see Auditory agnosia and auditory perceptual defects, later) was the patient's eventual ability to sing familiar songs and hymns with little hesitation and few errors of articulation, even though speaking remained very severely impaired. A remarkably similar postoperative course has been documented in a second patient (Burklund & Smith 1977). Other scattered examples in the literature are reviewed by Searleman (1977).

The rarity of such cases again makes it difficult to estimate how far the results may have been due to an unusual degree of bilaterality of language already present before operation, or how far new capacities to organise language were developed in the non-dominant hemisphere. The complex effects of hemispherectomy on language development following brain damage in childhood are described by Vargha-Khadem et al. (1991). A profile of right hemisphere language has been summarised as follows: reduced auditory–verbal short-term memory, better comprehension of speech than reading, and rudimentary phonology (affecting all tasks requiring grapheme–phoneme conversion).

Finally, there is now considerable evidence that the affective components of language, including prosody and emotional gesturing, appeciation of humour and metaphor, are the special prerogative of the right hemisphere (Ross & Mesulam 1979; Ross 1981; Benson & Zaidel 1985). Thus patients with right hemisphere strokes may lose the ability to express emotion by voice or gesture, or to perceive the affective colouring in the speech or gestures of others, while formal propositional aspects of language remain intact. Indeed, Ross (1981) suggests that the functional organisation of the affective components of language in the right hemisphere may closely mirror that of propositional language in the left, and has produced evidence of a similar range of 'aprosodic' subsyndromes to that encountered among the aphasias (motor aprosodia, sensory aprosodia, etc.).

The concept of 'auditory affective agnosia' in relation to language is considered later in the chapter (see under Auditory agnosia and auditory perceptual defects).

Localisation of language functions within the brain

We have little direct knowledge about the physiological mechanisms that underlie language functions in the healthy intact brain. Since language is unique to humans there is no paradigm which can be studied in animals, and evidence has had to accumulate slowly from the study of the damaged human brain. Inferences about normal function from studies of abnormal function are notoriously dangerous, and not

surprisingly numerous theories abound on psychological, physiological and anatomical levels. It is, however, useful to have a framework against which to view the phenomena of aphasia, and the theoretical background is therefore briefly reviewed before the clinical data are considered.

Early and primitive localisationist views postulated 'speech centres' for speaking, reading and writing, proposed by Lichtheim and Wernicke in the 1880s, which contained the repositories for word images and which could be disturbed either directly by lesions or by damage to various connecting pathways. Freud was one of the first to attack the 'diagram makers' and propose a more holistic view of the functions of the speech territory in the dominant hemisphere. Head further developed the dynamic concepts of Hughlings Jackson and proposed a classification that depended primarily on symptoms of deficit rather than locus of lesion. However, as noted above, there has been a resurgence of interest in those very diagrams which lend themselves to the information processing models favoured by contemporary cognitive neuropsychologists (Ellis and Young 1988). Indeed, the so-called Wernicke–Lichtheim model does rather well at making sense of disorders of spoken language and forms the basis of a useful classificatory scheme (see below). Disorders of across-language modalities have proved less tractable.

The classification of the aphasias must be seen in the light of the distinct aims of the clinician and the psycholinguist. The clinician is trained to recognise syndromes, collections of symptoms and signs that frequently cluster together. A syndrome so defined, if it is to have any utility, can then be related to aetiology, prognosis and possibly pathophysiology including anatomical localisation. Such syndromes tend to arise through the astute observational skills of an experienced clinician. Hence Broca's aphasia, a non-fluent disorder of the motoric aspects of speech with relative preservation of comprehension. The aetiology is often an occlusion of the left middle cerebral artery leading to an infarct of the lateral inferior frontal lobe. However, to the linguist or cognitive neuropsychologist, the pathology is of only peripheral interest in comparison to the nature of the language disorder itself. The non-fluency may be characterised more precisely as a reflection of 'agrammatism', the loss of syntactic structures or 'function words' linking verbs and nouns, such as prepositions, conjunctions and auxiliary verbs. This loss gives speech a telegraphic quality which nevertheless conveys meaning. It is the nature of the pure cognitive deficit that is of interest to the linguist and not the 'accidentally' coexistent features of the syndrome. Since comprehension, reading or writing may not be similarly affected, the cognitively minded observer argues that their presence or absence is not essential to the disorder and so can be set aside; if deficits were present in these modalities, it might point to a problem at the 'deeper' semantic level. Contrast this with the clinician, particularly the neurologist, who may use just such secondary aspects of the syndrome including even non-linguistic aspects such as a right Babinski reflex to form an impression of the extent of the patient's lesion as it affects the left hemisphere, possible causes and likely prognosis. Yet there is no psychological connection between retrieval of function words and extension of the great toe! The clinician is looking for the presence of associations between clinical features that have been noted by others to co-occur and which are probabilistic and can be supported by epidemiological evidence; the cognitive neuropsychologist is looking for patterns of deficits and abilities which relate to a theoretical model.

As a result of the above, classification of the aphasias can be confusing as it tries to represent these differing perspectives. The pure cognitive or linguistic account will tend to group language deficits according to the level of abnormality along the hierarchy shown below.

* Phonology (or orthography): the basic 'building blocks' of speech (written words).
* Syntax: the rules governing the grammatical forms of words and connections between words in sentences.
* Lexical semantics: word meaning.
* Pragmatics: to do with the intended meaning of language and conventional usage.

The broadest and most simplistic clinical classification is between motor, non-fluent, expressive Broca's aphasia on the one hand and sensory, fluent, receptive Wernicke's aphasia on the other. The Wernicke–Lichtheim model allows for these two broad types of language disorder, which are lesions to the motor word-representation and auditory word-representation centres respectively, the hypothetical centres sitting comfortably on defined neuroanatomical areas. Furthermore, the model both predicts and provides a framework to explain other language problems such as conduction aphasia (failure of repetition) and what became known as the transcortical aphasias in which repetition is preserved. Writing and reading are not included in this scheme. While a serious omission, this also reflects clinical practice at the bedside which, rightly or wrongly, tends to concentrate on spoken language.

Geschwind (1967) was an important heir to the likes of Wernicke and expanded the model to account for language in general, based on the learning and arousal of associative links. He pointed out that the distinctive element in human language, which is not present in animal communication, derives from our ability to form higher-order associations between one sensory stimulus and another. In subhuman primates the principal outflow from sensory association areas is to the limbic system, enabling the animal to learn which stimuli have importance with regard to drives for food, sex or aggression; interconnections between the sensory association regions for different sensory modalities are meagre by comparison. The impressive advance in the human brain lies in the expansion of the zone in the region of the angular gyrus at the junction of the temporal, parietal and occipital lobes, an area strategically situated with respect to the association cortices for hearing, touch and vision (heteromodal cortex). It is noteworthy that inputs to this part of the brain are almost exclusively from other cortical regions, and furthermore that it is one of the last brain regions to myelinate during development.

Neuroimaging and language

In general, structural neuroimaging has tended to support the traditional syndrome localisations for the main subvarieties (Broca's, Wernicke's and conduction aphasias), likewise for the principal subdivisions of alexia and agraphia (Benson & Ardila 1996). A large MRI study (Kreisler *et al.* 2000) examined 107 stroke patients and found that non-fluent disorders tended to be associated with frontal and putaminal lesions, repetition disorders to lesions of the insula–external capsule. Disorders of comprehension invariably involved lesions of the posterior parts of the temporal gyri, while fluent disorders with paraphasias were found with temporal lobe lesions with extension subcortically. Similarly, Bates *et al.* (2003) used a voxel-based method of matching MRI data with aphasia symptoms in 101 aphasic stroke patients and found that lesions within the left insula and deep parietal white matter affected fluency while more posterior lesions in the left middle temporal gyrus had the most impact on auditory comprehension (Fig. 2.1: see also Plate 2.1).

Such analyses shift between discussion of say 'Broca's area' as a fixed anatomical entity and as a theoretical construct. As neurologist Richard Wise (2003) concludes, neuroimaging allows more precise lesion location at the time of patient testing than was possible in the past and, as a result, syndromes have been described that may be associated with lesions at various locations. Rather than this being the result of individual differences, he suggests that it is likely that 'broadly similar clinical syndromes may result from very differently sited cortical, subcortical or tract lesions within distributed neural systems that are essentially similar between subjects'.

Non-invasive functional neuroimaging studies using PET and fMRI have contributed a great deal to illuminating the brain regions involved in language processing in the intact brain.

In what is now regarded as a classic study, Petersen *et al.* (1988) used PET to explore linguistic functions in an interesting experimental paradigm. Seventeen right-handed normal volunteers were given repeated brief PET scans, using ^{15}O-labelled water, under a succession of experimental conditions arranged hierarchically. By subtraction, the effects of each extra task demand on regional cerebral blood flow could be discerned. In the first comparison nouns were presented (visually or auditorily) without task demands, and compared with a control state of simple visual fixation. Involuntary word-form processing was targeted by this subtraction. Next the subject was required to speak each word, revealing areas involved in output coding and motor control. Finally, the subject was asked to give a use for each presented

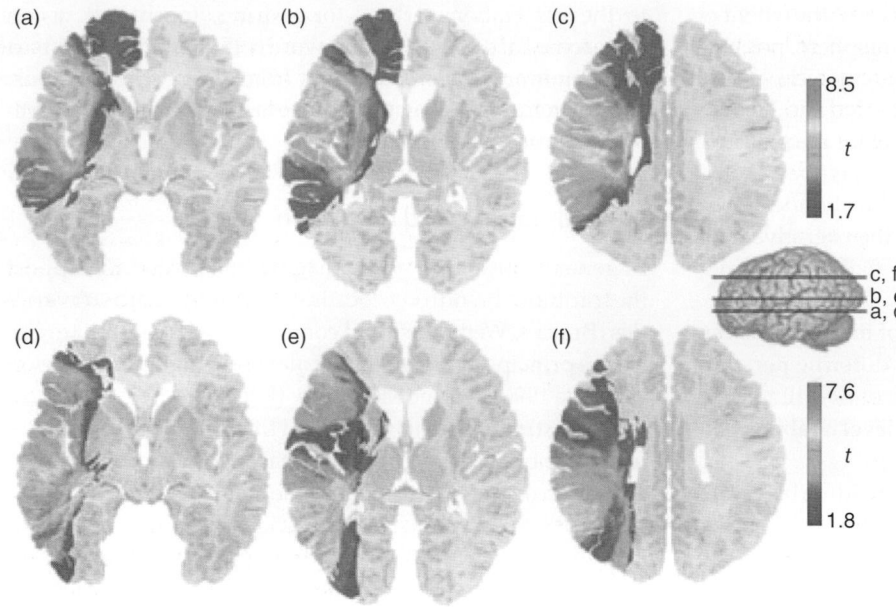

Fig. 2.1 Representative slices from VLSM maps computed for fluency and auditory comprehension performance of 101 aphasic stroke patients.

These maps are depictions of *t*-test results evaluating patients' performance on a voxel-by-voxel basis, for fluency (a–c) or auditory comprehension (d–f). High scores indicate that lesions to these voxels have a highly significant effect on behaviour. Low scores indicate that the lesions had relatively little impact on behaviour. From Bates *et al.* (2003), *Nature Neuroscience* **6**, 448–450. See also Plate 2.1.

word, revealing the cerebral substrate for noun–verb associations (semantic processing).

This work has been replicated and extended in numerous experiments since. Functional MRI has overtaken PET as the methodology of choice for functional neuroimaging and the combined body of work from both has been well reviewed for the general reader (Price 2000; Small and Burton 2002).

However, functional imaging techniques have shown additional complexities, revealing areas of hypometabolism extending beyond or even distant from the areas of known structural damage. Metter and Hanson (1994), for example, report PET studies which show that hypometabolism in the left temporoparietal cortex appears to be critical for the development of aphasia, being present in all the aphasics they studied irrespective of the location of structural damage. Recent work has attempted to shed light on the processes of recovery (Price & Crinion 2005): it appears that recovery of speech correlates with slowly evolving ipsilesional (left hemisphere) changes in activation. Right hemisphere homologous activation after, for example, left anterior hemisphere aphasia-producing stroke does not seem to correlate with recovery or preservation, so appears to be a reflection of non-functional (in the linguistic sense) changes. In terms of speech comprehension, the picture is more mixed and it seems that both the right and left temporal lobes contribute to recovery.

Clinical syndromes of language impairment

For the purposes of clinical evaluation it is useful to consider a broad division into defective understanding of speech or written material, and defective production of speech or writing. However, the great majority of patients with language disturbance show a complicated mixture of deficits.

For an extended presentation and discussion of the various disorders, Benson and Ardila (1996) should be consulted. At least partial support for the principal subvarieties and their anatomical localisation has come from neuroimaging studies, but with the caveats given by Wise and others. The syndromes outlined below are clearly to a considerable extent abstractions from a very complex whole.

Broca's aphasia (cortical motor aphasia, expressive aphasia)

The primary defect is on the effector side of speech, thus involving the mechanisms by which words are chosen and articulated and sentences constructed. Unlike pure word-dumbness, however, writing is affected in parallel with speaking, and while comprehension is relatively intact there may be difficulty in carrying out complex instructions. This may be on account of apraxia or because the instructions require complex internal verbalisation for their efficient execution.

Speech is characteristically sparse, slow and hesitant, with marked disturbances of rhythm, inflexion and articulation, unlike the fluent expressive speech of primary sensory dysphasia. Moreover, the patient is clearly under stress while trying to speak. Word-finding provides obvious difficulty, wrong words are often chosen and the words that are chosen are often mispronounced. Marked reiteration and perseveration are common. However, the patient usually recognises his mistakes, attempts to correct them and becomes impatient about them. Moreover, he can select the correct word when this is offered to him. There is a marked impairment of syntax (agrammatism; see under Localisation of language functions within the brain, earlier). This further impairs the patient's ability to transmit meaning. He often tries to compensate for his speech defects by means of pantomime and gesture, all again in contrast to the patient with primary sensory dysphasia.

The phrase length is short, and the style may be abbreviated and 'telegraphic' with omissions of words, but the speech that does emerge is meaningful. Ability to repeat what the examiner says to him may be an improvement on what the patient can produce spontaneously, but nevertheless is always profoundly impaired. In the most severe examples the patient may have only one or two words at his command, or there may be stereotyped repetition of some word or phrase (reiteration or 'recurring utterance'). However, total loss of ability to speak is not seen, and an occasional speech sound can usually be discerned.

Among these marked expressive difficulties it may be noted that the automatic repetition of serials, such as numbers or days of the week, is relatively well preserved even though they are not well articulated. If such lists are well articulated, an apraxia of speech may be suspected (see below). Also, in severe cases, emotional ejaculations may be surprisingly intact when voluntary utterance is reduced to the minimum. Sometimes an object exposed to view can be named when the same name cannot be found in spontaneous speech. Similarly, a habitual situation may call forth a word such as 'goodbye' when the patient is quite unable to produce it on request.

Comprehension of written and spoken instructions may be relatively intact but is rarely normal. Particular difficulty is encountered over the comprehension of grammatically significant structures. Quite often the patient may be well aware of the meaning of a word that he reads even though he cannot pronounce it aloud. Reading out loud will show a halting jerky flow, with slurring and occasional mispronunciations. Disturbances of writing may be closely similar to those of speaking. The lesion is in the posterior two-thirds of the third frontal convolution, i.e. the pars triangularis and operculum of the premotor cortex, the classic Broca's area. Sometimes this extends also onto the lower part of the precentral convolution.

Wernicke's aphasia (primary sensory/receptive aphasia)

The primary deficit is in the comprehension of spoken speech. There is defective appreciation of the meaning of words and in particular of meaning conveyed by grammatical relations. The patient has corresponding difficulty in repeating what is said to him and in responding to commands. In less severe examples the difficulty in responding to commands can be observed to increase with the complexity of instructions, though interestingly quite complex 'whole-body' commands can prove to be surprisingly well performed (Benson & Geschwind 1971). Other aspects of hearing are intact, as with pure word-deafness, but unlike the latter there are also impairments of spontaneous speech, writing and reading. These added difficulties are attributable to the fact that the cortical mechanisms for analysing incoming speech are directly implicated by the lesion, not merely cut off from input as in pure word-deafness.

Thus ability to speak is also impaired, presumably because auditory associations or schemata must first be aroused before the efferent speech mechanisms can produce speech in a normal manner. In this way the terms 'receptive' or 'sensory' may be misleading. Words are used wrongly, paraphasic errors and neologisms are frequent, and sentences tend to be poorly constructed with errors of grammar and syntax. However, the faulty speech is produced fluently and without effort. Normal rhythm and inflexion are preserved and there are no articulatory defects. The speech may even be excessive in flow or under pressure, perhaps because the effector mechanisms 'run on' to a large degree autonomously when freed from the control of higher functional levels.

> A patient reported by Brain (1965) responded as follows. When asked 'Do you have headaches?' he replied 'No. I've been fort in that way. I haven't been headache troubled not for a long time.' When shown a picture of an elephant he was unable to name it, but pointed to the mouth and said 'That's his sound, he is making his sound – seems to have got his voice opened there'. When shown a picture of a penguin he said 'A kind of little ver (bird) – machinery – a kind of animal do for making a sound'. When shown a tape measure he called it 'A kind of machinery', and when immediately afterwards shown a bunch of keys and asked to name it he said 'Indication of measurement of piece of apparatus or intimating the cost of apparatus in various forms'.

Reiterative errors are obvious in the above example, in that the speech is contaminated by words which the patient has once used but then cannot easily discard. The patient is usually unaware of his mistakes and makes no attempt to correct them. Unlike the patient with nominal aphasia (see below) he is often unable to recognise the correct name for an object when this is told to him.

Reading and writing are also impaired since these are presumably also dependent on the cortical areas involved in comprehending spoken speech (and developmentally they are learned in association with spoken language). Single words may be read aloud correctly, but reading out of sentences becomes jumbled and contaminated by paraphasic errors. Written instructions, even if correctly read, may not be carried out, indicating that the patient has failed to understand what he has read. Generally the degrees of disability in understanding spoken and written language parallel each other closely. The disturbances of writing also closely mirror those of spoken speech, except that a copious fluent flow is much less common in writing than in speaking.

The lesion is in the auditory association cortex of the superior and middle temporal gyri of the dominant hemisphere (Wernicke's area), presumably preventing the recoding of auditory messages for recognition, and debarring the arousal of auditory associations as a necessary step for reading, writing and the production of spoken speech.

Pure word-deafness (subcortical auditory aphasia, verbal auditory agnosia)

The patient can speak fluently and virtually without error, and similarly can write normally. He can also read and comprehend what he reads. The defect is restricted to the understanding of spoken speech, even though other aspects of hearing are intact. In fact the patient hears words as sounds but fails to recognise these sounds as words. Hemphill and Stengel's (1940) patient said 'Voice comes but no words. I can hear, sounds come, but words don't separate. There is no trouble at all with the sound. Sounds come. I can hear, but I cannot understand it.' As a result the patient cannot repeat words spoken to him and cannot write to dictation.

Such a defect can equally be regarded as an agnosia for spoken words. It is extremely rare, but there is general agreement that the lesion is in the dominant temporal lobe, closely adjacent to the primary receptive area for hearing, i.e. Heschl's gyrus of the first temporal convolution. Geschwind suggests that it is caused by interruption of the auditory pathway to the dominant temporal lobe together with a lesion of the corpus callosum. The patient can still hear because the auditory pathway to the non-dominant cortex is intact, but incoming auditory information cannot gain access to the speech-receiving mechanisms of the dominant lobe. The disorder is rare because a lesion in this situation will usually extend far enough to the surface to damage the speech-receiving mechanisms themselves, resulting in the more widespread disabilities of a primary sensory dysphasia.

Pure word-blindness (alexia without agraphia, agnosic alexia, subcortical visual aphasia, occipital alexia)

The patient can speak normally and has no difficulty with comprehension of the spoken word. His difficulties with language are entirely restricted to his understanding of what he reads. The patient can still describe or copy letters even though he cannot recognise them, showing that the defect is not due to loss of the visual images of the letters. Attempts at reading may betray a laborious letter-by-letter strategy. Some patients manage better with written script than printed material, presumably because they can more readily reproduce the letters in imagination with the right hand and thereby obtain kinaesthetic cues. Occasionally, numbers continue to be recognised when letters are not, perhaps again via kinaesthetic cues that are derived from early associations between counting and manual activities.

The patient can write spontaneously and to dictation, though subsequently he cannot read what he has written. The writing is usually entirely normal, though it may contain minor errors of reduplication or misalignment of letters. He may be able to copy written material slowly and laboriously.

An almost invariable accompaniment is a right homonymous hemianopia. Colours cannot be named, even though colour perception can be shown to be intact by sorting tests. Here it is probably significant that colour naming represents a purely visual–verbal association process and cannot derive support from other cues. Essentially, word-blindness is a failure to recognise the language values of the visual patterns which make up words, although there is no disturbance of the symbolic function of the words themselves. This is confirmed when the patient can spell out loud and recognise words that are spelled out loud. The lesion is of the left visual cortex together with the splenium of the corpus callosum; thus visual input is possible only to the right hemisphere, and cannot gain access to the language systems of the left. It is therefore a disconnection syndrome par excellence. The situation is analogous to that of the lesion causing pure word-deafness. However, pure word-blindness is commoner because the lesion does not so readily impinge on the language areas themselves. The usual cause is occlusion of the left posterior cerebral artery.

Pure word-dumbness (apraxic anarthria, subcortical motor dysphasia, aphemia)

The patient can comprehend both spoken speech and written material without difficulty, and shows this by his ability to respond to complex commands. He can express himself normally in writing, which also serves to demonstrate that inner speech is perfectly preserved. The defect is restricted to the production of spoken speech, which is marked by slurring and dysarthria. The patient cannot speak normally at will, cannot repeat words heard and cannot read aloud. In severe cases he may be totally unable to articulate. Yet for other purposes the muscles of the tongue and lips function without impairment.

The condition may thus be regarded as an apraxia restricted to the movements required for speech. The exact site of pathology is uncertain, but the lesion is probably beneath the region of the insula, interrupting the pathway from the cortical centres responsible for motor schemata for words to the motor systems used in articulated speech. It is extremely rare because the lesion usually also involves the former at the same time, resulting in a primary motor dysphasia. It has been claimed that Broca's original patient 'Tan' in fact had apraxia of speech and that his lesion (a cystic tumour) centred around the insula rather than what has become known as Broca's area (Dronkers *et al.* 1992).

Pure agraphia (agraphia without alexia)

Agraphia may accompany almost any form of generalised aphasia or be a component of generalised apraxia. As an isolated defect, however, it may be seen as the graphic equivalent of pure word-dumbness. Comprehension of written and spoken material is normal, and the patient's own speech is unimpaired. However, he is unable to write either spontaneously or to dictation, though he may fare rather better at the copying of written material.

Brain (1965) pointed out that writing is a considerably more complex process than articulated speech, since after the processes leading up to speech there must then be evocation of visual graphic schemata in the posterior parts of the brain, and of motor schemata in close relation to the motor cortex. The lesion in pure motor agraphia is thought to interrupt the pathway from the left angular gyrus to the hand area of the left motor cortex, and to lie usually in the second frontal gyrus anterior to the hand area or sometimes in the parietal lobe.

Nominal aphasia (amnesic aphasia, anomic aphasia)

Though this is one of the commonest forms of aphasia, it is the least understood in terms of pathophysiology. The principal difficulty lies in evoking names at will. This may vary from total inability to name any object on confrontation to a mild disorder demonstrable only where uncommon words are concerned. The patient can describe the object and give its use, even when the name eludes him, and like the patient with primary motor aphasia can usually recognise the correct name when this is offered to him. He can often use the same word without difficulty a moment later in spontaneous connected speech. Demonstration of knowledge of the concept behind the word in pure nominal aphasia is in contrast to the patient with semantic dementia, who has lost all the meanings attached to the word along with the word itself (see earlier in chapter under Amnesia in diffuse cerebral disease; also see Chapter 9: Frontotemporal dementia/Clinical features).

Conversational speech is fluent, with no difficulty in articulation and little or no paraphasic interference, but circumlocutions are used and word-finding pauses may be evident. 'Empty words' such as 'thing' or 'these' may be frequently employed, and there is a notable lack of substantive words. Otherwise, the grammatical structure of sentences is usually well preserved. The patient can repeat fluently what is said to him, and he usually performs relatively well on well-learned serials such as numbers or days of the week.

Comprehension is relatively preserved in most instances, but internal speech is often affected so there may be difficulty in understanding or executing some oral or written commands.

It is not generally agreed whether nominal dysphasia represents a distinct form of defect. Some view it merely as a mild form of primary sensory aphasia, since with expanding lesions one may merge progressively into the other. This is the type of aphasia which in mild degree has most often been attributed to diffuse rather than focal brain damage. Certainly it may occur with diffuse brain dysfunction due to toxic or degenerative conditions. However, it may also be found with focal brain lesions, perhaps particularly (though not exclusively) with dominant temporoparietal lesions in the neighbourhood of the angular gyrus. Acalculia and other components of Gerstmann's syndrome often occur as associated deficits.

Conduction aphasia (central dysphasia, syntactical dysphasia)

Essentially, conduction aphasia consists of a grave disturbance of language function in which speech and writing are impaired in the manner described above for primary sensory dysphasia, but in which comprehension of spoken and written material is nonetheless relatively well preserved, as shown for example by simple yes/no responses. Repetition of speech is very severely impaired.

According to Geschwind it results from a lesion that spares both Wernicke's and Broca's areas but disrupts the major connections between them. Thus Wernicke's area can function relatively well in analysing incoming information, though it can no longer act to guide the patient's own productions. There are contending views about the site of the responsible lesion (see Benson & Ardila 1996). One view, which accounts for the essential features of the disorder, blames a lesion of the arcuate fasciculus as it passes from the temporal to the frontal lobe by way of the parietal lobe. The more the lesion comes to implicate Wernicke's area itself, the more will comprehension be impaired and the closer will the picture approximate to that of primary sensory aphasia.

The repetition defect in conduction aphasia has come under closer scrutiny recently. Patients who show a marked repetition defect for verbal material presented in the auditory modality appeared on analysis to have a selective impairment of the immediate memory span for auditory verbal material that was directly related to the 'memory' load of the task. (Note that we routinely test repetition when we carry out the digit span test, but regard it as a test of immediate or short-term memory.) There is much less difficulty when comparable material is presented visually. Moreover, auditory verbal learning and verbal long-term memory are relatively intact, indicating that material can nonetheless gain access to the long-term memory store.

Syndromes of the isolated speech area

Under this title Goldstein (1948) and Geschwind *et al.* (1968) describe further variants of aphasia, which though rare demand an alternative explanation in terms of mechanism. Comprehension is profoundly disturbed, but in contrast to primary sensory dysphasia the patient can easily repeat what is said to him, and the ability to learn new verbal material is retained. Moreover, spontaneous speech is slow and laboured and lacks the fluency of primary sensory dysphasia. It is postulated that both Wernicke's and Broca's areas, and the connections between them, remain intact but the whole system is cut off from other parts of the cortex. It is the lack of these widespread connections that leads to impaired comprehension and defects of propositional speech.

Though in pure form the syndrome is extremely rare, two variants are well recognised. *Transcortical (or extrasylvian) motor aphasia* differs in that the patient can comprehend spoken speech, and is ascribed to a lesion anterior and/or superior to Broca's area, or in some cases in the supplementary area of the medial frontal cortex. *Transcortical (or extrasylvian) sensory aphasia* differs in that the fluency of output is preserved. Echolalia is often prominent. The facility with which the patient repeats the examiner's statements, and the fluent jumbled output of speech, stand in contrast to the patient's lack of comprehension. This may lead to misinterpretation of the syndrome as an acute psychotic disturbance, especially since obvious neurological deficits can be lacking (Benson & Ardila 1996). The lesion usually involves either the parieto-occipital or temporo-occipital border zone areas.

Aphasia and other aspects of intelligence

Opinion has differed about the extent to which aphasia can be regarded merely as 'loss of a linguistic tool' while other aspects of intellect remain intact. Language is, of course, an integral part of conceptual thinking and of problem-solving in many areas, but it may be that some aphasic patients retain in large degree the automatic and subconscious use of words in thinking processes. Impairment of the ordered perception of space or time may worsen aphasic difficulties, since a proper conception of such matters is essential for symbolic thought. Nevertheless, aspects of social cognition may remain highly attuned despite severe language impairments as may fine perceptual discriminations of people and places. The often difficult question of assessing legal competency in aphasic patients is discussed by Benson and Ardila (1996).

Subcortical aphasia

The possibility that subcortical pathology might contribute to, or even be responsible for, certain aphasic syndromes has a considerable history. Renewed attention has been directed to the issue now that neuroimaging is capable of revealing discrete subcortical infarcts, and certain syndromes such as 'thalamic' and 'striatal' aphasia have been proposed. Benson and Ardila (1996) review the still uncertain status of such syndromes, and the difficulty in deciding whether the language disturbance reflects the direct effects of the subcortical lesion or derives from distant effects induced elsewhere in the brain. Functional imaging techniques have shown that secondary involvement of cortical language areas is common,

presumably in consequence of 'diaschisis' subsequent to disruption of subcortical–cortical mechanisms (Perani *et al.* 1987). Instances of 'subcortical neglect' may similarly owe much to secondary effects on right hemisphere cortical activity.

The picture usually described is of mutism following an acute intracerebral haemorrhage, followed by hypophonia and slow amelodic output. This may evolve to a combination of severely paraphasic speech with relatively well-preserved capacity for repetition, which appears to be the characteristic pattern. The subcortical structures involved are virtually always situated in the hemisphere dominant for language.

Thalamic aphasia begins with mutism but generally changes to a fluent, paraphasic jargon output. Difficulty with naming is often dramatically severe, but comprehension and repetition are comparatively well preserved. In most cases the language disorder is transient, showing improvement over the course of weeks or months. The puzzling feature is the rarity of such a development among the considerable number of persons who develop thalamic lesions.

Striatal (striatocapsular) aphasia appears to derive chiefly from lesions of the putamen and internal capsule. The patients reported by Damasio *et al.* (1982a) had prominent involvement of the anterior limb of the capsule and also the head of the caudate nucleus. Speech remains sparse, fluent but hesitant, dysarthric and paraphasic, though again comprehension and repetition are usually good. The ability to name is better preserved than with thalamic dysphasia. Naeser *et al.* (1982) have pointed to subdivisions within the syndrome according to the precise site of the lesion and its extension into neighbouring territories. Perseveration was commonly associated with caudate lesions in the survey by Kreisler *et al.* (2000).

Alexia with agraphia (visual asymbolia, parietotemporal alexia)

The patient is unable to read as with pure word-blindness, but in addition he is unable to write. However, the execution and comprehension of spoken speech are substantially unimpaired.

The difficulty in reading is similar to that described for pure word-blindness. The difficulty in writing varies from complete inability to form letters to preservation of partial attempts at writing words. Copying is better than spontaneous writing, which is the converse of the situation in pure word-blindness. Moreover, the patient cannot understand words that are spelled out loud, revealing that he is truly illiterate, unlike the patient with pure word-blindness.

The condition may be the predominant symptom from the outset but this is rare. Usually it is found as the residual disturbance when a more global dysphasia clears up. It is usually accompanied by some degree of nominal dysphasia, dyscalculia, spatial disorganisation or visual object agnosia.

The defect results from disturbance of those parts of the brain which deal with the visual symbolic components of language. The lesion is usually extensive within the parietal or parietotemporal region of the dominant hemisphere, but the angular and supramarginal gyri are always involved.

Acquired alexias

The psycholinguistic classification of the dyslexias or alexias has been one of the successes of the cognitive neuropsychology approach (Shallice 1988). Intriguing forms of dyslexic error have been highlighted, for example in 'deep dyslexia' in which words are misread yet in a manner that betrays understanding at some level of their meaning (so-called 'semantic errors') (Marshall & Newcombe 1973). For example, 'dinner' may be read as 'food', 'close' as 'shut', or 'dog' as 'animal'. Such patients are unable to read even simple non-words and cannot 'sound them out'. Observations such as these have led to speculation and experimentation in attempts to clarify the various routes whereby the written word image is translated into meaning (Coltheart *et al.* 1987). Anatomically, patients with deep dyslexia tend to have extensive lesions, usually vascular, involving left perisylvian regions but extending into the frontal, parietal and temporal lobes. Hence additional language problems are common. The extent to which the intact right hemisphere might take on some of the left hemisphere's functions in this situation is hotly debated.

Phonological dyslexia is characterised by a selective impairment in the ability to read non-words but without the semantic errors of deep dyslexia. Anatomically, the lesions tend to involve the anterior perisylvian areas. In contrast 'surface dyslexia' is characterised by a tendency to read words according to how they ought to sound given grapheme–phoneme conversion rules (e.g. 'come' → 'comb', 'island' → 'izland'), known as regularisation errors. This pattern may be seen in semantic dementia. The responsible lesions tend to be left temporal, insula and putamen.

Developmental dyslexia (specific reading retardation)

Some children experience unusual difficulty in learning to read and to spell, despite normal or even superior intelligence and equivalent educational opportunities to their peers. The proportion so affected has varied in different surveys and according to the criteria employed, but has been judged to involve just under 4% of 10 year olds on the Isle of Wight compared with almost 10% in inner London boroughs (Rutter & Yule 1975). Such disorder has been labelled 'developmental dyslexia' or, alternatively, 'specific reading retardation' to distinguish it from the reading difficulties associated with generally poor intellectual endowment.

Important distinctions from the latter have emerged in group comparisons, including a threefold to fourfold preponderance in boys, an association with speech and language impairment as opposed to a wider range of developmental delays, and less frequent evidence of brain damage as judged from birth history, neurological examination or EEG (Rutter 1978; Maughan & Yule 1994). Rather strikingly, the Isle of Wight study showed that children with specific reading retardation made significantly less progress with reading or spelling than children with 'general reading backwardness', between the ages of 10 and 14, despite their superior intelligence, whereas their progress with mathematics was superior as expected (Yule 1973; Rutter *et al.* 1976). Distinctions between the two groups have traditionally relied on identifying the size of the discrepancy between reading attainment as predicted on the basis of age and IQ scores and the actual level of attainment observed. Though criticised because of the doubtful predictive value of IQ for literacy attainment, such a formula permits the identification of children with disproportionate reading difficulty across a wide range of levels of intelligence, including those whose intelligence is below the average.

The disorder is now increasingly recognised among those engaged in education, and specialist courses designed to upgrade the knowledge and expertise of teachers are slowly being established. However, the problems not uncommonly persist into adult life as a continuing source of handicap and social embarrassment. With effort and specialist teaching some affected individuals appear to overcome their reading problems, proceeding successfully to higher education, though poor spelling usually persists as an aftermath.

Different theories abound as to the basis of the condition. Genetic influences are quite strongly apparent from twin studies and more recent molecular genetic studies in which loci on chromosomes 6 and 18 have shown strong and replicable effects on reading abilities (Francks *et al.* 2002). Environmental influences such as poor family circumstances or inadequate schooling clearly also make a contribution.

Traditionally, the disorder has been viewed by neurologists as 'maturational' in nature, perhaps resulting from delayed myelination or other problems in crucial neural systems. However, recent studies have given support to the proposition that definable abnormalities of cerebral structure or function may sometimes persist even in adults who have largely compensated for their early deficits. These abnormalities include anomalous asymmetry, areas of architectonic dysplasia, disruption of the normal laminar organisation of the cortex, along with neuronal 'ectopias' consisting of abnormal nests of cells in the cortex and subjacent white matter. There may be an association with epilepsy.

MRI studies have confirmed that an unusual degree of symmetry of the planum is significantly more common in dyslexic subjects than controls (Larsen *et al.* 1990). Moreover, in Larsen *et al.*'s study of 19 adolescent dyslexics, there was a close relationship between abnormal symmetry of the planum and measures of phonological dysfunction. Hynd and Hiemenz (1997) summarise more recent interesting findings concerning posterior perisylvian morphology in dyslexia. Other regional abnormalities affecting the splenium of the corpus callosum, which connects the regions of the angular gyri of the two hemispheres, have been noted as well as abnormal connections to the left fusiform gyrus, thought by some to represent a 'word form' area (see Demonet *et al.* 2004 for a review). Along different lines, Livingstone *et al.* (1991) and others have pursued the hypothesis that there are problems with relatively 'early' perception of visual material. Finally, Uta Frith and her colleagues have devised elegant strategies for exploring the role of defective phonological decoding in dyslexia, using PET to detect the brain regions involved (Paulesu *et al.* 1996). Problems in the domain of phonology are currently strongly favoured as a core problem in developmental dyslexia (Snowling 1996), and phonological strategies appear to be especially effective with many dyslexics in attempts at remediation. Moreover, among those dyslexics who attain academic success, this is often largely achieved through acquiring a large 'sight vocabulary', and underlying deficits in phonology may persist throughout adulthood. An excellent review of the research in this area and its implications is provided by Vellutino *et al.* (2004).

Jargon aphasia

'Jargon aphasia' is the term used when speech is produced freely, volubly and clearly, but with such semantic jumble and misuse of words that meaning cannot be discerned. Typically there are phonetic distortions, neologisms, words put together in meaningless sequence, and sequences which are entirely irrelevant. The intonation and rhythm of formal speech are nevertheless preserved. Jargon aphasia is conventionally regarded as representing a severe example of primary sensory aphasia, perhaps with superadded difficulties due to pure word-deafness, or perhaps with a marked degree of generalised intellectual impairment. Kertesz and Benson (1970) have reported typical severe neologistic jargon in patients with both Wernicke's and conduction aphasia.

Weinstein *et al.* (1966) were led to conclude quite differently that jargon aphasia represents aphasia in conjunction with anosognosia, rather than a distinctive pattern of breakdown in the intrinsic speech structure. In their patients receptive difficulties were rarely severe, and the distinctive accompanying feature was disturbance of consciousness sufficient to produce confabulation, disorientation and reduplicative delusions. In conformity with their observations on anosognosia generally (see Anosognosia, later), the jargon often appeared selectively when the patient was questioned about his disabilities, and more coherent speech was produced in relation to neutral topics. The pathological basis was a lesion of the dominant hemisphere along with additional brain damage elsewhere, and all patients had bilateral cerebral involvement. However, in favour of the conventional view that jargon represents a primary receptive defect, with failure to monitor speech productions, is the finding that patients who display it are not disturbed in the normal fashion when made to listen to delayed auditory feedback of their own speech productions.

Psychiatric disturbance and aphasia

Benson and Geschwind (1971) and Benson (1973) summarise the common forms of reaction that may be seen in aphasic patients. These differ considerably in the different forms of language defect.

In primary motor aphasia (Broca's aphasia), frustration and depression are frequently seen, or more rarely the 'catastrophic reaction' in which tension and embarrassment culminate in a sudden outburst of weeping or anger with the patient's realisation of his failings. Indeed the absence of distress among such patients is usually indicative of widespread cerebral damage and consequent impairment of general intellectual ability. Both frustration and depression are considered to indicate a more favourable prognosis for recovery with therapy, representing as they do an awareness of the speech difficulties. On the other hand, angry negativism with hostile responses and refusal to participate in treament can sometimes emerge and seriously complicate rehabilitation.

In contrast, the patient with primary sensory (Wernicke's) aphasia typically shows a lack of interest in, or even unawareness of, his language problems. Such patients often act as though they believe their own speech to be normal and as though they feel that people around them fail to speak normally. Agitation and sometimes severe paranoid reactions may ensue, with suspicions that others are talking about them, plotting against them or deliberately using unintelligible jargon to prevent them from understanding. Outbursts of impulsive aggressive behaviour may be seen. In Benson's experience almost every patient who had needed custodial care during recovery from aphasia had suffered a paranoid reaction secondary to severe comprehension disability. Aphasia is frequently followed by calamitous alterations in lifestyle and economic status, along with disruption of simple pleasures such as conversation, reading or watching television. Social and family status are often undermined, irrespective of the presence of other handicaps such as hemiparesis, likewise confidence in sexual functioning.

Language and schizophrenia: the problem of 'thought disorder'

Thought disorder is the label that psychiatrists use to describe what is essentially an expressive disorder of spoken language, found in schizophrenia but not exclusive to that disorder. The distinction between the language disorder seen in certain schizophrenic and manic patients and the phenomena of aphasia due to brain damage needs to be very carefully distinguished. This can only be done by careful attention to the *form* of language output and by comprehensive tests of language function. Linguists who have studied schizophrenic speech have reached different conclusions, some arguing for a distinct disorder of language and others that such speech can be classified within the standard aphasia rubric. In one study that used speech transcripts from patients with schizophrenic thought disorder and (mostly) fluent aphasias, clinicians were poor at distinguishing the two (Faber *et al.* 1983). The 'word salad' of the chronically deteriorated schizophrenic may sometimes closely resemble aphasic speech; conversely, some patients with aphasia are mistakenly diagnosed as psychotic for long periods of time, especially those with primary sensory aphasia or transcortical sensory aphasia who produce a wealth of paraphasic neologisms. The neurological examination is often negative in such patients, their output is vague and apparently 'confused', and they may react negatively to the examiner's speech in a manner suggestive of psychosis. Any sudden onset of speech disorder must therefore always dictate caution, even in the established chronic schizophrenic patient.

Gerson *et al.* (1977) analysed tape-recorded interviews with groups of posterior aphasic and schizophrenic patients in order to determine the features most useful in making the clinical distinction. The length of verbal responses to open-ended questions was considerably shorter among the aphasics, and these did not show the bizarre reiterative themes frequently encountered among the schizophrenics. The aphasic patients showed at least some awareness of their language difficulties, and used gestures or pauses to enlist the examiner's aid, whereas the schizophrenic patients were impervious to the adequacy or otherwise of their communication. Vagueness of response arose from word-finding difficulties in the aphasic patients but was apparently attributable to shifts of attention in the schizophrenics. The 'circumlocution' of aphasia could thus often be contrasted with the 'circumstantiality' of schizophrenic speech. In Faber *et al.*'s (1983) study, paraphasias were equally distributed among the two patients groups but frank incoherence, idiosyncratic use of words and tangentiality were more common in the thought disorder group.

In a recent and fine-grained application of an aphasiological approach to schizophrenic thought disorder, Oh *et al.* (2002) compared a carefully selected group of six patients with thought disorder and a matched comparison group of seven patients without. They used a battery of tests including the Boston Diagnostic Aphasia Examination (BDAE) coupled with a quantitative analysis of patients' utterances, and in a subgroup the Psycholinguistic Assessment of Language Processing in Aphasia (PALPA) and the Test for the Reception of Grammar (TROG). They found that some of the abnormalities observed in the speech of patients with schizophrenia, including syntactic errors, may be accounted for by their general cognitive impairment. This implies that deficits in attention and concentration or working memory are at the root of such problems and that higher-level problems of discourse planning reflect problems with planning generally. Of particular interest was the finding that the thought-disordered group, even those with preserved cognitive functioning, showed most impairment at the level of semantics in their expressive speech. This was in contrast to high levels of visual confrontation naming and ability to comprehend complex material, for example '. . . working the mind can comfort the bathroot as well, so it can be growthful, understand?' elicited during conversation. Attempts to recount fairy tales elicited disorganised and tangential speech that lacked a global semantic structure, presumably because of the open-ended, unconstrained nature of these tasks. Putting all the results together the authors characterised 'schizophasia' as an expressive semantic abnormality with preserved naming. In line with the main locus of impairment as being at the semantic level, Rodriguez-Ferrera *et al.* (2001) also found ample evidence of semantic disorders in speech in their sample of 40 schizophrenia patients using the Pyramid and Palm Trees test, in which the subject is shown the written name of an object (e.g. an Egyptian pyramid) and then has to decide which of two other words is related to it, a palm tree or a pine tree. The thought-disordered patients' errors on this task revealed impairments at the level of semantic representations or concepts. This supported work by Kuperberg *et al.* (1998, 2000) which showed that thought-disordered patients (in comparison to non-thought-disordered controls) were less 'surprised' by linguistically anomalous endings to spoken sentences, indexed by relatively less prolongation in reaction time to press a button indicating they had heard a target word at the end of the sentence. They were less sensitive to linguistic (syntactic, semantic and pragmatic) violations because they were apparently unable to use linguistic context to form an overall semantic representation needed to process speech online.

Reduced expression

Poverty of speech and poverty of thought content are cardinal symptoms of schizophrenia normally assessed through the patient's spoken output. Reduced or slowed speech may reflect depressed mood and psychomotor retardation generally, as well as part of the negative schizophrenia syndrome. Non-fluency in this situation may occasionally need to be distinguished from a Broca's aphasia. Interestingly, reduced left prefrontal activation as measured by PET may accompany such deficits in both schizophrenia and depression (Dolan *et al.* 1994). Parkinsonism, either idiopathic or secondary to antipsychotic medication, may cause a similar clinical picture. Again, one might argue whether poverty of speech is truly a language disorder or a higher-level problem of initiation and planning. 'Dynamic aphasia' is the term sometimes given to the rare neurological syndrome in which spontaneous verbal output is much reduced but is normal when 'unlocked' by presentation of a picture or a simple question or a repetition task. It is initiation of speech that is compromised due to a left frontal lesion, perhaps localised to Brodmann's area 45.

The verbal fluency test may be used to quantify reduced speech in terms of a psychometric deficit. The patient can be asked to generate as many words as possible in a minute beginning with a given letter (F, A or S). This can be contrasted with semantic fluency in which the patient is asked to produce as many words as possible from a given category (e.g. four-legged animals). Generally, more items are produced in the latter situation, but where the semantic system is compromised (in Alzheimer's disease and, some would argue, schizophrenia) the pattern may be reversed.

Conversion disorders

It is only on rare occasions that difficulty arises in distinguishing between psychogenic and organic disturbances of language function. The most common hysterical speech disorder consists of complete aphonia or mutism, or if sounds are produced there are usually no recognisable words at all but repetitions of phonemes and babble reminiscent of 'speaking in tongues' found in some evangelical religious settings during trance. A very rare example of dyslexia and dysgraphia of psychogenic origin has been described by Master and Lishman (1984).

Executive (frontal lobe) syndromes

Certain clinical features have long been associated with damage to the frontal lobes. These are not unique to frontal lobe pathology, but they are seen more regularly and perhaps more strikingly than after damage to other cortical structures. This lack of one-to-one correspondence between behaviour and lesion location led Baddeley and Wilson (1986) to coin the term 'executive dysfunction' for what had previously been known as 'frontal lobe dysfunction'.

Clinical picture

Evidence about this syndrome has come from studies of patients with various types of brain pathology. These include patients with head injury or frontal lobe tumours. Evidence has also accumulated from studies of patients after surgical excisions of frontal lobe lesions and, in the past, from patients who had extensive frontal leucotomies. The consensus of evidence suggests that lesions of the convex lateral surface (dorsolateral cortex) are especially prone to mental slowing and a lack of spontaneity, whereas lesions to the orbital undersurface of the brain (ventromedial pathology) are liable to have adverse effects on personality and social behaviour. Bifrontal lesions appear particularly damaging. The most striking changes are often in terms of behaviour, social awareness, habitual mood, volition, and psychomotor activities.

Commonly, there are what might be described as 'negative' symptoms. These include a lack of initiative and spontaneity, usually coupled with a general diminution of motor activity. Responses are sluggish, tasks are left unfinished, and new initiatives rarely undertaken. In consequence, the capacity to function independently in daily life can be profoundly affected. Yet when vigorously urged, or constrained by a structured situation, the patient may function quite well. Hebb (1949) described how cognition and intellect can be apparently unaffected despite huge frontal lesions, and the patient may achieve virtually normal performance in situations in which the examiner provides the impetus, such as in many formal tests of intelligence. How far the impairment of initiative represents a true loss of interest, or an apparent loss due to impaired volition, is often hard to discern, but this apathy and inertia may closely mimic depression.

Other patients tend to show 'positive' symptoms. They are restless and hyperactive rather than sluggish, but again are likely to display a lack of purposive goal-directed behaviour. Their mood is often mildly euphoric and out of keeping with their situation. There may be rather empty high spirits, accompanied by a boisterous over-familiarity in manner. Such changes are rarely sustained, however, and when left to themselves these patients become inert and apathetic. Outbursts of irritability are also common and a childlike petulance may also be seen. The euphoria is sometimes elaborated into a tendency to joke or pun, to make facetious remarks or to indulge in pranks. Very occasionally, it extends to a state of excitement, pressure of speech, and ebullience, which can be termed 'secondary mania'.

Serious changes are observed in social awareness and behaviour. Typically, the patient is less concerned with the consequences of his acts than formerly. Loss of 'finer feelings' and social graces form part of a general coarsening of the personality. In interpersonal relationships, there is a lack of the normal adult tact and restraints, and a diminished appreciation of the impact of behaviour on others. Judgement may be markedly impaired. The patient shows little concern about his future and fails to plan ahead or to carry through ideas. Inability to forejudge the consequence of actions leads to foolish or irresponsible behaviour. Normal social restraints fail to exert control. Disinhibition is sometimes apparent in sexual behaviour, and may vary from lewd remarks to overt disinhibited behaviour that may even precipitate criminal charges.

These changes are seen to varying degree, sometimes merely as a blunting of the previous personality, but sometimes as a radical change of behaviour that is grossly disabling. The patient usually has little insight into the changes which have occurred. The component symptoms may be seen in different combinations, but there is a certain commonality from one patient to another, which has led to the continuing use of the terms 'dysexecutive' or 'frontal lobe' syndrome.

Classical case reports

Harlow (1868 [1993]) described the case of Phineas Gage, a railway engineer in New England. Gage's job was to bore a hole, lay explosive, cover it with sand, and then to use a fuse and a tamping iron to set off the explosive. However, on one occasion, he made a grave mistake, placing the tamping iron directly over the explosive, at which point there was an explosion that sent the iron through his skull and for a further 20 feet or so into the air. Remarkably, Gage did not lose consciousness, and he was able to walk to the cart which took him to hospital. In fact, he lived for another 20 years. He had little difficulty with language or memory, and his motor skills were unchanged. However, there was a pronounced change in personality and behaviour: whereas he had been considered an outstanding employee, he became unreliable, disrespectful and was lacking in social skills, and soon lost his job. Harlow (1868) attributed this altered behaviour to damage to the frontal lobes of Gage's brain. Gage's body was exhumed in 1866, and the skull and the offending tamping iron were preserved in a Harvard museum. This allowed Damasio *et al.* (1994) to carry out modern neuroimaging on the skull and to estimate the precise location of Gage's brain lesion. They concluded that his lesion would have principally involved the orbitofrontal and anterior medial frontal regions bilaterally.

Eslinger and Damasio (1985) described a somewhat similar patient. This man was chief accountant, a college graduate, who had been extremely successful in his early career, rapidly climbing his professional hierarchy. A large frontal meningioma was removed surgically, involving a large portion of the orbitofrontal cortex but also involving dorsolateral frontal cortex. Although his IQ and memory were well preserved, this man's professional life deteriorated strikingly. He set up business with a former coworker, but the business failed and he became bankrupt. He drifted through several jobs, but he was found to be disorganised and was dismissed from each of them. He would take two hours to get ready in the mornings; he was somewhat obsessional, and indecisive. Purchasing goods required lengthy consideration of brands, prices and methods of purchase.

Interestingly, Shimamura (2002) has described similar phenomena in the photographer Eadweard Muybridge. Muybridge, who was born in Kingston upon Thames, emigrated to North America as a young man, finding his way to California. However, he was caught up in a stagecoach robbery, in which he was thrown from the stagecoach injuring his head. Subsequently, Muybridge returned temporarily to the UK, where he was looked after by Sir William Gull of Guy's and St Thomas's hospitals during his convalescence. He returned to North America, and most of his photographic inventions and innovations, including his famous studies of people or racehorses in motion (which were the precursor of cine-photography), were carried out during the next 30 years. However, his behaviour was changed in ways which Shimamaura (2002) attributes to frontal lobe damage as a result of the head injury. During this period, Muybridge shot dead his wife's lover but managed to obtain an acquittal on the grounds of his brain injury.

A more specific deficit was described by Lhermitte (1986), who reported imitation and so-called 'utilisation behaviour' in patients with frontal lobe lesions. Lhermitte observed patients in complex everyday life situations, i.e. without the constraints normally imposed during clinical assessment. He noted behaviours which he proposed reflected a lack of personal autonomy, coupled with an excessive dependence on the social and physical environment ('environmental dependency syndrome'). Decisions concerning the patients' actions were not made for themselves, but the behaviours were called forth by surrounding external stimuli: 'For the patient, the social and physical environments issue the order to use them, even though the patient "himself" or "herself" has neither the idea nor the intention to do so.' Lhermitte suggested that a shift in the balance between personal autonomy and environmental influences reflected decreased control by frontal systems over the parietal sensorimotor systems linking the individual to the world around. From this might follow such classic features as disinhibited behaviour, distractibility, loss of flexibility of action, and loss of self-criticism.

Thus when taken into a room containing a buffet, Lhermitte's patient laid out the glasses and offered him food, spontaneously behaving like a hostess. Confronted with make-up, she used it immediately, and seeing wool and knitting needles began to knit. Another patient, when taken into a bedroom with the sheet turned back, got undressed, went to bed and prepared to go to sleep. On hearing the word 'museum' while in an apartment, he began methodically to examine the paintings on the wall, and walked from room to room inspecting various objects.

Neuropsychology of executive function

An enormous range of cognitive functions has been attributed to the frontal lobes. These include the initiation of responses, the maintenance of responses, the suppression of irrelevant or inappropriate responses, the planning and organisation of behaviour, abstract and conceptual thinking, monitoring and editing of responses, the temporal organisation of behaviour and memory, aspects of working memory, and the encoding and/or retrieval of new or remote episodic memories.

Consistent with this, a wide range of tests has been developed that purport to measure some aspect of executive function. Commonly employed are FAS verbal fluency, the Wisconsin or Modified card-sorting tests, cognitive estimates, Trailmaking, various tasks that require alternating patterns of behaviour or shifts in response, the Stroop test, working memory or continuous performance tests, prospective memory, and source or temporal context memory tasks. One view is that the commonality in such tests boils down to a single factor, akin to Spearman's 'g' (Duncan 1986, 2001), which guides activation of representations stored elsewhere in the brain. The alternative view is that, to varying degrees, these tasks reflect differing aspects of frontal lobe functioning. In practice, correlations between performance on these different tasks are relatively low, especially when IQ has been partialled out (Shoqeirat *et al.* 1990; Kopelman 1991). Moreover, patients with large frontal lesions can show significant behavioural impairments without this necessarily being reflected in their performance on any of these tests (Shallice & Burgess 1991a,b). More recently, 'ecologically valid' virtual reality tasks have been developed (Morris *et al.* 2005), but questions still arise as to how and to what degree these relate to the more traditional tasks, and whether frontal lobe function should be conceived as having an underlying unity or whether it is essentially fragmented.

In the light of this, attempts have been made to 'model' frontal lobe function. Wood and Grafman (2003) have reviewed some of these theories. These authors point out that the ventromedial prefrontal cortex has reciprocal connections with brain regions associated with emotional processing (amygdala), memory (hippocampus) and higher-order sensory processing (temporal visual association areas), as well as with dorsolateral prefrontal cortex. The dorsolateral prefrontal cortex has reciprocal connections with brain regions associated with motor control (basal ganglia, premotor cortex, supplementary motor area), performance monitoring (cingulate cortex) and higher-order sensory processing (association areas, parietal cortex). The ventromedial prefrontal cortex is therefore well suited to support functions involving the integration of information about emotion, memory and environmental stimuli, and the dorsolateral prefrontal cortex to support the regulation of behaviour and control of responses to environmental stimuli.

Perhaps the most popular model of executive or frontal lobe function is the *supervisory attentional system* model of Norman and Shallice (1980; see Shallice 1988). This model was based on two main premises: the first that the routine selection of routine operations is decentralised, and the second that non-routine selection is qualitatively different and involves a general-purpose supervisory system, which modulates rather than dictates the operation of the rest of the system. The model postulates that routine mental procedures are handled using processing modules, schemata linking these modules together for a particular task, and 'contention scheduling' which allows multiple routine tasks to occur together in an efficient way. For non-routine activities, the supervisory system was required to control the schemata and contention scheduling. A criticism of this model (and also of Baddeley's 'central executive' working memory model) is that it is essentially homuncular. However, more recently, an elaboration of this model has been proposed, which postulates at least six component processes that are recruited by the supervisory system in anticipation of, or early in, task performance (Stuss *et al.* 2005). These processes are energising schemata, task-setting, inhibiting task-irrelevant schemata, adjusting contention scheduling so that the automatic processes can work more smoothly, monitoring the level of activity in schemata, and controlling the 'if this, then that' logic required to move through the steps of a task. It is argued that these different higher-order processes, subcomponents within the unitary system, will allow the frontal lobes to perform a variety of 'anterior attentional' tasks, including focused attention, divided attention, sustained attention, inhibitory processes, switching attention, preparation in response to a signal, and setting an appropriate sequence of processes. Moreover, by careful architectonic localisation of brain lesions, Stuss *et al.* (2005) have begun to examine the critical sites for performance of these tasks, arguing that the energisation of schemata is sensitive to pathology in the medial superior frontal regions, whereas the monitoring of stimulus occurrence and response behaviour is sensitive to right lateral frontal pathology.

Recent work has also examined the functioning of the frontal poles or anterior prefrontal cortices (Burgess *et al.* 2005). This region can be activated in functional imaging studies independently of other frontal lobe regions and, again, lesions to this region do not necessarily result in impaired functioning on traditional executive tests. Most commonly, impairments are seen on tests involving multi-tasking or prospective memory. Burgess *et al.* (2005) have postulated that this region is particularly involved as a 'gateway mechanism' that controls switching between stimulus-orientated and stimulus-independent thought (compare Lhermitte, above). This cognitive control mechanism is used in a wide range of situations critical to competent behaviour in everyday life, ranging from straightforward 'watchfulness' to complex activities such as remembering to carry out intended actions after a delay, multi-tasking, and aspects of recollection. These are situations which require the person to be particularly alert to the environment, to concentrate deliberately on his thoughts, or to be involved in conscious switching between these states. The authors have speculated that damage to the functioning of this region might be relevant to psychiatric phenomena such as hallucinations and intrusive thoughts.

Other theories of frontal lobe functioning have been well reviewed by Wood and Grafman (2003); more specifically, the putative role of ventromedial frontal lesions in the genesis of spontaneous confabulation has been noted above. Neuropsychological research on executive functioning also has practical clinical implications in terms of the development of cognitive and behavioural rehabilitation strategies (e.g. goal management training; Levine *et al.* 2000) and in terms of examining the interaction with behavioural genetics, using contemporary techniques to identify genetic markers (e.g. O'Keefe *et al.* 2004).

Disorders of action and the apraxias

Apraxia refers, in essence, to an inability to carry out learned voluntary movements, or movement complexes, when this cannot be accounted for in terms of weakness, incoordination, sensory loss or involuntary movements. The patient cannot willingly set the movement in train or guide a series of consecutive movements in their correct spatial and temporal sequence, even though the same muscles can be used and analogous movements performed in other contexts.

Liepmann (1905) first established the validity of apraxia as a clinical entity in its own right, and that both unilateral and bilateral forms of the syndrome could occur. He showed that it could be differentiated from language disorders and paralysis, although he argued that apraxia was not a simple unitary disorder but that it could arise at a number of stages in the processes involved in organising a voluntary action. Geschwind and Damasio (1985) pointed out that apraxia is often overlooked on clinical examination since it is unlikely to be complained of by the patient or his family. The patient who is apraxic on testing will usually perform learned movements normally in a natural setting, and especially when he can see and manipulate objects in their proper environment. In consequence, the disorder is probably a good deal commoner than is usually appreciated.

The essential nature of apraxic disturbances is still poorly understood. Aphasia is an accompanying defect in the great majority of cases and deficient comprehension of commands may sometimes play a part. Agnosia for an object may hinder the patient from carrying out purposive movements appropriate to its use, while agnosia for spatial relationships will similarly interfere with the copying of a movement by imitation. Over and above such complications, however, there is usually a higher-order cognitive impairment with a specific bearing on motor function.

The difficulties for any explanatory system include the observation that movements which cannot be performed to command can sometimes be performed in imitation of the examiner, or a movement which cannot be initiated is performed a moment later when the patient's attention is not directed towards it. Sometimes simple discrete movements are affected, and sometimes complex coordinated sequences as in the use of a tool. Frequently, performance is much better in the actual presence of the tool than when the patient is asked to demonstrate its use in imagination. To a surprising degree, whole-body movements to command are often found to be perfectly preserved, while limb and facial movements are defective. Hence, simple hierarchies of difficulty do not provide an adequate explanation for these anomalies.

Apraxia is probably more often seen in diffuse than in strictly focal brain lesions so that other intellectual processes are often involved. With focal lesions, however, other cognitive processes may prove to be largely intact, even though at first sight the severely apraxic patient is sometimes misdiagnosed as having a dementia. Nevertheless, such patients are severely handicapped in many tasks requiring the demonstration of intelligence. It is likely that the schemata for purposive movement are so interwoven in cognitive processes that their disruption is bound to have a more general adverse effect.

Brain (1965) suggested that purposive movements are organised by 'schemata' that may or may not enter consciousness depending on the context of the movement. The more practised the act, and the more automatic it has become, the more it will be carried out without conscious awareness and conscious volition. Apraxia may be regarded as the result of disorganisation in such schemata and as taking place at various levels of complexity. At the highest level will be found disturbance where schemata are involved in the formulation of the idea of a movement; at the lowest, the schema consists of a motor pattern that regulates the selection of appropriate muscles. In contrast, Geschwind (1965) characteristically put forward a disconnection model, in which he postulated that lesions which disrupted connections between auditory association cortex and motor association cortex of the dominant hemisphere would result in an inability to carry out motor commands with the limbs on either side of the body. Lesions of the left motor cortex would produce a right hemiplegia together with apraxia limited to the left arm when the origin of the transcallosal pathway had been destroyed. Lesions of the corpus callosum would result in apraxia to command without dysphasia, and limited to the left arm and leg, since the motor cortex of the right hemisphere would now be isolated from the speech mechanisms of the left. More contemporary theories are discussed below.

Many varieties of apraxia have been postulated and these are briefly outlined below.

Limb kinetic apraxia: the skill and delicacy of movements is disturbed for both complex and simple actions. Thus the patient may have difficulty in doing up buttons or opening a safety pin. The difficulty the patient experiences reflects the degree of muscular complexity, rather than the psychomotor processes involved. It may be confined to particular muscle groups, and even to certain fingers of the hand. This form has characteristics intermediate between a paresis and apraxia, and therefore is often excluded from the apraxias proper. It results from a relatively small lesion of the contralateral premotor cortex.

Ideomotor apraxia refers to the inability to carry out a requested movement properly. It may be regarded as a disturbance of voluntary movement at a fairly low level of motor organisation or, alternatively, as a disturbance of the use of space centred on the body. The patient can often formulate to himself the idea of a movement that he wishes to perform but is unable to execute it. Thus the voluntary impulse does not evoke the appropriate organisation of the movement in space and time. For example, the patient cannot raise his hand or wave it to command, even though the instructions are understood. In some cases, he could copy a couple of movements, but this too may fail. Yet essentially the same movements can be performed automatically, as in signalling goodbye or in the course of other activities to which his attention is not directed. The disorder is usually bilateral and most commonly involves the arms. Unilateral apraxia almost always involves the left arm, and then is typically seen with right hemiplegia and aphasia.

Ideational apraxia: the patient is unable to carry out coordinated sequences of actions, such as taking a match from a box and striking it, or to perform the complex movements involved in using such tools as a comb or pair of scissors. Ideomotor apraxia may coexist or, in contrast, the patient may be capable of straightforward imitation of simple movements. Sometimes, performance is clearly better when the tool is held by the patient than when he attempts to demonstrate the action in the abstract. Variability may be seen from one task to another and on different occasions. In ideational apraxia, the conception of the required movements appears to be disturbed, together with planning of the acts to be accomplished. It may be regarded as a form of 'programming' apraxia, whereas ideomotor apraxia is a more basic executory defect. Ideational apraxia is always bilateral. If based on circumscribed pathology, the lesion usually involves the dominant hemisphere, usually in the parietal or temporal lobes. It is most commonly seen in diffuse brain lesions, usually accompanied by severe dysphasia or a considerable degree of generalised cognitive impairment.

Apraxia for dressing refers specifically to difficulty in putting on clothes. The patient cannot relate the spatial form of garments to that of his body, putting a jacket on back to front or the arm in the wrong sleeve. Buttons and laces present particular difficulties and are often left undone. The concept of dressing apraxia is useful clinically in drawing attention to a dramatic symptom when more refined tests of apraxia and agnosia have yet to be performed. However, it is improbable that it reflects a distinct form of apraxia, and the symptoms probably depend on a variety of deficits that differ from case to case. In many cases, right–left disorientation, unilateral inattention, neglect of the left limbs and other disturbances of body image are likely to contribute. The disorder is often seen in dementia, and more commonly in bilateral or right-sided parieto-occipital lesions than left-sided lesions.

Constructional apraxia refers to instances where the spatial disposition of actions is altered without any apraxia for individual movements. This becomes apparent in tasks involving the use or representation of space, e.g. in the constructional copying of patterns under visual control. The defect is clearly not purely motor in nature, but involves perceptual functions as well. This may be immediately apparent in the patient's satisfaction with a grossly imperfect copy of presented test material. Many authorities have interpreted constructional apraxia as a form of visuospatial agnosia.

The neuropsychology of action

McCarthy and Warrington (1990) argued that the classificatory systems for apraxia are confusing and inconsistent. They advocated a strictly empirical task-oriented framework rather than one based on particular theoretical perspectives.

They considered disorders of voluntary action in terms of the following.

1 Disorders of simple repetitive movements, involving either unimanual or bimanual coordination of repetitive movements. Unimanual movements can be damaged by lesions in either hemisphere, whereas bimanual coordination problems usually follow damage to the frontal lobes or the supplementary motor region.

2 Disorders of unfamiliar actions and action sequences can involve single hand positions, usually affected by damage to the left parietal lobe, whereas copying or executing unfamiliar action sequences can be affected by lesions in either the left frontal or the left parietal lobes.

3 Impairment can occur in the ability to carry out familiar gestures, such as saluting or waving goodbye. Impairment in producing meaningful gestures on command has consistently been shown to result from left parietal lesions.

4 Impairments can be seen in producing actions appropriate to objects or in patients' ability to mimic the use of a single or multiple objects. Such impairments result from left hemisphere damage, and it appears that regions around the parieto-temporal junction are most likely to be implicated.

5 Body-part specific actions can be affected, as in gait apraxia (difficulty walking) or oral apraxia, in which the patient may be unable to protrude the tongue, open the mouth or cough on command, although these gestures do occur spontaneously, for example when eating. Gait apraxia is associated with bilateral frontal lesions, and oral apraxia with highly specific lesions in the left central operculum and insula.

6 Constructional apraxia can involve either left-sided or right-sided lesions, but different patterns are observed. Left hemisphere lesions give rise to oversimplified drawings, whereas right hemisphere pathology results in distortions in the spatial arrangements between the parts or in hemispatial neglect.

An influential distinction, much cited in neuropsychological discussions of apraxia, was made by Milner and Goodale (1992). They reported the case of an agnosic patient (D.F.) who had a profound deficit in judgements of visual form, including the orientation of bars, yet was able to match the position of her hand successfully to post an object through a slit that was presented in a range of orientations. In other words, D.F. could not access visual information for perceptual analysis (in an experimental psychophysical task) but could nevertheless use perceptions in the control of action. This led to the postulation of two visual perceptual pathways: a 'ventral' stream, terminating in the temporal lobes, which was concerned with object representation and recognition (of 'what' was out there), and a more pragmatic 'dorsal' stream, terminating in the parietal cortex, which was concerned with describing the visual world for the purposes of acting upon it ('where'). Sometimes these pathways are conceived as being involved in vision-for-perception (semantic) and vision-for-action (pragmatic), respectively. This model has been criticised for not saying much about the control of action *per se* and the internal generation of willed action (Haggard 2001), and for underestimating the role of the parietal lobe in, on the one hand, allowing the perception of spatial relations among objects and, on the other, storing complex representations of actions in the form of schemata (Jeannerod & Jacob 2005). It also fails to take account of the different levels of awareness which may occur in motor performance (Johnson & Haggard 2005). Interestingly, recent functional imaging studies, reviewed by Blakemore and Frith (2005), have found that observing, imagining or in any way representing an action excites the same motor programmes used to execute that action; in humans, a proportion of the brain regions involved in executing actions are activated by the mere observation of the action (known as the 'mirror system'). A specific but particularly interesting topic of investigation involves functional imaging studies of differing aspects of musical performance (Parsons *et al.* 2005).

Chainay and Humphreys (2002) have attempted to integrate many of the observed clinical and neuropsychological phenomena into what they call a 'convergent route model for action'. They suggest that perceptual information interacts directly with semantic information in selecting the appropriate action to make to an object. Semantic input defines the appropriate category of action, whilst the direct perceptual input helps to determine the optimal parameters for the motor programme (e.g. the appropriate grip and plane of action). These authors argue further that actions are contingent on a network of cortical, and possibly also subcortical, structures that are recruited according to the modality of input. Tactile input may facilitate object use through a pragmatic dorsal cortical pathway, whereas a semantic route to action is contingent on activation of 'action semantics' involving left frontal and left parietal regions. The authors described two patients whose problem seemed to be in selecting actions within an action output lexicon; these patients both showed generally good object recognition and naming, but were impaired in discriminating whether objects were correctly used. The authors suggest that these two patients were impaired at retrieving from an 'action output lexicon' information about how objects should be used. A third patient had a central deficit in accessing semantic knowledge about objects. This deficit was generally consistent across items, and it arose irrespective of the modality in which objects were presented (e.g. visually or tactilely) and irrespective of the task (naming, gesturing) if access to semantic knowledge was required. Elsewhere, Humphreys (2001) has argued that there can be a 'direct route' to action from perceptual input, even where semantic knowledge of objects and their use is severely damaged. The convergent route model of action postulates converging and interacting routes to the execution of motor programmes.

Disorders of perception and the agnosias

The term 'agnosia' was introduced by Freud (1891), although the condition had been described much earlier than this. It may be defined as 'an impaired recognition of an object which is sensorially presented while at the same time the impairment cannot be reduced to sensory defects, mental deterioration, disorders of consciousness and attention, or to a non-familiarity with the object' (Frederiks 1969). Agnosia thus implies a disorder of perceptual recognition that takes place at a higher level than the processing of primary sensory information. Even though elementary sensory processes are themselves unimpaired, there is an inability to interpret sensory information, to recognise its significance and endow it with meaning on the basis of past experience. Lissauer (1890), on the basis of his early case, divided the process of recognition into two stages: first a stage of processing whereby elementary physical stimuli are integrated to form a conscious percept ('apperception'), then the stage of associating the percept with other notions such as memory traces which endow it with meaning ('association'). Thus distinct forms of apperceptive and associative agnosia have come to be recognised.

Clinically, the situation is identified when there is a failure of recognition that cannot be attributed to a primary sensory defect or to generalised intellectual impairment. A patient may, for example, fail to recognise an object by sight and be unable to name it, demonstrate its use or relate it to a matching picture, even though vision is intact for other purposes. Nevertheless, the same object is readily recognised by means of touch, showing that the patient is suffering from a modality-specific defect of higher cerebral function and not from aphasia or apraxia. The several types of agnosia related to vision have received most attention, but agnosias are also described in relation to hearing and touch.

Brain (1965) pointed out that the underlying disorder of function must have something in common with both aphasia and apraxia, since a patient can only demonstrate that he recognises an object by using speech or action; in effect agnosia represents an isolated aphasia and apraxia related to a particular object when it is perceived through a particular sensory channel.

In the sections that follow the classic agnosic syndromes are described, and also the more common forms of related perceptual defect.

Visual agnosias and visual perceptual defects

Visual object agnosia

In visual object agnosia an object cannot be named by sight but is readily identified by other means such as touch or hearing. There is equally failure to select a matching picture from a group or to indicate the appropriate use of the object, showing that this is not a naming defect alone. Sometimes the patient may describe a use appropriate to an incorrect recognition. The difficulty may vary from day to day, and sometimes an object may be recognised from other cues in its familiar surroundings but not elsewhere. Usually the problem is restricted to small objects, but in severe examples it may extend to larger objects, with consequent difficulty in finding the way about.

In general, the more complex the visual information, the more difficulty the patient experiences. Greater problems may be encountered with two-dimensional representations, such as line drawings or photographs, than with the actual objects themselves. Commonly, though not invariably, faces continue to be recognised. In many reported examples there has been difficulty in describing objects from memory and in drawing them (i.e. loss of visual images of objects), and also difficulty with colour recognition, dyslexia and dysgraphia.

In keeping with the distinction between apperceptive and associative forms of agnosia described earlier in this section, subdivisions have been attempted in the field of visual object agnosia (McCarthy and Warrington 1990, pp. 22–55). Patients with visual apperceptive agnosia are particularly sensitive to difficulties surrounding perceptual aspects of identification and fail when these are increased, for example when the perceptual characteristics of an object are partially obscured, or distorted by photographing it from unusual angles. In contrast, visual associative agnosics fail on tests where objects must be matched according to common functions as opposed to physical identity (e.g. a watch and a clock) or when asked to pick out clear pictures of objects that belong to a particular class (e.g. objects found in a kitchen). In this they betray a lack of recognition of the essential meaning of the objects. Interestingly, associative agnosia can sometimes appear to be category specific, with particular difficulty centring on animate or inanimate objects, pictorial representations of concrete or abstract items, or even categories as specific as animals or foods.

Apperceptive agnosics cannot copy objects or drawings unless they do so slavishly and very slowly, often producing frequent errors; associative agnosics can perhaps make reasonable drawings of objects even when they cannot identify them. A double dissociation can sometimes be shown between these two forms of deficit: on the one hand failure to organise a coherent percept, and on the other failure to endow an adequately organised percept with meaning. In many patients, however, the features of both apperceptive and associative agnosia occur together, suggesting that the two may form a continuum (Jankowiak & Albert 1994). Stringent exclusion of subtle deficits in vision and multiple scotomata, as may occur following carbon monoxide poisoning, is required before diagnosis of agnosia can be made.

Clear-cut cases of visual object agnosia are rare. Lesions in the posterior parts of the cerebral hemispheres, involving the occipital, parietal and posterior temporal regions, are almost invariably responsible. Warrington (1985) suggests that following basic sensory analysis, input to the right hemisphere achieves perceptual categorisation and input to the left hemisphere semantic (meaning) categorisation. Accordingly apperceptive agnosic deficits can occasionally be seen in unusually clear form with right hemisphere lesions and associative agnosia with left hemisphere lesions. However, Jankowiak and Albert's (1994) careful review makes it clear that bilateral pathology can be detected in the great majority of cases, even though PET activation studies suggest that object identification takes place predominantly in the left posterior hemisphere. Apperceptive agnosia tends to be associated with diffuse or multifocal lesions, whereas associative agnosia may occur with more focal pathology within the territories of the posterior cerebral arteries. It is noteworthy that the three cases of apperceptive agnosia studied by Grossman *et al.* (1996) showed bilateral occipitotemporal hypoperfusion on PET, even though the MRI appearances had been unremarkable in two. Finally, Riddoch and Humphreys (2003) review more recent work on the visual agnosias including their own detailed case studies which illustrate perhaps better than any other method the logic behind the different types of perceptual abnormalities and their fractionation.

Prosopagnosia

Inability to recognise familiar faces has been described as a distinct and separate defect, which may or may not be combined with visual object agnosia and is certainly much commoner than the latter (Hécaen & Angelergues 1962). In extreme form the patient cannot recognise his own face in a mirror (see below). Classically, the patient with prosopagnosia can readily identify others from their voices or from other cues including their gait. The defect has been reported to be commoner with right than with left hemisphere lesions but in most cases there is probably bilateral involvement (Walsh 1994). This was strongly supported by Damasio *et al.* (1982b) in their analysis of post-mortem and CT scan data; bilateral lesions of the central visual system, situated specifically in the medial occipitotemporal regions, proved to be crucial for the development of prosopagnosia. Functional neuroimaging has highlighted the fusiform gyrus (often referred to as the fusiform face area or FFA), part of the medial occipital junction, as the central hub for face identity processing while the superior temporal sulcus is implicated in such aspects as eye gaze and facial movements. Lesions to the fusiform and adjacent lingual gyrus, and sometimes more anteriorly in the temporal lobe, may cause prosopagnosia, even if unilateral, especially if right-sided (see Barton 2003 for review).

The precise nature of the defect remains uncertain, and it seems likely that prosopagnosia is not a unitary disorder. Warrington and James (1967) showed a distinction between impaired recognition of a previously well-known face, which depends on long-term storage of visual information, and impaired recognition of a previously unknown face from short-term memory. The former tended to be associated with right temporal lesions and the latter with right parietal lesions. De Renzi *et al.* (1991) propose a division into 'apperceptive' forms, in which a disorder in processing shape information prevents a sufficiently clear representation of the face to activate memory for it, and 'associative' forms in which the memory itself is defective. In some instances, however, the condition must be regarded as a 'face-specific disorder', as in the interesting example reported by McNeil and Warrington (1993); here a patient with severe and persistent prosopagnosia for human faces was still able to identify individual members of his flock of sheep from pictures of their faces alone! Neurophysiological recording from the human right temporal lobe has confirmed that there are discrete populations of neurones that are related to the perception and comparison of faces (Ojemann *et al.* 1992). Developmental cases have been described, sometimes with developmental anomalies such as occipital microgyria but by no means always (Barton 2003). Perceptual distortions applied to faces are discussed below.

Facial affect perception

Perception of facial expressions of emotion may be dissociable from facial identity. There is some debate as to whether the right hemisphere is 'dominant' for such expressions or perhaps those of negative valence. Most evidence points to a general role for the right hemisphere in affect perception (Kucharska-Pietura *et al.* 2003). However, some remarkably specific deficits in the perception of expressions of fear (with intact perception of other expressions, both negative and positive) have been described due to lesions of the amygdala, especially when bilateral (Brierley *et al.* 2004). Adolphs *et al.* (1994) have reported the patient S.M. with Urbach–Weithe diease, which manifested as a specific degeneration of the amygdala. The patient has also been shown to lack the normal emotional enhancement of memory and to be more trusting of unfamiliar faces than expected. Evidence from these clinical cases converges on functional imaging research. For example, Morris *et al.* (1996) carried out PET scans whilst subjects viewed photographs of happy or fearful faces that varied systematically in the intensity of the emotional expressions. The neuronal response in the left amygdala was significantly greater to fearful as opposed to happy expressions, and it increased with increasing intensity of fearfulness and decreased with increasing intensity of happiness. Moreover, this emerged without a requirement for explicit processing of the facial expressions; the subjects were merely asked to judge whether each face was male or female. Related work has suggested that the amygdala may even respond to expressions of fear presented too quickly for conscious awareness.

Disgust is another 'basic' emotion that can be detected reliably from facial expression alone. A few cases of lack of disgust recognition have been described and the lesions appears to be in the caudate nucleus and perhaps the insula (Calder *et al.* 2000), again corroborating functional imaging work (Phillips *et al.* 1997).

Facial expressions may convey a wealth of information, from simple emotional state to complex 'social' emotions such as embarrassment or sympathy. Patients with neuropsychiatric disorders such as traumatic brain injury or frontotemporal dementia may misinterpret or fail to recognise important cues from facial expressions, leading to inappropriate or insensitive behaviour. It has been argued that an acquired failure to perceive sadness or fear in another (i.e. signals of distress) could lead to psychopathic behaviour while failure to understand a person's expressions of anger may compromise safety (Blair *et al.* 1999). Similarly, a general insensitivity to facial affect may both reflect and lead to emotional blunting as seen in psychotic and mood disorders. People with autism and Asperger's syndrome may have grave difficulty in understanding the meanings conveyed in facial expressions. All these conditions may lead relatives and carers to describe a lack of empathy in those affected. The usual near-instantaneous perception of such expressions as a whole that we take for granted may not be available in such disorders, where the individual parts of the face seem equally salient and rather unconnected.

Self-face perception

Failure to recognise one's own face has been noted in people with severe prosopagnosia. However, the most common setting for this symptom is severe dementia, where perception of the entire visual world is degraded and combined with faulty reasoning and confusion. A few cases have been described in which impaired self-recognition, the so-called mirror sign, seemed to be out of proportion to other deficits (Phillips *et al.* 1996) and others where the viewer is convinced that an additional, usually inauthentic version of himself is captured when looking into the mirror (a type of reduplication with features of Capgras' delusion). Usually, though, such complaints indicate depersonalisation without concomitant intellectual or neurological dysfunction. On closer questioning, the essence of the complaint, while obviously provoked by gazing at the mirror, is that the individual is unsure of his identity and feels detached from it.

Colour agnosia

Patients with colour agnosia show defective appreciation of the differences between colours and fail to relate colours to objects correctly, even though their primary colour vision is intact as shown by normal performance on the Ishihara chart. Thus they have difficulty in sorting objects according to colour, ordering them in series or matching colours one with another. A dominant occipital lobe lesion is usually responsible and a right homonymous hemianopia is frequently present.

A closely associated though separable defect consists of 'colour anomia' in which the subject is unable to name colours or to point appropriately to named colours, in the absence of any impairment of colour sense. Thus he may use the word 'blue' when shown a picture of a banana, yet be capable of placing the correctly coloured chip next to it. Such problems may be unaccompanied by any other form of language difficulty, representing an unusually clear example of disruption of neural systems that mediate between specific concepts and their corresponding word forms (Damasio & Damasio 1992). The lesion in such cases appears to lie in the temporal segment of the left lingual gyrus.

In central 'achromatopsia' there is a more profound loss of colour sense, extending even to an inability to imagine colours. The concept of colour itself is abolished and the world around, though perceived normally in form and depth, is seen in shades of grey. Damage in such cases is situated in the occipital and subcalcarine portions of the lingual gyri bilaterally (Damasio & Damasio 1992).

Simultanagnosia

Classically the patient fails to recognise the meaning of a complex picture while details are correctly appreciated. However, this is not attributable to difficulty in forming meaningful concepts, since with auditory information there is prompt understanding. Moreover, if plenty of time is given, or every individual feature of the picture is pointed out, the patient ultimately comprehends the meaning. In a similar way, words cannot be read except by spelling out individual letters.

The key problem appears to be with the perception of more than a limited number of units or configurations at a time. Thus tachistoscopic studies have shown that such patients have normal thresholds for the perception of single shapes and letters, but greatly elevated thresholds when more than one stimulus is presented at a time.

Coslett and Saffran (1991), in a detailed analysis of a case, suggested that the fundamental difficulty lay in the integration between object identity and information concerning spatial location when multiple items of visual information needed to be processed. They point out that the processing of multiple targets in an array must be carried out serially beyond a certain level, with storage of both the products of identification and their positions as the 'spotlight on visual attention' moves from one location to another. The inability to maintain appropriate linkages during the process of visual search appeared to account for their patient's failure. Posterior lesions of the dominant lobe have been implicated in patients who display the complete syndrome.

Problems in fixating on an object or directing fixation to a part thereof in an array may be regarded as simultanagnosia but tend to be seen more as problems in visuospatial attention. The term 'Balint's syndrome' is applied to this situation where there are difficulties in voluntary shifts of gaze with concomitant problems in reaching and pointing. Bilateral posterior occipitoparietal lesions are to blame.

Visuospatial defects

After cerebral lesions a number of defects of visuospatial perception may be demonstrated. However, it remains uncertain whether failure to reproduce simple models and drawings depends on dyspraxic difficulties or failure of visuospatial analysis, likewise how far inability to draw from memory may further depend on defective visual imagery. Classic visuospatial agnosia is indeed widely regarded as broadly synonymous with constructional apraxia, as discussed below. Nevertheless, certain syndromes of localising value can be recognised as follows.

Visuospatial agnosia

Visuospatial agnosia is identified by failure on tasks which demand explicit analysis of the spatial properties of a visual display. This is most readily tested by asking the patient to reproduce simple designs under visual control: the copying of drawings or the construction of patterns with bricks or sticks. The Block Design and Object Assembly subtests of the Wechsler Adult Intelligence Scale will most readily indicate minor degrees of such a defect.

Usually the patient has no difficulty in finding his way about, though an itinerary on a map cannot be indicated and towns cannot be correctly located. In the most severe examples a loss of topographical memory (see later in section) may be present as well. An interesting fact, often noted, is that patients with marked visuospatial defects rarely make specific complaints about them. Thus visuospatial agnosia easily eludes routine examination and special tests are needed for its detection.

Visuospatial agnosia may affect drawing ability. Drawings made by patients with left parietal lesions tend to be coherent but simplified versions of the model, with omission of details but relative preservation of spatial relationships. Performance is notably improved when the patient is provided with a model to copy. Frequently associated defects include aphasia, apraxia, or components of Gerstmann's syndrome (see next section) such as right–left disorientation. Patients with right parietal lesions produce more elaborate drawings, but made hastily and without care, and the result is typically scattered and fragmented. Disorientation on the page is marked, the left side of the page is relatively neglected, and the drawings are often asymmetrical and show gross disorganisation of spatial relationships. The presence of a model is of little extra help.

Some therefore prefer to retain the term 'constructional apraxia' when the disorder results from dominant hemisphere lesions, and 'visuospatial agnosia' when it is due to non-dominant lesions, although the distinctions between the two are by no means universally acknowledged.

Some evidence has come from studies of patients after section of the corpus callosum that upholds the greater importance of the non-dominant hemisphere in tasks demanding visuospatial analysis. In brief, the left hand often out-performs the right on unimanual construction tasks. Again there is the difficulty in teasing apart constructional (praxic) difficulties from purely perceptual ones (Bogen & Gazzaniga 1965; LeDoux *et al*. 1977).

Visual disorientation

A further defect of visuospatial ability consists of difficulty in localising objects in space by vision alone. As a result the patient cannot point accurately to an object or estimate its distance. Such difficulty can occur in either half-field of vision alone, contralateral to the side of a lesion, or involve the whole visual field with bilateral lesions. When involving the whole field of vision the patient has difficulty in finding his way around objects or in learning the topography of a room.

Visual disorientation is usually seen in conjunction with impairment on more complex visuospatial tasks, and the lesions are situated posteriorly within the hemispheres. Warrington and colleagues have suggested that there may be areas within the occipital lobes that contribute to the absolute localisation in space of a single object, whereas the integration of several spatial stimuli necessary for the appreciation of spatial relations between two or more objects is impaired by unilateral lesions within the right parietal area (see McCarthy & Warrington 1990). De Renzi *et al*. (1971) reported a test of spatial judgement that appeared to demonstrate complete dominance for the post-rolandic region of the right hemisphere.

Loss of topographical memory

Patients with visual object agnosia or visuospatial agnosia may sometimes still be able to visualise familiar scenes or describe familiar routes. However, loss of topographical memory may occur, again in conjunction with lesions in the parietal lobes. Landis *et al*. (1986) and McCarthy and Warrington (1990, pp. 333–337) have reviewed 20 published and 16 new cases of loss of 'topographical familiarity'. While bilateral posterior lesions were common in the group, they concluded that unilateral right-sided posteromedial lesions were critical. Subsequent case reports and functional MRI research has confirmed that the right parahippocampal gyrus is critical for such abilities.

Hécaen (1962) studied the clinical evidence of loss of topographical memory for a previously familiar environment and found that in most cases the parietal lesions were bilateral, though more of the unilateral cases involved the right than the left hemisphere.

Topographical disorientation

Semmes *et al*. (1955) showed that on tasks of following routes from maps, patients with parietal lesions did worse than patients with lesions elsewhere. Ratcliff and Newcombe (1973) produced especially interesting findings from a study of men with penetrating missile wounds of the brain. Two tests were employed: a visually guided stylus maze task, and a locomotor map-reading task in which the subject was required to trace out a designated route on foot. These were designed to tap visuospatial agnosia and topographical disorientation, respectively. Patients with lesions in the posterior part of the right hemisphere were significantly worse than those with left posterior lesions on the maze-learning test, but a significant deficit on the map-reading test emerged only in those with bilateral posterior lesions. A clear dissociation between the two tasks could sometimes be observed. Ratcliff and Newcombe were led to conclude that while the right hemisphere has a special role in the perception of space, it does not bear an exclusive responsibility for the maintenance of spatial orientation. Bilateral lesions appeared to be necessary before route finding was impaired, perhaps because this involves a constant reorientation to stimuli as the subject moves around and alters his frames of reference. Further experiments on the topic are described by De Renzi (1982), along with a detailed discussion of the various deficits that may contribute to topographical disorientation. An up-to-date synthesis of neuropsychological and neuroimaging data is provided by Aguirre and D'Esposito (1999).

Visual neglect

Unilateral visual neglect (or unilateral spatial agnosia) may be seen in spontaneous drawings, copies, description of pictures, or use of paper when writing. When eating, the patient may ignore food on the left side of the plate. It may also lead the patient to fail to take turnings to the left and consequently he may lose his way on familiar routes. A hemianopia may or may not be present but does not account for the deficit. This is an agnosia for space as such, not merely an agnosia for spatial relations between visual objects. It may be seen in many degrees of severity. It is well confirmed that neglect of the left half of space is very much more common than that on the right, and depends on a right temporoparietal lesion (Heilman *et al*. 1985). In an interesting report Halligan and Marshall (1991) have described a patient who showed severe visuospatial neglect for near ('peripersonal') space but not for extrapersonal space. Following a right middle cerebral infarction he showed left visuospatial neglect, a left hemiparesis and an inferior homonymous quadrantanopia. On standard line bisection tests, performed with the paper immediately before him, he showed marked displacements to the right, but was able accurately to indicate the midpoint of lines and to direct darts accordingly when these were some 2.5 m away. Most current theories of neglect emphasise attentional processes, i.e. the failure to direct attention to one part of space such as the left side (or to disengage it from another). This has led to theoretically motivated rehabilitation programmes, for example involving attentional cueing to the neglected side, for what is a notoriously disabling syndrome (Pierce & Buxbaum 2002).

In an elegant yet simple study, Bisiach and Luzzati (1978; described in detail in McCarthy & Warrington 1990, pp. 77–97) showed that the neglect of hemispace may affect mental representations as well as perceived space. They asked their neglect patients to imagine standing in the Piazza del Duomo in Milan and to describe the scene from two vantage points: with the cathedral behind or in front of them. In either case it was the buildings on their left that were omitted though knowledge of them was clearly preserved. In an added twist, Marshall and Halligan (1988) showed that some implicit knowledge could affect behaviour despite being explicitly neglected. Flames drawn emerging from the left part of the roof of a picture of a house were 'not seen' by a neglect patient who nevertheless stated a preference for an otherwise identical house with no flames.

Auditory agnosia and auditory perceptual defects

In auditory agnosia hearing is unimpaired, as tested by pure tone thresholds, but the patient fails to recognise or distinguish the sounds that he hears. Thus in everyday life he may give the appearance of being 'deaf'. Typically the onset is with severe dysphasia, which then clears substantially to leave the auditory problem in evidence. The patient is unable to recognise speech, as in pure word-deafness (see earlier in chapter), but in addition cannot recognise non-speech sounds such as the pouring of water, crumpling of paper or jingling of keys. Usually there is also failure to recognise musical sounds. These three defects, word-deafness, auditory agnosia and 'sensory amusia', can occur together with varying degrees of severity.

The disorder is extremely rare and few convincing examples have been reported. Vignolo (1969) provides a detailed review, both of the phenomena observed and of their relationships to aphasia. Most examples have been associated with bilateral lesions of the posterior parts of the temporal lobes.

Less complete difficulty with the processing of auditory information may be demonstrated in some patients with brain lesions. Vignolo (1969) showed that patients with right hemisphere lesions fail relatively on tests of discriminating meaningless sounds, whereas patients with left-sided lesions have greater difficulty in identifying sounds to which meaning can be attached. This indicates that the auditory-receiving areas of the two hemispheres are to some extent specialised, that of the right being specifically concerned with grasping the acoustic structure of the auditory input (i.e. subtle perceptual discrimination) and that of the left with endowing the input with meaning by virtue of semantic associative links (i.e. semantic decoding). Analogous differences between the hemispheres have more recently been shown for tactile recognition as well (see under Tactile perceptual defects, next).

With regard to music, the right temporal lobe appears overall to be more important than the left. Right temporal lobectomy has been found to impair performance on tests of musical aptitude, whereas left temporal lobectomy does not (Kimura 1961; Milner 1962). Shankweiler (1966) played extracts of familiar songs to patients who had had temporal lobectomies and found that the group with left lesions had greater difficulty in recalling the titles or words, whereas the group with right lesions had greater difficulty in reproducing or recognising the melody. Using dichotic listening tasks, words fed to the right ear (and proceeding thence by crossed pathways predominantly to the left hemisphere) are reported better than words fed to the left ear, whereas with fragments of melodies the situation is reversed (Kimura 1961, 1964). Moreover, when dichotic tests are given to lobectomised patients it is found that left temporal lobectomy produces a more severe decrement in the contralateral ear where words are concerned, and right temporal lobectomy for the recognition of musical passages (Shankweiler 1966).

Gordon and Bogen (1974) also reported interesting effects when patients were asked to sing familiar songs during the course of unilateral intracarotid amobarbital injections. When the left hemisphere was sedated with the drug the words of the song were severely affected while the melody continued well; in contrast, when the right hemisphere was sedated the words remained relatively intact whereas the pitch and melodic line were severely disrupted.

It seems clear therefore that the right hemisphere is superior to the left in most people for the perception of 'structured' musical passages, perhaps with the temporal lobes taking a lead in melody and harmony and frontal areas more involved in pitch, rhythm and phrasing. However, detailed analysis of various components of musical perception (pitch, timbre, discrimination and rhythm) have often given conflicting results, suggesting that neither hemisphere alone is specialised for all aspects of musical cognition and that musical training may confound the results. Lezak (1995) reviews the more recent clinical and experimental evidence, indicating that while the right hemisphere is generally the more important in melodic recognition and chord analysis, the left tends to predominate in the processing of sequential and discrete tonal components of music.

Early functional imaging work showed changes in cerebral blood flow in the right temporal cortex during the perceptual analysis of melodies and of the right frontal cortex during pitch comparisons but, predictably, more recent work has revealed additional complexities implicating wider and more distributed neural networks depending on the nature of the task. Finally, structural MRI has shown that musicians with perfect pitch have greater leftward asymmetry of the planum temporale than non-musicians. Zatorre (2003) summarises the current state of knowledge on music and the brain.

Amusia may be defined as an impairment or loss of musical function deriving from acquired disease of the brain (Henson 1985). Amusia without aphasia has proved to be rare, but examples have been described following right temporal or right frontal lesions. In such examples the deficit usually involves loss of capacity to sing or hum a tune (oral-expressive amusia). Henson (1985) reviews the scattered literature on other amusia syndromes: musical agraphia, musical alexia and musical amnesia, and receptive amusia in which there is failure to discriminate pitch, intensity, timbre and rhythm. This latter disturbance is usually seen only as part of a more widespread auditory agnosia.

Finally, under the heading of 'auditory affective agnosia', Heilman *et al.* (1975) have drawn attention to deficits in the appreciation of the affective tone of speech in patients with right hemisphere lesions. After listening to tape-recorded sentences, patients were asked to judge either the content or the emotional tone in which each sentence had been spoken (happy, sad, angry or indifferent). Six patients had right temporoparietal lesions (with left unilateral neglect) and six had left temporoparietal lesions (with fluent aphasia). The responses were made by selection from a series of line-drawn pictures appropriate to the sentences and emotions concerned. All subjects achieved perfect scores with respect to content, but those with right hemisphere lesions were significantly impaired in judging affective tone (Kucharska-Pietura *et al.* 2003).

Tactile perceptual defects

In tactile agnosia the patient is unable to recognise an object by touch, even though the sensory functions of the hand being tested are normal. The same object is immediately recognised by other means, for example by touching it with the opposite hand or by vision.

There is uncertainty surrounding the distinction between tactile agnosia and the 'astereognosis' of cortical sensory loss, in which there is equally failure of tactile recognition. However, some claim that in tactile agnosia the patient can still distinguish the size, shape and texture of the object even though the object cannot be recognised, whereas in astereognosis the appreciation of these sensory elements is impaired as well.

Commonly, tactile agnosia is restricted to one hand and results from a lesion in the opposite parietal lobe. The supramarginal gyrus has been especially incriminated. Bilateral tactile agnosia is said to follow damage in this region in the dominant hemisphere, and it is possible that in such cases callosal fibres to the opposite lobe have also been destroyed by the lesion. Bottini *et al.* (1995) showed that tactile matching of meaningless shapes (apperceptive recognition) was more affected by right hemisphere lesions, whereas similar matching of meaningful objects was compromised by left hemisphere lesions (associative recognition).

Gerstmann's syndrome

The concept of a 'Gerstmann syndrome' resulting from dominant parietal lobe lesions has become firmly entrenched in the neurological and psychological literature. It consists of finger agnosia, right–left disorientation, dyscalculia and dysgraphia. As such it remains a useful venue for the discussion of these disorders, and yields a useful group of simple clinical tests when one is looking for subtle signs of a lesion in the dominant hemisphere. However, the essential clustering together of the defects has been seriously questioned, and it is now clear that they barely constitute a syndrome in the accepted sense of the word.

It is known that the four components are not always found together, one or more often being absent when the others can be demonstrated clearly. Similarly, one or more components can occur along with other disorders of cognitive function: dysphasia, dyslexia, constructional apraxia, visual disorientation or generalised intellectual impairment. Benton (1961) examined the intercorrelations on tests of the four Gerstmann symptoms and of three other functions related to the parietal lobes (constructional ability, reading and visual memory) in a large unselected series of brain-damaged subjects; it emerged that the correlations of the Gerstmann abilities with each other was no higher than with the three abilities not included in the syndrome. In a separate analysis of patients with damage restricted to the left parietal lobe, the Gerstmann defects again failed to cluster together. Heimburger *et al.* (1964) in a similar study found that as the number of Gerstmann components increased, the lesions tended to be larger in size. When all four defects did appear together they were usually accompanied by severe impairment of many other functions. Nevertheless pure cases do occur rarely. It has not seemed possible to establish a common fundamental disturbance underlying each of the four defects.

Finger agnosia

Finger agnosia is shown by loss of ability to recognise, name, identify, indicate or select individual fingers, either on the patient's own body or on that of another person. Traditionally, the patient is asked to point to named fingers or to name an individual finger, but the presence of dysphasia may confound this simple procedure. Kinsbourne and Warrington (1962) advocated a test in which two fingers are simultaneously touched by the examiner and the patient is asked to state the number of fingers between those touched, first in practice sessions with the eyes open and then with the eyes closed.

The disorder appears bilaterally. The patient does not report it spontaneously, and thus like constructional apraxia it is a defect usually only revealed by specific testing. A lesion in the left parieto-occipital area appears to be critical for its appearance, but it is possible that it can occur very occasionally with right hemisphere lesions. The angular gyrus and the second occipital convolution have been especially incriminated.

Gerstmann (1958) himself proposed that finger agnosia may represent a minimal form of whole-body autotopagnosia, in other words a defect of recognition of the body or appreciation of the interrelations of body parts (see under Autotopagnosia, later). He suggested that complete autotopagnosia is very rarely seen because those lesions sufficient to produce it also result in concomitant defects that obscure the picture, whereas in the restricted form of finger agnosia it can be recognised as a clear-cut entity. It has been argued (Frederiks 1985) that no other part of the body is verbally differentiated to so great a degree as the hand, and none has such an extensive cerebral representation, hence its special vulnerability that emerges in finger agnosia. A more recent report of 'toe agnosia' calls this appealing theory into question (Tucha *et al.* 1997).

Right–left disorientation

This defect shows as inability to carry out instructions that involve an appreciation of right and left. The patient fails to point on command to objects on his right and his left, to indicate parts of his body on the right and the left, or to perform more complex instructions in which these directions form an integral part of the task. It undoubtedly reflects several complex disorders of function. Gerstmann (1958) suggested that like finger agnosia it represented a restricted form of body image disturbance. Benton (1959) on the other hand stressed that language is likely to be intrinsically concerned with many forms of the disorder. Sauget *et al.* (1971) investigated the relationship between sensory dysphasia and various forms of disturbance including right–left disorientation and finger agnosia, using both verbal and non-verbal tests. They concluded that these disturbances are closely linked to impairment of language comprehension, but that in addition impairment of somatosensory functions is necessary for their appearance. Frederiks (1985) suggests that visual aspects of the body schema, and the relation between corporeal and extracorporeal space, are likely to be fundamentally involved.

Right–left disorientation can generally be accepted as a sign of left hemisphere dysfunction, but is of little value for more precise localisation within the hemisphere. Occasionally, moreover, it may emerge with right hemisphere dysfunction (Benton & Sivan 1993).

Dyscalculia

Dyscalculia is an impairment of the capacity for calculation in persons who have hitherto shown no disorder of their arithmetical faculties, although developmental forms are well recognised (for review see Ardila & Rosselli 2002). It is clear that detailed analysis of the nature of the calculation defect is necessary if the symptom is to have any localising value since there are many possible sources of failure. Arithmetical ability can be disturbed independently of language functions and general intelligence, but pure cases of this nature are rare. Secondary dyscalculia can result from defects of short-term memory, perseveration or simple impairment of concentration (Butterworth 1999; Cappaletti *et al.* 2005).

Boller and Grafman (1985) subdivide primary dyscalculia into four varieties. First, there may be loss of ability to appreciate the names and significance of numbers or to combine them syntactically to produce a meaningful digit notation. Second, there may be problems with the spatial organisation required in numerical operations. Third, there may be difficulties in carrying out the basic computational aspects of addition, subtraction, multiplication and division (anarithmetica). This last may be subdivided into two sources of failure: inability to retrieve mathematical facts normally stored in memory (e.g. 5+4=9), or inability to engage in mathematical thinking and reasoning and to understand the procedural rules that underlie mathematical operations.

Such a distinction was clarified by Warrington (1982) in a case study of a physician with a left parietal subdural haematoma. Simple calculations were performed laboriously and inaccurately, and on introspection he found that the processes of addition and subtraction could no longer be performed 'automatically'. He could define the concepts of addition, subtraction, multiplication and division quite well and his understanding of such operations was unimpaired. What he lacked was direct access to the semantic memories of arithmetical facts so that he had to revert to the slow counting processes observed in children. Other anarithmetic patients differ from this in that they lack all concept of the mathematical operations, or are unable to comprehend the significance of individual numbers or number facts (e.g. that there are 100 pence in a pound, or that 12 is greater than 11).

Dyscalculia has been found in one form or another with lesions of the frontal, temporal, parietal or occipital lobes of the brain, but the parietal lobes have been most frequently involved and the left lobe more often than the right. This is supported by Grafman *et al.*'s (1982) study in which patients with focal damage to either hemisphere performed significantly worse than controls, but the left posterior brain-damaged group was particularly impaired; this was largely independent of such additional factors as dysphasia or visuoconstructive difficulties. Again, neuroimaging has tended to refine these observations with reference to normal functioning (Dehaene *et al.* 2004).

Disorders of body image

The body image, or 'body schema', may be regarded as a subjective model of the body against which changes in its posture, in the disposition of its parts, and in its soundness or integrity can be appreciated. As such the body image is not static but changes constantly under the influence of internal and external sensory impressions. Moreover, it invariably includes important unconscious as well as conscious components, so cannot be viewed as a mere picture in the mind. Normally it exists on the fringe of awareness, but aspects can be brought into consciousness when subjective attention is focused on them.

The body image is thus an abstract conception, acquired during development and compounded of physiological and psychological elements. Schilder (1935) extended the concept and in particular stressed that data from a wide range of sources must be incorporated into any notion of the body image, including aspects of personality, emotion and social interaction. For him the postural model proposed by Head (1920) represented only a low level of body image organisation, whilst higher levels are built out of instinctual needs and personal interactions.

Disorders of the body image are implicit in a wide range of puzzling and often bizarre clinical states, around which a good deal of controversy exists. Some disturbances represent the influence of structural or physiological changes in the brain, as seen for example in the presence of cerebral disease or in the effects of drugs such as cannabis or lysergic acid diethylamide (LSD). Other disturbances may accompany severe sensory deprivation or psychiatric illnesses such as depression or schizophrenia, and then may appear to be mainly psychological in origin. In some particularly puzzling disorders, such as anosognosia, it is probably necessary to invoke both organic and psychogenic factors in an attempt at a complete explanation.

Body image disturbances associated with brain lesions can be broadly divided into those affecting half of the body only, and those which involve bilateral disturbances. Unilateral body image disturbances are commoner with right hemisphere lesions than left, and the left side of the body is therefore most often affected. They include unilateral inattention, neglect, feelings and beliefs that the left limbs are missing (hemisomatognosia), and lack of awareness or denial of disability (anosognosia). Bilateral body image disturbances are commoner with left cerebral lesions than right. They are usually restricted to finger agnosia (see previous section, under Finger agnosia) or right–left disorientation (see previous section, under Right–left disorientation), but very occasionally there is difficulty in naming or pointing to any body part (autotopagnosia). Complex illusions of bodily transformation or displacement are less closely tied to lesions in known locations and seem to be more intimately involved with non-organic psychopathology. Such non-organic psychopathology of body image invariably concerns symmetrical structures (e.g. breasts, buttocks) or those in the midline (e.g. nose, penis), contrasting starkly with their organic counterparts.

Unilateral unawareness and neglect

This represents perhaps the best-known and most frequently encountered change in the body image. For reasons incompletely understood the disorder affects the left limbs in the great majority of cases, and appears to derive particularly from lesions in the neighbourhood of the supramarginal and angular gyri of the right parietal lobe. A spectrum of disturbances is seen, ranging from inattention and unawareness to neglect. Somatic and extrasomatic neglect (e.g. visual neglect) usually occur together but need not do so. Unilateral neglect without visual neglect is rather rare while the reverse is somewhat less so.

The range and interrelationships of these phenomena have been excellently described by Critchley (1953). A minor degree of inattention to the left limbs may require special techniques of examination to reveal it, such as double simultaneous stimulation of both sides of the body together (see Chapter 1, Clinical picture in focal cerebral disorder/Parietal lobes). In unawareness the disorder is more obtrusive, the patient failing to utilise the left hand in bimanual activities or overlooking the left foot when pulling on his slippers. When attention is specifically drawn to the left limbs, however, they are used with normal efficiency, or if a degree of paresis exists the patient admits his difficulties. It is as though the limbs of this side were 'occupying a lower level in a hierarchy of personal awareness' (Critchley 1953).

The disorder may involve no more than this or may include the more elaborate symptoms of neglect. The limbs may be ignored in washing or dressing, one half of the face may be left unshaven or the hair uncombed. This is more likely in the presence of confusion or other impairment of intellect. Sometimes unawareness or neglect accompany the development of a hemiparesis, and when this is present the more florid features of anosognosia may be added (see Anosognosia, later).

Such disorders are seen more commonly after acute brain lesions and particularly after cerebrovascular accidents. The degree of unawareness or neglect appears to be related to the abruptness of the lesion, the clarity of consciousness and whether motor weakness is present. Usually these are transient phenomena, and changeable from time to time during clinical examination, but occasionally the disability persists in some form as an enduring defect.

As noted, there is a well-established association between neglect and right parietal lesions, yet typical syndromes of neglect have been reported following damage in other locations such as the basal ganglia and thalamus. More transient states of contralateral neglect may be seen with left hemisphere lesions. The relationship between visual and somatic neglect and their cognitive and neurological underpinnings are set out in detail in Kerkhoff (2001).

Hemisomatognosia (hemisomatoagnosia, hemidepersonalisation, asomatognosia)

In this much rarer phenomenon the patient feels as though the limbs on one side are missing, sometimes episodically but sometimes as a continuous subjective state. It may feature as part of an aura in a focal epileptic attack.

The disorder is accompanied by various degrees of loss of insight. The limbs may feel absent though the patient knows this is not so, or he may say they are absent but can be corrected in his belief, or he may have a fixed delusion that they are absent which cannot be corrected. When consciousness is clear the patient usually retains insight into the illusory nature of the condition, even though it may feel very vivid, and can reassure himself as to the presence of the limbs by feeling or looking at them. In the presence of confusion, however, he may proclaim that the limbs are missing, look for them under the bed, or accuse others of taking them away. The condition is typically due to a parietal lobe lesion of the minor hemisphere and essentially corresponds to the syndrome of unilateral unawareness and neglect described above.

> Sierra *et al.* (2002) describe a case of a woman who experienced a generalised sense of depersonalisation following a right subdural haematoma over the parietal lobe following haemorrhage from a carotid aneurysm. She made a good recovery except for mild left arm weakness but felt as if the fingers of her right hand 'did not belong', as if the limbs had disappeared. Furthermore, the patient had the distressing urge to touch or pour hot water over herself for reassurance of her existence. She said: 'Sometimes I do not seem to know who I am, I doubt my own existence. I feel like a piece of furniture.' There was no sensory loss or clouding of consciousness.

Anosognosia

Anosognosia implies lack of awareness of disease and is most commonly shown for left hemiplegic limbs. It may occur along with unilateral neglect, hemisomatognosia or with the illusions of transformation and displacement considered below. It can, rarely, occur in isolation (Jehkonen *et al.* 2000).

In its mildest form the patient merely shows a lack of normal concern for his disability, attaching little importance to it and not grasping its implications. Or when confronted by the disability and obliged to admit it, he belittles the problem and shows an inappropriately flat or facetious reaction (anosodiaphoria). In true anosognosia, however, the patient appears to be completely unaware of the hemiplegia, makes no complaints about it and ignores the inconvenience it causes. In extreme cases, the deficit may be vehemently denied.

Commonly, anosognosia is merely a transient state in the early days after acute hemiplegia has developed, and recedes along with the initial clouding of consciousness. However, it may persist and become more floridly developed with obstinate denial or bizarre elaboration on a delusional basis. When attention is firmly drawn to the hemiplegia, the patient makes some shallow rationalisation for not performing the task, perhaps explaining that he has been ill recently or that he is too tired. In more bizarre cases he insists that the paralysed limbs do not belong to him or attributes them to some neighbouring person (somatoparaphrenia). He may claim that the limbs are some mechanical object, or talk to them and fondle them as though they had an existence of their own (known as 'personification'). Feelings of anger or hatred may be expressed towards them (misoplegia).

> A woman of 39 with left hemiplegia, hemianaesthesia and hemianopia was garrulous and confused. She denied that she was paralysed and insisted that her left arm and leg belonged to her daughter Ann, who she said had been sharing her bed for the past week. When the patient's wedding ring was pointed out to her she said that Ann had borrowed it to wear. The patient was encouraged to talk to Ann and to tell her to move her arm; she then became confused and talked vaguely about Ann being asleep and not to be disturbed. When asked to indicate her own left limbs she turned her head and searched in a bemused way over her left shoulder.
>
> The left arm of a patient with a right parietal lesion kept wandering about in the blind homonymous half-field of vision. When the patient wrote, the left hand would wander across and butt in and rest on the right hand. Not recognising this as his own he would exclaim 'Let go my hand!' He would swear at it in exasperation 'You bloody bastard! It's lost its soul, this bloody thing. It follows me around and gets in the way when I read' (Critchley 1964).

Such highly colourful reactions are rare, and it is doubtful whether they occur in the absence of clouding of consciousness or generalised intellectual impairment. They can usually be understood most readily in terms of psychogenic elaboration of some partially perceived defect, sometimes illustrating in unusually clear form the common psychological mechanisms of defence.

Anosognosia is also used as a generic term for imperception of deficits other than hemiplegia. Here again it may range in degree from lack of concern and attention to explicit verbal denial, and again it is often uncertain how far the disturbance is intrinsically related to cerebral disorder alone or how far it reflects superadded psychogenic mechanisms. It is perhaps most commonly seen in relation to aphasic symptoms, classically with primary sensory aphasia when the patient seems not to appreciate his mistakes. Unawareness or denial of amnesic defects is common as part of Korsakoff's syndrome. Blindness, especially when due to lesions of the optic radiations or striate cortices, may be denied, the patient attempting to behave as though he can see and describing purely imaginary visual experiences when tested (Anton's syndrome). Deafness due to cerebral lesions may more rarely be denied. Unawareness of painful stimuli (pain asymbolia) is another incompletely understood example, in which the patient may perceive a painful stimulus but fails to recognise it as unpleasant, so that little or no defensive reaction is produced. This rare disorder can result from an acquired cerebral lesion, usually in the dominant hemisphere, while other aspects of sensation are unaffected. It has been regarded as a failure to integrate the awareness of pain with awareness of the body image or, alternatively, as a gross denial in the psychogenic sense of painful experience.

The term 'anosognosia' has also been applied in relation to the cognitive deficits in the dementias, both focal and diffuse (see Clare 2004), and to the behavioural problems and personality changes seen after other forms of brain injury (Prigatano 2005), and even movement disorders. Indeed, the similarities between forms of lack of insight commonly observed in people with psychotic disorders and anosognosia has been a major stimulus to research and cross-fertilisation between neuropsychiatry and general psychiatry (Amador & David 2004).

Anosognosia for hemiplegia has been more closely studied than these other forms of the disorder. Nevertheless, the mechanisms involved remain unclear and are the subject of controversy. In the majority of cases there are sensory as well as motor deficits in the limbs concerned, but the condition is not explainable in terms of perceptual deficit alone, since occasionally hemiplegia is denied while the patient remains fully aware of the existence of the limbs. The role of general intellectual disturbance is also disputed. Anosognosia can occur in the presence of strictly focal brain damage and when the patient is mentally clear, although some degree of cognitive impairment or clouding of consciousness is more common. Still others emphasise the psychogenic component, and see anosognosia essentially as a motivated desire to repress the unpleasant facts of a disability. Such primitive defensive behaviour may admittedly be brought to the fore by the presence of cerebral disease.

Weinstein and Kahn (1955) stressed this last point of view in their survey of a large population of brain-injured patients. In addition to denial of the defects already mentioned they noted denial of incontinence and impotence, and patients totally confined to bed might occasionally insist that they had recently returned from a walk. Some degree of mental confusion could always be detected in their patients when specially sought out, though it was often of a subtle nature. Weinstein and Cole (1963) continued these observations in a later study restricted to anosognosia for hemiplegia. Fre-

quently some degree of awareness of the defect was betrayed, and medication or operation was accepted without demur. Common mental mechanisms for defence against anxiety could be seen to operate. The premorbid personalities of the patients had often shown strong perfectionistic traits, tendencies to deny illness, and to view health as important for their self-esteem. Where verbal anosognosia was concerned this often appeared to be an artefact of the interview situation, and the attitudes of observers and of the patient's relatives were important in determining the degree and duration of the denial. The most recent systematic study of anosognosia with hemiplegia was carried out by Marcel et al. (2004) on 64 selected stroke patients. They made the distinction between unawareness of paralysis and of its consequences, the latter being more widespread and persistent. Some were unaware of movement failures when they occurred while others were aware but quickly forgot, perhaps due to a failure to update long-term body knowledge memory. Contrary to Weinstein and Kahn, they observed that patients did not generally overestimate other abilities, but they did note that some patients who overestimated current bilateral task ability (e.g. tying one's shoe-laces) when asked in the first-person form did not overestimate when asked how well the examiner, if he was in their current condition, could do each task. Marcel et al. concluded that anosognosia for hemiplegia is not a unitary phenomenon.

Against the view that psychogenic factors predominate in anosognosia is the rather obstinate fact that anosognosia, like uncomplicated unilateral neglect, has usually been found to be very much commoner for the left than for the right side of the body. In Starkstein et al.'s (1992) series of stroke patients, 38% with left-sided signs showed anosognosia compared with 11% of those with right-sided signs. Moreover, the lesion, when focal, appears to implicate the temporoparietal region rather than the pre-rolandic cortex or lower levels of motor organisation. One complication is that there is no agreed definition of anosognosia, especially where the penumbra of related phenomena are concerned, so assessing prevalence is problematic. This is further complicated in left hemisphere-damaged patients by the presence of aphasia, which might lead to an underestimate of the condition in right hemiplegics (Cutting 1978).

The published work on the cerebral localisation of anosognosia has been systematically reviewed by Pia et al. (2004). They concluded that while right hemisphere damage is the hallmark, bilateral damage is frequently reported. Furthermore, the deficit seems to be equally frequent when the damage is confined to frontal, parietal or temporal cortical structures, and may also emerge as a consequence of subcortical lesions. Interestingly, the probability of occurrence of anosognosia was noted to be highest when the lesion involved parietal and frontal structures in combination.

The rarity of anosognosia and related defects in the right limbs is very hard to explain by any theory. It has been suggested that since the left limbs are normally subordinate to the right, cerebral lesions merely exaggerate this tendency or, alternatively, that with lesions of the dominant hemisphere intellectual deficits and aphasia readily swamp these more subtle manifestations. Others have attempted to resolve the dilemma by proposing that the non-dominant hemisphere is prepotent where the body image is concerned, or at least that it contains special mechanisms for the recognition of unilateral inequalities.

Autotopagnosia

Autotopagnosia refers to an inability to recognise, name or point on command to various parts of the body both on the right and on the left. The defect may apply to other people's bodies as well as to the subject's own, yet other external objects are dealt with normally.

Autotopagnosia in any extensive sense is extremely rare. However, restricted forms are seen in conjunction with many other types of body image disorder, in that a tendency may occur to misidentify certain body parts. Such a defect confined to one body half is seen in patients with unilateral neglect or anosognosia. Finger agnosia (see under Gerstmann's syndrome, earlier) is sometimes regarded as a minimal degree of whole-body autotopagnosia, and to represent the only clear-cut example that cannot be better explained in terms of other defects.

Most examples which implicate the body bilaterally are explainable in terms of apraxia, agnosia, aphasia or disorder of spatial perception. De Renzi and Scotti (1970) described a case which perhaps illustrates essential mechanisms of another type. The patient, who had a tumour of the left parietal lobe, failed to point to body parts, but in contrast could promptly name all parts pointed to by the examiner. He could also correctly monitor the accuracy or otherwise of another person's pointing. The same dissociation between pointing himself and naming could be seen for parts of objects other than the human body, for example for parts of a bicycle. The defect thus appeared to be a part of a more general disturbance of failure to analyse a whole into parts. Autotopagnosia is usually seen in conjunction with diffuse bilateral lesions of the brain. Lesions of the left hemisphere alone can produce it, but must always involve the parieto-occipitotemporal region (Frederiks 1985).

Illusions of transformation, displacement or reduplication

A great variety of body image disturbances may be loosely grouped together under this heading. They are seen in many clinical settings. Some of the less dramatic, such as feelings of heaviness or enlargement of a limb, may occur in healthy subjects in states of extreme exhaustion, sensory deprivation or in the course of falling asleep. Others, like feelings of distortion or free floating of the body, occur with generalised cerebral disorder as in delirium or under the influence of drugs such as LSD. Many unilateral examples are seen with focal brain disturbance, particularly as part of an epileptic aura, and some of the most bizarre instances, including autoscopy, can occur in the course of migrainous attacks. A further group appear in association with static lesions, particularly those which have led to left hemiplegia and anosognosia, but here again the phenomena are usually short-lived even if recurrent.

Macrosomatognosia and microsomatognosia consist of feelings of abnormal largeness or smallness of parts, or of half or even the whole of the body. Most commonly a single limb or a hand is affected alone. Such changes may be accompanied by sensations of heaviness, distortion or displacement of the part concerned, or features such as these may constitute the sole abnormality. Feelings of swelling, elongation, shortening or twisting may be experienced, rather than a change that preserves the normal proportions of the part. Rarely the experience may be of physical separation of the part from the rest of the body. The following examples are reported by Lukianowicz (1967).

An epileptic girl sometimes had a somatic sensory aura during which she felt that:

my whole body grows very rapidly almost to the point of bursting. After a few seconds it collapses, like a deflated balloon, and then I lose consciousness and have a turn.

A lorry driver discovered to have epilepsy had attacks:

when everything seems to run away from me, and then I get the feeling in my eyes that they tear out of their sockets, and rush out from the cabin, till they touch the people and the houses and the lampposts along the road . . . Then everything rushes towards me again and my eyeballs hurry back into their sockets. At other times I might feel that my hands and arms grow long very rapidly, till they seem to reach miles ahead. A moment later they begin to shrink until they come back to their normal size. I may have such a feeling several times in a minute or two.

A woman with migraine complained:

Before the ache I see coloured zig-zag stripes appearing always from the left side. After a while I begin to feel that my head shrinks until it becomes not bigger than a small orange. At that time it always occurs to me that my head must look like the small dried-up heads of the head-hunters in Borneo, which I had once seen on TV. This sensation lasts about 1 minute and then my head at once comes back to its normal size. This feeling of my head shrinking and expanding goes on for some time, until I get my splitting headache.

The patient almost always retains insight into the alien nature of the experiences, describing the abnormality in 'as if' terms. A truly delusional or hallucinatory experience is rare in the absence of marked impairment of consciousness or psychotic illness. It is of course hard to discern, in cases such as those just quoted, how far the abnormal experience is due to a primary disturbance of the body schema or how far it represents an imaginative elaboration of simple kinaesthetic and vestibular sensory changes. Derangements of either right or left hemisphere function may lead to such phenomena, and when a focal lesion is responsible the parietotemporo-occipital region is said to be usually involved.

Reduplicative phenomena usually involve the limbs, and most often the hand or fingers alone. Such phantoms are usually transient, appearing with darkness and drowsiness. Many cases occur with anosognosia for left hemiplegia, and may lead to illusions of movement in the paralysed limbs. Insight is again usually preserved in large degree, and when the patient looks at the actual limbs the phantom promptly disappears. However, occasional cases are reported in which enduring phantoms prove an embarrassment and inconvenience, and the patient feels obliged to make the real limb coincide in position with the phantom. More dramatic instances of reduplication may involve the whole-body image (Lukianowicz 1967).

Weinstein *et al.* (1954) have reported a few patients with reduplicative phenomena all with cerebral lesions of rapid onset and producing some degree of generalised confusion. One patient with a left hemiplegia claimed to have an extra left hand; one with a left hemiparesis and a fracture of the right leg stated that he had four legs; and one with a severe head injury who had previously had an eye removed claimed to have several eyes. Another patient with a cerebellar astrocytoma and meningitis said that he had three heads and four bodies, one of each with him and the remainder upstairs in a closet. In all four cases the reduplications were accompanied by other forms of reduplication for time, place or person. The 'body image' disturbance therefore appeared to be but one manifestation of a general pattern of reduplicative delusions.

Autoscopy (doppelgänger phenomenon). There is 'a complex psychosensorial hallucinatory perception of one's own body image projected into external visual space' (Lukianowicz 1958). Usually the image is in front of the patient at a certain distance, mostly fleetingly but very occasionally lasting for days at a time. It may be transparent, or coloured and definite, or show expressive movements. It may consist of the whole or only a part of the body, but the face is usually included. Cases have been described in which the image occurs to one side of the midline in a hemianopic field of vision. The experience may be extremely realistic but is almost always recognised by the subject to be a pathological event. The emotional reaction may be of anxiety or quiet surprise, depending on the patient's mental state.

Usually the experience is visual, as the name implies, but sometimes the body image is experienced as projected into outside space by senses other than vision. A number of subdivisions of this striking phenomenon are recognised, as discussed by Brugger *et al.* (1996).

With *autoscopic hallucinations* only the visual part of the body image is split off, usually being perceived as a lifeless though multicoloured image of the patient's own person. In *heautoscopy*, somaesthetic elements are additionally projected into peripersonal space so that the subject both sees and feels awareness of the presence of his double. The image is then experienced as a living being. The patient may indeed have difficulty in deciding whether he should refer to the phenomenon as 'seeing' or 'being' his double. In an *out-of-body experience*, the core subjective experience is the illusion of being separated from one's body, and visual elements may play a minor role. *'Feeling of presence'* occurs without visual elements, the person having the illusion of being accompanied by an invisible being. Typical features include a distinct localisation for the 'presence', as a rule at a specific distance from the subject's own body, also a conviction that the invisible being is real. It is endowed with an intense sense of familiarity and affinity, and sometimes it dawns on the subject that the presence is in fact a replica of himself. Heautoscopy and 'feeling of presence' can occur in close temporal conjunction with one another in certain organic states.

Brugger *et al.* (1996) suggest that autoscopic hallucinations owe most to occipitotemporal lesions and heautoscopy proper to temporoparietal lesions. 'Feeling of presence' may be closely associated with parietal lobe impairment and is often seen along with a sensory hemisyndrome or hemispatial neglect. Commonly, however, the associated cerebral pathology is diffuse. With regard to laterality, Brugger *et al.* suggest that the visual doppelgängers (autoscopic hallucinations and heautoscopy) occur more often with right hemisphere lesions than left, whereas out-of-body experiences are projected more often towards the right and presumably reflect left hemisphere dysfunction. In their analysis of 31 cases of 'feeling of presence', Brugger *et al.* found that the presence was typically confined to one hemispace and was rather more often lateralised to the right than the left; of 12 cases with unilateral brain lesions, eight were in the left hemisphere and four in the right.

Phantom limb, which occurs after amputation or peripheral lesions of the nervous system, has a basis quite distinct from the supernumerary phantom that occurs with cerebral disease (Halligan *et al.* 1993). It is nonetheless in some ways the most decisive proof of the existence of the body schema. Phantom limbs are seen most commonly after amputation, but similar phenomena may follow severe nerve plexus lesions or lesions of the brainstem and thalamus. Equivalent phantom phenomena have also been reported after removal of the breast, the genitalia or the eye.

Halligan (2002) provides a comprehensive review of the phenomenon throughout history to the present day and its implications for cognitive neuropsychiatry. Distinction must be made between the perception of the missing limb itself, including its spatial characteristics, and the perception of phantom limb sensations such as paraesthesiae, heaviness, cold, cramp and pain. If the phantom is to develop, it usually does so immediately after amputation, persisting sometimes for several months and sometimes for the rest of the patient's life. It has a markedly realistic character, can usually be 'moved' at will, and may assume a relaxed or a cramped position. In the course of time it may appear only sporadically, or it may gradually telescope, the distal portion ultimately approaching the stump and disappearing into it.

Pain in the phantom limb can be distressing and intractable. It is typically paroxysmal, burning or shooting in character, sometimes occurring alone and sometimes with paraesthesiae. As with other phantom limb sensations the pain may be markedly affected by influences such as a change in the weather, use of a prosthesis, use of the contralateral limb, pain elsewhere in the body or firm efforts at mental concentration. A topographically organised sensory representation of the phantom limb may develop (remapping), for example on the face or chest, stimulation of which may be experienced in the phantom and which may be detected using functional neuroimaging in the corresponding sensory cortical region.

A psychogenic component thus undoubtedly exists, and has been interpreted in terms of loss of bodily integrity and reaction to disablement. The current emotional state may have a profound effect, depression contributing to such an extent that electroconvulsive therapy (ECT) has sometimes been found to abolish phantom limb pain. Psychotherapy and hypnosis have accordingly sometimes met with success in treatment, as has sensory distraction. However, a physiological component is also indicated by the efficacy, short-lived though it may be, of surgical procedures. Relief may follow the excision of a stump neuroma, chordotomy, or lesions in the thalamic radiation or sensory cortex.

Body image disturbances in non-organic psychiatric illness

This area has rarely been examined systematically, and Lukianowicz's (1967) survey of 200 consecutive admissions to a mental hospital, 31 of whom complained spontaneously of unusual sensations and experiences in various parts of their bodies, provides a valuable set of observations.

Disturbances of the shape of the body image were the commonest abnormality and took many forms. In schizophrenia patients there were examples of feelings of change of shape to that of another animal, the hands feeling shrunken like crab's claws or the whole body feeling as though transformed into a dog. Such changes appeared to be based essentially on

misinterpreted bodily sensations, combined often with hallucinations of the sense of smell. Insight into the unreality of the experiences was commonly retained, though sometimes incompletely expressed. In some cases complex sensory experiences appeared to underlie feelings that the body was changing into that of the opposite sex, likewise in some examples of transformation into Christ or other figures. Care was taken to distinguish as far as possible between mechanisms such as these, in which there was a discernible relationship to corresponding bodily sensations and hallucinations, and the more usual situation in which a delusional belief in a new identity or sex was purely ideational.

Feelings of change of position in space included levitation, floating and falling, sometimes as hypnagogic phenomena but sometimes occurring in the full waking state. In epileptic patients equivalent sensations were sometimes observed as a kinaesthetic aura preceding an epileptic attack.

Feelings of reduplication and splitting occurred in schizophrenia and in depression.

A schizophrenic student had the feeling of:

two bodies, one outside the other, only a bit larger than my actual body. I feel that the 'inner' body is the real one, and the 'outer' is more like something artificial, a sort of shell over a hermit crab although it has the shape and the appearance of my 'real' body.

A woman when depressed had a feeling:

as if my body was split into two halves, like a stem of a tree struck by lightning. They both feel a few inches apart and there is nothing between them, but a black empty hole; black and empty and dead.

Again, in epileptic patients such experiences could herald an attack. Experiences of autoscopic doubling were also seen in patients with schizophrenia and depression.

Feelings of additional body parts occurred in several bizarre forms, sometimes inviting a psychodynamic formulation which would see them as symbolically representing displaced sexual organs (but see Halligan *et al.* 1993).

A man whose potency was dwindling as a result of spinal injury developed recurrent depressive episodes. In one there were visual and haptic hallucinations of spurs and horns growing from his ankles, in another of a ball sticking out of his thigh, and in another of big screws growing from his abdomen and thighs. He retained insight into their unreal nature, and ECT was effective in banishing the phenomena along with the depression.

Change of size sometimes affected the whole body, and sometimes parts only, such as the ears, nose or limbs. Again, displaced sexual symbolism sometimes provided the most ready explanation, though analogous examples occurring in the course of epileptic and migrainous attacks may have rested primarily on disturbed cortical function. Lilliputian experiences were rare in comparison to feelings of enlargement, but one depressed woman had distressing hypnagogic experiences in which she felt her body shrink rapidly to the size of her little finger.

Changes in mass were usually manifest as feelings of emptiness and hollowness of body parts, particularly of the head. They were confined to patients with depressive illness or neurotic disorder, and often came close to nihilistic delusions. The following case illustrates the possible distinction.

A man with an anxiety disorder described a recurrent hypnopompic experience as follows:

Just after I wake up, but before I move, I have a terrifying feeling that my whole body consists of skin with nothing inside, like an empty blown-up balloon, or an empty shell, only pretending to be a human body. It is a very frightening feeling, which lasts only a few seconds and disappears immediately when I move any part of my body.

In general these various disturbances in psychiatric patients seemed to be an integral part of their mental illnesses, along with the more common hallucinations and related psychotic symptoms. Successful treatment of the psychiatric illness invariably resulted in resolution of the body image disturbances.

More recently, Cutting (1989) has analysed body image disturbances in a series of 100 schizophrenic patients. Rather surprisingly almost half had experienced some form of disorder, the predominant subjective change being alterations in structure, weight or shape. Other abnormalities included tactile hallucinations, feelings of additions to the body, or belief in the presence of localised devices within the body. As expected many of these changes were highly bizarre. Consonant with Cutting's (1985, 1990) view that right hemisphere dysfunction is important in the pathogenesis of schizophrenia, 13 of the 14 instances in which the disorder was lateralised concerned the left side of the body.

As noted earlier, however, non-organic and particularly non-psychotic disorders of body image frequently affect midline structures and probably relate to exaggerations or distortions of common, culturally influenced preoccupations. For example, personal appearance or an aspect of body image becomes the focus of obsessional rumination, or overvalued ideas, and may lead to requests for surgical intervention, or may dominate eating behaviour as in anorexia nervosa. Again, treatment should be aimed at the underlying disorder.

Non-cognitive disturbances and regional brain dysfunction

The forms of disability discussed above have all been more or less closely tied to cognitive or perceptual deficits, even though these have sometimes been of a rather subtle nature. There remain, however, certain abnormalities of emotion, behaviour and 'personality' that appear to be related to regional brain dysfunction yet do not necessarily have cognitive disturbance at the core. These are clearly of special interest to the psychiatrist. Certain examples have been selected for discussion.

Abnormalities of emotion and personality cannot be assessed with anything like the precision that is usually possible for cognitive defects. It has already been seen how much uncertainty surrounds our understanding of such measurable disorders as memory impairment, and such testable defects as aphasia or apraxia. With the body image disturbances there is an uncertain admixture of physiogenic and psychogenic mechanisms to be considered. Such problems are greatly extended in any analysis of disordered emotion or abnormalities of personality and social behaviour. Despite such difficulties important leads have been obtained, and interesting clinicopathological correlations have emerged in the examples discussed below.

Disordered control of aggression

Aggression is commonly divided into 'defensive' and 'predatory'. In extreme form this may be manifest as outbursts of uncontrollable violence. In some instances such disturbance is clearly attributable to focal cerebral pathology: in relation to epilepsy, certain cerebral tumours and other forms of brain disease. But the argument has been extended to suggest that in some habitually aggressive individuals, not showing overt signs of cerebral disorder, there may be abnormalities of the neural apparatus subserving aggressive responses. Attention has been directed particularly at possible dysfunction of the 'limbic brain' and especially of the amygdaloid nuclei within the temporal lobes. This remains a contentious area, not least because of the frequent difficulty in apportioning blame between pathophysiological and psychosocial influences in clinical situations, as discussed below.

In seeking correlates between aggressive behaviour and brain pathology, one is handicapped by the difficulty of defining in what circumstances and to what degree aggression must be displayed before it is regarded as abnormal. A variety of motivations may be involved, and many aspects of aggression are biologically valuable in humans as in other animals. Its determinants include environmental, social, cultural and intrapsychic factors, also learned components, any of which can emerge as crucial in individual instances. However, there appear to be persons who are subject to recurring and harmful outbursts of aggressive behaviour, sometimes on little or no provocation, and certain aggressive offenders whose episodes remain inexplicable in terms of personality, social adjustment and the situation at the time. Here it would seem that there may be important cerebral determinants of this pattern of behaviour: an abnormal triggering of aggressive responses based in disturbed cerebral functioning (Filley *et al.* 2001).

Neural substrate for aggressive responses

A neural substrate for the elaboration and display of aggression has been amply demonstrated in both animals and man. A large literature exists to show that in animals aggressive behaviour can be facilitated, decreased or abolished by cerebral lesions, mostly situated in or near the limbic system and hypothalamus. Bard (1928), for example, showed the importance of the caudal half of the hypothalamus for the elaboration of 'sham rage' in decorticate cats, and Klüver and Bucy (1939) demonstrated an abnormal absence of anger and fear after bitemporal lesions in monkeys. Downer (1962) elegantly showed how removal of the amygdaloid nucleus from a single temporal lobe would, after section of the cerebral commissures, allow the monkey to display normal aggressive behaviour when stimuli were fed to the sound hemisphere but unnatural tameness when fed to the lesioned side.

Delgado's work was particularly impressive in illustrating the need to take into account both intracerebral mechanisms and socioenvironmental factors in the understanding of aggressive behaviour in animals (Delgado 1969). Radio-stimulation via implanted electrodes in the amygdala, hypothalamus, septum and reticular formation allowed discrete areas of the brain to be stimulated while monkeys and chimpanzees were free-ranging and interacting with their fellows. Certain areas when stimulated produced a threatening display or social conflict, but this depended on the hierarchical position of the animal in the group; such responses could be observed when a submissive monkey was at hand as a target, but were inhibited in the presence of a dominant animal. Moreover, elicited behaviour that might be interpreted as aggressive by the experimenter was apparently not always perceived as such by the other animals in the colony.

Clinical evidence

Some of the principal evidence has come from studies of patients with epilepsy. This is set out in Chapter 6, where the question of a special association between temporal lobe epilepsy and aggressive behaviour is discussed (see Crime and epilepsy). A proportion of patients with temporal lobe epilepsy appear to show explosive aggressive tendencies, not only in relation to attacks but as an enduring trait of their per-

sonalities. Temporal lobectomy carried out for the relief of epilepsy may be followed by pronounced improvement in the control of such disorder.

When patients with and without 'affective aggression' are contrasted, the former generally turn out to have more cognitive impairments and other psychiatric symptoms. Using MRI, van Elst *et al.* (2000) showed that at least a subgroup of the aggressive patients did not show evidence of mesial temporal sclerosis, but had marked atrophy of the amygdala. A separate report from the same research group (Woermann *et al.* 2000) using voxel-based analysis of MRI showed more distant left frontal grey matter volume deficits in the aggressive group, presumably contributing to the behavioural manifestation.

Patients with cerebral tumours have occasionally been observed to show abnormal outbursts of rage and destructive behaviour. Poeck (1969) reviews the literature, showing the frequent involvement in such cases of the hypothalamus, septal regions and medial temporal structures including the hippocampus and amygdaloid nucleus. Some patients have described their condition as a feeling of rage building up in spite of themselves, others as waiting tensely for the first opportunity to release their accumulated aggression. However, Poeck stresses that the relation between symptoms and lesions is by no means strict and constant. Important additional factors derive from the premorbid emotional make-up, and the presence or absence of diffuse brain damage.

A patient reported by Sweet *et al.* (1969) showed in very striking fashion the possible relationship between a circumscribed tumour and the wildly aggressive behaviour that ultimately ensued. The case also illustrates the complex nature of 'aggressive' behaviour in humans in general, and the hazards of attempting a simplistic formulation of the nature of the link between such behaviour and cerebral pathology.

In August 1966 a young man murdered his mother and wife in their apartments, then ascended the University of Texas tower, stepped on to the parapet and killed by gunfire 14 people, wounding 24 others. In his personal diaries he had recorded over several months that something peculiar was happening to him, which he did not understand but which he was noting down in the hope that its mention would help others to do so. Five months before the mass murder he had consulted a psychiatrist, stating early in the interview that sometimes he became so mad he could 'go up to the top of that University tower and start shooting at people'. Autopsy disclosed a glioblastoma multiforme; the damage to the brain from the gunshot wounds that terminated his barrage led to uncertainty about the precise location of the walnut-sized tumour, but it was considered to be probably in the medial part of one of the temporal lobes.

Other examples of an association between a lowered threshold for aggression and brain pathology include patients who become seriously disturbed as a result of birth trauma, head injury and intracerebral infections. However, in such situations clinicopathological correlations are rarely exact enough to allow firm conclusions to be drawn about the role of circumscribed as opposed to diffuse brain damage. Moreover, there will often be intervening variables by way of affective disorder or paranoid psychosis, especially when serious violence is involved (Gunn 1993). Tonkonogy (1991) performed CT and MRI in a mixed group of patients with organic psychosyndromes who had shown repetitive violent behaviour; in 5 of 14 patients, focal lesions were observed in the anterior temporal lobe structures close to the amygdala, most often attributable to head injury. The questions of impaired control of aggression after head injury is further discussed in Chapter 4 see under Aggression and of antisocial conduct after encephalitis lethargica in Chapter 7.

Opportunities for assessing the effects of stimulating discrete brain structures in humans have occasionally appeared to yield direct evidence for the role of limbic structures in elaborating emotional responses, including short-lived feelings of rage. Heath *et al.* (1955) stimulated the amygdaloid nucleus via implanted electrodes in a chronic schizophrenic patient, resulting in a sudden rage response when the current reached a certain intensity. She was perfectly aware of her feelings and was able to discuss them objectively between stimulations. The result was unstable, however, and later stimulation of the same point produced feelings of fear in place of rage. Delgado *et al.* (1968) found that stimulation of the amygdala and hippocampus in patients with temporal lobe epilepsy produced a variety of effects including pleasant sensations, elation, deep thoughtful concentration, relaxation and colour visions. However, in one patient with postencephalitic brain damage and epilepsy, stimulation of the right amygdala led to episodes of assaultive behaviour reminiscent of her spontaneous outbursts of anger: 7 seconds after the stimulation she interrupted her activities, threw herself against the wall in a fit of rage, then paced around the room for several minutes before resuming her normal behaviour. During the elicited rage attack no seizure activity was evident on depth recording. The observation proved to be of crucial importance for selecting the appropriate site for a destructive lesion within the temporal lobe. Fenwick (1986) reviews other early studies of this nature.

Psychosurgery for aggression

It thus seems fair to conclude that pathological derangements affecting the limbic areas, and perhaps especially the amygdaloid nuclei, are capable of leading to abnormal tendencies towards aggressive behaviour in humans. The conclusion has led to attempts at modifying such behaviour by a variety of psychosurgical procedures. Unilateral temporal lobectomy can meet with success in patients with temporal lobe epilepsy, as already mentioned, but bilateral operations are contraindicated by the severe memory deficits that follow. However, Turner (1969, 1972) reported success with bilateral division of tracts within the temporal lobes and with posterior cingulectomy, mostly in patients with temporal lobe epilepsy but also in some abnormally aggressive patients who had never had seizures.

Attention has also been directed at stereotactic operations on the amygdaloid nuclei in patients with temporal lobe epilepsy and violent behaviour (Hitchcock *et al.* 1972; Mark *et al.* 1972). The results were reported as often markedly successful, and without disabling side effects. Narabayashi performed amygdalectomies on one or both sides in a large population of patients, some with epilepsy and some with 'severe behaviour disorders and hyperexcitability' (Narabayashi *et al.* 1963; Narabayashi & Uno 1966). Nearly all were mentally subnormal. Generally positive results were claimed. It is hard in these reports to discern how specific were the effects on aggressive behaviour, and how far the improvements may have been related to improved control of epilepsy. An enormous series has been reported by Ramamurthi (1988) in India of 481 cases of bilateral amygdalotomy and 122 with mostly secondary posteromedian hypothalamotomies for otherwise untreatable aggression. Good results are asserted on three-quarters of the cohort which, it is claimed, persisted in the majority at 3 years. Naturally, randomised and double-blind evaluation of such treatments are difficult to achieve but one cannot be confident that these results are generalisable to clinical practice in most parts of the world. Advances in psychopharmacology combined with the social controversy surrounding psychosurgical treatments, especially when applied to minors and to persons held in custody on account of offences, means that such approaches are likely to be seen increasingly as an absolute last resort.

Habitually aggressive offenders

We must now consider the situation in individuals who display persistently aggressive behaviour yet who lack overt evidence of brain pathology. These are the persons traditionally labelled as 'aggressive psychopaths' or as having an 'explosive personality disorder'. Their outbursts of violence are usually merely a part of wide-ranging personality and social maladjustments. They are notoriously resistant to efforts at therapeutic intervention, yet many seem to outgrow their aggressive propensities in middle years. It is obviously a matter of importance to attempt to clarify whether in some such persons there are definable abnormalities of the neural apparatus subserving aggressive responses, and to what degree such abnormalities are inherited or acquired.

It has been known for many decades that a high proportion of persons with disturbed personalities, especially those who show aggressive antisocial behaviour, have abnormal

EEGs. Such EEG abnormalities involve the temporal lobes particularly, are often of a type suggesting cerebral immaturity, and tend to decrease with age in parallel with improvements in behaviour. Hill (1944) found that the abnormalities in aggressive psychopaths were often bilateral, synchronous, and postcentral in location, suggesting dysfunction in subcortical centres or the deep temporal grey matter.

Williams (1969) reinforced the importance of earlier findings. In a review of EEGs carried out on over 300 men convicted of violent crimes, he found that of those who had a history of habitual aggression or explosive rage, 65% had abnormal EEGs. When persons with disabilities suggesting structural brain damage were excluded (i.e. those who were mentally subnormal, had epilepsy, or with a history of major head injury) the figure remained high at 57%, around four to five times higher than in infrequently violent people from the same sample.

Since the early EEG studies, the full armamentarium of neurological investigations has been applied to people with serious aggression. This has been thoroughly reviewed recently with an emphasis on frontal lobe dysfunction (Brower and Price 2001). The participants in such studies tend to be drawn from a variety of settings, from the community to specialist forensic psychiatric units. The nature of the sample has a great bearing on the results, as does the extent to which potential confounding factors, such as drug and alcohol abuse, psychosocial deprivation, psychiatric disorder, epilepsy and legal implications, are taken into account. Most neuropsychological studies do indeed show an association between violent behaviour and executive deficits but the association is rather non-specific. The review cites studies using MRI that have shown, for example, reduced prefrontal grey matter volume in a small group with antisocial personality disorder even in comparison to a substance-dependent control group. A further study using FDG-PET on 41 'murderers' revealed reduced metabolic activity in prefrontal (and left subcortical) structures and this seemed to apply most to those without psychosocial risk factors for aggression and whose pattern of behaviour was of the non-predatory type (Brower & Price 2001). There is insufficient evidence to point more precisely to areas in the cortex or even prefrontal cortex that might subserve aggressive behaviour, but the authors suggest that dorsolateral and medial frontal abnormalities may relate to aggression of the impulsive versus unempathic varieties, respectively.

Episodic dyscontrol (intermittent explosive disorder)

After excluding patients who have demonstrable epilepsy, brain damage or psychotic illness as a basis for their aggressive acts (also those pursuing a motivated career of premeditated crime for gain), one is left with a number of persons who may be victims of their disturbed cerebral physiology. The essence of the claim is that violent behaviour can, in effect, be the only overt symptom of brain disorder.

The great majority of such persons are male, from seriously disturbed family backgrounds, and with a history of repeated outbursts of violent behaviour dating back to adolescence or even childhood. Provocation for such outbursts has often been minimal. Evidence of minor neurological dysfunction is not uncommon and there is a high frequency of abnormal EEGs, often involving the temporal lobes and sometimes quasi-epileptic in nature. Many have symptoms reminiscent of epileptic phenomena, even when not suffering from seizures; in particular the outbursts may be preceded or followed by features akin to those seen with temporal lobe epilepsy. The implication is that such persons have functional abnormalities of the neural systems subserving aggressive responses, which set the threshold for the elicitation of outbursts at an unusually low level.

Such a 'syndrome' appears to stand at the borderland between what is conventionally regarded as psychopathic personality and what with more definite clinical evidence might be included as temporal lobe epilepsy. Clear definition of the syndrome, and estimates of its frequency, are rendered difficult by the elusive nature of the ancillary evidence of cerebral dysfunction, and the ever-present confounding evidence of social and interpersonal stresses in the group.

The status, and indeed the existence, of the syndrome remains a matter of controversy. Some regard the concept as useful in clinical practice, which may benefit from treatment in its own right (Olvera 2002), while recognising that it cuts across traditional diagnostic boundaries (Elliott 1992). Others regard it as serving no useful purpose. Lucas (1994) presents a detailed review of the evolution of the concept and concludes that its nosological status is invalid. He stresses that it lacks clear demarcation from allied forms of disordered behaviour, and suggests that it represents one extreme of a continuum rather than a distinct nosological category.

Schizophrenia

Schizophrenia has proved to be an increasingly fruitful arena for neuropsychiatric research. Ever since its earliest delineation from Kraepelin's time, an organic contribution to the disorder has been suspected and is now increasingly accepted. Some thinkers have even gone so far as to predict that schizophrenia will soon be seen as quintessentially neuropsychiatric, the first in a wave of classical psychiatric disorders to be reclassified in a brave new era of enlightenment and pathophysiologically based diagnoses. So far this has not happened. What has occurred is that following a massive if uncoordinated international research effort, the brain basis of schizophrenia has become an essential part of the tenets of mainstream general psychiatry no longer requiring the prefix 'biological' or 'neuro-'. Hence, some mention of the neuropsychology, neuroanatomy, neurophysiology, neurochemistry and neuropathology of schizophrenia is to be expected in any manual of psychiatry and even a cursory discussion of the current state of evidence in each of these areas could stretch to many volumes. It may be that, over the horizon, there will be a discovery that renders much of this information redundant, so that in the next edition of this textbook a few concise paragraphs will be all that is required to outline the genes, brain systems, neurotransmitters and proteins that cause schizophrenia, followed over the page by the cure. Alas, for the time being it not possible to predict what promising avenues will lead to dead ends and what marginal observations will turn out to be breakthroughs.

What follows therefore is a highly partial account of schizophrenia through the filter of clinical neuropsychiatry. This comprises, first, a picture of schizophrenia as a neurological disorder, with emphasis on its associated cognitive and neurological deficits (with heavy reliance on MRI). Next, the symptomatic schizophrenia concept is discussed. The latter presents regularly in clinical contexts, for instance when investigation of a patient diagnosed with schizophrenia brings to light a significant brain or toxic abnormality. Finally, some implications of research in schizophrenia for the rest of neuropsychiatry is outlined.

Schizophrenia and neuropsychological impairment

The earlier term for schizophrenia, 'dementia praecox' (premature dementia), makes it clear how central cognitive impairment was to the early conceptualisation of the disorder. What has remained contested is whether such impairment is confined to some functions while sparing others and what is its temporal sequence. That is, is it there premorbidly, at the onset of the illness and does it accumulate as the disorder progresses?

When patients with chronic schizophrenia are assessed with a 'standard' clinical neuropsychological battery, their performance does not distinguish them from other neurological cases, including those with amnesia (see Memory disorder in the psychoses). Furthermore, elderly patients with schizophrenia will, on average, perform as badly on neuropsychological tests as patients with moderate Alzheimer's disease, with only marginally superior memory and inferior executive and motor functions (Davidson et al. 1996). Unselected convenience samples of schizophrenia patients will usually show impairments on a range of cognitive test between 1 and 3 standard deviations below the population mean (equivalent to 15–45 IQ points) and recent work on patients in their first episode confirms that much of this impairment is present from the beginning (Heinrichs & Zakzanis 1998; Bilder et al. 2002). Consistent with this is the failure to find marked cognitive decline following the first episode up to 5 years later. The very latest research using serial structural MRI measures is beginning to challenge this. There appears to be a general loss of brain substance (grey more than white) in patients with schizophrenia after their first episode, which seems to represent an acceleration of the normal age-related decline. This may be a strand of evidence

in favour of a 'neurodegenerative' element to schizophrenia (see below) but currently attention is focusing on the possible effects of medications, particularly typical or first-generation antipsychotics (Lieberman et al. 2005).

Premorbid and illness- and symptom-related cognitive deficits

One of the few consistent findings in the literature is that people destined to develop schizophrenia show, as a group, delayed developmental milestones and social development, plus inferior academic performance at school and on cognitive tests, in comparison to their peers. Studies that have compared schizophrenic-to-be children with their siblings have confirmed patients' lower premorbid IQs but reveal a less marked discrepancy than when classmates are used for comparison. The greatest discrepancy arises when schizophrenic-to-be children are compared with population norms (Aylward et al. 1984).

Getting an accurate picture of premorbid deficits in routine clinical practice is difficult unless school reports over many years have been retained. Tests of reading ability, such as the National Adult Reading Test, have been shown to be relatively immune from acquired cognitive decline so may serve as a proxy for premorbid ability (Crawford et al. 1992).

By far the strongest evidence comes from longitudinal birth cohorts from the UK and conscript cohorts from Sweden and Israel. The National Survey of Health and Development (Jones et al. 1994) comprised a random sample of all UK births in a single week in March 1946 (approximately 5000) and was studied on 19 occasions between the ages of 2 and 43 years on a number of health and social variables. Cases of schizophrenia (30 meeting DSM-IIIR criteria) were identified in the course of these assessments and from a register of psychiatric hospital admissions. The cases tended to score lower on all tests of educational abilities carried out at ages 8, 11 and 15, the deficit increasing with age. The other cohort was started in 1958 and became known as the National Child Development Survey (Done et al. 1994). It too consisted of all births in a single week. Individuals were assessed at ages 7, 11 and 16 on a large variety of health, psychological and social variables. There were approximately 40 such cases who met 'narrow' schizophrenia criteria and these were contrasted with a comparable group of pre-affective disorder and pre-neurosis children. The pre-schizophrenics showed a stable pattern of psychometric test score deficits equivalent to around 8–9 IQ points.

A cohort of Swedish men conscripted into the armed forces in 1969 has been followed up to the age of 43. Of around 50 000, some 362 developed schizophrenia (Zammit et al. 2004). There was a strong linear trend which showed that the lower the IQ was at age 18, the greater the risk of schizophrenia, with an approximately 10-fold difference between a low-borderline IQ and a superior IQ. It was as though the whole population of pre-schizophrenics had an IQ shifted downwards by 5–10 IQ points. This pattern is not seen in bipolar disorder. When the individual tests were examined there was a hint that verbal tests and those which required a degree of planning and strategy were more sensitive to the cognitive problems associated with schizophrenia but the overall finding was of a non-specific cognitive impairment (David *et al.* 1997). Note that cognitive functioning could not be regarded as 'abnormal' at this time.

The Israeli conscript cohort studies comprised both men and women and involved 536 people with schizophrenia (Reichenberg *et al.* 2002). Again, the results were remarkably consistent, with those destined to develop schizophrenia scoring lower on a range of tests, be they non-verbal such as the Raven's Progressive Matrices, or verbal, arithmetic or abstract reasoning (speaking and reading being spared). The effect sizes were between 0.2 and 0.6, which can be roughly translated into a 4–8 IQ points deficit. It should be noted that these cohort studies made efforts to control for behavioural and social problems, which might have confounded the results, and for prodromal decline. Hence cognitive efficiency is clearly suboptimal prior to the onset of schizophrenia but not in a way that could easily be detected clinically because it is neither particularly marked nor unusual in its pattern. This raises the question as to how this subtle cognitive dysfunction turns into the large neuropsychological deficits affecting patients with the disorder. Very few longitudinal studies have spanned the premorbid and postmorbid phases of the illness, an exception being that by Caspi *et al.* (2003) on the Israeli conscripts. They showed that when individuals were retested after a single episode of schizophrenia on the same battery of tests they had when inducted into the army, they tended to show a drop in reasoning, mental speed and concentration; if not, they certainly failed as a group to show any improvement on the tasks, which, however minor, was seen in the healthy control conscripts.

The remaining illness-related neuropsychological deficits prominent in cross-sectional studies of patients is yet to be fully explained. As implied above, it applies to established cases, as well as first-onset and drug-free patients (Saykin *et al.* 1994) and there is surprisingly little resolution after the episode has abated (Censits *et al.* 1997). Nevertheless some of the decline can probably be put down to the unfortunate combination of lost opportunities, physical illness, substance misuse, medication, lack of motivation, social isolation and selection factors, although why a small number of patients show a massive decline in intellectual functioning, sometimes in spite of relatively good symptom control, remains a mystery.

Generalised or specific?

Prior to the onset of schizophrenia it is clear that most if not all cognitive functions show some compromise. The same is true in the full-blown disorder (Heinrichs & Zakzanis 1998) but it has repeatedly been claimed that some test scores seem

to be disproportionately impaired and others relatively spared, i.e. there are specific neuropsychological deficits. Visual perception, recognition, naming and procedural or motor learning are relatively spared while executive functions (including working memory, tasks of set shifting, ignoring irrelevance, forward planning) and memory (Aleman *et al.* 1999), especially verbal and semantic, tend to be the functions more obviously affected. Hence it is not unreasonable to begin to talk of a schizophrenia profile. The Wisconsin Card Sorting Test is widely regarded as a test of frontal lobe/executive functioning (see Chapter 3, under Frontal lobe ('executive function') tests) and has been used frequently in studies of schizophrenia. Patients tend to perform badly, and this is interpreted as evidence of a specific frontal/executive deficit. However, the counter-argument is that given the general intellectual demands of the task in terms of working memory and sustained attention, as well as set-shifting and response inhibition, such an inference may be questioned. Indeed Dickinson *et al.* (2004) showed that most of the cognitive impairment in patients could be explained by a single factor (cf. IQ).

One reason why more specificity has not emerged may be that the 'schizophrenias' are heterogeneous at the cognitive level and that separating patients according to symptom pattern or syndrome might clarify the matter. Liddle (1987) found that symptoms of schizophrenia aggregated into three broad clusters: psychomotor poverty (affecting speech and movement and blunting of affect); reality distortion (essentially positive symptoms, hallucinations and delusions); and finally disorganisation (including thought disorder and inappropriate affect). Using a battery of neuropsychological tests, he showed that psychomotor poverty was associated with poorer performance on abstract reasoning and long-term memory tests, disorganisation on impairments of attention and learning, while the reality distortion symptoms correlated with impaired figure–ground perception (traditionally temporoparietal tests). Subsequently, Liddle *et al.* (1992) employed functional neuroimaging techniques to corroborate these clusters. ^{15}O-PET indices of resting regional cerebral blood flow (rCBF) were measured in cohorts of chronic schizophrenic patients with contrasting patterns of symptomatology. Patients classified as having the *psychomotor poverty syndrome* (i.e. poverty of speech, flattened affect and decreased spontaneous movement) showed decreased rCBF in the left prefrontal and parietal cortex, along with increases in the caudate nuclei. The area of left prefrontal hypoperfusion coincided with that shown by Frith *et al.* (1991) to be activated by the internal generation of willed as compared with routine actions. Patients with the *disorganisation syndrome* (disordered thought and inappropriate affect) showed increased resting rCBF most markedly in the anterior cingulate region. This coincides with the area maximally activated during performance of the Stroop test, in which competing responses must be suppressed (see Chapter 3, under Stroop tests); hence it may reflect a struggle in such patients to suppress inappropriate mental activity. Patients with the *reality distortion syndrome* (delusions and hallucinations) showed increases in rCBF most prominently in the left parahippocampal gyrus and contiguous areas. In each syndrome the detailed patterns of blood flow indicated that distributed neuronal networks rather than specific loci were implicated in the underlying abnormalities of brain function.

Much work has been done along these lines. At the risk of not doing justice to this work, a broad summary might be that, in general, standard neuropsychological tests do not show noticeable correlations with key symptoms such as hallucinations and delusions. Experimental paradigms that involve signal detection, source monitoring or attribution processes, alone or in combination, have helped to conceptualise hallucinations in cognitive terms (David 2004) and probabilistic reasoning plays some role in delusions (Gilleen & David 2005; Freeman 2007). Thought disorder does appear to be related to semantic processes and abnormal syntax (see Language and schizophrenia: the problem of 'thought disorder', earlier). Negative or deficit symptoms map more easily onto those deficits familiar in neurologically damaged patients. Lack of motivation, motor slowing, loss of initiative and affective flattening may all be seen in neurological patients, particularly those with frontal–striatal dysfunction, and the corresponding neuropsychological tests usually reflect these impairments (for further reading see David & Cutting 1994; Sharma & Harvey 2000). Social cognitive deficits are of topical interest and it has been proposed that the inability to infer correctly the beliefs, feelings and intentions of others (to have a 'theory of [other] minds') may underlie paranoia as well as inappropriate social behaviours (Frith 1992; Gilleen & David 2005).

Neuropsychological function has been related to various indices of outcome and predictors of rehabilitation success. Indeed, such functioning is a much stronger predictor of global outcome than symptoms. In a thorough review of the literature, Green (1996) and Green *et al.* (2000) concluded that the most consistent finding was that verbal memory was associated with all types of functional outcome so that deficits in this function could limit the level of outcome. Vigilance was related to social problem-solving and skill acquisition while card sorting predicted functioning in the community.

Structural brain imaging

Pathology at the microscopic level is still held up as the defining characteristic of a disease. The application of neuropathology to schizophrenia is reviewed below but its influence on the efforts to understand schizophrenia as a brain disease has recently been overshadowed by *in vivo* neuroimaging, especially MRI. The reasons are obvious: high-level anatomical information can be gleaned from any and all types of patient; samples can be studied that begin to meet epidemiological standards in terms of representativeness and lack of

bias; associations with relevant aetiological factors such as family history, treatment response and phase of illness can all be studied systematically without the need to wait for death and to contend with post-mortem artefacts.

Studies of structural neuroimaging in schizophrenia have parallels with neuropsychology. Quantitative reviews of studies using CT (van Horn & McManus 1992) show clear evidence for generalised loss of tissue (large ventricles and smaller cortical thickness). The body of work relating to structural MRI is now vast and has been subjected to several meta-analyses. These studies, in demonstrating and indeed quantifying consistently observed effects, will inevitably downgrade findings relating to specific brain structures in individual studies. Hence it remains possible that a particular neuroanatomical structure (or network of structures) deemed key to schizophrenia would nevertheless, because of its size, location or difficulties in measurement, be submerged among the larger effect sizes highlighted by meta-analytic reviews.

The most striking finding from both CT and MRI is the increase in ventricular size, a 40% increase being the median value reported in a review of volumetric MRI studies by Lawrie and Abukmeil (1998). Nevertheless, the range of values in schizophrenia overlaps considerably with the normal population so this finding has little clinical utility. The same reviewers calculated that the average loss of brain tissue was a mere 3%, with an effect size (i.e. units of standard deviation) of 0.26. If there is a region that seems to attract more tissue loss than the brain as a whole it is the temporal lobes, with around 8% loss on average in the same review. A more sophisticated analytic approach was taken by Wright *et al.* (2000) in their summation of 58 MRI studies involving 1588 patients with schizophrenia in total. The overall loss of brain volume was 2% and the overall increase in ventricular volume was 26%, mostly accounted for by increase in the body of the lateral ventricles. Medial temporal structures stood out from the rest, with the amygdalae, hippocampi and parahippocampi down by about 6% on both sides; however, this was equivalent to effect sizes (for hippocampus and parahippocampus) of between 0.4 and 0.69, in the moderate range.

The origin of these changes has been illuminated by application of MRI to monozygotic twins discordant for schizophrenia (Suddath *et al.* 1990). As well as having larger ventricles, affected twins had smaller temporal lobes and hippocampi than their co-twins. This compelling work confirmed the association between medial temporal volume loss and the schizophrenia phenotype as well as implying a necessary role for non-genetic factors, obstetric complications being a prime suspect (Dalman *et al.* 2001; Thomas *et al.* 2001; Cannon *et al.* 2002). Subsequent research has shown that unaffected relatives of people with schizophrenia tend to have larger ventricles than non-related controls.

The frontal lobes, despite their obvious functional relevance to schizophrenia, do not show quite the same level of structural loss, with a mean reduction effect size of 0.36 in a meta-analysis of 22 structural imaging studies (Zakzanis & Heinrichs 1999). Most studies have shown that grey matter takes the brunt of volume changes (Zipursky *et al.* 1992), although this may be partly due to the difficulty in defining white matter tracts reliably enough for volumetric measurement. Large white matter tracts such as the corpus callosum are easy to define, especially in the sagittal plane. This has been shown to be reduced in size in a small meta-analysis (Woodruff *et al.* 1995). Voxel-based methods of analysis avoid the difficulty (and tedium) of tracing around predetermined anatomical regions and are increasingly being employed in structural neuroimaging research. First, each subject's volumetric dataset must be transformed into a standard space and then an average brain volume for one group may be compared (by computer), voxel by voxel, with another. When used in schizophrenia, both white and grey matter regions (medial temporal lobe again, plus insula and prefrontal regions) may be identified as having reduced density, which probably translates to reduced volume (Shapleske *et al.* 2002; Honea *et al.* 2005) (Fig. 2.2: see also Plate 2.2).

In contrast to the repeated finding of reduced cerebral volume, the striatum (particularly the caudate) has been found to be increased in size. This has been attributed to treatment with conventional neuroleptic drugs.

Associations with regional brain pathology

Neurologist Fred Plum (1972) was led to make the memorable remark that 'schizophrenia is the graveyard of neuropathologists'. Now there has been an upsurge of interest in neuropathology, fuelled in part by the findings from neuroimaging and molecular biology (Harrison 1999; Harrison & Weinberger 2005). Plum's remark has been interpreted in several ways: first as a warning to pathologists to steer clear of schizophrenia if they wish their careers to survive, but second that the brain in schizophrenia is like a graveyard, in the sense that all sorts of odd things may be found there – gliosis, infarctions, dysplasias and so on. This latter interpretation is at least empirically supportable. Classical reviews by Davison and Bagley (1969) and Davison (1983) should be consulted as summaries of the rich literature before the era of CT. The coexistence of brain lesions or pathology in people

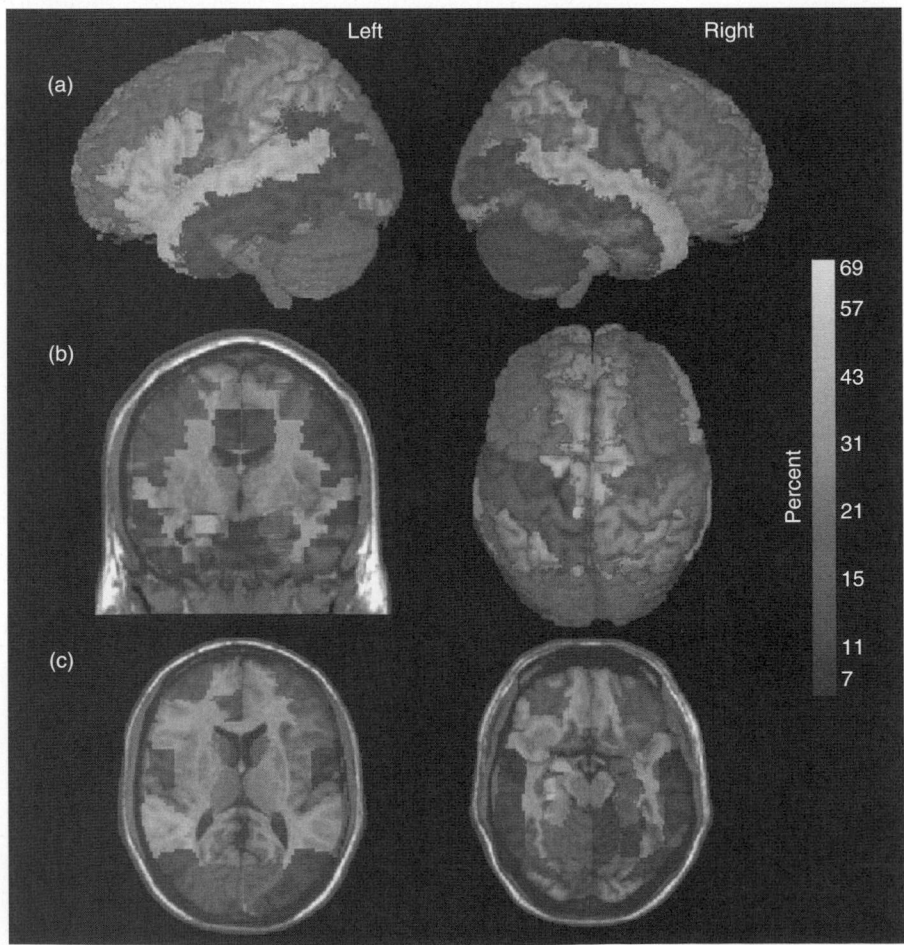

Fig. 2.2 Brain regions in which significant volume deficits in patients with schizophrenia were reported in voxel-based morphometry studies (*N*=15), by percentage of studies reporting the deficit. In row (a), left and right whole-brain three-dimensional images are overlaid with all regions in which significant volume deficits in patients with schizophrenia were reported. In row (b), a coronal view and an axial three-dimensional image are shown. In row (c), axial views are shown. From Honea *et al.* (2005), *American Journal of Psychiatry* **162**, 2233–2245. © 2005 American Psychiatric Association. See also Plate 2.2.

with schizophrenia raises nosological problems. For example, is any association with brain damage fortuitous or due to the unmasking of a genetic liability to the disorder, or more directly related by way of a causal influence of the brain lesion on the development of the schizophrenia? Harrison (1999) estimated from a thorough review of the neuropathology literature that up to 50% of brains from patients with schizophrenia contain non-specific focal degenerative abnormalities, such as small infarcts and white matter changes. He took these to be mostly if not always coincidental, since they were variable in distribution and nature, and reported as unrelated to the clinical picture occurring well after the onset of symptoms in some cases. Nevertheless, the conclusion emerges that lesions, particularly of the temporal lobes and diencephalon, appear to carry a small but definite risk of increasing the likelihood that a schizophrenia-like illness will develop. This hazard appears to exceed what would be expected in view of the known genetic propensities in the populations concerned. It has not yet been clarified whether such schizophrenias are identical in every respect with the naturally occurring idiopathic disorder, in particular with regard to the course followed. Phenomenologically, however, they appear to be indistinguishable from schizophrenias occurring in the absence of brain disease (Table 2.1).

Irrespective of such nosological refinements, the striking fact appears to be that psychotic illnesses with the major features of schizophrenia may coexist with cerebral lesions and may be generated in some fashion by them. The acute and chronic organic reactions described in Chapter 1 are by no means the exclusive hallmarks of mental disorder occasioned by cerebral dysfunction. The corollary implication is that while in the great majority of schizophrenias no clear-cut brain lesion will be revealed by routine investigation, in some patients there may be identifiable pathology that warrants careful appraisal.

The evidence incriminating the temporal lobes and diencephalon has come from diverse forms of cerebral pathology. That concerning head injuries is described in Chapter 4 (Psychoses), that for cerebral tumours in Chapter 5 (Temporal lobe tumours) and that for epilepsy in Chapter 6 (Postictal disorders). While far from satisfactory or entirely conclusive, for the reasons discussed above, the sum total of evidence begins to look impressive. Other clinical evidence has pointed to disease of the basal ganglia as having a special relationship with schizophrenia-like illnesses, for example in Huntington's disease (Chapter 9), Wilson's disease (Chapter 12) and the rare syndrome of idiopathic calcification of the basal ganglia (Chapter 10). Bowman and Lewis (1980) reinforced this association in their analysis of the site of major pathology in a large variety of cerebral disorders liable to show aspects of schizophrenic symptomatology.

It remains puzzling that frontal lesions are not more often incriminated, with the exception of occasional disorders such as metachromatic leucodystrophy (Chapter 14). Occasional anecdotal reports of schizophrenia following frontal damage are therefore of interest.

Table 2.1 Certainty and doubt in schizophrenia neuropathology. (From Harrison 1999.)

Macroscopic findings	
Enlarged lateral and third ventricles	++++
Decreased cortical volume	++++
Above changes present in first-episode patients	+++
Disproportionate volume loss from temporal lobe (including hippocampus)	+++
Decreased thalamic volume	++
Cortical volume loss affects grey rather than white matter	++
Enlarged basal ganglia secondary to antipsychotic medication	+++
Histological findings	
Absence of gliosis as an intrinsic feature	+++
Smaller cortical and hippocampal neurones	+++
Fewer neurones in dorsal thalamus	+++
Reduced synaptic and dendritic markers in hippocampus	++
Maldistribution of white matter neurones	+
Entorhinal cortex dysplasia	±
Disarray of hippocampal neurones	±
Miscellaneous	
Alzheimer's disease is not commoner in schizophrenia	++++
Pathology interacts with cerebral asymmetries	++

±, weak; +, moderate; ++, good; +++, strong; ++++, shown by meta-analysis.

A young man with a family history of depression suffered several episodes of bipolar affective illness over a 2-year period. He then sustained a head injury leading to a left frontal haematoma that necessitated a left frontal lobectomy. Nine months later he developed a classic schizophrenic illness which pursued a chronic course during 6 years' follow-up. A spike-discharging focus was detected 3 years after the injury when he developed epileptic seizures. The authors suggest that the transformation from bipolar affective disorder to schizophrenia, in a patient genetically predisposed to the former, was due to the unusual combination of damage to the left frontal lobe and an excitatory lesion in the left temporal lobe (Pang & Lewis 1996).

A boy sustained a blow to the head in the left frontal parietal region after being knocked from his bicycle by a car at the age of 14 years. There was no fracture, but he was unconscious for 3 or 4 hours and had a lowered level of consciousness for 2 weeks. EEGs at the time and 10 years later were normal. At the age of 16 he presented to psychiatric services following a suicide attempt. He had elaborate delusions of persecution, inappropriate affect and auditory hallucinations. Psychologically he was assessed to be in the bright normal range. An MRI scan carried out at the time of the report, when the patient was in his late twenties, showed generalised ventricular dilatation perhaps greater on the left. There was a family history of psychosis in a maternal cousin but no history of obstetric or perinatal complications. The patient responded to standard treatment (O'Callaghan et al. 1988).

A whole range of abnormalities not listed in Table 2.1 may also be found in the brains of people with psychotic disorder, namely those of developmental origin. These include agenesis of the corpus callosum (David et al. 1993), cavum septum pellucidum, aqueduct stenosis, arachnoid cysts, and so on (Shenton et al. 2001). Some of these would undoubtedly have gone unnoticed were it not for the widespread use of MRI. In clinical settings these disorders sometimes make atypical features of the patient's presentation more comprehensible, such as mild learning difficulty and motor clumsiness or minor physical anomalies. Anecdotally, such anomalies seem to confer a degree of treatment resistance. Statements on the aetiological relevance to schizophrenia requires a ratio to be calculated of the true rate of the abnormality in question in a representative sample of patients against that in the general population. We are beginning to see sufficient MRI research using 'healthy' or near-healthy controls to come up with just such figures. It turns out that of 1000 people, including some elderly, who had volunteered to be controls in

various research projects in the USA, 18% had abnormal MRI scans, although in just under 3% was this deemed to require a referral (Katzman et al. 1999). In some other surveys, confined to younger people, even higher levels of abnormalities have been reported. For example in a study of 98 controls, 152 with first-episode psychoses and 90 with chronic schizophrenia, 24%, 22% and 50% had abnormal MR scans, respectively, as judged by a radiologist blind to diagnosis (Lubman et al. 2002). Apart from possible evidence of demyelination, infarction, trauma, focal atrophy and white matter hyperintensities (see Chapter 3, White matter hyperintensities), developmental anomalies such as cerebellar ectopia, cavum septum pellucidum, pineal cysts and hamartomas were seen. Again, few required further investigation. Taking these findings together with numerous case reports, it is very likely that such abnormalities are more common in schizophrenia but only account for a small minority of cases. This may be taken as general evidence consistent with the view that disruption in neurodevelopment is a key aspect if not an essential part of the disorder.

While the widespread application of CT and MRI has uncovered cases of brain pathology that might otherwise have been missed, a thorough and systematic medical review will also reveal a small number of cases in whom a systemic disease may be of aetiological relevance. A cohort of 268 first-episode schizophrenia cases investigated by Johnstone et al. (1987) produced 15 patients (<6%) with relevant organic disease. These included three cases of syphilis, two of sarcoidosis, and one each of carcinoma of the lung, autoimmune multisystem disease, cerebral cysticercosis and thyroid disease. Substance abuse and previous head injury accounted for the rest.

Neuropathology

A detailed knowledge of the microscopic pathology in the brains of people with schizophrenia is beyond the scope of this book. For a summary of the current state of the art, it would be hard to better Harrison's comprehensive and accessible review (Harrison 1999). He concludes that the best explanation for the reduction in cerebral volume discussed above is reduced neuropil and neuronal size, rather than a loss of neurones. Such morphometric changes are, according to Harrison, suggestive of alterations in synaptic, dendritic and axonal organisation, a view supported by immunocytochemical and ultrastructural findings. Other cytoarchitectural features purported to be more frequent in schizophrenia, such as entorhinal cortex heterotopias and hippocampal neuronal disarray, remain to be confirmed. Importantly, Harrison does not view gliosis as an intrinsic feature, the implication of this being that the disordered brain in schizophrenia is not a response to an acquired insult or disease process as usually understood but rather it supports the hypothesis that schizophrenia is a disorder of prenatal neurodevelopment, and in this respect is quite unlike Alzheimer's disease for example. In another invaluable summary of this rapidly evolving field, Harrison and Weinberger (2005) summarise evidence linking neuropathology with the identification of several putative susceptibility genes (including neuregulin, dysbindin, *COMT, DISC1, RGS4, GRM3* and *G72*). The authors speculate that these genes may all converge functionally on schizophrenia risk via an influence on synaptic plasticity and the development and stabilisation of cortical microcircuitry. In a further attempt at integration, the authors try to link these findings with the known neurochemistry of schizophrenia and conclude that NMDA receptor-mediated glutamate transmission may be especially implicated, along with of course dopamine and possibly γ-aminobutyric acid (GABA) signalling (Table 2.2).

Functional brain imaging

Functional imaging studies effectively took origin from Ingvar and Franzen's (1974) demonstration of diminished cerebral blood flow to frontal regions in older chronic schizophrenic patients. Subsequent PET studies have given variable results, as reviewed by Bench *et al.* (1990) and Buchsbaum (1990), seemingly due to variations in technique and differences in the populations investigated. Nevertheless, most reports have shown lower metabolism in the frontal and temporal regions and basal ganglia than in posterior brain areas. With further experience, however, such hypometabolism appears to lack specificity in that it may also be seen in some degree in patients with depressive illness (see Executive (frontal lobe) syndromes, earlier). Weinberger *et al.*

(1991) concluded that in all studies which have used cognitive tasks demanding prefrontal activation, schizophrenia patients have tended to show a 'hypofrontal' pattern as measured by cerebral blood flow or glucose utilisation. This provides a tempting explanation for such common symptoms as affective blunting and impaired volition. Taking this further, Frith (1995) points out, for example, that 'self-monitoring' depends on a tight correspondence between anterior brain regions concerned with voluntary motor output and posterior regions concerned with the relevant sensory inputs. When normal subjects generate words there is an increase in blood flow to the dorsolateral prefrontal cortex and an associated decrease in the superior temporal cortex. In schizophrenic patients performing the same task, the dorsolateral prefrontal cortex increase was not associated with decreases in the left superior temporal cortex, implying a lack of connectivity between these two brain areas.

Despite the elegance of much functional MRI research in human subjects, its ability to reveal previously hidden truths about schizophrenia is limited. This stems from the problem in interpreting reduced activation in the light of virtually universally poorer performance. This is especially relevant to functional imaging of prefrontal deficits. When performance is equated, unusual patterns of activation may be seen, such as hyperfrontality, one interpretation being that patients are having to 'work harder' to produce adequate performance. Many researchers have grappled with this problem. Lahti *et al.* (2001) examined activation in deficit and non-deficit patients and showed that overall levels of activation

Table 2.2 Schizophrenia susceptibility genes and the strength of evidence in four domains. (From Harrison & Weinberger 2005.)

Gene	Locus	Strength of evidence (0 to +++++)* for			
		Association with schizophrenia	Linkage to gene locus	Biological plausibility	Altered expression in schizophrenia
COMT	22q11	++++	++++	++++	Yes, +
DTNBP1	6p22	+++++	++++	++	Yes, ++
NRG1	8p12–21	+++++	++++	+++	Yes, +
RGS4	1q21–22	+++	+++	+++	Yes, ++
GRM3	7q21–22	+++	+	++++	No, ++
DISC1	1q42	+++	++	++	Not known
G72	13q32–34	+++	++	++	Not known
DAAO	12q24	++	+	++++	Not known
PPP3CC	8p21	+	++++	++++	Yes, +
CHRNA7	15q13–14	+	++	+++	Yes, +++
PRODH2	22q11	+	++++	++	No, +
Akt1	14q22–32	+	+	++	Yes, ++

Note: Ratings are of course subjective and transient.
*Based on sample sizes and numbers of replications, not the magnitude of the relative risk; +++ is equivalent to at least three positive independent studies.

were similar between the patient groups and healthy controls on a control sensory motor task, but that only deficit patients failed to activate right middle frontal cortex in relation to a decision task. Cannon *et al.* (2005) made use of a visuospatial working memory task and variable memory load. It was the need to manipulate the visual material in mind that uncovered the patients' failure to increase activation in the dorsolateral prefrontal cortex and this was reflected in a falling off in performance.

Interesting attempts have also been made to explore differences on neuroimaging between schizophrenic patients with and without persistent auditory hallucinations. McGuire *et al.* (1993) obtained clear-cut results by arranging for each patient to serve as his own control, carrying out hexamethylpropyleneamine oxine (HMPAO)-SPECT scans (Chapter 3) first in the presence of ongoing auditory verbal hallucinations, then again some weeks later when these had largely resolved. On each occasion the patient was asked to signal the presence or absence of hallucinations immediately prior to the injection of HMPAO. Increased blood flow was demonstrated in Broca's area during the occurrence of hallucinations, i.e. the area that has been implicated in the subvocal rehearsal of inner speech (Paulesu *et al.* 1993). Such a finding supports the idea that hallucinations arise from the patient's failure to monitor his own thoughts and 'inner speech', which is therefore regarded as alien and perceived as emanating from others.

In a further study, schizophrenic patients liable to auditory verbal hallucinations were compared with those who were not, even though hallucinations were not occurring at the time of testing (McGuire *et al.* 1995). ^{15}O-PET scans were carried out while the subject imagined sentences being spoken in another person's voice. In normal subjects this task is associated with increased activity in such areas as the left inferior frontal gyrus, the supplementary motor area and the left temporal cortex (McGuire *et al.* 1996). Patients prone to hallucinations showed the expected increase in frontal activity, but reductions rather than increases in the supplementary motor area and left temporal regions. Thus it appeared that a predisposition to auditory verbal hallucinations was reflected in aberrant connectivity between the areas concerned with the generation and monitoring of inner speech.

Functional MRI (see Chapter 3) has also been used to explore the cerebral correlates of auditory verbal hallucinations (David *et al.* 1996). Images were obtained during periods of auditory stimulation (speech) and visual stimulation (flashing lights), both when the patient was hallucinating and when he was not. Activation to visual stimulation occurred in the visual cortex irrespective of the presence or absence of auditory hallucinations, whereas temporal lobe activation to auditory stimulation was almost completely suppressed while hallucinations were in progress. David *et al.* interpret this as reflecting physiological competition for a common neural substrate, normally activated by speech, by the ongoing verbal hallucinations. A similar explanation seems to apply to visual hallucinations (ffytche *et al.* 1998). There have now been over a dozen studies that have tried to 'capture' auditory hallucinations using fMRI. Activity in the superior temporal lobe has been the predominant finding, although left inferior frontal areas also emerge frequently (David 2004).

Hemispheric differences

A separate but perhaps complementary strand to the picture concerns evidence that aspects of cerebral dominance may bear a special relationship to schizophrenia. Historically, the schizophrenia-like psychoses seen with epilepsy tended to be associated with foci in the left hemisphere. Furthermore, neuropathological and neuroimaging investigations have drawn particular attention to changes in the left temporal lobe in the generality of schizophrenias. The prevalence of non-right-handedness in schizophrenia may be taken as further support for the left hemisphere hypothesis or more general evidence in favour of subtle maldevelopment. In neurological terms a lack of cerebral asymmetry has been noted and efforts have been made to capture this completely in terms of 'torque' or radius of gyration. Crow has inferred from this a more fundamental disturbance in laterality and language development which, along with other evidence from wide-ranging sources, he posits to be the basis of schizophrenia psychopathology and which he believes may be related to the speciation of *Homo sapiens* (Crow 2000).

Neurodevelopmental models

A convincing account of a cerebral basis to schizophrenia must try to encompass a number of clinical observations: genetic liability to the disorder, a tendency to appear in adolescence or early adult life, response to certain medications, and distinct associations in certain cases with pathology affecting the temporal lobes and limbic areas. Other findings almost as firm also need to be taken into account: 'season of birth effects' with an excess during the late winter and early spring months, vulnerability to life events and to 'expressed emotion', the presence of antecedent impairments from childhood onwards (Jones *et al.* 1994), and a host of tantalising relationships with aspects of cerebral laterality.

The neurodevelopmental theory of schizophrenia has gained prominence in the field and is argued persuasively by a number of authorities (Weinberger 1987, 1995; Murray *et al.* 1988; Allin and Murray 2002). It encompasses both genetic and environmental factors as having a causal relationship to the disease. Though not applicable in every case, the theory claims to account for a sizeable proportion of patients, particularly those with early onset of the illness and prominent negative symptoms.

It is suggested that many schizophrenic subjects harbour 'brain lesions', especially in the limbic system and frontal cortex, that have originated very early in life extending back even to the intrauterine period. Such lesions, which are of a subtle nature, predispose the affected person to develop schizophrenia later. They may be the product of genetic influences controlling early brain growth, infection, immune disorder, complications of pregnancy or abnormal patterns of neuronal migration. These last may be occasioned by damage to the fetus during pregnancy or may themselves be inherited directly. Important variables with respect to the risk of developing schizophrenia are likely to include the site and timing of the disturbances, and the presence or absence of a genetic predisposition to the disorder.

There are precedents for such a situation in both animal experimental work and humans (Weinberger 1987). Thus a lesion of the dorsolateral prefrontal cortex does not markedly affect the infant monkey's behaviour, but disrupts performance on delayed response tasks in adulthood. Similarly, perinatal hypoxia may lead to cerebral palsy in infancy but to athetosis and epilepsy some years later. Brain myelination is also known to continue well into postnatal life, particularly in areas such as the corpus callosum and the prefrontal cortex. Weinberger (1987) stresses that the dorsolateral prefrontal cortex is one of the last brain areas to myelinate, this continuing well into the second and third decades of life. In his model the declaration of symptoms may depend on the maturing of cortical–subcortical relationships.

Sex differences with regard to schizophrenia can be accommodated within the neurodevelopmental model. There is consistent evidence that the onset of the illness is earlier in males than females, and that males show poorer premorbid adjustment and tend to have a poorer outcome (Castle & Murray 1991). This accords with the evidence from neuroimaging and neuropathology that the male schizophrenic brain is more often abnormal than the female. Moreover, neurodevelopmental disorders are generally commoner in boys than girls, as with developmental dyslexia and autism, perhaps as a result of slower maturation or greater lateralisation of function that renders compensation for damage less successful.

References

Adolphs, R., Tranel, D., Damasio, H. & Damasio, A. (1994) Impaired recognition of emotion in facial expressions following bilateral damage to the human amygdala. *Nature* **372**, 669–672.

Aggleton, J.P. & Shaw, C. (1996) Amnesia and recognition memory: a re-analysis of psychometric data. *Neuropsychologia* **34**, 51–62.

Aggleton, J.P., McMackin, D., Carpenter, K. *et al.* (2000) Differential cognitive effects of colloid cysts in the third ventricle that spare or compromise the fornix. *Brain* **123**, 800–815.

Aguirre, G.K. & D'Esposito, M. (1999) Topographical disorientation: a synthesis and taxonomy. *Brain* **122**, 1613–1628.

Albert, M.S., Butters, N. & Levin, J. (1979) Temporal gradients in the retrograde amnesia of patients with alcoholic Korsakoff's disease. *Archives of Neurology* **36**, 211–216.

Albert, M.S., Butters, N. & Brandt, J. (1981) Patterns of remote memory in amnesic and demented patients. *Archives of Neurology* **38**, 495–500.

Aleman, A., Hijman, R., de Haan, E.H.F. & Kahn, R.S. (1999) Memory impairment in schizophrenia: a meta-analysis. *American Journal of Psychiattry* **156**, 1358–1366.

Alexander, G.E., Crutcher, M.D. & Delong, M.R. (1990) Basal ganglia–thalamocortical circuits: parallel substrates for motor, oculomotor, 'prefrontal' and 'limbic' functions. *Progress in Brain Research* **85**, 119–146.

Allin, M. & Murray, R. (2002) Schizophrenia: a neurodevelopmental or neurodegenerative disorder? *Current Opinion in Psychiatry* **15**, 9–15.

Amador, X.F. & David, A.S. (eds) (2004) *Insight and Psychosis: Awareness of Illness in Schizophrenia and Related Disorders*, 2nd edn. Oxford University Press, Oxford.

Anderson, M.C. & Green, C. (2001) Suppressing unwanted memories by executive control. *Nature* **410**, 366–369.

Anderson, M.C., Ochsner, K., Kuhl, B. *et al.* (2004) Neural systems underlying the suppression of unwanted memories. *Science* **303**, 232–235.

Ardila, A. & Rosselli, M. (2002) Acalculia and dyscalculia. *Neuropsychology Review* **12**, 179–231.

Aylward, E., Walker, E. & Bettes, B. (1984) Intelligence in schizophrenia: meta-analysis of the research. *Schizophrenia Bulletin* **10**, 430–459.

Baddeley, A.D. (1976) *The Psychology of Memory*. Harper & Row, New York.

Baddeley, A. & Wilson, B. (1986) Amnesia, autobiographical memory, and confabulation. In: Rubin, D.C. (ed.) *Autobiographical Memory*, pp. 225–252. Cambridge University Press, Cambridge.

Bard, P. (1928) A diencephalic mechanism for the expression of rage with special reference to the sympathetic nervous system. *American Journal of Physiology* **84**, 490–515.

Bartlett, F.C. (1932) *Remembering: A Study in Experimental and Social Psychology*. Cambridge University Press, Cambridge.

Barton, J.J.S. (2003) Disorders of face perception and recognition. *Neurologic Clinics* **21**, 521–548.

Bates, E., Wilson, S., Saygin, A. *et al.* (2003) Voxel-based lesion symptom mapping. *Nature Neuroscience* **6**, 448–450.

Bayley, P.J., Gold, J.J., Hopkins, R.O. & Squire, L.R. (2005) The neuroanatomy of remote memory. *Neuron* **46**, 799–810.

Becker, J.T., Bajulaiye, O. & Smith, C. (1992) Longitudinal analysis of a two-component model of the memory deficit in Alzheimer's disease. *Psychological Medicine* **22**, 437–445.

Bench, C.J., Dolan, R.J., Friston, K.J. & Frackowiak, R.S.J. (1990) Positron emission tomography in the study of brain metabolism in psychiatric and neuropsychiatric disorders. *British Journal of Psychiatry* **157** (suppl. 9), 82–95.

Benson, D.F. (1973) Psychiatric aspects of dysphasia. *British Journal of Psychiatry* **123**, 555–566.

Benson, D.F. & Ardila, A. (1996) *Aphasia. A Clinical Perspective*. Oxford University Press, New York.

Benson, D.F. & Geschwind, N. (1971) Aphasia and related cortical disturbances. In: Baker, A.B. & Baker, L.H. (eds) *Clinical Neurology*, pp. 51, 54, 102, 103 Harper & Row, New York.

Benson, D.F. & Zaidel, E. (1985) *The Dual Brain: Hemispheric Specialization in Humans.* The Guilford Press, New York.

Benton, A.L. (1959) *Right–Left Discrimination and Finger Localization.* Hoeber, New York.

Benton, A.L. (1961) The fiction of the 'Gerstmann Syndrome'. *Journal of Neurology, Neurosurgery and Psychiatry* **24**, 176–181.

Benton, A. & Sivan, A.B. (1993) Disturbances of the body schema. In: Heilman, K.M. & Valenstein, E. (eds) *Clinical Neuropsychology*, 3rd edn, ch. 6. Oxford University Press, New York.

Berlyne, N. (1972) Confabulation. *British Journal of Psychiatry* **120**, 31–39.

Bilder, R.M., Goldman, R.S., Volavka J. *et al.* (2002) Neurocognitive effects of clozapine, olanzapine, risperidone, and haloperidol in patients with chronic schizophrenia or schizoaffective disorder. *American Journal of Psychiatry* **159**, 1018–1028.

Bisiach & Luzzati 1978

Blair, R.J., Morris, J.S., Frith, C.D., Perrett, D.I. & Dolan, R.J. (1999) Dissociable neural responses to facial expressions of sadness and anger. *Brain* **122**, 883–893.

Blakemore, S. & Frith, C. (2005) The role of motor contagion in the prediction of action. *Neuropsychologia* **43**, 260–267.

Bogen, J.E. (1985) The callosal syndromes. In: Heliman, K. & Valenstein, E. (eds) *Clinical Neuropsychology*, pp. 295–338. Oxford University Press, New York.

Bogen, J.E. & Gazzaniga, M.S. (1965) Cerebral commissurotomy in man: minor hemisphere dominance for certain visuospatial functions. *Journal of Neurosurgery* **23**, 394–399.

Boller, F. & Grafman, J. (1985) Acalculia. In: Frederiks, J.A.M. (ed.) *Handbook of Clinical Neurology, Revised Series, vol. 1. Clinical Neuropsychology*, ch. 31. Elsevier Science Publishers, Amsterdam.

Bottini, G., Cappa, S.F., Sterzi, R. & Vignolo, L.A. (1995) Intramodal somaesthetic recognition disorders following right and left hemisphere damage. *Brain* **118**, 395–399.

Bowman, M. & Lewis, M.S. (1980) Sites of subcortical damage in diseases which resemble schizophrenia. *Neuropsychologia* **18**, 597–601.

Braak, H. & Braak, E. (1991) Neuropathological stageing of alzheimer-related changes. *Acta Neuropathologica* **82**, 239–259.

Brain, W.R. (1965) *Speech Disorders: Aphasia, Apraxia and Agnosia*, 2nd edn. Butterworths, London.

Brandt, J., Spencer, M., McSorley, P. & Folstein, M.F. (1988) Semantic activation and implicit memory in Alzheimer disease. *Alzheimer's Disease and Associated Disorders* **2**, 112–119.

Brierley, B., Medford, N., Shaw, P. & David, A.S. (2004) Emotional memory and perception dissociate in temporal lobectomy patients with amygdala damage. *Journal of Neurology, Neurosurgery and Psychiatry* **75**, 593–599.

Brierley, J.B. (1961) Clinico-pathological correlations in amnesia. *Gerontologia Clinica* **3**, 97–109.

Brierley, J.B. (1966) The neuropathology of amnesic states. In: Whitty, C.W.M. & Zangwill, O.L. (eds) *Amnesia*, ch. 7. Butterworth, London.

Brierley, J.B., Corsellis, J.A.N., Hierons, R. & Nevin, S. (1960) Subacute encephalitis of later adult life: mainly affecting the limbic areas. *Brain* **83**, 357–368.

Brower, M.C. & Price, B.H. (2001) Neuropsychiatry of frontal lobe dysfunction in violent and criminal behaviour: a critical review. *Journal of Neurology, Neurosurgery and Psychiatry* **71**, 720–726.

Bruce, D. (1985) On the origin of the term "neuropsychology". *Neuropsychologia* **23**, 813–814.

Brugger, P., Regard, M. & Landis, T. (1996) Unilaterally felt 'presences': the neuropsychiatry of one's invisible Doppelgänger. *Neuropsychiatry, Neuropsychology and Behavioral Neurology* **9**, 114–122.

Buchanan, T.W., Tranel, D. & Adolphs, R. (2005) Emotional autobiographical memories in amnesic patients with medial temporal lobe damage. *Journal of Neuroscience* **25**, 3151–3160.

Buchsbaum, M.S. (1990) The frontal lobes, basal ganglia, and temporal lobes as sites for schizophrenia. *Schizophrenia Bulletin* **16**, 379–389.

Burgess, P.W. & Shallice, T. (1996) Response suppression, initiation and strategy use following frontal lobe lesions. *Neuropsychologia* **34**, 263–273.

Burgess, P.W., Simons, J.S., Dumontheil, I. & Gilbert, S.J. (2005) The gateway hypothesis of rostral prefrontal cortex (area 10) function. In: *Measuring the Mind: Speed, Control and Age*, pp. 215–246. Oxford University Press, Oxford.

Burklund, C.W. & Smith, A. (1977) Language and the cerebral hemispheres. Observations of verbal and non-verbal responses during 18 months following left ('dominant') hemispherectomy. *Neurology* **27**, 627–633.

Butters, N. & Cermak, L.S. (1980) *Alcoholic Korsakoff's Syndrome: An Information-Processing Approach to Amnesia.* Academic Press, New York.

Butterworth, B. (1999) *What Counts: How Every Brain is Hardwired for Math.* Free Press, New York.

Cairns, H. & Mosberg, W.H. (1951) Colloid cysts of the third ventricle. *Surgery, Gynecology and Obstetrics* **92**, 545–570.

Calder, A.J., Keane, J., Manes, F., Antoun, N. & Young, A.W. (2000) Impaired recognition and experience of disgust following brain injury. *Nature Neuroscience* **3**, 1077–1078.

Cannon, M., Jones, P.B. & Murray, R.M. (2002) Obstetric complications and schizophrenia: historical and meta-analytic review. *American Journal of Psychiatry* **159**, 1080–1092.

Cannon, T.D., Glahn, D.C., Kim J. *et al.* (2005) Dorsolateral prefrontal cortex activity during maintenance and manipulation of information in working memory in patients with schizophrenia. *Archives of General Psychiatry* **62**, 1071–1080.

Caspi, A., Reichenberg, A., Weiser, M. *et al.* (2003) Cognitive performance in schizophrenia patients assessed before and following the first psychotic episode. *Schizophrenia Research* **65**, 87–94.

Castle, D.J. & Murray, R.M. (1991) The neurodevelopmental basis of sex differences in schizophrenia. *Psychological Medicine* **21**, 565–575.

Censits, D.M., Ragland, D., Gur, R.C. & Gur, R.E. (1997) Neuropsychological evidence supporting a neurodevelopmental model of schizophrenia: a longitudinal study. *Schizophrenia Research* **24**, 289–298.

Cermak, L.S. (1984) The episodic–semantic distinction in amnesia. In: Squire, L.R. & Butters, N. (eds) *The Neuropsychology of Memory*, pp. 55–62. Guilford Press, New York.

Cermak, L.S. & O'Connor, M. (1983) The anterograde and retrograde retrieval ability of a patient with amnesia due to encephalitis. *Neuropsychologia* **21**, 213–234.

Chainay, H. & Humphreys, G.W. (2002) Neuropsychological evidence for a convergent route model for action. *Cognitive Neuropsychology* **19**, 67–93.

Chan, D., Fox, N.C., Scahill, R. *et al.* (2001) Patterns of temporal lobe atrophy in semantic dementia and Alzheimer's disease. *Annals of Neurology* **49**, 433–442.

Christensen, H., Kopelman, M.D., Stanhope, N., Lorentz, L. & Owen, P. (1998) Rates of forgetting in Alzheimer's dementia. *Neuropsychologia* **36**, 547–557.

Cipolotti, L., Shallice, T., Chan, D. *et al.* (2001) Long-term retrograde amnesia: the crucial role of the hippocampus. *Neuropsychologia* **39**, 151–172.

Clare, L. (2004) Awareness in early-stage Alzheimer's disease: a review of methods and evidence. *British Journal of Clinical Psychology* **43**, 177–196.

Cohen, N.J., Poldrack, R.A. & Eichenbaum, H. (1997) Memory for items and memory for relations in the procedural/declarative memory framework. *Memory* **5**, 131–178.

Colchester, A., Kingsley, D., Lasserson, D., Kendall, B., Bello, F. & Rush, C. (2001) Structural MRI volumetric analysis in patients with organic amnesia. I: Methods and comparative findings across diagnostic groups. *Journal of Neurology, Neurosurgery and Psychiatry* **71**, 13–22.

Coltheart, M. (2004) Brain imaging, connectionism, and cognitive neuropsychology. *Cognitive Neuropsychology* **21**, 21–25.

Coltheart, M., Patterson, K. & Marshall, J.C. (eds) (1987) *Deep Dyslexia*, 2nd edn. Routledge & Kegan Paul, London.

Conway, M.A. & Tacchi, P.C. (1996) Motivated confabulation. *Neurocase* **2**, 325–328.

Corkin, S. (1968) Acquisition of motor skill after bilateral medial temporal lobe excision. *Neuropsychologia* **6**, 255–265.

Corkin, S. (1982) Some relationships between global amnesias and the memory impairments in Alzheimer's disease. In: *Alzheimer's Disease: A Report of Progress in Research, Aging*, vol. 19, Corkin, S., Davis, K.L., Growdon, J.H., Usdin, E. & Wurtman, R.J. (eds) pp. 149–164. Raven Press, New York [32].

Corkin, S., Amaral, D.G., Gonzalez, R.G., Johnson, K.A. & Hyman, B.T. (1997) H.M.'s medial temporal lobe lesion: findings from magnetic resonance imaging. *Journal of Neuroscience* **17**, 3964–3979.

Corsellis, J.A.N. (1970) The limbic areas in Alzheimer's disease and in other conditions associated with dementia. In: Wolstenholme, G.E.W. & O'Connor, M. (eds) *Alzheimer's Disease and Related Conditions*, pp. 32, 440. Churchill, London.

Coslett, B. & Saffran, E. (1991) Simultanagnosia. To see but not two see. *Brain* **114**, 1523–1545.

Crawford, J.R., Besson, J.A.O., Bremner, M., Ebmeier, K.P., Cochrane, R.H.B. & Kirkwood, K. (1992) Estimation of premorbid intelligence in schizophrenia. *British Journal of Psychiatry* **161**, 69–74.

Critchley, M. (1953) *The Parietal Lobes*. Edward Arnold, London.

Critchley, M. (1964) Psychiatric symptoms and parietal disease: differential diagnosis. *Proceedings of the Royal Society of Medicine* **57**, 422–428.

Crow, T.J. (2000) Schizophrenia as the price that homo sapiens pays for language: a resolution of the central paradox in the origin of the species. *Brain Research Reviews* **31**, 118–129.

Cutting, J. (1978) Study of anosognosia. *Journal of Neurology, Neurosurgery and Psychiatry* **41**, 548–555.

Cutting, J. (1979) Memory in functional psychosis. *Journal of Neurology, Neurosurgery and Psychiatry* **42**, 1031–1037.

Cutting, J. (1985) *The Psychology of Schizophrenia*. Churchill Livingstone, Edinburgh.

Cutting, J. (1989) Body image disorders: comparison between unilateral hemisphere damage and schizophrenia. *Behavioural Neurology* **2**, 201–210.

Cutting, J. (1990) *The Right Cerebral Hemisphere and Psychiatric Disorders*. Oxford University Press, Oxford.

Dalla Barba, G. (1993) Confabulation: knowledge and recollective experience. *Cognitive Neuropsychology* **10**, 1–20.

Dalla Barba, G. (2002) *Memory, Consciousness and Temporality*. Kluwer Academic Press, Boston.

Dalla Barba, G., Nedjam, Z. & Dubois, B. (1999) Confabulation, executive functions, and source memory in Alzheimer's disease. *Cognitive Neuropsychology* **16**, 3–5.

Dalman, C., Thomas, H.V., David, A.S., Gentz, J., Lewis, G. & Allebeck, P. (2001) Signs of asphyxia at birth and risk of schizophrenia. *British Journal of Psychiatry* **179**, 403–408.

Damasio, A.R. & Damasio, H. (1992) Brain and language. *Scientific American* **267**, 89–95.

Damasio, A.R., Damasio, H., Rizzo, M., Varney, N. & Gersh, F. (1982a) Aphasia with nonhemorrhagic lesions in the basal ganglia and internal capsule. *Archives of Neurology* **39**, 15–20.

Damasio, A.R., Damasio, H. & Van Hoesen, G.W. (1982b) Prosopagnosia: anatomic basis and behavioral mechanisms. *Neurology* **32**, 331–341.

Damasio, H., Grabowski, T., Frank, R., Galaburda, A.M. & Damasio, A.R. (1994) The return of Phineas Gage: clues about the brain from the skull of a famous patient. *Science* **264**, 1102–1105.

Davachi, L., Mitchell, J.P. & Wagner, A.D. (2003) Multiple routes to memory: distinct medial temporal lobe processes build item and source memories. *Proceedings of the National Academy of Sciences USA* **100**, 2157–2162.

David, A.S. (1992) Frontal lobology: psychiatry's new pseudoscience. *British Journal of Psychiatry* **161**, 244–248.

David, A.S. (2004) The cognitive neuropsychiatry of auditory verbal hallucinations: an overview. *Cognitive Neuropsychiatry* **9**, 107–123.

David, A.S. & Cutting, J.C. (eds) (1994) *The Neuropsychology of Schizophrenia*. Lawrence Erlbaum Associates, Hove, East Sussex.

David, A.S., Wacharasindhu, A. & Lishman, W.A. (1993) Severe psychiatric disturbance and abnormalities of the corpus callosum: review and case series. *Journal of Neurology, Neurosurgery and Psychiatry* **56**, 85–93.

David, A.S., Woodruff, P.W.R., Howard, R. *et al.* (1996) Auditory hallucinations inhibit exogenous activation of auditory association cortex. *NeuroReport* **7**, 932–93.

David, A.S., Malmberg, A., Brandt, L., Allebeck, P. & Lewis, G. (1997) IQ and risk for schizophrenia: a population-based cohort study. *Psychological Medicine* **27**, 1311–1323.

Davidson, M., Harvey, P., Welsh, K.A., Powchik, P., Putnam, K.M. & Mohs, R.C. (1996) Cognitive functioning in late-life schizophrenia: a comparison of elderly schizophrenic patients and patients with Alzheimer's disease. *American Journal of Psychiatry* **153**, 1274–1279.

Davison, K. (1983) Schizophrenia-like psychoses associated with organic cerebral disorders: a review. *Psychiatric Developments* **1**, 1–34.

Davison, K. & Bagley, C.R. (1969) Schizophrenia-like psychoses associated with organic disorders of the central nervous system: a review of the literature. In: Herrington, R.N. (ed.) *Current Problems in Neuropsychiatry.* British Journal of Psychiatry Special Publication No. 4. Headley Brothers, Ashford, Kent.

Dehaene, S., Molko, N., Cohen, L. & Wilson, A.J. (2004) Arithmetic and the brain. *Current Opinion in Neurobiology* **14**, 218–224.

Delgado, J.M.R. (1969) Offensive–defensive behaviour in free monkeys and chimpanzees induced by radio stimulation of the brain. In: Garattini, S. & Sigg, E.B. (eds) *Aggressive Behaviour*, p. 80. Excerpta Medica, Amsterdam.

Delgado, J.M.R., Mark, V., Sweet, W. *et al.* (1968) Intracerebral radio stimulation and recording in completely free patients. *Journal of Nervous and Mental Disease* **147**, 329–340.

Demonet, J.F., Taylor, M.J. & Chaix, Y. (2004) Developmental dyslexia. *Lancet* **363**, 1451–1460.

De Renzi, E. (1982) *Disorders of Space Exploration and Cognition.* John Wiley & Sons, Chichester.

De Renzi, E. & Scotti, G. (1970) Autotopagnosia: fiction or reality? *Archives of Neurology* **23**, 221–227.

De Renzi, E., Faglioni, P. & Scotti, G. (1971) Judgement of spatial orientation in patients with focal brain damage. *Journal of Neurology, Neurosurgery and Psychiatry* **34**, 485–495.

De Renzi, E., Liotti, M. & Nichelli, P. (1987) Semantic amnesia with preservation of autobiographic memory: a case report. *Cortex* **23**, 575–597.

De Renzi, E., Faglioni, P. & Nichelli, P. (1991) Apperceptive and associative forms of prosopagnosia. *Cortex* **27**, 213–221.

Deweer, B., Pillon, B., Michon, A. & Dubois, B. (1993) Mirror reading in Alzheimer's disease: normal skill learning and acquisition of item-specific information. *Journal of Clinical and Experimental Neuropsychology* **15**, 789–804.

Dickinson, D., Iannone, V.N., Wilk, C.M. & Gold, J.M. (2004) General and specific cognitive deficits in schizophrenia. *Biological Psychiatry* **55**, 826–833.

Dolan, R.J., Bench, C.J., Liddle, P.F. *et al.* (1993) Dorsolateral prefrontal cortex dysfunction in the major psychoses: symptom or disease specificity? *Journal of Neurology, Neurosurgery and Psychiatry* **56**, 1290–1294.

Done, D.J., Crow, T.J., Johnstone, E.C. & Sacker, A. (1994) Childhood antecedents of schizophrenia and affective illness: social adjustment at ages 7 and 11. *British Medical Journal* **309**, 699–703.

Dott, N.M. (1938) Surgical aspects of the hypothalamus. In: Clark, W.E.LeG., Beattie, J., Riddoch, G. & Dott, N.M. (eds) *The Hypothalamus*, p. 27. Oliver & Boyd, Edinburgh.

Downer, J.L. de C. (1962) Interhemispheric integration in the visual system. In: Mountcastle, V.B. (ed.) *Interhemispheric Relations and Cerebral Dominance*, ch. 6. Johns Hopkins Press, Baltimore.

Downes, J.J., Davis, E.J., Davies, P.M. *et al.* (1996) Stem-completion priming in Alzheimer's disease: the importance of target word articulation. *Neuropsychologia* **34**, 63–75.

Drachman, D.A. & Arbit, J. (1966) Memory and the hippocampal complex. *Archives of Neurology* **15**, 52–61.

Drachman, D.A., O'Donnell, B.F., Lew, R.A. & Swearer, J.M. (1990) The prognosis in Alzheimer's disease. *Archives of Neurology* **47**, 851–856.

Dragovic, M. & Hammond, G. (2005) Handedness in schizophrenia: a quantitative review of evidence. *Acta Psychiatrica Scandinavica* **111**, 410–419.

Dronkers, N.F., Shapiro, J.K., Redfern, B. & Knight, R.T. (1992) The role of Broca's area in Broca's aphasia. *Journal of Clinical and Experimental Neuropsychology* **14**, 52–53.

Duffy, L. & O'Carroll, R. (1994) Memory impairment in schizophrenia: a comparison with that observed in the alcoholic Korsakoff syndrome. *Psychological Medicine* **24**, 155–165.

Dunbar, G.C. & Lishman, W.A. (1984) Depression, recognition memory and hedonic tone: a signal detection analysis. *British Journal of Psychiatry* **144**, 376–382.

Duncan, J. (1986) Disorganisation of behaviour after frontal lobe damage. *Cognitive Neuropsychology* **3**, 271–290.

Duncan, J. (2001) An adaptive coding model of neural function in prefrontal cortex. *Nature Reviews. Neuroscience* **2**, 820–829.

Elliott, F.A. (1992) Violence. The neurologic contribution: an overview. *Archives of Neurology* **49**, 595–603.

Ellis, A.W. & Young, A.W. (1988) *Human Cognitive Neuropsychology.* Lawrence Erlbaum Associates, Hove, East Sussex.

Eslinger, P. & Damasio, A.R. (1985) Severe disturbance of higher cognition after bilateral frontal ablation. Patient, E.V.R. *Neurology* **35**, 1731–1741.

Eslinger, P.J. & Damasio, A.R. (1986) Preserved motor learning in Alzheimer's disease: implications for anatomy and behavior. *Journal of Neuroscience* **6**, 3006–3009.

Evans, J.J., Heggs, A.J., Antoun, N. & Hodges, J.R. (1995) Progressive prosopagnosia associated with selective right temporal lobe atrophy: a new syndrome? *Brain* **118**, 1–13.

Faber, R., Abrams, R., Taylor, M.A., Kasprison, A., Moris, C. & Weisz, R. (1983) Comparison of schizophrenic patients with formal thought disorder and neurologically impaired patients with aphasia. *American Journal of Psychiatry* **140**, 1348–1351.

Fenwick, P. (1986) Aggression and epilepsy. In: Trimble, M.R. & Bolwig, T.G. (eds) *Aspects of Epilepsy and Psychiatry*, ch. 4. John Wiley & Sons, Australia.

ffytche, D.H., Howard, R.J., Brammer, M.J., David, A.S., Woodruff, P.W.R. & Williams, S.C.R (1998) The anatomy of conscious vision: an fMRI study of visual hallucinations. *Nature Neuroscience* **1**, 738–742.

Filley, C.M., Price, B.H., Nell, V. *et al.* (2001) Toward an understanding of violence: neurobehavioral aspects of unwarranted physical aggression. Aspen Neurobehavioral Conference consensus statement. *Neuropsychiatry, Neuropsychology and Behavioral Neurology* **14**, 1–14.

Fletcher, P.C., Frith, C., Grasby, P.M., Shallice, T., Frackowiak, R.S.J. & Dolan, R.J. (1995) Brain systems for encoding and retrieval of auditory-verbal memory. *Brain* **118**, 401–416.

Flourens, J.P.M. (1824) *Recherches Experimentales sur les Proprietés et les Fonctions du Système Nerveux, dans les Animaux Vertébrés.* Crevot, Paris.

Francks, C., MacPhie, I.L. & Monaco, A.P. (2002) The genetic basis of dyslexia. *Lancet Neurology* **1**, 483–490.

Frederiks, J.A.M. (1969) Disorders of the body schema. In: Vinken, P.J. & Bruyn, G.W. (eds) *Handbook of Clinical Neurology*, vol. 4, ch. 11. North-Holland Publishing Co., Amsterdam.

Frederiks, J.A.M. (1985) Disorders of the body schema. In: Frederiks, J.A.M. (ed.) *Handbook of Clinical Neurology, Revised Series, vol.*

1. *Clinical Neuropsychology*, ch. 25. Elsevier Science Publishers, Amsterdam.

Freud, S. (1891) *On Aphasia: A Critical Study*. Translated by E. Stengel (1953), p. 78. Imago Publishing, London.

Frith, C. (1992) *Cognitive Neuropsychology of Schizophrenia*. Lawrence Erlbaum Associates, Hove, East Sussex.

Frith, C.D. (1995) Functional imaging and cognitive abnormalities. *Lancet* **346**, 615–620.

Frith, C.D., Friston, K.J., Liddle, P.F. & Frackowiak, R.S.J. (1991) Willed action and the prefrontal cortex in man: a study with PET. *Proceedings of the Royal Society of London* **244**, 241–246 (series B).

Fromholt *et al.* 2003

Gazzaniga, M.S. (1983) Right hemisphere language following brain bisection: a 20-year perspective. *American Psychologist* **38**, 525–537.

Gazzaniga, M.S. (1985) Some contributions of split-brain studies to the study of human cognition. In: Reeves, A.G. (ed.) *Epilepsy and the Corpus Callosum*, ch. 17. Plenum Press, New York.

Gazzaniga, M.S. & Sperry, R.W. (1967) Language after section of the cerebral commissures. *Brain* **90**, 131–148.

Gerson, S.N., Benson, F. & Frazier, S.H. (1977) Diagnosis: schizophrenia versus posterior aphasia. *American Journal of Psychiatry* **134**, 966–969.

Gerstmann, J. (1958) Psychological and phenomenological aspects of disorders of the body image. *Journal of Nervous and Mental Disease* **126**, 499–512.

Geschwind, N. (1965) Disconnexion syndromes in animals and man. *Brain* **88**, 237–294, 585–644.

Geschwind, N. (1967) Neurological foundations of language. In: Myklebust, H.R. (ed.) *Progress in Learning Disabilities*, pp. 182–198. Grune & Stratton, New York.

Geschwind, N. & Damasio, A.R. (1985) Apraxia. In: Frederiks, J.A.M. (ed.) *Handbook of Clinical Neurology, Revised Series, vol. 1. Clinical Neuropsychology*, ch. 28. Elsevier Science Publishers, Amsterdam.

Geschwind, N. & Levitsky, W. (1968) Human brain: left–right asymmetries in temporal speech region. *Science* **161**, 186–187.

Geschwind, N., Quadfasel, F.A. & Segarra, J.M. (1968) Isolation of the speech area. *Neuropsychologia* **6**, 327–340.

Gilboa, A., Winocur, G., Grady, C.L., Hevenor, S.J. & Moscovitch, M. (2004) Remembering our past: functional neuroanatomy of recollection of recent and very remote personal events. *Cerebral Cortex* **14**, 1214–1225.

Gilleen, J. & David, A.S. (2005) The cognitive neuropsychiatry of delusions: from psychopathology to neuropsychology and back again. *Psychological Medicine* **35**, 5–12.

Glisky, E.L., Reminger, S., Hardt, O., Hayes, S.M. & Hupbach, A. (2004) A case of psychogenic fugue: I understand, aber ich verstehe nichts. *Neuropsychologia* **42**, 1132–1147.

Golby, A.J., Poldrack, R.A., Brewer, J.B., Spencer, D., Desmond, J.E. & Aron, A.P. (2001) Material-specific lateralization in the medial temporal lobe and prefrontal cortex during memory encoding. *Brain* **124**, 1841–1854.

Goldstein, K. (1948) *Language and Language Disturbances*. Grune & Stratton, New York.

Gordon, H.W. & Bogen, J.E. (1974) Hemispheric lateralization of singing after intracarotid sodium amylobarbitone. *Journal of Neurology, Neurosurgery and Psychiatry* **37**, 727–738.

Grafman, J., Passafiume, D., Faglioni, P. & Boller, F. (1982) Calculation disturbance in adults with focal hemispheric damage. *Cortex* **18**, 37–50.

Grafman, J., Salazar, A.M., Weingartner, H., Vance, C. & Ludlow, C. (1985) Isolated impairment of memory following a penetrating lesion of the fornix cerebri. *Archives of Neurology* **42**, 1162–1168.

Graham, K.S. & Hodges, J.R. (1997) Differentiating the roles of the hippocampal complex and the neocortex in long-term memory storage: evidence from the study of semantic dementia and Alzheimer's disease. *Neuropsychology* **11**, 77–89.

Graybiel, A.M. & Rauch, S.L. (2000) Toward a neurobiology of obsessive-compulsive disorder. *Neuron* **28**, 343–347.

Green, M.F. (1996) What are the functional consequences of neurocognitive deficits in schizophrenia? *American Journal of Psychiatry* **153**, 321–330.

Green, R. & Kopelman, M.D. (2002) Contribution of recollection memory and familiarity judgements to forgetting rates in organic amnesia. *Cortex* **38**, 161–178.

Green, M.F., Kern, R.S., Braff, D.L. & Mintz, J. (2000) Neurocognitive deficits and functional outcome in schizophrenia: are we measuring the 'right stuff'? *Schizophrenia Bulletin* **26**, 119–136.

Greene, J.D., Hodges, J.R. & Baddeley, A.D. (1995) Autobiographical memory and executive function in early dementia of Alzheimer type. *Neuropsychologia* **33**, 1647–1670.

Grossman, M., Galetta, S., Ding, X.-S. *et al.* (1996) Clinical and positron emission tomography studies of visual apperceptive agnosia. *Journal of Neuropsychiatry, Neuropsychology, and Behavioral Neurology* **9**, 70–77.

Gudjonsson, G.H. & Taylor, P.J. (1985) Cognitive deficit in a case of retrograde amnesia. *British Journal of Psychiatry* **147**, 715–718.

Guinan, E.M., Lowy, C., Stanhope, N., Lewis, P.D. & Kopelman, M.D. (1998) Cognitive effects of pituitary tumours and their treatments: two case studies and an investigation of 90 patients. *Journal of Neurology, Neurosurgery and Psychiatry* **65**, 870–876.

Gunn, J. (1993) Non-psychotic violence. In: Gunn, J. & Taylor, P.J. (eds) *Forensic Psychiatry. Clinical, Legal and Ethical Issues*, ch. 12. Butterworth/Heinemann, Oxford.

Haggard, P. (2001) The psychology of action. *British Journal of Psychology* **92**, 113–128.

Haist, F., Bowden, G.J. & Mao, H. (2001) Consolidation of human memory over decades revealed by functional magnetic resonance imaging. *Nature Neuroscience* **4**, 1139–1145.

Halligan, P.W. (2002) Phantom limbs: the body in mind. *Cognitive Neuropsychiatry* **7**, 251–258.

Halligan, P.W. & Marshall, J.C. (1991) Left neglect for near but not far space in man. *Nature* **350**, 498–500.

Halligan, P.W., Marshall, J.C. & Wade, D.T. (1993) Three arms: a case study of supernumerary phantom limb after right hemisphere stroke. *Journal of Neurology, Neurosurgery and Psychiatry* **56**, 159–166.

Hamann, S.B., Squire, L.R. & Cahill, L. (1997) Emotional perception and memory in amnesia. *Neuropsychology* **11**, 104–113.

Harding, A., Halliday, G., Caine, D. & Kril, J. (2000) Degeneration of anterior thalamic nuclei differentiates alcoholics with amnesia. *Brain* **123**, 141–154.

Harlow, J. (1868) Recovery after severe injury to the head. *Publications of the Massachusetts Medial Society* **2**, 327–346.

Harlow, J.M. (1993) Recovery from the passage of an iron bar through the head. *History of Psychiatry* **4**, 271–281 [reprinted from 1868].

Harrison, P.J. (1999) The neuropathology of schizophrenia. A critical review of the data and their interpretation. *Brain* **122**, 593–624.

Harrison, P.J. & Weinberger, D.R. (2005) Schizophrenia genes, gene expression, and neuropathology: on the matter of their convergence. *Molecular Psychiatry* **10**, 40–68. [Erratum appears in *Molecular Psychiatry* 2005, **10**, 420.]

Head, H. (1920) *Studies in Neurology*, vol. 2. Oxford University Press, Oxford.

Heath, R.G., Monroe, R.R. & Mickle, W.A. (1955) Stimulation of the amygdaloid nucleus in a schizophrenic patient. *American Journal of Psychiatry* **111**, 862–863.

Hebb, D.O. (1949) *The Organization of Behaviour*. Chapman & Hall, New York.

Hécaen, H. (1962) Clinical symptomatology in right and left hemisphere lesions. In: Mountcastle, V.B. (ed.) *Interhemispheric Relations and Cerebral Dominance*, ch. 10. Johns Hopkins Press, Baltimore.

Hécaen, H. & Angelergues, R. (1962) Agnosia for faces (prosopagnosia). *Archives of Neurology* **7**, 24–32.

Heilman, K.M., Scholes, R. & Watson, R.T. (1975) Auditory affective agnosia. Disturbed comprehension of affective speech. *Journal of Neurology, Neurosurgery and Psychiatry* **38**, 69–72.

Heilman, K.M., Valenstein, E. & Watson, R.T. (1985) The neglect syndrome. In: Frederiks, J.A.M. (ed.) *Handbook of Clinical Neurology, Revised Series, vol. 1. Clinical Neuropsychology*, ch. 12. Elsevier Science Publishers, Amsterdam.

Heimburger, R.F., Demyer, W. & Reitan, R.M. (1964) Implications of Gerstmann's syndrome. *Journal of Neurology, Neurosurgery and Psychiatry* **27**, 52–57.

Heinrichs, R.W. & Zakzanis, K.K. (1998) Neurocognitive deficit in schizophrenia: a quantitative review of the evidence. *Neuropsychology* **12**, 426–445.

Hemphill, R.E. & Stengel, E. (1940) A study on pure word-deafness. *Journal of Neurology, Neurosurgery and Psychiatry* **3**, 251–262.

Henson, R.A. (1985) Amusia. In: Frederiks, J.A.M. (ed.) *Handbook of Clinical Neurology, Revised Series, vol. 1. Clinical Neuropsychology*, ch. 32. Elsevier Science Publishers, Amsterdam.

Hill, D. (1944) Cerebral dysrhythmia: its significance in aggressive behaviour. *Proceedings of the Royal Society of Medicine* **37**, 317–328.

Hitch, G.J. (1984) Working memory [editorial]. *Psychological Medicine* **14**, 265–271.

Hitchcock, E., Ashcroft, G.W., Cairns, V.M. & Murray, L.G. (1972) Preoperative and postoperative assessment and management of psychosurgical patients. In: Hitchcock, E., Laitinen, L. & Vaernet, K. (eds) *Psychosurgery*, ch. 14. Charles C. Thomas, Springfield, IL.

Hodges, J.R. & Carpenter, K. (1991) Anterograde amnesia with fornix damage following removal of IIIrd ventricle colloid cyst. *Journal of Neurology, Neurosurgery and Psychiatry* **54**, 633–638.

Hodges, J.R. & Oxbury, S.M. (1990) Persistent memory impairment following transient global amnesia. *Journal of Clinical and Experimental Neuropsychology* **12**, 904–920.

Hodges, J.R. & Ward, C.D. (1989) Observations during transient global amnesia. A behavioural and neuropsychological study of five cases. *Brain* **112**, 595–620.

Hodges, J.R. & Warlow, C.P. (1990) The aetiology of transient global amnesia. *Brain* **113**, 639–657.

Hodges, J.R., Patterson, K., Oxbury, S. & Funnell, E. (1992) Semantic dementia: progressive fluent aphasia with with temporal lobe atrophy. *Brain* **115**, 1783–1806.

Hodges, J.R., Davies, R., Xuereb, J. *et al.* (2004) Clinicopathological correlates in frontotemporal dementia. *Annals of Neurology* **56**, 399–406.

Holdstock, J.S., Mayes, A.R., Roberts, N. *et al.* (2002) Under what conditions is recognition spared relative to recall after selective hippocampal damage in humans? *Hippocampus* **12**, 341–351.

Honea, R., Crow, T.J., Passingham, D. & Mackay, C.E. (2005) Regional deficits in brain volume in schizophrenia: a meta-analysis of voxel-based morphometry studies. *American Journal of Psychiatry* **162**, 2233–2245.

Humphreys, G. (2001) Objects, affordances . . . action! *The Psychologist* **14**, 408–409.

Huppert, F.A. (1994) Memory function in dementia and normal aging: dimension or dichotomy? In: Huppert, F.A., Brayne, C. & O'Connor, D.W. (eds) *Dementia and Normal Aging*, ch. 15. Cambridge University Press, Cambridge.

Huppert, F.A. & Kopelman, M.D. (1989) Rates of forgetting in normal ageing: a comparison with dementia. *Neuropsychologia* **27**, 849–860.

Huppert, F.A. & Piercy, M. (1976) Recognition memory in amnesic patients: effects of temporal context and familiarity of material. *Cortex* **12**, 3–20.

Huppert, F.A. & Piercy, M. (1978a) The role of trace strength in recency and frequency judgements by amnesic and control subjects. *Quarterly Journal of Experimental Psychology* **30**, 347–354.

Huppert, F.A. & Piercy, M. (1978b) Dissociation between learning and remembering in organic amnesia. *Nature* **275**, 317–318.

Huppert, F.A. & Piercy, M. (1979) Normal and abnormal forgetting in organic amnesia: effect of locus of lesion. *Cortex* **15**, 385–390.

Hynd, G.W. & Hiemenz, J.R. (1997) Dyslexia and gyral morphology variation. In: Hulme, C. & Snowling, M. (eds) *Dyslexia: Biology, Cognition and Intervention*, ch. 3. Whurr Publishers, London.

Ingvar, D.H. & Franzen, G. (1974) Abnormalities of cerebral blood flow distribution in patients with chronic schizophrenia. *Acta Psychiatrica Scandinavica* **50**, 425–462.

Jackson, J.H. (1869) Certain points in the study and classification of diseases of the nervous system (Goulstonian Lectures). *Lancet* **i**, 307, 344, 379. Reprinted (1932) in Taylor, J. (ed.) *Selected Writings of John Hughlings Jackson*, vol. 2, p. 246. Hodder & Stoughton, London.

Jankowiak, J. & Albert, M.L. (1994) Lesion localization in visual agnosia. In: Kertesz, A. (ed.) *Localization and Neuroimaging in Neuropsychology*, ch. 14. Academic Press, San Diego.

Jeannerod, M. & Jacob, P. (2005) Visual cognition: a new look at the two-visual systems model. *Neuropsychologia* **43**, 301–312.

Jehkonen, M., Ahonen, J.-P., Dastidar, P., Laippala, P. & Vilkki, J. (2000) Unawareness of deficits after right hemisphere stroke: double-dissociations of anosognosias. *Acta Neurologica Scandinavica* **102**, 378–384.

Johnson, H. & Haggard, P. (2005) Motor awareness without perceptual awareness. *Neuropsychologia* **43**, 227–237.

Johnson, M.K., Hashtroudi, S. & Lindsay, D.S. (1993) Source monitoring. *Psychological Bulletin* **114**, 3–28.

Johnson, M.K., O'Connor, M. & Cantor, J. (1997) Confabulation, memory deficits, and frontal dysfunction. *Brain and Cognition* **34**, 189–206.

Johnstone, E.C., McMillan, J.F. & Crow, T.J. (1987) The occurrence of organic disease of possible or probable aetiological significance in a population of 268 cases of first episode schizophrenia. *Psychological Medicine* **17**, 371–379.

Jones, P., Rodgers, B., Murray, R. & Marmot, M. (1994) Child developmental risk factors for adult schizophrenia in the British 1946 birth cohort. *Lancet* **334**, 1393–1402.

Joyce, E.M., Collinson, S.L. & Crichton, P. (1996) Verbal fluency in schizophrenia: relationship with executive function, semantic memory and clinical alogia. *Psychological Medicine* **26**, 39–49.

Kandel, E.R. & Hawkins, R.D. (1992) The biological basis of learning and individuality. *Scientific American* **267**, 78–86.

Kapur, N. (1990) Transient epileptic amnesia: a clinically distinct form of neurological memory disorder. In: Markowitsch, H.J. (ed.) *Transient Global Amnesia and Related Disorders*, pp. 140–151. Hogrefe and Huber, Toronto.

Kapur, N. (2000) Focal retrograde amnesia and the attribution of causality: an exceptionally benign commentary. *Cognitive Neuropsychology* **17**, 623–637.

Kapur, N. & Brooks, D.J. (1999) Temporally specific retrograde amnesia in two cases of discrete bilateral hippocampal pathology. *Hippocampus* **9**, 247–254.

Kapur, N. & Coughlan, A.K. (1980) Confabulation and frontal lobe dysfunction. *Journal of Neurology, Neurosurgery and Psychiatry* **43**, 461–463.

Kapur, N., Ellison, D., Smith, M.P., McLellan, D.L. & Burrows, E.H. (1992) Focal retrograde amnesia following bilateral temporal lobe pathology. *Brain* **115**, 73–85.

Kaszniak, A.W., Garron, D.C. & Fox, J. (1979) Differential effects of age and cerebral atrophy upon span of immediate recall and paired associated learning in older patients suspected of dementia. *Cortex* **15**, 285–295.

Katzman, G.L., Dagher, A.P. & Patronas, N.J. (1999) Incidental findings on brain magnetic resonance imaging from 1000 asymptomatic volunteers. *JAMA* **282**, 36–39.

Kerkhoff, G. (2001) Spatial hemineglect in humans. *Progress in Neurobiology* **63**, 1–27.

Kertesz, A. & Benson, D.F. (1970) Neologistic jargon: a clinico-pathological study. *Cortex* **6**, 362–386.

Kimura, D. (1961) Some effects of temporal lobe damage on auditory perception. *Canadian Journal of Psychology* **15**, 156–165.

Kimura, D. (1964) Left–right differences in the perception of melodies. *Quarterly Journal of Experimental Psychology* **16**, 355–358.

Kinsbourne, M. & Warrington, E.K. (1962) A study of finger agnosia. *Brain* **85**, 47–66.

Klein, R. (1952) Immediate effects of leucotomy on cerebral functions and their significance. *Journal of Mental Science* **98**, 60–65.

Klüver, H. & Bucy, P.C. (1939) Preliminary analysis of functions of the temporal lobes in monkeys. *Archives of Neurology and Psychiatry* **42**, 979–1000.

Kopelman, M.D. (1985a) Rates of forgetting in Alzheimer-type dementia and Korsakoff's syndrome. *Neuropsychologia* **23**, 623–638.

Kopelman, M.D. (1985b) Multiple memory deficits in Alzheimer-type dementia: implications for pharmacotherapy. *Psychological Medicine* **15**, 527–541.

Kopelman, M.D. (1987a) Two types of confabulation. *Journal of Neurology, Neurosurgery and Psychiatry* **50**, 1482–1487.

Kopelman, M.D. (1987b) Amnesia: organic and psychogenic. *British Journal of Psychiatry* **150**, 428–442.

Kopelman, M.D. (1989) Remote and autobiographical memory, temporal context memory and frontal atrophy in Korsakoff and Alzheimer patients. *Neuropsychologia* **27**, 437–460.

Kopelman, M.D. (1991) Frontal dysfunction and memory deficits in the alcoholic Korsakoff syndrome and Alzheimer-type dementia. *Brain* **114**, 117–137.

Kopelman, M.D. (1995) The Korsakoff syndrome. *British Journal of Psychiatry* **166**, 154–173.

Kopelman, M.D. (2000) Focal retrograde amnesia and the attribution of causality: an exceptionally critical review. *Cognitive Neuropsychology* **17**, 585–621.

Kopelman, M.D. (2002) Invited Review: disorders of memory. *Brain* **125**, 2152–2190.

Kopelman, M.D. & Corn, T.H. (1988) Cholinergic 'blockade' as a model for cholinergic depletion: a comparison of the memory deficits with those of Alzheimer-type dementia and the alcoholic Korsakoff syndrome. *Brain* **111**, 1079–1110.

Kopelman, M.D. & Stanhope, N. (1997) Rates of forgetting in organic amnesia following temporal lobe, diencephalic, or frontal lobe lesions. *Neuropsychology* **11**, 343–356.

Kopelman, M.D., Wilson, B.A. & Baddeley, A.D. (1989) The autobiographical and personal semantic memory in amnesic patients. *Journal of Clinical and Experimental Neuropsychology* **11**, 724–744.

Kopelman, M.D., Christensen, H., Puffett, A. & Stanhope, N. (1994) The great escape: a neuropsychological study of psychogenic amnesia. *Neuropsychologia* **32**, 675–691.

Kopelman, M.D., Stanhope, N. & Kingsley, D. (1997) Temporal and spatial context memory in patients with focal frontal, temporal lobe and diencephalic lesions. *Neuropsychologia* **35**, 1533–1545.

Kopelman, M.D., Stanhope, N. & Kingsley, D. (1999) Retrograde amnesia in patients with diencephalic, temporal lobe or frontal lobe lesions. *Neuropsychologia* **37**, 939–958.

Kopelman, M.D., Lasserson, D., Kingsley, D., Bello, F., Rush, C. & Stanhope, N. (2001) Structural MRI volumetric analysis in patients with organic amnesia. 2. Correlations with anterograde memory and executive tests in 40 patients. *Journal of Neurology, Neurosurgery and Psychiatry* **71**, 23–28.

Kopelman, M.D., Lasserson, D., Kingsley, D. *et al.* (2003) Retrograde amnesia and the volume of critical brain structures. *Hippocampus* **13**, 879–891.

Kopelman, M.D., Bright, P., Buckman, J., Fradera, A., Haruo, Y. & Colchester, A.C.F. (2005) Recall and recognition memory in amnesia: patients with hippocampal, medial temporal, temporal lobe or frontal pathology. *Neuropsychologia* **45**, 1232–1246.

Korsakoff, S.S. (1889) Psychiatric disorder in conjunction with peripheral neuritis [translated]. Reprinted in Victor, M. & Yakovel, P.I. (1955) *Neurology* **5**, 394–406.

Kral, V.A. & Durost, H.B. (1953) A comparative study of the amnesic syndrome in various organic conditions. *American Journal of Psychiatry* **110**, 41–47.

Kreisler, A., Godefroy, O., Delmaire, C. *et al.* (2000) The anatomy of aphasia revisited. *Neurology* **54**, 1117–1123.

Kucharska-Pietura, K., Phillips, M.L., Gernand, W. & David, A.S. (2003) Perception of emotions from faces and voices following unilateral brain damage. *Neuropsychologia* **41**, 1082–1090.

Kuperberg, G., McGuire, P. & David, A.S. (1998) Reduced sensitivity to linguistic context in schizophrenic thought disorder: evidence from on-line monitoring for words in linguistically anomalous sentences. *Journal of Abnormal Psychology* **107**, 423–434.

Kuperberg, G.R., McGuire, P.K. & David, A.S. (2000) Sensitivity to linguistic anomalies in spoken sentences: a case study approach to understanding thought disorder in schizophrenia. *Psychological Medicine* **30**, 345–357.

Lahti, A.C., Holcomb, H.H., Medoff, D.R., Weiler, M.A., Tamminga, C.A. & Carpenter, W.T. Jr (2001) Abnormal patterns of regional cerebral blood flow in schizophrenia with primary negative symptoms during an effortful auditory recognition task. *American Journal of Psychiatry* **158**, 1797–1808.

Lambon, R. Matthew, A., Patterson, K. (2003) Homogeneity and heterogeneity in mild cognitive impairment and Alzheimer's disease: a cross-longitudinal study of 55 cases. *Brain* **126**, 2350–2362.

Landis, T., Cummings, J.L., Benson, F. & Palmer, E.P. (1986) Loss of topographical familiarity: an environmental agnosia. *Archives of Neurology* **43**, 132–136.

Larsen, J.P., Høien, T., Lundberg, I. & Ødegaard, H. (1990) MRI evaluation of the size and symmetry of the planum temporale in adolescents with developmental dyslexia. *Brain and Language* **39**, 289–301.

Lashley, K.S. (1937) Functional determinants of cerebral localization. *Archives of Neurology. Psychiatry* **38**, 371–387.

Lawrie, S.M. & Abukmeil, S.S. (1998) Brain abnormality in schizophrenia. A systematic and quantitative review of volumetric magnetic resonance imaging studies. *British Journal of Psychiatry* **172**, 110–120.

Laws, K.R. (1999) A meta-analytic review of Wisconsin Card Sort studies in schizophrenia: a generalised deficit in disguise. *Cognitive Neuropsychiatry* **4**, 1–35.

LeDoux, J.E., Wilson, D.H. & Gazzaniga, M.S. (1977) Manipulospatial aspects of cerebral lateralization: clues to the origin of lateralization. *Neuropsychologia* **15**, 743–750.

Lepage, M., Habib, R. & Tulving, E. (1998) Hippocampal PET activations of memory encoding and retrieval: the HIPER model. *Hippocampus* **8**, 313–322.

Levine, B., Robertson, I.H., Clare, L. *et al.* (2000) Rehabilitation of executive functioning: an experimental-clinical validation of Goal Management Training. *Journal of the International Neuropsychological Society* **6**, 299–312.

Lezak, M.D. (1995) *Neuropsychological Assessment*, 3rd edn. Oxford University Press, New York.

Lhermitte, F. (1986) Human autonomy and the frontal lobes. Part II. Patient behavior in complex and social situations: the environmental dependency syndrome. *Annals of Neurology* **19**, 335–343.

Liddle, P.F. (1987) The symptoms of chronic schizophrenia: a re-examination of the positive–negative dichotomy. *British Journal of Psychiatry* **151**, 145–151.

Liddle, P.F., Friston, K.J., Frith, C.D., Hirsch, S.R., Jones, T. & Frackowiak, R.S.J. (1992) Patterns of cerebral blood flow in schizophrenia. *British Journal of Psychiatry* **160**, 179–186.

Lieberman, J.A., Tollefson, G.D., Charles, C. *et al.* (2005) Antipsychotic drug effects on brain morphology in first-episode psychosis. *Archives of General Psychiatry* **62**, 361–370.

Liepmann, H. (1905) Die Linke Hemisphaere und das Handlen. *Muechner Medizinsche Wochenschrift* **49**, 2375–2378.

Lishman, W.A. (1972) Selective factors in memory. Part 1: age, sex and personality attributes. *Psychological Medicine* **2**, 121–138.

Lishman, W.A. (1974) The speed of recall of pleasant and unpleasant experiences. *Psychological Medicine* **4**, 212–218.

Lissauer, H. (1890) Ein Fall von Seelenblindheit nebst einem Beitrage zur Theorie derselben. *Archiv für Psychiatrie und Nervenkrankheiten* **21**, 222–270.

Livingstone, M.S., Rosen, G.D., Drislane, F.W. & Galaburda, A.M. (1991) Physiological and anatomical evidence for a magnocellular defect in developmental dyslexia. *Proceedings of the National Academy of Sciences USA* **88**, 7943–7947.

Lloyd, G.G. & Lishman, W.A. (1975) Effect of depression on the speed of recall of pleasant and unpleasant experiences. *Psychological Medicine* **5**, 173–180.

Lubman, D.I., Velakoulis, D., McGorry, P.D. *et al.* (2002) Incidental radiological findings on brain magnetic resonance imaging in first-episode psychosis and chronic schizophrenia. *Acta Psychiatrica Scandinavica* **106**, 331–336.

Lucas, P. (1994) Episodic dyscontrol: a look back at anger. *Journal of Forensic Psychiatry* **5**, 371–407.

Lukianowicz, N. (1958) Autoscopic phenomena. *Archives of Neurology and Psychiatry* **80**, 199–220.

Lukianowicz, N. (1967) 'Body image' disturbances in psychiatric disorders. *British Journal of Psychiatry* **113**, 31–47.

Luria, A.R. (1964) Neuropsychology in the local diagnosis of brain damage. *Cortex* **1**, 3–18.

Mabille, H. & Pitres, A. (1913) Sur un cas d'amnésie de fixation post-apoplectique ayant persisté pendant vingt-trois ans. *Revue de Médicine* **33**, 257–279.

McCarthy, R.A. & Warrington, E.K. (1990) *Cognitive Neuropsychology: A Clinical Introduction*. Academic Press, London.

McCarthy, R.A., Kopelman, M.D. & Warrington, E.K. (2005) Remembering and forgetting of semantic knowledge in amnesia: a sixteen-year follow-up investigation of RFR. *Neuropsychologia* **43**, 356–372.

McDowell, J. (1981) Effects of encoding instructions on recall and recognition on Korsakoff patients. *Neuropsychologia* **19**, 43–48.

McGuire, P.K., Shah, G.M.S. & Murray, R.M. (1993) Increased blood flow in Broca's area during auditory hallucinations in schizophrenia. *Lancet* **342**, 703–706.

McGuire, P.K., Silbersweig, D.A., Wright, I. *et al.* (1995) Abnormal monitoring of inner speech: a physiological basis for auditory hallucinations. *Lancet* **346**, 596–600.

McGuire, P.K., Silbersweig, D.A., Murray, R.M., David, A.S., Frackowiak, R.S.J. & Frith, C.D. (1996) Functional anatomy of inner speech and auditory verbal imagery. *Psychological Medicine* **26**, 29–38.

McKee, R.D. & Squire, L.R. (1992) Equivalent forgetting rates in long-term memory for diencephalic and medial temporal amnesia. *Neurosciences* **12**, 3765–3772.

McKenna, P.J., Tamlyn, D., Lund, C.E., Mortimer, A.M., Hammond, S. & Baddeley, A.D. (1990) Amnesic syndrome in schizophrenia. *Psychological Medicine* **20**, 967–972.

McKenna, P., Clare, L. & Baddeley, A.D. (1995) Schizophrenia. In: Baddeley, A.D., Wilson, B.A. & Watts, F.N. (eds) *Handbook of Memory Disorders*, ch. 11. John Wiley & Sons, Chichester.

McNeil, J.E. & Warrington, E.K. (1993) Prosopagnosia: a face-specific disorder. *Quarterly Journal of Experimental Psychology*, **46A**, 1–10.

Maguire, E.A., Henson, R.A., Mummery, C.J. & Frith, C.D. (2001) Activity in prefrontal cortex, not hippocampus, varies parametrically with the increasing remoteness of memory. *NeuroReport* **12**, 441–444.

Mair, W.G.P., Warrington, E.K. & Weiskrantz, L. (1979) Memory disorder in Korsakoff's psychosis: a neuropathological and neuropsychological investigation of two cases. *Brain* **102**, 749–783.

Manns, J.R., Hopkins, R.O., Reed, J.M., Kitchener, E.G. & Squire, L.R. (2003) Recognition memory and the human hippocampus. *Neuron* **37**, 171–180.

Marcel, A.J., Tegner, R. & Nimmo-Smith, I. (2004) Anosognosia for plegia: specificity, extension, partiality and disunity of bodily unawareness. *Cortex* **40**, 19–40.

Mark, V.H., Sweet, W.H. & Ervin, F.R. (1972) The effect of amygdalotomy on violent behavior in patients with temporal lobe epilepsy. In: Hitchcock, E., Laitinen, L. & Vaernet, K. (eds) *Psychosurgery*, ch. 12. Charles C. Thomas, Springfield, IL.

Markowitsch, H.J., Fink, G.R., Thone, A., Kessler, J. & Heiss, W.-D. (1997) A PET study of persistent psychogenic amnesia covering the whole life span. *Cognitive Neuropsychiatry* **2**, 135–158.

Marshall, J.C. & Gurd, J.M. (2003) Neuropsychology: past, present and future. In: Halligan, P.W., Kischka, U. & Marshall, J.C. (eds) *Handbook of Clinical Neuropsychology*, pp. 3–14. Oxford University Press, Oxford.

Marshall, J.C. & Halligan, P.W. (1988) Blindsight and insight in visuo-spatial neglect. *Nature* **336**, 766–767.

Marshall, J.C. & Newcombe, F. (1973) Patterns of paralexia: a psycholinguistic approach. *Journal of Psycholinguistic Research* **2**, 175–199.

Master, D.R. & Lishman, W.A. (1984) Seizures, dyslexia, and dysgraphia of psychogenic origin. *Archives of Neurology* **41**, 889–890.

Master, D.R., Lishman, W.A. & Smith, A. (1983) Speed of recall in relation to affective tone and intensity of experience. *Psychological Medicine* **13**, 325–331.

Maughan, B. & Yule, W. (1994) Reading and other learning disabilities. In: Rutter, M., Taylor, E. & Hersov, L. (eds) *Child and Adolescent Psychiatry. Modern Approaches*, 3rd edn, ch. 36. Blackwell Science, Oxford.

Mayes, A.R. (1988) *Human Organic Memory Disorders*. Cambridge University Press, Cambridge.

Mayes, A.R. & Downes, J.J. (1997) What do the theories of the functional deficit(s) underlying amnesia have to explain? *Memory* **5**, 3–36.

Mayes, A.R. & Meudell, P.R. (1981) How similar is immediate memory in amnesic patients to delayed memory in normal subjects? A replication, extension and reassessment of the amnesic cueing effect. *Neuropsychologia* **19**, 647–654.

Mayes, A.R., Meudell, P.R. & Pickering, A. (1985) Is organic amnesia caused by a selective deficit in remembering contextual information? *Cortex* **21**, 167–202.

Mayes, A.R., Meudell, P.R., Mann, D. & Pickering, A. (1988) Location of lesions in Korsakoff's syndrome: neurological and neuropathological data n two patients. *Cortex* **24**, 367–388.

Mayes, A.R., Montaldi, D., Spencer, T.J. & Roberts, N. (2004a) Recalling spatial information as a component of recently and remotely acquired episodic or semantic memories: an fMRI study. *Neuropsychology* **18**, 426–441.

Mayes, A.R., Holdstock, J.S., Isaac, C.L. *et al.* (2004b) Associative recognition in a patient with selective hippocampal lesions and relatively normal item recognition. *Hippocampus* **14**, 763–784.

Mechanic, M.D., Resick, P.A. & Griffin, M.G. (1998) A comparison of normal forgetting, psychopathology, and information processing models of reported amnesia for recent sexual trauma. *Journal of Consulting and Clinical Practice* **66**, 948–957.

Meeter, M. & Murre, J.M.J. (2004) Consolidation of long-term memory: evidence and alternatives. *Psychological Bulletin* **130**, 843–857.

Metter, E.J. & Hanson, W.R. (1994) Use of positron emission tomography to study aphasia. In: Kertesz, A. (ed.) *Localization and Neuroimaging in Neuropsychology*, ch. 5. Academic Press, San Diego.

Meudell, P.R., Mayes, A.R. & Neary, D. (1979) Is amnesia caused by a consolidation impairment? In: Oborne, D.J., Gruneberg, M.M. & Eiser, J.R. (eds) *Research in Psychology and Medicine*, vol. 1, pp. 323–330. Academic Press, London.

Miller, E. (1973) Short- and long-term memory in patients with presenile dementia. *Psychological Medicine* **3**, 221–224.

Miller, J.W., Petersen, R.C., Metter, E.J., Millikan, C.H. & Yanagihara, T. (1987) Transient global amnesia: clinical characteristics and prognosis. *Neurology* **37**, 733–737.

Milner, A.D. & Goodale, M.A. (1992) Separate visual pathways for perception and action. *Neurosciences* **15**, 20–25.

Milner, B. (1962) Laterality effects in audition. In: Mountcastle, V. (ed.) *Interhemispheric Relations and Cerebral Dominance*, ch. 9. Johns Hopkins Press, Baltimore.

Milner, B. (1966) Amnesia following operation on the temporal lobes. In: Whitty, C.W.M. & Zangwill, O. (eds) *Amnesia*, ch. 5. Butterworths, London.

Morris, J.S., Frith, C., Perrett, D.I. *et al.* (1996) A differential neural response in the human amygdala to fearful and happy facial expressions. *Nature* **383**, 812–815.

Morris, R.G., Kotitsa, M. & Bramham, J. (2005) Planning in patients with focal brain damage: from simple to complex task performance. In: Morris, R.G. & Ward, G. (eds) *The Psychology of Planning: Cognitive and Neuropsychological Perspectives*, 153–180. Psychology Press, Hove.

Moscovitch, M. & Melo, B. (1997) Strategic retrieval and the frontal lobes: evidence from confabulation and amnesia. *Neuropsychologia* **35**, 1017–1034.

Moss, H.E. & Kopelman, M.D. (2003) Lost for words or loss of memories: the hippocampi and autobiographical memory in semantic dementia. *Journal of the International Neuropsychological Society* **9**, 531.

Murray, R.M., Lewis, S.W., Owen, M.J. & Foerster, A. (1988) The neurodevelopmental origins of dementia praecox. In: Bebbington, P. & McGuffin, P. (eds) *Schizophrenia. The Major Issues*, ch. 8. Heinemann, Oxford.

Nadel, L. & Moscovitch, M. (1997) Memory consolidation, retrograde amnesia and the hippocampal complex. *Current Opinion in Neurobiology* **7**, 217–227.

Naeser, M.A., Alexander, M.P., Helm-Estabrooks, N., Levine, H.L., Laughlin, S.A. & Geschwind, N. (1982) Aphasia with predominantly subcortical lesion sites. Description of three capsular putaminal aphasia syndromes. *Archives of Neurology* **39**, 2–14.

Narabayashi, H. & Uno, M. (1966) Long range results of stereotaxic amygdalotomy for behaviour disorders. *Confinia Neurologica* **27**, 168–171.

Narabayashi, H., Nagao, T., Saito, Y., Yoshida, M. & Nagahata, M. (1963) Stereotaxic amygdalotomy for behaviour disorders. *Archives of Neurology* **9**, 1–16.

Nestor, P.J., Fryer, T.D., Ikeda, M. & Hodges, J.R. (2003) Retrosplenial cortex (BA 29/30) hypometabolism in mild cognitive impairment (prodromal Alzheimer's disease). *European Journal of Neuroscience* **18**, 2663–2667.

Newcombe, F. (1969) *Missile Wounds of the Brain: A Study of Psychological Deficits*. Oxford University Press, Oxford.

Norman, D.A. & Shallice, T. (1980) Attention to action: willed and automatic control of behaviour. In: Davidson, R.J., Schwartz, G.E. & Shapiro, D. (eds) *Consciousness and Self-regulation*. Centre for Human Information Processing, Technical report No. 99. Plenum Press, New York.

O'Callaghan, E., Larkin, C., Redmond, O., Stack, J., Ennis, J.T. & Waddington, J.L. (1988) Early-onset schizophrenia after teenage head injury. A case report with magnetic resonance imaging. *British Journal of Psychiatry* **153**, 394–396.

O'Connor, M., Butters, N., Miliotis, P., Eslinger, P. & Cermak, L.S. (1992) The dissociation of anterograde and retrograde amnesia in a patient with herpes encephalitis. *Journal of Clinical and Experimental Neuropsychology* **14**, 159–178.

Ogden, J.A. (1993) Visual object agnosia, prosopagnosia, achromatopsia, loss of visual imagery, and autobiographical amnesia following recovery from cortical blindness: case M.H. *Neuropsychologia* **31**, 571–589.

Oh, T.M., McCarthy, R.A. & McKenna, P.J. (2002) Is there a schizophasia? A study applying the single case approach to formal thought disorder in schizophrenia. *Neurocase* **8**, 233–244.

Ojemann, J.G., Ojemann, G.A. & Lettich, E. (1992) Neuronal activity related to faces and matching in human right nondominant temporal cortex. *Brain* **115**, 1–13.

O'Keeffe, F.M., Dockree, P.M. & Robertson, I.H. (2004) Poor insight in traumatic brain injury mediated by impaired error processing? Evidence from electrodermal activity. *Cognitive Brain Research* **22**, 101–112.

Olvera, R.L. (2002) Intermittent explosive disorder: epidemiology, diagnosis and management. *CNS Drugs* **16**, 517–526.

Osler, W. (1913) Spcialism in the general hospital. *Bulletin. Johns Hopkins Hospital* **24**, 167–171.

Pang, A. & Lewis, S.W. (1996) Bipolar affective disorder minus left prefrontal cortex equals schizophrenia. *British Journal of Psychiatry* **168**, 647–650.

Papez, J.W. (1937) A proposed mechanism of emotion. *Archives of Neurology and Psychiatry* **38**, 725–743.

Parkin, A.J. (1987) *Memory and Amnesia: An Introduction*. Basil Blackwell, Oxford.

Parkin, A.J. & Leng, N.R.C. (1988) Comparative studies of human amnesia: syndrome or syndromes? In: Markowitsch, H.J. (ed.) *Information Processing by the Brain*, pp. 107–123. Hans Hubber, Toronto.

Parsons, L.M., Sergent, J., Hodges, D.A. & Fox, P.T. (2005) The brain basis of piano performance. *Neuropsychologia* **43**, 199–215.

Paulesu, E., Frith, C.D. & Frackowiak, R.S.J. (1993) The neural correlates of the verbal component of working memory. *Nature* **362**, 342–345.

Paulesu, E., Frith, U., Snowling, M. *et al.* (1996) Is developmental dyslexia a disconnection syndrome? Evidence from PET scanning. *Brain* **119**, 143–157.

Perani, D., Vallar, G., Cappa, S., Messa, C. & Fazio, F. (1987) Aphasia and neglect after subcortical stroke. A clinical/cerebral perfusion correlation study. *Brain* **110**, 1211–1229.

Petersen, S.E., Fox, P.T., Posner, M.I., Mintun, M. & Raichle, M.E. (1988) Positron emission tomographic studies of the cortical anatomy of single-word processing. *Nature* **331**, 585–589.

Phillips, M.L., Howard, R. & David, A. (1996) Mirror, mirror on the wall, who . . . ? A case study of impaired visual self recognition. *Cognitive Neuropsychiatry* **1**, 153–174.

Phillips, M.L., Young, A.W., Senior C. *et al.* (1997) A specific neural substrate for perceiving facial expressions of disgust. *Nature* **389**, 495–498.

Pia, L., Neppi-Modona, M., Ricci, R. & Berti, A. (2004) The anatomy of anosognosia for hemiplegia: a meta-analysis. *Cortex* **40**, 367–377.

Pick, A. (1892) Ueber die Beziehungen der senilen Hirnatrophie zur Aphasie. *Prager Medizinische Wochenschrift* **17**, 165–167.

Pierce, S.R. & Buxbaum, L.J. (2002) Treatments of unilateral neglect: a review. *Archives of Physical Medicine and Rehabilitation* **83**, 256–268.

Plum, F. (1972) Prospects for research on schizophrenia. 3. Neuropsychology. Neuropathological findings. *Neurosciences Research Program Bulletin* **10**, 384–388.

Poeck, K. (1969) Pathophysiology of emotional disorders associated with brain damage. In: Vinken, P.J. & Bruyn, G.W. (eds) *Handbook of Clinical Neurology*, vol. 3, ch. 20. North-Holland Publishing Company, Amsterdam.

Press, G.A., Amaral, D.G. & Squire, L.R. (1989) Hippocampal abnormalities in amnesic patients revealed by high-resolution magnetic resonance imaging. *Nature* **341**, 54–57.

Price, C.J. (2000) The anatomy of language: contributions from functional neuroimaging. *Journal of Anatomy* **197**, 335–359.

Price, C.J. & Crinion, J. (2005) The latest on functional imaging studies of aphasic stroke. *Current Opinion in Neurology* **18**, 429–434.

Prigatano, G.P. (2005) Disturbances of self-awareness and rehabilitation of patients with traumatic brain injury: a 20-year perspective. *Journal of Head Trauma Rehabilitation* **20**, 19–29.

Pyszora, N.M., Barker, A.F. & Kopelman, M.D. (2003) Amnesia for criminal offences: a study of life sentence prisoners. *Journal of Forensic Psychiatry and Psychology* **14**, 475–490.

Ramamurthi, B. (1988) Stereotactic operation in behaviour disorders. Amygdalotomy and hypothalamotomy. *Acta Neurochirurgica Supplementum (Wien)* **44**, 152–157.

Ranganath, C., Yonelinas, A.P., Cohen, M.X., Dy, C.J., Tom, S.M. & D'Esposito, M. (2004) Dissociable correlates of recollection and familiarity within the medial temporal lobes. *Neuropsychologia* **42**, 2–13.

Rasmussen, T. & Milner, B. (1977) The role of early left-brain injury in determining lateralization of cerebral speech functions. *Annals of the New York Academy of Sciences* **299**, 355–369.

Ratcliff, G. & Newcombe, F. (1973) Spatial orientation in man: effects of left, right, and bilateral posterior cerebral lesions. *Journal of Neurology, Neurosurgery and Psychiatry* **36**, 448–454.

Reed, J.M. & Squire, L.R. (1997) Impaired recognition memory in patients with lesions limited to the hippocampal formation. *Behavioral Neuroscience* **111**, 667–675.

Reed, J.M. & Squire, L.R. (1998) Retrograde amnesia for facts and events: findings from four new cases. *Journal of Neuroscience* **18**, 3943–3954.

Reed, J.M., Marsden, P., Lasserson, D., Sheldon, N., Lewis, P. & Stanhope, N. (1999) FDG-PET analysis and findings in Wernicke–Korsakoff syndrome. *Memory* **7**, 599–612.

Reed, L.J., Lasserson, D., Marsden, P. *et al.* (2003) [18]FDG-PET findings in the Wernicke–Korsakoff syndrome. *Cortex* **39**, 1027–1045.

Reed, L.J., Lasserson, D., Marsden, P., Bright, P., Stanhope, N. & Kopelman, M.D. (2005) Correlations of regional cerebral metabolism with memory performance and executive function in patients with herpes encephalitis or frontal lobe lesions. *Neuropsychology* **19**, 555–565.

Reichenberg, A., Weiser, M., Rabinowitz, J. *et al.* (2002) A population-based cohort study of premorbid intellectual, language, and behavioral functioning in patients with schizophrenia, schizoaffective disorder, and nonpsychotic bipolar disorder. *American Journal of Psychiatry* **159**, 2027–2035.

Rempel-Clower, N.L., Zola, S.M., Squire, L.R. & Amaral, D.G. (1996) Three cases of enduring memory impairment after bilateral damage limited to the hippocampal formation. *Journal of Neuroscience* **16**, 5233–5255.

Ribot, T. (1882) *Diseases of Memory.* Appleton, New York.

Riddoch, M.J. & Humphreys, G.W. (2003) Visual agnosia. *Neurologic Clinics* **21**, 501–520.

Rodriguez-Ferrera, S., McCarthy, R.A. & McKenna, P.J. (2001) Language in schizophrenia and its relationship to formal thought disorder. *Psychological Medicine* **31**, 197–205.

Ross, E.D. (1981) The aprosodias: functional–anatomic organisation of the affective components of language in the right hemisphere. *Archives of Neurology* **38**, 561–569.

Ross, E.D. & Mesulam, M.-M. (1979) Dominant language functions of the right hemisphere. Prosody and emotional gesturing. *Archives of Neurology* **36**, 144–148.

Rubin, D.C. & Schulkind, M.D. (1997) Distributions of important and word cued autobiographical memory in 20-, 35-, and 70-year-old adults. *Psychology and Ageing* **12**, 524–535.

Rudge, P. & Warrington, E.K. (1991) Selective impairment of memory and visual perception in splenial tumours. *Brain* **114**, 349–360.

Rutter, M. (1978) Prevalence and types of dyslexia. In: Benton, A.L. & Pearl, D. (eds) *Dyslexia. An Appraisal of Current Knowledge*, ch. 1. Oxford University Press, New York.

Rutter, M. & Yule, W. (1975) The concept of specific reading retardation. *Journal of Child Psychology and Psychiatry* **16**, 181–197.

Rutter, M., Tizard, J., Yule, W., Graham, P. & Whitmore, K. (1976) Research report: Isle of Wight Studies 1964–1974. *Psychological Medicine* **6**, 313–332.

Ryan, L., Nadel, L., Keil, K., Putnam, K., Schnyer, D. & Trouard, T. (2001) Hippocampal complex and retrieval of recent and very remote autobiographical memories: evidence from functional magnetic resonance imaging in neurologically intact people. *Hippocampus* **11**, 707–714.

Sagar, H.J., Cohen, N.J., Sullivan, E.V., Corkin, S. & Growdon, J.H. (1988) Remote memory function in Alzheimer's disease and Parkinson's disease. *Brain* **111**, 185–206.

Sanders, H.I. & Warrington, E.K. (1971) Memory for remote events in amnesic patients. *Brain* **94**, 661–668.

Sauget, J., Benton, A.L. & Hécaen, H. (1971) Disturbances of the body schema in relation to language impairment and hemispheric locus of lesion. *Journal of Neurology, Neurosurgery and Psychiatry* **34**, 496–501.

Saykin, A.J., Gur, R.C., Gur, R.E. *et al.* (1991) Neuropsychological function in schizophrenia, selective impairment in memory and learning. *Archives of General Psychiatry* **48**, 618–624.

Saykin, A.J., Shtasel, D.L., Gur, R.E. *et al.* (1994) Neuropsychological deficits in neuroleptic naive patients with first-episode schizophrenia. *Archives of General Psychiatry* **51**, 124–131.

Schacter, D.L. (1987) Memory, amnesia, and frontal lobe dysfunction. *Psychobiology* **15**, 21–36.

Schacter, D.L. (2001) *The Seven Sins of Memory: How the Mind Forgets and Remembers.* Houghton Mifflin Company, New York.

Schacter, D.L. & Wagner, A.D. (1999) Medial temporal lobe activations in fMRI and PET studies of episodic encoding and retrieval. *Hippocampus* **9**, 7–24.

Schacter, D.L., Wang, P.L., Tulving, E. & Freedman, M. (1982) Functional retrograde amnesia: a quantitative case study. *Neuropsychologia* **20**, 523–532.

Schacter, D., Norman, K.A. & Koutstaal, W. (1998) The cognitive neuroscience of constructive memory. *Annu Rev Psychol* **49**, 289–318.

Schilder, P. (1935) *The Image and Appearance of the Human Body: Studies in the Constructive Energies of the Psyche.* Kegan Paul, Trench, Trubner, London.

Schnider, A. (2001) Spontaneous confabulation, reality monitoring, and the limbic system: a review. *Brain Research Reviews* **36**, 150–160.

Schnider, A., von Daniken, C. & Gutbrod, K. (1996) The mechanisms of spontaneous and provoked confabulations. *Brain* **119**, 1365–1375.

Scoville, W.B. (1954) The limbic lobe in man. *Journal of Neurosurgery* **11**, 64–66.

Scoville, W.B. & Milner, B. (1957) Loss of recent memory after bilateral hippocampal lesions. *Journal of Neurology, Neurosurgery and Psychiatry* **20**, 11–21.

Searleman, A. (1977) A review of right hemisphere linguistic capabilities. *Psychological Bulletin* **84**, 503–528.

Semmes, J., Weinstein, S., Ghent, L. & Teuber, H.-L. (1955) Spatial orientation in man after cerebral injury. 1: Analyses by locus of lesion. *Journal of Psychology* **39**, 227–244.

Semmes, J., Weinstein, S., Ghent, L. & Teuber, H.L. (1963) Correlates of impaired orientation in personal and extrapersonal space. *Brain* **86**, 747–772.

Serafetinides, E.A. & Falconer, M.A. (1962) Some observations on memory impairment after temporal lobectomy for epilepsy. *Journal of Neurology, Neurosurgery and Psychiatry* **25**, 251–255.

Shallice, T. (1988) *From Neuropsychology to Mental Structure*. Cambridge, Cambridge University Press.

Shallice, T. (2003) Functional imaging and neuropsychology findings: how can they be linked? *Neuroimage* **20** (suppl. 1), S146–S154.

Shallice, T. & Burgess, P.W. (1991a) Deficits in strategy application following frontal lobe damage in man. *Brain* **114**, 727–741.

Shallice, T. & Burgess, P.W. (1991b) Higher-order cognitive impairments and frontal lobe lesions in man. In: *Frontal Lobe Function and Dysfunction*, pp. 125–138. Oxford University Press, New York.

Shallice, T., Fletcher, P., Frith, C.D., Grasby, P., Frackowiak, R.S. & Dolan, R.J. (1994) Brain regions associated with acquisitions and retrieval of verbal episodic memory. *Nature* **368**, 633–635.

Shankweiler, D. (1966) Effects of temporal-lobe damage on perception of dichotically presented melodies. *Journal of Comparative and Physiological Psychology* **62**, 115–119.

Shapiro, B.E., Grossman, M. & Gardner, H. (1981) Selective musical processing deficits in brain damaged populations. *Neuropsychologia* **19**, 161–169.

Shapleske, J., Rossell, S., Woodruff, P. & David, A. (1999) The planum temporale: a systematic, quantitative review of its structural, functional and clinical significance. *Brain Research Reviews* **29**, 26–49.

Shapleske, J., Rossell, S.L., Chitnis, X.A. *et al.* (2002) A computational morphometric MRI study of schizophrenia: effects of hallucinations. *Cerebral Cortex* **12**, 1331–1341.

Sharma, T. & Harvey, P. (eds) (2000) *Cognitive Functioning in Schizophrenia*. Oxford University Press, New York.

Shenton, M.E., Dickey, C.C., Frumin, M. & McCarley, R.W. (2001) A review of MRI findings in schizophrenia. *Schizophrenia Research* **49**, 1–52.

Shimamura, A.P. (2002) Muybridge in motion: travels in art, psychology and neuropsychology. *History of Photography* **26**, 341–350.

Shimamura, A.P., Salmon, D.P., Squire, L.R. & Butters, N. (1987) Memory dysfunction and word priming in dementia and amnesia. *Behavioral Neuroscience* **101**, 347–351.

Shoqeirat, M.A., Mayes, A., MacDonald, C., Meudell, P. & Pickering, A. (1990) Performance on tests sensitive to frontal lobe lesions by patients with organic amnesia: Leng and Parkin revisited. *British Journal of Clinical Psychology* **29**, 401–408.

Sierra, M., Lopera, F., Lambert, M.V., Phillips, M.L. & David, A.S. (2002) Separating depersonalisation and derealisation: the relevance of the 'lesion method'. *Journal of Neurology, Neurosurgery and Psychiatry* **72**, 530–532.

Small, S.L. & Burton, M.W. (2002) Functional magnetic resonance imaging studies of language. *Current Neurology and Neuroscience Reports* **2**, 505–510.

Smith, A. (1966) Speech and other functions after left (dominant) hemispherectomy. *Journal of Neurology, Neurosurgery and Psychiatry* **29**, 467–471.

Smith, A. (1972) Dominant and non-dominant hemispherectomy. In: Smith, W.L. (ed.) *Drugs, Development and Cerebral Function*, ch. 3. Charles C. Thomas, Springfield, IL.

Snowden, J.S., Goulding, P.J. & Neary, D. (1989) Semantic dementia: a form of circumscribed cerebral atrophy. *Behavioural Neurology* **2**, 167–182.

Snowden, J.S., Griffiths, H.L. & Neary, D. (1996) Semantic–episodic memory interactions in semantic dementia: implications for retrograde memory function. *Cognitive Neuropsychology* **13**, 1101–1137.

Snowling, M.J. (1996) Dyslexia: a hundred years on. A verbal not a visual disorder, which responds to early intervention. *British Medical Journal* **313**, 1096–1097.

Sperry, R.W. (1966) Brain bisection and consciousness. In: Eccles, J.C. (ed.) *Brain and Conscious Experience*, ch. 13. Springer-Verlag, Berlin.

Sperry, R.W. & Gazzaniga, M.S. (1967) Language following surgical disconnection of the hemispheres. In: Darley, F.L. (ed.) *Brain Mechanisms Underlying Speech and Language*, pp. 41, 313. Grune & Stratton, New York.

Squire, L.R. (1986) Mechanisms of memory. *Science* **232**, 1612–1619.

Squire, L.R. (1987) Memory: neural organization and behavior. In: Mountcastle, V.B. (ed.) *Handbook of Physiology, Section I: The Nervous System V*, vol. 5, part I, pp. 295–371. American Physiological Society, Bethesda, MD.

Squire, L.R. & Alvarez, P. (1995) Retrograde amnesia and memory consolidation: a neurobiological perspective. *Current Opinion in Neurobiology* **5**, 169–177.

Squire, L.R. & Haist, F. (1989) The neurology of memory: quantitative assessment of retrograde amnesia in two groups of amnesic patients. *Journal of Neuroscience* **9**, 828–839.

Squire, L.R., Shimamura, A.P. & Graf, P. (1987) Strength and duration of priming effects in normal subjects and amnesic patients. *Neuropsychologia* **25**, 195–210.

Starkstein, S.E., Fedoroff, J.P., Price, T.R., Leiguarda, R. & Robinson, R.G. (1992) Anosognosia in patients with cerebrovascular lesions. A study of causative factors. *Stroke* **23**, 1446–1453.

Starr, A. & Phillips, L. (1970) Verbal and motor memory in the amnestic syndrome. *Neuropsychologia* **8**, 75–88.

Stefanacci, L., Buffalo, E.A., Schmolk, H. & Squire, R.L. (2000) Profound amnesia after damage to the medial temporal lobe: a neuroanatomical and neuropsychological profile of patient E.P. Journal of Neuroscience **20**, 7024–7036.

Stuss, D.T., Alexander, M.P., Lieberman, A. & Levine, H. (1978) An extraordinary form of confabulation. *Neurology* **28**, 1166–1172.

Stuss, D.T., Alexander, M.P., Shallice, T. *et al.* (2005) Multiple frontal systems controlling response speed. *Neuropsychologia* **43**, 396–417.

Suddath, R.L., Christison, G.W., Torrey, E.F., Casanova, M.F. & Weinberger, D.R. (1990) Anatomical abnormalities in the brain of monozygotic twins discordant for schizophrenia. *New England Journal of Medicine* **322**, 789–794.

Sweet, W.H., Ervin, F. & Mark, V.H. (1969) The relationship of violent behaviour to focal cerebral disease. In: Garattini, S. &

Sigg, E.B. (eds) *Aggressive Behaviour*, pp. 81, 82, 189. Excerpta Medica, Amsterdam.

Symonds, C.P. (1966) Disorders of memory. *Brain* **89**, 625–644.

Talland, G.A. (1965) *Deranged Memory: A Psychonomic Study of the Amnesic Syndrome*. Academic Press, New York.

Tamlyn, D., McKenna, P.J., Mortimer, A.M., Lund, C.E., Hammond, S. & Baddeley, A.D. (1992) Memory impairment in schizophrenia: its extent, affiliations and neuropsychological character. *Psychological Medicine* **22**, 101–115.

Taylor, P.J. & Kopelman, M.D. (1984) Amnesia for criminal offences. *Psychological Medicine* **14**, 581–588.

Teasdale, J.D. & Spencer, P. (1984) Induced mood and estimates of past success. *British Journal of Clinical Psychology* **23**, 149–150.

Teuber, H.-L. (1962) Effects of brain wounds implicating right or left hemisphere in man. In: Mountcastle, V.B. (ed.) *Interhemispheric Relations and Cerebral Dominance*. John Hopkins Press, Baltimore.

Thomas, H.V., Dalman, C., David, A.S., Gentz, J., Lewis, G & Allebeck, P. (2001) Obstetric complications and risk of schizophrenia. Effect of gender, age at diagnosis and maternal history of psychosis. *British Journal of Psychiatry* **179**, 409–414.

Tonkonogy, J.M. (1991) Violence and temporal lobe lesion: head CT and MRI data. *Journal of Neuropsychiatry and Clinical Neurosciences* **3**, 189–196.

Tranel, D. & Damasio, A.D. (1995) Neurobiological foundations of human memory. In: Baddeley, A.D., Wilson, B.A. & Watts, F.N. (eds) *Handbook of Memory Disorders*, ch. 2. John Wiley & Sons, Chichester.

Tucha, O., Steup, A., Smely, C. & Lange, K.W. (1997) Toe agnosia in Gerstmann syndrome. *Journal of Neurology, Neurosurgery and Psychiatry* **63**, 399–403.

Tucker, D.M., Roeltgen, D.P., Tully, R., Hartmann, J. & Boxell, C. (1988) Memory dysfunction following unilateral transection of the fornix: a hippocampal disconnection syndrome. *Cortex* **24**, 465–472.

Tulving, E. (1972) Episodic and semantic memory. In: Tulving, E. & Donaldson, W. (eds) *Organisation of Memory*, ch. 10. Academic Press, New York.

Tulving, E., Kapur, S., Craik, F.I.M., Moscovitch, M. & Houle, S. (1994) Hemispheric encoding/retrieval asymmetry in episodic memory: positron emission tomography findings. *Proceedings of the National Academy of Sciences USA* **91**, 2016–2020.

Turnbull *et al.* 2005

Turner, E.A. (1969) A surgical approach to the treatment of symptoms in temporal lobe epilepsy. In: Herrington, R.N. (ed.) *Current Problems in Neuropsychiatry*, ch. 17. British Journal of Psychiatry Special Publication No. 4. Headley Brothers, Ashford, Kent.

Turner, E.A. (1972) Operations for aggression: bilateral temporal lobotomy and posterior cingulectomy. Ch. 18 In: Hitchcock, E., Laitinen, L. & Vaernet, K. (eds) *Psychosurgery*, ch. 18. Charles C. Thomas, Springfield, IL.

Valenstein, E., Bowers, D., Verfaellie, M., Heilman, K.M., Day, A. & Watson, R.T. (1987) Retrosplenial amnesia. *Brain* **110**, 1631–1646.

Vallar, G. & Papagno, C. (1995) Neuropsychological impairments of short-term memory. In: Baddeley, A.D., Wilson, B.A. & Watts, F.N. (eds) *Handbook of Memory Disorders*, ch. 6. John Wiley & Sons, Chichester.

van Elst, L.T., Woermann, F.G., Lemieux, L., Thompson, P.J. & Trimble, M.R. (2000) Affective aggression in patients with temporal lobe epilepsy: a quantitative MRI study of the amygdala. *Brain* **123**, 234–243.

Van Horn, J.D. & McManus, I.C. (1992) Ventricular enlargement in schizophrenia. A meta-analysis of studies of the ventricle:brain ratio (VBR). *British Journal of Psychiatry* **160**, 687–697.

Vargha-Khadem, F., Isaacs, E.B., Papaleloudi, H., Polkey, C.E. & Wilson, J. (1991) Development of language in six hemispherectomized patients. *Brain* **114**, 473–495.

Vellutino, F.R., Fletcher, J.M., Snowling, M.J. & Scanlon, D.M. (2004) Specific reading disability (dyslexia): what have we learned in the past four decades? *Journal of Child Psychology and Psychiatry and Allied Disciplines* **45**, 2–40.

Verfaellie, M., Reiss, L. & Roth, H.L. (1995) Knowledge of New English vocabulary in amnesia: an examination of premorbidly acquired semantic memory. *Journal of the International Neuropsychology Society* **1**, 443–453.

Victor, M. (1964) Observations on the amnestic syndrome in man and its anatomical basis. In: Brazier, M.A.B. (ed.) *Brain Function, vol. II: RNA and Brain Function, Memory and Learning*, pp. 25, 30, 580. University of California Press, Berkeley and Los Angeles.

Victor, M., Angevine, J.B., Mancall, E.L. & Fisher, C.M. (1961) Memory loss with lesions of hippocampal formation. *Archives of Neurology* **5**, 244–263.

Victor, M., Adams, R.D. & Collins, G.H. (1971) *The Wernicke–Korsakoff Syndrome*. Blackwell Scientific Publications: Oxford.

Vignolo, L.A. (1969) Auditory agnosia: a review and report of recent evidence. In: Benton, A.L. (ed.) *Contributions to Clinical Neuropsychology*, ch. 7. Aldine Publishing Company, Chicago.

Viskontas, I.V., McAndrews, M.P. & Mosocovitch, M. (2000) Remote episodic memory deficits in patients with unilateral temporal lobe epilepsy and excisions. *Neurosciences* **20**, 5853–5857.

Wada, J. & Rasmussen, T. (1960) Intracarotid injection of sodium amytal for the lateralization of cerebral speech dominance: experimental and clinical observations. *Journal of Neurosurgery* **17**, 266–282.

Walsh, K. (1994) *Neuropsychology. A Clinical Approach*, 3rd edn. Churchill Livingstone, Edinburgh.

Warrington, E.K. (1975) The selective impairment of semantic memory. *Quarterly Journal of Experimental Psychology* **27**, 635–657.

Warrington, E.K. (1982) The fractionation of arithmetic skills: a single case study. *Quarterly Journal of Experimental Psychology* **34A**, 31–51.

Warrington, E.K. (1985) Agnosia: the impairment of object recognition. In: Frederiks, J.A.M. (ed.) *Handbook of Clinical Neurology, Revised Series, vol. 1. Clinical Neuropsychology*, ch. 23. Elsevier Science Publishers, Amsterdam.

Warrington, E.K. & Duchen, L.W. (1992) A re-appraisal of a case of persistent global amnesia following right temporal lobectomy: a clinico-pathological study. *Neuropsychologia* **30**, 437–451.

Warrington, E.K. & James, M. (1967) An experimental investigation of facial recognition in patients with unilateral cerebral lesions. *Cortex* **3**, 317–326.

Warrington, E.K. & Weiskrantz, L. (1968) New method of testing long-term retention with special reference to amnesic patients. *Nature* **217**, 972–974.

Warrington, E.K. & Weiskrantz, L. (1982) Amnesia: a disconnection syndrome? *Neuropsychologia* **20**, 233–248.

Weinberger, D.R. (1987) Implications of normal brain development for the pathogenesis of schizophrenia. *Archives of General Psychiatry* **44**, 660–669.

Weinberger, D.R. (1995) From neuropathology to neurodevelopment. *Lancet* **346**, 552–557.

Weinberger, D.R., Berman, K.F. & Daniel, D.G. (1991) Prefrontal cortex dysfunction in schizophrenia. In: Levin, H.S., Eisenberg, H.M. & Benton, A.L. (eds) *Frontal Lobe Function and Dysfunction*, ch. 14. Oxford University Press, New York.

Weinstein, E.A. & Cole, M. (1963) Concepts of anosognosia. In: Halpern, L. (ed.) *Problems of Dynamic Neurology*, p. 70. Hadassah Medical School, Jerusalem.

Weinstein, E.A. & Kahn, R.L. (1955) *Denial of Illness: Symbolic and Physiological Aspects*. Charles C. Thomas, Springfield, IL.

Weinstein, E.A., Kahn, R.L., Malitz, S. & Rozanski, J. (1954) Delusional reduplication of parts of the body. *Brain* **77**, 45–60.

Weinstein, E.A., Lyerly, O.G., Cole, M. & Ozer, M.N. (1966) Meaning in jargon aphasia. *Cortex* **2**, 165–187.

Westmacott, R., Leach, L., Freedman, M. & Moscovitch, M. (2001) Different patterns of autobiographical memory loss in semantic dementia and medial temporal lobe amnesia. *Neurocase* **7**, 37–55.

Wheeler, M.A., Stuss, D.T. & Tulving, E. (1995) Frontal lobe damage produces episodic memory impairment. *Journal of the International Neuropsychology Society* **1**, 525–536.

Whitty, C.W.M. & Lewin, W. (1960) A Korsakoff syndrome in the post-cingulectomy confusional state. *Brain* **83**, 648–653.

Williams, D. (1969) Neural factors related to habitual aggression: consideration of the differences between those habitual aggressives and others who have committed crimes of violence. *Brain* **92**, 503–520.

Williams, M. & Smith, H.V. (1954) Mental disturbances in tuberculous meningitis. *Journal of Neurology, Neurosurgery and Psychiatry* **17**, 173–182.

Wilson, B.A. & Wearing, D. (1995) Prisoner of consciousness: a state of just awakening following herpes simplex encephalitis. In: Campbell, R. & Conway, M.A. (eds) *Broken Memories*, pp. 14–30. Blackwell, Oxford.

Wilson, B.A., Kopelman, M.D. & Kapur, N. (2008) Prominent and persistent loss of past awareness in amnesia: delusion, impaired consciousness of coping strategy? *Neuropsychological Rehabilitation* **18**, 527–540.

Wilson, B.A., Cockburn, J. & Baddeley, A. (1985) The Rivermead Behavioural Memory Test. Thames Valley Test Company, Ely, UK.

Wise, R.J. (2003) Language systems in normal and aphasic human subjects: functional imaging studies and inferences from animal studies. *British Medical Bulletin* **65**, 95–119.

Woermann, F.G., van Elst, L.T., Koepp, M.J. *et al.* (2000) Reduction of frontal neocortical grey matter associated with affective aggression in patients with temporal lobe epilepsy: an objective voxel by voxel analysis of automatically segmented MRI. *Journal of Neurology, Neurosurgery and Psychiatry* **68**, 162–169.

Wood, J.N. & Grafman, J. (2003) Human prefrontal cortex: processing and representational perspectives. *Nature Reviews. Neuroscience* **4**, 139–147.

Woodruff, P.W.R., McManus, I.C. & David, A.S. (1995) Meta-analysis of corpus callosum size in schizophrenia. *Journal of Neurology, Neurosurgery and Psychiatry* **58**, 457–461.

Wright, I.C., Rabe-Hesketh, S., Woodruff, P.W.R., David, A.S., Murray, R.M. & Bullmore, E.T. (2000) Meta-analysis of regional brain volumes in schizophrenia. *American Journal of Psychiatry* **157**, 16–25.

Yakovlev, P.I. & Rakic, P. (1966) Patterns of decussation of bulbar pyramids and distribution of pyramidal tracts on two sides of the spinal cord. *Transactions of the American Neurological Association* **91**, 366–367.

Yule, W. (1973) Differential prognosis of reading backwardness and specific reading retardation. *British Journal of Educational Psychology* **43**, 244–248.

Zaidel, E. (1977) Unilateral auditory language comprehension on the token test following cerebral commissurotomy and hemispherectomy. *Neuropsychologia* **15**, 1–18.

Zaidel, E. (1978) Auditory language comprehension in the right hemisphere following cerebral commissurotomy and hemispherectomy: a comparison with child language and aphasia. In: Caramazza, A. & Zurif, E. (eds) *Language Acquisition and Language Breakdown*. Johns Hopkins University Press, Baltimore.

Zakzanis, K.K. & Heinrichs, R.W. (1999) Schizophrenia and the frontal brain: a quantitative review. *Journal of the International Neuropsychology Society* **5**, 556–566.

Zammit, S., Allebeck, P., David, A.S. *et al.* (2004) A longitudinal study of premorbid IQ score and risk of developing schizophrenia, bipolar disorder, severe depression and other non-affective psychoses. *Archives of General Psychiatry* **61**, 354–360.

Zangwill, O.L. (1966) The amnesic syndrome. In: Whitty, C.W.M. & Zangwill, O.L. (eds) *Amnesia*, ch. 3. Butterworth, London.

Zangwill, O.L. (1967) The Grunthal–Störring case of amnesic syndrome. *British Journal of Psychiatry* **113**, 113–128.

Zatorre, R.J. (2003) Music and the brain. *Annals of the New York Academy of Sciences* **999**, 4–14.

Zipursky, R.B., Lim, K.O., Sullivan, E.V., Brown, B.W. & Pfefferbaum, A. (1992) Widespread cerebral gray matter volume deficits in schizophrenia. *Archives of General Psychiatry* **49**, 195–205.

Zola-Morgan, S., Cohen, N.J. & Squire, L.R. (1983) Recall of remote episodic memory in amnesia. *Neuropsychologia* **21**, 487–500.

Zola-Morgan, S., Squire, L.R. & Amaral, D.G. (1986) Human amnesia and the medial temporal region: enduring memory impairment following a bilateral lesion limited to field CA1 of the hippocampus. *Journal of Neuroscience* **6**, 2950–2967.

Clinical Assessment

Anthony S. David

Institute of Psychiatry, King's College, London

The assessment of patients with organic psychiatric disorder follows the time-honoured principles of clinical practice generally. It is sometimes a time-consuming process, requiring a good deal of patience and persistence. A careful history is essential, the mental state must be systematically examined, and a thorough physical examination will be required as well. The picture will then often remain incomplete without evaluation by a clinical psychologist with neuropsychology skills and the undertaking of certain ancillary investigations. A period of observation in hospital in a specialised unit can do much to clarify the situation when the diagnosis is unclear, but may not be accessible. Similarly, direct observation of the patient's living circumstances can be highly illuminating. In many cases, the initial contact with the patient will merely serve to establish the major probabilities in diagnosis and allow more detailed planning for further enquiries.

No attempt is made in the present chapter to outline a comprehensive schema for psychiatric history-taking or examination. This is dealt with in textbooks of general psychiatry and related publications (Goldberg & Murray 2006). The purpose here is to focus on those aspects of clinical enquiry which assume particular importance when one suspects an organic disease process in the genesis of the patient's mental symptoms. The value of certain psychometric tests and other investigatory procedures is also discussed.

History-taking

The difference between a good neuropsychiatrist and a mediocre one is a good history, which must include an informant interview and information on previous medical contact (the 'old notes'). And be aware that a 'poor historian' is the description of someone who takes a poor history rather than one who gives it.

If the history is equivocal, certain features on examination usually soon indicate when there is likely to be an organic

basis for the disturbance. The main task thereafter is to refine the diagnosis by seeking to determine the nature of the pathological process. It is only in a minority of patients, albeit a vitally important group, that the presentation may be misleading, namely in the very early case or in cases with an abundance of 'functional' psychiatric features.

Time spent in obtaining a detailed history is almost always rewarded, and may yield more important leads to the correct diagnosis than a host of investigations. Certainly it will indicate what investigations, if any, need to be pursued. Moreover, the patient's account and his behaviour during interview will provide a wealth of information about his mental state and the intactness or otherwise of cognitive functions.

Statements derived from the patient alone frequently prove misleading, with regard to both the gravity of the symptoms and the time course of their evolution. This is clearly so when the patient is confused or suffering from obvious memory impairment, but can be equally important in other situations. The changes occasioned by brain damage can be hard for the patient to evaluate subjectively, even when insight is largely retained. Certainly, when asked to judge whether memory or other difficulties are worsening or improving, he will often seize on some recent instance that may have more to do with chance and circumstance than with the course of the clinical condition. In many cases there will be genuine loss of insight, and sometimes a desire to conceal from himself and from others that intellectual functions are failing. Sometimes, too, the early changes will be of a type more obvious to outsiders than to the patient himself: changes in mood, enthusiasms, habitual activities and attitudes. Such matters obviously require the detailed testimony of someone who has known the patient intimately throughout the evolution of the disorder.

Abnormalities are likely to include such matters as disordered behaviour, and disturbances of mood, memory and subjective experience. Physical symptoms will also often

Lishman's Organic Psychiatry: A Textbook of Neuropsychiatry, 4th edition.
© 2009 Blackwell Publishing.   ISBN 978-1-4051-1860-1

figure prominently. The full range of complaints and apparent defects of functioning must be carefully explored, with readiness to search beneath the immediately presenting picture. Physical symptoms may have come to serve as the focus of attention for the patient and his relatives, and the true extent of mental abnormalities may only be revealed by specific enquiry. On the other hand the physical components should not be lightly brushed aside; in particular complaints of headache, malaise or generalised weakness must not be underestimated. When there is a problem of differential diagnosis between organic and non-organic mental illness, it will be necessary to preserve a delicate balance in the enquiries until information begins to tip the balance in one direction or the other (Lishman 1992).

Particular attention must always be paid to the mode of onset of the disorder, the duration of symptoms and the way they have progressed. Where developments have been insidious the onset is often dated very imprecisely, even by relatives, with some striking incident serving as a screen for much that went before. Systematic enquiry about the level of functioning prior to the alleged onset can then be useful – behaviour on a previous holiday or at Christmas time for example – and serve to remind informants of the earlier evidence of disorder.

Enquiry should always be made for fluctuations in behaviour or changes that have been observed from one situation to another. Nocturnal worsening is an important indicator of minor degrees of clouding of consciousness. Behaviour which is relatively intact in the restricted field of domestic activities may be dramatically changed when new experiences need to be confronted. Episodic abnormal behaviour of sudden onset and ending will raise the suspicion of an epileptic component.

Other salient matters which deserve specific enquiry are outlined in Chapter 1 where differential diagnosis is discussed. These include not only features among the presenting symptoms, but also antecedent conditions such as head injury, alcoholism or drug abuse. A long list of medically unexplained symptoms cropping up periodically over a number of years, sometimes known only to the patient's general practitioner, is essential in formulating a diagnosis around somatisation or conversion. Tactful and careful enquiry may need to be made about sexual practices if any suspicion of AIDS arises. Any recent physical illness must be noted, or medications recently prescribed, or conditions predisposing to anoxia such as cardiac failure, respiratory inadequacy or the recent administration of an anaesthetic. Any history of dysphasia, paresis, fits or other transitory neurological disturbances must be ascertained.

It is perhaps worth emphasising that the formal psychiatric history remains important even when the presenting complaints have a markedly organic flavour. Where the question arises of a differential diagnosis between organic and non-organic mental illness, all parts of the standard psychiatric enquiry will need to be completed. Previous reactions to stress, and symptoms observed during previous episodes of ill health, may help to clarify the significance of the present clinical features. Of course when there is abundant evidence of a cerebral pathological process, some parts of the formal psychiatric history will be redundant. However, there is still a need to know about premorbid patterns of functioning, special vulnerabilities and details of the patient's social and family setting. Such information may throw light on the content of the illness and on special factors that will need to be borne in mind in management. Knowledge of the level achieved in education and at work can similarly be valuable in assessing present evidence of intellectual decline.

Physical examination

The more one suspects an organic basis for the patient's mental condition, the more important will be the physical examination. Often it is the latter that yields decisive information about the precise aetiology and the treatment required. In practice the dichotomy between the physical and the mental examination can tend to melt away, with each providing essential leads to the other. This is particularly evident in the examination of higher mental functions, where the neurological examination overlaps with the detailed assessment of cognitive status.

Special attention will usually need to be devoted to the neurological system, but other systems can be just as crucially important. Johnson (1968) found that among 250 consecutive admissions to a psychiatric hospital, 12% had some physical illness that was an important aetiological factor in the presenting mental disorder. The majority were diagnosable by routine physical examination and had been missed prior to admission. Among his examples were cases of myxoedema, neurosyphilis, cerebral anoxia due to cardiac failure, chest infections, anaemia, liver failure, carcinoma and cerebral vascular disease. In addition many other physical disorders were discovered that did not contribute directly to the presenting clinical picture. Even higher rates are seen in elderly patients admitted to psychiatric receiving wards. Koran *et al.* (1989), in a thorough evaluation of patients in the Californian mental health system, identified an important physical disease in almost 40% of cases. This was judged to be causal in 6% and to exacerbate the mental disorder in 9%. Relevant conditions included organic brain syndrome, epilepsy, migraine, head injury, diabetes, and thyroid and parathyroid disorders. One-sixth of the causal illnesses had been overlooked, also more than half of those which were exacerbating the picture. Some of the principal physical signs that must be sought with care are described in the following text. There are several reasons why physical and psychiatric illnesses may coincide (Box 3.1).

It is important, especially in the neurological examination, to interpret abnormal findings in relation to the total clinical picture. Among the elderly in particular, isolated neurological abnormalities can be without significance. Absent vibration sense, mild tremors, sluggish and irregular pupils, isolated abnormalities of tendon reflexes or a doubtfully positive plantar response may lack diagnostic significance, or be related to minor pathology without relevance to the present problem. On the other hand, when viewed against the total picture these can be just the features which lead eventually to the true diagnosis.

Gross neurological abnormalities will rarely be encountered in patients with diffuse cerebral impairment, but certain less striking features should be carefully observed. Some of these are not widely appreciated and can be important in raising suspicion of a degenerative brain process. Lack of manual precision, motor impersistence and perseveration of motor acts may emerge clearly in the course of neurological testing. A clumsy graceless walk or minor unsteadiness may betray cerebral pathology, even in the absence of definite pyramidal, extrapyramidal or cerebellar signs. This may be striking once attention has been directed towards it. In patients suspected of cerebral vascular disease, special attention should be paid to swallowing, speech and the jaw jerk as indicators of early pseudobulbar palsy. A wide-based gait has been stressed as an early indicator of normal-pressure hydrocephalus (see Chapter 9, Examination). Minor parkinsonian features, such as a stooping posture or lack of associated arm movements on walking, may also be noticed in diffuse cerebral disease. Table 3.1 sum-

marises important neurological signs that might be especially useful in the diagnosis of dementing conditions.

Neurological soft signs

As well as these general observations and the conventional neurological examination, a number of other signs may be elicited that may betray subtle neurological dysfunction. These include the so-called soft neurological signs, which comprise integrative sensory functions such as sensory extinction and graphaesthesia, motor sequencing acts such as the fist–edge–palm test, and the primitive reflexes such as the pout, snout, grasp and palmomental (unilateral contraction of the muscles of the chin producing a wince-like movement when the thenar eminence of the ipsilateral hand is stroked briskly). Mirror movements (movement provoked in the one hand during a complex unimanual action in the other) may be observed. These signs have low specificity, being found in patients with a variety of diffuse neurological disorders and dementias as well as developmental disorders and the psychoses, not to mention a small proportion of healthy subjects, especially the elderly; they have been shown to correlate with negative symptoms and cognitive impairments in schizophrenia (Bombin *et al.* 2005). Nevertheless, a prominent grasp reflex in a young adult with a history of personality change for example would raise suspicion of a frontal lobe syndrome.

The mental state

The evaluation of mental state provides a cross-sectional view that supplements the longitudinal view of the illness derived from the history. It also adds decisive information of its own. It is essential to realise that key features such as memory impairment may have to be sought diligently if they are to be properly displayed.

There are obviously certain aspects of the mental state which are of especial importance in organic psychiatric disease, and these are described in some detail below. In particular, the correct evaluation of cognitive functions is often central to the identification of cerebral pathology. However, too early or exclusive a preoccupation with the assessment of cognitive functions can be a mistake, and stands to leave much valuable information uncharted. Short-cuts should be avoided, the aim being always a systematic and comprehensive examination of the full range of mental phenomena. Often, for example, it is uncertain how much of the picture may be explained on the basis of non-organic rather than organic mental disturbance, and such a differentiation requires careful assessment of all aspects of the mental state. Even when cerebral pathology is abundantly obvious, it is still necessary to be thoroughly aware of the patient's affective state, the nature of his interpersonal reactions and the content of his subjective experiences. The emphasis in the following sections on certain aspects should therefore not

Table 3.1 Abnormal neurological signs and their significance in dementia. (From Cooper & Greene 2005 with permission of BMJ Publishing Group Ltd.)

Physical sign	Seen in
Ataxia	Paraneoplastic disease, cerebellar tumour, Whipple's disease, Creutzfeldt–Jakob disease, AIDS dementia complex, spinocerebellar ataxia, Wernicke–Korsakoff syndrome, Hallervorden–Spatz syndrome, ornithine transcarbamylase deficiency, Niemann–Pick disease, mitochondrial disorders, adrenoleucodystrophy, neurodegeneration with brain iron accumulation, lead poisoning
Involuntary movements	Huntington's disease, inherited metabolic disorders including Wilson's disease, Creutzfeldt–Jakob disease, corticobasal degeneration, systemic lupus erythematosus, Whipple's disease, Hallervorden–Spatz syndrome, Lesch–Nyhan syndrome
Myoclonus	Post-anoxia, Creutzfeldt–Jakob disease, Alzheimer's disease, subacute sclerosing panencephalitis, myoclonic epilepsies, Hashimoto's encephalopathy, dementia with Lewy bodies, corticobasal degeneration (CBD)
Extrapyramidal signs	Dementia with Lewy bodies, Parkinson's disease, progressive supranuclear palsy, vascular dementia, frontotemporal dementia, Creutzfeldt–Jakob disease, Wilson's disease, Huntington's disease, dentato-rubro-pallido-luysian atrophy, neuroacanthocytosis, cerebral autosomal dominant arteriopathy with subcortical infarcts and leucoencephalopathy (CADASIL), Niemann–Pick disease, mitochondrial disorders, neurodegeneration with brain iron accumulation
Pyramidal signs	Motor neurone disease, Creutzfeldt–Jakob disease, CBD, vitamin B_{12} deficiency, multiple sclerosis, spinocerebellar ataxia, multisystem atrophy, hydrocephalus, Alzheimer's disease, Hallervorden–Spatz syndrome, CADASIL, mitochondrial disorders, adrenoleucodystrophy, frontotemporal dementia
Optic disc pallor	Multiple sclerosis, vitamin B_{12} deficiency
Papilloedema	Tumour, subdural haematoma, hydrocephalus
Cortical blindness	Vascular disease, Alzheimer's disease, Creutzfeldt–Jakob disease
Anosmia	Subfrontal meningioma, head injury, Alzheimer's disease, Parkinson's disease, Huntington's disease
Abnormal eye movements	Progressive supranuclear palsy, Wernicke–Korsakoff syndrome, Whipple's disease, corticobasal degeneration, mitochondrial cytopathies, cerebellar tumours, causes of raised intracranial pressure, Creutzfeldt–Jakob disease, mitochondrial disorders, Huntington's disease, Niemann–Pick disease type C
Other cranial nerve signs	Sarcoidosis, tumours, neoplasia, tuberculous meningitis
Alien hand	Corticobasal degeneration
Visual field defect	Tumour, vascular disease, Creutzfeldt–Jakob disease
Pupillary abnormalities (Argyll Robertson pupil)	Neurosyphilis
Peripheral neuropathy	Vitamin B_{12} deficiency, paraneoplastic disorders, neuroacanthocytosis, spinocerebellar ataxia, Hallervorden–Spatz syndrome, adrenoleucodystrophy, neurodegeneration with brain iron accumulation, lead poisoning, systemic lupus erythematosus
Early onset incontinence	Tumour, hydrocephalus, progressive supranuclear palsy
Bulbar features	Frontal dementia (motor neurone disease)
Fasciculations	Frontal dementia (motor neurone disease), rarely Creutzfeldt–Jakob disease
Seizures	Vasculitis, neoplasia, primary angiitis of the nervous system, limbic encephalitis, AIDS dementia complex, neurosyphilis, subacute sclerosing panencephalitis, Hashimoto's encephalopathy
Grimacing facial expression	Wilson's disease

be taken to imply that other areas are necessarily of minor importance.

The mental state observed at interview must be evaluated against background information from others who have observed the patient in real-life situations. The interview has its own importance in allowing a systematic exploration of relevant areas of function, but is necessarily restricted in scope and is in many ways an artificial situation. For this reason admission to hospital for a period of observation often adds greatly to the assessment, although this is increasingly difficult to organise within modern community-orientated psychiatry services. Nurses' reports of behaviour in the ward, interactions with others and variability during the day can yield crucial information. Occupational therapy can provide the best setting of all when it comes to observing the detailed nature of the patient's difficulties over everyday tasks.

Appearance and general behaviour

Certain features obvious at a glance may raise suspicion of an organic basis for mental symptoms. Any evidence of physical ill health should be noted: pallor, loss of weight or indications of physical weakness. The facies can be very important: a certain laxness of the muscles of the lower face and lack of emotional play about the features can suggest a cerebral degenerative process in the absence of depression. Movements may be slow, sparse or tremulous. The appearance may be older than expected for the patient's age, or standards of self-care and general tidiness may be poor. A lapse of standards that cannot readily be explained on the basis of severe emotional disturbance can be a sensitive pointer to cerebral pathology.

Features which should be noted in the course of conversation include slowness, hesitancy, perseverative tendencies and defective uptake or grasp. This is the time to note whether the patient is alert and responsive or dull and apathetic, whether he is friendly and cooperative or distant and reserved. The adequacy with which attention can be held, diverted or shifted from one topic to another may be seen to be abnormal. Impulsiveness, disinhibition or blunted sensitivity to social interaction are other relevant features that may emerge during the interview. The patient may be noted to tire unusually quickly with mental effort.

Behaviour in the ward can also be revealing. The patient may prove to be indifferent to events and out of contact with his surroundings, sometimes with variability from one part of the day to another. Impaired awareness of the environment may be manifest in a puzzled expression, aimless wandering, restlessness or repetitive stereotyped behaviour. Responses to various requirements and situations may reveal defects not previously suspected. He may lose his way, misidentify people or betray serious lapses of memory. Interactions with those around may reveal paranoid tendencies, or he may be observed to react to hallucinatory experiences not previously disclosed. Competence over dressing, undressing and matters of hygiene can be assessed. Disordered feeding habits can occasionally reveal the inroads of dementia in a patient with an otherwise well-preserved social manner. Any episode of incontinence will of course be noted, along with the patient's reaction towards it.

Mood

A variety of abnormalities of mood can occur with organic cerebral dysfunction, depending partly on the nature of the cerebral pathology and partly on the premorbid personality. Some forms of reaction are particularly common and immediately raise suspicion.

Clouding of consciousness is often accompanied by an inappropriate placidity and lack of concern, coupled with some degree of disinhibition. The florid hostile or fearful moods of delirium are also characteristic, often changing rapidly from one moment to another. In early dementia a quiet wondering perplexity is often the predominant mood, or emotional lability in which signs of distress resolve as abruptly as they appear.

An empty shallow quality to the emotional display should always raise suspicion of organic cerebral disease, likewise apathy in which there is little discernible emotion, and euphoria in which a mild elevation of mood is unbacked by a true sense of happy elation. Emotional blunting and flattening are other characteristic signs. These classic forms are not invariable, however. Some patients with organic brain damage show heightened and sustained anxiety or marked depressive reactions.

Characteristic emotional responses may emerge when the patient is faced with problems that tax his ability. He may over-react in an anxious aggressive manner, or alternatively become quiet, sullen and withdrawn. Goldstein (1942) described the catastrophic reaction (*katastrophenreaktion*) that can be observed in such circumstances, occasionally without warning but usually heralded by increasing anxiety and tension. The patient looks dazed and starts to fumble. Whereas a moment before he was calm and amiable, he now shows an intense affective response, varying from irritability and temper to outbursts of crying and despair. Autonomic disturbance is seen in the form of flushing, sweating or trembling. He may become evasive where further questions are concerned, or show a sudden aimless restlessness.

Talk and content of thought

The patient's talk, both spontaneously and in response to questions, provides a wealth of important clues. Discursive tendencies may be noted, or minor incoherence, or perseverative and paraphasic errors. Perseveration is a sign of great importance in indicating cerebral pathology; having given a response the patient repeats this inappropriately to subsequent questions, as a consequence of difficulty with shifting his attention. Perseveration must be distinguished from reiteration, in which the patient continually repeats some word, phrase or question without intervention by the examiner. The formal examination for dysphasic disturbances is considered below (see Chapter 2, Disorders of language and the aphasias.

There may be pressure of talk, which serves as a screen to cover defects. The patient may employ denials or evasions when pressed for details about his history, or try to explain away failures with facile rationalisations. It can be important to push gently beneath a well-preserved social façade in order to determine the true extent of the inroads made by cerebral pathology.

Observation of the content of talk is the chief means of access to the patient's thought processes. A surprising poverty of thought may be revealed, or preoccupation with restricted themes. Associations may be found to be impoverished and reasoning power impaired.

Time should be spent in attempts to get as complete a picture as possible of any pathological ideas, experiences or attitudes that may be present. Paranoid tendencies are common in the presence of intellectual deterioration and ideas of reference may be marked. Delusional ideas may be stamped with certain characteristic features, as already described in Chapter 2.

Perceptual distortions, illusions and hallucinations must be noted. In organic psychiatric disorders these occur chiefly in the visual modality; they tend to be commoner when sensory cues diminish towards nightfall, and may be fleeting and changeable. Feelings of familiarity or unfamiliarity may be intrusive, with depersonalisation, derealisation or *déjà vu*. Body image disorders merit careful assessment.

The patient's attitude to his illness should always be ascertained. He may fail to recognise that he is unwell, deny any disability or take a surprisingly lighthearted view of his case. At the same time he may prove to be fully compliant over examination or admission to hospital. His own explanations for his symptoms should be determined. This alone can give important indications concerning his capacity for making realistic judgements.

Assessment of the cognitive state

The cognitive state examination can be crucial for producing evidence of an organic component in a mental illness. The number of tests and procedures available for assessing cognitive functions is rather bewildering, and it is therefore helpful to acquire a standard routine. This also has value in building up the clinician's experience of the different tests and the meaning to be put on failure in various situations. He can then formulate subjective judgements in cases where the evidence is not clear-cut; such judgements in turn are essential when deciding whether more detailed investigations should be undertaken.

Most of the brief shorthand tests employed by the psychiatrist lack adequate standardisation and validation. Indeed when their value has been tested they have often, taken individually, proved to be remarkably inefficient in distinguishing between organic and non-organic psychiatric illness. Many prove to be closely related to the patient's educational level and general intelligence, some are markedly affected by increasing age and others by emotional disturbance. Some of the more detailed psychometric procedures elaborated by psychologists are clearly superior for the task of identifying organic psychiatric disorder but are too cumbersome for use in every patient.

Nevertheless, the routine tests available to the clinician have a value of their own. They have the important virtue of throwing a wide net and touching on a number of facets of cognitive function in a reasonably concise manner. In the course of administering them the examiner also obtains numerous indirect clues; the patient's behaviour while attempting the tests, and the nature of his approach, provide important information in themselves. Thus when taken in conjunction with observations gleaned during the interview there is a substantial chance that cerebral impairment will be suspected when it exists. Such suspicions can then be followed up by more decisive means.

The fact that patients with non-organic psychiatric conditions sometimes show impaired performance on the tests is paradoxically of value as well. It is important, for example, to gauge how severely concentration is impaired in depressive illness, or to observe how little impact outside events have made in a patient with severe and sustained anxiety. The routine use of the tests in every patient is therefore seldom a waste of time.

The important matter is to recognise the limitations of the tests and to have a clear strategy for knowing how far to press the cognitive status examination in a given situation. A brief examination is described below for use in every psychiatric patient, and then a more extended battery for use when organic cerebral disease is definitely suspected.

Routine cognitive state examination

Orientation

Orientation for time is assessed by asking the patient to name the day of the week, date, month and year. Minor degrees of temporal disorientation may be identified by asking the patient to estimate the time of day, or to estimate how much time has elapsed since the interview was started. *Impaired appreciation of the flow of time* is sometimes surprisingly revealed and points strongly towards delirium. Orientation for place is assessed by asking the patient to name his present whereabouts and to give the address. Orientation for person is tested simply by asking the patient his name.

Common sense must obviously be used in administering these simple questions. It will usually have become apparent in the course of history-taking if the patient is correctly orientated for place and person and these questions can therefore often be omitted. However, orientation for time is worth testing in all patients, since this is commonly the first area to suffer in the course of mild impairment of consciousness or intellectual impairment. Latitude will obviously be required in interpreting errors with respect to date; Brotchie *et al.* (1985) showed that errors of a day or more occurred in 29% of healthy elderly subjects when orientation was accurate in other respects. Patients with chronic schizophrenia may underestimate their age (age disorientation) and this error tends to predict wider cognitive impairments. It points to a failure to update personal records with the entrenchment of the disorder and is claimed not to be a mere by-product of institutionalisation (Manschreck *et al.* 2000).

Attention and concentration

Marked difficulties with attention and concentration will usually have become apparent in the course of history-taking and examination. When so, it is important to record qualitative observations in full.

Note deficiencies in the way in which attention is *aroused* or *sustained*, whether the patient is readily *distracted* by extraneous or internal stimuli, and whether *attention fluctuates* from one moment to another. There may be difficulty in *shifting attention* from one topic or frame of reference to another, or attention may be *diffuse* so that it cannot be directed to a particular purpose. Note impairment of ability to *concentrate on a coherent line of thought or reasoning*, or undue readiness with which powers of concentration become *fatigued*.

Brief tests that can be used to record attention and concentration include asking the patient to give the days of the week or months of the year in reverse order; recording and timing his efforts to subtract serial sevens from 100; or asking him to perform other simple tests of mental arithmetic appropriate to his level of intelligence.

The ability to repeat digits forwards and backwards (digit span) provides another useful yardstick. The digits must be delivered in an even tone and at a rate of one per second if accurate comparisons are to be made. A start will usually be made with two or three digits forwards, increasing by one each time until the patient's limit is reached.

Memory

The ability to register, retain and retrieve information should be assessed by two or three simple tests. The patient's capacity for current memorising (new learning) has the most important clinical implications and warrants close attention.

Ask the patient to listen carefully while you tell him a name and address, then ask for its immediate reproduction. Record his answer verbatim, and repeat if necessary when the first response is unsatisfactory. Test retrieval 3–5 minutes later after interposing other cognitive tests, and again record the answer verbatim.

Test ability to repeat a sentence immediately after a single hearing. The sentence should be appropriate to the patient's intellectual level as in the following examples from the Stanford–Binet series.
- Year 13: 'The aeroplane made a careful landing in the space which had been prepared for it'.
- Average adult: 'The red-headed woodpeckers made a terrible fuss as they tried to drive the young away from the nest.'
- Superior adult: 'At the end of the week the newspaper published a complete account of the experiences of the great explorer.'

If suspicion of impairment has arisen, test the number of repetitions necessary for accurate reproduction of the eponymous Babcock sentences: 'One thing a nation must have to become rich and great is a large secure supply of wood' or 'The clouds hung low in the valley and the wind howled among the trees as the men went on through the rain'. Three repetitions of either of these sentences should allow word-perfect reproduction in a patient of average intelligence.

A technique similar to that of Irving *et al.* (1970) may be useful with patients of limited ability or when it is hard to be sure of cooperation. The patient is told he will be given the name of a flower and asked to repeat it ('The flower is – a daffodil – please repeat daffodil'), then a colour ('The colour is – blue – please repeat blue'), then a town ('The town is – Brighton'), and so on. The list may continue with makes of car, days of week, etc., until some six or ten items have been given according to the patient's ability. Recall is tested 3–5 minutes later, first without prompting, then if necessary after giving each category name. This provides the opportunity for testing free recall and cued recall separately, and will sometimes demonstrate good learning ability when other techniques have failed. Perseveration is sometimes clearly displayed on the test, likewise confabulatory tendencies.

Other aspects of memory assessment are necessarily largely subjective. Discrepancies may already have emerged between the patient's account of his illness and that given by informants. *Pay special attention to memory for recent happenings and in particular for the temporal sequence of recent events.* The circumstances surrounding the patient's admission to hospital and happenings in the ward thereafter should be briefly reviewed, since these are matters about which the examiner will have independent knowledge.

Retrieval from the remote past is more difficult to evaluate, but an attempt should be made to judge the adequacy of the patient's account of his earlier life, and to examine this for evidence of gaps or inconsistencies. Care must be taken in doubtful cases to frame questions in such a way that memory for the past is truly tested. Thus the question 'How old were you when you started school?' can produce an easy habitual response and secure a correct reply, whereas 'Can you describe your first day at school?' requires the mobilisation of actual memories.

Record any *selective impairments of memory* which become apparent in the interview for *special incidents, periods or themes* in the patient's life. *Retrograde and anterograde amnesia* must be specified in detail in relation to head injury or epileptic phenomena. Describe any evidence of *confabulation* or *false memories*. Note the patient's attitude to any memory difficulties which he displays.

General information

A brief estimate should be made of the patient's knowledge of current events, and of his ability to handle material from his long-term memory store (utilisation of old knowledge).

Ask about recent items of interest in the news, political, sporting or otherwise, in accordance with the patient's known interests and activities. Ask him to name key personalities: members of the Royal Family, prime ministers, members of the cabinet or well-known television performers. (Clearly such questions will only need to be pursued when reason has emerged to doubt the patient's competence.) In patients who disclaim any interest in political or sporting events, television soap operas can provide a useful vehicle for assessment, providing of course that the examiner is adequately informed about them! Surprisingly detailed knowledge may be forthcoming in patients who appear to be severely impaired.

Ask for the dates of the first and second world wars, and test for knowledge of capitals and countries. In the face of poor responses pursue the patient's general knowledge further by asking for names of cities in England, rivers, etc.

If reason has emerged to suspect a disturbance of abstract thinking, ask the patient to explain the difference between concepts such as 'child' and 'dwarf', 'poverty' and 'misery', 'river' and 'canal', 'lie' and 'mistake', and test ability to give the meaning behind well-known proverbs.

Intelligence

The patient's educational and occupational history, taken in conjunction with his own interests and activities, should allow a rough estimate to be made of the expected level of intelligence. *Any aspects of performance during testing which are at variance with this should be carefully noted.*

Orientation for time and place is closely bound up with current memorising ability and with clarity and coherence of thought. The tests of orientation as described above are nevertheless very useful, and have repeatedly emerged as among the most discriminating features in the mental state examination for distinguishing between organic and non-organic psychiatric disorders. Attention is not a clearly defined concept and overlaps with functions described as alertness, awareness and responsiveness. It is nonetheless widely accepted as a clinically useful concept, with particular relevance to general mental acuity and minor impairment of consciousness. Concentration is a similarly imprecise term, referring to capacity for focusing and sustaining mental activity on the task in hand. Both stand to be markedly affected by preoccupations or abnormalities of mood, and can therefore be disturbed in many forms of psychiatric illness. Equally, however, they can give important indications of clouding of consciousness or general intellectual impairment. It will be noted that simple tests of arithmetic form an integral part of the tests for attention and concentration, and this in itself can be valuable in revealing marked defects in numerical ability. The digit repetition test is included in this section, rather than in the assessment of memory, since it is well established that the immediate memory span is usually normal in amnesic subjects.

The assessment of memory is of the utmost importance, since memory failure is a particularly sensitive indicator of cerebral dysfunction. It is here that the most decisive evidence of an organic component in the illness will often be obtained. Fortunately for clinical practice, the aspect of memory that is most amenable to careful testing is also the aspect most vulnerable to cerebral dysfunction, namely the capacity for acquiring and retaining new information.

The section on general information extends the evaluation of memory, and at the same time brings added information against which to judge the likelihood of generalised intellectual impairment.

Mini-Mental State Examination

The Mini-Mental State Examination (MMSE) was elaborated by Folstein *et al.* (1975) as a simplified form of the routine cognitive status examination. It has the virtue of brevity, taking only 5–10 minutes to administer, yet test–retest reliability is high and it has been shown to discriminate well between patients with dementia and delirium (Anthony *et al.* 1982). The MMSE is widely used and provides a rough and ready index of cognitive functioning and can be used to track improvements and deterioration.

The first section covers orientation, memory and attention. Memory is tested by noting the number of trials required to learn three object names, then testing recall later. Attention is assessed by the serial subtraction of sevens or by spelling a word backwards. The second section tests ability to name common objects, follow verbal and written commands, write a sentence spontaneously and copy a simple figure (overlapping pentagons). The total score obtainable is 30, scores of less than 24 usually being indicative of cognitive impairment.

There are limitations to the MMSE, such as the relative paucity of memory and general knowledge items and those which tap into frontal-executive functions.

Extended cognitive state examination

The examination described above is adequate for routine psychiatric practice. The abnormalities that emerge will need to be evaluated against the total picture presented by the patient: sometimes they will raise the possibility of organic cerebral disorder, but quite often they will be attributable to factors such as low intelligence, emotional disturbance or psychotic thought disorder. More latitude will then be allowed for failure. However, when they raise a strong suspicion of organic psychiatric illness, more thoroughgoing evaluation will be required.

Some points of caution must be observed before embarking on the extended cognitive state examination.
1 The examination can be lengthy and fatigue may produce misleading results; the procedures should not be hurried, and several brief sessions are usually preferable to a single long drawn-out examination.
2 The examiner must remain sensitive to the patient's reactions to failure. A particular test must sometimes be set aside

for a while in the interests of sustaining cooperation; tests which are pressed too firmly may provoke 'catastrophic' reactions or bewilder the patient to the point where useful information is no longer obtained.

3 The tests must be adapted to the patient's intelligence and educational level, and to his particular difficulties.

4 It is essential to remain aware that one disability may have repercussions on performance at other tasks. Defective comprehension, for example, will cloud the issue when it comes to testing for dyspraxia. Allowance will need to be made for this in the selection of the tests, the order of their administration and the assessment of results.

Consequently, it is helpful to have a simple routine at the outset which allows the key area of function to be assessed in an abbreviated fashion, before proceeding to lengthier parts of the examination (Box 3.2).

A somewhat more systematic expansion of the MMSE has been proposed and this also serves as a bridge between initial assessment and formal neuropsychological assessment or between an extended clinical neuropsychiatric evaluation. The Addenbrooke's Cognitive Examination (ACE) (Mathuranath *et al.* 2000) takes about 20 minutes to administer. It consists of six components evaluating separate cognitive domains. A maximum score of 100 is weighted as follows: orientation (10), attention (8), memory (35), verbal fluency (14), language (28), and visuospatial ability (5). The orientation and attention components are as in the MMSE. The memory section involves the recall of three items from the MMSE, a name and address learning and delayed recall test, plus semantic memory. The language component includes naming 12 line drawings, comprehension, repeating words and sentences, reading regular and irregular words, and writing. Visuospatial testing consists of copying overlapping pentagons (from the MMSE) plus a wire cube, and drawing a clock face. Verbal fluency consists of 'P' words and animals and requires separate scoring. The ACE has good sensitivity and specificity and appears to be able to distin-

guish between 'functional' and 'organic' disorders reasonably well (Fig. 3.1) (Dudas *et al.* 2005). A cut-off of 88 has been proposed for screening purposes.

Even after this fairly comprehensive screening, individual areas of cognitive function must be systematically explored, with the aim of covering each of the sections described below. Those which require most careful assessment in the particular patient will by now be apparent since attention will have been directed towards them by the history, the neurological examination and the cognitive deficits already displayed.

Box 3.2 Initial assessment of cognitive function

1 Take careful note of the patient's *level of cooperation*: his willingness to apply himself to the test procedures will be fundamental to the amount of reliable information that can be obtained

2 Make a preliminary assessment of the *level of conscious awareness*: this must have an early priority since performance on all other tests may be affected by minor degrees of clouding of consciousness

3 Next assess *language functions*: much of what follows will depend on the accuracy of verbal communication. In addition to noting verbal ability, ask the patient to name a series of objects and to perform a series of simple commands

4 *Memory functions*, if not already tested, should be briefly examined as already described

5 *Visuospatial ability* should always be screened because non-verbal deficits of this nature may otherwise remain concealed. Ask the patient to copy simple designs (such as those in Visuospatial and constructional difficulties, later in chapter).

6 Test the integrity of *volitional movements* and at the same time of *right–left orientation* by asking the patient to point to various parts of the body. For example, 'Touch your left ear with your left hand', 'Touch your left knee with your right hand'.

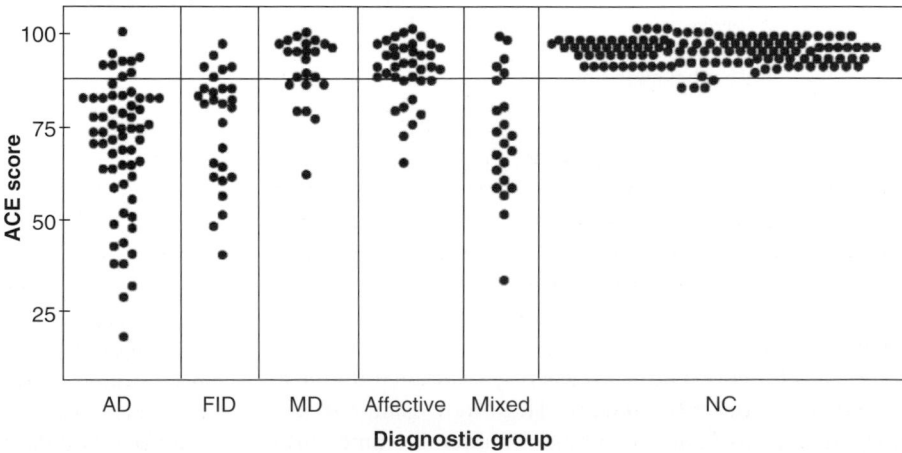

Fig. 3.1 Scatterplot of total scores in various diagnostic groups using Addenbrooke's Cognitive Examination (ACE). Reference line is a score of 88, the recommended cut-off score on the ACE for screening purposes. (From Dudas *et al.* 2005 with permission.)

Level of conscious awareness

Impairment of consciousness is obvious when there is frank drowsiness or somnolence during examination. It is the detection of minor degrees of impairment that causes difficulties. There are no pathognomonic signs or tests for minor impairment of consciousness, and its detection is largely a matter for subjective clinical judgement based on a variety of clues.

Record any obvious impairment in the form of drowsiness or diminished awareness of the environment. Note fluctuations during examination, and question relatives or nursing staff about changes which occur from time to time during the day. Impairment may only become obvious towards nightfall or when the patient is fatigued.

Minor impairment will be suspected when the patient is dull, inert and uncertain in behaviour even though he is not drowsy, or when responses to external events are diminished. There may be a vagueness and hesitancy about the manner of speaking. Once the examiner suspects a reduction in the level of consciousness it can be helpful to repeat questions concerning dates and names of places, with the object of seeing whether consistent answers are given. Tests of orientation, attention, concentration and memory may be poorly performed, often with variability from one occasion to another. Judgement of the passage of time will often be markedly inaccurate. Attention will usually be ill sustained and ill focused, and the patient may tend to lose the thread in conversation. Lucid intervals may emerge from time to time and form a marked contrast to the general tenor of behaviour. Even when seemingly alert it may be discovered that the patient has failed to register on-going experiences, including those of the interview itself.

Simple procedures may be employed to assess capacity for sustained attention or 'vigilance' over a period of time. The patient may be asked, for example, to raise his hand whenever an 'A' is spoken, and a series of letters are then delivered in an even tone and at a constant rate. A more difficult version consists of raising the hand whenever any vowel is spoken, or whenever two vowels succeed one another. A written form of the test can easily be made by asking the patient to cancel all letters of a designated type on a printed sheet or in a passage of prose material.

If somnolent, can the patient be roused to full or only partial awareness? If his attention cannot be sustained, does he drift back towards sleep or does his attention wander onto other topics? When consciousness is severely impaired describe the nature of the stimulus required to evoke a response (e.g. conversation, firm commands, commands following arousal by shaking, painful stimuli) and the character of the response produced (e.g. a correct verbal reply or motor act, an incorrect and muddled response, failure to respond to commands but accurate localisation of a painful stimulus, ill-coordinated and ineffectual motor movements). The Glasgow Coma Scale (see Chapter 4, under Measuring head injury severity) will prove of value for monitoring progress in patients with seriously impaired consciousness.

Evidence for delirium, stupor or coma should be specified in detail.

Language functions

Language functions are conveniently examined under the six headings described below. Thorough examination of dysphasic disturbances can take considerable time, but in the non-dysphasic subject screening need last only a few minutes. At the onset it is important to note whether the patient is *predominantly right- or left-handed*.

Motor aspects of speech

Note the quality of spontaneous speech and that in reply to questions. Minor expressive speech defects may only emerge when the patient is pressed to engage in conversation, to describe his work, his house, or some event in his life.

Is there any disturbance of articulation (dysarthria)? When slight dysarthria is suspected test ability to pronounce a phrase such as 'West Register Street'.

Is there slowness or hesitancy with speech production and is the output sparse? Conversely, is the output excessive with a definite pressure of speech (logorrhoea)?

Does he use wrong words, words which are nearly but not exactly correct, or words that do not exist? *Paraphasic errors* may be defined as 'substitutions within language' (Benson & Geschwind 1971) and exist in several forms; they may involve the substitution of one correct word for another, the distortion of one syllable within a word, or the production of a group of sounds with no specific meaning (neologisms).

Note whether words are omitted and sentences abbreviated (telegram style). Are there inaccuracies of grammatical construction (paragrammatisms)? Is the normal rhythm and inflexion of speech disturbed (dysprosody)? Is speech totally disorganised and incomprehensible (jargon aphasia)?

Observe carefully for perseverative errors of speech (see Chapter 2, Broca's aphasia, and Verbal fluency, later in chapter), also for reiteration of phrases just spoken (echolalia), of single words (pallilalia) or of a terminal syllable (logoclonia).

When defects are found, test whether automatic speech or the naming of serials is better preserved than conversational speech: ask him to repeat a well-known nursery rhyme or prayer, to count to 20, or to give the days of the week. Are emotional utterances or ejaculations preserved when formal speech is defective?

From the phenomenological point of view, Benson and Geschwind (1971) recommend a basic division into *fluent and non-fluent* forms of dysphasic speech, the former characterising posterior lesions and the latter anterior lesions. Fluent aphasias generally show clear articulation, the words are produced without effort, output is normal or excessive, paraphasic errors are frequent, phrase length is not curtailed, and normal rhythm and inflexion are preserved. Non-fluent aphasias show poor articulation, the speech is produced with obvious difficulty, output is sparse but nonetheless the content is meaningful when this can be discerned, phrase length is reduced to one or two words, and the rhythm and inflexion are disturbed.

Comprehension of speech

The understanding of speech must be separately assessed, whether or not production is defective. Even when the patient is mute or his utterances totally incomprehensible it is still necessary to determine whether he can understand what is said to him.

Can he point correctly on command to objects around him? Can he carry out simple orders on request, for example pick up an object, show his tongue? Failure can be misleading since it may be due to dyspraxia; thus if commands are not carried out, test whether he can signal his response to simple yes–no questions.

Can he respond to more complex instructions, for example walk over to the door and come back again, or take his spectacles from his pocket and put them on the table. Can he follow a series of commands sequentially, for example go to the window, tap it twice, turn around, then come back again.

Marie's Three Paper Test is widely employed for the rapid assessment of mild comprehension defects. Three pieces of paper of different sizes are put before the patient. He is told to take the largest and hand it to the examiner, take the smallest and throw it to the ground, and take the middle-sized piece and put it in his pocket.

The understanding of prepositional and syntactic aspects of speech can be a sensitive indicator of minor comprehension difficulties. It is readily tested by providing the patient with three objects such as a book, pen and coin, then issuing increasingly complex instructions as follows: 'Put the coin on the book; put the coin and the pen under the book; tap the book and then the coin with the pen; put the book between the pen and the coin; place the book over the coin then put the pen inside it', and so on.

If comprehension of spoken speech is defective, test whether understanding of written words and instructions is better preserved. Test whether other hearing functions are intact, for example the startle response to sudden noise. Test for auditory agnosia by noting whether the patient can recognise non-verbal noises (clapping hands, snapping fingers, jingling money) or copy the production of such sounds when they are made outside the field of vision.

Repetition of speech

Can the patient repeat digits, words, short phrases or sentences exactly as you give them? The classic phrase for testing repetition is 'No ifs, ands or buts'. Successful repetition involves both motor and sensory parts of the speech apparatus and also the connections between the two. Failure in repetition may occur despite adequate spontaneous articulation and good comprehension. Paraphasic errors often emerge most clearly in the testing of repetition.

Word finding

Does the patient have difficulty in finding words during conversation, or use circumlocutions? Test specifically for nominal aphasia by asking him to name both common and uncommon objects (for example the parts of a wrist watch, and other objects in the room). Include an examination of his ability to name colours.

Nominal aphasia may be the only language disturbance in patients with cerebral damage and must therefore always be tested with care. Ease of word finding is inversely related to the frequency of occurrence of the word in the language, and the detection of slight nominal aphasia requires testing with objects whose names occur relatively infrequently such as 'buckle', 'pointer' or 'dial', but not 'watch' or 'strap'; 'lapel' or 'knuckle', but not 'button' or 'finger'; 'radiator' or 'linoleum', but not 'picture' or 'carpet'.

Reading

Present the patient with the written names of objects in the room and ask him to point to them. If this is performed correctly, present him with written instructions to perform specific actions.

Test his ability to read aloud, and determine whether he understands what he has read. If the patient fails to read aloud it is still necessary to assess whether he has read, since some aphasics comprehend well even though they fail to read aloud.

Writing

Test ability to write spontaneously and to dictation. Examine written productions for substitutions, perseverations, spelling errors and letter reversals. Is copying better preserved than writing to dictation? Is spelling out loud better preserved than spelling on paper? Is the writing of habitual material (signature, address) relatively intact? Are numbers written more accurately than words or letters?

The main syndromes of language impairment can be distinguished by the pattern of breakdown in the above examination. Table 3.2 summarises performance on the different tests of language function in relation to the syndromes of aphasia described in the chapter on neuropsychology.

Verbal fluency

Verbal fluency must be separately assessed, even when there is no other form of language disturbance, since fluency is characteristically impaired with frontal lesions.

A simple technique is to ask the patient to give as many words as he can think of beginning with a certain letter of the alphabet, for example 1 minute for words beginning with F, then 1 minute for A and 1 minute for S (letter or phonological fluency). The total achieved on this 'FAS' test should be in excess of 30. Norms are available in relation to the patient's age and educational level (see Lezak 1995). Alternatively, the patient may be asked to give the names of animals or the names of objects found in a kitchen (semantic fluency).

The number of words accomplished will often be strikingly low even though there is no evidence of dysphasia. This accords with the impoverishment of spontaneous speech that may be observed with frontal lesions. It can be necessary to allow the patient a full minute over his attempts at each category, since words may be rapidly produced initially then tail off in noteworthy fashion. Frequent perseverations and out of category items are a distinctly 'frontal' feature. The effect is more pronounced with left frontal lesions than right. Most individuals will produce more animals than F, A or S words, although patients with loss of semantic knowledge (e.g. Alzheimer's disease or frontotemporal dementia) may show a reverse pattern. Corresponding deficits can also be demonstrated on a design fluency test, but in this case the task is more affected by right frontal lesions than left (Jones-Gotman & Milner 1977).

Number functions

Test the patient's ability to perform simple arithmetical operations – addition, subtraction, multiplication, division – in relation to his educational and occupational background. Assess his ability to handle money correctly.

Can he count objects and make a rough estimate of the number of matches laid before him? Can he give the average size and weight of a man? Can he estimate the size of various objects in the room?

Test his ability to read and write numbers of two and more digits.

Table 3.2 Performance on tests of language function in different varieties of dysphasia. (After Benson & Geschwind 1971.)

	Spontaneous speech	Comprehension	Repetition	Naming	Reading	Writing
Pure word-deafness	F	–	–	+	+	+(not to dictation)
Pure word-blindness (alexia without agraphia)	F	+	+	+	–	+
Pure word-dumbness	NF	+	–	±	+	+
Pure agraphia (agraphia without alexia)	F	+	+	+	+	–
Primary sensory (Wernicke's) dysphasia	F	–	–	±	–	–
Primary motor (Broca's) dysphasia	NF	±	–	±	Aloud – Compr ±	–
Nominal dysphasia	F	+	+	–	±	±
Conduction dysphasia	F	+	–	±	Aloud – Compr +	–
Isolation syndrome	NF	–	+	–	–	–
Transcortical motor dysphasia	NF	+	±	–	Aloud – Compr +	–
Transcortical sensory dysphasia	F	–	+	–	–	–
Alexia with agraphia (visual asymbolia)	F	+	+	+	–	–

Compr, comprehension; F, fluent speech productions; NF, non-fluent speech productions.

Memory

Full examination of memory will always be required along the lines already set out in Chapter 2 (Disorders of memory). Special attention should be directed at recent memory and new learning ability.

A convenient and sensitive method for supplementing the assessment of new learning ability consists of testing the patient's capacity for learning supra-span lists of digits (Drachman & Arbit 1966; Warrington 1970). The normal digit span is first determined (as in Memory, earlier in chapter), then ability to extend the list by one or two items is assessed by repeated presentations. Amnesic subjects can perform adequately on the straightforward digit span test, but show a dramatic breakdown in performance as soon as this is exceeded.

Simple paired-associate learning may also be tested, as outlined in Memory.

Non-verbal memory should be tested in addition to verbal memory by asking the patient to reproduce simple geometrical figures (such as those shown in the next section) after an interval of 5 minutes.

Visuospatial and constructional difficulties

Patients with visuospatial agnosia may make no complaints, thus failing to direct attention towards the problem. It is important therefore to include tests which betray such difficulties when a cerebral lesion is suspected.

Test the patient's ability to judge the relation between objects in space: to estimate distances, to say which of two objects is nearer to him, and which is larger. Can he with eyes closed indicate the spatial order of objects in the room around him?

Visuospatial agnosia is often associated with constructional dyspraxia and the distinction between the two defects is usually far from clear-cut (see Chapter 2, Visual object agnosia). Constructional dyspraxia is tested as follows.

Test ability to connect two dots by a straight line, and to find the middle of a straight line and of a circle. Test ability to draw simple figures such as a square, circle and triangle. Ask the patient to copy a series of line drawings of increasing complexity such as those shown below.

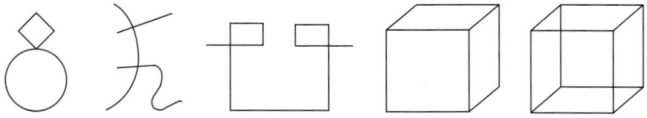

The test may be made more difficult by removing the model and asking the patient to draw the figure from immediate memory. Ask him to draw a house, a bicycle, a clock face and set the hands, and to indicate the principal towns on a rough map of England. Note particularly whether he shows neglect of one half of visual space or crowds material into one part of the paper. Test ability to construct simple figures when presented with sticks or matches. Can he construct a triangle and a square, or copy more complex designs? Can the patient assemble a simple jig-saw puzzle, or reassemble a piece of paper that has been cut into several fragments?

The copying of a range of geometrical figures has the virtue of being graded in difficulty and of providing a permanent record. Most normal subjects will succeed in copying at least the first four of the test figures illustrated earlier in this section. Free drawing of a house or bicycle has the advantage of being more natural and also more difficult. It often reveals more subtle forms of defect, but can be hard to interpret since normal individuals vary considerably in drawing skill. Sometimes highly characteristic defects may emerge, as when windows are placed in the roof or outside the main body of the building. The drawing of a clock is particularly useful in showing how accurately the figures can be spaced around the dial, or in revealing unilateral neglect of space by the omission of figures from one half of the dial. The use of sticks and other materials for constructional tasks gives

the opportunity to observe the patient's capacity to improve his performance and to alter mistakes. Similarly a standardised version of clock drawing (CLOX; see Fig. 3.2) enhances the reliability of the test and enables the comparison of performance to instruction versus copying. Only the former relates to specific cognitive impairment and executive function deficits.

Other agnosic disturbances

Other forms of agnosia are very rare. Before concluding that agnosia is present it is essential to try to exclude impairments of primary perception as the cause of failure on a test (such as impaired visual acuity, field defects or deafness). Firm

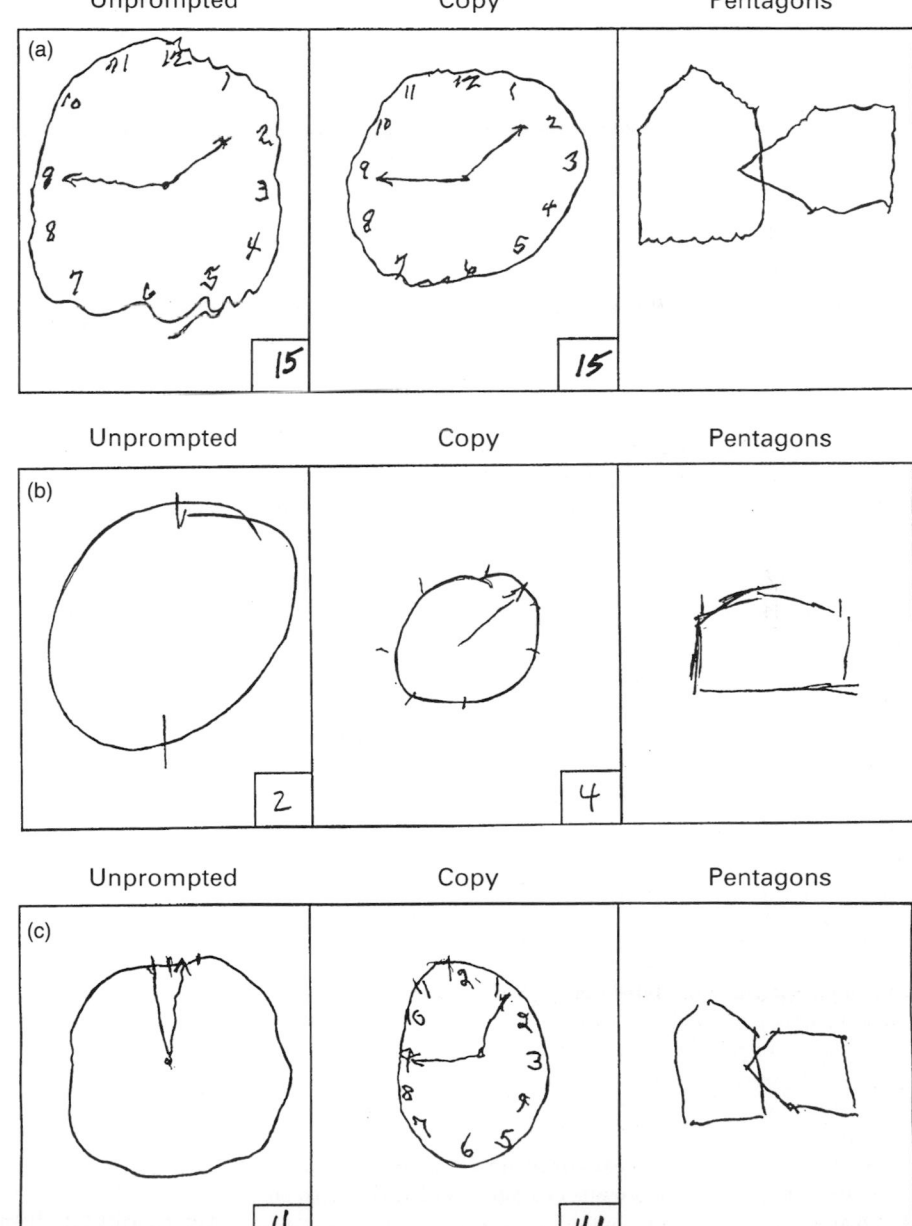

Fig. 3.2 Qualitative differences in CLOX performance in (a) a normal elderly control, (b) a patient with Alzheimer's disease and (c) a patient with non-cortical vascular disease. (a) An 82-year-old elderly control: EXIT25 score 8/50 (score greater than 5/50 indicates impairment); MMSE score 29/30. (b) A 74-year-old married white woman with Alzheimer's disease: EXIT25 score 21/50 (score of 24/50 is comparable with 6-year-old child or residents requiring skilled nursing); MMSE score 12/30. (c) A 74-year-old right-handed white man with a history of coronary artery disease (status post myocardial infarction), hypertension, non-insulin-dependent diabetes mellitus, and falls: EXIT22 score 24/50; MMSE score 28/30. (From Royall *et al.* 1998 with permission.)

indications of an agnosic problem will often be obtained by finding that an object which cannot be identified through one sensory modality is immediately identified through another.

Can the patient describe what he sees and identify objects and persons? Ask him to name a particular object in a group exposed to view and to describe its use, or if aphasic to indicate its use (*visual object agnosia*). If he fails, test whether he can identify the object by other senses such as touch. Ask him to name the colours of objects, to indicate their colour on a chart and to group objects according to their colour (*colour agnosia*). Ask him to describe a meaningful situation in a picture shown to him (*simultanagnosia*). Is his recognition of faces defective (*prosopagnosia*)? Ask him to point out a named person known to him among a group or to name photographs of relatives or of well-known public figures.

Auditory agnosia will already have been assessed (see under comprehension of speech, Chapter 2).

Tactile agnosia is tested by asking the patient to identify objects by touch with the eyes closed. Each hand must be tested separately. Care must be taken that other sensory information (such as the rattle of money) does not give the necessary clue for identification. Ask him to name the objects and to describe their shape, texture and use. In the event of failure, test whether the objects can then be identified by vision. If dysphasic, his responses must be assessed by testing selection from a group of objects exposed to view.

Dyspraxia and related disturbances

Before diagnosing dyspraxia it is essential to make sure that the patient's difficulties cannot be explained on the basis of muscular weakness, incoordination or profound sensory disturbance. Many dyspraxic patients are also dysphasic, so care must be taken to check whether instructions are understood. To prove the existence of dyspraxia it is necessary to show that a movement not made under one set of conditions (e.g. on command) can be performed under others (e.g. spontaneously), or that movements of equal or greater complexity can be made under other circumstances. It is also necessary to exclude simple unwillingness to cooperate. Because of the complexities of this area of dysfunction it is advisable in all cases to make a careful note of what the patient does, how he does it and what he fails to do (Critchley 1953). The examination should test the integrity of learned movements both to command and to imitation. It must also encompass the capacity for making familiar gestures, and for using objects in pantomime and in reality.

Test the patient's ability to carry out purposeful movements to command, such as holding out the arms, crossing legs, showing teeth, screwing up eyes or nodding the head. Test each hand separately for making a fist, opposition of thumb and little finger, pronation and supination (*ideomotor dyspraxia*).

Test ability to rise from a chair on command and to turn around (*whole body dyspraxia*).

Test ability to imitate postures of the hand and arm demonstrated by the examiner, and to adopt with one limb the posture imposed on the other.

Test expressive and make-believe movements such as knocking at a door or waving goodbye. Ask the patient to demonstrate how he would brush his teeth, use a hammer or kick a ball.

Test the patient's ability to carry out complex coordinated sequences of movements, such as taking a match from a box and striking it, winding a watch, cutting with scissors, or folding a piece of paper and putting it in an envelope (*ideational dyspraxia*).

Does the patient show undue difficulty with dressing and undressing, get muddled when inserting limbs into clothing, or try to put garments on the wrong way round (*dressing dyspraxia*)?

Tests of frontal lobe function

When frontal damage is suspected certain tests are specially indicated. Many of these tap 'executive functions' in that they examine the initiation, planning and regulation of goal-directed behaviours. Others assess capacities for abstract thinking, categorisation or judgement. Only some are suitable for bedside examination, which will therefore often need to be supplemented by neuropsychological tests as described in Chapter 2 [under Executive (frontal lobe) syndromes]. These have been helpfully combined and validated in the form of the Frontal Assessment Battery (FAB) (Box 3.3) (Dubois *et al.* 2000). It includes simple items on conceptual similarity; verbal fluency; Luria's motor tests; tests of alternating movements and response inhibition; and utilisation behaviour. Table 3.3 shows the comparative scores on the MMSE, a dementia rating scale and the FAB in groups of patients with a variety of neuropsychiatric conditions associated with executive function deficits, including Parkinson's disease, progressive supranuclear palsy, frontotemporal dementia, and corticobasal degeneration. The FAB is better able to distinguish the groups from controls than the MMSE. Another useful instrument designed to be incorporated into a clinical assessment is the Executive Interview (EXIT25) (Royall *et al.* 1992) According to the authors, it defines the behavioural sequelae of executive dyscontrol and provides a standardised clinical encounter in which they can be observed.

Other bedside tests include the *Cognitive Estimates Test* (see Cognitive Estimates Test, later in chapter), which assesses the patient's capacity for making realistic practical judgements of size and number.

Ask, for example, 'What is the largest object normally found in a house? What is the best paid job in Britain today? How fast do racehorses gallop? What it the length of the average man's spine?'

The idea is that a cognitively intact person would be able to answer these questions through reflection and common sense. Pathological responses are those that are way outside the limits of a reasonable guess. So in the question about a man's spine, a correct answer would obviously be somewhat less than the average height of a man but more than a couple of feet.

Behavioral observations can be equally important in pointing to frontal dysfunction. Note whether the patient is

Box 3.3 Content, instructions and scoring of the Frontal Assessment Battery (FAB)

1 Similarities (conceptualisation)
'In what way are they alike?'
A banana and an orange
A table and a chair
A tulip, a rose and a daisy

Score
Only category responses (fruits, furniture, flowers) are considered correct.
Three correct: 3
Two correct: 2
One correct: 1
None correct: 0

2 Lexical fluency (mental flexibility)
'Say as many words as you can beginning with the letter S, any words except surnames or proper nouns.'
The time allowed is 60 seconds.

Score
Word repetitions or variations (shoe, shoemaker), surnames or proper nouns are not counted as correct responses.
More than nine words: 3
Six to nine words: 2
Three to five words: 1
Less than three words: 0

3 Motor series (programming)
'Look carefully at what I'm doing.'
The examiner, seated in front of the patient, performs alone three times with his left hand the series of Luria (1966): fist–edge–palm. 'Now, with your right hand do the same series, first with me, then alone.' The examiner performs the series three times with the patient, then says to him 'Now, do it on your own.'

Score
Patient performs six correct consecutive series alone: 3
Patient performs at least three correct consecutive series alone: 2
Patient fails alone, but performs three correct consecutive series with the examiner: 1
Patient cannot perform three correct consecutive series even with the examiner: 0

4 Conflicting instructions (sensitivity to interference)
'Tap twice when I tap once.'
To be sure that the patient has understood the instruction, a series of three trials is run: 1-1-1.
'Tap once when I tap twice.'
To be sure that the patient has understood the instruction, a series of three trials is run: 2-2-2.
The examiner then performs the following series: 1-1-2-1-2-2-2-1-1-2.

Score
No error: 3
One or two errors: 2
More than two errors: 1
Patient taps like the examiner at least four consecutive times: 0

5 Go–no go (inhibitory control)
'Tap once when I tap once.'
To be sure that the patient has understood the instruction, a series of three trials is run: 1-1-1.
'Do not tap when I tap twice.' To be sure that the patient has understood the instruction, a series of three trials is run: 2-2-2.
The examiner then performs the following series: 1-1-2-1-2-2-2-1-1-2.

(continued)

Score

No error: 3

One or two errors: 2

More than two errors: 1

Patient taps like the examiner at least four consecutive times: 0

6 Prehension behavior ('utilisation') (Lhermitte 1983; Lhermitte *et al.* 1986)

'Do not take my hands.'

The examiner is seated in front of the patient. Place the patient's hands palm up on his knees. Without saying anything or looking at the patient, the examiner brings his or her hands close to the patient's hands and touches the palms of both the patient's hands, to see if he will spontaneously take them. If the patient takes the hands, the examiner will try again after asking him 'Now, do not take my hands.'

Score

Patient does not take the examiner's hands: 3

Patient hesitates and asks what he has to do: 2

Patient takes the hands without hesitation: 1

Patient takes the examiner's hand even after he has been told not to do so: 0

apathetic, disinhibited, unkempt or lacking in normal social graces.

Topographical sense and right–left orientation

Does the patient have difficulty in finding his way about the ward (topographical disorientation)? Does he confuse his bed with other people's? Can he describe the relations between parts of the ward or of his own house? Can he describe the route from home to hospital? If necessary test his ability to follow a simple route in the ward or hospital.

Can the patient point on command to objects around him on the right and on the left? Ask him to move on command right and left parts of the body, and to point to individual parts on the right and left side of his own body, and of the examiner sitting opposite him. Can he perform complex instructions like 'touch your right ear with your left hand' or 'pick up the left hand coin with your left hand and place it in my right hand'?

Body image disturbances

Body image disturbances will often be revealed by the patient's behaviour or his own subjective complaints, but sometimes special tests or questions will be required to elicit them. Asking the patient to make a rough drawing of a man will sometimes give the first indication of body image disorder (Cohn 1960).

Test for *finger agnosia*. Ask the patient to move on command or point to individual fingers, his own and the examiner's. Kinsbourne and Warrington (1962) describe various tests which have proved to be more sensitive indicators of finger agnosia than the conventional tests. In one such, two of the patient's fingers are touched simultaneously and he is asked to state how many fingers lie between them.

Test for disturbance of identification of other body parts (*autotopagnosia*). Ask the patient to move on command and to name various parts of his body, to point to them and to parts of the examiner's body.

Note any evidence of *unilateral unawareness or neglect* of the body. When present this will usually involve the left side. Does the patient utilise the left hand normally in bimanual activities? Is the left side of the body relatively neglected in washing, combing or dressing? When attention is drawn to such defects does he recognise them and correct them?

Table 3.3 Comparative scores on the Mini-Mental State Examination (MMSE), Dementia Rating Scale (DRS) (Mattis 1988) and Frontal Assessment Battery (FAB): study group characteristics. (From Dubois *et al.* 2000 with permission.)

Population	N	Age (years)	MMSE	Mattis DRS	FAB
Controls	42	58.0±14.4[a]	28.9±0.8[a]	141.0±2.4[a]	17.3±0.8[a]
Patients	121	64.4±9.3[a]	25.5±4.8[a]	118.0±19.1[a]	10.3±4.7[a]
PD	24	59.4±12.9[c,g]	28.0±1.9[i,j]	134.0±15.2[c,g,i]	15.9±3.8[c,g,i]
MSA	6	65.0±10.5	25.7±3.9[j]	127.0±16.2[e]	13.5±4.0[e,f]
CBD	21	67.4±8.1[b,c]	26.4±3.8[b]	123.7±15.0[b,e]	11.0±3.7[b,e,d]
PSP	47	66.9±7.0[g,h]	26.2±3.7[h]	117.7±15.2[g,h]	8.5±3.4[d,f,g]
FTD	23	60.3±8.5[b,h]	20.7±6.3[b,h,i]	101.5±20.0[b,e,h,i]	7.7±4.2[b,e,i]

Values are presented as mean ± SD. Significantly different at $P < 0.05$ for [a]controls and patients; [b]frontotemporal dementia (FTD) and corticobasal degeneration (CBD); [c]Parkinson's disease (PD) and CBD; [d]progressive supranuclear palsy (PSP) and CBD; [e]FTD and multiple system atrophy (MSA); [f]PSP and MSA; [g]PD and PSP; [h]FTD and PSP; [i]PD and FTD; [j]PD and MSA.

Determine whether he has unusual subjective sensations or beliefs about the limbs of one half of the body. Do they feel as though absent or changed, either intermittently or continuously (*hemisomatognosia*)?

Does the patient ignore or show lack of concern about an injured or functionally defective part of the body, for example a left hemiparesis or hemianopic field defect (*anosognosia*)? He may verbally deny the defect or deny ownership of the affected body part.

Other general indications of organic cerebral disorder

Note the ability of the patient to *sustain attention* during the above test procedures. Did he *fatigue unduly easily*? Was he able to *shift attention* readily from one task to another? Did he show *perseveration* in the use of words or in response to commands (Chapter 2) Note and describe any evidence of *lability of mood* or *euphoria*. Were emotional responses *exaggerated, flattened or lacking*? When confronted with a task beyond his ability did he show evidence of a *catastrophic reaction* (see Mood, under Mental state, earlier in this chapter)? Did he show *impulsiveness, disinhibition or over-familiarity* at any point during the testing? Did the patient *appreciate his failings* and show *appropriate concern*? Did he use *evasions* or *excuses* to cover up his deficits?

Examination of the mute or apparently inaccessible patient

States of mutism, stupor and apparent inaccessibility may be due to organic brain disease or to psychiatric disorders such as depression, catatonic schizophrenia or conversion hysteria. In all cases it is necessary to carry out a detailed neurological examination and to assess the apparent level of conscious awareness (as outlined above) before considering other aspects of the problem.

The differential diagnosis of stupor is considered in Chapter 1. In addition to the intracerebral causes it is essential to bear in mind the possibilities of physical illness, especially metabolic, and to examine for physical complications of stupor such as hypotension or retention of urine. It is also important to remember that in stupors due to non-organic psychiatric illness the patient's comprehension of remarks made in his presence may be intact despite appearances to the contrary.

Stupor, semicoma and hypersomnia

The definitions of these terms are not sufficiently precise to be used as the sole description of the phenomena they comprise. The following features should therefore be described separately.

To what extent does the patient dress, feed himself or cooperate with feeding, and attend to matters of hygiene and elimination?

Are the eyes open or shut? If open, are they apparently watchful and do they follow moving objects? If shut, do they open in response to stimulation, and is there resistance to passive opening?

Assess the patient's response to graded stimulation as outlined in Chapter 1. When aroused does he become briefly alert and verbally responsive?

Is the physical posture comfortable, constrained, awkward, bizarre, or in any way indicative of possible delusional beliefs? Does the patient resume a previous posture if moved or when placed in an awkward position? Do movements display special meaning, for example on a possible delusional basis or in response to hallucinatory experiences?

Is the facial expression constant or varying, alert or vacant, blank or meaningful? Is it secretive, withdrawn, indicative of sadness, hopelessness or ecstasy? Does it betray attention to hallucinatory experiences?

Is there any physical or emotional reaction to what is said or done to the patient or within his hearing? Does he show an emotional response when sensitive subjects are discussed? Does he show signs of irritation or annoyance when moved against his wishes?

Examine the state of the musculature. Is it relaxed or rigid? Is rigidity increased by passive movements? Examine for negativism, flexibilitas cerea, automatic obedience and echopraxia. Note evidence of resistiveness, irritability or defensive movements during examination.

In the neurological examination pay special attention to evidence of raised intracranial pressure or of diencephalic or upper brainstem disturbance: thus examine for papilloedema, observe equality and reactivity of pupils, note quality of respiration, look for evidence of long tract deficit in the limbs, and test for conjugate reflex eye movements on passive head rotation.

After recovery, examine for memory of events occurring during the abnormal phase and for fantasies or other subjective experiences occurring at the time.

Mutism

Mutism is a condition in which the person does not speak and makes no attempt at spoken communication despite preservation of an adequate level of consciousness. It may sometimes be the only abnormality in otherwise normal behaviour.

Is it elective, confined to some situations, or in relation to some persons but not others? Is the patient disturbed by it as shown by gesticulations or evidence of distress? Does he attempt to communicate by signs? When offered paper and pen does he communicate in writing?

Distinguish mutism from severe motor aphasia, anarthria, aphonia, poverty of speech or severe psychomotor retardation. Is partial vocalisation preserved, are emotional ejaculations possible, and can simple yes–no answers be given? Test separately for ability to articulate (to whisper or make the lip movements of speech) and ability to phonate (to produce coarse vocalisations or to hum). Can he cough? Does he speak very occasionally and briefly on restricted themes? Does he reply or signal responses to some questions but only after a long delay? In the distinction from aphasia it is important to remember that the most profoundly aphasic patient is never mute; he is always able to make some speech sounds, even if these are restricted to crude syllabic stereotypies or repeated expletives (Benson 1973).

A careful history from informants may sometimes enable distinctions to be made more readily than from examination alone.

Psychometric assessment

The clinical value of psychological testing in the field of organic psychiatry has been much debated. Overenthusiastic claims have sometimes followed the introduction of new tests and procedures for the identification of cerebral dysfunction, and have had to be tempered later in the light of experience. However, even when the claims themselves have been modest the psychiatrist has often misunderstood the situation, and has expected a degree of exactitude from psychometric testing that is unrealistic. Collaboration with clinical psychologists, especially those with special expertise in neuropsychology, is extremely helpful, both in diagnosis and in management, provided a jointly balanced view is taken of the situation. In the diagnosis of brain damage the psychiatrist's and the psychologist's approach are both in their own ways fallible, but each may usefully supplement the other.

The limitations of psychometric tests must be appreciated. There appears to be no single test that will differentiate brain-damaged patients from others without some degree of overlap, and even the most skilful selection of groups of tests will occasionally produce misleading results. Accordingly, test results should only be interpreted in conjunction with all other sources of information relevant to the issue in question. The worst service to psychometry, and to the patient, is likely to come from attempts to rely on test scores viewed in isolation. Similar disappointment would be expected to follow if any clinical diagnostic procedure were singled out and given unique importance. It is essential therefore to retain a general clinical impression as a back-up to the detailed findings.

Advantages

As diagnostic instruments, psychological tests have certain definite advantages over the ordinary procedures of clinical assessment. The tests can be given in strictly standardised form and the results are usually scored numerically. Hence they can be validated on large groups of patients, so that norms can be established and the extent of individual variation gauged with some precision. In these respects they represent a marked advance on the psychiatrist's assessment of the mental state. With their aid one can talk meaningfully in terms of *probabilities* where the presence or absence of brain damage is concerned, and the level of probability is often crucial in deciding what action to pursue. Similarly, the measures can be repeated on more than one occasion, permitting accurate comparisons over an interval of time. This can be invaluable when equivocal findings have emerged at the first consultation; after establishing a baseline the patient's progress can be charted with some accuracy, and any evidence of decline will be highlighted.

Psychological testing can also concentrate in detail on an individual area of functioning which has come under suspicion. Minor degrees of memory impairment or verbal disability, for example, can be pursued with much more thoroughness by psychometric tests than in the clinical interview. The structure of such deficits can also be explored in greater detail. It is here that the psychologist must sometimes be prepared to sacrifice the rigid standardisation of his

approach in order to follow the leads that emerge. Piercy (1959) has argued cogently that some kinds of evidence are better assessed by an experienced human observer than by a standardised procedure; the nature of the failure can be important and this is not always obvious from the score alone. In other words, the advantages of the standardised approach must not be allowed to become an unduly restrictive influence or valuable information will sometimes be lost.

Limitations
Sensitivity and specificity

Typically a test is standardised on groups of subjects known to be suffering from brain damage, and groups in whom this is known to be absent by independent criteria. Nevertheless, few tests are given to large representative populations of 'normal' individuals in which a certain level of 'abnormal' test results is to be expected. In clinical use the test will often be applied to borderline problems in which other evidence of brain damage is equivocal, and here it will not yet have established its credentials. The difficulty in establishing the sensitivity of the test in equivocal cases lies in the problem of obtaining a final arbiter of brain damage. Follow-up of disputed cases can help by displaying the *predictive value* of the test, but such studies have not been carried out extensively.

Attention and motivation

All tests require a certain level of attention and cooperation. Consequently they are vulnerable to emotional disturbance and other influences that have nothing to do with brain damage. Tests which distinguish well between brain-damaged and healthy subjects may therefore give misleading results when applied to certain psychiatric patients. Depression, for example, may disrupt performance on sensitive tests of memory, and schizophrenic thought disorder may lead to poor performance on tests of abstract thinking. Thus any test which is to be usefully employed for differential diagnosis between organic and non-organic psychiatric illness must first be standardised on patients suffering from a wide range of mental disorders.

Theoretical basis

Common misconceptions have also concerned the nature of brain damage itself, and the constancy of its relationship to the behavioural deficits that follow. Tests have sometimes relied heavily on unitary theories of cerebral dysfunction, and many of those put forward as global indicators of 'brain damage' pay little regard to what is known of regional cerebral organisation. Thus tests which sample a restricted aspect of cognitive activity may fail to identify cerebral lesions that are sufficiently circumscribed to leave that particular function intact. Purely verbal tests, for example, may fail to detect visuospatial difficulties resulting from a restricted lesion of the non-dominant hemisphere.

'Untestable' patients

Many patients may simply be too disturbed to undergo systematic psychometric testing, although obtaining meaningful test results from a disturbed patient will reflect the skill and ingenuity of the tester. Here the experienced clinician comes into his or her own: engaging the distractible patient for a few minutes to determine their level of orientation; using objects around them to test praxis, naming, and recognition. Can the patient recall something in the newspaper by his side? Can she report on what she has been watching on the TV? Does he recognise the person next to him and know his name? Given a pen, can she write her name or draw a picture? Patients are never untestable, although the clinician may be incapable of testing them.

Evidential status

Psychometric testing is sometimes regarded, erroneously, as objective. True, unlike bedside assessments, such testing is quantifiable. It should be transparent – the results must be interpreted but such interpretation is rational and governed by rules – valid and reliable. Good inter-rater reliability implies that the tester's characteristics should not influence the test results; standardising testing methods and high standards of clinical training ensure this. However, despite all this, psychometry is rarely objective since testing requires the cooperation of the subject. This may be important in medicolegal and some clinical contexts where a patient may wish to influence the results in one direction or another.

Applications

From the foregoing it will be clear that the questions asked of the psychologist must be realistic, and should reflect some knowledge both of the limitations and special advantages of the psychometric procedures available. It will usually be helpful to discuss the patient fully beforehand in order to focus on the problems to be solved. Requests that the psychologist should 'exclude the possibility of brain damage' or 'localise the lesion' will not yield unequivocal answers, but to ask for collaboration in assessing the *likelihood* of brain damage, focal or diffuse, may add valuable evidence to that already available. The job of lesion localisation is generally delegated to the neuroradiologist. Establishing a baseline level of ability prior to treatment or with a view to tracking decline is extremely valuable. Apart from diagnosis, psychometry can also be valuable where rehabilitation is concerned. Areas of relatively intact function can be identified, and problems highlighted on which re-education should be concentrated. Progress can be monitored with a fair degree of accuracy, enabling ultimate goals to be discerned.

In the sections that follow some of the available tests are briefly described. Some provide essentially qualitative information, although the great majority yield numerical scores. Some rely on profiles of comparison between different functional capacities, or help to demonstrate the fall from esti-mated levels of premorbid intelligence (e.g. the National Adult Reading Test). Others concentrate on certain areas alone, such as perception, language or memory, although obviously considerable overlap will often occur. Mention is also made of certain aptitude tests, often initially designed for healthy individuals, but also useful as a guide to the rehabilitation and resettlement of brain-damaged patients. Questionnaires and rating scales which have been employed with severely brain-damaged subjects are also discussed.

The tests themselves vary widely in the extent to which they have been validated and the adequacy with which norms have been established. This is not the place to attempt a thorough review of their respective credentials, but rather to give an outline for the clinician of commonly used tests, their aims and procedures. Details can be found in the compilations produced by Crawford *et al.* (1992a) and Lezak (1995).

Standardised tests of intelligence and memory

Wechsler Adult Intelligence Scale

The Wechsler Adult Intelligence Scale (WAIS), produced by the Psychological Corporation of America, is an extensively standardised instrument for the measurement of intelligence, providing separate scores for 'verbal' and 'performance' abilities. Possible deterioration from estimated or established premorbid levels can be assessed, and this alone can yield important information about the likelihood of brain damage. Qualitative interpretation of different subtest scores may indicate areas of special cognitive difficulty. The current version is WAIS-III (Wechsler 1997).

Verbal subtests (untimed except for arithmetic)

1 Information: 29 questions covering a wide variety of information and arranged in order of difficulty.
2 Comprehension: 16 items in which the subject must explain what should be done in certain circumstances, the meaning of proverbs, etc. This aims at measuring practical judgement and common sense.
3 Arithmetic: 14 mental arithmetic problems set in the context of everyday activities.
4 Similarities: 14 items in which the subject must say in what way two things are alike.
5 Digit Span: lists of 3–9 digits to be reproduced forwards and 2–8 digits to be reproduced backwards.
6 Vocabulary: 35 words graded in difficulty for which the subject must give the meaning.
7 Letter–Number Sequencing: the object is to extract separate sequences of letters and numbers from a mixed sequence containing both (optional).

Performance subtests (all timed except matrix reasoning)

1 Digit Symbol: the subject must follow a simple code in matching symbols to digits, as quickly as he can.
2 Picture Completion: the subject is shown 20 pictures of human features, familiar objects or scenes, and must say what important part is missing from each.

3 Block Design: this is similar to the Kohs' Block Design Test. The subject must reproduce designs with red and white blocks.
4 Picture Arrangement: 10 sets of cartoon pictures must be arranged in sequence so as to tell a sensible story.
5 Matrix Reasoning (replaces object assembly from WAIS-R): the subject chooses the next in a sequence of abstract coloured symbols.
6 Symbol Search: the subject has to look for either of two symbols in a sequence.

The raw score on each subtest is transmuted into a standard score (scaled score), which represents the individual's distance from the mean in terms of the distribution for that particular subtest. By this procedure all subtest scores are expressed in units that can be compared one with another. WAIS-III subtests may be grouped to form indices: verbal comprehension, perceptual organisation, working memory and processing speed. Abbreviated forms of the test are commonly used in clinical practice and the Psychological Corporation have an official version, the Wechsler Abbreviated Scale of Intelligence (WASI) comprising vocabulary, block design, similarities and matrix reasoning. The scores on the WAIS is standardised to give a mean IQ of 100 with one standard deviation equal to 15 IQ points; the 50% confidence limits range from 90 to 110 and the 95% confidence limits from 70 to 130. Below 70 is regarded as in the mental retardation range.

The current WAIS-III was intended to be of greater utility to neuropsychologists than its predecessors (see Tulsky & Haaland 2001). For example, measurement of letter–number span appears to be a good index of working memory and matrix reasoning (derived from Raven's Progressive Matrices, a non-verbal measure of IQ in adults and children; Raven *et al.* 1992), of 'fluid' intelligence, and is less contaminated by performance speed which tends to be affected non-specifically in many clinical groups. In general the battery has significant advantages over many 'proper' a priori neuropsychological tests: extensive population age-corrected norms, strictly operationalised procedures, and reasonable face validity in terms of underlying cognitive processes. The WAIS-III is designed to be allied to the Wechsler Memory Scale (WMS-III) so memory impairment can judged to be consistent with or disproportionate to general abilities (see below). It may also be administered by any non-specialist clinical psychologist. On the other hand, it is clearly sensitive to education, language and other ethnic and cultural factors (like many tests). It takes time to complete and while relating the WAIS-III to previous versions and the childhood version (WISC) is fairly straightforward, it is not without problems.

As a neuropsychological test, brain damage may be reflected in discrepancies between the verbal and performance IQs. In very general terms, verbal subtests will tend to be impaired by lesions in the dominant hemisphere, and those involving visuospatial functions by lesions in the non-dominant hemisphere, although verbal–performance discrepancies cannot be used as a reliable guide to laterality of brain damage. The likelihood of a verbal–performance discrepancy being pathological can be gleaned from the scoring manual. *Deterioration indices* involve comparisons between other contrasting groups of subtests. 'Hold' tests are identified which are found to be relatively impervious to the effects of brain damage, whereas 'Don't hold' tests show early decline. The former include subtests that reflect the use of old knowledge (e.g. vocabulary and information), whereas the latter require speed or the perception of new relations in verbal or spatial content (digit symbol and block design). One of the most useful applications of an IQ score derived from the WAIS is comparison with an earlier score (an index of premorbid IQ or at the very least a broad estimate of premorbid functioning from previous occupation or educational attainment) in providing prima facie evidence of decline as in a dementing condition or following a brain insult.

The application of the WAIS as a diagnostic instrument has been criticised on theoretical grounds, in that the reliability of subtests taken individually is not sufficiently high to allow a confident interpretation of any but the largest differences between them. Scatter can result not only from pathological processes but also from differences in educational, occupational and cultural factors. Nevertheless, qualitative interpretation of subtest scores may provide useful clinical information, yielding important pointers for verification by more detailed testing. In my opinion, the WAIS is undervalued as an assessment tool in neuropsychiatry.

National Adult Reading Test

A simple technique for yielding an approximate estimate of general intelligence consists in administering a series of words to be read aloud (Nelson 1982; Nelson & Willison 1991). Nelson and McKenna (1975) introduced this rapid method using words from the Schonell Graded Word Reading Test, and Nelson and O'Connell (1978) then modified it by drawing up a list of words spelled in an irregular manner (e.g. ache, bouquet, naive, sidereal). The level of word reading ability achieved by an adult has been shown to correlate highly with intelligence and, being well practised and overlearned, it proves to be relatively resistant to influences which impair other aspects of cognitive function.

It is this last aspect which makes the test especially useful. The authors showed that even in patients with dementia the ability to read words declined little if at all, at least in the patients used in the samples they examined. Thus subjects without evidence of brain disorder gave results closely comparable to patients with cerebral atrophy, even though in the latter the WAIS IQ had deteriorated considerably. It was possible to show that estimates of premorbid intelligence derived from the National Adult Reading Test (NART) were more stable even than those derived from the vocabulary subtest of the WAIS. The validity of the test in this regard has since been confirmed in further studies (Crawford *et al.* 1990) and use of the NART has spread to other clinical groups such as patients with schizophrenia and bipolar affective disorder. However, the test has come under criticism, with evidence that in patients with dementia of moderate severity it may yield an underestimate of premorbid competence (O'Carroll *et al.* 1995). Also, the NART is prone to floor effects.

After administering the NART, regression equations may be used to obtain an estimate of minimum premorbid intelligence, and discrepancies between this and current WAIS IQ. It may also be used to estimate premorbid levels of verbal fluency (Crawford *et al.* 1992b). The test has obvious limitations, however, especially for non-native speakers of English, subjects who were always poor readers, or who have acquired reading difficulties or dysarthria. Versions of the NART in other languages are available, although abundant irregular words are a special feature of English and simply do not arise in, for example, everyday Italian.

Memory tests
Wechsler Memory Scale (WMS-III)
Wechsler's battery of memory tests aims at measuring several different aspects of memory by rapid standardised procedures. As with the WAIS, it too was updated in 1997 and quite radically so. Two of the three visual subtests that had been in WMS-R (figural memory and visual paired associates) were deleted and the third (visual reproduction) was retained as optional. The WMS-III introduced the new Family Pictures and Faces subtests that use genuine stimuli such as photographs rather than just abstract shapes. The old 'attention/concentration' factor was reconceptualised as 'working memory'. This is assumed to be parallel to the WAIS-III working memory factor but there are different subtests: the spatial span, assumed to be a visual analogue of the digit span task (Tulsky 2004).

Clinicians routinely examine differences between an individual's performance on immediate and delayed memory tasks as a way of differentially diagnosing encoding versus retention deficits. In the WMS-III, evaluation of the Immediate Memory Index (IMI) and the General Memory Index (GMI) allows such a comparison. The logical memory story (A) is largely unchanged, and there is a new second story (B) which is now repeated a second time to assess the benefit of repetition. The test is also followed by a 30-item yes–no recognition memory subtest.

All the subtests except spatial span are given in immediate (1) and delayed (2) conditions. Altogether they form indices: Immediate Memory (composed of Logical Memory 1, Verbal Paired Associates 1, Faces 1, and Family Pictures 1); General Memory (composed of Logical Memory 2, Verbal Paired Associates 2, Faces 2, and Family Pictures 2); and Working Memory (composed of Letter–Number Sequencing and Spatial Span).
- Information and Orientation (optional).

- Logical Memory examines the immediate recall of two short stories, the second of which is presented twice. The subject is asked to retell the stories immediately or after a delay of around 30 minutes. After the delayed condition the subject is asked yes–no questions about the stories.
- Faces: 24 photographs are presented followed by 48 photos and the subject is asked to say which out of these he recognises.
- Family Pictures: photos of a family and a series of scenes. The subject has to remember information, such as who was doing what and where. Both Faces and Family Pictures have immediate and delayed presentations.
- Word Lists (optional): 12 semantically related words are presented orally to be recalled. There are four learning trials. Then a new 12-word list is presented as before. Then the subject has to recall as many words as he can from the first list. After delay, recall of the first list is again tested. Finally, 24 words are read and the subject indicates, one by one, if it was on the first list.
- Verbal Paired Associates: eight pairs of words are read to the subject. Then the first of each pair is read and the subject has to remember its pair. There are four trials of the list in different orders. All pairs are novel (compare the previous version, which had hard and easy (commonly associated) word pairs). In the delayed condition, the first of each pair is again read out and the corresponding word is sought. All words are then read and subject has to indicate whether each is old or new.
- Visual Reproduction (optional) involves the immediate recall of five geometrical figures. The subject must draw what he remembers after seeing each card for 10 seconds. In the delayed condition there are recall, recognition, copying and matching tests.
- Letter–Number Sequencing: a string of alternating letters and numbers are presented orally. The test is to repeat the numbers in ascending order followed by the letters in alphabetical order.
- Spatial Span: a series of patterns is shown on a three-dimensional board. The examiner points to them one by one. The subject then has to repeat this. Subsequently the subject points to the blocks in reverse order.
- Mental Control (optional), e.g. reciting days of the week.
- Digit Span (optional): forwards and backwards.

Neuropsychological tests
Detailed knowledge of the huge range of neuropsychological tests currently available is not required for the practising neuropsychiatrist. However, an idea of the nature and administration of a few commonly used tests is very useful in interpreting reports, recommending tests and discussing their results in an informed way with colleagues. Interested readers should consult Lezak (1995) and Anastasi & Urbina (1997). Table 3.4 lists the main classes of tests with examples not described above. Details of some of the more commonly used tests are given in the Appendix.

Special and ancillary investigations

Further investigations will often be required when an organic basis is suspected for psychiatric disorder. Certain routine tests should ideally be performed on all psychiatric inpatients, including estimation of haemoglobin,

Table 3.4 Neuropsychological tests.

Tests of perception/attention
Bender–Gestalt Test (Bender Visual Motor Gestalt Test)
Visual Object and Space Perception Battery (VOSP)
Behavioural Inattention Test (line bisection, star cancellation)
Tests of Everyday Attention (TEA)
Rey–Osterrieth Test (see under Memory)

Language tests
Boston Naming Test
Graded Naming Test
Token Test
Speed and Capacity of Language Processing Test
Speed of Comprehension Test
Spot-the-Word Test
Psycholinguistic Assessments of Language Processing in Aphasia
 (PALPA)

Memory tests
Paired associate learning tests
Object Learning Test
List learning tests
Rey Auditory Verbal Learning Test
California Verbal Learning Test
Recognition memory tests
 Camden Memory Test
Benton Visual Retention Test
Rey–Osterrieth Test
Adult Memory and Information Processing Battery
Rivermead Behavioural Memory Test
Autobiographical Memory Interview (AMI)

Frontal lobe ('executive function') tests
Verbal fluency tests
Wisconsin Card Sorting Test
Modified Wisconsin Card Sorting Test
Stroop tests
Cognitive Estimates Test
Strategy application tests
 Behavioural Assessment of Dysexecutive Syndrome (BADS)
 Hayling Test
 Brixton Test
Tower of London Test
Trail Making Test
Goldstein–Sheerer tests

Vigilance tests
Paced Auditory Serial Addition Test (PASAT)
Continuous Performance Test

'Batteries'
Halstead–Reitan Battery
Cambridge Neuropsychological Test Automated Battery (CANTAB)

Dementia questionnaires and rating scales
Blessed's Dementia Scale
Middlesex Elderly Assessment of Mental State (MEAMS)
Geriatric Mental State Schedule
Cambridge Examination for Mental Disorders of the Elderly
 (CAMDEX/CAMCOG)

Aptitude tests
Vineland Social Maturity Scale

erythrocyte sedimentation rate, urea, electrolytes and blood glucose, liver function tests, thyroid function, calcium and phosphate, serological tests for syphilis, chest radiograph and routine urine examination. The patient's temperature should always be taken, with 4-hourly recording if minor rises are suspected. These serve as screening tests for coincidental as well as causally related physical disorders. Other investigations will be indicated on the basis of the history and clinical examination when specific disorders are suspected. An important principle is that investigations should always be planned to give the maximum required information with the minimum of inconvenience to the patient. Investigations without discomfort or risk will obviously be more readily undertaken than those which carry the possibility of pain or complications. For example, skull radiography, electroencephalography (EEG) and computed tomography (CT) will sometimes be performed even when the level or suspicion of organic involvement is low, whereas lumbar puncture and other invasive procedures will be reserved until very specific and important questions need to be answered. The yield of abnormal CT results in psychiatric patients from various series has been described by Roberts and Lishman (1984).

Few of these tests have well-defined sensitivities and specificities for neuropsychiatric disorders and a great deal of judgement and consideration is required when embarking on elaborate investigations. Special investigations will only yield useful data if they have been discussed properly with the professional carrying them out. The indications for these and other investigations are detailed in the relevant chapters later in the book. The special investigations required in connection with some of the rarer causes of dementia are outlined in Chapter 9, and see Love 2005. Certain other investigations of particular relevance to cerebral dysfunction are discussed in detail below.

Electroencephalography

The EEG has the important advantage over many other procedures that it is safe and without discomfort to the patient. It is accordingly used extensively when organic psychiatric disorders are suspected. Furthermore, it remains the major non-invasive means of determining the physiological or functional state of the brain, as opposed to its anatomical status. However, certain marked limitations in its diagnostic usefulness must be borne in mind.

Characteristics
EEG rhythms are conventionally classified into four components according to their frequencies: delta (<4 Hz), theta (4–7 Hz), alpha (8–13 Hz) and beta (>13 Hz) (Storm van Leeuwen *et al.* 1966). The normal EEG has a well-developed alpha rhythm, maximal in the occipital and parietal regions, which attenuates on opening the eyes and reappears when they are closed again. It similarly attenuates when the patient engages in mental activity such as simple mental arithmetic. The

average voltage of the alpha rhythm is 30–50 μV with spindle-shaped modulations. Small amounts of other rhythms are allowable provided the alpha activity is well developed. Beta activity is seen mainly in the precentral regions, and low-voltage theta becomes more obvious with relaxation and drowsiness. Delta activity is normally seen only in very young children and during sleep.

Lambda waves are saw-toothed in form and characteristically situated over the occiput. They reflect small eyeball movements. Mu rhythm has a characteristic waveform and a frequency within the alpha range; it is commonly present in the rolandic area and is diminished by contralateral limb movement (Toone 1984). K complexes are brief bursts of high-voltage slow waves that may emerge during non-REM (rapid eye movement) sleep.

Abnormal EEG elements that can be important in diagnosis include the following.
• *Spikes* are high peaked discharges that rise and fall abruptly and stand out above the general amplitude of the other waves.
• *Sharp waves* rise steeply then fall more slowly, and may occupy the alpha, theta or delta range.
• Composite elements may consist of spikes alternating with delta waves (*spike-and-wave* or *wave-and-spike* discharges) or slow waves preceded by several spikes (*poly-spike and wave*). Wave-and-spike discharges occurring at a rhythm of 3 Hz constitute the classic EEG feature of simple absence attacks; those faster and slower than this may be referred to as *wave-and-spike variants*.
Abnormal rhythms and other elements can be generalised, unilateral or focal, and may be described as synchronous or asynchronous depending on the coincidence of their appearance in different leads.

Various activating procedures may be used to clarify marginal abnormalities, or to reveal those concealed in the resting record. Hyperventilation is used to increase the excitability of cortical cells, probably mainly as a result of hypocapnic constriction of cerebral vessels leading to cerebral hypoxia (Meyer & Gotoh 1960). Epileptic foci and other disturbances may emerge more clearly. Photic stimulation consists of repetitive light flashes of varying frequency. Within certain ranges of flash frequency (especially 8–15 Hz) the occipital alpha rhythm adjusts itself to the flash rate (occipital 'driving'), and paroxysmal abnormalities may emerge in the form of high-voltage complex elements spreading to the frontal and temporal regions. Seizure patterns may emerge, and a generalised seizure may even be provoked. Sleep may be induced by barbiturates if it does not occur naturally. This can be useful in activating the spike or sharp wave discharges of epilepsy, especially those arising within the temporal lobes. Thiopental may be given intravenously and typically induces beta activity, often in the form of discrete runs or spindles. The induced beta activity is commonly less well developed at the electrodes over the site of damage in the affected temporal lobe. Other drugs may occasionally be employed for the activation of seizure patterns but only

under skilled supervision in specialised centres. Anticonvulsant medication may be withdrawn prior to EEG and telemetry studies in people suspected of having non-epileptic attack disorders (see Chapter 6).

In addition to the normal electrode placements over the scalp, sphenoidal, nasopharyngeal or foramen ovale electrodes can be valuable for locating discharges from the antero-inferior portions of the temporal lobes. These are chiefly used when assessing the suitability of epileptic patients for temporal lobectomy. Much may also be gained from depth electrode studies, or by recording directly from the exposed cortex at operation (electrocorticography). These procedures can obviously be undertaken only in special centres.

Limitations

In many ways, EEG has failed to satisfy early expectations as a diagnostic aid for reasons discussed by Kiloh *et al.* (1981), although more quantitative methods of analysis can improve its yield as a test (see Hughes and John 1999 for review). Accordingly it must only be interpreted with its limitations clearly in mind. Moreover, much of its traditional advantage in being non-invasive has now been eroded by the introduction of modern brain imaging techniques (Toone 1984).

In the first place, the EEG can be normal in patients with obvious cerebral dysfunction, especially if only a single recording is relied on. It is probably true to say that a normal EEG never excludes any clinical condition, but can merely serve to diminish the probability of its existence. Conversely, a certain proportion of healthy individuals will exhibit abnormal EEGs. The EEG is particularly sensitive to such physiological variables as level of awareness, acid–base equilibrium and blood sugar level. Such physiological changes in the record are indistinguishable from those associated with many pathological states, and can readily be misinterpreted as evidence of disease.

Again, with rare exceptions, the patterns obtained have little diagnostic specificity, and the EEG should only be used as an additional source of information to add to the evidence of the history and clinical examination. It can be a valuable aid in localisation but is of little help in pathological diagnosis. Even with regard to localisation it is known that a focal lesion can occasionally be associated with disturbance some distance away, or alternatively give rise to generalised EEG abnormalities. For these reasons the most useful help will be obtained from the investigation when the person interpreting the record is fully acquainted with all relevant clinical information about the patient's illness.

There can be added difficulties in psychiatric patients, in that mental disorders of apparently non-organic origin are known to be associated with an increased incidence of abnormalities in the EEG. This can sometimes cloud the issue when it comes to the differential diagnosis between organic and non-organic psychiatric conditions. Whereas perhaps

10–15% of normal subjects show some abnormality on EEG, this figure has sometimes been found to be higher among patients with neurotic disorders. The abnormalities in such patients commonly lie just outside the normal range, with an excess of generalised theta or beta rhythms of rather low amplitude. Patients with bipolar affective disorder have been reported to show marginally abnormal records in up to 20% of cases, although again the finding is far from consistent. Schizophrenia is sometimes associated with more definite abnormalities, in perhaps one-quarter of cases. Catatonic schizophrenia shows abnormal records more commonly than other varieties. However, these changes are not constant, failing to appear in some patients and sometimes varying from one attack to another in the same patient.

In patients with disorders of behaviour and personality the incidence of abnormalities is perhaps highest of all. Classic studies by Hill and Watterson (1942) found that 48% of patients diagnosed as psychopathic had abnormal EEGs compared with 15% of controls, and among aggressive psychopaths the proportion rose to 65%. The majority of the abnormalities in patients with personality disorder appear to reflect cerebral immaturity, and are of a type that would be accepted as normal in a very much younger age group. Sometimes the so-called immaturity may be the result of past cerebral insults, even of birth injury, but the great majority appear merely to be associated with delayed maturation. Thus the abnormalities tend to decrease with age, and this may be accompanied by a parallel improvement in behaviour.

Another difficulty with psychiatric patients can be the result of treatments currently or recently given. Many of the widely prescribed drugs affect the EEG, in some individuals to a marked extent. Fenton (1974) and Kiloh et al. (1981) have reviewed the main changes that occur. Barbiturates and other sedatives increase fast activity and sometimes produce a small amount of diffuse theta or even delta activity. Most sedatives also tend to aggravate epileptic discharges. On the other hand, anticonvulsants other than barbiturates have little effect on the EEG. Chlorpromazine in low dosage may disturb alpha activity, with the occasional appearance of slow frequencies. In dosages much higher than tend to be used nowadays, it may produce generalised delta waves or hypersynchronous high-voltage discharges. Chlorpromazine also potentiates epileptic discharges. Clozapine has dose-related epileptogenic properties. Similar changes are produced by most other antipsychotics, tricyclic antidepressants and lithium. Benzodiazepines (e.g. diazepam) are usually associated with increased fast activity.

Electroconvulsive therapy can render the EEG hard to interpret for a time. Each fit is followed by generalised theta and delta activity, which becomes more persistent as successive treatments are given. After three or four treatments spaced at intervals of 2–3 days the abnormal rhythms may persist in the intervals between, often with frontal prepon-

derance. As the course of treatment proceeds the disturbance becomes more widespread and of higher voltage, and alpha activity may disappear. Individual patients differ in the severity of these effects and in the time taken for return to normality (around 1–3 months).

Uses

This brief description of some of the difficulties surrounding the interpretation of the EEG is necessary before discussing situations where it can serve a useful purpose (Smith 2005). In general terms, suspicions of abnormality of brain structure or function are confirmed by the EEG in more than 60% of cases with around 10% false positives, based on a large group of patients aged over 50 years investigated for organic disease (Leuchter et al. 1993). Hence it can bring added information in psychiatric patients when the question of an organic basis for the illness has arisen. In diagnostically obscure cases one can look for clues which may indicate the need for further investigation. A single focus of abnormally fast or slow activity will always suggest the presence of a cerebral lesion and must be followed up further, likewise gross asymmetries of normal or abnormal activity between the hemispheres. EEG also plays a part in the differentiation between organic and non-organic psychiatric illness, though caution must be observed. A normal record will be of little help in the distinction, but it will certainly be less easy to maintain a diagnosis of a purely psychogenic disturbance in the presence of a grossly abnormal record.

Epilepsy

The disturbances seen in epileptic subjects are considered in detail in Chapter 6. Characteristic epileptic discharges consist of spikes, sharp waves or wave-and-spike complexes. When recurrent these are very strong evidence in favour of an epileptic process. In primary generalised epilepsy, wave-and-spike complexes may consist of runs of classic 3-Hz spike and wave, but in the presence of grand mal attacks they are commonly somewhat faster or consist of variants with poly-spike and wave. Other abnormalities common in epileptics, but without the same degree of specificity, include paroxysms of symmetrical delta activity, bursts of theta, or a diffuse excess of delta and theta. Epilepsy that originates within the cortex shows a spike and sharp wave focus, or local spike discharges either singly or in groups. These often betray the point of origin of the seizures, although sometimes they are transmitted widely to other areas. Temporal lobe epilepsy often shows spike discharges over the temporal region, but occasionally the record can be normal until sleep is induced and sphenoidal or nasopharyngeal electrodes are employed.

The principal value of the EEG in epilepsy is to distinguish patients with a discharging cortical focus from those with primary generalised epilepsy. In patients without an aura to their grand mal attacks there may be no other means of making the distinction. The EEG can localise the cortical lesion, indicate its extent, and whether it is unilateral or bilateral, although this has become less important with the advent of magnetic resonance imaging (MRI).

On the broader question of the diagnosis of epilepsy, the EEG can be useful but is not an infallible guide. Epileptiform discharges are found in occasional normal persons, in many degenerative brain disorders and in some patients with psychosis or personality disorder. Conversely, in some 20–30% of patients with epilepsy, a single routine EEG will be normal. In exceptional cases the record can remain normal even during an attack, as in some cases of Jacksonian and psychomotor epilepsy when the foci are so discrete, and of such low voltage, that they fail to reach the surface electrodes. The recognition of the epileptic nature of a group of symptoms must therefore remain primarily a clinical task, but one which obtains firm confirmation from the EEG in the majority of cases. Where the clinical features are dubious this confirmation can have a decisive influence on the diagnosis and future management. Classic spike-and-wave discharges, for example, may resolve doubts when an adequate witnessed account of attacks is not forthcoming. And in temporal lobe epilepsy, the EEG can sometimes point directly to the diagnosis in patients who have hitherto been considered to suffer from 'hysteria', anxiety attacks or short-lived psychotic reactions. The EEG is particularly valuable in confirming or excluding non-convulsive status epilepticus, which can present as a confusional state.

Space-occupying lesions

Space-occupying lesions are revealed by the EEG in a high proportion of cases but is no longer used for this purpose. A focal delta wave focus will constitute strong presumptive evidence of a cerebral tumour, especially when combined with the other features outlined in Chapter 5. Alternatively, it may give the first indication of a developing cerebral abscess when this arises as a complication of a generalised infection. A subdural haematoma in the elderly sometimes presents with a psychiatric picture, and the EEG can be the factor that alerts one to the diagnosis. Typically, there is diminished amplitude or suppression of cerebral rhythms over the affected hemisphere, and some irregular slow activity on the affected side, although the contralateral hemisphere may be affected as well. One must also beware of the occasional cases with well-defined but utterly misleading foci, even sometimes locating the tumour or haematoma to the wrong side of the head.

Cerebral infarction

With cerebral infarctions the EEG can be of help in gauging prognosis. Patients with minimal changes during the acute episode can generally be expected to make a good recovery, and also patients in whom the EEG changes resolve steadily from an early date. However, an EEG that becomes normal while neurological deficits persist suggests that little further clinical improvement can be expected.

Head injury

After head injury the EEG may again sometimes help in gauging prognosis (see Chapter 4) or in pointing to an organic component in disturbances which have seemed to be purely psychological in origin. EEG changes may occasionally foreshadow the development of post-traumatic epilepsy, but the interseizure record remains normal in a high proportion of patients even when fits have already become established.

Encephalitis

In encephalitis the EEG, together with examination of the cerebrospinal fluid (CSF), can be a valuable means of following progress. Abnormalities consist of diffuse irregular slow waves and scattered sharp waves, with slowing or reduction in alpha activity. Seizure patterns (e.g. periodic epileptiform discharges) are not uncommon in the acute stage and if bilateral confer a poor prognosis on herpes simplex encephalitis (Fig. 3.3). There may be a warning of complications and of permanent brain damage when slow waves persist. The appearance of new spikes or spike-and-wave complexes raises the possibility that secondary epilepsy will develop. In subacute sclerosing panencephalitis the EEG changes described in Chapter 7 have high diagnostic value.

Metabolic disorders

In metabolic disorders the EEG is a sensitive indicator of cerebral insufficiency, and can reflect worsening or improvement of the clinical condition with a fair degree of accuracy. The changes lack specificity for the various metabolic disorders, being for example similar in hypoglycaemia, anoxia, hypokalaemia, carbon dioxide retention or vitamin B_{12} deficiency. Nevertheless, they can provide important information in patients who present with indefinite features in the mental state. They may help to confirm the organic basis for paranoid syndromes or disturbances of behaviour in patients who are only minimally confused. Alternatively, when organic features are well developed the EEG may help in the sometimes difficult distinction between reversible causes and progressive brain pathology. Obrecht *et al.* (1979) have demonstrated the value of the EEG in patients with acute confusional states in general hospital practice, particularly in helping to distinguish metabolic and other systemic disorders from intracranial pathologies.

The earliest changes are slowing of the alpha rhythm along with diminution of voltage. Later there is progressive slowing and disorganisation, with runs of theta that come to replace all other activity. Finally, in metabolic coma regular high-voltage delta activity appears, sometimes bilaterally synchronous and sometimes more random in distribution. In deep coma, when the patient is quite unresponsive, the

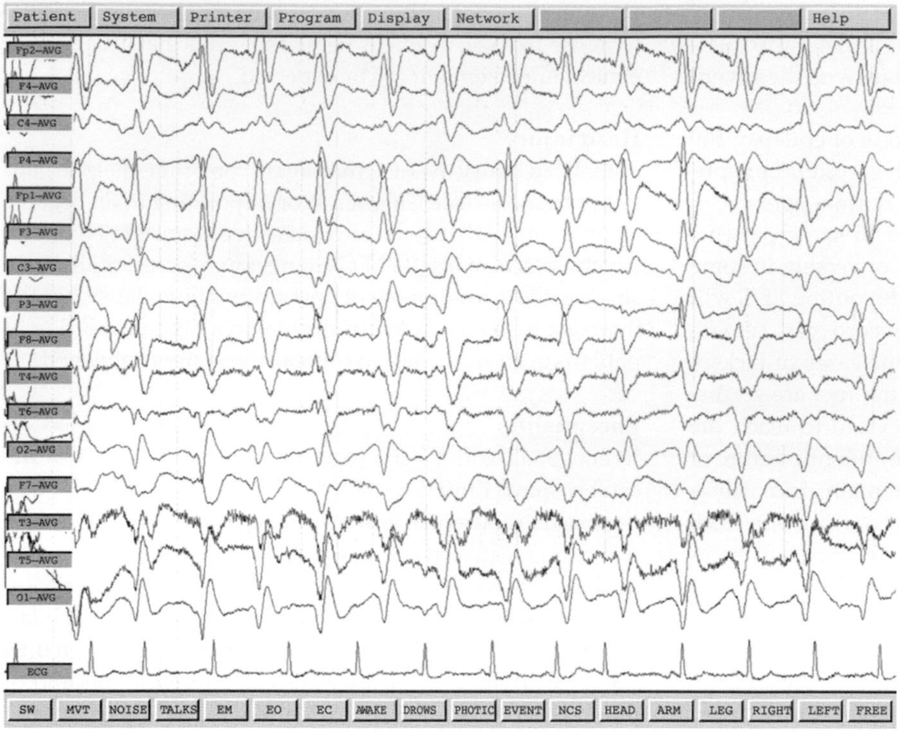

Fig. 3.3 Herpes simplex encephalitis: left-sided slow activity and repetitive periodic epileptiform discharges. (From Smith 2005 with permission of BMJ Publishing Group Ltd.)

amplitude of the EEG diminishes and ultimately the record becomes flat and featureless.

Disturbance of consciousness

Disturbance of consciousness will produce EEG slowing even when very mild and when cognitive difficulty can be hard to detect on clinical examination. This can be shown by serial recordings, and can occasionally be useful in the retrospective diagnosis of minimal degrees of clouding of consciousness. The absolute frequency of the dominant rhythm is less important than the degree of slowing. Thus 8–9 Hz may be abnormal if it has replaced alpha of a higher frequency. This explains why patients with clouding of consciousness can have an apparently normal EEG. When slowing has reached 5–6 Hz the characteristic disruption of activity on eye opening no longer occurs, representing the physiological correlate of the reduced impact of perceptions derived from the environment. Fluctuations in the severity of delirium, as reflected in outward behaviour, prove not to be related to changes in the underlying metabolic disturbance as reflected in the EEG, but to be more closely tied to psychological and environmental factors.

While there is often a relationship between the degree of EEG slowing and level of impairment of consciousness, this is not invariable. Delirium tremens is an obvious exception, in that during profound delirium the EEG may be normal or show fast activity of low to moderate voltage rather than slowing of rhythms. Lipowski (1990) suggests that slowing of the EEG is characteristic of delirium that presents with reduced alertness and wakefulness, whereas in hyperactive delirium fast activity may be superimposed on this, sometimes with features resembling those of REM sleep.

The EEG can be of some diagnostic help in comatose patients. Comas due to metabolic disturbance will show diffuse high-voltage delta activity as described above, whereas in barbiturate overdosage there will be augmented amplitude and an increase in fast frequencies. Space-occupying lesions may be indicated by focal abnormalities, or epileptic activity may be revealed. Pseudocoma due to conversion disorder, psychosis or affective disorder would be expected to give rise to a normal or near normal EEG. The record will show responsiveness to auditory and visual stimuli.

Presenile and senile dementias

In the dementias the degree of EEG abnormality appears to be more closely related to the rate of progression of the disorder than to the degree of intellectual impairment at a given point in time. Briefly, in dementia of the Alzheimer type the commonest abnormality is accentuation of the normal EEG changes with ageing, and may therefore be difficult to diagnose with confidence. Alpha activity is slowed in frequency and reduced in quantity, and diffuse theta or delta rhythms tend to appear. The vascular dementias show a similar picture, though often with focal features where local cerebral infarctions have occurred. Presenile Alzheimer's disease is associated with a particularly high incidence of abnormalities. Alpha activity tends to disappear, and is replaced

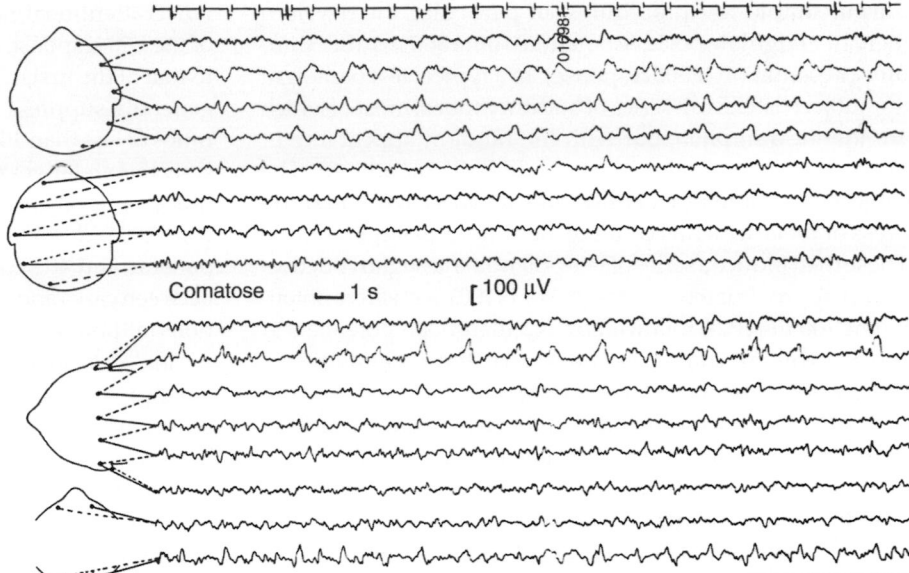

Comatose ⊢⎯⎯⊣ 1 s [100 µV

Fig. 3.4 Characteristic EEG findings in sporadic Creutzfeldt–Jakob disease: periodic complexes at approximately 1 per second, and very low amplitude featureless background between complexes. (From Smith 2005 with permission of BMJ Publishing Group Ltd.)

with irregular theta on which runs of delta activity may be superimposed. Pronounced flattening of the record will raise the possibility of Huntington's chorea, whereas repetitive spike discharges or characteristic triphasic sharp wave complexes may be indicative of Creutzfeldt–Jakob disease (CJD) (Fig. 3.4).

In all these conditions the EEG abnormalities may fail to develop in a significant proportion of mild to moderate cases, and even advanced dementia can occasionally exist alongside a normal EEG. Moreover, with some exceptions, the changes that occur lack specificity for the illnesses in question. Nevertheless, an EEG can be helpful in early and uncertain cases of dementia. In the previously mentioned study by Leuchter *et al.* (1993), 42% of patients with suspected dementia without clear impairment had an abnormal EEG, the figure rising to 65% in those with mild to moderate impairment. A normal EEG in such circumstances will make Alzheimer's disease unlikely, but will not exclude other varieties of dementia. The EEG may also help in the distinction between diffuse and focal lesions.

Finally, in elderly patients the EEG may aid differentiation between depressive pseudodementia and degenerative brain disease. A normal EEG in a patient who has been diagnosed as suffering from Alzheimer's disease or vascular dementia, and who shows features of depression, will at least suggest that the diagnosis should be reconsidered (Kiloh *et al.* 1981).

Event-related potentials (evoked potentials)

Incoming sensory stimuli are associated with brief changes in brain potentials, and these can be detected when suitable averaging methods are used to demarcate them from the background EEG activity. Successive epochs of EEG are summated and averaged by computer while repeated

visual, auditory or somatosensory stimuli are presented to the subject. The value of such techniques lies in their non-invasive nature and the minimal requirement for cooperation from the subject. Applied to almost any sensory modality, they can demonstrate abnormal sensory condition (Walsh *et al.* 2005). Moreover, certain late components of event-related potentials (ERPs), when coupled with minimal task demands, have proved to reflect psychological processes such as expectation and motivation, and to be abnormal in some psychiatric conditions.

The early components, generated within 20 ms or so from stimulus presentation, reflect neuronal activity in the sensory end organs and afferent pathways, and can be sensitive indicators of pathology in the auditory apparatus, optic pathways and brainstem. The value of visual pattern-evoked responses, brainstem auditory-evoked responses and somatosensory responses in the diagnosis of multiple sclerosis is described in Chapter 14) although yet again MRI is the main diagnostic tool. Wright *et al.* (1984) found that while pattern-evoked responses were normal in dementia, the major positive component (P2) to flash was considerably delayed, presumably because this is generated in association cortex rather than primary visual cortex.

However, the principal interest for psychiatry centres on the late components of ERPs elicited while the subject is engaged in some simple task (cognitive ERPs). Grey Walter *et al.* (1964) described *contingent negative variation* (CNV), observed when a subject was told to press a button in response to a flash of light which occurred 3 seconds after hearing a warning click. During the period of expectation a negative potential could be recorded from the scalp that increased steadily in amplitude until the button press was performed. Sutton *et al.* (1965) then showed that certain late potentials were a function of the uncertainty experienced by the subject during simple test procedures, in particular the development of a large late positive potential some 300 ms after stimulus presentation (P300 response). In a typical test paradigm the subject listens to a series of auditory tones, most of which are identical in pitch, but with the random appearance of rarer stimuli at another pitch ('odd-ball' paradigm). The subject must attend carefully, and respond with a button press or make a mental count of the abnormal target stimuli. These then induce a series of late potentials: a negative deflection at approximately 100 ms (N1 or N100), a positive potential at 200 ms (P2), followed by N2 then P300 potentials at 300 ms. This last component has been extensively studied in relation to dementia and schizophrenia.

The P300 is significantly delayed in a majority of patients with dementia, and in proportion to the severity of the dementia (Gordon *et al.* 1986; Neshige *et al.* 1988). Moreover, there are indications that differences can be discerned in different varieties of dementia. Goodin and Aminoff (1986) showed that patients with subcortical dementia (Parkinson's and Huntington's disease) showed more severe delays in the P300 than in those with Alzheimer's disease, also longer delays in the earlier N1 and P2 components. The patients with Parkinson's and Huntington's disease differed from one another by greater P2 delay in the latter group. Observations have also been made in parkinsonian patients during 'on' and 'off' phases, with significant decreases in P300 latency while motor ability is improved (Starkstein *et al.* 1989). Goodin *et al.* (1990) found delayed latencies in all four components in patients with AIDS dementia, and to a lesser extent in many HIV-positive men who were clinically asymptomatic and with normal EEGs. It remains to be determined how far this may indicate subclinical brain infection and be of prognostic significance.

P300 findings in schizophrenia are more variable, but a majority of investigators have found diminished amplitudes of response, with or without abnormal latencies. Blackwood and Muir (1990) summarise studies showing differences between schizophrenic and depressed patients, and which may hold promise for circumscribing the boundaries of schizophrenia more closely. The P300 changes appear to be largely independent of the state of relapse or remission, and have been detected in asymptomatic relatives of schizophrenic patients; hence it is a good candidate for an endophenotype. Bramon *et al.* (2005) performed a meta-analysis on the results of several studies, yielding data on 472 relatives and 513 controls. The P300 amplitude was significantly reduced and latency significantly delayed in the relatives of schizophrenia patients. In a more general systematic review and meta-analysis, Bramon *et al.* (2004) considered 46 studies, including 1443 patients and 1251 controls. The pooled standardised effect sizes for (reduced) P300 amplitude was 0.85 (95% CI 0.65–1.05; $P < 0.001$) and for (increased) P300 latency –0.57 (95% CI –0.75 to –0.38; $P < 0.001$).

The other evoked potential to have attracted interest is the P50, an early response to usually auditory stimuli thought to reflect attentional gating. The most useful variable is the ratio of the P50 response amplitude of the second or test stimulus to that of the first or conditioning stimulus. Normal subjects generally suppress the second response and typically have ratios of less than 40%. Subjects with schizophrenia and possibly their relatives show deficits in sensory gating, with P50 ratios generally greater than 50%. In the review by Bramon *et al.* (2004), 20 P50 studies were considered that included 421 patients and 401 controls. The effect size for the difference between cases and controls was just over 1.5 standard deviations (although latency did not differ).

Finally, a novel use of the P300 potential has been the attempt to distinguish between feigned and 'hysterical' sensory loss. By applying regular innocuous sensory stimuli and the occasional painful stimulus to the 'anaesthetic' area, Lorenz *et al.* (1998) found an attenuated P300 in the conversion patient but a normal response in a subject instructed to feign sensory loss.

Brain electrical activity mapping

Brain electrical activity mapping (BEAM) represents an attempt to gain maximal information from EEG and evoked potential data by displaying regional brain activity in the form of visual topographic maps. Several systems are now in use, the common aim being to extract visual information relevant to electrophysiological abnormality as a complement to structural and metabolic methods of brain imaging.

Duffy *et al.* (1979) introduced BEAM, using 24 scalp electrodes to record EEG and visual evoked responses. The EEG data were subjected to spectral analysis, and runs containing spike discharges were digitised. Extremely brief epochs of the evoked responses were displayed in quick succession. The spatiotemporal information obtained in this manner was displayed as colour-coded maps, interpolated values being calculated for points between electrode placements. Nowadays the input of many more electrodes is used and the system may be used to detect subtle changes during a cognitive task or at rest. Morihisa (1989) describes the strengths and limitations of such techniques and the findings that have emerged in relation to schizophrenia and developmental dyslexia, and uses have been described in relation to encephalopathies and attention deficit disorder. The value of BEAM in diagnosis has been largely superseded by the other brain imaging techniques.

Magnetoencephalography

Magnetoencephalography (MEG) has been developed during the past two decades as a method for studying brain electrical activity that is complementary to EEG. It aims to measure not the electrical activity directly but the minute magnetic fields which are a by-product of that activity. These are charted over extremely brief epochs of time, measured in milliseconds. The fundamentals of the technique are described by Reeve *et al.* (1989), Fagaly (1990) and Andrews (1996).

The advantage of charting magnetic fields is that they are not attenuated and distorted by passage through the brain tissue, skull and scalp as are the electrical currents which constitute the EEG. Consequently localisation, whether superficial or deep, stands to be enhanced. And since the EEG is partly derived from radially orientated current sources and MEG from tangential sources, the simultaneous recording of both can provide complementary information with regard to the intracranial origin of electrical activity.

In recording the magnetoencephalogram a detection coil is placed in close proximity to the head surface and feeds information to a SQUID sensor (superconducting quantum interference device). Both the detection coil and the SQUID must be kept at superconducting temperatures, either by enclosing them in liquid helium in a vacuum-insulated chamber or by using closed-cycle refrigeration. This 'magnetometer' is capable of measuring extremely small variations in magnetic flux. The resulting information is fed through appropriate electronics to a data acquisition system. Since the SQUID must be protected from major changes in environmental magnetic fields it is usually necessary to carry out the recordings in a magnetically shielded room.

Although still largely a research technique, MEG has shown its potential for answering both fundamental and clinical problems. A principal virtue is its capacity to localise the source of electrical signals, with the equivalent of 100–300 recording channels, whether in the form of epileptic discharges or during studies of sensory evoked potentials (Barkley & Baumgartner 2003). Detection of deep foci has been used to enhance presurgical assessment in epilepsy, often in combination with EEG (Parra *et al.* 2004).

Considerable technical problems remain to be resolved before MEG becomes widely available as a clinical or research instrument. Apart from cost and logistics, there is the problem of developing valid models for localisation deep within the brain in the presence of multiple dipole sources with differing orientations. However, it is likely that the technique will contribute importantly to the understanding of the genesis of signals related to perception, cognition and behavioural responses, and might possibly clarify the site of major electrophysiological disturbances associated with psychiatric disorders. It could ultimately find a valuable place in the clinical investigation of patients with epilepsy (Reite 1990; Parra *et al.* 2004).

Lumbar puncture

Examination of the CSF can give valuable information in many clinical situations. It is usually a safe procedure but should never be undertaken lightly. The principal hazard is in patients with raised intracranial pressure and particularly when an intracranial tumour is present. The abrupt reduction of pressure due to withdrawal of fluid can bring about

tentorial herniation or a medullary pressure cone with fatal results. Even when the needle is quickly removed there may be continued leakage from the puncture hole in the dura mater so that complications can follow some time later. Lumbar puncture is therefore strictly contraindicated in the presence of papilloedema or when there are symptoms suggestive of raised intracranial pressure, except under skilled supervision and when neurosurgical help is immediately to hand.

In the absence of raised intracranial pressure the risk attached to lumbar puncture is small. Conversely, the risk of withholding it can be high. In psychiatric practice it will sometimes be indicated in patients who show disturbance of consciousness or unexplained change of behaviour, even in the absence of definite neurological signs. It can be a dangerous mistake to postpone the investigation on account of the severity of illness or uncooperative behaviour, although it will often be wise to delay in such circumstances until a CT scan and a neurological opinion have been obtained.

Walton (1993) reviews the information to be obtained from lumbar puncture. The pressure is raised in the presence of tumour, haematoma, abscess or cerebral oedema. A moderate rise may be seen in patients with severe arterial hypertension. The pressure may also be raised in certain rare disorders such as lead poisoning or hypoparathyroidism.

A pleocytosis implies inflammatory changes in the meninges, either primary as in meningitis, or secondary to cerebral infection as in encephalitis or cerebral abscess. Polymorphonuclear leucocytes predominate with pyogenic infections and may number many thousands per cubic millimetre, rendering the fluid turbid. Virus encephalitis shows mainly lymphocytes, though with some varieties there may be polymorphs in the early stages. The number of cells is normally rather low. When present, pleocytosis can be an essential observation for confirming the diagnosis. A moderate cellular reaction can similarly be important in the diagnosis of cerebral abscess, usually with 20–200 cells/mm^3, most of which are polymorphs. In untreated general paresis, 5–50 lymphocytes/mm^3 are usual, and as described in Chapter 7 the monitoring of the cellular content of the CSF is essential for judging the adequacy of treatment and for the early detection of relapse. A slight pleocytosis, nearly always of lymphocytes, may be present in other conditions including primary and secondary cerebral tumours, cerebral infarctions or multiple sclerosis.

Blood is found in the CSF after subarachnoid haemorrhage or when a primary intracerebral haemorrhage has extended to the subarachnoid space. Xanthochromia may persist as a yellow discoloration for several weeks thereafter. Xanthochromia in the absence of frank blood is also sometimes found with subdural haematomas.

An increased protein content is common to many conditions and can be difficult to interpret. The protein rises with meningitic infections and this can persist for some time after the pleocytosis has resolved. A moderate increase to 1.0 g/L

(100 mg/dL), or a little more, may occur with encephalitis, cerebral abscess, cerebral infarction, neurosyphilis, cerebral tumours and multiple sclerosis. Similar levels can be seen with cervical spondylosis or with myxoedema. In the latter situation it can be particularly misleading. With certain tumours such as meningiomas or acoustic neuromas the level is often considerably higher. Very high levels of up to 10 g/L (1000 mg/dL) without an accompanying cellular reaction is characteristic of the polyneuropathy of Guillain–Barré syndrome, also of spinal blockage from any cause.

The globulin fraction is raised in relation to the albumin in many inflammatory conditions. The gamma globulins are abnormally high, with a selective increase in the IgG fraction in the majority of cases of multiple sclerosis. Increases in the major immunoglobulins (IgG, IgA and IgM) are estimated using radioimmunoassay, immunoelectrophoresis and isoelectric focusing. *Oligoclonal banding* reflects the typical pattern of such changes in multiple sclerosis, but is also found in various forms of meningoencephalitis, subacute sclerosing panencephalitis and Guillain–Barré syndrome. Thus it is indicative of an immunological response rather than being diagnostic of a particular condition (Walton 1993). Immunoassay for protein 14-3-3 appears to be highly specific for CJD (see Chapter 9).

The sugar content of the fluid is greatly lowered or abolished in pyogenic meningitis. A moderate fall is found in tuberculous meningitis and can be a valuable pointer in differentiating this from the various forms of aseptic meningitis due to viral infection. The chloride content is also low in tuberculous meningitis.

Examination of films and culture of the fluid are important for determining the responsible organism when infection is present. Modern virological studies are highly sophisticated and sensitive (see Chapter 7) (Kennedy 2005). However, considerable time is required before the results of culture become available. The development of polymerase chain reaction techniques for the detection of viral DNA or RNA in the CSF yields an immediate and specific diagnosis with some infections, for example herpes simplex virus. Tests may be negative within the first 3 days and subsequently after acyclovir treatment (Tyler 2004). Examination of films may also reveal neoplastic cells, especially in carcinomatosis and the medulloblastomas of childhood. Serological tests for syphilis are important since it is possible that they may be negative in the serum in active cases of general paresis.

Thus in many situations examination of the CSF provides important information that contributes to the diagnosis. In some conditions such as encephalitis, general paresis and cerebral abscess it may be crucial in alerting one to the diagnosis. However, a normal CSF does not mean that a pathological process within the central nervous system (CNS) can be excluded. The degenerative processes responsible for the presenile and senile dementias do not as a rule show changes, and a completely normal fluid may be found in occasional cases of encephalitis. Moreover, many pathological processes responsible for enduring brain damage and neuropsychiatric disturbance will have subsided by the time the patient is examined, and will have left a normal fluid in their wake.

Radiography of the skull

The chief indication for skull radiography is usually suspicion of a cerebral tumour, although cranial CT and MRI are invariably used as first-line investigations if available. There may be erosion or bony overgrowth over the vault due to a meningioma, or abnormal vascular markings indicative of a tumour or angioma. Special views may show erosion of the internal auditory meatus due to an acoustic neuroma. Osteolytic bone lesions may give the first indication of carcinomatosis or multiple myeloma. General thickening or 'woolliness' may indicate Paget's disease.

The next main focus of interest is the sella turcica. Decalcification or erosion of the posterior clinoid processes is an important indication of raised intracranial pressure, or the fossa may be enlarged due to a pituitary or suprasellar lesion.

Intracranial calcification provides other clues. The pineal is calcified in approximately 50% of adults and may display shifts of the midline structures. The choroid plexuses and the falx cerebri may occasionally be calcified as well. Calcification within the body of a tumour can be of direct localising value, similarly calcification within the walls of a large cerebral aneurysm. Other rare conditions include calcification within the basal ganglia in hypoparathyroidism (see Chapter 10), calcification within the nodules in tuberose sclerosis or in the cysts of cysticercosis.

Computed tomography

CT probably represents the most significant advance in the use of X-rays for diagnosis since their discovery and has established itself as invaluable in the diagnosis of cerebral disorder. The system is approximately 100 times more sensitive than conventional radiography systems, yet exposes the patient to no greater radiation dosage than a standard series of ordinary skull radiographs. There is no need for anaesthesia or any form of invasive procedure, rendering it entirely safe for patients who might be unfit for contrast neuroradiology.

The ventricular system is clearly shown along with certain of the basal cisterns. The cortical sulci are detectable, and readily so when enlarged. Within the cerebral substance variations in soft tissues of nearly similar absorption density may be displayed; thus the thalami and heads of the caudate nuclei are generally identifiable as discrete structures, also the internal capsule and optic radiations. The cortical grey matter mantle is visible over the surface of the cerebral hemispheres. Progressive refinements incorporated into more recent machines have considerably increased the amount of detail displayed.

In investigating cerebral pathology the scan may show displacements of normal intracranial contents, but in addition many focal pathological processes produce changes in brain absorption density that enable lesions to be displayed directly. Space-occupying lesions are readily shown, including tumours, abscesses and haematomas. Local cerebral oedema is demonstrated, and infarction is revealed as a region of low absorption density.

The nature as well as the location of a tumour can often be demonstrated – whether benign or malignant, solid or cystic – as well as the degree to which surrounding oedema infiltrates brain tissue. A diffuse increase in absorption density is seen with meningiomas, colloid cysts and pituitary adenomas, whereas gliomas and metastases may be hyperdense or hypodense. A special advantage is the capacity to distinguish tumours from infarctions at an early stage, and in cases where angiography might well have been contraindicated. Intravenous injection of sodium iothalamate (Conray) can be used in doubtful cases to enhance the contrast between the tumour and surrounding brain tissue. In the management of strokes the differentiation between infarction and haemorrhage is relatively simple. This can be especially important if the patient is taking or due to take anticoagulants (Sandercock et al. 1985). The location, size and direction of propagation of intracerebral haematomas can be defined. After head injuries various important forms of cerebral pathology are displayed (see Chapter 4). In the acute stage of injury, scanning can be invaluable in demonstrating intracranial haematomas before the patient's deterioration makes them obvious to the surgeon.

The cerebral vasculature can now be imaged with impressive detail using helical CT. High-speed imaging is performed during the bolus administration of intravenous contrast. From a single pass of contrast medium, a three-dimensional reconstruction of the cerebral vasculature (including aneurysms and malformations) may be obtained that may then be inspected from any angle (Mazziotta 2000).

Cerebral atrophy shows as enlargement of the ventricles, broadening of the sylvian and interhemispheric fissures, and widening of the cerebral sulci, much as after air encephalography. Areas of relative translucency may be shown in the cerebral white matter in demyelinating disorders such as multiple sclerosis (Chapter 14) and Schilder's disease (Chapter 14). White matter changes may also be found in a proportion of demented patients and even sometimes in the healthy elderly (so-called leucoaraiosis), although MRI is the method of choice for revealing white matter pathology.

Significance of cerebral atrophy

Sometimes neuroimaging shows changes that are hard to interpret, particularly where cerebral atrophy is concerned. It is often easier to assess distortion by a space-occupying lesion than to decide on the significance of minor ventricular enlargement. Occasionally, moreover, the ventricles may prove to be enlarged or the sulci prominent in patients who show no evidence of cerebral disorder. Such examples raise obvious diagnostic difficulties, and are a reminder that a range of normal variation must be allowed where the appearances of the brain are concerned.

It is now clear from CT that ventricular size increases with age even in healthy persons, and particularly so in the later decades of life. For example, Barron et al. (1976) examined 135 normal volunteers by CT, demonstrating a gradual increase from the first to the sixth decades followed by a dramatic increase from the age of 70 onwards. The range in ventricular size also became wider among the elderly subjects.

With regard to dementia there is usually an obvious association with evidence of atrophy, although this is not absolute in every case. Younger demented patients are more likely to show decisively abnormal findings, in comparison with their peers, whereas in the elderly there may be considerable overlap with healthy persons of equivalent age. Jacoby and Levy (1980) found on discriminant function analysis that CT measurements produced a correct prediction of dementia in 83% of elderly subjects, cortical atrophy being a rather better discriminator than ventricular size. Interestingly, however, patients over the age of 80 were significantly less likely to have large ventricles compared with those a decade or so younger, perhaps reflecting the more benign course of dementia in the very elderly. Hubbard and Anderson (1981) were able to show by detailed autopsy measurements that the ventricles were of normal size for age in approximately 40% of patients with senile dementia.

The severity of cognitive impairment in dementia has proved to be closely related to the degree of cerebral atrophy. Furthermore, Burns and Pearlson (1994) reviewed the many CT studies in this area, showing that significant correlations with cognition have emerged twice as often for ventricular as for cortical measurements and that cognitive deterioration on follow-up is paralleled by further ventricular enlargement. MRI is particularly valuable in the diagnosis of dementing illnesses and has more sensitivity than CT. There is a large body of work examining the diagnostic value of volumetric measures of particular anatomical structures, rather than the brain as a whole, such as the hippocampus, amygdala and entorhinal cortex. Such indices have good positive predictive value (around 70–80%) in the diagnosis of Alzheimer's disease even in comparison to mild cognitive impairment.

The advent of CT opened the flood-gates to volumetric studies in schizophrenia, starting with Johnstone et al. (1976) who confirmed the presence of cerebral atrophy (see Chapter 2) in historical post-mortem and air-encephalographic studies. Studies in affective disorder soon followed. CT and MRI studies are thus increasing our appreciation that a degree of cerebral disorder may play some part in

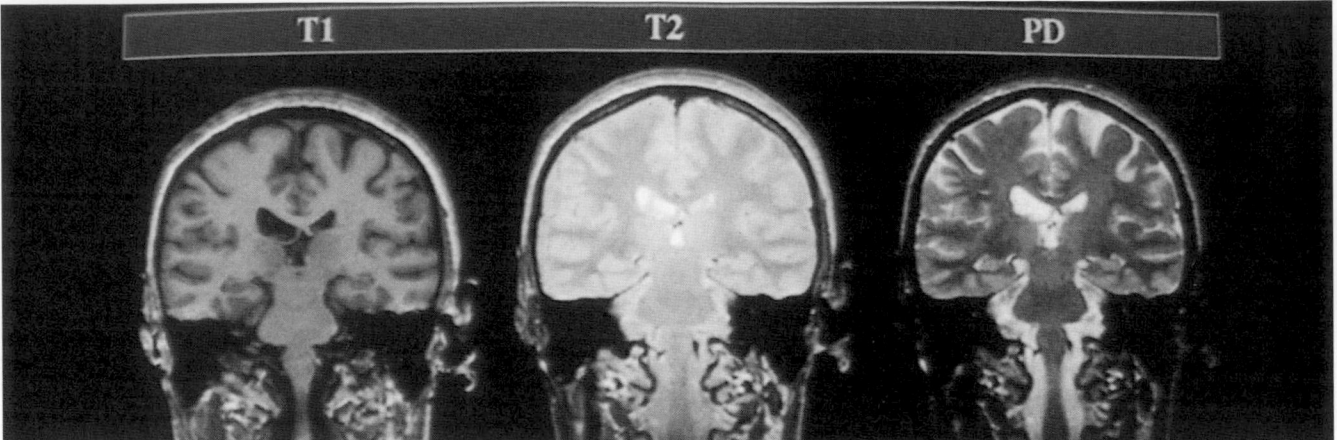

Fig. 3.5 Coronal magnetic resonance brain images illustrating different scanning sequences (see also Plate 3.1). T1, inversion recovery; T2, spin-echo; PD, proton density. (Courtesy of Dr Nancy Andreasen.)

contributing to a considerable range of mental illness. The degree of cerebral change encountered on CT will only rarely lead to difficulties with diagnosis, but on occasion it will be sufficient to call for detailed re-evaluation of the patient's illness. The cortical shrinkage and ventricular dilatation accompanying severe alcohol abuse will quite often be perplexing when the drinking history is unknown, likewise the appearances of atrophy that may accompany steroid administration (Bentson *et al.* 1978; Lagenstein *et al.* 1979). The latter appears to be largely reversible on discontinuation of the steroids. Minor reversible changes have also been reported in patients with anorexia nervosa (Palazidou *et al.* 1990).

Magnetic resonance imaging

The early 1980s saw the introduction of MRI and this has transformed diagnosis in neurology and neuropsychiatry (Besson 1990). It competes strongly with CT, yielding greatly superior anatomical and pathological information. Unlike CT it involves no X-irradiation but makes use of the magnetic properties of nuclei and their capacity to be excited by radiofrequency pulses.

Most routine MRI utilises the hydrogen nuclei of the tissues. In essence these are made to resonate in response to rapidly changing magnetic fields around them, and the signals they emit are then processed to yield a visual image based on their distribution and physicochemical state.

The patient is placed in a static magnetic field, varying in different machines from 0.5 to 4.0 T in strength. This produces a net alignment of the magnetic moments of the hydrogen nuclei in the tissues. Under such circumstances the nuclei 'precess' in a circular course about this axis, much as a spinning top will wobble. Brief bursts of radiofrequency pulses, applied at the appropriate frequency from a surrounding coil, augment the precession, and when the excitation pulse ends the nuclei return to their lower energy state. The electrical signals emitted from the tissues in the course of such energy changes can be detected and analysed by computer to reveal the distribution of the hydrogen nuclei involved. Techniques are used to 'scan' the tissues systematically, yielding visual images much as with CT.

A variety of scanning sequences can be selected in order to optimise the particular parameters used in image reconstruction. *Repeated free induction decay* or *saturation recovery* (RFID or SR) produce images that reflect proton density. *Inversion recovery* (IR) sequences reflect the longitudinal or spin-lattice relaxation time (T1) of the protons as they return to their previous equilibrium in line with the axis of the static magnetic field. *Spin echo* (SE) sequences are differently derived to display the transverse or spin–spin relaxation time (T2), during which the spinning protons are relaxing in phase with one another but interacting with the spins of other nuclei. These different scanning sequences are each suited to different purposes in visual imaging. In T1 images the CSF appears dark in relation to brain tissue; in T2 images the CSF is light, with grey matter also light and the white matter dark (as illustrated in Fig. 3.5: see also Plate 3.1).

Special sequences

Fluid-attenuated inversion recovery (FLAIR) produces a heavily weighted T2 image. This in turn suppresses CSF signal and renders lesions at the parenchyma–CSF interface more conspicuous. This is particularly useful in demyelinating disorders where there may be plaques close to the ventricles. Another use is in highlighting hippocampal sclerosis in patients with temporal lobe epilepsy and hippocampal involvement in limbic encephalitis (Fauser *et al.* 2005) (Fig. 3.6). However, caution is needed in interpreting these images since the healthy hippocampus may also show mildly increased signal intensity.

Diffusion-weighted imaging (DWI) employs SE-based sequences that are sensitised to diffusion by strong magnetic field-gradient pulses. The biggest contribution of DWI has been in the detection of acute cerebral infarction, since water diffusion drops to half its normal value early on, giving a region of hyperintensity on DWI scans (Brammer & Fazekas 2002).

Diffusion tensor imaging (DTI) and tractography: diffusion in the brain is hindered by biological tissue, being relatively less impeded along the axis of myelinated fibres. This asymmetry is known as diffusion anisotropy. DTI exploits this to image the consistency or otherwise of orientation of white matter tracts. It is therefore of most value in the

(a)

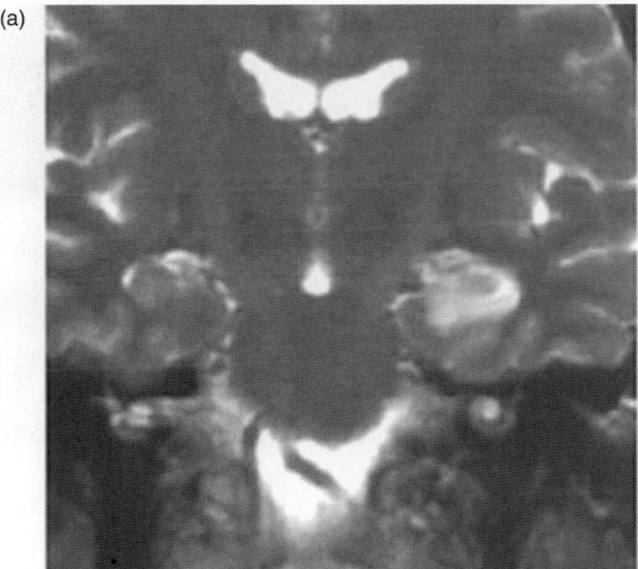

(b)

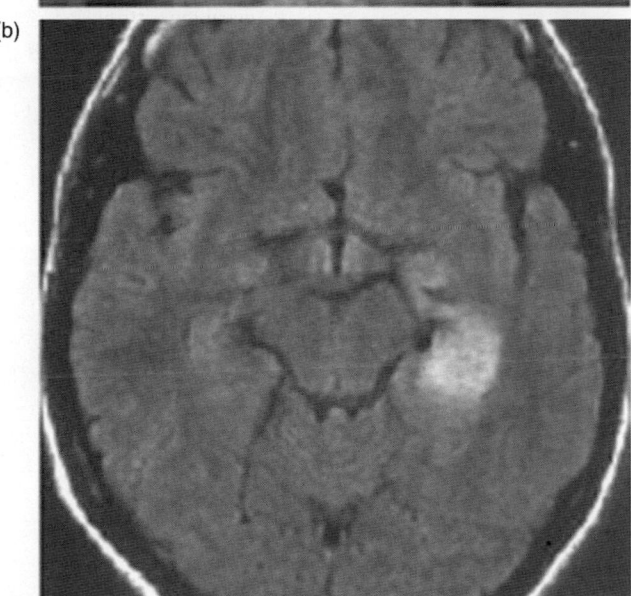

Fig. 3.6 Coronal T2-weighted sequence (a) and transverse FLAIR (b) showing hyperintensity and swelling of the left hippocampus (on the right of both images) and white matter oedema in the left parahippocampal gyrus. Scans are of a 32-year-old woman presenting with tonic–clonic seizures, diagnosed with voltage-gated potassium channel autoantibodies (non-neoplastic limbic encephalitis); 6 months after presentation the patient had some verbal and autobiographical memory impairment and showed atrophy of the left hippocampus. (From Fauser *et al.* 2005 with permission.)

investigation of white matter disease, including demyelination. Tractography is the rendering of information on white matter tract orientation and shape in three dimensions. The technique can be used to produce beautiful anatomical displays that expose the structural underpinnings for functional connectivity in the brain and has much promise in neuropsychiatric disorders where aberrant development is the presumed pathogenesis (Catani & ffytche 2005).

Magnetisation transfer (MT) refers to the magnetisation of hydrogen bonds bound to macromolecules such as cell membranes. A pulse is applied that results in the exchange of magnetisation between bound protons and free water protons. Signal intensity is reduced at the site where the transfer occurred. The upshot of this technique is to increase the contrast of liquids versus solids and is thus used to image the cerebral vasculature (including distal vessels) in magnetic resonance angiography (MRA), usually in conjunction with gadolinium contrast enhancement (Castillo & Mukherji 2001).

An outstanding feature of MRI is the exquisite level of soft tissue contrast obtained by scanning in the IR sequence (T1-weighted images). Grey and white matter are strongly differentiated, yielding fine anatomical detail. The cortical grey matter is shown clearly and the thalami and basal ganglia are demarcated from the surrounding white matter and ventricular system. Sagittal scans show the corpus callosum, the columns of the fornix and the brainstem. In the posterior fossa, the substantia nigra and the middle cerebral peduncles can be discerned.

MRI holds several pronounced advantages over CT. Improved detection of small demyelinating lesions is coupled with excellent visualisation of the posterior fossa and pituitary regions, since there is little or no bone artefact to intrude on the images obtained. The various scanning sequences available give versatility of choice, and the slices to be viewed are readily switched from transverse to coronal or sagittal planes without disturbing or moving the patient.

MRI's superiority over CT has emerged in many clinical settings: in the detection of cerebral tumours, small infarcts and other vascular disease of the brain, and in revealing the lesions responsible for epilepsy (Fig. 3.7). It is very much better at showing the residua of cerebral trauma (Chapter 8) and in the detection of cerebral infections including those due to HIV/AIDS (Chapter 7). MRI has produced a new diagnostic sign, the pulvinar sign (increased signal intensity on T2-weighted images), found in variant CJD (Fig. 3.8). FLAIR sequences are also of value in variant CJD, showing hyperintensity of the pulvinar and dorsomedial nuclei of the thalamus, the so-called hockey-stick sign (Zeidler *et al.* 2000). The value of MRI in relation to the dementias and other neurodegenerative disorders is described in the appropriate sections of this book but the regional atrophy that characterises the frontotemporal dementias is easily visualised with MRI (Cooper & Greene 2005) (Fig. 3.9). Routine examination may be supplemented by the intravenous administration of a paramagnetic contrast agent (gadolinium bound to the chelating agent diethylene triaminepentaacetic acid), which yields additional information about derangements of the blood–brain barrier in the vicinity of lesions. This can be valuable in the context of vascular disease and in distinguishing a tumour from the oedema that surrounds it. Developments in MRA have been noted above (Bradley 1992).

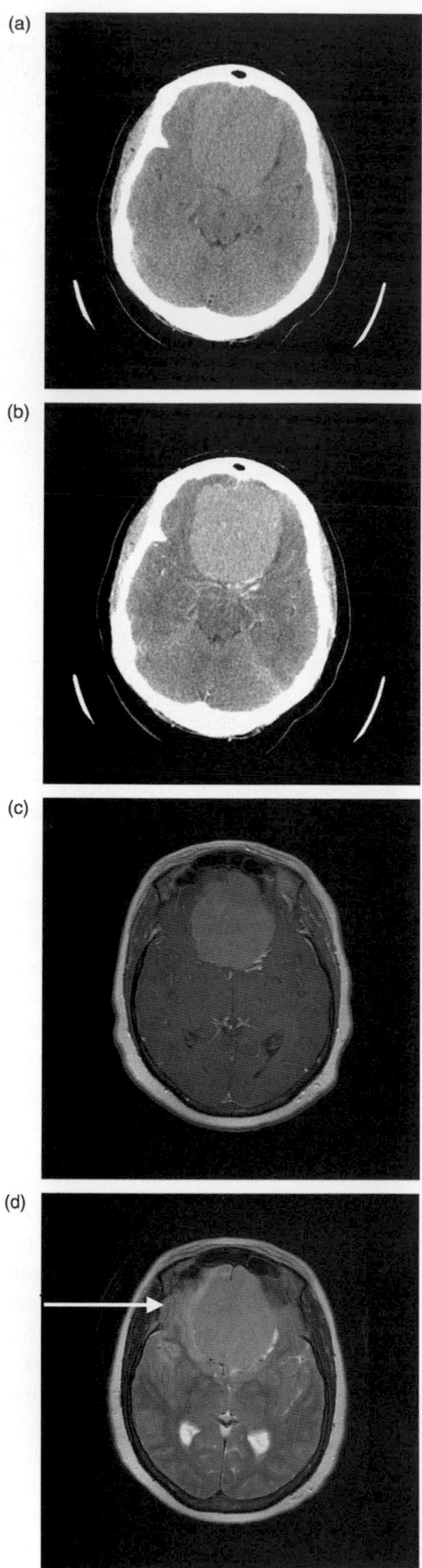

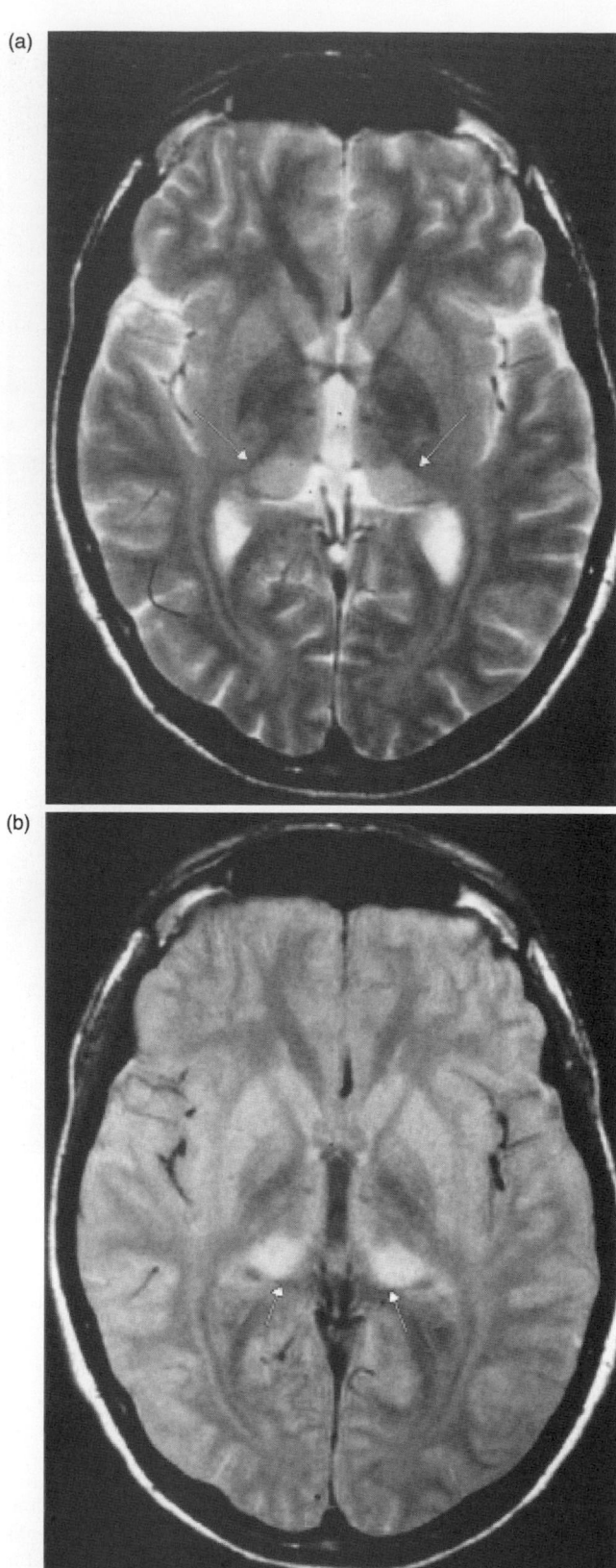

Fig. 3.7 A 55-year-old woman with a 2-year history of increasing self-neglect and deteriorating function at work, followed by acute onset of paranoid psychosis and unsteadiness. (a) CT without contrast and (b) CT with contrast, both showing large frontal meningioma with contrast enhancement. (c) T1-weighted MRI with contrast and (d) T2-weighted MRI showing meningioma plus right frontal infarction, presumed to be related to acute deterioration.

Fig. 3.8 The pulvinar sign in a histopathologically confirmed case of variant Creutzfeldt–Jakob disease. (a) T2-weighted axial MRI showing high signal in pulvinar of the thalamus (arrows). (b) Changes were consistently conspicuous on proton density-weighted images. (From Zeidler *et al.* 2000 with permission.)

Fig. 3.9 Axial MRI showing abnormalities in the spectrum of frontotemporal lobar degeneration. Frontotemporal dementia is associated with frontal and temporal atrophy. Progressive non-fluent aphasia typically presents with left-sided perisylvian atrophy, whereas semantic dementia is characterised by left-sided anterior temporal lobe atrophy. (From Van der Flier & Scheltens 2005 with permission of BMJ Publishing Group Ltd.)

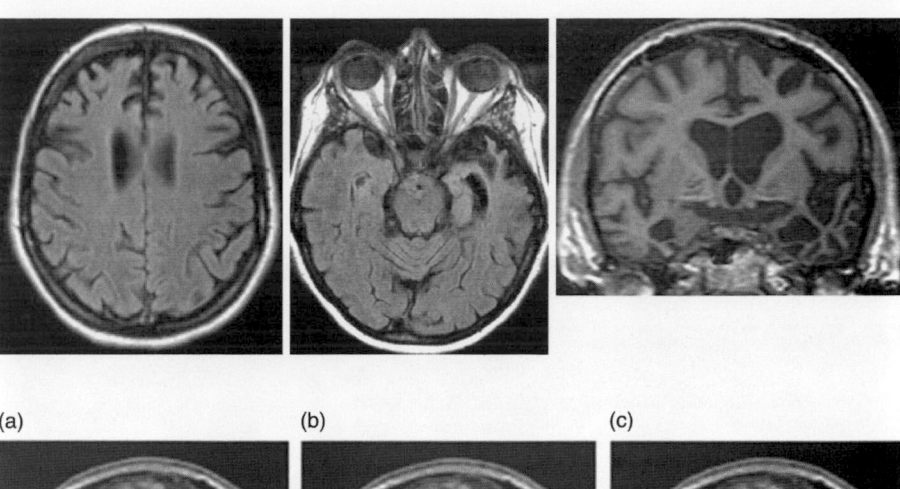

(a)   (b)   (c)

Fig. 3.10 Serially acquired T1-weighted MR scans from an initially asymptomatic patient destined to develop familial Alzheimer's disease. Scans were acquired over 4 years before criteria for dementia were met; the first symptoms were reported between scans (d) and (e). Each scan has been positionally registered to the baseline scan. See also Plate 3.2. (From Fox & Schott 2004 with permission.)

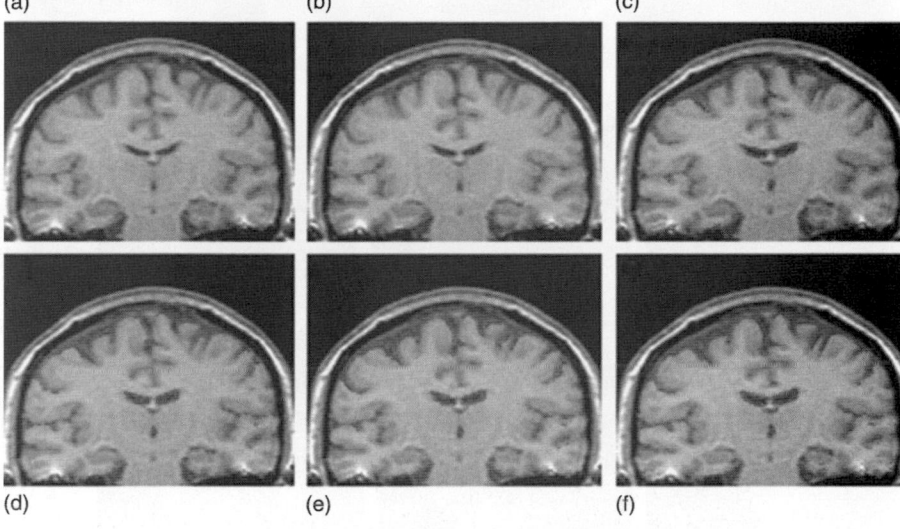

(d)   (e)   (f)

In all these settings MRI has the added advantage that repeat examinations are possible without hazard from radiation exposure. Use in relation to normal ageing and the diagnosis of Alzheimer's disease is an important clinical topic. It has been estimated that annual rates of cerebral atrophy are in the region of 0.2–0.5% in middle-aged healthy controls, rising to 3–5% at 70–80 years of age. This compares with rates of about 2–3% in Alzheimer's disease (Fox & Schott 2004). A 6-year longitudinal study showed that medial temporal lobe atrophy could be used to predict future cognitive decline in 45 participants aged over 60 years, with 91% specificity and 89% sensitivity (Rusinek *et al.* 2003) (Fig. 3.10: see also Plate 3.2). Schott *et al.* (2005) have used a method to coregister scans from individuals for the purposes of longitudinal comparisons using an automated technique known as the boundary shift integral method. They showed that this technique enabled more precise measurement of change. Changes in ventricular size – a 1-mL decrease in brain volume in Alzheimer's disease is on average accompanied by about 0.22 mL of ventricular expansion – showed even greater reliability. Presymptomatic change and progression are also visible on MRI in conditions such as Huntington's disease (Fig. 3.11).

With regard to safety of MRI, no adverse effects have been encountered, provided that patients with intracranial metallic foreign bodies, including aneurysmal clips, are excluded (the principal risk being the induction of heating in large metal objects such as skull prostheses), likewise patients with cochlear implants or cardiac pacemakers. Other potential exclusion criteria are discussed by Moseley (1994). Apart from feelings of claustrophobia and the noise of the machine (requiring ear protection), which some patients find distressing, the examination is without discomfort. Obese patients and those unable to lie still for several minutes may be better investigated with CT.

White matter hyperintensities

These are an example of an MRI-detected pathology, best seen on conventional dual-echo or T2-weighted images, or FLAIR sequences. They are frequently observed in the elderly but when multiple and confluent have definite pathological significance, being associated with increased risk of cerebrovascular and cardiovascular incidents, cognitive decline and depression (Launer 2003; Kales *et al.* 2005). Pathologically, the lesions show rarefaction of myelin sheaths and gliosis and are associated with microvascular

(a)   (b)

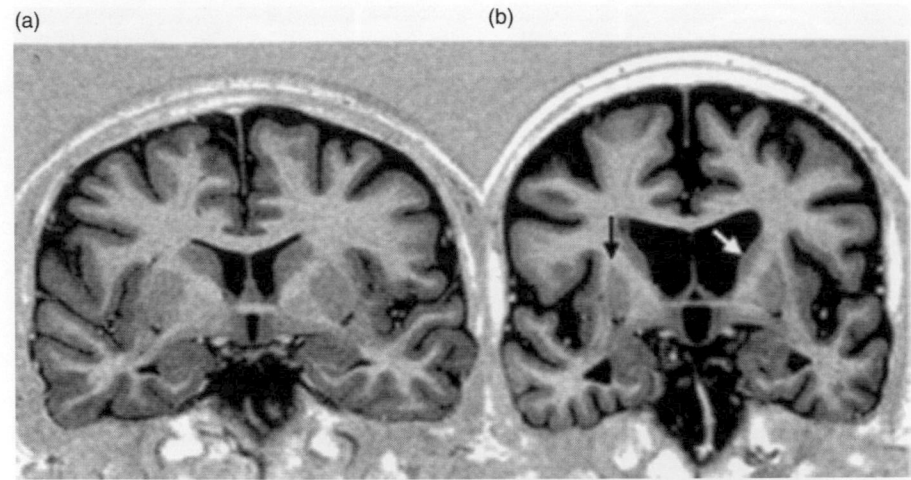

Fig. 3.11 Coronal T1-weighted inversion-recovery turbo spin-echo MRI: (a) healthy control subject; (b) Huntington's disease carrier with stage 2 disease showing thinning of the head of the caudate nucleus (white arrow) and the putamen (black arrow). (From Mascalchi *et al.* 2004 with permission.)

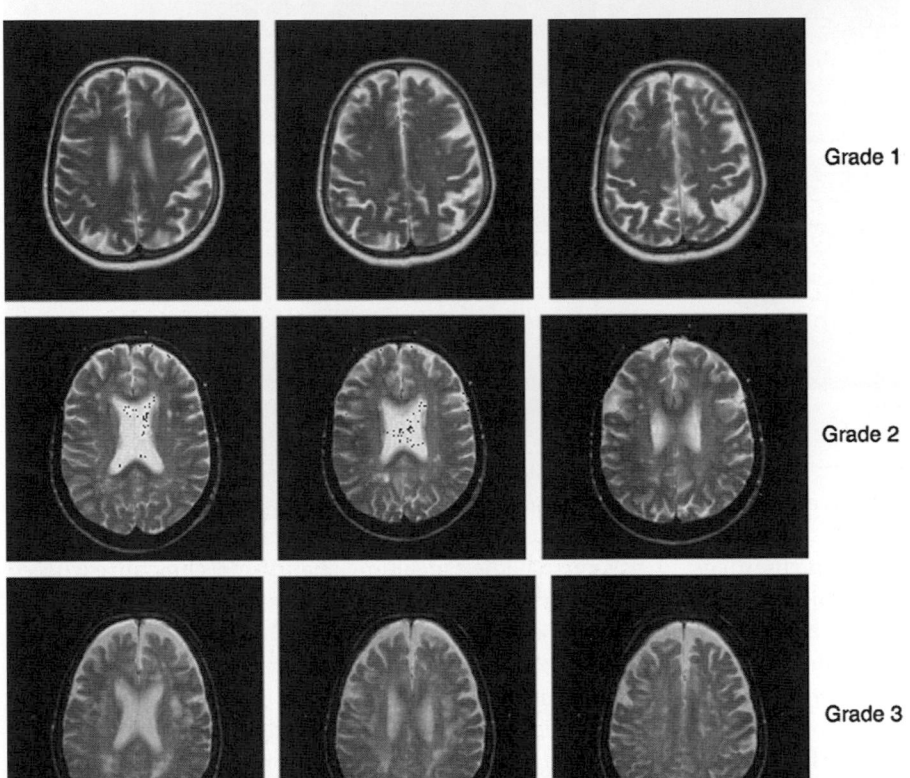

Grade 1

Grade 2

Grade 3

Fig. 3.12 T2-weighted MR scans showing punctuate (Grade 1), early confluent (Grade 2), and confluent (Grade 3) white matter hyperintensities. Grade 2 and 3 lesions have been shown histopathologically to be associated with microangiopathy. (From Kapeller *et al.* 2004 with permission.)

abnormalities. Taking their usually periventricular distribution into account, ischaemic injury from compromise to penetrating arterioles is a likely aetiology (Lee & Marcus 2006); similar pathology is seen in the brains of depressed patients with periventricular and deep white matter hyperintensities (WMHs) but with less emphasis on vascular occlusion, pointing perhaps towards hypotensive mechanisms. A frontal location was particularly associated with depression (Thomas *et al.* 2002). Similarly, 'silent' brain infarcts, revealed by MRI, confer a more than twofold increased risk of dementia and fivefold risk of stroke, discovered over periods of 3–4 years in the landmark Rotterdam study of over 1000 apparently healthy 60- to 90-year-olds (Vermeer *et al.* 2003). Based on MRI appearances, WMHs can be classified as punctuate (grade 1), patchy or beginning of confluence (grade 2), and confluent (grade 3). Periventricular hyperintensities may appear as caps around the frontal or posterior horns of the lateral ventricles (grade 1), bands along the lateral ventricles (grade 2), and irregular changes extending into deep white matter (grade 3) (Fig. 3.12) (Kapeller *et al.* 2004). For epidemiological research purposes the Rotterdam group rated the number and size of subcortical white matter lesions: small (<3 mm), medium (3–10 mm), and large (>10 mm). Periventricular white matter lesions were rated semiquantitatively per region: adjacent to frontal horn (frontal capping), adjacent to lateral wall of lateral ventricles, and occipital capping on a scale of 0 (no lesions), 1 (pencil thin periventricular lining), 2 (smooth halo or thick lining), or 3 (large confluent lesions). This was done for both hemispheres. The overall degree of periventricular white matter lesions was calculated by adding the scores for the three separate categories (range 0–9). A clear effect of 'normal' ageing can be seen in the graph (Fig. 3.13). This must be taken into account when judging whether a scan showing WMH is abnormal, and requires further investigation, or not. De Leeuw *et al.* (2001) found that in those aged over 60 years only 8% were free of subcortical white matter lesions, 20% had no periventricular white matter lesions and 5% had no white matter lesions in either location. Of subjects aged between 60 and 70 years, about 13% were completely free of subcortical white matter lesions and 32% were free of periventricular white matter

lesions, whereas for subjects aged between 80 and 90 years these percentages were 0 and 5, respectively.

A related pathology is punctate foci of signal loss on conventional T2 images, corresponding to microscopic intracerebral bleeds associated with hypertension. This can be highlighted with T2*-weighted images, which show focal deposits of haemosiderin as dark spots (Fig. 3.14) (Kapeller *et al.* 2004). Such lesions may also be seen in cerebral amyloid angiopathy and in cerebral autosomal dominant arteriopathy with subcortical infarcts and leucoencephalopathy (CADASIL).

Magnetic resonance spectroscopy

Magnetic resonance spectroscopy (MRS) is an important extension of MRI, in effect yielding information about certain chemical constituents of tissues. It depends on the principle that in a given magnetic field each distinct nuclear species spins at a unique frequency (Larmor frequency) that is altered slightly according to the chemical compound containing the element. This effect is called the *chemical shift*. When tissue within a static magnetic field is exposed to another competing field, by applying a radiofrequency pulse tuned to the Larmor frequency of the element in question, a spectrum can be obtained that reflects the various components in which the element is incorporated. By examining the spectrum the relative ratios of these components one to

(a)
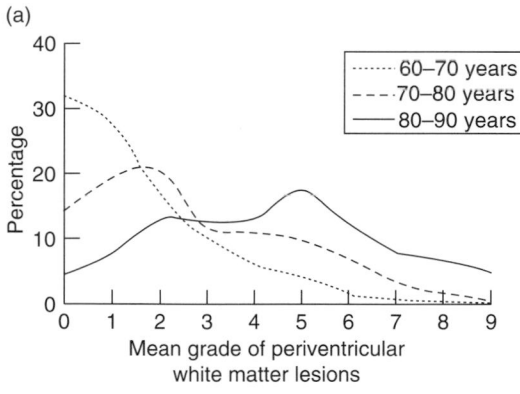

(b)
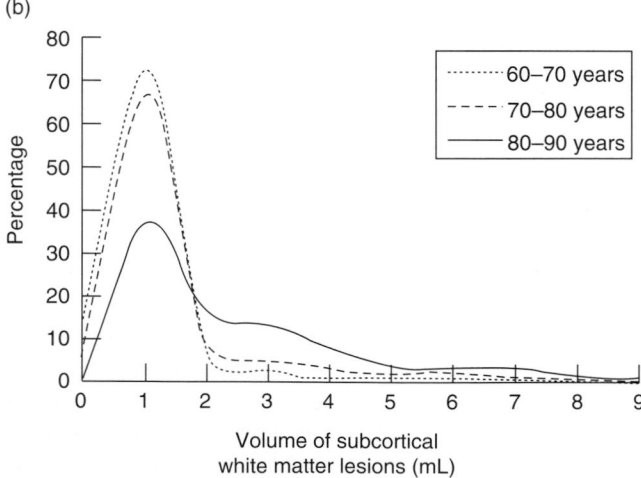

Fig. 3.13 Distribution of periventricular white matter lesions by 10-year age category. Note that the distribution of all subcortical white matter lesions is quite different showing marked skew with a peak around a mean score of 1 for all age groups. (From de Leeuw *et al.* 2001 with permission.)

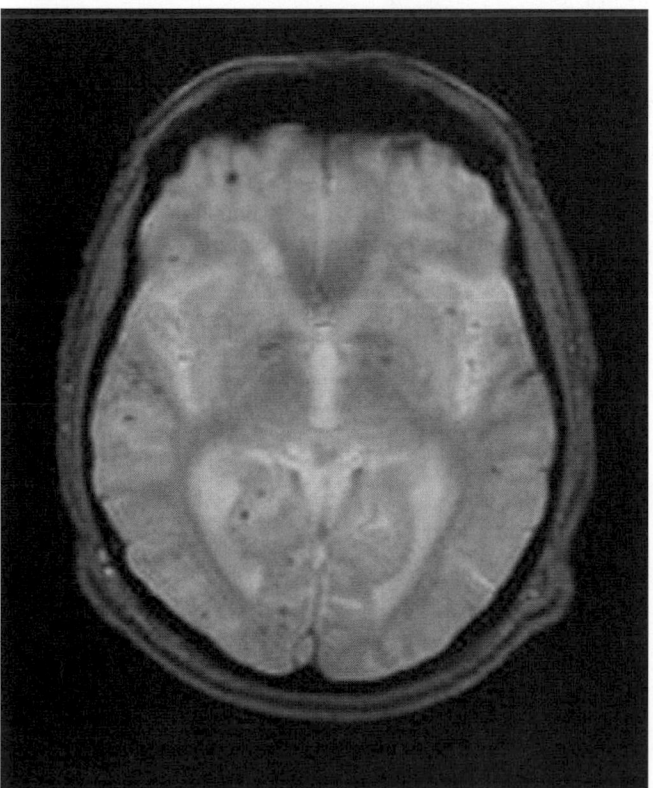

Fig. 3.14 T2*-weighted MRI scan showing microangiopathy-related haemosiderin deposits. (From Kapeller *et al.* 2004 with permission.)

another can be calculated. The biochemical information is necessarily obtained at the expense of spatial information, although techniques are available which seek a compromise between the two.

Technical details are described by Keshavan (1993) and Maier (1995), including applications of relevance for neuropsychiatry. In essence the patient is placed in an MRI scanner of strong magnetic capability (1.5 T or above) and a radiofrequency coil is centred over the area of the head to be sampled. By appropriate tuning of the coil, spectra can be obtained that reflect the hydrogen nucleus (^{1}H) or the phosphorus nucleus (^{31}P). A range of other nuclei are also accessible (^{19}F, ^{13}C, ^{23}Na, ^{7}Li), but for technical reasons have been less explored.

^{1}H MRS yields spectra representing the tissue content of water, choline, creatine, lactate and *N*-acetyl aspartate (NAA), also smaller peaks derived from amino acids such as glutamate and aspartate. The water peak must be suppressed by appropriate techniques to prevent it from overriding the others. ^{1}H MRS thus gives information about the metabolic status of amino acids, neurotransmitters and their derivatives. In addition, it has potential for investigating histological change, in that NAA appears to be located entirely within neurones and their processes. Van der Knaap *et al.* (1992) have shown that in cerebral degenerative conditions the ratio of NAA to creatine falls as the severity of neuronal damage increases, this sometimes being evident before structural change is demonstrable. With astrocytosis the relative concentrations of choline and creatine are increased, while creatine falls with membrane breakdown.

^{1}H MRS has been studied in relation to multiple sclerosis, epilepsy, inborn errors of metabolism and cerebrovascular disorders. In schizophrenia, Maier *et al.* (1995) have shown significant reductions of NAA, creatine and choline in the left hippocampus, with smaller losses on the right. Buckley *et al.* (1994) have detected decreases in NAA in the frontal cortex in schizophrenia patients. Decreases in glutamate and aspartate have also been found in the dorsolateral prefrontal cortex, indicative of early neuronal degeneration (Stanley *et al.* 1992, 1993).

^{31}P MRS yields spectra of particular relevance to impaired energy metabolism, showing peaks for adenosine triphosphate (ATP), phosphocreatine (PCr) and inorganic phosphate (Pi). Ratios of ATP and PCr to Pi provide a measure of tissue health, varying with ischaemia, metabolic disorders and drug therapy. ^{31}P resonances can also reflect membrane metabolism by revealing peaks for phosphomonoesters and diesters. ^{31}P MRS has been employed to study brain anoxia, trauma and demyelination, as well as Alzheimer's disease and AIDS dementia. In schizophrenia evidence has been obtained of metabolic hypoactivity and disturbed membrane phospholipid metabolism in the dorsolateral prefrontal cortex.

Other promising areas for neuropsychiatric research include the use of MRS to detect inborn errors of metabolism in which metabolic by-products accumulate in the brain; ^{19}F MRS for the study of fluorine-containing antipsychotics such as trifluoperazine and fluphenazine; and ^{7}Li MRS for follow-ing the pharmacokinetics of lithium (Keshavan *et al.* 1991). The labelling of glucose with ^{13}C has potential for brain metabolic investigations, and ^{23}Na MRS for differentiating the intracellular and extracellular pools of sodium. An excellent review of applications in psychiatry is provided by Malhi *et al.* (2002).

Functional magnetic resonance imaging

This still more recent development consists of ultra-fast imaging, whereby minute changes in regional cerebral blood flow can be detected and related to physiological activity occurring locally in the cortex. Brain changes can be charted in response to sensorimotor or cognitive activities, and it is possible even to capture alterations occurring with subjective events such as hallucinatory experiences (see later in section). Thus functional magnetic resonance imaging (fMRI) is a technique that can integrate structure with function by providing high-resolution mapping of the brain areas involved in discrete tasks and activities. Its promise for neuropsychiatry was spotted early (Binder & Rao 1994; David *et al.* 1994). Two main methods are used: fast low-angle shot (FLASH) and echoplanar imaging (EPI). FLASH depends on extremely brief intervals between successive radiofrequency pulses (5–15 ms), coupled with narrow 'flip angles' so that the proton nuclei return quickly towards their previous state of equilibrium. The resulting free induction decay images reveal any transient alterations of blood flow that occur. The EPI technique involves the encoding of free induction decay following a single radiofrequency excitation pulse, while a rapidly oscillating gradient is applied to generate a train of closely spaced signals from the tissue (gradient echoes).

Earlier studies used gadolinium enhancement, which increases the decay rate of the MRI signal (Belliveau *et al.* 1991), but Kwong *et al.* (1992) showed that it was possible to exploit the magnetic properties of haemoglobin when it changes from the oxyhaemoglobin to the deoxyhaemoglobin state (blood oxygenation-level-dependent contrast imaging or BOLD) (Ogawa *et al.* 1992). Changes in the relative proportions of oxyhaemoglobin and deoxyhaemoglobin, in response to local neuronal activity and the ensuing increased local blood flow, increases the relaxation time (T2* parameter), leading to a brightening of the magnetic resonance image in active regions. This completely non-invasive method of imaging transient changes in blood flow has obvious advantages over its precursors.

The earliest application of fMRI was in calcarine cortex activation in response to photic stimulation or chequerboard presentations, where the signal change may be around 2% or more; activation of contralateral and to some extent ipsilateral sensorimotor cortex on touching fingers to thumb; and activation of areas similar to those found with positron emission tomography (PET) on repetition of nouns and generation of verbs. Passive word listening activates the superior temporal gyri, especially on the left, and pattern recognition memory activates areas within the medial temporal and frontal lobes. The technique is used to study the cerebral correlates of auditory hallucinations in schizophrenia, as abnormal moods, compulsions, and specific fears have similarly proved tractable to fMRI research. Analytic and image acquisition has improved year on year to enable 'signals' of less than 1% to be distinguished from noise, so that the most subtle of mental states and cognitive processes, including for example recollective experience, regret, sexual attraction and moral outrage, can all be shown to have their own functional anatomy. Certain advantages are evident for fMRI over PET as an avenue for further studies, notably much higher resolution with fine localisation, and the ability to track cortical responses as brief as 1 second or less. The noninvasiveness of the procedure and its lack of radiation exposure readily permit repeat examinations and hence the mapping of developmental and degenerative processes. Disadvantages include the difficulty of adapting task paradigms to the restricted space available while the patient lies within the scanner and also the degree of signal 'drop-out' in certain regions of the brain due to magnetic susceptibility differences such as where brain is close to air-filled bone cavities such as the temporal lobes and inferior frontal lobes (Matthews & Jezzard 2004). These artefacts may be worsened at higher field strengths.

Despite the huge impact fMRI has had on cognitive neuroscience, so far its clinical applications have been limited. This is probably due to the sensitivity of the method, which tends to reduce test–retest reliability, and the reliance on computationally intensive post-processing to deal with movement artefacts and low signal to noise and in the selection of the appropriate task contrasts. After all, the technique is about brain function and is semiquantitative so only yields meaningful information in response to questions framed as follows: What is the brain doing when subject A is carrying out task x compared with task y, and is this different in subject B? fMRI in a single case, as required for clinical utility, is certainly feasible but most research relies on averaging across subjects and mapping onto a standard neuroanatomical brain space (rather than a person's actual brain). fMRI brain images may not align perfectly with structural images. Nevertheless, one application of fMRI likely to increase is lateralisation of language functions in pre-epilepsy surgery assessment since it is far less invasive than the Wada procedure (see Chapter 2) yet yields consistent results (Fig. 3.15: see also Plate 3.3). Localising eloquent cortex and indeed ictal activity in such patients is also possible with fMRI and much effort is being expended into integrating imaging across modalities, by using EEG or MEG concurrently or sequentially in the same patient (Matthews & Jezzard 2004). Obviously each technique has its own time window and none measures exactly the same phenomena. The future is bound to see the increasing use of fMRI in the early diagnosis and response to treatment of cognitive disorders and in the mapping of functional reorganisation after brain injury or stroke.

Positron emission tomography

PET is restricted to special centres, since a cyclotron must be close at hand for the manufacture of the short-lived isotopes involved. In essence, PET produces a cross-sectional image of brain radioactivity after the injection of a suitably labelled compound, yielding information about the site and rate of dynamic processes such as cerebral blood flow and metabolism. The principal value of the technique is its ability to reveal aspects of regional brain metabolism that are not otherwise accessible to study.

The principles involved are outlined by Bench *et al.* (1990) and Watson (1991). Compounds labelled with short-lived isotopes, for example ^{18}F or ^{15}O, are injected or inhaled and allowed to reach a

Fig. 3.15 Functional magnetic resonance imaging: differences in relative language lateralisation for a verbal fluency task can be found between patients with right or left temporal lobe epilepsy (TLE). Illustrative activation maps are shown here, co-registered with individual high-resolution structural MRI. Cluster detection was carried out on all voxels above $z = 2.3$ to determine clusters significantly activated (corrected $P < 0.01$) in the experimental task condition. The patient with right TLE has predominantly left hemisphere activation. In contrast, the activation map for the patient with left TLE shows bihemispheric activations. See also Plate 3.3. (From Matthews & Jezzard 2004 with permission.)

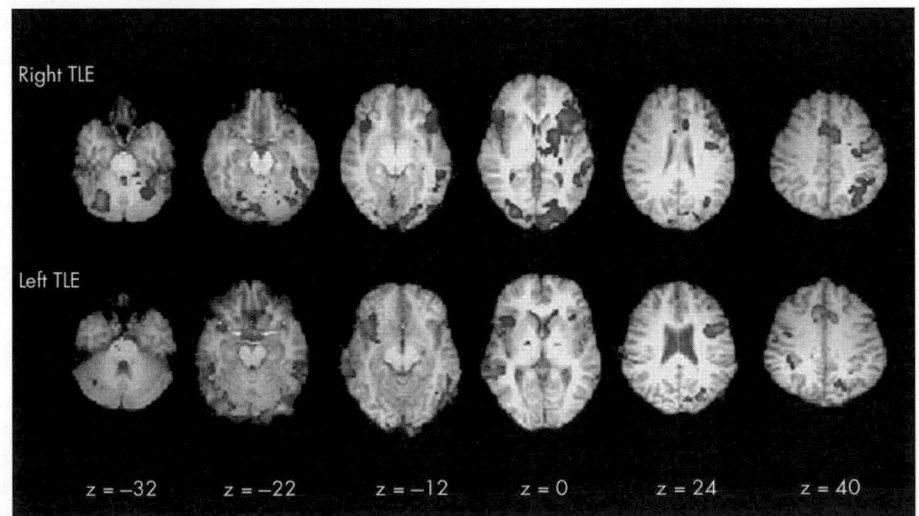

steady state in the tissues. The excess of protons over neutrons in such isotopes confers instability, leading to the emission of positrons (positively charged electrons). With the discharge of a positron, one of the protons in the nucleus becomes a neutron and stability is achieved again. An emitted positron has a range of only a few millimetres in the tissues before it encounters an ordinary electron and the two then annihilate each other. Their mass is converted into two gamma rays, which originate simultaneously and propagate in almost precisely opposite directions. This allows their point of origin to be determined by 'coincidence counting' with suitably placed detectors, and this point of origin will be very close to the point where the positron was released. Hence paired detectors arranged around the head can be used to compute the distribution of the isotope with a fair degree of accuracy. Algorithms similar to those used in CT can yield a visual image of its location within the brain. With the introduction of both single photon emission computed tomography (SPECT)/CT and PET/CT, multimodality imaging has entered routine clinical practice in some specialist centres, particularly in relation to neuro-oncology. Multiple slice spiral CT scanners have been incorporated with multiple detector gamma cameras or PET systems, allowing integration of structural and functional information on the same patient at the same time (Ell 2006).

The analysis of PET scan data using radiolabelled water, like fMRI, can be immensely complex, requiring numerous comparisons and the generation of extensive statistical data. In the identification of regional changes in blood flow, for example, regional shifts must be 'normalised' against global reductions elsewhere. Where activation paradigms are employed to assess changes in metabolism or blood flow consequent on cognitive or other activity, special care must be taken in this regard. 'Subtraction' techniques, whereby images generated in a given subject are compared while at rest and when engaged in some specific activity, were developed for PET and have now been adopted for fMRI. Similar methods have been developed for comparisons between different groups of subjects; the subtraction of common activity again allows display of an image that represents statistically significant differences on a pixel-by-pixel basis (statistical parametric maps) (Friston *et al*. 1991). fMRI has taken over from PET as the main tool of human cognitive neuroscience especially in healthy participants, since the need for radiopharmaceuticals and intravenous or intraarterial injection is avoided completely. Breakthroughs derived from PET studies in explicating the functional anatomy of complex sensory and cognitive processes in living humans (Haxby *et al*. 1991; Zeki *et al*. 1991) set the benchmark for fMRI, where findings have been largely replicated and extended.

The isotopes chiefly used are ^{15}O, ^{13}N, ^{11}C and ^{18}F, which have half-lives of approximately 2, 10, 20 and 110 minutes, respectively. ^{15}O may be inhaled and the arterial blood sampled to yield quantitative measurements of regional cerebral blood flow and regional cerebral oxygen utilisation. Alternatively, a bolus of ^{15}O-labelled water may be injected intravenously to obtain brief repeated images of cerebral blood flow, which serve as a marker of neuronal activity. ^{18}F may be incorporated into 2-deoxy-D-glucose (^{18}F-fluorodeoxyglucose or FDG), which is injected to measure local glucose metabolic rates. The compound enters the brain as though it were glucose, but cannot be degraded and remains trapped within the cells for several hours. Estimates of regional glucose utilisation can therefore be made by repeated venous sampling in conjunction with the scan. ^{11}C may be incorporated into deoxyglucose for similar purposes. The regional metabolic rate for glucose correlates strongly with synaptic activity.

The important PET studies carried out in relation to diseases and syndromes will be noted in their respective chapters. A useful recent monograph on the clinical and research uses of PET of relevance to neuropsychiatry, including Alzheimer's disease, movement disorders, depression and schizophrenia, is provided by Meltzer (2003), and Smith *et al*. (2003) also review applications of PET in these conditions plus anxiety disorders and obsessive–compulsive disorder.

PET studies with cerebral activation

PET can be used in two main ways. First, it can measure cerebral activity, inferred from changes in regional cerebral blood flow using radiolabelled water or regional cerebral metabolism using FDG. The other main use is to map the distribution of a physiologically relevant molecule or macromolecule (e.g. neurotransmitter, receptor or transporter) using radioligands (Pilowsky 1996). This may be used to elucidate disease mechanisms, to map degeneration in a group of pharmacologically active cells or to assist in pharmacotherapy. The first use is declining as a research tool but has a clearly defined clinical role in neuropsychiatry in the investigation of the dementias and movement disorders in particular. The second use is expanding as the chemical pathologies of disorders become better understood aided by the promise of novel drug development.

In Alzheimer's disease, the regional metabolic rate for glucose is reduced throughout the brain but particularly in the temporoparietal region, which may show 50% reductions in severe cases (Fig. 3.16: see also Plate 3.4);

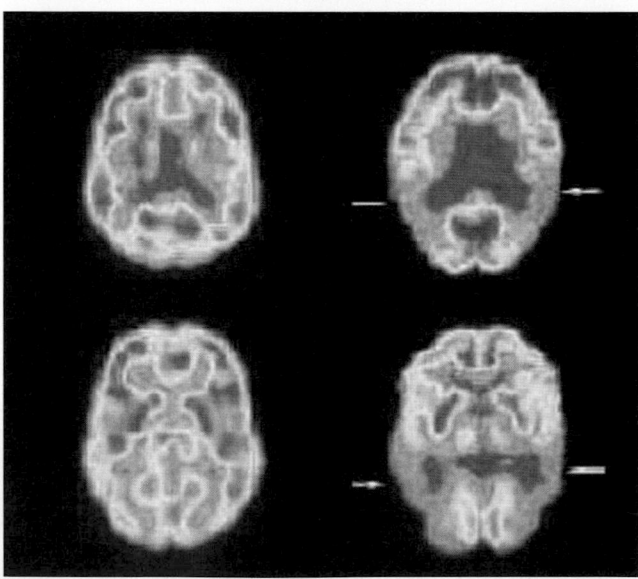

Fig. 3.16 Fluorodeoxyglucose positron emission tomography images in Alzheimer's disease: (left) normal brain; (right) Alzheimer's brain. Arrows point to area of posterior hypometabolism. See also Plate 3.4. Available at http://www.uhseastpetscan.com/zportal/portals/pat/brain/Alzheimers_Disease/pet_scans

frontotemporal dementias will tend to show the expected region-specific hypometabolism (Newberg *et al.* 2002). However, given the variations in normal ageing, PET cannot claim to be a diagnostic test at present. Early studies of Parkinson's disease indicated basal ganglia hypermetabolism against a background of general hypometabolism, especially in cases with cognitive impairment. These changes tend not to be reversible with standard treatment but are with successful fetal cell transplant. Hypometabolism in the caudate is a consistent finding in Huntington's disease. FDG-PET will show hypermetabolism in the region of an epileptic focus during seizures in up to 70% of cases and hypometabolism interictally in up to 80% (Newberg *et al.* 2002). Studies using PET (and SPECT, see later in chapter) have been able to demonstrate uncoupling of blood flow and metabolism following stroke, where blood flow may be disproportionately increased ('luxury' perfusion) or reduced ('misery' perfusion). Hence PET may be useful clinically in providing at least part of the explanation why a patient with a comparatively small structural lesion may nevertheless have profound deficits (Blake *et al.* 2003).

Radioligands and psychopharmacology

Most interest has centred on the dopaminergic system, in relation for example to movement disorders and schizophrenia as described in Chapters 12 and 2.

Postsynaptic D_2 receptors can be studied using raclopride labelled with ^{11}C. Presynaptic function is examined with ^{18}F-dopa which detects dopamine stores in nerve terminals, and with ^{11}C-nomifensine which labels presynaptic reuptake sites. The radiolabelled ligands include ^{11}C-flumazenil for central benzodiazepine receptors, ^{11}C-carfentanil for opiate receptors, ^{11}C-dexetimide for muscarinic cholinergic receptors, and ^{11}C-deprenyl for monoamine oxidase B. ^{11}C-N-methylspiperone binds to both D_2 and S_2 receptors, but the reversibility of its binding in the cortex can provide an index of serotonergic function there, although there are now radiotracers for 5-hydroxytryptamine receptors ($5HT_{2A}$) and transporters. Complex tracer kinetic models are utilised in certain studies to reveal subtle changes in receptor numbers and affinity, especially in the investigation of psychiatric disorders.

PET can be used to examine the influx of drugs into brain tissue and assess their interaction with receptors, to monitor receptor blockade in relation to clinical effect, or to observe responsivity of distinct neurochemical pathways to pharmacological agonists and antagonists. This last may be combined with simultaneous cognitive activation in order to reveal more clearly the differences between patients and controls. Some drugs may be labelled directly, such as the neuroleptics pimozide and clozapine and the anticonvulsants valproate and diphenylhydantoin. After injection in tracer amounts their distribution within the brain can be studied directly, also their affinities at specific receptor sites. Studies in relation to the neuroleptic treatment of schizophrenia are reviewed by List and Cleghorn (1993), with a more recent update provided by Frankle and Laruelle (2002). PET has been used to show the rapidity of D_2 receptor blockade in the striatum on commencing neuroleptics, and the time course of reversal of the blockade when they are discontinued. It has been suggested that rapid dissociation rates of binding to the D_2 receptor may underlie the low level of extrapyramidal side effects seen with the atypical antipsychotics. Dose-dependent relationships have been demonstrated between serum levels of neuroleptics and the degree of inhibition of striatal D_2 binding, and attempts have been made to detect differences in patients who are resistant to neuroleptic effects. Differences between typical and atypical antipsychotics have also been studied in this manner as well as 'regional selectivity' of effect, i.e. striatal versus extrapyramidal (Erritzoe *et al.* 2003).

Other molecules that may be labelled include amino acids, fatty acids, alcohols and sugars. A considerable variety of active metabolic processes are thus accessible to study.

PET in Parkinson's disease

Dopamine and dopaminergic neurones are central to the pathophysiology of Parkinson's disease. Applications of PET in the investigation of movement disorders is well reviewed by Piccini and Whone (2004), summarised below. Such neurones are susceptible to tagging by positron-emitting isotopes. This may involve the dopamine transporter (responsible for reuptake from the synaptic cleft), the vesicular monoamine transporter (VMAT)-2 (responsible for packaging dopamine into the synaptic vesicles), and the enzyme aromatic amino acid decarboxylase (responsible for transforming dopa to dopamine), which is located inside the synaptic terminal (Piccini & Whone 2004). The most extensively studied ligand in Parkinson's disease is ^{18}F-dopa which, as stated above, reflects predominantly presynaptic nigrostriatal activity. ^{18}F-Dopa shows reduced accumulation in the putamen, particularly the caudal region, in Parkinson's disease, and its distribution is frequently asymmetrical. Other parkinsonian syndromes may see similar reductions but not those of vascular origin. Essential tremor does not affect ^{18}F-dopa binding in the striatum (Fig. 3.17: see also Plate 3.5) (Brooks & Piccini 2006). The advantage of using radiotracers that interact with processes central to dopaminergic neurotransmission rather than those that act as direct measures of dopamine receptor occupancy (e.g. ^{11}C-raclopride) is that they are not so distorted by dopaminergic therapy and so may be more stable markers of disease (Brooks *et al.* 2003). D_2 binding is increased early in untreated Parkinson's disease.

Dopamine transporter ligands include ^{11}C-methylphenidate and the cocaine analogues ^{11}C-β-3β-(4-fluorophenyl) tropane (for PET) and ^{123}I-β-3β-(4-iodophenyl)tropane (CIT; for SPECT). Almost the entire VMAT-2 signal in the striatum is attributable to dopaminergic vesicular binding. Denervation is reflected in marked reductions in signal using the

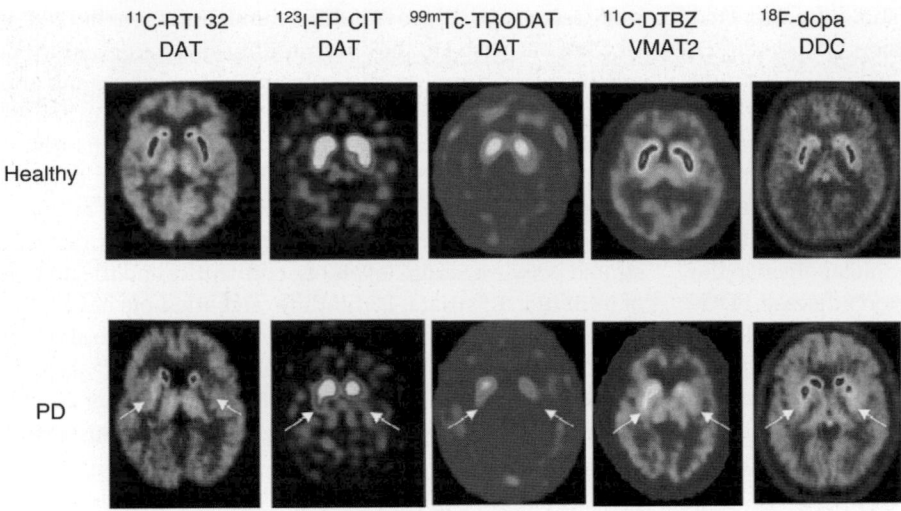

Fig. 3.17 Striatal uptake of dopamine transporter (DAT) ^{11}C-RTI-32, ^{123}I-β-CIT, ^{99m}Tc-TRODAT, vesicular monoamine transporter (VMAT2) ^{11}C-DTBZ, and dopa decarboxylase (DDC) ^{18}F-dopa in a healthy control subject and a patient with early Parkinson's disease (PD). In PD the putamens are targeted asymmetrically. See also Plate 3.5. (From Brooks & Piccini 2006 with permission.)

ligand ^{11}C-dihydrotetrabenazine (DTBZ), even in the early stages of Parkinson's disease and this is not affected by medication or disease-related compensatory changes (Bohnen & Frey 2003). ^{11}C-RTI-32 is an *in vivo* marker of both dopamine and noradrenaline (norepinephrine) transporter binding. In a small study in Parkinson's disease, anxiety inversely correlated with the binding in the limbic system including the anterior cingulate cortex, thalamus, amygdala and ventral striatum while apathy was inversely correlated with binding in the ventral striatum. The results suggest that depression and anxiety in Parkinson's disease may be associated with regionally specific loss of dopamine and noradrenaline innervation and that work in Parkinson's disease may have wide implications for the understanding of other neuropsychiatric disorders (Brooks & Piccini 2006).

Single photon emission computed tomography

SPECT has come into prominence more recently than PET, although in some respects its origins go back further. It is essentially an elaboration of radioisotope scanning brought about by the harnessing of computer technology analogous to that used in CT for reconstructing images of the brain. Though considerably less accurate than PET, and a good deal less amenable to quantitation, the images obtained with the most modern machines can be of remarkable quality (Fig. 3.18: see also Plate 3.6). Since the radioisotopes employed have much longer half-lives than those used for PET, there is no requirement to have a cyclotron close at hand. This accounts in large measure for the increasing attention devoted to the technique. SPECT can be available at any hospital where there is a nuclear medicine facility, and its greatly reduced cost in comparison with PET means that larger samples may be investigated and that it can be applied more readily in a clinical context. However, the range of normal variation encountered is considerable.

The procedure involves the administration of radiopharmaceuticals that emit not positrons but gamma rays (photons) directly. The tracers are taken up into the brain, and their regional concentration detected by focused collimators arranged around the head or by a rotating gamma camera. At each point the detector samples a cone of brain tissue, brain images then being obtained by summation according to the standard tomographic technique. Since the gamma rays are emitted directly from the radiotracers employed, there is no annihilation process as with PET. Coincidence counting is therefore precluded and the points of origin of the gamma rays are simply determined from their trajectories, consequently with less precision. Nevertheless, resolution approaches 8–10 mm with the most recent systems (cf. 5–7 mm with PET).

The tracers most frequently used are markers of cerebral blood flow. Glucose and oxygen uptake cannot be revealed directly by SPECT, but will normally be closely coupled to blood flow in the situations where SPECT is employed. With the continued development of tracer biochemistry, methods are also available for imaging a variety of neurotransmitters and their receptor sites as described below.

Xenon-133 (with a half-life of 5.3 days) may be administered by inhalation or injection for cerebral blood flow studies. Cerebral blood flow may then be measured without arterial blood sampling. However, isopropylamphetamine (IMP) labelled with ^{123}I is simpler to use. It has a half-life of 13 hours, and being lipophilic it penetrates brain tissue and becomes trapped within it, revealing patterns of distribution of blood flow that remain stable over a substantial period of time. Scanning is carried out after a single intravenous injection; higher resolution is obtained than with xenon but at the expense of longer scanning times. IMP has now been superseded by hexamethylpropyleneamineoxine (HMPAO) labelled with technetium-99m (^{99m}Tc), which is similarly lipophilic but has a shorter half-life (6 hours) and thus can be given in higher dosage, yielding improved definition and shorter scanning times. [99m]Tc is routinely available and can be obtained from a molybdenum-99 'generator' which has a shelf-life of 67 hours. The HMPAO is taken up in the brain in proportion to blood flow within a few minutes, yielding a 'frozen image' that remains stable for several hours. Scanning is normally undertaken some 20–30 minutes after injection. ^{99m}Tc-labelled ethyl cysteinate dimmer (ECD) is similar but is more stable *in vitro*.

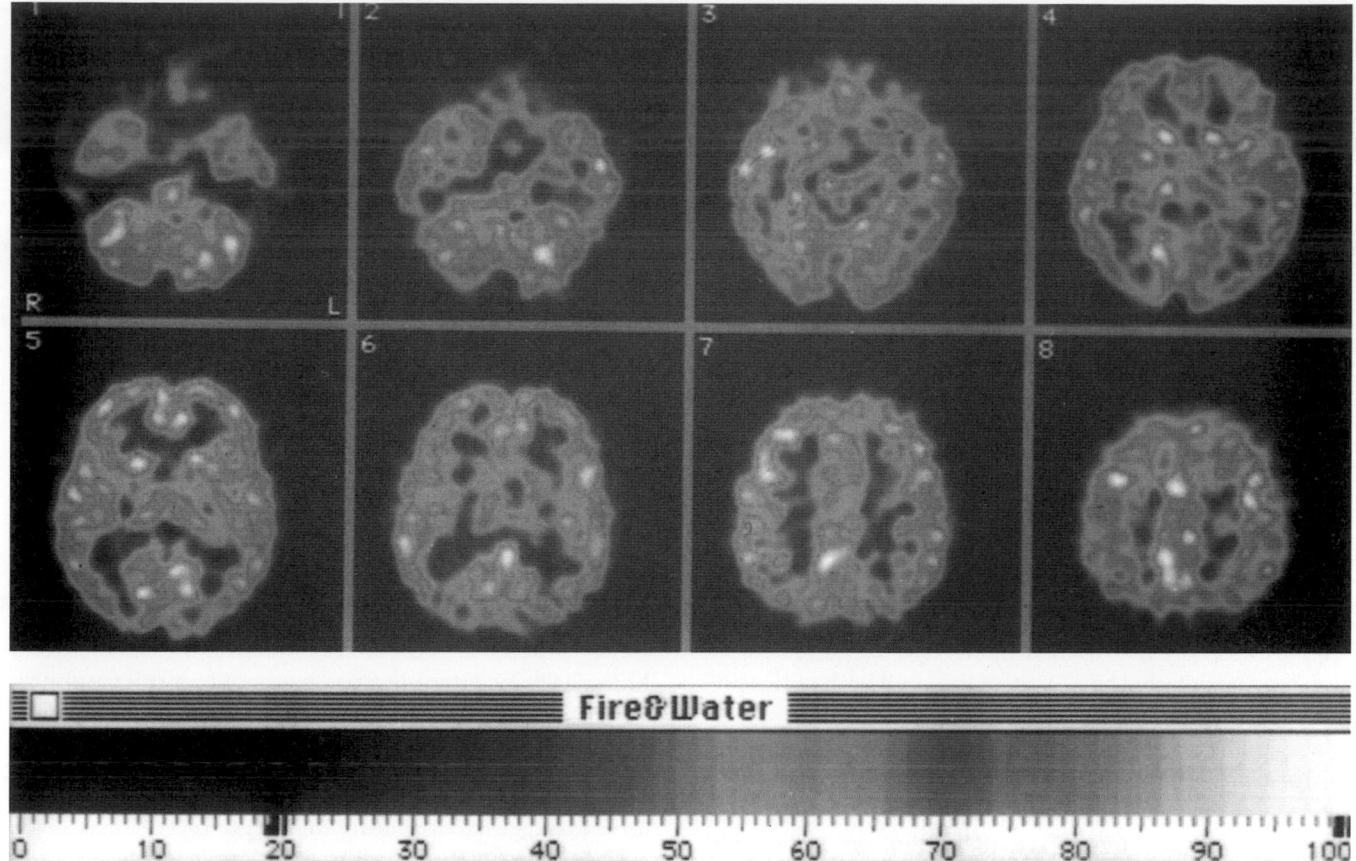

Fig. 3.18 An HMPAO-SPECT scan from a normal subject, using a Strichman Medical Equipment multislice, head-dedicated scanner. The slices are orientated parallel to the orbitomeatal plane. See also Plate 3.6. (Courtesy of the Department of Nuclear Medicine, King's College Hospital, London.)

SPECT has proved of clinical value in relation to strokes, and for the investigation of blood flow during migraine attacks. In the dementias, it can reveal the reductions of uptake in the temporoparietal regions typical of Alzheimer's disease, and has been used to demarcate the contrasting group of frontal lobe dementias (see Chapter 2, under Cerebral lobe localization). Multi-infarct dementia may be indicated by scattered focal deficits (see Chapter 8). In Huntington's disease changes may be detected in the heads of the caudate nuclei (Blake *et al.* 2003). Applications in the field of epilepsy and alcoholism are described in their respective chapters.

In a retrospective evaluation of 20 neuropsychiatric patients suffering from dementia, amnesic states, depression and personality disorder, Trzepacz *et al.* (1992) have shown the value of IMP SPECT in revealing clinically relevant brain abnormalities. Studies in schizophrenic patients have revealed hypoperfusion frontally much as in PET studies, and decreased blood flow has been reported in depression with significant increases on recovery (Sackheim *et al.* 1990). Musalek *et al.* (1989) have reported distinctive patterns in patients with auditory and tactile hallucinations. McGuire *et al.* (1993) used a split-dose technique with technetium-labelled HMPAO to provide a snapshot of brain function in patients experiencing auditory verbal hallucinations.

Neurotransmitter imaging

As with PET, SPECT make it possible to image certain neurotransmitter receptors. Most success has been achieved with the dopamine system: Crawley *et al.* (1986) used [77]Br-labelled spiperone and Pilowsky *et al.* (1994) iodobenzamide (IBZM) labelled with ^{123}I to explore D_2 receptor binding in a semi-quantitative manner. Quinuclidinyl-4-iodo-benzilate (QNB) labelled with ^{123}I may be used to detect muscarinic acetylcholine receptors, a decrease being revealed in the posterior temporal cortex in patients with Alzheimer's dementia (Holman *et al.* 1985; Weinberger *et al.* 1991). Other potential ligands include raclopride for D_2 receptors, IBZP for D_1 receptors and flumazenil for benzodiazepine receptors, all labelled with [123]I. As noted above, the dopamine transporter is amenable to SPECT radioimaging using ^{123}I-β-CIT, which can show 50% reductions at presentation. A fluoropropyl derivate has recently been developed, ^{123}I-FP-CIT, which has faster kinetics so that images can be acquired 3 hours after administration (compared with 24 hours) (Piccini & Whone

2004). Finally, ^{99m}Tc-TRODAT-1 is a convenient ligand for clinical use.

Other special investigations

Echoencephalography (ultrasound)

Echoencephalography is used to detect developmental anomalies of the brain and CNS *in utero* and in paediatric neurology (see Barnewolt & Estroff 2004 for review). It is a rapid procedure, without discomfort or risk to the patient.

Radioisotope scan (radionuclide scan, gamma encephalography)

Radioisotope scanning is a technique for the investigation of cerebral tumours and some cerebral infarctions. However, its use has declined very markedly since the introduction of CT and other scan procedures although it is still important where access to these is limited. An isotope preparation such as technetium-99 (^{99}Tc) is injected intravenously in a dose according to body weight. This is picked up by vascular tissue, especially neovascular tissue, and the gamma radiation may be detected by a 'scan' of the skull with radioactive counting equipment.

Isotope cisternography (isotope encephalography)

Isotope cisternography provides a means of obtaining a dynamic picture of the CSF circulation in conjunction with air encephalography in the investigation of patients with communicating hydrocephalus Since the advent of CT and MRI its usefulness has declined. Visualisation of the morphology and the dynamics of the CSF circulation may be achieved by intrathecal injection of metrizamide in conjunction with a CT scan (Isherwood 1983). However, modern dynamic MRI techniques can detect CSF flow patterns non-invasively.

Cerebral angiography

Cerebral angiography consists of taking X-ray films in rapid succession after an injection of contrast medium into the cerebral circulation. Injection of the common carotid artery displays the internal carotid and its area of supply by way of the anterior and middle cerebral arteries, and sometimes the posterior cerebral arteries also. Vertebral arteriography is more hazardous, but can be used to outline the vertebral, basilar and posterior cerebral arteries.

Because of the hazards, angiography has now been supplanted by CT (see Computed tomography, earlier in chapter) as a screening procedure for tumours. Furthermore, a range of new CT angiography and MRI applications such as MRA provide subsecond temporal resolution and three-dimensional techniques are rapidly developing (Coley *et al.* 2003). These may be used for investigation of a range of cerebrovascular disorders, including aneurysms and malformations. The precise delineation of vascular anomalies may still require X-ray angiographic techniques.

Air encephalography (pneumoencephalography)

Before CT became available, air encephalography was a technique of great importance for visualising intracranial pathology. For a while a place remained for the technique in a small minority of patients, chiefly for visualising small basal tumours near the optic or auditory nerves or in the brainstem, and for clarifying obstructions in the aqueductal region. Such areas are relatively inaccessible on CT but are now well visualised by MRI. MRI has also displaced the use of air encephalography for the investigation of patients with temporal lobe epilepsy, since coronal views allow detailed visualisation of the temporal horns of the lateral ventricles.

Nerve conduction studies and electromyography

Nerve conduction studies (NCS) are frequently carried out alongside electromyography (EMG). These tests are usually carried out by a clinical neurophysiologist and require some skill in their interpretation. Their main role is in the diagnosis and monitoring of disorders of the peripheral nervous and neuromuscular systems. Useful overviews of their role in clinical practice are provided by Mallik and Weir (2005) and Mills (2005a,b). Interested readers should consult the appropriate neurophysiological texts for more information.

NCS involve the application of depolarising square wave electrical pulses to the skin over a peripheral nerve producing (i) a propagated nerve action potential recorded at a distant point over the same nerve; and (ii) a compound muscle action potential arising from activation of muscle fibres in a target muscle supplied by the nerve. In both cases these may be recorded with surface or needle electrodes. Surface electrodes are designed to give information about the whole of a muscle stimulated, providing data for the time taken for the fastest axons to conduct an impulse to the muscle and the size of the response. Needle electrodes for NCS give very accurate conduction time information, but because they record from only a small area of muscle or nerve, they give poor or, in the case of nerves, more complex information making numerical analysis difficult. However, needle recordings are most appropriate when severe muscle wasting has occurred, or when the depth of a muscle under study makes a surface recording impossible (quoted from Mallik & Weir 2005).

EMG can detect abnormalities such as chronic denervation or fasciculations in clinically normal muscle. It can, by determining the distribution of neurogenic abnormalities, differentiate focal nerve, plexus, or radicular pathology; it can also provide supportive evidence of the pathophysiology of peripheral neuropathy, either axonal degeneration or demyelination. EMG is an obligatory investigation in motor neurone disease to demonstrate the widespread denervation and fasciculation required for secure diagnosis. Recordings are made with a disposable concentric needle electrode inserted into the muscle. A fine wire in the axis of the needle is insulated from the shaft, the end of the needle being cut at an acute angle. The area of the recording surface determines the volume of muscle that the needle can 'see'. Conventional EMG needles record from a hemisphere with radius of about 1 mm. Within this volume there are some 100 muscle fibres. The many hundreds of muscle fibres belonging to one motor unit are distributed widely throughout the cross-section of the muscle, and therefore within the detection region of the needle there may be just four to six fibres of a single motor unit. Analysis of the waveforms and firing rates of single motor or multiple motor units can give diagnostic information. Electromyographers are skilled at interpreting both the appearance of muscle activity and the sound of the activity transmitted through a loudspeaker. Normal resting muscle is silent (Mills 2005a).

Neurophysiology offers the most sensitive diagnostic tests for disorders of neuromuscular transmission. However, the tests are not absolutely specific. Repetitive nerve stimulation shows a decrementing response in myasthenia gravis, the decrement being more pronounced in proximal muscles. However, single-fibre EMG (SFEMG) is much more sensitive; SFEMG of facial muscles detects an abnormality in virtually all cases of myasthenia gravis. In Lambert–Eaton myasthenic syndrome, the compound muscle action potential evoked in hand muscles is small and increases dramatically after exercise. Decrement is seen on repetitive nerve stimulation, and stimulated SFEMG, if required, shows a frequency-dependent increase in jitter (Mills 2005b).

Since the peripheral nervous system may be affected as a component of a syndrome that also involves the CNS (e.g. toxic and metabolic disorders such as vitamin deficiencies and porphyria; peripheral and CNS demyelination as in multifocal leucoencephalopathy; degenerative disorders such as motor neurone disease; mitochondrial disorders affecting muscle and the CNS as in myoclonus epilepsy with ragged-red fibres) but is somewhat more accessible, such testing may be of great relevance to the neuropsychiatrist. NCS and EMG can clarify the causes of numbness, abnormal sensations, weakness, fatigue and muscle wasting, or at least help to exclude certain causes. This may be valuable in the investigation of conversion disorders and chronic fatigue syndromes. In the former, EMG may be combined with transcranial magnetic stimulation to demonstrate to the patient and clinician the integrity of the motor system or that 'the muscles and nerves are still working'. The main safety concern is the need for caution in patients with a cardiac pacemaker.

Appendix

Tests of perception

Bender–Gestalt Test (Bender Visual Motor Gestalt Test)
Bender produced what is primarily a copying test, independent of memory and learning ability, although it can be varied to examine reproduction from memory after a lapse of time if required.

Nine simple designs are presented to the subject, one at a time, and he is asked to copy them. The type and frequency of errors are noted, and serve as the basis for identifying neurotic, psychotic and brain-damaged subjects. Interpretation relies to a large extent on subjective intuitive procedures, but attempts have been made to standardise it for certain purposes.

It has been widely used as a rapid screening test, but the overlap between groups reduces its value when applied to the individual subject. Nevertheless its efficiency at detect-

ing brain damage has sometimes received surprisingly strong support compared with other long-established psychometric tests. Lezak (1995) reviews the now extensive literature of this simple test and the sometimes elaborate scoring procedures employed.

Visual Object and Space Perception Battery
Warrington and James (1991) have introduced a nine-test battery for exploring visual perception that can be given in parts or as a whole. Minimal motor response is required from the patient so that any praxic element is eliminated.

The first test screens for visual impairment, which might preclude proceeding further. A series of cards is shown with an all-over pattern and the patient must say which of them contains a degraded 'X'.

The next four tests show views of letters, animals or objects that have been rendered puzzling in various ways. In Incomplete Letters, the subject has to identify a series of randomly degraded letters. *Silhouettes* requires the subject to identify animals and inanimate objects depicted as black silhouettes and rotated through various degrees. In *Object Decision* the subject has to choose which of a group of silhouettes, again rotated, represents a real as opposed to an imaginary object. In *Progressive Silhouettes* the subject sees two series of silhouettes, each representing a single object, presented at a series of angles that gradually approach normality.

The final four tests deal with aspects of space perception. *Dot Counting* requires the subject to count the number of dots in a small array. In *Position Discrimination* the subject must decide which of two squares, presented side by side, has the dot exactly in the centre. *Number Location* consists of two squares one above the other; in the lower display there is a single dot, and the subject must say which number in the square above corresponds to its position. *Cube Analysis* requires the subject to count the number of cubes depicted in line drawings of three-dimensional displays.

Patients with right hemisphere lesions have been shown to perform less well than patients with left hemisphere lesions on all of these subtests.

Behavioural Inattention Test
This battery of tests is designed to examine unilateral visual neglect (Wilson *et al.* 1987). The first six subtests are traditional procedures for examining for neglect, and the next nine 'behavioural tests' aim to identify everyday problems likely to be faced by patients, thereby serving as a guide to rehabilitation.

The traditional tests include line crossing, letter cancellation, star cancellation, figure- and shape-copying tests, line bisection tests and free drawing of a clock, a man or woman and a butterfly.

The behavioural tests examine picture scanning, telephone dialling, menu reading, article reading, telling and setting the time on a clock face, coin sorting, address and sentence copying, map navigation and card sorting.

Halligan *et al.* (1991) have shown excellent test–retest reliabilities for the battery, and good correlations on each of the two subsets with occupational therapists' reports and measures of activities of daily living.

Test of Everyday Attention

The Test of Everyday Attention (Robertson *et al.* 1994, 1996) assesses three aspects of attention: selective attention, sustained attention, and attentional switching. The materials relate to everyday situations, making this instrument ecologically plausible and acceptable to patients. It is said to be sensitive enough to show age effects in the normal population while also showing specific types of attention disorders in patients with various types of neurological disorders. The subtests include the following.

- Map Search: looking at a large colour map of Philadelphia, patients search for symbols (selective attention).
- Elevator Counting (with and without distraction): listening to a series of tones, patients are asked to indicate a specific floor level (sustained attention).
- Visual Elevator: attentional switching and cognitive flexibility is measured by asking patients to count up and down as they follow a series of visually presented 'floors' in the imagined elevator (also in a fixed speed version presented on audio tape).
- Telephone Search: while looking at a simulated telephone directory patients are asked to identify key symbols (also presented as a dual task test: while searching through the directory the patient is asked to simultaneously count tones presented on tape).
- Lottery: patients are asked to listen for their 'winning number' presented on audio tape, then write down the two letters preceding a specified number.

The Test of Everyday Attention consists of parallel versions yielding nine percentile scores that can be used to track recovery of function following brain damage. Administration time is 45–60 minutes. The normative sample, composed of 154 normal individuals ranging from 18 to 80 years of age, is stratified by age and education.

Language tests

Boston Naming Test

This consists of 60 line drawings of objects that the patient must name (Kaplan *et al.* 1983). The items range in difficulty from common objects such as a tree or pencil to more difficult ones like a sphinx or a trellis. When the subject cannot name the picture he is given cues, first a stimulus cue (e.g. 'it's something to eat'), then a phonemic cue (i.e. the opening sound of the word). These help to identify whether the subject knew the word at all. The number of cues needed is noted.

Normative data on the test are provided by Van Gorp *et al.* (1986). It effectively elicits naming impairments in patients with aphasia, but is also sensitive to the language difficulties of patients with dementia (Margolin *et al.* 1990). Edith Kaplan (quoted in Lezak 1995) has noted that patients with right hemisphere damage, especially right frontal damage, may show responses indicative of perceptual fragmentation, for example identifying the mouth-piece of a harmonica as the line of windows on a bus.

Graded Naming Test

The subject is presented with 30 line drawings of items and asked to name them (McKenna & Warrington 1983). These vary with regard to frequency of usage and consequently in naming difficulty. It is possible to judge whether naming ability is in line with reading ability, as estimated by the NART or the Schonell Graded Word Reading Test, or with vocabulary scores as measured on the WAIS.

Token Test

De Renzi and Vignolo (1962) introduced a test especially sensitive to minor degrees of impairment of language comprehension. This can be of considerable value since routine examination often fails to detect slight receptive language disorder. Moreover a patient with aphasia may seem to have difficulties limited to verbal expression alone, and it can then be difficult to explore the more subtle aspects of language comprehension without taxing other cognitive functions as well.

The test uses a number of simple 'tokens' that are manipulated by the subject. He is given a series of verbal commands expressed in progressively more complex messages, in response to which he must perform simple manual tasks such as picking up, moving or touching the tokens. The tokens used are of two different shapes (circles and rectangles), two different sizes and five different colours. It is first necessary to ensure that the subject appreciates the meaning of circle and rectangle and that colour recognition is intact.

In the first part of the test the large circles and rectangles are displayed and the patient is asked to pick up each in turn by telling him to 'pick up the yellow rectangle', 'pick up the white circle', etc. Subsequent parts proceed in graded stages by introducing the small as well as the large tokens, by asking the subject to pick up two at a time, and by introducing more complex instructions that involve new grammatical elements. In the final part of the test, prepositions, conjunctions and adverbs are introduced so as to radically change the meaning of the action which the subject is required to perform. For example 'put the red circle on the green rectangle', 'touch the blue circle with the red rectangle', 'pick up all the rectangles except the yellow one', 'put the red circle between the yellow rectangle and the green rectangle', 'after picking up the green rectangle touch the white circle'.

Thus the test consists of messages that are conceptually elementary and short and easy to remember, but which make two kinds of demand on comprehension: the token must be identified by three independent features, and the subject must grasp the semantic complications which are later introduced. Deficits often become obvious only in the later stages of the test, and can then emerge clearly even among aphasics who have shown no evidence of difficulty with comprehension during normal conversation.

Boller and Vignolo (1966) found that the test was more impaired in aphasics than non-aphasics, as expected, but also that among non-aphasics it was more impaired by left-sided brain damage than right. The latent sensory aphasia thus identified was independent of non-language impairments as measured by Raven's Progressive Matrices, and appeared not merely to be a consequence of impaired general intelligence. The test was shown to be more sensitive for the detection of mild comprehension deficits than Marie's Three Paper Test, which has been widely employed for this purpose (see Comprehension of speech).

Speed and Capacity of Language Processing Test
In the first part, the Speed of Comprehension Test, the rate of processing of language is measured (Baddeley *et al.* 1992). The subject is required to read a number of statements that vary in content and syntactic structure, putting a tick against those which are true or sensible and a cross if they are false or silly. The subject must work as quickly as possible through the series.

The second part, the Spot-the-Word Test, is introduced to control for poor verbal skills *per se*, rather than slowed information processing. In this test the subject is presented with 60 pairs of items, each consisting of a word and an invented non-word, and must indicate which of the pair is real. The extent to which the subject's speed of comprehension falls behind performance on the Spot-the-Word Test indicates how far language comprehension skills have been impaired.

The Spot-the-Word Test may have another value in itself, in that it has proved to be a potentially useful method for estimating premorbid intelligence. Thus it has been shown to correlate highly with verbal intelligence as estimated by Mill Hill Vocabulary scores or performance on the NART, and performance seems not to decline with age even in the presence of intellectual impairment (Baddeley *et al.* 1993). In performing the task a number of parallel routes are available for making the lexical decisions – the meaning of the word, its orthographic appearance, its sound, or a general feeling of familiarity – and this may be what makes it relatively resistant to brain damage.

Psycholinguistic Assessments of Language Processing in Aphasia
The Psycholinguistic Assessments of Language Processing in Aphasia (PALPA) (Kay *et al.* 1992) consists of 60 tests of components of language structure such as orthography and phonology, word and picture semantics and morphology and syntax. The tests make use of simple procedures such as lexical decision, repetition and picture naming and have been designed to assess spoken and written input and output modalities. Guides are included that help to suggest which selection of test may be appropriate for each aphasic person.

Memory tests

Paired associate learning test
Paired associate learning involves mastery of the appropriate response when the first member of a pair of words is presented. It forms part of the Wechsler Memory Scale.

Three simple paired associates must be learned by repeated auditory presentation. In one form of the test, for example, the pairs are 'cabbage–pen', 'knife–chimney', and 'sponge–trumpet'. The examiner reads the list after telling the subject to remember the pairs that go together. The stimulus words are then given alone in random order, and repeated with appropriate corrections for errors until the subject achieves three consecutive correct responses on every one of the three different stimulus words. Any given stimulus word is dropped out as soon as its own criterion is reached. The score is the sum of the times the stimulus words must be presented before the total criterion is reached.

The test has proved to be a sensitive indicator of memory disorder in the elderly and to be independent of the patient's verbal intelligence. It is useful for measuring impairment in the acquisition phase of memory, but abnormally poor scores may be obtained in severely depressed and perplexed elderly subjects without evidence of brain damage (Post 1965). The test has been shown to correlate highly with the Modified Word Learning Test and the Synonym Learning Test (Kendrick *et al.* 1965; Bolton *et al.* 1967).

Isaacs and Walkey (1964) have prepared a simpler and shorter form that is less fatiguing and can be administered along with the clinical interview.

Three easy paired associates are given, and tested three times only in random order ('knife fork', 'east–west', 'hand–foot'). The procedure is then repeated with three rather harder associates ('cup–plate', 'cat–milk', 'gold–lead'), and the result is simply scored in terms of the number of errors from 0 to 18. Normal scores were judged to be in the range of 0–2, moderate impairment 3–9, and severe impairment 10–18.

The range of functions covered includes attention, registration, short-term recall and, to some extent, verbal learning. Motivational factors are clearly involved as well. Goldstein *et al.* (1988) investigated paired associate learning in patients who had undergone unilateral temporal lobectomy. A verbal paired associate task differentiated between left and right lobectomies better than did a test involving paired associate learning of designs, but when used together the two tests provided optimal discrimination between the two groups of patients.

Object Learning Test
Kendrick *et al.* (1979) have described an Object Learning Test that has proved more acceptable and less stressful to elderly patients than the Synonym Learning Test. This is again used in conjunction with the Digit Copying Test for aiding the distinction between the depressed and the demented elderly. The battery can be administered in approximately 10 minutes, and its reliability and validity have been examined on large samples of patients and controls.

Four cards are divided into 25 equal sections within which there are drawings of familiar objects (e.g. a comb and a teapot). The first card contains 10 items, the second 15, the third 20 and the fourth 25. Six of the items are repeated across all four cards and are always in the same position. Some items form a category across the cards. The cards are exposed to the subject for a standard length of time, and the score represents the total number of correct items recalled.

List learning tests

Tests examining the learning of word lists have a number of advantages. They provide information about the immediate memory span, the shape of the learning curve and the nature of the learning strategies employed (or their absence). In addition they give evidence of such matters as proactive interference and confabulation. Lezak (1995) reviews the two tests most widely used at present: the Rey Auditory Verbal Learning Test and the California Verbal Learning Test.

The *Rey Auditory Verbal Learning Test* consists of five presentations of a 15-word list, after each of which the subject must recall as many words as he can. A second 15-word list is then presented and tested for recall. The subject is then immediately asked to recall as much as he can of the first list, and retention is examined 30 minutes (or even 24 hours) later.

After each presentation the examiner writes down the words exactly as they are recalled. Scores are made of total words correctly recalled, of intrusions from one list to the other, and of errors made (i.e. words not on the lists). The shape of the learning curve over the repeated presentations of the first list can be examined, also retention after the period of delay. 'Primacy' and 'recency' effects (better recall of words towards the beginning and end of the list) are usually shown by normal subjects, but the primacy effect is often lacking when learning ability is defective. Extensive normative data are available for the test.

The *California Verbal Learning Test* is similar to the above, but includes 16 words which belong to four defined categories. This allows the subject's learning strategies to be examined more closely. Category-cued recall is tested as well as free recall, and a recognition trial is included.

Recognition memory tests

Warrington (1974, 1984) has described a simple technique for separately assessing verbal and non-verbal memory by means of an easily administered recognition memory task. A recognition paradigm is used in preference to free recall, since recognition tasks appear to be less vulnerable to anxiety and depression. Moreover, identical procedures can be followed for the verbal and non-verbal material, allowing direct comparisons between the two. It is sometimes claimed that poor performance on recognition memory tests along with only moderately impaired recall indicates feigned memory loss.

The material consists of 50 high-frequency words, each printed on a card, and 50 photographs of unknown faces. The words are presented to the subject at 3-second intervals, and he is asked to respond 'yes' or 'no' each time according to whether he judges the word to be pleasant or not pleasant. This strategy is adopted to ensure attention to the words. Recognition is tested immediately the presentation is complete by showing pairs of words, one of which is new and one of which has already been shown. A choice must be made each time between the two items.

The 50 photographs of faces are then shown at 3-second intervals, again with the requirement that the subject decides at each presentation whether the face is pleasant or unpleasant. Recognition is again tested as soon as presentation is complete by a similar forced-choice technique.

The Camden Memory Test Battery (Warrington 1996) is a shortened version of the above that probes recognition memory for words, faces and drawings. It is quick to and easy to administer but may be difficult for those patients who cannot keep up with the speed of presentation of material.

Benton Visual Retention Test

This visual recall test requires the reproduction of a series of geometrical figures shortly after their inspection (Sivan 1992).

The subject must draw the designs from memory after each card has been exposed for 10 seconds and then removed. The test can be varied by giving shorter exposures, or by imposing delays before reproduction is required. Copying of the designs while the card is in front of the subject allows separation of memory difficulties from visuoperceptual difficulties. Performance is scored in terms of the number of designs correctly reproduced and the number of errors made. Additional qualitative information may be derived from inspection of the type of errors committed: distortions, omissions, perseverations, rotations, misplacements and errors of size. Three parallel forms of the test are available.

Performance correlates highly with intelligence and chronological age, but normative data are available to make allowance for this. The value of the test in differentiating brain-damaged and non-brain-damaged groups has been repeatedly upheld, and it has proved to be sensitive to early cognitive decline (Lezak 1995). This is probably because the test involves so many different capacities: spatial perception, visual and verbal conceptualisation, short-term retention and recall, and visuoconstructive abilities. It is sensitive to left brain damage as well as right since many of the designs can be conceptualised verbally.

Rey–Osterrieth Test

This involves the copying of a single geometrical figure of complex design, then testing reproduction from memory some time later (Rey 1941; Osterrieth 1944). The initial copying phase therefore tests for attentional neglect and praxic skills.

The figure is too complex to be adequately verbalised, hence the test is of visual non-verbal memory. The subject is first asked to copy the design as accurately as he can with the original before him. Forty minutes later and without previous warning he is asked to draw the figure again, but this time from memory. The initial copying reflects any drawing disability or disorder of spatial perception, but the recall score reflects in addition any visual memory impairment.

The test usefully complements those which measure verbal memory functions. Patients with temporal lobe damage in the hemisphere dominant for speech tend to show little impairment with the Rey–Osterrieth Test, in contrast to their difficulties with verbal memory tests. However, right temporal lobectomy leads to a slight but significant defect on copying the figure, and a pronounced and disproportionate impairment when tested for delayed recall. Lezak (1995) reviews the extensive literature on the patterns of deficit seen with different brain lesions. Patients with parietal lobe lesions appear to show relatively stable retention despite having difficulty in copying the figure initially.

Adult Memory and Information Processing Battery
This brief battery of memory tests has British norms, stratified for age, and a parallel form is available (Coughlan & Hollows 1985). There are four memory subtests and two information-processing tests.

- Short Story Recall: recall is tested immediately after presentation and again after a 30-minute delay.
- Figure Copy and Recall: a complex two-dimensional figure is copied and recall is tested immediately and after a 30-minute delay.
- List Learning: a list of 15 words is presented in the same order for a maximum of five trials. A distracter trial is then presented, for which recall is tested, and then delayed recall of the original list is tested. The test assesses rote learning and susceptibility to interference.
- Design Learning: an abstract design must be learned, with up to five presentations. Recall of a distraction design is then followed by delayed recall of the original design. This again assesses rote learning and susceptibility to interference.
- Information Processing: tested by number cancellation and digit cancellation tasks.

Rivermead Behavioural Memory Test
This battery of tests was designed to be more 'ecologically' valid than most formal memory tests in that it emphasises skills needed in real-life situations (Wilson 1987; Wilson *et al.* 1991). It assesses memory impairment in terms of everyday memory functioning, thus bridging the gap between laboratory-based and naturalistic measures of memory. Four parallel forms of the test are available to allow repeat assessments during the course of rehabilitation. Good levels of correlation with standardised memory tests show that the battery is a valid indicator of memory functioning. Norms are available for adults and separately for elderly patients, and it may be adapted for use with children. A shortened form for use with aphasic patients has been shown to be sensitive to memory deficits rather than to the effects of language impairment (Cockburn *et al.* 1990). The several subtests include the following.

1 Orientation: tested for time and place and knowledge of the date.
2 Remembering a Name: the subject is told the first and second name that goes with a photograph, and recall of these is tested when the photograph is re-presented later in the session.
3 Picture Recognition: 10 line drawings of common objects are shown for 5 seconds each, and after a short delay the subject is asked to identify them from a set of 20.
4 Face Recognition: five photographs of faces seen a few minutes earlier must be identified out of a group of 10.
5 Story Recall: a short story similar to a newspaper item is read to the subject who is asked to repeat it immediately and again some 15 minutes later.
6 Route Memory: a short route around the room is demonstrated and copied immediately by the subject. Recall is required some 15 minutes later.
7 Prospective Memory: three innovative methods are used to test the subject's capacity to remember to do something.
  (a) At the start of the session an object (such as a comb or a key) is borrowed from the subject and hidden while the subject looks on; he must ask for it and remember where it was hidden at the end in response to a specific cue (e.g. 'We have now finished this test').
  (b) When an alarm rings the subject must remember to ask a specific question, told to him when the alarm was set 20 minutes earlier (e.g. about the next appointment).
  (c) He must remember an errand, e.g. to leave an envelope at a specific location along the route around the room.

Autobiographical Memory Interview
The Autobiographical Memory Interview (Kopelman *et al.* 1990) is a semi-structured interview consisting of two parts; the first assesses recall of facts from the patient's past life while the second assesses recall of specific incidents. Each part covers three epochs: childhood, early adulthood and the recent past. Administration time is 20 minutes and comparative data from amnesia patients and healthy controls are provided. The test is useful in the range of organic conditions especially dementia but is also of value in assessing fugue states.

Frontal lobe ('executive function') tests
Verbal fluency tests
A large number of tests can be used for assessing the reduction in verbal fluency associated with frontal brain lesions, especially left frontal lesions. These are reviewed by Lezak (1995). The 'FAS' test is briefly described earlier in the chapter (see Verbal fluency) and is part of the FAB. Written tests of word fluency have been devised, also tests of 'design fluency' which are somewhat more affected by right frontal damage than left.

Wisconsin Card Sorting Test
This complex sorting test has proved to be particularly sensitive to frontal lobe damage (Milner 1963). It has accordingly achieved considerable importance in neuropsychological testing, since frontal lesions may sometimes be difficult to detect by other psychometric procedures.

The material consists of 64 cards, each containing from one to four geometrical figures. These consist of any one of four shapes (triangles, stars, crosses and circles) in any one of four colours. Four stimulus cards are set out before the subject who must sort the remainder beneath them. His task is to discover by trial and error whether he is required to sort according to colour, form or number, the clue being the examiner's remark of 'right' or 'wrong' after each response is made. In administering the test the subject is required to sort first of all by colour, all other responses being called wrong; then when he has achieved 10 consecutive correct responses to colour, the required sorting principle shifts without warning to form. Later it shifts to number, then back again to colour, and so on. The test thus combines the requirement for shifting frames of reference with a need for empirical discovery of categories. A total score can be obtained, also scores for perseverative and non-perseverative types of error.

Nelson (1976) has reported a simplified and improved version of the test (Modified Wisconsin Card Sorting Test) in which those cards which share more than one attribute with a stimulus card have been eliminated. Possible ambiguities for the patient are thereby reduced and the time of administration considerably shortened. The total number of cards to be sorted in the modified test is reduced from 64 to 24.

Milner (1963) obtained clear evidence that impairment was closely related to lesions of the frontal lobes of either hemisphere, with no comparable effects from lesions in other areas of the brain. The impairment was chiefly seen with lesions of the dorsolateral convexities of the frontal lobe, rather than with inferior and orbital lesions. Moreover, the errors in the patients with frontal lobe lesions were chiefly of the perseverative type. These results were obtained in patients with focal cortical excisions for epilepsy. They were broadly confirmed by Drewe (1974) in a heterogeneous group of brain-damaged patients. Certain qualitative differences were found between the nature of the errors with left and right frontal lesions, the former producing the greater overall impairment. Grafman et al. (1990) confirmed an excess of perseverative errors in veterans with left dorsolateral frontal and left anterior temporal lobe penetrating head injuries.

Stroop tests

A variety of tests derive from the work of John Ridley Stroop (1935) on the interference that can arise between word reading and colour naming. Lezak (1995) reviews the several formats available. All are based on the observation that it takes longer to read printed colour names when they are printed in (and/or surrounded by) coloured ink different from the name of the colour word. This may be due to a variety of factors: response conflict, failure of response inhibition, or failure of selective attention. Studies have shown that the technique is sensitive to the effects of closed head injury, and that patients with left frontal lesions perform especially badly.

Pardo et al. (1990) carried out PET scans during performance on the test to reveal the brain areas involved in resolu-

tion of the interference effect. An extensive distributed network of regions was shown to be involved (left premotor, left post central, left putamen, supplementary motor area, right superior temporal gyrus and bilateral peristriate cortex), but the most robust responses were observed in the anterior cingulate region.

Tests vary in the number of words and colours employed, and whether the requirement is to read out the colour names or to report the colour in which each word is printed. Scoring may be by time, number of errors made, or number of items correctly performed within a designated time period. The Stroop Neuropsychological Screening Test (Trenerry et al. 1989) is conducted as follows.

Columns of four colour names are presented (red, blue, green and tan), all being printed in colours incongruent with the colour name. The subject must first read the colour names aloud as quickly as possible. In the second, crucial condition there are similar columns of colour names but this time the subject must say what colour ink the word is printed in. Thus, for example, if the word 'red' is printed in blue the subject must say 'blue'. The number completed correctly in 120 seconds is compared with two age bands of norms.

Cognitive Estimates Test

Shallice and Evans (1978) noted that a patient with selective frontal lobe damage showed gross inability to produce simple cognitive estimates despite having an IQ at the same level as prior to injury. In effect the patient was unable to select the appropriate cognitive plan for answering the question and failed to check the putative answer (see Chapter 2 and Tests of frontal lobe function).

The value of the procedure was checked on groups of patients with anterior and posterior cerebral lesions, by devising a series of questions such that the appropriate plan for answering them was not immediately apparent yet required no specialist knowledge. Scoring systems for the accuracy or bizarreness of the replies were established. The frontal lesion patients performed significantly worse than the posterior group, independently of the hemisphere involved. This persisted on partialling out scores on Raven's Matrices, indicating that the differences were not simply due to defects of reasoning or general intelligence. Examples of the questions used in the test are as follows.

- How tall is the average English woman?
- What is the best paid job in Britain today?
- What is the largest object normally found in a house?
- How fast do racehorses gallop?
- What is the height of the Post Office Tower?
- What is the age of the oldest person in Britain today?
- What is the length of an average man's spine?

Strategy application tests

Some patients with known frontal damage can be observed to perform surprisingly well on tests of frontal lobe function yet show marked organisational difficulties in everyday life.

Shallice and Burgess (1991) suggested that this might be due to the constraints incorporated in clinic-based tests where the subject has an explicit problem to be tackled, usually under guidance from the examiner. In most routine tests the patient rarely needs to organise and plan his behaviour over substantial periods of time, set a range of goals or deal with interleaving priorities. Yet 'executive' abilities of this nature are required in everyday activities.

Behavioural Assessment of Dysexecutive Syndrome
The Behavioural Assessment of Dysexecutive Syndrome (Wilson *et al.* 1996) contains a number of such tests desgined to have high 'ecological' validity and has been standardised in control subjects aged between 16 and 87 years. It has six subtests and a 20-item questionnaire known as the Dysexecutive Questionnaire, which is completed by the patient and a professional or informal carer. This assesses subjective awareness of cognitive problems such as abstract thinking problems, impulsivity, apathy, distractibility and unconcern for social rules, scored on a 5-point scale from 0 (never) to 4 (very often). The two versions enable a discrepancy score to be calculated: people with early Alzheimer's disease and traumatic brain injury frequently underestimate their problems in comparison to their carer. The other subtests include the following.

• Rule Shift: subjects first learn to respond 'yes' to a red card and 'no' to a black card. Subsequently, the rule changes and the subject has to respond 'yes' if the current card is the same as the previous one: red cards may not necessarily require a yes response.
• Action Program: this is a puzzle involving a number of objects (a beaker, a cork, some water, a tube, a hook, etc.). Abiding by certain rules, the subject has to get the cork out of the tube by floating the cork on the water and then emptying the water through the tube. The task requires novel problem solving and physical manipulation skills.
• Key Search: a square on a piece of paper stands for a field in which the subject has lost his keys. Starting from a point outside the field, the subject draws a line representing the route he would take to find his keys. A systematic search strategy which covers the area without doubling back scores the most marks.
• Temporal Judgement: this comprises four questions such as 'How long does it take to blow up a party balloon?' and 'How long do most dogs live for?' A sensible guess is requires, rather like the Cognitive Estimates Test.
• Zoo Map Test: this requires the patient to plan a route to visit six of twelve locations in a zoo, according to rules regarding the starting and finishing points, and using designated paths. In one scenario a planned route to follow is provided, while in another the patient has to plan a route, which requires forethought.
• Modified Six Elements: this requires the subject to carry out a group of six open-ended tasks in a fixed period of time (10 minutes) so as to maximise the overall score obtained. The tasks are divided into two sets of three: dictating details of a route to and from the hospital, carrying out arithmetical problems of increasing difficulty, and writing down the names of pictures of objects. Detailed written instructions are presented concerning rules to be followed in carrying out the tasks. Basically, the test involves devising a simple plan, scheduling the tasks

efficiently (not flitting from one to another), and keeping a check on time (a clock is placed in front of the subject).

Multiple Errands Test
The Multiple Errands Test is more complex, requiring the subject to complete a number of tasks away from the hospital in an unfamiliar shopping precinct. Thus it involves the dovetailing of multiple activities in a real-life situation where minor unforeseen events can occur. Again detailed 'rules' must be followed and the subject's behaviour is observed throughout.

The tasks principally involve buying specified items, but one requires more ingenuity and social judgement, namely to write on a card the name of the shop likely to contain the most expensive item on sale in the precinct, the price of a pound of tomatoes, the name of the coldest place in Britain and the rate of exchange of the French franc on the previous day. Thus a range of goals must be defined, actions planned, outcomes evaluated and appropriate adaptations made. Scores are made in terms of efficiency, rule breaks, misinterpretations and task failures. Qualitative aspects of performance are also charted. Goldstein *et al.* (1993) have reported impaired performance on the Multiple Errands Test in a patient with a circumscribed excision on the left frontal lobe, who showed preserved intelligence and memory and normal performance on other tests of frontal lobe function. The planning difficulties elicited by the test mirrored those that the patient experienced in everyday life.

Hayling Test
Patients complete 30 sentences, read by the examiner, from which the last word is omitted. In the first 15 sentences, the subject completes the sentence with a word that makes sense: 'The captain wanted to stay with the sinking . . . *ship*'. In the second set of sentences, the subject must come up with a final word that does not make sense in the sentence: 'London is a very busy . . . *ice-cream*'. Response latency is the main measure and the difference between the first and second phases of the test is an indicator of response suppression time.

Brixton Test
This measures the ability to detect rules in sequences of nonverbal stimuli. It usually takes between 5 and 10 minutes to perform. Errors are scored and converted to a scaled score of between 1 and 10. The subject is shown 10 circles on a page, one of which is filled. The object is to predict where the next filled circle will be after a short sequence (Burgess & Shallice 1997).

Tower of London Test
Shallice (1982) introduced this test, derived from the Tower of Hanoi oriental puzzle.

The subject must move a number of coloured beads placed on three upright poles so as to reproduce a pattern set by the examiner. It is a test of planning, in that the subject must look ahead and divide the task into a series of subtasks, and carry these out in the correct sequence in order to obtain the desired solution. Different grades of difficulty can be presented in terms of the minimum number of moves allowed to reproduce the pattern.

Shallice (1982) found that patients with left frontal lesions performed significantly worse than patients with brain lesions in other locations.

Trail Making Test

The Trail Making Test consists of 25 circles distributed over a sheet of paper. In the first part the circles are numbered, and the subject must draw a line connecting them in numerical sequence as quickly as possible. In the second part the circles contain both numbers and letters and the subject must alternate between numbers and letters as he proceeds in ascending sequence. The score is the time taken over the task. Errors must be corrected and are thus incorporated in the time scores.

Performance on the test requires spatial analysis, motor control, alertness, concentration and ability to shift attention between alternatives. In consequence, it is likely to be affected by brain damage in many locations. When the subject takes disproportionately longer to complete the second part than the first ('Trail B'), there are likely to be difficulties with complex conceptual tracking or with flexibly changing sets during ongoing activity. For this reason the test is sometimes employed when frontal damage is suspected. Impulsive errors may be noted, and perseverations revealed.

More generally, Reitan (1958) demonstrated excellent differentiation between brain-damaged and non-brain-damaged subjects, and this has since been repeatedly confirmed. However, both age and education have significant effects on performance, and depression has been shown to interact with the slowing produced by ageing (Lezak 1995).

Goldstein–Sheerer tests

Tests developed by Goldstein and Sheerer (1941) were formerly extensively employed for investigating capacity for abstract thinking and categorisation, but are now little used. Various tests in the group explore ability to abstract common properties of objects, to break up a whole into parts, and to shift from one frame of reference to another. Accordingly they can be particularly vulnerable to frontal lobe lesions.

This type of test relies heavily on qualitative observations, being concerned with the methods employed by the subject as well as with the end-point achieved, and it is difficult to obtain objective methods of scoring.

The Goldstein–Sheerer Cube Test consists of cubes with sides of different colours, which must be assembled to match printed designs. The Gelb–Goldstein Colour Sorting Test consists of woollen skeins of different colours and shades which must be selected by colour or brightness to go with chosen samples. The Gelb–Goldstein–Weigl–Sheerer

Object Sorting Test consists of a miscellaneous group of objects that must be sorted into designated groups (according to form, colour, use, etc.). The Colour Form Sorting Test utilises circles, squares and triangles in different colours that must be sorted according to one common property and then another. The Goldstein–Sheerer Stick Test requires the subject to copy geometrical designs with a number of sticks of different lengths.

Vigilance tests

A number of tests aim to measure the subject's capacity for the continuous monitoring of stimuli over relatively long periods of time. Such 'vigilance' tests come closer than most other procedures to measuring ability for sustained attention and concentration. They have been shown to be sensitive to brain damage, and can have special advantages for detecting minor degrees of clouding of consciousness.

In routine clinical practice the simple procedures outlined in Chapter 1 will often suffice for obtaining an estimate of sustained attention. More complex information processing tests, such as the Paced Auditory Serial Addition Test (PASAT), in which digits are presented auditorily at two speeds, may be employed in patients who can cooperate with the procedure.

A further series of tests requires the subject to react rapidly in response to signals that arrive in a preset random manner. Efficient performance requires the prolonged maintenance of a high level of attention, and rapid activation of perceptual and motor mechanisms. Their disadvantage is that special apparatus is required.

The simple estimation of reaction times has often shown good differentiation between brain-damaged subjects and controls (Blackburn & Benton 1955; Benton & Joynt 1959). De Renzi and Faglioni (1965) showed that measures of the reaction time to visual stimuli were more efficient than Raven's Matrices in discriminating between normal subjects and patients with focal cerebral lesions. However, Benton *et al.* (1959) found that reaction times were also significantly slowed in schizophrenic patients.

Rosvold *et al.* (1956) explored the value of a Continuous Performance Test in which letters were exposed by a revolving drum at 1-second intervals for periods of up to 10 minutes. The subject was required to press a button whenever the letter 'X' appeared, or in a more difficult version whenever an 'X' was preceded by an 'A'. Brain-damaged adults and children were shown to be significantly poorer at the test than normal controls. Other versions exist in which the repetition of a letter is the target. This may be sequential ('1-back') or separated by one or more intervening letters ('*n*-back'), which tests working memory.

Halstead–Reitan Battery

This extensive battery represents one of the most ambitious attempts to produce a comprehensive test for the investigation of brain damage. Reitan (1966) and Russell *et al.* (1970) describe its evolution and the attempts made to explore its diagnostic usefulness. The aim has been not only to detect brain damage but also to indicate whether this is likely to be focal or diffuse, lateralised to the right or left hemisphere, and whether acute and progressive or relatively static. Individual components of the battery are frequently used alone. Some of the principal tests involved are as follows.

- Halstead's Category Test consists of groups of pictures displayed on a screen, in response to which the subject must press one of four levers. The lever required at each exposure is determined by certain unifying concepts among the group of pictures, and the subject must discover the rules by repeated trial and error. It is thus a relatively complex concept formation test that requires the subject to note similarities and differences, to set up hypotheses and to test and modify them.
- The Critical Flicker Frequency Test measures the speed of flicker required before repeated brief exposures of light become fused.
- The Tactual Performance Test requires the subject to fit blocks into their spaces on a board while blindfolded and later to draw the board from memory. It requires tactile form discrimination, manual dexterity and coordination, and the visualisation of spatial configurations.
- The Rhythm Test requires the subject to differentiate between several pairs of rhythmic beats, and assesses alertness, ability for sustained attention and ability to perceive differing rhythmic sequences.
- The Speech Sounds Perception Test consists of a series of tape-recorded nonsense words that the subject must identify by selection from printed alternatives.
- The Finger Tapping Test is a simple measure of motor speed.
- The Time Sense Test requires the subject to observe the time taken for a hand to rotate around a dial, then after several practice trials to estimate the time from memory.
- The Halstead–Wepman Aphasia Screening Test contains items for testing ability to name objects, spell, identify single numbers and letters, read, write, calculate, name body parts and distinguish right from left.
- The Trail Making Test (described earlier) is added as a further part of the battery.
- Other tests include detailed assessments of the accuracy of sensory perception on each side of the body, and tests of finger recognition, graphaesthesia and stereognosis.

Computerised psychological tests

Tests that can be administered by computer have an obvious attraction for certain purposes, either to economise with the time of a psychologist when large numbers of patients need to be examined in research, or to allow very detailed exploration of specific psychological functions. In both contexts they have special advantages in permitting accurate recording of response times in addition to examining levels of performance.

Cambridge Neuropsychological Test Automated Battery (CANTAB)
An ingenious and sensitive group of automated tests was developed in the context of exploring deficits in patients with Alzheimer's dementia and Parkinson's disease (Morris

et al. 1987; Fray *et al.* 1996; Robbins *et al.* 1998; Robbins & Sahakian 2002). A laptop computer fitted with a touch-sensitive screen is used to record the patient's responses and reaction times. Component tests include the following, some of which are based on paradigms derived from animal work. The battery is used most in research contexts and also to evaluate new treatments. Since its introduction, it has frequently been updated and expanded. The original was rather limited in the coverage of human psychological functions (e.g. language and semantic memory).

Visual memory tests
Delayed match to sample (DMTS) assesses forced choice recognition memory for novel non-verbalisable patterns. This tests both simultaneous and short-term visual memory. Paired associate learning is a stringent test for episodic memory and associative learning. Pattern and spatial recognition memory are also part of the battery.

Executive function, working memory and planning
Intra/extra-dimensional (IED) shift task tests rule acquisition and attentional set shifting. This is a computerised analogue of the Wisconsin Card Sorting Test, and is sensitive to cognitive changes associated with schizophrenia, Parkinson's disease, and dopaminergic-dependent processes. The Stockings of Cambridge (SOC) is a version of the Tower of London Test and assesses spatial planning and motor control and is claimed to probe the dorsolateral prefrontal cortex. There are also spatial span (a visuospatial analogue of the Digit Span Test) and spatial working memory tests.

Attention tests
These tests measure different aspects of attention and reaction time. They include the simple and choice reaction time tasks with different response modes and increasing complexity.
- Match to Sample Visual Search (MTS) is a simultaneous visual search task with response latency dissociated from movement time. Efficient performance on this task requires the ability to search among the targets and ignore the distractor patterns that have elements in common with the target. This test may help to differentiate between primary movement disorders and dementing conditions.
- Rapid Visual Information Processing (RVP) is a test of sustained attention (similar to the Continuous Performance Task where a sequence of numbers has to be detected within a continuous stream).

Emotional decision-making tests
- Affective Go/No-go (AGN): this is a lexical decision test on words whose valence (positive and negative) is manipulated. Different reaction times to the word types is used in the analysis.
- Cambridge Gambling Task (CGT): this test has the appearance of a simple betting game. It requires the evaluation of risk and the ability to defer gratification. The likely neural substrate for this task is thought to be the orbitofrontal prefrontal cortex.

Semantic/verbal memory tests
These tests, which address semantic and/or verbal memory, are relatively new additions to the CANTAB battery. They include computerised versions of standard tests such as graded naming and verbal recognition memory.

Dementia questionnaires and rating scales

A number of questionnaires are available for making an approximate assessment of functions that tend to be impaired in dementing illnesses. These are not psychometric tests in the ordinary sense, but questionnaires filled in by doctors, nurses or relatives who have observed the patient closely. They often include questions relevant to social and emotional functioning in addition to observations about the patient's cognitive status.

Standardisation is often incomplete, but the questionnaires can give useful information in certain settings. Some have especial value in quantifying the degree of impairment when patients are too severely incapacitated to yield scores on formal psychometric tests. Others are useful for research purposes in allowing the separation of groups according to overall severity of disability. In clinical practice they can serve as an approximate screening device, or they can be repeated after an interval of time to gauge the rate of decline or improvement. Morris *et al.* (2000) discuss the principles behind psychometric assessment in the elderly and give some useful clinical pointers.

Blessed's Dementia Scale

Blessed *et al.* (1968) used a standard dementia scale in their study of the relationship between impairments of function and severity of neuropathological changes in the brains of old people.

The questionnaire is administered to a close relative or friend, who must answer the questions on the basis of the patient's level of performance during the preceding 6 months. One group of questions contains items concerning competence in personal, domestic and social activities, such as ability to perform household tasks, to cope with small sums of money, to find the way in familiar surroundings and to recall recent outings and visits. The next group concerns changes of habits, such as impairment of eating, dressing and sphincter control. The third is relevant to change in personality, interest and drive, such as increased rigidity, egocentricity, coarsening of affect, impaired emotional control or the abandonment of habitual interests.

Middlesex Elderly Assessment of Mental State (MEAMS)

This measures orientation and core neuropsychological functions in all 12 subtests covering perception, memory, language and executive functions. Each subtest is scored and a cut-off score determines pass or fail. The total number of subtests passed gives the global performance and outcome is classified into three ranges: impaired (0–7), borderline (8–9) and normal (10–12). It has reasonable validity and reliability (Golding 1989; Yaretzky *et al.* 2000) and can distinguish dementia from depression in most cases. However, it perhaps lacks sensitivity since it is predicated on the claim that all items should be passed by a 'normal' individual regardless of intellect, in both dementia and stroke (Cartoni & Lincoln 2005).

Geriatric Mental State Schedule

The Geriatric Mental State Schedule (GMS) is not simply a questionnaire but a standardised, semistructured interview for examining and recording the patient's mental state. It takes 30–40 minutes to administer and covers the period of a month prior to examination (Copeland *et al.* 1976). The GMS allows classification of elderly patients by symptom profile and can demonstrate changes in the profile over time. Good reliability between raters has been shown both for individual items and for diagnoses made on the basis of the schedule (Copeland *et al.* 1976). In a correlational procedure 21 factors were produced, including three dealing with cognitive impairment ('impaired memory', 'cortical dysfunction' and 'disorientation') and others concerned with depression, anxiety, somatic concerns, etc. The ability of these factors to discriminate between organic and non-organic disorders of the elderly has been demonstrated (Gurland *et al.* 1976).

The related Comprehensive Assessment and Referral Evaluation Schedule (CARE) (Gurland *et al.* 1977) contains psychiatric components largely derived from the GMS, along with questions covering medical disorders, social functioning and capacity to undertake activities of daily living. Henderson *et al.* (1983) have combined parts of both instruments to produce an interview for use in community surveys.

Further developments with the GMS have involved computerisation of the data to yield diagnostic information (Copeland *et al.* 1986). The system, known as AGECAT, summates symptom components and arrives at levels of confidence with which diagnoses of organic brain syndrome, schizophrenia, depression, for example, can be made. GMS-AGECAT diagnoses of dementia and depression have been shown to agree well with diagnoses made according to DSM-III criteria (Copeland *et al.* 1990). The addition of data from an informant interview (the History and Aetiology Schedule, HAS) allows further refinement and subdivision of diagnoses (HAS-AGECAT), including subdivision of dementia into senile dementia of the Alzheimer type, multi-infarct dementia and alcohol-related dementia. HAS-AGECAT is being used in ongoing studies of the prevalence and incidence of dementia in the elderly (Copeland *et al.* 1992).

Cambridge Examination for Mental Disorders of the Elderly (CAMDEX)

Published in 1988, this test has become widely influential (Roth *et al.* 1988) and has been updated and revised. It incorporates within a single standardised instrument all components needed to identify dementia in the elderly, even in the early stages. This is graded according to severity and subdivided into its main subcategories (senile dementia of Alzheimer type, vascular dementia, mixed forms, and dementia secondary to other causes). Items relevant to other confounding diagnoses are also included: delirium, depression, paranoid or paraphrenic illness, and anxiety and phobic disorders.

The schedule begins with a structured patient interview, incorporating questions about the present mental state, the previous personal and medical history, and the family history. A standardised assessment is made of a broad range of cognitive functions, also of other aspects of the mental state, appearance and demeanour. A brief physical and neurological examination is recorded along with the results of investigations. Finally, observations and information from a relative or other informant are systematically recorded. Administration involves approximately 60 minutes with the patient and a further 20 minutes with the informant. The items of information obtained from these multiple approaches are then assembled to produce diagnostic categories according to operational diagnostic criteria.

The subsection dealing with the cognitive examination (the CAMCOG; revised edition published in 1999) is particularly useful, being specially engineered to be 'user friendly' for non-psychologists. It incorporates tests of orientation, memory, language, perceptual abilities, praxis, attention and abstract thinking and is scored out of 107, with 80 used as a cut-off for dementia. Items contained within it comprise the MMSE (see Mini-Mental State Examination, earlier in chapter) but the CAMCOG is more thorough in its assessment. It can stand alone for certain purposes as a valuable brief means of performing a neuropsychological examination.

The Consortium to Establish a Registry for Alzheimer's Disease has has a neuropsychology battery that includes verbal fluency, naming, word list learning, word list recall, word list recognition, constructional praxis as well as the MMSE. This is available worldwide in many translations and appears to be useful as a screening test for dementia.

Aptitude tests

Vineland Social Maturity Scale
The Vineland Social Maturity Scale (Doll 1947) has been mainly used for studies in child development and mental retardation, but can also be useful in providing a measure of social functioning in brain-damaged adults. Repeat administration after an interval of time can reveal gains or losses in the social field, usefully supplementing measures of intellectual ability.

The scale consists of 117 items that sample various aspects of social ability: capacity for self-care, social independence in personal activities and social responsibility. The items are scored by interviewing someone closely acquainted with the patient. The chief categories of function measured by the scale are as follows.
• Self help general: for example 'cares for self at toilet', 'tells time to quarter hour'.

• Self help eating: for example 'drinks from cup or glass unaided', 'uses table knife for spreading'.
• Self help dressing: 'dresses self except for tying', 'bathes self assisted', 'bathes self unaided'.
• Self direction: 'makes minor purchases', 'uses money providently'.
• Occupation: 'uses tools or utensils', 'does simple creative work'.
• Communication: 'prints simple words', 'makes telephone calls', 'follows current events'.
• Locomotion: 'goes about neighbourhood unattended', 'goes about home freely', 'goes to distant places alone'.
• Socialisation: 'plays simple table games', 'assumes responsibilities beyond own needs', 'shares community responsibility'.

References

Anastasi, A. & Urbina, S. (1997) *Psychological Testing*, 7th edn. Prentice-Hall Inc., New Jersey.

Andrews, H. (1996) Magnetoencephalography. In: Lewis, S. & Higgins, N. (eds) *Brain Imaging in Psychiatry*, ch. 9. Blackwell Science, Oxford.

Anthony, J.C., Le Resche, L., Niaz, U., von Korf, M.R. & Folstein, M.F. (1982) Limits of the 'Mini-Mental State' as a screening test for dementia and delirium among hospital patients. *Psychological Medicine* **12**, 397–408.

Baddeley, A., Emslie, H. & Nimmo-Smith, I. (1992) *The Speed and Capacity of Language-Processing Test*. Thames Valley Test Company, Bury St Edmunds, UK.

Baddeley, A., Emslie, H. & Nimmo-Smith, I. (1993) The Spot-the-Word test: a robust estimate of verbal intelligence based on lexical decision. *British Journal of Clinical Psychology* **32**, 55–65.

Barkley, G.L. & Baumgartner, C. (2003) MEG and EEG in epilepsy. *Journal of Clinical Neurophysiology* **20**, 163–178.

Barnewolt, C.E. & Estroff, J.A. (2004) Sonography of the fetal central nervous system. *Neuroimaging Clinics of North America* **14**, 255–271, viii.

Barron, S.A., Jacobs, L. & Kinkel, W.R. (1976) Changes in size of normal lateral ventricles during aging determined by computerised tomography. *Neurology* **26**, 1011–1013.

Belliveau, J.W., Kennedy, D.N., McKinstry, R.C. *et al.* (1991) Functional mapping of the human visual cortex by magnetic resonance imaging. *Science* **254**, 716–719.

Bench, C.J., Dolan, R.J., Friston, K.J. & Frackowiak, R.S.J. (1990) Positron emission tomography in the study of brain metabolism in psychiatric and neuropsychiatric disorders. *British Journal of Psychiatry* **157** (suppl. 9), 82–95.

Benson, D.F. (1973) Psychiatric aspects of dysphasia. *British Journal of Psychiatry* **123**, 555–566.

Benson, D.F. & Geschwind, N. (1971) Aphasia and related cortical disturbances. In: Baker A.B. & Baker L.H. (eds) *Clinical Neurology*. Harper & Row, New York.

Benton, A.L. & Joynt, J. (1959) Reaction time in unilateral cerebral disease. *Confinia Neurologica* **19**, 247–256.

Benton, A.L., Jentsch, R.C. & Wahler, H.J. (1959) Simple and choice reaction times in schizophrenia. *Archives of Neurology and Psychiatry* **81**, 373–376.

Bentson, J., Reza, M., Winter, J. & Wilson, G. (1978) Steroids and apparent cerebral atrophy on computed tomography scans. *Journal of Computer Assisted Tomography* **2**, 16–23.

Besson, J.A.O. (1990) Magnetic resonance imaging and its applications in neuropsychiatry. *British Journal of Psychiatry* **157** (suppl. 9), 25–37.

Binder, J.R. & Rao, S.M. (1994) Human brain mapping with functional magnetic resonance imaging. In: Kertesz, A. (ed.) *Localization and Neuroimaging in Neuropsychology*, ch. 7. Academic Press, San Diego.

Blackburn, H.L. & Benton, A.L. (1955) Simple and choice reaction times in cerebral disease. *Confinia Neurologica* **15**, 327–338.

Blackwood, D.H.R. & Muir, W.J. (1990) Cognitive brain potentials and their application. *British Journal of Psychiatry* **157** (suppl. 9), 96–101.

Blake, P., Johnson, B. & van Meter, J.W. (2003) Positron emission tomography (PET) and single photon emission computed tomography (SPECT): clinical applications. *Journal of Neuro-ophthalmology* **23**, 34–41.

Blessed, G., Tomlinson, B.E. & Roth, M. (1968) The association between quantitative measures of dementia and of senile change in the cerebral grey matter of elderly subjects. *British Journal of Psychiatry* **114**, 797–811.

Bohnen, N.I. & Frey, K.A. (2003) The role of positron emission tomography imaging in movement disorders. *Neuroimaging Clinics of North America* **13**, 791–803.

Boller, F. & Vignolo, L.A. (1966) Latent sensory aphasia in hemisphere damaged patients: an experimental study with the Token Test. *Brain* **89**, 815–830.

Bolton, N., Savage, R.D. & Roth, M. (1967) The modified word learning test and the aged psychiatric patient. *British Journal of Psychiatry* **113**, 1139–1140.

Bombin, I., Arango, C. & Buchanan, R.W. (2005) Significance and meaning of neurological signs in schizophrenia: two decades later. *Schizophrenia Bulletin* **31**, 962–977.

Bradley, W.G. (1992) Recent advances in magnetic resonance angiography of the brain. *Current Opinion in Neurology and Neurosurgery* **5**, 859–862.

Brammer, R. & Fazekas, F. (2002) Diffusion imaging in multiple sclerosis. *Neuroimaging Clinics of North America* **12**, 71–77.

Bramon, E., Rabe-Hesketh, S., Sham, P., Murray, R.M. & Frangou, S. (2004) Meta-analysis of the P300 and P50 waveforms in schizophrenia. *Schizophrenia Research* **70**, 315–29.

Bramon, E., McDonald, C., Croft, R.J. *et al.* (2005) Is the P300 wave an endophenotype for schizophrenia? A meta-analysis and a family study. *Neuroimage* **27**, 960–968.

Brooks, D.J. & Piccini, P. (2006) Imaging in Parkinson's disease: the role of monoamines in behaviour. *Biological Psychiatry* **59**, 908–918.

Brooks, D.J., Frey, K.A., Marek, K.L. *et al.* (2003) Assessment of neuroimaging techniques as biomarkers of the progression of Parkinson's disease. *Experimental Neurology* **184** (suppl. 1), S68–S79.

Brotchie, J., Brennan, J. & Wyke, M.A. (1985) Temporal orientation in the pre-senium and old age. *British Journal of Psychiatry* **147**, 692–695.

Buckley, P.F., Moore, C., Long, H. *et al.* (1994) [1]H-magnetic resonance spectroscopy of the left temporal and frontal lobes in schizophrenia: clinical, neurodevelopmental, and cognitive correlates. *Biological Psychiatry* **36**, 792–800.

Burgess, P.W. & Shallice, T. (1997) *The Hayling and Brixton Tests.* Thames Valley Test Company, Bury St Edmunds, UK.

Burns, A. & Pearlson, G. (1994) Computed tomography. In: Burns, A. & Levy, R. (eds) *Dementia*, ch. 23. Chapman & Hall, London.

Cartoni, A. & Lincoln, N.B. (2005) The sensitivity and specificity of the Middlesex Elderly Assessment of Mental State (MEAMS) for detecting cognitive impairment after stroke. *Neuropsychological Rehabilitation* **15**, 55–67.

Castillo, M. & Mukherji, S.K. (2001) Clinical applications of FLAIR, HASTE and magnetization transfer in neuroimaging. *Neuroimaging Clinics of North America* **11**, 461–472.

Catani, M. & ffytche, D.H. (2005) The rises and falls of disconnection syndromes. *Brain* **128**, 2224–2239.

Cockburn, J., Wilson, B., Baddeley, A. & Hiorns, R. (1990) Assessing everyday memory in patients with dysphasia. *British Journal of Clinical Psychology* **29**, 353–360.

Cohn, R. (1960) *The Person Symbol in Clinical Medicine.* Thomas, Springfield, IL.

Coley, S.C., Wild, J.M., Wilkinson, I.D. & Griffiths, P.D. (2003) Neurovascular MRI with dynamic contrast-enhanced subtraction angiography. *Neuroradiology* **45**, 843–850.

Cooper, S. & Greene, J.D.W. (2005) The clinical assessment of the patient with early dementia. *Journal of Neurology, Neurosurgery and Psychiatry* **76** (suppl. 5), 15–24.

Copeland, J.R.M., Kelleher, M.J., Kellett, J.M. *et al.* (1976) A semistructured clinical interview for the assessment of diagnosis and mental state in the elderly: the Geriatric Mental State Schedule. *Psychological Medicine* **6**, 439–449.

Copeland, J.R.M., Dewey, M.E. & Griffith-Jones, H.M. (1986) Computerised diagnostic system and case nomenclature for elderly subjects: GMS and AGECAT. *Psychological Medicine* **16**, 89–99.

Copeland, J.R.M., Dewey, M.E. & Griffith-Jones, H.M. (1990) Dementia and depression in elderly persons: AGECAT compared with DSM III and pervasive illness. *International Journal of Geriatric Psychiatry* **5**, 47–51.

Copeland, J.R.M., Davidson, I.A., Dewey, M.E. *et al.* (1992) Alzheimer's disease, other dementias, depression and pseudodementia: prevalence, incidence and three-year outcome in Liverpool. *British Journal of Psychiatry* **161**, 230–239.

Coughlan, A.K. & Hollows, S.E. (1985) *The Adult Memory and Information Processing Battery.* A.K. Coughlan, Psychology Department, St James University Hospital, Leeds.

Crawford, J.R., Hart, S. & Nelson, H.E. (1990) Improved detection of cognitive impairment with the NART: an investigation employing hierarchical discriminant function analysis. *British Journal of Clinical Psychology* **29**, 239–241.

Crawford, J.R., Parker, D.M. & McKinlay, W.W. (1992a) *A Handbook of Neuropsychological Assessment.* Lawrence Erlbaum, Hove, UK.

Crawford, J.R., Moore, J.W. & Cameron, I.M. (1992b) Verbal fluency: a NART-based equation for the estimation of premorbid performance. *British Journal of Clinical Psychology* **31**, 327–329.

Crawley, J.W.C., Crow, T.J., Johnstone, E.C. *et al.* (1986) Uptake of [77]Br-spiperone in the striata of schizophrenic patients and controls. *Nuclear Medicine Communications* **7**, 599–607.

Critchley, M. (1953) *The Parietal Lobes.* Edward Arnold, London.

David, A., Blamire, A. & Breiter, H. (1994) Functional magnetic resonance imaging. A new technique with implications for psychology and psychiatry. *British Journal of Psychiatry* **164**, 2–7.

de Leeuw, F.E., de Groot, J.C., Achten, E. *et al.* (2001) Prevalence of cerebral white matter lesions in elderly people: a population based magnetic resonance imaging study. The Rotterdam Scan Study. *Journal of Neurology, Neurosurgery and Psychiatry* **70**, 9–14.

De Renzi, E. & Faglioni, P. (1965) The comparative efficiency of intelligence and vigilance tests in detecting hemispheric cerebral damage. *Cortex* **1**, 410–433.

De Renzi, E. & Vignolo, L.A. (1962) The token test: a sensitive test to detect receptive disturbances in aphasics. *Brain* **85**, 665–678.

Doll, E.A. (1947) *Vineland Social Maturity Scale. Manual of Directions*. Educational Test Bureau, Division of American Guidance Service, Minneapolis.

Drachman, D.A. & Arbit, J. (1966) Memory and the hippocampal complex. *Archives of Neurology* **15**, 52–61.

Drewe, E.A. (1974) The effect of type and area of brain lesion on Wisconsin Card Sorting test performance. *Cortex* **10**, 159–170.

Dubois, B., Slachevsky, A., Litvan, I. & Billon, B. (2000) The FAB: a frontal assessment battery at bedside. *Neurology* **55**, 1621–1626.

Dudas, R.B., Berrios, G.E. & Hodges, J.R. (2005) The Addenbrooke's Cognitive Examination (ACE) in the differential diagnosis of early dementias versus affective disorder. *American Journal of Geriatric Psychiatry* **13**, 218–226.

Duffy, F.H., Burchfiel, J.L. & Lombroso, C.T. (1979) Brain electrical activity mapping (BEAM): a method for extending the clinical utility of EEG and evoked potential data. *Annals of Neurology* **5**, 309–321.

Ell, P.J. (2006) The contribution of PET/CT to improved patient management. *British Journal of Radiology* **79**, 32–36.

Erritzoe, D., Talbot, P., Frankle, W.G. & Abi-Dargham, A. (2003) Positron emission tomography and single photon emission CT molecular imaging in schizophrenia. *Neuroimaging Clinics of North America* **13**, 817–832.

Fagaly, R.L. (1990) Neuromagnetic instrumentation. *Advances in Neurology* 54, 11–32.

Fauser, S., Talazko, J., Wagner, K. *et al.* (2005) FDG-PET and MRI in potassium channel antibody-associated non-paraneoplastic limbic encephalitis: correlation with clinical course and neuropsychology. *Acta Neurologica Scandinavica* **111**, 338–343.

Fenton, G. (1974) The straightforward EEG in psychiatric practice. *Proceedings of the Royal Society of Medicine* **67**, 911–919.

Folstein, M.F., Folstein, S.E. & McHugh, P.R. (1975) 'Mini-mental state'. A practical method for grading the cognitive state of patients for the clinician. *Journal of Psychiatric Research* **12**, 189–198.

Fox, N.C. & Schott, J.M. (2004) Imaging cerebral atrophy: normal ageing to Alzheimer's disease. *Lancet* **363**, 392–394.

Frankle, W.G. & Laruelle, M. (2002) Neuroreceptor imaging in psychiatric disorders. *Annals of Nuclear Medicine* **16**, 437–446.

Fray, P., Robbins, T.W. & Sahakian, B.J. (1996) Neuropsychiatric applications of CANTAB. *International Journal of Geriatric Psychiatry* **11**, 329–336.

Friston, K.J., Frith, C.D., Liddle, P.F. & Frackowiak, R.S.J. (1991) Comparing functional (PET) images: the assessment of significant change. *Journal of Cerebral Blood Flow and Metabolism* **11**, 690–699.

Goldberg, D. & Murray R.M. (2006) *Maudsley Handbook of Practical Psychiatry*, 5th edn. Oxford University Press, Oxford.

Golding, E. (1989) *Middlesex Elderly Assessment of Mental State*. Thames Valley Test Company, Bury St Edmunds, UK.

Goldstein, K. (1942) *After Effects of Brain Injuries in War*. Grune & Stratton, New York.

Goldstein, K. & Sheerer, M. (1941) Abstract and concrete behaviour. An experimental study with special tests. *Psychological Monographs* **53** (2), 1–151.

Goldstein, L.H., Canavan, A.G.M. & Polkey, C.E. (1988) Verbal and abstract designs paired associate learning after unilateral temporal lobectomy. *Cortex* **24**, 41–52.

Goldstein, L.H., Bernard, S., Fenwick, P.B.C., Burgess, P.W. & McNeil, J. (1993) Unilateral frontal lobectomy can produce strategy application disorder. *Journal of Neurology, Neurosurgery and Psychiatry* **56**, 274–276.

Goodin, D.S. & Aminoff, M.J. (1986) Electrophysiological differences between subtypes of dementia. *Brain* **109**, 1103–1113.

Goodin, D.S., Aminoff, M.J., Chernoff, D.N. & Hollander, H. (1990) Long latency event-related potentials in patients infected with human immunodeficiency virus. *Annals of Neurology* **27**, 414–419.

Gordon, E., Kraiuhin, C., Harris, A., Meares, R. & Howson, A. (1986) The differential diagnosis of dementia using P300 latency. *Biological Psychiatry* **21**, 1123–1132.

Grafman, J., Jonas, B. & Salazar, A. (1990) Wisconsin Card Sorting Test performance based on location and size of neuroanatomical lesion in Vietnam veterans with penetrating head injury. *Perceptual and Motor Skills* **71**, 1120–1122.

Grey Walter, W., Cooper, R., Aldridge, V.J., McCallum, W.C. & Winter, A.L. (1964) Contingent negative variation: an electric sign of sensori-motor association and expectancy in the human brain. *Nature* **203**, 380–384.

Gurland, B.J., Fleiss, J.L., Goldberg, K. *et al.* (1976) A semistructured clinical interview for the assessment of diagnosis and mental state in the elderly: the Geriatric Mental State Schedule. II A factor analysis. *Psychological Medicine* **6**, 451–459.

Gurland, B.J., Kuriansky, J., Sharpe, L., Simon, R., Stiller, P. & Birkett, P. (1977) The Comprehensive Assessment and Referral Evaluation (CARE): rationale, development and reliability. *International Journal of Aging and Human Development* **8**, 9–42.

Halligan, P.W., Cockburn, J. & Wilson, B. (1991) The behavioural assessment of visual neglect. *Neuropsychological Rehabilitation* **1**, 5–32.

Haxby, J.V., Grady, C.L., Ungerleider, L.G. & Horwitz, B. (1991) Mapping the functional neuroanatomy of the intact human brain with brain work imaging. *Neuropsychologia* **29**, 539–555.

Henderson, A.S., Duncan-Jones, P. & Finlay-Jones, R.A. (1983) The reliability of the Geriatric Mental State Examination. Community survey version. *Acta Psychiatrica Scandinavica* **67**, 281–289.

Hill, D. & Watterson, D. (1942) Electroencephalographic studies of psychopathic personalities. *Journal of Neurology, Neurosurgery and Psychiatry* **5**, 47–65.

Holman, B.L., Gibson, R.E., Hill, T.C., Eckelman, W.C., Albert, M. & Reba, R.C. (1985) Muscarinic acetylcholine receptors in Alzheimer's disease: in vivo imaging with iodine 123-labelled 3-quinuclidinyl-4-iodobenzilate and emission tomography. *Journal of the American Medical Association* **254**, 3063–3066.

Hubbard, B.M. & Anderson, J.M. (1981) Age, senile dementia, and ventricular enlargement. *Journal of Neurology, Neurosurgery and Psychiatry* **44**, 631–635.

Hughes, J.R. & John, E.R. (1999) Conventional and quantitative electroencephalography in psychiatry. *Journal of Neuropsychiatry and Clinical Neurosciences* **11**, 190–208.

Irving, G., Robinson, R.A. & McAdam, W. (1970) The validity of some cognitive tests in the diagnosis of dementia. *British Journal of Psychiatry* **117**, 149–156.

Isaacs, B. & Walkey, F.A. (1964) A simplified paired-associate test for elderly hospital patients. *British Journal of Psychiatry* **110**, 80–83.

Isherwood, I. (1983) Principles of neuroradiology. In: Weatherall, D.J., Ledingham, J.G.G. & Warrell, D.A. (eds) *Oxford Textbook of Medicine*, vol. 2, pp. 21.4–21.9. Oxford University Press, Oxford.

Jacoby, R.J. & Levy, R. (1980) Computed tomography in the elderly. 2. Senile dementia: diagnosis and functional impairment. *British Journal of Psychiatry* **136**, 256–269.

Johnson, D.A.W. (1968) The evaluation of routine physical examination in psychiatric cases. *Practitioner* **200**, 686–691.

Johnstone, E.C., Crow, T.J., Frith, C.D., Husband, J. & Kreel, L. (1976) Cerebral ventricular size and cognitive impairment in chronic schizophrenia. *Lancet* **ii**, 924–926.

Jones-Gotman, M. & Milner, B. (1977) Design fluency: the invention of nonsense drawings after focal cortical lesions. *Neuropsychologia* **15**, 653–654.

Kales, H.C., Maixner, D.F. & Mellow, A.M. (2005) Cerebrovascular disease and late-life depression. *American Journal of Geriatric Psychiatry* **13**, 88–98.

Kapeller, P., Schmidt, R. & Fazelas, F. (2004) Qualitative MRI: evidence of usual aging in the brain. *Topics in Magnetic Resonance Imaging* **15**, 343–347.

Kaplan, E., Goodglass, H. & Weintraub, S. (1983) *Boston Naming Test*. Lea & Febiger, Philadelphia.

Kay, J., Lesser, R. & Coltheart, M. (1992) *Psycholinguistic Assessments of Language Processing in Aphasia (PALPA)*. Psychology Press, Hove, UK.

Kendrick, D.C., Parboosingh, R.-C. & Post, F. (1965) A synonym learning test for use with elderly psychiatric subjects: a validation study. *British Journal of Social and Clinical Psychology* **4**, 63–71.

Kendrick, D.C., Gibson, A.J. & Moyes, I.C.A. (1979) The revised Kendrick battery: clinical studies. *British Journal of Social and Clinical Psychology* **18**, 329–340.

Kennedy, P.G. (2005) Viral encephalitis. *Journal of Neurology* **252**, 268–272.

Keshavan, M.S. (1993) Magnetic resonance spectroscopy. *Schizophrenia Monitor* **3** (3), 1–3.

Keshavan, M.S., Kapur, S. & Pettegrew, J.W. (1991) Magnetic resonance spectroscopy in psychiatry: potential, pitfalls and promise. *American Journal of Psychiatry* **148**, 976–985.

Kiloh, L.G., McComas, A.J., Osselton, J.W. & Upton, A.R.M. (1981) *Clinical Electroencephalography*, 4th edn. Butterworth, London.

Kinsbourne, M. & Warrington, E.K. (1962) A study of finger agnosia. *Brain* **85**, 47–66.

Kopelman, M., Wilson, B. & Baddeley, A. (1990) *The Autobiographical Memory Interview*. Thames Valley Test Company, Bury St Edmunds, UK.

Koran, L.M., Sox, H.C., Marton, K.I. *et al.* (1989) Medical evaluation of psychiatric patients. *Archives of General Psychiatry* **46**, 733–740.

Kwong, K.K., Belliveau, J.W., Chesler, D.A. *et al.* (1992) Dynamic magnetic resonance imaging of human brain activity during primary sensory stimulation. *Proceedings of the National Academy of Sciences USA* **89**, 5675–5679.

Lagenstein, I., Willig, R.P. & Kuhne, D. (1979) Reversible cerebral atrophy caused by corticotrophin. *Lancet* **i**, 1246–1247.

Launer, L.J. (2003) Epidemiology of white-matter lesions. *International Psychogeriatrics* **15** (suppl. 1), 99–103.

Lee, J.-M. & Marcus, H.S. (2006) Does the white matter matter in Alzheimer disease and cerebral amyloid angiopathy? *Neurology* **66**, 6–7.

Leuchter, A.F., Daly, K.A., Rosenberg-Thompson, S. & Abrams, M. (1993) Prevalence and significance of electroencephalographic abnormalities in patients with suspected organic mental syndromes. *Journal of the American Geriatrics Society* **41**, 605–611.

Lezak, M.D. (1995) *Neuropsychological Assessment*, 3rd edn. Oxford University Press, New York.

Lhermitte, F. (1983) 'Utilization behaviour' and its relation to lesions of the frontal lobes. *Brain* **106**, 237–255.

Lhermitte, F., Pillon, B. & Serdaru, M. (1986) Human autonomy and the frontal lobes. Part I. Imitation and utilization behavior: a neuropsychological study of 75 patients. *Annals of Neurology* **19**, 326–334.

Lipowski, Z.J. (1990) *Delirium: Acute Confusional States*, 2nd edn. Oxford University Press, Oxford.

Lishman, W.A. (1992) Neuropsychiatry. A delicate balance. *Psychosomatics* **33**, 4–9.

List, S.J. & Cleghorn, J.M. (1993) Implications of positron emission tomography research for the investigation of the actions of antipsychotic drugs. *British Journal of Psychiatry* **163** (suppl. 22), 25–30.

Lorenz, J., Kunze, K. & Bromm, B. (1998) Differentiation of conversive sensory loss and malingering by P300 in a modified oddball task. *Neuroreport* **9**, 187–191.

Love, S. (2005) Neuropathological investigation of dementia: a guide for neurologists. *Journal of Neurology, Neurosurgery and Psychiatry* **76** (suppl. V), 8–14.

Luria, A.R. (1966) *Higher Cortical Functions in Man*. Tavistock Publications, London.

McGuire, P.K., Shah, G.M.S. & Murray, R.M. (1993) Increased blood flow in Broca's area during auditory hallucinations in schizophrenia. *Lancet* **342**, 703–706.

McKenna, P. & Warrington, E.K. (1983) *Graded Naming Test*. NFER-Nelson, Windsor, UK.

Maier, M. (1995) In vivo magnetic resonance spectroscopy. Applications in psychiatry. *British Journal of Psychiatry* **167**, 299–306.

Maier, M., Ron, M.A., Barker, G.J. & Tofts, P.S. (1995) Proton magnetic resonance spectroscopy: an in vivo method of estimating hippocampal neuronal depletion in schizophrenia. *Psychological Medicine* **25**, 1201–1209.

Malhi, G.S., Valenzuela, M., Wen, W. & Sachdev, P. (2002) Magnetic resonance spectroscopy and its applications in psychiatry. *Australian and New Zealand Journal of Psychiatry* **36**, 31–43.

Mallik, A. & Weir, A.I. (2005) Nerve conduction studies: essentials and pitfalls in practice. *Journal of Neurology, Neurosurgery and Psychiatry* **76**, ii23–ii31.

Manschreck, T.C., Maher, B.A., Winzig, L., Candela, S.F., Beaudette, S. & Boshes, R. (2000) Age disorientation in schizophrenia: an indicator of progressive and severe psychopathology, not institutional isolation. *Journal of Neuropsychiatry and Clinical Neurosciences* **12**, 350–358.

Margolin, D.I., Pate, D.S., Friedrich, F.J. & Elia, E. (1990) Dysnomia in dementia and in stroke patients: different underlying cognitive deficits. *Journal of Clinical and Experimental Neuropsychology* **12**, 597–612.

Mascalchi, M., Lolli, F., Nave, R.D. *et al.* (2004) Huntington disease: volumetric, diffusion-weighted, and magnetization transfer MR imaging of brain. *Radiology* **232**, 867–873.

Mathuranath, P.S., Nestor, P.J., Berrios, G.E., Rakowicz, W. & Hodges, J.R. (2000) A brief cognitive test battery to differentiate Alzheimer's disease and frontotemporal dementia. *Neurology* **55**, 1613–1620.

Matthews, P.M. & Jezzard, P. (2004) Functional magnetic resonance imaging. *Journal of Neurology, Neurosurgery and Psychiatry* **75**, 6–12.

Mattis, S. (1988) *Dementia Rating Scale*. Psychological Assessment Resources Inc., Odessa, FL.

Mazziotta, J.C. (2000) Imaging: window on the brain. *Archives of Neurology* **57**, 1413–1421.

Meltzer, C.C. (2003) (guest ed.) Neurological applications of PET. *Neuroimaging Clinics of North America* **13**, 653–871.

Meyer, J.S. & Gotoh, F. (1960) Metabolic and electroencephalographic effects of hyperventilation. *Archives of Neurology* **3**, 539–552.

Mills, K.R. (2005a) The basics of electromyography. *Journal of Neurology, Neurosurgery and Psychiatry* **76**, 32–35.

Mills, K.R. (2005b) Specialised electromyography and nerve conduction studies. *Journal of Neurology, Neurosurgery and Psychiatry* **76**, 36–40.

Milner, B. (1963) Effects of different brain lesions on card sorting. *Archives of Neurology* **9**, 90–100.

Morihisa, J.M. (1989) Computerized EEG and evoked potential mapping. In: Andreasen, N.C. (ed.) *Brain Imaging: Applications in Psychiatry*, ch. 3. American Psychiatric Press, Washington, DC.

Morris, R.G., Evenden, J.L., Sahakian, B.J. & Robbins, T.W. (1987) Computer-aided assessment of dementia: comparative studies of neuropsychological deficits in Alzheimer-type dementia and Parkinson's disease. In: Stahl, S.M., Iversen, S.D. & Goodman, E.C. (eds) *Cognitive Neurochemistry*, ch. 2. Oxford University Press, Oxford.

Morris, R.G., Worsley, C. & Matthews, D. (2000) Neuropsychological assessment in older people: old principles and new directions. *Advances in Psychiatric Treatment* **6**, 362–372.

Moseley, I. (1994) Safety and magnetic resonance imaging. *British Medical Journal* **308**, 1181–1182.

Musalek, M., Podreka, I., Walters, H. *et al.* (1989) Regional brain function in hallucinations: a study of regional cerebral blood flow with 99m-Tc-HMPAO-SPECT in patients with auditory hallucinations, tactile-hallucinations, and normal controls. *Comprehensive Psychiatry* **30**, 99–108.

Nelson, H.E. (1976) A modified card sorting test sensitive to frontal lobe defects. *Cortex* **12**, 313–324.

Nelson, H.E. (1982) *The National Adult Reading Test Manual*. NFER-Nelson, Windsor, UK.

Nelson, H.E. & McKenna, P. (1975) The use of current reading ability in the assessment of dementia. *British Journal of Social and Clinical Psychology* **14**, 259–267.

Nelson, H.E. & O'Connell, A. (1978) Dementia: the estimation of premorbid intelligence levels using the new adult reading test. *Cortex* **14**, 234–244.

Nelson, H.E. & Willison, J.R. (1991) *National Adult Reading Test*, 2nd edn. NFER-Nelson, Windsor, UK.

Neshige, R., Barrett, G. & Shibasaki, H. (1988) Auditory long latency event related potentials in Alzheimer's disease and multi-infarct dementia. *Journal of Neurology, Neurosurgery and Psychiatry* **51**, 1120–1125.

Newberg, A., Alavi, A. & Reivich, M. (2002) Determination of regional cerebral function with FDG-PET imaging in neuropsychiatric disorders. *Seminars in Nuclear Medicine* **32**, 13–34.

Obrecht, R., Okhomina, F.O.A. & Scott, D.F. (1979) Value of EEG in acute confusional states. *Journal of Neurology, Neurosurgery and Psychiatry* **42**, 75–77.

O'Carroll, R.E., Prentice, N., Murray, C., van Beck, M., Ebmeier, K.P. & Goodwin, G.M. (1995) Further evidence that reading ability is not preserved in Alzheimer's disease. *British Journal of Psychiatry* **167**, 659–662.

Ogawa, S., Tank, D.W., Menon, R. *et al.* (1992) Intrinsic signal changes accompanying sensory stimulation: functional brain mapping with magnetic resonance imaging. *Proceedings of the National Academy of Science USA* **89**, 5951–5955.

Osterrieth, P.-A. (1944) Le test de copie d'une figure complexe. Contribution à l'étude de la perception et de la mémoire. *Archives de Psychologie* **30**, 206–353.

Palazidou, E., Robinson, P. & Lishman, W.A. (1990) Neuroradiological and neuropsychological assessment in anorexia nervosa. *Psychological Medicine* **20**, 521–527.

Pardo, J.V., Pardo, P.J., Janer, K.W. & Raichle, M.E. (1990) The anterior cingulate cortex mediates processing selection in the Stroop attention of conflict paradigm. *Proceedings of the National Academy of Sciences USA* **87**, 256–259.

Parra, J., Kalitzin, S., da Silva, N. & Lopes, F.H. (2004) Magnetoencephalography: an investigational tool or a routine clinical technique? *Epilepsy and Behavior* **5**, 277–285.

Piccini, P. & Whone, A. (2004) Functional brain imaging in the differential diagnosis of Parkinson's disease. *Lancet Neurology* **3**, 284–290.

Piercy, M. (1959) Testing for intellectual impairment: some comments on the tests and the testers. *Journal of Mental Science* **105**, 489–495.

Pilowsky, L.S. (1996) Imaging receptors in psychiatry. In: Lewis, S. & Higgins, N. (eds) *Brain Imaging in Psychiatry*, ch. 7. Blackwell Science, Oxford.

Pilowsky, L.S., Costa, D.C., Ell, P.J., Verhoeff, N.P.L.G., Murray, R.M. & Kerwin, R.W. (1994) D_2 dopamine receptor binding in the basal ganglia of antipsychotic-free schizophrenic patients: an ^{123}I-IBZM single photon emission computerised tomography study. *British Journal of Psychiatry* **164**, 16–26.

Post, F. (1965) *The Clinical Psychiatry of Late Life*. Pergamon, Oxford.

Raven, J.C., Court, J.H. & Raven, J. (1992) *Manual for Raven's Progressive Matrices and Vocabulary Scales. Section 3: Standard Progressive Matrices*. H.K. Lewis, London.

Reeve, A., Rose, D.F. & Weinberger, D.R. (1989) Magnetoencephalography. Applications in psychiatry. *Archives of General Psychiatry* **46**, 573–576.

Reitan, R.M. (1958) Validity of the trail making test as an indicator of organic brain damage. *Perceptual and Motor Skills* **8**, 271–276.

Reitan, R.M. (1966) A research program on the psychological effects of brain lesions in human beings. In: Ellis, N.R. (ed.) *Inter-*

national Review of Research in Mental Retardation, vol. 1. Academic Press, New York.

Reite, M. (1990) Magnetoencephalography in the study of mental illness. *Advances in Neurology* **54**, 207–222.

Rey, A. (1941) L'examen psychologique dans les cas d'encéphalopathie traumatique. *Archives de Pathologie* **28**, 286–340.

Robbins, T.W. & Sahakian, B.J. (2002) Computer methods of assessment of cognitive function. In: Copeland, J.R.M., Abou-Saleh, M.T. & Blazer, D.G. (eds) *Principles and Practice of Geriatric Psychiatry*, pp. 147–151. John Wiley & Sons, Chichester.

Robbins, T.W., James, M., Owen, A.M. *et al.* (1998) A study of performance on tests from the CANTAB battery sensitive to frontal lobe dysfunction in a large sample of normal volunteers: implications for theories of executive functioning and cognitive ageing. *Journal of the International Neuropsychological Society* **4**, 474–490.

Roberts, J.K.A. & Lishman, W.A. (1984) The use of the CAT head scanner in clinical psychiatry. *British Journal of Psychiatry* **145**, 152–158.

Robertson, I.H., Ward, T., Ridgeway, V. & Nimmo-Smith, I. (1994) *Test of Everyday Attention*. Thames Valley Test Company, Bury St Edmunds, UK.

Robertson, I.H., Ward, T., Ridgeway, V. & Nimmo-Smith, I. (1996) The structure of normal human attention: the Test of Everyday Attention. *Journal of the International Neuropsychological Society* **2**, 525–534.

Rosvold, H.E., Mirsky, A.F., Sarason, I., Bransome, E.D. & Beck, L.H. (1956) A continuous performance test of brain damage. *Journal of Consulting Psychology* **20**, 343–350.

Roth, M., Huppert, F.A., Tym, E. & Mountjoy, C.Q. (1988) *CAMDEX. The Cambridge Examination for Mental Disorders of the Elderly*. Cambridge University Press, Cambridge.

Royall, D.R., Mahurin, R.K. & Gray, K. (1992) Bedside assessment of executive cognitive impairment: the executive interview (EXIT). *Journal of the American Geriatrics Society* **40**, 1221–1226.

Royall, D.R., Cordes, J.A. & Polk, M. (1998) CLOX: an executive clock drawing task. *Journal of Neurology, Neurosurgery and Psychiatry* **64**, 588–594.

Rusinek, H., De Santi, S., Frid, D. *et al.* (2003) Regional brain atrophy rate predicts future cognitive decline: 6-year longitudinal MR imaging study of normal aging. *Radiology* **229**, 691–696.

Russell, E.W., Neuringer, C. & Goldstein, G. (1970) *Assessment of Brain Damage*. Wiley, New York.

Sackheim, H.A., Prohovnik, I., Moeller, J.R. *et al.* (1990) Regional cerebral blood flow in mood disorders: 1. Comparison of major depressives and normal controls at rest. *Archives of General Psychiatry* **47**, 60–70.

Sandercock, P., Molyneux, A. & Warlow, C. (1985) Value of computed tomography in patients with stroke: Oxfordshire Community Stroke Project. *British Medical Journal* **290**, 193–197.

Schott, J.M., Price, S.L., Frost, C., Whitwell, J.L., Rossor, M.N. & Fox, N.C. (2005) Measuring atrophy in Alzheimer disease: a serial MRI study over 6 and 12 months. *Neurology* **65**, 119–124.

Shallice, T. (1982) Specific impairments of planning. In: Broadbent, D.E. & Weiskrantz, L. (eds) *The Neuropsychology of Cognitive Function*, pp. 199–209. Royal Society, London.

Shallice, T. & Burgess, P.W. (1991) Deficits in strategy application following frontal lobe damage in man. *Brain* **14**, 727–741.

Shallice, T. & Evans, M.E. (1978) The involvement of the frontal lobes in cognitive estimation. *Cortex* **14**, 294–303.

Sivan, A.B. (1992) *Benton Visual Retention Test*, 5th edn. Psychological Corporation, San Antonio, TX.

Smith, G.S., Koppel, J. & Goldberg, S. (2003) Applications of neuroreceptor imaging to psychiatry research. *Psychopharmacology Bulletin* **37**, 26–65.

Smith, S.J.M. (2005) EEG in neurological conditions other than epilepsy: when does it help, what does it add? *Journal of Neurology, Neurosurgery and Psychiatry* **76** (suppl. II), 8–12.

Stanley, J.A., Williamson, P.C., Drost, D.J., Carr, T., Rylett, J. & Merskey, H. (1992) In vivo proton magnetic resonance spectroscopy in never treated schizophrenics. New Research Abstracts 10. American Psychiatric Association, Washington, DC.

Stanley, J.A., Williamson, P.C., Drost, D.J., Carr, T., Rylett, J. & Merskey, H. (1993) The study of schizophrenia via in vivo ^{31}P and ^{1}H MRS. *Schizophrenia Research* **9**, 210.

Starkstein, S.E., Esteguy, M., Berthier, M.L., Garcia, H. & Leiguarda, R. (1989) Evoked potentials, reaction time and cognitive performance in on and off phases of Parkinson's disease. *Journal of Neurology, Neurosurgery and Psychiatry* **52**, 338–340.

Storm van Leeuwen, W., Bickford, R., Brazier, M. *et al.* (1966) Proposal for an EEG terminology by the terminology committee of the International Federation for Electroencephalography and Clinical Neurophysiology. *Electroencephalography and Clinical Neurophysiology* **20**, 306–310.

Stroop, J.R. (1935) Studies of interference in serial verbal reactions. *Journal of Experimental Psychology* **18**, 643–662.

Sutton, S., Braren, M., Zubin, J. & John, E.R. (1965) Evoked-potential correlates of stimulus uncertainty. *Science* **150**, 1187–1188.

Thomas, A.J., O'Brien, J.T., Davis, S. *et al.* (2002) Ischemic basis for deep white matter hyperintensities in major depression: a neuropathological study. *Archives of General Psychiatry* **59**, 785–792.

Toone, B. (1984) The electroencephalogram. In: McGuffin, P., Shanks, M.F. & Hodgson, R.J. (eds) *The Scientific Principles of Psychopathology*. Grune & Stratton, London.

Trenerry, M.R., Crosson, B., Deboe, J. & Leber, W.R. (1989) *Stroop Neuropsychological Screening Test Manual*. Psychological Assessment Resources, Odessa, FL.

Trzepacz, P.T., Hertweck, M., Starratt, C., Zimmerman, L. & Adatepe, M.H. (1992) The relationship of SPECT scans to behavioral dysfunction in neuropsychiatric patients. *Psychosomatics* **33**, 62–71.

Tulsky, D.S. (2004) A new look at the WMS-III: new research to guide clinical practice. *Journal of Clinical and Experimental Neuropsychology* **26**, 453–458.

Tulsky, D.S. & Haaland, K. (2001) Exploring the clinical utility of WAIS-III and WMS-III. *Journal of the International Neuropsychological Society* **7**, 860–862.

Tyler, K.L. (2004) Update on herpes simplex encephalitis. *Reviews in Neurological Diseases* **1**, 169–178.

Van der Flier, W.M. & Scheltens, P (2005) Use of laboratory and imaging investigations in dementia. *Journal of Neurology, Neurosurgery and Psychiatry* **76** (suppl. 5), 45–52.

Van der Knaap, M.S., van der Grond, J., Luyten, P.R., Den Hollander, J.A., Nauta, J.J.P. & Valk, J. (1992) ^{1}H and ^{31}P magnetic resonance spectroscopy of the brain in degenerative cerebral disorders. *Annals of Neurology* **31**, 202–211.

Van Gorp, W.G., Satz, P., Kiersch, M.E. & Henry, R. (1986) Normative data on the Boston Naming Test for a group of normal older adults. *Journal of Clinical and Experimental Neuropsychology* **8**, 702–705.

Vermeer, S.E., Prins, N.D., den Heijer, T., Hofman, A., Koudstaal, P.J. & Breteler, M.M. (2003) Silent brain infarcts and the risk of dementia and cognitive decline. *New England Journal of Medicine* **348**, 1215–1222.

Walsh, P., Kane, N. & Butler, S. (2005) The clinical role of evoked potentials. *Journal of Neurology, Neurosurgery and Psychiatry* **76** (suppl. II), 16–22.

Walton, J. (1993) Disorders of function in the light of anatomy and physiology. In: Walton, J. (ed.) *Brain's Diseases of the Nervous System*, 10th edn, ch. 1. Oxford University Press, Oxford.

Warrington, E.K. (1970) Neurological deficits. In: Mittler, P. (ed.) *The Psychological Assessment of Mental and Physical Handicaps*. Methuen, London.

Warrington, E.K. (1974) Deficient recognition memory in organic amnesia. *Cortex* **10**, 289–291.

Warrington, E.K. (1984) *Manual for Recognition Memory Test for Words and Faces*. NFER-Nelson, Windsor, UK.

Warrington, E.K. (1996) *The Camden Memory Test Battery*. Psychology Press, Hove, UK.

Warrington, E.K. & James, M. (1991) *The Visual Object and Space Perception Battery*. Thames Valley Test Company, Bury St Edmunds, UK.

Watson, J.D.G. (1991) The current state of positron emission tomography. *British Journal of Hospital Medicine* **46**, 163–166.

Wechsler, D. (1997) *Wechsler Adult Intelligence Scale – 3rd Edition (WAIS-3)*. Harcourt Assessment, San Antonio, TX.

Weinberger, D.R., Gibson, R., Coppola, R. *et al.* (1991) The distribution of cerebral muscarinic acetylcholine receptors in vivo in patients with dementia: a controlled study with [123]IQNB and single photon emission computed tomography. *Archives of Neurology* **48**, 169–176.

Wilson, B.A. (1987) *Rehabilitation of Memory*. Guilford Press, New York.

Wilson, B.A., Cockburn, J. & Halligan, P. (1987) *Behavioural Inattention Test*. Thames Valley Test Company, Fareham, UK.

Wilson, B.A., Cockburn, J. & Baddeley, A. (1991) *The Rivermead Behavioural Memory Test*, 2nd edn. Thames Valley Test Company, Bury St Edmunds, UK.

Wilson, B.A., Alderman, N., Burgess, P.W., Emsliè, H. & Evans, J.J. (1996) Behavioural Assessment of Dysexecutive Syndrome. Thames Valley Test Company, Bury St Edmunds, UK.

Wilson, B.A., Kopelman, M.D. & Kapur, N. (2008) Prominent and persistent loss of past awareness in amnesia: delusion, impaired consciousness or coping strategy? *Neuropsychological Rehabilitation* **18**, 527–540.

Wright, C.E., Harding, G.F.A. & Orwin, A. (1984) Presenile dementia: the use of the flash and pattern VEP in diagnosis. *Electroencephalography and Clinical Neurophysiology* **57**, 405–415.

Yaretzky, A., Lif-Kimchi, O., Finkeltov, B. *et al.* (2000) Reliability and validity of the Middlesex Elderly Assessment of Mental State (MEAMS) among hospitalised elderly in Israel as a predictor of functional potential. *Clinical Gerontologist* **21**, 91–98.

Zeidler, M., Sellar, R.J., Collie, D.A. *et al.* (2000) The pulvinar sign on magnetic resonance imaging in variant Creutzfeldt–Jakob disease. *Lancet* **355**, 1412–1418.

Zeki, S., Watson, J.D.G., Lueck, C.J., Friston, K.J., Kennard, C. & Frackowiak, R.S.J. (1991) A direct demonstration of functional specialisation in human visual cortex. *Journal of Neuroscience* **11**, 641–649.

PART 2

Specific disorders

CHAPTER 4

Head Injury

Simon Fleminger

Maudsley Hospital, London

The size of the problem presented by head injuries to medical services and to the economy generally is immense. About 200 per 100 000 population per year suffer a head injury (Bruns & Hauser 2003). In the majority of these the head injury is classified as mild (Sorenson & Kraus 1991), yet perhaps as many as 100 per 100 000 per year go on to suffer significant disability at 1 year (Thornhill *et al.* 2000). Many of these people are young and will suffer long-term disability. As noted by Headway, the UK national head injury association, a 'head injury is for life'. In 1991 the economic cost in the USA was put at more than $48 billion per year (Krauss & Chu 2005). However, in the developed world, head injuries may be declining, probably reflecting better road safety, at least in part. Thus in the USA over the period 1980–1995 there was a 50% reduction in hospitalisation for head injury (Thurman & Guerrero 1999). The outlook in the developing world may be less encouraging. High levels of two-wheeled vehicle use, rapidly increasing car ownership but poorly developed road safety infrastructure, and lack of ambulances mean that disability due to head injury is on the increase (Gururaj 2002). The vast majority of head injuries in civilian life are closed injuries and result from acceleration/deceleration forces. When the term 'head injury' is used in this chapter it will by and large refer to closed head injury. Risk factors for sustaining a traumatic brain injury (TBI), synonymous with head injury, include male sex, younger age (peak at 15–24 years with a smaller peak in the elderly), alcohol, lower socioeconomic status and a psychiatric history (Fann *et al.* 2004).

Early mortality has been considerably improved as a result of advances in the management of the early acute stages. However, the chronic sequelae remain as a serious challenge to medical care and communal resources, and this can only be reflected very approximately in statistics. Quite apart from the physical sequelae, the psychiatric consequences and their social repercussions may be judged to be signifi-cant in upwards of one-quarter of patients who survive. Precise figures are hard to obtain because it is clear that many patients, even with severe incapacities, do not present them-selves for continuing medical attention. What is virtually certain is that the mental sequelae outstrip the physical as a cause of difficulty with rehabilitation, hardship at work and social incapacity generally, and in terms of the strain thrown on the families to whom the head-injured patient returns (Thomsen 1984).

Fahy *et al.*'s (1967) follow-up of a small group of very severe civilian head injuries vividly illustrates the amount of distur-bance enduring 6 years later. Only 5 of 22 patients were free from psychiatric sequelae, and psychiatric disturbance was a prominent cause of incapacity for work. Problems in the home included affective outbursts, chronic irritability, epileptiform and hallucinatory episodes and paranoid developments, in addition to impairment of intellectual processes. Yet only two of the patients had been referred for psychiatric advice during the follow-up period. It appears therefore that the psychiatrist sees only a small proportion of the problem (Deb *et al.* 1999a).

The acute phases of care following a head injury are pri-marily the province of the casualty officer, neurologist or neurosurgeon. Rehabilitation teams composed of thera-pists, with medical input usually from a rehabilitation physician or neurologist, manage the sequelae. However, neuropsychologists and psychiatrists are increasingly taking a central role in the rehabilitation phase, helping to ensure that the important long-term neuropsychiatric sequelae are properly managed. The greater part of this chapter is devoted to the long-term mental sequelae of head injury. Nevertheless, correct evaluation of the mechanisms which underlie the longer-term disturbances needs to be based on a proper understanding of the acute effects of head injury.

Lishman's Organic Psychiatry: A Textbook of Neuropsychiatry, 4th edition.
© 2009 Blackwell Publishing.   ISBN 978-1-4051-1860-1

Pathology and pathophysiology

Biomechanics of concussion and traumatic brain injury

Concussion may be defined as an immediate and transient alteration or loss of consciousness, or other disturbance of neurological function, when sudden mechanical forces are applied to the head. Using video analysis of concussions in football players (Pellman *et al.* 2003) and data from accelerometers placed in their helmets (Duma *et al.* 2005), it has been possible to estimate the acceleration/deceleration of the head during concussive head injuries as of the order of 80–100 *g* over 15 ms.

Loss of consciousness is particularly likely to follow acceleration/deceleration injuries where there is a rotational component. Rotations round a coronal axis, i.e. with the head moving from side to side, are probably more likely to produce loss of consciousness than rotation around the sagittal axis as in a nodding movement of the head (Smith & Meaney 2000). This may explain why impacts to the temporoparietal area are most likely to produce concussion (McIntosh *et al.* 2000). Presumably rotational forces are particularly likely to produce the swirling movement of the brain that has been observed in monkeys after acceleration injury (Pudenz & Shelden 1946). Side impacts in car accidents are possibly more likely to be associated with severe head injury, perhaps because of the side-to-side forces as the head hits the pillar between the front and rear doors (Nirula *et al.* 2003). It was suggested that if the force is applied to the face, causing facial fractures, this acts as a buffer reducing the brain injury (Löken 1959). However, a more recent study suggests this is not the case and that, in those presenting to accident and emergency departments, a facial fracture increases the likelihood of brain injury (Keenan *et al.* 1999).

Static crush closed head injuries, in which there is no acceleration/deceleration of the brain, are relatively unlikely to produce loss of consciousness (Russell & Schiller 1949). This was confirmed in a series of bitemporal crush injuries (Gonzalez Tortosa *et al.* 2004); less than half had loss of consciousness whereas all had basal skull fractures, pneumocephalus and otorrhagia. The majority also had injury to cranial nerves VI and VII and diabetes insipidus.

In open head injuries the dura is breached and laceration of brain tissue is present at the site of impact but contrecoup is slight or even absent. The extent of the damage in open head injuries depends on the velocity of the object. Penetrating injury from a knife or spike causes localised damage around the track. Shrapnel injuries tend to be quite low velocity, producing localised damage. However, bullet wounds, particularly from modern high-velocity rifles, produce massive shock waves throughout the brain causing widespread damage and usually death.

Pathology of head injury

The more severe injuries that come to post-mortem examination show a variety of pathological changes. Some are the result of direct physical damage to the brain parenchyma, and some the result of complicating factors such as vascular disturbances, cerebral oedema and anoxia. In penetrating injuries infection may be superadded.

Contusions

Severe contusions comprise a mixture of haemorrhage and necrosis, typically near the surface of the brain, due to severe localised forces. In an individual injury, determining where the head was hit, and the direction of the forces, is often difficult. For example, in a road traffic accident there may be more than one blow to the head in quick succession. Thus the concept of contrecoup injury, with contusions occurring on the side opposite the injury, is often not a reliable predictor of contusion location. What is more telling is that there are certain sites of predilection: the orbital surface of the frontal lobes, particularly medially, and the underside and tips of the temporal lobe (Fig. 4.1). Presumably these are the sites where the brain is most at risk of being traumatised by the hard skull. When the head is at rest at the time of injury, as in assault, the lesion will be maximal at the site of impact, but when in motion, as in falls or traffic accidents, the contrecoup effect is likely to be most pronounced (Bloomquist & Courville 1947; Löken 1959).

Diffuse axonal injury

As already described, acceleration/deceleration injuries produce swirling movements throughout the brain. The resulting rotational and linear stresses tear and damage nerve fibres throughout the brain. The diffuse interruption and degeneration of nerve fibres, with breakdown and resorption of myelin and the formation of retraction balls, is called diffuse axonal injury. First reported in patients dying after very severe brain injuries, it is likely that similar changes occur in some patients with mild closed injuries as well (Strich 1956, 1969; Teasdale & Mendelow 1984). The changes are mainly confined to the parasagittal central white matter and the grey–white matter interface of the hemispheres (Fig. 4.2), the corpus callosum, and the long tracts in the brainstem. With more severe injuries small haemorrhages are seen, particularly in the corpus callosum and the parasagittal white matter.

In the longer term, severe diffuse axonal injury produces ventriculomegaly with thinning of the corpus callosum, often in the absence of sulcal enlargement. Clinically, it may present with prolonged loss of consciousness in the absence of intracerebral contusions, and later result in neurological sequelae related to damage to white matter tracts in the brainstem, particularly the superior cerebellar peduncle, with for example slurring of speech and ataxia. Diffuse axonal injury is now sometimes used to describe a clinical

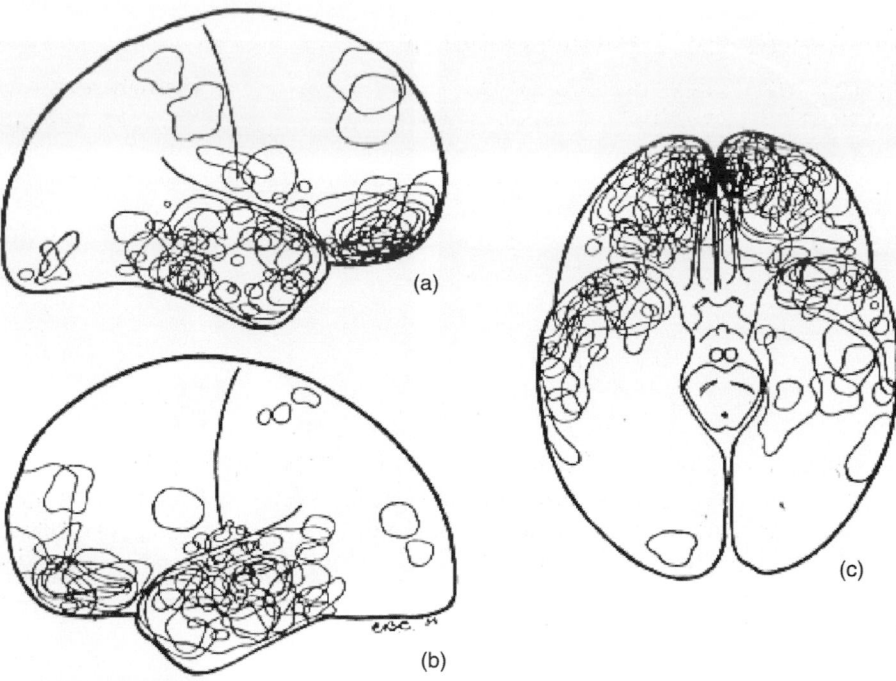

Fig. 4.1 Contusions after closed head injury: composite from 50 post-mortem cases. (From Courville 1937 with permission.)

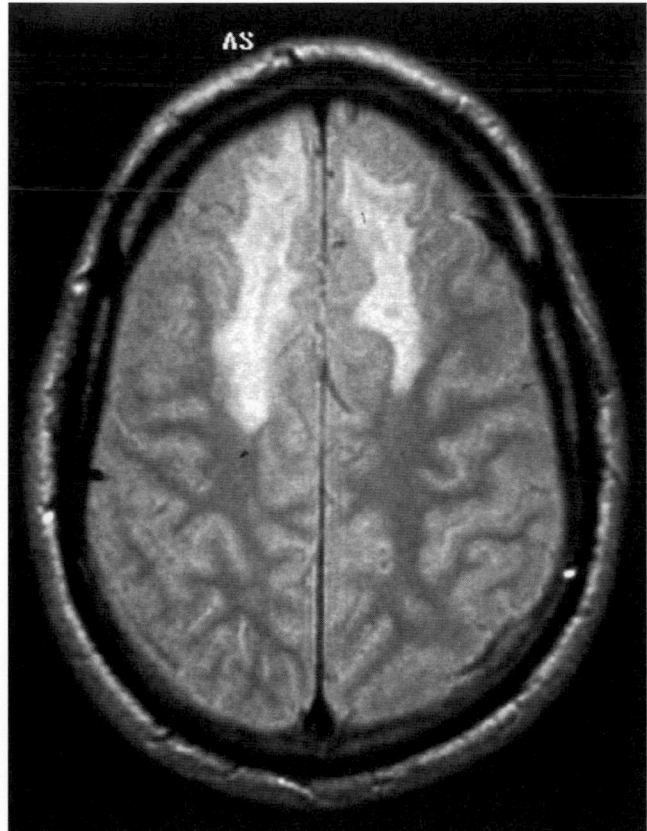

Fig. 4.2 Diffuse axonal injury shown as high signal in white matter on MRI T2 image several months after a closed head injury with about 30 minutes loss of consciousness. Posteriorly, the white matter appears normal, dark grey on T2. Anteriorly, there is high signal in the white matter. Note the flame-shaped appearance, partly because the highest signal tends to be near the white–grey matter interface, as is typical of diffuse axonal injury.

syndrome of diffuse injury where loss of consciousness is not explained by focal lesions. For example, Katz and Alexander (1994) defined patients with diffuse axonal injury as those with (i) acceleration/deceleration injury, (ii) immediate loss of consciousness and (iii) computed tomography (CT) and magnetic resonance imaging (MRI) findings of petechial white matter haemorrhages, isolated intraventricular or subarachnoid haemorrhage, diffuse swelling or normal scan. However, the use of what is essentially a neuropathological term to define a clinical syndrome in the absence of histological confirmation needs to be treated with a little circumspection.

Other sequelae

Vascular lesions

Vascular lesions include scattered punctate haemorrhages throughout the brain, along with large and small infarcts. Sometimes the whole or part of the territory of a major cerebral artery may become necrotic. Such vascular lesions probably result from a combination of factors: reduced cerebral blood flow immediately after the injury, hypotension, embolism, pre-existing atheroma, rise of intracranial pressure sufficient to occlude the arteries, and spasm of vessels due to mechanical strain at the junction of brain and vessel (Strich 1969; Graham & Adams 1971). Posterior cerebral artery strokes occur when tentorial herniation, due to brain swelling, compresses the artery (Fig. 4.3). Dissection of the major cerebral arteries, both carotid and vertebrobasilar, is a recognised complication; for example unexpected subintimal dissection of the middle cerebral artery was found in three cases with massive cerebral infarction (Rutherfoord *et al.* 1996).

(a)

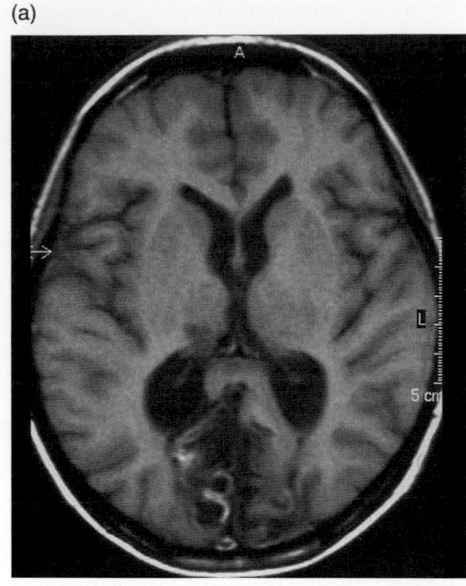

(b)

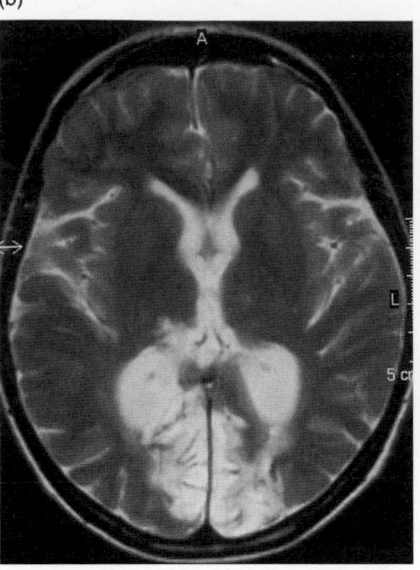

Fig. 4.3 Posterior cerebral artery infarct following head injury. (a) T1-weighted and (b) T2-weighted MRI brain scans of a woman in her fifties several months after a severe head injury with several days' coma. On recovery of consciousness she was blind. She initially denied any problems with her eyesight, but gradually acknowledged that she was unable to see. However, she developed the persistent delusion, which lasted several years, that her eyesight would recover fully if she kept to a special high-protein diet. She would become very angry and querulous if the diet that she demanded was not offered. She required long-term residential care, partly because of moderate cognitive impairment, but also because she always refused to accept any rehabilitation or aids to help her cope with her blindness.

Patients, particularly children (Kieslich *et al.* 2002), are therefore at risk of stroke in the days following injury.

Extensive bleeding may occur into the subarachnoid space, with the appearance of blood in the cerebrospinal fluid (CSF). Subdural haematomas may collect and become organised over the cerebral hemispheres. Blood collecting in the basal cisterns or over the surface of the brain may later lead to organised adhesions that obstruct the flow of CSF and lead to hydrocephalus. Bleeding into the brain tissue itself may result in an intracerebral haematoma.

Cerebral oedema

Cerebral oedema may develop in the acute stages and further complicate the picture. It is especially liable to occur in the region of contusions, lacerations, infarcts and haematomas. Cellular mechanisms, rather than breakdown of the blood–brain barrier, may be predominantly responsible (Marmarou *et al.* 2000). Diffuse cerebral swelling is more common in children (Kazan *et al.* 1997). The raised intracranial pressure that results can have serious consequences in terms of herniation of brain tissue through the tentorium and under the falx cerebri. If severe, such 'coning' may be fatal. Less severe cases can be followed by focal necrosis and haemorrhage in the medial temporal lobe structures and brainstem around the aqueduct and fourth ventricle (Duret's haemorrhages).

Cerebral anoxia

Cerebral anoxia is a common consequence of head injury. The anoxia will derive not only from cerebral oedema and other local changes, but also from hypotension, blood loss, disturbances in regulation of the cerebral circulation, and ventilatory insufficiency in the acute stages. In the 'golden

hour' after injury, maintenance of arterial oxygenation and blood pressure are crucial to management. Neuronal damage from anoxia will be aggravated by increased metabolic demand and accounts for various pathological findings, such as cortical necrosis in the depths of the cortical sulci, lesions in Ammon's horn and the basal ganglia, and the disappearance of Purkinje cells from the cerebellum. Cases studied early after injury show widespread chromatolysis in neurones both in the brainstem and throughout the cortex. The importance of early metabolic and neurochemical derangements in leading to brain damage is also increasingly recognised (see below).

In children after non-accidental brain injury it has been proposed that in many the brain injury is due to global hypoxia as a result of apnoea following damage to the craniocervical junction (Geddes *et al.* 2001); relatively few children dying from 'shaken baby' syndrome showed evidence of diffuse axonal injury, whereas the most common finding was global hypoxic damage.

Open head injuries

In open head injuries the skull and dural coverings are perforated. Extensive local laceration may lead to large cystic cavities and ventricular dilatations. Haemorrhage may occur locally, and infection is an ever-present risk. Small fractures in the neighbourhood of the nasal sinuses may pave the way for meningitis or local abscess formation. Following gunshot wounds, cerebral artery spasm (associated with subarachnoid bleeding) may be seen (Kordestani *et al.* 1997). The fibroglial scar that follows open head injury and which may produce distortion and traction on the brain may explain the high risk of late epilepsy.

Pathophysiology: biochemical and physiological changes

Though they share much in common, particularly in the case of more severe injury, it is useful to consider on the one hand the processes that result in loss of consciousness and on the other those which result in cell damage (Nortje & Menon 2004). In the latter, it may be valuable to distinguish between the mechanisms involved in diffuse axonal injury (white matter) and those causing neuronal cell death (grey matter). These issues are reviewed in Povlishock and Katz (2005).

Loss of consciousness and coma

The pathophysiology of loss of consciousness is poorly understood, particularly for milder head injuries (McCrory et al. 2001). The cardinal symptoms of concussion point to a major involvement of brainstem centres. In addition to loss of consciousness there is respiratory arrest, generalised vasoconstriction, loss of corneal reflexes and paralysis of deglutition. Concussive convulsions, i.e. non-epileptic seizures immediately following the impact (McCrory et al. 1997), may arise in the brainstem, supporting the argument for brainstem involvement. Experimental concussion in monkeys produces surprisingly little effect on cortical electroencephalographic (EEG) rhythms and far more disturbance in the medial reticular formation (Ward 1966). Studies suggesting that cholinergic systems may be involved (Hayes et al. 1989) perhaps point to brainstem structures. On the other hand, it has been proposed that the forces and resulting injury usually spread centripetally, from the cortex to the brainstem (Ommaya & Gennarelli 1974), in which case only more severe head injuries affect the brainstem. However, it is probable that this hypothesis best explains the consequences of head injury that result in permanent physical damage to the brain, which may be rather different from effects that produce transient unconsciousness at milder levels of injury. Others have argued that mechanically induced cellular depolarisation, perhaps localised to the brainstem or a more diffuse cortical effect, is critical. One plausible mechanism, perhaps of greater relevance to injury resulting in coma of more than a few minutes, is that the trauma results in massive and rapid release of potassium into the extracellular space (Maroon et al. 2000). This is associated with excessive glutamate release and produces depolarisation of neurones and unconsciousness. This is then followed by a hypermetabolic state as Na^+/K^+ pumps are activated to restore extracellular potassium levels to normal.

Histological studies can provide only indirect evidence of the mechanism of loss of consciousness, especially since mild concussion may represent loss of function without structural alteration. Neuronal changes have been shown in the brainstem of animals in proportion to the strength of the blows inflicted (Windle & Groat 1944; Groat & Simmons 1950), but these may be secondary to cervical cord damage occasioned by bending and stretching of the neck (Friede 1961). The MRI evidence discussed under Neuroimaging and head injury (later in chapter) suggests that hemisphere damage may be associated with loss of consciousness, with brainstem mechanisms suffering secondarily. However, prolonged coma and death is associated with pathology in the upper brainstem (Jellinger & Seitelberger 1969; Firsching et al. 2002; Wedekind et al. 2002) and thalamus (Maxwell et al. 2004), and with severe diffuse axonal injury (Jennett et al. 2001). Unsurprisingly, raised intracranial pressure early after injury predicts poor prognosis (Signorini et al. 1999a) and is likely to be one factor contributing to coma.

Diffuse axonal injury

Experimental models of injury have indicated that the changes of diffuse axonal injury take hours to develop (Povlishock & Coburn 1989). At the moment of impact there is little evidence of axons being torn apart, but their axolemma is damaged by the stretching and compression forces. This allows calcium to enter the axon, activating proteases that damage the intracellular structures (neurofilaments and microtubules) necessary for axoplasmic transport. Transport products accumulate, resulting in axonal swelling, lobulation, and ultimately transection with formation of the classic *retraction ball* over the course of the first day or two. Over the ensuing weeks and months attempts at regrowth and regeneration can be observed, with sprouting from the proximal segment. Damaged axons can be seen lying adjacent to intact fibres. The observation that diffuse axonal injury takes hours to develop, rather than being an irreversible effect of the impact itself, lends support to the maxim that care of the patient in the first few hours following a severe injury is critical to outcome.

The β-amyloid precursor protein (βAPP) is transported along axons but only becomes detectable by immunocytochemical staining when the axonal transport systems are disrupted and it accumulates. It has been used as a sensitive marker for diffuse axonal injury; βAPP staining is evident within 1–2 hours of injury and can then be used to track the axonal swelling and formation of axonal bulbs over the first few hours after injury (McKenzie et al. 1996; Wilkinson et al. 1999). High levels are found following closed head injury, for example due to falls (Abou-Hamden et al. 1997). βAPP staining has broadened the concept of diffuse axonal injury; it is observed before changes are observed on routine histopathology using silver staining (Geddes et al. 2000). However, the greater sensitivity of βAPP staining has come at the expense of less specificity; it is to be found in many patients without TBI, for example in those dying from opiate overdose (Niess et al. 2002). This may be explained by the finding that anoxic brain injury produces βAPP staining, although the pattern of staining is probably different from that in TBI (Kaur et al. 1999). Therefore some now distinguish traumatic diffuse axonal injury from other causes of diffuse axonal injury.

Neuronal death

To understand the processes leading to cell death after TBI it is useful to distinguish necrotic from apoptotic mechanisms (Povlishock & Katz 2005), although the cellular mechanisms involved probably overlap and elevated intracellular calcium is common to both. Both involve neurones and glia. Necrotic cell death is produced by cellular disruption, either from the destructive forces of the trauma on the cell membrane or due to ischaemia for example related to intracerebral contusion/haemorrhage. Necrotic cell death is rapid and relatively passive, with swelling of cytoplasm and mitochondria. Various processes may contribute, including the toxic effects of excitatory neurotransmitters, particularly glutamate (Faden *et al.* 1989), mitochondrial dysfunction (Robertson 2004), calcium activation of proteases and phospholipases, formation of toxic free radicals and low intracellular magnesium. Immunological processes may also be involved (Schmidt *et al.* 2005), including activation of interleukins (Tasci *et al.* 2003).

On the other hand, apoptosis, or programmed cell death, is a much more active process with a variety of triggers, including ligand binding to specific cell death receptors on the surface of the cell (e.g. FAS), resulting in alterations of the balance within the cell of pro- and anti-apoptotic pathways, in particular the Bcl-2 family of proteins. Caspases, which cleave proteins, are central to the pathways causing cell death, one of which involves the activation of endonucleases that attack the cell's DNA, producing DNA fragments. Terminal deoxynucleotide transferase-mediated nick end labelling (TUNEL) of DNA fragments allows apoptotic cells to be identified histochemically. Evidence of apoptosis is seen in the majority of patients after severe injury, much of it within white matter as early as 45 minutes after injury, maximal at a few days and sometimes lasting over a year (Smith *et al.* 2000; Williams *et al.* 2001; Hausmann *et al.* 2004; Wilson *et al.* 2004). Studies examining tissue taken in the course of therapeutic evacuation of severe contusions have demonstrated changes in the pro-apoptotic proteins Bax and caspase, and the anti-apoptotic protein Bcl (Ng *et al.* 2000; Nathoo *et al.* 2004); patients lacking Bcl had worse outome. Tissue taken at surgery has also demonstrated upregulation of the FAS receptor death-inducing signalling complex within a few hours of injury (Qiu *et al.* 2002), and expression of c-Fos and c-Jun mRNA, which may relate to activation of apoptotic pathways, with greater expression associated with worse outcome at 1 year (Whitfield & Pickard 2000).

Both necrotic and apoptotic cell death are seen in focal injury, e.g. contusions, with necrotic cell death being predominant in the core of the damaged area, and apoptotic cell death being observed in the pericontusional zone (Liou *et al.* 2003; Hausmann *et al.* 2004). Of special interest is the diffuse neuronal death seen throughout the brain but particularly in the cortex, hippocampus (Maxwell *et al.* 2003) and diencephalon. This may be due to anoxia associated with the trauma, but animal models suggest that mechanical disruption to the membrane is also involved, triggering both necrotic and apoptotic pathways. However, axonal transection, due to diffuse axonal injury, does not necessarily cause the neuronal soma to die. On the other hand, neurotrophic factors may counter the effects facilitating cell death (Chiaretti *et al.* 2003).

Other sequelae
Ventriculomegaly

Enlargement of the lateral ventricles, and to a lesser extent the third and fourth ventricles, is common after severe TBI (Mazzini *et al.* 2003). Usually regarded as due to cerebral atrophy, particularly of white matter, a key clinical question is whether ventriculomegaly is in fact, in that particular patient, due to blockage of the free flow of CSF, with or without elevated intracranial pressure. This is discussed further in the section on neuroimaging.

Effects on cerebral metabolism

In the immediate aftermath of brain injury, post-traumatic biochemical changes (see above) are likely to increase metabolic demand. Alcoholics will be particularly at risk; in hospital they will effectively be in an alcohol withdrawal state, known to increase the metabolic activity of the brain, in the first few days after injury. It has been suggested that a common pattern after head injury is for there to be normal or low flow rates in the first 24 hours, succeeded by relative hyperaemia ('luxury' perfusion) that may persist for many days (Overgaard & Tweed 1974). Correspondingly, increased cerebral glucose uptake is found in the first 3–4 days after severe brain injury (Bergsneider *et al.* 1997). This is then followed by somewhat reduced uptake 1–3 weeks after injury and then gradual recovery over the course of 1 year (Bergsneider *et al.* 2001). However, similar changes in glucose uptake are seen in mild head injury (Bergsneider *et al.* 2000), suggesting that the causes of the changes in glucose uptake are multifactorial. For example, intraparenchymal haemorrhagic lesions may produce increased or reduced uptake.

Global reductions in blood flow after head injury are associated with worse outcome (Bouma *et al.* 1991). Oxygen delivery is further jeopardised by poor diffusion from the capillary to the cell (Menon *et al.* 2004). Disordered autoregulation (Nortje & Menon 2004) may contribute to a mismatch between cerebral blood flow and metabolism. Patients with very severe injury show reduced oxygen and glucose utilisation in grey matter (Glenn *et al.* 2003). Those with lower cerebral metabolic rates have worse outcomes, and reductions in deep structures relate to prolonged coma. In white matter, a mismatch between increased glucose metabolism but without increased oxygen consumption may be seen (Wu *et al.* 2004).

Aβ peptide deposition

Of interest to the proposal that head injury may be a risk factor for Alzheimer's disease (see Chapter 9) is the observation that Aβ peptides, which are produced by cleavage of βAPP (see above) and which aggregate to form β-amyloid protein, have been found to accumulate in about 30% of patients after TBI and may form plaques (Roberts *et al.* 1994; Ikonomovic *et al.* 2004), similar to those seen in Alzheimer's disease. However, some groups have failed to find elevated Aβ after head injury (Adle-Biassette *et al.* 1996; Macfarlane *et al.* 1999).

The ε4 allele of apolipoprotein E (ApoE) is known to be a risk factor for Alzheimer's and other neurological diseases, perhaps related to effects on Aβ metabolism. Several studies have therefore looked at the relationship between ApoE ε4 status and head injury outcome. Most studies that have examined this have found that ε4-positive status (whether homozygous or heterozygous) is associated with worse outcome (Table 4.1). Two large prospective studies have failed to find an effect in both mild (Chamelian *et al.* 2004) and more severe (Teasdale *et al.* 2005) head injuries, but in moderate to severe injury the evidence overall does suggest that those who are ApoE ε4 positive do worse, both in terms of early and late outcomes.

Cell regeneration/plasticity

It is now evident that cells in the adult mammalian brain can divide and develop into new neurones, particularly in the hippocampus and subventricular zones, but also in the neocortex (Magavi *et al.* 2000) and that these cells can form long-distance corticothalamic connections. There is evidence of cell proliferation in rat brain after TBI, although no evidence of development of neurones was found (Chirumamilla *et al.* 2002). These findings are of interest to human recovery from

Table 4.1 Apolipoprotein (Apo)E status and outcome after head injury.

	Mild	Mixed/uncertain	Moderate/severe
Early effects	Worse on speed measures (PASAT and Pegboard) at 3 weeks* (1)	No difference on GOS[†] (17)	Longer loss of consciousness* (2) Increased haematoma volume on CT brain scan* (3)
Intermediate outcome months post injury	No difference on various measures including GOS, neuropsychological battery, RPCSQ[†] (11)	Greater disability scores on motor items of FIM but not cognitive* (6)	Fewer with good outcome at 6 months (1 of 27 vs 13 of 42)* (2) More severe disability* (2) More poor outcome (dead/severe disability) (10 of 19 vs 21 of 81) (note more alcohol at time of injury)* (7) Late post-traumatic seizures: relative risk 2.4 (95% CI 1.15–5.07)* (12) No difference GOSE[†] (14)
Late outcome years post injury	Do worse on divided attention, recognition of faces and recall of actions* (4) More chronic traumatic encephalopathy in high-exposure boxers* (5) More older active football players in impaired range on general cognitive functioning (3 of 5 vs 1 of 11)* (16)	Worse impairment of memory but not executive function* (8) More dementia* (9, 15) No difference in risk of dementia[†] (13, 14)	Trend towards fewer with good late outcome (22% vs 30%; P = 0.084)* (10)

* Patients who are positive for the ApoE ε4 allele do worse than those who are ApoE ε4 negative. Note that patients who are ApoE ε4 positive can be heterozygous or homozygous.

[†] Patients who are ApoE ε4 positive do not have a different outcome from those who are ApoE ε4 negative.

References: (1) Liberman *et al.* (2002); (2) Friedman *et al.* (1999); (3) Liaquat *et al.* (2002); (4) Sundstrom *et al.* (2004); (5) Jordan *et al.* (1997); (6) Lichtman *et al.* (2000); (7) Chiang *et al.* (2003); (8) Crawford *et al.* (2002); (9) Koponen *et al.* (2004); (10) Millar *et al.* (2003); (11) Chamelian *et al.* (2004); (12) Diaz-Arrastia *et al.* (2003); (13) O'Meara *et al.* (1997); (14) Mehta *et al.* (1999); (15) Mayeux *et al.* (1995); (16) Kutner *et al.* (2000); (17) Teasdale *et al.* (2005).

GOS, Glasgow Outcome Score; GOSE, Glasgow Outcome Score, extended; FIM, Functional Independence Measure; PASAT, Paced Auditory Serial Addition Task; RPCSQ, Rivermead Post Concussion Symptom Questionnaire; CI, confidence interval.

TBI, suggesting the potential for improved recovery if these regenerative pathways can be facilitated.

In animal models of TBI, neurones demonstrate plasticity, in terms of sprouting of new dendrites but also in terms of synaptic reorganisation involving both pruning and new synapse formation.

Neurotransmitters

The effects of head injury on catecholamine pathways are not well defined. Animal models have suggested greater reductions in dopamine than noradrenaline (norepinephrine) function particularly in frontal lobes. A clinical study of the positive effect of a dopamine agonist on executive function supports this suggestion (McDowell *et al.* 1998). In patients with very severe brain injury it has been suggested that lesions around the substantia nigra may cause parkinsonism (Matsuda *et al.* 2003). Single photon emission computed tomography (SPECT) has found evidence of dopamine transporter loss in striatum after TBI, indicating presynaptic dopamine loss (Donnemiller *et al.* 2000). Evidence for involvement of serotonergic systems in humans is inconsistent, with elevated and/or reduced levels of serotonin metabolites being found in CSF.

A more consistent story is emerging for acetylcholine. Elevated levels are consistently found in CSF early after injury. In the long term, reductions in choline acetyltransferase, the presynaptic marker of cholinergic neurones, are found in cortex (Murdoch *et al.* 1998) without changes in postsynaptic nicotinic or muscarinic receptors. These findings tally with histological evidence of damage to the nucleus basalis of Meynert (Murdoch *et al.* 2002) and more recently with MRI evidence of reduced grey matter density of basal forebrain (Salmond *et al.* 2005), the basal forebrain being the location of the nucleus basalis of Meynert and the septal nuclei, the main cholinergic nuclei and source of presynaptic neurones.

Peripheral markers of cell damage

It would be useful, particularly for those with milder injuries, to have a serum or plasma assay that was a marker of the degree of cerebral damage after a head injury and which could thereby help predict outcome. Several have been proposed but it seems that S-100B, a protein derived from glial cells, is the best candidate. Blood levels of S-100B taken within a few hours or days after injury may be a useful marker of the degree of cerebral damage. There is certainly good evidence in moderate to severe head injury that higher S-100B levels predict worse outcome in terms of both morbidity (Dimopoulou *et al.* 2003; Pelinka *et al.* 2004) and disability measures between 1 month and 1 year after injury (Raabe & Seifert 2000; Rothoerl *et al.* 2000; Townend *et al.* 2002). For mild head injury the picture is more equivocal, with several studies failing to find an early outcome effect (Ingebrigtsen *et al.* 1999, 2000; de Boussard *et al.* 2005; Stapert *et al.* 2005), whereas others find that higher S-100B levels are associated with neuroimaging evidence of brain injury (Ingebrigtsen *et al.* 1999, 2000) or symptoms/handicap in the first few weeks or months (De Kruijk *et al.* 2002a; Stranjalis *et al.* 2004) or as late as 1 year after injury (Waterloo *et al.* 1997; Stalnacke *et al.* 2005). Despite these largely positive associations between S-100B levels and outcome, it is possible that levels are associated with extracranial injury rather than brain injury. For example, elevated levels have been found in those with severe extracranial injury without good evidence of head injury (Savola *et al.* 2004); one study has shown elevated levels after running a marathon (Hasselblatt *et al.* 2004). In conclusion, as it stands, S-100B measured in the blood is not a useful marker of brain injury severity in the individual patient; in those with mild head injury the results are too inconsistent; and in those with more severe injury the extent of the injury will be self-evident from standard clinical measures and there is no evidence that S-100B level adds value to these observations.

The importance of these discoveries lies in the promise they offer for the development of neuroprotective agents, several of which have been found to be effective in animal studies. However, clinical studies have been disappointing, perhaps reflecting the much greater heterogeneity, both of the head injury and the nature and timing of treatment, found in the clinical setting compared with the well-controlled and optimised laboratory setting. For example, steroids early after injury might be expected to be effective given the evidence for the deleterious effects of activation of inflammatory pathways. However, in practice steroids do not work (Edwards *et al.* 2005). At present early sedation and ventilation, with good control of blood gases, blood pressure and intracranial pressure, seem to be the most important acute treatment strategies for severe head injury.

Electroencephalogram after head injury

Bickford and Klass (1966) review the EEG alterations seen after head injury. One of the most sensitive changes is local suppression of alpha rhythm in the region of a localised blow or in the contrecoup area. The degree of impairment of alpha rhythm in the early days after injury may predict outcome (Vespa *et al.* 2002). With severe injury, delta waves at 1–3 Hz appear and may persist for several weeks or months. During recovery there is a gradual trend towards increase of frequency and normality over the weeks and months that follow.

The EEG can be helpful in the differential diagnosis of the unconscious patient, chiefly by pointing to causes other than head injury that might be overlooked. Fast activity may suggest drug overdosage, marked localised delta activity will point to a primary intracerebral lesion, and spike-and-wave bursts will indicate an epileptic process. The EEG can also draw attention to complications following head injury.

With regard to prognosis, less can be said with certainty. The degree of overall EEG abnormality is not a firm guide and must always be taken in conjunction with other clinical data. Some suggest that cognitive event-related potentials or quantified EEG may be useful in determining the organic contribution to symptoms after mild brain injury (Gaetz & Bernstein 2001). However, most have not found these investigations to be clinically useful. This is perhaps not surprising given the evidence that a normal EEG may be associated with worse prognosis in those with persistent symptoms after less severe head injury (Williams 1941; Muller 1969). Nevertheless, serial recordings may be helpful, especially in revealing the organic component in cases thought to be due entirely to psychogenic factors. The EEG is unreliable as a guide to the later development of epilepsy, some 50% of patients who develop post-traumatic epilepsy having normal or only minimally abnormal EEGs initially. Jennett (1975) found no consistent correlation between EEG abnormalities during the first year after injury and the development of late epilepsy. However, a persistent EEG focus 1 month after injury is a risk factor for post-traumatic epilepsy (Angeleri et al. 1999).

Neuroimaging and head injury

Computed tomography has proved invaluable in the hours and days after injury in displaying the neuropathological effects of head injury and in serving as a guide to surgical intervention. Acute mass effects are revealed by shift of the midline structures or compression of the midbrain cisterns. Extradural, subdural and intracerebral haematomas as well as areas of contusion and oedema are shown. In the later stages ventricular enlargement may become apparent, along with focal or generalised atrophy. With severe injuries only some 5% yield scans that can be considered normal in all respects (Eisenberg & Levin 1989). Findings on a CT brain scan may contribute to the assessment of head injury severity (Marshall et al. 1991).

Compared with CT, MRI is more sensitive at revealing brain pathology but is less suited to the investigation of patients in the acute stages, especially when on life support equipment. Moreover, the superiority of MRI does not lie in matters likely to influence acute surgical management (Fiser et al. 1998). Nonetheless, the yield from MRI greatly exceeds that from CT; this partly reflects the intrinsically greater sensitivity of MRI, but also the location of lesions in TBI. Contusions tend to occur at the brain–bone interface, the soft brain becoming traumatised against the bone (see Fig. 4.1). Bone is very much more radiodense than soft tissue and this may result in imaging artefacts adjacent to the inner surface of the skull, making it difficult to detect lesions at this interface (see Fig. 4.7). Given that these contusions may have important implications for later neuropsychiatric sequelae, MRI is the preferred imaging technique in this situation. In the chronic stages MRI is also superior to CT in the detection of white matter changes consequent on diffuse axonal injury (Kelly et al. 1988; Mittl et al. 1994). However, it is important to bear in mind that as the sensitivity of imaging increases, so too the likelihood that a subtle abnormality will be found that is unrelated to the injury. For example, on T2-weighted imaging, non-specific white matter hyperintensities are found in healthy control subjects; the older the subject, the more likely they are to be seen.

Certain clinicopathological correlations have emerged. Severity of injury, as judged by degree and duration of consciousness, is related to both the number and location of MRI lesions (Jenkins et al. 1986). Their depth from the cortical surface was found to increase with severity, reinforcing the view that the brain is injured concentrically inwards from the surface in closed head injury. Only one of 50 patients showed a brainstem lesion, compared with 46 showing hemisphere damage, suggesting that white matter hemispheric lesions may be the primary event in traumatic loss of consciousness. Similarly in children, deeper lesions are seen with more severe injuries (Grados et al. 2001).

Levin et al. (1987a) noted the frequency of MRI lesions in the frontal and temporal regions, both areas that are often neurologically silent. Deficits on neuropsychological testing in the acute stage were related to size and location of such abnormalities, for example perseveration with frontal involvement, and memory difficulties with temporal lesions. At follow-up, MRI in individual patients could be informative, for example in a patient whose left frontal haematoma and diminished verbal fluency were observed to resolve together.

Wilson et al. (1988) examined the relationship between MRI lesions and outcome. Patients were scanned in the acute stages and then at follow-up 5–18 months later. Measures of neuropsychological outcome showed a strong correlation with the abnormalities that persisted, especially those in the deeper brain regions. Ventricular enlargement on follow-up correlated strongly with residual neuropsychological disability. Cerebral atrophy, as demonstrated by ventricular enlargement or reduction in brain volume, in the chronic phase after injury has consistently been found to be associated with poor outcome, both using CT (Levin et al. 1981; Timming et al. 1982; Reider-Groswasser et al. 1993) and MRI (Blatter et al. 1997). At least some of the atrophy that follows severe TBI may be due to hypoxia in the immediate post-injury period (Ariza et al. 2004).

Volumetric measurements of grey and white matter have enabled more detailed analysis of the contributions of atrophy of different regions to outcome. Atrophy of corpus callosum is frequently found (Levin et al. 1990a), sometimes with high signal on fluid-attenuated inversion recovery (FLAIR) sequences (Ashikaga et al. 1997), and is associated with more severe injury (Yount et al. 2002; Tomaiuolo et al. 2004) and worse outcome (Takaoka et al. 2002). An attempt to demonstrate an association between slowed interhemispheric transfer of information and the extent of corpus callosal atrophy was not successful (Mathias *et al.* 2004a), although generalised white matter atrophy was associated with slowed information processing. Enlargement of the third ventricle predicts poor outcome (Bigler *et al.* 1999; Henry-Feugeas *et al.* 2000; Groswasser *et al.* 2002), perhaps because it is a marker of severe frontal white matter injury. Much of the ventriculomegaly and sulcal enlargement is explained by white matter atrophy (Bigler *et al.* 2002); thus temporal horn enlargement may be explained more by white matter atrophy in the temporal lobe than by hippocampal atrophy. Yet hippocampal atrophy is a fairly consistent finding (Bigler *et al.* 1997; Arciniegas *et al.* 2001) and correlates with memory impairment (Tomaiuolo *et al.* 2004). Studies of grey matter have found generalised cortical atrophy as well as more specific atrophy or reduced grey matter density of cingulate gyrus, thalamus and basal forebrain, as well as hippocampal and cerebellar atrophy (Gale *et al.* 2005; Salmond *et al.* 2005).

There is some evidence that atrophy is likely to be greater in those with drug or alcohol abuse (Bigler *et al.* 1996; Barker *et al.* 1999; Wilde *et al.* 2004), which is unsurprising given the potential for alcohol itself to produce cerebral and cerebellar atrophy. However, in one of these studies the group with drug and alcohol abuse had more severe injury as measured by the Glasgow Coma Scale (GCS) than those without abuse, and once this was controlled for there was no evidence for greater atrophy in the drug and alcohol group. In this case it might be argued that one reason those with alcohol abuse had more severe GCS scores was because they were more likely to be intoxicated at the time of injury, and that it was the intoxication rather than greater injury severity that produced the lower GCS scores. A history of prior alcohol abuse may produce selective reduction of frontal grey matter volume (Jorge *et al.* 2005).

While reasonable correlations between cerebral atrophic changes and injury severity and outcome are found consistently, it is less certain that they add much to outcome prediction over and above standard clinical measures; for example van der Naalt *et al.* (1999a) found that when it came to predicting outcome at 1 year, once the duration of post-traumatic amnesia (PTA) had been taken into account, findings on CT and MRI were not particularly helpful.

It has been even more difficult to demonstrate clear associations between lesion location and outcome (Markowitsch & Calabrese 1996; Azouvi 2000). This may well reflect the high degree of intercorrelation between lesions (Wilson, J.T. *et al.* 1992), the diffuse nature of the injury in closed head injuries, and that brain which appears normal on neuroimaging may nevertheless be damaged (see studies on diffusion-weighted imaging at the end of this section). Bigler (2001) described three cases with left frontal injuries but all with very different neuropsychological outcomes. In a review of brain imaging findings that relied heavily on CT studies, Wilson (1990)

showed that greater damage to left hemisphere was associated with greater impairment on measures of intellectual damage, particularly for verbal material. Injury was almost always more severe anteriorly, and this frontal injury was best at predicting outcome (van der Naalt *et al.* 1999a; Pierallini *et al.* 2000). The adverse effects of frontal and temporal injury have been documented using CT imaging. Levin *et al.* (1987b), using the Neurobehaviour Rating Scale in patients with closed head injury, showed that symptoms which clinicians attribute to frontal injury (e.g. disinhibition, poor insight and unrealistic planning) were more common in patients with CT evidence of frontal lesions compared with those with lesions confined to the extrafrontal region. Those with frontotemporal lesions show more executive impairment (Lehtonen *et al.* 2005), although this did not result in any worse community participation at 1-year follow-up.

Early agitation (van der Naalt *et al.* 2000), aggression (Tateno *et al.* 2003) and behavioural problems (Wallesch *et al.* 2001) have been found to be associated with frontal injury. However, in mild TBI it may be more difficult to relate MRI findings to the effects of the injury (Hughes *et al.* 2004). Abnormalities on MRI were found in 26 of 80 patients with mild TBI, but in only five of the patients were they definitely post-traumatic; there was no significant correlation with outcome.

The discussion thus far has focused largely on MRI findings using routine T1, T2 and FLAIR sequences. Despite being more sensitive than CT brain imaging, the routine MRI brain scan may nevertheless be normal, or only show limited focal injury, in somebody whose symptoms suggest quite widespread cerebral injury. Are there other magnetic resonance techniques and imaging sequences that enable the detection of brain injury in the normal-appearing brain? Gradient echo sequences are particularly good at picking up the signal from paramagnetic material, including iron. It is therefore a sensitive technique for detecting haemosiderin left behind after intracerebral haemorrhage (Fig. 4.4; see also Fig. 3.14), identifying lesions not seen on routine T2 sequences (Di Stefano *et al.* 2000; Wardlaw & Statham 2000). This is particularly the case for small haemorrhages of diffuse axonal injury, where three times as many lesions are found on gradient echo as routine T2 images (Scheid *et al.* 2003), and at least some of these probably have functional consequences (Yanagawa *et al.* 2000). Lesion load measured using gradient echo may be a better predictor of PTA duration than standard T2 sequences (Gerber *et al.* 2004). Therefore gradient echo sequences should be requested, particularly in cases of mild injury where the evidence of diffuse axonal injury might otherwise be missed. However, it should not be forgotten that small intracerebral haemorrhages may be observed using gradient echo in perhaps 5% of otherwise healthy elderly patients (Symms *et al.* 2004). On the other hand, 20% of low-signal foci, consistent with intracerebral haemosiderin deposits from old haemorrhage, identified

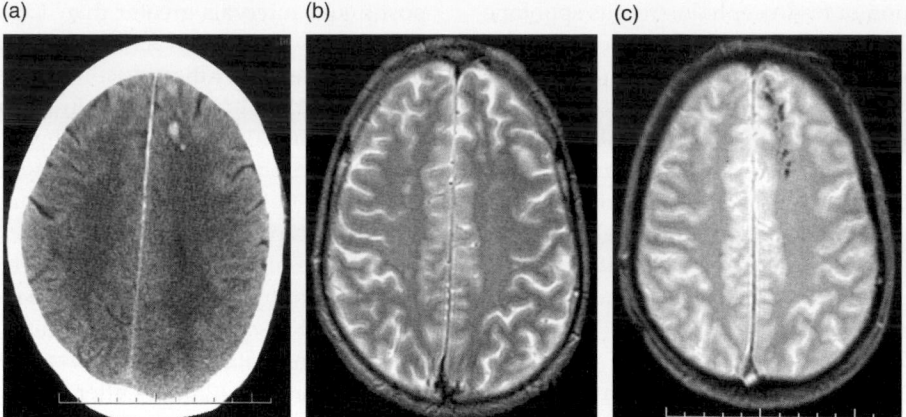

(a)   (b)   (c)

Fig. 4.4 Gradient-echo MRI images identify old haemorrhage. A 62-year-old man fell 4 metres and hit his head. There was possibly no loss of consciousness, but he was sedated and ventilated for 4 hours, and confused and agitated for several days. His post-traumatic amnesia lasted about 2 weeks. He made a good recovery by 2 months, although he was left with personality change such that he was slightly less aware of safety. A CT brain scan was performed on the day on the injury and an MRI brain scan 2 months later. (a) CT brain scan shows left frontal haemorrhages; (b) MRI T2 image shows some probable high signal in left frontal white matter and small low signal further anteriorly; (c) MRI gradient-echo image with easily visible low signal at sites of old haemorrhage.

in the first year after injury using gradient echo MRI, are no longer detected 2 years after injury (Messori *et al.* 2003). Therefore normal gradient echo scans, particularly some time after injury, cannot exclude previous haemorrhage.

Magnetisation transfer imaging (MTI) and diffusion-weighted imaging (DWI) have found abnormal signal in normal-appearing white matter after TBI (reviewed in Symms *et al.* 2004). In patients with mild TBI and normal MRI, as well as others with more severe injury, abnormalities of corpus callosum and other white matter tracts may be found (Sinson *et al.* 2001; Arfanakis *et al.* 2002; Inglese *et al.* 2005). DWI is particularly useful for studying white matter tract integrity. Apparent diffusion coefficient (ADC) may be reduced early after injury in the corpus callosum, perhaps reflecting cellular oedema (Liu *et al.* 1999). Increases in diffusivity have been found in professional boxers, of whom more than 50% had normal routine MRI scans (Zhang *et al.* 2003), and in two patients with severe TBI in normal-appearing white matter (Rugg-Gunn *et al.* 2001). In those with more severe injury, abnormalities detected by DWI in the early days after injury may predict outcome, worse outcome being associated with reduced fractional anisotropy (Ptak *et al.* 2003). Changes in ADC, either measured using the mean value for whole brain (Shanmuganathan *et al.* 2004) or lesion volume detected using ADC maps (Schaefer *et al.* 2004), were better predictors of injury severity and outcome respectively than were standard MRI measures.

Development of ventriculomegaly and hydrocephalus
One question of interest is the evolution of neuroimaging changes over time. Early CT brain imaging over the first few hours and days after injury may show the gradual bleeding into contusions, which become larger and more radiodense.

However, of more interest to the assessment of late symptoms is the distinction between those changes that occur with normal recovery and those which may reflect secondary complications. In particular it is important to know the time course of the ventriculomegaly that accompanies cerebral atrophy: are increases in ventricular volume due to the development of post-traumatic hydrocephalus, which requires shunting, or can they be accepted as the changes normally observed due to atrophy as brain tissue dies and is resorbed? Unfortunately, there is uncertainty as to whether later enlargement, after the first few weeks, is more likely to represent hydrocephalus that may require shunting, or ventriculomegaly due to progressive cerebral atrophy. One study has suggested that early enlargement, before 1 month, is more likely to be due to obstruction of CSF (Meyers *et al.* 1983), whereas another (Marmarou *et al.* 1996) suggested that later enlargement, progressing beyond 1 month, was more likely to be associated with hydrocephalus than atrophy. Subarachnoid or intraventricular bleeding and meningitis at the time of the trauma are risk factors for hydrocephalus.

Very divergent rates are offered for the proportion of patients whose ventricular enlargement is due to hydrocephalus as opposed to atrophy (Guyot & Michael 2000). In one study 45% of patients with ventriculomegaly within 3 months of a severe head injury were found to have hydrocephalus, defined by increased resistance to CSF outflow or raised intracranial pressure (Marmarou *et al.* 1996). However, in other series of severe head injuries less than 2–3% were diagnosed as having post-traumatic hydrocephalus (Lee *et al.* 1998; Matsushita *et al.* 2000). This latter figure is perhaps more consistent with the finding that surgery for post-traumatic ventriculomegaly may not improve outcome (Fu *et al.* 2002). It must also be remembered that a good proportion of hydrocephalus remits spontaneously (Front *et al*. 1972). Therefore most would not proceed to surgery unless there was good clinical evidence (e.g. deteriorating clinical state) that hydrocephalus was pathogenic. The estimate of Cardoso and Galbraith (1985) that about 0.5% of severe head injuries may benefit from shunting may be more realistic than the 10% that some authors have suggested (Mazzini *et al*. 2003). Nevertheless, hydrocephalus needs to be excluded before a diagnosis of vegetative state is made and here CSF studies may be critical in determining who will benefit from shunting (Pickard *et al*. 2005).

The clinical syndrome of a post-traumatic progressive dementia, with or without deteriorating incontinence and gait ataxia, that responds to shunting is very rare but needs occasionally to be considered, particularly if there are risk factors for hydrocephalus. Brain imaging not only excludes a subdural haemorrhage but also allows the present state of the ventricles to be compared with previous findings, or act as a baseline to determine any future change in ventricular size.

However, a moderate progressive increase in size of the ventricles, months and even years after injury, does not necessarily indicate the presence of hydrocephalus as a secondary complication. Progressive atrophy may take place over many years. Blatter *et al*. (1997) studied 123 patients, mostly with moderate to severe injury, who had MRI brain scans at different time intervals after injury; based on the injury to scan interval they were divided into five groups with different post-injury intervals, and the mean scores for each group plotted against their mean time after injury. Correcting for age, sex and head size, the images were analysed to determine the volumes of CSF spaces and total brain and these were then compared with controls without head injury. On the time-dependent plot of standardised brain volume the greatest reduction was seen between the groups measured at a mean of 13 and 42 days after injury, respectively (Fig. 4.5). This was matched by proportionally larger increases in CSF volume, most evident in temporal horn. Further increases in ventricular volume were not observed in the groups with

post-injury intervals greater than 136 days. Reductions in brain volume were seen across the later groups, but beyond 310 days after injury the reductions were hardly greater than those predicted by reductions in brain volume seen with normal ageing (0.26% per year). Whereas reductions in brain volume were only of the order of 2–3%, increases in ventricular volume (lateral, third and temporal horn) were of the order of twofold to threefold. Despite the limitations of this study it does match clinical experience; the vast majority of cerebral atrophy is to be found within the first 6 months after injury. MacKenzie *et al*. (2002) examined repeat MRI scans in seven patients with mild to moderate head injury; on average the first scan was 125 days after injury and the second 350 days, although there was a large range of post-injury intervals. The rate of reduction in brain volume over time was three to four times faster than seen in four controls with repeat scans. Neither of these studies reported whether the patients were abusing alcohol or drugs, which could have been a confounder.

Functional neuroimaging: studies of cerebral blood flow and metabolism

Single photon emission computed tomography scanning, usually using hexamethylpropyleneamine oxine (HMPAO) to measure blood flow, has been shown to complement the information obtained with CT or MRI, and indeed to reveal additional areas of cerebral damage that correlate with clinical signs (Newton *et al*. 1992). Nineteen patients undergoing rehabilitation between 3 months and 3 years after injury were subjected to all three investigations. A total of 43 perfusion deficits were shown by SPECT, compared with 21 focal lesions on MRI and 13 on CT. Of these 43 lesions, 31 were not apparent on either CT or MRI. The number of SPECT lesions correlated significantly with the Glasgow Outcome Score. Lesions shown by SPECT, but not apparent on CT or MRI, sometimes revealed important clinical correlations. One patient, for example, was left with reading difficulties 5 months after injury; the only abnormal finding was on SPECT which showed a perfusion defect in the left poste-

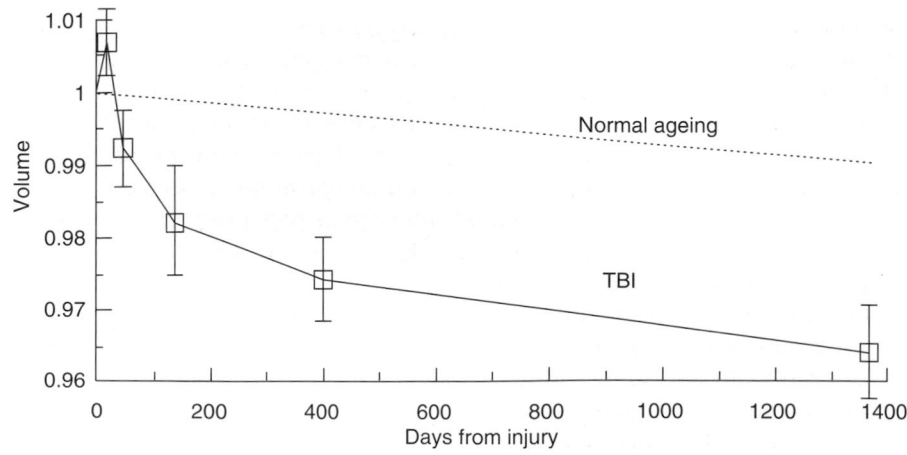

Fig. 4.5 Changes in normalized brain volume measured using MRI. Changes over time are corrected for differences in age, sex and head size using data from a normative database. Note that this is not a longitudinal study but consists of multiple cohorts each at different times after injury. (From Blatter *et al*. 1997 with permission.)

rior parietal region. Similar findings have been reported more recently, with hypoperfusion in the frontal lobes being associated with personality change (Kinuya *et al.* 2004). However, not all studies have found SPECT to be more sensitive than MRI (Stamatakis *et al.* 2002), perhaps because some of the hypoperfusion evident in early SPECT scans will resolve, whereas structural changes are more enduring. Nevertheless, several studies have demonstrated areas of hypoperfusion using SPECT in patients with mild TBI and persistent symptoms and with little evidence of injury on CT or MRI (Kant *et al.* 1997; Umile *et al.* 2002; Bonne *et al.* 2003; Korn *et al.* 2005). For example, one study found almost 60% of such patients to have abnormalities on SPECT (Abu-Judeh *et al.* 1999). A recent study prospectively examined patients within 72 hours of a mild head injury and found 63% to have abnormalities on technetium-99m ethylcysteinate dimer (^{99m}Tc-ECD) SPECT (Gowda *et al.* 2006), although there was also a surprisingly high rate (34%) of patients with CT scan lesions. In patients with anosmia after trauma, SPECT (Varney & Bushnell 1998) or positron emission tomography (PET) (Varney *et al.* 2001) may demonstrate hypoperfusion of the orbitofrontal cortex, although these studies both come from the same research group and await confirmation.

Ruff *et al.* (1989) attempted to demonstrate the value of PET when neuropsychological deficits persisted in the presence of normal CT and MRI scans. Six such patients were scanned 3–5 years after injury, and anterior frontal hypometabolism was shown in five. Some of the patients in this study had suffered minimal injuries and the significance of the hypometabolism in such cases should perhaps be viewed with caution. Although these findings may be taken to indicate evidence of brain injury only disclosed by SPECT or PET, it is important to remember that cerebral hypoperfusion may be found in patients without brain injury but with for example depression or schizophrenia.

Studies with PET, using either $H_2^{15}O$ to measure blood flow or ^{18}F-FDG (fluorodeoxyglucose) to measure cerebral metabolic rate, generally corroborate these SPECT findings. For example, reductions in cerebral metabolic rate in thalamus and brainstem in the days after injury are greater in those who remain in coma (Hattori *et al.* 2003; Nakayama *et al.* 2006), many of these patients showing no abnormality on CT or MRI. One study by Fontaine *et al.* (1999) has suggested that the localisation of hypometabolism detected using FDG PET in the resting state in patients with severe TBI, but without major focal abnormalities on MRI, correlates with their mental state. Those with executive and memory difficulties were more likely to demonstrate hypometabolism in lateral and medial prefrontal areas, whereas medial prefrontal and cingulate areas were affected in those with behavioural disorder. A single case study found reduced hippocampal and anterior cingulate metabolism in a patient with a relatively isolated prolonged retrograde amnesia (RA) (Mattioli *et al.* 1996). Patients with mild TBI may (Gross *et al.* 1996) or may not (Chen *et al.* 2003) show changes in cerebral

metabolic rate in the resting state, although in the latter study smaller increases in cerebral blood flow were found on a spatial working memory task. Patients with more severe injury also show changes in the pattern of cerebral metabolic response to task demand. For example, on a memory retrieval task they showed more widespread activation with less asymmetry of cerebral activation and less activation of dorsomedial thalamus, known to be involved in normal memory retrieval (Levine *et al.* 2002). Whether or not patients show greater or lesser activation than controls may depend on the task. Smaller increases in regional cerebral blood flow in the frontal lobe were seen during free recall on a verbal memory task, whereas during the recognition phase of the same task there was greater activation than seen in controls (Ricker *et al.* 2001).

Functional MRI (fMRI) studies provide support for the thesis that cortical activation in response to cognitively demanding tasks tends to be more widespread after TBI. McAllister *et al.* (1999), studying patients with mild TBI, were the first to demonstrate this effect. Subjects performed the '*n*-back' working memory task in which they listened to a string of letters and were asked to indicate when a currently presented letter matched a letter they had heard 0, 1 or 2 letters back in the string. Although the injured patients performed almost as well as controls, they showed a different pattern of cerebral activation. With the more demanding task (2-back), comparing it with the 1-back task, the brain-injured patients showed more extensive activation of frontal and parietal areas. A similar pattern was found in a single case with severe injury (Scheibel *et al.* 2003). In an fMRI study of patients with severe TBI using a modified version of the Paced Auditory Serial Addition Task (PASAT), patients made more errors and showed a more dispersed activation of cerebral cortex in frontal and temporal areas (Christodoulou *et al.* 2001).

The value of functional imaging in the assessment of individual cases is yet to be established, although the findings can be of interest. For example, Langfitt *et al.* (1986) showed how areas of hypometabolism often extend beyond the structural abnormalities.

A student was unconscious for 20 minutes after a fall, and MRI examination showed right frontal and temporal lobe contusions; CT showed the right frontal contusion only. PET scan 17 days later, when he was alert but slowed, demonstrated impaired glucose metabolism in the frontal poles and orbital cortex of *both* hemispheres and in both anterior temporal lobe regions. Six months later the right frontal and temporal damage was still evident on structural scans; metabolism had improved in both frontal lobes but the right was still impaired. The left but not the right temporal abnormality had recovered. At this stage he still complained of difficulty with concentration, and though performing well on IQ tests he was inattentive and slowed in conversation.

Magnetic resonance spectroscopy can give some insight into cerebral metabolism. For example, a low N-acetylaspartate to creatinine ratio is thought to be a marker of neuronal/axonal loss or damage. Several studies have measured this in white matter, including corpus callosum, in the days and months after TBI and found a reduced ratio (Cecil *et al.* 1998), which was associated with worse outcome (Friedman *et al.* 1998; Garnett *et al.* 2000; Sinson *et al.* 2001). Reductions in N-acetylaspartate in grey matter may also correlate with outcome (Brooks *et al.* 2000).

Acute effects of head injury

The most constant of the acute effects of head injury is impairment of consciousness, ranging from momentary dazing to prolonged coma. This is usually succeeded during recovery by a variable period of confusion, and the whole episode proves later to be surrounded by characteristic amnesic defects. These three features form the cardinal symptoms of the early effects of head injury. They provide important information about the severity of brain damage that is likely to have occurred, and must therefore be taken carefully into account when assessing prognosis. In addition, of course, there may be added effects due to damage to specific parts of the brain, and as a result of the various complications outlined above.

Impairment of consciousness

A good deal of debate has surrounded the definition of concussion. That given by Caveness and Walker (1966) is reproduced here: 'a clinical syndrome characterised by immediate and transient impairment of neural function, such as alteration of consciousness, disturbances of vision, equilibrium, due to mechanical forces'. Concussion can refer to any severity of head injury, from the mildest without loss of consciousness to the most severe with prolonged coma. However, in common usage concussion often implies a milder injury with absent or short-duration loss of consciousness and in which irreversible damage to neurones is slight or non-existent though neuronal dysfunction may last days or weeks.

Impairment of consciousness, however transient, follows all but the mildest blow in closed head injuries, and especially when the head is free to move at impact. There may be no detectable impairment of consciousness, but merely transient symptoms including muddled thinking, or disturbance of equilibrium and dizziness, or of vision or hearing; professional sportsmen refer to this constellation of symptoms as a 'ding' (Yarnell & Lynch 1973). Alternatively, there may be no outward sign of impairment of consciousness to onlookers, yet the patient has no recollection of the injury, showing that registration was failing to occur at the time. Loss of consciousness after penetrating head injuries is considerably less common, also in static crushing injuries as already discussed.

In the typical case loss of consciousness is complete. The patient falls to the ground, displays no response to stimuli, and for a moment shows arrest of respiration, profound fall of blood pressure, pallor, dilated pupils, loss of corneal reflexes and paralysis of deglutition. There may be a period of flaccid paralysis with loss of tendon reflexes. With recovery, shallow sighing respiration is resumed and the circulatory state gradually returns to normal. Consciousness returns after a variable interval depending on the severity of injury. Usually this is followed by a period of confusion, drowsiness and headache, and sometimes by vomiting and dizziness. The duration of complete unconsciousness is often overestimated by the patient, because of the confusion that follows and the PTA which may greatly outlast the resumption of outwardly normal behaviour. Conversely, the patient may sometimes underestimate the period of unconsciousness or deny any knowledge of it.

In some, within 2 seconds of impact and lasting a few seconds there is mass contraction of the limbs often with arms held forward in a 'bear-hug' posture; this tonic phase may be followed by myoclonic jerking for a few seconds (McCrory *et al.* 1997). These concussive convulsions resemble epileptic seizures but there is uncertainty about their pathophysiology. They are not associated with an increased risk for post-traumatic epilepsy. By and large they are benign and some patients quickly regain consciousness and have little to show for the dramatic event.

Periods of unconsciousness lasting several hours are occasionally compatible with uneventful and complete recovery. However, the longer its duration and the deeper the level of coma, the more probable it is that permanent brain damage will have been sustained. Prolonged unconsciousness is more likely to be accompanied by evidence of brain damage on neurological examination, by evidence of raised intracranial pressure and by the presence of blood in the CSF. It is also more likely to be followed by a considerable period of post-traumatic confusion and by both physical and mental long-term sequelae.

The prolonged post-traumatic coma may be profound from the outset, or may deepen rapidly in the early stages due to intracerebral or subarachnoid bleeding. Decerebrate rigidity is common, with tonic fits, stertorous breathing, tachycardia and hyperpyrexia. Anoxia is a special hazard, resulting from obstruction of the airways or damage to the respiratory and vasomotor centres in the brainstem. Ominous signs of brainstem compression include muscular flaccidity, failing respiration, falling blood pressure and fixed dilated pupils. Skilled nursing and watchful medical supervision are therefore essential, with readiness to operate for extradural, subdural and intracerebral haematomas. Artificial aids to sustain respiration may be required for considerable periods of time, and electrolyte imbalance or anaemia due to blood loss may need correction. In severe cases unconsciousness may persist for weeks or even months, and here permanent after-effects are to be expected. Lewin (1959) assessed the quality of recovery in 102 patients who had remained unconscious for over a month; 39 died, 15 were left very severely disabled, 29 made partial recoveries and 19 were ultimately well enough to return to their former work. If a good recovery was to be made, then some improvement was usually seen within the first month after injury: not necessarily return of consciousness but certainly increased responsiveness to pain or diminution of spasticity.

Post-traumatic delirium (post-traumatic confusional state) and post-traumatic amnesia

Post-traumatic delirium

As unconsciousness recedes the patient passes through a phase of impairment of consciousness with disorientation and impaired cognitive ability. This post-traumatic delirium (confusional state) shows much variation, depending on the severity of the injury and its complications, and coloured also by aspects of the patient's personality and present surroundings. In this stage there is always some degree of failure to retain new information. Accordingly, the period of post-traumatic delirium comes to be incorporated within the post-traumatic amnesic gap.

After momentary concussion a return to normal may be expected within a few minutes. After unconsciousness lasting several hours the ensuing disturbance may last for some days or weeks. In the most severe injuries, where permanent disablement is to follow, the phase of acute confusion may last for many months and ultimately shade into the picture of post-traumatic dementia. Thus there exists a fairly close relationship between severity of injury and duration of disorientation (Alderso & Novack 2002). However, exceptions are seen, since the severity of the delirium often depends on complicating factors such as anoxia, electrolyte disturbance, systemic infection or severe blood loss that need not lead to enduring brain damage. The disturbance is usually more prolonged and severe in the elderly, those with cerebrovascular disease or with alcohol dependence.

The form which the disturbance takes is variable, ranging from apathetic withdrawal, through restless irritability, to florid delirious states. Fear, persecutory beliefs, and perplexity as in any delirium are common. There may be suspicious disbelief of the role and purpose of those around, such that nurses and other patients are thought to be spies or gaolers. More openly expressed delusions often originate in sensory falsifications and poverty of grasp. They are usually highly charged with emotion, changeable and unsystematised, and paranoid in content. Disorientation for time and place is marked at first. Cognitive dysfunction is also shown in difficulty with simple mental tests and obvious inability to concentrate or sustain mental effort. In many cases outward behaviour is little disturbed beyond obvious lethargy and failure of cognitive function. In these cases progress usually follows a torpid apathetic course until consciousness is fully regained.

As the confusional state improves, confabulations may come to dominate the mental state, almost always accompanied by lack of insight into the injury and its effects, and disorientation. The confabulating patient may be surprisingly upbeat and some are quite euphoric. Confabulation is often associated with misinterpretation of surroundings and misidentification of people. It is not unusual for patients to believe that staff or other patients on the ward are familiar to them, for example that their doctor is well known to them or that other patients are old friends. Very occasionally the misidentifications are described only on recovery. A bizarre state of double orientation may be maintained, or there may be reduplicative paramnesia with reduplications of place. Patients may believe they are still at work, even when they have not worked for many years before the injury. Alternatively, they may believe they are somewhere with emotional significance for them (see case study below). Such confabulatory delusional disorientation is particularly common in those with a history of alcohol dependence.

Confabulation and reduplicative paramnesia
(Bach *et al.* 2000)

G.O., aged 59, suffered a head injury in south London, probably due to an assault, with unknown duration of loss of consciousness. GCS score on admission was 11 and CT scan showed bilateral frontal contusions, particularly involving the orbitofrontal cortex, and anterior temporal lobe contusions. G.O. had spent much time in England but was resident in Italy living quite close to his daughter. At the time of the interview 6 months after the injury, in July, he had been an inpatient at the Maudsley Hospital in Camberwell in south London, England, for about 3 months. There was some impairment of intellectual functioning, with a verbal IQ of 95 and performance IQ of 85, with moderate to severe impairments in memory and on executive tasks. He showed poor orientation to time and lacked insight into his impairment. For a period he had developed persecutory delusions, believing staff were plotting to kill him. About 2 weeks before the interview he had developed the belief that he was in hospital in Italy, and would occasionally speak to staff in Italian.

S.F.   What has led to your being in hospital now?

G.O.   I personally believe I was hit by a car in an alleyway where I was parked up behind my friend's flat.

S.F.   And how long ago was that?

G.O.   In the first week of May, 16 to 18 weeks ago.

S.F.   And where did the accident happen?

G.O.   It happened in England.

S.F.   And where are we now?

G.O.   We are now in Italy in a hospital.

S.F.   Where in Italy?

G.O.   Well I have tried over a dozen times to buy maps in order to ascertain this thoroughly for myself exactly where we are. Yes and everyone claims they don't have them, though they are eager for my custom, but once they have established what I want they send me down to the *caserma* [police station]. Because all the police there are English the police will sell me these or pass me on to the Italian equivalent of the Automobile Association.

S.F.   So this is all some sort of charade, masquerade?

G.O.   It's a charade, but a political charade.

S.F.   So we're somewhere in north, south Italy?

G.O.   In the north of Italy.

S.F.   And the evidence?

G.O.   Well now I know it because the ambulances are British. I have seen foot patrol on a couple of occasions of carabinieri.

S.F.   Just near here?

G.O.   Yes. But I have now heard on I suppose half a dozen times the sirens going as only an English one goes.

S.F.   So all the evidence is that we're in England, not Italy.

G.O.   Well it is now. I am totally convinced we're in a province of England.

S.F.   Yet located somewhere in north Italy?

G.O.   Yes.

S.F.   So we're not in south London?

G.O.   No.

S.F.   And are we in the Maudsley?

G.O.   We are in the Maudsley but at Italia. Yes.

S.F.   In Italy, not in Camberwell, south London where it's well known to be located?

G.O.   No, I would say that this part is the first cousin of the original.

S.F.   Similar or quite different?

G.O.   From what I understand I would say that it is nowhere near as modern as its true English equivalent. But let me say that I have been very impressed with what I have seen here and I would suggest that the British National Health Service would be well advised to send foraging and investigative teams to Italy proper, including this building, to ask questions and to observe them carrying out their duties.

Hallucinatory experiences may be troublesome; visual hallucinations are most evident, perhaps because they can often be inferred from the patient's behaviour, for example as they are seen to pluck at imaginary objects on their bedlinen.

Weston and Whitlock (1971) describe an example in which delusions apparently stemmed from a vivid hallucinatory experience occurring as part of the early post-traumatic delirium. The patient related an episode in which he believed he saw his parents being shot by Chinese communists. Thereafter when his family visited him he believed them to be impostors who had assumed their exact appearance in order to trick him. The profound memory disturbance from which the patient was suffering at the time had prevented him from realising that the head injury had occurred, or from reintegrating his vivid fantasy into normal daily experience.

These early psychotic states with confabulations, delusions and hallucinations are almost certainly a result of the generalised disturbance of brain function. They usually remit spontaneously, although once recovery has taken place amobarbital may produce a return of symptoms (Weinstein & Kahn 1951).

Post-traumatic agitation

During the post-traumatic delirium some patients pass through an excitable and overactive phase with florid disturbance of behaviour that can pose serious problems of management. Sometimes this is attributable to the abnormal experiences and delusional misinterpretations of a post-traumatic delirium, but sometimes it proves to foreshadow enduring changes of temperament and behaviour occasioned by the injury. The patient may be abusive, aggressive, sexually disinhibited and markedly uncooperative. This phase of agitated behaviour occurs in about 10% of patients with severe brain injury (Brooke *et al.* 1992). For most patients it will only last a few days and for the vast majority the agitation resolves spontaneously within a few weeks. Sexually disinhibited behaviour, when present, often follows the same pattern of recovery. Agitation almost invariably disappears before resolution of PTA. This is consistent with the observation that agitation and attentional deficits tend to go hand in hand (Corrigan *et al.* 1992). Agitated behaviour is associated with frontotemporal injury and doubles the risk of later emotional sequelae (van der Naalt *et al.* 2000). In some patients with post-traumatic agitation, for example following orbitofrontal injury (Silver & Yablon 1996), the constant pacing resembles akathisia seen in patients on antipsychotic drugs.

Post-traumatic amnesia

The period of PTA, which includes the period of unconsciousness and post-traumatic delirium when these are present, may be defined as the amnesic gap from the moment of injury to the time of resumption of normal continuous memory. It ends at the time from which the patient can later give a clear and consecutive account of what was happening around him.

Towards the end of PTA there may be a period when outward behaviour appears to have returned to normal, so that observers are easily misled into thinking that full recovery has occurred, but which the patient subsequently fails to recollect. During this period some degree of temporal disorientation is almost always in evidence if opportunities arise to test for it with care, but even questions designed to test short-term memory may sometimes be answered adequately. Memory functions may have recovered but not yet enough to lay down a permanent record. It is only when this period ends that the patient has recovered from their PTA. Some would argue that it is therefore only in retrospect that the true duration of PTA can be determined with certainty.

With milder injuries there may be no significant post-traumatic delirium; on recovery of consciousness the patient becomes alert and orientated. However, in some of these patients for a time events fail to be recorded in memory and the injury is therefore followed by an amnesic gap. PTA may even be seen in those without loss of consciousness. The classic example is that of the schoolboy struck during a game of football but not rendered unconscious. He may then continue to play, but later proves to have no recollection of the part of the game which immediately followed the injury. Similar examples are sometimes seen in boxers. Usually performance is noted to be substandard during the continuation of activity.

Occasionally some brief isolated experiences, islets of memory, are recalled immediately after the injury, usually in an inaccurate and confused way, and thereafter the dense amnesic period begins.

> A boy of 18 skidded in a car and hit a telegraph pole, sustaining a fractured skull and broken leg. He clearly recalled switching off the engine and forcing open the jammed car door, both of which were subsequently corroborated. Thereafter he could recall nothing until he came round in hospital some 48 hours later (Whitty & Zangwill 1966).

A more delayed onset to the amnesic phase may of course be seen when complications such as extradural haemorrhage lead to a second period of unconsciousness after full recovery has been attained; here events may be recalled from the lucid interval preceding the haemorrhage, and this may be of several hours' duration.

Patients are described as 'being in PTA' as a convenient shorthand to describe the acute recovery period from recovery of consciousness until the end of PTA. During this period patients gradually emerge from a state of impaired consciousness to a period where they are disorientated and amnesic but alert, with the whole episode ending, often gradually, as continuous day-to-day memory is achieved. Impairments of attention, orientation, memory and psychomotor speed are to be found throughout this period. There is no evidence that attentional problems are confined to a distinct confusional state (delirium) within the amnesic gap. There is therefore an argument for describing the whole of PTA, once consciousness is regained, as a post-traumatic confusional state.

There have been several detailed studies of patients during the course of the PTA. Levin and colleagues have made a number of interesting observations. Tests of remote memory have revealed a marked temporal gradient (Levin *et al.* 1985). Events from primary school days were, for example, better remembered than events from young adult life. The same technique applied to patients after resolution of PTA showed no such gradient, but demonstrated equivalent levels of recall for all life periods. A study of orientation during PTA showed that the usual sequence of recovery was for person, then place, then time (Levin 1990). The date was characteristically displaced backwards, for up to 5 years in severe injuries, then the discrepancy diminished as orientation improved.

Ewert *et al.* (1989) made an interesting comparison between procedural and declarative (episodic) memory during the course of PTA. Patients can acquire and retain new skills (mirror reading, maze learning and a pursuit–rotor task) during the PTA, while remaining disorientated and amnesic for ongoing events. Stuss *et al.* (1999) found gradual recovery of attention (e.g. months backwards), memory (e.g. recalling three words after 24 hours), and orientation, with easier tasks recovering before more demanding and effortful tasks. There was considerable overlap in the timing of recovery, but in general with attention recovering before memory. Wilson *et al.* (1999) also observed a gradual recovery of function; across a battery of neuropsychological tests of memory and attention there was no evidence of any sudden improvement across all tests as PTA ended, and the pattern of recovery was different for one patient compared with another. Slowing of reaction time and speed of information processing was prominent. This slowing was found to distinguish patients in PTA from those with a long-term amnesic syndrome (Wilson, B.A. *et al.* 1992).

Of interest is the relationship between recovery of orientation to time, person and place, and recovery of memory, as measured by the ability to remember items after a 24-hour delay. Gronwall and Wrightson (1980) showed that many patients are orientated but still show memory problems, an observation supported by Stuss *et al.* (1999) who showed, on average, orientation recovering before memory. However, Tate *et al.* (2000) suggested that the pattern they observed, with amnesia resolving before disorientation in 94% of cases, was because they had only studied patients with severe TBI.

In many, the termination of PTA is abrupt. The amnesic phase may have lasted from several minutes to several weeks, yet finally ends sharply with the return of normal continuous memory. It is for this reason that many patients can retrospectively give a firm end-point to their PTA. However, in others brief islands of memory at first emerge, vaguely recalled and jumbled in temporal sequence, before the continuity of memory is gradually restored. In those very severe injuries where enduring memory difficulties are to supervene, it is not possible to define the end of PTA.

False memories

The confabulatory state, often with delusional disorientation, that is found during PTA has been described above. Patients are usually subsequently found to be amnesic for the period and have no recollection of their psychotic experiences.

Occasionally the circumstances of the injury are recalled in a confused and muddled manner. This can have important medicolegal repercussions. Russell (1935) reported a patient who had a motorcycle accident and subsequently ascribed his injuries to an attack by the dog which had caused it. He later elaborated this by maintaining that the dog's owner had attacked him directly. In this case the delusions were short-lived and cleared as the post-traumatic confusion receded. A similar case was cited in which a doctor took home a boy who had fallen off his bicycle and was later accused by the boy of having run him down.

False memories, which at first sight are convincing enough, have sometimes been found to centre on a previous injury.

> A dispatch rider was concussed in a motorcycle accident. Following a period of complete unconsciousness he was confused and drowsy for 2–3 days, and after treatment at a local hospital was transferred to a special head injury unit 10 days later. When seen at that time he gave details of the accident, including its locale and the incident leading up to it, and recounted his journey from the first hospital. He gave his name and army number correctly, but persistently underestimated his age by 2 years. At clinical examination he appeared to be rational and fully orientated. It finally transpired, however, that he was giving details of an accident he had had before joining the army some 2 years previously, and that the description of his journey to the second hospital was also a false reminiscence. His final PTA was assessed as 12 days. It involved the period of false reminiscence and the first 2 days of his stay in the second hospital (Whitty & Zangwill 1966).

Some patients, when describing their memories of the trauma months or years later, will admit that they are uncertain how much of what they remember is in fact their own recollection of what they experienced and encoded at the time, and how much is in fact a reconstruction based on what they have been told of what happened. Harvey and Bryant (2001) reported that 40% of patients with mild TBI who early on had no recollection of the trauma, when asked 2 years later remembered the accident. How much of this recovery of memory was due to shrinkage of RA due to improved recall processing, and how much was in fact a reconstruction, is uncertain.

Retrograde amnesia

The duration of RA is measured as the time between the moment of injury and the last clear memory from before the injury which the patient can recall. The patient can often indicate with fair precision the last event which he can clearly recollect.

The RA is usually dense, even for events of high emotional significance and of course involving details of the accident itself. Usually the RA is much shorter than the PTA (Russell & Nathan 1946), although in rare exceptions the reverse is seen. Long retrograde gaps are generally seen only with more severe injuries, and these may be of many days' or weeks' duration. Conversely, examples of mild injury are seen in which no RA occurs whatever, and full details of the injury can be recalled up to the moment of loss of consciousness.

The organic basis for very long RA has come under suspicion, and certainly prolonged RA following mild head injury has often proved to be psychogenic in origin with, for example, functional imaging with SPECT being entirely normal (Di Renzi et al. 1997). Here the emotional shock of the accident is principally to be blamed. Nevertheless, long RA may be seen with other forms of organic brain damage, and experienced observers have agreed that after severe head injury a long RA may sometimes be directly attributable to organic factors. For example, Symonds (1962) reported a permanent RA of 1 year for which there was no indication other than that organic factors were at work. Russell and Nathan (1946) investigated the effect of thiopental narcosis on the duration of amnesias, and found a reduction in only 12 of 40 cases investigated. The reductions were mostly trivial in amount, and did not include material likely to have been repressed by psychological mechanisms. Moreover, the recovered material always bordered the fringes of the amnesic gap, suggesting again that it was substantially organic in origin. More recently, hypoactivation of an area of the right frontal lobe involved in episodic memory retrieval has been described in a patient with a prolonged RA (Levine et al. 1998), whereas another showed bilateral reduction in ^{18}F-FDG metabolism in anterior cingulate cortex and hippocampus (Mattioli et al. 1996).

The RA as determined shortly after injury may prove to be misleading. At first it may be very long, then shrink in the days or weeks that follow as normal orientation is regained. The final estimate should therefore not be made until the patient has emerged from the period of PTA and the fullest possible recovery of cerebral function has occurred.

Measuring head injury severity

Clinical methods

Perhaps the first stage in the neuropsychiatric assessment of a patient with a head injury is to determine the severity of the injury to the brain (Box 4.1). There are three useful clinical measures of head injury severity as predictors of long-term outcome: the GCS measured in the immediate or early aftermath of the injury, the duration of loss of consciousness, and the duration of PTA. In addition it is necessary to consider whether the injury has resulted in any neurological symptoms and signs, e.g. pupillary changes, or a hemiparesis, or alteration of behaviour in the immediate aftermath suggestive of a delirium, or whether there has been a skull fracture or other findings on neuroimaging. Although abnormalities on EEG correlate with injury severity, such findings are rarely used as part of the neuropsychiatric assessment to determine injury severity. The period of RA, i.e. the period leading up to the injury for which memories have been lost, does not correlate very well with injury severity.

Marshall *et al.* (1991) proposed that findings of diffuse injury on early CT brain imaging could contribute to head injury classification, particularly for those who on clinical measures seemed at low risk but where the CT scan showed brain injury. However, their method does not rate the presence or absence of subarachnoid haemorrhage, an important determinant of injury severity. A simple grading of CT scans, which includes whether subarachnoid haemorrhage is present, may do better as a predictor of outcome (Wardlaw *et al.* 2002).

Glasgow Coma Scale

The GCS (Teasdale & Jennett 1974) is routinely used in the management of acutely head-injured patients. The patient's clinical state is charted regularly on three graded parameters: motor responsiveness (no response, extensor response to pain, flexor response, withdrawal response, localising response, obeying commands), verbal performance (nil, without recognisable words, no sustained exchange possible, confused conversation, orientated for person, place and time) and eye opening (nil, in response to pain, in response to speech, spontaneously). Numerical scores are summated for the best responses obtained under each category at a defined point in time. In this way useful predictions can be made, often within 24 hours of injury.

Given that in any one patient serial ratings are usually taken, there is uncertainty about the timing of the recording that should be used as the best measure of injury severity. Some recommend the score on arrival in the emergency room, but if this is to be valuable as a measure to compare one patient with another, or one cohort with another, it does depend on the injury to hospital interval being reasonably consistent; in the UK this is usually about 30–60 minutes. The WHO Task Force (see below and Box 4.2) recommend using

---

Box 4.1 Indicators of head injury severity

- Depth of unconsciousness as assessed by GCS in the immediate aftermath of the injury. A score of 3 indicates absent responses, i.e. deep coma; 15 is normal conscious level
- Duration of loss of consciousness/coma
- Evidence of behavioural/cognitive change in the immediate aftermath suggestive of delirium
- Neurological symptoms and signs
- Evidence of skull fracture and/or other abnormalities on neuroimaging
- Blood in the CSF
- Duration of PTA: interval between the injury and return of normal day-to-day memories

Less useful indicators

- Duration of RA: the period leading up to the injury for which memories have been lost
- Abnormalities on EEG
- Markers of cell damage (e.g. S-100B)
- Evidence of injury to head, e.g. lacerations, bruising, bleeding from ears, fracture of maxilla/zygoma

---

Box 4.2 Definition of mild traumatic brain injury recommended by the WHO Collaborating Task Force (Carroll *et al.* 2004a,b)

Mild traumatic brain injury is an acute brain injury resulting from mechanical energy to the head from external physical forces. Operational criteria for clinical identification include the following.
- One or more of: confusion or disorientation, loss of consciousness for 30 minutes or less, PTA for less than 24 hours, or other transient neurological abnormalities such as focal signs, seizure, and intracranial lesion not requiring surgery.
- GCS score of 13–15 at 30 minutes after injury or later on presentation to hospital.

These manifestations of mild traumatic brain injury must not be due to drugs, alcohol or medications, caused by other injuries or treatment for other injuries, caused by other problems (e.g. psychological trauma, language barriers or coexisting medical conditions), or caused by penetrating craniocerebral injury.

the score at 30 minutes, or at the first opportunity after this. Others suggest that the worst GCS score should be used (Levin *et al.* 1990b) (see below). If the patient is sedated and ventilated, the GCS rating must have been taken before any sedation is offered. It may not matter which single measure of GCS is used, initial or lowest, since both have about the same, rather poor, ability to predict outcome (Zafonte *et al.* 1996). Katz and Alexander (1994), studying a cohort of very severely injured patients (the great majority had PTA greater than 1 week), used the highest (most responsive/alert) GCS score in the first few hours after injury, arguing that this was the best indication of the severity of diffuse injury, and was less vulnerable to the effects of focal injury or medication or very early effects before cardiopulmonary resuscitation. Using the highest early score is only applicable to those with very severe injury and has generally not been adopted.

Duration of loss of consciousness

It should come as no surprise to find that the duration of loss of consciousness following a closed head injury is a good marker of injury severity. However, in the very mild injury severity range, for example concussion in sport, whether or not someone has lost consciousness may not be critical. Loss of consciousness is often absent in concussive injuries in sport, and when present rarely lasts longer than 5 minutes. In this setting it has been difficult to demonstrate that those who sustain loss of consciousness do worse than those with no loss of consciousness in terms of reduced speed of information processing over the days following the head injury (see Mild TBI, Loss of consciousness and outcome, later in chapter). However, when it comes to comparing those who have sustained very brief loss of consciousness with those with prolonged loss of consciousness, then quite strong correlations between duration of loss of consciousness and outcome are found (Asikainen *et al.* 1998). Where serial GCS scores have been measured, the end of loss of consciousness is best defined by time to follow commands, i.e. the time when the patient scores 6 on the motor scale ('responds to commands') (Temkin *et al.* 1995; Whyte *et al.* 2001). A total GCS score of 9 or below usually indicates unconsciousness.

Duration of post-traumatic amnesia

The importance of the duration of amnesia as a guide to the severity of injury and prognosis for recovery was first clearly shown by Russell (1932). The duration of PTA shows close correlations with objective evidence of damage to brain tissue, as reflected in neurological residua such as motor disorder, dysphasia or anosmia, or enduring defects of memory and calculation (Russell & Smith 1961; Smith 1961). Moreover, the PTA is a permanent index of severity, and available to the clinician who enquires long after the injury. Measurement of PTA has now become a well-attested part of clinical practice, hence the importance of striving to record in every case the precise details of the post-traumatic gaps in memory.

The early descriptions of the use of PTA as a measure of injury severity suggest that it be used as a retrospective measure (Russell & Nathan 1946); the patient is asked what he or she remembers of events in the post-injury period and in this way the time until the return of continuous day-to-day memories can be determined. Subsequently, it has been argued that a more reliable estimate of PTA duration, only relevant to those with severe injuries, requires prospective assessment. Once the patient is conscious, regular testing enables the clinician to determine when he or she is reliably able to lay down memories from one day to the next (Shores *et al.* 1986). The end of PTA is usually defined by three consecutive days of perfect scores on simple memory tests, although there is ongoing debate about the best criterion to use (Tate *et al.* 2006). This debate rests heavily on the premise that PTA has an objective end-point. Some would argue that there is little consistency in the pattern of recovery of PTA, which consists of gradual recovery of different domains of memory and orientation at different times (see discussion above). Therefore as one makes the task or criterion used to define the end of PTA more difficult, the measured PTA duration will be longer; what criterion is set is somewhat arbitrary. Despite such complexities, good agreement between retrospective and prospective assessments of the duration of PTA are to be found (McMillan *et al.* 1996). This is useful clinically. In the absence of prospective measures of PTA it is still possible in the clinic, months or years after the injury, to assess the duration of PTA and use this as a measure of injury severity.

Classifying head injury severity

Despite the uncertainty about when to measure the GCS score for grading injury severity (see above), there is more consistent standardisation of head injury classification based on GCS than for either of the other two measures (Carroll *et al.* 2004a). It is now generally accepted that a GCS score of 13–15 defines mild TBI, 9–12 moderate brain injury, and 8 or less severe brain injury. Some define very severe as a GCS score of less than 6 (Table 4.2) while others state that those with a GCS score of 13 are more like those with a score of 12 than those with a score of 14/15, and that therefore it may be better to restrict mild TBI to GCS scores 14 and 15.

There is little consistency in the classification of head injury severity using loss of consciousness. It has been suggested that thresholds for minor, moderate, severe and very severe injury should be 15 minutes or less, more than 15 minutes but less than 6 hours, between 6 and 48 hours, and greater than 48 hours, respectively (Medical Disability Society 1988).

Russell and Smith (1961) proposed a classification of head injury severity according to duration of PTA: PTA <1 hour, slight concussion; PTA 1–24 hours, moderate concussion; PTA 1–7 days, severe concussion; PTA >7 days, very severe concussion. Jennett and Teasdale (1981) extended the range

Table 4.2 Proposed classification of severity of traumatic brain injury.*

	Mild	Moderate[†]	Severe	Very severe[‡]
GCS	13–15	9–12	6–8	3–5
LoC	<30 min	>30 min to 6 hours	>6 hours to 7 days	>7 days
PTA	≤24 hours	>24 hours to 14 days	>14 days to 8 weeks	>8 weeks

* The correspondence for the three measures, GCS (Glasgow Coma Scale), LoC (loss of consciousness) and PTA (post-traumatic amnesia), in terms of injury severity is based on data from Asikainen *et al.* (1998). Note that for any given LoC the length of PTA, on average, increases with age. For patients over 40, compared with those less than 40, the PTA is likely to be about 50% longer for any given LoC.

[†] Given that a GCS score >10 is usually associated with recovery of consciousness and that GCS is measured on arrival in the emergency room, which is usually within 1 hour of injury, the criteria for GCS and LoC will not always match. With regard to the threshold between moderate and severe injury, Bishara *et al.* (1992) found that about 50% of those with PTA duration of 1–4 weeks had GCS score 6–8 while the rest had GCS score of 9 and above, suggesting that the GCS threshold 8/9 is about equivalent to PTA threshold of 2 weeks. Stuss *et al.* (1999) suggested the best cut-off between moderate and severe to be a PTA of 16 days. An alternative classification according to PTA duration might be: moderate, >24 hours to 1 week; severe, >1 week to 4 weeks; very severe, >4 weeks.

[‡] GCS score 3–5 is commonly used as a category of very severe within the severe range. The equivalence of LoC >7 days to PTA >8 weeks is based on Katz and Alexander (1994). Bishara *et al.* (1992) found that all those with GCS score 3–8 had PTA >4 weeks while about half of those with PTA >4 weeks had GCS score 6–8; this is compatible with a threshold of GCS 5/6 as being equivalent to PTA of 8 weeks.

by defining very severe injury as PTA of 8–28 days and extremely severe injury as PTA >28 days. Two subsequent studies demonstrated the value of extending the classification to PTA durations greater than 7 days; van Zomeren and van den Burg (1985) found that those with PTAs of greater than 2 weeks had markedly higher rates of failure to return to work than those with PTAs of less than 2 weeks, and Bishara *et al.* (1992) found that those with a PTA of less than 8 weeks were quite likely to do well, whereas if the PTA was greater than 8 weeks a poor outcome with considerable disability was likely.

Carroll *et al.* (2004a) reviewed the various criteria that have been used in different studies to define mild TBI, in other words the boundary between mild and moderate injury. The criteria for loss of consciousness ranged from less than 5 to less than 30 minutes, and for PTA studies tended to use either less than 1 hour or less than 24 hours as the criterion. For GCS there was much greater consistency, with the majority using GCS scores of 13–15 to define mild TBI. Based on this review the WHO Task Force recommended that mild TBI be defined by a GCS score or 13–15, loss of consciousness of less than 30 minutes, and PTA of less than 24 hours (see Box 4.2), although it was noted that these criteria were not necessarily congruent, i.e. a patient might have a GCS score of 13 but a PTA of a few days. However, for the boundary between moderate to severe injury there is no consensus as to what combination of GCS, loss of consciousness and PTA duration to use.

Given the lack of evidence for any stepwise changes in the effect of increasing injury severity on outcome, the decision as to what thresholds to use to classify injuries as mild, moderate or severe is essentially arbitrary. What is required is a classification that ensures the best internal consistency of the three measures, GCS, loss of consciousness and PTA. Empirical data on the equivalence of these three measures is needed to determine the most internally consistent thresholds. For example, Katz and Alexander (1994) demonstrated that in severe diffuse traumatic injury the best fit between a patient's loss of consciousness and PTA was defined by the following equation:

$$PTA\ (weeks) = 0.4 \times LOC\ (days) + 3.6$$

where LOC is loss of consciousness. Norrman and Svahn (1961) obtained very similar results in an unselected series of 24 cases of severe head injury with loss of consciousness greater than 1 week. PTA duration was predicted by the equation:

$$PTA\ (weeks) = 0.44 \times LOC\ (days) + 0.2$$
correlation coefficient $r = 0.69$

This tallies with clinical experience; on average the duration of PTA is several times longer than the duration of loss of consciousness. This relationship is perhaps most consistent for diffuse injuries. Katz and Alexander (1994) found that in patients with focal injuries it was more difficult to demonstrate correlations between PTA and loss of consciousness. Those with relatively long PTA durations compared with loss of consciousness may have more extensive damage to the cerebral hemispheres compared with central brain areas (Wilson *et al.* 1994).

The data from Asikainen *et al.*'s (1998) study looking at predictors of outcome may be used to inform the selection of thresholds for the three measures. Using their data on the rates of good outcome according to severity in a large cohort, then the outcome of patients defined by a GCS score, on admission to hospital, of 13–15 (mild injury; about two-thirds good outcome) matches quite well with those with loss of consciousness less than 30 minutes and PTA duration less than 24 hours. Those with GCS scores of 9–12 (moderate injury; about 28% good outcome) have very similar outcomes to those with loss of consciousness between 30 minutes and 6 hours and PTA durations between 24 hours and 14 days. Finally, the generally poor outcome of those with GCS scores of 8 or less (severe injury; only about 10% good outcome) tallied with the outcome of all those with loss of consciousness of 6 hours or more or with PTA of 14 days or more. The criteria of Table 4.2 are based on these data.

Predicting outcome based on measures of head injury severity

On the neurosurgical unit for patients with very severe injury, the GCS score, often in combination with pupillary signs and measures of raised intracranial pressure, helps to predict whether somebody is likely to survive the first year, and if so with severe disability or with reasonable recovery (Levin *et al.* 1990b; Signorini *et al.* 1999b). However, changes in neurosurgical practice over recent years, for example greater use of early elective ventilation and sedation, may mean that the GCS score has lost its predictive power in this situation (Balestreri *et al.* 2004).

GCS scores are generally not as good as loss of consciousness or PTA at predicting who is likely to achieve good recovery and who is likely to be left with significant disability (Bishara *et al.* 1992; Katz & Alexander 1994). Asikainen *et al* (1998) did get reasonable correlations of functional outcome with GCS, but loss of consciousness and PTA were better at predicting the important outcome of return to work.

There is some uncertainty as to whether loss of consciousness or PTA is better at predicting longer-term outcome. One would expect loss of consciousness, being more proximal to the trauma, to be a better marker of the severity of the impact and the damage sustained. PTA is more likely to be responsive to the effects of early interventions; neurosurgeons may even use it as a surrogate outcome measure (Ellenberg *et al.* 1996). One advantage that PTA may have over loss of consciousness when used to predict longer-term outcome is that PTA is at least partly due to executive and memory impairments, and it is these impairments that are important determinants of outcome. There may also be commonality between those systems, particularly involving frontal and temporal lobes, that if damaged contribute to prolonged PTA and those which result in behavioural changes that will disadvantage a person in the workforce. Psychiatric disablement shows an important relationship to the duration of PTA, particularly where organic mental disabilities such as intellectual impairment, euphoria,

disinhibition or aspects of 'frontal lobe syndrome' are concerned (Lishman 1968). In Steadman and Graham's (1970) series the mean duration of PTA was significantly increased in patients who showed post-traumatic change of personality. These changes handicap a person's employability.

Reasonably high correlations between PTA duration and likelihood of return to work have been found ($r = 0.54$) in patients with severe injury (van Zomeren & van den Burg 1985). However, in head-to-head comparisons it has been difficult to demonstrate that PTA is a better predictor of outcome than is loss of consciousness (Asikainen *et al.* 1998).

In the individual patient clinical common sense is needed to interpret the head injury severity measures. For any given GCS, loss of consciousness or PTA, various factors if present will result in overestimation of injury severity. These include alcohol or drug intoxication at the time of injury, eye swelling, ventilation and sedation and other prescribed drugs, particularly analgesics. Malingering should occasionally be considered, for example if there is a surprisingly long PTA compared with other injury severity measures. In patients who develop a persistent anterograde amnesia, the PTA duration will be prolonged indefinitely and is no longer particularly valuable as an injury severity measure.

Injury severity measures are fairly weak predictors of outcome. At best they are perhaps able to explain 50% of the variance in outcome at 1–2 years. The wise clinician will be wary of offering firm predictions of outcome, particularly in the early post-injury period. They will have seen patients who, despite having suffered a PTA of many weeks, successfully return to intellectually demanding work. Yet others, without any suggestion of pre-injury vulnerability or concerns about compensation that might complicate recovery, do badly despite clinically trivial injury. Bearing these caveats in mind, Table 4.3 provides a rough guide to the likely

Table 4.3 Likely outcome for given duration of PTA.*

PTA duration	Likely outcome
<1 hour	Usually return to work within 1 month
<1 day	Usually return to work within 2 months
<1 week	Usually return to work within 4 months
>1 week	Often followed by invalidism extending over the greater part of a year
>2 weeks	Almost inevitable measurable residual cognitive problems, of variable impact
>1 month	At best a reduced work capacity, at worst some community supervision
>3 months	Makes voluntary or subsidised work a likely best outcome, while at worst residential placement may be needed

* This summary is based on the data and estimates of Steadman and Graham (1970) and on Greenwood (2002). Note that as age increases, poor outcome is more likely.

outcomes of patients; when interpreting these results it is important to remember the vital contribution of age to outcome. Predictions of prognosis may be helped using other measures. For example, measures of early cognitive status on emergence from PTA help predict outcome even after taking PTA duration into account (Sherer *et al.* 2002).

A sophisticated pathway analysis has combined measures of pre-injury status, for example age and drug abuse, with injury severity and status at 6 months after injury to predict outcome at 1 year in patients with severe injury (Novack *et al.* 2001). Once cognitive status at 6 months had been taken into account, head injury severity had little predictive power, suggesting that much of the effect of head injury severity on outcome (e.g. community integration and employment at 1 year) is effected through cognitive impairments. Emotional status at 6 months, measured with the Neurobehavioural Rating Scale, did not correlate with outcome at 1 year, yet premorbid status did. Although this analysis helps us understand the pathways underlying the multivariate contributions to outcome, its complexity militates against it being taken up as a clinically useful tool.

An important, though not overriding qualification to the above concerns the situation in open as opposed to closed head injuries. In penetrating injuries, particularly those due to high-velocity missiles, there is a tendency for the PTA to be very short or even absent in up to 50% of cases (Russell 1951). Nevertheless, even among penetrating head injuries a close relationship exists between the length of PTA and the amount of psychiatric disability or intellectual impairment as assessed in general terms 1–5 years later (Lishman 1968).

Chronic sequelae of head injury

With recovery from the acute stages, a mild head injury is quite compatible with return to full efficiency, both physically and mentally. This important fact is not always appreciated by the patient and his relatives for whom the very term 'concussion' can have ominous overtones. Nevertheless, head injury does account for a great deal of chronic disability. Common physical defects include cranial nerve lesions such as anosmia, oculomotor pareses, visual field defects and motor disorders resulting from cortical or brainstem lesions. Slurred speech, ataxia and paresis of the limbs are the common physical sequelae. Peripheral sensory defects are seen less frequently. In penetrating injuries, or after complications due to intracranial bleeding, such focal neurological defects will be more common. Generally the recovery of the physical sequelae tends to reach a plateau by 1 or 2 years after injury, although there are reports of for example hemiplegia improving over many years. Dysphasia is particularly likely to improve in the long term (Thomsen 1984).

The clinical importance of the mental aftermaths cannot be overstressed. Observers are uniformly agreed that problems such as cognitive incapacity or change of personality far outstrip the physical sequelae as obstacles to rehabilitation and as a source of long-term disability (Bond 1976; Field 1976; Jennett *et al.* 1981). Decline in employment is more likely to be associated with mental than physical factors (Roberts 1976; Brooks, D.N. *et al.* 1987), likewise the strain imposed on families and those responsible for care (McKinlay *et al.* 1981; Thomsen 1984; Florian *et al.* 1989).

Recovery and long-term outcome

Several studies have attempted to chart the pattern and speed of recovery in patients followed prospectively. All agree that the major gains are usually made during the first post-injury year, the most substantial improvement occurring in the first 6 months. The Glasgow workers (Bond & Brooks 1976; Jennett *et al.* 1977, 1981) have used broad categories of social outcome rather than focusing on cognitive defects alone; using the Glasgow Outcome Score, patients were classified in terms of remaining dependent on daily support, being able to travel and work in sheltered environments, or resuming normal life even in the face of minor continuing deficits (Jennett & Bond 1975). They found that only a minority of severely injured patients changed from one major grade of social outcome to another after the first post-injury year. However, more recent studies suggest a less certain future for the patient. Some have found that during subsequent years continuing improvement can be encountered to an extent that would probably not have been predicted. Others have found that a significant proportion of patients may in fact deteriorate compared with how they were in the early months after injury (see below).

Psychometric testing has shown that different components of cognitive function tend to plateau at different periods. Thus Mandleberg and Brooks (1975) found that scores on verbal subtests of the Wechsler Adult Intelligence Scale (WAIS) tended to approach those of a non-injured control group after 1 year, whereas recovery on performance subtests continued for about 3 years. The slower restitution on performance items no doubt depends on their complex nature, requiring a synthesis of numerous capacities such as perception, attention, learning and psychomotor speed. The recovery of memory functions has been investigated similarly (Brooks 1976; Parker & Serrats 1976), again with indications that most of the improvement takes place during the first year.

However, even over the first year or two of recovery there may be quite different patterns of recovery. Two studies have shown that in a proportion of patients, early improvement in the first 6 months may be followed by a deterioration in memory (Ruff *et al.* 1991) or behaviour (Dunlop *et al.* 1991) within 12 months. Depression, alcohol and social factors predicted who was likely to deteriorate over the 6–12 months after injury; this scenario may be similar to the post-concussion syndrome (see below).

Therefore in all but the mildest cases a firm prognosis should not be attempted until 2 or 3 years have elapsed from the time of injury. And even after this there may be improvement in social functioning probably due to adaptation and adjustment to the deficits which persist. For example, Thomsen (1984) found that half the patients who could not be left alone at 2.5 years were living independently when followed up 10–15 years later. She suggested that improvement in psychosocial functioning can continue for many years. Wilson (1994, 1995) found that 8 of 25 patients with head injury that she had seen for memory rehabilitation 5–12 years before had improved.

Corkin *et al.*'s (1989) study of soldiers surviving penetrating head injury in the Second World War suggested a less optimistic outcome in the long term, possibly due to accelerated decline with ageing in consequence of depleted neuronal reserves.

Corkin *et al.* (1989) traced 50 or so soldiers who had had penetrating head injuries and compared them with 27 controls who had suffered peripheral nerve injuries. The groups were matched for age, education and premorbid intelligence. All subjects had already undergone extensive neuropsychological investigation 30 years earlier, and changes in performance on these same tests could now be accurately assessed. Head injury had led to accelerated decline on total scores from the Army General Classification Test (AGCT), and on its arithmetic subtest, when head-injured and non-head-injured subjects were compared. Means were in the same direction for the vocabulary and the block-counting subscales, and on a hidden figures test. Exacerbated decline was greatest among older subjects, and was common rather than restricted to a small subsample, affecting for example some 75% of persons where the AGCT total scores were concerned. The head-injured patients were not demented, and Corkin *et al.* made the important clinical point that before diagnosing dementia in a patient with a history of head trauma, one should consider the possibility that exacerbated cognitive decline is the responsible factor rather than a new pathological process.

These findings from detailed psychometry support the impressionistic report from Walker and Blumer (1989) that mental deterioration appeared to affect one-quarter of the head-injured soldiers they followed up after the Second World War, starting at around 25 years after injury; they had all suffered from post-traumatic epilepsy. The changes, often not recognised by the subjects themselves but apparent to their wives and friends, took the form of forgetfulness, inattention, mental fatigue and confusion. The tendency to deteriorate did not correlate with the persistence of any type of seizure. In contrast to these findings, Newcombe (1996) has been unable to find evidence of accelerated cognitive decline from her extensive survey of British soldiers sustaining focal brain injuries in the Second World War.

Recent studies of closed head injury, in civilian cohorts, also point to the risk that a proportion of survivors of head injury will deteriorate over time. Perhaps the first indication of this came from Glasgow (Brooks *et al.* 1986), where comparison of relatives' reports at 1 year with their reports at 5 years after injury found that many were reporting greater problems at 5 years, for example disturbed behaviour and threats of violence. In Australia a study comparing patient reports at 2 years with 5 years after injury was a little more optimistic (Olver *et al.* 1996), with improvements in some ratings. However, this optimism was qualified by the observation that there was an increase over the 3-year interval in the number out of work. In the USA a study based on a database of several rehabilitation centres has examined outcome measures collected longitudinally up to 5 years after injury (Hammond *et al.* 2004). As expected the majority of patients (75%), comparing their status at 1 year after injury with that at 5 years, were unchanged. Of those who changed by more than one point on the Disability Rating Scale, twice as many improved (18%) as deteriorated (7%). However, when Millar *et al.* (2003) compared outcome, measured using the Glasgow Outcome Score, at 6 months after injury with that on average almost 18 years later, they found twice as many had deteriorated (32%) as improved (15%). The deterioration was not predicted by ApoE ε4 status. Whitnall *et al.* (2006) recruited patients from several general hospitals with a broad range of severity but with mild injury comprising the majority. Scores on the Glasgow Outcome Score at 1 year after injury were compared with those about 5 years later. As many patients had deteriorated (rated 'good recovery' at 1 year but 'disabled' at 5 years) (12%) as had improved (13%). Of particular interest to the neuropsychiatrist was the observation that at 5–7 years those who deteriorated, compared with those who improved, were more depressed and anxious, had lower self-esteem and had more problems with alcohol.

Himanen *et al.* (2006) did find evidence of long-term decline. They followed up patients on average 30 years after their initial assessment, which was typically about 2.5 years after injury. Over half were severe head injuries and the mean age at follow-up was 60. A pattern of slight general decline was seen, particularly in men and tending to involve visuospatial functioning and visual memory. Younger patients tended to be spared and more severely affected patients showed greater decline on some tests. On a general measure of mild deterioration, 56% did worse while 23% did better at 30-year follow-up.

It is perhaps of interest that of these studies, those with the better long-term outcome (Thomsen 1984; Wilson 1994, 1995; Hammond *et al.* 2004) tended to come from follow-up of patients who had been through rehabilitation. This may be an ascertainment effect; only those likely to do well in the long term turn up for rehabilitation in the first place. However, perhaps early rehabilitation does place the patient and carers in a better position to cope, over the longer term, with the sequelae of head injury.

When interpreting long-term follow-up studies it is important to remember that in general the rates of follow-up are quite low, with only a few studies achieving better than 50%

follow-up. Those with less education, those who are more socially deprived or from ethnic minorities, those who acquire the injury because of violence, or those who have a history of alcohol or drug abuse are less likely to be followed up (Sullivan & Corkin 1984; Corrigan *et al.* 2003). So it is likely that studies with low follow-up rates are going to report better outcome than those that have been able to achieve a more comprehensive evaluation at follow-up.

Finally, it is worth noting that these long-term studies consistently find high levels of mortality. Accidents, alcohol and suicide contribute to the late mortality after head injury (Pentland *et al.* 2005), particularly in those with mild injury.

Head injury as a risk for dementia

Roberts (1976, 1979) focused particular attention on the question of late dementia in his follow-up of 291 survivors from very severe injuries. Careful enquiry 10–25 years later yielded evidence of worsening in 31 patients, and in 10 the possibility was raised of a progressive dementia. However, taking all associated factors into account, such as age, alcoholism, epilepsy and hydrocephalus, there was little to support the notion that a single head injury could set in train a progressive dementing process. Some patients may have had Alzheimer's disease unrelated to the injury, but a more general explanation seemed to lie with the natural processes of ageing affecting a brain already depleted of its functional reserves. Nevertheless, occasional patients have been reported who have demented exceptionally early, for example the man described by Rudelli *et al.* (1982) who had a severe head injury at 22, began to dement at 30, and died of Alzheimer's disease at 38 years.

The possibility that there may be a statistical link between Alzheimer's disease and earlier head trauma remains intriguing. This could be explained by increased β-amyloid deposition in the cortex in the wake of trauma (see above). An alternative explanation is that the reduced neuronal reserve brought about by the head injury brings forward the clinical presentation of dementia in those patients who would have developed a dementia anyway, regardless of the head injury. A study of Second World War Navy and Marine veterans found that those who suffered a non-penetrating head injury during the war, compared with those with an unrelated medical condition, were at increased risk of dementia when assessed over 40 years later (Plassman *et al.* 2000). There seemed to be a dose–response effect: mild head injury did not increase the risk, but the hazard ratio for those with moderate head injury was 2.3 (CI 1.04–5.17) and for severe head injury 4.5 (CI 1.77–11.47).

The relationship between head injury and dementia has largely been studied using case–control methodology; the proportion of patients with Alzheimer's disease with a history of head injury is compared with the proportion of normal controls, of the same age and sex, who report having had a head injury. These studies are of course exposed to reporting bias so the better studies ensure that a matched informant, e.g. a spouse, is used to obtain the history of head injury, both in the case of the patient and the control. It is also necessary to ensure that the controls do not suffer dementia. A meta-analysis of 15 such studies, replicating one of 10 years before (Mortimer *et al.* 1991), found evidence to support the link but the effect was confined to men (Fleminger *et al.* 2003a). For men the odds ratio (OR) of having a history of head injury, for patients with Alzheimer's disease compared with controls, was about 2.

It has been suggested that the risk is related to ApoE status, with those who are ε4 positive being at greater risk (Mayeux *et al.* 1995), although this finding is not consistent (O'Meara *et al.* 1997). Another study using a different methodology also found an effect of ApoE ε4 status (Koponen *et al.* 2004); at 30-year follow-up of 60 patients with head injury, all six patients with dementia were ApoE ε4 positive, whereas only 32% of the total sample were. In the study of Second World War veterans described above there was a non-significant trend towards a stronger association between Alzheimer's disease and head injury in men with more ε4 alleles (Plassman *et al.* 2000).

The special situation with regard to repeated mild head injuries, as sustained during boxing, is discussed later (see Boxing, under Head injuries in sport, later in chapter). For a single head injury it seems likely that the injury does confer a slight increased risk of Alzheimer's disease, particularly in men and probably partly related to the ApoE status of the patient. However, the attributable risk for Alzheimer's disease, as a result of head injury, is small. At most only a small proportion of Alzheimer's disease could be prevented by eliminating head injury.

Aetiology of psychiatric disability after head injury

Over and above any obvious brain damage there are a multitude of factors, constitutional and environmental, that can decisively shape the psychiatric picture in the individual. Such a situation is, of course, common in psychiatric illness, and head-injured patients illustrate particularly well the interplay of many contributory factors rebounding on each other. Confronted with an individual case, clinicians must nevertheless try to decide which are the causal factors presently operating and the relative weights to be given to each, before they can hope to tackle the problem effectively or make a reasoned estimate at prognosis. It will therefore be useful first to review the range of aetiological factors that may contribute to post-traumatic psychiatric disability before describing the common clinical pictures that result. The case in which any one of them operates alone will be rare, and in particular one cannot expect a firm dichotomy between physiogenic and psychogenic causes. Most often the two will be found to be inextricably combined. However, each aetiological factor will first be considered individually since this is the process that clinical enquiry must follow in seeking to clarify the determinants of disability in an individual case.

Some factors, such as the influence of environmental difficulties, have been readily shown to exert a powerful effect; others, including the effects of brain damage itself, have been more difficult to demonstrate, certainly where symptoms other than cognitive deficits are concerned. However, it is important to avoid the fallacy of concluding that where aetiological factors are easy to demonstrate they are necessarily most potent in action. In particular it is difficult to demonstrate minor degrees of brain damage during life, and one must therefore be wary of dismissing the physiogenic contribution. On the other hand, we must not cling to the possibility that 'subclinical' brain damage is responsible in the face of overwhelming evidence that psychogenesis leads the field.

In the discussion that follows it is equally important to remember that even very large series of head-injured patients are liable to special selection, i.e. ascertainment effects, because of the settings in which they are studied and the populations from which they are drawn. Series derived from acute sources will differ substantially from patients referred later for treatment in rehabilitation units. Patients seen solely in connection with claims for compensation will be different again. All such factors may strongly bias interpretations concerning causal factors. Also the people who suffer head injuries are, to a certain extent, a select group (Haas *et al.* 1987). Premorbid factors may not be determining the outcome of injury as much as the fact that the person got injured in the first place. For example, psychiatric illness increases the risk of suffering a head injury (Fann *et al.* 2002, 2004).

In general, larger effects are found when the series has been selected from late ascertainment after injury; it seems likely that those with chronic sequelae, particularly where there is less in the way of severe injury, will be selectively recruited into these studies, and it is these patients who are more likely to have pre-injury character traits that put them at risk of developing psychological sequelae.

Mental constitution and premorbid personality

The effects of mental constitution and premorbid personality may be manifest in terms of global outcome, or there may be specific effects such that a specific attribute predicts a particular response to injury. An example of this is the common observation that brain injury tends to exacerbate premorbid personality traits. For example, somebody with antisocial personality traits before injury now presents with an antisocial personality disorder after injury, or the presence of obsessional personality traits before injury makes survivors of brain injury vulnerable to obsessive–compulsive disorder (OCD). However, reliable assessments of premorbid mental constitution and personality are hard to make (Ruff *et al.* 1996a) and it is therefore not surprising that different studies have placed differing emphasis on their importance.

Two studies from the 1940s (Lewis 1942; Ruesch & Bowman 1945) looked at the importance of constitutional factors by comparing head-injured patients with non-head-injured patients with neurosis and found a remarkable degree of similarity in constitutional background between the two. Lewis concluded that the 'long-lasting relatively intractable post-concussional syndrome is apt to occur in much the same person as develops a psychiatric syndrome anyway', whereas Ruesch and Bowman noted that the longer the disability persisted, the less likely was it to be the expression of brain damage. Slater's (1943) classic study of 2000 neurotic soldiers also showed the importance of constitutional factors, but here a contribution due to brain damage also emerged; it was clearly shown that soldiers who had sustained brain damage scored lower than average on most items of constitutional vulnerability. Head injury, in effect, appeared to contribute something additional to disturb the overall balance that could be discerned between stress and predisposition in the genesis of neurotic symptoms.

Dencker (1958, 1960) collected 118 twin pairs in which only one of the twins had been injured. The head-injured twins were inferior to their controls on a variety of tests of intellectual function, although the deficits were usually subtle and unobtrusive in everyday life. However, no significant differences were found where emotional and other psychiatric symptoms were concerned. The monozygotic pairs were more concordant than the dizygotic where certain post-traumatic symptoms were concerned – headache, dizziness, impaired memory, sensitivity to noise and decreased alcohol tolerance – suggesting that these at least were founded in genetic constitution rather than in any brain damage that had occurred. Several patients were found to have undergone a 'change of personality' since the injury, with increased tension, fatiguability or lessened ability to work, but where monozygotic partners were available for comparison they proved to be closely similar for the traits concerned. Therefore constitutional factors may explain disability that would otherwise have been ascribed to the head injury itself. However, it should be noted that the patients studied by Dencker were examined on average 10 years after injury by which time many of the more specific consequences had probably become submerged. Nevertheless, the findings underline the misleading impression that can be obtained from a cursory psychiatric history. An example of this is a case report of a 9-year-old boy with a history of restlessness and concentration difficulties following a head injury (Nylander & Rydelius 1988). These symptoms were initially attributed to the head injury but examination of his identical twin brother demonstrated very similar behavioural problems.

More recent studies have tended to find less evidence for the role of constitutional factors on outcome after brain injury. This is perhaps best illustrated by Tate's (1998) study in which she examined Symonds' aphorism: 'it is not only the kind of injury that matters, but the kind of head' (Symonds 1937, p. 1092). In two carefully controlled studies, though with relatively small numbers (total of 20 with poor pre-injury psychosocial functioning), she looked at outcome on average 6 years and 6 months respectively after injury. She found no evidence that those with a history of for example delinquency, criminal convictions or substance abuse did worse following severe head injury, outcome being defined by psychosocial integration and neuropsychometry. In a similar study, Hall et al. (1998) examined patients ascertained by admission to inpatient rehabilitation following severe head injury (average length of coma 5–6 days) and also found no difference between those who were at high risk from constitutional factors (N = 39) and those who were not (N = 43). And in the same year Corrigan et al. (1998) showed that it was difficult to predict outcome in the first 5 years after injury, based on pre-injury characteristics, again in those who had been admitted to inpatient rehabilitation.

Some studies have found effects of pre-injury status on outcome. Pre-injury socioeconomic status was found to predict outcome in severe TBI 14 years after injury (Hoofien et al. 2002). Novack et al. (2001) undertook a sophisticated pathway analysis of contributions from premorbid, injury severity and recovery variables on outcome 1 year after injury in 107 patients with severe head injury recruited from an inpatient rehabilitation unit. Premorbid factors were found to have very significant effects on outcome, partly mediated through their effects on cognitive and functional status at 6 months. However, the premorbid factor was a composite of several measures including age at injury, well known to have a powerful effect on outcome.

There is an impression that it may be easier to demonstrate the effect of mental constitution on the prediction of persistent problems after less severe injury. Thus in a follow-up of Vietnam veterans, which examined those who had suffered head injuries since discharge from the armed forces (Luis et al. 2003), there was an effect of pre-injury psychiatric problems on outcome after their mainly mild head injuries. Those with anxiety, depression, mania or psychosis before age 20 were less likely to be in employment when assessed, on average several years after injury, than those without such a history, and more likely to have persistent symptoms of post-concussion syndrome. Ponsford et al. (2000), again looking at mild head injury, found that psychiatric problems antedating the injury were more common in those with post-concussion symptoms at 3 months after injury, although the effect was not seen at 1 month after injury. One study in which 60% had a mild head injury found that those due to violence were associated with worse psychosocial functioning before injury, as defined by for example a criminal record or alcohol abuse, and with worse outcome at 1 year (Machamer et al. 2003). Deb et al. (1999b) following up head injury (82% with mild head injury) found that a history of less education and psychiatric illness before the injury pre-

dicted the presence of a psychiatric illness at 1 year after injury. Other studies looking at mild head injury have failed to find a convincing effect of pre-injury factors, although some of these were weakened by ascertainment effects (Karzmark et al. 1995; Cicerone & Kalmar 1997, Savola & Hillbom 2003; Rush et al. 2004).

Despite suggestions that particular personality attributes make a person vulnerable to the effects of a head injury (Kay et al. 1992), empirical evidence for this idea is limited. Classification into personality types such as psychopathic or neurotic does not add much additional information (Kozol 1945, 1946), although studies with the Minnesota Multiphasic Personality Inventory (MMPI) have indicated that high scores on the hysterical, depressive and hypochondriacal scales are associated with the long persistence of neurotic complaints (Walker & Erculei 1969). Two recent studies have attempted to identify the effects of specific pre-injury personality traits, using the revised NEO Personality Inventory rated by an informant immediately after injury, and found only very limited effects on outcome for both moderate to severe head injury (Malec et al. 2004) and mild TBI (Rush et al. 2004).

What is the evidence that specific personality features will tend to influence the form that post-traumatic disability takes? Good evidence that a severe head injury will exacerbate prior personality traits or personality disorder is lacking. Malia et al. (1995) attempted to objectively demonstrate an effect of four pre-injury personality attributes ('loss of control', 'humour', 'optimism', and 'easy-going disposition') measured retrospectively at the time of admission for neurological rehabilitation. The majority had suffered a severe head injury, but about 20% of the 74 patients studied had brain injury from other causes. Only 'easy-going disposition' before injury was found to have an effect on outcome defined as better psychosocial functioning, and the effect was weak and only observed in those studied within a year of injury. Using the revised NEO Personality Inventory, Kurtz et al. (1998) looked for systematic changes in personality by comparing pre-injury scores with post-injury scores, both measured by an informant after injury. No systematic changes were observed; in other words it was not possible to define change in personality based on pre-injury personality.

There is therefore a dissonance between these empirical findings and common clinical observation and opinion which would have us believe that pre-injury personality has a specific effect on outcome. This opinion was enunciated by Kay et al. (1992) who anecdotally suggested there were specific patterns of pre-injury personality styles that put patients at risk of a poor response. For example:

> The overachiever, who is often obsessive–compulsive and derives his or her sense of self from driven accomplishment, is at risk for a catastrophic reaction.

Grandiose persons get into trouble by being so unable to acknowledge their decrease in ability that they deny it to themselves and others and continue to blunder into situations that evoke failure. The crash of self-esteem, when it comes, is usually catastrophic.

Ruff *et al.* (1996a) presented four case reports to support this line of reasoning. One explanation for the failure of empirical data to validate clinical wisdom could be that the empirical methods used to identify the personality effects are too weak. They almost invariably rely on post-injury assessment of pre-injury characteristics, a method known to be vulnerable to bias. Alternatively, the measures used are simply not tuned to the personality effects that clinicians observe to have predictive value. Possibly clinical wisdom is based on a few convincing cases, but these good exemplars, being few and far between, are not sufficient to produce statistically significant effects when analysed in large cohorts where the majority show little if any effect. Or perhaps clinical wisdom is at fault, and is based on clinicians and informants incorrectly attributing the consequences of brain injury to the kind of head that was injured.

The adverse effects of alcohol abuse before injury are discussed later in this section (see Alcohol and drug abuse and head injury).

The effects of pre-injury IQ are of interest to a resource capacity model of outcome after brain injury (Satz 1993) which proposes that those with greater redundancy of cognitive processing will be less vulnerable to the effects of brain injury. However, inconsistent effects of educational achievement on likelihood of return to work are found. Of more interest, though not easy to interpret, are the findings from the Vietnam Head Injury Study (Grafman *et al.* 1988). An effect of pre-injury IQ was found, but only when post-injury intelligence scores were compared with control subjects who had not suffered a head injury but who were also followed up over 15 years. When head-injured subjects were compared with controls of equivalent IQ, those head-injured subjects with lower pre-injury IQ did worse than their head-injured peers with higher IQ, i.e. they made less gains over their IQ-matched controls than did their more intelligent peers over their controls.

Age at time of injury

Finally, under the heading of constitution it is important to note that many aspects of post-traumatic disability, and especially cognitive impairments, increase with age at the time of injury. This is probably due to the rising incidence of complicating factors such as cerebrovascular disease, the diminishing reserve of neurones, and the general loss of resilience and adaptability among older persons. Mortality also rises sharply. In Kerr *et al.*'s (1971) series of civilian head injuries, a steady rise in mortality occurred after the age of 50, this appearing to be due to age-related factors such as medical complications or pre-existing disease. Pentland *et al.* (1986)

showed that patients over 65 admitted to the head injury unit in Edinburgh with severe injuries were twice as likely to die (77%) as younger patients with the same severity of injury (39%). The elderly with moderately severe injuries were more than twice as likely to remain severely disabled or in a vegetative state (35% vs 14%). Pennings *et al.* (1993) obtained very similar figures in terms of both mortality and disability.

For any given severity of injury, measured by GCS score or length of coma, older patients have longer PTA and worse functional outcome (Katz & Alexander 1994). This effect seemed to begin at about age 40. Stuss *et al.* (2000) confirmed the effect of age on PTA; in those with loss of consciousness of more than 30 hours, those less than 26 years old had a mean PTA of just over 3 weeks whereas for those aged 26 and older the PTA was more likely to be 5–7 weeks. Russell (1932) found that memory difficulties increased regularly with age and were three times as common among patients over 40 as in younger patients. It is therefore not surprising that increasing age is consistently found to have a marked adverse effect on a patient's chances of returning to work. For example, in Heiskanen and Sipponen's (1970) group of severe brain injuries, less than 30% of the survivors aged 50 or over were able to return to their former work, whereas more than 70% of those under 20 were able to do so. Less optimistic figures were found by Brooks, N. *et al.* (1987a) with only 12% of patients older than 45 years returning to work compared with about 40% in those aged 17–30 years. Adler (1945) found that neurotic symptoms, mainly anxieties and fears, were more frequent as age at time of injury advanced, and attributed this to the increased problems of occupational and financial adjustment which had to be faced by older people.

Circumstances of the injury

The circumstances of the accident may have important effects on outcome, as when a reckless driver has injured his family or a workman has been forced against his will to use faulty equipment. The setting may have been peculiarly conducive to fear, anger or resentment as in the following case.

A man aged 48 was coshed on the way to bank his firm's takings and rendered briefly unconscious. For 12 months thereafter he showed enduring symptoms of anxiety and depression despite full physical and intellectual recovery. His ability to function at work appeared to be unaccountably impaired. It ultimately emerged that after a series of frustrating setbacks he had come to be employed in a humble capacity by his successful younger brother who ran a flourishing business. Years of suppressed resentment and hostility were now focused on the injury, and the full significance to him of being attacked while banking the firm's profits immediately became apparent (Lishman 1973).

The concept of cryptotrauma was introduced by Pilowsky (1985) to describe instances in which exploration of the details surrounding the accident can be rewarding in revealing circumstances of special significance. And even ignoring individual determinants of this nature, it is possible to show that disability tends to differ from one broad category of accident to another, whether on the roads, at work or in the home (Brain 1942; Adler 1945; Miller 1966). This may relate to the harmful effects of perception of fault (Rutherford 1989; Wood 2004); those patients who blamed a person or organisation for their injury were more likely to have symptoms. Early emotional reactions after injury (Brenner *et al.* 1944; King 1996), or when the injury has occurred in an emotionally loaded setting (Guttmann 1946), also increase the risk of later problems.

Emotional reaction to the trauma may be one reason why violence-related injury is associated with worse outcome (Wenden *et al.* 1998). However, as noted above, it seems likely that part of this effect is because many of the factors that increase the risk of suffering violence are the same as those that have a negative effect on later outcome, for example alcohol and drug abuse and lower social class (Bogner *et al.* 2001; Bushnik *et al.* 2003; Gerhart *et al.* 2003; Machamer *et al.* 2003).

The emotional repercussions of the accident may be more influential than was supposed at first sight. This is particularly likely when psychiatric disability is disproportionate to the likely severity of brain damage incurred, or when it outstrips expectations derived from a knowledge of previous mental stability:

> A woman of 45 was disabled for many months by a number of neurotic complaints after surviving intact from a car crash. The head injury had been mild but her vision had been threatened for a time. Her persistent neurotic reaction was surprising in view of her excellent previous mental health and stability. She eventually confessed to a long-standing secret liaison with the husband of a friend, in whose company the accident had occurred. She had made a fervent resolve to end the relationship by way of atonement if her sight should be spared, and this she was now striving to do. Here the injury served as a focus for long-standing conflict and guilt, in addition to providing ongoing emotional distress of a deeply disturbing kind (Lishman 1973).

In the early stages after injury the patient is vulnerable and often highly suggestible. In particular, he may be strongly influenced by what he hears from fellow patients, the treatment received and how much is or is not explained to him. Protracted investigations can sometimes stir up enduring anxiety.

> A policewoman of 22 sustained a minor blow on the head when travelling on duty in a car. Continuing headache led to skull X-ray which showed some increased convolutional markings. A CT scan was therefore undertaken in case a pre-existing hydrocephalus had been exacerbated. This was normal but the foramen magnum seemed enlarged. A myelogram was therefore carried out to exclude any possibility of abnormality at the craniocervical junction and was also normal. Throughout the 6 weeks of investigation her headaches steadily worsened and were still troublesome some 3 years later when she was referred for a second opinion. Her attention had indeed been firmly focused on her early symptoms (Lishman 1988).

Environmental and social difficulties encountered during convalescence and thereafter must always be carefully evaluated because they may be accessible to remediation. Threats to family or personal security and occupational difficulties are likely to be much more difficult for the patient, with their physical or intellectual deficits, to cope with. Fear of returning to a dangerous occupation where the accident has occurred can have a powerful influence in determining prolonged invalidism. Likewise an unstable domestic background or oversolicitude on the part of the family. Tarsh and Royston (1985) have documented the influence of changes within the family in contributing to prolongation of disability, especially overprotection from family members and changes in the normal family hierarchies and roles. Children are particularly vulnerable to the effects of the family environment (see under Head injury in childhood, later in chapter).

Sometimes the problems have been present from before the injury. Selzer *et al.* (1968) were able to show an excess of personal conflicts and stresses in the lives of drivers causing fatal accidents during the 12 months preceding these events, many of which were still affecting the driver at the time. No less than 20% had had an acutely disturbing experience during the preceding 6 hours. An excess of life events in the recent lives of victims of accidental injury has been found (Whitlock *et al.* 1977; Fenton *et al.* 1993).

Compensation, litigation, secondary gain and attribution bias

The important aspects of medicolegal assessment of head injury are dealt with later in this chapter (see Medicolegal considerations). Here it will suffice to note that impending litigation can strongly motivate the aggravation and prolongation of disability. That the compensation issue, like other conflicts, can operate at many levels of consciousness should be no cause for surprise. In some, probably rare cases, there will be entirely conscious simulation for gain, but in the great majority the compensation issue colours the picture in more subtle ways. Once the possibility of compensation is raised the patient finds himself in complex legal dealings; there are frustrations due to delay, anxieties due to conflicting advice and often capital outlay. In effect the injured person is invited to complain and, having done so, finds he must complain repeatedly, often over years to a number of specialists (Cole 1970).

It is sometimes reported that disability continues until the compensation issue is settled, then clears abruptly whether or not financial reward has been forthcoming (Miller 1961). Even so, improvement on settlement need not imply that the patient has been 'manufacturing' his symptoms: genuine uncertainty and worry have been decisively removed (Merskey & Woodforde 1972). Examples of abrupt resolution on settlement are, in fact, much rarer than is commonly supposed. Steadman and Graham (1970) found that patients whose claims were rejected took a long time to recover or return to work, and 'neurotic resentment' seemed a possible explanation for this. Kelly and Smith (1981) traced 43 of 100 patients to determine the long-term outcome of the post-traumatic syndrome when the compensation issue was at stake; of 26 who had failed to return to work by the settlement date, only one was at work 18 months later, yet all but four had considered the settlement adequate. Rutherford (1989) followed 44 consecutive patients referred for medicolegal reports. At the time of writing the reports 57% had symptoms, but this had fallen to 39% at the time of settlement; there was little further fall in the proportion still complaining (34%) when followed up 1 year later.

Miller (1961, 1966) in reviewing 200 patients seen for medicolegal assessment after head injury estimated that the compensation issue contributes to disability in one-quarter to one-third of all patients. Neurotic disability was twice as common after industrial accidents as after road traffic accidents, and employees of large organisations or nationalised concerns were affected more commonly than those of small intimate firms. Additional evidence of the importance of litigation has been deduced from the fact that post-concussional symptoms are less frequent after injuries at sport or in the home where compensation is not payable (Miller 1969; Rutherford *et al.* 1977). However, before attributing this effect to secondary gain, the possible noxious effects of 'perception of fault' need to be considered (Wood 2004). It is psychologically more traumatic if injury is perceived as being the fault of somebody else, rather than one's own fault or an act of God. And these psychological effects are likely to be even more harmful if there was wanton negligence or a directed assault.

In a clever meta-analysis, Binder and Rohling (1996) compared symptom severity in those who were pursuing compensation with those who were not across 17 studies. The symptoms of those pursuing compensation were worse by on average half a standard deviation (median effect size 0.47). The effect was greater in those with milder injuries. Since then studies have demonstrated that the effect is seen

from as early as a few days or weeks after mild head injury (Feinstein *et al.* 2001; Paniak *et al.* 2002a). However, it must be remembered that only those with symptoms will pursue compensation; those with good outcome will be filtered out of the compensation-seeking cohort, leaving behind only those with worse outcome. Therefore even if the pursuit of compensation does not cause symptoms, the compensation-seeking cohort will always be more symptomatic. And even if compensation is found to causally increase symptoms, this does not necessarily mean that claimants are exaggerating their symptoms. Repeated questioning from lawyers and doctors not only focuses the patient's attention on early symptoms that perhaps were due to recede, but in addition reinforces the prospect of their continuance or of worse to come. Cassidy *et al.* (2004) showed that changes in the law from an adversarial tort system to one of no fault improved outcome as measured by the faster resolution of compensation claims. Nevertheless, some would argue that faster resolution of compensation claims is not in fact a good proxy measure for speedier recovery of symptoms.

If compensation does cause a worse outcome, several mechanisms may be at work. Most difficult to evaluate is the possibility of malingering, a diagnosis perhaps better left to lawyers than physicians (Halligan *et al.* 2003). Nevertheless, patients do sometimes knowingly deceive their doctors, claiming severe disability when little or none exists. In one survey, neuropsychologists estimated that almost 30% of personal injury cases involved probable malingering (Mittenberg *et al.* 2002). Miller and Cartlidge (1972) rather brusquely criticise the unwillingness of doctors to consider simulation, and report a vivid example as follows.

> A 30-year-old labourer had sustained a mild head injury without loss of consciousness. During the ensuing months he developed anxiety, depression and stammering, unrelieved by psychotropic drugs, and after a course of electroconvulsive therapy he became totally mute. At the time of examination he had not been heard to utter for nearly 2 years. Numerous referrals had led to a multitude of diagnoses, but 11 psychiatric reports had failed to mention the possibility of malingering.
>
> As can be imagined, examination presented considerable difficulty. The case was well documented and the patient's wife most informative. His own contribution consisted in grimly nodding his head in affirmation or negation of questions and of written notes passed across the table. This he accomplished fluently and accurately. In this manner he registered complaints of frequent headaches, dizziness on change of posture, forgetfulness, and intermittent severe depression. From the beginning of this remarkable consultation it was difficult to escape the impression that the patient was malingering. He was tense, evasive, suspicious

and defensive – and his wife's attitude was very similar. The examiner's conviction that the patient was endeavouring to deceive was so strong that he telephoned a colleague and arranged for him to accompany the claimant unobserved on his mainline train back to the Midlands. The patient exchanged his first remarks with his wife as the train drew out of Newcastle station, and by the time his companion left the train at Durham the whole compartment was engaged in uninhibited and cheerful conversation on matters of the day.

As in this case, malingering often involves two related processes. On the one hand patients lie about the degree to which they are undertaking activities; in other words they are in fact performing activities, e.g. working, but tell their doctor they are not. Only very rarely does this come to light. On the other hand, there may be deliberate simulation; they do very little and pretend to be disabled, whereas in fact they are quite capable of undertaking activities were they inclined to do so. It is this that the clinician is likely to observe at interview. However, confidently distinguishing this pretence from unconscious exaggeration of disability as a result of a conversion disorder (dissociative disorder/hysteria) will often be difficult if not impossible. The parties contesting the claim for compensation will sometimes arrange for covert surveillance of the claimant in order to determine his true level of functioning; this is scarcely appropriate in the context of clinical evaluation, but it is well to be aware that such evidence may be produced.

Motivation factors probably operate at various levels of consciousness. It seems unlikely that the 12 patients with mild head injury examined by Keller *et al.* (2000) in whom there were no unsettled liability claims willfully underperformed on a test of divided attention. Yet the patients' performance improved after they were told that the test result might influence their ability to drive. Neuropsychological evidence that a person's pattern of poor performance on cognitive testing is unlikely to be due simply to brain injury and seems psychologically motivated may be helpful in the evaluation of symptoms (Iverson & Binder 2000). The most convincing demonstration of this comes from forced choice recognition tests, in which the subject has to choose the correct answer from two or more possibilities presented to him. For example, from two faces he has to choose the one that was shown earlier from the one he has not seen before. When a subject chooses significantly fewer correct responses than would be predicted by chance, then this is evidence that the patient probably knows which is the correct one but is, possibly deliberately, choosing the other. Other examples of patterns of responding that suggest underperformance or exaggeration or poor effort include failing on easy tests yet doing relatively well on more difficult tests, or demonstrating greater variation in performance from one test to another or across the same test measured on different occasions than expected (Strauss *et al.* 1999). Another inconsistency that may be identified is performance on neuropsychological testing that is quite contrary with the patient's performance in everyday life.

If a patient's performance on psychological testing deteriorates over time after injury, quite contrary to the pattern of normal recovery, this suggests psychological forces at work or possibly malingering. However, cognitive decline over time is observed in a small proportion of cases after head injury (see above) for reasons that are not well understood. Sometimes the cognitive decline is attributed to the onset of depression. The effect of depression on cognitive function in patients involved in litigation after a head injury may be measurable but minimal (Sherman *et al.* 2000). Where it was observed it was in the domains of memory and speed of information processing and in those with milder impairments. Others have found the effect of depression to be on executive function (Jorge *et al.* 2004) as well as processing speed and memory (Rapoport *et al.* 2005). However, the interpretation of such cross-sectional studies is undermined by ascertainment effects and issues of cause and effect: does worse cognition make you more depressed, or does being depressed impair cognitive performance? The longitudinal studies discussed in the section on long-term outcome (see above) are therefore of interest. Depression was found to be associated with deteriorating performance both over the first year and over subsequent years. The observation that treating depression after a mild head injury will improve cognition awaits confirmation (Fann *et al.* 2001).

When pursuing compensation it is not sufficient for claimants to demonstrate that they are disabled after the injury. It must be shown that the injury caused the disability. Claimants may therefore be motivated to overestimate their previous health. Indeed this has been demonstrated in patients pursuing compensation after a head injury. They may claim greater academic success before the injury than was in fact achieved (Greiffenstein *et al.* 2002a) and may underestimate the degree to which they were symptomatic before injury (Lees-Haley *et al.* 1996, 1997). As such, patients overestimate the degree to which the head injury is a cause of symptoms. This misattribution may be compounded by 'expectation as aetiology' (Mittenberg *et al.* 1992) whereby people's expectation of the symptoms experienced after a head injury plays a part in determining outcome. Transcultural studies on mild head injury find that far fewer symptoms are reported in Lithuania, a country where there are minimal possibilities for economic gain from a head injury and where the general population do not expect patients to suffer persisting symptoms, than in Canada where personal injury claims are common (Ferrari *et al.* 2001). However, this story is complicated by the observation that the effect of overestimating one's pre-injury health is common to all patients with a head injury (Hilsabeck *et al.* 1998; Ferguson *et al.* 1999), not just those in litigation, and indeed is common to injured patients, not just those with a head injury (Hilsabeck *et al.* 1998), regardless of cause. As such, it seems that the 'good old days' hypothesis, though less specific, may be more important than 'expectation as aetiology' (Gunstad & Suhr 2001).

Development of epilepsy

Post-traumatic epilepsy develops in about 2–5% of closed head injuries and in over 30% when the dura mater has been penetrated (D'Ambrosio & Perucca 2004). Those with a history of alcohol abuse are particularly vulnerable (Frey 2003). It is also worth remembering that not all seizures after head injury are due to epilepsy (Westbrook *et al.* 1998; Hudak *et al.* 2004), and that prolonged seizures after a mild head injury should particularly raise suspicion of non-epileptic seizures (Barry *et al.* 1998). On the other hand, some head injuries may be due to epilepsy (Zwimpfer *et al.* 1997). The general question of post-traumatic epilepsy is considered in Chapter 6.

The development of seizures represents a serious complication and stands to aggravate the psychiatric disability ensuing from the injury. First there is the socially disruptive effect of the epilepsy, which increases self-concern, hinders rehabilitation and brings special problems in readaptation to daily life. The fits may make their appearance when the patient is on the point of regaining confidence, and represent an added hurdle to be overcome. In addition, the physiological disturbance underlying the epilepsy may add to the effects of brain damage already present. After closed head injury temporal lobe epilepsy is the commonest form (Jennett 1962), and this is the type most frequently incriminated in leading to psychiatric disturbance. However, it has been difficult to demonstrate adverse effects of post-traumatic epilepsy in patients with closed head injury if controls are matched for severity of injury (Haltiner *et al.* 1996), although those with epilepsy tend to require higher levels of nursing care after discharge from rehabilitation (Armstrong *et al.* 1990). Given the potential adverse effects of phenytoin and phenobarbital on cognition and behaviour, it is probably wise that patients with post-traumatic epilepsy taking these drugs are changed to carbamazepine (Wroblewski *et al.* 1989) or valproate. And if these drugs are being used prophylactically to prevent post-traumatic epilepsy, the patient should generally be weaned off them given that there is no evidence for the value of prophylactic therapy (Schierhout & Roberts 1998).

Lishman (1968) found that epilepsy occurred during the ensuing 5 years in 45% of patients with penetrating injuries, and there was a highly significant relationship between its development and the degree of overall psychiatric disability. Epilepsy that developed during the first year after injury was

mainly responsible for the association. The relationship remained significant after controlling for the differing amounts of brain damage sustained among the epileptic and non-epileptic patients. Increased psychopathology in patients with post-traumatic epilepsy was also found in the Vietnam Head Injury Study, though there were no effects of seizure type (Swanson *et al.* 1995). Patients with post-traumatic epilepsy after penetrating injuries may be at greater risk of late cognitive impairment many years post injury (Salazar *et al.* 1987; Walker & Blumer 1989).

Amount of brain damage incurred

The main difficulty in estimating the contribution of brain damage to different forms of post-traumatic psychiatric disability lies in the problem of detecting minor degrees of damage while the patient is alive. The available techniques of neuroimaging, EEG and psychometry cannot be expected always to reflect small amounts of neuronal loss or focal brain dysfunction. A common approach has been to examine the nature and severity of post-traumatic symptoms against clinical indices known to reflect severity of brain damage, such as length of coma, length of PTA, and other clinical features seen shortly after injury. Thus increasing PTA has been found to correlate with increasing evidence of neurological disorder and memory and/or calculation defect, whereas the incidence of anxiety and depression, dizziness sans vertigo, and headache was unaffected by duration of PTA (Russell & Smith 1961).

Intellectual impairment after head injury is readily attributed to brain damage, although even here it is important to be wary of inferring brain damage because of complaints of intellectual impairment and even poor performance on cognitive testing, when all the objective indices suggest a very mild or trivial head injury. When brain damage has resulted in severe cognitive impairment there will of necessity be a significant effect on personality. It is therefore not surprising that personality change has been found to be commoner after the more severe injuries (Steadman & Graham 1970). Patients with moderate to severe dementia after a brain injury are almost invariably impulsive, demanding to have their wants met immediately, at least somewhat thoughtless of others, and often quite suspicious. They will usually prefer routines and are often inflexible. Slow thought processing, poor judgement and lack of spontaneous thought and activity contributes to social withdrawal. The overlap between cognitive impairment and personality change is best illustrated by the dysexecutive syndrome in which the disorder of higher cognition is associated with the presence of persistent behavioural change (Burgess *et al.* 1998). However, even here it may be difficult to be certain that the presence of a reported personality change is due to brain injury, particularly if associated with emotional symptoms and common somatic symptoms, such as headache and dizziness, and where the symptoms show marked variation over time, e.g. from hour to hour or day to day.

The relationship of overall psychiatric disability to injury severity is less convincing. In Walker and Jablon's (1959) large series the severity of injury appeared to bear some relation to many aspects of psychiatric disorder: impaired judgement, mentation, memory, alterations of personality and even the post-traumatic syndrome. However, in a study of patients 2 years post injury, severity of injury correlated only with impairment of intellectual functions and very little, if at all, with emotional instability or post-traumatic headache and dizziness (Norrman & Svahn 1961). Indeed self-reports of emotional sequelae, measured using the MMPI, have been shown to be more common in those with mild compared with severe head injury (Leininger et al. 1991). There may be a complex relationship between injury severity and likelihood of psychiatric sequelae; those with moderate to severe TBI have higher initial risk in the first year, whereas mild TBI is associated with more persistent illness still evident at 3 years (Fann et al. 2004).

Lishman's (1968) investigation of 670 soldiers with penetrating injuries used objective measures including X-ray data and surgeons' operating notes to allow direct estimation of the extent of brain tissue destruction. A wide spectrum of psychiatric disabilities was investigated, including intellectual, affective and behavioural changes, also persistent somatic complaints for which no physical basis could be discovered. It was readily shown that simple measures of the amount of brain damage incurred were related to the amount of psychiatric disorder encountered 1–5 years later. This relationship was broadly maintained when allowance was made for effects due solely to intellectual impairment. When PTA was used as an index of diffuse as opposed to focal brain damage, again regular correlations were seen with the severity of eventual psychiatric disability. The components of psychiatric disability that were particularly closely tied to the indices of brain damage included apathy, euphoria, and behavioural disorders such as disinhibition, facile or childish behaviour and lack of judgement and consideration for others. Among symptoms which had apparently contributed little if at all to the relationships with brain damage were difficulty in concentration, depression, anxiety, irritability, and somatic complaints such as headache, dizziness, fatigue and sensitivity to noise. Difficulty with memory occupied an intermediate position, suggesting a more variable aetiology: some patients suffered principally from organic disturbance of memory and some from psychogenic elaboration of minimal defects.

Nevertheless, the correlations between brain damage and psychiatric disability, while highly significant statistically, were relatively small (correlation coefficients in the region of 0.25). In other words, brain damage could be shown to con-tribute little more than one-fifteenth part of the total causation of psychiatric disability in the material.

Alcohol and drug abuse and head injury

Waller (1968), investigating road deaths in California, found that 58% of drivers, 47% of passengers and 36% of pedestrians had alcohol in the blood, most with levels exceeding the legal maximum for drivers. Moreover, 75% of the drivers could be classified as problem drinkers. In the UK it has been estimated that one-quarter of all road accident deaths are associated with alcohol (Raffle 1989). In an urban trauma centre perhaps 40% of head injuries are in those with a history of heavy drinking (Kolakowsky-Hayner et al. 1999). The prevalence of head injury in alcoholic subjects is some two to four times that of the general population (Hillbom & Holm 1986). Alcohol, particularly binge drinking, is associated with assaults and falls (Savola et al. 2005), whereas drug abuse may have a more particular association with assaults (Corrigan et al. 1995).

The ways in which acute alcohol intake can increase the extent of brain injury, and chronic intake can delay reparative processes within the nervous system, are now appreciated from laboratory experimental studies (Albin & Bunegin 1986). There are many other reasons why those with a history of alcohol dependence might do worse after a head injury including the known effects of alcohol dependence in the absence of a head injury to produce cognitive impairment. However, not all studies find that an elevated blood alcohol at the time of injury predicts a worse outcome once injury severity measures of depth or length of unconsciousness have been controlled (Nath et al. 1986; Alexander et al. 2004). This may be because those who are intoxicated will, for any given severity of TBI, have deeper and more prolonged unconsciousness; their conscious level is suppressed by the sedative effects of alcohol. Thus when matched for injury severity using measures of conscious level, intoxicated patients may have similar outcomes, despite potential deleterious effects of alcohol on outcome. As a group, patients who are blood alcohol positive on admission tend to have lower GCS scores (Chatham-Showalter et al. 1996).

Nevertheless many studies do demonstrate the adverse effects of alcohol on functional outcomes. This may be explained by greater cerebral atrophy in patients with either a history of alcohol dependence or a positive blood alcohol at admission (see Neuroimaging and head injury, earlier in chapter), and there is evidence that for any given level of physical trauma those who are intoxicated have more severe evidence of brain injury on CT (Cunningham et al. 2002). Patients who resume alcohol abuse have less medial frontal grey matter, impaired performance in executive tasks, and are less likely to return to work (Jorge et al. 2005).

Brooks et al. (1989) found that alcohol intake at injury was a significant predictor of the severity of memory impairment

2–6 years later. Moreover, there was an interaction between the severity of the injury and amount of alcohol consumed on the size of the memory deficit; to have a short PTA and to have drunk heavily led to a worse outcome than occurred in patients with a considerably longer PTA who had drunk lightly or not at all.

In Brooks *et al.*'s (1989) study the deleterious effects of drinking at the time of the accident emerged more clearly than the effects of habitual consumption, although the two were strongly interrelated. However, Rönty *et al.* (1993) have shown the effects of habitual excessive consumption on CT measures of brain damage in 56 consecutive patients with mild or moderate injury, including 15 alcohol abusers and 41 without alcohol problems. The groups were comparable in terms of age and severity of injury. The alcohol group showed markedly larger initial volumes of brain injury on CT. On rescanning 6 months and 1 year later the alcohol groups had developed more local brain atrophy, and greater ventricular and sulcal enlargement, despite equivalence on these measures with the non-alcoholic group at the time of injury. Only 40% of the alcohol group returned to work after the injury compared with 73% of the remainder. A deleterious effect of alcohol intoxication at the time of injury on neuropsychological test performance in the months after injury, independent of the effects of a history of pre-injury alcohol abuse, has been found (Tate & Broe 1999). Over 50% were intoxicated at the time of injury and these patients did worse on tests of memory and block design, after controlling for injury severity and history of alcohol abuse. Alcohol and drug misuse before injury increase the risk of mood disorder after injury (Dikmen *et al.* 2004; Jorge *et al.* 2005).

In view of the close association of head injury with alcoholism, it is worth having a low index of suspicion for its role in many of the sequelae of head injury. It is associated with subdural haemorrhage (Sonne & Tonnesen 1992). Agitation requiring restraint in the early post-injury period is more common in those with a history of alcohol use (Edlund *et al.* 1991) and may be related to an alcohol withdrawal syndrome. It is easy to miss Wernicke–Korsakoff syndrome in a patient recovering from head injury, yet treatment with thiamine might ameliorate at least some of the cognitive impairment. There is therefore something to be said for routinely prescribing thiamine in patients with a head injury with a history of alcohol dependence (Ferguson *et al.* 1997).

It is not uncommon to observe patients with a prolonged and severe history of alcohol dependence before injury to be apparently cured of alcohol dependence while on an inpatient rehabilitation unit. For many months after the injury they show no sign of craving or interest in alcohol. However, this happy state of affairs does not always last. As former cues are reintroduced when they begin to take visits into the community past pubs and off-licenses, and re-establish former friendships and generally become more active, drinking behaviour often returns. Nevertheless, there may be a tendency for the proportion of patients with drinking problems to decrease after brain injury (Kreutzer *et al.* 1990). Bombardier *et al.* (2003) compared subjects' drinking habits in the year before and the year after a head injury. In the year before 41% were rated as heavy drinkers, but this had reduced to 17% in the year following injury. They found little evidence of new cases of alcohol dependence arising in the post-injury year. However, when followed up for 30 years almost 12% of patients were found to have developed alcohol abuse not previously present (Koponen *et al.* 2002). In a study looking particularly at drug abuse, there is evidence that there may be some who only take to drug abuse after the injury, and might not have done so had they not been injured (Hibbard *et al.* 1998).

Location of brain damage incurred

Many investigations have sought to determine how far psychiatric disability depends on the location of damage within the brain. Studies examining the correlations between neuroimaging and outcome in closed head injury are discussed in Neuroimaging and head injury, earlier in chapter. However, closed head injury is not a good model for predicting brain–behaviour relationships because of the diffuse nature of the insult. On the other hand, penetrating injuries are more suitable for analysis, though even here it must be recognised that damage may exist where it is unsuspected.

Teuber (1959, 1962) and coworkers investigated cognitive and perceptual defects in a large series of penetrating injuries with regional brain damage. Patients with left parietotemporal lesions showed significant losses on the AGCT of general intelligence when pre- and post-traumatic scores were compared. No such losses were found after lesions elsewhere. The differences persisted after excluding patients with dysphasia.

Hillbom's (1960) important investigation surveyed a large number of wartime head injuries, of which 415 were randomly selected for special study. Among unilateral wounds, the left were associated with more psychiatric disturbance than the right, particularly where dementias and psychoses were concerned. Patients with parietal, occipital and cerebellar lesions were relatively free from psychiatric disturbance.

Lishman (1968) also found left hemisphere lesions to be more closely associated with overall psychiatric disability than right hemisphere lesions and patients with injury to the left temporal lobe were particularly at risk. However, intellectual disorders were found more commonly after left hemisphere damage, while affective disorders, behavioural disorders and somatic complaints were more frequent after right hemisphere damage (Table 4.4). Intellectual disorders were especially associated with damage to the parietal and temporal lobes, whereas affective disorders, behavioural disorders and somatic complaints were more frequent after frontal lobe damage. Sexual disturbances were seen only after frontal wounds, and with one exception this was also

Table 4.4 Symptoms and symptom groups seen 1–5 years after penetrating injury in relation to location of brain damage. (After Lishman 1968.)

	No. of cases (total 345)	Hemisphere		Lobe(s) (right, left or both)			
		Left	Right	Frontal	Parietal	Temporal	Occipital
Any intellectual disorder	117	*			*	*	?*
General intellectual impairment	32	*				*	?*
Dysphasia	24	*			*	*	
Impairment of memory	50	*			*		*
Difficulty in concentration	87		*				*
Any affective disorder	113		*	*			
Depression	58		*	*	*		
Anxiety	40						*
Irritability	72		*	*	*		
Aggression	10			*			
Apathy	35		*				
Euphoria	10			*			
Any behavioural disorder	40		*	*			
Crime or misdemeanours	5			*			
Sexual disturbance	8			*			
Lack of judgement, etc.	20			*			
Facile or childish behaviour	17		*	*			
Disinhibition	13			*			
Somatic complaints	71		*	*			
Headache or dizziness	62			*			
Fatigue	16				*		
Sensitivity to noise	24			*			
'Frontal lobe syndrome'	32		*	*			

* Indicates strong evidence of special association.

true of criminal behaviour. The 'frontal lobe syndrome' (recorded for patients who showed euphoria, lack of judgement, facile or childish behaviour or disinhibition) was especially common after frontal wounds, but 9 of 32 examples were found after wounds which did not apparently involve the frontal lobes at all.

In the Vietnam Head Injury Study, right orbitofrontal injury was associated with increased edginess, anxiety and depression, whereas left dorsolateral frontal lesions showed greater anger and hostility (Grafman *et al.* 1986a). The literature on the behavioural consequences of patients suffering head injuries in the world wars, which also demonstrated locaton-specific effects, will be reviewed in detail below.

There is therefore support for the broad generalisation that lesions in some areas provide a greater psychiatric hazard than others, and that this involves emotional and behavioural disturbances as well as cognitive defects. Nevertheless, it seems likely that in general the amount of brain damage incurred is more important than its location in determining outcome (Grafman *et al.* 1986b).

Categories of post-traumatic psychiatric disorder

The many different forms of post-traumatic psychiatric disablement cannot be rigidly classified, and complex admixtures of symptoms are frequently seen. For example, changes of temperament may occur along with intellectual impairment, or paranoid developments may arise in association with neurotic disability. Quite often, however, specific features or a combination of related features are outstanding, or even seen in relative isolation. For this reason the four main categories of psychiatric disturbance are examined separately: cognitive impairment, change of personality, psychosis, and affective disorders. The problem of the so-called post-concussion syndrome will be dealt with separately, alongside a discussion of outcome after mild head injury.

The relative frequency of these changes may be gauged from the analysis of two large series of patients in which these broad divisions have been observed. Hillbom's (1960) follow-up of 3552 wartime injuries, of which 1505 were penetrating, showed cognitive impairment in 2%, changes of character in 18%, psychoses in 8% and severe neuroses in 11%. Ota's (1969) large series of 1168 closed head injuries among Japanese civilians showed cognitive impairment in 3%, changes of character in 6%, psychoses in 5% and neuroses in 22%. The frequency of cognitive impairment will depend heavily on the severity of brain injury studied. For example, half of patients with severe head injury will have memory impairment (Levin 1990).

More recently, standardised diagnostic assessments have ascertained the frequency of Axis 1 mental disorders after closed head injury. High rates of depression and anxiety disorders were identified in patients with a head injury attending a brain injury rehabilitation outpatient clinic; 26% had a major depressive disorder and 24% generalised anxiety disorder (Fann *et al.* 1995). Using the Structured Clinical Interview for DSM-IV Diagnoses (SCID) in community-dwelling survivors of head injury on average 7 years post injury, strikingly high rates of depression and anxiety disorders have been found (Hibbard *et al.* 1998): 80% were diagnosed as suffering any Axis 1 disorder, with 61% having major depression and 9–19% one or other of the anxiety disorders; 28% had a substance use disorder. Using a robust method of subject ascertainment, Deb *et al.* (1999b) found that in a consecutive series of 120 patients aged 18–64 years admitted to a hospital following a TBI, at 1 year post injury 14% had an International Classification of Diseases (ICD)-10 diagnosis of depressive illness and 9% panic disorder, higher rates than in the general population. Comorbidity is common; in one study half of patients with major depression also had generalised anxiety disorder (van Reekum *et al.* 1996). Patients with TBI, compared with age- and sex-matched controls, have more psychiatric illness both before and after the head injury (Fann *et al.* 2004). The database of the NIMH Epidemiologic Catchment Area Study has been analysed to compare lifetime rates of psychiatric illness in those who reported that they had suffered a head injury with loss of consciousness, with controls (Silver *et al.* 2001). Increased rates of depression (11% vs 5%), anxiety disorders (e.g. panic disorder 3.2% vs 1.3%), alcohol (24% vs 10%) and drug abuse (11% vs 5%) were seen. It was not possible to say if these disorders antedated or postdated the head injury. What is perhaps surprising from these studies is the relative lack of reporting of post-traumatic stress disorder.

Cognitive impairment

More severe head injuries are likely to be followed by persisting cognitive impairment of a degree proportional to the amount of brain damage incurred. In closed head injuries a PTA of 24 hours may be taken as a very approximate clinical guide; below this, complete intellectual recovery may be expected in a fair proportion of cases, but with durations in excess of 24 hours the patient will be fortunate to escape

without some intellectual impairment. With penetrating injuries the length of PTA is a less reliable guide. In these cases concussion and amnesia may then be brief or absent, yet focal cognitive defects can be severe, especially if haemorrhage or infection have occurred. With increasing age intellectual impairment becomes more likely. Damage to the dominant hemisphere will generally produce more severe effects on intellectual function than damage to the non-dominant hemisphere (Teuber 1959, 1962; Piercy 1964).

As in almost all cases of diffuse brain damage, the hallmarks of the cognitive impairment of closed head injury are psychomotor slowing, difficulties with attention and concentration and memory, and impairment of executive function. In cases where the only finding was diffuse axonal injury the most frequent impairments were in memory and executive function, but no cognitive domain was consistently spared (Scheid *et al.* 2006).

Impairments of speed of information processing, capacity for information processing, attention and executive function go hand in hand and many of the common cognitive symptoms of closed head injury can be understood as arising from their selective vulnerability. The result is slowness over tasks, inattention due to overload, and distractibility due to lack of spare capacity for the monitoring of irrelevant stimuli; working memory is impaired (McDowell *et al.* 1997). These symptoms overlap with those described as part of the dysexecutive syndrome: lack of fluency and problems with dual-task processing and multi-tasking, organising, planning and prioritising, switching from one task to another, inhibiting behaviour and adapting to novel situations, abstract reasoning and judgment, and with monitoring.

Dissecting out the contribution of the psychological processes underlying these various symptoms is not easy. For example, the attentional problems that follow brain injury are multifaceted and overlapping. They include alterations in alertness, psychomotor slowing, distractibility, impaired sustained attention and difficulties switching attention (van Zomeren *et al.* 1984; Gronwall 1987, 1989; Stuss *et al.* 1989). The degree to which these various facets of attention share common processing impairments is uncertain. It seems likely that while slowed speed of information processing is central to many attentional problems (Ponsford & Kinsella 1992), it cannot account for all (Whyte *et al.* 1995). So, for example, impairments of those aspects of attention related to executive function (Spikman *et al.* 1996) are observed independent of slowing.

Simple reaction times are not a good indicator of injury severity and more complex tasks are more likely to show evidence of psychomotor slowing. The PASAT taps many of the cognitive processes related to slowing of information and working memory and is particularly sensitive to head injury (Tombaugh 2006). It has been suggested that delayed processing speed is particularly likely when interhemispheric information procession is required (Mathias *et al.* 2004b).

Likewise dual-task processing impairments may be particularly vulnerable to diffuse brain injury (Vilkki *et al*. 1996), suggesting that it is damage to the white matter tracts that interferes with the networks necessary for information processing and attention.

Executive disorder after head injury is also multifaceted and the tests used to measure it overlap with tests of 'frontal lobe function'. No one single measure of executive function seems adequate to capture the various impairments and behaviours that may be described as being part of the dysexecutive syndrome (Bamdad *et al*. 2003). The Behavioural Assessment of Dysexecutive Syndrome (BADS) (Wilson *et al*. 1996), which has tests requiring the subject to impose a plan to solve the task rather than simply having to follow rules, was developed as a sensitive measure. In fact, multiple tests, including more traditional tests of frontal executive disorder such as Wisconsin Card Sorting Test (WCST), Trails B, verbal fluency and the Stroop, as well as BADS, may be necessary to detect all patients with evidence of executive problems (Bennett *et al*. 2005).

As a general rule, patients after closed head injury may show impairments on frontal lobe tests or tests of executive function, in the absence of any evidence of impairment of IQ; it is therefore essential to have undertaken tests of frontal or executive function, for example BADS, before ruling out evidence of cognitive impairment. Some patients with good evidence in day-to-day life of disorganised thinking due to brain injury will nevertheless perform well on standard frontal executive tests. Impairments may only be evident for tests which replicate the unstructured demands of everyday life (Shallice & Burgess 1991); tests of shopping performance seem to be particularly telling (Alderman *et al*. 2003) (Fig. 4.6).

The growing literature on the cognitive processes, located particularly in medial orbitofrontal lobe, involved in decision-making in relation to goal-directed behaviour (Kringelbach & Rolls 2004) helps explain how impairments of cognition overlap with changes in behaviour and personality (Damasio 1996). For example, central executive deficits measured using dual-task processing may be related to

(a)   (b)

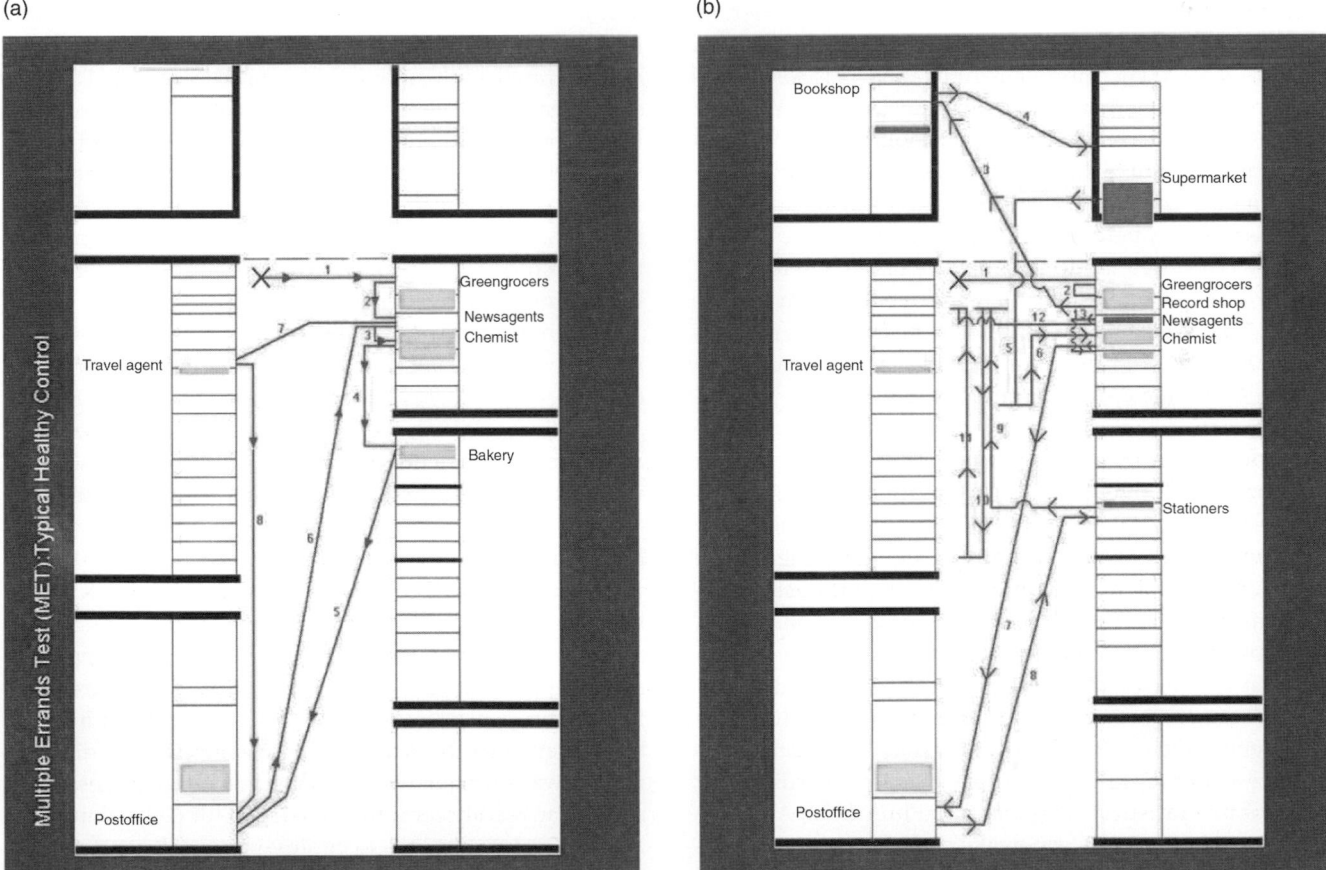

Fig. 4.6 Multiple Errands Test. Patients are given the task of buying items in a certain order, with additional rules that they have to follow. (a) The systematic path of a healthy control patient undertaking the task in a pedestrianised street. (b) The disorganized path of a patient with a dysexecutive syndrome who undertakes the task in an inefficient manner and breaks the rules. (Courtesy of Professor Paul Burgess.)

behavioural dyscontrol (Alderman 1996). Abnormal performance on a gambling test may be associated with personality change (Levine *et al.* 2005).

Memory is also disproportionately affected in relation to intellectual function (Levin *et al.* 1988). Several problems are characteristic of the memory impairment of closed head injury (Baddeley *et al.* 2002). Inaccurate recall of memories is probably partly related to problems with source memory, in other words identifying the context in which a memory is embedded. One consequence is intrusions, for example recalling a word from the wrong word list. Confabulations are common and lack of insight for the memory disorder is almost universal if confabulation is marked. Problems with executive function probably partly explain why patients have problems with memory recall (Vanderploeg *et al.* 1994), perhaps because of a failure to apply active strategies to help recall. Impairments in executive function may also contribute to the impairments seen in prospective memory, i.e. the ability to remember to do something (Kinsella *et al.* 1996).

Language and communication problems are quite common, though pure aphasic syndromes are not. Many patients complain of word-finding difficulties. Deficits in executive function and social cognition contribute to the communication difficulties, for example patients often show impairments in understanding of metaphor or faux pas (Milders *et al.* 2003). Improvement in aphasia is sometimes quite marked, whether after penetrating injury (Walker & Blumer 1989) or closed head injury (Thomsen 1984). Verbal IQ is more resistant to the effects of closed head injury than is performance IQ and it is therefore not unusual to see a significant discrepancy between verbal and performance IQ, particularly for those measures which are timed. On the other hand, insight into any cognitive impairment and any accompanying behavioural change tends to be lost early, and this often has a marked bearing on the patient's capacity to manage their finances and affairs for example.

All gradations are seen, ranging from established severe post-traumatic dementia to minimal degrees of intellectual impairment that may come to light only when the patient returns to work. After very severe closed head injury the impairment of intellect is usually global, affecting a wide range of cognitive functions together. Marked post-traumatic dementia is usually accompanied by hemiparesis, quadriparesis or other striking neurological disablement. In the most severe cases the patient remains mute and immobile on recovery from coma, persisting thus until death supervenes, often within a year. This is the *persistent vegetative state*, which represents the most severe form of disability compatible with survival (Jennett & Plum 1972; Andrews 1999; Bates 2005). The sleep–wake cycle is preserved, indicating that the patient is no longer comatose, but all mental function appears to be lost. The eyes may be open and blink to menace or follow moving objects, but they are not attentive. Liquids placed in the mouth may be swallowed. Beyond this, however, responsiveness is usually limited to primitive postural and reflex movements of the limbs. Such a condition represents essentially a state of wakefulness without awareness. The similarity to akinetic mutism is obvious, though in the latter the potential for responding may be considerably greater. The most important differential diagnosis is a locked-in syndrome. In these patients the ability to communicate is lost, yet conscious awareness and thought is relatively spared. Therefore every attempt to establish communication with the patient, for example using eye blink to indicate 'yes/no', needs to be explored. PET scanning may demonstrate reduced cerebral cortex blood flow (Menon *et al.* 1998). The difficult ethical and legal problems surrounding the point at which life-sustaining treatment might possibly be withdrawn are discussed by Howard and Miller (1995). The responsible lesions may lie in the cortex, thalamus or brain stem, with diffuse white matter damage being universal at autopsy.

Short of this, the patient is profoundly slow and apathetic, frequently with incontinence and gross dysarthria. All intellectual processes are severely affected and even recognition of relatives may be long delayed. These patients are described as being in a minimally conscious state (Giacino & Whyte 2005). Further recovery often brings evidence of emotional lability, with episodes of uncontrolled weeping or laughing, or more rarely with outbursts of poorly coordinated aggressive behaviour. The 'catastrophic reaction' may be called forth when the patient is confronted with a task beyond his ability, with sudden flushing, restless overactivity and either explosive anger or weeping. In one very severely injured patient, eye-contact caused dramatic distress and opisthotonic posturing, and was associated with a decline in the overall condition (Fleminger *et al.* 1996).

Slow improvement over many months or sometimes years may be expected in all but the most severe examples. Apathy or empty euphoria may remain as persistent features. Logical and abstract thinking will be most markedly affected as in other forms of dementia. Blunting of affect and loss of libido is the rule, and paranoid developments are not uncommon.

Focal cognitive impairment

A focal emphasis of brain pathology may result in focal cognitive deficits, which either stand out against a background of general intellectual impairment or on occasion appear in highly circumscribed form. Strictly focal deficits are more likely after penetrating injuries than closed head injuries, but nonetheless the search for focal emphasis in disorder must always be pursued. A dysphasic or an amnesic syndrome can readily come to be mistaken for global dementia. Areas of relatively intact cognitive function must always be demarcated so that they can be used to the full in rehabilitation.

Selective impairment of memory may persist despite excellent restitution of other intellectual functions. This may be sufficiently marked to constitute a 'post-traumatic Korsakoff syndrome', and presumably depends on circumscribed damage to structures in the diencephalon or medial temporal lobe structures.

It is unfortunately true that when focal deficits are very marked and persistent, in patients with closed head injury the likelihood of impairment in other areas of intellectual function is high. However, in penetrating injuries, for example due to high-velocity missiles, highly selective impairments in language, visual perception and spatial orientation persisting 20 years after injury, yet without any evidence of generalised intellectual deterioration, may be seen (Newcombe 1969).

Change of personality

Change of personality implies an alteration in the patient's habitual attitudes and patterns of behaviour, so that his reactions to events and to people are different from what they were before. This may occur as a persistent sequel of head injury and is undoubtedly one of the most distressing aftereffects for the families of the victims. The patient may be aware of the change in himself, though quite often he is completely oblivious of it. Sometimes the alterations are gross and obvious, or sometimes detectable only to those who knew him well beforehand.

The term is used to cover a wide variety of disturbances that can be hard to evaluate or to classify with precision. Such disturbances may overlap with changes in cognition, or with persistent changes in mood. Accordingly, this area of post-traumatic change is particularly difficult to interpret. Aspects of the pre-traumatic personality will usually be found to colour the picture, and many of the changes will represent intensification of traits that were present all along. Sometimes, however, as with frontal lobe damage, there will be elements of change that are new and broadly similar in all individuals affected. Sometimes the changes will be determined by brain damage, sometimes by psychogenic factors and sometimes by a combination of the two. Where brain damage is insubstantial, the stress of the accident and its subsequent repercussions will often be found to be the factors mainly responsible, acting on special vulnerabilities in the person concerned.

Alexander (1982) points out that head injury is particularly prone to damage the neocortical portions of the limbic system: the frontopolar, orbitofrontal and anterior temporal regions (see Fig. 4.1). Few other pathologies routinely damage such areas in a symmetrical fashion while largely sparing the rest of the neocortex. This may explain why behavioural problems are often greatly out of proportion to the severity of neurological defects, and why profound changes in behaviour, affect and emotion can occur even when there is little by way of long-term cognitive impairment.

Nevertheless, the personality change after brain injury is heterogeneous. Lezak (1978), on the basis of her extensive experience, suggested five broad and overlapping categories of personality change:
- impaired capacity for social perceptiveness;
- impaired capacity for control and self-regulation;
- stimulus-bound behaviour producing difficulties in initiating and planning behaviour;
- emotional alterations, particularly apathy, silliness and lability;
- inability to profit from experience.

However, when standard criteria are applied to describe typical personality disorders following head injury, a somewhat different picture emerges. For example, of 60 patients with head injury (half of whom had severe or very severe injuries) followed up 30 years after injury, 23% were found to have a personality disorder (Koponen *et al.* 2002). The most frequent were avoidant (15.0%), paranoid (8.3%) and schizoid (6.7%). Another study rated two-thirds of patients to have a personality disorder, the most frequent being borderline, avoidant, paranoid, obsessive–compulsive and narcissistic disorder (Hibbard *et al.* 2000). The association with borderline personality disorder is in keeping with the finding that 40% of men presenting with borderline personality disorder give a history of head injury, compared with only 4% of controls (Streeter *et al.* 1995).

In Roberts' (1976, 1979) survey of the long-term outcome of severe head injuries, the commonest pattern of personality change had a distinctly frontal character. This he termed 'fronto-limbic dementia', a combination of disabling euphoria, disinhibition or anergia, associated in the majority of cases with intense irritability. Marked examples were seen only after very severe injuries. Memory was usually also very defective. Less commonly, the frontal personality change was present without undue irritability. Occasional patients indeed could be said to have shown *improvement* in personality, in that they were now less prone to worry and were more outgoing and sociable.

Personality change and location of injury
Frontal lobe lesions remain the best-known example of the effects of regional cerebral damage on personality. However, two important questions emerge. First is there evidence that frontal injury, either bilateral or unilateral, as opposed to injury to other parts of the brain, is particularly likely to cause a change in personality? If so, is it possible to determine any associations between the sort of personality change observed and the localisation of the lesion within the frontal lobe?

The first observation that indicated that personality change might be particularly likely after frontal as opposed to other brain injuries was perhaps the case report of Phineas Gage. He was injured by an iron bar which passed through his frontal lobes and caused profound personality change (Harlow 1868). Then, in a study of historical importance,

Phelps (1898) investigated the site of laceration of the brain at autopsy and compared this with the presence or absence of mental abnormalities immediately before death in a series of head-injured patients. Among 225 autopsies, mental change had existed in only four cases where lacerations had spared the left frontal lobe. Furthermore, among 28 cases with frontal lobe laceration, abnormalities had been noted only when the left lobe was damaged.

Since then extensive series of patients with penetrating head injuries have been investigated after each world war. Unfortunately, many of these studies relied heavily on impressionistic statements. Nevertheless, Feuchtwanger's (1923) study provides strong support for the selective effects of injuries that are frontal as opposed to non-frontal. He compared 200 frontal gunshot wounds with 200 cases where bullets had penetrated other parts of the skull. The outstanding changes in the frontal group included euphoria, facetiousness, irritability, apathy and defects of attention. There was often an incapacity for planning ahead, tactlessness and moral defects. Where intellect was disturbed this seemed usually to be secondary to disorders of emotion and volition. Support for these findings came from Hillbom (1960); character change was observed in 43% of those with frontal injury as opposed to 25% across the whole group of brain injured. Lishman (1968) identified 32 patients who showed euphoria, lack of judgement, facile or childish behaviour or disinhibition; this 'frontal lobe syndrome' was especially common after frontal wounds, but 9 of the 32 appeared to have no involvement of frontal lobes at all. Grafman et al. (1996) found that patients from the Vietnam Head Injury Study with injuries only involving frontal lobe, compared with those with injuries not involving frontal lobe, were more likely to show aggression; for example 19% as opposed to 8% were rated as having threatened to injure others. Others have noted the liability of frontal lesions to produce changes of character that led to criminality (Lindenberg 1951; Mutschler 1956). Kleist (1934) added loss of initiative, aspontaneity of motor activity, lack of ideation and mutism as characteristic of frontal injuries.

We can therefore confidently assert that injury to the frontal lobes carries a particular risk of personality change, and that the personality change tends to have particular characteristics. However, consistent effects of laterality of lesion have not been found. The special psychiatric hazard of bifrontal injuries has been noted (Heygster 1949), although this may at least in part be because medial and orbital frontal lesions are particularly likely to be bilateral.

Are there any selective effects of the site of injury within the frontal lobe? Differences have been described between wounds of the convex lateral surface and wounds of the orbital parts of the lobe, the former producing mainly intellectual and motor changes while the latter had more serious effects on the personality (Kleist 1934; Faust 1955, 1960; Walch 1956). Walch was able to compare 117 cases with orbit-ofrontal injuries with 185 frontal injuries not involving orbitofrontal cortex. Disinhibition was common to both but those with orbitofrontal injuries remained 'indifferent to every attempt at guidance' and a high proportion showed changes in 'the more highly developed qualities of personality'. On the other hand, lack of drive was more associated with convexity lesions. Faust similarly stressed the lack of productive thinking, indifference and incapacity for decisions with convexity lesions. Patients with orbital lesions often failed to show defects on formal intelligence testing, but were prone to develop marked personality changes.

In line with these observations Blumer and Benson (1978) proposed two types of personality change after frontal injury. One in which apathy and indifference were marked was termed 'pseudodepressed'. This was associated with convexity lesions, and also injury to basal ganglia and thalamus and their connections. On the other hand, orbitofrontal lesions might produce a 'pseudopsychopathic' personality with changes in the direction of puerility and euphoria. The patient lacked adult tact and restraint and might be coarse, facetious, hyperkinetic or promiscuous. Irritability and impulsive antisocial behaviour could be seen. More recent investigations into social cognition, decision-making and control of goal-directed behaviour lend support to the notion that damage to orbitofrontal or ventromedial cortex might result in such disturbance of social behaviour (see below).

In view of the close proximity of the cribriform plate to the medial orbitofrontal cortex, it is not surprising that some patients with disturbance of social cognition associated with damage to medial orbitofrontal cortex also have anosmia (Cicerone & Tanenbaum 1997) (Fig. 4.7). Anosmia is associated with injury to orbitofrontal cortex (Yousem et al. 1999). Anosmia may be associated with impairment of executive function (Callahan & Hinkebein 1999), and with hypoperfusion of orbitofrontal cortex (Varney et al. 2001). However, the observation that anosmia is particularly associated with antisocial personality change after head injury (Varney 1988) has not been replicated (Greiffenstein et al. 2002b).

The picture just described has obtained recognition on account of the uniformity of the changes seen from case to case. Frontal lobe personality change bears a definitive stamp which in large measure cuts across differences in premorbid personality. However, less is known about specific personality changes that may follow circumscribed lesions of other parts of the brain. Temporal lobe injuries appear to show a special frequency of personality disorder, both in their own right and by virtue of the temporal lobe epilepsy which may accompany them (Ajuriaguerra & Hecaen 1960).

Injury to the basal parts of the brain also attracted special attention. Kretschmer (1949, 1956) described a 'basal syndrome' which found wide support in the German literature. This results from lesions of the midbrain, hypothalamus and orbitofrontal cortex. It is characterised by sluggishness and apathy along with fluctuations of mood and sudden outbursts of irritability, typically coupled with disturbance of fundamental drives and instincts – appetite, thirst and sleep rhythm – and varied sexual pathologies. Hoheisel and Walch (1952) described five patients with marked bipolar fluctuations of mood persisting for a long time after head injury; one such case had a shell splinter in the hypothalamus and the other four showed clinical signs that indicated diencephalic injury.

Personality change and cognitive impairment

In those with severe brain injury the personality change will often be but one aspect of the global dementia which follows injury, and cognitive deficits of some degree will be in evidence. With more severe dementia there will be slowing, impairment of motivation, loss of libido and withdrawal of interest in surrounding events and people. Emotional changes include blunting, instability, apathy or euphoria.

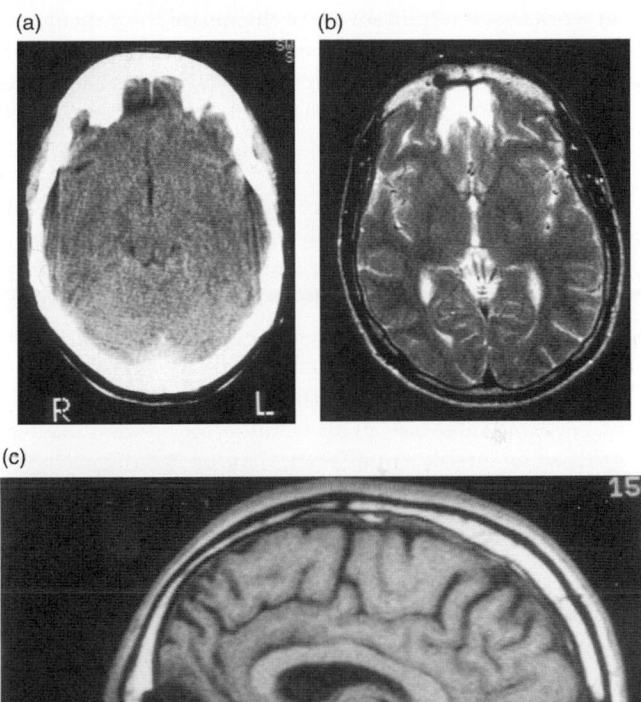

Fig. 4.7 Personality change after head injury associated with medial orbitofrontal damage. A 33-year-old plumber was involved in a fight and was knocked to the ground. He was unconscious for about 5 minutes and was admitted to hospital for a few days. He was never able to return to his job. He became disorganised and lacking initiative and drive. He came to rely entirely on his girlfriend and a good friend for support, e.g. to manage his finances and get him to appointments. He developed a severe constant headache and threatened violence against his doctors for not being able to help him. The CT brain scan (a) was reported as normal and he was turned down for both Disability Living Allowance and by the Criminal Injuries Compensation Authority; his disability was regarded as a gross over-reaction to a mild and relatively trivial head injury. At 5 years post injury he had a full neuropsychiatric assessment which noted that he had been anosmic ever since the injury, and that in the first few days in hospital after the injury he was confused and occasionally walked around the ward naked. MRI identified a lesion of the medial orbitofrontal lobe bilaterally: (b) T2 weighted; (c) sagittal section T1 weighted; (d) coronal section T1 weighted. This had in fact been evident on the CT scan as a hypodense area, but was presumably regarded as artefact. Because it was now evident that his personality change and dysexecutive disorder was due to a traumatic lesion of the brain, he was successful in appealing for disability allowance and compensation. Five years later, 10 years after the injury, he continues to lead a dependent life, is unemployed, only going on holiday when taken by his friends, has split with his girlfriend and now lives with his mother. He gets quite depressed at times but remains grateful that the cause of his problems has been properly established.

Irritability and explosive anger occur in some cases and paranoid developments in others. A passive and childish dependence may develop, with petulant behaviour and egocentricity. In very severe examples the essential individuality of the person may be to a large extent obscured.

The changes that accompany intellectual impairment may be no more than a loss of refinement or lessened vitality of behaviour, sometimes seen only as transient disturbances which gradually recede over the months that follow. Even so these may combine with adverse circumstances in marriage or at work to set in train severe problems for the patient and his family. With minor degrees of intellectual loss the change may be understandable in terms of the patient's reaction to awareness of minor degrees of cognitive impairment. This may call forth anxiety and depression, especially when the previous personality has been marked by traits of insecurity or feelings of personal inadequacy. Much will depend on the demands made by the environment, and on the handling which the patient receives during the early post-traumatic phase.

In other cases, however, circumscribed brain damage may operate more directly by disruption of cerebral systems upon which the synthesis of the personality depends. The latter situation is compatible with excellent preservation of intellect to formal testing, yet the personality change is nonetheless 'organic' in origin.

A 34-year-old man was referred for psychiatric rehabilitation 7 years after head injury. A fall at work had resulted in fractures of the frontal bones of the skull and these had opened up pathways of infection from the frontal sinuses to the brain. Over the ensuing years extensive chronic abscess formation had caused much brain destruction in both frontal lobes. Prior to the accident he had been a stable thoughtful man, happily married and interested in his family. Now he was talkative, restless and grossly disinhibited. His wife had divorced him on account of his preoccupation with pornographic material and his irresponsibility generally. Twelve thousand pounds awarded to him by way of compensation had been spent within a few months, partly on extravagant presents for relatives and acquaintances, and partly on the reckless purchase of a business which soon went bankrupt. He showed no concern or insight into his disabilities, and made jocular comments about the troubles which had befallen him. Full psychometric testing showed a level of intelligence within the average range and consistent with his previous education and work record. No memory or learning deficits could be detected (Lishman 1973).

A 24-year-old guardsman shot himself through both frontal lobes while playing Russian roulette. He was in coma for 10 days, and mute, incontinent and profoundly anergic for many months thereafter. When seen 3 years later he was permanently hospitalised and appeared to have reached a plateau where improvement was concerned. Apart from dysarthria there were no neurological abnormalities. He was polite and friendly, and on first acquaintance there was little abnormal to detect. Conversation revealed a rather off-hand manner with some degree of euphoria, but he was reasonably well informed about current events. In his daily life, however, he was profoundly lacking in initiative and needed supervision to care for his appearance. When left to his own devices he preferred to lie in bed for most of the day. He was inclined to indulge in childish pranks, and to buy pin-up magazines and talk of women though libido was totally lacking. He was extremely easily led into mischief and had twice been convicted for breaking and entering while on leave from hospital. The only change he recognised in himself was that nothing worried him any more. He showed no remorse about the recent convictions and no concern about his future. When asked about the game of Russian roulette he replied that it had been 'a bit silly, I suppose'. Psychological testing showed intelligence in the average to superior range with no disturbance of memory. But perseverative tendencies were marked and there was considerable difficulty in shifting attention from one task to another.

Though formal tests of intellect may be normal, patients with these sorts of personality change often do badly on tests of social cognition, decision-making and control of goal-directed behaviour. The cognitive impairment and personality change may be two sides of the same coin. This was proposed by Tate (1999) with respect to executive dysfunction and characterological change after head injury. She found greater loss of emotional control, a measure of characterological change, was predicted by more rule-breaking errors in a test of verbal fluency, a test of executive function.

It seems likely that damage to orbitofrontal or ventromedial frontal cortex is central to both the impairment of higher cognition (social cognition, decision-making and control of goal-directed behaviour) and the personality. Damasio (1996) uses a 'somatic marker' hypothesis to explain the link between damage to medial orbitofrontal lobe and impaired social decision-making. It is proposed that normal social behaviour depends on a somatic marker, linked to the limbic system, guiding social decisions based on experience of the outcome of previous similar situations. Decisions which in the past have resulted in poor outcomes are suppressed by the somatic marker. This process is critically dependent on the medial orbitofrontal cortex, where limbic system responses, thought to underpin the somatic marker, are able to influence decisions that depend on cortical processing.

Damasio suggests that failure to recognise and understand emotional signals and social cues is not the problem. The problem lies in the ability to decide and act appropriately despite good social understanding. However, not all agree that social understanding is intact. Patients with ventromedial frontal lesions show impaired ability to interpret nonverbal emotional expression, e.g. from body posture or facial expression (Mah *et al.* 2005); this impairment correlated with greater scores on the Neurobehavioural Rating Scale. Similarly, impairments of recognition of expressions of emotion have been found in a patient with orbitofrontal injury and acquired sociopathy (Blair & Cipolotti 2000). Others have emphasised the role of ventral frontal cortex in the extinction of previously rewarded behaviour (Rolls *et al.* 1994). Patients with ventral frontal lesions, half of whom had suffered a head injury, were unable to alter their behaviour appropriately despite being aware that the situation had changed. Their scores on a questionnaire rating disinhibition or other socially inappropriate behaviours correlated with failure to switch responses.

Milders *et al.* (2003) were able to demonstrate that patients after head injury had problems recognising facial expressions and detecting social faux pas, but the impairment did not correlate with ratings of behavioural problems, although there were trends in the direction of greater impairment being associated with greater behavioural problems. Tests of gambling behaviour may weakly predict the failure of patients to regulate behaviour according to internal goals (Levine *et al.* 2005).

It therefore seems likely that the personality change many describe as the frontal lobe syndrome is due to subtle but disabling impairments of higher cognitive function, particularly as they relate to social understanding and decision-making especially in complex unstructured situations to meet internal goals.

Aggression

The symptom of reduced control over aggression deserves special consideration (see Chapter 2, Disordered control of aggression). This is seen with sufficient frequency after head injury, and often enough in relative isolation, to suggest a particular association with head injury. Three times as many head-injured patients showed significant aggression during the first 6 months post injury as did a control group with multiple trauma but without head injury (33.7% vs 11.5%) (Tateno *et al.* 2003). This difference was not explained by greater alcohol use or depression in the head injured. And problems with aggression continue for many years in a proportion of cases. Indeed relatives tend to report increasing problems with temper outbursts over the years post injury

(Brooks *et al.* 1986; Hall *et al.* 1994). Using a fairly conservative estimate of aggressive behaviour, measured using the Overt Aggression Scale (Yudofsky *et al.* 1986), about one-quarter of patients are found to display aggressive behaviour at 6, 24 and 60 months after discharge from an inpatient rehabilitation unit (Baguley *et al.* 2006). At each time point it was not simply the same patients who displayed aggression; a good proportion of patients moved from being aggressive to not aggressive and vice versa in no particular pattern.

It is customary to distinguish verbal aggression from physical aggression towards either objects or people. Though this is important for risk management, there is little evidence that these different behaviours can be teased apart. Agitation, on the other hand, with marked restlessness and distractibility, is usefully considered separately even though aggression may be present. Agitation is particularly likely to be seen in the early post-injury period in the context of the post-traumatic delirium. Sexually aggressive behaviour, often with evidence of other sexually disinhibited behaviour, may be seen in relative isolation from other forms of aggression and is considered in detail later in this chapter (see Sexuality, social adaptation and effects on the family).

Predictors of aggression include alcohol (Tateno *et al.* 2003), younger age at injury (Greve *et al.* 2001; Baguley *et al.* 2006), being depressed (Tateno *et al.* 2003; Jorge *et al.* 2004; Baguley *et al.* 2006), frontal injury (Tateno *et al.* 2003; and see discussion on frontal injury and personality change above), and a pre-injury history of antisocial behaviour (Greve *et al.* 2001; Tateno *et al.* 2003).

One question of interest is whether a particular pattern of aggressive behaviour tends to be seen in patients after TBI. Hooper *et al.* (1945) described 12 cases of 'episodic rage' with sudden explosions of violent behaviour under minor provocation, sometimes bringing the individuals before the courts repeatedly. The authors stressed that the condition was very different from the more common symptom of post-traumatic irritability, especially in its explosive quality. It could occur, moreover, without evidence of irritability between attacks. In general the problem was found to follow severe head injury, although in a few cases the blow had been quite mild. Such behaviour has been described as the *organic aggression syndrome* (Silver *et al.* 2005) (Box 4.3). The term 'episodic dyscontrol syndrome' has also been used (Eames & Wood 2003). In some patients small amounts of alcohol will trigger the attacks. Very occasionally it may represent an epileptic phenomenon. Short of this, EEG studies may reveal focal temporal lobe disturbance, and on theoretical grounds suspicion falls heavily on brain damage implicating the periamygdaloid region within the temporal lobes (Eames & Wood 2003). The argument that an epileptic disturbance may be involved is difficult to confirm but receives gentle support from the observation that carbamazepine may be effective.

However, good empirical evidence that brain injury does result in a specific syndrome of aggressive behaviour is

> **Box 4.3 Characteristic features of organic aggression syndrome** (Silver *et al.* 2005)
>
> - Reactive: triggered by modest or trivial stimuli
> - Non-reflective: usually does not involve premeditation or planning
> - Non-purposeful: aggression serves no obvious long-term aims or goals
> - Explosive
> - Periodic: long periods of relative calm
> - Ego-dystonic: afterwards patients show remorse and are upset; behaviour is out of character; do not blame others or justify behaviour

lacking. Some clinicians would argue that in the majority of cases troublesome aggression is observed in those who were inclined to aggression before their injury, and in whom there is a background level of increased irritability, intolerance of frustration, and mood swings. There may well be alcohol and drug abuse in the background. Aggressive behaviour in such patients is sometimes a means to obtaining what they want, though at other times may serve no purpose. It seems likely that cases of aggression after head injury do not form a homogeneous group. Indeed, careful enquiry may show that aggressive outbursts have characterised the individual from childhood and adolescence onwards, and that the head injury is merely being blamed for a pre-existing condition (Lishman 1978).

However, other habitually aggressive persons may show true worsening. In some the explosive diathesis will have emerged as a new disorder, out of character for the individual and relevant directly to the injury. The more severe the injury, the more likely that brain damage is responsible. Frontal lobe damage may be particularly significant (Grafman *et al.* 1996) on account of its disinhibiting effects on the personality. One must remain alert, nonetheless, to the possibility that current life stresses, affective disorder or paranoid developments are the factors principally operating to aggravate the situation.

In many cases it is the family who are particularly at risk. In some cases this may be because of conspicuous jealousy within the marital context, or it may reflect high levels of expressed emotion. Burgess and Wood (1990) describe a patient whose uncontrollable behavioural outbursts could easily be triggered by the ward staff, but were immediately inhibited when the doctor appeared on the scene. They argued that this was because of a failure of contention scheduling by the patient. Once anger was triggered, the patient was unable to switch to a behavioural schema that was able to inhibit the anger. However, the appearance of the doctor, perhaps because of what he or she represented, caused automatic selection of a new behavioural schema and an end to the outburst.

Sometimes psychogenic factors may emerge in the end as playing the most important part.

> A man of 21 had shown repeated episodes of markedly aggressive behaviour, chiefly directed towards the police, since a road traffic accident 2.5 years earlier. These had led to repeated convictions and several brief periods of imprisonment. He had previously been a police cadet and there was ample evidence that his conduct prior to the injury had been entirely satisfactory. Detailed investigations failed to show any evidence of brain damage; full EEG studies revealed no abnormality, psychological testing indicated good intelligence without evidence of intellectual impairment, and prolonged fasting showed no evidence of hypoglycaemia. The injury itself had been mild, without neurological sequelae and with a PTA of only 20 minutes.
>
> The great majority of aggressive outbursts occurred after excessive drinking, and when the patient felt that he had been provoked in some degree. Excessive drinking had set in during a phase of severe depression following the loss of a friend in the accident, and continued as the patient became progressively embittered and disgruntled at his failure to find a new career. He now found himself in a vicious circle as a result of repeated convictions, and much of his aggressive behaviour could be seen as bravado in attempts to regain his self-esteem. His hatred of the police force was overt, and he felt their rejection keenly. When drunk, encounters with the police led immediately to the release of explosive outbursts of violence.

Studies of violent offenders have also demonstrated the link between aggression and head injury. For example, moderate to severe head injury was found in 6 of 20 men convicted of domestic violence compared with only one of 20 controls (Turkstra *et al.* 2003). Others have found associations with crime in general. High rates of reported head injury, antedating their forensic history, have been found in convicted felons (Sarapata *et al.* 1998). Men who have committed murder before age 18 are very likely to have suffered a serious head injury in childhood (Lewis *et al.* 2004). One study identified 152 men who had suffered a head injury before age 15 from a prospective study of 12 000 born in Finland in 1966. These men had an increased risk of being in the national register for criminal offences committed after age 15 (OR 1.6); in about 30% of cases this was associated with alcohol abuse (Timonen, Miettunen *et al.* 2002). In the majority of cases the head injury was probably mild, being defined as 'concussion', i.e. without evidence of contusion or skull fracture. This suggests that at least part of the association between suffering a head injury and engaging in a criminal career was because of personality characteristics that are risk factors for both. In other words those who are likely to lead antisocial lives are also likely to suffer a head injury as a child or adolescent.

Personality change without brain damage

Changes of temperament less likely to be based on brain pathology include fluctuating depression, morbid anxiety, obsessional traits and persistent irritability. All are common, and frequently come to be included under the rubric of personality change. Often they represent an intensification of previous personality traits and will have emerged on other occasions under different conditions of stress. They may emerge as responses to physical defects or minor cognitive impairments, certainly in the early stages of convalescence, but when persistent they can more commonly be traced to stresses consequent upon the injury. They are, in fact, often more accurately to be regarded as neurotic reactions than as changes of personality. In some cases detailed enquiry will show that they conform to the picture of post-traumatic stress disorder (PTSD), with intrusive thoughts concerning the accident and avoidance of situations related to it. PTSD can be long-lasting as a source of chronic disability, with reports of it persisting even several decades after wartime stresses. Such patients may readily come to be labelled as suffering from personality change.

Psychoses

The psychosis that can occur during the period of acute post-traumatic delirium has already been described. Psychotic episodes may develop later in association with post-traumatic epilepsy, and here also an organic basis can be discerned. The problem is more complex when chronic psychoses, of a schizophreniform or affective nature, develop in a patient whose head has been injured. The causal role of the injury may then be far from clear, especially if some considerable time has elapsed between the trauma and the onset of the illness. Frequently the patient or his relatives will seize upon the injury in retrospect as an acceptable and understandable cause, and the issue may become a matter of medicolegal importance.

Various possibilities exist. Brain disturbance may itself contribute directly to such developments; or the injury may have acted as a non-specific stress to precipitate the psychosis. Alternatively, factors associated with the psychotic illness caused the head injury (reverse causality). For example, the head injury occurred during the prodromal phase of the psychosis, or personality characteristics which increase the risk of psychosis also increase the risk of suffering a head injury. Finally, of course, the possibility of simple coincidence must also be considered.

These matters have not been disentangled to a satisfactory extent and the rigorous review of David and Prince (2005) lays out the complex issues. Large numbers of cases are hard to assemble, and comparisons between different series raise special difficulties, not least with regard to diagnostic criteria. In general, the longer the lapse of time between the injury and the onset of the psychosis, the more likely that the relationship is coincidental. However, even with a lapse of many years it can be very difficult to discount the injury entirely as a contributory factor, especially if there is clear evidence of persisting brain damage with symptoms derived therefrom in the interim. Both organic disturbances and psychological aftermaths can sometimes be expected to operate over long periods of time in contributing to psychotic developments, for example the long interval characteristically observed between the onset of epilepsy and the onset of the schizophrenia-like psychoses related to it (see Chapter 6).

Nevertheless, a constitutional predisposition to the psychosis is probably a major factor in many cases of psychotic illness following head injury. Tennent (1937) found evidence of special vulnerability in five cases of schizophrenia where the psychotic illness followed directly on the head injury and became manifest as soon as the delirium subsided. All had shown evidence of schizoid traits in the premorbid personality, and the illnesses followed the course of ordinary schizophrenia. Among four depressive psychoses, three had been treated previously for similar affective disorder. The injuries therefore appeared to have made manifest, at a particular point in time, what would in all probability have followed other stressful situations in that particular person.

What is the evidence that head injury can cause a chronic psychotic illness, a schizophrenia or schizophreniform psychosis, not secondary to hypomania or depression? Sometimes in a particular patient it is difficult to refute the argument that had he not suffered the head injury he would not have become psychotic. The argument tends to rest heavily on the observation that the psychotic illness appears to have evolved from symptoms that were seen in the post-traumatic delirium, particularly confabulations or perceptual distortions. Delusional misidentification may be a central feature of the psychosis in these patients (Marshall *et al.* 1995). Delusional misidentification, for example reduplicative paramnesia, is characteristic of the post-traumatic amnesic period but in rare cases can extend beyond this period and last for several years. Derealisation may play a part and Young *et al.* (1992) describe a case where derealisation seemed to play a part in the development of Cotard's syndrome, as it did in the following case.

Four years earlier, a 33-year-old man had suffered a very severe head injury requiring over 6 months inpatient treatment and rehabilitation. A sense of derealisation began within a few months of the accident. Initially it was intermittent and cyclical but in the past 2 years had become constant. He found it impossible to accept the world was real, instead believing that he had died and was living in the 'afterlife'. He believed that people he knew, in particular his wife, had been replaced by imposters using the 'shells' of his previous family and friends. Minor happenings would support his conviction, for example an error in a newspaper article 'would not have happened in the real world'. The beliefs were very distressing and he had almost no insight into them. He became rigid, irritable, cold and aloof and unable to manage the family finances. At times he had become depressed and suicidal and had attempted to harm himself on two occasions. MRI (Fig. 4.8) showed ventriculomegaly with atrophy of the corpus callosum and evidence of old haemorrhage into the cerebral white matter, findings consistent with diffuse axonal injury.

Another example of the phenomenology of the psychosis supporting the notion that the psychosis is a direct consequence of the head injury is to be found in patients with severe cognitive impairment with amnesia and poor insight. Some of these patients may show persecutory delusions centred on the belief that belongings of theirs have been stolen; such delusions are typical of, for example, Alzheimer's dementia. It is also of interest to consider whether patients who are psychotic after head injury have special characteristics. On the one hand, are they different from psychotic patients without a head injury? On the other, are they different in some way from head-injured patients who are not psychotic?

There have been two case–control studies comparing head-injured patients with chronic psychosis with head-injured control (non-psychotic) patients to see if there is anything particular about head-injured patients who develop psychosis. Sachdev et al. (2001) ensured that the controls were age and sex matched to the psychotic patients, but ascertainment bias and relatively small numbers limit con-

fidence in the findings in both studies. Moreover, given their methodology neither study allows any direct conclusion as to whether psychosis is more common after head injury. One-third of the patients of Fuji and Ahmed (2001) were taking illicit drugs that might induce psychosis, compared with about 10% of those without psychosis. Both studies found that, unlike those without psychosis, more than half of psychotic patients were below the age of 21 when injured. The mean interval between injury and psychosis was about 4–5 years. Epilepsy was if anything more frequent in the non-psychotic patients. The vast majority of the Fuji and Ahmed (2001) series suffered mild head injury, and this was less severe than in controls, whereas in the Sachdev et al. (2001) series more severe injury was observed in those who were psychotic. Sachdev et al. found higher rates of family history of psychosis in a first-degree relative in the psychotic group, confirming this as one of the best-established risk factors for the development of psychosis after head injury (Achté et al. 1969; Davison & Bagley 1969). Both studies considered whether the chronic psychosis they observed in these head-injured patients differed from that seen in patients with schizophrenia, and suggested there was less evidence of negative symptoms in those with psychosis following head injury. However, no telling differences were seen.

More convincing evidence that rates of chronic psychosis may be increased after head injury comes from the study of cohorts of head-injured patients that have been followed up. These are usefully reviewed in David and Prince (2005). Many of the studies come from series of soldiers with open head injuries and using criteria for psychosis that are difficult to interpret. Achté et al. (1967, 1969) produced one of the most comprehensive studies of psychotic illness after head injury by following 3552 Finnish soldiers who fought in the Second World War for 22–26 years; the majority had suffered closed head injury, although injury was often due to shrapnel. During this period 92 patients (2.6%) developed

(a)

(b)

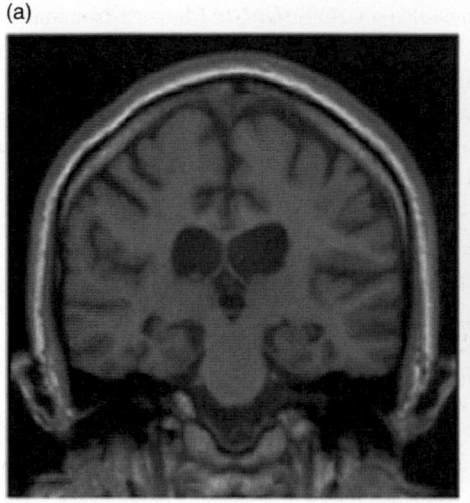
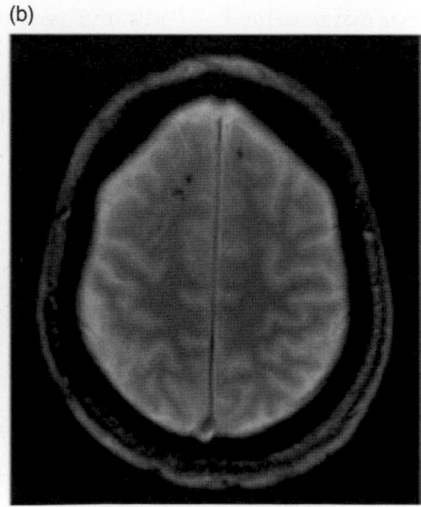

Fig. 4.8 A 33-year-old man with 10 days loss of consciousness after head injury left him with mild to moderate cognitive impairment. Some months after the injury he developed the belief that his wife had been replaced by an imposter and that the whole world was unreal and that he was dead. (a) Coronal section T1 weighted MRI shows mild ventriculomegaly and atrophy of corpus callosum and hippocampi. (b) Gradient-echo axial MRI shows old small haemorrhages in frontal lobes.

psychoses resembling schizophrenia, which is well above the incidence to be expected in the general population. They found that patients with mild injuries developed schizophrenia more frequently than those with severe injuries, and suggested that factors independent of the injury usually played a decisive role.

Civilian cohorts tend to be smaller and unfortunately, though they hint at increased rates of chronic psychosis, many are also jeopardised by poor definition of psychosis. Roberts (1979) described seven cases of paranoid dementia plus two with a schizophrenia-like psychosis developing 10–24 years after severe head injury in 291 civilian patients, suggesting a fivefold relative risk compared to those without a head injury. The findings of De Mol *et al.* (1987), suggesting a threefold to fourfold relative risk are not easy to interpret given that in 80% the psychosis occurred within 6 months of the injury. Two smaller studies are of potential interest. Thomsen (1984), a speech pathologist, describes eight cases of 'post-traumatic psychosis' in 40 patients with very severe head injury followed up over 10–15 years; these eight cases tended to be younger, with no patient over 25 and five in their teens when they suffered the head injury. Unfortunately, from the description of the cases it is not clear that they were in fact suffering with psychotic symptoms, for example two patients were sexually disinhibited and fits of rage attacks were seen in three, but there is no description of the patients suffering delusions or hallucinations. Lezak (1987) describes eight patients, from a cohort of 42 men with very severe head injury (the majority had loss of consciousness of more than 2 weeks) followed up every year for about 5 years, who on at least three occasions displayed hallucinatory or delusional ideation, paranoia or both. None had any prior psychiatric history. In their study of psychiatric illness 1 year after a head injury, the majority being mild, Deb *et al.* (1999b) found one patient to have developed schizophrenia, equivalent to an annual incidence of 0.8%, more than would have been expected in the normal population. Koponen *et al.* (2002) in their study of 60 patients followed up 30 years after injury found psychotic disorder with onset after TBI in four male patients (6.7%; CI 1.9–16). Two of them had moderate brain injuries and the other two severe. Three of the four had delusional disorder and two also had dementia. In two cases the onset was within 1 year of injury but in the other two delusional disorder did not appear until 10 years post injury.

It is therefore difficult to draw any consistent conclusions from these cohort studies. There is an impression that younger patients at the time of injury are more vulnerable to developing psychosis, though of course it is people in their late teens and early twenties who are most vulnerable to developing schizophrenia anyway. Many of the studies hint at an increased rate of psychosis compared with the normal population and this is not far different from Davison and Bagley's (1969) estimate of a twofold to threefold relative risk. However, for many studies the numbers are small and the confidence intervals large and the definition of what constitutes a psychotic illness is weak. They rely on independent assessment of rates of psychosis in the normal population to draw any conclusions about the relative risk.

Large surveys of the total population, including all those who are or are not psychotic and who have or have not had a head injury, do allow direct assessment of the relative risk of head injury in those who develop psychosis. One such cross-sectional survey is the National Epidemiologic Catchment Area Study in the USA. Silver *et al.* (2001) analysed the survey data and found that 361 of 5034 participants indicated that they had suffered a head injury causing loss of consciousness or confusion; 73 of the total sample developed schizophrenia, 3.4% of the head-injured group and 1.9% of those without a head injury (after adjusting for several variables including age, sex and alcohol abuse). The OR of 1.8, controlling for age, sex, marital status and socioeconomic status, was just significant, indicating almost twice the rate of schizophrenia in those with a history of head injury. However, the OR was no longer significant after also adjusting for alcohol use (OR 1.7, CI 0.9–3.0). In summary the study suggests there may be a less than twofold increase in the rate of schizophrenia.

Case–control studies also allow direct comparison of the association between head injury and psychosis. The standard retrospective case–control takes patients who have developed psychosis and asks them if they have ever suffered a head injury to see if there is an excess rate in those who are psychotic compared with controls. Two studies have examined this in terms of childhood head injury as a risk factor for later schizophrenia. One looked at this question from the point of view of childhood head injury in those admitted to hospital with mental illness or for surgery (Wilcox & Nasrallah 1987). Compared with surgical controls, those admitted with schizophrenia had a much higher, and statistically significant, rate of reported head injury in childhood (OR 16). This was greater than for those with bipolar disorder (OR 7), although given the large confidence intervals this was not statistically significant. Recall bias could have had a marked effect in this study, weakening one's confidence in the conclusion. AbdelMalik *et al.* (2003) used unaffected family members (*N* = 102), from 23 families in whom more than one had schizophrenia, as controls. In these multiply affected families, 16 of 67 who suffered schizophrenia reported having had a head injury before age 11 compared with 12 of 102 unaffected controls. The OR of 2.3 was just significant. However, in almost all cases the head injury was mild, of whom probably a good proportion suffered no loss of consciousness.

Another study that used unaffected family members from schizophrenia pedigrees as controls is the case–control study of Malaspina *et al.* (2001). Subjects from families in whom at least two members had schizophrenia or two members had bipolar disorder were asked whether they had ever had a head injury. The controls were the unaffected family members. Those with schizophrenia reported having had more head injuries than the unaffected family members (OR 3.3) and this was slightly, but not statistically significantly, more than for bipolar disorder (OR 2.2). Those who came from a schizophrenia pedigree and suffered a head injury were more likely to develop schizophrenia than bipolar disorder, whereas this was not the case with bipolar disorder; there may be a pathoplastic effect of familial predisposition to schizophrenia on the outcome of head injury. Of particular interest was the finding that those at risk of developing schizophrenia have a greater risk of suffering a head injury.

The case–control studies described thus far have all relied on retrospective reporting of a history of head injury. More recent studies have used large databases of health records to enable direct comparison between those recorded, at the time, as being admitted with a head injury and subsequently recorded as suffering a psychotic illness. Fann *et al.* (2004) interrogated the records of a health maintenance organisation covering 450 000 people in Washington state. Every person aged 15 or older with a head injury in 1993, diagnosed using ICD coding in the emergency department or inpatient wards or outpatient clinic ($N = 939$ of whom 136 were moderate/severe), was tracked to see whether they developed a psychiatric illness in the 3 years following the injury (classified either by diagnosis or antipsychotic use). The psychiatric health of the subjects during the year before the head injury was also assessed. For each person, three age- and sex-matched controls without head injury were likewise followed up. In those without a preceding history of psychosis, and with a moderate to severe head injury, in the second and third years post injury there was an elevated risk of psychosis (OR 5.9 and 3.6 respectively, both just statistically significant). However, the interpretation of this finding is not straightforward. It is based on small numbers, so the confidence intervals are large. The majority of those with moderate and severe head injuries were over 65. It seems that merely being prescribed an antipsychotic was sufficient for a person to be labelled as suffering a psychotic illness. And as David and Prince (2005) point out, those subjects with apparent new-onset psychosis in the 3 years post injury may well have had a history of psychosis in the more distant past. In fact the most striking finding from analysis of this database is that having a mental illness makes a person at increased risk of suffering a head injury within 1 year (Fann *et al.* 2002).

Nielsen *et al.* (2002) used the Danish national health record databases. In this study the cases studied were 8288 patients having their first admission for schizophrenia. They were compared with 82 880 age- and sex-matched controls without schizophrenia. The register of all admissions to Danish general hospitals was then searched to see if these cases and controls had suffered a head injury requiring admission to hospital in the 15 years before the admission for schizophrenia (or in the case of controls an equivalent risk period). To try to control for accident proneness, the database was also searched to see if the subjects had been admitted for a fracture but without head injury. Compared with controls, patients with schizophrenia were not at increased risk of head injury. For example, 2.2% of patients with schizophrenia compared with 2.4% of controls had suffered a 'severe' head injury in the at-risk period. Closer analysis of the data did suggest that in men there was a relative excess of head injury compared with fractures, but it is difficult to interpret exactly what this finding means. The effect was greatest in the year before diagnosis of schizophrenia; this was the time the patients seemed to be at greatest risk, over and above controls, of suffering a head injury. This is compatible with reverse causality; during the prodrome of the schizophrenia the risk of head injury is increased. However, this explanation does not sit comfortably with the observation that risk of fractures was not increased in the year before schizophrenia. The study design was limited by the ascertainment method to determine schizophrenia; patients had to have been both admitted to hospital and given an ICD-8 diagnosis of schizophrenia. Nevertheless, it can be argued that a patient who is significantly disabled after a head injury, compared with a previously fit person, is likely to take a different pathway to care when becoming psychotic for the first time. These patients might also be expected to be diagnosed with an organic psychosis rather than schizophrenia. Both effects could result in underreporting of the number of patients who develop a non-affective psychosis after a head injury. And these effects would be most evident in those with the severest injuries, perhaps those most at risk of developing a psychotic illness. More recently, Harrison *et al.* (2006) using similar methods found no excess risk of schizophrenia after head injury, but did find a small increased risk of non-schizophrenic non-affective psychoses (OR 1.37). This finding is combatible with the argument that there is a slight increased risk of non-affective psychoses after head injury.

From this review of the evidence it can be seen that it is not possible to come to any definite conclusion about whether head injury can cause a chronic psychotic illness, a schizophrenia or schizophreniform psychosis, not secondary to hypomania or depression. Nevertheless, across a range of study designs there is a fairly consistent message that there may be an increased risk of schizophrenia-like illness after head injury. However, in many of these studies the head injury was mild, probably making the studies more vulnerable to spurious reporting and ascertainment effects, and also hinting that the head injury was acting as a non-specific psychological stressor, rather than brain injury explaining the link. Two other conclusions emerge from the review. First, those with a predisposition to psychosis are at greatest risk of developing psychosis after head injury. This suggests that those who develop psychosis after head injury might well have become psychotic even if they had not been injured. Second, those at risk of developing a psychotic illness are probably also at greater risk of suffering a head injury, an example of reverse causality. Some will suggest that the methods and size of Nielsen *et al.*'s (2002) study trump all others and that this study is the only one to trust. Others will suggest that though large and apparently robust, even this study is open to question, and that a reasonable conclusion to draw is that head injury does increase the risk of psychosis, perhaps doubling it. Nevertheless, probably the majority of those who become psychotic after head injury, particularly if it is a mild head injury, would have developed a chronic psychosis anyway. Furthermore, it is quite likely that in fact these patients only had a head injury in the first place because their predisposition to psychosis was associated with being accident prone. Given this tentative conclusion that head injury causes chronic psychosis, more specific conclusions, for example that psychosis is especially linked to temporal lobe damage (Davison & Bagley 1969), must be regarded as somewhat speculative.

Another question of interest is the effect of head injury on the course of schizophrenia. It is not uncommon for patients with schizophrenia to suffer a head injury, either accidental or due to deliberate self-injury. Is this likely to make their psychotic illness worse? Or will the head injury aggravate the negative symptoms of schizophrenia? At present there is no evidence to answer these questions. Of interest is the case report of Pang and Lewis (1996) suggesting that damage to the left prefrontal and temporal cortex following a head injury changed the pattern of symptoms in an individual with past history of bipolar affective disorder, such that the patient developed typical schizophrenia 9 months later.

Mood and anxiety disorders

Mood disorders (affective disorders) following TBI are an important focus for diagnosis and treatment (Evans & Levine 2002; Fleminger *et al.* 2003b). However, two important questions about the nosological status of these disorders in somebody with a brain injury emerge (Eames 2001). First, to what extent should emotional reactions that are easily understandable in terms of the adverse effects of the injury on the person be diagnosed as depression? Second, what is one to make of symptoms of mood disorders, for example anhedonia and apathy, when these symptoms may also be a direct consequence of brain injury? Frontal lobe injury may produce states where fatuous jocularity is prominent, not dissimilar to changes sometimes seen in hypomania. Bilateral high brainstem or internal capsule lesions may produce the syndrome of pseudobulbar palsy, with dramatic brief-lived pathological laughter and crying. Is this a disorder of the affect such that the patient feels like laughing or feels sad, or a disorder of the expression of emotion but in the absence of any subjective change in affect? On the other hand, it is quite possible, particularly in those with severe injury, that any subjective mood state is masked because the patient lacks the ability to express feelings.

For these reasons standard diagnostic schema, like the *Diagnostic and Statistical Manual of Mental Disorders* (DSM), should be interpreted with care when applied to the brain-injured person. This is particularly the case if information is collected by self report in response to standard questions, rather than by interview with somebody familiar with psychiatric diagnosis. Rating scales, like the Hamilton Rating Scale or the Beck Depression Inventory or Hospital Anxiety and Depression Scale, are even less reliable ways to identify clinical syndromes. Such methods will fail to distinguish symptoms like concentration impairment that may be a direct consequence of brain injury from bona fide symptoms of a depressive illness. The typical emotional sequelae of head injury overlap with changes of personality, including moodiness and dysthymia, and normal reactions to life events. Symptoms of anxiety are often prominent. Symptoms such as feeling miserable, powerless, frustrated and dissatisfied, being irritable and moody do not sit happily in any nosology. The propensity for individual clinicians to rate such symptoms as evidence of a mental illness probably varies markedly, and this may partly explain the large differences in reported rates of depression following head injury.

Bipolar affective disorder including manic–depressive psychosis and mania

Psychotic symptoms associated with mood disorders
Chronic psychotic illness not secondary to hypomania or depression has already been discussed. An early suggestion that head injury can result in a psychosis associated with a mood disorder came from Symonds' (1937) description of two patients with depressive psychosis in whom the symptoms developed before they had recovered from their acute post-traumatic confusion. Symonds proposed that as the patients could not appreciate the effects of the injury at the time, this was evidence favouring the view that the illness was the direct result of organic brain disturbance.

Occasional case reports of psychosis associated with mood disorder are to be found (McLay *et al.* 2004), sometimes associated with nihilistic delusions related to a sense of derealisation (Butler 2000) (see Fig. 4.8). On the other hand, Hibbard *et al.* (1998) found 23% of those diagnosed with major depression after head injury to have psychotic symptoms. This was based on a survey of 100 community-dwelling patients at least 1 year, and on average 7 years, after a head injury; 61% were identified, using a structured interview by a psychologist, to have major depression. Given this very high rate of depression, the finding that about 12 of the 100 patients had psychotic features should be interpreted with caution.

Bipolar affective disorder
Mania may occur early after head injury. In one study of six patients who developed mania (9% of all cases with a head injury), all but one had resolved by 6 months post injury

(Jorge *et al.* 1993a). However, symptoms of mania will overlap with symptoms typically seen in the period of PTA, when agitation, distractibility, irritability and disinhibition are common, and this may lead to diagnostic confusion. An example of this diagnostic dilemma is to be found in the case report of Mustafa *et al.* (2005) of a woman developing increased psychomotor activity and decreased need for sleep 23 days after a head injury and almost certainly in the period of PTA. Mania developing later after injury is relatively uncommon and point prevalence studies, for example at 1 year (Deb *et al.* 1999b), may fail to identify any patients who are manic. Achté *et al.* (1967) found 47 cases of affective disorder (1.3% of their series) of whom only three were typically manic–depressive. Mortensen *et al.* (2003) used a case–control methodology to interrogate the Danish medical and psychiatric databases to see whether head injury was a risk factor for later bipolar affective disorder. Those with bipolar affective disorder were 1.5 times as likely to have suffered a previous head injury requiring admission. The increased risk was confined to head injury occurring within 5 years of the bipolar illness and only accounted for a small proportion of bipolar disorder.

Much of the literature has tended to rely on case studies. Bracken (1987) found 20 cases in the literature and reported a striking example of his own as follows.

A 48-year-old woman fell from a trapeze sustaining multiple injuries. She lost consciousness for 10 minutes and had a PTA of approximately 3 days. On recovery from her physical injuries she was confused and disorientated, and over the next few days became overactive and grandiose. This was 3 weeks after her fall. The CT scan was normal. On transfer to a psychiatric unit she was fully orientated but with marked pressure of speech and flight of ideas. She reported feeling very happy and 'very strong' and said she was writing a book which would be a best seller. There was no previous personal or family history of psychiatric disorder.

With chlorpromazine and haloperidol she gradually settled over the next 8 weeks. She then developed a depressive episode which responded to mianserin. Psychological tests suggested possible residual deficits in visual and verbal memory, and there was persistent diplopia due to fourth cranial nerve palsies. She was well again 3 months after the accident.

Clark and Davison (1987) reported two further cases, one beginning 2 months after closed head injury and the other 6 months after operation for post-traumatic subdural haematomas. Shukla *et al.* (1987) assembled 20 cases, the mania following closed head injury by a mean of 2.8 years (range

0–12 years). No patient had a family history of bipolar illness, though six had one or more relatives with histories of depression. Epilepsy had developed in half of the patients and appeared to be a predisposing factor. Among phenomenological features, they stressed that irritable moods were commoner than euphoria and that assaultive behaviour was common. Fourteen patients experienced recurrent mania without depression, and the sample as a whole showed an excess of manic over depressive episodes.

A study of 12 patients who developed mania after a variety of brain lesions (tumours, strokes and head injuries) was presented by Starkstein *et al.* (1988). Of the two head injuries in the series, one developed repeated manic episodes after an interval of 18 months, and the other became manic 2 years after frontal injury associated with marked change of personality. There have been a few case reports of rapid cycling manic–depressive illness developing after head injury (Zwil *et al.* 1993; Monji *et al.* 1999; Murai & Fujimoto 2003).

Although a story has emerged that seconday mania is more common with brain lesions involving the right hemisphere, there is little convincing evidence of any laterality effect after head injury. Mania is probably more common in those who have suffered head injury with damage to frontal, particularly orbitofrontal, and temporal cortex. Hoheisel and Walch (1952) suggested that hypothalamic damage might also play a part.

Major depression

Major depression is quite common after head injury, and remains so for many years after injury. Perhaps the first study to use standard criteria to diagnose depression was that of Jorge *et al.* (1993b) who found that major depression seen shortly after head injury may owe something to lesion location, whereas later-onset depression, nevertheless in the first year post injury, was more closely tied to psychosocial factors.

Of 66 consecutive patients admitted to hospital with closed head injury, 17 (26%) met DSM-III criteria for major depression at examination 1 month later. When compared with non-depressed patients they showed an increased past history of psychiatric disorder and a higher frequency of alcohol or drug abuse. Severity of injury was not significantly different, but analysis of lesion location from CT scans showed an excess of left anterior brain damage in the depressed group. Of those who were not depressed at 1 month, 27% went on to become depressed at 3, 6 or 12 months. At any one time, about 20–25% of patients were depressed, with over 40% of the cohort suffering depression at some point over the first year. Direct comparisons between early and later-onset depression groups confirmed the importance of lesion location in the former (frequently subcortical involvement) and of poorer social functioning in the latter.

Depression is found to be quite mobile in the first year after head injury. Those who are depressed often recover within a few months, and their place in the group found to be depressed at a later time will have been taken by a patient not previously depressed. Thus less than one-fifth of those depressed at 12 months had been depressed at 1 month, and of those not depressed at 1 year almost half had been depressed at some stage earlier in the year. Other studies also find rates of clinically diagnosed depression of the order of 20–30% over the first year (Kersel *et al.* 2001; Jorge *et al.* 2004). Bowen *et al.* (1999) used a self-report measure to identify clinically significant mood disorders and found higher rates (39% at 6 months and 35% at 1 year). Deb *et al.* (1999b) offer a more conservative estimate for the rate of major depression observed at 1 year. Patients were interviewed by a psychiatrist using a standardised structured interview; 14% met ICD-10 criteria for major depression. When comparisons have been made, depression after head injury seems to be more common than in other patients without central nervous system involvement but with comparable injury or disability.

Longer-term prevalence studies suggest even higher rates of depression. Two studies from Kreutzer and colleagues, using different cohorts, find similar rates of depression. Their earlier study (Kreutzer *et al.* 2001) took 722 patients referred for outpatient assessment at a regional trauma centre on average 2.5 years post injury. Using items from a self-report measure that were regarded as diagnostically relevant to a DSM, they diagnosed 42% as suffering major depression. The second study (Seel *et al.* 2003) took 666 patients admitted for rehabilitation across several centres who were followed up. Using the same technique as in their first study, 27% met criteria for major depression. Hibbard *et al.* (1998) (see above) offer higher rates of depression. Hoofien *et al.* (2001) only studied patients with severe injury and found 45% to be depressed 14 years after injury. Rather similar figures are emerging for the rates of depression more than two decades after injury. Major depression was present in 27% of those injured 30 years before (Koponen *et al.* 2002). However, more conservative estimates were found by Holsinger *et al.* (2002) studying veterans of the Second World War 50 years after closed head injury and compared with men without head injury. The lifetime prevalence of depression was 18.5% compared with 13.4% for the controls.

These large variations in prevalence of depression some time after head injury may partly reflect the different psychosocial circumstances of the cohorts. There is an impression that later depression is more related to psychosocial adversity (Seel *et al.* 2003) and worse psychosocial outcome (Hibbard *et al.* 2004). On the other hand, selective ascertainment might partly explain some of the excess in depression; it is those patients who are depressed who are most likely to be referred for rehabilitation some time after injury.

One question of theoretical interest is the extent to which the depression seen in a person with a head injury is different in terms of phenomenology from depression in the absence of head injury. Aloia *et al.* (1995) found little difference between the two depression syndromes. Nevertheless,

apathy is probably more evident in depressed head-injured patients, Kant *et al.* (1998a) finding that 60% of their cohort of 83 head-injured patients were both depressed and apathetic; 20% had either apathy or depression alone and less than 20% were spared. A question of more practical interest given the potential difficulties diagnosing depression in somebody with a head injury is which symptoms best differentiate those who are depressed after a head injury from those who are not. Kreutzer *et al.* (2001) found that the most frequently endorsed symptoms of depression were fatigue (46%), frustration (41%) and poor concentration (38%), but these would be common in patients not depressed after a head injury. The best discriminators of those who are depressed from those who are not are probably symptoms such as lack of confidence, feelings of hopelessness, and self-deprecation (Jorge *et al.* 1993c). Biological symptoms, such as sleep disturbance, were not of much value early post injury. In fact sleep disturbance is common after head injury, regardless of depression. For example, 30% of patients attending a rehabilitation centre have been found to have insomnia, particularly problems with getting off to sleep (Fichtenberg *et al.* 2002). Hypopituitarism may contribute to depressive symptoms (Ghigo *et al.* 2005). Several studies have shown that depression is associated with anxiety, aggression and alcohol and substance abuse. It is more common in those with a history of affective disorder (Jorge *et al.* 2004; Rapoport *et al.* 2005).

After a severe injury patients often become increasingly aware of their disability as they recover, i.e. their insight improves. This may be one reason why patients seen after 6 months post injury demonstrate greater emotional reactions than do those seen within 6 months (Fordyce *et al.* 1983). As insight improves, depression increases (Morton & Wehman 1995). In a longitudinal study, Godfrey *et al.* (1993) found that improved insight into behavioural and cognitive impairments was associated with onset of emotional dysfunction. Wallace and Bogner (2000) used a cross-sectional approach. Patients on average 2 years post injury who lacked insight into their impairments were less likely to report anxiety and depression. These effects might partly reflect the observation in those without a head injury for depressed mood to be associated with better insight ('sadder but wiser').

A related question is the extent to which depressed mood can exacerbate cognitive impairment. This was studied by Rapoport *et al.* (2005) in 74 patients attending an outpatient TBI clinic many months following mild and moderate injury; 28% were diagnosed, using the Structured Clinical Interview for Depression, to have major depression. Controlling for effects of age and injury severity, these 21 patients showed greater cognitive impairment, particularly in terms of processing speed, working memory and verbal memory and executive function. For example, mean processing speed on WAIS was reduced from 19 to 14; the depressed patients made twice as many perseverative errors on WCST. A second study found that subjective memory complaints were more likely in those who were depressed, and those with milder head injuries (Chamelian & Feinstein 2006).

Major depression is probably more common in those with pathological laughing or crying, otherwise called emotional lability or incontinence, or pseudobulbar affect. Pathological laughing or crying occurs in perhaps 5% of patients with head injury, and is associated with more severe injuries especially if there are neurological features of brainstem injury (Zeilig *et al*. 1996).

Mixed states of depression and anxiety

Post-traumatic states with mixed anxiety and depression represent the commonest of the psychiatric sequelae of head injury, in some series outnumbering all other forms of disability together (Ota 1969; Morton & Wehman 1995). Minor depression and states of tension and anxiety are frequently accompanied by irritability, phobic symptomatology and social avoidance. Biological features, for example anorexia, insomnia and early-morning waking, are rarely marked. The depression often fluctuates in severity, and may be responsive to change of activity and surroundings. Sometimes it proves to be no more than a readiness to be cast down by the troubles of daily life, and sometimes it is more accurately described as a state of gloomy and morose preoccupation. Symptoms of an anxiety disorder, in particular agoraphobia, travel phobia or PTSD, are common and sometimes the anxiety disorder is the outstanding problem (see below). When anxiety and depression are accompanied by somatic symptoms, particularly fatigue, headache, sensitivity to noise and dizziness, then the condition may be labelled post-concussion syndrome (see Post-concussion syndrome, later in chapter). Somatic symptoms are frequently the subject of anxious introspection and hypochondriacal concern.

Irritability is among the most common of the emotional consequences of injury and shows strong associations with depression and anxiety. The patient is more short-tempered than usual, more inclined to be snappy and stricter in matters of discipline. High levels of irritability persist for many years after injury (Brooks *et al*. 1986). All grades are seen, extending to the serious loss of control of aggression already considered above. It can be difficult to decide how far this represents an affective disturbance, or alternatively a personality change due to brain damage. Among patients with severe irritability persisting more than 1 year after injury, Lishman (1968) found little evidence to suggest that brain damage was an important factor in the group as a whole.

The failure of some classificatory systems, such as DSM-IV, to include a state of mixed anxiety and depression, or cothymia as it has been called (Tyrer *et al*. 2001), in their classificatory systems probably explains why recent studies using formal psychiatric classification may be a little misleading. A state of mixed anxiety and depression is rarely diagnosed, although authors may refer to a 'dual diagnosis'

or 'comorbidity' of an anxiety disorder and a depressive disorder.

Methods of assessment which use symptom questionnaires are probably better at capturing the spectrum of emotional reactions after head injury. For example, Fordyce *et al*. (1983) used the MMPI and the Katz Adjustments Scale (KAS) to identify the enhanced emotional reactions of head-injured patients. Those more than 6 months post injury were more anxious and depressed and more socially withdrawn. Curran *et al*. (2000) found that the presence of anxiety, measured using the State–Trait Anxiety Inventory (Spielberger 1983), was strongly correlated with the presence of depressive symptoms measured using the Beck Depression Inventory (Pearson's $r = 0.75$). Symptoms of anxiety and depression were more strongly associated with coping style than with severity or even the presence of brain injury. Those who dealt with problems in an active manner had fewer symptoms than those with a non-productive coping style characterised by, for example, self-blame and ignoring problems. Morris *et al*. (2005) used qualitative research methods to explore the content of symptoms of anxiety and depression after head injury. They identified some concerns that are often overlooked. For example, in some patients social anxiety was related to feelings of self-consciousness because of scars. Many suffered a persisting sense of loss due to failure to fulfil their dreams. Some described negative reactions from others. Often these were felt to be due to a lack of understanding of the consequences of head injury. Other participants mentioned feeling ignored or overlooked by others or feeling patronised.

Constitutional factors may be important in some cases. Neurotic reactions like those just described are probably more likely to occur in those prone to develop these symptoms anyway (see section on pre-traumatic factors above). The range of symptoms in a series of cases diagnosed as 'neurotics' (Slater 1943) was very similar regardless of whether the cohorts had suffered a head injury or not, as was the degree of vulnerability as judged by family and personal history. Nevertheless, Slater's study of soldiers subject to breakdown in war appeared to indicate that organic factors did play some part, although such factors are probably less important in those who develop chronic symptoms.

Anxiety disorders

Generalised anxiety disorders

Anxiety may coexist with depression or stand alone. Persistent states of anxiety and tension are particularly common after accidents of an especially frightening nature. In a survey of 188 consecutive victims of road traffic accidents, Mayou *et al*. (1993) found that one-fifth suffered from an acute stress syndrome as an aftermath, with mood disturbance and horrific memories of the accident. At follow-up 3 months and 1 year later, one-tenth of the series showed persisting mood disorder with anxiety as the major component. The acute stress syndrome was significantly related to neuroticism in the premorbid personality; continuing emotional distress was also especially likely in those who were psychologically and socially vulnerable, but was additionally strongly associated with chronic medical disability and social, financial and work problems. Harvey and Bryant (2000) found that those who develop symptoms of acute stress are at high risk of later PTSD. Concerns about cognitive performance contribute to anxiety and this often becomes evident as the patient returns to work. Problems with memory may be particularly difficult for the patient to evaluate. These concerns facilitate the development of behaviours such as indecisiveness, checking, avoidance of activities and a reluctance to take on new tasks. Similarly, anxiety is linked to somatic symptoms, for example headache when concentrating. Fear of walking unaided, because of feelings of dizziness or unsteadiness when walking, may be seen ('phobic imbalance'). This may reflect vestibular damage.

A man of 30 was seen 18 months after a head injury occasioned by a falling ladder. He had been only briefly concussed, but immediately afterwards became dizzy and vomited several times. Thereafter he experienced vertigo and nausea on sudden head movement, persisting on occasion 1 month later. During this time he became acutely phobic of enclosed spaces and travelling and gave in his notice at work. The dizziness subsided but the phobias persisted and intensified. He began drinking heavily. Detailed examination showed no evidence of brain damage, and it was strongly argued by the defendants that his present condition owed much to alcohol and little, if anything, to the injury. The genuineness of the phobias themselves was called into question.

However, examination revealed two striking signs. On tilting him backwards to a horizontal position with the head to one side he developed bursts of nystagmus, indicative of labyrinthine damage. Furthermore, on persuading him to enter the hospital lift he developed obvious signs of autonomic distress, with the pulse rate rising from 84 to 120 per minute. Subsequent neuro-otological examination showed that the right labyrinth was completely non-functioning. Crucial evidence was thus available to demonstrate labyrinthine damage accruing from the injury, and to confirm the genuine nature of his phobias (Lishman 1978).

However, in some patients anxiety aggravates the sense of unsteadiness.

Warden and Labbate (2005) describe a man who suffered a mild brain injury and fractured femur whose recovery of walking was slow. He developed a fear of falling and constant dizziness and blurred vision while walking, and later panic attacks with vertigo. He felt unable to walk without a stick even though his physiotherapists thought he should be able to walk unaided. He started abusing alcohol. His girlfriend noted that he was becoming increasingly dependent on her to help him walk, and that he walked *better* after drinking a few beers. With treatment, including sertraline, his symptoms subsided.

Estimates of the prevalence of anxiety disorders after head injury vary (Warden & Labbate 2005) and high rates have been reported after childhood head injury (Vasa *et al.* 2002). A reasonable estimate of the rate of generalised anxiety disorder at 1 year is 10–15% (Salazar *et al.* 2000). On the other hand, Deb *et al.* (1999b), also at 1 year post injury, found only 2% with generalised anxiety disorder but 9% with panic disorder; it is possible that small differences in classification of a patient into one diagnosis or the other may explain the difference with Salazar *et al.* (2000). In other words, about 10% probably suffer generalised anxiety with or without panic. Koponen *et al.* (2002) found 8% suffering panic disorder many years post injury. However, rates of anxiety, as defined by adjustment reactions, after TBI may not be much different from estimates of the pre-injury status (Fann *et al.* 2004).

Phobic disorders

Travel phobia is one of the commonest of phobic disorders after head injury and, not surprisingly, is seen particularly in those injured in an accident involving some means of transportation. Nervousness and travel avoidance are seen. The symptoms are often seen alongside more generalised symptoms of anxiety and it is not unusual to find heightened concerns for the safety of themselves and their loved ones in a variety of situations apart from travel. Understandably, the symptoms tend to be greatest in the form of transport where the injury was suffered, often the car. Typical symptoms of car travel phobia are a fear of speed, a need to maintain distance from the car in front, jumpiness and hyperarousal. The startle response may be exaggerated. As such there is often an overlap with PTSD. Symptoms are often worse when patients are being driven than when they are driving. Mayou *et al.* (2000) found that of those with mild head injury after a road traffic accident, 20% suffered travel anxiety 1 year later, not significantly different from the 16% observed in those who were injured in a road traffic accident but without a head injury. The authors note that there was probably less travel anxiety in those who had suffered major head injury.

Agoraphobia is not an unusual consequence of head injury. It is the commonest phobic disorder in the general population and therefore in a good proportion of cases might have been seen regardless of the head injury. However, in some cases anxiety related to, for example, difficulties coping with hustle and bustle, or concerns around falling if accidentally pushed in a crowd, or fears about losing one's way, seem to be instrumental in the development of agoraphobia. On the other hand, social avoidance, a common symptom after head injury, is rarely associated with a specific social phobia. Koponen *et al.* (2002) report that 5 of 60 patients assessed 30 years post injury had a specific phobia but give no further detail about the type of phobia.

Post-traumatic stress disorder

It is not unusual after a head injury for the patient to dwell on the circumstances of the injury or relive it in terrifying dreams. There may be marked startle responses and phobic avoidance of situations that bring the accident to mind. These are the typical symptoms of PTSD. It is now clear that symptoms of PTSD must be sought with care, in that patients may not always vouchsafe them directly. The disturbance can be long-lasting and disabling, and in chronic form the patient may merely present with non-specific complaints of irritability, insomnia, depression and general inability to cope.

Although many patients may report some of the symptoms of PTSD, far fewer meet full diagnostic criteria for PTSD. This requires that the patient is exposed to a terrifying experience and that symptoms from three domains should be present. The first consists of reliving the trauma, with nightmares, intrusive daytime recollections and sudden 'flashbacks' in which the traumatic event is re-experienced with realistic intensity. The second comprises avoidance behaviours in relation to reminders of the trauma. Closely related to avoidance there may be emotional numbing and detachment. The third includes heightened arousal and startle responses. Other non-specific symptoms include irritability and difficulties with memory and concentration. Using self-report measures to diagnose PTSD is not recommended and this is particularly the case after head injury because some of the symptoms of PTSD may be seen in head-injured patients regardless of any heightened emotional reaction to the injury. Sumpter and McMillan (2005) showed that whereas more than 40% of their 34 head-injured cases were classified as PTSD using self-report, e.g. with the Impact of Events Scale, only one was diagnosed as a case of PTSD using clinical interview.

In Mayou *et al.*'s (1993) survey of road traffic accidents, many of whom had not suffered a head injury, one-tenth of the victims were judged to meet criteria for PTSD during the subsequent year. The development of PTSD was not associated with a history of previous psychological problems; the principal and very strong predictor was the rating of 'horrific' memories of the accident at interview shortly after it

occurred. PTSD did not occur in subjects who had been unconscious and were amnesic for the accident. Similarly, Warden *et al.* (1997) were unable to find patients who met the full criteria for PTSD among 47 head-injured veterans who had sustained substantial PTA.

Others have demonstrated that PTSD symptoms may be found in those with severe head injury. Williams *et al.* (2002) used the Impact of Events Scale and found that 18% of 66 patients with a severe head injury and significant period of PTA had symptoms of PTSD. PTSD was diagnosed in over one-quarter of patients attending a brain injury rehabilitation unit after a severe head injury (Bryant *et al.* 2001) and was associated with worse outcome, suggesting that it was important not to overlook the diagnosis. However, others have found much lower rates for PTSD diagnosis. For example, of the 120 patients studied by Deb *et al.* (1999b) 1 year post injury, seven suffered nightmares and four were described as suffering symptoms of PTSD but in no case was a diagnosis of PTSD made. Only 3% of over 300 cases of mild head injury in McMillan's (1996) series were diagnosed with PTSD.

In a study of 307 patients admitted to a trauma centre, the rate of PTSD at 1 year of just over 10% was no different in those with mild TBI compared with those without a head injury (Creamer *et al.* 2005). Furthermore, within the group with mild TBI the prevalence of PTSD was about the same regardless of whether there was amnesia for the event. On the other hand, several studies have shown that greater amnesia for the event or injury severity is protective. Gil *et al.* (2005) diagnosed PTSD in 14% of 120 patients with mild TBI 6 months post injury and found that memory for the event made PTSD more likely. In a series of patients assessed on average about 8 weeks after injury, Feinstein *et al.* (2002) found that those with PTA greater than 1 hour were less likely to have symptoms of PTSD than those with PTA of less than 1 hour. Glaesser *et al.* (2004), studying 46 patients attending a neurological rehabilitation clinic after a head injury, found much higher rates of PTSD in those who were not unconscious for an extended period (27%) compared with those who were unconscious for more than 12 hours (3%; 1 of 31 patients). Intrusive memories were more frequent in patients who had not been unconscious.

It seems clear that aspects of the typical picture of PTSD can sometimes develop when the patient has lost consciousness after head injury, and in the presence of PTA. However, the symptom content of PTSD is probably a little different in those with head injury, compared with those without (Harvey *et al.* 2003). Though nightmares are quite common after head injury (Deb *et al.* 1999a), the content is not always directly related to images of the accident itself. There is less evidence of symptoms of re-experiencing; for example, six (13%) of Warden *et al.*'s (1997) patients met the avoidance and arousal criteria for PTSD while lacking the re-experiencing criteria. The following case is instructive (McMillan 1991).

A girl of 18 sustained a severe head injury in a road traffic accident and was unconscious for 3 or 4 days. She initially had a mild right hemiparesis, dysphasia, euphoria and poor memory, and spent 3 months in a rehabilitation unit. The duration of PTA was about 6 weeks. After 7 months she returned to her job as a bank clerk.

Fourteen months after the accident she was referred with symptoms of fatigue, poor concentration, dizziness, headache and difficulty in coping at work. There was a good deal of evidence of depression. However, other symptoms were not consistent with low mood or a post-concussion syndrome. She had intrusive thoughts several times a day about her friend who had died in the accident, and could not prevent these from entering her mind. They were triggered by situations where the two might conceivably have met, such as in the local supermarket. In addition she showed cognitive and physical avoidance of reminders of the accident, including hospitals in general. The thought of entering the rehabilitation unit where she had been treated was particularly anxiety-provoking. She did not talk about the accident to anyone, and continually postponed visiting the grave of her friend. She suffered from continual and irrational guilt, believing that she had somehow caused or failed to prevent the accident. Treatment involved cognitive–behavioural exposure techniques and resulted in marked improvement.

Co-morbidity. Post-traumatic stress disorder is associated with worse psychosocial outcome (Bryant *et al.* 2001). This probably partly reflects the fact that PTSD is often associated with anxiety and depression (Warden *et al.* 1997; Bryant *et al.* 2001; Levin *et al.* 2001). There is a marked overlap of PTSD with symptoms that are diagnosed as post-concussion syndrome (Bryant & Harvey 1999) and it is noteworthy that both conditions are predicted by early emotional reactions post injury, and may be prevented by early post-injury psychological treatments.

Mechanisms. King (1997) suggested that brief islands of memory, some of which were perhaps reconstructions, was one possible explanation for the emergence of PTSD after head injury. In other patients because the peritraumatic amnesia is negligible, there is no reason why a typical PTSD picture should not emerge. In those with significant amnesia implicit memory mechanisms may be at work. The following case illustrates the possible role of implicit memory.

A 30-year-old man was injured while unloading pallets of wood off a lorry. A laden pallet fell from the hoist and hit his head. He was unconscious for several hours and had an RA of about 2 days and a PTA of about 3 weeks. On recovery from his PTA he suffered unpleasant derealisation experiences. For a period he became convinced that the whole event had been some sort of strange masquerade, played out by the hospital and others for an unknown purpose, but that in fact the accident had never happened. He recovered from this delusion but for many months symptoms of fatigue and poor concentration prevented him returning to work. During this period he and his wife spontaneously noted that when in the car, being driven by his wife, if they passed a lorry laden with pallets and carrying a hoist, he would become tense and suffer symptoms of anxiety. Yet he said that he did not remember that the accident had been caused by a falling pallet.

Conversion disorders

Hysterical symptoms have figured prominently in some series of head-injured patients, perhaps especially those admitted to army neurosis centres during times of war (Anderson 1942). The usual range of dissociative states may occur: fits, fugues, amnesias, Ganser states, motor paralyses, anaesthesias, and disturbances of speech, sight or hearing. The onset is usually soon after the injury, although later developments may occur in association with depression or when complex neurotic states emerge in relation to compensation issues. For example, Dalfen and Anthony (2000) identified four patients with a Ganser syndrome characterised by approximate answers (*vorbeigehen*) in a series of 513 cases of mild TBI followed up over the first year post injury; in three of the cases the syndrome was associated with an acute stress reaction. Only one was pursuing compensation.

Whitlock (1967) compared 56 patients admitted to psychiatric units with hysterical conversion symptoms, with a group of controls matched for age and sex but suffering from depressive or anxiety states. Almost two-thirds of the patients with hysterical disorders had suffered significant preceding or coexisting brain disorder, compared with only 5% of the controls. Head injury had preceded the onset of hysterical phenomena within 6 months in 21% of the hysterical patients but in none of the controls. It would seem therefore that head injury may be a more frequent antecedent of the clinical picture of hysteria than is commonly supposed. A significant proportion of the cases described by Eames (1992) as suffering hysteria after brain injury had suffered a head injury.

Obsessive–compulsive disorder

Obsessive–compulsive symptoms may emerge in susceptible individuals, usually as a colouring to pictures of depression or anxiety. However, OCD is not a common sequelae, Deb *et al.* (1999b) for example finding only 2 of 120 patients at 1 year to have OCD, probably not much greater than population norms. This is probably a more realistic estimate than the 9% rate reported by Hibbard *et al.* (1998). Hillbom (1960) reported 14 examples among 415 cases (3.4%), of whom almost two-thirds had epilepsy, three times the prevalence among the patients generally.

McKeon *et al.* (1984) have reported four patients with severe OCD following directly from head injuries of moderate severity. Three were from a consecutive series of 25 patients suffering from obsessive–compulsive neurosis, the fourth from a pair of monozygotic twins discordant for the disorder. The prompt onset of symptoms, usually within 24 hours of injury, and the absence of premorbid obsessional traits in all but one case suggested that the brain trauma may have contributed directly to the neurosis by some physiogenic mechanism rather than acting as a non-specific stress. More recently, Berthier *et al.* (2001) described 10 cases of OCD secondary to head injury; six were mild, two moderate and two severe head injuries. Two patients were premorbidly indecisive and perfectionist and two had a history of PTSD related to sexual abuse. In all but one case the symptoms of OCD developed within 1 month of injury and, particularly in those with mild TBI, were associated with generalised anxiety or symptoms of PTSD. The symptoms of OCD were fairly typical although all 10 patients showed quite marked aggressive behaviour. Most showed both obsessions and compulsions. Common obsessions included fears of contamination and thoughts about symmetry and exactness. The most frequent compulsions were checking, cleaning and washing, and repeating rituals. Six of the patients showed obsessional slowness. Significant impairment of executive function was common.

Unlike the most common neuroses, Hillbom (1960) found that compulsive disorders tended to occur after reasonably severe rather than mild injuries. Of all the anxiety disorders, OCD is perhaps the most closely linked to changes in brain function, particularly involving the frontal lobes and their connections (Lucey *et al.* 1997). It is therefore not surprising that some case reports suggest a particular role of frontal injury (Bilgic *et al.* 2004; Ogai *et al.* 2005). On the other hand, psychosurgery for severe OCD also involves interrupting frontal connections. In the following case a patient previously seen in a general psychiatric clinic because of symptoms of OCD presented several years later to a specialist brain injury clinic following a head injury.

This lawyer presented in his early thirties with symptoms of OCD. Over several months he had developed gradually deteriorating symptoms of excessive checking and safety fears. He also had obsessional thoughts of harming those who were close to him. These symptoms had a very adverse effect on his marriage and for a period of time he was off work. He was successfully treated with cognitive–behaviour therapy but retained many obsessional and perfection-istic personality traits. Several years later he fell and suffered a severe head injury with moderate bilateral frontal contusions. He attended the brain injury outpatient clinic for advice about his memory impairment. Neuropsychological testing showed significant but mild memory impairment and some evidence of executive impairment. Nevertheless, he was able to return to his job. In passing he noted that his tendency to worry excessively and his perfectionism no longer troubled him. If anything, his wife complained that he was a little too laid back.

Suicide

Death by suicide is considerably increased after head injury, occurring in about 1% of patients over the first 15 years or so after injury (Achté *et al.* 1971; Tate *et al.* 1997; Teasdale & Engberg 2001). Thus completed suicides have accounted for up to 14% of all deaths in the medium-term mortality studies, i.e. 20–25 years (Vaukhonen 1959; Achté & Anttinen 1963; Pentland *et al.* 2005). Increased levels of suicide relative to the general population have been reported among both brain-injured war veterans and civilian populations. Achté *et al.* (1971) identified 85 suicides in a cohort of 6498 Finish brain-injured veterans from the Second World War followed up over a 25-year period and estimated the suicide rate to be twice that of the general population. More recently, Teasdale and Engberg (2001) conducted a population study of suicide among patients admitted to any hospital in Denmark over a 15-year period with a diagnosis of head injury. The standard mortality ratio for suicide among people with cerebral contusions/traumatic intracranial haemorrhages (characterised as a severely injured group) was found to be four times greater than for the general population. The risk of suicide among people sustaining concussion or cranial fractures was also elevated, approximately double that of the general population. For all three groups, the risk of suicide was constant over the 15-year period, with no particular time period after injury being of significantly greater risk.

Epidemiological studies also suggest higher lifetime prevalence rates for suicide attempts, with Silver *et al.* (2001) reporting a rate of 8.1% among people with head injury in comparison to the general population (1.9%). This elevated risk was still significant after controlling for demographics, socioeconomic status, quality of life, alcohol abuse and the presence of any co-morbid psychiatric disorder. In an examination of the clinical features of suicide attempts, Simpson and Tate (2005) found that overdoses accounted for 62% of 80 suicide attempts committed by 45 people with head injuries, followed by cutting (17%) and miscellaneous other means. Precipitating factors included depression/hopelessness, relationship breakdown or conflict, social isolation and other stressors, e.g. lack of finances or work difficulties. Almost half (48%) went on to make one or more further attempts, typically within 1 year of the index attempt. Two reviews of people who completed suicide after head injury identified post-injury rates of suicide attempt of 25% and 62.5% respectively (Achté *et al.* 1971; Tate, Simpson *et al.* 1997).

The relative contribution of premorbid, injury and post-injury factors to suicide and suicide attempts is still unclear. One major difficulty is that suicide and head injuries share a number of antecedent risk factors, including the predominance of young adult males, a history of substance abuse or psychiatric illness, and aggressive personality traits. In the case of mild head injuries, Teasdale and Engberg (2001) have suggested that these type of factors, present premorbidly or concomitant to the head injury, may be of more significance than the brain damage *per se* in the subsequent suicides. Further to this issue, Oquendo *et al.* (2004) found initial evidence that mild TBI may have a common antecedent risk factor to suicidal acts (i.e. suicide attempts) in non-brain-damaged populations, namely traits of hostility and aggression. In the study, the authors reported that these traits were the stronger predictors of suicide attempts, and that the mild TBI may have either been incidental or, at most, acted to exacerbate existing aggressive behaviour patterns.

In contrast, after severe injuries it is likely that the pattern of neuropathology, residual adaptive abilities, psychological reactions to the injury and the presence of psychiatric disorders play a significant role, both in completed suicide (Teasdale & Engberg 2001) and suicide attempts (Simpson & Tate 2005). In the case of suicides, lesions were commonly found in the frontal and temporal lobes of the brain (Vaukhonen 1959). The presence of a depressive psychosis or substance abuse has been identified as a significant risk factor in 5–40% of cases (Achté *et al.* 1971; Tate *et al.* 1997). Clinically, studies have also reported the presence of adaptive problems, including financial difficulties, vocational problems, relationship disputes and stress in marital relations, and personality change (Vaukhonen 1959; Hillbom 1960; Achté *et al.* 1971; Tate *et al.* 1997). Risk factors for suicide attempts include a post-injury history of psychiatric/emotional disturbance or substance abuse, as well as clinically significant levels of suicide ideation (Simpson & Tate 2002, 2005). There was a powerful interaction between risk factors such that patients with both a post-injury history of psychiatric disturbance and substance abuse were 21 times more likely to have made a post-injury suicide attempt than patients with neither (Simpson & Tate 2005). Premorbid risk factors cannot be discounted, even in those with more severe injuries. With regard to treatment, practice options suggested by current research include reducing the lethality of the environment, following published guidelines in the prescription and administration of medication, treatment of comorbid substance abuse or depressive disorders, and increased monitoring/support for at least 1 year following a suicide attempt.

Mild TBI

Observations on the sequelae of mild TBI are intimately linked to the discussion of the post-concussion syndrome (see below), one possible outcome of mild TBI. However, because post-concussion syndrome may also follow moderate and severe injuries, it is discussed separately. This first section concentrates on what is known about the outcome of mild TBI in terms of neuropathological and imaging findings, symptoms, cognitive impairment and recovery of disability and handicap. Some of these matters have already been considered, but with reference to the full range of head injury severity. Over the last decade many studies have focused on mild TBI in an attempt to define its natural history. Studies of concussion in sport have provided unique opportunities for observation.

Definition of mild TBI

It has been noted that there is much greater consensus on the definition of mild TBI than for moderate and severe TBI (Classifying head injury severity, earlier in chapter). There is general agreement that the core criterion, in terms of defining the boundary between mild and moderate head injury, is that the GCS score should not be less than 13. In terms of the boundary between no significant head injury and mild head injury, most will allow any disturbance of consciousness, not necessarily loss of consciousness, such that the patient meets the criterion of having suffered a concussion (see Impairment of consciousness, under Acute effects of head injury, earlier in chapter). This therefore distinguishes mild TBI from what might be called a trivial head injury, in which there was a blow to the head, but with no subjective effects on the mental state or neurological function. Whether a person can suffer a TBI in the absence of a blow to the head, simply on the basis of acceleration/deceleration forces transmitted to the head by the neck (e.g. whiplash injury), is uncertain. More recently there has been interest in the potential effects of blast injury, and there is uncertainty as to the extent of any brain damage caused by the air pressure wave of an explosion. Some definitions of mild TBI will exclude those with a skull fracture or focal neurological signs whose injury is regarded as at least moderate. Even more restrictive are those definitions that do not allow focal intracranial abnormalities on brain imaging. However, for the purposes of the discussion here, these more restrictive definitions are not used. Most definitions exclude those with penetrating injury.

Two observations from study of the outcome of mild TBI have a bearing on the definition. On the one hand there appears to be no stepwise effect of loss of consciousness on outcome (see below). On the other, comparing those with GCS scores of 15 with those whose GCS score is 14 or 13, there is a gradient of effect. For example, Kraus *et al.* (1984) found that those with a GCS score of 15 stayed on average 2 days in hospital, whereas those with a GCS score of 13 or 14 stayed on average 3 days. Hsiang *et al.* (1997) reported good outcome at 6 months in 98%, 93% and 76% of those with GCS scores of 15, 14 and 13, respectively. The outcome for patients with a GCS score of 15 and with acute radiographic abnormalities was about the same as all those with GCS scores of 13 and 14, and worse than those with a score of 15 but without any findings on CT. When considering these findings it must be acknowledged that one explanation is that lower GCS scores are probably associated with more severe injury generally. McCullagh *et al.* (2001) did not find an effect of GCS score within the range 13–15 on outcome about 6 months post injury, but the study was based on clinic referrals and therefore exposed to ascertainment effects.

Thus the definition of mild TBI in fact covers quite a range of injury. For example, the definition will include the injury suffered by a footballer who suffers a 'ding' when hit on the side of the head and is momentarily dazed. It will also cover somebody who is unconscious for 20 minutes after a fall from 10 metres and is still a little confused 12 hours later in casualty. Yet the outcome from these two patients is likely to be rather different.

Evidence for permanent damage to the brain in mild TBI

Two questions arise in relation to pathological sequelae of mild head injury. What are the risks of developing significant focal brain injury, e.g. intracranial haematoma, that is evident clinically or on neuroimaging? The second question is much more difficult to answer and therefore contentious: how many suffer diffuse axonal injury, perhaps invisible on neuroimaging, which nevertheless explains some of the post-concussional symptoms?

The first question is of most interest to the neurosurgeon or emergency physician in relation to triage and follow-up of patients presenting after a mild head injury. A meta-analysis (af Geijerstam & Britton 2003) concluded that:

> Of 1000 patients arriving at hospital with mild head injury, 1 will die, 9 will require surgery or other intervention, and about 80 will show pathological findings on CT. At least these 8% of patients will probably need in-hospital care.

This is in keeping with the more recent series of Fabbri *et al.* (2004); of over 5000 patients, 6% had an intracranial lesion on CT brain scan and 1% required neurosurgery. Patients at higher risk of complications are those with neurological signs, older age, alcohol abuse or a GCS score of 13 or 14 (Culotta *et al.* 1996; Gomez *et al.* 1996; Servadei *et al.* 2001). For example, CT abnormalities are found in 5% of those with a GCS score of 15 but in 30% of those with a GCS score of 13 (Borg *et al.* 2004). For those with a GCS score of 15 when this is associated with severe headache, nausea or vomiting there is a higher risk of an abnormality on CT brain imaging (Batchelor & McGuiness 2002). It is worth noting that although only a very small proportion suffer complications, because mild head injury is so much more common than moderate and severe head injury, a significant proportion of those who do suffer complications requiring surgery have mild injuries. For example, more than 40% of all patients with depressed fractures have never lost consciousness (Jennett 1989). Definite post-traumatic MRI abnormalities were found in 5 of 80 patients with mild head injury, with some abnormality in a further 21. Abnormalities on MRI did not predict outcome, except for early attentional problems (Hughes, Jackson *et al.* 2004).

Thus some sequelae will be readily evident on brain imaging. In the majority of patients with mild head injury, even using the sensitive structural MRI techniques (see below), the brain appears normal. However, a normal MRI scan does not rule out the possibility of diffuse axonal injury. Three lines of evidence suggest that diffuse axonal injury may occur after mild head injury.

1 Anecdotal studies describe evidence of diffuse axonal injury at post-mortem in patients who have had a mild head injury and died shortly after from other causes (Oppenheimer 1968). Using more sensitive techniques, which are however probably less specific and therefore run the danger that they may be sensitive to effects other than trauma, Blumbergs *et al.* (1994) found evidence of axonal damage using staining to amyloid precursor protein in five elderly patients, average age 77 years, dying mostly from respiratory causes between 2 and 99 days after mild head injury.

2 Povlishock and Coburn (1989) argue that brain injury in the cat produced by fluid-percussion is an appropriate model of human mild head injury. When given a very brief anaesthetic to cover the procedure, cats recover in minutes with no residual signs evident at 1 day and usually no macroscopic findings in the brain. Yet there is widespread evidence of diffuse axonal injury, particularly involving long tracts.

3 Specialised neuroimaging techniques suggest that white matter injury may be seen in patients with mild head injury: diffusion tensor imaging and magnetisation transfer imaging on MRI may show abnormalities in normal-appearing corpus callosum after mild head injury (see under Neuroimaging and head injury, earlier in chapter).

However, even if neurones are not permanently damaged after mild head injury, is there good evidence for neuronal dysfunction? If so, for how long? Various methods have been used to look for evidence of significant brain dysfunction after a mild injury. One critical issue is whether the studies have been performed in unselected patients, which usually requires recruitment from a casualty department at a time close to the injury, or in selected cases, for example from patients attending an outpatient clinic to which they have been referred. Studies on selected cohorts are at risk of overestimating any association between mild head injury and abnormal findings. Thus for example several studies using functional imaging in symptomatic patients have shown areas of hypometabolism after mild head injury (see Functional neuroimaging: studies of cerebral blood flow and metabolism, earlier in chapter) but this may have more to do with the fact that they have symptoms than because they have suffered a head injury. On the other hand, the findings of McAllister *et al.* (1999), which show convincing changes in the organisation of cerebral function in the early weeks after a mild head injury, were on unselected cases of mild head injury.

Most would agree that the routine EEG is not helpful. There has been greater interest in evoked potentials, including brainstem auditory-evoked potentials and visual-evoked potentials and event-related potentials like the P300. However, perhaps because some of these are highly specialist techniques requiring careful interpretation, early findings have not always been replicated and have not become part of routine clinical practice. Gaetz and Bernstein (2001) (and see below) in their review of electrophysiological procedures for the assessment of mild TBI conclude that cognitive event-related potentials seem to be more sensitive to injury than evoked potentials. There is some evidence that these effects may be long-lasting (Bernstein 2002). Whether cognitive event-related potentials have any value in the work-up of patients with mild head injury or post-concussion syndrome will depend very much on whether they are able to distinguish the effects of the head injury from any comorbid condition such as depression.

Two studies of motor control have found mild impairments in patients after mild head injury despite an absence of neurological signs. Postural control abnormalities were found in a highly selected group of 15 patients who complained of imbalance after mild head injury (Geurts *et al.* 1999). These patients had larger centre of pressure fluctuations, i.e. swayed more, when standing on a balance platform than did controls. The changes correlated with a speed of information processing task not with measures of emotional well-being, suggesting that they reflected some underlying brain dysfunction. Heitger *et al.* (2004) found subtle impairments of oculomotor control and visuomotor arm movement control in 30 patients within 10 days of mild head injury. The findings were interpreted as evidence of impairment in visuomotor networks linking visual input to motor output. Impairments did not correlate with neuropsychological findings, suggesting that the effects were independent of any generalised psychomotor slowing seen early after mild head injury. However, these findings need to interpreted alongside the observation that the pattern of motor impairment in some patients after mild head injury may not correspond with physiological pathways (Greiffenstein *et al.* 1996), suggesting that non-organic factors are responsible.

Cognitive impairment after mild head injury

Cognitive impairment is likely to be the direct result of the damage to the brain tissue. Minor injuries are compatible with full intellectual recovery, in the sense that the patient feels himself to be unimpaired and psychometric tests reveal no deficits in performance, even when indubitable loss of

consciousness has occurred. Levin *et al.* (1987c) followed a group of patients with minor head injury. Patients with a previous history of alcohol or drug abuse, previous head injury or a history of neurological or psychiatric disorder were excluded. Tests of memory, attention and information processing showed impairments at 1 week, but these generally resolved during the next 3 months. Somatic complaints and affective symptoms also diminished but cleared less completely. It was concluded that a single uncomplicated minor head injury produces no permanent neurobehavioural sequelae in the great majority of patients, provided they have been free from pre-existing neuropsychiatric disorder. It is possible nevertheless that subtle changes, too minor to be detected, may still exist.

Over recent years there have been several systematic reviews that have used metaanalysis to describe the neuropsychological outcome of mild TBI. The meta-analyses are based on the effect size comparing injured with control subjects. The effect size is the size of the difference between two groups as a proportion of the standard deviation of the scores. Thus an effect size of 0.5 indicates that one group did worse or better by half a standard deviation. As an approximation, effect sizes of 0.2 are usually considered to be small, 0.5 is moderate and 0.8 is large. The advantage of using the effect size is that it can be used as a common metric to compare studies that have used very different neuropsychological tests.

Quality is ensured by criteria that exclude studies on cohorts recruited from clinics or medicolegal practice because the ascertainment of such patients is strongly determined by the presence of symptoms. On the other hand, for example, a study recruiting all patients with mild head injuries presenting to an emergency department would be allowed. Some of the reviews (Binder *et al.* 1997; Frencham *et al.* 2005) have demanded at least 50% of the sample are followed up, to minimise the risk that the measured sample is not representative of all injuries. Using these criteria Binder *et al.* (1997) only examined papers with follow-up intervals of longer than 3 months post injury and found little evidence of neuropsychological impairment. There was some evidence that measures of attention were slightly impaired. Frencham *et al.* (2005) used the Binder *et al.* criteria to identify studies published since 1996 and therefore not included in the earlier review. They also included studies with shorter post-injury intervals to determine what impairments might be seen early after injury. The overall effect size for the 12 studies of less than 3 months was 0.33, which was statistically significant. On the other hand, the effect size for the 17 studies greater than 3 months was non-significant at 0.11. Thus early post-injury impairments are largely resolved by 3 months. The authors also examined whether any particular psychological domain was particularly vulnerable. The largest effects sizes were for speed of information processing (0.47), memory and executive function (both 0.3), and tests of attention (0.25); all were statistically significant. However, measures of intelligence, both verbal and performance IQ, were not significantly impaired. They noted that even for the test with the biggest difference between controls and injured (speed of information processing), the effect size of 0.45 meant that only one-third of head-injured patients would be worse than any of the control subjects; in other words, two-thirds of the cohorts would overlap in their scores. Schretlen and Shapiro (2003) identified 16 studies many of which were different from the Frencham review, and obtained very similar results. Effects sizes at less than 7 days, 7–29 days, 30–89 days and greater than 90 days were about 0.5, 0.3, 0.1 and 0 respectively.

Belanger *et al.* (2005) took a slightly different approach in their meta-analysis. They wanted to examine the effects on outcome of litigation or being seen in a clinic, so they included all studies and then collated them according to the source of ascertainment. A dramatic effect of ascertainment was seen for the studies of patients after 3 months. For the eight studies with unselected samples assessed after 3 months the effect size was 0.04; in other words, in agreement with the findings described above, there was no evidence for neuropsychological impairment after 3 months. This compared with an overall effect size of 0.63 for the 23 unselected sample studies assessed within 3 months after injury, and in whom the most vulnerable domains were delayed memory and fluency (1.03 and 0.89 respectively). However, for both selected groups, litigation and clinic based, effect sizes after 3 months were 0.78 and 0.74 respectively, and there was a fairly consistent effect across all psychological domains. Across eight litigation studies there was a hint that impairments deteriorated over time; the overall effect size for the two studies before 3 months was 0.52, and for the six studies after 3 months was 0.78. It is worth noting that these patients who had mild head injuries but who were involved in litigation did almost as badly as unselected patients with moderate/severe head injury in whom an effect size of about 0.8 was found in the meta-analysis of Schrelten and Shapiro (2003). Despite this, it is important not to conclude from these findings that litigation causes this level of symptoms. At least part of the explanation will be a large ascertainment effect, such that the litigant cohorts will have selected, i.e. not included, those who do well. In other words, it is only those with a lot of problems who are recruited into the litigation cohort; for those who do not have any problems, there is no point seeking compensation.

These reviews suggest that there may be some slight enduring impairment in some after mild head injury. Vanderploeg *et al.* (2005) have used follow-up of over 4000 Vietnam veterans about 15 years after they had been discharged from the military in order to examine the effects of mild head injury; 254 veterans said that they had suffered a head injury with loss of consciousness since discharge which had not required hospitalisation. These veterans with a history of mild head injury, on average about 8 years before testing, were slightly impaired on PASAT and on a measure of proactive interference of memory, although on many tests no impairment was seen.

Head injuries in sport provide a unique opportunity to consider the effects of very mild injury. They are relatively homogeneous, with only exceptional cases having more than a few minutes of loss of consciousness. They are relatively predictable. For example, an American footballer has about a 5–15% chance of sustaining a concussion during the course of a season. Those who are not concussed can act as a ready source of controls. And they are relatively easy to capture. Many of them occur during competitive play with trainers, medics and sometimes television crews to observe what happened.

In an interesting study Barth *et al.* (1989) investigated very mild head injuries (loss of consciousness less than 2 minutes) among university football players, comparing PASAT scores at 24 hours and thereafter with pre-injury performance. Players with mild orthopaedic injuries served as controls. When tested at 24 hours after head injury, PASAT scores failed to improve as they did in controls due to practice effect. Thereafter, serial testing showed resolution of the impairment. Symbol–digit decoding revealed a similar pattern of transient deficits. Symptom scores for headache, dizziness, nausea, weakness and difficulty with memory were also increased at 24 hours, and then subsided to normal by 10 days. Thus a single very mild head injury caused cognitive/information-processing deficits that could be documented at 24 hours, and which were accompanied and followed by subjective complaints.

These findings have been backed up by a recent meta-analysis of 21 studies (Belanger & Vanderploeg 2005), which confirmed that by 7 days post injury it was difficult to identify much cognitive impairment compared with controls. In the first 24 hours after injury the average effect size was 0.97, with the greatest impact on memory and tailor-made test batteries (effect sizes of about 1.5). For studies between 1 and 7 days the effect size was down to 0.43, and for most assessments longer than 1 week after the injury there was little if any impairment. The effects of sports injuries will be discussed in more detail below, including a discussion of the possible confounding effects of practice, prior cognitive impairment and multiple concussions. However, it is safe to conclude that only the occasional head injury sustained in sport will produce cognitive impairment beyond 2 weeks after the injury, yet in the first 24 hours after injury many will have significant difficulties with memory and slowing of information processing.

This survey therefore indicates that the majority of the athletes are asymptomatic within a day or two, whereas many of those seen in casualty will require several weeks to recover. Much of this difference is simply because the sports injuries are milder. Although there are exceptions (Raisanen *et al.* 1999), most athletes with concussion never get to hospital, would have a GCS score of 15 were it measured 20–30 minutes post injury (i.e. at about the same time after injury as the GCS is measured in casualty), and lose consciousness if at all only very briefly. However, it is also possible that other factors also determine the athletes' better outcome. Physical factors may be relevant. The athlete's head and brain may be more resilient and the physical blows suffered in sport generally less harmful. Psychological factors probably also play a part; most athletes are highly motivated to return to playing and are unlikely to regard anybody to blame for the injury.

In summary, studies of neuropsychological functioning after mild head injury point to some disturbances in cognitive functioning shortly (i.e. in the first few days or weeks) after injury, with these impairments typically most apparent on tasks with an attentional and/or processing speed component (Cicerone & Azulay 2002). However, evidence for persisting impairments following mild head injury from prospective longitudinal studies is somewhat weaker.

Loss of consciousness and outcome

It is sometimes said that, within the spectrum of mild head injury, whether or not somebody loses consciousness is immaterial to the outcome. In other words, those who are concussed but do not lose consciousness do as badly as those who lose consciousness. For example, Sharma *et al.* (2001) found that a history of unconsciousness did not correlate very well with the risk of intracranial complications. This story starts with the finding of Lidvall *et al.* (1974) that concussional intensity is not a good predictor of the cognitive impairment found in the days after injury. In a similar study based on patients attending casualty with a mild head injury, but not including those with a GCS score of 13, Lovell *et al.* (1999) compared the 60% who had loss of consciousness with the 20% who definitely did not. They were tested on average 1–2 days post injury on a range of neuropsychological tests and no differences were found between those with and those without loss of consciousness. Further support came from studies of concussion in sport. McCrory *et al.* (2000) studied 23 players concussed during a game of Australian rules football, of whom three had lost consciousness. Loss of consciousness did not predict slower information processing, measured using the digit–symbol substitution test, within 15 minutes of injury (the data are not given). Erlanger *et al.* (2003) assessed 47 concussed college American footballers, of whom 12 had suffered loss of consciousness. At the sideline of the playing field in the minutes after injury, those who had lost consciousness had more symptoms. However, when assessed 2 days later, loss of consciousness did not predict who had more symptoms. Somewhat more ambivalent is the study of 78 concussed

high school and college amateur athletes (69% American football) (Collins *et al.* 2003); 15 suffered loss of consciousness, which in 11 lasted less than 1 minute. When assessed on average 1–2 days post injury, 34 cases had poor outcome, in terms of symptoms and memory difficulties; 21% of the poor outcome group compared with 12% of the good outcome group had suffered loss of consciousness (not statistically significant). One study has suggested that the timing of the measures may be critical in determining whether loss of consciousness has an effect on outcome (McCrea *et al.* 2002). Of 91 college athletes who suffered a concussion, when tested 15 minutes later using a brief battery of tests of orientation, memory and concentration, by far the greatest impairment was seen in the seven patients who had suffered loss of consciousness. However, by 48 hours there was no difference.

Therefore when loss of consciousness lasts only a few seconds or at most a minute or so, effects are seen when testing is done within about 15 minutes of the injury; brief loss of consciousness does produce greater impairment than concussion without loss of consciousness. However, this effect of brief loss of consciousness is quickly lost and within about 24 hours can no longer be reliably detected.

Multiple concussions and outcome

Discussion of the effects of multiple concussions is most relevant to the sequelae from mild head injury; it is rare for an individual to suffer multiple moderate to severe head injuries, but multiple mild head injuries, particularly in sport, are not all that uncommon. Gronwall and Wrightson (1975) were able to find 20 cases and, using PASAT, they demonstrated that rates of information processing were slower after a second mild head injury than after a single injury of equivalent severity, despite a mean of 4.5 years between the two. The time taken to recover to normal levels of functioning was also significantly delayed. Teasdale and Engberg (2003) studied the cognitive test scores of young men aged about 18 drafted into the Danish army. National health records were used to identify those conscripts who had suffered a mild head injury, requiring at most 24 hours admission, when younger. Those with a history of concussion did worse than control uninjured men; their chances of scoring in the 'dysfunctional range' were raised, with an OR of about 1.4. More men (27%) of those who had suffered two or more concussions scored in the dysfunctional range than those who had only suffered one head injury (23%). This trend was not significant; however, if only those with injuries before age 11 years were analysed, men with double concussion did significantly worse (27% vs 21%). The study therefore provides gentle support for the hypothesis that two mild head injuries in childhood are worse than one. However, an equally plausible explanation for the findings is that those of lower IQ are more injury prone.

This reverse causality explanation also has to be considered in studies of sport injury. There is little doubt that certain athletes are injury prone. The proportion of athletes with multiple concussions exceeds that predicted by chance. The relative risk of sustaining a concussion over a two-season follow-up of American football players if that person had already suffered one or more head injuries was 16% compared with 3% for those with no history of concussion (Zemper 2003). However, some of this may be because one concussion leads to another. Guskiewicz et al. (2003) identified 12 within-season repeat concussions in athletes, and in 11 the second injury occurred within 10 days of the first. Several studies on athletes have examined the hypothesis that multiple concussions are associated with worse outcome, but none have prospectively followed athletes from before their first ever concussion to see if their worse performance in fact antedated any head injury. In general, those with a history of previous concussion do worse after the index concussion (Collins et al. 1999; Iverson et al. 2004; Moser et al. 2005). One study found more loss of consciousness (~10% vs ~4%) and slower rates of recovery in those with previous concussion (Guskiewicz et al. 2003). In a study of 698 jockeys, 108 said that they had suffered a head injury and of these 27 reported two or more (Wall et al. 2006). Those with repeat injury did worse than both single injury and those with no injury on the Stroop test of response inhibition. However, two studies of athletes have failed to find any differences between those with two previous concussions and those with one (Macciocchi et al. 2001; Iverson et al. 2006). The special case of boxing is discussed under Head injuries in sport, later in chapter.

Two studies have considered the possibility that subtle cognitive effects of a mild head injury may only become manifest when the reduced cognitive reserves have to be called upon. Ewing et al. (1980) showed impairment on tests of memory and vigilance under conditions of hypoxic stress 1–3 years later, although there was no suggestion that this was related to the presence or absence of post-concussional symptoms. On the other hand, Klein et al. (1996) argued that involutional change would expose any reduced reserve and therefore tested 25 older people who had suffered a mild head injury many years before and compared their performance with 20 age-matched controls. They found no difference.

Typical post-concussion symptoms after mild head injury

Organic contributions to the picture in the days following injury are suggested by the frequency of headache, dizziness, fatigue, difficulties with concentration and memory, and noise sensitivity. Within 1 week of injury, headache, dizziness, fatigue and sensitivity to noise and light are commoner after minor head injury than after injury to the limbs (McMillan & Glucksman 1987). The three symptoms

showing the greatest discrimination between the head injured and the control group within 1 month of injury have been found to be fatigue, doing things slowly and poor balance (all much more common in the head injured group) (Paniak et al. 2002b). By 1 month, and certainly by 3 months, many of these somatic symptoms of concussion will have recovered and if the patient remains symptomatic, emotional symptoms are likely to have become more evident. Lidvall et al. (1974) found that patients tended not to report anxiety and irritability in the first 2 weeks, but that by 3 months anxiety was one of the most common symptoms. Headache improves rapidly over the first few days and weeks, but remains high on the list of most frequent symptoms in many studies, even as late as 1 year. However, headache is quite common in the general population, so it is difficult in many cases to confidently predict that late headache is due to the head injury (see below for more detailed discussion of headache and dizziness). Common symptoms at 3 months and 1 year include irritability, fatigue, anxiety and poor sleep (Lidvall et al. 1974). When compared with control populations, those who have suffered mild head injury still report more somatic post-concussional symptoms late after injury. Depression after mild head injury is more likely in those with early depressive symptoms and who are older (Levin et al. 2005). Because depression is associated with poor outcome (Rapoport et al. 2003), those who do badly after mild head injury are sometimes described as the 'miserable minority' (Ruff et al. 1996b).

Recovery of symptoms after mild head injury

Time course of recovery

It is less easy to come to any firm conclusions about the time course of the recovery of symptoms after mild head injury than it is for the recovery of cognitive impairment. The reported rates of symptoms vary widely from one study to another. Also it may be much more difficult to confidently attribute any symptoms that are found to the head injury (see below). However, the trajectory of the recovery of symptoms after concussion in sport is relatively easy to follow. Few sportsmen describe symptoms attributable to the concussion beyond a week or two (McCrory et al. 2000). This is consistent with Lowdon et al. (1989) who studied the most minor head injuries seen in casualty, those with a PTA of less than 15 minutes. Although 90% had symptoms in the aftermath, by 2 weeks the majority of patients were symptom free. The median time off work was 1 week.

However, if all mild head injuries, defined by a GCS score of 13–15, presenting to casualty are followed up, then symptoms lasting weeks and months will be found in a significant proportion. The picture is probably worse if those with complicated injuries, for example with abnormalities on CT brain scan or with skull fractures, and those with previous head injuries or psychiatric problems are included. Cohorts that have been subject to ascertainment bias may suggest even greater morbidity. While this bias is readily apparent if the patients are recruited from clinics to which they have been referred because they are symptomatic, even those agreeing to take part in prospective studies recruited in casualty may be biased towards those with more severe injuries compared with those who do not consent (McCullagh & Feinstein 2003).

In Lidvall *et al*.'s (1974) prospective study there was a marked and continuing decline in the percentage of patients displaying one or more post-concussional symptom, from 73% at 2 days to 24% at 3 months, the fall being particularly marked during the first post-injury week. In the longer term such changes doubtless continue. Reviews of the literature (Iverson 2005; McAllister 2005) indicate the wide variation in the proportion of patients reporting symptoms at time points during the first year after a mild head injury. The figures from the review by Jacobson (1995) are worth quoting: persistent complaints are observed in 25–65% at 3 months, in 21–24% at 6 months, and in 14–18% at 1 year.

Perhaps of more interest is the proportion of cases with significant disability. Some indication of this is the presence of multiple symptoms. Of the 83 patients followed up by Lidvall *et al*. (1974), nine had numerous complaints at each time point over the first 3 months, with some tending to get worse over time. Ingebrigtsen *et al*. (1998) estimated that at 3 months 40% had three or more symptoms. Of those followed up by Deb *et al*. (1998), 17% at 1 year were diagnosed as psychiatric cases; they had to have loss of consciousness or abnormal findings on radiology or neurological examination to be included. On the other hand, only about 2–5% of those with uncomplicated mild head injury followed up by Alves *et al*. (1993) had multiple symptoms at 1 year, a figure which tallies with the 5% of Rutherford *et al*. (1979). Jones (1974) found that only 1% of patients were still symptomatic after 1 year, but this low rate is probably because the study was designed to detect neurosurgical complications rather than neuropsychiatric sequelae, and because very mild injuries were included.

Estimates of overall outcome have also been diverse. Hsiang *et al*. (1997) found good outcome in over 90%, but in the series by Deb *et al*. (1998) only 70% had good outcome as defined by the Glasgow Outcome Scale. Even worse are the figures from Glasgow, where 47% were disabled at 1 year (Thornhill *et al*. 2000). This figure, the same as those with severe injury, perhaps reflects the high levels of morbidity in the sample before the injury; alcohol was involved in about 60% of the injuries and only 35% were employed, a housewife or in further education before the injury. Van der Naalt *et al*. (1999b) identified 12% with moderate disability at 1 year in a follow-up of patients with GCS score 13 or 14, while the rest (88%) had good outcome; 79% had returned to work. This latter figure is consistent with that of Symonds and Russell (1943) who found that 88% went back

to work, all within 6 months, with 75% of the total sample being rated fully fit. However, the figures from Ruffolo *et al*. (1999) are less optimistic; only 21 of their 50 patients (42%) who suffered a mild head injury in a motor vehicle accident and who were in work at the time of the injury had returned to work when followed up on average 7 months after the accident.

Interpretation of these findings is complicated by the possibility of high rates of morbidity in those who suffer injuries other than head injury. High rates of post-concussional symptoms are found in those with chronic pain (Iverson & McCracken 1997) and even in the general population (Chan 2001), particularly those who are depressed (Iverson & Lange 2003). Indeed in a study comparing those with and without a head injury and with and without depression it was depression, rather than a head injury, that largely accounted for symptoms on the MMPI (Aloia *et al*. 1995). Some studies on mild head injury have addressed these concerns using a control population as a comparator. Within 1 month after injury Paniak *et al*. (2002b) were able to demonstrate greater morbidity in those with mild head injury than in controls without any injury. Kraus *et al*. (2005) compared over 235 patients with mild head injury (72% of those eligible) with 235 patients with injuries of comparable severity but not involving the head, recruited from casualty and followed up at 6 months. Fatigue was one of the commonest symptoms in both cohorts (about 43%). Headaches, dizziness, blurred or double vision and memory problems were more common in those with head injury. However, in terms of morbidity there was little to choose between the two groups. In fact more of the head-injured cohort had returned to work. Two studies have examined consecutive admissions to casualty following a motor vehicle accident 6–9 months after the accident to see whether those who had suffered a mild head injury in the accident did worse than those who had not. Friedland and Dawson (2001) found that on average scores on the Sickness Impact Profile, which measures perceived changes in daily activities and behaviour, were doubled in those with mild head injuries, although on several other measures, including rate of return to work and scores on the General Health Questionnaire, no differences were found. Bryant and Harvey (1999) found no differences in reporting rate across several symptoms including fatigue, dizziness and headache, but did find at least double the rate of irritability in those with head injury 6 months after the accident. Jurkovich *et al*. (1995) examined all those with lower limb fractures as the index population, and found that those who also had a head injury did almost twice as badly on a measure of psychosocial disability both at 6 months and 1 year. Those with severe head injury were excluded from the study. However, two studies comparing mild head injury with those who suffer injuries but not to the head, with follow-up at 1 year, have been more equivocal: Mickevičiene *et al.* (2004) found some evidence for greater symptoms of memory and concentration problems and dizziness and fatigue; Hanks *et al.* (1999) used the Katz Adjustment Scales and found no evidence for greater emotional problems. Studying patients attending pain clinics as opposed to a brain injury follow-up clinic, Smith-Seemiller *et al.* (2003) found more evidence of noise and light sensitivity and concentration problems in the head-injured cohort, with a trend for them also to have more headaches.

In summary, patients weeks and months after a mild head injury probably do suffer more symptoms than those with other injuries and compared with the general population, but the effect is not large. There is considerable overlap of symptoms across these groups, although those with mild head injury tend to have more symptoms that are typically associated with head injury, including concentration problems, headache, dizziness and noise and light sensitivity. Those who are depressed tend to report more symptoms, whether or not they have a head injury.

Predictors of symptoms

An understanding of the risk factors for doing badly after mild head injury may allow early therapeutic interventions aimed at preventing the development of a persistent post-concussion syndrome in those at risk. Identification of risk factors is best achieved using prospective follow-up of patients attending casualty, and this is what is discussed here. Case–control studies which compare those who are recruited into the study because they are symptomatic with others who are not are more exposed to bias. Nevertheless, case–control studies do add to a better understanding of the post-concussion syndrome and are discussed below.

It is probably useful to distinguish predictors of symptoms within weeks of injury from predictors of symptoms present months and years after injury. Almost all studies that examine the effects of age find that being older is a risk factor for symptoms both early and late after injury. In some studies women do worse (Alves *et al.* 1993; Ponsford *et al.* 2000; McCauley *et al.* 2001) but this is not an entirely consistent finding (Savola & Hillbom 2003). It is probably the case that organic factors are best at predicting early post-injury symptoms. For example, post-concussional symptoms at 1 week may be more common in those with CT brain scan or SPECT abnormalities within the first 3 days (Gowda *et al.* 2006). Perhaps those with the dopamine D_2 receptor T allele are at greatest risk (McAllister *et al.* 2005); they had worse performance at about 5 weeks post injury on a measure of response latency. Poor performance on two or more of a battery of neuropsychological tests performed within 24 hours of injury was found to predict post-concussional symptoms up to 3 months after injury, but not at 6 months (Bazarian *et al.* 1999). Two studies, both with reasonable follow-up rates (De Kruijk *et al.* 2002a; Savola & Hillbom 2003), found elevated S-100B and

the presence of dizziness or headache in casualty to predict the presence of post-concussional symptoms around 1–6 months later. It is possible that a normal HMPAO-SPECT within 4 weeks of a mild head injury excludes poor outcome at 1 year (Jacobs *et al.* 1996). Rutherford *et al.* (1977) were able to show an association between the prevalence of symptoms at 6 weeks and the presence of diplopia, anosmia or other neurological abnormalities during the first 24 hours after injury. The effect was still present at 1-year follow-up (Rutherford *et al.* 1979).

However, emotional factors are probably the best predictors of poor outcome, particularly when symptoms become more persistent. Their effects can be discerned even within a few weeks. Rutherford *et al.* (1977) found that the symptom rate was significantly higher at 6 weeks in those who blamed their employers for their accidents compared with those who blamed themselves. Lidvall *et al.* (1974) found that patients with post-concussional symptoms during the early months had suffered more anxiety about the accident from the earliest stages, more worries about other ailments and more fears that they had sustained serious and possibly permanent brain damage. King *et al.* (1999) showed that those who reported more anxiety and depression and who had higher scores on the Impact of Events Scale within the first few weeks were more likely to have symptoms at 3 and 6 months. Similarly, McCauley *et al.* (2001) found depression at 1 month was a predictor of post-concussion syndrome at 3 months. Post-concussional symptoms are more often seen in those who are depressed (Rapoport *et al.* 2003) or have symptoms of PTSD (Bryant & Harvey 1999). The role of motivational factors and litigation is considered below.

Pre-traumatic factors also have a role in outcome. In general, the milder the injury and the longer symptoms last, the more likely that constitutional factors will be found to explain who remains symptomatic. Thornhill *et al.* (2000) found that pre-existing physical limitations or brain illness predicted problems at 1 year. However, even as early as 3 months, Ponsford *et al.* (2000) found that the 24% of patients whose lives were significantly disrupted by symptoms were more likely to have a history of psychiatric problem, or a head injury or other neurological problems. Keshavan *et al.* (1981) showed that premorbid 'neuroticism' scores were influential at 3 months. In a study of veterans who were assessed many years after discharge from the military (Luis *et al.* 2003), they were asked if in the meantime they had suffered a mild head injury. A post-concussion symptom complex was more common in those with a mild head injury, especially if associated with loss of consciousness. However, the best predictors of the presence of the post-concussion symptom complex were early-life psychiatric difficulties such as anxiety or depression, limited social support, and lower intelligence. Nevertheless, not all studies find effects of pre-injury emotional factors (Cicerone & Kalmar 1997).

Post-concussion syndrome

A 50-year-old man was referred for assessment 6 years after an injury which had occurred when his lorry was involved in an accident. He had not been rendered unconscious at the time, and indeed the likelihood of trauma to the head had been very slight indeed. He had, however, been exposed to severe emotional shock. During the early months after the accident he had been extremely depressed and lacking in confidence, afraid to meet people and afraid to leave the house.

During the second year after injury he continued to be severely disabled with depression, insomnia and inability to concentrate. His wife described episodes at night in which he would wet the bed, wander from the house, or wake in fear claiming that spiders, frogs and snakes were biting him in bed. She was noted to be excessively overprotective and to smother him with affection. At a medical interview in connection with a claim for compensation it was virtually impossible to get coherent statements from him. He continued to deteriorate, becoming increasingly retarded and vague. Five years after injury it was reported that he could not answer simple questions about his name, age or address. He exhibited a gross tremor of the hands, and his general demeanour now suggested an element of psychogenic elaboration.

Six years after injury he was hospitalised at a considerable distance from his home. Gradually he improved with encouragement. At times he would converse normally, display full orientation and reasonable memory for the events of the past 6 years. During his wife's visits, however, he relapsed into his earlier vague manner, became childishly dependent and expressed irrational fears about being abandoned or subjected to unnecessary operations. By the end of his 4-week stay in hospital it was obvious that he was capable of functioning at a normal level, and comprehensive investigations, including full psychometric testing, failed to reveal any evidence of brain damage. He expressed a desire to return to work, and viewed the previous 6 years as 'blown out of all proportion' and 'being caught up in a network of problems'. Unfortunately, his wife insisted on removing him from hospital before definitive steps could be taken to secure his return to work.

In this case the appearance of severe and progressive dementia proved ultimately to be a response to the psychological trauma of the accident. There was abundant evidence that his wife had colluded and reinforced this aspect of the situation, and in many ways the compensation motive appeared to be more active where his wife was concerned than with the patient himself.

A young professional suffered brief concussion when hit on the head by a falling object; there was no loss of consciousness. She suffered transient dizziness lasting a few days and felt 'spaced out' for about a week with intermittent headaches. Nevertheless, after 5 days she returned to work to a demanding workload. She immediately noticed that she had difficulties concentrating and that working exacerbated her headache. She found it difficult to keep up with her commitments and became increasingly anxious. She suffered a panic attack and at times had depersonalisation experiences. After a month she stopped work and started doing less and less because of symptoms of fatigue and headache when she exerted herself.

By 3 months after the injury she was disabled by symptoms of depression, fatigue, headache and anxiety and was referred for specialist treatment. MRI brain scan was normal. Treatment included telling her company that she would not be returning to work for at least 3 months, an explanation for her symptoms and their prognosis, and guidance on a slow graded return to activities, starting with physical activity. Her activity levels improved and symptoms abated. By 6 months she returned to work part time with strict instructions to her and her employers that she was initially not to work more than 16 hours a week. By 9 months post injury she was working full time with no symptoms.

A journalist fell from a horse and was still unconscious when she arrived in hospital by ambulance. She soon regained consciousness but was vomiting for most of that day. She was kept in hospital overnight and by the next morning was still 'woozy'. Two days later at home she was very disabled by symptoms and in pain. An MRI scan about 2 weeks after the injury showed some evidence of an intracranial bleed. When she attempted to return to work within a few weeks of injury, fatigue was problematic and she had problems doing two things at once. By 1 year after the injury she was still limited to a maximum of 3 days work a week and notes that 'I feel exhausted much of the time, I am more sensitive to noise and I sometimes have difficulty in doing two things at once' (Sieghart 2000).

These three patients describe three very different stories yet all might have been diagnosed as post-concussion syndrome, at least at some stage during their illness. Therefore the diagnosis 'post-concussion syndrome' may be regarded as unsatisfactory. In the past it has rarely been clearly defined and different authors include different symptoms under the heading. Central to most definitions are headache and dizziness, but to these may be added fatigue, intolerance of noise and light, irritability, emotional instability, insomnia, difficulty with memory, difficulty with concentration or simply 'mental symptoms'. Anxiety and depression are seen in many, and other common emotional symptoms include travel phobia and PTSD. Some patients have marked fatigue akin to chronic fatigue syndrome, and it is possible that the similarities between post-concussion syndrome and the somatisation disorders (Wessely *et al.* 1999) may outweigh any differences between them. Minor degrees of overt intellectual impairment or of change in personality have sometimes also been included, which complicates the picture further. It is not surprising that the concept lacks clarity, and that its aetiology has remained in doubt. Lewis (1942) referred to it as 'that common dubious psychopathic condition – the bugbear of the clear-minded doctor and lawyer'.

The term 'post-concussion syndrome' does not necessarily imply that the head injury was mild. The diagnostic criteria are disinterested as to whether the head injury is mild or severe. However, DSM-IV excludes those with a dementia due to the head injury. It is generally recognised that the symptoms of post-concussion syndrome are more likely to be the cause of disability in a patient after mild head injury than in a patient with more severe injury in whom cognitive impairment and personality change, clearly attributable to brain damage, are the disabling symptoms.

The syndrome may follow injuries of markedly different severity. Numerous different symptoms can be found, cognitive, somatic and emotional, with the pattern varying greatly from one person to another. There is therefore no unique syndrome and some recommend that we employ the term used by DSM-IV: *post-concussional disorder* (Ruff 2005). The criteria used by DSM-IV for post-concussional disorder are stricter than those used by ICD-10 to diagnose post-concussion syndrome (Boake *et al.* 2005). DSM-IV requires 'significant cerebral concussion', symptoms that last longer than 3 months and begin or worsen after injury, and some evidence of cognitive deficits. ICD-10 merely requires a head injury and three or more of eight common post-concussional symptoms.

A second problem is the difficulty linking residual symptoms to the head injury. As noted above, post-concussional symptoms are common in those who have never had a head injury. A further criticism is that post-concussion syndrome is overdiagnosed because some patients with this diagnosis in fact have a collection of symptoms each with their own diagnosis. For example, somebody with dizziness, headache and irritability might be diagnosed as having post-concussion syndrome, but in fact has a combination of benign positional vertigo, migraine and episodic dyscontrol respectively (Eames 2001).

The diagnosis is also plagued by uncertainty about its cause. When easily demonstrable causes for post-concussion syndrome cannot be found, we are left uncertain how much is physiogenic and how much psychogenic. Some see symptoms as founded in subtle cerebral pathology, while others argue that their roots lie in conflict and anxiety. Much may depend on whether the symptoms under observation are early or late after injury (Lishman 1988). Different populations of patients with post-concussional symptoms will be encountered according to whether they are studied weeks or years after the injury has occurred. Lishman (1988) suggests that organic influences may be operative in the early stages, but that psychogenic mechanisms may often be prepotent when the symptoms are long-lasting. This observation has been confirmed in more recent reviews of the sum total of evidence (Ryan & Warden 2003; Carroll *et al.* 2004b; McAllister 2005). The diverse evidence related to predictors of poor outcome, based on unselected cohorts of patients with mild head injury, has been reviewed above. Here the evidence related to studies on patients with persistent post-concussion syndrome, often recruited from medicolegal practice, is discussed.

Many studies have looked for a physiogenic basis for symptoms in patients with post-concussion syndrome. Those who are symptomatic are more likely to have problems with speed of information processing, and divided and sustained attention, both in the first few months and in the year or two after injury (Gronwall & Wrightson 1974; Leininger *et al.* 1990; Bohnen *et al.* 1992; Chan *et al.* 2003).

Several studies have found changes in cerebral metabolism or blood flow in patients with persistent post-concussion syndrome. Three have looked at ^{99m}Tc-HMPAO-SPECT brain imaging in the resting state. Anterior mesial temporal hypoperfusion (Varney *et al.* 1995), frontal lobe abnormalities (Kant *et al.* 1997), and more widespread hypoperfusion, particularly involving frontal lobes (Bonne *et al.* 2003), have been found. Rates of abnormality on MRI are probably much less, for example 9% abnormal findings on MRI compared with 50% abnormal findings on SPECT in one study (Kant *et al.* 1997). When PET is used to examine glucose metabolism in symptomatic patients with normal structural brain imaging, frontal and temporal abnormalities may be observed (Ruff *et al.* 1994), although this is not consistently seen. Chen *et al.* (2003) found no group differences when comparing five patients with persistent symptoms after mild head injury with five uninjured controls using FDG-PET. However, using $H_2^{15}O$-PET to measure regional cerebral blood flow, these five patients did have smaller increases in blood flow during a spatial working memory task. Interpretation of these observations on cerebral blood flow and metabolism needs to be tempered by consideration of a report of dramatic reduction in mesial temporal and frontal metabolism on FDG-PET in a patient with psychogenic amnesia after psychic trauma but no head injury (Markowitsch *et al.* 1998). Changes in cerebral blood flow and metabolism may be found in depression and PTSD.

Patients with persistent symptoms may show altered electrophysiological responses, including the P50 (Arciniegas *et al.* 2001). The event-related potential to the second of paired auditory stimuli is normally suppressed, but in those with persistent symptoms there was less suppression. There may be changes in other event-related potentials (Gaetz & Weinberg 2000), for example a P300 that is reduced in amplitude and slightly delayed. It has been suggested that delayed brainstem auditory-evoked responses are associated with the development of persistent symptoms (Montgomery *et al.* 1984, 1991), but these findings have not been consistently replicated (Gaetz & Bernstein 2001).

Such observations support the notion of some alteration of cerebral function in those with persistent symptoms after mild head injury. However, if altered cerebral function was the cause of post-concussion syndrome, then one might expect it to be more common in those with severe head injury compared with mild, but the component symptoms lack demonstrable relationship to extent or severity of brain damage (Norrman & Svahn 1961; Lishman 1968). For example, Russell and Smith (1961) showed that longer-duration PTA is associated with more neurological sequelae but did not affect the incidence of anxiety, depression, dizziness sans vertigo and headache. Keshavan *et al.* (1981) showed that whereas the degree of disability was directly related to injury severity, the number of symptoms reported by patients was better explained by psychological factors. Those with mild injury, compared with severe injury, are more likely to have pain and depression (Beetar *et al.* 1996; Kolb & Wishaw 2003). Kay *et al.* (1971) examined patients who had failed to make a good recovery from a head injury. Those without evidence of residual brain damage, i.e. without neurological sequelae, gross personality change or cognitive impairment, were more likely to describe post-concussional symptoms, particularly headache. Furthermore, across those with mild head injuries, some symptoms of post-concussion syndrome are perhaps more common the milder the injury (Lidvall *et al.* 1974).

Non-organic contributions become much easier to discern when patients are still complaining of symptoms after the first few months have elapsed. At 3–6 months after injury, Kay *et al.* (1971) found that psychosocial factors were influential in distinguishing between patients with post-concussional symptoms and those without, i.e. marital status, social class, type of accident and previous history of psychiatric illness. No measure of severity of injury did so. Interestingly, however, as in Rutherford's study, disturbances of vision and anosmia persisting after the acute stages

were commoner in the group with post-concussional symptoms. When persisting beyond 1 year, the evidence becomes overwhelming that such long-lasting post-concussional symptoms in the majority with mild head injury rest principally on psychogenic mechanisms. They figure with great frequency among litigants for compensation (see Compensation, litigation, secondary gain and attribution bias, earlier in chapter, for full discussion of effects of secondary gain, compensation and attribution bias). Symptoms may indeed sometimes set in only after a latent interval following injury, and sometimes the fully-fledged syndrome follows an injury in which there has been no physical trauma to the head but merely severe emotional shock (Walshe 1958). Finally, such symptoms are remarkably rare, as long-continued and disabling features, in the presence of marked intellectual impairment or neurological disability. Nevertheless, as shown in Fig. 4.7, it is important to remain open to the possiblity that long-lasting symptoms in those with a mild head injury are due to the direct effects of brain injury.

Thus it may be concluded that the post-concussion syndrome has a complex aetiology in which numerous factors come to play a part. A model is proposed (Lishman 1988) whereby the cerebral dysfunction engendered by head injury, even mild head injury, commonly yields a nuclear group of symptoms, headache, dizziness and fatigue being prominent among them. At the outset these are largely organic in origin, but they are destined to recede by a natural process of healing towards the status quo. If the patient is able to feel untroubled by them, and if left undisturbed by his environment, recuperation will in favourable cases be complete.

However, obstacles to their resolution may arise, and it seems likely that these are mainly of a psychological nature. They may lie in the patient's tendency to worry unduly and to build anxiety around the symptoms, in the handling he receives from those around and the attention he is encouraged to focus on them. Obstacles may arise from other sources of distress: domestic difficulties, resentment about the accident, the need to cope too early or to face an uncongenial job. He may become significantly depressed, and there may be conflict over compensation. What has initially been based in physiogenic disturbance readily thereafter becomes prolonged, and nonetheless disabling, by virtue of a complicated interplay of psychogenic factors. Such a model would appear to apply to the great majority of patients.

Jacobson (1995) presents a more complex model that attempts to avoid a rigid distinction between physiological disorder and psychological disturbance in the genesis and maintenance of symptoms. Cognitive–behavioural factors, including social stresses, personal resources and coping processes, are seen as influential over the entire time course of the syndrome, much also depending on individual differences in sensory sensitivity and psychophysiological reactivity. Analogies are drawn with the large range of factors known to be important in relation, for example, to persistent pain. Again, the model serves as an important focus around which to explore treatment options in the individual patient. Ruff (2005) concisely summarises the evidence: 'PCD [post-concussional disorder] can be caused by (1) neuropathology, (2) psychopathology, (3) secondary gain in the form of consciously reduced effort or malingering, and (4) any combination thereof'.

Post-traumatic headache

Chronic post-traumatic headache tends to be more troublesome in those with mild head injury than in those whose injury is severe (Alexander 1992; Beetar *et al.* 1996). A significant minority report disabling headache, resistant to every therapeutic attempt, for months and years after injury.

Headache early after injury carries a different prognosis. Headache is present in the majority of patients attending casualty with a mild head injury, but by 48 hours only 52% still complained of headache and by 1 week only 27% (Coonley-Hoganson *et al.* 1984). Lidvall *et al.* (1974) showed the marked decline in headache over the first 3 months. Jones (1974) found that 57% continued to suffer headache, dizziness or both for at least 2 months but the vast majority appeared to be asymptomatic by the 1-year follow-up.

Persistent headache must raise the possibility of subdural haematoma and requires full and careful neurological examination, supplemented by CT or MRI. It may derive from pathology in the upper cervical spine, especially after whiplash injuries. Examination may reveal focal areas of tenderness in the occipital muscles or in relation to healed scalp lacerations. Occipital neuralgia seemed to explain the headache of 10 patients reported by Hecht (2004). The headaches responded to nerve block of the greater occipital nerve. Abnormal vasospastic responses of the arteries of the scalp, or tension headache due to muscle contraction, must also be considered. Friedman (1969) reviewed the numerous theories about the pathogenesis of chronic post-traumatic headache and concluded that there was no specific type.

A more recent review confirms that the exact pathophysiology of headache after trauma is still unknown in many cases (Packard 1999). Commonly, when headache has persisted for many months after injury, no demonstrable physical basis will be discovered. Headache that is diffuse, vaguely described and unremitting throughout the day immediately raises the possibility of a psychogenic basis. The lack of clear precipitants causing it to worsen, and resistance to analgesics, also bias the diagnosis in this direction. Frequently, post-traumatic headache is found along with other components of neurotic disability, and may be noted to fluctuate in severity along with tension or depression. The literature on chronic post-traumatic headache overlaps with that on whiplash injury; whiplash victims make up a good proportion of many cohorts of post-traumatic headache (Martelli, Grayson *et al.* 1999).

Walker and Erculei (1969) analysed the features of post-traumatic headache seen in men 14–17 years after injury. The onset and termination of episodes was usually gradual, and the headache was commonly bilateral and referred to frontal regions. Precipitants, in order of frequency, included noise, nervousness, work, eye strain and lack of sleep. Aggravating factors, in order of frequency, were noise, movement, light, coughing or sneezing and breathing. The descriptions used by the patients were of dull ache, throbbing, pressure, sharp pain or scalp soreness. The headaches were occasionally coupled with nausea and visual disturbances, possibly representing migraine.

Headaches after trauma are rather similar to those seen in patients without a head injury (Haas 1996); 75% were tension type headaches, 21% had migraine without aura and the remainder could not be classified. In comparison to others with chronic headache, but without a head injury, those with post-traumatic headache tend to be more disabled (Marcus 2003; Tatrow *et al.* 2003). This may partly reflect the observation that post-traumatic headache, even in cases of mild head injury or whiplash, seems to be associated with cognitive impairment (Martelli *et al.* 1999).

Dizziness and vertigo

As in the case of headache there is some evidence that dizziness in the absence of vertigo is more common with less severe injury (Russell & Smith 1961). This suggests that dizziness is not merely a reflection of physical injury related to head injury severity, and must be carefully distinguished from true vertigo. Vertigo is probably more common after moderate than mild head injury, and in perhaps 50% of cases, especially if the injury is more than mild, objective vestibular disorder may be found often associated with hearing loss (Berman & Fredrickson 1978). Comprehensive tests of vestibular function may be of value in doubtful cases (Toglia 1969). Harrison (1956) stressed the frequency after head injury of positional nystagmus of the benign paroxysmal type, found in 17 of 108 post-traumatic subjects. However, most of these patients reported a true rotational component to their dizziness, and they were seen within 2 weeks of injury. Care must also be taken to exclude orthostatic hypotension, which may lead to feelings of syncope.

Dizziness that persists for many months will, like headache, often be found to have no demonstrable physical basis. Careful enquiry often shows that it is no more than uncertainty of balance, light-headedness or subjective unsteadiness of gait. It is frequently associated with headache, likewise with other neurotic complaints. The syndrome of 'phobic imbalance', which may be traceable to early vestibular damage but then persists as a disabling neurosis, is described in Anxiety disorders (Generalized anxiety disorders), earlier in chapter. However, dizziness is one of the post-concussive symptoms that best distinguishes patients with a head injury from the general population (Paniak *et al.*

2002b). Furthermore, even though it was associated with psychological distress, dizziness was an independent predictor of failure to return to work at 6 months after mild to moderate injury (Chamelian & Feinstein 2004). This suggests that dizziness should not simply be seen as a marker of psychological problems. In those who complain of imbalance months and years after mild injury, but without vertigo, there may be objective evidence of impairment of postural control (Geurts, Knoop *et al.* 1999).

Whiplash injuries

Whiplash injury results from a sudden unexpected jolt to the body while the head is free to move at the time of impact. The common cause is a road accident collision from behind. There is therefore no warning and since the normal protective reflexes that splint the neck cannot come into operation, the neck is subjected to abrupt hyperextension/flexion or rotational stresses. The result is damage and bruising to the ligaments and other soft tissues of the neck. By any strict definition bony injuries, dislocations or disc protrusions of the spine are excluded, likewise direct trauma to the head.

The condition has attracted a great deal of attention on account of the sometimes prolonged sequelae, which include local pain and stiffness along with considerable invalidism due to headache and nervous complaints. Characteristically such patients become more disabled, and handicapped for longer periods of time, than would be anticipated from the mild character of their accidents. Given that the victim's car is usually stationary when struck from behind, there is almost invariably the possibility of a compensation claim (*res ipse loquitur*). Many patients are soon involved in litigation, and it is often a matter of dispute whether enduring symptoms are determined by organic or psychological factors. When complaints of difficulty with concentration and memory are prominent, it may be further suggested that brain damage has been sustained, despite the lack of any direct trauma to the head.

The immediate sequelae are acute shock and bewilderment, and there may be momentary dazing and confusion. 'Concussion' has been reported in 20–60% of cases, i.e. momentary loss of consciousness followed by feeling stunned and out of contact with surroundings. In many cases, however, it will be hard to judge whether this represents a true impairment of consciousness or a transient episode of dissociation occasioned by stress. Pain and stiffness in the neck, often with headache, develop within minutes or hours, but may be delayed until the following day. In an analysis of 190 acute cases, Balla and Iansek (1988) reported neck ache in 90%, headache in 75% and limitation of neck movement in 50%. Tenderness and spasm of the neck muscles is often severe, with pain spreading to the shoulders and back and into the occipital region. Sharp radicular pain may radiate to the lower jaw, arms and upper anterior chest.

Treatment with rest, analgesics and temporary immobilisation in a soft collar allows resolution of symptoms over the following weeks in favourable cases. The remainder, varying in different reports from 25% to 50% (Radanov *et al.* 1994a), progress to development of *late whiplash syndrome*, in which neck and head pain persist for many months along with symptoms reminiscent of the post-concussion syndrome. The headache is mainly occipital but can be generalised or frontal. It may be dull, sharp or throbbing, and is often accompanied by dizziness. Additional symptoms include prominent fatigue and decreased tolerance to light and sound. Difficulty with sleeping may be due to distressing dreams of the accident. The disability engendered is often remarkably severe, with inability to work and curtailment of social life in as many as 10%. In unfavourable cases the syndrome may persist for several years.

The genesis of this chronic syndrome is open to much uncertainty. Organic components may underlie pain referred from strains to ligaments and the small apophyseal joints of the spine, aggravated no doubt by spasm of the cervical muscles. Disinclination on the part of the patient to attempt gradual mobilisation may lead to a vicious circle of continuing tension from efforts to guard and splint the spine. Much of the psychological distress may stem from the pain and disability engendered in this manner. The possibility that brain damage of a subtle nature may sometimes make a contribution is hard to rule out with certainty. Alexander (1998) concludes that the evidence for brain damage, in the absence of any direct blow to the head, is interesting but not substantive, despite suggestive evidence from animal studies (Ommaya *et al.* 1968).

Possibilities of brain damage are also raised by reports of momentary 'concussion' in a proportion of cases, as already described. An example of amnesia lasting for 72 hours was reported by Fisher (1982).

A woman of 67 was struck from behind while a passenger in a stationary car, sustaining a whiplash injury but no direct trauma to the head. When asked immediately if she was hurt she replied 'What am I doing here?', and proved to be muddled and to have no idea of the purpose of the journey. She was nevertheless fully alert. When examined 2.5 and 10 hours later she was still disorientated and unable to retain any new information. She could not recall anything of the past 4 days and showed faulty recall of the previous weeks and months. She repeatedly asked where she was and what time it was. There was horizontal nystagmus to the left but no other neurological abnormality. By 72 hours after the accident her memory had returned to normal. She could finally recall the car being struck but remained amnesic for the 48 hours that followed. Suggested explanations included shear stresses in the brain or interference with circulation in the vertebral arteries.

However, there has been little else to support the presence of brain damage in the generality of whiplash patients. MRI was normal in the four patients examined by Maimaris (1989). Several studies have examined cerebral metabolism and blood flow using FDG-PET and HMPAO-SPECT respectively in patients with chronic whiplash. One study hinted at the possibility of parieto-occipital abnormalities (Otte *et al.* 1997), but a subsequent more rigorous study suggested that any parieto-occipital changes could be accounted for by differences in cortical thickness as measured by MRI (Bicik *et al.* 1998). Instead, frontotemporal hypometabolism was found that was highly correlated with depression, suggesting it was related to the known effects of depression on cerebral blood flow. Neuropsychological testing has occasionally appeared to uphold the presence of mild brain damage (Bohnen *et al.* 1993). However, poor cognitive performance is associated with high levels of anxiety, rather than changes in cerebral blood flow and metabolism (Radanov *et al.* 1999).

Psychogenic factors are strongly suspected of making an important contribution in many of the prolonged cases. In the first place, symptoms often worsen steadily over several weeks after the accident, which seems inconsistent with organic pathological factors (Gotten 1956). Moreover, psychological sequelae are understandable in terms of the sudden shock attaching to the acute experience, especially since consciousness is usually fully retained throughout. The spasm and tension in the neck muscles may themselves owe much to emotional tension. Mayou *et al.* (1993) found a strong relationship between emotional disorder 1 year after whiplash injury and scores of neuroticism in the premorbid personality.

A few studies have attempted to explore the relative importance of organic and non-organic factors in the aftermath of whiplash injuries. There is good evidence that being female and older are risk factors for chronic symptoms (Cote *et al.* 2001a). Radanov *et al.* (1994b) published a series of studies on up to 117 patients followed up over 1 year. Litigation was not a factor because of the Swiss insurance and legal systems. At all follow-up examinations (3, 6 and 12 months), the outcome was strongly related to the severity of the neck injury, as reflected in initial symptoms of radicular irritation and intensity of neck pain. These proved in effect to be the most reliable indicators of recovery. Other predictors of poor outcome at 6 and 12 months were indicative of the initial reaction to the injury, namely severity of sleep disturbance and scores of 'nervousness', both of which may have been attributable to pain. Better scores across a range of psychosocial measures favoured those with better outcome, though none were statistically significant.

Others have also found that early measures of the severity of neck injury and pain are good predictors of late outcome (Kasch *et al.* 2001; Gun *et al.* 2005; Pobereskin 2005), although estimates of the force of the injury (e.g. as measured by the speed of impact) are not (Richter *et al.* 2004; Pobereskin 2005). On the other hand, when patients are assessed with a quality-of-life questionnaire early after injury, those who report being more distressed are more likely to have symptoms 1 year later (Richter *et al.* 2004; Gun *et al.* 2005).

The role of litigation will often be thought to be important, and prospective follow-up studies have highlighted the deleterious effects of litigation on outcome (Gun *et al.* 2005; Pobereskin 2005). Among patients seen for medicolegal assessment, Pearce (1989) reported spurious weakness of grip in over half and non-anatomical sensory loss in one-third. Schmand *et al.* (1998) found that patients with chronic post-whiplash syndrome, the majority of whom were in litigation, did badly on a memory test that is in fact very easy even for patients with organic amnesia. The 60% of patients who scored below cut-off on this test also did badly across a range of other tests of cognition. Cassidy *et al.* (2000) studied claims following motor vehicle accidents in Saskatchewan before and after a tort insurance system was changed to a no-fault system. Under the no-fault system the average time to closure of claims was halved to about 200 days. The authors suggested that time to closure of claims was a valid marker of recovery, and therefore claimants recover faster if compensation for pain and suffering is not available. Faster claim closure was associated with a more favourable health status (Cote *et al.* 2001b). However, it is difficult to find the published data on which they base their conclusion that 'recovery from neck pain, physical disability, and depression occurred twice as fast under the no-fault system as under the tort system' (Cassidy *et al.* 2000). On the other hand, some patients remain symptomatic after settlement of all compensation issues (Maimaris *et al.* 1988; Newman 1990), and the chronic syndrome can be seen when litigation has not been at issue.

In Lithuania, where compensation for whiplash is not generally available, surprisingly low rates of chronic whiplash have been reported (Obelieniene *et al.* 1999); 98 (47%) of 210 victims of a rear-end collision, consecutively identified from the records of the traffic police, reported initial neck pain and/or headache. However, by about 3 weeks all had completely recovered from their accident-induced neck pain or headache. The authors argue that in Lithuania there is little notion that rear-end collisions can cause chronic symptoms. Based on this and other observations, Ferrari and Schrader (2001) propose a biopsychosocial model for chronic whiplash syndrome. This account refutes the notion that whiplash is the result of a chronic physical injury, but acknowledges that there were originally, early after injury, physical and psychological sources for the somatic symptoms. They suggest that the driving force behind the development of symptoms is patients' expectation that they are likely to suffer chronic symptoms. Problems are then amplified by the behaviour of professionals and the effects of litigation. As with post-concussion syndrome, attribution also plays a large part; symptoms that the patient might well have had anyway are attributed to the injury.

Head injuries in sport

Various aspects of head injury in sport have already been discussed in the section on mild head injury, including the time course of recovery of symptoms, the relationship of outcome to loss of consciousness, and the effects of multiple concussions. Post-traumatic convulsions were considered in Acute effects of head injury (Impairment of consciousness), earlier in chapter. The majority of athletes concussed while playing sport have significant slowing of information processing for a few hours after injury, but this has usually resolved after a few days. Ice hockey and rugby have the highest rates of concussion for team sports, but even cheerleaders are vulnerable (Boden *et al.* 2003). Estimates of the probability that any individual athlete will be injured playing ice hockey or rugby during one season are quite diverse, with figures ranging from 3% to 20% (Koh *et al.* 2003). Sometimes even higher figures are quoted, perhaps indicating that it may be difficult to define the lower limit of concussion. High rates of concussion are seen in amateurs as well as professional athletes. In several sports the rules have been changed over recent years to minimise the risk of injury, for example by outlawing dangerous tackles or by enforcement of helmets, and as such lower rates are probably now being recorded (Powell & Barber-Foss 1999). In many sports it is unusual for the injury to be more than very mild, but in horse riding and skiing, and of course motorsports, a higher proportion, though still a minority, will suffer severe head injuries.

Much attention has been paid to guidelines for management in the immediate aftermath of concussion, particularly with regard to whether the athlete should cease playing and for how long. It is hoped that those at risk of further injury can be identified. It might be that continuing impaired coordination and reaction times render them at risk of sustaining further injury. This concern is heightened by the possibility that a second impact following shortly after the first is particularly dangerous. It is also important to identify those at risk of a neurosurgical emergency, for example due to an acute subdural haemorrhage. Validated guidelines on return to play do not exist but the consensus is that symptoms of concussion, both at rest and on exertion, should have completely resolved before the athlete is allowed to resume participation (Johnston *et al.* 2001). Special consideration may be needed for those with a history of multiple concussions and for boxing. Computerised assessments are probably better than pen-and-paper tests at detecting the slight impairments of psychomotor speed which might indicate that complete recovery from a recent head injury has not yet been achieved (Collie *et al.* 2006).

It has been suggested that the occasional person who sustains a second head injury before the symptoms of the first have fully cleared goes on to suffer catastrophic cerebral oedema, usually followed by death. This *second impact syndrome* is ascribed to a failure of cerebral vascular autoregulation, causing vascular congestion (Bailes & Cantu 2001). The evidence that the syndrome exists rests on only a few case reports. Most of the cases are children or adolescents; it is known that massive cerebral oedema is more common in childhood head injury regardless of any second impact (see below). One review identified only five probable cases in the world literature and suggested there was insufficient evidence to conclude that the syndrome exists (McCrory & Berkovic 1998). Nevertheless, as noted above, all concur that the athlete must be asymptomatic before returning to play. Anybody who returns to play while still groggy is at risk of much more severe injury, for example because of impaired righting reflexes.

It has been noted that in some sports a single athlete is quite likely to experience multiple concussions during their career. The possible cumulative effect of multiple concussions has been discussed above. Indeed the possibility that multiple blows to the head, each insufficient to produce concussion, can cause irreversible cumulative brain injury has been raised by surveys of professional soccer players. A series of studies of retired soccer players found cognitive deficits that were attributed to a history of heading the ball, though with little attempt to exclude alcohol as an alternative explanation. Two studies (Matser *et al.* 2001; Witol & Webbe 2003) found a dose–response relationship between estimates of the number of times footballers had headed the ball during their career and cognitive impairment. In a review of the evidence, McCrory (2003) concludes that head-to-ball contact is unlikely to cause injury, but head-to-head contact, which often occurs as two footballers go to head a ball, might.

Boxing

The question of chronic traumatic encephalopathy in boxers is of special interest, because here serious sequelae appear to follow repeated mild head injuries, each in itself leading to no more than brief concussion. Roberts' (1969) extensive survey, described below, was important in establishing the syndrome as a valid entity, and in providing clear indications that the boxing career had been responsible. The unusual combination of neurological features provides a characteristic picture, and suggests that a distinctive pathological process is responsible. The disabilities usually set in towards the end of the boxing career while the patient is still relatively young. Sometimes the onset is acute and can be traced to a series of particularly hard fights, thereafter dictating retirement. Most examples date from the protracted boxing careers that were pursued before the Second World War when medical control over boxing was less rigorous than at present. New cases are now rarely seen probably because since the

1930s the average number of career bouts has dropped from over 300 to 13 (Clausen *et al.* 2005).

In its fully developed form the syndrome, otherwise know as dementia pugilistica, consists of cerebellar, pyramidal and extrapyramidal features, along with a varying degree of intellectual deterioration. In mild examples there is dysarthria, facial immobility and poverty and slowness of movement. Unsteadiness of gait may not be present, but evidence of asymmetrical pyramidal lesions is common from an early stage. At its most severe there is disabling ataxia, disequilibrium, a festinant gait, tremor of the hands and head, and spasticity or rigidity of the limbs.

Roberts (1969) carefully traced a random sample of 250 professional boxers who had held a professional licence for at least 3 years between 1929 and 1955; 224 were available for examination, of whom 37 (17% of the total) showed evidence of the characteristic syndrome. Approximately one-third of the 37 were judged to be affected severely enough to be recognisable by a layperson as 'punch drunk'. The clinical picture, while varying in degree, was remarkably constant from one case to another. Moreover, the prevalence of the syndrome increased with increasing exposure to boxing as judged from the history. Epilepsy occurred no more frequently than in the general population. The majority of cases remained static once boxing was discontinued. Occasionally, the condition had become more obvious with advancing age, but it was hard to distinguish this from the changes associated with ageing generally. However, undoubted progression was seen in four cases.

Almost half of Roberts' 37 cases showed intellectual and personality changes indicative of dementia in addition to their neurological disablement. This occurred with all degrees of severity. The incidence of personality change was hard to assess, but the boxers' wives often described progressive apathy and irritability with liability to outbursts of temper. Severe paranoid illness appeared to be common, particularly in subjects who showed intellectual deterioration. Johnson (1969) paid special attention to the psychiatric features in 17 ex-boxers with chronic traumatic encephalopathy. The neurological features had usually appeared before the psychological manifestations, and each could then follow an independent course. Four main areas of psychiatric disturbance were apparent: a chronic amnesic state in 11 patients; progressive dementia with disorganisation of intellect and personality in three; morbid jealousy in five; and rage reactions in three. In addition, five patients had shown evidence of psychotic illness.

Studies of boxers in the modern era

The debate now centres on whether the medical controls now in place, and the more limited boxing careers, have rendered boxing safe. In the field of amateur boxing, negative as well as positive findings are found. More worrying evidence is to be found in surveys of professional boxers. The consensus of recent evidence from brain imaging and psychometry is that chronic as well as acute brain damage is still prone to occur, even in comparatively young boxers who are pursuing successful careers. The preliminary observation of Jordan *et al.* (1997) suggests that this is particularly likely in those who are APOE ε4 positive. Of 30 professional boxers, those who were both positive for APOE ε4 and had been in more than 11 bouts were most at risk of neurological manifestations of chronic traumatic encephalopathy.

Neuroimaging

Earlier studies, while giving grounds for concern, suffered from lack of control comparisons. However, more recent studies generally find fewer abnormalities. Jordan and Zimmerman (1988) found no abnormalities on MRI in nine amateurs who had been suspended after knockouts or excessive head blows. In contrast, 7 of 21 amateurs and professionals referred for examination showed white matter changes and focal contusions on CT and MRI (Jordan & Zimmerman 1990). Jordan *et al.* (1992) performed CT brain scanning in 338 active professional boxers. In only 22 (6.5%) was 'borderline' brain atrophy found, and in a further three cases focal low-attenuation lesions were consistent with the effects of previous TBI. There were no definite effects of the number of bouts or knockouts, whereas those with large cavum septum pellucidum were more likely to show atrophy.

The Swedish study of Haglund and Bergstrand (1990) (see below) on former amateur boxers failed to find evidence of brain damage on MRI or CT. However, Zhang *et al.* (2003) did find evidence of cerebral atrophy on MRI in 24 professional boxers as well as evidence of white matter disease both on routine MRI and using DWI to detect higher diffusion constants. Higher diffusion constants correlated with more frequent boxing injuries that required transfer to hospital.

Kemp *et al.* (1991, 1995) have investigated the situation using functional imaging, arguing that by the time CT scans are abnormal the brain damage is likely to be irreversible. In this study, 34 amateur boxers were compared with 34 controls using HMPAO-SPECT, all scans being compared with an 'atlas of normality'. The boxers showed a significantly greater number of perfusion abnormalities than the controls.

Neuropsychology

The 18 boxers tested by Casson *et al.* (1984), of whom 13 were professionals, were without a history of drug or alcohol abuse and had been active only since the Second World War. Neuropsychological testing revealed deficits in several areas of functioning, performance being particularly poor on tests of short-term memory. McLatchie *et al.* (1987) restricted attention to active amateur boxers, aged 18–49 years, and found subtle evidence such as upgoing plantar responses or a degree of manual incoordination, suggestive of brain injury in 7 of 20 individuals; 9 of 15 were impaired on tests of verbal and non-verbal learning. However, only one had an abnormal CT scan with ventricular dilatation. The presence of abnormalities on neurological examination correlated significantly with the number of bouts fought.

More thorough-going investigations have used carefully selected controls, usually sportsmen from other fields or prospective boxers in training who have not yet been involved in bouts. Here the evidence has sometimes been conflicting. Drew *et al.* (1986) compared young professional boxers with control athletes and found inferior performance on a memory test and on several subtests from the Halstead–Reitan battery that was highly correlated with the number of bouts fought. Ravdin *et al.* (2003) tested professional boxers before and on three occasions within the first month after a bout. Those with high exposure to competitive bouts showed impairment of the normal practice effect on a verbal learning test. In contrast, Levin *et al.* (1987d) found little difference on psychometry between 13 young professionals early in their careers and matched controls involved with other sports. Similarly, Brooks, N. *et al.* (1987b) found essentially negative results on psychological tests in a group of active amateur boxers. However, only half of those invited took part in testing; those refusing may have been subjectively aware of impairments. Moriarty *et al.* (2004) followed over 100 amateur boxers during the course of a boxing tournament during which each boxer had, on average, two bouts. There was no deterioration in cognitive performance as a result of participation in the tournament with the exception of seven boxers whose bout was stopped by the referee, who showed significant slowing in simple and choice reaction time.

Of all neuropsychological tests, speed of finger tapping may be selectively vulnerable. In a thorough investigation of 50 former amateur boxers randomly selected from the boxing register and compared with soccer players and track and field athletes (Haglund & Bergstrand 1990; Haglund & Persson 1990; Murelius & Haglund 1991), the sole difference from controls was on a test of finger tapping. Porter and Fricker (1996) studied 20 amateur boxers and compared them with 20 men who trained in the same gym but did not compete. The boxers were quicker on Trials A and B, but showed slightly slower finger tapping that was if anything worse when followed up, on average after a further 12 bouts, about 16 months later. However, there was no evidence of further deterioration when they were followed up over 9 years (Porter 2003).

Thus, with certain exceptions, surveys would appear to suggest that amateur as opposed to professional boxing is relatively safe with respect to the risk of long-term brain damage. Some findings, however, still raise concern.

Pathology

In those with chronic traumatic encephalopathy, cerebral atrophy is commonly revealed on CT, with dilatation of the ventricles, sulcal shrinkage and sometimes obvious cerebellar atrophy. A characteristic finding is perforation of the septum pellucidum (cavum septum pellucidum), rarely seen in other conditions but occasionally found in otherwise healthy people. It is thought to be a direct result of rupture of the walls of the septum consequent upon recurrent abrupt rises of intracerebral pressure.

At post-mortem, cerebral atrophy and ventricular enlargement are often obvious to the naked eye, and ragged holes may be seen in the septum pellucidum. The most obvious abnormalities are in the deep midline structures, with tearing of the septal region and atrophy of the fornices (Corsellis *et al.* 1973; Corsellis 1989). On microscopy, severe gliosis is seen in such regions, also in the thalamus and hypothalamus. The cerebellum is affected, with gliosis and loss of Purkinje cells. In the substantia nigra there is loss of pigmented neurones similar to that seen in Parkinson's disease.

The cerebral cortex shows extensive loss of neurones, many of those surviving showing neurofibrillary degeneration of the Alzheimer type. Such changes are particularly obvious in the temporal grey matter. However, the senile plaques typical of Alzheimer's disease do not occur. This combination of histological abnormalities forms a pattern apparently unique to the effects of boxing. Additional findings include tearing of axons in the white matter and distorted axonal swellings, also evidence of previous perivascular, meningeal and subpial haemorrhages (Adams & Bruton 1989). The findings by Roberts *et al.* (1990) are of considerable interest. In a re-examination of the material reported by Corsellis *et al.* (1973), using immunocytochemical methods it was shown that though congophilic plaques were absent there was accumulation of amyloid β protein in the brain. All cases with substantial neurofibrillary tangle formation showed extensive immunoreactive deposits of β protein, not congregated in plaques as in Alzheimer's disease but distributed more diffusely. The observation that those who are APOE ε4 positive are more vulnerable to clinical manifestations of traumatic encephalopathy (Jordan *et al.* 1997; see above) lends support to the notion that amyloid β protein deposition plays a part in the pathogenesis.

Helmets and headgear

Wearing a crash helmet may dramatically reduce the risk of head and facial injuries for bicyclists involved in a crash, even if it involves a motor vehicle (Thompson *et al.* 2000). However, this conclusion is derived from case–control studies in which the injuries of cyclists wearing a helmet when involved in an accident are compared with those not wearing a helmet. Head and brain injuries are about two-thirds less in those who wear helmets. However, this result does not necessarily imply that helmets reduce brain injuries. The behaviour of helmet-wearing cyclists is likely to be different from those who choose not to wear a helmet, with the former likely to be more safety conscious and consequently have less severe accidents. In view of this uncertainty there is a continuing, and polarised, debate on the value of cycle helmets. There is more general agreement that motorcycle helmets are valuable. A systematic review of the evidence, again largely dependent on case–control studies, concluded that they appear to reduce the risk of mortality, and are associated with a 72% risk reduction in head injuries (Liu *et al.* 2004). Helmets were also found to reduce the risk of facial injuries. These favourable effects did not seem to come at the expense of a greater risk of neck injuries. Studies of ice-hockey players also hint at the value of helmets, particularly those with full face-guards, in reducing face and head injuries with no extra risk to the neck (Stuart *et al.* 2002).

In rugby football, the size and type of any helmet is limited by the rules, which effectively only allow the use of soft helmets or headgear. However, it seems likely that this type of headgear is ineffective at reducing the likelihood of concussion. McIntosh and McCrory (2001) randomly selected the under-15 rugby teams of nine schools to wear headgear, whereas the teams from seven schools formed the non-headgear controls. Concussion rates were the same with or without headgear. A laboratory analysis of the impact energy attenuation of rugby headgear showed that they were unlikely to be effective at reducing concussion (McIntosh & McCrory 2000). Likewise, headgear designed to lessen the blow to the head when heading a soccer ball are probably ineffective (Naunheim, Ryden *et al.* 2003).

Head injury in childhood

The after-effects of head injury in children differ from those in adults in certain important respects (Box 4.4). The reasons are to be sought in several different factors. On the one hand, the neural apparatus as a whole appears to be more resilient to damage in childhood. Yet, conversely, certain functions are particularly vulnerable when they are damaged during the course of development. The issues involved, and the complex balance between advantageous and disadvantageous effects when the brain is damaged before maturity, are discussed by Rutter (1993). The social setting of the child is also different to the adult's and will have important influences: the compensation motive is likely to be absent, whereas the cognitive and emotional aftermaths of injury are likely to hamper school work and call forth interactions with the parents that may have important effects.

There is general agreement that the overall incidence of sequelae is lower in children than adults, particularly for mild and moderate injury (Adelson & Kochanek 1998). In physical terms this can partly be attributed to the greater pliability of the skull and intracranial structures in childhood. The pressure effects of the blow will be better absorbed and vessels less readily ruptured. On the other hand, weak neck musculature, a larger head-to-body weight ratio and lack of myelination may all make the child more vulnerable

---

Box 4.4 Head injury in children

- Shaken baby syndrome present
- Cerebral oedema more likely
- Intracranial haematoma less likely
- Standard measures of injury severity less reliable
- More post-traumatic epilepsy within first week
- Less late post-traumatic epilepsy
- Of those with severe injury the very young probably do worse
- Greater effects of (i) pre-injury status and (ii) family/other psychosocial factors
- Relatively stereotyped personality change of emotional lability, hyperkinesis and reduced attention span, irritability with outbursts or aggression and rage, and impaired social judgement
- Less evidence of post-concussional symptoms
- Potential for more plasticity
- Generally better outcomes after mild and moderate injury
- Strokes immediately following injury more likely

---

to diffuse axonal injury. Flexion/extension deformity of the brainstem may cause respiratory arrest and consequent hypoxic brain injury; as noted in Cerebral anoxia (under Pathology and pathophysiology, earlier in chapter) this may be particularly relevant to shaken baby syndrome. Cerebral oedema is more common in the young, and it is noteworthy that cases of second impact syndrome, in which it is proposed that catastrophic cerebral oedema follows two Relatively minor head injuries occurring in close succession (see section on sports injury), are found almost always in children and adolescents. On MRI, lesions deep in the brain, for example basal ganglia, thalamus and brainstem, are more common with more severe injuries (Grados *et al.* 2001). However, depth of lesion is not a good predictor of outcome; during recovery children with deeper lesions were able to catch up with their peers with more superficial injuries (Blackman *et al.* 2003). Very young children, less than 3 years old, may be more likely to develop early post-traumatic seizures within the first week after injury (Hahn, Chyung *et al.* 1988). However, children are probably less likely to develop late (after the first week) post-traumatic epilepsy; for example this was found in only 9% of children with very severe injuries requiring inpatient rehabilitation (Appleton & Demellweek 2002).

The powers of restitution and compensation seem to be greater in the young nervous system. However, it is important not to conclude that greater plasticity of the young brain necessarily results in better outcome. The compensatory potential of the young brain in response to focal injuries, as for example used in many animal studies of plasticity, is probably jeopardised in TBI. The diffuse injury of trauma will mean that the areas of the brain that might have taken over new functions are likely to be themselves compromised. Early damage to the brain may also compromise brain growth (Kolb & Wishaw 2003). For example, there is less growth of corpus callosum after severe TBI in childhood (Levin *et al.* 2000).

Accurate comparisons between groups of child and adult patients are difficult. Though the GCS remains valid for middle and older children, in young children the verbal and eye scores are not easily assessed. The length of PTA cannot be measured accurately in young children, and it is uncertain that it carries the same implications for severity as in adults. Nevertheless, it seems that surprisingly good outcomes are seen in a proportion of children despite days or even weeks of coma (Bawden *et al.* 1985); however, in these children the clinician needs to be alert to the possibility that later development, particularly social development during teenage years, will have been affected. Very young patients with severe injuries are more likely to do badly than older children and adults with equivalent severity of injury (Taylor & Alden 1997; Anderson *et al.* 2000). They suffer a 'double hazard' (Anderson *et al.* 2005) with loss of acquired skills plus interference with further development, such that the child may show little evidence of recovery over time and considerable problems at school (Ewing-Cobbs *et al.* 2004).

The form that residual disturbance takes is also rather different in children. Cognitive disturbances will be influenced by the stage of development that has been reached. While in adults somatic symptoms such as headache and dizziness are the most frequent and long-lasting effects, these are rarely disabling in children. Instead, certain serious disorders of behaviour may be much in evidence, and tend to take distinctive forms.

The greatest problems tend to be seen in those with 'severe TBI, socioeconomic disadvantage, and preinjury behavioural concerns' (Schwartz *et al.* 2003). It is therefore important to evaluate the pre-injury state. Adverse psychosocial factors are not only associated with worse outcome (Anderson *et al.* 2004), but are quite likely to have been responsible for the injury, whether accidental or nonaccidental, in the first place (Demellweek *et al.* 2002). Those who suffer non-accidental injury tend to do worse (Prasad *et al.* 2002). The behaviour of the child themselves is also a risk factor. Although the literature is not entirely consistent, it is likely that children who sustain injuries, not just head injuries, are those with more behavioural problems; for example, Bijur *et al.* (1988) found that boys aged 5 with high aggression scores had over twice the rate of injuries over the age range 5–10 years as those with low aggression scores. Children who have suffered multiple mild head injuries show evidence of poorer performance on measures of intelligence (Teasdale & Engberg 2003). However, this is no different from children with multiple injuries but not to the head (Bijur *et al.* 1996), suggesting that the lower IQ was a cause of the multiple head injuries rather than a consequence. Bloom *et al.* (2001) found that despite attempts to exclude children with pre-injury neuropsychiatric disorders, careful inquiry 1 year post injury showed that 35% (16 of 46) had suffered pre-injury psychiatric problems; 10 had attention deficit hyperactivity disorder (ADHD) and six had anxiety disorders. Care is therefore needed before attributing any post-injury intellectual or behavioural problems to the injury itself (Ponsford *et al.* 1999; Donders & Strom 2000).

Cognitive defects have different implications compared with adults, since mental skills are in the process of development. The child stands not only to lose what has already been acquired, but also to prejudice chances of future intellectual growth. In practice profound intellectual disablement appears to be distinctly rare as a result of head injuries. However, occasional examples of severe dementia do occur in children, usually in association with spasticity and other marked neurological defects.

More commonly, the child is observed to be set back only temporarily, and to make good in the months that follow. Recently acquired abilities to walk or talk may be lost, or school work is found to be impaired for a time in relation to his fellows. For a while he may appear to be more backward than is truly the case, as a result of ill-sustained attention, sluggishness or ready mental fatigue. While they persist, however, such factors can hamper education to a serious degree. Behavioural changes are sometimes even more disruptive of progress at school, leading to persistent under-achievement even when no intellectual loss can be identified.

The precise effects of childhood injury on intellectual function are incompletely understood. Clearly, the dynamics of cerebral organisation change during the course of development, so that functions which are crucial at one stage can later be supplemented by others, or deficits which at first remain latent may later be revealed. When considering recovery of IQ after childhood injury it is worth remembering that if the child's actual score on a task remains unchanged over time, this will be registered as a drop in their IQ, because the score of their peers with normal development will have improved.

Chadwick *et al.* (1981) have reported one of the few prospective studies of the cognitive sequelae of head injury in school-age children. Groups of 29 children with 'mild' injuries (PTA <7 days) and 31 with 'severe' injuries (PTA >7 days) were followed with repeat testing for up to 27 months; 28 non-head-injured children served as controls. When the PTA had been less than 24 hours in duration there was no convincing evidence of intellectual impairment, even transient in nature. Others have also shown that children with mild head injury usually have no measurable enduring cognitive deficits (Anderson *et al.* 2001; Teasdale & Engberg 2003; Roncadin *et al.* 2004). However, Chadwick *et al.* (1981) found that deficits were common when the PTA had exceeded 3 weeks, and in some cases could still be detected at the final follow-up examination. In general visuospatial and visuomotor skills tended to be more severely affected than verbal skills. Improvement was most rapid during the early months, but further gains were observed for a year and sometimes continued into the second post-injury year as well. A definitely adverse effect on school performance was observed only in children with the most severe injuries, where the PTA had exceeded 3 weeks in duration.

Subsequent studies have further defined the impairments seen (Middleton 2001) and demonstrated that the majority of children with severe head injury will suffer significant effects on their progress at school, on social function, and on cognition (Emanuelson *et al.* 1998; Ewing-Cobbs *et al.* 1998; Max *et al.* 1998a; Teasdale & Engberg 2003). As in adults working memory and speed of information processing, for example as measured by performance on the *n*-back task, is affected in proportion to the severity of the injury (Levin *et al.* 2002; Roncadin *et al.* 2004). Attention and memory are also particularly vulnerable, with the degree of memory impairment correlating with the volume of frontal lesions (Di Stefano *et al.* 2000). Frontal injury also contributes to executive impairment. This common sequela is associated with changes in behaviour (Levin & Hanten 2005), and worse psychosocial outcome (Levin *et al.* 2004). However, compared with adults there may be a greater contribution of non-frontal lesions, compared with frontal, to executive impairment (Slomine *et al.* 2002). This may be because, compared with the adult, the child's brain can compensate for isolated frontal injury, but not if there is in addition more global injury.

Among focal defects, dysphasia has been most closely investigated. A change in cerebral dominance is possible after unilateral brain injury in early life, and this plasticity appears to persist in some degree in later childhood. Communication and social skills are affected, as in adults, by poor understanding of social cues and metaphor (Dennis *et al.* 2001).

Psychiatric sequelae, particularly behaviour disturbances, are repeatedly stressed as the commonest and most disruptive of the sequelae of head injury in children (Max 2005). After both mild (Massagli *et al.* 2004) and severe (Max *et al.* 1998b) head injury, rates of psychiatric illness, particularly oppositional defiant disorder and conduct disorder (Max *et al.* 1998c), are raised. The most common picture is a mixture of restless overactivity ('hyperkinesis'), impulsive disobedience at home and at school, and explosive outbursts of anger and irritability. Marked delinquency may appear by way of stealing, cruelty and destructiveness. Black *et al.* (1969) followed up an unselected cohort of 105 children injured between the ages of 2 and 14. At 1 year after injury approximately 20% of the children showed behaviour disorders that had not been present before. The most disruptive effects on adjustment were produced by hyperkinesis (present in 32% and appearing as a new phenomenon in 15%) and problems with anger control (present in 20% and a new development in 13%). Problems of discipline such as lying, stealing or

destructiveness were a major problem in 10%, and excessive lethargy or passivity had persisted since the accident in 8%. Sleep disturbances and problems with appetite were also occasionally observed. Hyperkinesis was commoner in younger than older children, and behaviour disturbance generally was more frequent in boys than girls. A similar picture, though with higher rates of disturbance, was found by Max *et al.* (2001) studying 37 children with severe head injury; 49% showed personality change with affective instability and the majority of these 18 children also showed recurrent outbursts of aggression or rage, and markedly impaired social judgement. Again apathy and indifference were less frequent, being present in five children (14%).

Brown *et al.*'s (1981) careful prospective study of 50 school-age children demonstrated that the development of new behavioural disorder was related to severity of injury. The group with PTA of less than 1 week showed a raised level of *pre*-accident psychiatric disturbance compared with controls, but no increase following injury. In contrast, approximately half of those with PTA exceeding 1 week developed new behavioural disorders, this being commoner the more severe the injury. Max *et al.* (2006) also found that injury severity was a predictor for personality change in 177 children with a range of injury severities followed up over 2 years. The proportion of children with a change in personality declined from 22% at 6 months to a stable rate of about 12% over the 1–2 year follow-up period. These 12% were more likely to have frontal injuries and to be rated has having shown worse pre-injury behaviour, but showed no differences on other psychosocial measures. Nevertheless, several studies have demonstrated that the family environment does predict long-term outcome, particularly for behavioural problems (Max *et al.* 1998c; Stanton 1999; Taylor *et al.* 1999, 2002).

Hyperkinesis with reduced attention span is a well-recognised sequela of head injury in children and often fulfils ADHD diagnostic criteria; in a series of 99 children with moderate and severe injury, 20 were found to have antecedent ADHD and 15, when assessed at 1 year post injury, had developed ADHD post injury (Gerring, Brady *et al.* 1998). These 15 children had significantly greater preinjury psychosocial problems, and were more likely to have other behavioural problems, than those without ADHD. Though there was no significant effect of injury severity, as measured by lower IQ, other studies have demonstrated that new onset ADHD is more likely in those with more severe injury, and have confirmed the association with preinjury factors (Gerring *et al.* 1998; Max *et al.* 1998d). Children with secondary ADHD are not only more likely to have suffered a severe injury but, as in ADHD in the absence of head injury, also show response inhibition on a stop-signal task (Max *et al.* 2004).

Whatever its origin, post-traumatic behaviour disturbance can have serious consequences in terms of school achievement, which may be markedly impaired despite good preservation of intellect on formal testing. Hill (1989) discusses the serious impact that personality changes after severe head injury can have on schooling and social development; blunting of emotional responsiveness may make continuing social education extremely difficult, and loss of tact and judgement may lead to social isolation, particularly in adolescents. Considerable adverse effects on personality may accrue from changes in self-appraisal and self-identity during a vulnerable phase of development. Turning to other psychiatric sequelae (Max 2005), PTSD is occasionally seen after childhood head injury. Children with depression or anxiety after head injury have often had these symptoms before injury. Psychosis is a very rare consequence, and it is interesting to note that autism seems to be absent after head injury.

Although parents tend to report problems with conduct and attention after head injury, it is, if anybody, the injured children themselves who report post-concussional symptoms in the early weeks after mild to moderate injury, similar to those described by adults (Mittenberg *et al.* 1997). Persistent disabling post-concussion syndrome is not a recognised sequela of mild head injury in childhood. However, one study has found that, compared with children with fractures to the legs, children after a mild head injury report more headaches, dizziness, fatigue and memory problems 2 years after injury (Overweg-Plandsoen *et al.* 1999). However, these findings run counter to clinical experience that headache is rarely prolonged and that dizziness is likewise very rare after injuries early in life.

Medicolegal considerations

The majority of head injuries result from either road traffic accidents or accidents at work and therefore frequently become an issue before the courts. Motor insurance covers road traffic accidents, and personal accident insurance covers many accidents which occur in other settings. Legal problems may involve the proof of prime responsibility or of negligence. With industrial injuries the employee will need to show that the employer was negligent or in breach of a statutory duty. The no-fault system operative in New Zealand has attracted considerable interest, in that injured persons have no need to take legal action. Instead there is a statutory body, with responsibility for compensation, rehabilitation and accident prevention.

Whatever the setting of the accident, a medical report usually comes to form an important part of the proceedings. However, psychiatrists should probably decline requests from solicitors to write reports on patients they are treating. It can be difficult for the doctor to marry the requirements of the court report, with its demand for a disinterested approach, with his/her therapeutic alliance with the patient. It is usually better to appoint an independent expert witness.

The defendant in the case, usually an insurance company, will often wish to seek another independent opinion. In some instances the doctors from the two sides meet and agree on a report for the court, but this is not always the happy solution. Legal proceedings may become burdensome and prolonged. Nevertheless, in the interests of justice to all parties the situation must be accepted, and a proper skill in the presentation of evidence must be acquired.

The court will need to make its decision on three main aspects of the situation where the medical evidence is concerned: (i) on the nature and degree of disablement that has followed the injury; (ii) on the likely duration and future course of such disablement, and the impact it will make on the quality of the patient's life; and (iii) fundamental to all the rest, the causative relationship between the disability and the injury which preceded it. All three can in some circumstances be the subject of uncertainty and open to argument.

Nature and degree of disablement

The nature of the disablement and its severity are decided from clinical examination, supplemented wherever possible by objective test procedures. With many areas, however, it is necessary to depend largely on the patient's own account, that of his friends and relatives and sometimes that of his employers. Evidence from observation in hospital or rehabilitation units is invaluable, since the other sources can hardly be expected to be free from bias once litigation is under way. Very important information can often be obtained from the records of the patient's general practitioner, particularly where premorbid levels of functioning are concerned.

All too often it is necessary to accept unsubstantiated evidence and to make a reasoned interpretation of its reliability. Evidence of altered disposition or of emotional instability, for example, must often be derived from accounts of behaviour furnished by others. The situation can be particularly difficult when subjective complaints form the main burden of the patient's disability, as with persistent headache, dizziness, fatigue or inability to concentrate.

The impression made at interview, and equally that made before the court, can be misleading in both directions. The patient with intellectual impairment or frontal lobe damage may cheerfully disclaim any symptoms whatever, and the likely impact of the injury on his life may be revealed only by an informant, skilled examination or psychological testing. Conversely, the patient may greatly exaggerate his symptoms, and claim unfitness for work or inability for enjoyment when objective evidence of disability is slight.

As noted earlier (see effects of compensation, under Compensation, litigation, secondary gain and attribution bias, earlier in chapter), a diagnosis of deliberate simulation must be made with extreme caution. Careful note should be made of the patient's attitude to detailed history-taking, and of any striking inconsistencies which emerge. For example, the vigour with which he pursues the claim and the detail with which he recounts events connected with it may be at variance with his complaints of torpor, failing memory or difficulty in sustaining concentration. His appearance may belie complaints of insomnia or constant headache. The medical advice that the patient has sought in the interim, and the regularity with which he has attended and followed the treatment prescribed, may also give important indications of the true extent of his suffering. It is fair and just to tell him on occasion of conflicts in his evidence, and to reassess this further in the light of his response and explanations.

Estimate of prognosis

The question of prognosis will certainly be considered by the court. Here it is usually possible to do no more than give a reasoned expectation and to be frank about the measure of uncertainty which surrounds it. It could be argued that after head injury of any severity the patient's condition is never likely to reach stability, and that full justice could only be met by a lifetime's follow-up (Miller 1969). In practice, however, a compromise must be accepted, since compensation is likely to be paid as a lump sum on the basis of shorter-term assessment, usually within 2–3 years of the accident, together with prediction of the likely future course.

Follow-up studies of patients coming before the courts, which would help estimation of prognosis, are remarkably few. However, here the frustrating delays which so commonly attend legal proceedings can sometimes prove to be an indirect advantage, especially when the patient has remained under regular surveillance and when repeated detailed examinations have been carried out. Even severe post-traumatic dementias are known to be compatible with improvement over long periods of time, and serial testing may already have indicated the course that is likely to be followed in the present instance. Moreover, a truly confident prognosis can sometimes only be given when the patient has returned to work. Examination may have failed to reveal much in the way of intellectual loss, yet impaired judgement and irresponsibility may later prove to make him totally unsuitable for his former occupation.

On the other hand, where the compensation motive is suspected to be active, it may be felt that until litigation is ended the future course will remain uncertain. If the compensation issue is thought to play a part in determining the prolongation of symptoms, this should be clearly stated in the report. However, sometimes it is better not to venture too firm a forecast but merely to state the uncertainties which surround the patient's future course. It is the decision of the court which will be operative, and where present medical knowledge is insufficient to help in this decision it must not be allowed to bias it unfairly.

The question of post-traumatic epilepsy should be considered in every case, and when epilepsy has not already occurred the possibility of its future development should be kept in mind, given the possible impact on future disability.

Other possible late effects of head injury – post-traumatic parkinsonism or the development of multiple sclerosis or Alzheimer's disease – are probably too rare and too controversial to warrant mention unless they have already made an appearance.

In all questions of prognosis, and particularly where mental symptoms are concerned, the patient's age, general physical and mental health, and the intelligence which he may bring to bear on adjusting to his disability should be fully considered. The court will strive to make a just award on the basis of loss of earnings and impairment of the quality of life to be followed, rather than on the actual severity of individual symptoms. Therefore the social setting must also be carefully evaluated. For example, the patient who relies on his intellect for pursuing his career may be especially handicapped by even slight disturbance of cognitive function.

Relationship to injury

With regard to the causative relationship between the injury and the disability that follows, we are liable to find that the further we move away from purely physical disabilities, the more causation is likely to be open to question. Cosmetic, orthopaedic and neurological defects can usually be directly blamed on the injury, but psychiatric sequelae with their multifactorial aetiologies can raise very special problems.

The physician must not always expect to find a strict concordance between what is accepted as causal medically and what is viewed as causal in the legal sense of the term (Trimble 1981). The medical definition of causation embraces all the things which have contributed to the result, not only the proximate events but also pre-existing conditions such as special vulnerability in the individual. On the other hand, the juridical definition of causation is almost wholly absorbed in whether some specified event, in this case an injury, can be shown to have contributed to the result.

This is particularly important for consideration of predisposing factors. What is of interest to the court is whether a similar result could have occurred with a high probability at any time or in other circumstances, even had the injury not occurred. Thus a patient long subject to recurring neurotic disability may receive scant sympathy from the court when injury is seen to lead once more to a situation which has often occurred before. The correctness or otherwise of such views could be the subject of long debate. However, it is the legal decision which carries force, and the duty of the medical referee is to place before the court the sum total of evidence in the individual case.

When complicating factors follow injury the court will similarly need to decide what weight to put on them. Sometimes the injury will be seen to have set in motion a whole chain of circumstances that contribute towards the psychiatric disability. Thus the break-up of a marriage or the loss of a career may be traceable directly to the injury, and may be factors of great importance in prolonging affective disorder or neurotic forms of reaction. The injury itself may have been mild, even when repercussions have been severe. On the other hand, independent intervening life events, e.g. the death of a spouse from cancer, may need to be considered in terms of their contribution to psychiatric disability.

It is therefore essential for the physician to formulate all aetiological factors that have a clear bearing on the case, in addition to the restricted role of the trauma itself. Unfortunately, in the determination of psychiatric sequelae, some of the contributory factors will be idiosyncratic to the individual concerned.

Finally, when the clinical picture agrees closely with what would have been expected from the severity or location of known brain damage, this concordance should be stressed. For example, egocentricity, irresponsibility or coarseness of personality will be more readily attributed to head injury when damage has involved the frontal lobes, even if the premorbid personality was poorly integrated beforehand. Similarly, the auras of post-traumatic epileptic attacks may conform to the site of penetrating injury, and confirm that a new disorder has been produced even though the patient has experienced epilepsy before.

The court report

A first essential in undertaking examinations for the courts is to obtain the patient's consent for the report to be sent to the solicitors who request it. Adequate time should be devoted to the interview and examination, or to a series of examinations if these are indicated. Full notes must be kept of all the information obtained since medical documents may be called before the court. Bell (1992) gives detailed advice about the evidence to be gathered and the preparation of the report.

Time should be spent in obtaining the fullest possible information about details of the injury itself, from which to judge the likely severity and distribution of brain damage. The duration of unconsciousness, confusion, RA and PTA should be carefully assessed, along with the extent of early neurological defects. Complications such as skull fracture, raised intracranial pressure, blood in the CSF, haematomas or intracranial infection should be noted, also early episodes of fainting or other transient disorders that may prove to be the prelude to post-traumatic epilepsy. Drugs, particularly analgesic and sedative, administered in the early days after injury should be documented; they may prolong the period of reduced conscious level so that if their effects are ignored the severity of injury may be overestimated.

Any deficiency in investigations which come to light should be remedied. Careful psychometric testing is almost always needed. It is rarely possible to compare the results of psychological testing with results obtained before the injury occurred, but valuable interpretations can often be made when results are judged against previous educational and occupational attainments. The results of psychological testing should not be given unbacked by the general clinical impression of severity of impairment, since dementia may be manifest in behaviour and personality deterioration as well as in cognitive dysfunction. Some understanding of the psychological test methods used to detect poor effort or malingering may be required. MRI scanning may be needed.

The report should embody the date and place of examination and specify the length of contact with the patient and his illness. Additional sources of information that have contributed to the material in the report should be listed: reports from informants, general practitioners and other hospitals, and the results of special investigations performed. The patient's symptoms and all objective evidence of deficits should be described in detail, and only thereafter should any tentative opinion be expressed about the reliability or otherwise with which the patient's complaints can be taken to represent the true state of his disability. In other words, full descriptive evidence should always be presented before matters of interpretation. The question of prognosis should be handled with caution, and expressed in probabilities rather than certainties.

Finally, the formulation of aetiology will embrace the likely role of trauma in relation to the picture presented by the patient, together with such constitutional and other antecedent circumstances that may have conferred special vulnerability. In cases where there is evidence of antecedent vulnerability it may be useful to consider the likely natural history of the patient had the injury not occurred. Where causal chains of circumstances have followed in the wake of injury and added to the disability, these should also be clearly and simply explained. Full supporting data must always be given to help define the contribution due to injury and that due to other additional factors.

The report should be as concise as possible and should avoid technical jargon, or where this is inevitable a simple explanation may need to be included. It is sometimes necessary to bear in mind that the patient may himself have access to the report, although this should not be allowed to dictate any alteration in material content. Finally, it is perhaps worth mentioning that in the interests of justice it behoves doctors to re-read their reports with scrupulous attention to the overall impression that it makes. Their evidence will have a powerful influence, even though the final decision regarding compensation will be made by others. It is all too easy for the doctor to identify with the patient's wish for compensation, especially when this is to be forthcoming from a large impersonal body. Conversely, when the patient has been importunate, dilatory or difficult to treat, a careful re-reading of the report may indicate that the writer has come to be unfairly biased against him.

Rehabilitation and psychological therapies

The treatment of the acute stages and early complications of head injury are not dealt with here, nor the important matter of prevention of head injuries. Nevertheless, it should be noted that clinicians are well placed to inform the public and government about the consequences of head injury and the value of measures aimed at reducing the risk of head injury.

Early management
Prevention of post-concussion syndrome
Guidelines for management of head injuries in the accident and emergency room of a severity that may or may not require admission tend to focus on early detection of neurosurgical complications. What is often lacking is guidance for the patient with less severe injury on how to manage over the days and weeks that follow, back at home and trying to get back to work.

The majority of patients with mild head injury are going to do well without any intervention and, for example, early enforced bed rest of a few days is probably not helpful (De Kruijk *et al.* 2002b). Strategies to identify patients at high risk of problems may be useful. Wade, King and colleagues, using randomised controlled trial (RCT) methodology, demonstrated that there was not much value in offering additional information, advice and support 7–10 days after injury to all patients with mild head injury (Wade *et al.* 1997). However, for those whose injury was severe enough to require admission to hospital this intervention did reduce postconcussional symptoms and social disability at 6 months (Wade *et al.* 1998). Others, using similar strategies aimed at providing guidance on how to manage symptoms, have found similar effects (Mittenberg *et al.* 1996; Ponsford *et al.* 2002). It seems that a single session of assessment and advice may be sufficient (Paniak *et al.* 2000).

Early rehabilitation for severe injury
Rehabilitation should be planned and supervised with care from the early stages of recovery. The initial convalescent period is usually undertaken in hospital, and ideally in an atmosphere as free from stress as possible. Physical activity should be encouraged, provided certain limits are imposed, and the value of early mobilisation has come to be generally recognised (Lewin 1968). Graduated exercises and games help to restore the patient's physical self-confidence, and morale is improved by opportunities for social interaction. It is essential that the patient and family know that a full assessment has been made of any possible damage to his brain, and feel confident that the advice given is soundly based. Time devoted to exploration of anxieties is always well spent. However, early estimates of prognosis should be given cautiously, offering a broad window of possible outcomes.

Explanation should be given about residual symptoms at an early date – fatigue, mental slowing, headache, dizziness – but difficulties not already present should not be implanted in the patient's mind. Depending on the severity of the injury, strategies for return to work or for more intensive rehabilitation, possibly in a residential unit, will need to be considered. The first step must always be the systematic evaluation of residual disabilities and assessment of the causes operating in the individual case.

Neurological sequelae
The main areas that require evaluation are locomotion, upper extremity function and impairment of communication. Visual acuity and visual field defects must also be assessed. Hemiparesis requires physiotherapy when more than mild and transient, similarly paraparesis or ataxia of gait. Occupational therapy has a special place in restoring useful function to the upper limbs, and speech therapy in assessing that food and drink can be safely swallowed and in helping the resolution of dysphasia or dysarthria. When treatment is undertaken in hospital or in rehabilitation units the nursing staff can contribute usefully in these areas, likewise the relatives when patients are treated on an outpatient basis.

Cognitive impairment
Full psychometric assessment is a first essential, and serves to highlight both areas of deficit and areas of preserved function on which to capitalise. Memory functions are of crucial importance and should be comprehensively evaluated from the outset.

Some general principles should underlie the planning of the therapeutic programme. First, the confidence, and where possible the full cooperation, of the patient must be secured. The relatives also must be kept informed of aims, progress and necessary limitations. Second, an optimistic and positive approach is required in order to instil enthusiasm, with ready allowance for fatigue and tolerance of shortcomings. The personalities of the therapists can therefore be of great importance. Third, the programme must be graded, with goals at any stage that are realisable, rational and acceptable to the patient (Wilson *et al.* 2002). Self-esteem is bolstered by the setting of tasks that can be mastered, however simple these may need to be at first. Success then serves as a catalyst which encourages and maintains endeavour. The tasks must also be suited to the patient's needs and inclinations. Finally, throughout the course of rehabilitation careful attention must be paid to basic matters such as the maintenance of optimal physical health. It is vital to detect depression, and to make due allowance for matters of personality change as well as intellectual impairment.

Reviews of the efficacy of cognitive rehabilitation suggest that some treatments may be effective (Cicerone *et al.* 2000). However, there has been a tendency to concentrate on outcomes that are closely linked to the intervention, for example a measure of speed of information processing in a study aimed at improving attention, rather than outcomes that patients themselves will be aware of, for example in terms of improved quality of life or reduced handicap (Carney *et al.* 1999). It is important to use outcome measures that as well as being reliable are relevant to the patient or carer (Fleminger & Powell 1999).

To understand the targets of rehabilitation it is useful to consider the framework of the World Health Organisation International Classification of Impairments, Disabilities and Handicaps (ICIDH) (WHO 1980). Whereas *impairment* refers to the direct effects of the disease on physiological or psychological performance, *disability* refers to the consequences of impairments on the ability of the person to undertake activities. *Handicap* extends the concept of disability to take into account the fact that the social effects of a disability may depend heavily on the person's circumstances. An example of this latter effect is the dramatic differences in handicap experienced by a professional violinist compared with a right-handed painter, when both suffer the same disability due to a left hemiplegia.

Cognitive rehabilitation can be broadly categorised into those strategies that attempt to reduce the impairment and those that attempt to reduce the disability and handicap through compensatory techniques (Ylvisaker *et al.* 2002). For example, in patients with amnesia, rehabilitation might aim to reduce the degree of memory impairment by the use of memory exercises or drills aimed at improving memory, or it might look at compensatory strategies to help them cope with memory impairment and enable them to remain independent at home. Compensatory strategies could include electronic memory aids, errorless learning strategies, mnemonics, and cooking with an electric cooker with a timer rather than gas. A good example is Neuropage, an electronic paging device that is programmed according to the needs of the individual patient to bleep several times during the course of the day to remind the patient to undertake various activities. This was found not only to reduce memory failures but to improve planning (Wilson *et al.* 2001). Such compensatory techniques are readily aligned with goal planning, which almost invariably forms the basis for planning and implementing rehabilitation. The research evidence suggests that rehabilitation aimed at reducing cognitive impairments may not be as effective as techniques aimed at improving disability and handicap (Wilson 2002).

It is sometimes argued that rehabilitation does not necessarily require a full theoretical understanding of the psychological processes underpinning the cognitive function that is impaired; and that a simple functional analysis of the consequences of the impairment is adequate to guide the rehabilitation strategy to be used. Evidence in support of this was presented in a meta-analysis examining studies aimed at improving attention (Park & Ingles 2001). Attention retraining techniques typically involve repetitive exercises or drills requiring a response to visual or auditory stimuli and are often informed by the theoretical ideas of cognitive neuroscience. These were compared with approaches that concentrated on helping the patient with attention deficits to perform specific functional skills. The latter approaches were generally found to be more effective. However, theory-driven rehabilitation may be effective, as demonstrated in a study to improve problem-solving skills (Hewitt *et al.* 2006). An autobiographical cueing system, in which patients are prompted to think of specific examples from memory of when they did something similar in the past, was shown to be effective. This intervention was derived from research on executive function. However, it must be admitted that the dysexecutive syndrome is often very difficult to treat, probably because it is often associated with limited insight.

Behavioural disorder

Strategies for managing behavioural problems after brain injury will usually go hand in hand with the methods described above for managing cognitive impairment. Services for head-injured patients need to be able to address all areas of difficulty, including emotional problems. Techniques derived from cognitive therapy, aimed at helping the patient alter maladaptive patterns of thinking, may be needed. However, programmes of treatment aimed at improving behavioural problems tend to rest heavily on techniques involving reinforcement or inhibition of specific behaviours. Such behaviour therapy is particularly relevant to those with severe cognitive impairment, or with poor insight or poor motivation.

Behaviour therapy starts with a behavioural analysis. A baseline diary is kept to document the frequency of behaviours, as well as their antecedents and consequences. In this way the therapist can draw up a programme aimed at reducing the occurrence of situations that trigger the behaviour and the responses of others that seem to reinforce it. Many models of behaviour therapy are based on the assumption that social interaction is a potent reinforcer of behaviour (Hollon 1973). Antisocial behaviours are therefore easily reinforced because of the attention they evoke. This results in learned maladaptive patterns of behaviour that are best treated with programmes based on ignoring the challenging behaviour. Imposed periods of social isolation ('time out') may also be required, or abrupt 'on the spot' withdrawal of staff attention ('time out on the spot', also known as TOOTS), all against a background of positive reinforcement when things are going well. Thus more constructive responses are shaped and encouraged using differential reinforcement of other (DRO) behaviour (Hegel & Ferguson 2000). Other strategies to be considered include star charts, with rewards being gained for absence of unwanted behaviour. Some units use a token economy regime carefully adapted to the circumstances of each individual patient. Tokens are earned or forfeited in relation to key aspects of the day's behaviour, then exchanged for privileges within the unit. To be effective these techniques must be implemented in a unit where all the staff are trained to provide a consistent approach (Eames & Wood 1985). Though there have been no RCTs demonstrating the efficacy of such behavioural programmes, well-controlled single case studies provide convincing evidence that they work, at least in some patients (Alderman *et al.* 1999).

Once behaviours have come under control in a particular setting it will be necessary to ensure that the success can be generalised to other, probably less structured, settings. This is likely to involve working with the family and carers so that they understand the principles involved, e.g. in order to reduce the risk of reinforcing unwanted behaviours. This may involve educating the family about the potential deleterious effects of expressed emotion and the importance of providing a non-confrontational ambiance that is predictable and supportive. Patients are likely to do badly in a turbulent setting where carers and family vacillate between displays of affection on the one hand and critical comments and anger on the other. Psychotherapy at a relatively superficial level can be of benefit if a working relationship can be established. It should aim at helping the patient to achieve some insight when this is lacking, at least into the more disturbing aspects of his behaviour. A measure of control may sometimes be achieved in such matters as disinhibition, impulsiveness or emotional outbursts, though progress is usually limited. Discussion can also usefully centre on problems that arise day to day in consequence of the patient's altered disposition, and here group therapy may be effective (Delmonico *et al.* 1998).

Short of such decisive intervention, much may still be required by way of clinical surveillance. This may be particularly the case for patients with personality disorder, this usually being resistant to psychological treatment. In many patients there will be enduring concerns about their safety and the safety of others. When irresponsibility is a marked feature, close supervision may be needed over matters of finance, and the patient's family must be brought fully into the picture. Indeed post-traumatic personality change is often the area in which the relatives most require advice, explanation and support. Ongoing contact with a social worker or case manager can prove invaluable in helping to avoid domestic, financial and occupational crises.

Rehabilitation services: from post-traumatic amnesia to return to work

Head-injured patients often present a combination of physical handicap with disturbances of intellect, mood and behaviour. They are therefore liable to fall between the two stools of adequate provision for physical therapy and adequate facilities for psychiatric supervision (Lishman 1983). Properly organised rehabilitation units allow a multidisciplinary approach, both in evaluation and in the supervision of treatment. Neurologists, rehabilitation physicians, psychologists and psychiatrists may need to work together alongside physiotherapists, occupational therapists, speech therapists and social workers. Exactly what services are needed for the individual patient will be determined by the severity of injury, the nature of the sequelae and the stage of recovery.

Inpatient and day-patient intensive rehabilitation

For those with more severe disability a period spent in a rehabilitation unit is often valuable for assessing the full extent of the patient's difficulties and limitations, and may help towards the elimination of socially disruptive behaviour. If possible this should take place as soon as the patient is medically and surgically stable. If patients remain on the medical or surgical ward, they are likely to get bored, frustrated and agitated and to need sedation. Transfer to a rehabilitation unit may therefore be an important step in preventing behavioural problems escalating. Depending on the nature of the patient's disability, it may be more appropriate to arrange transfer to a specialist neurophysical rehabilitation unit. On the other hand, a unit for patients with cognitive and behavioural problems may be more suitable, particularly if there are problems with insight and reduced safety awareness, as often found in these early stages.

It has been suggested that such interventions, delivered early, will reduce subsequent disability and indeed pay for themselves as a result of reduction in subsequent health-care costs (Cope & Hall 1982). Many units take a holistic approach, embedding cognitive rehabilitation in a therapeutic programme that addresses all aspects of recovery including the behavioural and emotional sequelae (Prigatano *et al.* 1984; Ben-Yishay *et al.* 1985). One study found that even among severely injured and behaviourally disturbed patients who would normally be considered to have a poor prognosis, intensive rehabilitation can be effective (Burke *et al.* 1988). The majority had been unconscious for over 6 weeks and showing evidence of diffuse or frontal brain damage. Almost 90% had been referred because of emotional and behavioural problems, and one-third were admitted directly from secure psychiatric settings. Follow-up 3–12 months later showed that half were living independently, and half were maintaining successful employment, albeit often in supported settings.

Therefore intensive rehabilitation seems to be effective for some patients. However, the only RCT to evaluate inpatient cognitive rehabilitation found that, for the majority of patients after a moderate to severe head injury, a low-intensity home-based programmes was as effective (Salazar *et al.* 2000). It must be acknowledged that a select group of patients was studied; they were all active-duty military personnel with family support. For those with more severe injury, unconscious for more than 1 hour, the inpatient programme did seem to be more effective. Therefore for many, particularly if support is available at home, rehabilitation in the community is appropriate. On the other hand, some will need inpatient cognitive rehabilitation, particularly those with little safety awareness, behavioural problems or limited support at home. Some of these patients will need to move on to a transitional living unit, a halfway house, so that they can improve their independent living skills in a more demanding setting, before finally returning to live in the community.

Community rehabilitation and return to work

For those living in the community, rehabilitation often works best if the therapist goes to the patient's home. This makes it easier to ensure that therapy is tailored to the patient and his situation. One RCT has shown that such outreach programmes are effective at reducing disability even years after injury (Powell *et al.* 2002). A goal-planning approach is likely to be used, with most goals getting the patient doing more with less support. Some of the action plans to achieve these goals will require one-to-one support, with a therapist or care worker being with the patient for perhaps a few hours a day. Others will require independent work both within the home and outside. Setting a structured timetable to the week is likely to be a crucial element. Once reasonable independent living skills have been mastered, strategies to look at return to work will be an important consideration for many patients.

An essential part of rehabilitation lies in the help and guidance offered when the time comes for preparation for return to work (Yasuda *et al.* 2001). The strategies to consider when post-concussional symptoms are present are discussed in the next section. However, the ideal of return to the original occupation may have to be changed on account of persistent physical or mental handicaps. In practice the chief hindrances usually prove to be of a psychological kind: poor timekeeping, inadequacy of memory, slowness and weakness of attention, early fatigue, irritability and poor social judgement. Therefore a thorough assessment will be needed to ensure that employment targets that are reasonably achievable are selected. Sometimes specialist return-to-work programmes will be needed. These are usually day programmes to mimic the demands of getting to work daily (Box 4.5). In the longer term, job retention is as important as getting back to work. Those who are unable to manage under ordinary working conditions may need entry to a sheltered workshop or day centre. Alternative targets include unpaid work such as homemaker, volunteer or student.

McMillan *et al.* (1988) argue for the benefits of introducing case management for severely head-injured patients. A designated case manager should be in a position to establish a continuous link among the various service providers, build up knowledge of what is available locally, and coordinate input to the patient and the family. However, RCT evaluation of the usefulness of such a role in the UK has given inconclusive results, largely it seems because of difficulties in augmenting contact with the scarce rehabilitation services available (Greenwood *et al.* 1994).

Post-concussion syndrome

Treatments to thwart the development of post-concussional symptoms have already been discussed. There is less research

---

> **Box 4.5 Components of a vocational rehabilitation programme** (Yasuda *et al.* 2001)
>
> - Training to secure prerequisite stamina, work competencies and behaviour, and productivity levels
> - Job development and analysis to identify which jobs are likely to be most suitable
> - Placement in a supportive employment setting with a job coach to improve the individual's stamina, work competencies and behaviour, and productivity levels, and to identify problems (e.g. for 3–4 months)
> - Substantive job placement in which job coach/counsellor provides support to secure employment through working with the employer and person with TBI
> - Short-term support and long-term follow-up in which job coach/counsellor provides limited, on-the-job support and follow-up by phone

---

evidence to guide the treatment of symptoms once they have become persistent. Most would agree that a thorough evaluation aimed particularly at understanding the contribution of brain injury, and in addition other causative factors, is the foundation for a therapeutic alliance. Education about the aetiology of symptoms will follow. This will pay particular attention to the possibility that psychological factors can result in physical and cognitive symptoms; much can be learnt from the reattribution model used in somatisation disorder (Goldberg *et al.* 1989). Patients also need to understand that management is the same regardless of whether symptoms are due to brain injury or psychological processes; there is therefore no value, in the face of a normal MRI, in an endless search for conclusive evidence of brain damage. Once the possibility of brain damage has been fully assessed, further physical investigations are best kept to a minimum. A preliminary study of the effectiveness of cognitive–behaviour therapy for persistent post-concussional symptoms is encouraging; 11 patients randomly allocated to 3 months of cognitive–behaviour therapy suffered less psychological distress at the end of treatment than the nine patients allocated to waiting list control (Tiersky *et al.* 2005).

A key issue may be return to work. Symptoms will often have deteriorated alongside attempts at returning to work, and the patient is likely to be troubled because the pressure to return to work quickly conflicts with the need to allow symptoms to resolve, sometimes quite slowly. With the patient's permission, and usually after discussion with family, the employers should be contacted with a return to work strategy. This is likely to include an initial period off work; how long for will depend on clinical common sense, which will be guided by how long symptoms have been present. A firm medical recommendation that the patient requires a prolonged period off work may be needed; if patients are apprehensive about tight deadlines for returning to work, this is likely to aggravate symptoms. Symptoms that have been present for months are not likely to improve in a few days or weeks, so a medical certificate of 3 months is a starting point, perhaps with guidance to the employers that depending on progress this may need to be extended. It is usually better to overestimate the time that will be needed, so that the employer and the patient are pleased should the latter be fit to start before the target date, rather than disappointed that the target date has passed and the patient has failed to return. On the other hand, it is important not to make blanket recommendations that all patients, including those with mild symptoms, have long periods of convalescence; for some this will cause frustration and may consequently aggravate symptoms, quite apart from the financial problems that may result, or the possibility that the job is jeopardised as a result.

Mood disorder and PTSD

Mood and anxiety disorders call for careful evaluation especially when long continued after injury, with readiness to explore the detailed factors operating in the individual case. The situation of the patient, including his family setting, must be comprehensively reviewed; where litigation is in progress liaison with the lawyers representing the case can be helpful. Antidepressant medication and the minor tranquillisers are valuable aids, but for many patients the mainstay of treatment lies in psychotherapy and in attention to the social problems that exist. Psychotherapy may need to consist of little more than ongoing support, reassurance and the ventilation of anxieties. More sophisticated psychotherapeutic interventions will need to take account of any cognitive impairment (Borgaro et al. 2003). Some patients may benefit from relaxation therapy, and this is often used alongside a formal anger management programme for patients with marked irritability and episodic loss of temper. If litigation is present, its speedy resolution is in general to be desired, certainly in cases where brain damage does not play an identifiable part.

PTSD is likely to require trauma-focused cognitive–behaviour therapy, shown to be effective in patients with PTSD without a brain injury. The cognitive–behaviour therapy may need to be adjusted and set within the context of a neurorehabilitation programme for those with significant cognitive impairment (Williams et al. 2003). It may be possible to prevent the development of PTSD by targeting those with an acute stress reaction and offering them early cognitive–behaviour therapy (Bryant et al. 2003); the proportion of patients with PTSD symptoms at 6 months was reduced from 58% to 17%.

Post-traumatic headache

Long-continued and disabling post-traumatic headache can pose a difficult therapeutic problem. Frequently a number of simple remedies will have been tried without success, and the headache will be found to be inextricably intertwined with a variety of other complaints. Evaluation and treatment must give full attention to both organic and psychological factors. The range of organic causes that need to be considered has already been outlined in the Post-traumatic headache section (under Post-concussion syndrome) earlier in chapter. A recent review of treatment is not encouraging (Lew et al. 2006). The prognosis of post-traumatic headache that has lasted more than a few months is poor. One case series of 20 does suggest that cognitive–behaviour therapy may be useful (Gurr & Coetzer 2005).

Pharmacotherapy

Cognitive impairment

Two main classes of drugs have been used to improve cognition, including memory impairment, after head injury: drugs that enhance catecholamine transmission and drugs that enhance cholinergic transmission. In both cases it is useful to distinguish early effects to promote concentration and recover and reduce confusion, from late effects once cognitive impairments are static.

A systematic review of the value of the catecholamine agonists amantadine, amphetamine and methylphenidate for acute TBI concluded that there is insufficient evidence to support the routine use of these agents to promote recovery from TBI (Forsyth & Jayamoni 2003). Nevertheless, two small RCTs did find that both early amantadine (Meythaler et al. 2002) and methylphenidate (Plenger et al. 1996) may hasten recovery. More recently, a small RCT comparing methylphenidate and sertraline with placebo, 1 month post injury, tentatively concluded that methylphenidate seemed to be better at improving cognitive function (Lee et al. 2005). Whyte et al. (2004) studied the effects of methylphenidate, on average over 3 years after injury, on numerous measures of attention and memory. Over the 6 weeks of the study patients received alternate weeks of methylphenidate or placebo. Using a rigorous methodology they identified three measures of psychomotor speed, concentration and memory that were improved by methylphenidate. Bromocriptine may be able to improve executive function, including dual-task processing (McDowell et al. 1998).

Early case studies, including one small RCT (Cardenas et al. 1994) suggested that physostigmine, a short-acting cholinesterase inhibitor, might improve memory and reduce confusion after head injury (Goldberg et al. 1982; Eames & Sutton 1995). The newer generation of cholinesterase inhibitors, like donepezil, are much more convenient to administer. Numerous small case series have suggested that they seem safe, and may be effective for both early confusion (Walker et al. 2004) and late concentration and memory impairment (Morey et al. 2003; Tenovuo 2005). Two RCTs have assessed the effectiveness of donepezil and rivastigmine, respectively. Twenty patients with cognitive impairments, on average about 4 months after a head injury, entered a placebo-controlled cross-over trial comparing 10 weeks' treatment with donepezil, mostly at 10 mg/day, with 10 weeks' placebo (Zhang *et al.* 2004). Measures of short-term memory and attention improved more quickly during donepezil treatment. However, in a study of rivastigmine (3–6 mg/day) and placebo over 12 weeks in 157 patients on average several years after a head injury with average duration of loss of consciousness of 3 weeks, no effects on a visual attention task or a memory task were found (Silver *et al.* 2006). A subgroup analysis hinted at improvements in those with more severe memory impairment on rivastigmine. Rivastigmine was shown to be safe and well tolerated. Therefore cholinesterase inhibitors may be useful, but should probably only be carefully tried in those with significant memory impairment. Practical aspects of treatment have been addressed in a useful review (Blount *et al.* 2002).

Behavioural problems

Although agitation and aggression are common problems after head injury, there is little good evidence to guide the clinician on which drug to use, and indeed whether any are in fact effective (Fleminger *et al.* 2003c). The literature is replete with case reports or small case series advocating the effectiveness of different drugs, but given that agitation tends to resolve spontaneously and that aggression is often very changeable, carefully controlled studies are needed. In this setting of uncertainty it is essential to ensure that medication is definitely necessary, to choose drugs with minimum potential for interactions and side effects, and to attend to the principles of drug treatment illustrated in Box 4.6.

Drug treatment for agitation is probably best avoided. Because agitation is often associated with the period of post-traumatic delirium, anything which increases confusion, and that includes almost all psychotropics, may increase agitation. In addition, any akathisia from antipsychotic medication will make agitation worse. There is therefore a good case for waiting, or for trying amantadine or methylphenidate.

For aggression the anticonvulsants carbamazepine and valproate have a strong track record, and given that they may have positive effects on mood are often a reasonable first choice, particularly if epilepsy is present. The observation that valproate does not appear to jeopardise cognitive function is reassuring (Dikmen *et al.* 2000). On the other hand, if there is evidence of psychosis or fear or mania, then an antipsychotic should probably be tried. However, there are indications from animal studies that antipsychotics may hinder neuronal recovery, and the risk of tardive dyskinesia, and probably neuroleptic malignant syndrome, is increased in people with a brain injury. Given these concerns and the fact that there is no definitive research evidence of efficacy in this situation, for each patient the clinician needs to be confident that antipsychotic medication has helped and continues to be necessary, if it is to be prescribed long term. Because they are probably less likely to produce side effects, atypical antipsychotics are generally used, but their potential for sedation and weight gain may limit their value.

It is worth considering a trial of a benzodiazepine, being mindful of the potential for disinhibition of behaviour and for tolerance. Short-acting benzodiazepines are particularly likely to be addictive, and if given 'as required' may reinforce unwanted behaviour. Therefore it is probably best to use regular dosing with diazepam. Interestingly, the class of drugs that have been best studied are the beta-blockers. Several small RCTs suggest they may be effective. However, large doses were used in these studies, with many patients suffering side effects. An alternative is to try an antidepressant, for example trazodone, before considering a beta-blocker. One case series found treatment with sertraline to be associated with reduced irritability and aggression (Kant *et al.* 1998b).

Sexually disinhibited behaviour may respond to antipsychotic medication. Sometimes an anti-androgen is needed (Emory *et al.* 1995). However, it is important to remember that sexually disinhibited behaviour that occurs during the early stages of recovery is likely to resolve spontaneously as the period of post-traumatic confusion resolves. In this setting simple behavioural and environmental manipulations may be more appropriate.

Dopamine agonists probably have a specific role in the treatment of apathy (Marin & Wilkosz 2005). The only properly controlled study has looked at bromocriptine, which was found to improve motivation (Powell *et al.* 1996). In some patients the improvements in motivation seemed to persist even after bromocriptine was stopped, and this is in line with anecdotal observations in clinical practice. Bromocriptine had a selective effect on motivation, having no effect on depression.

Mood and anxiety disorders

The selective serotonin reuptake inhibitors (SSRIs) are probably the first choice for treating depression after head injury, not least because they tend to have few side effects and may help symptoms that commonly accompany depression, particularly anxiety and irritability (Alderfer *et al.* 2005).

Box 4.6 Principles of drug treatment

- No knee-jerk reactions
- Start low, go slow, add one at a time
- Beware cocktails and interactions
- Beware chasing your tail
- Beware 'as required' short-acting anxiolytics
- Trial of treatment: if it does not work, stop it – slowly

Choose drugs with less

- Potential for lowering seizure threshold
- Extrapyramidal and anticholinergic side effects
- Potential for drug interactions

However, there is little evidence on which to make recommendations. Two uncontrolled studies have used sertraline, one in patients with mild head injury (Fann *et al*. 2000) and the other in patients with acquired brain injury including head injury (Turner-Stokes *et al*. 2002), both finding that patients with major depression generally improved. Citalopram, like sertraline, has little propensity for drug interactions and is therefore a reasonable alternative. Drugs that interact with other drugs commonly used after head injury need to be managed carefully.

A 40-year-old man suffered two post-traumatic epileptic seizures in the first year after a severe head injury, but had not had any further seizures since starting carbamazepine 3 years ago. He had been on a combination of fluoxetine and carbamazepine for 2 years and depression-free for over 18 months. Within 1 week of stopping fluoxetine he had a seizure. Carbamazepine levels were found to be subtherapeutic. Because of deteriorating symptoms of depression, he was started back on the fluoxetine. Repeat carbamazepine levels, with no change in dose, were now in the therapeutic range. He had no further epilepsy.

However, depression in those who have suffered a head injury may be more difficult to treat than depression in the absence of brain injury (Dinan & Mobayed 1992). Therefore other classes of antidepressants may need to be considered if depression fails to respond to an SSRI. One uncontrolled case series suggests that moclobemide may be an alternative (Newburn *et al*. 1999). Trazodone, which has the advantage of being relatively sedative but with few anticholinergic side effects, is sometimes used, particularly if depression is accompanied by anxiety, insomnia or aggression. Electroconvulsive therapy is not contraindicated when other measures have failed (Kant *et al*. 1999), and can occasionally be dramatically effective in cases of severe depression or prolonged stupor following head injury (Silverman 1964).

Pathological laughing or crying, or emotional lability, sometimes responds dramatically to an SSRI (Sloan *et al*. 1992). One study found that citalopram seemed to be as good as paroxetine, but possibly had fewer side effects (Muller *et al*. 1999).

The management of patients with anxiety disorders, including obsessive–compulsive disorder and PTSD, following head injury must be guided by the principles of treatment used in patients without brain injury. For the postconcussion syndrome, if depression or anxiety is prominent then it is probably worth trying an SSRI.

Post-traumatic headache
There have been few thorough evaluations of what might help post-traumatic headache and the good results observed

in uncontrolled studies of valproate, propranolol and/or amitriptyline, and sumatriptan, are not always observed in clinical practice (Lew *et al*. 2006). Non-addictive analgesics have a place. Ergotamine preparations may be tried when episodic headache is suspected to have a vascular basis (McBeath & Nanda 1994). Antidepressants can sometimes produce results, but it is worth remembering that they themselves may cause headache.

Physical treatments often tried include local heat, and local anaesthetic injections to tender sites and to the upper cervical spine. These have a useful place (Hecht 2004), but when overemployed carry the danger of focusing attention exclusively on one aspect of the problem alone.

Mania, psychosis and confabulation
Psychoses, including mania, which develop after head injury generally require the same psychiatric management as the equivalent illnesses occurring in other settings. Of the mood stabilisers, the anticonvulsant valproate is likely to be the first option when treating mania, partly because of reports that lithium may exacerbate confusion and ataxia and reduce seizure threshold in patients with brain injury (Silvey *et al*. 2005).

Some patients will require an antipsychotic, in which case it is probably best to choose an atypical antipsychotic, taking into account the cautions described above. There are no systematic evaluations of antipsychotic use in patients who are psychotic after head injury. There have been case reports suggesting that risperidone is effective (Silvey *et al*. 2005), but depending on the circumstances olanzapine, quetiapine and aripiprazole are reasonable alternatives. It is perhaps worth considering clozapine in patients who have failed to respond to other antispychotics and whose behaviour remains very difficult to manage (Michals *et al*. 1993). Because the occasional patient will suffer epilepsy as a side effect, some clinicians routinely add valproate when using clozapine in somebody with a head injury.

Clinical experience suggests that confabulations may be less likely to respond to antipsychotic medication than delusions. Cholinesterase inhibitors might be considered an alternative to an antipsychotic. Given that confabulations are often short-lived, there is often an argument for not offering drug treatment.

Children
A small RCT found that ADHD symptoms in children with head injury improved with methylphenidate treatment (Mahalick *et al*. 1998), although other studies have been less encouraging (Williams *et al*. 1998). Amantadine may improve behaviour and executive function (Beers *et al*. 2005).

Sleep
Insomnia at night is often associated with excessive sleep during the day. Therefore strategies to improve sleep at night

as well as maintain wakefulness during the day are likely to be required. For nocturnal insomnia, good sleep hygiene measures need to be put in place. Treatment with hypnotics is generally guided by the same principles as for insomnia in those without a head injury. Cautious use of benzodiazepine hypnotics is required and the non-benzodiazepine hypnotics like zopiclone are probably a better starting point. Sedative antidepressants should be considered, particularly trazodone. One small RCT comparing melatonin and low-dose amitriptyline (25 mg) with placebo in patients with chronic insomnia after head injury found small beneficial effects (Kemp *et al.* 2004). There was a tendency for melatonin to improve daytime alertness and amitriptyline to improve night-time sleep. For severe daytime sleepiness modafanil seems safe and may be appropriate (Teitelman 2001).

Post-traumatic epilepsy

This important complication needs to be managed along the same lines as epilepsy due to other causes. There may be a place, in carefully selected cases, for operative removal of an epileptogenic scar. Prophylactic medication for post-traumatic seizures occurring after the first week following closed head injury probably does not work (Schierhout & Roberts 1998). Patients who have been started on anticonvulsants but who have not suffered seizures after the first week generally need to be weaned off the medication by 6 months, unless the anticonvulsant is being used as a mood stabiliser or analgesic. Exceptions would include patients who had required neurosurgery, or with an open head injury or depressed skull fracture or epilepsy antedating the head injury.

Sexuality, social adaptation and effects on the family

Disturbances in sexual functioning and sexual relationships are widespread after head injury. Reduced levels of sexual drive, increased levels of erectile problems, ejaculatory and orgasmic difficulties and diminished frequency of intercourse have been reported at rates ranging from 30% to 60% in both civilian and veteran populations (Walker & Jablon 1959; Kreuter *et al.* 1998; Ponsford *et al.* 2003). For established couples, at least half report substantial dysfunction in their sexual relationship (O'Carroll *et al.* 1991). Sexual problems are not related to the gender of the patient but are associated with depression (Hibbard *et al.* 2000). This may be partly explained by the observation that SSRIs are often associated with side effects including decreased libido, erectile difficulties, delayed ejaculation and anorgasmia (Dolberg *et al.* 2002).

Many drugs impair sexual function and therefore the first stage of management is a thorough review of medication. If the patient is taking an SSRI, an antidepressant of another class with less propensity for causing sexual dysfunction should be considered. Sildenafil has proved effective in treating organic and psychogenic erectile disorders among head-injured patients, although significant care is required in

assessing the potential consequences of successful treatment on existing marital relationships. Existing sex therapy techniques for the treatment of ejaculatory disorders, modified to compensate for the motorsensory and cognitive sequelae of head injuries, have also been a useful approach (Simpson *et al.* 2003). National head injury consumer associations have developed information resources about the impact of head injury on sexual function. Finally, because many sexual problems are a reflection of broader relationship problems, they may need to be treated alongside marital therapy.

Sexually disinhibited behaviour is not uncommon after very severe head injuries during the period of recovery from post-traumatic delirium. In the majority of such cases the problem resolves spontaneously quite quickly. However, in a survey of outpatients admitted to a regional brain injury rehabilitation service, frotteurism, exhibitionism and coercive sexual behaviours were identified among 7% of a series of 445 patients (Simpson *et al.* 1999). Only 2 of 29 patients had a premorbid history of sexual offences.

Behavioural approaches employing techniques such as time out, dating skill training, self-monitoring of sexual urges, and scheduled staff feedback have been shown to be effective in treating mild to moderate levels of disinhibited behaviour (Zencius *et al.* 1990). In more severe cases of hypersexuality, often resulting in criminal sexual assaults, medroxyprogesterone acetate was found to be an effective management approach in one case series (Emory *et al.* 1995). The authors highlighted the importance of patient compliance with the medication, the necessity of providing cognitive–behaviour counselling as an adjunct to the pharmacotherapy, and the difficulties in preventing recidivism over the long term in cases where the patient had a comorbid substance abuse disorder.

Consideration of the sequelae of head injury is incomplete without mention of the broad effects on the quality of the patient's life and that of his family. It is abundantly clear that leisure and social activities are often profoundly disrupted, sometimes in the long term, quite apart from the consequences in terms of employment and finance. Family relationships can come under considerable strain. In all these respects the mental aftermaths, and particularly changes in personality, can prove more disruptive than the purely physical disabilities.

It was apparent in Thomsen's (1974) follow-up of severely head-injured patients that loss of social contact featured prominently among their problems. Most had lost touch with previous friends, and possibilities for making new acquaintances were few. Intellectual deficits, but even more so changes in personality, created the major problems in daily living. A prospective follow-up by Oddy and Humphrey (1980) reinforced these findings: leisure activities were still impaired 2 years after injury in half of their patients, this rarely being due to physical problems alone. Weddell *et al.* (1980) demonstrated marked changes in the social milieu of young adults followed 2 years later, in terms of changes in work, leisure activities, contact with friends and family life. Working capacity was affected by neurophysical status, memory difficulties and personality problems; it was the last, however, which contributed most to loss of friendships and to dependence on the family.

Families make an extremely important contribution to the ongoing recovery of people with head injury. Most patients are discharged to the family home after acute hospitalisation or rehabilitation, where close relatives continue to provide long-term support. The impact of a relative sustaining a head injury on the broader family system has been extensively documented. Very strikingly, Rosenbaum and Najenson (1976) compared the wives of 10 patients suffering from severe head injury with those of paraplegic controls who had sustained no loss of cognitive function. At 1 year follow-up, the wives of the head-injured patients were significantly more depressed, had experienced greater changes in their lives and had suffered greater social restriction.

In family members, high rates of distress and disruption, ranging from 25% to 52%, have been reported for a range of indicators including depression and anxiety (Livingston *et al.* 1985) and subjective burden (Brooks, D.N. *et al.* 1987). In addition, there may be changes in family functioning such as reduced levels of communication, affective involvement general functioning, and role change (Anderson *et al.* 2002). Florian *et al.* (1989) highlighted a number of the particular challenges that arise for families in respect to head injuries. Lack of comprehension of the patient's behaviour and its origins can lead to unhelpful responses on the part of those around. Anger may arise from a suspicion that the patient is not making proper effort, or guilt that disappointing progress reflects the carer's own inadequacy. This circle of anger and guilt can lead to emotional distancing. Denial by parents or spouses of the severity of the impact of the injury may persist for many years, along with unrealistic expectations of progress; and with eventual disappointment this can turn to anger directed at those responsible for rehabilitation. The wives of patients often need to adjust to regressive child-like behaviour, to altered sexual behaviour, and to facing the burden of child care alone (Lezak 1978).

Investigations of the causes of distress in families and carers have focused on three broad domains.

1 The characteristics of the person with TBI: the most commonly identified predictors are behavioural and emotional sequelae of the injury, for example irritability, aggression, anger outbursts, depression, and self-centredness (Brooks & McKinlay 1983; Kreutzer *et al.* 1994), followed by cognitive impairments, such as memory problems or slowed information processing (McKinlay *et al.* 1981; Hall *et al.* 1994; Wallace *et al.* 1998). There is little association between physical impairments and distress of the family or carer.

2 The characteristics of the relatives: reliance on non-adaptive coping mechanisms (Sander *et al.* 1997), an at-risk psychosocial history (Hall *et al.* 1994), and the degree of

change between pre- and post-injury social roles (Leathem *et al.* 1996) correlate with the degree of distress experienced by the carers of the patient. A number of reports suggest that spouses experience greater distress than parents, but others have not found this to be the case.

3 The presence of social support for relatives has been identified as a mitigating factor (Ergh *et al.* 2002). The critical ingredient is that the relative should feel supported, rather than for example the size of their social network (Hall *et al.* 1994; Sander *et al.* 1997; Ergh *et al.* 2002). Other types of support, such as access to professional information and financial support, are also important (Leathem *et al.* 1996; Ergh *et al.* 2002).

Despite the extensive literature, there have been few studies evaluating the efficacy of family treatment. Long-term support often falls to self-help groups and charities, who provide counselling, support and social activities for patients and their families. For reasons such as these, the National Head Injuries Association (Headway) has been established as a voluntary charitable trust, with the aim of providing counselling, support and social activities for patients handicapped in the long term and for their families.

Acknowledgements

The editors thank Dr Grahame Simpson, Rehabilitation Studies Unit, University of Sydney, Australia, for his help in writing the sections on Suicide and on Sexuality, social adaptation and effects on the family.

References

AbdelMalik, P., Husted, J. *et al.* (2003) Childhood head injury and expression of schizophrenia in multiply affected families. *Archives of General Psychiatry* **60**, 231–236.

Abou-Hamden, A., Blumbergs, P.C. *et al.* (1997) Axonal injury in falls. *Journal of Neurotrauma* **14**, 699–713.

Abu-Judeh, H.H., Parker, R. *et al.* (1999) SPET brain perfusion imaging in mild traumatic brain injury without loss of consciousness and normal computed tomography. *Nuclear Medicine Communications* **20**, 505–510.

Achté, K.A. & Anttinen, E.E. (1963) Suizide bei Hirngeschädigten des Krieges in Finland. *Fortschritte der Neurologie, Pychiatrie* **31**, 645–667.

Achté, K.A., Hillbom, E. *et al.* (1967) *Post-traumatic Psychoses Following War Brain Injuries*. Reports from the Rehabilitation Institute for Brain-injured Veterans in Finland. Helsinki.

Achté, K.A., Hillbom, E. *et al.* (1969) Psychoses following war brain injuries. *Acta Pychiatrica Scandinavica* **45**, 1–18.

Achté, K.A., Lonnquist, J. *et al.* (1971) Suicide following war brain injuries. *Acta Psychiatrica Scandinavica* **225**, 1–94.

Adams, C.W.M. & Bruton, C.J. (1989) The cerebral vasculature in dementia pugilistica. *Journal of Neurology, Neurosurgery and Psychiatry* **52**, 600–604.

Adelson, P.D. & Kochanek, P.M. (1998) Head injury in children. *Journal of Child Neurology* **13**, 2–15.

Adle-Biassette, H., Duyckaerts, C. et al. (1996) Beta AP deposition and head trauma. *Neurobiology of Aging* **17**, 415–419.

Adler, A. (1945) Mental symptoms following head injury. *Archives of Neurology and Psychiatry* **53**, 34–43.

af Geijerstam, J.L. & Britton, M. (2003) Mild head injury. Mortality and complication rate: meta-analysis of findings in a systematic literature review. *Acta Neurochirurgica (Wien)* **145**, 843–50; discussion 850.

Ajuriaguerra, J.D. & Hecaen, H. (1960) *Le Cortex Cerebral: Étude Neuro-psycho-pathologique*. Masson, Paris.

Albin, M.S. & Bunegin, L. (1986) An experimental study of craniocerebral trauma during ethanol intoxication. *Critical Care Medicine* **14**, 841–845.

Alderfer, B.S., Arciniegas, D.B. et al. (2005) Treatment of depression following traumatic brain injury. *Journal of Head Trauma Rehabilitation* **20**, 544–562.

Alderman, N. (1996) Central executive deficit and response to operant conditioning methods. *Neuropsychological Rehabilitation* **6**, 161–186.

Alderman, N., Davies, J.A. et al. (1999) Reduction of severe aggressive behaviour in acquired brain injury: case studies illustrating clinical use of the OAS-MNR in the management of challenging behaviours. *Brain Injury* **13**, 669–704.

Alderman, N., Burgess, P.W. et al. (2003) Ecological validity of a simplified version of the multiple errands shopping test. *Journal of the International Neuropsychological Society* **9**, 31–44.

Alderso, A.L. & Novack, T.A. (2002) Measuring recovery of orientation during acute rehabilitation for traumatic brain injury: value and expectations of recovery. *Journal of Head Trauma Rehabilitation* **17**, 210–219.

Alexander, M.P. (1982) Traumatic brain injury. In: Benson, D.F. & Blumer, D. (eds) *Psychiatric Aspects of Neurologic Disease*, ch. 11. Grune & Stratton, New York.

Alexander, M.P. (1992) Neuropsychiatric correlates of persistent postconcussive syndrome. *Journal of Head Trauma Rehabilitation* **7**, 60–69.

Alexander, M.P. (1998) In the pursuit of proof of brain damage after whiplash injury. *Neurology* **51**, 336–340.

Alexander, S., Kerr, M.E. et al. (2004) The effects of admission alcohol level on cerebral blood flow and outcomes after severe traumatic brain injury. *Journal of Neurotrauma* **21**, 575–583.

Aloia, M.S., Long, C.J. et al. (1995) Depression among the head-injured and non-head-injured: a discriminant analysis. *Brain Injury* **9**, 575–583.

Alves, W., Macciocchi, S.N. et al. (1993) Post concussive symptoms after uncomplicated mild head injury. *Journal of Head Trauma Rehabilitation* **8**, 48–59.

Anderson, C. (1942) Chronic head cases. *Lancet* **ii**, 1–4.

Anderson, M.I., Parmenter, T.R. et al. (2002) The relationship between neurobehavioural problems of severe traumatic brain injury (TBI), family functioning and the psychological well-being of the spouse/caregiver: path model analysis. *Brain Injury* **16**, 743–757.

Anderson, V., Catroppa, C. et al. (2000) Recovery of intellectual ability following traumatic brain injury in childhood: impact of injury severity and age at injury. *Pediatric Neurosurgery* **32**, 282–290.

Anderson, V., Catroppa, C. et al. (2001) Outcome from mild head injury in young children: a prospective study. *Journal of Clinical and Experimental Neuropsychology* **23**, 705–717.

Anderson, V., Catroppa, C. et al. (2005) Functional plasticity or vulnerability after early brain injury? *Pediatrics* **116**, 1374–1382.

Anderson, V.A., Morse, S.A. et al. (2004) Thirty month outcome from early childhood head injury: a prospective analysis of neurobehavioural recovery. *Brain* **127**, 2608–2620.

Andrews, K. (1999) The vegetative state: clinical diagnosis. *Postgraduate Medical Journal* **75**, 321–324.

Angeleri, F., Majkowski, J. et al. (1999) Posttraumatic epilepsy risk factors: one-year prospective study after head injury. *Epilepsia* **40**, 1222–1230.

Appleton, R.E. & Demellweek, C. (2002) Post-traumatic epilepsy in children requiring inpatient rehabilitation following head injury. *Journal of Neurology, Neurosurgery and Psychiatry* **72**, 669–672.

Arciniegas, D.B., Topkoff, J.L. et al. (2001) Reduced hippocampal volume in association with p50 nonsuppression following traumatic brain injury. *Journal of Neuropsychiatry and Clinical Neuroscience* **13**, 213–221.

Arfanakis, K., Haughton, V.M. et al. (2002) Diffusion tensor MR imaging in diffuse axonal injury. *American Journal of Neuroradiology* **23**, 794–802.

Ariza, M., Mataro, M. et al. (2004) Influence of extraneurological insults on ventricular enlargement and neuropsychological functioning after moderate and severe traumatic brain injury. *Journal of Neurotrauma* **21**, 864–876.

Armstrong, K.K., Sahgal, V. et al. (1990) Rehabilitation outcomes in patients with posttraumatic epilepsy. *Archives of Physical Medicine and Rehabilitation* **71**, 156–160.

Ashikaga, R., Araki, Y. et al. (1997) MRI of head injury using FLAIR. *Neuroradiology* **39**, 239–242.

Asikainen, I., Kaste, M. et al. (1998) Predicting late outcome for patients with traumatic brain injury referred to a rehabilitation programme: a study of 508 Finnish patients 5 years or more after injury. *Brain Injury* **12**, 95–107.

Azouvi, P. (2000) Neuroimaging correlates of cognitive and functional outcome after traumatic brain injury. *Current Opinion in Neurology* **13**, 665–669.

Bach, L.J., Happe, F., Fleminger, S. & Powell, J. (2000) Theory of mind: independence of executive function and the role of the frontal cortex in acquired brain injury. *Cognitive Neuropsychiatry* **5**, 175–192.

Baddeley, A.D., Kopelman, M.D. et al. (2002) *Handbook of Memory Disorders*. John Wiley & Sons, Chichester.

Baguley, I.J., Cooper, J. et al. (2006) Aggressive behavior following traumatic brain injury: how common is common? *Journal of Head Trauma Rehabilitation* **21**, 45–56.

Bailes, J.E. & Cantu, R.C. (2001) Head injury in athletes. *Neurosurgery* **48**, 26–45; discussion 45–46.

Balestreri, M., Czosnyka, M. et al. (2004) Predictive value of Glasgow Coma Scale after brain trauma: change in trend over the past ten years. *Journal of Neurology, Neurosurgery and Psychiatry* **75**, 161–162.

Balla, J. & Iansek, R. (1988) Headache arising from disorders of the cervical spine. In: Hopkins, A. (ed.) *Headache: Problems in Diagnosis and Management*, ch. 10. Saunders, London.

Bamdad, M.J., Ryan, L.M. et al. (2003) Functional assessment of executive abilities following traumatic brain injury. *Brain Injury* **17**, 1011–1020.

Barker, L.H., Bigler, E.D. et al. (1999) Polysubstance abuse and traumatic brain injury: quantitative magnetic resonance imaging and neuropsychological outcome in older adolescents and young adults. *Journal of the International Neuropsychological Society* **5**, 593–608.

Barry, E., Krumholz, A. *et al.* (1998) Nonepileptic posttraumatic seizures. *Epilepsia* **39**, 427–431.

Barth, J.T., Alves, W.M. *et al.* (1989) Mild head injury in sports: neuropsychological sequelae and recovery of function. In: Levin, H.S., Eisenberg, H.M. & Benton, A.L. (eds) *Mild Head Injury*, ch. 17. Oxford University Press, Oxford.

Batchelor, J. & McGuiness, A. (2002) A meta-analysis of GCS 15 head injured patients with loss of consciousness or post-traumatic amnesia. *Emergency Medicine Journal* **19**, 515–519.

Bates, D. (2005) The vegetative state and the Royal College of Physicians guidance. *Neuropsychological Rehabilitation* **15**, 175–183.

Bawden, M.T., Levine, S.C. *et al.* (1985) Speeded performance following head injury in children. *Journal of Clinical and Experimental Psychology* **7**, 39–54.

Bazarian, J.J., Wong, T. *et al.* (1999) Epidemiology and predictors of post-concussive syndrome after minor head injury in an emergency population. *Brain Injury* **13**, 173–189.

Beers, S.R., Skold, A. *et al.* (2005) Neurobehavioral effects of amantadine after pediatric traumatic brain injury: a preliminary report. *Journal of Head Trauma Rehabilitation* **20**, 450–463.

Beetar, J.T., Guilmette, T.J. *et al.* (1996) Sleep and pain complaints in symptomatic traumatic brain injury and neurologic populations. *Archives of Physical Medicine and Rehabilitation* **77**, 1298–1302.

Belanger, H.G. & Vanderploeg, R.D. (2005) The neuropsychological impact of sports-related concussion: a meta-analysis. *Journal of the International Neuropsychological Society* **11**, 345–357.

Belanger, H.G., Curtiss, G. *et al.* (2005) Factors moderating neuropsychological outcomes following mild traumatic brain injury: a meta-analysis. *Journal of the International Neuropsychological Society* **11**, 215–227.

Bell, D.S. (1992) *Medico-legal Assessment of Head Injury*. Charles C. Thomas, Springfield, IL.

Bennett, P.C., Ong, B. *et al.* (2005) Assessment of executive dysfunction following traumatic brain injury: comparison of the BADS with other clinical neuropsychological measures. *Journal of the International Neuropsychological Society* **11**, 606–613.

Ben-Yishay, Y., Rattok, J. *et al.* (1985) Neuropsychological rehabilitation: quest for a holistic approach. *Seminars in Neurology* **5**, 252–258.

Bergsneider, M., Hovda, D.A. *et al.* (1997) Cerebral hyperglycolysis following severe traumatic brain injury in humans: a positron emission tomography study. *Journal of Neurosurgery* **86**, 241–251.

Bergsneider, M., Hovda, D.A. *et al.* (2000) Dissociation of cerebral glucose metabolism and level of consciousness during the period of metabolic depression following human traumatic brain injury. *Journal of Neurotrauma* **17**, 389–401.

Bergsneider, M., Hovda, D.A. *et al.* (2001) Metabolic recovery following human traumatic brain injury based on FDG-PET: time course and relationship to neurological disability. *Journal of Head Trauma Rehabilitation* **16**, 135–148.

Berman, J.M. & Fredrickson, J.M. (1978) Vertigo after head injury: a five year follow-up. *Journal of Otolaryngology* **7**, 237–245.

Bernstein, D.M. (2002) Information processing difficulty long after self-reported concussion. *Journal of the International Neuropsychological Society* **8**, 673–682.

Berthier, M.L., Kulisevsky, J.J. *et al.* (2001) Obsessive compulsive disorder and traumatic brain injury: behavioral, cognitive, and neuroimaging findings. *Neuropsychiatry, Neuropsychology and Behavioral Neurology* **14**, 23–31.

Bicik, I., Radanov, B.P. *et al.* (1998) PET with 18fluorodeoxyglucose and hexamethylpropylene amine oxime SPECT in late whiplash syndrome. *Neurology* **51**, 345–350.

Bickford, R.G. & Klass, D.W. (1966) Acute and chronic EEG findings after head injury. In: Caveness, W.F. & Walker, A.E. (eds) *Head Injury: Conference Proceedings*, ch. 6. Lippincott, Philadelphia.

Bigler, E.D. (2001) Neuropsychological testing defines the neurobehavioural significance of neuroimaging-identified abnormalities. *Archives of Clinical Neuropsychology* **16**, 227–236.

Bigler, E.D., Blatter, D.D. *et al.* (1996) Traumatic brain injury, alcohol and quantitative neuroimaging: preliminary findings. *Brain Injury* **10**, 197–206.

Bigler, E.D., Blatter, D.D. *et al.* (1997) Hippocampal volume in normal aging and traumatic brain injury. *American Journal of Neuroradiology* **18**, 11–23.

Bigler, E.D., Johnson, S.C. *et al.* (1999) Head trauma and intellectual status: relation to quantitative magnetic resonance imaging findings. *Applied Neuropsychology* **6**, 217–225.

Bigler, E.D., Anderson, C.V. *et al.* (2002) Temporal lobe morphology in normal aging and traumatic brain injury. *American Journal of Neuroradiology* **23**, 255–266.

Bijur, P., Golding, J. *et al.* (1988) Behavioral predictors of injury in school-age children. *American Journal of Diseases of Children* **142**, 1307–1312.

Bijur, P.E., Haslum, M. *et al.* (1996) Cognitive outcomes of multiple mild head injuries in children. *Journal of Developmental and Behavioral Pediatrics* **17**, 143–148.

Bilgic, B., Baral-Kulaksizoglu, I. *et al.* (2004) Obsessive-compulsive disorder secondary to bilateral frontal damage due to a closed head injury. *Cognitive and Behavioral Neurology* **17**, 118–120.

Binder, L.M. & Rohling, M.L. (1996) Money matters: a meta-analytic review of the effects of financial incentives on recovery after closed-head injury. *American Journal of Psychiatry* **153**, 7–10.

Binder, L.M., Rohling, M.L. *et al.* (1997) A review of mild head trauma. Part I: meta-analytic review of neuropsychological studies. *Journal of Clinical and Experimental Neuropsychology* **19**, 421–431.

Bishara, S.N., Partridge, F.M. *et al.* (1992) Post-traumatic amnesia and Glasgow Coma Scale related to outcome in survivors in a consecutive series of patients with severe closed-head injury. *Brain Injury* **6**, 373–380.

Black, P., Jeffries, J.J. *et al.* (1969) The post-traumatic syndrome in children. In: Walker, A.E., Caveness, W.F. & Critchley, M. (eds) *The Late Effects of Head Injury*, ch. 14. Charles C. Thomas, Springfield, IL.

Blackman, J.A., Rice, S.A. *et al.* (2003) Brain imaging as a predictor of early functional outcome following traumatic brain injury in children, adolescents, and young adults. *Journal of Head Trauma Rehabilitation* **18**, 493–503.

Blair, R.J. & Cipolotti, L. (2000) Impaired social response reversal. A case of 'acquired sociopathy'. *Brain* **123**, 1122–1141.

Blatter, D.D., Bigler, E.D. *et al.* (1997) MR-based brain and cerebrospinal fluid measurement after traumatic brain injury: correlation with neuropsychological outcome. *American Journal of Neuroradiology* **18**, 1–10.

Bloom, D.R., Levin, H.S. *et al.* (2001) Lifetime and novel psychiatric disorders after pediatric traumatic brain injury. *Journal of the American Academy of Child and Adolescent Psychiatry* **40**, 572–579.

Bloomquist, E.R. & Courville, C.B. (1947) The nature and incidence of traumatic lesions of the brain: a survey of 350 cases with autopsy. *Bulletin of the Los Angeles Neurological Society* **12**, 174–183.

Blount, P.J., Nguyen, C.D. *et al.* (2002) Clinical use of cholinomimetic agents: a review. *Journal of Head Trauma Rehabilitation* **17**, 314–321.

Blumbergs, P.C., Scott, G. *et al.* (1994) Staining of amyloid precursor protein to study axonal damage in mild head injury. *Lancet* **344**, 1055–1056.

Blumer, D. & Benson, D.F. (1978) Personality changes with frontal and temporal lobe lesions. In: Benson, D.F. & Blumer, D. (eds) *Psychiatric Aspects of Neurologic Disease*, pp. 151–170. Grune & Stratton, New York.

Boake, C., McCauley, S.R. *et al.* (2005) Diagnostic criteria for postconcussional syndrome after mild to moderate traumatic brain injury. *Journal of Neuropsychiatry and Clinical Neuroscience* **17**, 350–356.

Boden, B.P., Tacchetti, R. *et al.* (2003) Catastrophic cheerleading injuries. *American Journal of Sports Medicine* **31**, 881–888.

Bogner, J.A., Corrigan, J.D. *et al.* (2001) A comparison of substance abuse and violence in the prediction of long-term rehabilitation outcomes after traumatic brain injury. *Archives of Physical Medicine and Rehabilitation* **82**, 571–577.

Bohnen, N., Jolles, J. *et al.* (1992) Neuropsychological deficits in patients with persistent symptoms six months after mild head injury. *Neurosurgery* **30**, 692–695; discussion 695–696.

Bohnen, N., Jolles, J. *et al.* (1993) Persistent neuropsychological deficits in cervical whiplash patients without direct headstrike. *Acta Neurologica Belgica* **93**, 23–31.

Bombardier, C.H., Temkin, N.R. *et al.* (2003) The natural history of drinking and alcohol-related problems after traumatic brain injury. *Archives of Physical Medicine and Rehabilitation* **84**, 185–191.

Bond, M.R. (1976) Assessment of the psychosocial outcome of severe head injury. *Acta Neurochirurgica* **34**, 57–70.

Bond, M.R. & Brooks, D.N. (1976) Understanding the process of recovery as a basis for the investigation of rehabilitation for the brain injured. *Scandinavian Journal of Rehabilitation Medicine* **8**, 127–133.

Bonne, O., Gilboa, A. *et al.* (2003) Cerebral blood flow in chronic symptomatic mild traumatic brain injury. *Psychiatry Research* **124**, 141–152.

Borg, J., Holm, L. *et al.* (2004) Diagnostic procedures in mild traumatic brain injury: results of the WHO Collaborating Centre Task Force on Mild Traumatic Brain Injury. *Journal of Rehabilitation Medicine* **43** (suppl.), 61–75.

Borgaro, S., Caples, H. *et al.* (2003) Non-pharmacological management of psychiatric disturbances after traumatic brain injury. *International Review of Psychiatry* **15**, 371–379.

Bouma, G.J., Muizelaar, J.P. *et al.* (1991) Cerebral circulation and metabolism after severe traumatic brain injury: the elusive role of ischemia. *Journal of Neurosurgery* **75**, 685–693.

Bowen, A., Chamberlain, M.A. *et al.* (1999) The persistence of mood disorders following traumatic brain injury: a 1 year follow-up. *Brain Injury* **13**, 547–553.

Bracken, P. (1987) Mania following head injury. *British Journal of Psychiatry* **150**, 690–692.

Brain, W.R. (1942) Discussion on rehabilitation after injuries to the central nervous system. *Proceedings of the Royal Society of Medicine* **35**, 302–305.

Brenner, C., Riedman, A.P. *et al.* (1944) Post-traumatic headache. *Journal of Neurosurgery* **1**, 379–391.

Brooke, M.M., Questad, K.A. *et al.* (1992) Agitation and restlessness after closed head injury: a prospective study of 100 consecutive admissions. *Archives of Physical Medicine and Rehabilitation* **73**, 320–323.

Brooks, D.N. (1976) Wechsler Memory Scale performance and its relationship to brain damage after severe closed head injury. *Journal of Neurology, Neurosurgery and Psychiatry* **39**, 593–601.

Brooks, D.N. & McKinlay, W. (1983) Personality and behavioural change after severe blunt head injury: a relative's view. *Journal of Neurology, Neurosurgery and Psychiatry* **46**, 336–344.

Brooks, D.N., Campsie, L. *et al.* (1987) The effects of severe head injury on patient and relative within seven years of injury. *Brain Injury* **2**, 1–13.

Brooks, N., Campsie, I.. *et al.* (1986) The five year outcome of severe blunt head injury: a relative's view. *Journal of Neurology, Neurosurgery and Psychiatry* **49**, 764–770.

Brooks, N., McKinlay, W., Beattie, A. & Campsie, L. (1987a) Return to work within the first seven years of severe head injury. *Brain Injury* **1**, 5–19.

Brooks, N., Kupshik, G., Wilson, L., Galbraith, S. & Ward, R. (1987b) A neuropsychological study of active amateur boxers. *Journal of Neurology, Neurosurgery, and Psychiatry* **50**, 997–1000.

Brooks, N., Symington, C., Beattie, A. *et al.* (1989) Alcohol and other predictors of cognitive recovery after severe head injury. *Brain Injury* **3**, 235–246.

Brooks, W.M., Stidley, C.A. *et al.* (2000) Metabolic and cognitive response to human traumatic brain injury: a quantitative proton magnetic resonance study. *Journal of Neurotrauma* **17**, 629–640.

Brown, G., Chadwick, D. *et al.* (1981) A prospective study of children with head injuries. III. Psychiatric sequelae. *Psychological Medicine* **11**, 63–78.

Bruns, T.J. & Hauser, W.A. (2003) The epidemiology of traumatic brain injury: a review. *Epilepsia* **44** (suppl. 10), 2–10.

Bryant, R.A. & Harvey, A.G. (1999) Postconcussive symptoms and posttraumatic stress disorder after mild traumatic brain injury. *Journal of Nervous and Mental Disease* **187**, 302–305.

Bryant, R.A., Marosszeky, J.E. *et al.* (2001) Posttraumatic stress disorder and psychosocial functioning after severe traumatic brain injury. *Journal of Nervous and Mental Disease* **189**, 109–113.

Bryant, R.A., Moulds, M. *et al.* (2003) Treating acute stress disorder following mild traumatic brain injury. *American Journal of Psychiatry* **160**, 585–587.

Burgess, P.W. & Wood, R.L. (1990) Neuropsychology of behaviour disorders following brain injury. In: Wood, R.L. (ed.) *Neurobehavioural Sequelae of Traumatic Brain Injury*, pp. 110–113. Taylor and Francis, New York.

Burgess, P.W., Alderman, N. *et al.* (1998) The ecological validity of tests of executive function. *Journal of the International Neuropsychological Society* **4**, 547–558.

Burke, W.H., Wesolowski, M.D. *et al.* (1988) Comprehensive head injury rehabilitation: an outcome evaluation. *Brain Injury* **2**, 313–322.

Bushnik, T., Hanks, R.A. *et al.* (2003) Etiology of traumatic brain injury: characterization of differential outcomes up to 1 year postinjury. *Archives of Physical Medicine and Rehabilitation* **84**, 255–262.

Butler, P.V. (2000) Diurnal variation in Cotard's syndrome (copresent with Capgras delusion) following traumatic brain injury. *Australian and New Zealand Journal of Psychiatry* **34**, 684–687.

Callahan, C.D. & Hinkebein, J. (1999) Neuropsychological significance of anosmia following traumatic brain injury. *Journal of Head Trauma Rehabilitation* **14**, 581–587.

Cardenas, D.D., McLean, A. Jr *et al.* (1994) Oral physostigmine and impaired memory in adults with brain injury. *Brain Injury* **8**, 579–587.

Cardoso, E.R. & Galbraith, S. (1985) Posttraumatic hydrocephalus: a retrospective review. *Surgical Neurology* **23**, 261–264.

Carney, N., Chesnut, R.M. *et al.* (1999) Effect of cognitive rehabilitation on outcomes for persons with traumatic brain injury: a systematic review. *Journal of Head Trauma Rehabilitation* **14**, 277–307.

Carroll, L.J., Cassidy, J.D. *et al.* (2004a) Methodological issues and research recommendations for mild traumatic brain injury: the WHO Collaborating Centre Task Force on Mild Traumatic Brain Injury. *Journal of Rehabilitation Medicine* **43** (suppl.), 113–125.

Carroll, L.J., Cassidy, J.D. *et al.* (2004b) Prognosis for mild traumatic brain injury: results of the WHO Collaborating Centre Task Force on Mild Traumatic Brain Injury. *Journal of Rehabilitation Medicine* **43** (suppl.), 84–105.

Cassidy, J.D., Carroll, L.J. *et al.* (2000) Effect of eliminating compensation for pain and suffering on the outcome of insurance claims for whiplash injury. *New England Journal of Medicine* **342**, 1179–1186.

Cassidy, J.D., Carroll, L. *et al.* (2004) Mild traumatic brain injury after traffic collisions: a population-based inception cohort study. *Journal of Rehabilitation Medicine* **43** (suppl.), 15–21.

Casson, I.R., Siegel, O. *et al.* (1984) Brain damage in modern boxers. *Journal of the American Medical Association* **251**, 2663–2667.

Caveness, W.F. & Walker, A.E. (1966) Appendix: head injury glossary. In: Caveness, W.F. & Walker, A.E. (eds) *Head Injury: Conference Proceedings*. Lippincott, Philadelphia.

Cecil, K.M., Hills, E.C. *et al.* (1998) Proton magnetic resonance spectroscopy for detection of axonal injury in the splenium of the corpus callosum of brain-injured patients. *Journal of Neurosurgery* **88**, 795–801.

Chadwick, O., Rutter, M. *et al.* (1981) A prospective study of children with head injuries. II. Cognitive sequelae. *Psychological Medicine* **11**, 49–61.

Chamelian, L. & Feinstein, A. (2004) Outcome after mild to moderate traumatic brain injury: the role of dizziness. *Archives of Physical Medicine and Rehabilitation* **85**, 1662–1666.

Chamelian, L. & Feinstein, A. (2006) The effect of major depression on subjective and objective cognitive deficits in mild to moderate traumatic brain injury. *Journal of Neuropsychiatry and Clinical Neuroscience* **18**, 33–38.

Chamelian, L., Reis, M. *et al.* (2004) Six-month recovery from mild to moderate traumatic brain injury: the role of APOE-epsilon4 allele. *Brain* **127**, 2621–2628.

Chan, R.C. (2001) Base rate of post-concussion symptoms among normal people and its neuropsychological correlates. *Clinical Rehabilitation* **15**, 266–273.

Chan, R.C., Hoosain, R. *et al.* (2003) Are there sub-types of attentional deficits in patients with persisting post-concussive symptoms? A cluster analytical study. *Brain Injury* **17**, 131–148.

Chatham-Showalter, P.E., Dubov, W.E. *et al.* (1996) Alcohol level at head injury and subsequent psychotropic treatment during trauma critical care. *Psychosomatics* **37**, 285–288.

Chen, S.H., Kareken, D.A. *et al.* (2003) A study of persistent post-concussion symptoms in mild head trauma using positron emission tomography. *Journal of Neurology, Neurosurgery and Psychiatry* **74**, 326–332.

Chiang, M.F., Chang, J.G. *et al.* (2003) Association between apolipoprotein E genotype and outcome of traumatic brain injury. *Acta Neurochirurgica (Wien)* **145**, 649–653; discussion 653–654.

Chiaretti, A., Piastra, M. *et al.* (2003) Correlation between neurotrophic factor expression and outcome of children with severe traumatic brain injury. *Intensive Care Medicine* **29**, 1329–1338.

Chirumamilla, S., Sun, D. *et al.* (2002) Traumatic brain injury induced cell proliferation in the adult mammalian central nervous system. *Journal of Neurotrauma* **19**, 693–703.

Christodoulou, C., DeLuca, J. *et al.* (2001) Functional magnetic resonance imaging of working memory impairment after traumatic brain injury. *Journal of Neurology, Neurosurgery and Psychiatry* **71**, 161–168.

Cicerone, K.D. & Azulay, J. (2002) Diagnostic utility of attention measures in postconcussion syndrome. *Clinical Neuropsychologist* **16**, 280–289.

Cicerone, K.D. & Kalmar, K. (1997) Does premorbid depression influence post-concussive symptoms and neuropsychological functioning? *Brain Injury* **11**, 643–648.

Cicerone, K.D. & Tanenbaum, L.N. (1997) Disturbance of social cognition after traumatic orbitofrontal brain injury. *Archives of Clinical Neuropsychology* **12**, 173–188.

Cicerone, K.D., Dahlberg, C. *et al.* (2000) Evidence-based cognitive rehabilitation: recommendations for clinical practice. *Archives of Physical Medicine and Rehabilitation* **81**, 1596–1615.

Clark, A.F. & Davison, K. (1987) Mania following head injury: a report of two cases and a review of the literature. *British Journal of Psychiatry* **150**, 841–844.

Clausen, H., McCrory, P. *et al.* (2005) The risk of chronic traumatic brain injury in professional boxing: change in exposure variables over the past century. *British Journal of Sports Medicine* **39**, 661–664; discussion 664.

Cole, E.S. (1970) Psychiatric aspects of compensable injury. *Medical Journal of Australia* **1**, 93–100.

Collie, A., Makdissi, M. *et al.* (2006) Cognition in the days following concussion: comparison of symptomatic versus asymptomatic athletes. *Journal of Neurology, Neurosurgery and Psychiatry* **77**, 241–245.

Collins, M.W., Grindel, S.H. *et al.* (1999) Relationship between concussion and neuropsychological performance in college football players. *Journal of the American Medical Association* **282**, 964–970.

Collins, M.W., Iverson, G.L. et al. (2003) On-field predictors of neuropsychological and symptom deficit following sports-related concussion. *Clinical Journal of Sport Medicine* **13**, 222–229.

Coonley-Hoganson, R., Sachs, N. et al. (1984) Sequelae associated with head injuries in patients who were not hospitalized: a follow-up survey. *Neurosurgery* **14**, 315–317.

Cope, D.N. & Hall, K. (1982) Head injury rehabilitation: benefit of early intervention. *Archives of Physical Medicine and Rehabilitation* **63**, 433–437.

Corkin, S., Rosen, J. et al. (1989) Penetrating head injury in young adulthood exacerbates cognitive decline in later years. *Journal of Neuroscience* **9**, 3876–3883.

Corrigan, J.D., Mysiw, W.J. et al. (1992) Agitation, cognition and attention during post-traumatic amnesia. *Brain Injury* **6**, 155–160.

Corrigan, J.D., Rust, E. et al. (1995) The nature and extent of substance abuse problems in persons with traumatic brain injury. *Journal of Head Trauma Rehabilitation* **10**, 29–46.

Corrigan, J.D., Smith-Knapp, K. et al. (1998) Outcomes in the first 5 years after traumatic brain injury. *Archives of Physical Medicine and Rehabilitation* **79**, 298–305.

Corrigan, J.D., Harrison-Felix, C. et al. (2003) Systematic bias in traumatic brain injury outcome studies because of loss to follow-up. *Archives of Physical Medicine and Rehabilitation* **84**, 153–160.

Corsellis, J.A.N. (1989) Boxing and the brain. *British Medical Journal* **298**, 105–109.

Corsellis, J.A.N., Bruton, C.J. & Freeman-Browne, D. (1973) The aftermath of boxing. *Psychological Medicine* **3**, 270–303.

Cote, P., Cassidy, J.D. et al. (2001a) A systematic review of the prognosis of acute whiplash and a new conceptual framework to synthesize the literature. *Spine* **26**, E445–E458.

Cote, P., Hogg-Johnson, S. et al. (2001b) The association between neck pain intensity, physical functioning, depressive symptomatology and time-to-claim-closure after whiplash. *Journal of Clinical Epidemiology* **54**, 275–286.

Courville, C.B. (1937) *Pathology of the Central Nervous System*, Part IV. Pacific Press, Mountain View, CA.

Crawford, F.C., Vanderploeg, R.D. et al. (2002) APOE genotype influences acquisition and recall following traumatic brain injury. *Neurology* **58**, 1115–1118.

Creamer, M., O'Donnell, M.L. et al. (2005) Amnesia, traumatic brain injury, and posttraumatic stress disorder: a methodological inquiry. *Behaviour Research and Therapy* **43**, 1383–1389.

Culotta, V.P., Sementilli, M.E. et al. (1996) Clinicopathological heterogeneity in the classification of mild head injury. *Neurosurgery* **38**, 245–250.

Cunningham, R.M., Maio, R.F. et al. (2002) The effects of alcohol on head injury in the motor vehicle crash victim. *Alcohol and Alcoholism* **37**, 236–240.

Curran, C.A., Ponsford, J.L. et al. (2000) Coping strategies and emotional outcome following traumatic brain injury: a comparison with orthopedic patients. *Journal of Head Trauma Rehabilitation* **15**, 1256–1274.

Dalfen, A.K. & Anthony, F. (2000) Head injury, dissociation and the Ganser syndrome. *Brain Injury* **14**, 1101–1105.

Damasio, A.R. (1996) The somatic marker hypothesis and the possible functions of the prefrontal cortex. *Philosophical Transactions of the Royal Society of London B* **351**, 1413–1420.

D'Ambrosio, R. & Perucca, E. (2004) Epilepsy after head injury. *Current Opinion in Neurology* **17**, 731–735.

David, A.S. & Prince, M. (2005) Psychosis following head injury: a critical review. *Journal of Neurology, Neurosurgery and Psychiatry* **76** (suppl. 1), i53–i60.

Davison, K. & Bagley, C.R. (1969) Schizophrenia-like psychoses associated with organic disorders of the central nervous system: a review of the literature. In: Herrington, R.N. (ed.) *Current Problems in Neuropsychiatry*, pp. 113–184. Headley Brothers, Ashford, Kent.

Deb, S., Lyons, I. et al. (1998) Neuropsychiatric sequelae one year after a minor head injury. *Journal of Neurology, Neurosurgery and Psychiatry* **65**, 899–902.

Deb, S., Lyons, I. et al. (1999a) Neurobehavioural symptoms one year after a head injury. *British Journal of Psychiatry* **174**, 360–365.

Deb, S., Lyons, I. et al. (1999b) Rate of psychiatric illness 1 year after traumatic brain injury. *American Journal of Psychiatry* **156**, 374–378.

De Boussard, C.N., Lundin, A. et al. (2005) S100 and cognitive impairment after mild traumatic brain injury. *Journal of Rehabilitation Medicine* **37**, 53–57.

De Kruijk, J.R., Leffers, P. et al. (2002a) Prediction of post-traumatic complaints after mild traumatic brain injury: early symptoms and biochemical markers. *Journal of Neurology, Neurosurgery and Psychiatry* **73**, 727–732.

De Kruijk, J.R., Leffers, P. et al. (2002b) Effectiveness of bed rest after mild traumatic brain injury: a randomised trial of no versus six days of bed rest. *Journal of Neurology, Neurosurgery and Psychiatry* **73**, 167–172.

Delmonico, R.L., Hanley-Peterson, P. et al. (1998) Group psychotherapy for persons with traumatic brain injury: management of frustration and substance abuse. *Journal of Head Trauma Rehabilitation* **13**, 10–22.

Demellweek, C., Baldwin, T. et al. (2002) A prospective study and review of pre-morbid characteristics in children with traumatic brain injury. *Pediatric Rehabilitation* **5**, 81–89.

De Mol, J., Violon, A. et al. (1987) Post-traumatic psychoses: a retrospective study of 18 cases. *Archivio di Psicologia, Neurologia e Psichiatria* **48**, 336–350.

Dencker, S.J. (1958) A follow-up study of 128 closed head injuries in twins using co-twins as controls. *Acta Psychiatrica et Neurologica Scandinavica Supplementum* **123**, 1–125.

Dencker, S.J. (1960) Closed head injury in twins. *Archives of General Psychiatry* **2**, 569–575.

Dennis, M., Purvis, K. et al. (2001) Understanding of literal truth, ironic criticism, and deceptive praise following childhood head injury. *Brain and Language* **78**, 1–16.

Diaz-Arrastia, R., Gong, Y. et al. (2003) Increased risk of late post-traumatic seizures associated with inheritance of APOE epsilon4 allele. *Archives of Neurology* **60**, 818–822.

Dikmen, S.S., Machamer, J.E. et al. (2000) Neuropsychological effects of valproate in traumatic brain injury: a randomized trial. *Neurology* **54**, 895–902.

Dikmen, S.S., Bombardier, C.H. et al. (2004) Natural history of depression in traumatic brain injury. *Archives of Physical Medicine and Rehabilitation* **85**, 1457–1464.

Dimopoulou, I., Korfias, S. et al. (2003) Protein S-100b serum levels in trauma-induced brain death. *Neurology* **60**, 947–951.

Dinan, T.G. & Mobayed, M. (1992) Treatment resistance of depression after head injury: a preliminary study of amitriptyline response. *Acta Psychiatrica Scandinavica* **85**, 292–294.

Di Renzi, E., Lucchelli, F. *et al.* (1997) Is memory loss without anatomical damage tantamount to a psychogenic deficit? The case of pure retrograde amnesia. *Neuropsychologia* **35**, 781–794.

Di Stefano, G., Bachevalier, J. *et al.* (2000) Volume of focal brain lesions and hippocampal formation in relation to memory function after closed head injury in children. *Journal of Neurology, Neurosurgery and Psychiatry* **69**, 210–216.

Dolberg, O.T., Klag, E. *et al.* (2002) Relief of serotonin selective reuptake inhibitor induced sexual dysfunction with low-dose mianserin in patients with traumatic brain injury. *Psychopharmacology* **161**, 404–407.

Donders, J. & Strom, D. (2000) Neurobehavioral recovery after pediatric head trauma: injury, pre-injury, and post-injury issues. *Journal of Head Trauma Rehabilitation* **15**, 792–803.

Donnemiller, E., Brenneis, C. *et al.* (2000) Impaired dopaminergic neurotransmission in patients with traumatic brain injury: a SPECT study using 123I-beta-CIT and 123I-IBZM. *European Journal of Nuclear Medicine* **27**, 1410–1414.

Drew, R.H., Templer, D.I. *et al.* (1986) Neuropsychological deficits in active licensed professional boxers. *Journal of Clinical Psychology* **42**, 520–525.

Duma, S.M., Manoogian, S.J. *et al.* (2005) Analysis of real-time head accelerations in collegiate football players. *Clinical Journal of Sport Medicine* **15**, 3–8.

Dunlop, T.W., Udvarhelyi, G.B. *et al.* (1991) Comparison of patients with and without emotional/behavioral deterioration during the first year after traumatic brain injury. *Journal of Neuropsychiatry and Clinical Neuroscience* **3**, 150–156.

Eames, P. (1992) Hysteria following brain injury. *Journal of Neurology, Neurosurgery and Psychiatry* **55**, 1046–1053.

Eames, P. (2001) Distinguishing neuropsychiatric, psychiatric and psychological consequences of acquired brain injury. In: Wood, R.L. & McMillan, T. (eds) *Neurobehavioural Disability and Social Handicap Following Traumatic Brain Injury*, pp. 29–45. Psychology Press, Hove.

Eames, P. & Sutton, A. (1995) Protracted post-traumatic confusional state treated with physostigmine. *Brain Injury* **9**, 729–734.

Eames, P. & Wood, R. (1985) Rehabilitation after severe brain injury: a follow-up study of a behaviour modification approach. *Journal of Neurology, Neurosurgery and Psychiatry* **48**, 613–619.

Eames, P. & Wood, R.L. (2003) Episodic disorders of behaviour and affect after acquired brain injury. *Neuropsychological Rehabilitation* **13**, 241–258.

Edlund, M.J., Goldberg, R.J. *et al.* (1991) The use of physical restraint in patients with cerebral contusion. *International Journal of Psychiatry in Medicine* **21**, 173–182.

Edwards, P., Arango, M. *et al.* (2005) Final results of MRC CRASH, a randomised placebo-controlled trial of intravenous corticosteroid in adults with head injury-outcomes at 6 months. *Lancet* **365**, 1957–1959.

Eisenberg, H.M. & Levin, H.S. (1989) Computed tomography and magnetic resonance imaging in mild to moderate head injury. In: Levin, H.S., Eisenberg, H.M. & Benton, A.L. (eds) *Mild Head Injury*, ch. 8. Oxford University Press, Oxford.

Ellenberg, J.H., Levin, H.S. *et al.* (1996) Posttraumatic amnesia as a predictor of outcome after severe closed head injury. Prospective assessment. *Archives of Neurology* **53**, 782–791.

Emanuelson, I., von Wendt, L. *et al.* (1998) Late outcome after severe traumatic brain injury in children and adolescents. *Pediatric Rehabilitation* **2**, 65–70.

Emory, L.E., Cole, C.M. *et al.* (1995) Use of Depo-Provera to control sexual aggression in persons with traumatic brain injury. *Journal of Head Trauma Rehabilitation* **10**, 47–58.

Ergh, T.C., Rapport, L.J. *et al.* (2002) Predictors of caregiver and family functioning following traumatic brain injury: social support moderates caregiver distress. *Journal of Head Trauma Rehabilitation* **17**, 155–174.

Erlanger, D., Kaushik, T. *et al.* (2003) Symptom-based assessment of the severity of a concussion. *Journal of Neurosurgery* **98**, 477–484.

Evans, J.J. & Levine, B. (2002) Mood disorders: issues of prevalence, misdiagnosis, assessment and treatment. *Neuropsychological Rehabilitation* **12**, 167–174.

Ewert, J., Levin, H.S. *et al.* (1989) Procedural memory during posttraumatic amnesia in survivors of severe closed head injury. Implications for rehabilitation. *Archives of Neurology* **46**, 911–916.

Ewing, R., McCarthy, D. *et al.* (1980) Persisting effects of minor head injury observable during hypoxic stress. *Journal of Clinical Neuropsychology* **2**, 147–155.

Ewing-Cobbs, L., Fletcher, J.M. *et al.* (1998) Academic achievement and academic placement following traumatic brain injury in children and adolescents: a two-year longitudinal study. *Journal of Clinical and Experimental Neuropsychology* **20**, 769–781.

Ewing-Cobbs, L., Barnes, M. *et al.* (2004) Modeling of longitudinal academic achievement scores after pediatric traumatic brain injury. *Developmental Neuropsychology* **25**, 107–133.

Fabbri, A., Servadei, F. *et al.* (2004) Prospective validation of a proposal for diagnosis and management of patients attending the emergency department for mild head injury. *Journal of Neurology, Neurosurgery and Psychiatry* **75**, 410–416.

Faden, A.I., Demediuk, P. *et al.* (1989) The role of excitatory aminoacids and NMDA receptors in traumatic brain injury. *Science* **244**, 798–800.

Fahy, T.J., Irving, M.H. *et al.* (1967) Severe head injuries: a six-year follow-up. *Lancet* **ii**, 475–479.

Fann, J.R., Katon, W.J. *et al.* (1995) Psychiatric disorders and functional disability in outpatients with traumatic brain injuries. *American Journal of Psychiatry* **152**, 1493–1499.

Fann, J.R., Uomoto, J.M. *et al.* (2000) Sertraline in the treatment of major depression following mild traumatic brain injury. *Journal of Neuropsychiatry and Clinical Neuroscience* **12**, 226–232.

Fann, J.R., Uomoto, J.M. *et al.* (2001) Cognitive improvement with treatment of depression following mild traumatic brain injury. *Psychosomatics* **42**, 48–54.

Fann, J.R., Leonetti, A. *et al.* (2002) Psychiatric illness and subsequent traumatic brain injury: a case control study. *Journal of Neurology, Neurosurgery and Psychiatry* **72**, 615–620.

Fann, J.R., Burington, B. *et al.* (2004) Psychiatric illness following traumatic brain injury in an adult health maintenance organization population. *Archives of General Psychiatry* **61**, 53–61.

Faust, C. (1955) Zur Symptomatik frischer und alter Stirnhirnverletzungen. *Archiv für Psychiatrie und Nervenkrankheiten* **193**, 78–97.

Faust, C. (1960) Die psychischen Störungen nach Hirntraumen: Akute traumatische Psychosen und psychische Spätfolgen nach

Hirnverletzungen. In: Gruhle, H.W., Jung, R., Mayer-Gross, W. & Miller, M. (eds) *Psychiatrie Der Gegenwart: Forschung Und Praxis*, vol. 2, pp. 552–645. Springer-Verlag, Berlin.

Feinstein, A., Ouchterlony, D. *et al.* (2001) The effects of litigation on symptom expression: a prospective study following mild traumatic brain injury. *Medicine, Science and the Law* **41**, 116–121.

Feinstein, A., Hershkop, S. *et al.* (2002) Posttraumatic amnesia and recall of a traumatic event following traumatic brain injury. *Journal of Neuropsychiatry and Clinical Neuroscience* **14**, 25–30.

Fenton, G., McClelland, R. *et al.* (1993) The postconcussional syndrome: social antecedents and psychological sequelae. *British Journal of Psychiatry* **162**, 493–497.

Ferguson, R.J., Mittenberg, W. *et al.* (1999) Postconcussion syndrome following sports-related head injury: expectation as etiology. *Neuropsychology* **13**, 582–589.

Ferguson, R.K., Soryal, I.N. *et al.* (1997) Thiamine deficiency in head injury: a missed insult? *Alcohol and Alcoholism* **32**, 493–500.

Ferrari, R. & Schrader, H. (2001) The late whiplash syndrome: a biopsychosocial approach. *Journal of Neurology, Neurosurgery and Psychiatry* **70**, 722–726.

Ferrari, R., Obelieniene, D. *et al.* (2001) Symptom expectation after minor head injury. A comparative study between Canada and Lithuania. *Clinical Neurology and Neurosurgery* **103**, 184–190.

Feuchtwanger, E. (1923) *Die Funktionen des Stirnhirns: ihre Pathologie und Psychologie*. Springer-Verlag, Berlin.

Fichtenberg, N.L., Zafonte, R.D. *et al.* (2002) Insomnia in a post-acute brain injury sample. *Brain Injury* **16**, 197–206.

Field, J.H. (1976) *Epidemiology of Head Injuries in England and Wales*. HMSO, London.

Firsching, R., Woischneck, D. *et al.* (2002) Brain stem lesions after head injury. *Neurological Research* **24**, 145–146.

Fiser, S.M., Johnson, S.B. *et al.* (1998) Resource utilization in traumatic brain injury: the role of magnetic resonance imaging. *American Surgeon* **64**, 1088–1093.

Fisher, C.M. (1982) Whiplash amnesia. *Neurology* **32**, 667–668.

Fleminger, S. & Powell, J. (1999) Editorial. *Neuropsychological Rehabilitation* **9**, 225–230.

Fleminger, S., Murphy, L. *et al.* (1996) Malignant distress on eye contact after severe head injury. *Journal of Neurology, Neurosurgery and Psychiatry* **61**, 114–115.

Fleminger, S., Oliver, D.L. *et al.* (2003a) Head injury as a risk factor for Alzheimer's disease: the evidence 10 years on. A partial replication. *Journal of Neurology, Neurosurgery and Psychiatry* **74**, 857–862.

Fleminger, S., Oliver, D.L. *et al.* (2003b) The neuropsychiatry of depression after brain injury. *Neuropsychological Rehabilitation* **13**, 65–87.

Fleminger, S., Greenwood, R.J. *et al.* (2003c) Pharmacological management for agitation and aggression in people with acquired brain injury. *Cochrane Database of Systematic Reviews* 1, CD003299.

Florian, V., Katz, S. *et al.* (1989) Impact of traumatic brain damage on family dynamics and functioning: a review. *Brain Injury* **3**, 219–233.

Fontaine, A., Azouvi, P. *et al.* (1999) Functional anatomy of neuropsychological deficits after severe traumatic brain injury. *Neurology* **53**, 1963–1968.

Fordyce, D.J., Roueche, J.R. *et al.* (1983) Enhanced emotional reactions in chronic head trauma patients. *Journal of Neurology, Neurosurgery and Psychiatry* **46**, 620–624.

Forsyth, R. & Jayamoni, B. (2003) Noradrenergic agonists for acute traumatic brain injury. *Cochrane Database of Systematic Reviews* **1**, CD003984.

Frencham, K.A., Fox, A.M. *et al.* (2005) Neuropsychological studies of mild traumatic brain injury: a meta-analytic review of research since 1995. *Journal of Clinical and Experimental Neuropsychology* **27**, 334–351.

Frey, L.C. (2003) Epidemiology of posttraumatic epilepsy: a critical review. *Epilepsia* **44**, 11–17.

Friede, R.L. (1961) Experimental concussion acceleration: pathology and mechanics. *Archives of Neurology* **4**, 449–462.

Friedland, J.F. & Dawson, D.R. (2001) Function after motor vehicle accidents: a prospective study of mild head injury and posttraumatic stress. *Journal of Nervous and Mental Disease* **189**, 426–434.

Friedman, A.P. (1969) The so-called post traumatic headache. In: Walker, A.E., Caveness, W.F. & Critchley, M. (eds) *The Late Effects of Head Injury*, ch. 5. Charles C. Thomas, Springfield, IL.

Friedman, G., Froom, P. *et al.* (1999) Apolipoprotein E-epsilon4 genotype predicts a poor outcome in survivors of traumatic brain injury. *Neurology* **52**, 244–248.

Friedman, S.D., Brooks, W.M. *et al.* (1998) Proton MR spectroscopic findings correspond to neuropsychological function in traumatic brain injury. *American Journal of Neuroradiology* **19**, 1879–1885.

Front, D., Beks, J.W. *et al.* (1972) Abnormal patterns of cerebrospinal fluid flow and absorption after head injuries; diagnosis by isotope cisternography. *Neuroradiology* **4**, 6–13.

Fu, L., Tang, Y. *et al.* (2002) Effect of nonoperative treatment on the outcome of patients with posttraumatic hydrocephalus. *Chinese Journal of Traumatology* **5**, 7–11.

Fujii, D.E. & Ahmed, I. (2001) Risk factors in psychosis secondary to traumatic brain injury. *Journal of Neuropsychiatry and Clinical Neuroscience* **13**, 61–69.

Gaetz, M. & Bernstein, D.M. (2001) The current status of electrophysiologic procedures for the assessment of mild traumatic brain injury. *Journal of Head Trauma Rehabilitation* **16**, 386–405.

Gaetz, M. & Weinberg, H. (2000) Electrophysiological indices of persistent post-concussion symptoms. *Brain Injury* **14**, 815–832.

Gale, S.D., Baxter, L. *et al.* (2005) Traumatic brain injury and grey matter concentration: a preliminary voxel based morphometry study. *Journal of Neurology, Neurosurgery and Psychiatry* **76**, 984–988.

Garnett, M.R., Blamire, A.M. *et al.* (2000) Early proton magnetic resonance spectroscopy in normal-appearing brain correlates with outcome in patients following traumatic brain injury. *Brain* **123**, 2046–2054.

Geddes, J.F., Whitwell, H.L. *et al.* (2000) Traumatic axonal injury: practical issues for diagnosis in medicolegal cases. *Neuropathology and Applied Neurobiology* **26**, 105–116.

Geddes, J.F., Vowles, G.H. *et al.* (2001) Neuropathology of inflicted head injury in children. II. Microscopic brain injury in infants. *Brain* **124**, 1299–1306.

Gerber, D.J., Weintraub, A.H. *et al.* (2004) Magnetic resonance imaging of traumatic brain injury: relationship of T2*SE and T2GE to clinical severity and outcome. *Brain Injury* **18**, 1083–1097.

Gerhart, K.A., Mellick, D.C. *et al.* (2003) Violence-related traumatic brain injury: a population-based study. *Journal of Trauma* **55**, 1045–1053.

Gerring, J.P., Brady, K.D. *et al.* (1998) Premorbid prevalence of ADHD and development of secondary ADHD after closed head injury. *Journal of the American Academy of Child and Adolescent Psychiatry* **37**, 647–654.

Geurts, A.C., Knoop, J.A. *et al.* (1999) Is postural control associated with mental functioning in the persistent postconcussion syndrome? *Archives of Physical Medicine and Rehabilitation* **80**, 144–149.

Ghigo, E., Masel, B. *et al.* (2005). Consensus guidelines on screening for hypopituitarism following traumatic brain injury. *Brain Injury* **19**, 711–724.

Giacino, J. & Whyte, J. (2005) The vegetative and minimally conscious states: current knowledge and remaining questions. *Journal of Head Trauma Rehabilitation* **20**, 30–50.

Gil, S., Caspi, Y. *et al.* (2005) Does memory of a traumatic event increase the risk for posttraumatic stress disorder in patients with traumatic brain injury? A prospective study. *American Journal of Psychiatry* **162**, 963–969.

Glaesser, J., Neuner, F. *et al.* (2004) Posttraumatic stress disorder in patients with traumatic brain injury. *BMC Psychiatry* **4**, 5.

Glenn, T.C., Kelly, D.F. *et al.* (2003) Energy dysfunction as a predictor of outcome after moderate or severe head injury: indices of oxygen, glucose, and lactate metabolism. *Journal of Cerebral Blood Flow and Metabolism* **23**, 1239–1250.

Godfrey, H.P., Partridge, F.M. *et al.* (1993) Course of insight disorder and emotional dysfunction following closed head injury: a controlled cross-sectional follow-up study. *Journal of Clinical and Experimental Neuropsychology* **15**, 503–515.

Goldberg, D., Gask, L. *et al.* (1989) The treatment of somatization: teaching techniques of reattribution. *Journal of Psychosomatic Research* **33**, 689–695.

Goldberg, E., Gerstman, L.J. *et al.* (1982) Effects of cholinergic treatment on posttraumatic anterograde amnesia. *Archives of Neurology* **39**, 581.

Gomez, P.A., Lobato, R.D. *et al.* (1996) Mild head injury: differences in prognosis among patients with a Glasgow Coma Scale score of 13 to 15 and analysis of factors associated with abnormal CT findings. *British Journal of Neurosurgery* **10**, 453–460.

Gonzalez Tortosa, J., Martinez-Lage, J.F. *et al.* (2004) Bitemporal head crush injuries: clinical and radiological features of a distinctive type of head injury. *Journal of Neurosurgery* **100**, 645–651.

Gotten, N. (1956) Survey of one hundred cases of whiplash injury after settlement of compensation. *Journal of the American Medical Association* **162**, 865–867.

Gowda, N.K., Agrawal, D. *et al.* (2006) Technetium Tc-99m ethyl cysteinate dimer brain single-photon emission CT in mild traumatic brain injury: a prospective study. *American Journal of Neuroradiology* **27**, 447–451.

Grados, M.A., Slomine, B.S. *et al.* (2001) Depth of lesion model in children and adolescents with moderate to severe traumatic brain injury: use of SPGR MRI to predict severity and outcome. *Journal of Neurology, Neurosurgery and Psychiatry* **70**, 350–358.

Grafman, J., Vance, S.C. *et al.* (1986a) The effects of lateralized frontal lesions on mood regulation. *Brain* **109**, 1127–1148.

Grafman, J., Salazar, A. *et al.* (1986b) The relationship of brain-tissue loss volume and lesion location to cognitive deficit. *Journal of Neuroscience* **6**, 301–307.

Grafman, J., Jonas, B.S. *et al.* (1988) Intellectual function following penetrating head injury in Vietnam veterans. *Brain* **111**, 169–184.

Grafman, J., Schwab, K. *et al.* (1996) Frontal lobe injuries, violence, and aggression: a report of the Vietnam Head Injury Study. *Neurology* **46**, 1231–1238.

Graham, D.I. & Adams, J.H. (1971) Ischaemic brain damage in fatal head injury. *Lancet* **i**, 265–266.

Greenwood, R. (2002) Head injury for neurologists. *Journal of Neurology, Neurosurgery and Psychiatry* **73** (suppl. 1), i8–i16.

Greenwood, R.J., McMillan, T.M. *et al.* (1994) Effects of case management after severe head injury. *British Medical Journal* **308**, 1199–1205.

Greiffenstein, M.F., Baker, W.J. *et al.* (1996) Motor dysfunction profiles in traumatic brain injury and postconcussion syndrome. *Journal of the International Neuropsychological Society* **2**, 477–485.

Greiffenstein, M.F., Baker, W.J. *et al.* (2002a) Actual versus self-reported scholastic achievement of litigating postconcussion and severe closed head injury claimants. *Psychological Assessment* **14**, 202–208.

Greiffenstein, F.M., Baker, W.J. *et al.* (2002b) Brief report: anosmia and remote outcome in closed head injury. *Journal of Clinical and Experimental Neuropsychology* **24**, 705–709.

Greve, K.W., Sherwin, E. *et al.* (2001) Personality and neurocognitive correlates of impulsive aggression in long-term survivors of severe traumatic brain injury. *Brain Injury* **15**, 255–262.

Groat, R.A. & Simmons, J.Q. (1950) Loss of nerve cells in experimental cerebral concussion. *Journal of Neuropathology and Experimental Neurology* **9**, 150–163.

Gronwall, D. (1987) Advances in the assessment of attention and information processing after head injury. In: Levin, H.S., Grafman, J. & Eisenberg, H.M. (eds) *Neurobehavioral Recovery From Head Injury*, ch. 24. Oxford University Press, Oxford.

Gronwall, D. (1989) Cumulative and persisting effects of concussion on attention and cognition. In: Levin, H.S., Eisenberg, H.M. & Benton, A.L. (eds) *Mild Head Injury*, ch. 10. Oxford University Press, Oxford.

Gronwall, D. & Wrightson, P. (1974) Delayed recovery of intellectual function after minor head injury. *Lancet* **ii**, 605–609.

Gronwall, D. & Wrightson, P. (1975) Cumulative effect of concussion. *Lancet* **ii**, 995–997.

Gronwall, D. & Wrightson, P. (1980) Duration of post-traumatic amnesia amnesia after mild head injury. *Journal of Clinical and Experimental Neuropsychology* **2**, 51–60.

Gross, H., Kling, A. *et al.* (1996) Local cerebral glucose metabolism in patients with long-term behavioral and cognitive deficits following mild traumatic brain injury. *Journal of Neuropsychiatry and Clinical Neuroscience* **8**, 324–334.

Groswasser, Z., Reider II, G. *et al.* (2002) Quantitative imaging in late TBI. Part II. Cognition and work after closed and penetrating head injury: a report of the Vietnam head injury study. *Brain Injury* **16**, 681–690.

Gun, R.T., Osti, O.L. *et al.* (2005) Risk factors for prolonged disability after whiplash injury: a prospective study. *Spine* **30**, 386–391.

Gunstad, J. & Suhr, J.A. (2001) Expectation as etiology versus the good old days: postconcussion syndrome symptom reporting in athletes, headache sufferers, and depressed individuals. *Journal of the International Neuropsychological Society* **7**, 323–333.

Gurr, B. & Coetzer, B.R. (2005) The effectiveness of cognitive-behavioural therapy for post-traumatic headaches. *Brain Injury* **19**, 481–491.

Gururaj, G. (2002) Epidemiology of traumatic brain injuries: Indian scenario. *Neurological Research* **24**, 24–28.

Guskiewicz, K.M., McCrea, M. *et al.* (2003) Cumulative effects associated with recurrent concussion in collegiate football players: the NCAA Concussion Study. *Journal of the American Medical Association* **290**, 2549–2555.

Guttmann, E. (1946) Late effects of closed head injuries: psychiatric observations. *Journal of Mental Science* **92**, 1–18.

Guyot, L.L. & Michael, D.B. (2000) Post-traumatic hydrocephalus. *Neurological Research* **22**, 25–28.

Haas, D.C. (1996) Chronic post-traumatic headaches classified and compared with natural headaches. *Cephalalgia* **16**, 486–493.

Haas, J.F., Cope, D.N. *et al.* (1987) Premorbid prevalence of poor academic performance in severe head injury. *Journal of Neurology, Neurosurgery and Psychiatry* **50**, 52–56.

Haglund, Y. & Bergstrand, G. (1990) Does Swedish amateur boxing lead to chronic brain damage? 2. A retrospective study with CT and MRI. *Acta Neurologica Scandinavica* **82**, 297–302.

Haglund, Y. & Persson, H.E. (1990) Does Swedish amateur boxing lead to chronic brain damage? 3. A retrospective clinical neurophysiological study. *Acta Neurologica Scandinavica* **82**, 353–360.

Hahn, Y.S., Chyung, C. *et al.* (1988) Head injuries in children under 36 months of age. Demography and outcome. *Childs Nervous System* **4**, 34–40.

Hall, K.M., Karzmark, P. *et al.* (1994) Family stressors in traumatic brain injury: a two-year follow-up. *Archives of Physical Medicine and Rehabilitation* **75**, 876–884.

Hall, K.M., Wallbom, A.S. *et al.* (1998) Premorbid history and traumatic brain injury. *NeuroRehabilitation* **10**, 3–12.

Halligan, P.W., Bass, C. *et al.* (2003) *Malingering and Illness Deception.* Oxford University Press, London.

Haltiner, A.M., Temkin, N.R. *et al.* (1996) The impact of posttraumatic seizures on 1-year neuropsychological and psychosocial outcome of head injury. *Journal of the International Neuropsychological Society* **2**, 494–504.

Hammond, F.M., Grattan, K.D. *et al.* (2004) Five years after traumatic brain injury: a study of individual outcomes and predictors of change in function. *NeuroRehabilitation* **19**, 25–35.

Hanks, R.A., Temkin, N. *et al.* (1999) Emotional and behavioral adjustment after traumatic brain injury. *Archives of Physical Medicine and Rehabilitation* **80**, 991–997.

Harlow, J.M. (1868) Recovery from the passage of an iron bar through the head. *Publications of the Massachussetts Medical Society* **2**, 327–347. Cited in Damasio, H., Grabowski, T., Frank R. *et al.* (1994) The Return of Phineas Gage: clues about the brain from the skull of a famous patient. *Science* **264**, 1102–1105.

Harrison, G., Whitley, E. *et al.* (2006) Risk of schizophrenia and other non-affective psychosis among individuals exposed to head injury: case control study. *Schizophrenia Research* **88**, 119–126.

Harrison, M.S. (1956) Notes on the clinical features and pathology of post-concussional vertigo, with especial reference to positional nystagmus. *Brain* **79**, 474–486.

Harvey, A.G. & Bryant, R.A. (2000) Two-year prospective evaluation of the relationship between acute stress disorder and post-traumatic stress disorder following mild traumatic brain injury. *American Journal of Psychiatry* **157**, 626–628.

Harvey, A.G. & Bryant, R.A. (2001) Reconstructing trauma memories: a prospective study of amnesic trauma survivors. *Journal of Traumatic Stress* **14**, 277–282.

Harvey, A.G., Brewin, C.R. *et al.* (2003) Coexistence of posttraumatic stress disorder and traumatic brain injury: towards a resolution of the paradox. *Journal of the International Neuropsychological Society* **9**, 663–676.

Hasselblatt, M., Mooren, F.C. *et al.* (2004) Serum S100beta increases in marathon runners reflect extracranial release rather than glial damage. *Neurology* **62**, 1634–1636.

Hattori, N., Huang, S.C. *et al.* (2003) Correlation of regional metabolic rates of glucose with Glasgow Coma Scale after traumatic brain injury. *Journal of Nuclear Medicine* **44**, 1709–1716.

Hausmann, R., Biermann, T. *et al.* (2004) Neuronal apoptosis following human brain injury. *International Journal of Legal Medicine* **118**, 32–36.

Hayes, R.L., Lyeth, B.G. *et al.* (1989) Neurochemical mechanisms of mild and moderate head injury: implications for treatment. In: Levin, H.S., Eisenberg, H.M. & Benton, A.L. (eds) *Mild Head Injury*, pp. 54–79. Oxford University Press, New York.

Hecht, J.S. (2004) Occipital nerve blocks in postconcussive headaches: a retrospective review and report of ten patients. *Journal of Head Trauma Rehabilitation* **19**, 58–71.

Hegel, M.T. & Ferguson, R.J. (2000) Differential reinforcement of other behavior (DRO) to reduce aggressive behavior following traumatic brain injury. *Behavior Modification* **24**, 94–101.

Heiskanen, O. & Sipponen, P. (1970) Prognosis of severe brain injury. *Acta Neurologica Scandinavica* **46**, 343–348.

Heitger, M.H., Anderson, T.J. *et al.* (2004) Eye movement and visuomotor arm movement deficits following mild closed head injury. *Brain* **127**, 575–590.

Henry-Feugeas, M.C., Azouvi, P. *et al.* (2000) MRI analysis of brain atrophy after severe closed-head injury: relation to clinical status. *Brain Injury* **14**, 597–604.

Hewitt, J., Evans, J.J. *et al.* (2006) Theory driven rehabilitation of executive functioning: improving planning skills in people with traumatic brain injury through the use of an autobiographical episodic memory cueing procedure. *Neuropsychologia* **44**, 1468–1474.

Heygster, H. (1949) Über doppelseitige Stirnhirnverletzungen. *Pychiatrie, Neurologie und Medizinische Psychologie* **1**, 114–123.

Hibbard, M.R., Uysal, S. *et al.* (1998) Axis I psychopathology in individuals with traumatic brain injury. *Journal of Head Trauma Rehabilitation* **13**, 24–39.

Hibbard, M.R., Bogdany, J. *et al.* (2000) Axis II psychopathology in individuals with traumatic brain injury. *Brain Injury* **14**, 45–61.

Hibbard, M.R., Ashman, T.A. *et al.* (2004) Relationship between depression and psychosocial functioning after traumatic brain injury. *Archives of Physical Medicine and Rehabilitation* **85** (4 suppl. 2), S43–S53.

Hill, P. (1989) Psychiatric aspects of children's head injury. In: Johnson, D.A., Uttley, D. & Wyke, M. (eds) *Children's Head Injury. Who Cares?*, ch. 11. Taylor & Francis, London.

Hillbom, E. (1960) After-effects of brain-injuries. *Acta Psychiatrica et Neurologica Scandinavica Supplementum* **142**, 1–195.

Hillbom, M. & Holm, L. (1986) Contribution of traumatic head injury to neuropsychological deficits in alcoholics. *Journal of Neurology, Neurosurgery and Psychiatry* **49**, 1348–1353.

Hilsabeck, R.C., Gouvier, W.D. *et al.* (1998) Reconstructive memory bias in recall of neuropsychological symptomatology. *Journal of Clinical and Experimental Neuropsychology* **20**, 328–338.

Himanen, L., Portin, R. *et al.* (2006) Longitudinal cognitive changes in traumatic brain injury: a 30-year follow-up study. *Neurology* **66**, 187–192.

Hoheisel, H.P. & Walch, R. (1952) Über manisch-depressive und verwandte Verstimmungszustände nach Hirnverletzung. *Archiv für Psychiatrie und Nervenkrankheiten* **188**, 1–25.

Hollon, T.H. (1973) Behaviour modification in a community hospital rehabilitation unit. *Archives of Physical Medicine and Rehabilitation* **54**, 65–68.

Holsinger, T., Steffens, D.C. *et al.* (2002) Head injury in early adulthood and the lifetime risk of depression. *Archives of General Psychiatry* **59**, 17–22.

Hoofien, D., Gilboa, A. *et al.* (2001) Traumatic brain injury (TBI) 10–20 years later: a comprehensive outcome study of psychiatric symptomatology, cognitive abilities and psychosocial functioning. *Brain Injury* **15**, 189–209.

Hoofien, D., Vakil, E. *et al.* (2002) Comparison of the predictive power of socio-economic variables, severity of injury and age on long-term outcome of traumatic brain injury: sample-specific variables versus factors as predictors. *Brain Injury* **16**, 9–27.

Hooper, R.S., McGregor, J.M. *et al.* (1945) Explosive rage following head injury. *Journal of Mental Science* **91**, 458–471.

Howard, R.S. & Miller, D.H. (1995) The persistent vegetative state. Information on prognosis allows decisions to be made on management. *British Medical Journal* **310**, 341–342.

Hsiang, J.N., Yeung, T. *et al.* (1997) High-risk mild head injury. *Journal of Neurosurgery* **87**, 234–238.

Hudak, A.M., Trivedi, K. *et al.* (2004) Evaluation of seizure-like episodes in survivors of moderate and severe traumatic brain injury. *Journal of Head Trauma Rehabilitation* **19**, 290–295.

Hughes, D.G., Jackson, A. *et al.* (2004) Abnormalities on magnetic resonance imaging seen acutely following mild traumatic brain injury: correlation with neuropsychological tests and delayed recovery. *Neuroradiology* **46**, 550–558.

Ikonomovic, M.D., Uryu, K. *et al.* (2004) Alzheimer's pathology in human temporal cortex surgically excised after severe brain injury. *Experimental Neurology* **190**, 192–203.

Ingebrigtsen, T., Waterloo, K. *et al.* (1998) Quantification of postconcussion symptoms 3 months after minor head injury in 100 consecutive patients. *Journal of Neurology* **245**, 609–612.

Ingebrigtsen, T., Waterloo, K. *et al.* (1999) Traumatic brain damage in minor head injury: relation of serum S-100 protein measurements to magnetic resonance imaging and neurobehavioral outcome. *Neurosurgery* **45**, 468–475; discussion 475–476.

Ingebrigtsen, T., Romner, B. *et al.* (2000) The clinical value of serum S-100 protein measurements in minor head injury: a Scandinavian multicentre study. *Brain Injury* **14**, 1047–1055.

Inglese, M., Makani, S. *et al.* (2005) Diffuse axonal injury in mild traumatic brain injury: a diffusion tensor imaging study. *Journal of Neurosurgery* **103**, 298–303.

Iverson, G.L. (2005) Outcome from mild traumatic brain injury. *Current Opinion in Psychiatry* **18**, 301–307.

Iverson, G.L. & Binder, L.M. (2000) Detecting exaggeration and malingering in neuropsychological assessment. *Journal of Head Trauma Rehabilitation* **15**, 829–858.

Iverson, G.L. & Lange, R.T. (2003) Examination of postconcussion-like symptoms in a healthy sample. *Applied Neuropsychology* **10**, 137–44.

Iverson, G.L. & McCracken, L.M. (1997) 'Postconcussive' symptoms in persons with chronic pain. *Brain Injury* **11**, 783–790.

Iverson, G.L., Gaetz, M. *et al.* (2004) Cumulative effects of concussion in amateur athletes. *Brain Injury* **18**, 433–443.

Iverson, G.L., Brooks, B.L. *et al.* (2006) No cumulative effects for one or two previous concussions. *British Journal of Sports Medicine* **40**, 72–75.

Jacobs, A., Put, E. *et al.* (1996) One-year follow-up of technetium-99m-HMPAO SPECT in mild head injury. *Journal of Nuclear Medicine* **37**, 1605–1609.

Jacobson, R.R. (1995) The post-concussional syndrome: physiogenesis, psychogenesis and malingering. An integrative model. *Journal of Psychosomatic Research* **39**, 675–693.

Jellinger, K. & Seitelberger, F. (1969) Protracted post-traumatic encephalopathy: pathology and clinical implications. In: Walker, A.E., Caveness, W.F. & Critchley, M.T. (eds) *The Late Effects of Head Injury*, ch. 18. Charles C. Thomas, Springfield, IL.

Jenkins, A., Teasdale, G. *et al.* (1986) Brain lesions detected by magnetic resonance imaging in mild and severe head injuries. *Lancet* **ii**, 445–446.

Jennett, B. (1975) *Epilepsy After Non-missile Head Injuries*. Heinemann, London.

Jennett, B. (1989) Some international comparisons. In: Levin, H.S., Eisenberg, H.M. & Benton, A.L. (eds) *Mild Head Injury*, pp. 23–34. Oxford University Press, New York.

Jennett, B. & Bond, M. (1975) Assessment of outcome after severe brain damage: a practical scale. *Lancet* **i**, 480–484.

Jennett, B. & Plum, F. (1972) Persistent vegetative state after brain damage. A syndrome in search of a name. *Lancet* **i**, 734–737.

Jennett, B. & Teasdale, G. (1981) *Management of Head Injuries*. F.A. Davis, Philadelphia.

Jennett, B., Teasdale, G. *et al.* (1977) Severe head injuries in three countries. *Journal of Neurology, Neurosurgery and Psychiatry* **40**, 291–298.

Jennett, B., Snoek, J. *et al.* (1981) Disability after severe head injury: observations on the use of the Glasgow Coma Scale. *Journal of Neurology, Neurosurgery and Psychiatry* **44**, 285–293.

Jennett, B., Adams, J.H. *et al.* (2001) Neuropathology in vegetative and severely disabled patients after head injury. *Neurology* **56**, 486–490.

Jennett, W.B. (1962) *Epilepsy After Blunt Head Injuries*. Heinemann, London.

Johnson, J. (1969) Organic psychosyndromes due to boxing. *British Journal of Psychiatry* **115**, 45–53.

Johnston, K.M., McCrory, P. *et al.* (2001) Evidence-based review of sport-related concussion: clinical science. *Clinical Journal of Sport Medicine* **11**, 150–159.

Jones, R.K. (1974) Assessment of minimal head injuries: indications for in-hospital care. *Surgical Neurology* **2**, 101–104.

Jordan, B.D. & Zimmerman, R.D. (1988) Magnetic resonance imaging in amateur boxers. *Archives of Neurology* **45**, 1207–1208.

Jordan, B.D. & Zimmerman, R.D. (1990) Computed tomography and magnetic resonance imaging comparisons in boxers. *Journal of the American Medical Association* **263**, 1670–1674.

Jordan, B.D., Jahre, C. *et al.* (1992) CT of 338 active professional boxers. *Radiology* **185**, 509–512.

Jordan, B.D., Relkin, N.R. *et al.* (1997) Apolipoprotein E epsilon4 associated with chronic traumatic brain injury in boxing. *Journal of the American Medical Association* **278**, 136–140.

Jorge, R.E., Robinson, R.G. *et al.* (1993a) Secondary mania following traumatic brain injury. *American Journal of Psychiatry* **150**, 916–921.

Jorge, R.E., Robinson, R.G. *et al.* (1993b) Depression following traumatic brain injury: a 1 year longitudinal study. *Journal of Affective Disorders* **27**, 233–243.

Jorge, R.E., Robinson, R.G. *et al.* (1993c) Are there symptoms that are specific for depressed mood in patients with traumatic brain injury? *Journal of Nervous and Mental Disease* **181**, 91–99.

Jorge, R.E., Robinson, R.G. *et al.* (2004) Major depression following traumatic brain injury. *Archives of General Psychiatry* **61**, 42–50.

Jorge, R.E., Starkstein, S.E. *et al.* (2005) Alcohol misuse and mood disorders following traumatic brain injury. *Archives of General Psychiatry* **62**, 742–749.

Jurkovich, G., Mock, C. *et al.* (1995) The Sickness Impact Profile as a tool to evaluate functional outcome in trauma patients. *Journal of Trauma* **39**, 625–631.

Kalsbeek, W.D., McLaurin, R.L. *et al.* (1980) The national head and spinal cord injury survey: major findings. *Journal of Neurosurgery* **53**, S19–S31.

Kant, R., Smith-Seemiller, L. *et al.* (1997) Tc-HMPAO SPECT in persistent post-concussion syndrome after mild head injury: comparison with MRI/CT. *Brain Injury* **11**, 115–124.

Kant, R., Duffy, J.D. *et al.* (1998a) Prevalence of apathy following head injury. *Brain Injury* **12**, 87–92.

Kant, R., Smith-Seemiller, L. *et al.* (1998b) Treatment of aggression and irritability after head injury. *Brain Injury* **12**, 661–666.

Kant, R., Coffey, C.E. *et al.* (1999) Safety and efficacy of ECT in patients with head injury: a case series. *Journal of Neuropsychiatry and Clinical Neuroscience* **11**, 32–37.

Karzmark, P., Hall, K. *et al.* (1995) Late-onset post-concussion symptoms after mild brain injury: the role of premorbid, injury-related, environmental, and personality factors. *Brain Injury* **9**, 21–26.

Kasch, H., Bach, F.W. *et al.* (2001) Handicap after acute whiplash injury: a 1-year prospective study of risk factors. *Neurology* **56**, 1637–1643.

Katz, D.I. & Alexander, M.P. (1994) Traumatic brain injury. Predicting course of recovery and outcome for patients admitted to rehabilitation. *Archives of Neurology* **51**, 661–670.

Kaur, B., Rutty, G.N. *et al.* (1999) The possible role of hypoxia in the formation of axonal bulbs. *Journal of Clinical Pathology* **52**, 203–209.

Kay, D.W.K., Kerr, T.A. *et al.* (1971) Brain trauma and the postconcussional syndrome. *Lancet* **ii**, 1052–1055.

Kay, T., Newman, B. *et al.* (1992) Toward a neuropsychological model of functional disability after mild traumatic brain injury. *Neuropsychology* **6**, 371–384.

Kazan, S., Tuncer, R. *et al.* (1997) Post-traumatic bilateral diffuse cerebral swelling. *Acta Neurochirurgica (Wien)* **139**, 295–301; discussion 301 302.

Keenan, H.T., Brundage, S.I. *et al.* (1999) Does the face protect the brain? A case-control study of traumatic brain injury and facial fractures. *Archives of Surgery* **134**, 14–17.

Keller, M., Hiltbrunner, B. *et al.* (2000) Reversible neuropsychological deficits after mild traumatic brain injury. *Journal of Neurology, Neurosurgery and Psychiatry* **68**, 761–764.

Kelly, A.B., Zimmerman, R.D. *et al.* (1988) Head trauma: comparison of MR and CT-experience in 100 patients. *American Journal of Neuroradiology* **9**, 699–708.

Kelly, R. & Smith, B.N. (1981) Post-traumatic syndrome: another myth discredited. *Journal of the Royal Society of Medicine* **74**, 275–277.

Kemp, P.M., MacLeod, M.A. *et al.* (1991) Cerebral perfusion in amateur boxers. Is there evidence of brain damage? [Abstract] *Nuclear Medicine Communications* **12**, 279.

Kemp, P.M., Houston, A.S. *et al.* (1995) Cerebral perfusion and psychometric testing in military amateur boxers and controls. *Journal of Neurology, Neurosurgery and Psychiatry* **59**, 368–374.

Kemp, S., Biswas, R. *et al.* (2004) The value of melatonin for sleep disorders occurring post-head injury: a pilot RCT. *Brain Injury* **18**, 911–919.

Kerr, T.A., Kay, D.W.K. *et al.* (1971) Characteristics of patients, type of accident, and mortality in a consecutive series of head injuries admitted to a neurosurgical unit. *British Journal of Preventive and Social Medicine* **25**, 179–185.

Kersel, D.A., Marsh, N.V. *et al.* (2001) Psychosocial functioning during the year following severe traumatic brain injury. *Brain Injury* **15**, 683–696.

Keshavan, M.S., Channabasavanna, S.M. *et al.* (1981) Post-traumatic psychiatric disturbances: patterns and predictors of outcome. *British Journal of Psychiatry* **138**, 157–160.

Kieslich, M., Fiedler, A. *et al.* (2002) Minor head injury as cause and co-factor in the aetiology of stroke in childhood: a report of eight cases. *Journal of Neurology, Neurosurgery and Psychiatry* **73**, 13–16.

King, N.S. (1996) Emotional, neuropsychological, and organic factors: their use in the prediction of persisting postconcussion symptoms after moderate and mild head injuries. *Journal of Neurology, Neurosurgery and Psychiatry* **61**, 75–81.

King, N.S. (1997) Post-traumatic stress disorder and head injury as a dual diagnosis: islands of memory as a mechanism. *Journal of Neurology, Neurosurgery and Psychiatry* **62**, 82–84.

King, N.S., Crawford, S. *et al.* (1999) Early prediction of persisting post-concussion symptoms following mild and moderate head injuries. *British Journal of Clinical Psychology* **38**, 15–25.

Kinsella, G., Murtagh, D. *et al.* (1996) Everyday memory following traumatic brain injury. *Brain Injury* **10**, 499–507.

Kinuya, K., Kakuda, K. *et al.* (2004) Role of brain perfusion single-photon emission tomography in traumatic head injury. *Nuclear Medicine Communications* **25**, 333–337.

Klein, M., Houx, P.J. *et al.* (1996) Long-term persisting cognitive sequelae of traumatic brain injury and the effect of age. *Journal of Nervous and Mental Disease* **184**, 459–467.

Kleist, K. (1934) *Kriegverletzungen des Gehirns in ihrer Bedeutung für Hirnlokalisation und Hirnpathologie.* Barth, Leipzig. Quoted by Tow, P.M. (1955) *Personality Changes Following Frontal Leucotomy.* Oxford University Press, Oxford.

Koh, J.O., Cassidy, J.D. *et al.* (2003) Incidence of concussion in contact sports: a systematic review of the evidence. *Brain Injury* **17**, 901–917.

Kolakowsky-Hayner, S.A., Gourley, E.V. III *et al.* (1999) Pre-injury substance abuse among persons with brain injury and persons with spinal cord injury. *Brain Injury* **13**, 571–581.

Kolb, B. & Wishaw, I.Q. (2003) *Fundamentals of Human Neuropsychology.* Freeman Worth, New York.

Koponen, S., Taiminen, T. *et al.* (2002) Axis I and II psychiatric disorders after traumatic brain injury: a 30-year follow-up study. *American Journal of Psychiatry* **159**, 1315–1321.

Koponen, S., Taiminen, T. *et al.* (2004) APOE-epsilon4 predicts dementia but not other psychiatric disorders after traumatic brain injury. *Neurology* **63**, 749–750.

Kordestani, R.K., Counelis, G.J. *et al.* (1997) Cerebral arterial spasm after penetrating craniocerebral gunshot wounds: transcranial Doppler and cerebral blood flow findings. *Neurosurgery* **41**, 351–359; discussion 359–360.

Korn, A., Golan, H. *et al.* (2005) Focal cortical dysfunction and blood–brain barrier disruption in patients with postconcussion syndrome. *Journal of Clinical Neurophysiology* **22**, 1–9.

Kozol, H.L. (1945) Pretraumatic personality and sequelae of head injury. *Archives of Neurology and Psychiatry* **53**, 358–364.

Kozol, H.L. (1946) Pretraumatic personality and psychiatric sequelae of head injury. *Archives of Neurology and Psychiatry* **56**, 245–275.

Kraus, J., Schaffer, K. *et al.* (2005) Physical complaints, medical service use, and social and employment changes following mild traumatic brain injury: a 6-month longitudinal study. *Journal of Head Trauma Rehabilitation* **20**, 239–256.

Krauss, J.F. & Chu, L.D. (2005) Epidemiology. In: Silver, J.M., McAllister, T.W. & Yudofsky, S.C. (eds) *Textbook of Traumatic Brain Injury,* pp. 279–308. American Psychiatric Publishing, Washington DC.

Kraus, J.F., Black, M.A. *et al.* (1984) The incidence of acute brain injury and serious impairment in a defined population. *American Journal of Epidemiology* **119**, 186–201.

Kretschmer, E. (1949) Die Orbitalhirn-und Zwischenhirnsyndrome nach Schädelbasisfrakturen. *Allgemeine Zeitschrift für Psychiatrie* **124**, 358–360.

Kretschmer, E. (1956) Lokalisation und Beurteilung psychophysischer Syndrome bei Hirnverletzten. In: Rehwald, E. (ed.) *Das Hirntrauma,* pp. 155–158. Thieme, Stuttgart.

Kreuter, M., Dahllof, A.G. *et al.* (1998) Sexual adjustment and its predictors after traumatic brain injury. *Brain Injury* **12**, 349–368.

Kreutzer, J.S., Doherty, K. *et al.* (1990) Alcohol use among persons with traumatic brain injury. *Journal of Head Trauma Rehabilitation* **11**, 58–69.

Kreutzer, J.S., Gervasio, A.H. *et al.* (1994) Primary caregivers' psychological status and family functioning after traumatic brain injury. *Brain Injury* **8**, 197–210.

Kreutzer, J.S., Seel, R.T. *et al.* (2001) The prevalence and symptom rates of depression after traumatic brain injury: a comprehensive examination. *Brain Injury* **15**, 563–576.

Kringelbach, M.L. & Rolls, E.T. (2004) The functional neuroanatomy of the human orbitofrontal cortex: evidence from neuroimaging and neuropsychology. *Progress in Neurobiology* **72**, 341–372.

Kurtz, J.E., Putnam, S.H. *et al.* (1998) Stability of normal personality traits after traumatic brain injury. *Journal of Head Trauma Rehabilitation* **13**, 1–14.

Kutner, K.C., Erlanger, D.M. *et al.* (2000) Lower cognitive performance of older football players possessing apolipoprotein E epsilon4. *Neurosurgery* **47**, 651–657; discussion 657–658.

Langfitt, T.W., Obrist, W.D. *et al.* (1986) Computerized tomography, magnetic resonance imaging, and positron emission tomography in the study of brain trauma. Preliminary observations. *Journal of Neurosurgery* **64**, 760–767.

Leathem, J., Heath, E. *et al.* (1996) Relatives' perceptions of role change, social support and stress after traumatic brain injury. *Brain Injury* **10**, 27–38.

Lee, H., Kim, S.W. *et al.* (2005) Comparing effects of methylphenidate, sertraline and placebo on neuropsychiatric sequelae in patients with traumatic brain injury. *Human Psychopharmacology* **20**, 97–104.

Lee, T.T., Galarza, M. *et al.* (1998) Diffuse axonal injury (DAI) is not associated with elevated intracranial pressure (ICP). *Acta Neurochirurgica (Wien)* **140**, 41–46.

Lees-Haley, P.R., Williams, C.W. *et al.* (1996) Response bias in self-reported history of plaintiffs compared with nonlitigating patients. *Psychological Reports* **79**, 811–818.

Lees-Haley, P.R., Williams, C.W. *et al.* (1997) Response bias in plaintiffs' histories. *Brain Injury* **11**, 791–799.

Lehtonen, S., Stringer, A.Y. *et al.* (2005) Neuropsychological outcome and community re-integration following traumatic brain injury: the impact of frontal and non-frontal lesions. *Brain Injury* **19**, 239–256.

Leininger, B.E., Gramling, S.E. *et al.* (1990) Neuropsychological deficits in symptomatic minor head injury patients after concussion and mild concussion. *Journal of Neurology, Neurosurgery and Psychiatry* **53**, 293–296.

Leininger, B.E., Kreutzer, J.S. *et al.* (1991) Comparison of minor and severe head injury emotional sequelae using the MMPI. *Brain Injury* **5**, 199–205.

Levin, H.S. (1990) Memory deficit after closed head injury. *Journal of Clinical and Experimental Neuropsychology* **12**, 129–153.

Levin, H.S. & Hanten, G. (2005) Executive functions after traumatic brain injury in children. *Pediatric Neurology* **33**, 79–93.

Levin, H.S., Meyers, C.A. *et al.* (1981) Ventricular enlargement after closed head injury. *Archives of Neurology* **38**, 623–629.

Levin, H.S., High, W.M. *et al.* (1985) Impairment of remote memory after closed head injury. *Journal of Neurology, Neurosurgery and Psychiatry* **48**, 556–563.

Levin, H.S., Amparo, E. *et al.* (1987a) Magnetic resonance imaging and computerized tomography in relation to the neurobehavioural sequelae of mild and moderate head injuries. *Journal of Neurosurgery* **66**, 706–713.

Levin, H.S., High, W.M. *et al.* (1987b) The neurobehavioural rating scale: assessment of the behavioural sequelae of head injury by the clinician. *Journal of Neurology, Neurosurgery and Psychiatry* **50**, 183–193.

Levin, H.S., Mattis, S. *et al.* (1987c) Neurobehavioral outcome following minor head injury: a three-center study. *Journal of Neurosurgery* **66**, 234–243.

Levin, H.S., Lippold, S.C. *et al.* (1987d) Neurobehavioural functioning and magnetic resonance imaging findings in young boxers. *Journal of Neurosurgery* **67**, 657–667.

Levin, H.S., Goldstein, F.C. *et al.* (1988) Disproportionately severe memory deficit in relation to normal intellectual functioning after closed head injury. *Journal of Neurology, Neurosurgery and Psychiatry* **51**, 1294–1301.

Levin, H.S., Williams, D.H. *et al.* (1990a) Corpus callosal atrophy following closed head injury: detection with magnetic resonance imaging. *Journal of Neurosurgery* **73**, 77–81.

Levin, H.S., Gary, H.E. Jr *et al.* (1990b) Neurobehavioral outcome 1 year after severe head injury. Experience of the Traumatic Coma Data Bank. *Journal of Neurosurgery* **73**, 699–709.

Levin, H.S., Benavidez, D.A. *et al.* (2000) Reduction of corpus callosum growth after severe traumatic brain injury in children. *Neurology* **54**, 647–653.

Levin, H.S., Brown, S.A. *et al.* (2001) Depression and posttraumatic stress disorder at three months after mild to moderate traumatic brain injury. *Journal of Clinical and Experimental Neuropsychology* **23**, 754–769.

Levin, H.S., Hanten, G. *et al.* (2002) Working memory after traumatic brain injury in children. *Annals of Neurology* **52**, 82–88.

Levin, H.S., Zhang, L. *et al.* (2004) Psychosocial outcome of TBI in children with unilateral frontal lesions. *Journal of the International Neuropsychological Society* **10**, 305–316.

Levin, H.S., McCauley, S.R. *et al.* (2005) Predicting depression following mild traumatic brain injury. *Archives of General Psychiatry* **62**, 523–528.

Levine, B., Black, S.E. *et al.* (1998) Episodic memory and the self in a case of isolated retrograde amnesia. *Brain* **121**, 1951–1973.

Levine, B., Cabeza, R. *et al.* (2002) Functional reorganisation of memory after traumatic brain injury: a study with H₂¹⁵O positron emission tomography. *Journal of Neurology, Neurosurgery and Psychiatry* **73**, 173–181.

Levine, B., Black, S.E. *et al.* (2005) Gambling task performance in traumatic brain injury: relationships to injury severity, atrophy, lesion location, and cognitive and psychosocial outcome. *Cognitive and Behavioral Neurology* **18**, 45–54.

Lew, H.L., Lin, P.H. *et al.* (2006) Characteristics and treatment of headache after traumatic brain injury: a focused review. *American Journal of Physical Medicine and Rehabilitation* **85**, 619–627.

Lewin, W. (1959) The management of prolonged unconsciousness after head injury. *Proceedings of the Royal Society of Medicine* **52**, 880–884.

Lewin, W. (1968) Rehabilitation after head injury. *British Medical Journal* **1**, 465–470.

Lewis, A.J. (1942) Discussion on differential diagnosis and treatment of post-contusional states. *Proceedings of the Royal Society of Medicine* **35**, 607–614.

Lewis, D.O., Yeager, C.A. *et al.* (2004) Ethics questions raised by the neuropsychiatric, neuropsychological, educational, developmental, and family characteristics of 18 juveniles awaiting execution in Texas. *Journal of the American Academy of Psychiatry and the Law* **32**, 408–429.

Lezak, M.D. (1978) Living with the characterologically altered brain injured patient. *Journal of Clinical Psychiatry* **39**, 592–598.

Lezak, M.D. (1987) Relationships between personality disorders, social disturbances, and physical disability following traumatic brain injury. *Journal of Head Trauma Rehabilitation* **2**, 57–69.

Liaquat, I., Dunn, L.T. *et al.* (2002) Effect of apolipoprotein E genotype on hematoma volume after trauma. *Journal of Neurosurgery* **96**, 90–96.

Liberman, J.N., Stewart, W.F. *et al.* (2002) Apolipoprotein E epsilon 4 and short-term recovery from predominantly mild brain injury. *Neurology* **58**, 1038–1044.

Lichtman, S.W., Seliger, G. *et al.* (2000) Apolipoprotein E and functional recovery from brain injury following postacute rehabilitation. *Neurology* **55**, 1536–1539.

Lidvall, H.F., Linderoth, B. *et al.* (1974) Causes of the post-concussional syndrome. *Acta Neurologica Scandinavica Supplementum* **56**, 1–144.

Lindenberg, W. (1951) Hirnverletzung, organische Wesensänderung Neurose. *Nervenarzt* **22**, 254–260.

Liou, A.K., Clark, R.S. *et al.* (2003) To die or not to die for neurons in ischemia, traumatic brain injury and epilepsy: a review on the stress-activated signaling pathways and apoptotic pathways. *Progress in Neurobiology* **69**, 103–142.

Lishman, W.A. (1968) Brain damage in relation to psychiatric disability after head injury. *British Journal of Psychiatry* **114**, 373–410.

Lishman, W.A. (1973) The psychiatric sequelae of head injury: a review. *Psychological Medicine* **3**, 304–318.

Lishman, W.A. (1978) Psychiatric sequelae of head injuries: problems in diagnosis. *Journal of the Irish Medical Association* **71**, 306–314.

Lishman, W.A. (1983) *Brain Damage and Psychiatric Disability*. Royal Hospital and Home for Incurables, Booklet 1/83. Putney, London.

Lishman, W.A. (1988) Physiogenesis and psychogenesis in the 'post-concussional syndrome'. *British Journal of Psychiatry* **153**, 460–469.

Liu, A.Y., Maldjian, J.A. *et al.* (1999) Traumatic brain injury: diffusion-weighted MR imaging findings. *American Journal of Neuroradiology* **20**, 1636–1641.

Liu, B., Ivers, R. *et al.* (2004) Helmets for preventing injury in motorcycle riders. *Cochrane Database of Systematic Reviews* 2, CD004333.

Livingston, M.G., Brooks, D.N. *et al.* (1985) Patient outcome in the year following severe head injury and relatives' psychiatric and social functioning. *Journal of Neurology, Neurosurgery and Psychiatry* **48**, 876–881.

Löken, A.C. (1959) The pathologic-anatomical basis for late symptoms after brain injuries in adults. *Acta Psychiatrica et Neurologica Scandinavica Supplementum* **137**, 30–42.

Lovell, M.R., Iverson, G.L. *et al.* (1999) Does loss of consciousness predict neuropsychological decrements after concussion? *Clinical Journal of Sport Medicine* **9**, 193–198.

Lowdon, I.M., Briggs, M. *et al.* (1989) Post-concussional symptoms following minor head injury. *Injury* **20**, 193–194.

Lucey, J.V., Burness, C.E. *et al.* (1997) Wisconsin Card Sorting Task (WCST) errors and cerebral blood flow in obsessive-compulsive disorder (OCD). *British Journal of Medical Psychology* **70**, 403–411.

Luis, C.A., Vanderploeg, R.D. *et al.* (2003) Predictors of postconcussion symptom complex in community dwelling male veterans. *Journal of the International Neuropsychological Society* **9**, 1001–1015.

McAllister, T.W. (2005) Mild brain injury and the post concussion syndrome. In: Silver, J.M., McAllister, T.W. & Yudofsky, S.C. (eds) *Textbook of Traumatic Brain Injury*, pp. 279–308. American Psychiatric Publishing Inc., Washington, DC.

McAllister, T.W., Saykin, A.J. *et al.* (1999) Brain activation during working memory 1 month after mild traumatic brain injury: a functional MRI study. *Neurology* **53**, 1300–1308.

McAllister, T.W., Rhodes, C.H. *et al.* (2005) Effect of the dopamine D2 receptor T allele on response latency after mild traumatic brain injury. *American Journal of Psychiatry* **162**, 1749–1751.

McBeath, J.G. & Nanda, A. (1994) Use of dihydroergotamine in patients with postconcussion syndrome. *Headache* **34**, 148–151.

McCauley, S.R., Boake, C. *et al.* (2001) Postconcussional disorder following mild to moderate traumatic brain injury: anxiety, depression, and social support as risk factors and comorbidities. *Journal of Clinical and Experimental Neuropsychology* **23**, 792–808.

Macciocchi, S.N., Barth, J.T., Littlefield, L. *et al.* (2001) Multiple concussions and neuropsychological functioning in collegiate football players. *Journal of Athletic Training* **36**, 303–306.

McCrea, M., Kelly, J.P. *et al.* (2002) Immediate neurocognitive effects of concussion. *Neurosurgery* **50**, 1032–1040; discussion 1040–1042.

McCrory, P.R. (2003) Brain injury and heading in soccer. *British Medical Journal* **327**, 351–352.

McCrory, P.R. & Berkovic, S.F. (1998) Second impact syndrome. *Neurology* **50**, 677–683.

McCrory, P.R., Bladin, P.F. *et al.* (1997) Retrospective study of concussive convulsions in elite Australian rules and rugby league footballers: phenomenology, aetiology, and outcome. *British Medical Journal* **314**, 171–174.

McCrory, P.R., Ariens, T. *et al.* (2000) The nature and duration of acute concussive symptoms in Australian football. *Clinical Journal of Sport Medicine* **10**, 235–238.

McCrory, P.R., Johnston, K.M. *et al.* (2001) Evidence-based review of sport-related concussion: basic science. *Clinical Journal of Sport Medicine* **11**, 160–165.

McCullagh, S. & Feinstein, A. (2003) Outcome after mild traumatic brain injury: an examination of recruitment bias. *Journal of Neurology, Neurosurgery and Psychiatry* **74**, 39–43.

McCullagh, S., Oucherlony, D. *et al.* (2001) Prediction of neuropsychiatric outcome following mild trauma brain injury: an examination of the Glasgow Coma Scale. *Brain Injury* **15**, 489–497.

McDowell, S., Whyte, J. *et al.* (1997) Working memory impairments in traumatic brain injury: evidence from a dual-task paradigm. *Neuropsychologia* **35**, 1341–1353.

McDowell, S., Whyte, J. *et al.* (1998) Differential effect of a dopaminergic agonist on prefrontal function in traumatic brain injury patients. *Brain* **121**, 1155–1164.

Macfarlane, D.P., Nicoll, J.A. *et al.* (1999) APOE epsilon4 allele and amyloid beta-protein deposition in long term survivors of head injury. *Neuroreport* **10**, 3945–3948.

Machamer, J.E., Temkin, N.R. *et al.* (2003) Neurobehavioral outcome in persons with violent or nonviolent traumatic brain injury. *Journal of Head Trauma Rehabilitation* **18**, 387–397.

McIntosh, A.S. & McCrory, P. (2000) Impact energy attenuation performance of football headgear. *British Journal of Sports Medicine* **34**, 337–341.

McIntosh, A.S. & McCrory, P. (2001) Effectiveness of headgear in a pilot study of under 15 rugby union football. *British Journal of Sports Medicine* **35**, 167–169.

McIntosh, A.S., McCrory, P. *et al.* (2000) The dynamics of concussive head impacts in rugby and Australian rules football. *Medicine and Science in Sports and Exercise* **32**, 1980–1984.

MacKenzie, J.D., Siddiqi, F. *et al.* (2002) Brain atrophy in mild or moderate traumatic brain injury: a longitudinal quantitative analysis. *American Journal of Neuroradiology* **23**, 1509–1515.

McKenzie, K.J., McLellan, D.R. *et al.* (1996) Is beta-APP a marker of axonal damage in short-surviving head injury? *Acta Neuropathologica* **92**, 608–613.

McKeon, J., McGuffin, P. *et al.* (1984) Obsessive-compulsive neurosis following head injury. A report of four cases. *British Journal of Psychiatry* **144**, 190–192.

McKinlay, W.W., Brooks, D.N. *et al.* (1981) The short-term outcome of severe blunt head injury as reported by relatives of the injured persons. *Journal of Neurology, Neurosurgery and Psychiatry* **44**, 527–533.

McLatchie, G., Brooks, N. *et al.* (1987) Clinical neurological examination, neuropsychology, electroencephalography and computed tomographic head scanning in active amateur boxers. *Journal of Neurology, Neurosurgery and Psychiatry* **50**, 96–99.

McLay, R.N., Drake, A. *et al.* (2004) Major depressive disorder with psychotic features in an aviator after head trauma. *Aviation Space and Environmental Medicine* **75**, 175–179.

McMillan, T.M. (1991) Post-traumatic stress disorder and severe head injury. *British Journal of Psychiatry* **159**, 431–433.

McMillan, T.M. (1996) Post-traumatic stress disorder following minor and severe closed head injury: 10 single cases. *Brain Injury* **10**, 749–758.

McMillan, T.M. & Glucksman, E.E. (1987) The neuropsychology of moderate head injury. *Journal of Neurology, Neurosurgery and Psychiatry* **50**, 393–397.

McMillan, T.M., Greenwood, R.J. *et al.* (1988) An introduction to the concept of head injury case management with respect to the need for service provision. *Clinical Rehabilitation* **2**, 319–322.

McMillan, T.M., Jongen, E.L. *et al.* (1996) Assessment of post-traumatic amnesia after severe closed head injury: retrospective or prospective? *Journal of Neurology, Neurosurgery and Psychiatry* **60**, 422–427.

Magavi, S.S., Leavitt, B.R. *et al.* (2000) Induction of neurogenesis in the neocortex of adult mice. *Nature* **405**, 951–955.

Mah, L.W., Arnold, M.C. *et al.* (2005) Deficits in social knowledge following damage to ventromedial prefrontal cortex. *Journal of Neuropsychiatry and Clinical Neuroscience* **17**, 66–74.

Mahalick, D.M., Carmel, P.W. *et al.* (1998) Psychopharmacologic treatment of acquired attention disorders in children with brain injury. *Pediatric Neurosurgery* **29**, 121–126.

Maimaris, C. (1989) Neck sprains after car accidents. *British Medical Journal* **299**, 123.

Maimaris, C., Barnes, M.R. *et al.* (1988) 'Whiplash injuries' of the neck: a retrospective study. *Injury* **19**, 393–396.

Malaspina, D., Goetz, R.R. *et al.* (2001) Traumatic brain injury and schizophrenia in members of schizophrenia and bipolar disorder pedigrees. *American Journal of Psychiatry* **158**, 440–446.

Malec, J.F., Brown, A.W. *et al.* (2004) Personality factors and injury severity in the prediction of early and late traumatic brain injury outcomes. *Rehabilitation Psychology* **49**, 55–61.

Malia, K., Powell, G. *et al.* (1995) Personality and psychosocial function after brain injury. *Brain Injury* **9**, 697–712.

Mandleberg, I.A. & Brooks, D.N. (1975) Cognitive recovery after severe head injury. I. Serial testing on the Wechsler Adult Intelligence Scale. *Journal of Neurology, Neurosurgery and Psychiatry* **38**, 1121–1126.

Marcus, D.A. (2003) Disability and chronic posttraumatic headache. *Headache* **43**, 117–121.

Marin, R.S. & Wilkosz, P.A. (2005) Disorders of diminished motivation. *Journal of Head Trauma Rehabilitation* **20**, 377–388.

Markowitsch, H.J. & Calabrese, P. (1996) Commonalities and discrepancies in the relationships between behavioural outcome and the results of neuroimaging in brain-damaged patients. *Behavioural Neurology* **9**, 45–55.

Markowitsch, H.J., Kessler, J. *et al.* (1998) Psychic trauma causing grossly reduced brain metabolism and cognitive deterioration. *Neuropsychologia* **36**, 77–82.

Marmarou, A., Foda, M.A. *et al.* (1996) Posttraumatic ventriculomegaly: hydrocephalus or atrophy? A new approach for diagnosis using CSF dynamics. *Journal of Neurosurgery* **85**, 1026–1035.

Marmarou, A., Portella, G. *et al.* (2000) Distinguishing between cellular and vasogenic edema in head injured patients with focal lesions using magnetic resonance imaging. *Acta Neurochirurgica Supplementum* **76**, 349–351.

Maroon, J.C., Lovell, M.R. *et al.* (2000) Cerebral concussion in athletes: evaluation and neuropsychological testing. *Neurosurgery* **47**, 659–669; discussion 669–672.

Marshall, J.C., Halligan, P.W. *et al.* (1995) Reduplication of an event after head injury? A cautionary case report. *Cortex* **31**, 183–190.

Marshall, L.F., Marshall, S.B. *et al.* (1991) A new classification of head injury based on computerized tomography. *Journal of Neurosurgery* **75**, S14–S20.

Martelli, M.F., Grayson, R.L. *et al.* (1999) Posttraumatic headache: neuropsychological and psychological effects and treatment implications. *Journal of Head Trauma Rehabilitation* **14**, 49–69.

Massagli, T.L., Fann, J.R. *et al.* (2004) Psychiatric illness after mild traumatic brain injury in children. *Archives of Physical Medicine and Rehabilitation* **85**, 1428–1434.

Mathias, J.L., Bigler, E.D. *et al.* (2004a) Neuropsychological and information processing performance and its relationship to white matter changes following moderate and severe traumatic brain injury: a preliminary study. *Applied Neuropsychology* **11**, 134–152.

Mathias, J.L., Beall, J.A. *et al.* (2004b) Neuropsychological and information processing deficits following mild traumatic brain injury. *Journal of the International Neuropsychological Society* **10**, 286–297.

Matser, J.T., Kessels, A.G. *et al.* (2001) A dose–response relation of headers and concussions with cognitive impairment in professional soccer players. *Journal of Clinical and Experimental Neuropsychology* **23**, 770–774.

Matsuda, W., Matsumura, A. *et al.* (2003) Awakenings from persistent vegetative state: report of three cases with parkinsonism and brain stem lesions on MRI. *Journal of Neurology, Neurosurgery and Psychiatry* **74**, 1571–1573.

Matsushita, H., Takahashi, K. *et al.* (2000) [A clinical study of posttraumatic hydrocephalus.] *No Shinkei Geka* **28**, 773–779.

Mattioli, F., Grassi, F. *et al.* (1996) Persistent post-traumatic retrograde amnesia: a neuropsychological and (18F)FDG PET study. *Cortex* **32**, 121–129.

Max, J.E. (2005) Children and adolescents. In: Silver, J.M., McAllister, T.W. & Yudofsky, S.C. (eds) *Textbook of Traumatic Brain Injury*, pp. 477–494. American Psychiatric Publishing Inc., Washington, DC.

Max, J.E., Koele, S.L. *et al.* (1998a) Adaptive functioning following traumatic brain injury and orthopedic injury: a controlled study. *Archives of Physical Medicine and Rehabilitation* **79**, 893–899.

Max, J.E., Koele, S.L. *et al.* (1998b) Psychiatric disorders in children and adolescents after severe traumatic brain injury: a controlled study. *Journal of the American Academy of Child and Adolescent Psychiatry* **37**, 832–840.

Max, J.E., Castillo, C.S. *et al.* (1998c) Oppositional defiant disorder symptomatology after traumatic brain injury: a prospective study. *Journal of Nervous and Mental Disease* **186**, 325–332.

Max, J.E., Arndt, S. *et al.* (1998d) Attention-deficit hyperactivity symptomatology after traumatic brain injury: a prospective study. *Journal of the American Academy of Child and Adolescent Psychiatry* **37**, 841–847.

Max, J.E., Robertson, B.A. *et al.* (2001) The phenomenology of personality change due to traumatic brain injury in children and adolescents. *Journal of Neuropsychiatry and Clinical Neuroscience* **13**, 161–170.

Max, J.E., Lansing, A.E. *et al.* (2004) Attention deficit hyperactivity disorder in children and adolescents following traumatic brain injury. *Developmental Neuropsychology* **25**, 159–177.

Max, J.E., Levin, H.S. *et al.* (2006) Predictors of personality change due to traumatic brain injury in children and adolescents six to twenty-four months after injury. *Journal of Neuropsychiatry and Clinical Neuroscience* **18**, 21–32.

Maxwell, W.L., Dhillon, K. *et al.* (2003) There is differential loss of pyramidal cells from the human hippocampus with survival after blunt head injury. *Journal of Neuropathology and Experimental Neurology* **62**, 272–279.

Maxwell, W.L., Pennington, K. *et al.* (2004) Differential responses in three thalamic nuclei in moderately disabled, severely disabled and vegetative patients after blunt head injury. *Brain* **127**, 2470–2478.

Mayeux, R., Ottman, R. *et al.* (1995) Synergistic effects of traumatic head injury and apolipoprotein-epsilon 4 in patients with Alzheimer's disease. *Neurology* **45**, 555–557.

Mayou, R.A., Bryant, B. *et al.* (1993) Psychiatric consequences of road traffic accidents. *British Medical Journal* **307**, 647–651.

Mayou, R.A., Black, J. *et al.* (2000) Unconsciousness, amnesia and psychiatric symptoms following road traffic accident injury. *British Journal of Psychiatry* **177**, 540–545.

Mazzini, L., Campini, R. *et al.* (2003) Posttraumatic hydrocephalus: a clinical, neuroradiologic, and neuropsychologic assessment of long-term outcome. *Archives of Physical Medicine and Rehabilitation* **84**, 1637–1641.

Medical Disability Society (1988) *The Management of Traumatic Brain Injury*. Development Trust for the Young Disabled, London.

Mehta, K.M., Ott, A. *et al.* (1999) Head trauma and risk of dementia and Alzheimer's disease: the Rotterdam Study. *Neurology* **53**, 1959–1962.

Menon, D.K., Owen, A.M. *et al.* (1998) Cortical processing in persistent vegetative state. Wolfson Brain Imaging Centre Team. *Lancet* **352**, 200.

Menon, D.K., Coles, J.P. *et al.* (2004) Diffusion limited oxygen delivery following head injury. *Critical Care Medicine* **32**, 1384–1390.

Merskey, H. & Woodforde, J.M. (1972) Psychiatric sequelae of minor head injury. *Brain* **95**, 521–528.

Messori, A., Polonara, G. *et al.* (2003) Is haemosiderin visible indefinitely on gradient-echo MRI following traumatic intracerebral haemorrhage? *Neuroradiology* **45**, 881–886.

Meyers, C.A., Levin, H.S. *et al.* (1983) Early versus late lateral ventricular enlargement following closed head injury. *Journal of Neurology, Neurosurgery and Psychiatry* **46**, 1092–1097.

Meythaler, J.M., Brunner, R.C. *et al.* (2002) Amantadine to improve neurorecovery in traumatic brain injury-associated diffuse axonal injury: a pilot double-blind randomized trial. *Journal of Head Trauma Rehabilitation* **17**, 300–313.

Michals, M.L., Crismon, M.L. *et al.* (1993) Clozapine response and adverse effects in nine brain-injured patients. *Journal of Clinical Psychopharmacology* **13**, 198–203.

Mickeviciene, D., Schrader, H. *et al.* (2004) A controlled prospective inception cohort study on the post-concussion syndrome outside the medicolegal context. *European Journal of Neurology* **11**, 411–419.

Middleton, J.A. (2001) Practitioner review: psychological sequelae of head injury in children and adolescents. *Journal of Child Psychology and Psychiatry* **42**, 165–180.

Milders, M., Fuchs, S. *et al.* (2003) Neuropsychological impairments and changes in emotional and social behaviour following severe traumatic brain injury. *Journal of Clinical and Experimental Neuropsychology* **25**, 157–172.

Millar, K., Nicoll, J.A. *et al.* (2003) Long term neuropsychological outcome after head injury: relation to APOE genotype. *Journal of Neurology, Neurosurgery and Psychiatry* **74**, 1047–1052.

Miller, H. (1961) Accident neurosis. *British Medical Journal* **1**, 919–925, 992–998.

Miller, H. (1966) Mental after-effects of head injury. *Proceedings of the Royal Society of Medicine* **59**, 257–261.

Miller, H. (1969) Problems of medicolegal practice. In: Walker, A. E., Caveness, W.F. & Critchley, M. (eds) *The Late Effects of Head Injury*, ch. 42. Charles C. Thomas, Springfield, IL.

Miller, H. & Cartlidge, N. (1972) Simulation and malingering after injuries to the brain and spinal cord. *Lancet* **i**, 580–585.

Mittenberg, W., DiGiulio, D.V. *et al.* (1992) Symptoms following mild head injury: expectation as aetiology. *Journal of Neurology, Neurosurgery and Psychiatry* **55**, 200–204.

Mittenberg, W., Tremont, G. *et al.* (1996) Cognitive-behavioral prevention of postconcussion syndrome. *Archives of Clinical Neuropsychology* **11**, 139–145.

Mittenberg, W., Wittner, M.S. *et al.* (1997) Postconcussion syndrome occurs in children. *Neuropsychology* **11**, 447–452.

Mittenberg, W., Patton, C. *et al.* (2002) Base rates of malingering and symptom exaggeration. *Journal of Clinical and Experimental Neuropsychology* **24**, 1094–1102.

Mittl, R.L., Grossman, R.I. *et al.* (1994) Prevalence of MR evidence of diffuse axonal injury in patients with mild head injury and normal head CT findings. *American Journal of Neuroradiology* **15**, 1583–1589.

Monji, A., Yoshida, I. *et al.* (1999) Brain injury-induced rapid-cycling affective disorder successfully treated with valproate. *Psychosomatics* **40**, 448–449.

Montgomery, A., Fenton, G.W. *et al.* (1984) Delayed brainstem conduction time in post-concussional syndrome. *Lancet* **i**, 1011.

Montgomery, E.A., Fenton, G.W. *et al.* (1991) The psychobiology of minor head injury. *Psychological Medicine* **21**, 375–384.

Morey, C.E., Cilo, M. *et al.* (2003) The effect of Aricept in persons with persistent memory disorder following traumatic brain injury: a pilot study. *Brain Injury* **17**, 809–815.

Moriarty, J., Collie, A. *et al.* (2004) A prospective controlled study of cognitive function during an amateur boxing tournament. *Neurology* **62**, 1497–1502.

Morris, P.G., Prior, L. *et al.* (2005) Patients' views on outcome following head injury: a qualitative study. *BMC Family Practice* **6**, 30.

Mortensen, P.B., Mors, O. *et al.* (2003) Head injury as a risk factor for bipolar affective disorder. *Journal of Affective Disorders* **76**, 79–83.

Mortimer, J.A., van Duijn, C.M. *et al.* (1991) Head trauma as a risk factor for Alzheimer's disease: a collaborative re-analysis of case-control studies. EURODEM Risk Factors Research Group. *International Journal of Epidemiology* **20** (suppl. 2), S28–S35.

Morton, M.V. & Wehman, P. (1995) Psychosocial and emotional sequelae of individuals with traumatic brain injury: a literature review and recommendations. *Brain Injury* **9**, 81–92.

Moser, R.S., Schatz, P. *et al.* (2005) Prolonged effects of concussion in high school athletes. *Neurosurgery* **57**, 300–306.

Muller, G.E. (1969) Early clinical history, EEG controls, and social outcome in 1,925 head injury patients. In: Walker, A.E., Caveness, W.F. & Critchley, M. (eds) *The Late Effects of Head Injury*, pp. 414–422. Charles C. Thomas, Springfield, IL.

Muller, U., Murai, T. *et al.* (1999) Paroxetine versus citalopram treatment of pathological crying after brain injury. *Brain Injury* **13**, 805–811.

Murai, T. & Fujimoto, S. (2003) Rapid cycling bipolar disorder after left temporal polar damage. *Brain Injury* **17**, 355–358.

Murdoch, I., Perry, E.K. *et al.* (1998) Cortical cholinergic dysfunction after human head injury. *Journal of Neurotrauma* **15**, 295–305.

Murdoch, I., Nicoll, J.A. *et al.* (2002) Nucleus basalis of Meynert pathology in the human brain after fatal head injury. *Journal of Neurotrauma* **19**, 279–284.

Murelius, O. & Haglund, Y. (1991) Does Swedish amateur boxing lead to chronic brain damage? 4. A retrospective neuropsychological study. *Acta Neurologica Scandinavica* **83**, 9–13.

Mustafa, B., Evrim, O. *et al.* (2005) Secondary mania following traumatic brain injury. *Journal of Neuropsychiatry and Clinical Neuroscience* **17**, 122–124.

Mutschler, D. (1956) Neurosebildende Faktoren bei Hirnverletzten. In: Rehwald, E. (ed.) *Das Hirntrauma*. Thieme, Stuttgart.

Nakayama, N., Okumura, A. *et al.* (2006) Relationship between regional cerebral metabolism and consciousness disturbance in traumatic diffuse brain injury without large focal lesions: an FDG-PET study with statistical parametric mapping analysis. *Journal of Neurology, Neurosurgery and Psychiatry* **77**, 856–862.

Nath, F.P., Beastal, G. et al. (1986) Alcohol and traumatic brain damage. *Injury* **17**, 150–153.

Nathoo, N., Narotam, P.K. et al. (2004) Influence of apoptosis on neurological outcome following traumatic cerebral contusion. *Journal of Neurosurgery* **101**, 233–240.

Naunheim, R.S., Ryden, A. et al. (2003) Does soccer headgear attenuate the impact when heading a soccer ball? *Academic Emergency Medicine* **10**, 85–90.

Newburn, G., Edwards, R. et al. (1999) Moclobemide in the treatment of major depressive disorder (DSM-3) following traumatic brain injury. *Brain Injury* **13**, 637–642.

Newcombe, F. (1969) *Missile Wounds of the Brain: A Study of Psychological Deficits*. Oxford University Press, Oxford.

Newcombe, F. (1996) Very late outcome after focal wartime brain wounds. *Journal of Clinical and Experimental Neuropsychology* **18**, 1–23.

Newman, P.K. (1990) Whiplash injury. *British Medical Journal* **301**, 395–396.

Newton, M.R., Greenwood, R.J. et al. (1992) A study comparing SPECT with CT and MRI after closed head injury. *Journal of Neurology, Neurosurgery and Psychiatry* **55**, 92–94.

Ng, I., Yeo, T.T. et al. (2000) Apoptosis occurs after cerebral contusions in humans. *Neurosurgery* **46**, 949–956.

Nielsen, A.S., Mortensen, P.B. et al. (2002) Is head injury a risk factor for schizophrenia? *Schizophrenia Research* **55**, 93–98.

Niess, C., Grauel, U. et al. (2002) Incidence of axonal injury in human brain tissue. *Acta Neuropathologica* **104**, 79–84.

Nirula, R., Mock, C. et al. (2003) Correlation of head injury to vehicle contact points using crash injury research and engineering network data. *Accident Analysis and Prevention* **35**, 201–210.

Norrman, B. & Svahn, K. (1961) A follow-up study of severe brain injuries. *Acta Psychiatrica Scandinavica* **37**, 236–264.

Nortje, J. & Menon, D.K. (2004) Traumatic brain injury: physiology, mechanisms, and outcome. *Current Opinion in Neurology* **17**, 711–718.

Novack, T.A., Bush, B.A. et al. (2001) Outcome after traumatic brain injury: pathway analysis of contributions from premorbid, injury severity, and recovery variables. *Archives of Physical Medicine and Rehabilitation* **82**, 300–305.

Nylander, I. & Rydelius, P.A. (1988) Post-concussion syndrome. Brain damage, constitutional characteristics and environmental reactions. *Acta Paediatrica Scandinavica* **77**, 475–477.

Obelieniene, D., Schrader, H. et al. (1999) Pain after whiplash: a prospective controlled inception cohort study. *Journal of Neurology, Neurosurgery and Psychiatry* **66**, 279–283.

O'Carroll, R.E., Woodrow, J. et al. (1991) Psychosexual and psychosocial sequelae of closed head injury. *Brain Injury* **5**, 303–313.

Oddy, M. & Humphrey, M. (1980) Social recovery during the year following severe head injury. *Journal of Neurology, Neurosurgery and Psychiatry* **43**, 798–802.

Ogai, M., Iyo, M. et al. (2005) A right orbitofrontal region and OCD symptoms: a case report. *Acta Psychiatrica Scandinavica* **111**, 74–76; discussion 76–77.

Olver, J.H., Ponsford, J.L. et al. (1996) Outcome following traumatic brain injury: a comparison between 2 and 5 years after injury. *Brain Injury* **10**, 841–848.

O'Meara, E.S., Kukull, W.A. et al. (1997) Head injury and risk of Alzheimer's disease by apolipoprotein E genotype. *American Journal of Epidemiology* **146**, 373–384.

Ommaya, A.K. & Gennarelli, T.A. (1974) Cerebral concussion and traumatic unconsciousness. Correlation of experimental and clinical observations of blunt head injuries. *Brain* **97**, 633–654.

Ommaya, A.K., Faas, F. et al. (1968) Whiplash injury and brain damage. An experimental study. *Journal of the American Medical Association* **204**, 285–289.

Oppenheimer, D. (1968) Microscopic lesions in the brain following head injury. *Journal of Experimental Neurology* **26**, 77–84.

Oquendo, M.A., Friedman, J.H. et al. (2004) Suicidal behavior and mild traumatic brain injury in major depression. *Journal of Nervous and Mental Disease* **192**, 430–434.

Ota, Y. (1969) Psychiatric studies on civilian head injuries. In: Walker, A.E., Caveness, W.F. & Critchley, M. (eds) *The Late Effects of Head Injury*, ch. 9. Charles C. Thomas, Springfield, IL.

Otte, A., Ettlin, T.M. et al. (1997) PET and SPECT in whiplash syndrome: a new approach to a forgotten brain? *Journal of Neurology, Neurosurgery and Psychiatry* **63**, 368–372.

Overgaard, J. & Tweed, W.A. (1974) Cerebral circulation after head injury. Part 1. Cerebral blood flow and its regulation after closed head injury with emphasis on clinical correlations. *Journal of Neurosurgery* **41**, 531–541.

Overweg-Plandsoen, W.C., Kodde, A. et al. (1999) Mild closed head injury in children compared to traumatic fractured bone: neurobehavioural sequelae in daily life 2 years after the accident. *European Journal of Pediatrics* **158**, 249–252.

Packard, R.C. (1999) Epidemiology and pathogenesis of post-traumatic headache. *Journal of Head Trauma Rehabilitation* **14**, 9–21.

Pang, A. & Lewis, S.W. (1996) Bipolar affective disorder minus left prefrontal cortex equals schizophrenia. *British Journal of Psychiatry* **168**, 647–650.

Paniak, C., Toller-Lobe, G. et al. (2000) A randomized trial of two treatments for mild traumatic brain injury: 1 year follow-up. *Brain Injury* **14**, 219–226.

Paniak, C., Reynolds, S. et al. (2002a) A longitudinal study of the relationship between financial compensation and symptoms after treated mild traumatic brain injury. *Journal of Clinical and Experimental Neuropsychology* **24**, 187–193.

Paniak, C., Reynolds, S. et al. (2002b) Patient complaints within 1 month of mild traumatic brain injury: a controlled study. *Archives of Clinical Neuropsychology* **17**, 319–334.

Park, N.W. & Ingles, J.L. (2001) Effectiveness of attention rehabilitation after an acquired brain injury: a meta-analysis. *Neuropsychology* **15**, 199–210.

Parker, S.A. & Serrats, A.F. (1976) Memory recovery after traumatic coma. *Acta Neurochirurgica* **34**, 71–77.

Pearce, J.M.S. (1989) Whiplash injury: a reappraisal. *Journal of Neurology, Neurosurgery and Psychiatry* **52**, 1329–1331.

Pelinka, L.E., Kroepfl, A. et al. (2004) GFAP versus S100B in serum after traumatic brain injury: relationship to brain damage and outcome. *Journal of Neurotrauma* **21**, 1553–1561.

Pellman, E.J., Viano, D.C. et al. (2003) Concussion in professional football: reconstruction of game impacts and injuries. *Neurosurgery* **53**, 799–812; discussion 812–814.

Pennings, J.L., Bachulis, B.L. et al. (1993) Survival after severe brain injury in the aged. *Archives of Surgery* **128**, 787–793; discussion 793–794.

Pentland, B., Jones, P.A. et al. (1986) Head injury in the elderly. *Age and Ageing* **15**, 193–202.

Pentland, B., Hutton, L.S. *et al.* (2005) Late mortality after head injury. *Journal of Neurology, Neurosurgery and Psychiatry* **76**, 395–400.

Phelps, C. (1898) *Traumatic Injuries of the Brain and its Membranes.* Kimpton, London.

Pickard, J.D., Coleman, M.R. *et al.* (2005) Hydrocephalus, ventriculomegaly and the vegetative state: a review. *Neuropsychological Rehabilitation* **15**, 224–236.

Pierallini, A., Pantano, P. *et al.* (2000) Correlation between MRI findings and long-term outcome in patients with severe brain trauma. *Neuroradiology* **42**, 860–867.

Piercy, M. (1964) The effects of cerebral lesions on intellectual function: a review of current research trends. *British Journal of Psychiatry* **110**, 310–352.

Pilowsky, Y., I. (1985) Cryptotrauma and 'accident neurosis'. *British Journal of Psychiatry* **147**, 310–311.

Plassman, B.L., Havlik, R.J. *et al.* (2000) Documented head injury in early adulthood and risk of Alzheimer's disease and other dementias. *Neurology* **55**, 1158–1166.

Plenger, P.M., Dixon, C.E. *et al.* (1996) Subacute methylphenidate treatment for moderate to moderately severe traumatic brain injury: a preliminary double-blind placebo-controlled study. *Archives of Physical Medicine and Rehabilitation* **77**, 536–540.

Pobereskin, L.H. (2005) Whiplash following rear end collisions: a prospective cohort study. *Journal of Neurology, Neurosurgery and Psychiatry* **76**, 1146–1151.

Ponsford, J. & Kinsella, G. (1992) Attentional deficits following closed-head injury. *Journal of Clinical and Experimental Neuropsychology* **14**, 822–838.

Ponsford, J., Willmott, C. *et al.* (1999) Cognitive and behavioral outcome following mild traumatic head injury in children. *Journal of Head Trauma Rehabilitation* **14**, 360–372.

Ponsford, J., Willmott, C. *et al.* (2000) Factors influencing outcome following mild traumatic brain injury in adults. *Journal of the International Neuropsychological Society* **6**, 568–579.

Ponsford, J., Willmott, C. *et al.* (2002) Impact of early intervention on outcome following mild head injury in adults. *Journal of Neurology, Neurosurgery and Psychiatry* **73**, 330–332.

Ponsford, J., Olver, J. *et al.* (2003) Long-term adjustment of families following traumatic brain injury where comprehensive rehabilitation has been provided. *Brain Injury* **17**, 453–468.

Porter, M.D. (2003) A 9-year controlled prospective neuropsychologic assessment of amateur boxing. *Clinical Journal of Sport Medicine* **13**, 339–352.

Porter, M.D. & Fricker, P.A. (1996) Controlled prospective neuropsychological assessment of active experienced amateur boxers. *Clinical Journal of Sport Medicine* **6**, 90–96.

Povlishock, J.T. & Coburn, T.H. (1989) Morphopathological change associated with mild head injury. In: Levin, H.S., Eisenberg, H.M. & Benton, A.L. (eds) *Mild Head Injury*, pp. 37–53. Oxford University Press, New York.

Povlishock, J.T. & Katz, D.I. (2005) Update of neuropathology and neurological recovery after traumatic brain injury. *Journal of Head Trauma Rehabilitation* **20**, 76–94.

Powell, J., Heslin, J. *et al.* (2002) Community based rehabilitation after severe traumatic brain injury: a randomised controlled trial. *Journal of Neurology, Neurosurgery and Psychiatry* **72**, 193–202.

Powell, J.H., al-Adawi, S. *et al.* (1996) Motivational deficits after brain injury: effects of bromocriptine in 11 patients. *Journal of Neurology, Neurosurgery and Psychiatry* **60**, 416–421.

Powell, J.W. & Barber-Foss, K.D. (1999) Traumatic brain injury in high school athletes. *Journal of the American Medical Association* **282**, 958–963.

Prasad, M.R., Ewing-Cobbs, L. *et al.* (2002) Predictors of outcome following traumatic brain injury in young children. *Pediatric Neurosurgery* **36**, 64–74.

Prigatano, G.P., Fordyce, D.J. *et al.* (1984) Neuropsychological rehabilitation after closed head injury in young adults. *Journal of Neurology, Neurosurgery and Psychiatry* **47**, 505–513.

Ptak, T., Sheridan, R.L. *et al.* (2003) Cerebral fractional anisotropy score in trauma patients: a new indicator of white matter injury after trauma. *American Journal of Roentgenology* **181**, 1401–1407.

Pudenz, R.H. & Shelden, C.H. (1946) The lucite calvarium: a method for direct observation of the brain. *Journal of Neurosurgery* **3**, 487–505.

Qiu, J., Whalen, M.J. *et al.* (2002) Upregulation of the Fas receptor death-inducing signaling complex after traumatic brain injury in mice and humans. *Journal of Neuroscience* **22**, 3504–3511.

Raabe, A. & Seifert, V. (2000) Protein S-100B as a serum marker of brain damage in severe head injury: preliminary results. *Neurosurgical Review* **23**, 136–138.

Radanov, B.P., Sturzenegger, M. *et al.* (1994a) Relationship between early somatic radiological, cognitive and psychosocial findings and outcome during a one-year follow-up in 117 patients suffering from common whiplash. *British Journal of Rheumatology* **33**, 442–448.

Radanov, B.P., Di Stefano, G. *et al.* (1994b) Common whiplash: psychosomatic or somatopsychic? *Journal of Neurology, Neurosurgery and Psychiatry* **57**, 486–490.

Radanov, B.P., Bicik, I. *et al.* (1999) Relation between neuropsychological and neuroimaging findings in patients with late whiplash syndrome. *Journal of Neurology, Neurosurgery and Psychiatry* **66**, 485–489.

Raffle, P.A.B. (1989) Interrelation between alcohol and accidents. *Journal of the Royal Society of Medicine* **82**, 132–138.

Raisanen, J., Ghougassian, D.F. *et al.* (1999) Diffuse axonal injury in a rugby player. *American Journal of Forensic Medicine and Pathology* **20**, 70–72.

Rapoport, M.J., McCullagh, S. *et al.* (2003) The clinical significance of major depression following mild traumatic brain injury. *Psychosomatics* **44**, 31–37.

Rapoport, M.J., McCullagh, S. *et al.* (2005) Cognitive impairment associated with major depression following mild and moderate traumatic brain injury. *Journal of Neuropsychiatry and Clinical Neuroscience* **17**, 61–65.

Ravdin, L.D., Barr, W.B. *et al.* (2003) Assessment of cognitive recovery following sports related head trauma in boxers. *Clinical Journal of Sport Medicine* **13**, 21–27.

Reider-Groswasser, I., Cohen, M. *et al.* (1993) Late CT findings in brain trauma: relationship to cognitive and behavioral sequelae and to vocational outcome. *American Journal of Roentgenology* **160**, 147–152.

Richter, M., Ferrari, R. *et al.* (2004) Correlation of clinical findings, collision parameters, and psychological factors in the outcome of whiplash associated disorders. *Journal of Neurology, Neurosurgery and Psychiatry* **75**, 758–764.

Ricker, J.H., Muller, R.A. *et al.* (2001) Verbal recall and recognition following traumatic brain injury: a ^{15}O-water positron emission tomography study. *Journal of Clinical and Experimental Neuropsychology* **23**, 196–206.

Roberts, A.H. (1969) *Brain Damage in Boxers*. Pitman, London.

Roberts, A.H. (1976) Sequelae of closed head injuries. *Proceedings of the Royal Society of Medicine* **69**, 137–141.

Roberts, A.H. (1979) *Severe Accidental Head Injury: An Assessment of Long-term Prognosis*. Macmillan, London.

Roberts, G.W., Allsop, D. *et al.* (1990) The occult aftermath of boxing. *Journal of Neurology, Neurosurgery and Psychiatry* **53**, 373–378.

Roberts, G.W., Gentleman, S.M. *et al.* (1994) Beta amyloid protein deposition in the brain after severe head injury: implications for the pathogenesis of Alzheimer's disease. *Journal of Neurology, Neurosurgery and Psychiatry* **57**, 419–425.

Robertson, C.L. (2004) Mitochondrial dysfunction contributes to cell death following traumatic brain injury in adult and immature animals. *Journal of Bioenergetics and Biomembranes* **36**, 363–368.

Rolls, E.T., Hornak, J. *et al.* (1994) Emotion-related learning in patients with social and emotional changes associated with frontal lobe damage. *Journal of Neurology, Neurosurgery and Psychiatry* **57**, 1518–1524.

Roncadin, C., Guger, S. *et al.* (2004) Working memory after mild, moderate, or severe childhood closed head injury. *Developmental Neuropsychology* **25**, 21–36.

Rönty, H., Ahonen, A. *et al.* (1993) Cerebral trauma and alcohol abuse. *European Journal of Clinical Investigation* **23**, 182–187.

Rosenbaum, M. & Najenson, T. (1976) Changes in life patterns and symptoms of low mood as reported by wives of severly brain-injured soldiers. *Journal of Consulting and Clinical Psychology* **44**, 881–888.

Rothoerl, R.D., Woertgen, C. *et al.* (2000) S-100 serum levels and outcome after severe head injury. *Acta Neurochirurgica Supplementum* **76**, 97–100.

Rudelli, R., Strom, J.O. *et al.* (1982) Post traumatic premature Alzheimer's disease. *Archives of Neurology* **39**, 570–575.

Ruesch, J. & Bowman, K.M. (1945) Prolonged post-traumatic syndromes following head injury. *American Journal of Psychiatry* **102**, 145–163.

Ruff, R. (2005) Two decades of advances in understanding of mild traumatic brain injury. *Journal of Head Trauma Rehabilitation* **20**, 5–18.

Ruff, R.M., Buchsbaum, M.S. *et al.* (1989) Computerized tomography, neuropsychology, and positron emission tomography in the evaluation of head injury. *Neuropsychiatry, Neuropsychology, and Behavioral Neurology* **2**, 103–123.

Ruff, R.M., Young, D., Gautille, T. *et al.* (1991) Verbal learning deficits following severe brain injury: heterogeneity in recovery over 1 year. *Journal of Neurosurgery* **75**, S50–S58.

Ruff, R.M., Crouch, J.A. *et al.* (1994) Selected cases of poor outcome following a minor brain trauma: comparing neuropsychological and positron emission tomography assessment. *Brain Injury* **8**, 297–308.

Ruff, R.M., Mueller, J. *et al.* (1996a) Estimation of premorbid functioning after traumatic brain injury. *NeuroRehabilitation* **7**, 39–53.

Ruff, R.M., Camenzuli, L. *et al.* (1996b) Miserable minority: emotional risk factors that influence the outcome of a mild traumatic brain injury. *Brain Injury* **10**, 551–565.

Ruffolo, C.F., Friedland, J.F. *et al.* (1999) Mild traumatic brain injury from motor vehicle accidents: factors associated with return to work. *Archives of Physical Medicine and Rehabilitation* **80**, 392–398.

Rugg-Gunn, F.J., Symms, M.R. *et al.* (2001) Diffusion imaging shows abnormalities after blunt head trauma when conventional magnetic resonance imaging is normal. *Journal of Neurology, Neurosurgery and Psychiatry* **70**, 530–533.

Rush, B., Malec, J. *et al.* (2004) Preinjury personality traits and the prediction of early neurobehavioral symptoms following mild traumatic brain injury. *Rehabilitation Psychology* **49**, 275–281.

Russell, W.R. (1932) Cerebral involvement in head injury. *Brain* **55**, 549–603.

Russell, W.R. (1935) Amnesia following head injuries. *Lancet* **ii**, 762–763.

Russell, W.R. (1951) Disability caused by brain wounds. *Journal of Neurology, Neurosurgery and Psychiatry* **14**, 35–39.

Russell, W.R. & Nathan, P.W. (1946) Traumatic amnesia. *Brain* **69**, 280–300.

Russell, W.R. & Schiller, F. (1949) Crushing injuries to the skull. *Journal of Neurology, Neurosurgery and Psychiatry* **12**, 52–60.

Russell, W.R. & Smith, A. (1961) Post-traumatic amnesia in closed head injury. *Archives of Neurology* **5**, 4–17.

Rutherfoord, G.S., Dada, M.A. *et al.* (1996) Cerebral infarction and intracranial arterial dissection in closed head injury. *American Journal of Forensic Medicine and Pathology* **17**, 53–57.

Rutherford, W.H. (1989) Postconcussion symptoms: relationship to acute neurological indices, individual differences, and circumstances of injury. In: Levin, H.S., Eisenberg, H.M. & Benton, A.L. (eds) *Mild Head Injury*, ch. 14. Oxford University Press, Oxford.

Rutherford, W.H., Merrett, J.D. *et al.* (1977) Sequelae of concussion caused by minor head injuries. *Lancet* **i**, 1–4.

Rutherford, W.H., Merrett, J.D. *et al.* (1979) Symptoms at one year following concussion from minor head injuries. *Injury* **10**, 225–230.

Rutter, M. (1993) An overview of developmental neuropsychiatry. In: Besag, F.M. & Williams, R.T. (eds) *The Brain and Behaviour: Organic Influences on the Behaviour of Children*. Educational and Child Psychology, pp. 4–11. Special supplement to *Educational and Child Psychology*, **10**.

Ryan, L.M. & Warden, D.L. (2003) Post concussion syndrome. *International Review of Psychiatry* **15**, 310–316.

Sachdev, P., Smith, J.S. *et al.* (2001) Schizophrenia-like psychosis following traumatic brain injury: a chart-based descriptive and case-control study. Psychological Medicine **31**, 231–239.

Salazar, A.M., Grafman, J. *et al.* (1987) Epilepsy and cognitive loss after penetrating head injury. *Advances in Epileptology* **16**, 627–631.

Salazar, A.M., Warden, D.L. *et al.* (2000) Cognitive rehabilitation for traumatic brain injury: a randomized trial. Defense and Veterans Head Injury Program (DVHIP) Study Group. *Journal of the American Medical Association* **283**, 3075–3081.

Salmond, C.H., Chatfield, D.A. *et al.* (2005) Cognitive sequelae of head injury: involvement of basal forebrain and associated structures. *Brain* **128**, 189–200.

Sander, A.M., High, W.M. Jr *et al.* (1997) Predictors of psychological health in caregivers of patients with closed head injury. *Brain Injury* **11**, 235–249.

Sarapata, M., Herrmann, D. *et al.* (1998) The role of head injury in cognitive functioning, emotional adjustment and criminal behaviour. *Brain Injury* **12**, 821–842.

Satz, P. (1993) Brain reserve capacity and symptom onset after brain injury: a formulation and review of evidence for threshold theory. *Neuropsychology* **7**, 273–295.

Savola, O. & Hillbom, M. (2003) Early predictors of post-concussion symptoms in patients with mild head injury. *European Journal of Neurology* **10**, 175–181.

Savola, O., Pyhtinen, J. *et al.* (2004) Effects of head and extracranial injuries on serum protein S100B levels in trauma patients. *Journal of Trauma* **56**, 1229–1234; discussion 1234.

Savola, O., Niemela, O. *et al.* (2005) Alcohol intake and the pattern of trauma in young adults and working aged people admitted after trauma. *Alcohol and Alcoholism* **40**, 269–273.

Schaefer, P.W., Huisman, T.A. *et al.* (2004) Diffusion-weighted MR imaging in closed head injury: high correlation with initial Glasgow Coma Scale score and score on modified Rankin scale at discharge. *Radiology* **233**, 58–66.

Scheibel, R.S., Pearson, D.A. *et al.* (2003) An fMRI study of executive functioning after severe diffuse TBI. *Brain Injury* **17**, 919–930.

Scheid, R., Preul, C. *et al.* (2003) Diffuse axonal injury associated with chronic traumatic brain injury: evidence from T2-weighted gradient-echo imaging at 3 T. *American Journal of Neuroradiology* **24**, 1049–1056.

Scheid, R., Walther, K. *et al.* (2006) Cognitive sequelae of diffuse axonal injury. *Archives of Neurology* **63**, 418–424.

Schierhout, G. & Roberts, I. (1998) Prophylactic antiepileptic agents after head injury: a systematic review. *Journal of Neurology, Neurosurgery and Psychiatry* **64**, 108–112.

Schmand, B., Lindeboom, J. *et al.* (1998) Cognitive complaints in patients after whiplash injury: the impact of malingering. *Journal of Neurology, Neurosurgery and Psychiatry* **64**, 339–343.

Schmidt, O.I., Heyde, C.E. *et al.* (2005) Closed head injury: an inflammatory disease? *Brain Research Reviews* **48**, 388–399.

Schretlen, D.J. & Shapiro, A.M. (2003) A quantitative review of the effects of traumatic brain injury on cognitive functioning. *International Review of Psychiatry* **15**, 341–349.

Schwartz, L., Taylor, H.G. *et al.* (2003) Long-term behavior problems following pediatric traumatic brain injury: prevalence, predictors, and correlates. *Journal of Pediatric Psychology* **28**, 251–263.

Seel, R.T., Kreutzer, J.S. *et al.* (2003) Depression after traumatic brain injury: a National Institute on Disability and Rehabilitation Research Model Systems multicenter investigation. *Archives of Physical Medicine and Rehabilitation* **84**, 177–184.

Selzer, M.L., Rogers, J.E. *et al.* (1968) Fatal accidents: the role of psychopathology, social stress, and acute disturbances. *American Journal of Psychiatry* **124**, 1028–1036.

Servadei, F., Teasdale, G. *et al.* (2001) Defining acute mild head injury in adults: a proposal based on prognostic factors, diagnosis, and management. *Journal of Neurotrauma* **18**, 657–664.

Shallice, T. & Burgess, P.W. (1991) Deficits in strategy application following frontal lobe damage in man. *Brain* **114**, 727–741.

Shanmuganathan, K., Gullapalli, R.P. *et al.* (2004) Whole-brain apparent diffusion coefficient in traumatic brain injury: correlation with Glasgow Coma Scale score. *American Journal of Neuroradiology* **25**, 539–544.

Sharma, P., Dahiya, R.S. *et al.* (2001) How important is history of unconsciousness in head injury patients? *Journal of the Indian Medical Association* **99**, 81–83.

Sherer, M., Sander, A.M. *et al.* (2002) Early cognitive status and productivity outcome after traumatic brain injury: findings from the TBI model systems. *Archives of Physical Medicine and Rehabilitation* **83**, 183–192.

Sherman, E.M., Strauss, E. *et al.* (2000) Effect of depression on neuropsychological functioning in head injury: measurable but minimal. *Brain Injury* **14**, 621–632.

Shores, E.A., Marosszeky, J.E. *et al.* (1986) Preliminary validation of a clinical scale for measuring the duration of post-traumatic amnesia. *Medical Journal of Australia* **144**, 569–572.

Shukla, S., Cook, B.L. *et al.* (1987) Mania following head trauma. *American Journal of Psychiatry* **144**, 93–96.

Sieghart, M.A. (2000) What they didn't tell you about mild head injury. *The Times*, 21 March 2000, 12–13.

Signorini, D.F., Andrews, P.J. *et al.* (1999a) Adding insult to injury: the prognostic value of early secondary insults for survival after traumatic brain injury. *Journal of Neurology, Neurosurgery and Psychiatry* **66**, 26–31.

Signorini, D.F., Andrews, P.J. *et al.* (1999b) Predicting survival using simple clinical variables: a case study in traumatic brain injury. *Journal of Neurology, Neurosurgery and Psychiatry* **66**, 20–25.

Silver, B.V. & Yablon, S.A. (1996) Akathisia resulting from traumatic brain injury. *Brain Injury* **10**, 609–614.

Silver, J.M., Kramer, R. *et al.* (2001) The association between head injuries and psychiatric disorders: findings from the New Haven NIMH Epidemiologic Catchment Area Study. *Brain Injury* **15**, 935–945.

Silver, J.M., Yudofsky, S.C. *et al.* (2005) Aggressive disorders. In: Silver, J.M., McAllister, T.W. & Yudofsky, S.C. (eds) *Textbook of Traumatic Brain Injury*, pp. 259–278. American Psychiatric Publishing Inc., Washington, DC.

Silver, J.M., Koumaras, B. *et al.* (2006) Effects of rivastigmine on cognitive function in patients with traumatic brain injury. *Neurology* **67**, 748–755.

Silverman, M. (1964) Organic stupor subsequent to a severe head injury treated with ECT. *British Journal of Psychiatry* **110**, 648–650.

Silvey, J.M., Arciniegas, D.B. *et al.* (2005) Psychopharmacology. In: Silver, J.M., McAllister, T.W. & Yudofsky, S.C. (eds) *Textbook of Traumatic Brain Injury*, pp. 609–640. American Psychiatric Publishing Inc., Washington, DC.

Simpson, G. & Tate, R. (2002) Suicidality after traumatic brain injury: demographic, injury and clinical correlates. *Psychological Medicine* **32**, 687–697.

Simpson, G. & Tate, R. (2005) Clinical features of suicide attempts after traumatic brain injury. *Journal of Nervous and Mental Disease* **193**, 680–685.

Simpson, G., Blaszczynski, A. *et al.* (1999) Sex offending as a psychosocial sequela of traumatic brain injury. *Journal of Head Trauma Rehabilitation* **14**, 567–580.

Simpson, G., McCann, B. *et al.* (2003) Treatment of premature ejaculation after traumatic brain injury. *Brain Injury* **17**, 723–729.

Sinson, G., Bagley, L.J. *et al.* (2001) Magnetization transfer imaging and proton MR spectroscopy in the evaluation of axonal injury: correlation with clinical outcome after traumatic brain injury. *American Journal of Neuroradiology* **22**, 143–151.

Slater, E. (1943) The neurotic constitution: a statistical study of 2000 neurotic soldiers. *Journal of Neurology and Psychiatry* **6**, 1–16.

Sloan, R.L., Brown, K.W. *et al.* (1992) Fluoxetine as a treatment for emotional lability after brain injury. *Brain Injury* **6**, 315–319.

Slomine, B.S., Gerring, J.P. *et al.* (2002) Performance on measures of executive function following pediatric traumatic brain injury. *Brain Injury* **16**, 759–772.

Smith, A. (1961) Duration of impaired consciousness as an index of severity in closed head injuries: a review. *Diseases of the Nervous System* **2**, 69–74.

Smith, D.H. & Meaney, D.F. (2000) Axonal damage in traumatic brain injury. *The Neuroscientist* **6**, 483–495.

Smith, F.M., Raghupathi, R. *et al.* (2000) TUNEL-positive staining of surface contusions after fatal head injury in man. *Acta Neuropathologica* **100**, 537–545.

Smith-Seemiller, L., Fow, N.R. *et al.* (2003) Presence of post-concussion syndrome symptoms in patients with chronic pain vs mild traumatic brain injury. *Brain Injury* **17**, 199–206.

Sonne, N.M. & Tonnesen, H. (1992) The influence of alcoholism on outcome after evacuation of subdural haematoma. *British Journal of Neurosurgery* **6**, 125–130.

Sorenson, S.B. & Kraus, J.F. (1991) Occurrence, severity, and outcomes of brain injury. *Journal of Head Trauma Rehabilitation* **6**, 1–10.

Spielberger, C.D. (1983) *Manual for the State-Trait Anxiety Inventory (STAI)*. Consulting Psychologists Press, Palo Alto, CA.

Spikman, J.M., van Zomeren, A.H. *et al.* (1996) Deficits of attention after closed-head injury: slowness only? *Journal of Clinical and Experimental Neuropsychology* **18**, 755–767.

Stalnacke, B.M., Bjornstig, U. *et al.* (2005) One-year follow-up of mild traumatic brain injury: post-concussion symptoms, disabilities and life satisfaction in relation to serum levels of S-100B and neurone-specific enolase in acute phase. *Journal of Rehabilitation Medicine* **37**, 300–305.

Stamatakis, E.A., Wilson, J.T. *et al.* (2002) SPECT imaging in head injury interpreted with statistical parametric mapping. *Journal of Nuclear Medicine* **43**, 476–483.

Stanton, B.R. (1999) Does family functioning affect outcome in children with neurological disorders? *Pediatric Rehabilitation* **3**, 193–199.

Stapert, S., de Kruijk, J. *et al.* (2005) S-100B concentration is not related to neurocognitive performance in the first month after mild traumatic brain injury. *European Neurology* **53**, 22–26.

Starkstein, S.E., Boston, J.D. *et al.* (1988) Mechanisms of mania after brain injury: 12 case reports and review of the literature. *Journal of Nervous and Mental Disease* **176**, 87–100.

Steadman, J.H. & Graham, J.G. (1970) Head injuries: an analysis and follow-up study. *Proceedings of the Royal Society of Medicine* **63**, 23–28.

Stranjalis, G., Korfias, S. *et al.* (2004) Elevated serum S-100B protein as a predictor of failure to short-term return to work or activities after mild head injury. *Journal of Neurotrauma* **21**, 1070–1075.

Strauss, E., Hultsch, D.F. *et al.* (1999) Using intraindividual variability to detect malingering in cognitive performance. *Clinical Neuropsychology* **13**, 420–432.

Streeter, C.C., Van Reekum, R. *et al.* (1995) Prior head injury in male veterans with borderline personality disorder. *Journal of Nervous and Mental Disease* **183**, 577–581.

Strich, S.J. (1956) Diffuse degeneration of the cerebral white matter in severe dementia following head injury. *Journal of Neurology, Neurosurgery and Psychiatry* **19**, 163–185.

Strich, S.J. (1969) The pathology of brain damage due to blunt head injuries. In: Walker, A.E., Caveness, W.F. & Critchley, M.T. (eds) *The Late Effects of Head Injury*, ch. 51. Charles C. Thomas, Springfield, IL.

Stuart, M.J., Smith, A.M. *et al.* (2002) A comparison of facial protection and the incidence of head, neck, and facial injuries in Junior A hockey players. A function of individual playing time. *American Journal of Sports Medicine* **30**, 39–44.

Stuss, D.T., Stethem, L.L. *et al.* (1989) Reaction time after head injury: fatigue, divided and focused attention, and consistency of performance. *Journal of Neurology, Neurosurgery and Psychiatry* **52**, 742–748.

Stuss, D.T., Binns, M.A. *et al.* (1999) The acute period of recovery from traumatic brain injury: posttraumatic amnesia or posttraumatic confusional state? *Journal of Neurosurgery* **90**, 635–643.

Stuss, D.T., Binns, M.A. *et al.* (2000) Prediction of recovery of continuous memory after traumatic brain injury. *Neurology* **54**, 1337–1344.

Sullivan, E.V. & Corkin, S. (1984) Selective subject attrition in a longitudinal study of head-injured veterans. *Journal of Gerontology* **39**, 718–720.

Sumpter, R.E. & McMillan, T.M. (2005) Misdiagnosis of post-traumatic stress disorder following severe traumatic brain injury. *British Journal of Psychiatry* **186**, 423–426.

Sundstrom, A., Marklund, P. *et al.* (2004) APOE influences on neuropsychological function after mild head injury: within-person comparisons. *Neurology* **62**, 1963–1966.

Swanson, S.J., Rao, S.M. *et al.* (1995) The relationship between seizure subtype and interictal personality. Results from the Vietnam Head Injury Study. *Brain* **118**, 91–103.

Symms, M., Jager, H.R. *et al.* (2004) A review of structural magnetic resonance neuroimaging. *Journal of Neurology, Neurosurgery and Psychiatry* **75**, 1235–1244.

Symonds, C.P. (1937) Mental disorder following head injury. *Proceedings of the Royal Society of Medicine* **30**, 1081–1092.

Symonds, C.P. (1962) Concussion and its sequelae. *Lancet* **i**, 1–5.

Symonds, C.P. & Russell, W.R. (1943) Accidental head injuries. *Lancet* **i**, 7–10.

Takaoka, M., Tabuse, H. *et al.* (2002) Semiquantitative analysis of corpus callosum injury using magnetic resonance imaging indicates clinical severity in patients with diffuse axonal injury. *Journal of Neurology, Neurosurgery and Psychiatry* **73**, 289–293.

Tarsh, M.J. & Royston, C. (1985) A follow-up study of accident neurosis. *British Journal of Psychiatry* **146**, 18–25.

Tasci, A., Okay, O. *et al.* (2003) Prognostic value of interleukin-1 beta levels after acute brain injury. *Neurological Research* **25**, 871–874.

Tate, R.L. (1998) It is not only the kind of injury that matters, but the kind of head: the contribution of premorbid psychosocial factors to rehabilitation outcomes after severe traumatic brain injury. *Neuropsychological Rehabilitation* **8**, 1–18.

Tate, R.L. (1999) Executive dysfunction and characterological changes after traumatic brain injury: two sides of the same coin? *Cortex* **35**, 39–55.

Tate, R.L. & Broe, G.A. (1999) Psychosocial adjustment after traumatic brain injury: what are the important variables? *Psychological Medicine* **29**, 713–725.

Tate, R.L., Simpson, G.K. *et al.* (1997) Completed suicide after traumatic brain injury. *Journal of Head Trauma Rehabilitation* **12**, 16–28.

Tate, R.L., Pfaff, A. *et al.* (2000) Resolution of disorientation and amnesia during post-traumatic amnesia. *Journal of Neurology, Neurosurgery and Psychiatry* **68**, 178–185.

Tate, R.L., Pfaff, A. *et al.* (2006) A multicentre, randomised trial examining the effect of test procedures measuring emergence from post-traumatic amnesia. *Journal of Neurology, Neurosurgery and Psychiatry* **77**, 841–849.

Tateno, A., Jorge, R.E. *et al.* (2003) Clinical correlates of aggressive behavior after traumatic brain injury. *Journal of Neuropsychiatry and Clinical Neuroscience* **15**, 155–160.

Tatrow, K., Blanchard, E.B. *et al.* (2003) Posttraumatic headache: biopsychosocial comparisons with multiple control groups. *Headache* **43**, 755–766.

Taylor, H.G. & Alden, J. (1997) Age-related differences in outcomes following childhood brain insults: an introduction and overview. *Journal of the International Neuropsychological Society* **3**, 555–567.

Taylor, H.G., Yeates, K.O. *et al.* (1999) Influences on first-year recovery from traumatic brain injury in children. *Neuropsychology* **13**, 76–89.

Taylor, H.G., Yeates, K.O. *et al.* (2002) A prospective study of short- and long-term outcomes after traumatic brain injury in children: behavior and achievement. *Neuropsychology* **16**, 15–27.

Teasdale, G. & Jennett, B. (1974) Assessment of coma and impaired consciousness: a practical scale. *Lancet* **ii**, 81–84.

Teasdale, G. & Mendelow, D. (1984) Pathophysiology of head injuries. In: Brooks, N. (ed.) *Closed Head Injury. Psychological, Social and Family Consequences*, ch. 2. Oxford University Press, Oxford.

Teasdale, G.M., Murray, G.D. *et al.* (2005) The association between APOE epsilon4, age and outcome after head injury: a prospective cohort study. *Brain* **128**, 2556–2561.

Teasdale, T.W. & Engberg, A.W. (2001) Suicide after traumatic brain injury: a population study. *Journal of Neurology, Neurosurgery and Psychiatry* **71**, 436–440.

Teasdale, T.W. & Engberg, A.W. (2003) Cognitive dysfunction in young men following head injury in childhood and adolescence: a population study. *Journal of Neurology, Neurosurgery and Psychiatry* **74**, 933–936.

Teitelman, E. (2001) Off-label uses of modafinil. *American Journal of Psychiatry* **158**, 1341.

Temkin, N.R., Holubkov, R. *et al.* (1995) Classification and regression trees (CART) for prediction of function at 1 year following head trauma. *Journal of Neurosurgery* **82**, 764–771.

Tennent, T. (1937) Discussion on mental disorder following head injury. *Proceedings of the Royal Society of Medicine* **30**, 1092–1093.

Tenovuo, O. (2005) Central acetylcholinesterase inhibitors in the treatment of chronic traumatic brain injury-clinical experience in 111 patients. *Progress in Neuropsychopharmacology and Biological Psychiatry* **29**, 61–67.

Teuber, H.-L. (1959) Some alterations in behaviour after cerebral lesions in man. In: Bass, A.D. (ed.) *Evolution of Nervous Control*, pp. 157–194. American Association for the Advancement of Science, Washington, DC.

Teuber, H.-L. (1962) Effects of brain wounds implicating right or left hemisphere in man. In: Mountcastle, V.B. (ed.) *Interhemi-spheric Relations and Cerebral Dominance*, pp. 131–157. Johns Hopkins Press, Baltimore.

Thompson, D.C., Rivara, F.P. *et al.* (2000) Helmets for preventing head and facial injuries in bicyclists. *Cochrane Database of Systematic Reviews* 2, CD001855.

Thomsen, I.V. (1974) The patient with severe head injury and his family: a follow-up study of 50 patients. *Scandinavian Journal of Rehabilitation Medicine* **6**, 180–183.

Thomsen, I.V. (1984) Late outcome of very severe blunt head trauma: a 10–15 year second follow-up. *Journal of Neurology, Neurosurgery and Psychiatry* **47**, 260–268.

Thornhill, S., Teasdale, G.M. *et al.* (2000) Disability in young people and adults one year after head injury: prospective cohort study. *British Medical Journal* **320**, 1631–1635.

Thurman, D. & Guerrero, J. (1999) Trends in hospitalization associated with traumatic brain injury. *Journal of the American Medical Association* **282**, 954–957.

Tiersky, L.A., Anselmi, V. *et al.* (2005) A trial of neuropsychologic rehabilitation in mild-spectrum traumatic brain injury. *Archives of Physical Medicine and Rehabilitation* **86**, 1565–1574.

Timming, R., Orrison, W.W. *et al.* (1982) Computerized tomography and rehabilitation outcome after severe head trauma. *Archives of Physical Medicine and Rehabilitation* **63**, 154–159.

Timonen, M., Miettunen, J. *et al.* (2002) The association of preceding traumatic brain injury with mental disorders, alcoholism and criminality: the Northern Finland 1966 Birth Cohort Study. *Psychiatry Research* **113**, 217–226.

Toglia, J.U. (1969) Dizziness after whiplash injury of the neck and closed head injury: electronystagmographic correlations. In: Walker, A.E., Caveness, W.F. & Critchley, M. (eds) *The Late Effects of Head Injury*, ch. 6. Charles C. Thomas, Springfield, IL.

Tomaiuolo, F., Carlesimo, G.A. *et al.* (2004) Gross morphology and morphometric sequelae in the hippocampus, fornix, and corpus callosum of patients with severe non-missile traumatic brain injury without macroscopically detectable lesions: a T1 weighted MRI study. *Journal of Neurology, Neurosurgery and Psychiatry* **75**, 1314–1322.

Tombaugh, T.N. (2006) A comprehensive review of the Paced Auditory Serial Addition Test (PASAT). *Archives of Clinical Neuropsychology* **21**, 53–76.

Townend, W.J., Guy, M.J. *et al.* (2002) Head injury outcome prediction in the emergency department: a role for protein S-100B? *Journal of Neurology, Neurosurgery and Psychiatry* **73**, 542–546.

Trimble, M.R. (1981) *Post-traumatic Neurosis: from Railway Spine to the Whiplash.* John Wiley & Sons, Chichester.

Turkstra, L., Jones, D. *et al.* (2003) Brain injury and violent crime. *Brain Injury* **17**, 39–47.

Turner-Stokes, L., Hassan, N. *et al.* (2002) Managing depression in brain injury rehabilitation: the use of an integrated care pathway and preliminary report of response to sertraline. *Clinical Rehabilitation* **16**, 261–268.

Tyrer, P., Seivewright, H. *et al.* (2001) Prospective studies of cothymia (mixed anxiety-depression): how do they inform clinical practice? *European Archives of Psychiatry and Clinical Neuroscience* **251** (suppl. 2), II53–II56.

Umile, E.M., Sandel, M.E. *et al.* (2002) Dynamic imaging in mild traumatic brain injury: support for the theory of medial temporal vulnerability. *Archives of Physical Medicine and Rehabilitation* **83**, 1506–1513.

van der Naalt, J., Hew, J.M. *et al.* (1999a) Computed tomography and magnetic resonance imaging in mild to moderate head injury: early and late imaging related to outcome. *Annals of Neurology* **46**, 70–78.

van der Naalt, J., van Zomeren, A.H. *et al.* (1999b) One year outcome in mild to moderate head injury: the predictive value of acute injury characteristics related to complaints and return to work. *Journal of Neurology, Neurosurgery and Psychiatry* **66**, 207–213.

van der Naalt, J., van Zomeren, A.H. *et al.* (2000) Acute behavioural disturbances related to imaging studies and outcome in mild-to-moderate head injury. *Brain Injury* **14**, 781–788.

Vanderploeg, R.D., Schinka, J.A. *et al.* (1994) Relationships between measures of auditory verbal learning and executive functioning. *Journal of Clinical and Experimental Neuropsychology* **16**, 243–252.

Vanderploeg, R.D., Curtiss, G. *et al.* (2005) Long-term neuropsychological outcomes following mild traumatic brain injury. *Journal of the International Neuropsychological Society* **11**, 228–236.

van Reekum, R., Bolago, I. *et al.* (1996) Psychiatric disorders after traumatic brain injury. *Brain Injury* **10**, 319–327.

van Zomeren, A.H. & van den Burg, W. (1985) Residual complaints of patients two years after severe head injury. *Journal of Neurology, Neurosurgery and Psychiatry* **48**, 21–28.

van Zomeren, A.H., Broumer, W.H. *et al.* (1984) Attentional deficits: the riddles of selectivity, speed, and alertness. In: Brooks, N. (ed.) *Closed Head Injury. Psychological, Social and Family Consequences*, ch. 5. Oxford University Press, Oxford.

Varney, N.R. (1988) Prognostic significance of anosmia in patients with closed-head trauma. *Journal of Clinical and Experimental Neuropsychology* **10**, 250–254.

Varney, N.R. & Bushnell, D. (1998) NeuroSPECT findings in patients with posttraumatic anosmia: a quantitative analysis. *Journal of Head Trauma Rehabilitation* **13**, 63–72.

Varney, N.R., Bushnell, D.L. *et al.* (1995) NeuroSPECT correlates of disabling mild head injury: preliminary findings. *Journal of Head Trauma Rehabilitation* **10**, 18–28.

Varney, N.R., Pinkston, J.B. *et al.* (2001) Quantitative PET findings in patients with posttraumatic anosmia. *Journal of Head Trauma Rehabilitation* **16**, 253–259.

Vasa, R.A., Gerring, J.P. *et al.* (2002) Anxiety after severe pediatric closed head injury. *Journal of the American Academy of Child and Adolescent Psychiatry* **41**, 148–156.

Vaukhonen, K. (1959) Suicide among the male disabled with war injuries to the brain. *Acta Psychiatrica et Neurologica Scandinavica Supplementum* **137**, 90–91.

Vespa, P.M., Boscardin, W.J. *et al.* (2002) Early and persistent impaired percent alpha variability on continuous electroencephalography monitoring as predictive of poor outcome after traumatic brain injury. *Journal of Neurosurgery* **97**, 84–92.

Vilkki, J., Virtanen, S. *et al.* (1996) Dual task performance after focal cerebral lesions and closed head injuries. *Neuropsychologia* **34**, 1051–1056.

Wade, D.T., Crawford, S. *et al.* (1997) Does routine follow up after head injury help? A randomised controlled trial. *Journal of Neurology, Neurosurgery and Psychiatry* **62**, 478–484.

Wade, D.T., King, N.S. *et al.* (1998) Routine follow up after head injury: a second randomised controlled trial. *Journal of Neurology, Neurosurgery and Psychiatry* **65**, 177–183.

Walch, R. (1956) Orbitalhirn und Charakter. In: Rehwald, E. (ed.) *Das Hirntrauma*, pp. 203–213. Thieme, Stuttgart.

Walker, A.E. & Blumer, D. (1989) The fate of World War II veterans with posttraumatic seizures. *Archives of Neurology* **46**, 23–26.

Walker, A.E. & Erculei, F. (1969) *Head Injured Men Fifteen Years Later*. Charles C. Thomas, Springfield, IL.

Walker, A.E. & Jablon, S. (1959) A follow-up of head-injured men of World War II. *Journal of Neurosurgery* **16**, 600–610.

Walker, W., Seel, R. *et al.* (2004) The effects of Donepezil on traumatic brain injury acute rehabilitation outcomes. *Brain Injury* **18**, 739–750.

Wall, S.E., Williams, W.H. *et al.* (2006) Neuropsychological dysfunction following repeat concussions in jockeys. *Journal of Neurology, Neurosurgery and Psychiatry* **77**, 518–520.

Wallace, C.A. & Bogner, J. (2000) Awareness of deficits: emotional implications for persons with brain injury and their significant others. *Brain Injury* **14**, 549–562.

Wallace, C.A., Bogner, J. *et al.* (1998) Primary caregivers of persons with brain injury: life change 1 year after injury. *Brain Injury* **12**, 483–493.

Waller, J.A. (1968) Holiday drinking and highway fatalities. *Journal of the American Medical Association* **206**, 2693–2697.

Wallesch, C.W., Curio, N. *et al.* (2001) Outcome after mild-to-moderate blunt head injury: effects of focal lesions and diffuse axonal injury. *Brain Injury* **15**, 401–412.

Walshe, F.M.R. (1958) The role of injury, of the law and of the doctor in the aetiology of the so-called traumatic neurosis. *Medical Press* **239**, 493–496.

Ward, A.A. (1966) The physiology of concussion. In: Caveness, W.F. & Walker, A.E. (eds) *Head Injury: Conference Proceedings*, ch. 16. Lippincott, Philadelphia.

Warden, D.L. & Labbate, L.A. (2005) Posttraumatic stress disorder and other anxiety disorders. In: Silver, J.M., McAllister, T.W. & Yudofsky, S.C. (eds) *Textbook of Traumatic Brain Injury*, pp. 231–244. American Psychiatric Publishing Inc., Washington, DC.

Warden, D.L., Labbate, L.A. *et al.* (1997) Posttraumatic stress disorder in patients with traumatic brain injury and amnesia for the event? *Journal of Neuropsychiatry and Clinical Neuroscience* **9**, 18–22.

Wardlaw, J.M. & Statham, P.F. (2000) How often is haemosiderin not visible on routine MRI following traumatic intracerebral haemorrhage? *Neuroradiology* **42**, 81–84.

Wardlaw, J.M., Easton, V.J. *et al.* (2002) Which CT features help predict outcome after head injury? *Journal of Neurology, Neurosurgery and Psychiatry* **72**, 188–192; discussion 151.

Waterloo, K., Ingebrigtsen, T. *et al.* (1997) Neuropsychological function in patients with increased serum levels of protein S-100 after minor head injury. *Acta Neurochirurgica (Wien)* **139**, 26–31; discussion 31–32.

Weddell, R., Oddy, M. *et al.* (1980) Social adjustment after rehabilitation: a two year follow-up of patients with severe head injury. *Psychological Medicine* **10**, 257–263.

Wedekind, C., Hesselmann, V. *et al.* (2002) Trauma to the pontomesencephalic brainstem: a major clue to the prognosis of severe traumatic brain injury. *British Journal of Neurosurgery* **16**, 256–260.

Weinstein, E.A. & Kahn, R.L. (1951) Patterns of disorientation in organic brain disease. *Journal of Neuropathology and Clinical Neurology* **1**, 214–226.

Wenden, F.J., Crawford, S. et al. (1998) Assault, post-traumatic amnesia and other variables related to outcome following head injury. Clinical Rehabilitation 12, 53–63.

Wessely, S., Nimnuan, C. et al. (1999) Functional somatic syndromes: one or many? Lancet 354, 936–939.

Westbrook, L.E., Devinsky, O. et al. (1998) Nonepileptic seizures after head injury. Epilepsia 39, 978–982.

Weston, M.J. & Whitlock, F.A. (1971) The Capgras syndrome following head injury. British Journal of Psychiatry 119, 25–31.

Whitfield, P.C. & Pickard, J.D. (2000) Expression of the immediate early genes c-Fos and c-Jun after head injury in man. Neurological Research 22, 138–144.

Whitlock, F.A. (1967) The aetiology of hysteria. Acta Psychiatrica Scandinavica 43, 144–162.

Whitlock, F.A., Stoll, J.R. et al. (1977) Crisis, life events and accidents. Australian and New Zealand Journal of Psychiatry 11, 127–132.

Whitnall, L., McMillan, T.M. et al. (2006) Disability in young people and adults after head injury: 5–7 year follow up of a prospective cohort study. Journal of Neurology, Neurosurgery and Psychiatry 77, 640–645.

Whitty, C.W.M. & Zangwill, O.L. (1966) Traumatic amnesia. In: Whitty, C.W.M. & Zangwill, O.L. (eds) Amnesia, ch. 4. Butterworths, London.

WHO (1980) International Classification of Impairments, Disabilities and Handicaps. A Manual of Classification Relating to the Consequence of Disease. World Health Organisation, Geneva.

Whyte, J., Polansky, M. et al. (1995) Sustained arousal and attention after traumatic brain injury. Neuropsychologia 33, 797–813.

Whyte, J., Cifu, D. et al. (2001) Prediction of functional outcomes after traumatic brain injury: a comparison of 2 measures of duration of unconsciousness. Archives of Physical Medicine and Rehabilitation 82, 1355–1359.

Whyte, J., Hart, T. et al. (2004) Effects of methylphenidate on attention deficits after traumatic brain injury: a multidimensional, randomized, controlled trial. American Journal of Physical Medicine and Rehabilitation 83, 401–420.

Wilcox, J.A. & Nasrallah, H.A. (1987) Childhood head trauma and psychosis. Psychiatry Research 21, 303–306.

Wilde, E.A., Bigler, E.D. et al. (2004) Alcohol abuse and traumatic brain injury: quantitative magnetic resonance imaging and neuropsychological outcome. Journal of Neurotrauma 21, 137–147.

Wilkinson, A.E., Bridges, L.R. et al. (1999) Correlation of survival time with size of axonal swellings in diffuse axonal injury. Acta Neuropathologica 98, 197–202.

Williams, D. (1941) The electro-encephalogram in chronic post-traumatic states. Journal of Neurology, Neurosurgery and Psychiatry 4, 131–146.

Williams, S., Raghupathi, R. et al. (2001) In situ DNA fragmentation occurs in white matter up to 12 months after head injury in man. Acta Neuropathologica 102, 581–590.

Williams, S.E., Ris, M.D. et al. (1998) Recovery in pediatric brain injury: is psychostimulant medication beneficial? Journal of Head Trauma Rehabilitation 13, 73–81.

Williams, W.H., Evans, J.J. et al. (2002) Brief report: prevalence of post-traumatic stress disorder symptoms after severe traumatic brain injury in a representative community sample. Brain Injury 16, 673–679.

Williams, W.H., Evans, J.J. et al. (2003) Neurorehabilitation for two cases of post-traumatic stress disorder following traumatic brain injury. Cognitive Neuropsychiatry 8, 1–18.

Wilson, B.A. (1994) Life after brain injury: long-term outcome of 101 people seen for rehabilitation 5–12 years earlier. In: Fourez, J. & Page, N. (eds) Treatment Issues and Long-term Outcomes. Proceedings of the 18th Annual Brain Impairment Conference, pp. 1–6. Australian Academic Press, Bowen Hills, Queensland.

Wilson, B.A. (1995) Long-term prognosis of patients with severe memory disorders. Neuropsychological Rehabilitation 1, 117–134.

Wilson, B.A. (2002) Towards a comprehensive model of cognitive rehabilitation. Neuropsychological Rehabilitation 12, 97–110.

Wilson, B.A., Baddeley, A.D. et al. (1992) How does post traumatic amnesia differ from the amnesic syndrome and from chronic memory impairment. Neuropsychological Rehabilitation 2, 231–243.

Wilson, B.A., Alderman, N., Burgess, P., Emslie, H. & Evans, J.J. (1996) Behavioural Assessment of Dysexecutive Syndrome. Thames Valley Test Company, Bury St Edmunds.

Wilson, B.A., Evans, J.J. et al. (1999) Measuring recovery from post traumatic amnesia. Brain Injury 13, 505–520.

Wilson, B.A., Emslie, H.C. et al. (2001) Reducing everyday memory and planning problems by means of a paging system: a randomised control crossover study. Journal of Neurology, Neurosurgery and Psychiatry 70, 477–482.

Wilson, B.A., Evans, J.J. et al. (2002) Cognitive rehabilitation: a goal-planning approach. Journal of Head Trauma Rehabilitation 17, 542–555.

Wilson, J.T. (1990) The relationship between neuropsychological function and brain damage detected by neuroimaging after closed head injury. Brain Injury 4, 349–363.

Wilson, J.T., Hadley, D.M. et al. (1992) Intercorrelation of lesions detected by magnetic resonance imaging after closed head injury. Brain Injury 6, 391–399.

Wilson, J.T., Teasdale, G.M. et al. (1994) Post-traumatic amnesia: still a valuable yardstick. Journal of Neurology, Neurosurgery and Psychiatry 57, 198–201.

Wilson, J.T.L., Wiedmann, K.D. et al. (1988) Early and late magnetic resonance imaging and neuropsychological outcome after head injury. Journal of Neurology, Neurosurgery and Psychiatry 51, 391–396.

Wilson, S., Raghupathi, R. et al. (2004) Continued in situ DNA fragmentation of microglia/macrophages in white matter weeks and months after traumatic brain injury. Journal of Neurotrauma 21, 239–250.

Windle, W.F. & Groat, R.A. (1944) Experimental structural alterations in the brain during and after concussion. Surgery, Gynecology and Obstetrics 79, 561–572.

Witol, A.D. & Webbe, F.M. (2003) Soccer heading frequency predicts neuropsychological deficits. Archives of Clinical Neuropsychology 18, 397–417.

Wood, R.L. (2004) Understanding the 'miserable minority': a diathesis-stress paradigm for post-concussional syndrome. Brain Injury 18, 1135–1153.

Wroblewski, B.A., Glenn, M.B. et al. (1989) Carbamazepine replacement of phenytoin, phenobarbital and primidone in a rehabilitation setting: effects on seizure control. Brain Injury 3, 149–156.

Wu, H.M., Huang, S.C. et al. (2004) Subcortical white matter metabolic changes remote from focal hemorrhagic lesions suggest diffuse injury after human traumatic brain injury. *Neurosurgery* **55**, 1306–1315; discussion 1316–1317.

Yanagawa, Y., Tsushima, Y. *et al.* (2000) A quantitative analysis of head injury using T2-weighted gradient-echo imaging. *Journal of Trauma* **49**, 272–277.

Yarnell, P.R. & Lynch, S. (1973) The 'ding': amnestic states in football trauma. *Neurology* **23**, 196–197.

Yasuda, S., Wehman, P. *et al.* (2001) Return to work for persons with traumatic brain injury. *American Journal of Physical Medicine and Rehabilitation* **80**, 852–864.

Ylvisaker, M., Hanks, R. *et al.* (2002) Perspectives on rehabilitation of individuals with cognitive impairment after brain injury: rationale for reconsideration of theoretical paradigms. *Journal of Head Trauma Rehabilitation* **17**, 191–209.

Young, A.W., Robertson, I.H. *et al.* (1992) Cotard delusion after brain injury. *Psychological Medicine* **22**, 799–804.

Yount, R., Raschke, K.A. *et al.* (2002) Traumatic brain injury and atrophy of the cingulate gyrus. *Journal of Neuropsychiatry and Clinical Neuroscience* **14**, 416–423.

Yousem, D.M., Geckle, R.J. *et al.* (1999) Posttraumatic smell loss: relationship of psychophysical tests and volumes of the olfactory bulbs and tracts and the temporal lobes. *Academic Radiology* **6**, 264–272.

Yudofsky, S.C., Silver, J.M. *et al.* (1986) The Overt Aggression Scale for the objective rating of verbal and physical aggression. *American Journal of Psychiatry* **143**, 35–39.

Zafonte, R.D., Hammond, F.M. *et al.* (1996) Relationship between Glasgow Coma Scale and functional outcome. *American Journal of Physical Medicine and Rehabilitation* **75**, 364–369.

Zeilig, G., Drubach, D.A. *et al.* (1996) Pathological laughter and crying in patients with closed traumatic brain injury. *Brain Injury* **10**, 591–597.

Zemper, E.D. (2003) Two-year prospective study of relative risk of a second cerebral concussion. *American Journal of Physical Medicine and Rehabilitation* **82**, 653–659.

Zencius, A., Wesolowski, M.D. *et al.* (1990) Managing hypersexual disorders in brain-injured clients. *Brain Injury* **4**, 175–181.

Zhang, L., Ravdin, L.D. *et al.* (2003) Increased diffusion in the brain of professional boxers: a preclinical sign of traumatic brain injury? *American Journal of Neuroradiology* **24**, 52–57.

Zhang, L., Plotkin, R.C. *et al.* (2004) Cholinergic augmentation with donepezil enhances recovery in short-term memory and sustained attention after traumatic brain injury. *Archives of Physical Medicine and Rehabilitation* **85**, 1050–1055.

Zwil, A.S., McAllister, T.W. *et al.* (1993) Ultra-rapid cycling bipolar affective disorder following a closed-head injury. *Brain Injury* **7**, 147–152.

Zwimpfer, T.J., Brown, J. *et al.* (1997) Head injuries due to falls caused by seizures: a group at high risk for traumatic intracranial hematomas. *Journal of Neurosurgery* **86**, 433–437.

CHAPTER 5

Cerebral Tumours

Nuria Mellado-Calvo and Simon Fleminger

Maudsley Hospital, London

Tumours involving the central nervous system (CNS) form a diverse group as regards their pathology and clinical course. In one study, the incidence rate for glial tumours was 6.7 per 100 000 population per year, accounting for approximately 51% of all CNS primary neoplasms (Bondy *et al.* 2005). However, brain metastases, predominantly originating in the lung and breast, are commoner than primary cerebral tumours by a ratio of 10 : 1 (Culine *et al.* 1998). Over two-thirds (70%) of all tumours are supratentorial and their distribution by lobe and age of onset are influenced to some extent by histology (Price *et al.* 2005) (Tables 5.1 and 5.2). For example, medulloblastomas are most common in the posterior fossa and in children, whereas gliomas predominate in the middle-aged population and meningiomas and metastatic disease are more frequent in the elderly (Price *et al.* 2005) (Table 5.3).

There is little good evidence for the role of electromagnetic fields, cell phones producing non-ionising radiation, diet, alcohol, tobacco, exposure to industrial chemicals, or medications as aetiological factors in the pathogenesis of brain tumours. Ionising radiation (Grayson 1996), electromagnetic radiation (Hardell *et al.* 2000) and viruses may play a role in some. For example, SV40 and JC viruses have been found in paraffin-embedded cerebral tissue of children with medulloblastoma (Khalili 2001). There could be a negative association between varicella-zoster herpesvirus and the development of glioma in adults; those with gliomas have been found to have higher levels of anti-varicella-zoster IgG (Wrensch *et al.* 2005).

Genetic susceptibility

The association of hereditary syndromes with cerebral malignancies is well known. Turcot's syndrome is characterised by the presence of adenomatous polyposis of the large intestine and high-grade astrocytomas and medulloblastomas. In the neurofibromatoses, increased rates of glioma are seen in neurofibromatosis (NF)-1, and multiple meningiomas and bilateral vestibular schwannomas in NF-2. The nevoid basal cell carcinoma syndrome has been linked with medulloblastoma and Gardner's syndrome with glioma (Bondy *et al.* 2005). In Li–Fraumeni syndrome, individuals present with sarcomas and multiple cancers affecting the breast and brain (Li *et al.* 1998).

The possible contribution of alterations in the genetic material to tumour formation has been reviewed by Hill *et al.* (1999). Mutations in tumour-suppressor genes may be responsible. Examples include (i) p53, located on chromosome 17p, and found in 40% of astrocytic tumours of all grades; (ii) CDKN2 (cyclin-dependent kinase, involved in the cell cycle) mutation on chromosome 9p in high-grade astrocytomas; and (iii) deletions of chromosome 10, which occur frequently in astrocytic tumours. There is evidence for the presence of tumour-suppressor genes on chromosome 10 (Ichimura *et al.* 1998).

In some cases there is activation of an oncogene leading to increased cell proliferation, for example epithelial growth factor receptor (EGFR) is amplified in malignant astrocytomas. As noted above patients with NF-2 are at risk of meningiomas and schwannomas. The *NF2* gene is located on chromosome 22q12. Its protein product, merlin, is a cytoskeletal protein. It is truncated when mutated, resulting in structural abnormalities that presumably lend themselves to tumour formation. Deletion of loci on chromosome 22q occurs in approximately 30% of sporadic meningiomas.

Other mechanisms that may be involved in the development of oncogenicity include abnormalities in signal transduction pathways. For instance, 55% of meningiomas express the *ROS1* tyrosine kinase oncogene. Platelet-derived growth factor receptor (PDGFR) overexpression has been observed in gliomas. Intracellular second messengers such as Ras (a monomeric GTPase named after the *ras* gene first identified in viruses that cause rat sarcomas) have been

Lishman's Organic Psychiatry: A Textbook of Neuropsychiatry, 4th edition.
© 2009 Blackwell Publishing.   ISBN 978-1-4051-1860-1

Table 5.1 Relative frequency of intracranial cerebral tumours according to location in the adult. (From Price *et al.* 2005 with permission.)

Location	Frequency (%)
Frontal lobe	22
Temporal lobe	22
Parietal lobe	12
Occipital lobe	40
Pituitary area	10
Posterior fossa	30

Table 5.2 Topographical distribution of intracranial tumours in the adult. (Modified from Price *et al.* 2005 with permission.)

Location	Tumour type
Cerebral hemispheres	Glioma
	Meningioma
	Oligodendroglioma
	Ependymoma
	Metastatic carcinoma
Corpus callosum	Astrocytoma
Optic chiasm and nerve	Astrocytoma
Lateral ventricle	Ependymoma
	Meningioma
	Choroid plexus papilloma
Third ventricle	Colloid cyst
	Ependymoma
Pituitary region	Pituitary adenoma
	Craniopharyngioma
	Meningioma
	Germ cell neoplasm
Fourth ventricle	Ependymoma
	Choroid plexus papilloma
	Meningioma
Pineal region	Germ cell neoplasm
Cerebellum/posterior fossa	Medulloblastoma
	Astrocytoma
	Metastatic carcinoma
	Haemangioblastoma
Cerebellopontine angle	Acoustic schwannoma
	Meningioma
	Choroid plexus papilloma
	Epidermoid cyst
	Glomus jugulare tumour
	Glioma
	Oligodendroglioma
	Lipoma
	Astrocytoma

Table 5.3 Relative frequencies of common histological types of cerebral tumour. (From Price *et al.* 2005 with permission.)

Tumour type	Frequency (%)
Gliomas	40–55
Astrocytomas	10–15
Glioblastomas	20–25
Others	10–20
Meningiomas	10
Pituitary adenomas	10
Neurilemmomas (acoustic neuromas mainly)	5–8
Medulloblastomas and pinealomas	5
Miscellaneous	5

implicated; increased activity is found in high-grade gliomas and correlates with the rapid proliferation of these tumours. Increased *in vitro* activity of protein kinase C (PKC), another intracellular messenger, is associated with high growth rate in gliomas (Martin & Hussaini 2005). There may be important genetic influences on treatment of cerebral tumours. In low-grade gliomas, the allelic loss of chromosomes 1p and 19q renders them chemosensitive (Rees 2002).

General characteristics of neuropsychiatric symptoms

Patients with brain tumours typically present with headaches, papilloedema, seizures, focal neurological deficits, or non-specific cognitive or personality changes. The clinical constellation of symptoms varies depending on the location, histology and tumoral rate of growth (Wen *et al.* 2005). Occasionally, the earliest manifestations may consist of mental symptoms alone. When mental disturbance is the most prominent feature, the patient may come first to the attention of the psychiatrist. It is, of course, comparatively rare for the psychiatrist to find a cerebral tumour in a patient with mental disorder. Parry's (1968) finding of 1 per 200 patients admitted to a psychiatric unit is probably higher than average. However, the converse is extremely common and many patients with cerebral tumours show pronounced mental symptoms at some time in their course. The frequency has been reported variously as 10% to virtually 100% of cases, depending on the care with which psychological symptoms are sought. Two of the larger series of tumour patients studied personally by the authors, and with psychological symptoms in mind, were those of Keschner *et al.* (1938) and Hécaen and Ajuriaguerra (1956). Keschner *et al.* reported mental symptoms in 78% of 530 cases, Hécaen and Ajuriaguerra in 52% of 439 cases (Table 5.4).

From the clinical point of view, mental symptoms are generally of little use as a guide to the location or nature of the tumour. Neurological signs are greatly superior in this regard, and neuroimaging has diminished the importance

Table 5.4 Prevalence of mental symptoms with cerebral tumours.

Location of tumour	Study 1 (Keschner *et al.* 1938)*			Study 2 (Hécaen & Ajuriaguerra 1956)[†]		
	No. of cases	Mental symptoms (%)	'Early' mental symptoms (%)	No. of cases	Mental symptoms (%)	Onset with mental symptoms (%)
All tumours	530	78	15	439	52	18
Supratentorial	401	87	18	354	56	19
Infratentorial	129	47	5	85	40	12
Frontal	68	85	25	80	68	20
Temporal	56	93	29	75	68	28
Parietal	32	81	19	75	52	16
Occipital	11	82	9	25	52	32

* Excluding paroxysmal disturbances.
[†] Including paroxysmal disturbances.

even of those mental symptoms which might have been of value. Tumour material has also proved disappointing for the study of the cerebral basis of mental phenomena. It is often hard to disentangle the effects of the lesion itself from remote pressure effects, circulatory disturbances or the generalised effects of raised intracranial pressure. Nevertheless, the psychological effects of cerebral tumours show many features of interest, and can occasionally be of crucial clinical importance, affecting the quality of life of the patient. Although fatigue, emotional and existential issues are common in all cancer patients, the presence of depressive symptoms was the single most important predictor of quality of life in a cohort of 73 brain tumour patients (Pelletier *et al.* 2002).

Changes may be seen in any aspect of psychological function, and may be localised to one aspect or quite widespread. Alterations in level of consciousness, cognition, the affective state and other functions that may be described as 'change of personality' are not infrequent. Complex psychological symptoms such as hallucinations and delusions may also appear, and the picture can be complicated by paroxysmal disorders consequent on an epileptogenic focus. Occasionally, frank psychotic illnesses are seen or more frequently stress-related disturbances occasioned by the constitution of the individual. In the exceptional case the tumour will present with psychiatric symptoms, but more usually the psychiatric symptoms accompany a tumour that is already known to be present. Minski's (1933) report of psychiatric symptomatology among patients from the Maudsley Hospital is typical: 25 of 58 patients with cerebral tumour showed 'functional' mental illness, and in almost half of these physical signs were absent. Fourteen patients displayed severe depression, seven excitements, and one each showed schizophrenia, an anxiety state, an obsessional disorder and hysteria.

In very general terms it may be said that slow-growing tumours tend to produce changes of personality, and allow premorbid tendencies to manifest themselves; more fast-growing tumours lead to cognitive defects, whereas the most rapid lead to acute organic reactions with obvious impairment of consciousness.

Cognitive changes

Disturbance of cognitive function is the most commonly noted psychological change. In minor degree it shows as diminished capacity to attend and concentrate, faulty memory and easy fatiguability. These rather subtle changes may be the first manifestation of the lesion, and sometimes provide the sole indication of disease for long periods of time. The cognitive changes may encompass changes in memory, attention, problem-solving, psychomotor speed and visuospatial functioning, among other deficits (Garofalo & Baum 2001).

More severe cognitive impairment may present in the form of dementia, with slowed and concrete thinking, impoverished associations, defective judgement and obvious difficulty with memory. Perseveration is sometimes marked. Speech may be slowed and incoherent, even in the absence of dysphasia and even with tumours of the non-dominant hemisphere. Such changes can be steadily progressive, but more characteristically tend to fluctuate in severity from one occasion to another.

Focal cognitive changes are commoner than generalised dementia as befits the focal nature of the lesion. Or a focal emphasis may be detected even when global deterioration is present. A circumscribed amnesic syndrome may appear while other functions remain well preserved, with markedly defective memory for recent events, disorientation and even confabulation. All varieties of dysphasia can be seen, also apraxia, visuospatial defects and topographical disorder, and serve as a guide to location. Certain cognitive disturbances characteristic of tumours are considered in the following text.

Disturbance in the level of consciousness/delirium will add to the cognitive changes, again tending to fluctuate with periods of lucidity. Later, drowsiness and somnolence appear, and as the lesion extends the level of consciousness declines progressively, ending, if untreated, in coma.

Cognitive function is an important marker of prognosis. In patients with glioma those with poor cognitive function have a worse prognosis (Meyers *et al*. 2000a; Klein *et al*. 2003). This is probably partly explained by the observation that tumour regrowth (local or diffuse) or leptomeningeal metastases may induce cognitive deficits (Taphoorn & Klein 2004). Importantly, cognitive deterioration may indicate tumour progression before there is evidence of recurrence on computed tomography (CT) or magnetic resonance imaging (MRI), as evidenced by Meyers and colleagues after evaluating 56 patients with recurrent brain tumours in which cognitive deterioration preceded radiographic changes by 6 weeks (Meyers *et al*. 2000a; Meyers & Hess 2003).

The effects on cognition of the treatment of cerebral tumours may have important repercussions for quality of life in both children and adults. This is particularly relevant given the improvements in survival time that are now being seen. Whereas the cognitive dysfunction following surgery appears to be less significant in adults (Tucha *et al*. 2001), provided it does not damage eloquent tissue, a moderate level of neuropsychological morbidity has been reported in children (Carpentieri *et al*. 2003). In addition radiation-induced neurotoxicity in the brain is a well-known phenomenon and a cause for concern (see also section on Management of the tumour; Radiotherapy). Its complications may be acute and reversible or delayed and permanent (New 2001). Neurological complications have been described with the use of chemotherapy and biological therapies (Hildebrand 2006), ranging from headache to cognitive slowing and even encephalopathy.

Lower non-verbal memory scores have been found in patients with low-grade glioma treated with chemotherapy and radiotherapy compared with those receiving no treatment (40 patients, 24 receiving no treatment) (Correa *et al*. 2007). In 28 patients with primary CNS lymphoma, those receiving more aggressive forms of treatment showed deficits in the memory and attention executive domains, especially those who received radiotherapy as opposed to those treated with methotrexate-based chemotherapy (Correa *et al*. 2004).

Therefore it has been suggested that a comprehensive assessment of cognitive functions, activities of daily living and quality of life can provide insights into the degree of impairment due to the tumour and neurotoxicity following its treatment (Weitzner & Meyers 1997).

Affective and anxiety disorders

Anxiety, sleep difficulties and depressive illness are common in patients with brain tumours (Stark *et al*. 2002). Depressive symptoms may have an overall incidence of 20–25%. Organic factors, such as tumour location, may play a small part in the aetiology. Other significant stressors include the disability caused by the tumour, and being diagnosed with a life-threatening illness. The majority of those at more advanced stages of the disease or with severe disability and/or pain are likely to have significant depressive symptoms. The Karnofski score, a measure of performance status in cancer patients (with lower scores indicating greater disability), is inversely correlated with the severity of depressive symptoms (Bukberg *et al*. 1984).

Affective changes rarely occur in isolation, but frequently accompany other mental manifestations. With intellectual impairment there tends to be emotional dullness, apathy and aspontaneity; alternatively, euphoria may stand in striking contrast to what would be expected in view of the patient's physical defects and disabilities. However, depression and anxiety are also common with cerebral tumours, sometimes as understandable adjustment reactions and sometimes pathological in degree. Irritability can be a prominent feature particularly early on (Henry 1932), or there may be emotional lability with marked and evanescent swings of mood. Sustained elation is rarely seen. Suicidal tendencies occur in perhaps 10% of cases.

Pringle *et al*. (1999), in their prospective study of 109 patients, reported that 16% were depressed preoperatively and 6% postoperatively. Of the cohort of 40 patients with gliomas or meningiomas studied by Anderson *et al*. (1999), 15% reported depression following surgical treatment. The same rate of depression has been reported by physician ratings of depression following surgical treatment for glioma; this increased to 22% over the 6-month postoperative period (Litofsky *et al*. 2004). In this study a much higher rate (93%) of patients reported symptoms consistent with depression. One interpretation is that physicians miss depression in these patients. On the other hand, it is easy to overestimate rates of depression if the diagnostic instrument used fails to distinguish between demoralisation and major depression (Pace & Pompili 2005). Using *Diagnostic and Statistical Manual of Mental Disorders* (DSM)-IV criteria, Wellisch *et al*. (2002) found that 28% of their sample of 89 ambulatory patients fulfilled the diagnosis of major depressive disorder, key predictors being frontal location, family history and combined sadness and lack of motivation. As many as 50% of patients with brain tumours face existential issues akin to patients with cancer (Pelletier *et al*. 2002). In this study of 73 patients with primary brain tumours, depression, fatigue, emotional distress and existential issues correlated with one another, but it was depression that best predicted quality of life. Tumour laterality may have an effect on patients' perception of their quality of life. In their study of 101 patients, Salo *et al*. (2002) found that patients with tumours located on the right or in the anterior region reported poorer quality of life than those with a tumour on the left side or posteriorly.

Rates of anxiety disorders may be increased in cerebral tumours and location may be of significance. In their cohort of 101 patients, Mainio and colleagues found that, preoperatively, patients with a tumour in the right hemisphere had statistically significant mean anxiety scores compared with those who had a tumour in the left hemisphere. These scores declined after 3 months and 1 year after surgery on the patients with a right-sided tumour (Mainio *et al.* 2003). Mainio *et al.* (2005) studied 59 patients with primary brain tumours and assessed their obsessionality preoperatively and postoperatively. Whereas there was no significant difference preoperatively, obsessionality scores were higher in the patients with a tumour in the left anterior region of the brain, measured at 3 months postoperatively and predominantly in women ($P = 0.036$), as compared with other regions of the brain. Peterson *et al.* (1996) identified three children, from more than 800 presenting to their speciality obsessive–compulsive disorder (OCD)/Tourette clinic over 10 years, in whom symptom progression of OCD or tics seemed to be related to progression of a primary cerebral tumour. One had an optic chiasm glioma that involved hypothalamus, thalami, ventral striatum and nucleus accumbens; one had a left parietal glioma involving corpus callosum, cingulate gyrus and caudate nuclei; and one had a midbrain glioma with hydrocephalus and involvement of periaqueductal grey matter and the thalamus. The authors suggested that involvement of the limbic system was common to all three cases.

Psychotic symptoms

Hallucinations may occur in any modality, commonly as part of an epileptic disturbance but also without evidence of paroxysmal activity. The nature of the hallucinations will depend on the location of the tumour. Occipital tumours are associated with simple visual hallucinations; temporal lobe tumours with more complex formed visual and auditory hallucinations, also gustatory and olfactory hallucinations; and parietal lobe tumours with localised tactile and kinaesthetic hallucinations. However, the distinctions are not absolute. Circumscribed frontal lobe tumours may sometimes produce visual, auditory or even gustatory hallucinations, presumably through effects on the neighbouring temporal lobe. Medial frontal lesions can also discharge directly to the temporal lobe and produce hallucinations and other phenomena by this means. Peduncular hallucinosis caused by brainstem compression has been described in a variety of posterior fossa tumours (Roser *et al.* 2005; Mocellin *et al.* 2006). These are usually self-limited and resolve spontaneously. Visual perseveration (palinopsia) and auditory perseveration (palinacousis) in the context of ictal activity have been reported in a patient with a left temporoparietal astrocytoma (Auzou *et al.* 1997).

Any form of delusional illness may accompany cerebral tumour, either early or late in its evolution. Depressive, schizophrenic, paranoid and hypomanic illnesses have all been reported, usually but not always in association with evidence of organic brain dysfunction. When they occur, delusions may have a characteristic organic colouring, being poorly elaborated, shallow or fleeting.

Factors governing symptom formation

In terms of the nature of the tumour, by and large the main factors related to symptom formation are its rate of growth, the presence or absence of raised intracranial pressure, and the size of the tumour. It has not been possible to identify precise relations between tumour location or histological type and the likelihood of mental sequelae. In addition, the role of individual differences in symptom formation is often overlooked, partly because it may be difficult to study. However, it should be remembered that in patients with a special predisposition to mental disorder, the tumour may act as little more than a precipitating factor in the psychiatric disturbance that develops.

Raised intracranial pressure and cerebral oedema

A good deal of the neuropsychiatric symptomatology is a consequence of raised intracranial pressure. Resolution of confusion, drowsiness, apathy and even coma have followed lowering of intracranial pressure, either by decompression or dexamethasone. The pathophysiology of these effects may lie largely with disturbance of the brainstem reticular formation and its rostral projection to the cortex, or with direct compression of brain tissue, impeded circulation and impaired flow of cerebrospinal fluid (CSF). After long-continued elevation of pressure there may be extensive parenchymal damage resulting from such factors, and the mental impairments will then remain even after the pressure is lowered. Focal effects in the region of the tumour may also be aggravated by increased pressure, as seen for example when dysphasic symptoms recede as the pressure is lowered.

Even when intracranial pressure is not raised, there are likely to be other important factors at work leading to the appearance of mental symptoms. Of these, localised cerebral oedema in the neighbourhood of the tumour is clearly of special importance. Psychiatric sequelae of meningiomas were found to correlate with the extent of peritumoral oedema rather than the size of the tumour itself (Lampl *et al.* 1995). The pathophysiological mechanism implicated in the appearance of psychiatric symptoms in the context of cerebral oedema could be attributed to the disruption of intracerebral pathways rather than the single pressure effect *per se*.

Nature of the tumour

It seems likely that the rapidity of growth of a tumour is one of the most important factors determining the incidence and

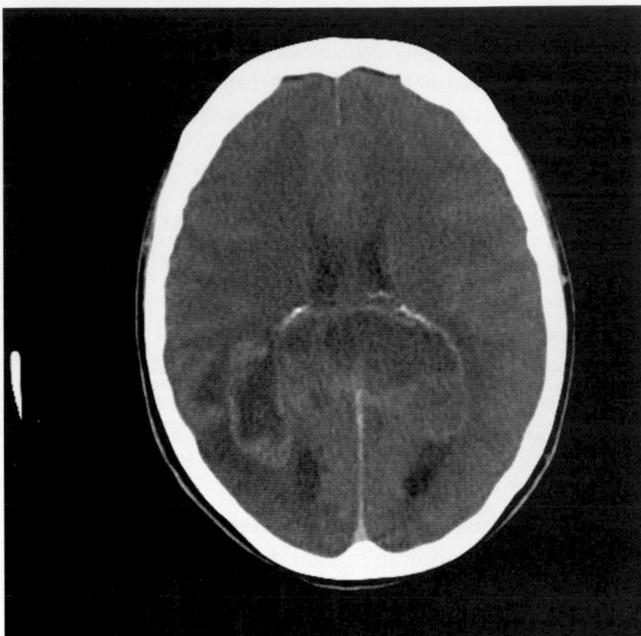

Fig. 5.1 Glioblastoma multiforme. Axial post-contrast CT shows a large rim-enhancing tumour involving and causing marked expansion of the splenium of the corpus callosum. The tumour extends into both adjacent cerebral hemispheres. This appearance may also be described as a butterfly glioma.

severity of mental symptoms, and tumour volume and rapidity of growth appear to be better predictors of impaired cognitive function than histology alone (Kayl & Meyers 2003). Keschner *et al.* (1938) found that tumours which produced no mental symptoms whatsoever were mainly of the slow-growing type. The observation that symptoms were more frequent with malignant tumours than benign (Busch 1940) may be explained by rate of tumour growth. This might also be one of the reasons why gliomas have repeatedly been found to produce a higher incidence of mental disturbance than meningiomas. In Hécaen and Ajuriaguerra's (1956) series, for example, mental disturbances were noted in 61% of gliomas compared with 43% of meningiomas. Furthermore, within the group of gliomas, rapidity of growth appears to be important; Busch (1940) found much higher rates of symptoms in patients with glioblastomas (70–80%) (Fig. 5.1) than in those with lower-grade astrocytomas (25–35%).

Poorer quality of life has been reported in patients with the most malignant (WHO grades III and IV) gliomas compared with those with less aggressive histology (Salo *et al.* 2002). Metastatic tumours with several deposits scattered throughout the brain have proven to be associated with a larger prevalence of mental disturbance than any variety of primary intracerebral tumour (Keschner *et al.* 1938).

Location of the tumour

The importance of tumour location in relation to mental symptoms has been much debated. Many observations concerning special regional effects can be offset by negative findings. Bleuler (1951), reviewing 600 unselected tumours from the Zurich neurosurgical clinic, suggested that the psychopathological picture was in fact very uniform; 83% of his patients showed mental symptoms, but there were no significant differences according to the site of the tumour. Only two mental syndromes could be reliably differentiated: clouding of consciousness in the acute stage, and a 'chronic amnesic syndrome' in the chronic stage. The latter embraced more than memory defects alone, also including widespread cognitive disturbances, emotional instability and impairment of personality. However, it seems likely that local effects may be seen, for example focal cognitive deficits with parietal tumours and focal amnesic syndromes with diencephalic tumours. Hallucinations also clearly derive from focal lesions of the brain.

When considering more than such relatively elementary symptoms, it becomes harder to demonstrate the role of focal cerebral disorder in the pictures that result. Thus disturbances of affect and personality cannot be tied convincingly to tumours in specific parts of the brain, and psychotic illness appears to be largely determined by other factors. Frontal and temporal lobe tumours show a somewhat higher frequency of mental disturbances than do tumours of the parietal or occipital lobes (Keschner *et al.* 1938; Hécaen & Ajuriaguerra 1956).

Frontal lobe tumours

Frontal lobe tumours are notorious for their ability to present under guises that may lead to the mistaken diagnosis of a primary dementing illness. This is partly due to the paucity of striking neurological signs accompanying frontal lesions, and partly to the frequency with which mental disturbances appear from an early stage. When considering the effects of frontal lobe tumours it is useful to remember the clinical syndromes that may be observed following orbitofrontal lesions compared with lesions affecting dorsolateral prefrontal lobe or anterior cingulate (Cummings 1993).

Impairment of consciousness and intellectual deterioration were found more frequently with frontal lobe tumours than with tumours of any other location in Hécaen and Ajuriaguerra's (1956) series. Sachs (1950), in a large series of patients with meningiomas, found eight who presented with dementia before any symptoms indicative of tumour had appeared, and in six the tumours were frontal in location. Sometimes dramatically successful results can follow the removal of such a tumour.

A woman of 64 was admitted to hospital in a deteriorated state and unable to give an account of herself. Her husband stated that the illness began 2 years previously when she became excessively preoccupied with the ills of her pet dog. For 3 months there had been episodes of trembling all over, but not associated with any loss of consciousness. She had gradually become forgetful and muddled and had lost all initiative. For 3 weeks she had been confined to bed and was too confused to dress herself. She was doubly incontinent. There had been no headache, fits or vomiting.

On examination she showed a profound dementia with disorientation in time and place. She lay inert in bed but was not difficult to rouse. There was no dysphasia or apraxia, but she could not cooperate with detailed tests of intellectual function. The only neurological signs were a persistent tremor of the outstretched hands and an equivocal left plantar response. The sense of smell was intact. Electroencephalography (EEG) showed evidence of a lesion in the left frontotemporal region, and skull radiography showed erosion of the posterior clinoid processes. At operation a left frontal parasagittal meningioma was removed.

Two months postoperatively her mental state was judged to be entirely normal and she said she felt better than for several years. She recalled little of her preoperative condition except that she had been distressed over her incontinence (Sachs 1950).

A woman developed grand mal epileptic fits at the age of 40, and at 53 was admitted to a psychiatric hospital because she had become apathetic, inert, incontinent and bedridden. She was aggressive when approached and deteriorated in habits. Skull radiography was interpreted as showing hyperostosis frontalis interna. After 12 years in hospital she remained severely demented, was somnolent and showed little response to questions. She sat with the tongue protruded to the right, and making purposeless repetitive movements of the right arm and leg. She was anosmic, could only just distinguish between light and dark, and showed a left-sided facial weakness. There was no obvious weakness of the limbs but she could neither stand nor walk.

Investigations revealed a massive bifrontal meningioma, probably attached to the crista galli. After its removal she made a remarkable improvement, regained some degree of spontaneity, speech and sight and was able to get about. She recognised and talked with relatives for the first time in 12 years. She had a dense amnesia for the 15–20 years before the operation and misjudged events and ages accordingly (Hunter *et al*. 1968).

According to Lampl *et al*. (1995), tumours of the left frontal lobe appear to be associated with greater cognitive disturbance than tumours of the right. In their study of 50 patients with meningioma, those with tumours in the base of the skull were free of psychiatric symptoms, whereas 44% of the patients with convexity meningiomas presented with psychiatric morbidity consisting of major depression in nine (four with psychotic features), atypical depression in four, and unspecified psychosis in three. Smith's (1966) careful analysis of psychometric tests showed greater losses in both verbal and performance abilities in left compared with right frontal tumours, the difference still persisting when aphasic patients were excluded. Bilateral involvement, as with tumours originating in the midline, produce more disturbance than when a single lobe is implicated alone (Strauss & Keschner 1935).

Generalised dementia is the most frequent picture, but disturbance of memory can occasionally be seen in relative isolation. The disturbances of affect most characteristic of frontal lobe tumours appear to be irritability, depression, euphoria and apathy. Occasionally, anxiety and obsessional symptoms may coexist (John *et al*. 1997). Irritability is repeatedly stressed and may occur as a presenting symptom. Some of the patients reported by Direkze *et al*. (1971) had initially been admitted to psychiatric units on account of depression, which then proved to be unresponsive to electroconvulsive therapy. Euphoria and apathy generally occur along with intellectual enfeeblement, or in conjunction with other organically determined changes of personality. Chee *et al*. (1985) have charted improvement in six patients with frontal meningiomas who presented with dementia, sometimes with recovery postoperatively to normal intellectual function as confirmed by psychometry.

Frontal lobe tumours may present with changes of disposition and behaviour, even in the absence of intellectual deficits or neurological signs. This appears to be characteristic of slow-growing meningiomas. In Strauss and Keschner's (1935) series of frontal tumours, for example, change of personality was one of the earliest manifestations in almost one-quarter of patients. Irresponsibility, childishness and lack of reserve are changes stressed most frequently.

The wife of a 60-year-old man was surprised to find that her husband had forgotten to buy her a birthday present one year, and that he seemed quite unconcerned about this oversight. This was quite out of character for him. Around the same time he lost his job as a bus driver, because of concerns from his managers that he was behaving unreasonably when asked to take on work. Over the next few weeks and months he became increasingly apathetic and thoughtless. He would sit around at home doing nothing. He became unreliable, socially disinhibited and no longer took proper care of household belongings. At no time was he obviously depressed nor did he complain of headaches nor suffer any seizures. Over the course of the next few months he developed urinary incontinence.

MRI brain scan revealed an enhancing lesion in the midline consistent with a meningioma (Fig. 5.2). The tumour was removed and found to be a grade 2 meningioma. Postoperatively he was left with executive impairment, verbal and physical aggression, and a confabulatory state. These symptoms gradually improved but he was left with persisting cognitive impairment.

Of 25 patients reported by Direkze *et al.* (1971), 11 presented with subtle personality alterations.

A 53-year-old clergyman began outlining rather smutty jokes, a greengrocer was charged on five occasions for speeding, all within 3 weeks, and a pharmacist became forgetful, easily provoked and asked his wife to play cowboys and Indians with him. All proved to have astrocytomas.

Disinhibition sometimes leads to striking social lapses or minor misdemeanours as the first obvious sign of change:

A man of 58 presented with a 12-month history of extravagance, boastfulness, excessive drinking, marital discord, unrealistic planning and several changes of job. He had held a responsible job in a senior position. He showed a happy confident manner and believed he was rich, but was self-neglectful and lacking in insight. The plantar reflexes were upgoing and there was papilloedema on the left with reduced visual acuity. A left olfactory groove meningioma was discovered (Avery 1971).

On the other hand, frontal tumours may present with mania. Starkstein *et al.* (1988) found that of six patients with tumours who developed mania either before or after surgical removal, all but one were frontal or temporal in location; there also appeared to be a special relationship with right hemisphere involvement.

Severe urgency, frequency and incontinence are often presented early in the course of a frontal tumour, and can occur in the absence of dementia, indifference or lack of social concern (Andrew & Nathan 1964; Maurice-Williams 1974). The ability to inhibit the micturition reflex appears to be impaired, likewise ability to stop the flow once it has begun. A similar disorder of defecation may develop, though less often and less severely. Contrary to common teaching, the patients are usually upset and embarrassed by their incontinence at this stage, although later on it may emerge in the context of general indifference and self-neglect.

(a)　　　　　　　　　　(b)

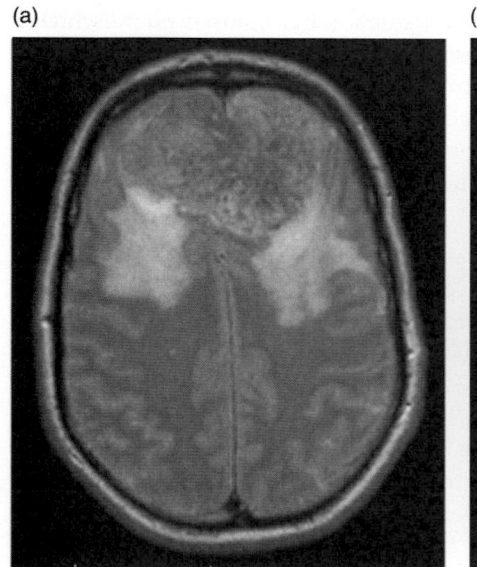 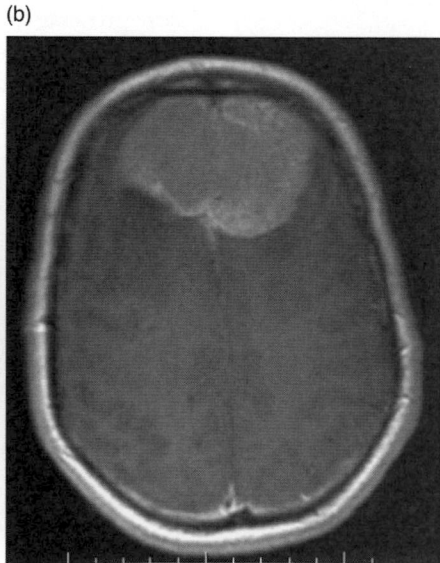

Fig. 5.2 There is a T2 isointense, homogeneously enhancing, extra-axial tumour arising from the falx and extending laterally on both sides to distort the frontal lobes. T2 hyperintensity reflecting vasogenic oedema is noted in the frontal white matter bilaterally. (a) Axial T2-weighted image; (b) Axial T1 post-gadolinium image.

Corpus callosum tumours

Tumours originating within the corpus callosum are notorious for the severity of the mental disturbances that follow. A large series was reported by Schlesinger (1950), who found mental changes in 92% when the rostrum was involved, in 57% with mid-callosal tumours and in 89% with tumours of the splenium. In a small consecutive series, Selecki (1964) confirmed the special frequency of mental symptoms with anterior and posterior tumours compared with those arising from the middle portion. Anterior tumours tended to lead to rapid mental deterioration before the appearance of neurological sign, headache or other evidence of raised intracranial pressure. Rudge and Warrington (1991) have drawn attention to the special tendency for tumours of the splenium to present with marked deficits of memory and visual perception, sometimes while other aspects of intellectual function are relatively well preserved.

The usual picture is of a rapidly progressive impairment of intellectual functions, beginning with marked memory difficulties. Sometimes there is striking blocking of thought and action which may resemble that seen with catatonic schizophrenia. Alpers (1936) thought that the clinical picture was often sufficiently characteristic for the diagnosis to be made directly.

> A man of 64 had a 4-week history of behaving strangely at work, seeming oblivious of questions and unable to focus his attention. At home, he would sit in the same place for hours at a time, once wound a clock for 3 hours on end, and once lathered his face for 2 hours. On examination there was bilateral spasticity but no papilloedema. He sat staring ahead oblivious of his surroundings, or with his eyes closed picking aimlessly at the bed clothes. Sometimes he lay for long periods tapping his head with his hand. It was hard to make contact with him, and most questions met with no response. He was disoriented, but at times seemed to recognise people. Perseveration was extremely marked. He proved to have a glioblastoma practically confined to the genu of the corpus callosum (Alpers 1936).

Personality changes may also be an early feature, similar in all respects to those seen with frontal lobe tumours. Florid psychotic symptoms have also been reported (Murthy *et al*. 1997). In his comprehensive review, Elliott (1969) suggests that the combination of delusions and stupor can come to resemble schizophrenia closely. A large part of the mental disturbance is probably due to the tendency for tumours of the corpus callosum to involve adjacent structures. Almost all involve the third ventricle and diencephalon at some stage, which presumably accounts for the somnolence, akinesis and stupor which ultimately appear.

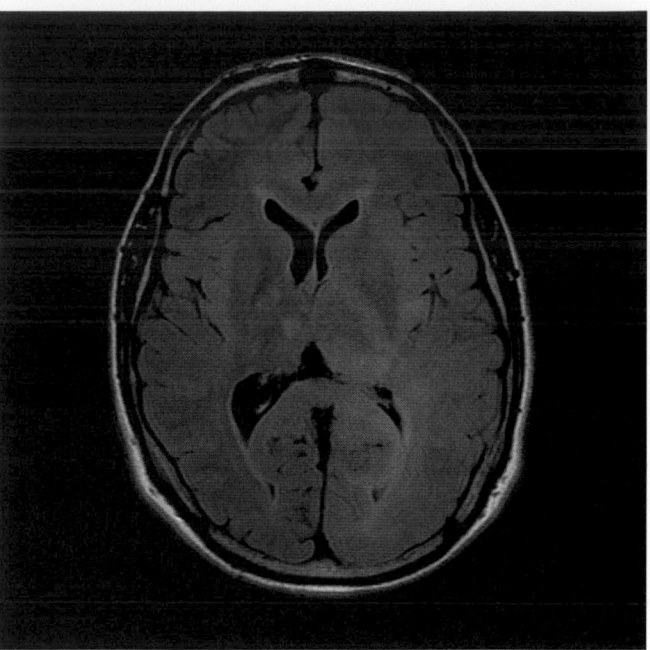

Fig. 5.3 Gliomatosis cerebri. Axial FLAIR (fluid-attenuated inversion recovery) image shows subtle and diffuse hyperintensity throughout much of the white matter of the left cerebral hemisphere. Apart from slight effacement of the cerebral sulci, there is little distortion of the brain architecture. Signal abnormality is also shown within the right thalamus.

Gliomatosis cerebri (Fig. 5.3) is a rare neoplasm in which individual neoplastic cells diffusely permeate the brain, usually starting with extensive infiltration of the white matter including the corpus callosum, with later involvement of basal ganglia, other cerebral nuclei and cerebral cortex (Filley *et al*. 2003). It has been suggested that the dementia syndrome seen in gliomatosis cerebri resembles that found in other diseases with selective involvement of cerebral white matter, for example multiple sclerosis or HIV dementia. Early on there are subtle cognitive and emotional changes, which are then followed by deficits in sustained attention, memory retrieval, visuospatial skills and frontal lobe function but with sparing of language for example. This picture is said to be characteristic of white matter dementia (Filley 1998).

Temporal lobe tumours

Temporal lobe tumours (Fig. 5.4) produce perhaps the highest frequency of mental disturbances (Table 5.5). In part this may be ascribed to the paroxysmal phenomena occasioned by temporal lobe epilepsy. Apart from features particular to temporal lobe epilepsy, there does not seem to be any form of mental disturbance specific enough to be of localising value. Non-dominant temporal lobe tumours can be clinically silent until they are very large, whereas tumours on the dominant side tend to produce the greater cognitive disturbances in both verbal and non-verbal functions (Bingley 1958).

Often the symptoms of temporal lobe tumours are akin to those of frontal lobe tumours, for example slowing and aspontaneity of speech and movement are seen in both. Memory disturbances may likewise feature prominently, including occasional cases that present with a florid Korsakoff syndrome or pure amnesia (Umemura *et al.* 1997). Impairment of semantic memory with preservation of autobiographical memory has been reported in a meningioma

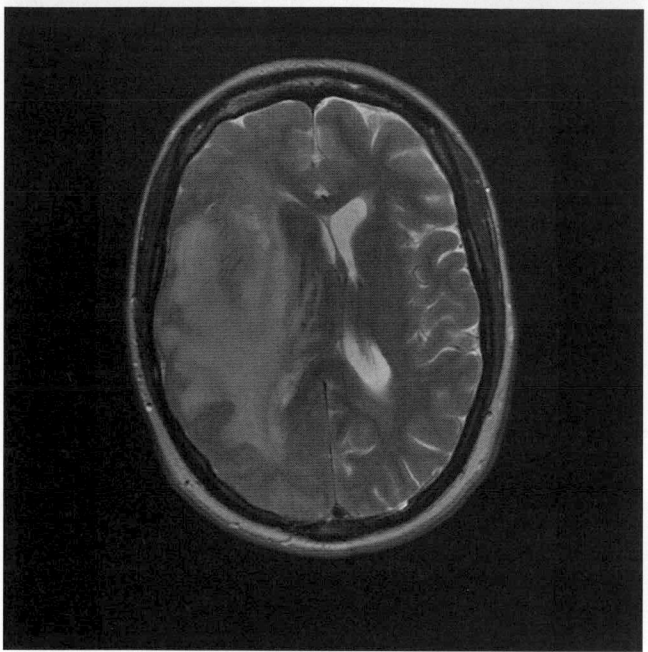

Fig. 5.4 Temporal high-grade astrocytoma. Axial T2 image shows an extensive area of T2 hyperintensity in the right temporal lobe.

producing bilateral damage of the anterior part of the middle region of the temporal lobe (Yasuda *et al.* 1997).

Affective disturbances are common. Paroxysms of anxiety or anger have been described, and occasional cases have presented with mania or hypomania. Exacerbation of mania, previously stabilised pharmacologically, has been described in a patient with a right temporal lobe astrocytoma (Sokolski & Denson 2003).

In their review, Gupta and Kumar (2004) reported personality changes with left frontal and left temporal meningiomas. However, there does not appear to be a form of personality change specific for temporal lobe tumours. A change towards facetiousness, foolish joking and childish behaviour may be indistinguishable from that seen in frontal lesions, and has been reported to be just as common. Strobos (1953) observed marked personality alterations in 7 of 62 patients with temporal lobe tumours, including psychopathic and paranoid trends, hypochondriasis and extreme irritability.

Occasionally, patients with temporal lobe tumours develop psychotic illnesses resembling schizophrenia, which may be the initial manifestation. Such cases are rare, but were drawn together in a review of the literature by Davison and Bagley (1969). The location of the tumour in 77 cases of 'schizophrenia' from 42 published reports was compared with two large unselected series of tumours. A significantly higher proportion of temporal lobe and pituitary tumours were present in the 'schizophrenic' group. There was insufficient information to indicate whether such patients had been genetically predisposed to schizophrenia, or whether temporal lobe pathology might have played a more direct aetiological role.

Some isolated clinical examples rather strongly suggest that the temporal lobe pathology may itself be responsible: see following case vignettes.

Table 5.5 Prevalence of forms of mental disturbance with cerebral tumours.

Location of tumour	Study 1 (Keschner *et al.* 1938)*					Study 2 (Hécaen & Ajuriaguerra 1956)[†]		
	No. of cases	Disturbance of consciousness (%)	Change of intellect (%)	Disturbance of memory and orientation (%)	Disturbance of affect (%)	No. of cases	Intellectual disturbance (%)	Affective and personality disturbance (%)
Frontal	68	65	47	50	59	80	60	38
Temporal	56	75	50	57	61	75	43	24
Parietal	32	69	38	25	38	75	35	19
Occipital	11	64	36	45	45	25	24	20
Mesodiencephalic	–	–	–	–	–	61	26	21
All supratentorial	401	69	44	45	54	–	–	–
All infratentorial	129	37	12	8	23	85	22	12

*Excluding paroxysmal disturbances.
[†]Including paroxysmal disturbances.

A 53-year-old woman with a previous sociable and outgoing personality was admitted to hospital after attacking her husband with a knife. She felt persecuted by her family, believing that they were attempting to harm her and that her son was turned into a dog. She complained of severe headache and thoraco-epigastric pain. On examination, her speech was incoherent and she displayed bizarre facial mannerisms and sudden unpredictable behaviour. She became stuporose and died. A glioblastoma in the right temporal lobe was found (Haberland 1965).

A 51-year-old woman without a psychiatric background presented with a 15-year history of attacks of visual disturbance in the right visual field and 1-year history of grand mal epilepsy. A left temporal astrocytoma was partially removed and she made an excellent recovery. Two years later, she became depressed for several weeks after her husband suffered a stroke. Her depressive symptoms improved, but she gradually developed a number of odd ideas and occasional hallucinations in the right half visual field. She was admitted to hospital several months later. At that time, she obviously displayed first-rank schizophrenic symptoms and persecutory delusions. On examination, there was evidence of thought disorder, with preservation of personality with warm affect. She had relative insight into the abnormal nature of her beliefs and experiences. A return of her dysphasia was observed as well as an upper quadrantic field defect and slight dropping of the outstretched right arm. The EEG showed an increase in slow activity in the left frontotemporal region. She was commenced on chlorpromazine and her psychotic symptoms and neurological deficits improved, regaining full recovery within 2 months. The EEG improved to its baseline state. Residual dysphasic symptoms manifested, especially when tired with occasional grand mal fits, minor epileptic attacks and a persistent deficit of recent memory. Unfortunately, 1 year later, she died after gradual neurological deterioration. The post-mortem revealed a recurrence of the tumour in the left frontotemporal region.

In addition to patients who present with symptoms of schizophrenia, the complex hallucinations of temporal lobe tumours may lead to diagnostic confusion. Visual and auditory hallucinations can be either simple or complex, the latter being especially liable to lead to a mistaken diagnosis of psychotic illness. Visual hallucinations occurring within a hemianopic field of vision are particularly characteristic of temporal lobe disturbance. Olfactory and gustatory hallucinations may arise from the uncinate region. It has been suggested that the patient accepts such hallucinatory

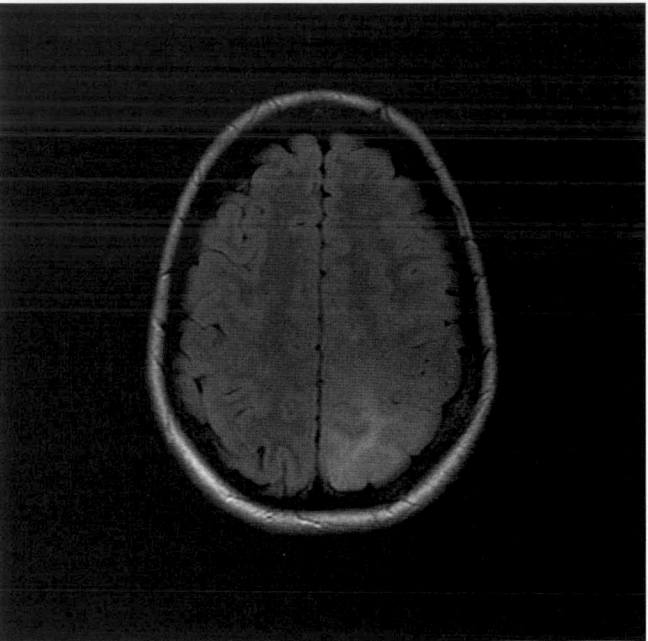

Fig. 5.5 Parietal oligodendroglioma. Axial FLAIR image shows a hyperintense lesion in the left parietal lobe involving cortex and subjacent white matter. Histology revealed a grade II oligodendroglioma.

experiences as real at the time of their occurrence, but thereafter rapidly regains insight into their abnormal nature.

Epilepsy occurs in approximately 50% of patients with temporal lobe tumours, which is commoner than with tumours in other locations (Paillas & Tamalet, 1950; Strobos 1953). In addition to hallucinatory experiences, the epileptic auras may contain a variety of abnormal subjective experiences that lead to diagnostic difficulty, including unreality, *déjà vu*, dreamy states, forced thoughts, overwhelming fears and other sudden emotional changes.

Parietal tumours

Tumours of the parietal lobe (Fig. 5.5) are less likely than frontal or temporal lobe tumours to produce psychological changes, including personality change, and more likely to lead to early neurological signs in motor and sensory systems. Erroneous diagnosis of primary psychiatric disorder is therefore uncommon. Nevertheless, depression has been noted with considerable frequency (Hécaen & Ajuriaguerra 1956). Hallucinatory experiences consist of tactile or kinaesthetic hallucinations confined to the opposite half of the body, also 'tactile perseveration' as when the patient continues to perceive a contact long after the stimulus has been removed.

The principal psychiatric interest attached to parietal lobe tumours lies in the complex and fascinating cognitive disturbances that may occur (see Chapter 2). At first sight these may very occasionally be mistaken for hysteria; for example unilateral inattention or neglect with anosognosia, associated with non-dominant tumours, might look like a conversion disorder. Critchley (1964) stressed other similarities between hysteria and parietal disease: difficulties with communication may make it hard to secure the patient's attention and cooperation, and performance may show marked inconsistencies such that the patient succeeds in a task which a moment before had appeared to be beyond him. The epileptic manifestations that accompany parietal lobe tumours, and which may antedate the appearance of neurological signs, sometimes consist of transient disturbances of body image. These again may be sufficiently bizarre to suggest a non-organic psychiatric disorder. Examples reported by Hécaen and Ajuriaguerra (1956) included the spasmodic feeling of someone standing close by, absence or displacement of a part of the body, transformation of a limb into a mechanical object, and the phantom appearance of a third limb. On the other hand, when the cognitive disturbances of parietal lobe are accompanied by marked indifference or social withdrawal the presentation may raise the possibility of dementia.

Occipital tumours

Patients with occipital lesions tend to be spared psychiatric sequelae, although they are at increased risk of raised intracranial pressure causing a disturbance of consciousness. Amnesic difficulties and dementia can occasionally be striking. Visual agnosic defects can be valuable in localising features.

Diencephalic tumours

Tumours originating in the deep midline structures of the diencephalon (i.e. thalamus, hypothalamus and other structures in the neighbourhood of the third ventricle) may produce striking disturbances with important localising significance. The most important of these are memory impairment, often with confabulation, hypersomnia and akinetic mutism. Particularly in children, hyperphagia with obesity may be the presenting symptom.

Marked amnesic difficulties, often with confabulation, are typical of tumours located in the neighbourhood of the third ventricle (Sprofkin & Sciarra 1952; Delay *et al.* 1964). Of the 180 patients with cerebral tumours systematically studied by Williams and Pennybacker (1954), 26 had impairment of memory as the outstanding cognitive defect. More than half of these 26 patients had tumours involving the region of the third ventricle. The four patients with a classic amnesic–confabulatory syndrome all had localised lesions directly involving the floor or walls of the third ventricle.

Burkle and Lipowski (1978) describe a patient in whom memory deficits were accompanied by such prominent psychiatric disorder that the organic nature of her troubles was at first overlooked. The lesion, a colloid cyst (Fig. 5.6, though not in the patient described) of the third ventricle, was eventually removed with excellent results.

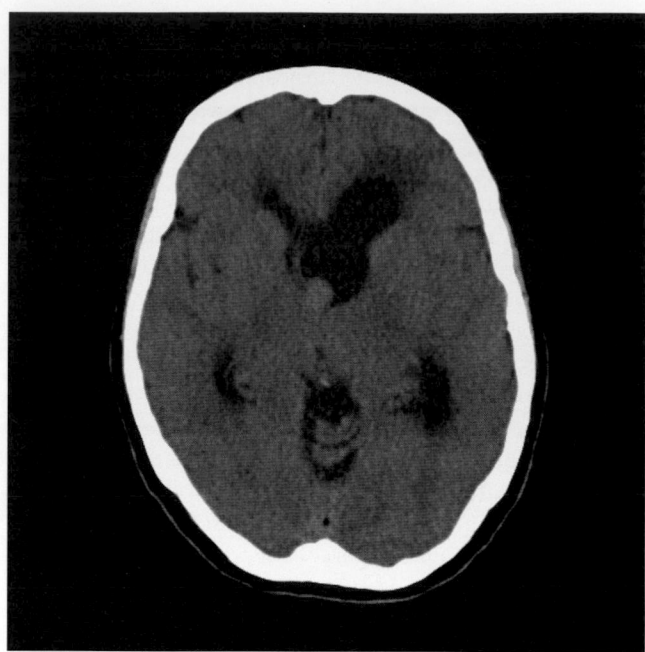

Fig. 5.6 Colloid cyst. CT shows a hyperdense rounded lesion in the left foramen of Monro causing a localised obstructive hydrocephalus, mainly of the left lateral ventricle.

A woman of 24 complained of increasing depression, sleepiness, loss of interest and memory lapses. Her depression had been coming on gradually over several months. On examination she was disoriented for the day of the week, showed poor recall of objects, but had no neurological abnormalities. She was apathetic, spoke slowly and stared impassively. A diagnosis was made of severe depression. Further examination confirmed marked impairment of judgement and recent memory, and she was considered to be affectively flat rather than depressed. The possibility was raised of hysteria or an organic brain syndrome. Skull radiography surprisingly showed evidence of raised intracranial pressure, and a CT scan showed dilated lateral ventricles and a spherical mass in the third ventricle. A colloid cyst was removed and she ultimately made a full recovery (Burkle & Lipowski 1978).

Somnolence and hypersomnia are frequent with diencephalic tumours and consequently have some localising value, for example in a patient with disturbances of memory or intellect. It is necessary to distinguish true hypersomnia from the impairment of consciousness that results from raised intracranial pressure. The hypersomnia due to diencephalic lesions is essentially an excess of normal sleep, and when roused the patient awakens normally and fully; patients with torpor due to raised intracranial pressure may similarly be roused, but usually display muddled awareness and obvious intellectual impairment. Very rarely, attacks virtually undistinguishable from idiopathic epilepsy or cataplexy occur, with uncontrollable drowsiness and weakness of the limbs. These may be provoked by laughter or other sudden emotional reactions.

Frequently, but not invariably, the sleep disturbances are accompanied by other evidence of hypothalamic disorder, such as amenorrhoea, diabetes insipidus or voracious appetite. Disturbances of thermoregulation may cause pyrexia and lead to a mistaken diagnosis of an infective process. Tumours affecting the hypothalamus or third ventricular region in childhood, such as pinealomas or craniopharyngiomas, can lead to delayed sexual development or occasionally to precocious puberty. These varied disturbances may occur in the absence of somnolence.

Akinetic mutism, first described by Cairns *et al.* (1941) in a patient with an epidermoid cyst of the third ventricle (see case study below), is another syndrome seen with lesions of the posterior diencephalon or upper midbrain (see Chapter 1, under Diencephalon and brainstem, and Causes of stupor). When caused by a cystic tumour that can be aspirated, the akinetic mutism can be potentially reversible. A dense amnesic gap is then left for the duration of the episode. It may occasionally need to be distinguished from depressive or catatonic stupor.

The patient sleeps more than normally, but he is easily roused. In the fully developed state he makes no sound and lies inert, except that his eyes regard the observer steadily, or follow the movement of objects, and they may be diverted by sound. Despite his steady gaze, which seems to give promise of speech, the patient is quite mute or answers only in whispered monosyllables. Oft-repeated commands may be carried out in a feeble, slow and incomplete manner, but usually there are no movements of a voluntary character, no restless movements, struggling or evidence of negativism. Emotional movement also is almost in abeyance. A painful stimulus produces reflex withdrawal of the limb and, if the stimulus is sustained, slow feeble voluntary movements of the limbs may occur in an attempt to remove the source of stimulation, but usually without tears, noise or other manifestations of pain or displeasure.

Personality change may be the most striking mental symptom. In some there will be features of frontal lobe disturbance: carelessness, fatuous serenity, disinhibition and lack of concern for those around. Indifference to the gravity of the condition may be striking, with affirmation of well-being and denial of illness. Complex disturbances of personality have also been reported.

A patient of 39 was found at post-mortem to have a teratoma of the third ventricle which had destroyed the hypothalamus, but without evidence of hydrocephalus or cortical damage. For a year before the signs of the tumour developed he had become irritable, hypersensitive, aggressive, unreasonable and stubborn, in contrast to his previous personality. He had shown periods of great excitement, and frequently flew into a rage over trivial matters. Meanwhile, his business judgement had become impaired and he had become careless of responsibilities. Ultimately he exhibited severe loss of memory (Alpers 1937).

Thalamic tumors

Patients with thalamic tumors have been reported to show early and severe dementia, which may run a rapid course (Lagares *et al.* 2004). Smyth and Stern (1938) reported six such cases. In two, severe dementia coexisted with little evidence of raised intracranial pressure or ventricular dilatation, and at post-mortem examination the tumour had not extended widely into the surrounding white matter. The focal lesion may therefore be significant in itself in causing intellectual disturbance. Abnormalities of pupillary reflexes were common in Smyth and Stern's cases. However, neurological signs may be absent, as in the case of a 65-year-old woman with bilateral thalamic glioma who presented with personality changes and progressive cognitive deterioration (Kouyialis *et al.* 2004), or only appear late.

Hamartomas

Hamartomas (Fig. 5.7) are malformations consisting of hyperplastic neuronal tissue in an ectopic area. Reeves and Plum (1969) reported a patient whose dementia was accompanied by outbursts of rage and marked hyperphagia; at post-mortem, a circumscribed hamartoma was found in the hypothalamus.

It is now recognised that hypothalamic hamartomas may present with aggression, precocious puberty and gelastic seizures (Weissenberger *et al.* 2001). Laughing attacks may be seen as early as the first year of life with other epileptic attacks, sometimes of multiple forms, being seen often before age 10. By this time behavioural problems and cognitive impairment are often evident (Berkovic *et al.* 1988). Cognitive impairments are seen in the majority of patients and it has been suggested that this is at least partly due to epilepsy (Deonna & Ziegler 2000). This may be explained to some extent by the adverse effects of antiepileptic medication on cognition. Frattali *et al* (2001) also found greater cognitive impairment in those with more severe seizures, and proposed that the deficits in long-term retrieval and processing speed are associated with conduction pathways involving the amgydala and hippocampal formation.

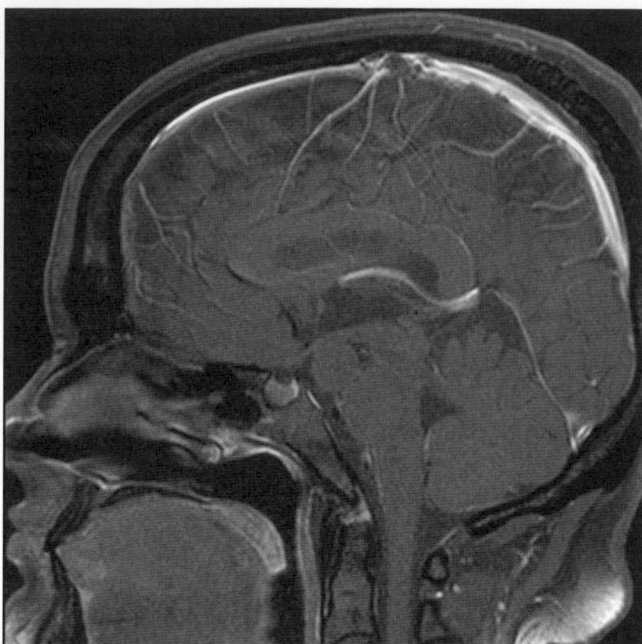

Fig. 5.7 Hypothalamic hamartoma. Sagittal T1 post-gadolinium image shows a large pedunculated non-enhancing mass arising from the hypothalamus and extending inferiorly into the interpeduncular cistern.

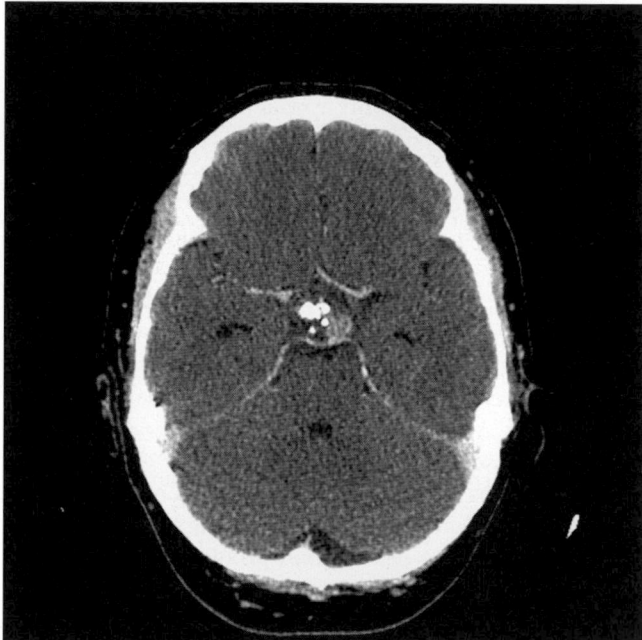

Fig. 5.8 Craniopharyngioma. CT shows a part solid, part calcified cystic mass in the suprasellar region.

Ali *et al* (2006) studied psychiatric morbidity in 10 patients with hypothalamic hamartomas and found high rates of mood and anxiety disorders. Eight patients had a past or present diagnosis of at least one anxiety disorder; of these,

social anxiety disorder was the most common. Six patients had a current or past history of an affective disorder. They proposed that involvement of limbic structures with their connections to the hypothalamic–pituitary–adrenal axis might account for some of the symptoms.

Craniopharyngiomas

Craniopharyngiomas (Fig. 5.8), when coming to light in middle or old age, may present with failing intellect and memory in the absence of obvious neurological signs (Russell & Pennybacker 1961). This excess of memory defects remains even after the effects of raised intracranial pressure are controlled for. One of Williams and Pennybacker's patients illustrates the distinction that can at times be made between the general mental changes of raised intracranial pressure and the specific memory changes related to the focal lesion.

A young man of 22 was found to have a craniopharyngioma involving the floor of the third ventricle. It had interrupted circulation of the CSF and caused a marked rise in intracranial pressure, producing some local brainstem signs, severe confusion, drowsiness and intermittent coma. Ventricular tapping relieved these symptoms and he became alert and cooperative. However, a marked memory deficit for recent events then emerged, with elaborate and detailed confabulation. Part of the tumour was cystic and was directly tapped, thereby reducing local pressure on the hypothalamus. Following this he became fully orientated and his confabulation ceased. As the cyst again filled up, the amnesic–confabulatory syndrome reappeared. As the CSF circulation was again interrupted and general tension rose, so drowsiness and mental confusion supervened. These sequences were repeated on several occasions.

The clue in such diencephalic dementias may lie in somnolence or other symptoms of hypothalamic disturbance, but these are not obvious in every case. These tumours are strategically situated so as to compress the optic chiasma, and therefore often produce visual symptoms and signs that the patient is often unaware of. Spence *et al.* (1995) describe a patient with a craniopharyngioma who presented with a major depression. Here the clues to the presence of the tumour lay in hypersomnia and hyperphagia, in contrast to the insomnia and anorexia that had characterised previous bouts of depression. Another feature, always deserving of note, was the failure to respond to antidepressant medication. Hyperphagia may be particularly problematic in children with craniopharyngioma. One explanation is that the hypothalamus becomes insensitive to leptin, a hormone that binds to the satiety centre of the hypothalamus and which thus controls food intake (Roth *et al.* 1998).

Temper outbursts have been described. A relationship between hypothalamic lesions and intermittent explosive disorder was found in two case reports of craniopharyngioma with involvememt of the hypothalamo-hypophyseal region (Tonkonogy & Geller 1992). However, one carefully designed study failed to demonstrate any excess neuropsychiatric morbidity in 18 patients after surgery for craniopharyngioma compared with control subjects who had been operated on for pituitary tumours (Bellhouse *et al.* 2003). This lack of effect may be explained by the fact that the authors were only able to interview those who were less symptomatic; only about half of the patients who were still alive after surgery, on average about 5–10 years before, were available or agreed to be interviewed.

Pituitary tumours

Tumours arising from the pituitary gland may present with raised intracranial pressure, pituitary dysfunction or visual failure. Mental changes may be found at an early stage and well before these other features are marked.

With some forms of pituitary tumours the psychiatric picture may be partly attributable to the endocrine disturbances that result, for example when Cushing's disease develops with basophil tumours or acromegaly with acidophil tumours. The common prolactin-secreting adenoma may be accompanied by marked depression, which resolves when prolactin levels are corrected. It is therefore hard to apportion the blame between the effects of hormonal changes and the effects of the CNS lesion, but there is general agreement that much of the psychiatric disturbance is due directly to extensions of the tumour beyond the sella turcica. Upward extension occurs in the direction of the third ventricle and will cause the mental symptoms typical of diencephalic tumours. Forward extension may occur between the frontal lobes, or laterally into the temporal lobe, all of which will contribute to the picture that ensues. They are also well situated to cause obstruction to the circulation of the CSF, with additional effects on the mental state due to raised intracranial pressure.

A range of disturbances are seen: hypothalamic disturbances with somnolence, polyuria and obesity, circumscribed amnesic states, deterioration of personality, and epilepsy including the uncinate fits of temporal lobe epilepsy. Dullness, apathy and passivity appear to be particularly characteristic, with mental slowing out of proportion to changes in intracranial pressure. Lack of concern may be striking, even in the face of progressive blindness. Emotional instability is also stressed, with liability to episodes of irritability and sudden rage.

Korali *et al.* (2003) studied 93 patients with pituitary adenoma presenting to an endocrine clinic. Half had a non-functioning adenoma. Using the Composite International Diagnostic Interview and a symptom checklist (SCL 90R), they found no good evidence of an increased risk of psycho-

pathology compared with a population sample of 481 subjects. There was a suggestion of an increased risk of somatoform disorders, and in men an increased risk of depression. However, another study investigated 33 women with growth hormone deficiency due to pituitary disease (Bulow *et al.* 2002). The majority had been operated on for pituitary tumours and had received radiotherapy. Approximately half of them had visual dysfunction. Compared with population-based controls, higher rates of mental symptoms including somatisation, anxiety and depression were found. There was evidence of intellectual impairment as well; the cases had lower scores in four of seven neuropsychological tests.

Lower quality of life has been reported even in patients with non-functioning pituitary adenomas. One case–control study of 99 patients in long-term remission following surgical treatment of a non-functioning pituitary adenoma found that patients reported higher levels of fatigue, changes in emotional reaction and limitation of role compared with the controls (Dekkers *et al.* 2006).

Posterior fossa tumours

Under this heading are included tumours of the cerebellum, cerebellopontine angle and brainstem (Fig. 5.9). As already seen, tumours originating below the tentorium cerebelli have a considerably lower incidence of mental symptoms than those originating above, despite the fact that raised

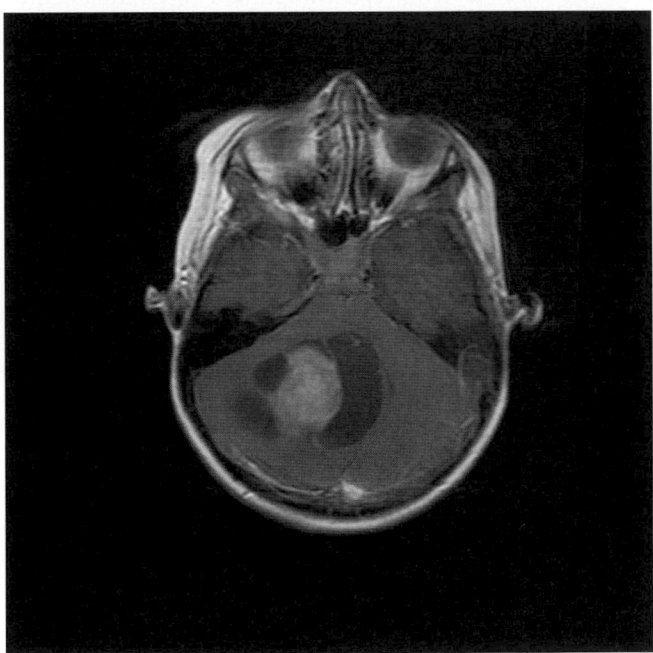

Fig. 5.9 Pilocytic astrocytoma in a 10-year-old male. Axial T1 post-gadolinium image shows a part cystic, part solid enhancing mass in the right cerebellar hemisphere resulting in complete effacement of the fourth ventricle. There is an associated obstructive hydrocephalus (not shown).

intracranial pressure is much commoner and tends to occur earlier.

Cognitive disturbances are often closely tied to evidence of raised intracranial pressure. The intellectual impairment is usually global, and amnesic defects or other focal cognitive deficits rarely appear in isolation. The impairments usually develop insidiously, and parallel the development of internal hydrocephalus caused by obstruction to flow of CSF. For example, Aarsen *et al.* (2004) found a significant relationship between the severity of preoperative hydrocephalus and impairment of visuospatial skills in children after surgical treatment for cerebellar pilocytic (low-grade) astrocytoma. Very slow-growing subtentorial tumours sometimes result in profound ventricular dilatation before they present for attention, and by then dementia may be severe.

It is easy to understand how hydrocephalus secondary to a posterior fossa tumour might cause significant cognitive and behavioural sequelae. Similarly, such sequelae might occur when the tumour, or its treatment, involves areas in the brainstem serving cortical arousal. However, over recent years there has also been interest in the possibility that damage confined to the cerebellum might have non-motor sequelae and produce a *cerebellar cognitive affective syndrome*. This was first described by Schmahmann and Sherman (1998) in adults with a variety of cerebellar lesions, including strokes, hypoplasia and tumours. It was posited that cognitive sequelae observed in these patients included executive, verbal, visuospatial, and attentional and memory deficits and that these were often accompanied by disinhibited or inappropriate behaviour and flattening of affect. These findings are consistent with those of Wilson and Rupp (1946) over half a century before; 5 of 21 patients had initially been admitted to psychiatric units with symptoms of memory disturbance, confusion, retardation of thinking and emotional instability; in these cases evidence of raised intracranial pressure was sometimes absent at the time of presentation.

Evidence of cognitive and affective sequelae following discrete cerebellar damage has also emerged from the study of children with posterior fossa tumours. Levisohn *et al.* (2000) studied 19 children who had only received surgery for their cerebellar tumour, and in whom the damage was therefore probably confined to the cerebellum. They were tested on average 5 months after surgery. A range of cognitive impairments was seen and there was a tendency for extensive lesions involving the cerebellar vermis to be associated with abnormal regulation of affect, for example irritability, disinhibition and lability of affect. These findings have been corroborated in a study that compared cognitive outcomes in young adults who had been treated, on average about 15 years previously when they were children, for either low-grade cerebellar astrocytomas (12 cases) or posterior fossa medulloblastoma (11 cases) (Ronning *et al.* 2005). Because the astrocytoma group only received surgical treatment, the authors suggested that in this group the damage was limited

to the cerebellum, whereas the medulloblastoma group, who received surgery, chemotherapy and radiotherapy, had more widespread damage. The astrocytoma group fared better than the medulloblastoma group, but both had impaired scores on measures of motor speed, attention and executive function.

It has been suggested that not only are lesions of the cerebellar vermis particularly likely to be associated with changes in affect, but that right cerebellar lesions are more likely to be associated with verbal deficits and left-sided lesions with non-verbal deficits, presumably reflecting the crossed cerebellar connections (Gottwald *et al.* 2004). However in a study of 103 children with cerebellar astrocytomas, tested on average 108 days after surgery, no evidence of an effect of lesion location was found, although the study did confirm the presence of cognitive impairment across the group as a whole (Beebe *et al.* 2005).

In children recovering after surgery for posterior fossa tumours, a syndrome of mutism and other behavioural problems in the early postoperative days is sometimes seen. This is sometimes referred to as cerebellar mutism, or the syndrome of cerebellar mutism and subsequent dysarthria, and sometimes as the *posterior fossa syndrome*. There is thus uncertainty as to the extent this acute syndrome is related specifically to cerebellar effects, or to problems elsewhere within the posterior fossa. It was labelled the posterior fossa syndrome in a study of 142 children following resection of posterior fossa tumours (Pollack 1997); 12 children, of whom seven had a medulloblastoma, developed transient mutism and in each case the tumour involved the cerebellar vermis. In general mutism developed 1–4 days postoperatively and typically was associated with neurobehavioural abnormalities including emotional lability, reduced initiation of movement and poor oral intake. The changes were generally transient, resolving after weeks or months. Because this neurobehavioural syndrome was generally associated with bilateral pontine oedema, the authors suggested that any of a number of sites within the posterior fossa might have been affected and therefore labelled it posterior fossa syndrome. Similarly, in a study of over 250 children with posterior fossa tumours who underwent surgical resection, 20 cases (8%) of posterior fossa syndrome were identified (Doxey *et al.* 1999). The most frequent postoperative findings included mutism, lasting on average about 10 weeks, as well as more permanent neurological sequelae such as ataxia and hemiparesis. In 16 of the 20 cases the tumour was a medulloblastoma. On the other hand, a similar constellation of symptoms, centred on acquired mutism lasting between 1 day and 5 months, was observed in 12 of 42 children following surgery to tumours localised to the cerebellum (Catsman-Berrevoets *et al.* 1999); it was labelled as the syndrome of cerebellar mutism and subsequent dysarthria. Again, children with medulloblastoma, often involving the cerebellar midline/vermis, were at greatest risk, as were those with tumours greater than 5 cm in diameter. More recently, a study of patients seen in a psychiatric liaison service has highlighted changes in mood and behaviour (Turkel *et al.* 2004); 19 children mostly with midline lesions, 17 with tumours and two with arteriovenous malformations were found within days of posterior fossa surgery to be dysphoric, inattentive, to have psychomotor retardation or be withdrawn and apathetic, or be agitated and irritable; 10 were transiently mute and 14 required ventriculoperitoneal shunting for hydrocephalus. The changes were regarded as similar but more acute to those seen in the cerebellar cognitive affective syndrome.

The effects just described are found after the child has presented with neurological symptoms. However, occasionally, posterior fossa tumours appear to lead to early and pronounced changes of behaviour. In Hécaen and Ajuriaguerra's (1956) series there were four cases of cerebellar tumour in children that had produced anxiety, withdrawal, and deterioration in school work, hyperactivity and problems of control. Cairns (1950) reported three children with astrocytomas of the pons in whom the initial symptoms included irritability, fretfulness, cruelty and obstinacy. In two of these, symptoms were sufficiently pronounced to constitute a complete change of character, and in all three they antedated the appearance of headache or the development of physical signs.

Some mental sequelae can be understood as reactions to the neurological disability. For example, Bristow's (1991) two patients with tumours of the brainstem had reacted to dizziness, loss of balance and other minor symptoms by becoming depressed or anxious, and had initially been diagnosed as neurotic. However, in other cases mental symptoms can be traced to direct effects of the tumour on brainstem pathways or to raised intracranial pressure. Shepherd and Wadia (1956) reported six patients with acoustic neuromas in whom chronic hydrocephalus produced confusion, impaired memory, change of personality and lack of insight. In two the mental changes were the presenting feature. Woodcock (1967) found mental changes including personality deterioration, impairment of memory and intellect, confusion, depression, euphoria and neurotic traits in 7 of 30 cases and concluded that these were attributable to vascular disturbances consequent on brainstem distortion.

Psychotic symptoms have been reported in a surprising number of cases, chiefly depressive or paranoid psychoses occurring in clear consciousness (Dobrokhotova & Faller 1969; Scott 1970). Manic or mixed states have been described in three adults with acoustic neuroma (Kalayam *et al.* 1994). Visual hallucinations may occur with subtentorial tumours, presumably via pressure effects transmitted through the tentorium to the adjacent occipital cortex (see above).

Investigations

When there are grounds for seriously suspecting the existence of a tumour, neurological or neurosurgical help should be obtained without delay. In the meantime preliminary investigations will need to include a full medical examination, including a neurological examination, and chest radiography to exclude metastatic disease. Neurological examination may need to be augmented by quantitative evaluation of visual fields using a combination of Goldman kinetic perimetry and Humphries static perimetry, particularly if there is suspicion of a tumour in the vicinity of the pituitary. Audiometry may be a useful screening test for the diagnosis of cerebellopontine angle tumours, for example 98% of patients with vestibular schwannoma have sensorineural hearing loss on pure tone audiometry.

Haematological, biochemical and immunological tests should form part of the basic diagnostic armamentarium. Endocrinological evaluation to assess the functioning of the hypothalamic–pituitary axis before and after treatment is important in the management of tumours in this region as well as in brain tumour patients treated with radiotherapy, as these patients frequently develop hormonal deficits.

An MRI brain scan (see below) will be the most important investigation, except in those in whom there are contraindications to MRI, in which case CT brain scanning will be required. Neither skull radiography nor EEG are particularly useful investigations. Although seizures are the presenting symptoms in about one-third of patients, in approximately 20% of cases a normal EEG is obtained, so the investigation cannot be relied upon to exclude the possibility of a tumour. Malignant tumours produce more EEG abnormalities than benign; in fact meningiomas may occasionally yield abnormal tracings only several years after the onset of clinical symptoms. Evoked potentials, such as brainstem auditory-evoked potentials and visual-evoked potentials, have a role in the diagnosis and monitoring of neurological function during surgical resection of tumours.

Ultrasonography may be the screening procedure of choice for infant and fetal brain tumours. Cytology may be useful in the diagnosis of pineal region tumours, often difficult to biopsy. It may be an asset in the postoperative staging of tumours as the presence of leptomeningeal involvement influences prognosis and treatment. Pineal germ-cell tumours secrete biological markers such as α-fetoprotein, the β-subunit of human chorionic gonadotrophin and placental alkaline phosphatase into the CSF. Their detection assists in the diagnosis and monitoring of the tumours (Wen *et al.* 2005). It should be emphasised that a lumbar puncture carries risks for patients with raised intracranial pressure and should be avoided in these circumstances (Wen *et al.* 2005).

Neuroimaging (see Chapter 2)

Structural neuroimaging using MRI is the mainstay of the investigation of suspected tumours; CT may be an adequate alternative. MRI and CT can be expected to give firm indications as to site, and the nature of the tumour may also be disclosed. The capacity to distinguish tumours from infarction at an early stage is particularly useful, and in cases of doubt repetition after an interval of 2–3 weeks will usually clarify the issue. In addition to direct visualisation of the tumour mass, important information is obtained from brain displacements, surrounding oedema and changes in the overlying bone.

With CT, a meningioma is shown as an extra-axial lesion of immediate or slightly increased density, whereas gliomas and metastases may be either hypodense or hyperdense. Calcification, which is quite common in meningiomas, craniopharyngiomas and oligodendrogliomas, or bleeding within the tumour may be detected. If there is suspicion of a mass on CT, then post-contrast scans are required to characterise it further. Cystic or necrotic areas may also be clearly displayed.

MRI is the gold standard for the diagnosis of brain tumours. Its increased sensitivity, excellent tissue contrast and good resolution allow the detection of very small lesions. The images are not degraded by artefact from overlying bone, and the capacity to image in multiple planes can yield extra information about tumour size, shape and position. MRI frequently shows that the tumour and its associated brain response is more extensive than suspected on CT, and gadolinium enhancement helps delineate the tumour margins from surrounding oedema. The typical changes on T1 and T2 sequences, according to tumour type, are shown in Table 5.6 (Nabors 2005). Variants of standard MRI sequences, including perfusion and diffusion MRI, magnetic resonance spectroscopy or magnetic resonance angiography, and functional MRI, may occasionally be useful supplementary investigations. They may help define tumour characteristics, evaluate blood flow and measure volume, and thus improve management and assessment of prognosis (Nabors 2005). Nevertheless, MRI does have its limitations with respect to cerebral tumours (Box 5.1).

Positron emission tomography (PET) and single-photon emission computed tomography (SPECT) allow the detection of tumours as the result of their neurochemical and physiological responses, such as increased blood flow to the tumour, protein production or glucose consumption (Nabors 2005). They can be combined with other techniques to improve diagnostic accuracy and it has for example been suggested that these techniques allow radiation necrosis to be distinguished from tumour, which is often difficult with CT or MRI (Taphoorn & Bromberg 2005). Chao *et al.* (2001) studied 47 patients treated with stereotactic radiosurgery and followed them with MRI and ^{18}F-fluorodeoxyglucose (FDG)-PET to determine the ability of these investigations to distinguish radionecrosis from recurrent tumour. For brain metastases FDG-PET was able to diagnose recurrent tumour with a sensitivity of 65% and a specificity of 80%, using follow-up MRI or pathological conformation as the gold standard, whereas MRI coregistration with FDG-PET increased the sensitivity to 86% and a specificity at 80%.

Box 5.1 Limitations of MRI (Nabors 2005)

- Patient limitations (pacemakers, foreign metallic objects, claustrophobia)
- Lower sensitivity for calcified tumours
- Treatment (i.e. corticosteroids) may influence enhancement
- Enhancement does not always correlate with histological grade or definition of tumour borders
- Prior radiotherapy and surgery may influence T2 signal and extent of post-contrast enhancement
- Low specificity (i.e. infections and abscesses)

Computed tomography angiography is useful for excluding the presence of an aneurysm which may resemble a tumour in the sellar region. Catheter angiography may be required to evaluate vascular tumours such as meningiomas, with a view to preoperative embolisation.

Problems with misdiagnosis

Over the last 30 years more ready access to neuroimaging has dramatically reduced the likelihood that a cerebral tumour will be missed. Nevertheless, in the past, surveys of post-mortem material from psychiatric hospitals gave cause for concern. About 1 in 30 patients was found to have a cerebral tumour: Patton and Sheppard (1956) found 3.7% to have a cerebral tumour, Raskin (1956) 3.5% and Andersson (1970) 3%. In non-mental hospitals the rates are probably lower: Patton and Sheppard (1956) found cerebral tumours in 2.4% of those dying in a general hospital. Moreover, this difference was significantly greater for benign meningiomas, which constituted 33% of the tumours in mental hospitals but only 14% in non-mental hospitals.

Further evidence that benign meningiomas appear to be over-represented in psychiatric patients comes from a comparison of Raskin's (1956) series from the Boston State Psychiatric Hospital with two large series from neurological units as reported by Sumner (1969). Gupta and Kumar (2004) carried out a 5-year retrospective study of case records selecting patients whose psychiatric symptoms antedated the diagnosis of brain tumour. This study demonstrates the propensity for meningiomas to present with psychiatric symptoms; 80% of the 79 patients had presented with affective symptoms in the guise of anxiety or depression.

Dumas-Duport (1970) suggests that when tumour types are studied in a living psychiatric population the frequencies approach much more closely those of the general population; it is only when post-mortem psychiatric material is studied that the proportion of meningiomas rises and the proportion of gliomas falls so markedly. This is probably because post-mortem surveys deal mostly with chronically hospitalised patients, and meningiomas tend to produce chronic pictures of mental disorder and therefore tend to be missed. The predilection of meningiomas for the anterior

Table 5.6 Summary of imaging features of brain tumours. (Modified from Nabors 2005 with permission.)

Pilocytic astrocytoma (WHO grade I)
Cerebral, cerebellar, thalamic, ventricular location
Tumour nodules show intense enhancement
Hypointense to isointense on T1-weighted images
Hyperintense on T2-weighted images

Astrocytoma (WHO grade II)
Well-defined homogeneous masses
Calcification present in up to 50%, although not always evident
Hypointense on T1-weighted images
Hyperintense on T2-weighted images

Anaplastic astrocytoma (WHO grade III)
Heterogeneous images, less well-defined borders, greater mass effect, vasogenic oedema and
    enhancement
Heterogeneous signal intensity on non-contrast T1- and T2-weighted images

Glioblastoma multiforme (WHO grade IV)
Poorly defined with mass effect and vasogenic oedema. Haemorrhage is common
Heterogeneous signal intensity on both T1- and T2-weighted images
Signature: large region of high signal on T2-weighted images (oedema + microscopic tumour
    infiltration)
Good visualisation on T2 FLAIR

Oligodendroglioma
Calcification frequent
Heterogeneous in signal intensity
Predominantly isointense with grey matter on T1-weighted images and hyperintense on
    T2-weighted images

Medulloblastoma
Calcification frequent
Heterogeneous in signal intensity
Predominantly isointense with grey matter on T1-weighted images and hyperintense on
    T2-weighted images

Ependymoma
Posterior fossa in children, spinal cord in adults
Hypointense to isointense on T1-weighted images, hyperintense on T2-weighted images

Meningioma
Extra-axial
Hypointense to isointense on T1-weighted images, isointense on T2-weighted images
Homogeneous enhancement

Craniopharyngioma
Sellar to suprasellar location
Calcifications present on CT
Cystic components may contain cholesterol and may be hyperintense on T1-weighted images
Mixed signal on T2-weighted images
Solid portion shows enhancement with contrast

Primary central nervous system lymphoma
Immunocompetent: single lesion, peripheral location
Immunosuppressed: multiple lesions with deeper location (basal ganglia)
Hypointense to isointense on T1-weighted images
Isointense to mildly hypointense on T2-weighted images
Intense enhancement with contrast

Metastases
Hypointense on T1-weighted images, hyperintense on T2-weighted images (although variable)

Paraneoplastic limbic encephalitis
Medial temporal lobe
Hyperintense on T2-weighted images

basal parts of the skull often allows them to grow large without clinical findings other than, for example, progressive failure of intellect. Hunter *et al.* (1968) were able to report three patients with frontal meningiomas who had been mentally ill for 3, 25 and 43 years, respectively, before the correct diagnosis was made. Focal neurological signs of great importance may easily be missed owing to the intellectual enfeeblement of the patient; in particular it is difficult to assess visual fields or unilateral anosmia without the patient's full cooperation.

Most if not all these tumours would now be identified quite early in the course of the illness using CT or MRI brain scans. Nevertheless, it is instructive to consider the incorrect diagnoses that were made when clinicians did not have access to neuroimaging, and the cerebral tumour was missed. In many cases the patient was incorrectly diagnosed as suffering Alzheimer's disease or one of the other progressive dementing illnesses. This misdiagnosis is of course a special hazard in the elderly in whom dementing illness is more common. This hazard is probably compounded by the involutional cerebral atrophy of the older person. As a result, compared with a young person, space-occupying lesions can grow to a larger size before causing an increase in intracranial pressure, and so will be more easily missed (McMenemey 1941).

Cerebrovascular disease was anther common misdiagnosis. In Raskin's (1956) series all 10 of the patients with meningiomas that had been missed during life were incorrectly diagnosed as suffering 'cerebral arteriosclerosis'. Evidence of arteriosclerosis on clinical examination, or a past history of focal cerebrovascular accidents, may lead the examiner to undervalue the significance of focal symptoms and signs when these exist. In addition, some tumours first declare themselves with an episode of infarction, and further investigation may then not be pursued.

Alcoholism may also be misleading. When a clear history of alcohol abuse is obtained, persistent amnesic difficulties will often be ascribed to this. Similarly, episodes of confusion in the early stages of a tumour may be mistaken for intoxication. In the following case study the diagnosis was only made because of the patient's request for a CT scan.

A man of 34 was referred because of his concern over impaired concentration and memory. He had been a severe alcoholic until 2 years previously, but since then had abstained completely. Problems with memory had been marked when drinking and had improved considerably since he stopped, but this improvement had reached a plateau. He was also aware of ready mental fatigue, and was eager to know whether brain damage due to alcoholism had persisted. His only other complaint was of episodes of vertigo and nausea for the past 3 months, ascribed by his general practitioner to labyrinthitis. Examination showed positional nystagmus but no other neurological signs. There was no evidence of cognitive impairment on examining his mental state.

He was strongly reassured that there was little likelihood of alcoholic brain damage. Psychometric testing reinforced this conclusion, showing superior intelligence and intact memory functions. By way of further reassurance his request for a CT scan was granted. A large cystic lesion was revealed in the cerebellum, compressing the fourth ventricle and causing dilatation of the third and lateral ventricles. By the time of the scan, 1 month after presentation, he had developed ataxia of gait and papilloedema was apparent. This had not been present before. At operation a low-grade cystic astrocytoma was removed and he made an excellent recovery.

Toth *et al.* (2002) described a case in which a 46-year-old man presented with an amnesic confabulatory syndrome in the context of heavy alcoholism. The patient did not respond to intravenous thiamine. Neuroimaging revealed an enhancing mass located within the third ventricle and involving cortical and subcortical regions. Histology proved it to be a primary CNS lymphoma. There was considerable radiological reduction of the lesions following administration of dexamethasone, which unfortunately was not accompanied by clinical improvement.

Epileptic seizures may be misinterpreted as due to idiopathic epilepsy. Approximately 20% of tumours are estimated to present with epilepsy, mostly of a focal nature (see below). In psychiatric practice temporal lobe epilepsy will present a special hazard, since even the epileptic nature of the phenomena may be missed. Malamud (1967) reviewed the case histories of 18 patients coming to post-mortem in psychiatric hospitals with tumours of the limbic areas of the brain; all had been diagnosed as suffering from non-organic psychiatric illnesses, although much of the symptomatology appeared to be based in temporal lobe epilepsy that had been overlooked.

A special source of error is the readiness with which the patient's family, and his physician, are liable to interpret early symptoms in terms of current stress in the life situation. Minski (1933) found that 19 of 58 patients with cerebral tumours admitted to the Maudsley Hospital had a clear history of stress antedating admission in the form of recent accidents, bereavements or occupational difficulties. Sometimes the stress may have served to focus attention on early symptoms, or sometimes the patient's attempt to cope with the problem may have unmasked his reduced adaptability.

A man of 37 was referred by a neurologist for psychiatric treatment on account of depression and irritability of recent onset, together with panicky feelings when travelling. He had developed epilepsy 4 years earlier, after a mild head injury, but this remained well controlled by anticonvulsant medication. He also complained of intermittent headache and difficulty in concentrating on his job, but in fact was coping well and had recently been promoted. Neurological examination was entirely normal. He had always been of an anxious, pedantic disposition and prone to take his responsibility very seriously. His wife was expecting the birth of a second child and they were due to face considerable financial difficulties. He was treated with minor tranquillisers and supportive psychotherapy for 6 months, and showed improvement. Suddenly, however, he developed a hemianopia and a sixth nerve palsy, and was admitted to hospital in semicoma. A slow-growing astrocytoma in the non-dominant temporal lobe was discovered.

Dissociative and conversion disorders are a well-known source of error. Neurological signs of a puzzling or unconvincing nature readily invite this label, especially in patients with an unstable background. Certain symptoms, such as somnolence, may be viewed with suspicion when they are unsupported by physical findings. The patient who has displayed conversion symptoms in the past is especially at risk (see Chambers 1955).

Management of brain tumours

Medical management

Acute treatment may be needed to stabilise the patient with regard to peritumoral oedema and raised intracranial pressure, seizures or delirium. Other medical issues likely to need attention include managing side effects of chemotherapy and immunosupression, and prophylaxis of venous thromboembolism. When the hypophysis is affected, endocrine deficiencies may need to be treated. Additionally, a package of supportive care aimed at providing a good quality of life should be considered.

Seizures are the presenting symptom of brain tumours in approximately 20% of patients and may be present at some stage of the illness in 62% or more of patients (Wen & Marks 2002). Supratentorial tumours located within or near the cortex tend to have a higher incidence of seizure activity; younger patients and those with more aggressive tumours or malignancies are most at risk. Treatment is with standard antiepileptic drugs, acknowledging that the epilepsy is focal or secondary generalised. Given that the patient is likely to be on other drugs that are metabolised by the hepatic microsomal cytochrome P450 system, including dexamethasone and some of the chemotherapeutic agents, antiepileptics with less interaction with the cytochrome system, like levetiracetam and gabapentin (Vecht et al. 2003), may be preferred. Patients with a brain tumour are likely to be sensitive to the effects of antiepileptic drugs. The cognitive impairments that may result from antiepileptic drugs, such as slowing of mental performance, sedation and fatigue, are common symptoms of brain tumours per se. Therefore the lowest effective dose and monotherapy, as opposed to polytherapy, are preferred (Meador 1994). Prophylactic use of antiepileptics in patients with brain tumour who are asymptomatic is unnecessary; even in patients who have had a craniotomy, the value of prophylactic antiepileptic medication to reduce the frequency of seizures is unclear (Glantz et al. 2000).

For the management of peritumoral oedema and raised intracranial pressure, dexamethasone is the preferred high-potency steroid. It has little mineralocorticoid activity and possibly a lower risk of infection and cognitive impairment compared with other corticosteroids (Wen & Marks 2002). The dose will depend on tumour histology, location, size and amount of peritumoral oedema, and may be limited by the development of complications of steroid treatment. These include peptic ulceration, particularly in the elderly and those with a history of peptic ulcers. Steroid myopathy occurs in 2–21% of brain tumour patients on treatment; again the elderly are more at risk. The clinician also needs to be aware of the risk of Pneumocystis carinii pneumonia (PCP), a risk that will be aggravated by other immunosuppressant treatment. Some recommend monitoring of CD4+ cells as a marker of risk, and for those patients at greatest risk prophylactic anti-PCP treatment (Kumar & Krieger 1998). Other complications of dexamethasone include sleep disturbance, delirium or psychosis, and osteopenia.

All oncological patients have an increased risk of thromboembolism (deep vein thrombosis) and pulmonary embolism. For patients with brain tumours, the risk of deep vein thrombosis and pulmonary embolism is higher than in the general cancer population (Hamilton et al. 1994; Deitcher & Gomes 2003). It may be appropriate for some patients to receive prophylactic low-molecular-weight heparins, although any benefit may be outweighed by the increased risk of intracranial bleeding (Wen & Marks 2002).

A variety of endocrine deficits may be seen in patients with tumours located in the hypothalamo-pituitary area and in patients treated with radiotherapy. When present these will require expert assessment and treatment (Swensen & Kirsch 2002). Apathy, fatigue and low mood not amounting to depression may coexist and be the result of the hemispheric and diencephalic dysfunction accompanying the pituitary disease. It has been suggested that in such patients it is important to identify any abnormalities of the hypothalamic–pituitary axis and treat it accordingly (Weitzner et al. 2005).

Management of psychiatric sequelae

Many patients with brain tumours will need treatment for their depression and anxiety. Appropriate treatment of a depressive illness may improve quality of life and functional outcome (Mainio *et al.* 2003). Attention should be paid to suicidal ideation and risk, as cancer patients are at increased suicidal risk compared with the general population, especially when in pain and during the end-stages of the illness (Breitbart 1995). Once the diagnosis of depression is established, the choice of antidepressant will depend heavily on the propensity for side effects. Generally, the selective serotonin reuptake inhibitors (SSRIs) are the drugs of choice (Pirl & Roth 1999; Schwartz *et al.* 2002). Psychological interventions such as supportive psychotherapy and cognitive–behaviour techniques in combination with pharmacotherapy have been recommended, although the evidence base for effectiveness is not robust (Newell *et al.* 2002). Anxiety is common and is often associated with depression. Exacerbation of premorbid traits may become manifest. Behavioural interventions such as relaxation training, systematic desensitisation and imagery techniques may be of benefit for some patients (Redd *et al.* 2001). Pharmacotherapy, for example benzodiazepines, may be indicated when the levels of anxiety and distress are high.

Cognitive impairment is an important indicator of prognosis and may also help the clinician to choose the treatment of choice with regard to the risks and benefits of new treatment regimens and their potential neurotoxicity (Meyers *et al.* 2000a). As noted above, cognitive deterioration may be an early marker of tumour progression. Serial neuropsychological testing may therefore be necessary, bearing in mind that patients with cerebral tumours are unlikely to tolerate prolonged testing (Meyers 2000). The choice of cognitive test will depend on the setting and will range from the Mini-Mental State Examination to more comprehensive functional tests. A hierarchical approach, taking about 1 hour to complete, has been proposed (Taphoorn & Klein 2004).

It has been suggested that methylphenidate may improve cognition. In a controlled trial of 30 patients, improvements in stamina, bladder control and cognitive function were seen in about half while on methylphenidate (Meyers *et al.* 1998). This was despite the fact that in some there was progressive tumour growth documented on MRI. A randomised, double-blind, cross-over study of children who had been treated with chemotherapy or radiotherapy to the CNS for brain tumour (*N* = 43) or acute lymphoblastic leukaemia (*N* = 40) found beneficial effects of methylphenidate on attentional and social deficits reported by teachers and parents (Mulhern *et al.* 2004). Unfortunately, the results are not presented in such a way that it is possible to single out only those with brain tumours.

Palliative care will be an important aspect of management. Disabling neurological symptoms like dysphagia will need careful attention, and adequate pain control needs to be available. Carers will need support. Hospice care provision may be needed for some terminally ill patients. All will require conscientious attention to the ethical, existential and spiritual matters at the end of life.

Management of the tumour

The specific management of brain tumours goes beyond the scope of this chapter. However, some of the recent therapeutic developments are discussed, placing special emphasis on the neuropsychiatric consequences of receiving such treatments.

Chemotherapy

The sensitivity of the cerebral tumour to chemotherapy depends on the histology. Medulloblastomas, lymphomas, oligodendrogliomas and germ cell tumours are significantly chemosensitive. Recently, the alkylating agent temozolamide has been shown to be effective in ologodendroglial tumours, oligoastrocytic tumours and anaplastic astrocytomas in terms of both progression-free and overall survival (Taphoorn & Klein 2004). Chemotherapy is more effective when there is less tumour present and therefore it is usually administered following radiotherapy or surgery; however, it can be used either concurrently or as initial therapy depending on the functional status of the patient (Mathieu & Fortin 2006). Aggressive tumours may require combination chemotherapy.

Neurotoxicity is a troublesome side effect of chemotherapy and is more likely when drugs are administered intravenously, and especially intrathecally. For example, intrathecal methotrexate can produce a necrotising encephalopathy (Brock & Jennings 2004). Temozolamide may produce headaches, seizures and neurological deterioration. Cisplatin may cause encephalopathy as well as peripheral neuropathy (Steeghs *et al.* 2003). Intra-arterial carmustine may cause central neurotoxicity with imaging and pathological features similar to late radiation necrosis (Taphoorn & Klein 2004). The risk of developing cognitive side effects is increased when radiotherapy precedes or is given concomitantly with chemotherapy (Taphoorn & Klein 2004).

Surgery

Neurosurgical treatment may be needed at an early stage to establish the histological diagnosis. In some cases it will be necessary to reduce the size of the tumour to alleviate symptoms of raised intracranial pressure, whereas in others the neurosurgeon will attempt complete resection. However, neurosurgery may result in damage to otherwise healthy peritumoral tissue, as well as tissue along the path of access to the tumour. The neurosurgeon may therefore be reluctant to operate if the tumour is near eloquent areas of the brain (Taphoorn & Klein 2004). However, Duffau *et al.* (2003) oper-

Box 5.2 Factors associated with radiation-induced deficits

- Radiation factors: total dose, fractional dose, total duration of therapy, volume of brain irradiated
- Patient factors: age, genetic predisposition, pre-existing neurological diseases (e.g. multiple sclerosis), systemic diseases and concomitant radiotherapy
- Endocrine dysfunction secondary to radiation damage to the hypothalamic–pituitary axis, resulting in adrenal, thyroid and growth-hormone deficits

Box 5.3 Mechanisms of radiation neurotoxicity

- Ionising damage to the genetic structure of cells, particularly oligodendrocyte progenitor cells. Radiation breaks the DNA strands and attacks RNA, proteins and lipids (Abrey & Correa 2005). Because radiation-induced damage leads to demyelination in the white matter, oligodendrocytes might be a potential target. Damage to the ability of oligodendrocyte progenitors to reproduce and replace mature myelin-producing oligodendrocytes may have a pathogenetic effect (Van der Maazen et al. 1991)
- Vascular endothelial damage, with subsequent ischaemia. However, the degree of necrosis of the neural tissue is often greater than expected for the amount of vascular damage
- Radiation interrupts cellular proliferation and kills dividing cells. This occurs particularly in rapidly dividing cells rather than cells in S phase (New 2001). It may also lead to apoptotic cell death (Peissner et al. 1999)

ated on 77 patients with low-grade gliomas who did not have apparent clinical deficits despite the fact that there was evidence of tumour invasion of primary sensory and/or motor areas or language areas. All patients showed clinical deficits postoperatively, although complete recovery occurred within 3 months in 73 cases. In patients whose cerebral blood flow may be compromised by raised intracranial pressure, the neurosurgeon will be concerned about the general risks of anaesthesia.

As mentioned above, some children undergoing resection of posterior fossa tumours suffer a syndrome of cognitive impairment and affective symptoms. The postoperative cognitive dysfunction in children with cerebral tumours has been delineated in a study of 106 children within 3 months after surgery for different tumours (craniopharyngioma, low-grade glioma, ependymoma and optic glioma) prior to stereotactic radiotherapy. A discrepancy between verbal and performance IQ scores, with performance IQ being consistently lower than verbal IQ, was detected in 45% of the patients and lower performances in the language, visuospatial and motor domains in 20–30% (Carpentieri et al. 2003).

Radiotherapy

Cognitive deficits attributed to radiotherapy have been reported in children receiving radiotherapy to the brain for acute leukaemia or brain tumours; greater impairment is found in females (Sarkissian 2005). Problems are also observed in adults years after prophylactic irradiation of the brain for gliomas, brain metastases, primary CNS lymphoma, nasopharyngeal malignancies or small-cell lung carcinoma (Taphoorn & Klein 2004). The factors associated with radiation-induced deficits are shown in Box 5.2.

Vascular damage and demyelination are the main features of radiation damage. Vascular abnormalities initially consist of transient perivascular lymphocytic infiltrations which then lead to progressive vascular alterations with haemorrhage and necrosis. Demyelination with subsequent breakdown of the myelin sheath occurs when oligodendrocytes are damaged (Peissner et al. 1999; Belka et al 2001). Various pathophysiological hypotheses have been proposed to explain the damage (Box 5.3).

Some patients develop an acute radiation encephalopathy within 2 weeks, caused by vasogenic oedema and disruption of the blood–brain barrier. Characteristic symptoms include headache, somnolence, and worsening of neurological symptoms that were already present. This acute encephalopathy improves with corticosteroids. About 1–6 months after completion of radiotherapy, patients may develop an early-delayed radiation encephalopathy which may be difficult to distinguish from early tumour progression. Drowsiness, worsening of neurological symptoms and transient cognitive deficits consisting of short-term memory and attentional deficits are seen. It may resolve completely after 6–12 months (Lewanski et al. 2000; Armstrong et al. 2002; Taphoorn & Bromberg 2005). Late-delayed encephalopathy is serious and irreversible. It may take the form of local radionecrosis or diffuse leucoencephalopathy and cerebral atrophy (Taphoorn & Klein 2004). There is an association between the severity of cognitive deficits and imaging abnormalities such as cerebral atrophy and leucoencephalopathy (Postma et al. 2002). Memory, attention and new learning, as well as processing speed are sensitive to radiotherapy. Common neurological sequelae include urinary incontinence, ataxia, and pyramidal as well as extrapyramidal signs. MRI may show diffuse atrophy with ventricular enlargement as well as severe confluent white matter abnormalities on T2-weighted MRI (Monje & Palmer 2003; Taphoorn & Klein 2004). Meyers et al. (2000b) followed 19 patients with basal skull tumours who had received paranasal sinus radiotherapy between 20 months and 20 years earlier. More than half of the patients had difficulty in learning new information and 80% displayed accelerated forgetting over time. Additionally, one-third of the patients displayed deficits of visuomotor speed, frontal lobe executive function and fine motor coordination. Two of the patients had severe necrosis with ensuing dementia and blindness (Meyers *et al.* 2000b). Klüver–Bucy syndrome has been described in a 58-year-old woman who received postoperative radiotherapy for a craniopharyngioma, with extensive bilateral mesial temporal necrotic lesions (Benito-León & Domínguez 1998).

Improvements in technology aim to deliver high doses of radiation to the tumour while significantly sparing the surrounding healthy structures. Intensity-modulated radiation therapy (IMRT) generates small modulated radiation beams that strike a tumour with varying intensities and from many angles to attack the target in a complete three-dimensional manner. Stereotactic surgery combines the principles of stereotactic localisation with precise delivery of radiation to an imaging-defined target. The gamma knife uses emitted photons that are directed precisely through circular channels drilled into a high-density metal helmet. Linear accelerator-based radiosurgery (LINAC) uses a stereotactic head frame and a 6-MeV linear accelerator, while the cyberknife has a compact lightweight linear accelerator mounted on a robotic arm. These methods are all efficacious and offer a more circumscribed approach to the treatment of brain tumours (Brown & Pollock 2005).

New therapeutic modalities

Novel therapeutic approaches targeted at the aetiological factors that may be responsible for tumours, especially gliomas, have been developed. They are being used as adjuvant therapy in combination with other treatments.

• Gene therapy (Hutterer *et al.* 2006): viral genes are delivered to the malignant cells, rendering them susceptible to the effects of antiviral drugs, which block their proliferation.

• Signal transduction inhibitors (Sathornsumetee & Rich 2006) aim to reverse the abnormal activation or suppression responsible for the resistance to radiotherapy.

• Immunotherapy, particularly the use of monoclonal antibodies directed against antigens expressed by glioma cells (Akabani *et al.* 2005). Interferons are also being used (Hoang-Xuan & Delattre 1996).

• Tamoxifen, a hormonal treatment that inhibits and modulates PKC (an enzyme involved in cellular signal transduction), may have a role (Mastronardi *et al.* 1998).

• Stem cell therapy (Yuan *et al.* 2006) aims to deliver molecules capable of enhancing antitumour immunity or altering their genetic structure.

These are all promising strategies in the earlier stages of development for clinical practice.

References

Aarsen, F.K., Van Dongen, H.R., Paquier, P.F., Van, M.M. & Catsman-Berrevoets, C.E. (2004) Long-term sequelae in children after cerebellar astrocytoma surgery. *Neurology* **62**, 1311–1316.

Abrey, L.E. & Correa, D.D. (2005) Neurologic complications of radiation therapy. In: Schiff, D. & O'Neill B.P. (eds) *Principles of Neuro-oncology*, pp. 711–727. McGraw-Hill, New York.

Akabani, G., Reardon, D.A., Coleman, R.E. *et al.* (2005) Dosimetry and radiographic analysis of ^{131}I-labeled anti-tenascin 81C6 murine monoclonal antibody in newly diagnosed patients with malignant gliomas: a phase II study. *Journal of Nuclear Medicine* **46**, 1042–1051.

Ali, S., Moriarty, J., Mullatti, N. & David, A. (2006) Psychiatric comorbidity in adult patients with hypothalamic hamartoma. *Epilepsy and Behavior* **9**, 111–118.

Alpers, B.J. (1936) A note on the mental syndrome of corpus callosum tumours. *Journal of Nervous and Mental Disease* **84**, 621–627.

Alpers, B.J. (1937) Relation of the hypothalamus to disorders of personality. *Archives of Neurology and Psychiatry* **38**, 291–303.

Anderson, S.I., Taylor, R. & Whittle, I.R. (1999) Mood disorders in patients after treatment for primary intracranial tumours. *British Journal of Neurosurgery* **13**, 480–485.

Andersson, P.G. (1970) Intracranial tumours in a psychiatric autopsy material. *Acta Psychiatrica Scandinavica* **46**, 213–224.

Andrew, J. & Nathan, P.W. (1964) Lesions of the anterior frontal lobes and disturbances of micturition and defaecation. *Brain* **87**, 233–262.

Armstrong, C.L., Hunter, J.V., Ledakis, G.E. *et al.* (2002) Late cognitive and radiographic changes related to radiotherapy: initial prospective findings. *Neurology* **59**, 40–48.

Auzou, P., Parain, D., Ozsancak, C., Weber, J. & Hannequin, D. (1997) [EEG recordings during episodes of palinacousis and palinopsia.] *Revue Neurologique (Paris)* **153**, 687–689.

Avery, T.L. (1971) Seven cases of frontal tumour with psychiatric presentation. *British Journal of Psychiatry* **119**, 19–23.

Beebe, D.W., Ris, M.D., Armstrong, F.D. *et al.* (2005) Cognitive and adaptive outcome in low-grade pediatric cerebellar astrocytomas: evidence of diminished cognitive and adaptive functioning in National Collaborative Research Studies (CCG 9891/POG 9130). *Journal of Clinical Oncology* **23**, 5198–5204.

Belka, C., Burdach, W., Kortmann, R.D. & Bamberg, M. (2001) Radiation induced CNS toxicity: molecular and cellular mechanisms. *British Journal of Cancer* **85**, 1233–1239.

Bellhouse, J., Holland, A. & Pickard, J. (2003) Psychiatric, cognitive and behavioural outcomes following craniopharyngioma and pituitary adenoma surgery. *British Journal of Neurosurgery* **17**, 319–326.

Benito-León, J. & Domínguez, J. (1998) Kluver–Bucy syndrome in late delayed postirradiation encephalopathy. *Journal of Neurology* **245**, 325–326.

Berkovic, S.F., Andermann, F., Melanson, D., Ethier, R.E., Feindel, W. & Gloor, P. (1988) Hypothalamic hamartomas and ictal laughter: evolution of a characteristic epileptic syndrome and diagnostic value of magnetic resonance imaging. *Annals of Neurology* **23**, 429–439.

Bingley, T. (1958) Mental symptoms in temporal lobe epilepsy and temporal lobe gliomas. *Acta Psychiatrica et Neurologica Scandinavica Supplementum* **120**, 1–151.

Bleuler, M. (1951) Psychiatry of cerebral diseases. *British Medical Journal* **2**, 1233–1238.

Bondy, M.L., El-Zein, R. & Wrensch, M. (2005) Epidemiology of brain cancer. In: Schiff, D. & O'Neill B.P. (eds) *Principles of Neuro-oncology*, pp. 3–16. McGraw-Hill, New York.

Breitbart, W. (1995) Identifying patients at risk for, and treatment of major psychiatric complications of cancer. *Support Care Cancer* **3**, 45–60.

Bristow, M.F. (1991) Posterior fossa tumours presenting to psychiatrists. *Behavioral Neurology* **4**, 249–253.

Brock, S. & Jennings, H.R. (2004) Fatal acute encephalomyelitis after a single dose of intrathecal methotrexate. *Pharmacotherapy* **24**, 673–676.

Brown, P.D. & Pollock, B.E. (2005) Principles of radiotherapy and radiosurgery. In: Schiff, D. & O'Neill B.P. (eds) *Principles of Neuro-oncology*, pp. 143–161. McGraw-Hill, New York.

Bukberg, J., Penman, D. & Holland, J.C. (1984) Depression in hospitalized cancer patients. *Psychosomatic Medicine* **46**, 199–212.

Bulow, B., Hagmar, L., Orbaek, P., Osterberg, K. & Erfurth, E.M. (2002) High incidence of mental disorders, reduced mental well-being and cognitive function in hypopituitary women with GH deficiency treated for pituitary disease. *Clinical Endocrinology* **56**, 183–193.

Burkle, F.M. & Lipowski, Z.J. (1978) Colloid cyst of the third ventricle presenting as psychiatric disorder. *American Journal of Psychiatry* **135**, 373–374.

Busch, E. (1940) Physical symptoms in neurosurgical disease. *Acta Psychiatrica et Neurologica Scandinavica* **15**, 257–290.

Cairns, H. (1950) Mental disorders with tumours of the pons. *Folio Psychiatrica, Neurologica et Neurochirurgica Neerlandica* **53**, 193–203.

Cairns, H., Oldfield, R.C., Pennybacker, J.B. & Whitterbridge, D. (1941) Akinetic mutism with an epidermoid cyst of the 3rd ventricle. *Brain* **64**, 273–290.

Carpentieri, S.C., Waber, D.P., Pomeroy, S.L. *et al.* (2003) Neuropsychological functioning after surgery in children treated for brain tumor. *Neurosurgery* **52**, 1348–1356.

Catsman-Berrevoets, C.E., Van Dongen, H.R., Mulder, P.G., Geuze, D., Paquier, P.F. & Lequin, M.H. (1999) Tumour type and size are high risk factors for the syndrome of 'cerebellar' mutism and subsequent dysarthria. *Journal of Neurology, Neurosurgery and Psychiatry* **67**, 755–757.

Chambers, W.R. (1955) Neurosurgical conditions masquerading as psychiatric diseases. *American Journal of Psychiatry* **112**, 387–389.

Chao, S.T., Suh, J.H., Raja, S., Lee, S.Y. & Barnett, G. (2001) The sensitivity and specificity of FDG PET in distinguishing recurrent brain tumor from radionecrosis in patients treated with stereotactic radiosurgery. *International Journal of Cancer* **96**, 191–197.

Chee, C.P., David, A., Galbraith, S. & Gillham, R. (1985) Dementia due to meningioma: outcome after surgical removal. *Surgical Neurology* **23**, 414–416.

Correa, D.D., DeAngelis, L.M., Shi, W., Thaler, H., Glass, A. & Abrey, L.E. (2004) Cognitive functions in survivors of primary central nervous system lymphoma. *Neurology* **62**, 548–555.

Correa, D.D., DeAngelis, L.M., Shi, W., Thaler, H.T., Lin, M. & Abrey, L.E. (2007) Cognitive functions in low-grade gliomas: disease and treatment effects. *Journal of Neuro-oncology* **81**, 175–184.

Critchley, M. (1964) Psychiatric symptoms and parietal disease: differential diagnosis. *Proceedings of the Royal Society of Medicine* **57**, 422–428.

Culine, S., Bekradda, M., Kramar, A., Rey, A., Escudier, B. & Droz, J.P. (1998) Prognostic factors for survival in patients with brain metastases from renal cell carcinoma. *Cancer* **83**, 2548–2553.

Cummings, J.L. (1993) Frontal–subcortical circuits and human behavior. *Archives of Neurology* **50**, 873–880.

Davison, K. & Bagley, C.R. (1969) Schizophrenia-like psychoses associated with organic disorders of the central nervous system: a review of the literature. In: Herrington, R.N. (ed.) *Current Problems in Neuropsychiatry*. British Journal of Psychiatry Special Publication No. 4, pp. 113–184. Headley Brothers, Ashford, Kent.

Deitcher, S.R. & Gomes, M.P. (2003) Hypercoagulable state testing and malignancy screening following venous thromboembolic events. *Vascular Medicine* **8**, 33–46.

Dekkers, O.M., van der Klaauw, A.A., Pereira, A.M. *et al.* (2006) Quality of life is decreased after treatment for nonfunctioning pituitary macroadenoma. *Journal of Clinical Endocrinology and Metabolism* **91**, 3364–3369.

Delay, J., Brion, S. & Derouesné, C. (1964) Syndrome de Korsakoff et étiologie tumorale. *Revue Neurologique (Paris)* **111**, 97–133.

Deonna, T. & Ziegler, A.L. (2000) Hypothalamic hamartoma, precocious puberty and gelastic seizures: a special model of 'epileptic' developmental disorder. *Epileptic Disorders* **2**, 33–37.

Direkze, M., Bayliss, S.G. & Cutting, J.C. (1971) Primary tumours of the frontal lobe. *British Journal of Clinical Practice* **25**, 207–213.

Dobrokhotova, T.A. & Faller, T.O. (1969) Concerning the psychopathological symptomatology in tumours of the posterior brain cavity. *Zhurnal Neuropatologi i Psikhiatrii* **8**, 1225–1230.

Doxey, D., Bruce, D., Sklar, F., Swift, D. & Shapiro, K. (1999) Posterior fossa syndrome: identifiable risk factors and irreversible complications. *Pediatric Neurosurgery* **31**, 131–136.

Duffau, H., Capelle, L., Denvil, D. *et al.* (2003) Functional recovery after surgical resection of low grade gliomas in eloquent brain: hypothesis of brain compensation. *Journal of Neurology, Neurosurgery and Psychiatry* **74**, 901–907.

Dumas-Duport, C. (1970) Tumeurs cerebrales chez les malades mentaux. Thesis for Doctorate of Medicine, Faculté de Médicine de Paris.

Elliott, F.A. (1969) The corpus callosum, cingulate gyrus, septum pellucidum, septal area and fornix. In: Vinken, P.J. & Bruyn, G.W. (eds) *Handbook of Clinical Neurology*, vol. 2, ch. 24. North-Holland Publishing Co., Amsterdam.

Filley, C.M. (1998) The behavioral neurology of cerebral white matter. *Neurology* **50**, 1535–1540.

Filley, C.M., Kleinschmidt-DeMasters, B.K., Lillehei, K.O., Damek, D.M. & Harris, J.G. (2003) Gliomatosis cerebri: neurobehavioral and neuropathological observations. *Cognitive and Behavioral Neurology* **16**, 149–159.

Frattali, C.M., Liow, K., Craig, G.H. *et al.* (2001) Cognitive deficits in children with gelastic seizures and hypothalamic hamartoma. *Neurology* **57**, 43–46.

Garofalo, J.P. & Baum, A. (2001) Neurocognitive sequelae of cancer therapies. *Current Opinion in Psychiatry* **14**, 575–583.

Glantz, M.J., Cole, B.F., Forsyth, P.A. *et al.* (2000) Practice parameter: anticonvulsant prophylaxis in patients with newly diagnosed brain tumors. Report of the Quality Standards Subcommittee of the American Academy of Neurology. *Neurology* **54**, 1886–1893.

Gottwald, B., Wilde, B., Mihajlovic, Z. & Mehdorn, H.M. (2004) Evidence for distinct cognitive deficits after focal cerebellar lesions. *Journal of Neurology, Neurosurgery and Psychiatry* **75**, 1524–1531.

Grayson, J.K. (1996) Radiation exposure, socioeconomic status, and brain tumor risk in the US Air Force: a nested case-control study. *American Journal of Epidemiology* **143**, 480–486.

Gupta, R.K. & Kumar R. (2004) Benign brain tumours and psychiatric morbidity: a 5-year retrospective data analysis. *Australian and New Zealand Journal of Psychiatry* **38**, 316–319.

Haberland, C. (1965) Psychiatric manifestations in brain tumours. *Bibliotheca Psychiatrica et Neurologica* **127**, 65–86.

Hamilton, M.G., Hull, R.D. & Pineo, G.F. (1994) Prophylaxis of venous thromboembolism in brain tumor patients. *Journal of Neuro-oncology* **22**, 111–126.

Hardell, L., Nasman, A., Pahlson, A. & Hallquist, A. (2000) Case–control study on radiology work, medical x-ray investigations, and use of cellular telephones as risk factors for brain tumors. *Medscape General Medicine* **2**, E2.

Hécaen, H. & Ajuriaguerra, J.D.E. (1956) *Troubles Mentaux au cours des Tumeurs Intracraniennes*. Masson, Paris.

Henry, G.W. (1932) Mental phenomena observed in cases of brain tumour. *American Journal of Psychiatry* **89**, 415–473.

Hildebrand, J. (2006) Neurological complications of cancer chemotherapy. *Current Opinion in Oncology* **18**, 321–324.

Hill, J.R., Kuriyama, N., Kuriyama, H. & Israel, M.A. (1999) Molecular genetics of brain tumors. *Archives of Neurology* **56**, 439–441.

Hoang-Xuan, K. & Delattre, J.Y. (1996) Biological and monoclonal antibody therapy for high-grade gliomas. *Baillieres Clinical Neurology* **5**, 395–411.

Hunter, R., Blackwood, W. & Bull, J. (1968) Three cases of frontal meningiomas presenting psychiatrically. *British Medical Journal* **3**, 9–16.

Hutterer, M., Gunsilius, E. & Stockhammer, G. (2006) Molecular therapies for malignant glioma. *Wiener Medizinische Wochenschrift* **156**, 351–363.

Ichimura, K., Schmidt, E.E., Miyakawa, A., Goike, H.M. & Collins, V.P. (1998) Distinct patterns of deletion on 10p and 10q suggest involvement of multiple tumor suppressor genes in the development of astrocytic gliomas of different malignancy grades. *Genes, Chromosomes and Cancer* **22**, 9–15.

John, G., Eapen, V. & Shaw, G.K. (1997) Frontal glioma presenting as anxiety and obsessions: a case report. *Acta Neurologica Scandinavica* **96**, 194–195.

Kalayam, B., Young, R.C. & Tsuboyama, G.K. (1994) Mood disorders associated with acoustic neuromas. *International Journal of Psychiatry in Medicine* **24**, 31–43.

Kayl, A.E. & Meyers, C.A. (2003) Does brain tumor histology influence cognitive function? *Neuro-Oncology* **5**, 255–260.

Keschner, M., Bender, M.B. & Strauss, I. (1938) Mental symptoms associated with brain tumour: a study of 530 verified cases. *Journal of the American Medical Association* **110**, 714–718.

Khalili, K. (2001) Human neurotropic JC virus and its association with brain tumors. *Disease Markers* **17**, 143–147.

Klein, M., Postma, T.J., Taphoorn, M.J. *et al.* (2003) The prognostic value of cognitive functioning in the survival of patients with high-grade glioma. *Neurology* **61**, 1796–1798.

Korali, Z., Wittchen, H.U., Pfister, H., Hofler, M., Oefelein, W. & Stalla, G.K. (2003) Are patients with pituitary adenomas at an increased risk of mental disorders? *Acta Psychiatrica Scandinavica* **107**, 60–68.

Kouyialis, A.T., Boviatsis, E.J., Prezerakos, G.K., Korfias, S. & Sakas, D.E. (2004) Complex neurobehavioural syndrome due to bilateral thalamic glioma. *British Journal of Neurosurgery* **18**, 534–537.

Kumar, S.D. & Krieger, B.P. (1998) CD4 lymphocyte counts and mortality in AIDS patients requiring mechanical ventilator support due to *Pneumocystis carinii* pneumonia. *Chest* **113**, 430–433.

Lagares, A., de Toledo, M., Gonzalez-Leon, P. *et al.* (2004) [Bilateral thalamic gliomas: report of a case with cognitive impairment.] *Revista de Neurologia* **38**, 244–246.

Lampl, Y., Barak, Y., Achiron, A. & Sarova-Pinchas I. (1995) Intracranial meningiomas: correlation of peritumoral edema and psychiatric disturbances. *Psychiatry Research* **58**, 177–180.

Levisohn, L., Cronin-Golomb, A. & Schmahmann, J.D. (2000) Neuropsychological consequences of cerebellar tumour resection in children: cerebellar cognitive affective syndrome in a paediatric population. *Brain* 123, 1041–1050.

Lewanski, C.R., Sinclair, J.A. & Stewart, J.S. (2000) Lhermitte's sign following head and neck radiotherapy. *Clinical Oncology* **12**, 98–103.

Li, Y., Millikan, R.C., Carozza, S. *et al.* (1998) p53 mutations in malignant gliomas. *Cancer Epidemiology, Biomarkers and Prevention* **7**, 303–308.

Litofsky, N.S., Farace, E., Anderson, F. Jr *et al.* (2004) Depression in patients with high-grade glioma: results of the Glioma Outcomes Project. *Neurosurgery* **54**, 358–366.

McMenemey, W.H. (1941) A critical review: dementia in middle age. *Journal of Neurology, Neurosurgery and Psychiatry* **4**, 48–79.

Mainio, A., Hakko, H., Niemela, A., Tuurinkoski, T., Koivukangas, J. & Rasanen, P. (2003) The effect of brain tumour laterality on anxiety levels among neurosurgical patients. *Journal of Neurology, Neurosurgery and Psychiatry* **74**, 1278–1282.

Mainio, A., Hakko, H., Niemela, A., Salo, J., Koivukangas, J. & Rasanen, P. (2005) Level of obsessionality among neurosurgical patients with a primary brain tumor. *Journal of Neuropsychiatry and Clinical Neurosciences* **17**, 399–404.

Malamud, N. (1967) Psychiatric disorder with intracranial tumours of limbic system. *Archives of Neurology* **17**, 113–123.

Martin, P.M. & Hussaini, I.M. (2005) PKC eta as a therapeutic target in glioblastoma multiforme. *Expert Opinion on Therapeutic Targets* **9**, 299–313.

Mastronardi, L., Puzzilli, F. & Ruggeri, A. (1998) Tamoxifen as a potential treatment of glioma. *Anticancer Drugs* **9**, 581–586.

Mathieu, D. & Fortin, D. (2006) The role of chemotherapy in the treatment of malignant astrocytomas. *Canadian Journal of Neurological Sciences* **33**, 127–140.

Maurice-Williams, R.S. (1974) Micturition symptoms in frontal tumours. *Journal of Neurology, Neurosurgery and Psychiatry* **37**, 431–436.

Meador, K.J. (1994) Cognitive side effects of antiepileptic drugs. *Canadian Journal of Neurological Sciences* **21**, S12–S16.

Meyers, C.A. (2000) Neurocognitive dysfunction in cancer patients. *Oncology (Williston Park)* **14**, 75–79.

Meyers, C.A. & Hess, K.R. (2003) Multifaceted end points in brain tumor clinical trials: cognitive deterioration precedes MRI progression. *Neuro-Oncology* **5**, 89–95.

Meyers, C.A., Weitzner, M.A., Valentine, A.D. & Levin, V.A. (1998) Methylphenidate therapy improves cognition, mood, and function of brain tumor patients. *Journal of Clinical Oncology* **16**, 2522–2527.

Meyers, C.A., Hess, K.R., Yung, W.K. & Levin, V.A. (2000a) Cognitive function as a predictor of survival in patients with recurrent malignant glioma. *Journal of Clinical Oncology* **18**, 646–650.

Meyers, C.A., Geara, F., Wong, P.F. & Morrison, W.H. (2000b) Neurocognitive effects of therapeutic irradiation for base of skull tumors. *International Journal of Radiation Oncology, Biology and Physics* **46**, 51–55.

Minski, L. (1933) The mental symptoms associated with 58 cases of cerebral tumour. *Journal of Neurology and Psychopathology* **13**, 330–343.

Mocellin, R., Walterfang, M. & Velakoulis, D. (2006) Neuropsychiatry of complex visual hallucinations. *Australian and New Zealand Journal of Psychiatry* **40**, 742–751.

Monje, M.L. & Palmer, T. (2003) Radiation injury and neurogenesis. *Current Opinion in Neurology* **16**, 129–134.

Mulhern, R.K., Khan, R.B., Kaplan, S. *et al.* (2004) Short-term efficacy of methylphenidate: a randomized, double-blind, placebo-controlled trial among survivors of childhood cancer. *Journal of Clinical Oncology* **22**, 4795–4803. [Erratum appears in *Journal of Clinical Oncology* 2005, **23**, 248.]

Murthy, P., Jayakumar, P.N. & Sampat, S. (1997) Of insects and eggs: a case report. *Journal of Neurology, Neurosurgery and Psychiatry* **63**, 522–523.

Nabors, B.L. (2005) Neuroimaging. In: Schiff, D. & O'Neill, B.P. (eds) *Principles of Neuro-oncology*, pp. 53–80. McGraw-Hill, New York.

New, P. (2001) Radiation injury to the nervous system. *Current Opinion in Neurology* **14**, 725–734.

Newell, S.A., Sanson-Fisher, R.W. & Savolainen, N.J. (2002) Systematic review of psychological therapies for cancer patients: overview and recommendations for future research. *Journal of the National Cancer Institute* **94**, 558–584.

Pace, A. & Pompili, A. (2005) Depression in patients with high-grade glioma: results of the Glioma Project. *Neurosurgery* **56**, E873.

Paillas, J.-E. & Tamalet, J. (1950) Les tumeurs temporales. *Presse Medicale* **58**, 550–554.

Parry, J. (1968) Contribution a l'etude des manifestations des lesions expansives observees dans un hopital psychiatrique. Thesis, Faculté de Médicine de Paris.

Patton, R.B. & Sheppard, J.A. (1956) Intracranial tumors found at autopsy in mental patients. *American Journal of Psychiatry* **113**, 319–324.

Peissner, W., Kocher, M., Treuer, H. & Gillardon, F. (1999) Ionizing radiation-induced apoptosis of proliferating stem cells in the dentate gyrus of the adult rat hippocampus. *Brain Research Molecular Brain Research* **71**, 61–68.

Pelletier, G., Verhoef, M.J., Khatri, N. & Hagen, N. (2002) Quality of life in brain tumor patients: the relative contributions of depression, fatigue, emotional distress, and existential issues. *Journal of Neuro-oncology* **57**, 41–49.

Peterson, B.S., Bronen, R.A. & Duncan, C.C. (1996) Three cases of symptom change in Tourette's syndrome and obsessive–compulsive disorder associated with paediatric cerebral malignancies. *Journal of Neurology, Neurosurgery and Psychiatry* **61**, 497–505.

Pirl, W.F. & Roth, A.J. (1999) Diagnosis and treatment of depression in cancer patients. *Oncology* **13**, 1293–1301.

Pollack, I.F. (1997) Posterior fossa syndrome. *International Review of Neurobiology* **41**, 411–432.

Postma, T.J., Klein, M., Verstappen, C.C. *et al.* (2002) Radiotherapy-induced cerebral abnormalities in patients with low-grade glioma. *Neurology* **59**, 121–123.

Price, T.R.P., Goetz, K.L. & Lovell, M.R. (2005) Neuropsychiatric aspects of brain tumours. In: Yudofsky, S.C. & Hales, R.E. (eds) *Textbook of Neuropsychiatry and Clinical Neurosciences*, 4th edn, pp. 753–782. American Psychiatric Publishing Inc., Washington, DC.

Pringle, A.M., Taylor, R. & Whittle, I.R. (1999) Anxiety and depression in patients with an intracranial neoplasm before and after tumour surgery. *British Journal of Neurosurgery* **13**, 46–51.

Raskin, N. (1956) Intracranial neoplasms in psychotic patients. *American Journal of Psychiatry* **112**, 481–484.

Redd, W.H., Montgomery, G.H. & DuHamel, K.N. (2001) Behavioral intervention for cancer treatment side effects. *Journal of the National Cancer Institute* **93**, 810–823.

Rees, J.H. (2002) Low-grade gliomas in adults. *Current Opinion in Neurology* **15**, 657–661.

Reeves, A.G. & Plum, F. (1969) Hyperphagia, rage and dementia accompanying a ventromedial hypothalamic neoplasm. *Archives of Neurology* **20**, 616–624.

Ronning, C., Sundet, K., Due-Tonnessen, B., Lundar, T. & Helseth, E. (2005) Persistent cognitive dysfunction secondary to cerebellar injury in patients treated for posterior fossa tumors in childhood. *Pediatric Neurosurgery* **41**, 15–21.

Roser, F., Ritz, R., Koerbel, A., Loewenheim, H. & Tatagiba, M.S. (2005) Peduncular hallucinosis: insights from a neurosurgical point of view. *Neurosurgery* **57**, E1068.

Roth, C., Wilken, B., Hanefeld, F., Schroter, W. & Leonhardt, U. (1998) Hyperphagia in children with craniopharyngioma is associated with hyperleptinaemia and a failure in the downregulation of appetite. *European Journal of Endocrinology* **138**, 89–91.

Rudge, P. & Warrington, E.K. (1991) Selective impairment of memory and visual perception in splenial tumours. *Brain* **114**, 349–360.

Russell, R.W.R. & Pennybacker, J.B. (1961) Craniopharyngioma in the elderly. *Journal of Neurology, Neurosurgery and Psychiatry* **24**, 1–13.

Sachs, E. (1950) Meningiomas with dementia as the first and presenting failure. *Journal of Mental Science* **96**, 998–1007.

Salo, J., Niemela, A., Joukamaa, M. & Koivukangas, J. (2002) Effect of brain tumour laterality on patients' perceived quality of life. *Journal of Neurology, Neurosurgery and Psychiatry* **72**, 373–377.

Sarkissian, V. (2005) The sequelae of cranial irradiation on human cognition. *Neuroscience Letters* **382**, 118–123.

Sathornsumetee, S. & Rich, J.N. (2006) New treatment strategies for malignant gliomas. *Expert Review of Anticancer Therapy* **6**, 1087–1104.

Schlesinger, B. (1950) Mental changes in intracranial tumours, and related problems. *Confinia Neurologica* **10**, 225–263, 322–355.

Schmahmann, J.D. & Sherman, J.C. (1998) The cerebellar cognitive affective syndrome. *Brain* **121**, 561–579.

Schwartz, L., Lander, M. & Chochinov, H.M. (2002) Current management of depression in cancer patients. *Oncology* **16**, 1102–1110.

Scott, M. (1970) Transitory psychotic behaviour following operation for tumours of the cerebello-pontine angle. *Psychiatria, Neurologia, Neurochirurgia* **73**, 37–48.

Selecki, B.R. (1964) Cerebral mid-line tumours involving the corpus callosum among mental hospital patients. *Medical Journal of Australia* **2**, 954–960.

Shepherd, R.H. & Wadia, N.H. (1956) Some observations on atypical features in acoustic neuromas. *Brain* **79**, 282–318.

Smith, A. (1966) Intellectual functions in patients with lateralised frontal tumours. *Journal of Neurology, Neurosurgery and Psychiatry* **29**, 52–59.

Smyth, G.E. & Stern, K. (1938) Tumours of the thalamus: a clinicopathological study. *Brain* **61**, 339–374.

Sokolski, K.N. & Denson, T.F. (2003) Exacerbation of mania secondary to right temporal lobe astrocytoma in a bipolar patient previously stabilized on valproate. *Cognitive and Behavioral Neurology* **16**, 234–238.

Spence, S.A., Taylor, D.G. & Hirsch, S.R. (1995) Depressive disorder due to craniopharyngioma. *Journal of the Royal Society of Medicine* **88**, 637–638.

Sprofkin, B.E. & Sciarra, D. (1952) Korsakoff psychosis associated with cerebral tumours. *Neurology* **2**, 427–434.

Stark, D., Kiely, M., Smith, A., Velikova, G., House, A. & Selby, P. (2002) Anxiety disorders in cancer patients: their nature, associations, and relation to quality of life. *Journal of Clinical Oncology* **20**, 3137–3148.

Starkstein, S.E., Boston, J.D. & Robinson, R.G. (1988) Mechanisms of mania after brain injury: 12 case reports and review of the literature. *Journal of Nervous and Mental Disease* **176**, 87–100.

Steeghs, N., de Jongh, F.E., Sillevis Smitt, P.A. & van den Bent, M.J. (2003) Cisplatin-induced encephalopathy and seizures. *Anticancer Drugs* **14**, 443–446.

Strauss, I. & Keschner, M. (1935) Mental symptoms in cases of tumour of the frontal lobe. *Archives of Neurology and Psychiatry* **33**, 986–1005.

Strobos, R.R.J. (1953) Tumours of temporal lobe. *Neurology* **3**, 752–760.

Sumner, D. (1969) The diagnosis of intracranial tumours. *British Journal of Hospital Medicine* **2**, 489–494.

Swensen, R. & Kirsch, W. (2002) Brain neoplasms in women: a review. *Clinical Obstetrics and Gynecology* **45**, 904–927.

Taphoorn, M.J.B. & Bromberg, J.E.C. (2005) Neurological effects of therapeutic irradiation. *Continuum: Lifelong Learning in Neurology* **11**, 93–115.

Taphoorn, M.J. & Klein, M. (2004) Cognitive deficits in adult patients with brain tumours. *Lancet Neurology* **3**, 159–168.

Tonkonogy, J.M. & Geller, J.L. (1992) Hypothalamic lesions and intermittent explosive disorder. *Journal of Neuropsychiatry and Clinical Neurosciences* **4**, 45–50.

Toth, C., Voll, C. & Macaulay, R. (2002) Primary CNS lymphoma as a cause of Korsakoff syndrome. *Surgical Neurology* **57**, 41–45.

Tucha, O., Smely, C. & Lange, K.W. (2001) Effects of surgery on cognitive functioning of elderly patients with intracranial meningioma. *British Journal of Neurosurgery* **15**, 184–188.

Turkel, S.B., Shu, C.L., Nelson, M.D. *et al.* (2004) Case series: acute mood symptoms associated with posterior fossa lesions in children. *Journal of Neuropsychiatry and Clinical Neurosciences* **16**, 443–445.

Umemura, A., Yamada, K., Masago, A., Tanigawa, M., Nakaaki, S. & Hamanaka, T. (1997) Pure amnesia caused by bilateral temporal lobe astrocytoma: case report. *Neurologia Medico-chirurgica (Tokyo)* **37**, 556–559.

Van der Maazen, R.W., Kleiboer, B.J., Verhagen, I. & van der Kogel, A.J. (1991) Irradiation in vitro discriminates between different O-2A progenitor cell subpopulations in the perinatal central nervous system of rats. *Radiation Research* **128**, 64–72.

Vecht, C.J., Wagner, G.L. & Wilms, E.B. (2003) Treating seizures in patients with brain tumors: drug interactions between antiepileptic and chemotherapeutic agents. *Seminars in Oncology* **30** (6 suppl. 19), 52.

Weissenberger, A.A., Dell, M.L., Liow, K. *et al.* (2001) Aggression and psychiatric comorbidity in children with hypothalamic hamartomas and their unaffected siblings. *Journal of the American Academy of Child and Adolescent Psychiatry* **40**, 696–703.

Weitzner, M.A. & Meyers, C.A. (1997) Cognitive functioning and quality of life in malignant glioma patients: a review of the literature. *Psychooncology* **6**, 169–177.

Weitzner, M.A., Kanfer, S. & Booth-Jones, M. (2005) Apathy and pituitary disease: it has nothing to do with depression. *Journal of Neuropsychiatry and Clinical Neurosciences* **17**, 159–166.

Wellisch, D.K., Kaleita, T.A., Freeman, D., Cloughesy, T. & Goldman, J. (2002) Predicting major depression in brain tumor patients. *Psychooncology* **11**, 230–238.

Wen, P.Y. & Marks, P.W. (2002) Medical management of patients with brain tumors. *Current Opinion in Oncology* **14**, 299–307.

Wen, P.Y., Teoh, S.K., Gigas, D.C. & MacDonald, L. (2005) Presentatiom and approach to the patient. In: Schiff, D. & O'Neill, B.P. (eds) *Principles of Neuro-oncology*, pp. 37–51. McGraw-Hill, New York.

Williams, M. & Pennybacker, J. (1954) Memory disturbances in third ventricle tumours. *Journal of Neurosurgery and Psychiatry* **17**, 115–123.

Wilson, G. & Rupp, C. (1946) Mental symptoms associated with extramedullary posterior fossa tumours. In: *Transactions of the American Neurological Association, 71st Annual Meeting*, pp. 104–107. William Byrd Press, Richmond, VA.

Woodcock, S.M. (1967) Mental symptoms in patients with acoustic neuromas. *Journal of Neurology, Neurosurgery and Psychiatry* **30**, 587.

Wrensch, M., Weinberg, A., Wiencke, J. *et al.* (2005) History of chickenpox and shingles and prevalence of antibodies to varicella-zoster virus and three other herpesviruses among adults with glioma and controls. *American Journal of Epidemiology* **161**, 929–938.

Yasuda, K., Watanabe, O. & Ono, Y. (1997) Dissociation between semantic and autobiographic memory: a case report. *Cortex* **33**, 623–638.

Yuan, X., Hu, J., Belladonna, M.L., Black, K.L. & Yu, J.S. (2006) Interleukin-23-expressing bone marrow-derived neural stem-like cells exhibit antitumor activity against intracranial glioma. *Cancer Research* **66**, 2630–2638.

CHAPTER 6

Epilepsy

John D.C. Mellers

Maudsley Hospital, London

The manifestations of epilepsy include facets of equal importance to the psychiatrist and the neurologist. Some aspects indeed stand firmly at the junction between the two disciplines. The seizure itself may take the form of the classic motor convulsion or consist instead of complex abnormalities of behaviour and subjective experience. Associated disorders may sometimes include cognitive difficulties, personality disturbances or psychotic illnesses of various types and durations. In all these respects the study of patients with epilepsy has played an important part in advancing our knowledge of brain function and dysfunction, and in indicating something of the pathophysiological basis for certain forms of psychological disorder.

The accent in this chapter is on those aspects most relevant to the work of the psychiatrist. It is now clear that the great majority of people with epilepsy suffer little or no mental disturbance, but those who do can present difficult and complicated problems. Psychosocial and organic factors are often inextricably mixed in causation, and assessment of all the evidence available in the individual patient can be a complex and time-consuming matter.

Classification of seizures and epilepsies

Chadwick (1994) recommends defining an *epileptic seizure* as 'an intermittent, stereotyped disturbance of consciousness, behaviour, emotion, motor function or sensation that on clinical grounds is believed to result from cortical neuronal discharge'. This definition conveys three important principles: (i) that the core presenting feature, the seizure, is a transient abnormality of neurological function that is highly uniform from one episode to the next; (ii) that the diagnosis depends primarily on clinical judgement; and (iii) that the underlying mechanism of an epileptic seizure is an abnormal cortical discharge. The term *epilepsy* denotes a condition in which there are recurrent epileptic seizures (unless they arise in the context of a reversible toxic or metabolic state). Although a diagnosis of epilepsy implies that symptoms are the result of abnormal electrical activity, this may in turn have many different causes. Thus, epilepsy must always be regarded as a symptom rather than a disease. It is a sign of abnormality within the central nervous system (CNS) that requires further elucidation.

The current classification of epilepsy (Commission on Classification and Terminology of the International League Against Epilepsy 1981, 1989) approaches the subject at two levels: (i) there is a system for classifying seizures based on clinical signs and symptoms (i.e. semiology), and (ii) there is a classification of epileptic syndromes. The latter is derived from the classification of seizures, but in addition takes into account patterns of signs and symptoms, age at onset, electrophysiological findings, natural history and factors of potential aetiological significance, including background and family history and pathology where known. It represents an attempt to define syndromes that are homogeneous with respect to aetiology and which have practical implications for treatment and prognosis. It is an imperfect and evolving nosology. With advances in our understanding of pathophysiology, and perhaps the genetics of epilepsy in particular, future refinements to this system are both inevitable and desirable.

Classification of seizures

The International League Against Epilepsy (ILAE) system for classifying epileptic seizures is shown in Table 6.1. The most important division distinguishes between seizures that arise from epileptic discharges beginning in a circumscribed brain region (*partial seizures*) and seizures that have no detectable focal onset and seemingly involve the cortex bilaterally from the start (*generalised seizures*). A third category of unclassified or mixed seizure types is included in recognition of

Lishman's Organic Psychiatry: A Textbook of Neuropsychiatry, 4th edition.
© 2009 Blackwell Publishing.   ISBN 978-1-4051-1860-1

Table 6.1 International classification of epileptic seizures. (Adapted from Commission on Classification and Terminology of the International League Against Epilepsy 1981 with permission.)

I	*Partial seizures*
A	Simple partial seizures
B	Complex partial seizures
C	Partial seizures evolving to secondarily generalised seizures
II	*Generalised seizures*
A1	Absence seizures
A2	Atypical absence seizures
B	Myoclonic seizures
C	Clonic seizures
D	Tonic seizures
E	Tonic–clonic seizures
F	Atonic seizures
III	*Unclasssified epileptic seizures*

rare cases in which classification is uncertain. A description of the main clinical characteristics of seizure types is given in the next section to provide an overview of seizure semiology. Further detail about specific semiological features and their localising value is given in the section covering the localisation-related epilepsy syndromes. A glossary of terms used to describe seizures is provided by the ILAE (Blume *et al.* 2001).

Partial seizures

The term 'partial' in the current classification system replaces the older terms 'focal' and 'focal-onset'. Partial seizures occur when an epileptic discharge arises from a localised region of a single cerebral hemisphere. Partial seizures are subclassified according to whether consciousness is fully retained throughout (*simple partial*) or impaired (*complex partial*) and whether they evolve to become a generalised seizure.

Simple partial seizures

During a simple partial seizure the patient remains fully conscious and is therefore usually able to provide a description of the attack. The symptoms at the beginning of the seizure are of great importance as they may indicate which area of the brain is involved at the onset of the epileptic discharge. Any neurological function may be affected but motor signs are the most frequent. The most common form of simple partial seizure is a motor seizure arising from the primary motor cortex. This gives rise to regular, rhythmical, jerking (clonic) movements in the group of muscles corresponding to the affected area in the cortex. If the seizure discharge spreads, it does so along the motor strip moving between adjacent regions of the motor homunculus. This phenomenon was first described by Hughlings Jackson and focal motor seizures of this type are known as *Jacksonian motor seizures*. The progression to adjacent muscle groups is known as

a *Jacksonian march*. Other motor signs, including dystonic posturing and complex behavioural automatisms, are more common in complex partial seizures. A special variety of dystonic posturing in which there is sustained rotation of the head and neck, sometimes accompanied by version of the eyes into lateral gaze, may be referred to as an *adversive seizure*. The direction in which the head and eyes move at seizure onset is a moderately reliable lateralising sign, with both moving away from the hemisphere in which the discharge begins. Partial motor seizures may sometimes be followed by a transient paralysis (*Todd's paresis*), which may last from minutes to several hours. Vocalisations and sudden cessation of speech are further examples of motor phenomena. With respect to sensory experiences, an important principle is that when the epileptogenic focus is sited in primary sensory cortex, the patient experiences elementary sensory symptoms. In contrast, seizures arising in neocortical regions with a higher-order integrating sensory function, for example temporoparietal areas, result in more complex illusions and hallucinations. Thus, seizures arising in the first postcentral gyrus evoke somatosensory symptoms such as tingling, pins and needles, electrical sensations and numbness which, like their motor counterpart, may show Jacksonian progression. Similarly, seizures arising in the primary visual or auditory cortex are associated with elemental hallucinations: in the case of the primary visual cortex, flashing lights, simple shapes and patterns are commonly described, while buzzing and hissing sounds are examples of symptoms associated with epileptic foci in the primary auditory cortex (middle temporal gyrus). Olfactory and gustatory experiences are usually unpleasant (burning, metallic) or difficult for the patient to characterise, and are associated with seizures arising in the limbic system. A relatively common symptom, sometimes known as a *cephalic aura*, is the experience of an indescribable sensation in the head. Symptoms classified as autonomic by the ILAE include some of the most common epileptic symptoms. Most notably, the classic *epigastric aura*, which comprises a sensation of 'butterflies in the stomach', beginning in the epigastrium and then rising up the chest. This is most commonly associated with medial temporal lobe foci. Other autonomic symptoms include changes in heart rate, blood pressure, perspiration, piloerection, 'goosebumps' and mydriasis. These symptoms arise when midline basal brain structures are involved in seizure discharge.

Of particular interest to psychiatrists are the symptoms described as psychic in the ILEA classification. Cognitive symptoms include dysphasia and various distortions of memory (dymnesic symptoms) such as *déjà vu*, a vivid sense that everything has happened before, *jamais vu*, a sense that everything suddenly seems unfamiliar and new, and *panoramic memory*, in which the patient relives an experience from their past played back rapidly in the mind's eye. Patients may experience distortions of thought such as *forced thinking*, which describes a feeling of being compelled to think about a specific topic or word; or *crowding of thoughts*, which describes a feeling of racing, disorganised thoughts. Subtle but disturbing changes in the quality of perception are reported, including derealisation and depersonalisation, distortions in the perception of time and changes in the significance of objects. These latter are often impossible for patients to describe but may involve a sense that a specific object in their environment seems changed and has a heightened but mysterious personal relevance. Affective symptoms are usually unpleasant and include fear, dysphoria, sadness and feelings of unworthiness or guilt. Occasionally mood changes are pleasurable. Illusions and complex fully formed hallucinations in all modalities may occur. Patients usually retain insight into the illusory nature of their misperceptions.

Simple partial seizures are brief, usually lasting for a few seconds only and rarely for more than 2 minutes. Scalp electroencephalography (EEG) during a simple partial seizure (ictal EEG) is usually entirely normal (Devinsky *et al.* 1988) and thus is usually not helpful in differentiating simple partial seizures from psychiatric presentations such as dissociative seizures, panic attacks or psychotic symptoms.

Complex partial seizures

Complex partial seizures are partial seizures that involve some degree of impaired consciousness. In most complex partial seizures, however, the patient is fully aware for a few seconds at seizure onset. In these cases patients experience symptoms at the beginning of a complex seizure, known as an *aura*, that may include any of those associated with simple partial seizures described above. In some 20% of cases patients report no aura, indicating either that consciousness was impaired from the start or that the patient has no memory of any premonitory symptoms after the seizure. Subtle degrees of impaired consciousness may be difficult to determine, especially in the presence of dysphasia or overwhelming affective experiences and indeed this is a criticism that has been levelled at the current system of classification. Although the defining characteristic of complex partial seizures is that consciousness is impaired at some stage of the seizure, unconsciousness – with loss of axial muscle tone, a fall and complete unresponsiveness – is not implied. Rather there is clouding of consciousness during which the patient will appear confused, disoriented and preoccupied but may interact with people and handle objects in their immediate environment, albeit in a disorganised manner and in ways that are inappropriate to the immediate social context. To the observer there is an inconspicuous and gradual transition from normal alertness to impaired responsiveness. Recovery, likewise, is almost never abrupt. During the phase of impaired consciousness the patient commonly engages in repetitive semi-purposeful activities known as *automatisms* [Classification of epilepsy syndromes (Anatomically defined localisation-related epilepsy syndromes) and Epileptic automatisms (under Classification of psychiatric syndromes in epilepsy)]. The most common are oro-alimentary automatisms, which include lip-smacking, chewing and swallowing movements. Repetitively picking at, or adjusting, clothing or handling objects within easy reach are also frequent (gestural automatisms). Vocal automatisms may include perseverative utterances (sometimes called epileptic pallilalia), humming, singing and laughing (*gelastic seizures*). The laughter in gelastic seizures typically has an unusual quality, is not infectious and seems mirthless. Wandering is common (ambulatory automatisms) and may seem semi-purposeful, as if the patient is searching for something or trying to escape, or may involve walking in circles (*cursive seizures*) or running. Although impairment of consciousness has conventionally been regarded as a necessary condition for the emergence of automatisms, isolated cases have been reported in which automatisms have occurred while the patient remained fully alert and responsive during clearly documented simple partial seizures (Alarcon *et al.* 1998; Biraben *et al.* 2001). The ictal EEG in complex partial seizures reveals unilateral or frequently bilateral epileptiform discharges most commonly in the temporal or frontotemporal regions.

Partial seizures with secondary generalisation

Approximately 60% of patients with partial seizures will experience a secondary generalised seizure at some point. Occasionally, patients have secondarily generalised seizures with almost every partial seizure. In such cases the generalised convulsion may be so dramatic that it overshadows the preceding partial seizure. For this reason, when a patient presents with apparent generalised seizures, care must always be taken to search for any evidence of a partial seizure onset: from the patients themselves, who should be questioned about aura symptoms, and from witnesses who should be asked about blank staring episodes or brief automatisms occurring before the convulsion.

Generalised seizures

The defining characteristic of generalised seizures is that they have no detectable focal onset: the abnormal electrical discharges that accompany clinical seizures involve the cerebral cortex bilaterally at onset. Competing hypotheses have proposed that the primary abnormality, conceived of as hyperexcitability, might lie in the cortex or in a subcortical 'centrencephalic' system (i.e. brainstem reticular formation and the nuclei of the diffuse thalamic projection system), a debate that has not yet been resolved (Avoli *et al.* 2001). Generalised seizures are divided into six sharply differing forms: absence (petit mal), myoclonic, tonic–clonic, tonic, clonic and atonic, as described below. This classification is based on the marked clinical differences between each type of seizure, but each seizure type is also accompanied by characteristic EEG findings. This presumably reflects distinct underlying pathophysiology, but the nature of this is poorly understood, as indeed are the mechanisms that link EEG abnormalities with clinical semiology.

Absence (petit mal) seizures

Absence (petit mal) seizures begin in childhood or adolescence and dissappear in 80% of cases by adulthood, or are replaced by generalised tonic–clonic seizures. They rarely occur *de novo* in adults (see Generalised epilepsy and Nonconvulsive status epilepticus (Absence status) later in chapter). Without warning the patient loses contact with the environment, usually for 4 or 5 seconds but occasionally for as long as half a minute. To the onlooker the patient appears momentarily dazed, stops speaking and becomes immobile. The face is pale, the eyes assume a glazed appearance and the pupils may be observed to be fixed and dilated. Posture and balance are usually well maintained, though muscular relaxation may allow the head to slump forward. Brief muscular twitches may be seen around the eyes, occasionally extending to brief myoclonic jerks of the limbs. Such movements are bilateral and symmetrical. Consciousness is typically deeply impaired during the attack, though in rare cases subjects may remain dimly aware of what is happening around them. There are usually no after-effects. The patient may later be aware of the attack as a momentary break in the continuity of events, but quite often does not know it has occurred and continues immediately with the sentence or activity that was interrupted. While each attack is brief, runs of attacks sometimes occur in rapid succession. The frequency of episodes is commonly five to ten per day, but sometimes hundreds may be noted in the course of a single day. In such cases individual seizures may be so fleeting and inconspicuous that the disorder only comes to light because of a decline in a child's performance at school. Lennox (1960) suggested that if attacks do not occur daily, the diagnosis should be questioned.

Atypical absences show more protean manifestations, yet are accompanied in the main by the EEG features of simple absences. They begin and end abruptly like typical absences but the duration of attacks is likely to be longer, and they are often accompanied by prominent increases or decreases in muscle tone and tonic activity (Holmes *et al.* 1987). They are more likely to occur in patients with developmental delay and additional seizure types, and the interictal EEG is more frequently abnormal. However, typical and atypical absences seem not to be discrete entities, but rather form parts of a continuum. In 'absence with automatism' there may be lip-smacking, chewing, mouthing or fumbling movements, even brief aimless walking, and vocalisations may occur. Such automatisms can present difficulty over clinical differentiation from brief temporal lobe seizures, particularly when the latter are partially controlled by drugs. Close observation of the content of the attacks and the EEG picture usually serve to make the distinction, but sometimes even the latter will yield inconclusive results. In such circumstances one may ultimately be forced to a trial of different medications (Marsden & Reynolds 1982).

Tonic–clonic seizures

Tonic–clonic seizures (formerly known as grand-mal seizures) of the primary generalised type occur without immediate warning and consciousness is lost abruptly. However, some subjects may be aware that a fit is imminent on account of ill-defined symptoms (the *prodrome*, see Pre-ictal disorders, later in chapter) present for hours or even days before the seizure, such as irritability, sleep disturbance, anxiety, nausea or headache. In subjects liable to myoclonic jerks these may increase in frequency for some hours before the tonic–clonic seizure. The seizure consists of a tonic followed by a clonic phase that involves all parts of the body symmetrically and from the same moment. During the tonic phase there is first flexion then extension of the axial muscles, rapidly spreading to the limbs. Forced exhalation may be accompanied by vocalisation in the form of a moan or cry. Disruption of respiration may lead to cyanosis. Eyes remain open, are deviated upwards and the pupils dilated. As the clonic phase begins, muscular ridgidity is gradually replaced by generalised jerking movements that are regular and synchronous in all four limbs. Initially, the convulsive movements are fast (8 Hz) and appear tremulous but they gradually slow to around 4 Hz. Respiration becomes laboured and saliva may be extruded through closed teeth, giving the appearance of frothing at the mouth. Patients may injure themselves by falling at seizure onset, may bite their tongue or inside of their cheek at the beginning of the clonic phase, and may be incontinent during either the tonic phase or in the immediate postictal period. Compression fractures of the vertebrae may occur in the tonic phase but are often asymptomatic. The seizure is usually followed by a deep sleep, which may then be succeeded by nausea, vomiting and headache. If sleep does not occur, a period of confusion is usually seen before full consciousness is regained. During this period the patient is disorientated, often restless, rambling and incoherent, and sometimes unaware of his personal identity. On recovery there is total amnesia for the content of the attack and frequently for a period of several seconds extending in a retrograde direction. Most tonic–clonic seizures last for less than 1 minute. Occaisionally, especially with treatment, very brief seizures are followed by rapid recovery with little postictal confusion.

Tonic and clonic seizures

Tonic and clonic seizures may occur in isolation. Tonic seizures simply resemble the tonic phase of a tonic–clonic seizure as described above. They most commonly occur in sleep and recovery is typically abrupt with little postictal confusion. Slowly evolving changes in tone are occasionally seen as are versive movements. Isolated clonic seizures begin with a sudden loss of consciousness, loss of muscle tone and a fall.

Myoclonic seizures

The term 'myoclonus' may be used in a generic sense and refers to shock-like involuntary movements arising through a variety of neurological mechanisms which, in addition to epilepsy, may include disorders of the spinal cord, cerebellum and brainstem. In the context of epilepsy, myoclonic seizures are sudden shock-like movements, lasting for only a fraction of a second, affecting mainly the neck, arms and shoulders. Objects that are being held may be dropped or flung violently. If the trunk or legs are affected, the patient may be thrown off balance. Seizures are often bilateral but not necessarily so and a single limb or even a single muscle group may be affected. It is uncertain whether consciousness is lost or retained, since the seizures last for so very short a time, but myoclonic seizures occurring in rapid succession may be associated with impaired awareness and responsiveness. Single myoclonic jerks frequently occur in subjects suffering from absences or atonic seizures. Benign myoclonic jerks may also be seen in normal individuals when falling asleep. Myoclonic seizures are a defining characteristic of juvenile myoclonic epilepsy (see below). They may also be symptomatic of several serious brain diseases. They are a characteristic feature of subacute encephalitis, the cerebral lipoidoses and Creutzfeldt–Jakob disease. Rare progressive forms of myoclonic epilepsy, which may be associated with progressive ataxia or dementia, include Unverricht–Lundborg disease and Lafora body disease (Epilepsy occurring in hereditary disorders, later in chapter).

Atonic seizures

Atonic seizures involve a sudden loss or diminution of muscle tone, resulting in precipitate muscular relaxation affecting the head, trunk, jaw or limbs. Attacks occur without warning and last for a few seconds only. After-effects, other than those due to bruising or emotional shock, do not occur. *Astatic seizure* is a term that has come into widespread use since the 1981 ILAE classification. It refers to seizures in which the main, if not only, manifestation is loss of erect posture and a fall. The term reflects a growing realisation that such attacks occur in different forms of epilepsy and that pure atonic seizures as defined in the classification system are uncommon (Egli *et al.* 1985). Thus, sudden hypotonic falls may follow generalised myoclonic seizures (myoclonic–astatic seizures) or brief tonic seizures or may occur in patients with tonic–clonic seizures, when they represent unusually brief and abortive forms of major seizure discharges. Finally, astatic seizures have been documented as a late development in patients with intractable temporal lobe epilepsy (Gambardella *et al.* 1994). The term 'drop attack' is sometimes regarded as synonymous with astatic seizure, but the former may be used as a generic term to describe a sudden fall without conspicuous impairment of consciousness that may have causes other than epilepsy such as certain forms of syncope and cataplexy (see Differential diagnosis of epilepsy, later in chapter, covering the differential diagnosis of epilepsy).

Unclassifiable and mixed forms of epileptic seizures

In some patients the most careful investigation will fail to clarify the precise nature of attacks and seizures will defy attempts at classification. Certain neonatal seizures fall into this category.

Classification of epilepsy syndromes

The ILAE classification of epilepsy is an attempt to classify epileptic syndromes by aetiology (Table 6.2). Two levels of classification are employed. Firstly, syndromes are divided into *localisation-related* or *generalised* depending on whether underlying pathology is known or suspected to be focal or general. Secondly, a classification based on known, presumed or likely aetiology is made. In relation to the first level of classification, the term 'localisation-related' is preferred to 'partial' to avoid connotations that a syndrome is incomplete in some way. Although this aspect of the syndromic classification mirrors the division of seizures into partial and generalised, it should be emphasised that it is intended as a definition based on whether or not pathology is focal, not simply on whether the seizures seen in the syndrome are partial or generalised: partial seizures may occur in patients with a symptomatic generalised epilepsy and partial seizures may secondarily generalise in localisation-related epilepsy. The second level of classification defines three classes of aetiology: 'symptomatic' denotes an identified aetiology; 'idiopathic' denotes unknown aetiology; and 'cryptogenic' is used in relation to syndromes that seem so strikingly uniform that a specific aetiology is suspected or presumed. The idiopathic designation is more precisely defined as epilepsy arising as a primary or autochthonous disorder (arising of itself) and includes syndromes known or likely to have a genetic basis. The system of classifying epilepsy syndromes is widely recognised as imperfect and evolving, with substantial revisions expected in the near future. Revisions are especially likely with developments in our understanding of the genetic basis of epilepsy (Engel 2001). Nevertheless, in clinical practice the current classification represents a valuable framework against which an individual patient's clinical history should be considered in order to guide treatment decisions and advice about prognosis.

Localisation-related epilepsy syndromes

Modern investigations, particularly magnetic resonance imaging (MRI), will identify a specific aetiology in the majority of patients with partial seizures, who may therefore be classified as having symptomatic localisation-related epilepsy. In most patients without an identifiable lesional basis for their epilepsy, a combination of localising semiological features and/or focal electrophysiological findings will lead to the assumption that a cause is present but eludes identification. These cases would therefore be regarded as cryptogenic. In relation to the idiopathic syndromes, it should be noted that a number of inherited syndromes of localisation-related epilepsy, for example autosomal dominant nocturnal frontal lobe epilepsy (see Genetic basis of epilepsy, later in

Table 6.2 International classification of epilepsies and epileptic syndromes. (Modified from Commission on Classification and Terminology of the International League Against Epilepsy 1989 with permission.)

---

1 Localisation-related (local, focal, partial) epilepsies and syndromes
1.1 Idiopathic
Benign childhood epilepsy with centrotemporal spikes
Childhood epilepsy with occipital paroxysms
Primary reading epilepsy

1.2 Symptomatic
Chronic epilepsia partialis continua of childhood (Kojewnikoff's syndrome)
Syndromes characterised by seizures with specific modes of precipitation
Temporal lobe epilepsy
Frontal lobe epilepsy
Parietal lobe epilepsy
Occipital lobe epilepsy

1.3 Cryptogenic

2 Generalised epilepsies and syndromes
2.1 Idiopathic (with age-related onset)
Benign neonatal familial convulsions*
Benign neonatal convulsions*
Benign myoclonic epilepsy in infancy*
Juvenile absence epilepsy (pyknoepilepsy)
Childhood absence epilepsy
Juvenile myoclonic epilepsy (impulsive petit mal)
Epilepsy with grand mal seizures on awakening
Other generalised idiopathic epilepsies
Epilepsies with seizures precipitated by specific modes of activation

2.2 Cryptogenic or symptomatic
West syndrome
Lennox–Gastaut syndrome
Epilepsy with myoclonic–astatic seizures
Epilepsy with myoclonic absences

2.3 Symptomatic
2.3.1 Non-specific etiology
Early myoclonic encephalopathy*
Early infantile epileptic encephalopathy with suppression-burst*
Other symptomatic generalised epilepsies not defined above
2.3.2 Specific syndromes
Epileptic seizures complicating other disease states

3 Epilepsies and syndromes undetermined, whether focal or generalised

4 Special syndromes
4.1 Situation-related seizures
Febrile convulsions
Isolated seizures or isolated status epilepticus
Seizures occurring only when there is an acute metabolic or toxic event due to factors such as alcohol, drugs, eclampsia, non-ketotic hyperglycaemia

---

* Syndromes confined to the neonate or early infancy are not considered further here.

chapter), are not included in the current classification as they had not been described when it was published.

Idiopathic localisation-related epilepsy
Benign childhood epilepsy with centrotemporal spikes (also known as benign partial epilepsy of childhood and benign rolandic epilepsy). This syndrome is characterised by infrequent highly characteristic partial seizures with onset between age 3 and 12 years. Affected children are neurologically and intellectually normal. Seizures usually arise in sleep, are simple partial in form, and typically begin in facial and orobuccal areas with clonic movements, speech arrest, drooling and dysarthria, sometimes evolving to unilateral tonic or clonic seizures. Secondary generalisation may occur. Up to 10% of patients will have experienced a prior febrile convulsion and 40% have a family history of epilepsy. While a variety of pathological changes have been reported in patients who otherwise meet criteria for this syndrome, such findings probably suggest the diagnosis should be revised. The EEG reveals focal spikes, most commonly in the central and mid-temporal region. It should be noted that centrotemporal spikes may be seen in healthy children, the vast majority of whom will never develop epilepsy (Verrotti *et al.* 1999). The syndrome is almost invariably benign with seizures disappearing by the late teens. Treatment does not alter the natural history of the disorder and may only be indicated when there are secondarily generalised seizures or frequent daytime seizures. Counselling for families about the benign nature of the disorder is effective in preventing the psychosocial morbidity that may be associated with the diagnosis of epilepsy (Lerman & Kivity, 1975). Variations from the characteristic clinical presentation are associated with a less favourable outcome (Fejerman *et al.* 2000) and have been referred to as atypical 'benign' localisation-related epilepsy.

Childhood epilepsy with occipital paroxysms. A clinical presentation with onset between 1 and 16 years of age comprising partial seizures arising from the occipital lobes associated with occipital epileptiform abnormalities on the EEG. Panayiotopoulos (1999a) has argued that two syndromes should be distinguished within this group. Early-onset benign childhood occipital epilepsy is a common childhood epilepsy with peak age of onset of about 5 years. It is a benign disorder and seizures are very infrequent; one-third of children have a single seizure only and the median number of seizures is two or three. The characteristic semiology is that of a complex partial seizure featuring eye deviation and vomiting progressing to a unilateral or generalised convulsion. In contrast, late childhood epilepsy with occipital paroxysms is a rare disorder with mean age at onset of around 8 years. Seizures are frequent and characteristically diurnal. A variety of visual phenomena dominate the semiology. Elementary visual hallucinations may be the principal feature early on but the semiology may evolve to include ictal blindness, complex hallucinations, illusions, ocular pain as well as oculomotor features including eye deviation and eyelid fluttering. A postictal headache closely resembling migraine is common. Seizures often resolve by the late teens but up to 40% of patients may have ongoing occipital lobe seizures requiring treatment.

Reading epilepsy. This is an uncommon syndrome characterised by seizures precipitated by reading either silently or aloud (Koutroumanidis *et al.* 1998; Ramani 1998) (see also discussion of seizures with specific modes of precipitation, later in chapter). Other language-related activities (e.g. writing, mental calculations, reading music) may sometimes trigger seizures and the term *language-related epilepsy* has been suggested. Onset is typically postpubertal but may be as young as 10. Males are affected twice as commonly as females. A family history of similar seizures is found in up to one-quarter of patients. Consciousness is apparently preserved during the seizures, although patients may report subjective impairments of concentration such as mental blocking or getting stuck on a word. The characteristic form of seizure in most patients is myoclonic-like jerking of the jaw and tongue. This may spread to the upper limbs and a secondarily generalised seizure is likely if the patient persists with reading after seizure onset. Less commonly, the seizures are more clearly partial in form, involving paroxysms of alexia without motor features. The classification of the syndrome poses difficulties: in a few patients the seizures are clearly partial with localised unilateral onset, but in the majority the seizures are myoclonic with ictal EEG recordings demonstrating distributed discharges with a left anterior predominance. Using functional MRI to localise spike discharges, Archer *et al.* (2003) have postulated that spikes originating in working memory areas of the dorsolateral prefrontal cortex spread to activate a cortical–subcortical circuit.

Symptomatic and cryptogenic localisation-related epilepsy

The syndrome of *epilepsia partialis continua of childhood* (Kojewnikoff's syndrome) is given special status in the current classification syndrome. Epilepsia partialis continua (EPC) is defined as continuous clonic muscular twitching lasting for hours, days or even longer. Thus it is a form of partial status epilepticus involving protracted simple partial motor seizures. A review of 36 patients presenting with this clinical picture revealed two who had myoclonus of subcortical origin and recommended that such cases be termed 'myoclonia continua', reserving the label of EPC for continuous muscle jerks of cortical origin (Cockerell *et al.* 1996; Placidi *et al.* 2001). The ictal EEG may show focal epileptiform discharges or slowing, but is often normal. Causes include structural lesions such as cerebrovascular disease, tumours and trauma but in up to half of patients structural imaging is normal. Metabolic disturbances, including hyperglycaemia, hyponatraemia and hepatic encephalopathy,

may also present with EPC (Schomer 1993). In children, the term Kojewnikoff's syndrome is associated with two different clinical pictures: (i) recurrent infrequent episodes of EPC without any underlying progressive neurological disorder; and (ii) EPC occurring in the context of a variety of progressive disorders. In the latter group, the most important association is with Rasmussen's encephalitis, a rare immune-mediated encephalitis of unknown aetiology that leads to progressive cerebral hemiatrophy and associated neurological dysfunction (Bien *et al.* 2005). In this condition the localisation of focal motor seizures migrates as the disease progresses. Other disorders associated with EPC include inborn errors of metabolism and infective and paraneoplastic encephalitides.

Anatomically localised syndromes

The 1998 ILAE classification proposal also described four anatomically defined localisation-related syndromes: temporal, frontal, parietal and occipital lobe epilepsies. These syndromes are thus set apart from the remainder of the classification system which is based on aetiology. However, they are of the utmost importance in clinical practice as they account for at least two-thirds of adults with epilepsy. The clinical features of these syndromes are therefore considered in detail later in Anatomically defined epilepsy syndromes.

Generalised epilepsy
Idiopathic generalised epilepsy

Three of the idiopathic generalised epilepsy syndromes occur in the neonatal period or infancy and are not considered further here. The remaining syndromes are childhood and juvenile absence epilepsy, juvenile myoclonic epilepsy and epilepsy with generalised tonic–clonic seizures on awakening (Duncan 1997a; Janz 1997; Andermann & Berkovic 2001). Diagnosis at syndrome level has critical implications for choice of treatment and for the likelihood of remission. However, there is considerable overlap between these syndromes and they may best be viewed as part of a continuum. Typical absence seizures that begin before the age of 8 have a good chance of remitting by early adulthood. With later onset, absences are more likely to be associated with other seizure types and the prognosis becomes less favourable. At the opposite end of the continuum, when onset occurs later in childhood, the predominant seizure types are likely to be myoclonic or tonic–clonic (usually seen on awakening). In this group, the response to medication, specifically valproate, is excellent but there is an extremely high chance of relapse if treatment is withdrawn.

Childhood absence epilepsy is characterised by the appearance of absence seizures in early childhood, typically between the ages of 4 and 8. The annual incidence is 6–8 per 100 000. There is a slight female preponderance and a strong genetic predisposition: a twin study found concordance rates in monozygotic and dizygotic twin pairs of 75% and 5%, respectively,

(Gedda & Tatarelli 1971). Up to 40% of patients will develop generalised tonic–clonic seizures, often 5–10 years after the onset of absences. The disorder is usually benign: neurological and intellectual development is normal, there is an excellent response to medication (over 70% completely remit) and 80% of patients may be withdrawn from medication and remain seizure-free by early adulthood. The ictal EEG is characteristic, showing 3-Hz spike-and-wave discharges. Absence seizures are reliably triggered by hyperventilation, which can easily be performed during EEG recording allowing the diagnosis to be established with certainty. With a later age at onset, there is increased likelihood of atypical features and overlap with other syndromes. Such atypical features include a faster spike-and-wave pattern on EEG, associated myoclonic or tonic–clonic seizures and a greater chance that seizures will not remit. Cognitive and behavioural problems are also more likely in this group.

Juvenile absence epilepsy is arbitrarily defined as absence seizures with onset after the age of 10. It is less common than the childhood form of the disorder but also has a strong genetic predisposition. Up to 80% of patients will develop generalised tonic–clonic seizures and around 15% will develop myoclonic seizures.

Juvenile myoclonic epilepsy (JME) accounts for about 10% of all epilepsy. Up to 50% of patients have a family history of epilepsy with variable patterns of inheritance. Gentic heterogeneity is likely. Males and females are equally affected and the disorder presents in the early teenage years (80% between 12 and 18). Myoclonic jerks are the defining clinical feature and a necessary criterion for the diagnosis. They occur in isolation in less than 5% of patients. Generalised tonic–clonic seizures are seen in 95% and absence seizures in about 40%. When absence seizures occur they usually precede myoclonic seizures by years. Such patients will therefore initially be classified as having absence epilepsy, being reclassified as having JME when myoclonic jerks appear. However, most patients with JME present after their first tonic–clonic seizure. The diagnosis is often missed because many patients do not volunteer a history of myoclonic jerks, which usually precede the first tonic–clonic seizure by months or years. Specific enquiry about shakiness, clumsiness, twitches and 'nervousness' is often required to elicit this distinctive history. Sometimes the jerks may only be noticed by the patient's family. A characteristic feature of the myoclonic and tonic–clonic seizures in JME is that they tend to occur first thing in the morning just after awakening. A cluster of myoclonic jerks may sometimes give the patient a useful warning that a tonic–clonic seizure is impending. Sleep deprivation and alcohol intake the night before are common triggers for seizures. Up to 30% of patients with JME are photosensitive. The interictal EEG shows 4–6 Hz polyspike and slow-wave discharges that last up to 20 seconds. Sleep deprivation is a

useful procedure for increasing the sensitivity of EEG and discharges may be provoked by hyperventilation and photic stimulaton. Over 50% of patients have focal EEG abnormalities including asymmetry of generalised discharges, focal slow waves, spikes or sharp waves. Over 80% of patients become seizure-free with valproate monotherapy. Lamotrigine, topiramate and levetiracetam are effective second-line drugs. Carbamazepine and phenytoin typically increase seizure frequency. Lifelong treatment is widely held to be necessary because of a very high relapse rate on treatment withdrawal. The specificity of this treatment response and requirement for lifelong treatment underline the importance of correctly identifying this disorder.

Epilepsy with generalised tonic–clonic seizures on awakening is distinguished from JME either by the absence of myoclonic jerks in a patient with early-morning tonic–clonic seizures (usually defined as occurring within 2 hours of awakening) or when myoclonic seizures make their first appearance some time after tonic–clonic seizures. In practice this distinction may be very difficult to make and there is considerable overlap between the two syndromes in terms of age of onset, seizure precipitants and EEG findings. As with JME, valproate is the treatment of choice (although perhaps with a slightly less favourable outcome) and there is a very high relapse rate if treatment is withdrawn.

Other idiopathic generalised epilepsy syndromes. Typical absence seizures occurring in association with conspicuous eyelid or perioral myoclonus are not currently recognised as discrete syndromes but may have distinct implications for prognosis (Panayiotopoulos 2005). In eyelid myoclonia with absences, brief absences are associated with striking rhythmic jerking of the eyelids, often with jerky upward deviation of the eyes and retropulsion of the head. There is a strong association with photosensitivity. In perioral myoclonia, brief absences are associated with similar myoclonic jerking involving the perioral facial and masticatory muscles. There is no association with photosensitivity (see below). In both conditions, there may be a poor response to treatment and perioral myoclonia with absences is associated with a high incidence of absence status.

Syndromes characterised by seizures with specific modes of precipitation

Reflex seizures. The old term 'reflex seizures' is still widely used to denote seizures that occur in response to some specific precipitating stimulus. The current classification system includes categories for both localisation-related and generalised syndromes characterised by such seizures. Visual stimuli are the most frequent trigger for reflex seizures (Ferlazzo *et al.* 2005). Flickering light, as encountered with sunlight through trees, disco lighting, television and videogames, is the most common visual trigger but pattern sensitivity, typically related to strongly lined patterns such as escalator steps, is also seen. Seizures are usually generalised, although photosensitive partial seizures in patients with and without occipital lesions have been described. Pure photosensitive epilepsy, in which seizures occur exclusively in response to visual stimulation, accounts for some 40% of cases. Most of the remaining 60% will have idiopathic generalised epilepsy, especially JME in which photosensitivity is seen in 40–90%. Photosensitivity is seen in up to 10% of epilepsy arising in late childhood. It is more common in females. EEG recording usually reveals a prolonged spike (or polyspike)-and-wave photoparoxysmal response (PPS) to intermittent photic stimulation (typically 10–30 flashes per second). Photosensitivity is inherited, either as an autosomal dominant trait with incomplete penetrance or through multiple susceptibility genes. Up to 50% of healthy siblings of patients with photosensitive epilepsy will demonstrate PPS. The antiepileptic of first choice is valproate, but preventive measures may be very helpful. Avoiding the stimulus by covering one eye and wearing polarised or tinted glasses may be effective. Television sets with high refresh rates (100 Hz as opposed to 50 Hz) are less likely to trigger photosensitivity. Cognitive tasks, both verbal (reading epilepsy) and non-verbal, are probably the next most frequent stimuli to be associated with reflex seizures. Reading epilepsy (Koutroumanidis *et al.* 1998; Ramani 1998) is currently classified as a localisation-related syndrome but a proportion of patients have generalised epilepsy, as evidenced by seizure semiology and EEG findings, including the presence of PPS in some 9%. Non-verbal tasks, such as mental calculation and spatial tasks, are also associated with reflex generalised seizures (Goossens *et al.* 1990). Reflex partial seizures have been described with a wide variety of tiggers. Somatosensory stimulation and sudden voluntary movement of the limbs may in rare cases trigger partial seizures in patients with cerebral lesions. Musicogenic seizures usually have a temporal lobe lesional basis (Zifkin & Zatorre 1998). Other examples include eating, proprioceptive stimuli and hot water. The chief importance of reflex epilepsy for the psychiatrist is that attacks may easily be suspected of being functional in origin until their reflex epileptic basis is recognised. The existence of such clear-cut examples is also a reminder of the importance of searching for possible precipitating factors in other patients.

Self-induced seizures. Patients with reflex epilepsy may induce seizures by deliberately exposing themselves to triggering stimuli (Ng 2002). Over 90% of such cases involve children with photosensitive epilepsy who pass their hand repeatedly in front of their eyes, blink rapidly, stare at a television from a short distance, or jump up and down in front of venetian blinds. A more recently recognised triggering manoeuvre involves extreme upward deviation of the eyes with slow eyelid closure. Self-induced seizures are notoriously difficult to treat. Some children appear to derive pleasure from self-induction; in others it may represent a form of compulsion or a wilful means of gaining attention or avoiding stress.

Cryptogenic or symptomatic generalised syndromes

This category includes a number of clinical syndromes in which generalised seizures are associated with profound intellectual impairment. In many cases an underlying cause can be identified. In others, however, the aetiology remains unknown; a proportion of these may represent as yet unidentified genetic syndromes and thus might better be regarded as 'idiopathic'. The syndromes are described in order of their age of onset.

West syndrome consists of the triad of infantile spasms, arrest of psychomotor development and the characteristic EEG finding of hypsarrhythmia. The latter consists of almost continuously abnormal electrical activity, with irregularly recurring spikes and slow waves of high amplitude in all leads. The typical spasms consist of brief repeated flexor, or more rarely extensor, spasms of the trunk and limbs. 'Salaam attacks', with bowing of the head and trunk, are a common but not constant manifestation. Spasms may be asymmetrical and there may be associated partial seizures. The onset peaks at 4–7 months of age and almost all cases present during the first year of life. Boys are affected more often than girls. In the great majority of cases an underlying cause can be identified (birth hypoxia, the presence of cerebral malformations or metabolic disorders) and developmental abnormality has been obvious since birth (symptomatic group). With modern neuroimaging the proportion of patients in whom no cause is found has fallen as low as 10%. The term 'idiopathic West syndrome' is sometimes reserved for the very small proportion of patients who recover spontaneously after a brief period of infantile spasms. In this group, spasms set in after normal development and no aetiology is discovered. For the majority of symptomatic cases, however, the prognosis is grave. Although the spasms rarely persist beyond 3 years of age, other seizures supervene in some 50% of children, particularly in the form of Lennox–Gastaut syndrome (see below). Learning difficulties are observed in up to 85% of cases (Aicardi 1986). Controlling seizures and suppressing EEG abnormalities, both of which interfere with normal function and development, are the main focus of treatment. Conventional antiepileptic treatment is usually without effect. Adrenocorticotrophic hormone (ACTH) or steroids can be successful in suppressing the spasms and the EEG abnormalities. Vigabatrin may be helpful but clear guidelines for its use are still required, especially in view of the potential for retinal toxicity associated with this drug (Hrachovy & Frost 2003).

Lennox–Gastaut syndrome (Markand 2003). Like the above, this is an age-related epileptic encephalopathy of varied aetiology. The onset is typically between 1 and 8 years of age, mainly in preschool children. The syndrome is characterised by multiple seizure types, intellectual failure and/or behavioural disturbance and by EEG abnormalities comprising diffuse slow spike-and-wave discharges set against an abnormal background with paroxysms of fast 10–12 Hz rhythms that may be associated with a tonic seizure. In one-third of patients, no aetiology is identified and these cases are referred to as cryptogenic Lennox–Gastaut syndrome. The causes identified in the symptomatic cases are diverse and similar to those found in West syndrome. Indeed, in many symptomatic cases the syndrome represents a progression from West syndrome, in which case infantile spasms are either gradually replaced by tonic and other seizure types or there is a seizure-free period with improvement in psychomotor function brought to a halt by the onset of Lennox–Gastaut syndrome. The seizures in Lennox–Gastaut syndrome are frequent, severe and hard to control, consisting of mixed seizure types: tonic attacks occurring particularly during sleep and affecting the axial musculature, atonic and myoclonic attacks and atypical absences. Episodes of non-convulsive status are frequent. In consequence, much of the child's waking life may be spent in an obtunded state. The seizures commonly persist into adult life, and less than 10% of cases make a full recovery. Continuing intellectual impairment is common. As with West syndrome, cases in which no aetiology is found have a better prognosis. Valproate and benzodiazepines have been the mainstay of treatment but more recently introduced drugs, particularly lamotrigine and topiramate, now have a recognised role in treatment as they have established efficacy and a good safety profile. ACTH, prednisolone, ketogenic diet and vagal nerve stimulation (VNS) may also be of benefit (Lee & Ong 2004). Corpus callosotomy is an effective treatment for atonic seizures, which may be very frequent and extremely disabling, but VNS is being evaluated as an alternative surgical procedure (Frost *et al*. 2001).

Epilepsy with myoclonic astatic seizures (Guerrini & Aicardi 2003). This syndrome arises in early childhood (from 7 months to 8 years), usually in a child who has previously developed normally. Up to 80% of patients are boys. There is a strong genetic component with a family history of epilepsy in up to one-third of affected children. Evidence for other aetiologies is usually not found. Thus, the syndrome may be better classified as idiopathic. Onset is typically with tonic–clonic seizures, which may be febrile. Other seizure types appear over time and include myoclonus, astatic seizures, atypical absence seizures, nocturnal tonic seizures and episodes of non-convulsive status. Prognosis is variable, with seizures disappearing completely after 2 or 3 years in two-thirds of patients in whom intellectual functioning may be normal. Outcome seems to be strongly related to seizure

control and a poor prognosis is predicted by the occurrence of episodes of non-convulsive status.

Epilepsy with myoclonic absences (Bureau & Tassinari 2005). This is a rare disorder of middle childhood with a mean age at onset of 7 years. Boys are more commonly affected. The defining characteristics of the syndrome are absence seizures that are associated with dramatic bilateral myoclonic jerks which can be demonstrated to be synchronous with a 3-Hz ictal EEG discharge. Intellectual development is abnormal in approximately 50%. Aetiology can be identified in one-third of patients, including perinatal insult and karyotypic abnormalities. Additional seizure types including absence and tonic–clonic seizures are seen in 40% of patients. Frequent tonic–clonic seizures predict a poor response to treatment and poor long-term prognosis.

Epilepsy syndromes undetermined whether focal or generalised

This group of disorders includes syndromes in which both generalised and partial seizures occur and in which underlying aetiology is poorly understood. Certain neonatal syndromes are included in this category and are considerd only briefly.

Severe myoclonic epilepsy in infancy (Dravet's syndrome) is a progressive epileptic encephalopathy that develops in the first year of life after a short period of normal development. Initial seizures are usually febrile convulsions but mixed seizure types soon appear. Associations with mutations in the sodium channel gene *SCN1A* have recently been described (Guerrini & Aicardi 2003).

Epilepsy with continuous spike–waves in slow-wave sleep describes syndromes characterised by specific cognitive deficits associated with almost continuous high-frequency spike-and-wave discharges during slow-wave sleep. The most common presentation is better known as Landau–Kleffner syndrome (acquired epileptic aphasia), a rare childhood disorder that may present with either seizures or aphasia. Patients with *acquired epileptic opercular syndrome* present with progressive loss of voluntary movement of the mouth including kissing, oral expression and eating, often associated with drooling. There is overlap between presentations and some regard Landau–Kleffner syndrome and epilepsy with continuous spike–waves in slow-wave sleep as the same condition (Shafrir & Prensky 1995). Onset is usually before the age of 5 years. The child loses comprehension of speech after seemingly normal development, and rapidly ceases to use speech to communicate. The cognitive deficits may sometimes extend beyond auditory comprehension, and behaviour disorder with agitation, echopraxia and frontal characteristics may develop. Seizures are usually mild and infrequent, and may be partial motor or tonic–clonic in form. In some 20% of cases of Landau–Kleffner syndrome, obvious seizures remain in abeyance, although close inspection may reveal minor episodes. The striking EEG abnormality is the presence of almost continuous spike-and-wave discharges during slow-wave sleep, which may be relatively localised to bilateral rolandic areas in the opercular variant of the syndrome. The EEG during wakefulness shows spikes or spike-and-wave complexes, usually generalised or multifocal bilaterally in the temporal and parietal regions. The seizures are typically resistant to treatment but usually remit before the age of 15 years. Language difficulties may persist even into adult life. The surgical procedure of multiple subpial transection is effective in controlling seizures and improving the EEG and may be associated with dramatic improvements in language function (Selway & Dardis 2004). Further research is required to define more clearly the indications for this approach. The cause of the condition is unknown, although symptomatic cases with acquired lesions or neurodevelopmental abnormalities have been reported.

Special syndromes: situation-related seizures

The current classification system lists a number of situation-related syndromes; disorders in which isolated or recurrent seizures occur in the presence of an identifiable triggering event. Childhood febrile convulsions are included in this category, as are seizures arising as a consequence of an acute metabolic or toxic event (see Causes of acute symptomatic seizures). Febrile convulsions are of considerable significance because they are common and because of their association with epilepsy in later life.

Febrile convulsions are seizures occurring in childhood in association with a febrile illness not caused by a CNS infection (Waruiru & Appleton 2004; Sadleir & Scheffer 2007). They are the most common form of epilepsy, affecting 2–5% of children. Most febrile convulsions start in the second year of life, with a range from 2 months to 7 years. Approximately one-third of children will experience a second episode, usually within 3 years of the first. The risk of a recurrent febrile convulsion is increased if the first seizure occurs before 18 months of age, if there is a family history of febrile convulsions, or if the first seizure occurred early in the course of a febrile illness or with a relatively low fever. Most febrile seizures are generalised and of short duration (90% under 10 minutes). Overall, 2–4% of children will experience at least one unprovoked seizure following a single febrile convulsion, a risk up to four times that in the general population. This modestly increased risk for later epilepsy applies to both generalised and localisation-related epilepsy (Trinka et al. 2002). An increased risk of epilepsy following febrile convulsions has most consistently been associated with a family history of epilepsy, the presence of early-onset

neurodevelopmental abnormalities and 'complex' features present during the febrile convulsion. These complex features are prolonged duration (greater than 10–15 minutes), recurrent febrile seizures within a single febrile illness and the presence of focal neurological features during or after the seizure. Annegers et al. (1987) found that the risk of unprovoked seizures rose from 2.4% following a 'simple' febrile convulsion to 6–8% for those with a single complex feature, 17–22% with two complex features and 49% with all three complex features. There is a rapidly expanding literature on the genetics of febrile convulsions. Between 25% and 40% of patients have a family history of febrile convulsions. Polygenic inheritance most likely contributes to the majority of cases, but a small number of families inherit the disorder as an autosomal dominant condition, and a number of genes have recently been identified (Audenaert et al. 2006). The controversial relationship between febrile convulsions, hippocampal sclerosis and temporal lobe epilepsy is discussed under Aetiology of temporal lobe epilepsy.

Anatomically defined localisation-related epilepsy syndromes

Seizures originating in different anatomical locations take characteristic forms but there is considerable overlap. The symptoms at the very beginning of a seizure generally provide the most critical clue to localisation, but a focal epileptic discharge may spread to adjacent brain regions so rapidly (within milliseconds) that the clinical manifestations of seizures arising in functionally quite distinct cortical regions become indistinguishable. Nevertheless, typical modes of presentation that correspond to anatomical location are now recognised and are of considerable importance in clinical practice. Skilled appraisal of clinical semiology will help determine which hemisphere and which cortical region are involved. With respect to aetiology, the syndromes have more in common than otherwise. In the following section the primary aim is therefore to describe the semiological features of each syndrome. Aetiological factors, where distinctive, are mentioned but are dealt with in greater detail elsewhere in the chapter.

Temporal lobe epilepsy

Temporal lobe epilepsy (TLE) is the most common of the anatomically defined syndromes, accounting for around 60% of all patients with localisation-related epilepsy. Temporal lobe seizures produce the most varied and complex auras of all. They are of particular interest to the psychiatrist because they often contain elements that echo symptoms seen in psychiatric disorder.

The most frequent cause of TLE is hippocampal sclerosis, also known as mesial temporal sclerosis or Ammon's horn sclerosis, accounting for 50–70% of cases in temporal lobectomy series (Bruton 1988). Hippocampal sclerosis is strongly associated with a history of childhood febrile convulsions

Table 6.3 Auras of partial seizures.

Symptom	Frequency in TLE* (%)	Specificity: the relative frequency of aura by localisation syndrome			
		Temporal	Frontal	Parietal	Occipital
Epigastric aura	30–53	+++	–	–	–
Cephalic aura	23–30	++	++	–	–
Anxiety/fear	14–24	++	+	–	–
Hallucinations/illusions					
Visual	16–18	+	–	+	+++
Elementary	5–7	+	–	+	+++
Complex	3	++	–	++	–
Auditory	8–16	+++	–	+	–
Elementary	1–12	+++	–	–	–
Complex	3–4	+++	–	–	–
Olfactory	8–12	+++	+	–	–
Gustatory	3–11	+++	+	–	–
Somatosensory	2–19	+	++	+++	–
Dysmnesic/*déjà vu*	7–18	+++	–	–	–
No aura	10–51				

–, uncommon (though may occur)/not a specific feature for that localisation, ranging to +++, relatively common and/or specific.
* Figures for the prevalence of these symptoms in temporal lobe epilepsy (TLE) are derived from series reported by Currie *et al.* (1971), King and Ajmone Marsan (1977), Taylor and Lochery (1987) and Palmini and Gloor (1992). Estimates of the relative frequency in different lobar epilepsies are derived from King and Ajmone Marsan (1977) and Palmini and Gloor (1992).

but the causal direction of this association has not been established: hippocampal sclerosis may be the pathological signature of severe febrile convulsions or there may be underlying disorders that predispose to both febrile convulsions and TLE (see Aetiology of temporal lobe epilepsy). Other causes of TLE include dysembryoplastic neuroepithelial tumours, cavernous angiomas, gliomas, cortical dysplasia and gliosis secondary to encephalitis or meningitis.

Temporal lobe seizures may take the form of simple and complex partial seizures, with both occurring in some 70% of patients (Janszky *et al.* 2004a). Compared with extratemporal seizures, those arising in the temporal lobes characteristically have a gradual onset, usually feature a conspicuous motionless stare and are relatively prolonged, with automatisms often continuing for 2 minutes, occasionally even longer. A wide variety of auras occur in TLE and many are highly characteristic (Table 6.3).

Auras of temporal lobe epilepsy. A variety of autonomic features and visceral sensations figure prominently in temporal lobe auras. The epigastric aura is the most common, being reported by up to 50% of patients with TLE (Henkel *et al.* 2002). It consists of ill-defined sensations rising from the epigastrium towards the throat, typically described as churning, 'butterflies' or a feeling of nervousness. Also frequent are inexplicable odd sensations in the head (cephalic aura), although these have less specificity for TLE. Other autonomic effects include changes in skin colour, blood pressure, heart rate, perspiration, salivation and piloerection. Subjective dizziness is common. True vertigo accompanied by tinnitus and changes in auditory perception is rare.

Affective experiences are a feature of approximately one-quarter of temporal lobe auras. The most common is anxiety, which is often intense (ictal fear) and wells up suddenly without provocation. Other unpleasant affects include depression, guilt and, rarely, anger. Pleasurable affects of joy, elation or ecstasy occur less frequently (Stefan *et al.* 2004). Ictal emotional experiences may be very intense and tend to have a unique, though often difficult-to-describe, quality that makes them unlike anything else in the patient's experience: they are usually stereotyped and crude, lacking the subtlety of normal emotions. Affective auras are an intrinsic part of the seizure, and not merely a reaction to some other aspect of the aura. The emotional content of the aura may nevertheless colour hallucinatory experiences or occasionally be associated with disturbed behaviour. Biraben *et al.* (2001) have drawn attention to the behavioural features that accompany intense ictal fear, which may include a call for help, marked agitation or frightened immobility. These authors and others have described an association between ictal fear and non-dominant medial temporal foci (Hermann *et al.* 1992; Sazgar *et al.* 2003).

Biraben *et al.* (2001) report a detailed investigation of eight patients with ictal fear. All but one were fully conscious throughout their seizures and the remaining patient had only questionable and momentary impairment. Despite preserved awareness, clear oro-alimentary automatisms (lip-smacking, chewing, swallowing) were seen in all but one patient and dystonic posturing or fleeting localised clonic movement were almost as common. The patients were thoroughly investigated with ictal EEG, including depth recordings, MRI and single-photon emission computed tomography (SPECT). In seven cases the epileptogenic lesion was in the temporal lobe (three on the left, three on the right and one bilateral; six involved the non-dominant hemisphere); the remaining patient had a frontal lobe focus. Seizure onset in medial temporal lobe structures was associated with mild subjective mood changes only. As the emotional experience escalated to one of fear accompanied by autonomic and behavioural features, there was an associated spread of EEG abnormalities to frontal regions. The authors propose that the syndrome of intense ictal fear is associated with functional involvement of a distributed limbic network involving medial temporal lobe, orbito-prefrontal cortex and anterior cingulate.

Cognitive abnormalities include disturbances of speech, memory and thought. Vocalisation is seen in approximately 50% of temporal lobe seizures. It is usually non-verbal, in which case it may be associated with either dominant or non-dominant foci and has no lateralising value. However, speech automatisms (recurrent, irrelevant or emotionally toned utterances), which can be thought of as evidence of preserved speech during the seizure discharge, are strongly related to a non-dominant temporal lobe focus (Williamson *et al.* 1998). Disturbances of memory (*dysmnestic aura*) range from sudden difficulty with recall to compulsive reminiscence on topics, scenes or events from the past. The essential quality of recognition may change, with strong feelings of familiarity or unfamiliarity leading to *déjà vu* and *jamais vu*. *Presience* is a related phenomenon in which patients describe a profound sense of 'knowing' what is about to happen (Sadler & Rahey 2004). In the rare panoramic memory, the patient feels that whole episodes from his past life are lived again in a brief period of time as complex organised experiences. Indeed, distortion of time sense is often an integral part of the experience of the aura, time appearing to rush by precipitately or alternatively to stand quite still.

The purely subjective disorders of thinking constitute some of the most striking auras. They are rare and have less specificity for TLE, having also been described in frontal lobe seizures (Mendez *et al.* 1996). Patients may become abruptly aware of difficulty in thinking coherently, of mixing things up, or of great confusion and turmoil in their mind. There may be a compulsion to think on certain restricted topics (forced thinking), or there may be intrusion of thoughts or of stereotyped words or phrases against the subject's will (evocation of thoughts). A sudden cessation in the stream of thought may occur and later be described in a manner indistinguishable from schizophrenic 'blocking'.

Altered perceptual experiences include both distortions of real perceptions (illusions) and spontaneous hallucinations.

Hallucinations of taste (gustatory) and smell (olfactory) derive from medial temporal lobe structures, particularly the amygdala, and are of considerable significance for the diagnosis of TLE (Acharya *et al.* 1998). They are nevertheless uncommon, accounting for less than 10% of temporal lobe auras, and may also be seen in frontal lobe seizures. The smells and tastes are usually described as unpleasant. Tumours are the most common aetiology associated with olfactory auras (Acharya *et al.* 1998). Sounds may seem suddenly remote or intensely loud. Auditory hallucinations, associated with foci in the superior lateral temporal gyrus, may be simple or complex, ranging from ringing and buzzing noises to organised experiences such as music or voices. Visual illusions may include objects appearing larger (macropsia) or smaller (micropsia), inclined at an angle (plagiopsia), elongated or flattened (dysplatopsia), drained of colour (achromatopsia) or infused with a specific colour (erythropsia, red; xanthopsia, blue). There may be distorted perception of distance, objects may be seen in multiples (monocular diplopia, polyopia), or there may be image persistence or perseveration in the form of an after-image (paliopsia). Visual hallucinations may consist of the simple elements described for occipital seizures, but more characteristically involve complex formed hallucinations of scenes, faces or visions of past experiences. Hallucinations that appear to involve some replay of memory clearly overlap with dysmnestic phenomena and indeed such aura are often associated with *déjà vu* phenomena and an odd 'dreamy state' (Vignal *et al.* 2007). It is therefore not surprising that complex visual hallucinations have been described with both medial temporal lobe foci (Bien *et al.* 2000; Vignal *et al.* 2007) and lateral temporal lobe foci (Wieser 2000). Negative visual symptoms are more typical of occipital lobe epilepsy but are sometimes seen in TLE, and a concentric constriction of the visual field (tunnel vision) may be specific for temporal lobe aura (Bien *et al.* 2000). The emotional quality of perceptual experiences may change, so that objects, sounds or events suddenly acquire a peculiar and vivid significance. The patient may alternatively feel suddenly remote from the environment, and feelings of derealisation and depersonalisation may be marked.

These varied aspects of the auras can occur in any combination. There is often a characteristic 'march', passing for example from an initial epigastric sensation to gustatory hallucinations to forced thinking, or from intense *déjà vu* to an overwhelming sense of fear. Sometimes various aspects of the aura appear to occur simultaneously, or the content is so rich and strange that the patient lacks the vocabulary to describe the experiences. Many are extremely bizarre, particularly those which involve disturbance of appreciation of reality and of the self. Williams (1966) pointed out that the temporal lobes perform the function of integrating sensations of all kinds, and in addition probably contain the neural substrates for emotion itself:

It is the integration of the whole of exteroceptive and proprioceptive sensations with emotions and moods which culminates in the
ultimate sense of 'I am', so that it is not at all surprising that disintegration of this organisation, with retention of sensation, leads to so
many of the bizarre disturbances of self which disturb the patient
with temporal lobe epilepsy.

The precise content of the auras may sometimes change with
the passage of time, and scrutiny of the patient's notes may
reveal well-documented phenomena earlier in the illness of
which the patient now has no recollection. This tendency can
sometimes increase the risk of the patient being regarded as
suffering from a psychogenic disorder.

Ictal semiology and automatisms in TLE. The motor manifestations of TLE have often been overlooked yet they are common
and in some instances provide reliable lateralising signs.
Dystonic posturing, most commonly of the hand or arm,
occurs in up to 70% of temporal lobe seizures and strongly
suggests a contralateral focus. Versive movements of the
head, eyes and even trunk are also common. At seizure
onset they are perhaps associated with an ipsilateral focus
(Williamson *et al.* 1998). A more reliable lateralising sign is
versive movement occurring late in the seizure, immediately
prior to secondary generalisation, at which point it is
strongly associated with a contralateral focus (head, eyes
and/or trunk turn away from the side of seizure origin)
(Marks & Laxer 1998; Williamson *et al.* 1998). Unilateral
clonic movements also indicate a contralateral focus but are
less common.

The most frequent automatisms are oro-alimentary (lip-
smacking, chewing, swallowing) and gestural (fumbling,
picking, rubbing movements). Unilateral gestural automatisms are suggestive of an ipsilateral focus, probably because
of ictal paresis of the contralateral limb. Other common
automatisms include ictal speech, grimacing, wandering
and searching behaviour. Automatisms involving the lower
limbs in pedalling or kicking movements are rare in TLE
and more often associated with frontal lobe seizures. The
prolonged nature of automatisms in TLE has already been
mentioned. Slow gradual recovery with postictal delirium
extending over several minutes is characteristic and headache is common. Postictal dysphasia suggests a focus in the
dominant hemisphere but care must be taken to distinguish
this from non-specific aspects of impaired communication
associated with delirium. Postictal nose-rubbing is common
and is ipsilateral to the seizure focus in 90% of cases (Geyer
et al. 1999). Todd's paresis is rare in TLE but lateralises seizure
onset to the contralateral hemisphere. Patients are usually
amnesic for the ictal period covering the blank stare and
automatisms. Secondary generalisation is less common than
with extratemporal partial seizures.

The clinical features that are most helpful in lateralising
temporal lobe seizures are summarised in Table 6.4. Seizures
arising in the lateral neocortical temporal lobe are more likely

Table 6.4 Clinical features of temporal lobe seizures with lateralising value.

Lateralising value	Semiological feature
Ipsilateral	Unilateral gestural automatisms
	Postictal nose rubbing
Contralateral	Dystonic posturing
	Late versive movement (preceding secondary generalisation)
	Unilateral clonic activity (uncommon)
	Todd's paresis (uncommon)
Dominant hemisphere	Postictal dysphasia
Non-dominant hemisphere	Ictal speech

Note that the aura of temporal lobe epilepsy have little lateralising value with the possible exception of ictal fear, which may suggest a focus in the non-dominant hemisphere.

to feature complex auditory and visual aura with relatively
prolonged preservation of awareness at seizure onset. Motor
phenomena are also more common with foci in this area
(Wieser 2000).

Frontal lobe epilepsy

Frontal lobe epilepsy (FLE) probably accounts for 20–30%
of localisation-related epilepsy (Manford *et al.* 1992; Jallon
et al. 2001). Post-traumatic aetiology is common, although
tumours and cortical dysplasia are more frequent in surgical
series (Manford *et al.* 1996a). *Autosomal dominant nocturnal
frontal lobe epilepsy* is a rare but distinctive disorder characterised by autosomal dominant inheritance with high penetrance and frequent nocturnal frontal seizures with complex
hyperkinetic behavioural automatisms (Scheffer *et al.* 1995).
Mutations in the neuronal nicotinic acetylcholine receptor
α_4 and β_2 subunits have been identified (Phillips *et al.* 2001)
(see Genetic basis of epilepsy, later in chapter). After TLE,
patients with FLE are the second largest group to receive surgical treatment for epilepsy. With improvements in neuroimaging and depth EEG techniques, the proportion of operable
FLE seems likely to increase. Considerable effort has therefore been devoted to more precisely defining the semiology
of frontal lobe seizures. Overall, frontal lobe seizures tend to
begin and end abruptly, are brief (usually less than 1 minute
in duration), often frequent, and show a tendency to occur at
night and in clusters. Motor phenomena, which may include
complex posturing and behavioural automatisms, are
usually the most conspicuous feature. A number of syndromes corresponding to anatomical localisation within the
frontal lobe have now been delineated (Williamson & Jobst
2000; McGonigal & Chauvel 2004). Some, such as simple
partial motor seizures of the Jacksonian type, are relatively
common, well recognised and present few diagnostic difficulties. Other presentations have been described relatively

recently and still remain unfamiliar to those not working in the field of epilepsy. These syndromes are of particular importance to psychiatrists as their bizarre nature means they are often mistaken for non-epileptic dissociative seizures. The anatomical classification of these syndromes is approximate and there is considerable overlap between them (Manford *et al*. 1996a).

Focal clonic motor seizures clearly implicate involvement of the contralateral primary motor cortex in the pre-rolandic gyrus. They may occasionally be seen in association with seizure discharges spreading to this region from elsewhere in the frontal lobe. Focal motor seizures may occur as a special form of status epilepticus (epilepsia partialis continua), in which case the underlying pathology may be focal, diffuse (e.g. Rasmussen's encephalitis) or be associated with metabolic disturbance.

Unlike other frontal lobe seizures, those arising in the supplementary motor area (SMA) are sometimes preceded by an aura that is usually somatosensory (Morris *et al*. 1988). The sensations are vague, distributed and less well defined compared with those associated with parietal foci. More often, SMA seizures begin with the abrupt onset of complex motor postures usually involving the upper limbs. The 'fencing posture', in which the contralateral arm is raised above the head and flexed at the elbow, is the classic example. Versive movements of the eyes and head are also common and, as described above for TLE, when they occur late in the seizure prior to secondary generalisation they lateralise seizure onset to the contralateral hemisphere. Postures are typically bilateral and may evolve to writhing twisting movements. Consciousness is usually preserved throughout the seizure. Another rare form of dorsolateral frontal seizure is the so-called 'frontal absence', which consists of behavioural arrest accompanied by spike-and-wave rather than tonic discharge on EEG.

The most bizarre frontal lobe seizures are those involving complex behavioural automatisms. The anatomical localisation within the frontal lobes is less certain for these seizures but current evidence suggests that prefrontal origin, perhaps especially from the orbitomedial cortex, is likely (Williamson *et al*. 1985; Waterman *et al*. 1987; So *et al*. 1998; Jobst *et al*. 2000; Kotagal *et al*. 2003). These must surely rank as some of the most dramatic presentations in neurology. They are often referred to as *hypermotor seizures*, a term that usefully evokes the core features. Seizures begin very abruptly. There is often intense grimacing, with the patient seemingly gripped by some overwhelming emotion. Typically, however, patients do not describe ictal fear. Complex behavioural automatisms then follow. These are typically frantic, bilateral and often overtly sexual. Pedalling, thrashing, kicking movements are common and may be of such a degree that patient appear to thrust themselves out of bed. The upper limbs may be involved in vigourous clapping, finger-clicking, grasping, rubbing and pounding movements. Sexual automatisms often appear aggressive and include pelvic thrusting, undressing and genital manipulation. Speech arrest is a feature of dominant hemisphere frontal seizures but speech automatisms accompanying hypermotor seizures arising from the non-dominant hemisphere may also be dramatic, with screaming and swearing. Patients often report partial awareness during these seizures. Brief duration (mean 20–40 seconds) is a characteristic feature and they typically end as abruptly as they begin.

Clearly, there is scope for confusion between frontal lobe seizures and non-epileptic events yet the syndromes have now been so well described that experienced clinicians are often able to make a diagnosis after witnessing a seizure. The bizarre nature of the automatisms, preservation of awareness during bilateral motor involvement and abrupt termination of the seizures are features particularly likely to raise doubts about diagnosis. Diagnostic difficulties are compounded by the fact that interictal and ictal scalp EEG is often normal (Bautista *et al*. 1998). Helpful pointers include the highly stereotyped nature of the attacks, brief duration and, during EEG telemetry, their occurrence during electrographically documented sleep.

Parietal lobe epilepsy

Parietal lobe epilepsy is rare, probably accounting for less than 5% of localisation-related epilepsy (Sveinbjornsdottir & Duncan 1993; Siegel & Williamson 2000). Tumours are the most common aetiology. Somatosensory auras are reported by some 80% of patients, with elementary paraesthesiae by far the most common feature. These may be described as tingling, numbness, prickling, crawling or electrical sensations and implicate the primary somatosensory region in the postcentral gyrus. The paraesthesiae are usually contralateral to the epileptic focus but may rarely be bilateral or ipsilateral. Pain, which may be intense, is less common but quite specific for parietal foci, and thermal sensations rarer still. Paraesthesiae may spread in a Jacksonian manner and be accompanied by focal clonic or tonic motor phenomena. Seizures arising on the medial surface from the paracentral lobule may give rise to genital sensations that are usually unilateral and not necessarily described as pleasurable. These tactile sensations are distinct from the orgasmic aura occasionally described in TLE (Janszky *et al*. 2004b) but there may be sexual elements in the ensuing seizure semiology. Foci in posterior regions of the parietal convexity give rise to a variety of complex though uncommon aura. These include distortions of body image, in which parts of the body seem altered in shape or size or even to be absent, illusions that parts of the body are moving or have changed posture, and ictal ideomotor apraxia (ictal paroxysmal paralysis). Panic has been described as a feature but is now more closely associated with TLE. Epileptogenic lesions that lie across the boundaries of the parietal lobe may obviously present with features more characteristic of the adjacent brain region. Similarly, following the aura, ictal spread is usually rapid and the semiology of automatisms in parietal complex partial seizures is non-specific. In a series of 82 patients with parietal lobe epilepsy, 57% exhibited unilateral clonic activity (suggesting spread to precentral cortex), 28% tonic posturing (suggesting involvement of the SMA) and 17% demonstrated oral or gestural automatisms (compatable with temporal lobe involvement) (Salanova *et al.* 1995).

Occipital lobe epilepsy

Occipital lobe epilepsy accounts for around 5–7% of localisation-related epilepsy but is probably under-recognised (Manford *et al.* 1992; Jallon *et al.* 2001). Childhood syndromes are frequently misdiagnosed as migraine (Panayiotopoulos 1999b) and in adults occipital lobe seizures notoriously mimic other partial seizures because of rapid propagation to temporal and frontal lobes. Elementary visual hallucinations are the hallmark of occipital seizures but are not seen in all cases (Sveinbjornsdottir & Duncan 1993; Blume & Wiebe 2000). The hallucinations consist mainly of bright, coloured spots, circles, balls or blobs. They typically appear in the contralateral hemifield and move, flash or twinkle. Negative phenomena, such as scotoma, 'black or white outs', and ictal amaurosis are less common. Complex visual illusions and hallucinations are associated with temporal lobe seizures but may be seen with occipitotemporal foci. Primary occipital motor phenomena include eye deviation, both tonic and oculoclonic, forced eyelid closure and palpebral jerks. In young children, vomiting, pallor and headache are often prominent features. While elementary visual auras are highly characteristic of occipital seizures, the ensuing semiology, like that seen in parietal epilepsy, reflects spread to the temporal and frontal lobes and these features may dominate the clinical presentation leading to false localisation. Postictal blindness may be prolonged and provides an important clue to occipital lobe onset.

Common causes of occipital lobe epilepsy include tumours, trauma and developmental malformations. In a comprehensive review of aetiology in occipital lobe epilepsy, Taylor *et al.* (2003) emphasise the importance of developmental malformations but also highlight certain distinctive syndromes that have specific implications for management. Occipital lobe seizures may be the presenting feature of reversible posterior leucoencephalopathy, seen in acute hypertensive encephalopathy, eclampsia and during immunosuppressant treatment. The characteristic MRI appearance of bilateral T2 signal hyperintensity in occipitoparietal white matter is believed to reflect oedema secondary to disrupted autoregulation of the posterior cerebral circulation. Other clinical features include headache, confusion, vomiting and visual disturbance. It is typically completely reversible with treatment of the underlying cause (Hinchey *et al.* 1996). Another syndrome, epilepsy with bilateral occipital calcifications, is notable because of its association with coeliac disease. Seizures usually begin in the first decade of life. The typical appearances of bilateral calcification on computed tomography (CT) may not be seen at first presentation and screening for coeliac disease should therefore be considered in all idiopathic cases of occipital lobe epilepsy. A gluten-free diet may have a dramatic effect on seizure control. Occipital seizures are also seen in the progressive myoclonic epilepsies (see Epilepsy occurring in inherited disorders). Finally, three syndromes of idiopathic childhood epilepsy have now been recognised. Early- and late-onset syndromes of childhood epilepsy with occipital spikes are both relatively benign conditions, although the latter not infrequently requires longer-term antiepileptic drug treatment. Idiopathic photosensitive occipital epilepsy presents between 5 and 17 years of age with complex partial seizures (featuring prominent visual aura) triggered by television and videogames. The prognosis is excellent and simple measures taken to avoid triggering factors may make medical treatment unnecessary.

Other syndromes

Other rare forms of epilepsy that can produce puzzling clinical pictures are mentioned briefly.

Gelastic epilepsy. This is a term used for seizures preceded or accompanied by laughter. The laughter may very occasionally be accompanied by a subjective experience of mirth, but is most typically without affect and is of a hollow quality. Some patients report a 'pressure to laugh' which is vaguely pleasurable and may be accompanied by lacrimation (*dyscrastic seizure*) (Sturm *et al.* 2000). Gelastic seizures are closely associated with hypothalamic hamartomas, although there are occasional reports of seizures accompanied by laughter in patients with temporal and frontal lobe lesions. The classical view of the syndrome has been that most patients with hypothalamic hamartomas present with gelastic seizures in infancy or early childhood. In such cases, multiple seizure types, both partial and generalised, rapidly supervene and the clinical picture is one of a progressive epileptic encephalopathy with intractable seizures, behavioural disturbance and cognitive decline. However, it is now recognised that some patients, especially those with small hamartomas, may not present until adulthood in which case the clinical picture is distinctly mild and compatible with normal intellect (Mullatti *et al.* 2003). It is thought that the hamartoma is itself epileptogenic, discharges propagating through neighbouring thalamocortical connections to produce generalised seizures, and through limbic pathways to produce partial seizures. Although surgical approaches to the lesion may be difficult, seizures are usually halted following resection of the hamartoma and anecdotal reports suggest cognitive decline may be arrested and behaviour improved (Berkovic *et al.* 2003). Recent evidence from cerebral electical stimulation studies suggest that gelastic seizures may represent activation of a hypothetical motor component of laughter in the anterior cingulate cortex, the emotional content of laughter being subserved by temporal regions (Sperli *et al.* 2006).

Transient epileptic amnesia. This distinctive syndrome of recurrent episodes of amnesia has been described relatively recently (Butler 2006). Based on a description of 10 cases and a review of previous reports, Zeman *et al.* (1998) have recommended criteria for the diagnosis: (i) recurrent witnessed episodes of amnesia; (ii) evidence that other cognitive functions are intact during the episodes; and (iii) support for a diagnosis of epilepsy based on EEG findings, the presence of other epileptic semiology and/or a response to antiepileptic drugs. The disorder typically begins in later life. The amnesic episodes are recurrent (average of three per year), characteristically occur on waking, and usually last less than an hour. In 60% of cases there are other clinical features suggestive of TLE, such as olfactory aura or oral automatisms. In the remainder, amnesia is the only ictal manifestation. During the episode the patient displays a dense retrograde amnesia that may extend back in time for days or years. There is usually anterograde amnesia during the episode but the patient may have recall for the episode after recovery, i.e. they may 'remember forgetting'. An intriguing aspect of the syndrome is that it is strongly associated with two specific interictal disturbances of memory, present between episodes of transient amnesia: firstly, accelerated forgetting of newly learned material and, secondly, a characteristic patchy loss of autobiographical memory. Most patients with transient epileptic amnesia spontaneously complain of the latter problem, which involves forgetting emotionally salient episodes (holidays, weddings) from the remote past, events that usually predate the first episode of transient amnesia by many years. Underlying aetiology is typically not identified and the episodes usually resolve completely with antiepileptic medication.

Diencephalic (autonomic) epilepsy is characterised by autonomic symptoms that predominate during attacks. It is likely that most reported examples represent partial seizures arising from the medial temporal lobe. Indeed, the epigastic aura of TLE is regarded, in part at least, as reflecting autonomic dysfunction (Blume *et al.* 2001). Fox *et al.* (1973) reported a patient whose attacks consisted of episodic flushing and sweating, lasting 10–20 minutes, followed by feeling cold and shivering. Slight confusion could sometimes ensue. The rectal temperature fell during attacks and was recorded as low as 34°C. In other cases seizures may take the form of a sudden desire to urinate or defecate, sensations of heat or cold, flushing, hyperpnoea, difficulty with breathing, salivation, lacrimation or abnormal gastric sensations. It may be hard to distinguish such symptoms from those of an anxiety state, although the sudden onset and ending and the regular stereotyped nature of the attacks may give the clue.

Prevalence and aetiology of epilepsy

Prevalence

The prevalence of epilepsy is approximately 7 per 1000 in the developed world (Haerer *et al.* 1986; Keranen *et al.* 1989; Hauser *et al.* 1991). The annual incidence is around 50 per 100 000 and approximately 1 in 30 individuals will develop epilepsy at some point in their lives (Hauser *et al.* 1993; MacDonald *et al.* 2000). Most studies report a slight preponderance of males relative to females, although the difference is rarely statistically significant. Age of onset shows the highest rate in the first year of life and in the elderly, with the lowest incidence in people in their thirties. Epilepsy is more prevalent in areas of lower socioeconomic status (Morgan *et al.* 2000) and a primary-care based study in the south-east of England (Heaney *et al.* 2002) has shown an association between measures of socioeconomic deprivation and the incidence of new cases of epilepsy, suggesting that this relationship is not just a reflection of downward social drift secondary to epilepsy but that factors related to socioeconomic deprivation may be causally related to epilepsy. Of the different types of epilepsy, the great majority appearing in the first 20 years of life are generalised epileptic syndromes, while after this age the proportion of localisation-related epilepsies rapidly increases.

Aetiology

In clinical practice, epilepsy should be viewed as a symptom rather than a disease in itself. A great variety of causes may underlie the occurrence of seizures and need to be carefully investigated. When this is done, however, a considerable number of cases remain in which no cause is discernible. The proportion of such cases has been remarkably constant across studies, representing approximately two-thirds of patients in several large populations (Alstrom 1950; Juul-Jensen 1964; Gudmundsson 1966; Sander *et al.* 1990; Hauser *et al.* 1993; Forsgren *et al.* 1996; Olafsson *et al.* 1996). Aetiological factors identified in three representative studies are shown in Table 6.5. The relative incidence of different causes varies with age. Among children with epilepsy in whom a cause is found, congenital factors account for 60%, while tumours and trauma are the leading causes in young adults. Among older adults the likelihood of identifying a cause for seizures is higher overall, with the proportion of vascular causes rising to over 50%.

Genetic basis of epilepsy

Based on the epidemiological evidence reviewed above it has been estimated that some 30% of epilepsy has a largely genetic basis (designated idiopathic epilepsy in the current classification system) (Berkovic *et al.* 2006). Acquired causes are identified in a further 30%, the so-called symptomatic

Table 6.5 Aetiological factors in three studies of new-onset epilepsy (figures are percentages).

Aetiology	UK (Sander et al. 1990)	USA (Hauser et al. 1993)	France (Jallon et al. 2001)	Range
Vascular	15	11	3	3–15
Trauma	3	6	3	3–6
Neoplasm	6	4	1	1–6
Infection	2	3	1	1–3
Degenerative	–	4	1	1–4
Congenital	–	8	4	4–8
Other	13	–	5	5–13
Total symptomatic	39	35	18	18–39
Total unknown	61	65	81	61–81
Presumed cryptogenic	–	–	49	
Presumed idiopathic	–	–	32	

The UK and USA studies were community (general practice)-based and population-based respectively. The French study recruited subjects through specialists working in hospital and community settings. Many worked in private practice and the authors note that this may have biased their study in favour of younger subjects, a factor that might account for the lower proportion of cases in which aetiology was found. The study is included here as it is the only one to have estimated the proportion of cryptogenic and idiopathic aetiological categories.

epilepsies. The remaining cases are those in which a cause is suspected but cannot be identified, the cryptogenic epilepsies. Twin studies have demonstrated that a genetic contribution is strongest in the generalised epilepsies but is also significant for localisation-related epilepsies (Berkovic *et al.* 1998; Vadlamudi *et al.* 2004). Likewise, family studies have shown that the risk of epilepsy in first-degree relatives of patients with idiopathic epilepsy is higher than that in those with symptomatic epilepsy, which is still greater than in relatives of controls (Ottman *et al.* 1996). Thus, there is clear evidence that genetic factors play a role even in symptomatic epilepsy. These findings have led to the view that the relationship between genetic and acquired ('environmental' in genetic parlance) factors in the aetiology of epilepsy is best conceived of as a continuum (Sander *et al.* 1990; Berkovic *et al.* 2006). At one end of the spectrum are the relatively rare epilepsy syndromes for which single gene defects have been found. At the other are cases in which acquired lesions are the overriding factor and genetic predisposition may have little influence. In the middle lie the vast majority of patients for whom some interaction between genetic and environmental factors is operative.

Like any other common medical disorder the most important genetic factors in epilepsy are likely to be polygenic, with multiple susceptibility genes contributing to overall risk. Individual susceptibility genes may confer risk for epilepsy in general and/or for certain epilepsy syndromes specifically, with the final phenotype being the result of a complex interaction between genes and environment (Johnson & Sander 2001). As yet, no susceptibilty genes have been clearly identified. However, promising avenues for identifying such genes stem from studies of rare families with inherited epilepsy syndromes in which specific mutations have been discovered. Almost all the genes identified so far have been related to ion channel function and it seems likely that susceptibility genes will act, either directly or as modifiers, through similar mechanisms.

Identified genes

Epilepsy syndromes for which mutations have been identified are shown in Table 6.6. Comprehensive reviews have been provided by Steinlein (2004) and Berkovic *et al.* (2006). Only a brief description of the more common syndromes affecting adults is given here. *Generalised epilepsy with febrile seizures plus*, now widely referred to as GEFS+, includes a spectrum of clinical phenotypes. The core features are febrile seizures and febrile seizures that persist into later childhood (FS+). Otherwise the prominent seizure type is usually generalised, although partial seizures may also be seen and a clinical picture consisting of TLE alone in some family members has been reported recently (Scheffer *et al.* 2007). Familial *autosomal dominant lateral temporal lobe epilepsy with auditory features* is characterised by neocortical temporal lobe seizures that are usually simple partial and feature auditory, sometimes visual, aura. The clinical characteristics of *autosomal dominant nocturnal frontal lobe epilepsy* are as implied by its name. Specific mutations in this disorder have been differentially associated with response to carbamazepine treatment, raising the prospect that increased understanding of the genetic basis for these syndromes may shed light on the mechanisms underlying response and resistance to antiepileptic drug treatment (Sisodiya 2005).

Table 6.6 Epilepsy syndromes for which genetic mutations have been identified. (Adapted fom Berkovic *et al.* 2006 with permission.)

Monogenic idiopathic epilepsy	Associated genes
Voltage-gated channelopathies	
Benign familial neonatal seizures	K$^+$ channel genes: *KCNQ2, KCNQ3*
Benign familial neonatal–infantile seizures	Na$^+$ channel genes: *SCN2A*
Generalised epilepsy with febrile seizures plus (GEFS+)	Na$^+$ channel genes: *SCN1B, SCN1A*
Severe myoclonic epilepsy of infancy	Na$^+$ channel genes: *SCN1A*
Autosomal dominant lateral temporal lobe epilepsy with auditory features	K$^+$ channel subunit: *LG/1*
Ligand-gated channelopathies	
Autosomal dominant nocturnal frontal lobe epilepsy	Nicotinic acetylcholine receptor subunit genes: *CHRNA4, CHRNB2*
Idiopathic generalised epilepsy with GEFS+	GABA receptor subunit gene: *GABRG2*
Familial juvenile myoclonic epilepsy	GABA receptor subunit gene: *GABRG1*

Table 6.7 Principal causes of progressive myoclonic epilepsy. (Adapted from Shahwan *et al.* 2005 with permission.)

	Age onset	Seizure type	Ataxia	Dementia	Genetic basis	Diagnostic test
Unverricht–Lundborg disease	6–15	Myoclonus +++ Other generalised seizures	Mild and late	Mild and late	Autosomal recessive	Genetic testing
Lafora body disease	12–17	Myoclonus, generalised seizures and occipital seizures	Early	Rapidly progressive	Autosomal recessive	Skin biopsy
MERFF	Adolescence to early adulthood	Myoclonus	Variable	Variable	Mitochondrial	Muscle biopsy
NCL	Infant to adult	Variable	Variable	Rapidly progressive	Autosomal recessive, except adult form (Kufs) which is autosomal dominant	Electron microscopy for intracellular inclusions in eccrine secretory cells, muscle and rectal biopsy
Sialidoses	Juvenile to adult	Myoclonus	Gradual	Variable	Autosomal recessive	Fundoscopy/urinary and white cell enzyme assays
DRPLA	Variable	Myoclonus and other generalised seizures	Progressive	Progressive	Autosomal dominant	Genetic testing

DRPLA, dentatorubral-pallidoluysian atrophy; MERFF, myoclonic epilepsy with ragged red fibres; NCL, neuronal ceroid lipofuscinosis.

Epilepsy occurring in hereditary disorders

A great number of inherited disorders are associated with seizures (Beghi 2004). These include chromosomal abnormalities (e.g. Down's syndrome and fragile X), genetic syndromes with multiorgan effects (e.g. neurofibromatosis and tuberous sclerosis), neurodevelopmental disorders, and certain neurodegenerative disorders. In most cases, seizures probably arise through structural cerebral abnormalities or systemic metabolic effects, rather than through direct genetic epileptogenic mechanisms. Abnormalities of cortical devel-

opment are described in the subsequent section. Seizures are a cardinal feature of a number of rare inherited metabolic disorders known collectively as the progressive myoclonic encephalopathies (PMEs), described briefly below.

The PMEs are a group of rare disorders characterised by myoclonic seizures, tonic–clonic seizures and progressive neurological deterioration, typically with ataxia and dementia (Table 6.7). Most of the underlying disorders have a genetic component. Well-characterised causes include Unverricht–Lundborg disease, Lafora body disease, myoclonic epilepsy with ragged red fibres, neuronal ceroid lipofuscinosis, sialidoses, and dentatorubral-pallidoluysian atrophy (Shahwan *et al.* 2005). Myoclonus in PME is often multifocal and stimulus-sensitive, being precipitated by posture, action or specific external stimuli such as light, sound and touch. The face and extremities are typically affected and massive bilateral myoclonus affecting the limbs may cause falls and injury.

Unverricht-Lundorg disease is the most common cause of PME. It presents between 6 and 15 years of age with stimulus-sensitive myoclonus and other generalised seizures. Ataxia and mild dementia may develop later.

Lafora body disease presents between 12 and 17 years of age and may initially be indistinguishable from idiopathic generalised epilepsy. In addition to myoclonus and generalised seizures, occipital seizures with transient blindness and visual hallucinations are seen and provide a clue to the correct diagnosis. Cognitive decline, often with prominent emotional disturbance, and ataxia are seen early in the course of the disorder. Most patients die within 10 years of onset.

Myoclonic epilepsy with ragged red fibres is a mitochondrial disorder that presents in adolescence or early adulthood with proximal muscle weakness, neuropathy, ataxia, deafness, seizures and intellectual decline. Other clinical features may include short stature, cardiomyopathy, lipomas and diabetes. There is some overlap with a related disorder, mitochondrial encephalopathy with lactic acidosis and stroke-like episodes (MELAS). MELAS presents in early childhood with shortness of stature and any one of the core features within the acronym. Lactic acidosis may be provoked by exercise or intercurrent illness and is associated with nausea, vomiting and coma leading to an episodic presentation of symptoms.

Neuronal ceroid lipofuscinoses are characterised by accumulation of abnormal lipopigments in lysosomes. Infantile, juvenile and adult-onset (Kufs disease) forms are seen, each with distinct genetic causes. Most are autosomal recessive, although Kufs disease may be autosomal dominant. Two forms of sialidosis are rare causes of PME. They are associated with a variety of autosomal recessive mutations affecting the lysosomal sialidase enzyme and have a variable onset from neonatal to early adult. The cherry-red spot myoclonus syndrome (sialidosis type I) is associated with characteristic appearances on fundoscopy.

Dentatorubral-pallidoluysian atrophy is an autosomal dominant disorder that may present with ataxia, choreoathetosis, myoclonus, epilepsy, dementia and psychiatric disorder. It may closely resemble Huntington's chorea. It is caused by an unstable CAG expansion on chromosome 12p13.31.

Other very rare causes of PME. These include the juvenile form of Huntington's disesase, early-onset Alzheimer's disease, Hallervorden–Spatz disease and coeliac disease.

Epilepsy due to birth injury or congenital malformations

Complications of pregnancy and delivery may damage the brain and lead to epilepsy. Most often the seizures will be declared in infancy or date from very early in childhood. Anoxia is an important cause of damage, likewise direct trauma leading to cerebral haemorrhage. However, the risk of epilepsy associated with complications of pregnancy and birth have probably been overstated in the past. The National Collaborative Perinatal Project (Nelson & Ellenberg 1986) examined hundreds of perinatal factors in 2000 children, around 1% of whom had developed epilepsy by 7 years of age. The only significant factors concerning perinatal history were neonatal seizures and being small for gestational age. Congenital malformations (cerebral and non-cerebral) and a family history of certain neurological disorders were the major predictors of epilepsy. A large proportion of children with spasticity, infantile hemiplegia or severe mental defect will suffer from seizures. Covert brain injury without such gross defects is likely to account for seizures in many more. Overall, epilepsy occurs in some 50% of patients with cerebral palsy and the risk rises to over 70% if there is coexistent learning difficulty (Wallace 2001). Both partial and generalised seizures are seen.

Congenital disorders and developmental defects may likewise be found in epilepsies of early onset, and are increasingly demonstrated in cases of adult onset as well. The types of pathology responsible are legion, including porencephaly, tuberous sclerosis and arteriovenous malformations (Sturge–Weber and von Hippel–Lindau syndromes). Particular attention has recently been focused on malformations due to abnormal cortical development, formerly known as cortical dysgenesis. A system of classifying these cerebral malformations has been proposed that divides the disorders into three main categories depending on which aspect of neurodevelopment is primarily affected: cell proliferation, neuronal migration or cortical organisation (Barkovich *et al.* 2001). In many cases a genetic basis for these disorders is either suspected or has been established and sporadic genetic abnormalities (mutations) have also been identified. Other cases may derive from environmental insults to the brain.

The advent of high-resolution MRI has enabled some forms of cortical developmental abnormality to be detected by neuroimaging. It is now clear that these disorders are an important cause of intractable localisation-related epilepsy and are likely to account for many cases that might previously have been regarded as cryptogenic. In a survey of 341 adults with chronic partial epilepsy from the National Hospital, Queens Square, London, cortical dysgenesis emerged as the second most common cause of epilepsy after hippocampal sclerosis, accounting for 12% of cases (Li *et al*. 1995). In a study of 100 adults with refractory epilepsy associated with cortical maldevelopment, the median age at onset was 10 years but in 30 patients the onset was in adulthood (Raymond *et al*. 1995). The great majority of these patients had previously been labelled as suffering from 'cryptogenic' epilepsy. In three-quarters the dysgenesis was established by MRI, and in the remainder by histological examination of surgical or post-mortem material.

Sisodiya (2004) discusses the malformations of cortical development most commonly identified in patients with epilepsy.

Focal cortical dysplasia is probably the most common malformation reported in MRI series and is an important cause of non-familial partial epilepsy arising in the first decade. Seizures are usually unresponsive to drug treatment, and surgery after appropriate investigation may result in freedom from seizures in up to 50% of carefully selected patients.

Periventricular heterotopia. In this malformation, nodules of grey matter representing groups of neurones that have failed to migrate are seen. Most cases are attributable to an X-linked disorder but sporadic cases and non-sex-linked forms have also been described. The typical patient is female and of normal intellect with seizures beginning in the second decade. Surgical treatment is usually not possible and specialist genetic counselling may be appropriate.

Polymicrogyria. This denotes the presence of an area of multiple abnormally small gyri. The abnormality may be unilateral or bilateral and may occur on its own or as part of a syndrome with multiple congenital abnormalities. Polymicrogyria may occur in association with schizencephaly, an abnormality characterised by the presence of a transcortical cleft. Surgical resection of polymicrogyral abnormalities is rarely successful in controlling epilepsy, probably because neighbouring areas of cortex are also abnormal and implicated in epileptogenesis.

Subcortical band heterotopia. A layer of neurones that failed to migrate fully to the cortex is found in the white matter just under the cortical mantle. More severe disruption of neuronal migration may result in the complete failure of neurones to reach the cortex, giving the cortex an abnormally smooth appearance (lissencephaly) with gyri being either flat and few (pachygyria) or absent (agyria). X-linked and autosomal genetic causes have been identified. Female carriers of the X-linked disorder may have learning difficulties and epilepsy but lack subcortical band heterotopias. Surgery is usually unhelpful and genetic counselling is an important aspect of management.

Dysembryoplastic neuroepithelial tumours (DNETs). These are some of the commonest types of tumour in epilepsy (Daumas-Duport *et al*. 1988; Raymond *et al*. 1994). They are classified as malformations arising from abnormal cell proliferation. DNETs are associated with partial seizures with onset before age 20, usually much younger. The lesions are predominantly intracortical, usually involving the frontal or temporal lobes, and the MRI picture of a cystic well-circumscribed lesion of mixed signal characteristics is sometimes sufficiently distinctive to be diagnostic. Characteristics of the tumour include a multinodular architecture, calcification, and cellular polymorphism with an admixture of glial cells, neuronal cells and sometimes germinal matrix components. DNETs may sometimes be difficult to distinguish from low-grade gliomas, even with histology, and long-term monitoring with MRI may be indicated. Malignant transformation of DNETs is currently thought to be very rare. DNETs may be associated with other epileptogenic lesions, including other malformations of cortical development and mesial temporal sclerosis. Seizures are often refractory to medical treatment but surgery, after appropriate detailed presurgical assessment, offers an excellent chance of seizure freedom.

Post-traumatic epilepsy

Head injury is a common cause of epilepsy in young adults. The underlying pathology may be a small cicatrix due to organisation of a circumscribed and superficial haemorrhage, or a more extensive glial reaction with focal atrophy and distortion of brain tissue demonstrable on neuroimaging (see Chapter 4).

The development of post-traumatic epilepsy can be profoundly disabling and has important medicolegal implications. Guidance towards the likelihood of its appearance in an individual case is therefore important. Because seizures arising at different times after head injury have different implications for prognosis, in particular for the likelihood of developing epilepsy, it is useful to distinguish between immediate seizures (occurring within seconds or minutes of the injury), early seizures arising during the period when the patient is recovering from the acute injury (by convention usually regarded as the first week), and late seizures (Frey 2003). Immediate seizures may go unobserved and the underlying mechanisms and implications remain uncertain. They are widely regarded as benign. Approximately 90% of seizures arising in the first 4 weeks after head injury do so in the first week (Annegers *et al*. 1998). These early seizures have a better prognosis with a lessened tendency to persist than late seizures (Jennett, W.B. 1969; Jennett, B. 1975; Annegers *et al*. 1998). Early seizures are commonly focal motor attacks and, in contrast to seizures which develop later, temporal lobe seizures are rare.

In an important population-based study, Annegers *et al*. (1998) report the incidence of unprovoked seizures in 4541 adults and children with traumatic brain injury, characterised by loss of consciousness, post-traumatic amnesia (PTA) or skull fracture, followed for over 10 years. Unprovoked seizures were defined as those occurring after recovery from

Table 6.8 Standardised incidence ratios of unprovoked seizures following brain injury. (From Annegers *et al.* 1998.)

Number of years after brain injury	Standardised incidence ratio for unprovoked seizures (95% CI)
Mild injury (LoC or PTA <30 min)	
<1	3.1 (1.0–7.2)
1–4	2.1 (1.1–3.8)
5–9	0.9 (0.3–2.6)
≥10	1.1 (0.5–2.1)
Moderate injury (LoC or PTA 30 min to 24 hours and/or skull fracture)	
<1	6.7 (2.4–14.1)
1–4	3.1 (1.4–6.0)
5–9	3.0 (1.2–6.2)
≥10	1.8 (0.8–3.6)
Severe injury (LoC or PTA >24 hours, intracranial haematoma or brain contusion)	
<1	95.0 (58.4–151.2)
1–4	16.7 (8.4–32.0)
5–9	12.0 (4.5–26.6)
≥10	4.0 (1.1–10.2)

LoC, loss of consciousness; PTA, post-traumatic amnesia.

the acute effects of injury (over 1 week from injury) in the absence of an acute CNS insult. Head injuries were classified by severity into three groups. Mild injuries were those in which the duration of loss of consciousness or PTA was less than 30 minutes. Moderate injuries were those accompanied by loss of consciousness or PTA of between 30 minutes and 24 hours or associated with skull fracture. Severe injuries were characterised by loss of consciousness or PTA of more than 24 hours, intracranial haematoma or brain contusion (based on the presence of focal neurological signs or observation during surgery). Incidence rates for unprovoked seizures were compared with rates for the general population. In line with previous reports (Jennett 1975), the main finding was that severity of injury was strongly correlated with the risk of subsequent epilepsy and also with the length of time following injury for which the patient remained at elevated risk of seizures (Table 6.8). Over the follow-up period the incidence of unprovoked seizures was 1% following mild injury, 2% following moderate injury and 12% in the severe injury group. Patients with mild injury had a marginal 1.5-fold increased risk of seizures compared with the general population and were not at any appreciably greater risk of epilepsy 5 years after injury if seizures had not developed by that time. In contrast, patients with severe brain injury had a 17-fold increased risk of seizures and remained at increased risk of new-onset seizures beyond 10 years after the injury. The strongest predictors of seizures were, in descending order, brain contusion, subdural haematoma, skull fracture, loss

of consciousness or PTA of more than 24 hours, and age over 65. Early seizures (in the first week after injury), often regarded as predictive of subsequent epilepsy, were associated with subsequent unprovoked seizures but when other risk factors were taken into account the presence of early seizures was no longer a significant prognostic indicator. This latter point was underlined by the observation that of 36 patients with mild head injury who had an early seizure, none subsequently developed epilepsy.

These findings are broadly consistent with the earlier study by Jennett (1975), although he did find that seizures in the first week were significant predictors of subsequent epilepsy. In his detailed examination of risk factors, Jennett found the incidence of epilepsy after head injury to be 1%. He found that a seizure occurring within the first week raised the incidence of subsequent epilepsy to 25%. The occurrence of a depressed skull fracture raised the incidence to 15%, and an intracranial haematoma to 31%. A depressed fracture associated with a PTA in excess of 24 hours led to an incidence of 32%. If in addition these features were associated with a seizure within the first week, the incidence was 57%.

Penetrating injuries carry a much higher incidence of post-traumatic epilepsy, reported as being 30–50% (Russell & Whitty 1952; Walker & Jablon 1961; Salazar *et al.* 1985). The risk of seizures after penetrating injury, as with closed head injury, is highest in the first year but remains elevated for 10 years or more. In Russell and Whitty's series, the highest incidence was from wounds in the central regions of the brain (parietal 65%, motor and premotor cortex 55%), with a diminished incidence towards the poles (prefrontal 39%, temporal 38%, occipital 38%). Multilobar injuries are associated with the highest incidence of epilepsy (Caveness *et al.* 1979).

Caveness *et al.* (1979), reviewing studies from the First and Second World Wars and the Korean and Vietnam wars, showed that the incidence of post-traumatic epilepsy had remained substantially the same despite marked improvements in the management of acute head injuries. With regard to prognosis, experience from the Korean campaigns shows that approximately half of the patients with seizures had ceased to have them within 5–10 years, and that in half of the remainder the fits proved to be intractable. Prophylactic treatment with antiepileptic drugs may reduce the incidence of early seizures after closed or penetrating head injury but is not effective in preventing late seizures and is likely to exacerbate cognitive deficits and impede rehabilitation (Beghi 2003).

Postinfective epilepsy

Infections of the brain and its meningeal coverings may lead to seizures in the acute stage, or produce scarring that becomes the source of seizures some considerable time later. Encephalitis is more likely to be followed by epilepsy than meningitis. In a population-based follow-up study,

Annegers *et al.* (1988) found that the risk of epilepsy was dependent on the type of infection and the presence of seizures during the acute illness. Thus, the 20-year risk of seizures following encephalitis with early seizures was 22% (10% if there were no early seizures). The corresponding figures for bacterial meningitis were 13% with early seizures and 2.4% without them. Seizures most frequently occurred in the first 5 years after the initial illness but the risk remained elevated for at least 15 years. The risk of epilepsy following aseptic meningitis was not increased compared with the general population. Over one-third of patients will develop epilepsy after a cerebral abscess (Koszewski 1991). The incidence of epilepsy due to covert brain involvement during the course of mumps, whooping cough and other infectious diseases of childhood is impossible to determine. Epidemiological studies have failed to demonstrate any association between vaccination and epilepsy (Gale *et al.* 1994). Neurosyphilis must not be overlooked as a cause of late-onset epilepsy. Parasitic cysts within the brain are an important cause of seizures in certain parts of the world (see Chapter 7).

Epilepsy due to cerebrovascular disease

Stroke is an important cause of epilepsy beginning in later adult life, and asymptomatic cerebral infarction is likely to account for many cases of cryptogenic epilepsy in the elderly. Between 2% and 4% of patients will experience a seizure within 24 hours of a stroke (So *et al.* 1996; Burn *et al.* 1997). The risk of later seizures is highest in the first year after stroke, but remains elevated compared with the general population for over 5 years, at which time 7–11% will have experienced a seizure. Approximately half of these seizures are isolated events. When seizures recur they are usually infrequent and rarely pose a major problem. The risk of seizures is greater following intracerebral or subarachnoid haemorrhage than following cerebral infarction, with the exception of total anterior circulation infarction following which up to one-third of patients will suffer a seizure (Burn *et al.* 1997). The likelihood of recurrent seizures (epilepsy) is increased in those with seizures occurring in the first 24 hours and if there is a further stroke (So *et al.* 1996).

Other vascular abnormalities

Approximately 20% of patients with arteriovenous malformations will develop seizures (Crawford *et al.* 1986a). The risk of seizures is higher in younger patients and following haemorrhage. In Crawford's series, the risk of seizures was doubled in those who had been treated neurosurgically (Crawford *et al.* 1986b). Cavernous haemangiomas have been associated with a similar risk of seizures (Kondziolka *et al.* 1995). These hamartomatous vascular lesions are relatively well circumscribed and the outcome after surgical resection may be better than for arteriovenous malformations (Kitchen *et al.* 2004).

Epilepsy due to cerebral tumour

A space-occupying lesion may first declare itself with seizures and must be suspected in late-onset epilepsy. Tumours in the so-called silent regions of the brain naturally present a special hazard in this regard. Approximately 40% of patients with fits due to tumour will have seizures as the first symptom (Chadwick 1993). Low-grade tumours are more likely to present with seizures than rapidly invasive tumours (Cascino 1990). Both primary and secondary tumours can be responsible.

Epilepsy due to degenerative disorders

In a population-based study from the Rochester Epidemiology Group, Alzheimer's disease was associated with a sixfold increased risk of unprovoked seizures (Hesdorffer *et al.* 1996). Generalised seizures predominate, although there is also an increased risk of partial seizures. Myoclonus is a late manifestation in up to 10% of patients with Alzheimer's disease confirmed at post-mortem (Hauser *et al.* 1986). Seizures may occur as early as 3 months after Alzheimer's disease is diagnosed, but the incidence rises as the disease progresses. In a prospective study of 44 patients with mild probable Alzheimer's disease, Romanelli *et al.* (1990) reported a cumulative incidence of 16% over 7.5 years. Seizures tend to be infrequent (average of about two annually), and are rarely associated with significant problems (McAreavey *et al.* 1992). The Rochester study quoted above found that patients with dementia other than Alzheimer's disease had an eightfold increased risk of seizures, although associations with specific diagnoses in this group were not specified. Patients with multi-infarct dementia were underrepresented in this sudy as subjects with a history of stroke were excluded, but it seems likely that this condition is associated with a relatively high risk of seizures.

Epilepsy due to drugs and toxins

Chronic alcohol use is a well-established risk factor for epileptic seizures. In the UK general practitioner-based epidemiological study of epilepsy, alcohol was judged to be a significant factor in 6% of cases (Sander *et al.* 1990). There is a dose-dependent relationship between daily intake of alcohol and the relative risk of seizures. The increased risk (in men) begins with a daily consumption of about 50 g of alcohol (about 4 units), rising to a 16-fold increased risk with an intake of greater than 200 g/day (Ng *et al.* 1988; Leone *et al.* 1997). Victor and Brausch (1967) reported that 88% of seizures in chronic alcohol abusers occurred within 48 hours of stopping drinking and were therefore related to alcohol withdrawal. Others have been unable to replicate this finding (Ng *et al.* 1988), with 50% of seizures in some series seemingly unrelated to withdrawal (Bartolomei *et al.* 1997). Bartolomei *et al.* (1997) found that such seizures were associated with the presence of other alcohol-related neurological sequelae, and suggested that the seizures may themselves be secondary to a cumulative neurotoxic effect of chronic alcohol misuse. Heroin use has been associated with a small increased risk of unprovoked seizures in one study (Ng *et al.* 1990). However, most drugs and toxins are associated with acute seizures rather than epilepsy and are therefore considered in the section below describing provoked seizures.

Other causes

Seizures may occur in connective tissue disorders and vasculitides involving the brain. Multiple sclerosis is associated with a threefold increased risk of seizures: Olafsson *et al.* (1999) found that the cumulative incidence of seizures 10 years after diagnosis was 1.9%.

Aetiology of temporal lobe epilepsy

A good deal of interest has centred on the pathological substrate of TLE, since this may be examined in resected brain tissue obtained at temporal lobectomy. A variety of lesions are found: scars, infarcts, small benign tumours of developmental origin (hamartomas) or *mesial temporal lobe sclerosis*. The latter is by far the commonest lesion found at operation, occurring in some 50% of cases, and appears to be the commonest single finding in any epileptic patient who dies a natural death (Falconer & Taylor 1968). The pathogenesis of mesial temporal lobe sclerosis is thus a subject of considerable importance.

The sclerosis consists of dense glial infiltration of Ammon's horn and adjacent structures such as the amygdala and uncus in the medial part of the temporal lobe. It is usually unilateral. The associated epilepsy commonly sets in during the first decade of life, is frequently severe and responds particularly well to surgical resection of the lesion. Initially it was thought to result from birth injury, either through generalised hypoxia or as a result of herniation and compression of the posterior cerebral arteries against the tentorial opening. However, careful studies suggest that this is not so (Ounsted *et al.* 1966; Falconer & Taylor 1968; Falconer 1974). Neither high birth weight nor prematurity predisposes to TLE, and the incidence of birth injury in patients with medial temporal lobe sclerosis has usually been found to be no higher than in other groups with TLE. Nonetheless, Bruton (1988), in an analysis of a large series of resected temporal lobe specimens, found a weakly significant relationship between the presence of the lesion and a history of birth injury, suggesting that the latter may be operative in a small proportion of cases.

A factor that has emerged as especially common is a history of febrile convulsions, often with status epilepticus, occurring in early childhood. This was confirmed in Bruton's study. It was suggested that the anoxia deriving from such episodes, if sufficiently prolonged at this vulnerable period, may cause irreversible damage to the medial temporal lobe structures and result in due course in the sclerotic epileptogenic lesion. A similar lesion can be produced experimentally in adolescent baboons by inducing serial epileptic attacks or status epilepticus, and as in humans the resulting lesion is usually unilateral (Meldrum *et al.* 1973, 1974).

However, the relationship between febrile convulsions and TLE remains one of the most controversial areas in epilepsy (Waruiru & Appleton 2004). While an association between hippocampal sclerosis and febrile convulsions, particularly prolonged convulsions with focal features, has been a consistent finding (Trinka *et al.* 2002), a causal relationship has not been established. There are three possible explanations for the association: (i) febrile convulsions may cause hippocampal damage in a previously normal individual; (ii) febrile convulsions arising because of some pre-existing genetic or structural predisposition to epilepsy may cause hippocampal sclerosis; or (iii) hippocampal pathology, occurring in isolation or with more widespread cerebral pathology, may precede and predispose to the development of febrile seizures, which are therefore an epiphenomenon of the underlying cause of the epilepsy. Although studies with animal models, mentioned above, support a causal role for febrile convulsions, prospective studies in children have been unable to identify hippocampal sclerosis following prolonged febrile seizures (Scott *et al.* 2003; Tarkka *et al.* 2003). However, larger studies may be required to resolve this issue. In support of the third possibility, recent neuropathological data from 33 children with intractable TLE found cortical dysplasia in three-quarters of those patients with a history of febrile convulsions (Porter *et al.* 2003). Also, in an MRI study of adults with TLE, of those with hippocampal sclerosis, two-thirds had no history of febrile convulsions and 15% had additional evidence of cortical dysgenesis (Kuks *et al.* 1993).

Causes of acute symptomatic seizures

Acute symptomatic, or provoked, seizures have many different causes. Among acute CNS insults, the most frequent causes are head trauma, cerebrovascular disease and infection (Annegers *et al.* 1995). Delanty *et al.* (1998) have reviewed the large number of systemic medical conditions in which seizures may arise. Important causes include renal and hepatic failure, ischaemic hypoxia, endocrine disorder and electrolyte disturbance. Examples of the latter include hyponatraemia and hypernatraemia, hypomagnesaemia and hypocalcaemia, and hypoglycaemia and hyperglycaemia. Seizures may be the presenting feature of hypertensive encephalopathy. This disorder is associated with oedema in the parietal and occipital lobes caused by a failure of autoregulation of the posterior cerebral circulation. A characteristic posterior leucoencephalopathy, which is reversible, is seen on MRI. A great number of drugs may cause seizures (Garcia & Alldredge 1994). Drugs were implicated in 1.7% of all seizure-related patients attending San Francisco General Hospital over a 10-year period (Messing *et al.* 1984). The most frequent culprits were psychotropics (35%), isoniazid (20%), bronchodilators (10%), stimulants (10%) and insulin (10%). Most, if not all, antidepressant and antipsychotic drugs are associated with a significant risk of seizures following overdose. However, with the exception of clozapine, the risk of seizures at therapeutic doses is low (Alldredge 1999). Clozapine is associated with a 4% risk of seizures at doses of 600–900 mg daily. The hazards of psychotropics in people with epilepsy have probably been exaggerated (see Psychotropic medication in epilepsy, later in chapter). Organic solvents and poisoning with heavy metals such as lead, mercury and tungsten may also cause seizures.

Aggravating and precipitating factors in epilepsy

Whatever the underlying cause of seizures, certain factors may operate to facilitate attacks. Some are largely idiosyncratic to the individual concerned, as seen in extreme degree in reflex epilepsy (see Syndromes characterised by seizures with specific modes of precipitation, earlier in chapter). Others may be of more general relevance. Some two-thirds of patients with epilepsy report seizure precipitants (Spatt *et al.* 1998; Frucht *et al.* 2000). The most commonly reported trigger is stress (in around 30%) followed closely by fatigue and sleep deprivation. Other precipitants emerging from these self-report studies have been fever or intercurrent illness, alcohol, fasting, caffeine and many more. Changes in the weather were identified as the second most important trigger (30%) in an Austrian study (Spatt *et al.* 1998), while less than 10% of patients attending a tertiary referral centre in the USA identified 'heat and humidity' as significant (Frucht *et al.* 2000). These discrepant findings serve to emphasise that an individual's perception of relevant triggers will be strongly coloured by the many factors, personal and cultural, that shape beliefs concerning illness attribution. Exacerbations of seizures related to the menstrual cycle (*catamenial seizures*) have been identified in careful prospective studies in up to one-third of women (Herzog *et al.* 1997).

The relationship between stress and seizures was investigated by Stevens (1959), who found that an emotionally stressful interview could have a markedly adverse effect on the stability of EEG patterns in a large proportion of epileptics, but was without effect in normal controls. More specifically, Barker and Wolf (1947) illustrated the highly individual triggering that could occur in relation to certain conflict situations. They presented a detailed psychological study of a patient whose epileptic attacks appeared to be related to occasions when his anger broke through customary inhibitory restraints. When interviewed under amobarbital (Sodium Amytal), he expressed mounting rage against his mother, culminating in a seizure with coincident epileptic discharges on the EEG.

Psychiatric disability among people with epilepsy

The majority of patients with newly diagnosed epilepsy will have their seizures fully controlled with antiepileptic drug treatment and are probably not at increased risk of psychiatric disorder. For example, Jacoby *et al.* (1996) studied depression in a community sample of people with epilepsy, nearly half of whom had been free of seizures for over 2 years. In this seizure-free group the prevalence of depression was only 4%, comparable to what might have been expected in the general population. Depression was found in 10% of patients who reported less than one seizure per month and in 21% of those with more frequent seizures. Time and again, studies of the association between epilepsy and various psychiatric disorders have identified some measure of seizure severity as one of the most important risk factors, and psychiatric disorder is undoubtedly over-represented in people with chronic intractable epilepsy. Among patients being evaluated for epilepsy surgery, for example, over one-third will have a current psychiatric diagnosis and a further third will have a significant past psychiatric history (Manchanda *et al.* 1996). In light of these findings, it is not surprising that studies of the prevalence of psychiatric morbidity in epilepsy have produced widely varying estimates depending on the population studied, as well as the measures and definitions used. Clearly, patients presenting to a psychiatrist, or requiring institutional care, will have a higher frequency of psychiatric and social problems than people with epilepsy attending only their general practitioner (Edeh *et al.* 1990). Equally, patients under supervision in tertiary referral services will be unrepresentative of the wider population.

Some representative data comes from surveys conducted in general practice. Pond and Bidwell (1960) collected information on 245 patients from 14 practices in south-east England. They found that 29% showed conspicuous mental problems and 7% of the total had already had psychiatric inpatient care, which was twice the rate expected in the general population. Edeh and Toone (1987) conducted the Clinical Interview Schedule in 88 patients in general practices in south London; 31% had a history of psychiatric referral and 48% were identified as having significant psychiatric morbidity. The great majority of psychiatric problems were minor affective disorders.

Graham and Rutter's (1968) survey dealt with schoolchildren between the ages of 5 and 14 on the Isle of Wight, and showed a high prevalence of psychiatric disturbance. The entire population of children on the island was screened and 85 cases of epilepsy were discovered (7.2 per 1000); 29% of those with epilepsy, but with no other evidence of a brain lesion ('uncomplicated epilepsy'), showed some psychiatric disorder. When in addition to epilepsy there was other independent evidence of brain damage, the figure rose to 58%. Children with TLE showed significantly more disturbance than children with other epileptic syndromes. These figures could be compared with the prevalence of psychiatric disorder among the rest of the schoolchildren of the island, which emerged at 6.8%. The type of psychiatric disorder shown by the children with 'uncomplicated epilepsy' was closely similar to that seen in other children with psychiatric problems, mainly neurotic disorders or antisocial conduct. Teachers' ratings showed that they were more restless and fidgety and more inclined to aggression than the generality of schoolchildren, but again these characteristics applied to children with psychiatric disorder even in the absence of epilepsy.

In a careful analysis of causes it was shown that lowered intelligence was unlikely to be a factor. The uncomplicated epileptic group showed a normal distribution of intelligence, likewise the subgroup with TLE. The ongoing handicap of epilepsy alone was unlikely to be responsible, since less than 12% of children with other chronic handicaps (asthma, heart disease, diabetes) showed psychiatric disorder, and in any case many of the children with epilepsy were little incapacitated by it. Widespread community prejudice against epilepsy was thought to be an adverse factor in the epileptic child's development, though many of the sample had nocturnal seizures only and psychiatric disability was not especially frequent in children whose teachers knew of their condition. Thus by exclusion it seemed that an important factor was probably the dysfunction occurring specifically within the brain. In addition the influence of parental handling appeared to be important; an adverse family background, measured in terms of the mother's emotional stability, was significantly more common among the epileptic children with psychiatric disability than in those without.

A number of case–control studies have compared the prevalence of psychiatric disorder in epilepsy and other patient groups. Overall, epilepsy has been associated with higher rates of psychiatric morbidity. However, the differences have not been striking and it seems likely that the chronic disability associated with intractable epilepsy is an important determinant of psychiatric sequelae. Mendez *et al.* (1986) surveyed 503 individuals with epilepsy and 186 with other disabilities attending vocational services for the disabled. Depressive symptoms were more common in the epileptic group, who were also more likely to have received psychiatric treatment. An additional finding was that a history of attempted suicide was four times more common in those with epilepsy (see Epilepsy and suicide, later in chapter). However, this study had considerable problems with selection bias; only one-third of survey questionnaires were returned. In a hospital-based study, Fiordelli *et al.* (1993) used the same Clinical Interview Schedule as Edeh and Toone (1987) to assess 100 outpatients but found a much lower prevalence of 'caseness' (19%), this differing little from controls attending hospital for minor surgical procedures. Depression and anxiety were the commonest problems. The lower prevalence of psychiatric disturbance compared with Edeh and Toone's survey may have reflected the exclusion of patients with IQs below 80, and the exclusion of those with evidence of brain lesions. To the extent that the latter might explain the difference, it would suggest that some of the psychiatric disability encountered in patients with epilepsy is attributable to brain damage rather than to the epilepsy *per se*. Most patients were on monotherapy, usually with carbamazepine, and it was possible to show that polypharmacy carried increased risk of psychiatric disorder. In a population-based case–control study from Iceland, Stefansson *et al.*

(1998) compared International Classification of Diseases (ICD)-9 psychiatric diagnoses among 241 disability claimants with epilepsy and 482 age- and gender-matched disability claimants with cardiorespiratory disease or arthropathy. Patients with learning disability and autism were excluded from the study. The prevalence of psychiatric disorder in the epilepsy group (35%) was not significantly higher than in the non-epileptic disability claimants (30%), although some specific diagnoses, notably non-affective psychoses, were more prevalent in those with epilepsy. Most recently, Ettinger *et al.* (2004) conducted a large postal survey comparing patients with self-reported diagnoses of epilepsy or asthma with healthy controls. Both patient groups had higher rates of depressive symptoms than controls but differences between the patient groups fell short of statistical significance when demographic variables were controlled for in the analysis. However, those with epilepsy were more likely to be unemployed and to report lower quality of life.

Thus, while in the majority of people epilepsy is compatible with normal mental health, psychiatric disturbance is far from uncommon and appears to outstrip that seen in the general population. It is found from a very early age and is accompanied by a great deal of chronic social disability, underlining the importance with which it must be viewed. The genesis of such disability is clearly a complex matter, partly psychological, partly social and partly pathophysiological in origin. In the sections that follow an attempt is made to explore in further detail the forms which psychiatric disability may take, its aetiology and its association with different varieties of epilepsy.

Classification of psychiatric symptoms and syndromes in epilepsy

Fenton (1981) proposed a system for classifying psychiatric disorder in epilepsy that has found widespread use (Table 6.9). Psychiatric presentations in epilepsy may be clearly attributable to the underlying cause of seizures. If this is not the case, there is often an obvious temporal relationship between episodic psychiatric symptoms and seizures. Thus, certain psychiatric presentations may precede seizures, arise as a direct manifestation of an epileptic discharge, or follow seizures. Finally, some patients with epilepsy develop persistent or recurrent psychiatric disorders that appear to be independent of seizure activity, or to at least show a variable relationship to the occurrence of seizures. Most of the presentations in the peri-ictal category are more or less unique to epilepsy (e.g. prodromal symptoms, epileptic aura and postictal psychosis). In contrast, the interictal category includes disorders that would meet standard diagnostic criteria for psychiatric conditions such as depression or schizophrenia, although the prefix 'organic' might be used in recognition of a presumed causal association with epilepsy, e.g. organic depressive disorder, organic psychosis.

Table 6.9 Classification of psychiatric presentations and disorders in epilepsy.

Disorders clearly attributable to the brain disorder causing epilepsy
Learning disability
Specific epileptic syndromes
  West syndrome
  Lennox–Gastaut syndrome
  Epilepsy with continuous spike-and-wave during slow-wave sleep
  Progressive myoclonic epilepsies
Cognitive and behavioural manifestations of other acquired causes of
  epilepsy

Disorders strictly related in time to seizure occurrence
Pre-ictal
Ictal: psychiatric manifestations of seizure activity
  Aura
  Automatisms
  Non-convulsive status epilepticus
Postictal
  Delirium
  Psychosis

Interictal psychiatric disorders
Affective disorder
Schizophrenia-like psychosis
Personality disorder/behaviour disorder
Dementia
Dissociative seizures

Disorders clearly attributable to the underlying brain disorder causing epilepsy

This category includes patients who have epilepsy of known aetiology in whom the underlying brain pathology is itself associated with psychiatric, cognitive or behavioural manifestations. The neurobehavioural manifestations are judged to be a consequence primarily of the underlying brain disorder rather than of epilepsy. Examples include a number of syndromes affecting children presenting with epilepsy associated with cognitive and behavioural problems. These include West and Lennox–Gastaut syndromes (see Cryptogenic or symptomatic generalised epilepsy syndromes, earlier in chapter) and the PMEs (see Epilepsy occurring in inherited disorders). The psychiatric disorders seen in children with learning difficulties and epilepsy also fall into this category, as do the cognitive and behavioural sequelae of dementias, focal brain pathologies and other causes of epilepsy in adults not considered further in this chapter.

Disorders temporally related to the occurrence of seizures

Pre-ictal disorders
The term 'prodrome' refers to a variety of subjective symptoms occurring in the hours or even days leading up to a seizure. They herald seizure onset but do not form part of it (Blume *et al.* 2001). Prodromal symptoms are distinguished from the aura of partial seizures by their gradual onset and prolonged duration. Non-specific, ill-defined feelings of malaise with headache, tiredness, irritability and dysphoria are typical but there may be more pronounced affective symptoms, in particular depression. Prodromal symptoms are reported by 7–20% of patients and are more common among patients with localisation-related epilepsy (Hughes *et al.* 1993; Schulze-Bonhage *et al.* 2006). It is important to note, however, that prodromes are also described by patients with generalised epilepsy syndromes and they should not be interpreted as evidence of focal brain disorder. The prodrome phenomenon has been little studied and the pathophysiological basis for these symptoms is not understood.

Ictal disorders

Epileptic aura
The many varieties of epileptic aura and their regional affiliations have been described in the section on the anatomically defined localisation-related epilepsy syndromes. Just as an epileptogenic lesion in the primary motor cortex may give rise to focal clonic muscle jerking, so other discharges, especially those arising in the temporal lobes, may result in purely mental phenomena. In a simple partial seizure such ictal psychiatric phenomena may be the only manifestation of the seizure, while in complex partial seizures they constitute the aura that precedes clouding of consciousness and loss of awareness. They are not, of course, psychiatric disorders at all. Their importance lies in the fact that they may occasionally be mistaken for the paroxysmal symptoms of functional psychiatric illness. Hallucinations and odd abberrations of thought, such as forced thinking or crowding of thoughts, may raise the possibility of psychosis. A diagnosis of primary depersonalisation disorder might be entertained if this is the principal symptom. Most commonly of all, ictal anxiety may be mistaken for panic disorder.

In most cases the distinction between epileptic aura and psychiatric symptoms is straightforward if the cardinal features of epileptic phenomena are borne in mind: they are brief, paroxysmal and highly stereotyped. In taking a history, the presence of other more obviously epileptic phenomena should be sought. The patient should be questioned carefully about the precise sequence of events during the attacks and asked specifically about other subective experiences. Two or more aura symptoms often occur together, for example anxiety and an epigastric aura, in which case it is the stereotyped combination and sequence of events that gives the diagnosis. An informant history is essential and often provides crucial evidence. It is important to ask specifically about motor features such as subtle dystonic posturing and automatisms. These may go entirely unnoticed by the patient even if remaining fully alert throughout the seizure (Biraben *et al.* 2001). There may also be brief periods of clouding of consciousness for which the patient has no memory but which are quite obvious to an observer. Additional features helpful in distinguishing ictal anxiety from panic disorder are (i) the autochthonous nature of ictal fear which arises 'of itself', independent of situational triggers; (ii) the intense and unique quality of the emotion, which is typically quite distinct from the patient's experience of 'normal' anxiety; and (iii) the cognitive symptoms of panic, such as a fear of dying or of suffocation, are usually absent in ictal fear.

Epileptic automatisms

Automatisms have conventionally been regarded as the behavioural concomitants of ictal or postictal delirium and indeed in most cases this is exactly what they appear to be. However, clear-cut examples of oro-alimentary automatisms (lip-smacking, swallowing movements) have now been documented during simple partial seizures in patients who show no evidence of clouding of consciousness (Alarcon *et al.* 1998; Biraben *et al.* 2001). These observations suggest a more sophisticated model of automatisms is required. They also explain the rather qualified tone of the definition recently put forward by the ILAE (Blume *et al.* 2001), which states that an automatism is 'a more or less coordinated, repetitive motor activity usually occurring when cognition is impaired and for which the subject is usually amnesic afterwards'. The terms used to describe automatisms are listed in Table 6.10. It is noteworthy that two descriptive terms, hypokinetic and dysphasic, included in the current ILAE glossary represent

something of a departure from the usual meaning of automatism (and indeed the ILAE's own definition) in that they describe neurological deficits rather than positive motor activity.

The great majority of automatisms are brief, lasting from a few seconds to several minutes, although occasional examples have lasted for up to 1 hour. Knox (1968) found that 80% occupied less than 5 minutes, and another 12% less than 15 minutes. Automatisms may range from simple movements, such as the oro-alimentary features mentioned above, to more complex semi-purposeful actions. These may be relatively self-contained and stereotyped, or be influenced by environmental factors and therefore variable from one occasion to the next. The subject may merely continue with what he was doing, a dazed expression and sudden inaccessibility being the only indications of the seizure. Or there may be no more than some regular stereotyped manoeuvre such as pulling at the clothes, passing a hand over the face or fumbling with objects near at hand. Brief automatisms can in fact pass unnoticed by onlookers. In more extended attacks patients perform a whole sequence of related actions: walking about the room, searching in drawers, moving objects or attempting to remove their clothing. The actions tend to be repetitive, fumbling and clumsy, but are sometimes reasonably well coordinated. The apparent purposefulness behind the movements also varies considerably. Intentions are usually poorly conceived and executed, but

Table 6.10 Terms describing automatisms.

Oro-alimentary	Lip-smacking, lip-pursing, chewing, licking, tooth grinding or swallowing
Mimetic	Facial expression suggesting an emotional state, often fear
Manual or pedal	Indicates principally distal components, bilateral or unilateral Fumbling, tapping, manipulating movements
Gestural (often unilateral)	Fumbling or exploratory movements with the hand directed toward self or environment Movements resembling those intended to lend emotional tone to speech
Hyperkinetic	Involves predominantly proximal limb and axial muscles producing irregular sequential ballistic movements such as pedalling, pelvic thrusting, thrashing, rocking movements Increase in rate of ongoing movements or inappropriately rapid performance of a movement
Hypokinetic	Decrease in amplitude and/or rate or arrest of ongoing motor activity
Dysphasic	Impairment of language without dysfunction of relevant primary motor or sensory pathways, manifested as impaired comprehension, anomia, paraphasic errors or a combination of these
Gelastic	Bursts of laughter or giggling, usually without an appropriate affective tone
Dyscrastic	Bursts of crying
Vocal	Single or repetitive utterances consisting of sounds such as grunts or shrieks
Verbal	Single or repetitive utterances consisting of words, phrases or brief sentencses
Spontaneous	Stereotyped, involve only self, virtually independent of environmental influences
Interactive	Not stereotyped, involve more than self, environmentally influenced

are sometimes successfully carried through even though inappropriate to the situation. The following examples described by Lennox (1960) are typical.

> A woman abruptly ceased her conversation, assumed a strained worried expression and walked away. Led into an adjoining room, she walked quickly from place to place saying 'I must get my coat'. After 5 minutes she consented to sit down and converse, asking what she should do about her affairs, but seemingly not satisfied with the answers because her questions would be repeated again and again. She had no recollection of this seizure or of the postictal conversation nor, in fact, of anything until after she awoke the next day.

> While in a physician's office a patient suddenly stopped talking and stared into space. He slumped in his chair for a brief moment, then sat up and began to rub his abdomen with both hands. A flashlight was shone into his eyes and he turned away. He began to rummage about the desk as if looking for something. When questioned as to what he wanted, he said 'I wanna, I wanna'. At this point he took a cigarette from his packet, lit it and started to smoke. He then got up from his chair, walked out of the office and wandered down the hall, opening all the doors and saying 'I want a toilet'. Next, he walked down the hall but could not be distracted by any outside contact. He then lay on the bed and appeared to regain contact gradually.

> A policeman directing traffic walked to a waiting car, opened the door, opened and examined the contents of the woman driver's handbag, then returned the bag and went back to his post. The woman reported the occurrence and the policeman denied knowledge of it. Subsequent seizures were predominantly convulsive.

To the onlooker, in the great majority of automatisms, the subjects are clearly out of touch with their surroundings. Typically they look somewhat dazed and vacant, and often anxious and tense. When spoken to there may be no response or they may mumble incoherently or answer quite irrelevantly. Attempts at distraction are likely to be resisted, and interference may meet with opposition amounting on rare occasions to combative behaviour. Only very rarely are patients reported in whom judgement and awareness were seemingly maintained during attacks. Hughlings Jackson (1889) recorded the case of a physician who apparently persisted with reasonably competent behaviour during some of his automatisms: in one he continued to write a prescription though the details of dosage were incorrect, and in another he correctly diagnosed a case of pneumonia during an episode for which he was afterwards completely amnesic. Such examples are exceptional and should perhaps be accepted with reserve. It is now widely agreed that behaviour is unlikely ever to be entirely normal, or conversation rational, while the attack is in progress (Jasper 1964; Fenton 1972). Even when complex coordinated activities are maintained, these are usually inappropriate in some respects to the immediate situation, and judgement will be seen to have been impaired. Subjectively the main feature noted by the patient is amnesia for the period of the automatism, and sometimes for a period after its termination as well. The amnesia is usually total, though a vague and muddled awareness of some parts may occasionally be retained.

Non-convulsive status epilepticus

Non-convulsive status epilepticus is a term used to denote conditions in which prolonged electrographic seizure activity results in non-convulsive seizure symptoms (Shorvon 1994; Walker *et al.* 2005). In epidemiological studies prolonged duration is usually operationally defined as over 30 minutes, although this time limit is arbitrary. Non-convulsive status epilepticus is under-recognised but probably accounts for around 40% of all status epilepticus. In older children and adults the most common forms are complex partial status and absence status. Mental state abnormalities and behavioural disturbance may be the most conspicuous features and these forms of status are not infrequently mistaken for psychiatric disorder.

Partial non-convulsive status epilepticus. Complex partial status is the most common form of non-convulsive status. It usually arises in a patient known to have epilepsy or in the context of an acute cerebral insult (Drislane *et al.* 1999). A recognised pattern in patients with intractable localisation-related epilepsy is for complex partial status to follow on from a secondarily generalised seizure. The classical picture is one of fluctuating delirium with motor automatisms. Patients characteristically cycle between a state of partial responsiveness and one of more severely impaired consciousness, with behavioural arrest and motor features. Sometimes the fluctuating nature of the delirium is obviously attributable to repeated complex partial seizures with incomplete recovery between seizures. In other cases, however, there is a more or less continuous state of impaired consciousness. Motor signs are focal and usually intermittent, with dystonia or myoclonic jerking that may be confined to a hand or foot, or may involve complex posturing and automatisms. Adversion of the head and eyes is common. Spontaneous nystagmus may be a helpful clinical sign. Behavioural changes range from psychomotor retardation to states of marked agitation and affective disturbance. The usual picture, however, is of a patient who seems relatively composed but withdrawn and inaccessible. Speech and behaviour seem sluggish, restless, repetitive and disorganised. Anxiety is the most common affective change and may be intense, accompanied by severe agitation. There may be psychotic symptoms including visual or auditory hallucinations and paranoid ideation and a clinical picture resembling catatonia has been described (Toone 1981; Lim *et al.* 1986). However, the presence of delirium is usually unmistakable and the distinction between complex partial status and functional psychiatric disorder should rarely be difficult. In this respect, prolonged seizures without impairment of consciousness, as found in simple partial status epilepticus, are potentially more problematic from a diagnostic point of view.

Simple partial status most commonly involves focal motor seizures in the syndrome epilepsia partialis continua (actually a convulsive form of partial status). Neurological deficits occurring as the sole manifestation of simple partial non-convulsive status are rare and include ictal aphasia (Kirshner *et al.* 1995) and ictal blindness (Barry *et al.* 1985). Instances of simple partial status involving subjective experiential phenomena in the absence of impaired consciousness (sometimes called *aura continua*) are the most likely to be confused with psychiatric disorder. Fortunately, such presentations seem to be very uncommon. Well-documented case reports have included patients with protracted epigastric, olfactory and gustatory aura (Wieser *et al.* 1985; Manford & Shorvon 1992) lasting from 30 minutes to several days. Manford and Shorvon considered that longer durations were possible and that cases were more common in clinical practice than the scarcity of case reports would seem to suggest. Most recently, Seshia and McLachlan (2005) have suggested that subtle forms of simple partial status with elementary sensory aura may even continue for years. In a brief report, these authors describe six patients who had ongoing symptoms that were similar to, though less intense than, their usual aura and lasted for 2–8 years. Anxiety as the only manifestation of simple partial status has been reported by McLachlan and Blume (1980). These authors describe a 21-year-old woman with episodes of fear lasting up to 12 hours during which she remained fully alert. She also had nocturnal complex partial seizures. EEG recordings demonstrated rhythmic discharges in the right anterior temporal region during episodes of fear. The onset of an episode was not captured but on one occasion ictal symptoms and EEG abnormalities disappeared simultaneously. Complex sensory phenomena have also been described in simple partial status epilepticus. However, protracted complex experiential symptoms that are demonstrably epileptic in origin and which occur in clear consciousness are exceptionally rare. Wieser (1980) describes a young woman who experienced recurrent episodes of non-convulsive status during depth-EEG recording. Two episodes began with protracted musical hallucinations in which the patient heard a familiar song (that was, however, different on each occasion) repeated over and over again. She was fully alert for at least 3 hours at the beginning of each episode, which thereafter evolved to complex partial status. The musical hallucinations were associated with a seizure discharge in right Heschl's gyrus. Consciousness became impaired as the discharge spread to involve medial temporal lobe structures bilaterally. There have also been single case reports of patients with episodes of complex visual (Sowa & Pituck 1989) and auditory (Blanke *et al.* 2003) hallucinations but both cases probably fall short of status because individual hallucinatory episodes were brief (minutes), albeit recurrent, and neurophysiological evidence of status was dubious.

Overall, it seems likely that our view of the clinical spectrum of non-convulsive status will broaden. Non-convulsive status should be suspected in any patient known to have epilepsy who presents with a protracted alteration in behaviour or mental state, especially if there is any suggestion of clouding of consciousness. On the current evidence it seems that epigastric aura and elementary sensory symptoms may sometimes occur in protracted form as simple partial status. However, when more complex psychiatric symptoms, including complex hallucinations, occur as protracted ictal phenomena it is almost always in the context of complex partial status, in which case clouding of consciousness and motor signs will suggest the correct diagnosis. EEG should be performed but a scalp recording is likely to be normal during simple partial status. In these cases a dramatic response to parenteral benzodiazepines supports, though does not prove, an epileptic aetiology.

Absence status. Absence status is a prolonged state of impaired consciousness associated with continuous 3-Hz spike-and-wave EEG abnormality (Shorvon & Walker 2005; Walker *et al.* 2005). It is usually seen in a child or adolescent known to have generalised epilepsy. The initial episode typically occurs a few years after epilepsy is first diagnosed but may occasionally be the first clinical presentation. Episodes are recurrent in over 80% of cases. Absence status has also recently been described in elderly patients, occurring either in patients with a history of generalised epilepsy or arising *de novo* in the context of metabolic disturbance and benzodiazepine withdrawal (Thomas *et al.* 1992; Agathonikou *et al.* 1998). The clinical features of absence status are sometimes surprisingly inconspicuous and the diagnosis may go unrecognised (Toone 1981; Shorvon & Walker 2005). Episodes usually start and stop abruptly, characteristically finishing with a tonic–clonic seizure or with sleep. They may last from several minutes to several hours or even days, during which the subject is confused, uncoordinated, slowed and perseverative. The degree of clouding of consciousness varies: at its slightest there is simply slowing of ideation and expression, but more commonly there is marked disorientation, confusion and automatic behaviour. The patient may be virtually stuporose, remaining motionless and apathetic, but if partially aroused is usually capable of limited voluntary action and may sometimes even respond to simple commands. In contrast with complex partial status, cycling between different states of consciousness is not seen. Motor features, present in about half of cases, are bilateral and myoclonic, involving periocular and periorbital regions or the upper limbs. Eyelid myoclonus is a particularly valuable sign in differentiating absence from complex partial status. Sometimes environmental stimulation will interrupt the condition, both in its clinical and EEG manifestations (Landolt 1958). Subsequently, there is complete amnesia for the episode or only a blurred and fragmentary memory. Abnormal mental states other than clouding of consciousness are very uncommon. Early descriptions of psychotic states have not been confirmed in more recent series and probably represent cases of complex partial status that were misidentified as absence status (Toone 1981).

Postictal disorders

Delirium

While epileptic seizures characteristically begin abruptly, recovery of normal function is usually gradual. In a complex partial seizure the transition from a state of unresponsiveness and confusion to one of alertness typically takes place over minutes. To an observer the impression is not unlike that of someone coming slowly to their senses after being awoken from sleep. The patient slowly becomes aware of where he is and gradually interacts more appropriately. The duration of clouding of consciousness and automatisms is characteristically more prolonged in temporal lobe seizures, whereas recovery may be surprisingly abrupt following frontal lobe seizures. Consciousness is more profoundly impaired following a generalised tonic–clonic seizure and recovery more protracted. Typically, patients are alert and responsive within 15 minutes or so, although they will often complain of headache, drowsiness and mental slowing. Even when overt delirium resolves relatively quickly, it is quite common for patients to report that they do not feel fully restored to their normal selves in terms of mental function for a day or two after a tonic–clonic seizure. On occasions, full recovery of consciousness may take much longer, especially in the elderly or in patients with learning difficulties. In such cases the distinction between prolonged postictal delirium and non-convulsive status may be very difficult (Fagan & Lee 1990). In patients with an established history of epilepsy, any pronounced deviation from their habitual pattern of recovery will obviously raise concerns. Careful observation for motor signs is important and an EEG will usually clarify the diagnosis.

Psychosis

The term 'postictal psychosis' refers to brief self-limiting episodes of psychosis that are of abrupt onset and follow seizures. The syndrome has now been well described in a number of case series (Logsdail & Toone, 1988; Savard *et al.* 1991; Devinsky *et al.* 1995; Umbricht *et al.* 1995; Kanner *et al.* 1996; Alper *et al.* 2001).

Clinical features. Postictal psychosis is probably the most common psychotic disorder seen in epilepsy. Prevalence rates of around 6% have been reported in two telemetry series (Kanner *et al.* 1996; Alper *et al.* 2001). Most patients have TLE, but the disorder may occur in other localisation-related syndromes and in generalised epilepsy: 3 of 14 patients reported by Logsdail and Toone (1988) fell into the latter category. Epilepsy has usually been present for over 10 years before the first episode. The precipitating event is an exacerbation of seizures, usually either a cluster of complex partial seizures or a secondarily generalised seizure. This is characteristically followed by a lucid interval (Logsdail & Toone 1988), lasting up to 24 hours, during which the patient appears to recover fully from the after-effects of seizures. The onset of psychotic symptoms is then often sudden and dramatic, accompanied by marked agitation and behavioural disturbance. The phenomenology is pleomorphic with a mixed picture including paranoid, grandiose and religious delusions, auditory, visual and somatic hallucinations, and prominent variable affective changes. While some have reported intermittent delirium, it is important to emphasise that these are true psychotic disorders with psychotic symptoms occurring mainly in the absence of impaired consciousness. A representative estimate of the mean duration of the psychotic episode is 3.5 days, with a range from 16 hours to 18 days (Devinsky *et al.* 1995). EEG obtained during an episode of postictal psychosis may show diffuse background slowing or an increase in interictal epileptifom abnormalities (Logsdail & Toone 1988; So *et al.* 1990), changes that are typical of post-seizure recordings in general.

In clinical practice, postictal psychosis must be differentiated from non-convulsive status. In most cases the distinction will be straightforward. Periods of impaired consciousness and intermittent motor signs will help identify patients with ongoing partial seizures. However, there is some potential overlap. Psychotic symptoms, agitation and behavioural disturbance may feature in both disorders. Impaired consciousness points to a diagnosis of status but subtle degrees of clouded consciousness may be impossible to exclude in a severely agitated psychotic patient. Furthermore, intermittent delirium is said to be a feature in some individuals with postictal psychosis. In this situation, the occurrence of a lucid interval is particularly helpful. In most cases of postictal psychosis, careful history-taking from an informant will establish a period of normal functioning between termination of seizure activity and psychosis.

As the episodes are self-limiting, treatment with antipsychotic medication is usually not indicated. However, the degree of agitation and behavioural disturbance may be such that hospital admission and sedation with benzodiazepines are required. Postictal psychoses have a tendency to recur and repeated episodes are often relatively stereotyped (Tarulli *et al.* 2001). Between 14% and 20% of patients with postictal psychosis will eventually develop chronic interictal psychoses, often after several years and recurrent episodes of postictal psychosis (Logsdail & Toone 1988; Tarulli *et al.* 2001). In the majority of such cases, Tarulli *et al.* found that the phenomenology of the chronic psychoses contained elements seen in preceding episodes of postictal psychosis. It is often stated that the main focus of treatment should be improved seizure control. In practice, however, this may be difficult. Most patients with postictal psychosis have epilepsy that has already proved unresponsive to several antiepileptic drugs. In those with TLE, the possibility of surgical treatment will often arise. However, postictal psychosis is strongly associated with bilateral temporal lobe pathology (see below), which must be carefully excluded before proceeding to lobectomy. There is a potential role for neuroleptics in preventing recurrent episodes of postictal psychosis and even reducing the risk of progression to chronic psychosis. Unfortunately, there is no evidence on which to base decisions about such treatment.

Risk factors. In a case–control study of psychiatric risk factors, Alper *et al.* (2001) found the only factor associated with postictal psychosis to be a family history of affective disorder. With regard to neurological variables, patients with postictal psychosis tend to have more frequent seizure clustering and secondary generalisation (Devinsky *et al.* 1995; Umbricht *et al.* 1995). Among those with TLE, the most consistent finding has been an association with bilateral temporal lobe pathology: bilateral EEG abnormalities are overrepresented, as are aetiologies that are associated with diffuse damage such as encephalitis and head injury. These findings have emerged from case series (Logsdail & Toone 1988; Savard *et al.* 1991), case–control studies (Devinsky *et al.* 1995; Umbricht *et al.* 1995) and also from case reports of a small but interesting subgroup of patients who first develop postictal psychosis after temporal lobectomy (Manchanda *et al.* 1993; Christodoulou *et al.* 2002). Christodoulou *et al.* (2002) report three such patients, all of whom had postoperative seizures arising from either the side contralateral to the operation (two cases) or bilaterally (one case). These three patients represented 5.5% of those with postoperative seizures, but one-third of those (nine patients in total) who developed contralateral or bilateral postoperative seizures. In patients being considered for temporal lobe surgery, a history of postictal psychosis should therefore raise a strong suspicion of bilateral pathology.

Finally, Briellmann *et al.* (2000) have reported quantitative MRI and histopathological findings in 51 patients with refractory TLE, six of whom had postictal psychosis. Postictal psychosis was associated with a relative preservation of anterior hippocampal volume and more frequent temporal lobe dysplasia. Bilateral abnormalities were not noted in this series but all patients were undergoing presurgical work-up and this may have led to a selection bias favouring those with unilateral disease.

In summary, postictal psychoses are the most common form of psychosis in patients with epilepsy. The clinical presentation is distinctive, with a sudden onset of mixed psychotic and affective features, most notably agitation, following a brief lucid interval after seizures. Individual episodes resolve within days but they tend to recur and a significant minority of patients will eventually develop chronic interictal psychoses. Postictal psychosis occurs most frequently in patients with TLE in whom the syndrome is associated with bilateral temporal lobe pathology. The pathophysiology of postictal psychosis is not understood but it is distinct, on clinical and electrophysiological grounds, from non-convulsive status. Postictal psychosis presumably reflects some transient physiological disturbance superimposed on a substrate of epileptogenic abnormality.

Interictal disorders

Depression

Depression and anxiety are the most frequently encountered interictal psychiatric disorders in epilepsy (Lambert & Robertson 1999; Harden 2002; Kanner 2003). However, exactly how common they are remains uncertain. Estimates of the prevalence and incidence of depression in epilepsy have varied up to tenfold. A familiar list of methodological considerations, especially those relating to sample characteristics and case definition, account for this variability. Community-based studies have found symptoms of depression (as distinct from depressive disorder) in 4–37% of people with epilepsy (Edeh & Toone 1987; Jacoby *et al.* 1996; O'Donoghue *et al.* 1999; Ettinger *et al.* 2004). Of the many studies that have investigated depression in patients attending specialist clinics, those that have used ICD or *Diagnostic and Statistical Manual of Mental Disorders* (DSM) diagnostic criteria are most easily interpreted. The prevalence of major depression in such settings has been estimated as 17–21% (Brookes & Crawford 2002; Jones *et al.* 2005). Further studies have examined patients with epilepsy admitted for presurgical evaluation. Such samples are of course highly selected, with the overwhelming majority of patients having medically refractory TLE. In these patient groups the lifetime prevalence of depression meeting DSM criteria has been estimated at 24–35% (Victoroff *et al.* 1994; Altshuler *et al.* 1999;

Glosser *et al.* 2000). Estimates of the point prevalence of DSM major depression in similar series have ranged from 3% over the past month (Manchanda *et al.* 1996) to 22% over the previous year (Devinsky *et al.* 2005). Bipolar disorder does not appear to be over-represented in epilepsy: even in presurgical series prevalence rates of below 1% are reported.

Relatively few studies have compared the prevalence of depression in epilepsy with other medical disorders. Most have used symptom measures rather than case definitions of depression. Mendez *et al.* (1986) sent postal questionnaires to individuals presenting to vocational services for the disabled. People with epilepsy reported more depressive symptoms than those with other disabilities despite similar ratings of disability. Two studies have reported higher rates of depression in patients attending specialist epilepsy centres compared with controls with insulin-dependent diabetes (Perini *et al.* 1996; Beghi *et al.* 2002). A further study found higher rates of depression in epilepsy compared with a mixed group of neurological disorders (Kogeorgos *et al.* 1982). Ettinger *et al.* (2004) conducted a large postal survey comparing the prevalence of depressive symptoms in people with epilepsy, asthma and controls. Symptoms of depression were most commonly reported by those with epilepsy, but differences between the epilepsy and asthma groups fell short of statistical significance when demographic variables were taken into account. Using similar survey methods, the same investigators have reported higher rates of bipolar symptoms (as distinct from bipolar disorder) in people with epilepsy compared with various medical control groups (Ettinger *et al.* 2005). Although half of those with bipolar symptoms reported being given a past diagnosis of bipolar disorder, it is possible that these findings reflect atypical forms of depression that some authorities have said are common.

Clinical presentation of depression in epilepsy
The possibility that depression in epilepsy may take atypical forms has attracted considerable interest. Several investigators have been struck by the fact that depressive symptoms in people with epilepsy often fall short of standard diagnostic criteria and yet are associated with significant morbidity (Mendez *et al.* 1986; Glosser *et al.* 2000). The terms 'interictal dysphoric disorder' (Blumer 1991) and 'dysthymia-like disorder of epilepsy' (Kanner 2003) have been proposed to describe these presentations. Essentially, the clinical picture is one of chronic dysthymia which is interrupted at frequent intervals by brief periods of normal mood. Affective symptoms are pleomorphic, with prominent irritability and endogenous somatic symptoms. Patients would meet standard diagnostic criteria for chronic dysthymia were it not for the intermittent course of the disorder (Kanner 2003). Blumer (1991) has described a more elaborate complex of symptoms including labile depressive symptoms (depressed

mood, with somatic symptoms including anergia, insomnia and pain), other affective symptoms (anxiety and phobias) and 'specific symptoms' of paroxysmal irritability and brief episodes of euphoric mood. It has been suggested that 30–70% of patients with epilepsy and depression have these atypical features. The syndrome is said to respond to antidepressant treatment perhaps in combination with low-dose neuroleptics (Blumer *et al.* 1995). Most clinicians will recall patients who seem to fit these descriptions but much work needs to be done to establish the validity of the concept. In particular, phenomenological comparisons with the spectrum of affective presentations in people without epilepsy are required to establish whether the syndrome is truly specific to epilepsy. The atypical nature of these presentations is cited as one reason why depression in epilepsy often goes unrecognised and untreated. Controlled trials demonstrating that such symptoms respond to treatment would help support the assertion that patients with atypical presentations represent a significant unmet need.

Risk factors for depression
A relationship between depression and poorly controlled epilepsy was most clearly demonstrated in the community-based study by Jacoby *et al.* (1996) already referred to in this chapter. Information on 696 patients was collected from general practice records and by postal questionnaires. Around half of the patients had been free of seizures for over a year, 27% were experiencing one or less seizures per month and 20% had more frequent seizures. Among seizure-free patients, 4% were found to have significant depression scores on the Hospital Anxiety and Depression Scale. The figure rose to 10% in those experiencing less than one seizure per month and to 21% in those with more frequent seizures. O'Donoghue *et al.* (1999) replicated these findings in their study: corresponding figures for depression in the three groups were 6% (seizure-free group), 11% (less than one seizure per month) and 33% (greater than one seizure per month). Studies based in tertiary referral centres are naturally biased in favour of patients with poorly controlled epilepsy. In these settings, a relationship with seizure frequency is generally not found (Mendez *et al.* 1986; Altshuler *et al.* 1999). However, when such patients undergo temporal lobectomy, becoming seizure-free is associated with an improvement in depressive symptoms (Reuber *et al.* 2004; Devinsky *et al.* 2005).

Depression is often believed to be especially common in patients with TLE (Lambert & Robertson 1999). This view has found some support from direct comparisons between epilepsy syndromes. Thus, Perini *et al.* (1996) identified depression in 11 of 20 patients with TLE, compared with 3 of 18 patients with JME. A larger study comparing 150 patients with localisation-related epilepsy and 70 with idiopathic generalised epilepsy found higher measures of depression and anxiety in the former group (Piazzini & Canger 2001). However, the mean seizure frequency in those with generalised epilepsy was less than one per year, while those with partial seizures averaged six per month. This was not controlled for in the analyses and may well have confounded the results. In contrast, a number of recent studies have found similar rates of depression across epilepsy syndromes (Manchanda *et al.* 1996; Beghi & Cornaggia 2002; Wrench *et al.* 2004; Jones *et al.* 2005). For example, Jones *et al.* (2005) found no relationship between major depressive disorder and epilepsy syndrome among 174 outpatients with chronic epilepsy, 55% of whom had localisation-related and 41% idiopathic generalised epilepsy. Underlining the fact that patients with generalised epilepsy are at risk of depression, Cutting *et al.* (2001) have described a series of 42 patients with adult-onset idiopathic generalised epilepsy. Overall, outcome was favourable, with seizures completely controlled in two-thirds and 90% in full employment. Despite this, one-quarter of these patients had a history of depression.

Flor-Henry (1969) originally suggested that depression, particularly depressive psychosis, was associated with right-sided TLE. Subsequent findings have been inconclusive, if anything marginally in favour of an association with left-sided TLE (Lambert & Robertson 1999). Recent temporal lobectomy series have cast further doubt on the issue: most, including the largest series published to date (Devinsky *et al.* 2005), have found no relationship with laterality (Ring *et al.* 1998; Altshuler *et al.* 1999); others have reported differences favouring an association with left-sided pathology (Quigg *et al.* 2003) or right-sided pathology (Glosser *et al.* 2000). If there is an effect of laterality on depression in epilepsy, it must surely be a small one.

No consistent relationships have emerged for other demographic and epilepsy-related variables including age, gender, age of onset or duration of epilepsy. A family history of psychiatric illness was found in 50% of patients with epilepsy and depression by Robertson *et al.* (1987) but Mendez *et al.* (1986) found that such a family history was less common in patients with depression and epilepsy than in a non-epileptic depressed control group. Adverse psychiatric reactions are well recognised with a number of antiepileptic drugs (Schmitz 1999). In most cases symptoms are mild, comprising non-specific features such as dysphoria, irritability and anxiety. More severe reactions, including psychosis, are less common. There are limited data concerning newer antiepileptic drugs but these 'neurobehavioural' symptoms are now routinely reported in preclinical trials. Often, however, the extent to which a particular drug is associated with adverse effects is not clear until it has been in clinical use for several years. No drug can be said to be free of adverse psychiatric effects. Those most frequently implicated include levetiracetam, tiagabine, topiramate and vigabatrin. Folic acid depletion may be caused by antiepileptic drugs, especially by those that induce hepatic enzymes, and

is a treatable cause of depression (Froscher *et al.* 1995). Overall, temporal lobectomy is associated with a reduction in psychiatric morbidity, especially when seizures are abolished. However, approximately one-third of patients will suffer a short-lived episode of depression, typically accompanied by anxiety, and emotional lability arising *de novo* a few weeks after their operation (Ring *et al.* 1998; Wrench *et al.* 2004). Those with a history of depression are at greatest risk but these reactions may occur in the absence of a past psychiatric history. Early recognition and treatment are important as symptoms may be severe, with a risk of suicide. On current evidence the natural history of these disorders seems to be for resolution within 6 months or so. These episodes may be more common after right-sided temporal lobectomies, and are less frequent following surgery for FLE. They are equally likely to occur in those with and without seizure recurrence and appear to be a biological consequence of temporal lobe surgery.

Overall, depression is undoubtedly common in people with epilepsy, especially those with poorly controlled seizures attending specialist services. Patients with TLE are particularly likely to fall into this category. However, earlier impressions of a specific association with TLE, and with right- or left-sided pathology, have not been substantiated. Depression may arise as a direct consequence of medical and surgical treatment. For most patients, however, psychosocial factors related to poorly controlled epilepsy are undoubtedly important. Ongoing seizures are associated with far-reaching effects on people's lives. In addition to the practical consequences of disability, including unemployment, dependence, social limitations and driving restrictions, epilepsy is still a stigmatised disorder. People whose epilepsy is in remission have a quality of life that is no different from the general population. They are also at no substantially increased risk of depression. For those with ongoing seizures, depression is the single most important predictor of a poor quality of life (Boylan *et al.* 2004). Freedom from seizures must clearly be the aim of epilepsy treatment, and the recognition and treatment of depression must be a high priority for all those involved in caring for people with epilepsy.

Anxiety

Anxiety arising as a direct manifestation of an epileptic discharge has been discussed in the preceding section on ictal psychiatric symptoms. In relation to interictal psychiatric disorders, anxiety and depression are probably equally common. Many studies have in fact found slightly higher rates of anxiety symptoms (Jacoby *et al.* 1996; Manchanda *et al.* 1996; O'Donoghue *et al.* 1999; Jones *et al.* 2005). Risk factors for anxiety have received far less attention but there is clearly considerable overlap with depression. Certainly, the relationship between anxiety and the presence of ongoing seizures is exactly the same as for depression (Jacoby *et al.* 1996; O'Donoghue *et al.* 1999).

The most frequent diagnoses are agoraphobia, generalised anxiety disorder and social phobia (Jones *et al.* 2005). Obsessive–compulsive disorder is not over-represented in epilepsy. The term 'seizure phobia' is sometimes used to refer to the situation in which a patient's fear of having a seizure is more disabling than the seizures themselves. The fear may be one of injury or embarrassment and is disproportionate to objective risk. The clinical picture has much in common with agoraphobia, patients engaging in a range of safety and avoidant behaviours that maintain their anxiety. Striking examples are sometimes encountered in patients who have had a successful outcome following epilepsy surgery. Despite becoming free of seizures such patients may remain virtually housebound through fear of having a seizure which, of course, becomes increasingly irrational as the period of seizure freedom extends. Such cases represent an archetypal paradigm for the role of avoidance in perpetuating phobia and respond well to cognitive–behaviour treatment. The situation may be more complex in the presence of ongoing seizures. Entrenched beliefs about epilepsy and what it means to be 'epileptic' may foster highly charged reactions of horror and disgust to seizures. In relation to the likelihood of injury, the boundaries between maladaptive safety behaviour and calculated risk-taking may be difficult to define. The clinical picture may be further complicated by benzodiazepine dependence. Benzodiazepines prescribed as rescue medication for prolonged seizures are likely to be taken inappropriately, either in response to supposed prodromal symptoms (for which the patient becomes increasingly vigilant) or as self-medication for anxiety. Newsom-Davis *et al.* (1998) give a detailed description of the application of cognitive–behaviour therapy in such a case.

Epilepsy and suicide

The risk of suicide is higher in people with epilepsy compared with that in the general population. However, reported rates of suicide have varied considerably between studies depending on the characteristics of the patient populations being considered. In an early review Barraclough (1981) concluded that epilepsy was associated with a fivefold increased risk of suicide, but noted that a 25-fold increase had been described in some highly selected samples. In contrast, two population-based studies of mortality in epilepsy have found no increased risk (Hauser *et al.* 1980; Cockerel *et al.* 1994). Most recently, in a careful cohort study involving over 9000 patients who had been admitted to hospital at one stage for epilepsy, Nilsson *et al.* (1997) reported a standardised mortality ratio for suicide of 3.5.

By far the most important risk factors for completed suicide in epilepsy are psychiatric history and previous suicide attempts. In this, patients with epilepsy who take their own lives are no different from other cases of suicide.

Obviously this highlights the importance of identifying psychiatric disorder in people with epilepsy. Of particular interest, however, is whether any specific clinical aspects of epilepsy are associated with greater risk. This question has been addressed in a careful case–control study reported by Nilsson *et al.* (2002). These authors compared psychiatric and neurological variables in 49 patients with epilepsy who had committed suicide (or probable suicide) and 171 epilepsy controls. A psychiatric history was associated with a ninefold risk of suicide. Less expectedly, early-onset epilepsy, especially epilepsy beginning during adolescence, was an important risk factor. The estimated relative risk of suicide was 16 (95% CI 4.4–58.3) for onset of epilepsy before 18 years of age, compared with onset after 29 years. There was a trend for patients with more frequent seizures and for those taking multiple antiepileptic drugs to be at increased risk but this fell short of significance. Incomplete neurological clinical records were more common in the cases of suicide, which led the authors to speculate that inadequate neurological follow-up, perhaps through non-attendance, could be a contributory factor. No relationship emerged between suicide and a range of other epilepsy-related variables, including type of epilepsy, localisation or lateralisation of the epileptogenic focus, the presence of neurological deficit or any specific antiepileptic medication.

Schizophrenia-like psychosis

The interictal schizophrenia-like psychoses of epilepsy are psychotic disorders that would meet diagnostic criteria for schizophrenia were it not for the coexistence of epilepsy. Implicit in this definition is that the psychotic episodes are of relatively long duration and show either no, or a variable, relationship to the occurrence of individual seizures.

Most early studies reported an excess of schizophrenia-like psychosis in people with epilepsy (see reviews by Sachdev 1998; Lancman 1999). A study by Mendez *et al.* (1993a) is noteworthy because it included a control group and used standard diagnostic criteria. These authors compared the prevalence of psychosis among 1611 patients attending an epilepsy clinic and 2167 patients attending a migraine clinic. A history of psychosis was found in 9.25% of the epilepsy group and 1.06% of the migraine patients. The prevalence of more narrowly defined schizophrenia in the epilepsy group was 4.72% once cases meeting DSM-III-R criteria for schizoaffective or undifferentiated psychosis were excluded. More recently, two epidemiological studies have provided support for the association. Stefansson *et al.* (1998) reported the prevalence of ICD-9 psychiatric diagnoses among disability claimants in Iceland, comparing 241 patients with epilepsy (patients with learning disability were excluded) and 482 subjects with non-neurological causes of disability. The overall prevalence of psychiatric disorder was similar in the two groups (35% and 30%, respectively) but schizophrenia and paranoid psychosis were significantly more common in the epilepsy group (3% compared with 0.6%). However, the most convincing evidence comes from a study of the Danish population registers (Qin *et al.* 2005). These authors examined the health registers for 2.7 million people born between 1950 and 1987, including data gathered up until 2002. ICD definitions of schizophrenia and epilepsy were used. The relative risk of schizophrenia in individuals with a history of epilepsy was 2.48 (95% CI 2.20–2.80). The relative risk for non-affective psychosis, including schizophrenia, was 2.93 (95% CI 2.69–3.20). As impressive as these findings are, one caveat should be noted. Cases of epilepsy were identified by hospital admission records, raising a question about the extent to which these findings might apply overall to individuals with epilepsy. The authors argue that their figures are representative as, they say, over 80% of patients with new-onset epilepsy are admitted to hospital in Denmark and prevalence rates for epilepsy derived from their data are similar to those from other large epidemiological studies.

It is therefore now reasonable to conclude that epilepsy is indeed associated with an increased risk of schizophrenia. The evidence for this association is most robust for patients who have chronic epilepsy associated with significant disability or requiring specialist medical attention. Patients in this group are two to three times more likely to develop schizophrenia than the general population.

Nature of the psychosis

The modern era of our understanding of the epileptic psychoses began with the influential study by Slater *et al.* (1963) who described 69 patients with epilepsy and a diagnosis of schizophrenia. This remains the most detailed description of a large series of such patients. Their observations rested essentially on clinical judgement. The mean age of onset of schizophrenia was 30 after a mean duration of epilepsy of 14 years. All the cardinal symptoms of schizophrenia were exhibited and Slater *et al.* stressed that it would not be possible to diagnose these patients, on psychiatric symptomatology alone, as suffering from anything other than a schizophrenic psychosis. However, they noted that certain combinations of symptoms differed slightly from the usual schizophrenic patterns. Personality abnormalities before the onset of psychosis were not prominent. Catatonic phenomena were rare and the loss of affective response did not occur so early or become so marked as in primary schizophrenia. They commented that by and large the patients were friendlier, more cooperative and less suspicious towards hospital staff.

Subsequent reports have confirmed an interval of approximately 10–15 years between the onset of epilepsy and psychosis. However, the subtle phenomenological differences observed by Slater *et al.* have not been replicated. Although Kristensen and Sindrup (1979) commented on retention of affective warmth, neither Perez and Trimble (1980) nor Toone

et al. (1982) were able to demonstrate any significant distinguishing phenomenological features using objective symptom measures. Likewise, although Toone *et al.* (1982) found that psychotic epileptic patients tended to have less premorbid personality abnormality, this was not confirmed by Mendez *et al.* (1993a) who compared 62 psychotic epileptics with 62 age- and gender-matched schizophrenic controls.

Nearly half of Slater *et al.*'s series had a chronic course. When the onset had been acute the prognosis was better, sometimes with improvement to the point of recovery. Those with an episodic onset sometimes pursued a fluctuating course thereafter. Follow-up at a mean interval of 8 years from onset showed that one-third had achieved remission, and a further third had improved with regard to psychotic manifestations. Onuma *et al.* (1991) found that 64% followed a chronic course over a 10-year period. Toone *et al.* (1982) found little difference between outcome in their series of 69 patients who had been admitted to hospital with psychosis and epilepsy compared with 53 non-epileptic consecutive admissions matched for ICD diagnosis. Their epileptic patients had slightly more frequent and longer admissions and were more likely to have their diagnosis changed over time.

Risk factors

A considerable amount of research has focused on risk factors for developing schizophrenia-like psychosis in epilepsy. The most consistent finding has been an association between psychosis and various indices of epilepsy severity, including seizure frequency, measures of seizure severity, multiple seizure types, a history of status, and the number of epilepsy-related hospital admissions (Mendez *et al.* 1993a; Schmitz *et al.* 1999; Adachi *et al.* 2000; Qin *et al.* 2005).

No consistent relationship has emerged between psychosis and age at onset of epilepsy, with some studies finding younger age of onset of epilepsy to be a risk factor (Umbricht *et al.* 1995; Adachi *et al.* 2000) and others reporting a significant relationship with later age at onset of epilepsy (Mendez *et al.* 1993a). Qin *et al.* (2005) demonstrated that the risk of psychosis increased linearly with increasing age at first admission for epilepsy.

Slater *et al.* noted a preponderance of patients with TLE in their series and an association between localisation-related epilepsy and psychosis has been reported by most large case–control studies (Mendez *et al.* 1993a; Adachi *et al.* 2000), although there have been negative findings (Schmitz *et al.* 1999). However, given that seizures are more likely to be medically intractable in localisation-related epilepsy than in idiopathic generalised epilepsy, on the present evidence it is not possible to distinguish between the effect of epilepsy syndrome and severity. Furthermore, in the epidemiological study by Qin *et al.* (2005), patients with localisation-related epilepsy were only slightly over-represented among those who were psychotic and this difference fell short of statistical significance. Related to the question of an association between type of epilepsy and psychosis, three studies have reported an increased rate of experiential epileptic auras among psychotic epileptics (Kristensen & Sindrup 1978a; Mendez *et al*. 1993a; Schmitz *et al*. 1999).

Perhaps the most controversial findings concern the relationship between psychosis and laterality of epileptic focus. Flor-Henry (1969) reported that among psychotic temporal lobe epileptics, those with schizophrenia were more likely to have dominant rather than non-dominant epileptic foci. Although this finding has received some support (Taylor 1975; Sherwin 1981; Perez *et al*. 1985), most findings have been negative (Kristensen & Sindrup 1978b; Jensen & Larsen 1979a; Umbricht *et al*. 1995; Schmitz *et al*. 1999). Most persuasively, two large case–control series have found no relationship between psychosis and the laterality of EEG abnormalities (Mendez *et al*. 1993a; Adachi *et al*. 2000). Functional neuroimaging studies have been divided, with evidence of both lateralised temporal lobe and more generally distributed abnormalities. Positron emission tomography (PET) in a small series revealed indications of reduced metabolism, especially in frontal, temporal and basal ganglia regions (Gallhofer *et al*. 1985). Marshall *et al*. (1993), in a small pilot study, obtained evidence from SPECT of lowered cerebral blood flow in the left medial temporal region in psychotic epileptic patients, and also in both thalami. In a larger SPECT investigation, Mellers *et al*. (1998) observed a significant *decrease* in blood flow in the left superior temporal gyrus during verbal activation, in contrast to non-psychotic epileptics and non-epileptic schizophrenic controls.

Structural imaging studies have found no consistent association with either regional or lateralised brain abnormalities. While Marchetti *et al*. (2003) found that left hippocampal volumes were smaller in 36 patients with epilepsy and psychosis compared with healthy (non-epileptic) controls, three studies have reported no differences in hippocampal volume between psychotic epileptics and epilepsy controls (Maier *et al*. 2000; Marsh *et al*. 2001; Tebartz van Elst *et al*. 2002). Instead, psychosis in epilepsy has been associated with a global reduction in cerebral volume (Marsh *et al*. 2001; Tebartz van Elst *et al*. 2002). The view that widespread cerebral damage rather than regional abnormality is relevant finds support from a number of other sources. Kristensen and Sindrup (1978a,b, 1979) reached this conclusion after they found that patients with epilepsy and psychosis were more likely to have generalised or multifocal EEG abnormalities, have a history of CNS insult, demonstrate abnormal neurological signs and have lower IQ measures than non-psychotic epilepsy controls. Umbricht *et al*. (1995) also found lower IQ measures in psychotic epileptics. Mellers *et al*. (2000) found that patients with schizophrenia-like psychosis of epilepsy showed an almost identical pattern of neuropsychological deficits compared with a matched group of patients with schizophrenia, with evidence of memory and executive impairments on a background of attentional and IQ deficits that suggested global cerebral dysfunction. Finally, in the only post-mortem study so far, Bruton *et al*. (1994) compared 19 patients with epilepsy and psychosis with 36 non-psychotic epilepsy controls. TLE and mesial temporal sclerosis occurred with equal frequency in the psychotic and control subjects. The psychotic group were distinguished from the controls by the presence of distributed cerebral pathology. The pathological findings included increased ventricular size, periventricular gliosis, more focal brain abnormalities and perivascular white-matter softening.

An additional finding is that where patients with schizophrenia-like psychoses have come to temporal lobectomy, mesial temporal lobe sclerosis has seemed less common than in TLE generally, and small cryptic tumours (hamartomas) have been particularly common (Taylor 1972; Falconer 1973). Taylor (1975) compared 47 patients whose resected specimens showed 'alien tissue' (small tumours, hamartomas and focal dysplasia) with 41 showing mesial sclerosis; 23% of the former but only 5% of the latter had been psychotic. In contrast, Roberts *et al*. (1990), in a further analysis of the material, found that mesial sclerosis was not uncommon in the presence of a schizophrenia-like psychosis but a second form of pathology (alien tissue ganglioglioma) was significantly more common in those who developed psychoses postoperatively. The lesions arise early in fetal or neonatal life and were associated with a particularly early onset of seizures. Where lesions were found in the resected specimens from patients with schizophrenia-like psychoses, they always involved the medial temporal lobe structures (amygdala, hippocampus and parahippocampal gyrus), the lateral parts of the lobe being rarely affected. Shaw *et al*. (2004) examined a further series of 11 patients with postoperative schizophrenia-like psychosis, comparing them to 33 postoperative non-psychotic controls. In agreement with the above findings, lesions other than mesial temporal sclerosis were over-represented in the psychotic group. Other risk factors were bilateral (preoperative) EEG abnormalities and a smaller amygdala on the unoperated side. Onset of psychosis was typically within 1 year of the operation, suggesting that the operation may have acted as a trigger for psychosis in vulnerable individuals.

A marked effect of left-handedness was seen in Taylor's patients (described above), 7 of 13 psychotic patients being left-handed compared with only 11 of 75 non-psychotic patients. In the alien tissue group, females, particularly left-handed females, were especially likely to have developed a schizophrenia-like psychosis. However, neither gender (Qin *et al*. 2005) nor left-handedness (Oyebode & Davison 1990) have been implicated as risk factors in other studies.

Finally, a number of authors have investigated family history of psychosis as a risk factor. Unfortunately, none of these studies have used a formal family interview approach.

Compared with epilepsy controls, patients with psychosis and epilepsy have an increased rate of family history of psychiatric disorder (Jensen & Larsen 1979b; Adachi *et al.* 2000). Compared with patients who have schizophrenia, psychotic epileptics have been reported as having similar (Toone *et al.* 1982) or less (Mendez *et al.* 1993a) family psychiatric history. Qin *et al.* (2005) examined the medical database for first-degree relatives of cases identified in their epidemiological study. They concluded that a family history of psychosis contributed to the risk of psychosis among patients with epilepsy and that the effect of a personal history of epilepsy on the risk of psychosis was greatest in those without a family psychiatric history. Interestingly, they also found that a family history of epilepsy was associated with a small but significant increased risk of psychosis.

Aetiology

Mechanisms behind the association between epilepsy and chronic schizophrenia-like psychoses have been considered in some detail (Symonds 1962; Slater *et al.* 1963; Sachdev 1998). Chance association may be operative, or precipitation in individuals genetically predisposed to schizophrenia. The psychosocial burden imposed by epilepsy or the effects of antiepileptic drug treatment may be important. Or there may be more direct links of a physiological nature.

A merely chance association appears unlikely. There is now robust evidence that intractable epilepsy is associated with a twofold to threefold increased risk of schizophrenia. However, it should be noted that if this figure is correct, then given the prevalence of schizophrenia, up to one in two patients with schizophrenia and epilepsy do have the two disorders by chance coincidence alone. This constitutes an important methodological problem for any investigation of specific aetiological links between epilepsy variables and psychosis.

Precipitation in individuals genetically predisposed to schizophrenia similarly appears unlikely to account for most cases. Patients with psychosis and epilepsy probably have a genetic diathesis for psychosis that lies between that found in the general population (and non-psychotic patients with epilepsy) and that found in patients with schizophrenia. Qin *et al.* (2005) have shown that a personal history of epilepsy increases the risk of schizophrenia in the absence of a family history of psychosis.

An increased risk of schizophrenia is best established for individuals who suffer from intractable and disabling epilepsy. However, disability alone does not appear to account for the increased incidence of psychosis. Stefansson *et al.*'s (1998) comparison of disability claimants with epilepsy and a group of non-neurological disability claimants found similar rates of psychiatric morbidity in the two groups but an increased risk of psychosis in the epilepsy group alone.

Psychosis has been reported as a rare complication of treatment with nearly every antiepileptic drug (Schmitz 1999). However, such psychoses usually resolve once the offending drug is withdrawn. Drug effects alone therefore seem unlikely to account for the recurrent or chronic psychoses most commonly associated with epilepsy. Furthermore, specific drugs have not been implicated in case–control studies (Mendez *et al.* 1993a). In a consecutive series of 44 patients with epilepsy and a variety of psychoses, Matsuura (1999) noted seven (16%) that followed the introduction of an add-on antiepileptic drug. In most cases the drug appeared to act as a trigger for psychosis in patients with a history of recurrent psychotic episodes. In some patients, notably in children treated with ethosuxamide, the appearance of psychosis may coincide with cessation of seizures (*alternative psychosis*) and the loss of paroxysmal abnormalities on EEG (*forced normalisation*) (Krishnamoorthy & Trimble, 1999). Thus, while epilepsy and psychosis are associated, within this association, at least in some individuals, there appears to be a biological antagonism between seizures and psychosis.

Overall, the evidence favours direct aetiological links between epilepsy (or its attendant brain dysfunction) and psychosis. The latter may be viewed as a 'symptomatic schizophrenia' analogous to that emerging with other brain lesions or with amphetamine abuse. The aetiological link with epilepsy could be via the seizures themselves, or by way of the underlying disorder of cerebral function that manifests itself as epilepsy.

Favouring the view that seizure activity might be important is the observation that epilepsy has usually been present for many years before the psychosis supervenes, also that various indices of seizure severity are associated with psychosis. The link between seizures and psychosis is most compelling in the case of the postictal psychoses (see Postictal disorders, earlier), in which there is, by definition, a clear temporal relationship between seizures or seizure clusters and psychotic symptoms. Furthermore, some 15% of patients with postictal psychosis will eventually develop chronic interictal psychosis (Tarulli *et al.* 2001), supporting the notion that seizure-related mechanisms have a role in the latter group.

Evidence that the underlying brain pathology or dysfunction is of primary importance stems from observations made regarding psychosis in patients undergoing temporal lobectomy (Taylor 1972; Roberts *et al.* 1990; Shaw *et al.* 2004). Patients who are psychotic before operation are likely to remain so, whether they become seizure-free or not. Of equal interest, patients may develop psychosis for the first time *after* the operation and, again, this may happen regardless of whether the operation successfully halted seizures. These observations suggest that factors related to epilepsy, but independent of the occurrence of seizures, are important. Possible factors in this category include pathological abnormalities of a developmental origin mentioned above and the functional burden imposed by distributed cerebral structural abnormalities that have been identified by neuroimaging and neuropathological studies.

A number of authors have speculated about possible psychological links between experiences during seizures and psychosis. The patients in Slater *et al.*'s series had often experienced complex aura symptoms, and a number explained them in a delusional way; the symptoms in fact came to enter into the content of the delusional psychoses. Pond (1962) suggested that there may sometimes be a causal relationship of a psychological kind between seizures and psychosis, the latter arising from abnormal emotional experiences, physically caused, which then become integrated into the totality of psychic life as a psychodynamic process. However, there are difficulties in accepting such a mechanism as a general explanation. Although some studies have reported an association between epileptic aura and psychosis, a substantial proportion of psychotic epileptics have generalised epilepsy and therefore do not experience auras. Furthermore, while a psychological explanation might be plausible for the derivation of delusional symptoms, or at least their content, it would be hard to account for psychotic features such as hallucinations, thought disorder or volitional disturbance on such a basis.

A physiological formulation of the link was put forward by Symonds (1962). In this view, both the epilepsy and the psychosis are manifestations of the same basic disorder of cerebral function within the temporal lobes, the epilepsy being an earlier and intermittent manifestation, and the psychosis a later product. Symonds postulated that this abnormality might consist not so much of the static lesion responsible for the epilepsy, but rather of the disordered electrophysiological activity which spreads within the temporolimbic system. At peaks of such disorder seizures are likely to occur, but the background disturbance may persist between attacks, with far-reaching effects on psychological function. In effect Symonds suggested that

> the temporal lobe includes within its boundaries circuits concerned with the physiological basis of the psychological disorder we call schizophrenia . . . it is not the loss of neurones in the temporal lobe that is responsible for the psychosis, but the disorderly activity of those that remain.

Stevens (1992) put forward a not dissimilar formulation. Brain damage is known to provoke regenerative sprouting of axons and synaptic proliferation, even in adults, and resected specimens from patients with TLE have shown sprouting of cells in the dentate gyrus and expansion of postsynaptic receptor sites in the parahippocampal gyrus. The functional consequences of such changes are largely unknown, but reorganisation of this nature, as a consequence of insults from seizures, could be associated with the onset of schizophrenia.

In summary, patients with intractable epilepsy have a twofold to threefold increased risk of schizophrenia. Psychotic symptoms typically begin some 15 years after the onset of epilepsy. Early observations suggesting subtle phenomenological differences between these psychoses and primary schizophrenia have not been confirmed. The prognosis is similar to primary schizophrenia. A family history of psychosis is a risk factor but a direct aetiological link between epilepsy and psychosis is likely to account for most cases. There is evidence to suggest that this link may be mediated through cumulative effects of recurrent seizures and by static effects of underlying brain pathology. Thus, patients with frequent severe seizures associated with distributed cerebral dysfunction and structural change are at greatest risk. A close association with TLE and with left-sided seizure foci now seems less likely. Certain pathological lesions originating early in neurodevelopment may be over-represented.

Personality in epilepsy

The notion that epilepsy might be associated with specific and enduring personality difficulties has fallen into disrepute. It is now recognised that these ideas arose from, and perpetuated, the stigma that has burdened people with epilepsy since ancient times. Descriptions of epileptic personalities in the medical literature of the nineteenth century were often pejorative and demonstrably fostered social discrimination. To take one example, Devinsky and Najjar (1999) point out that eugenic laws in the USA barring people with epilepsy from marriage were influenced by the prevailing medical view that epilepsy was associated with 'mental and moral weakness'. It is disquieting to learn that such laws remained in force in a few States as recently as 1966. Fortunately, medical opinion and legislation have moved on. As previously noted in this chapter, it is now clear that the overwhelming majority of people with epilepsy suffer no mental disorder. Yet there is a risk that the controversy surrounding links between epilepsy and personality might lead us to overlook some genuine associations and potentially useful insights into the relationship between brain and behaviour.

The subject of personality and epilepsy has been reviewed by a number of authors (Trimble 1983; Benson 1991; Blumer 1999; Devinsky & Najjar 1999). The idea that TLE, rather than epilepsy in general, was specifically implicated in personality disturbance began with Gibbs (1951) who reported clinical observations in 275 patients with 'psychomotor' epilepsy. He found that psychiatric disorder, which he divided into either 'severe personality disorder' or 'psychosis (all types)', was three times more common in patients with an anterior temporal lobe focus compared with those who had foci elsewhere. Gibbs' influential conclusion was that 'the sylvian fissure is one of the chief boundaries between neurology and psychiatry'. In 1975, Waxman and Geschwind proposed a syndrome of interictal behavioural changes they believed to be common in TLE. Geschwind syndrome, as it came to be known, comprised alterations in sexual behaviour (principally hyposexuality), religiosity and a tendency towards extensive, and in some cases compulsive, writing and drawing (hypergraphia). Waxman and Geschwind believed this behavioural syndrome was sufficiently distinct and common to be of diagnostic value. They also proposed the syndrome as a paradigm for linking human behaviour with a precise cerebral localisation. Bear and Fedio (1977) subsequently incorporated these traits with others gleaned from earlier descriptions in their 18-trait Bear and Fedio Index (BFI). In a small study involving 27 patients with presumed TLE, they found that the great majority of the chosen traits differentiated the epileptic patients from healthy controls and subjects with neuromuscular disorder. Particularly striking differences were seen with humourlessness, circumstantiality, dependence, sense of personal destiny and preoccupation with philosophical concerns. The profiles of traits tended to differ according to the hemisphere primarily involved. Patients with right temporal foci showed an excess of overt emotional traits (deepened emotionality, sadness, hypermoralism), whereas those with left temporal foci showed ruminative intellectual tendencies (religiosity, philosophical interests, humourlessness, sense of personal destiny).

However, further studies have thrown doubt on many of these associations. Bear and Fedio's initial study failed to include patients with other forms of epilepsy, nor did it control for the presence or absence of psychiatric disorder. Hermann and Riel (1981) compared patients with TLE and patients with primary generalised epilepsy, and found that only four of the traits differentiated them significantly (sense of personal destiny, philosophical interests, dependence and paranoia). Mungas (1982) found that no trait discriminated between patients with TLE and patients with psychiatric disorder; indeed when examined in a separate group of patients, a large proportion of the variance in the trait scores seemed attributable to the presence or absence of psychiatric illness. Master *et al.* (1984), in a thorough study, compared patients with TLE, other forms of epilepsy, psychiatric disorder and normal volunteers. The results again underlined the prominent effect of psychiatric disturbance. TLE made no discernible contribution of its own, and no differences in trait scores were observed between patients with right or left temporal lobe foci. In a critical review of the area, Devinsky & Najjar (1999) drew a number of conclusions. First, patients with epilepsy obtain higher scores on the BFI than healthy controls. Second, BFI scores do not discriminate between individuals with epilepsy and patients with psychiatric disorder who do not have epilepsy: the BFI is to some extent simply a marker of general psychopathology. Third, studies that have compared the BFI in patients with different forms of epilepsy have been inconclusive. In summary, while these studies contribute to the evidence that patients with epilepsy have higher rates of psychiatric morbidity than the general population, they have not identified behavioural traits that are specific to epilepsy. The BFI does not define an epileptic behavioural syndrome.

Yet the possibility remains that a subgroup of patients with TLE may display significant clustering of some components of the syndrome, perhaps especially in the presence of psychiatric disorder. The search for clearly definable traits, and their detailed associations, still has much to commend it. Considerable interest still attaches to phenomena such as hypergraphia. Sachdev and Waxman (1981) wrote to patients inviting them to describe their current state of health. Patients with TLE responded more frequently and extensively (mean 1301 words) compared with other epileptic patients (mean 106 words). Hermann *et al.* (1983) replicated the higher response rate in patients with TLE. Further associations have been described between hypergraphia in TLE and measures of general psychopathology (Hermann *et al.* 1988; Okamura *et al.* 1993), right-sided epileptic foci (Roberts *et al.* 1982) and brain damage (Okamura *et al.* 1993). Other phenomena may prove better accounted for by disorders well recognised outside the field of epilepsy. Viscosity, for example, refers to a tendency for prolonged social contacts, talking repetitively, circumstantially, pedantically, and not ending conversations after a socially appropriate interval. It is essentially an abnormality of language and social communication that might suggest a diagnosis of autistic spectrum disorder, especially if it were associated with other 'temporal lobe personality' features such as obsessionality.

The possibility that other epilepsy syndromes may be associated with specific personality features has received less attention. Janz's (1969) original description of JME included a variety of behavioural traits that he felt were characteristic. These included such features as irresponsibility, impulsivity, self-centredness, and emotional instability. This suggestion has not been systematically investigated and many of these characteristics might simply be attributable to adolescence. However, some indirect support comes from a study by Gelisse *et al.* (2001) who found 11 patients meeting DSM-IV criteria for borderline personality disorder among a consecutive series of 170 patients with JME. This finding is in marked contrast with those from studies of TLE that have not reported high rates of borderline personality disorder (see below). Borderline personality disorder is characterised by a number of traits reminiscent of Janz's description including impulsivity and emotional instability.

Juvenile absence epilepsy has traditionally been regarded as benign, in terms of both seizure outcome and psychiatric comorbidity. This view has recently been challenged in a thorough study by Wirrell *et al.* (1997). These authors compared psychosocial outcome in 65 patients with juvenile absence epilepsy and 76 patients with juvenile rheumatoid arthritis. The mean age at assessment was 23 years. Patients with juvenile absence epilepsy had significantly greater difficulties in terms of academic achievement, interpersonal relationships and behavioural problems. Outcome was least favourable in those (33%) who had ongoing seizures. At present, whether these problems reflect higher rates of formal psychiatric diagnoses, including personality disorder, is not known.

The relationships between personality and localisation-related epilepsies other than TLE have not been investigated. This seems particularly surprising in the case of FLE, which might be expected to be associated with distinct behavioural characteristics. Early descriptions of the syndrome (Williamson *et al.* 1985) noted that the majority of patients had a psychiatric history but the nature of this comorbidity has yet to be fully described.

The development of modern classification systems for mental disorders has provided a new framework for investigating personality in epilepsy. Two studies using DSM-III-R criteria have estimated the prevalence of personality disorder among epilepsy patients undergoing presurgical evaluation to be 18% and 22% (Manchanda *et al.* 1996, Lopez-Rodruigez *et al.* 1999). Neither study had a control group. However, these figures represent approximately twice the expected prevalence in the general population. Patients with dependent and avoidant personality disorder were particularly over-represented in both studies. In a detailed investigation of neurological variables, Lopez-Rodriguez *et al.* found a highly significant relationship between personality disorder and epileptic aura. No patient who did not experience an aura had a personality disorder. There were no associations with type of epilepsy or laterality, and no relationship with age at onset, duration of epilepsy or seizure frequency. These authors discuss possible explanations for the excess of dependent/avoidant personality disorders. Their findings may reflect an understandable reaction by patients to the psychosocial consequences of their illness, including the perceived stigma, and the loss of a sense of self-control that might be a consequence of unpredictable and disabling seizures. They also suggest biological mechanisms, citing evidence from animal studies linking meso-limbic lesions with social cohesiveness, fearfulness and avoidance. The association between personality disorder and epileptic aura is an intriguing one and mirrors earlier reports of an association between aura and both depression and psychosis. Again, the link could have a psychological basis. Avoidant or dependent traits might develop as a reaction to frightening and unwanted experiences. Or there may be some (unknown) difference in the biological substrate of seizures with and without aura that influences behaviour and personality. Such studies, using established diagnostic criteria and validated diagnostic interviews, offer a promising way forward in our attempt to understand the relationship between epilepsy, behaviour and personality.

Epilepsy and sexual dysfunction

Reduced libido and disorders of sexual function are over-represented in people with epilepsy (Lambert 2001). Men with epilepsy report less sexual interest than healthy controls and a history of erectile dysfunction is found in up to 57% (Toone *et al.* 1989; Montouris & Morris 2005). In women, hyposexuality has been a less consistent finding, but abnormalities of arousal and orgasmic dysfunction are relatively common (Harden 2005). In both men and women, psychosocial factors are undoubtedly important causes in many cases. Thus, sexual difficulties may be one consequence of the more general impact intractable epilepsy may have on confidence, self-esteem, social activity and interpersonal relationships. Occasionally, sexual difficulties may relate specifically to a fear of having a seizure during sex. However, some sexual problems in epilepsy undoubtedly have an organic basis. In particular, abnormalities of sex hormone metabolism, secondary to antiepileptic drug treatment, are an important and potentially reversible cause. Direct physiological links with TLE have also been suggested.

Antiepileptic drugs that induce hepatic enzymes (most notably phenobarbital, phenytoin and carbamazepine) increase circulating sex hormone-binding globulin. Consequently, the level of physiologically active (unbound and loosely bound) testosterone is reduced. Several studies have demonstrated that sexual dysfunction in men with epilepsy is associated with reduced levels of biologically active testosterone (Toone *et al.* 1983; Macphee *et al.* 1988; Isojarvi *et al.* 1995). In a more recent study of men with localisation-related epilepsy, those taking lamotrigine (which has little effect on hepatic enzymes) were found to have similar sexual functioning to normal controls and had significantly higher levels of free testosterone compared with men taking either carbamazepine or phenytoin who in turn had higher rates of sexual dysfunction (Herzog *et al.* 2005). A similar association between low free testosterone levels and sexual dysfunction has recently been reported in women with epilepsy (Herzog *et al.* 2003).

Higher rates of sexual disorder have been reported in patients with localisation-related epilepsy compared with generalised epilepsy (Gastaut & Collomb, 1954; Shukla *et al.* 1979; Toone *et al.* 1989). A specific association with right-sided temporal lobe foci has also been reported (Herzog *et al.* 1990; Daniele *et al.* 1997). Physiological disturbance of limbic brain regions implicated in sexual function, such as the amygdala and cingulate cortex, is a plausible mechanism for these findings but other differences between epilepsy syndromes, including the likelihood of remission and the type of drugs prescribed, may also be important.

Crime and epilepsy

Early writers such as Lombroso (1911) came to the unfortunate view that epilepsy and criminality were intimately related. Most criminals were even thought to have an 'epileptoid' constitution: 'If fully developed epileptic fits are often lacking in the born criminal, this is because they remain latent, and only show themselves later under the influence of the causes assigned (anger, alcoholism), which bring them to the surface.' Violent crimes were believed to be particularly characteristic. Maudsley (1873, 1906) thought that epilepsy should always be considered in aggressive crimes, and felt that crimes committed suddenly and in a 'blind fury' were often due to some form of epileptic process.

These views were decisively altered when careful surveys were carried out. Alstrom (1950) found no excess of criminal records compared with the population generally in 897 patients with epilepsy attending a Swedish clinic, provided they were not mentally affected. Those with psychiatric complications did show a significant excess, though the figure was not strikingly high (12% vs 5%). Major aggression was not observed in the sample, and the acts of violence that had occurred were usually trivial and closely connected with abuse of alcohol. Juul-Jensen's (1964) large Danish survey of 1020 adults with epilepsy substantially confirmed these findings. Both surveys, however, were largely confined to patients attending hospitals and clinics. Gudmundsson's (1966) attempt to survey all people with epilepsy resident in Iceland (987 individuals) produced rather different results: the men with epilepsy had been convicted three times as often as the male population generally.

Gunn approached the problem by an extensive survey of the prevalence of epilepsy among the prison and borstal populations of England and Wales (Gunn 1969; Gunn & Fenton 1971). At a conservative estimate, seven to eight prisoners per 1000 were found to be suffering from epilepsy, which is considerably higher than the prevalence of epilepsy in the general population. Young prisoners in particular were more likely to be suffering from epilepsy than persons of a similar age in the community. It seems therefore that people with epilepsy do have a higher probability of being committed to prison than other members of the population.

A representative sample of prisoners with epilepsy was then examined to see whether the types of crime committed differed from those of matched controls (Gunn & Bonn 1971). The great majority had been convicted for non-violent larceny, as with prisoners generally. There was no suggestion that epilepsy was associated with any particular form of offence, and no support for the view that crimes of violence were over-represented. Whitman *et al.* (1984) confirmed these findings in a survey of men entering the Illinois prison system; the prevalence of epilepsy was again raised, but there was no excess of more serious or violent crimes.

Nevertheless, the question arises whether violence may occur as a direct consequence of seizures or postictal automatisms. Most now agree that although this may happen it is very rare indeed. For example, Gunn and Fenton (1971), in a survey of 158 prisoners with epilepsy, found five who had seizures just after committing a crime, four who had seizures just before committing a crime, and four others in whom a possible association with automatism could be considered. In only one case was there evidence that murder had been committed during the course of an epileptic seizure or its immediate sequelae (Gunn 1978). Moreover, among 32 patients with epilepsy committed to Broadmoor Special Hospital, Gunn and Fenton (1971) found only two who had probably committed their crimes during a postictal state. Treiman (1986) reviewed 75 legal cases from the USA in which epilepsy had been used as a defence against charges of violent crime. The defence was accepted by the courts in only one case, a man who it was subsequently concluded had almost certainly never had epilepsy.

However, aggressive behaviour during ictal automatisms is occasionally reported. The patient may continue with an act in progress at the time and do harm by virtue of a confused state of mind. A patient mentioned by MacDonald (1969) was filling a kettle with a view to placing it on the fire when her seizure commenced, and she placed her baby on the fire instead. Such situations are, however, exceedingly rare, and acts of violence have emerged as distinctly unusual in reviews of patients subject to automatisms (Knox 1968; Treiman 1986). Most ictal or postictal aggressive behaviour is reactive or 'resistive', arising in the context of agitation and delirium as a response to confinement, restraint or some other interference by bystanders. Delgado-Escueta *et al.* (1981) reviewed video recordings of 33 seizures in 19 patients, selected from over 5000 as showing possible aggressive behaviour. Only seven were rated as showing substantial aggression, usually in the form of struggling when restrained or kicking out in fear, but three showed elements of physical attack with spitting, shouting or scratching and three attempted to destroy property. Gerard *et al.* (1998) have described six cases of postictal aggression. Postictal psychosis clearly accounted for aggression in two patients. In three cases, a period of recovery from postictal delirium lasting several hours preceded prolonged episodes of aggressive behaviour lasting up to 3 days. Athough psychotic symptoms were not documented in these cases, the occurrence of a lucid interval (see Postictal disorders) suggests some overlap with postictal psychosis. In the final case, however, aggressive behaviour arose after a brief period of postictal sleep. In this patient aggression had some resistive qualities but was also directed, relatively stereotyped, recurred frequently and was prolonged.

A 32-year-old man developed complex partial seizures aged 8. Seizures were initially well controlled with phenobarbital. In his teenage years he began using marijuana and cocaine. At this time his family noticed a change in his postictal behaviour. Following a seizure, complex partial with or without secondary generalisation, he would routinely sleep for 10–15 minutes. He would then awaken and often wander around aimlessly. If approached, even if only verbally, he would direct obscenities towards the person, and would often use physical force to push the person away. If the patient's mother was in the vicinity, he would actively seek her out, and display physical and verbal aggressive behaviour towards her alone. On one such occasion he held a knife to her throat. This aggressive behaviour typically lasted from 20 minutes to 1 hour, with gradual resolution to his baseline mild-mannered temperament. Interictally, he had no recollection of these events and showed considerable remorse afterwards. His postictal disturbance continued for 6 years despite not using alcohol or illicit substances. Anterior left temporal lobectomy was performed. Pathology showed mesial temporal sclerosis. Two seizures in the first 6 months following lobectomy were also accompanied by postictal aggression towards his mother.

Violence arising as a direct consequence of seizures is thus very rare. It usually represents a confused defensive reaction to attempts by others to restrain or assist the patient, actions that the patient appears to misconstrue as threatening. Such behaviour is brief, lasting only for the duration of postictal delirium. More prolonged aggressive episodes appearing after a period of recovery from seizures are sometimes associated with postictal psychosis. As detailed above, careful studies of people with epilepsy who have committed crimes have identified very few cases in which criminal acts have occurred during a seizure. The majority of criminal behaviour in people with epilepsy is therefore interictal and has little to do with the occurrence of seizures *per se* (Marsh & Krauss 2000). Furthermore, such criminal behaviour is no more likely to be violent than crime committed by people without epilepsy. Many factors that coexist with epilepsy are likely to underlie the association. Sociodemographic factors associated with offending behaviour in the general population, including various indices of social deprivation, are over-represented in people with epilepsy and undoubtedly underlie much of the association between epilepsy and criminal behaviour (Treiman 1986). Among medical variables, by far the most important factors are the presence of underlying brain damage and cognitive impairment (Stevens & Hermann 1981). Interictal psychopathology, particularly psychosis, may also be significant (Mendez *et al.* 1993b).

It can be important in medicolegal work to have guidelines for assessing the probability that a crime may have been committed during an episode of ictal or postictal confusion. In legal terms, an automatism occurs if an act is committed but was neither intended nor the result of recklessness (i.e. there is *actus rea* but no *mens rea*). In the UK legal automatisms are categorised as 'sane' if they arise from extrinsic causes (e.g. an acute head injury) or 'insane' if they arise through intrinsic causes (e.g. epilepsy). Prior to the 1991 Criminal Procedure Act, the defence of insane automatism attracted mandatory detention under Sections 37 and 41 of the Mental

Health Act, a situation that was obviously inappropriate for criminal acts committed in the context of epileptic or sleep automatisms. The Act gave the courts freedom to choose from a range of outcomes, including hospital treatment, guardianship, supervision and treatment, or absolute discharge (Brown & Bird 2001). A number of authorities have discussed criteria that may be applied in mounting a defence of automatism (Walker 1961; Knox 1968; Fenton 1972; Treiman 1999).

First of all, the patient should have a past history of unequivocal epileptic seizures. There need not necessarily be a previous history of aggression during automatism as such, though clearly when this is elicited it will strengthen the confidence with which the present example is so diagnosed. The diagnosis must always be made on clinical grounds, for epilepsy can occur in the presence of a normal EEG and, conversely, abnormal records may be obtained in patients who have never had a clinical attack. Nevertheless, an EEG compatible with the type of clinical disorder presumed to be present will constitute important additional evidence. Clearly video-EEG documentation of automatisms and associated aggressive behaviour will greatly strengthen the case.

With regard to the circumstances of the crime itself, this will always have been sudden, obvious motives will be lacking and there should be no evidence of planning or premeditation. The crime will appear to be senseless, there will typically have been little or no attempt at concealment and often no attempt at escape. The abnormal behaviour will usually have been of short duration, lasting minutes rather than hours, and will never have been entirely appropriate to the circumstances. Witnesses may have noted evidence of impairment of awareness, for example inappropriate actions or gestures, stereotyped movements, unresponsiveness or irrelevant replies to questions, aimless wandering around, or a dazed and vacant expression. However, these features may not be readily apparent to the untrained eye. Amnesia for the crime is the rule, but there should be no continuing anterograde amnesia for events following the resumption of conscious awareness. The more that these criteria are not fulfilled, the more will an epileptic basis for the act be regarded with suspicion.

Cognitive function in epilepsy

Although most people with epilepsy function within the normal range of cognitive ability, comparisons with appropriate control groups consistently demonstrate deficits (Motamedi & Meador 2003; Elger *et al.* 2004). There is now good evidence that such cognitive deficits are present at the time epilepsy is first diagnosed and may even precede the onset of seizures. This is hardly surprising when seizures are symptomatic of gross underlying brain disease. However, evidence of early cognitive deficits has also emerged from studies of patients with idiopathic and cryptogenic epilepsy. For example, Hermann *et al.* (2006) compared 53 children with epilepsy with 50 healthy controls (age- and gender-matched first cousins of the patients). Patients were included only if neurological examination and clinical MRI were normal and the patient group included almost equal numbers of subjects with generalised and localisation-related epilepsy. Neuropsychological testing, conducted on average 10 months after the onset of seizures, demonstrated a broad range of mild cognitive impairments that were present in both epilepsy syndromes. Of the children with epilepsy, 26% had a history of academic problems (compared with 4% of controls) and in the majority of cases these were identified by educational services before the first recognised seizure. Strong correlations between neuropsychological performance and morphometric brain measurements (white-matter volumes measured with MRI) were seen in the healthy controls but not in the patients in this study. This loss of normal structure–function relationships might have a number of explanations, including pathological disturbance of white matter connections or an overriding influence of other epilepsy-related variables on cognition.

Cognitive profiles and epilepsy syndrome

The pattern of cognitive impairment in chronic epilepsy varies according to the underlying epilepsy syndrome. TLE is the most common localisation-related syndrome and also the most common type of epilepsy treated surgically. The neuropsychological profile of TLE is therefore well characterised. While patients with TLE may show significant impairments across all cognitive domains, selective deficits in episodic memory are characteristic (Hermann *et al.* 1997). Left-sided TLE is associated with deficits in verbal episodic memory. Non-verbal memory deficits are associated with right-sided TLE, although findings are less consistent (Gleissner *et al.* 1998). The lateralisation of language dominance has a strong influence on these material-specific memory deficits. Thus, Kim *et al.* (2003) found clear evidence of the expected pattern of lateralised deficits in patients with left hemisphere language dominance. However, in patients with right or mixed hemisphere language dominance these associations were not seen. Hemispheric language dominance was determined by testing after intracarotid amobarbital in this study. The authors comment that failure to specify hemispheric language dominance, or using less stringent definitions of language dominance, might account for some of the many inconsistent findings in the literature. Memory deficits in TLE are most conspicuous in patients with evidence of hippocampal atrophy on MRI (Alessio *et al.* 2004). More generalised cognitive deficits in TLE have recently been correlated with measures of extratemporal anatomical abnormalities (Hermann *et al.* 2003).

There have been fewer investigations of cognitive function in FLE and most studies have included a large proportion of patients with acquired frontal lobe lesions. Whether frontal lobe seizures have a specific effect on cognition, independent of underlying pathology, has therefore not been established. Overall, there is an impression that FLE may be associated with relatively little in the way of cognitive deficits, especially when there is no demonstrable lesion. Where deficits are found, the profile is what might be expected in association with frontal lobe damage, with impairments in psychomotor speed, attention, working memory, response-inhibition and planning, set against a background of variable general impairment (Helmstaedter *et al.* 1996; Upton & Thompson 1996; Exner *et al.* 2002).

The conventional view that the idiopathic epilepsy syndromes are benign in terms of cognitive outcome has recently been challenged (Wirrell *et al.* 1997; Hommet *et al.* 2006). Studies of children and adults with idiopathic generalised epilepsy have demonstrated mild cognitive deficits that are present early in the natural history of the disorder (Pulliainen *et al.* 2000; Hermann *et al.* 2006). Whether abnormalities persist after seizures have resolved in the benign idiopathic syndromes has not been established. Overall, subtle general deficits have been described, but selective dysexecutive problems in areas such as concept formation, reasoning, planning, mental flexibility and working memory implicating frontal lobe abnormality have been demonstrated in patients with JME (Swartz *et al.* 1996; Devinsky *et al.* 1997). In view of the overlap between idiopathic generalised epilepsy syndromes it seems possible that similar deficits occur in other syndromes but this has not been systematically explored. Among idiopathic localisation-related syndromes, cognitive deficits have been demonstrated in benign childhood epilepsy with centrotemporal spikes (Weglage *et al.* 1997; Metz-Lutz *et al.* 1999; Northcott *et al.* 2006) and in idiopathic occipital lobe epilepsy (Gulgonen *et al.* 2000). The deficits in childhood epilepsy with centrotemporal spikes may correlate with the frequency of interictal EEG abnormalities. These disorders have an excellent outcome in terms of seizure resolution but there is some preliminary evidence that subtle cognitive problems may persist (Northcott *et al.* 2006).

Progressive cognitive impairment

An important question is whether epilepsy may cause progressive cognitive impairment. Just over a century ago, Berkley (1901) wrote

> The most numerous class of epileptics show, after the lapse of years, a slowly progressive dimming of the active perceptions of the mind, a loss of memory, a blunting of the affections, a permanent mental obtuseness which increases and grows, until, if the patient lives long enough, there is a more or less absolute annihilation of all the faculties.

This statement, which today seems so wide of the truth, perhaps serves as a reminder of just how profound the impact of modern epilepsy treatment has been. Yet a small proportion of people with epilepsy do appear to suffer some progressive cognitive impairment and many studies have attempted to define the extent of this. Cross-sectional studies are unable to distinguish clearly between the static effects of underlying brain abnormality and deficits acquired over time. Longitudinal studies are required to properly investigate whether intellectual impairments are progressive and to elucidate their causes. Over 20 such studies have now been published (reviewed by Dodrill 2004; Vingerhoets 2006). Early studies are difficult to interpret because epilepsy syndromes were not well defined and seizure frequency was often poorly documented. Among more recent investigations, surprisingly few have used appropriate comparison groups to control for test–retest effects on neuropsychological assessments. In reviewing the evidence, it is logical to consider studies of children and adults separately. The former seek to investigate the impact of epilepsy on intellectual development while studies of adults are concerned with the question of intellectual deterioration.

In a study of 83 preschool children with relatively infrequent seizures, Ellenberg *et al.* (1986) found no decline in IQ measures over a 3-year period. However, two studies (Bourgeois *et al.* 1983; Aldenkamp *et al.* 1990) of slightly older children (of primary school age) with more active epilepsy found that 11 and 24% respectively showed a decline in IQ measures of 9 points or more over an interval of approximately 4 years. Bourgeois and colleagues found the impaired group was characterised by more frequent seizures, toxic drug levels and younger age at onset of epilepsy. In a small controlled study, Neyens *et al.* (1999) investigated 11 children with epilepsy aged 7–15 years and 39 controls on three occasions over 18 months. The patient group showed lower IQ levels at baseline and less improvement in test performance over time. Most recently, Oostrom *et al.* (2005) compared 42 children with newly diagnosed idiopathic or cryptogenic epilepsy and 30 healthy gender-matched classmates over a 3.5-year interval on a comprehensive neuropsychological battery and behavioural checklist. Most of the children became seizure-free within the first 2 years of the study. A minority of the patient group (19%) had persistent cognitive difficulties. This group was no different in terms of epilepsy variables, including whether they became seizure-free, from those with better cognitive functioning, but psychosocial measures, such as poor parental adjustment to their child's diagnosis, adverse family situations and the prior existence of behavioural problems, were over-represented.

In adults, longitudinal studies have involved patients with localisation-related epilepsy, mainly TLE. A consistent finding has been that measures of global IQ remain relatively stable. However, there is growing evidence of progressive memory impairment. Helmstaedter *et al.* (2003) found a significant deterioration in tests of verbal and visual memory in 50% of 102 patients with intractable TLE over an average time interval just short of 5 years. Andersson-Rosswall *et al.* (2004) compared IQ and memory tests in 36 patients with partial seizures and 36 controls over 3–4 years. IQ and memory function were lower in the patients at baseline. IQ scores did not deteriorate, although they failed to show the improvement (presumably due to practice effects) seen in controls. However, 25% of patients demonstrated a deterio-

ration in verbal memory that was not seen in the controls. In another controlled study, Dodrill (2002) was unable to demonstrate a deterioration in the epilepsy group but did show less improvement in scores in patients compared with controls over an interval of 10 years. The pathological substrate for these memory deficits may be progressive medial temporal lobe damage secondary to ongoing seizure activity. Progressive hippocampal atrophy has been reported by some recent longitudinal MRI studies of TLE (Briellmann *et al.* 2005), although there have also been negative findings (Holtkamp *et al.* 2004).

In summary, longitudinal studies suggest that a minority of children with epilepsy, perhaps 10–20%, will suffer impaired intellectual development manifest as persistent or progressive cognitive deficit. Those with poorly controlled epilepsy appear most at risk but psychosocial variables may be equally important predictors of cognitive outcome. In adults, progressive decline in memory has been described in up to 50% of patients with poorly controlled TLE and this may be related to progressive hippocampal atrophy secondary to intractable seizures.

Causes of intellectual deterioration in poorly controlled epilepsy

Cognitive deficits in epilepsy, whether static or progressive, may have a number of causes. They may reflect the underlying cerebral disorder of which epilepsy is also a symptom. Alternatively, cognitive decline may be due to a number of factors directly related to epilepsy. Potential causes in this category include possible cumulative effects of neuronal damage incurred through repeated seizures, brain injury secondary to trauma or status epilepticus, the effects of drug treatment and, finally, the psychosocial impact of the disorder.

The majority of studies have found a relationship between cognitive impairment and measures of seizure frequency. However, there have been many negative findings, leading Dodrill (2004) to conclude that overall the evidence favours a relatively weak relationship between seizures and cognitive decline. Secondary generalised tonic–clonic seizures may be a more important factor than the frequency of partial seizures. Evidence for an association between duration of epilepsy and cognitive deterioration is similarly inconsistent and may only be demonstrable after a relatively long history (over 30 years) of intractable seizures (Jokeit & Ebner 1999). Prolonged or recurrent status epilepticus may result in permanent brain injury but there is little evidence concerning the impact of a history of status, or of seizure-related head injury, on cognitive outcome in epilepsy (Dodrill 2002).

Related to the issue of an association between seizures and cognitive decline is the observation that subclinical epileptiform discharges (demonstrated on EEG but not associated with overt clinical seizures) may be accompanied by transitory cognitive impairment (TCI) (Binnie 2003; Aldenkamp &

Arends 2004). The paradox of defining this condition by demonstrating a clinical effect (cognitive dysfunction) during an event which is designated subclinical has led to some debate about semantics, and clearly TCI could be regarded as a form of simple partial seizure whose sole manifestation is cognitive. The cognitive impairments are best demonstrated with tasks that involve high information-processing demands. The epileptiform discharges in question are typically around 3 seconds in duration, longer discharges being more likely to be accompanied by an overt clinical seizure. TCI is a relatively rare phenomenon and is demonstrable in less than 2% of patients with epilepsy. Cases in which TCI is a primary cause of ongoing cognitive or functional disability are likely to be much rarer still. A few case reports suggest that treatment aimed at reducing subclinical discharges may improve function in patients with carefully documented TCI. However, further research is required to assess the functional impact of TCI, including whether there are cumulative effects on cognitive function, and to establish management guidelines.

Antiepileptic drugs are an important cause of cognitive problems in people with epilepsy (see reviews by Vermeulen & Aldenkamp 1995; Kwan & Brodie 2001; Meador 2002). Deficits in psychomotor speed and attention are characteristic, with secondary effects on other cognitive domains. Adverse cognitive effects are especially likely in patients taking two or more antiepileptic drugs. This may be due to pharmacokinetic interactions, or to additive pharmacodynamic effects. The cognitive effects of antiepileptic drugs are typically dose related and may appear in association with other symptoms of neurotoxicity. However, idiosyncratic responses are sometimes encountered in which individual patients are intolerant of even low doses of specific drugs. Cognitive side effects are especially likely in patients with learning disability and in the elderly. Patients commonly develop tolerance to the adverse cognitive effects of antiepileptic drugs and an important strategy in clinical practice is to slow the rate at which drug dosage is increased. This is especially important when prescribing an antiepileptic drug as add-on treatment. Many studies have attempted to compare the cognitive profiles of different antiepileptic drugs. The field is beset with methodological difficulties but some conclusions have emerged. Phenobarbital is generally agreed to be associated with the worst cognitive effects. Phenytoin, carbamazepine, valproate and clonazepam probably have similar profiles. Among benzodiazepines, clobazam may be preferable to clozepam. Of the newer antiepileptic drugs, lamotrigine and gabapentin have a favourable cognitive profile compared with older drugs. Topiramate may cause severe cognitive effects and has been associated with specific deficits in word-finding and verbal fluency. However, cognitive problems with topiramate are less likely, and may even be avoided, when the dose is titrated slowly. There are insufficient data on other more recently introduced antiepileptic drugs, although there is a general impression that they have a relatively favourable cognitive profile compared with older drugs.

Finally, psychosocial factors have an important moderating influence on the relationship between cognitive ability in children with epilepsy and educational achievement. Persistent cognitive difficulties in children with epilepsy are associated with measures of poor parental adjustment and adverse family circumstances (Fastenau et al. 2004; Oostrom et al. 2005). The relationship between these factors is undoubtedly complex; cause and effect are difficult to determine. However, there is some evidence that emotionally supportive and well-organised families may ameliorate the negative impact of neuropsychological impairment on educational achievement (Fastenau et al. 2004). Psychosocial interventions for families struggling to cope with their child's epilepsy may prove to be important in determining long-term outcome.

Dissociative seizures

In ICD-10, the term 'dissociative convulsions' is used to refer to paroxysmal episodes of behaviour that resemble epileptic seizures and which are believed to be due to unconscious psychological processes. These episodes may imitate any form of epilepsy and the term *dissociative seizures* is probably more accurate because convulsions are often not present. Dissociative seizures are distinguished from factitious disorder on the grounds that the latter represents a wilful, conscious attempt to simulate illness for reasons that are understandable in terms of the individual's psychological state. Factitious disorder is in turn differentiated from malingering (not actually a medical diagnosis), in which illness is simulated to achieve some practical gain (e.g. financial compensation, avoidance of criminal responsibility or military service). In practice, the distinction between these three entities can be very difficult. Conscious fabrication may sometimes be suspected but a diagnosis cannot be made confidently unless the patient admits deliberately enacting the symptoms, or is 'caught out' by some form of covert surveillance (not, however, recommended). Even then, there is potential overlap: what begins as unconscious may become deliberate over time, and vice versa. Another difficult area concerns the boundaries of malingering: in many countries there is considerable financial reward (in the form of social security benefits) attached to the sick role, and this obviously represents a significant practical gain. Judging motivation is every bit as subjective, and difficult, as assessing the extent to which symptoms are under voluntary control.

By consensus most episodes are regarded as unconsciously motivated and therefore dissociative. However, some clinicians are not persuaded (Slavney 1994). The distinction between dissociative and factitious disorder implies a dichotomy that is undoubtedly an oversimplification. The two are better thought of as opposite ends of a spectrum of conscious awareness, with 'self-deception' occupying the middle ground. The concept of self-deception, which at a trivial level most people can relate to (e.g. how young/slim we look, procrastinating about a work deadline), provides a useful paradigm for understanding unconscious mechanisms and how subjective experience, and even quite complex behaviour, are prone to influences that are not always fully conscious, even in healthy individuals. Three observations provide some objective evidence that dissociative seizures are, at some level, unconscious: (i) most patients are compliant with antiepileptic drugs before the correct diagnosis is made; (ii) when patients are admitted for telemetry, the majority have a seizure in a setting which they must surely recognise involves sophisticated monitoring; and (iii) the seizures are usually a poor imitation of epilepsy. None of these points is by any means conclusive, but if deception is involved it is of a kind that eludes simple understanding.

Before leaving the subject of definition and nosology, it must be acknowledged that there is no consensus about what these episodes should be called. Terms such as 'pseudoseizures' and 'hysterical seizures' are seen as pejorative and have largely been abandoned. Others like 'non-epileptic seizures/events', 'non-epileptic attack disorder' and 'psychogenic non-epileptic seizures' are widely used but appear to define the condition by what it is not, and may therefore be interpreted by patients as suggesting that 'the doctors think I don't have epilepsy but they don't know what I've got'. Some of these terms are also used ambiguously. For example, 'psychogenic non-epileptic seizures' may be used to refer to dissociative seizures alone or to the group of psychiatric disorders (including panic attacks, psychosis, temper tantrums) that can be mistaken for epilepsy. Likewise, 'non-epileptic seizures' is often used to refer to the range of conditions, organic and otherwise, that may be mistaken for epilepsy, but on other occasions may be used as a form of shorthand to denote dissociative seizures. The term *functional seizures* overcomes many of these objections, is acceptable to patients (Stone *et al.* 2003) and also has the advantage of remaining neutral with respect to any assumptions about conscious or unconscious processes. However, it has not found widespread acceptance so far.

Demographic features

The clinical problem of dissociative seizures has generated a substantial literature and there have been a number of reviews (Krumholz 1999; Gates 2002; Reuber & Elger 2003; Mellers 2005). Approximately one in five patients referred to specialist centres for evaluation of apparently intractable epilepsy are found to have dissociative seizures. A similar proportion has also been reported in a community-based survey of new-onset seizure disorders (Kotsopoulos *et al.* 2003). Over two-thirds of patients are female. Seizures typically begin in the late teens or early twenties, but there is a wide range. In a minority (less than 20%) a history of epilepsy precedes the onset of dissociative seizures.

Unfortunately, there is often considerable delay in recognising the disorder and it is common for seizures to have been present, and treated as epileptic, for over 3 years before diagnosis. This of course represents a missed opportunity for appropriate treatment. In addition, patients are exposed to significant iatrogenic risks including antiepileptic drug toxicity, teratogenic risk and the risk, in up to 10%, of receiving emergency treatment for supposed 'status'. Unfortunately, the longer the patient and family live with an incorrect diagnosis of epilepsy, the more entrenched their adaption to a life of disability and the less likely that treatment will be effective.

Dissociative seizures must be distinguished from epilepsy and other paroxysmal disorders of consciousness and neurological function. The clinical features of dissociative seizures, and the role of special investigations are therefore detailed in the following sections on assessment and differential diagnosis.

Psychiatric assessment: aetiological formulation

Psychiatric assessment aims to detect any comorbid psychiatric disorder and to determine likely aetiological factors. Table 6.11 lists predisposing, precipitating and maintaining factors that may be relevant. Many of the factors are common to other somatoform disorders and indeed up to 80% of patients with dissociative seizures have a history of previous unexplained medical presentations (Bowman & Markand 1996). Variable rates of psychiatric comorbidity, including personality disturbance, depression and anxiety, have been reported. Adverse or traumatic experiences, particularly in childhood, are a common underlying theme. An association with sexual, physical and emotional abuse has been highlighted but other traumatic experiences or situations that foster enduring low self-esteem, for example being bullied at school or unrecognised learning difficulties, or a more general association with poor family functioning, may be equally important. Abnormal personality traits, dysfunctional coping styles and putative somatising or dissociative traits may be a consequence of adverse experiences at a stage of development when personality attributes are formed. Biological factors, including genetic influences on personality, are plausible but as yet hypothetical. None of these features, however, is unique to patients with dissociative seizures; they are seen in patients with other psychiatric disorders and other somatoform presentations. Why some individuals exposed to grossly abnormal experiences develop psychiatric disorder but not others, and what determines the form the illness takes, is not understood.

Triggers for the onset of the disorder are often not apparent, but an increased incidence of adverse life events in the year prior to onset has been reported. Sometimes the clinical history strongly suggests that the initial event may have been

Table 6.11 Predisposing, precipitating and maintaining factors in dissociative seizures. (Modified from Binzer *et al.* 2004 with permission.)

	Biological	Psychological	Social

Predisposing	Learning difficulties
	?Genetic influence on personality
	?Biological effect of early
	    adversity on CNS
	    development
		Perception of childhood experience as adverse
		Somatising trait
		Dissociative trait
		Avoidant coping style
		Personality disorder
		Mood disorder
			Adverse (abusive) experiences in childhood
			Poor family functioning
			Traumatic experiences in adulthood
			Modelling of attacks on others with epilepsy

Precipitating		Perception of life events as negative/ unexpected Acute panic attack/syncope	Adverse life events

Maintaining		Perception of symptoms as being beyond
		    personal control/due to disease
		Agoraphobia: avoidant and safety behaviour
		Angry/confused/anxious reaction to diagnosis
			Angry/confused/anxious reaction of carers
			    to the illness and to medical encounters
			Fear of responsibilities of being well/
			    benefits of being ill

a panic attack or an episode of vasovagal syncope. Once the disorder is established a number of maintaining factors become important. An agoraphobic pattern of avoidant and safety behaviour may serve to perpetuate anxiety about seizures, which in turn makes them more likely. Patients typically receive conflicting advice from many doctors and may encounter unsympathetic reactions in a variety of medical settings, all of which contribute to their anxiety, confusion and anger. Finally, for some individuals at least, the benefits of the sick role may provide an acceptable alternative to the responsibilities of healthy life, and carers, unwittingly or otherwise, may play an important role in perpetuating disability. The stigma attached to mental illness undoubtedly has an important role in shaping the medical presentation of somatoform disorders and contributes to the reluctance some patients have in accepting psychiatric treatment.

There is no widely agreed model for dissociative seizures. As already mentioned, studies of underlying aetiological factors reveal much that is common to other somatoform disorders. Dissociation can be thought of as a psychologically mediated, altered state of awareness or control over neurological function. It encompasses a range of mental processes including normal phenomena, such as focused and divided attention, as well as pathological states involving perceptual, cognitive and motor function (see Holmes *et al.* 2005). Dissociation may be encountered as an acute response to trauma, as chronic persistent symptoms (e.g. amnesia or paresis) or as recurrent paroxysmal events in dissociative seizures. Some two-thirds of patients with dissociative seizures report symptoms of autonomic arousal preceding their seizures (Goldstein & Mellers 2006). A dissociative response to arousal triggered by perceptual or cognitive cues, perhaps related to previous traumatic experiences in a manner akin to post-traumatic stress disorder (Ehlers & Clark 2000), is thus one possible mechanism. The pathophysiological basis of disso-

ciation is unknown. While it cannot be assumed that the processes underlying normal dissociative phenomena are active in pathological states, as a hypothesis this provides a useful starting point for further investigation. The concept of dissociation, and in particular the assumption of some continuity between normal and abnormal dissociative states, also provides a very useful model for discussing dissociative seizures with patients and carers.

The treatment of dissociative seizures is discussed under Treatment of psychosis, later in chapter. Reuber and Elger (2003) have reviewed naturalistic outcome studies. Overall, seizures persist for over 3 years in approximately two-thirds of patients. Even if seizures remit, patients tend to remain unemployed and dependent on social security. By far the most important predictor of outcome, as in other somatoform disorders (Couprie *et al.* 1995), is a short duration of illness at the time of diagnosis.

Assessment and investigation

It has often been said that epilepsy is a clinical diagnosis. A carefully elicited history and particularly an eyewitness description are the cornerstones of assessment, and diagnosis is said to be straightforward in expert hands (Chadwick & Smith 2002). Yet outside specialist settings, and perhaps even within them, diagnostic errors are frequent. In one study of patients referred to an epilepsy specialist, 26% of those already taking antiepileptic treatment had been misdiagnosed (Smith *et al.* 1999). Such mistakes have serious consequences. Firstly, they represent a missed opportunity for appropriate treatment. The two most common differential diagnoses, syncope and psychogenic attacks, account for the overwhelming majority of diagnostic errors. While most cases of syncope are vasovagal and have a relatively benign course, failure to recognise syncope due to cardiac arrhythmia has potentially fatal consequences. In the case of dissociative seizures, a missed diagnosis represents a lost opportunity for intervention early in the course of the disorder, when it is most effective. Secondly, misdiagnosis incurs the risks of inappropriate treatment, including drug toxicity and the hazards of emergency interventions for supposed status epilepticus. Patients misdiagnosed with epilepsy will also needlessly suffer driving and occupational restrictions. Finally, there are implications for health-care resources. Smith *et al.* (1999) estimated the cost of misdiagnosed epilepsy to the National Health Service to be around £125 million pounds annually. Overall, the consequences of a mistaken diagnosis probably outweigh the small risk of delaying treatment in epilepsy (Chadwick 1994; Manford 2001). A trial of treatment is seldom justified (see also discussion of injury and sudden death in epilepsy in Treatment, later in chapter).

The first task of assessment is to distinguish between epilepsy and other causes of transient loss of consciousness or paroxysmal neurological disturbance. Epileptic seizures are brief stereotyped disturbances of neurological function that may involve mental, autonomic, sensory and motor features. While the clinical manifestations of epileptic seizures are protean, the *sequence* of events will be similar from one episode to the next and will conform to a relatively small number of well-established patterns. These patterns, set out in the ILAE classification of seizures, provide the key to recognising an event as epileptic. If attacks are judged to be epileptic, seizures that have been provoked by some extrinsic factor must be differentiated from those likely to recur. Once the type of seizure has been recognised, clinical features and further investigation will help identify underlying aetiology and the epilepsy syndrome.

Clinical assessment

Are the seizures epileptic?

An eyewitness description should always be sought and will often provide the most important clues to diagnosis. The patient and informant need to be questioned closely about events before, during and after seizures. It is helpful to ask at the outset how many types of attack there are and then to determine the sequence of events for each type. The relationship between different types of seizures must also be established. For each phase of symptoms three questions are important: what happens, how long does it last and is it usually the same? Prodromal symptoms may precede the seizure by hours. The patient should be asked about any 'warning' at the onset of the attack before enquiry is made about specific types of aura. Epileptic aura usually last less than a minute or two. Symptoms preceding syncope may also be brief, but migrainous aura typically evolve more slowly. Does the patient lose awareness and at what point? It is important to obtain an informant history even when patients say they are aware throughout their seizures. Occa-

sionally, it becomes clear that consciousness is impaired only after speaking to an eyewitness. Equally, when patients say they are unaware throughout their seizures, this should be checked with an informant. If someone tries to assist or speaks to the patient in the middle of an attack, what happens? Does the patient respond? Does seizure activity change or stop (suggesting dissociative episodes)? The informant must be asked specifically about the subtle motor features of partial seizures as these may be very helpful diagnostically and are often not reported spontaneously. Examples include oral automatisms, facial twitching, dystonic posturing and the repetitive fumbling hand movements associated with gestural automatisms. Where the history suggests generalised seizures, it is important to check carefully for the presence of aura (which will suggest secondarily generalised seizures) and other generalised seizure types, specifically absences and myoclonic seizures which may otherwise go unreported. Absences may be put down to daydreaming or inattentiveness, and myoclonic jerks dismissed as clumsiness first thing in the morning. If there is a fall, it is important to establish if there is a rigid (tonic) crash to the ground, a sudden loss of tone with collapse and pallor (suggestive of syncope), or a 'swoon' (suggesting psychogenic aetiology). Careful attention needs to be paid to the nature, progression, timing and distribution of any convulsive movements. In a tonic–clonic seizure there will be a tonic phase of general stiffening followed by fine, symmetrical and synchronous clonic movements that increase subtly in amplitude and slow down as the seizure comes to an end. Thrashing, flailing, combative movements are unusual in epilepsy and will strongly suggest dissociative seizures, especially if they last for more than a minute or two. The most important feature of the recovery phase is how quickly normal function is restored. Slow recovery over several minutes with confusion is typical in epilepsy. However, abrupt recovery is seen after absence seizures and in some patients with FLE. Rapid recovery without confusion is characteristic of syncope and is seen in many dissociative seizures. Postictal tiredness, confusion and headache do not help differentiate dissociative and epileptic seizures. A clear description of postictal dysphasia will sometimes help identify partial onset epilepsy. Incontinence and injury are relatively non-specific: they are common in epilepsy but not uncommon in syncope or dissociative seizures. The type of injury may be a more helpful diagnostic clue. Recurrent dislocation of the shoulder (especially posterior dislocation) and vertebral body fractures almost always suggest epilepsy. Tongue-biting in epilepsy usually involves the lateral aspect of the tongue. In dissociative seizures, bites are more commonly to the tip of the tongue, the cheek or the lips, and carpet burns to the face or limbs are also common. It is important to examine the tongue if a history of bite injuries emerges: a severely scarred tongue is seldom seen in non-epileptic presentations. It is also important to ask if attacks occur in sleep and, if so, at what stage of the night and whether such attacks are the same as daytime episodes. Patients with dissociative seizures will report attacks during sleep as often as patients with epilepsy, but ictal EEG recordings will establish that, in dissociative seizures, the patient wakes before seizure onset (Duncan *et al.* 2004). Attacks occurring only at night will raise the possibility of a parasomnia. The timing of attacks and any circumstances that seem to be associated with a greater likelihood of their occurrence should be noted. Seizures occurring first thing in the morning after waking are characteristic of some syndromes of idiopathic generalised epilepsy. Situational triggers are probably more common in syncope and dissociative seizures than in epilepsy.

Differential diagnosis of epilepsy

Syncope

Syncope refers to a transient loss of consciousness caused by a sudden disruption of global cerebral blood flow (Table 6.12) (Mathias *et al.* 2001; Soteriades *et al.* 2002; Fitzpatrick & Cooper 2006). An atonic fall, marked pallor and rapid recovery are the core clinical features. *Vasovagal syncope* is by far the most common form and is experienced at some stage by up to half the population. Recurrent episodes are less common but still account for the majority of syncopal presentations to seizure clinics. Episodes occur when the patient is standing and emotional triggers are usually obvious. Common examples include receiving an injection or having blood taken, witnessing a distressing event or suffering pain or injury. There is often an agoraphobic flavour to the circumstances of the attack, with patients reporting an urgent

Table 6.12 Causes of syncope. (Adapted from Brignole *et al.* 2004 with permission.)

Neurally mediated (reflex)
Vasovagal: fainting following a distressing experience
Situational: micturition, defecation, Valsalva, eating, etc.
Carotid sinus hypersensitivity

Orthostatic
Autonomic dysfunction
   Complex autonomic dysfunction, e.g. multisystem atrophy
   Autonomic neuropathy, e.g. diabetes, amyloid, alcohol related
   Drugs, e.g. antihypertensives, diuretics, alcohol
Volume depletion

Cardiac
Arrythmias
   Tachyarrhythmias, e.g. ventricular tachycardia, supraventricular tachycardia, long QT syndrome
   Bradyarrhythmias, e.g. atrioventricular block, sinus node disease
Structural, e.g. valvular disease, hypertrophic cardiomyopathy, ischaemic left ventricular disease, left atrial myxoma, pulmonary embolism

Other
Vascular steal syndromes, e.g. subclavian steal syndrome

---

need to escape from crowded, enclosed and hot situations. Less commonly, syncope may be triggered by micturition, defecation and activities involving the Valsalva manoeuvre. Vasovagal syncope is usually identified by the combination of an emotional trigger and the characteristic symptoms of *presyncope* (Brignole *et al.* 2004). These include light-headedness, a feeling of detachment, visual blurring, altered hearing with a sense of noises receding and sometimes tinnitus, profuse perspiration (described as a 'cold sweat') and nausea (which may have a rising epigastric quality) (Sheldon *et al.* 2006). To the observer there is conspicuous pallor ('ashen' or 'deathly white') and a flaccid crumple to the ground brought about by a sudden loss of muscle tone. Consciousness is lost for a matter of seconds only and full alertness returns quickly. During the period of unconsciousness, muscle jerking is evident in 90% of cases when episodes are induced experimentally (Lempert *et al.* 1994) and will be reported by some 15% of informants (Sheldon *et al.* 2002). This takes the form of irregular myoclonic movements that are typically multifocal, asynchronous and asymmetrical. Incontinence and injury, including tongue-biting, are less common than in epilepsy but are reported.

Presyncopal symptoms are much less helpful in identifying other forms of syncope. Syncope due to arrhythmias may be preceded by palpitations but in most cases there are no warning symptoms of any kind. A family history of early cardiac death and a personal history of cardiac disease should raise suspicion. Syncope associated with exertion raises the possibility of structural cardiac disease and requires urgent investigation, although most cases will prove to be vasovagal. *Orthostatic syncope* occurs when rising from a recumbent to a standing position and presyncopal symptoms are often absent. Drugs are a common cause, but autonomic failure may be due to neuropathy or degenerative neurological disease. Carotid sinus hypersensitivity, which presents as syncope triggered by neck pressure (head turning, tight collar), is believed to be a common cause of reflex syncope and falls in the elderly (Humm & Mathias 2006; Kerr *et al.* 2006). Syncope precipitated by upper limb exercise will suggest a vascular steal syndrome. Intermittent obstructive hydrocephalus, caused by space-occupying lesions in the third ventricle, may present with headache and episodes of sudden loss of consciousness which are syncopal and secondary to brainstem compression.

The differentiation of epilepsy and syncope is further complicated by the fact that partial epileptic seizures may rarely cause syncope. Sinus tachycardia occurs in at least two-thirds of partial seizures and is probably of no consequence. However, ictal bradycardia is potentially of great importance. It is believed to be rare, occurring in less than 1% of partial seizures (Zijlmans *et al.* 2002) but is probably underrecognised (Tinuper *et al.* 2001). Ictal bradycardia and asystole may lead to syncope during the seizure, which can be mistaken for secondary generalisation (Rossetti *et al.* 2005).

Table 6.13 Comparative semiology of dissociative and epileptic seizures. (Adapted from Mellers 2005 with permission.)

	Dissociative seizures	Epileptic seizures
Helpful features		
Duration over 2 minutes	Common	Rare
Motor features		
Gradual onset	Common	Rare
Fluctuating course	Common	Very rare
Eyes closed	Common	Rare
Thrashing, violent movements	Common	Rare
Side-to-side head movement	Common	Rare
Asynchronous clonic movements	Common	Very rare
Pelvic thrusting	Occasional	Rare
Opisthotonus, *arc de cercle*	Occasional	Very rare
Automatisms	Rare	Common
Weeping	Occasional	Very rare
Recall for period of unresponsiveness	Common	Very rare
Unhelpful features (often misinterpreted as evidence for epilepsy)		
Stereotyped attacks	Common	Common
Incontinence	Occasional	Common
Injury		
Biting inside of mouth	Occasional	Common
Severe tongue-biting	Very rare	Common
Nocturnal occurrence ('in sleep')	Common	Common

Figures for frequency of these features are approximate: common, >30%; occasional, 10–30%; rare, <10%; very rare, <5%.

Dissociative seizures

The distinction between epilepsy and dissociative seizures has received a great deal of attention in the literature (Reuber & Elger 2003; Mellers 2005). Some useful features, and others that are often misinterpreted as suggesting epilepsy, are listed in Table 6.13. No single symptom or sign discriminates dissociative and epileptic seizures with complete certainty. Overall, the clinician must be familiar with the clinical forms epilepsy may take, and it is any variation from these patterns – an atypical sequence of events – that raises the possibility of dissociative seizures (Meierkord *et al.* 1991). The most useful distinguishing characteristics of dissociative seizures are probably long duration, eye closure, fluctuating motor activity, and recall following a period of unresponsiveness, especially if there were associated bilateral convulsive movements. A prolonged period (greater than 5 minutes) of motionless unresponsiveness (from which the patient recovers) almost never has an organic cause. Dissociative seizures are often accompanied by symptoms of arousal, including hyperventilation, peripheral paraesthesiae, dry mouth, palpitations and perspiration (Goldstein & Mellers 2006) and there is therefore some overlap with the symptoms of presyncope. These symptoms may precede the seizure or be noticed only on recovery. Sometimes hyperventilation will only be apparent from an eyewitness description. Patients typically deny emotional symptoms during their attacks, reporting instead symptoms of derealisation, including feeling 'cut-off' and in 'their own world'. Emotional triggers are also usually denied. A relationship with stress may be apparent, at least to eyewitnesses and the clinician if not to patients themselves, but precipitation by stress is also common in epilepsy, syncope and migraine. An agoraphobic pattern of avoidant behaviour is more commonly associated with dissociative seizures than with epilepsy.

Patients with dissociative seizures often have attacks at clinic appointments or in accident and emergency departments, and a carefully conducted examination during a seizure is invaluable. Video recordings of seizures obtained by witnesses (often these days with a mobile phone) may also be extremely helpful. The key points to note on observation are the timing and distribution of any motor activity and whether the eyes are closed. Prolonged violent thrashing movements that fluctuate over the course of the seizure will suggest dissociative disorder. If clonic-like movements are present, careful observation will be required to determine if these are regular and synchronous in each limb (as in epilepsy) or not (suggesting dissociative seizures). On examination, the clinician should establish whether patients are unresponsive by calling out to them. Inflicting painful stimuli is not helpful and ethically questionable. A simple test to establish avoidance of a (mildly) noxious stimulus is to hold the patient's hand over his face and drop it: during a dissociative seizure, on the second occasion this is done, the patient may be seen to control the movement so that the hand falls to one side. If the eyes are shut, an attempt to open the eyelids will usually be met with some resistance in dissociative seizures. If the eyes are open, two additional tests may be helpful. The first involves rolling the patient on to his side. In patients with dissociative seizures the eyes will often be deviated to the ground. If this is the case, the patient should be rolled on to the other side to see if the eyes are still directed towards the ground, the so-called Henry and Woodruff sign (Henry & Woodruff 1978). A second useful test is to hold a small mirror in front of the patient and look for evidence of convergent gaze and fixation on the reflection. This procedure will also often stop the seizure. Following a generalised tonic–clonic seizure the corneal reflex will usually be absent and plantar responses extensor. Pupils will be unresponsive to light in organic states of impaired consciousness.

Paroxysmal neurological disorders

Paroxysmal symptoms occurring as part of other psychiatric disorders may be mistaken for epilepsy. The most common problem concerns panic disorder (see Epileptic aura, earlier in chapter). The brief stereotyped nature of affective and perceptual epileptic aura, together with the presence of impaired consciousness and other epileptiform semiology, mean that distinguishing these ictal presentations from primary psychiatric disorder (panic disorder, psychosis, derealisation disorder) is usually straightforward. The rare occurrence of simple partial non-convulsive status with prominent experiential symptoms (aura continua) is discussed under Non-convulsive status epilepticus, earlier in chapter. Juvenile absence epilepsy may present with academic failure and complaints of inattentiveness at school that might raise the possibility of attention deficit disorder.

Other paroxysmal neurological disorders are listed in Table 6.14 and discussed below.

Transient ischaemic attacks. The clinical features of transient ischaemic attacks typically involve a loss of function (as

Table 6.14 Paroxysmal neurological disorders that may be mistaken for epilepsy.

Transient ischaemic attacks
Migraine
Vertigo
Hyperekplexia
Paroxysmal movement disorders
Sleep disorders
Narcolepsy
Cataplexy
Non-REM disorders
REM sleep behaviour disorder

REM, rapid eye movement.

distinct from the positive phenomenology of epilepsy) and are usually of relatively prolonged duration. Impaired consciousness is not a feature of neocortical ischaemia but may occur in vertebrobasilar ischaemic episodes.

Classical migraine with aura followed by headache, photophobia and nausea seldom causes any diagnostic difficulties. However, migrainous aura may occur in isolation (acephalgic migraine or migraine equivalent). Visual disturbances are the most common form of aura, but sensory, motor, speech and cognitive disturbance, including clouding of consciousness, are seen occasionally (Al Twaijri & Shevell 2002; Young & Silberstein 2006). The visual aura of migraine typically involve scintillating, monochromatic, zig-zag lines that evolve slowly over tens of minutes. In contrast, visual aura in occipital lobe epilepsy are of sudden onset, brief duration and of coloured, round, often moving shapes. Overall, the characteristic pattern of symptoms, slow onset and gradual resolution help identify the various presentations of migraine.

Vertigo is an illusion of rotation due to a disorder of the vestibular system (Halmagyi 2005). True vertigo must be distinguished from symptoms of dizziness and light-headedness, which are non-specific and often reported as prodromal symptoms in epilepsy, and in association with syncope and dissociative seizures. Vertigo has been described with frontal and parietal seizures but is such an uncommon feature of epilepsy that it should immediately call other diagnoses to mind (Altay *et al.* 2005). The underlying disturbance of vestibular function in recurrent vertigo is almost always peripheral, the most common cause being benign positional vertigo. This condition is readily identified by a history of symptoms precipitated by head movement. Consciousness is preserved but the sensation of disorientation can be so profound that patients may report diminished awareness. Nausea and vomiting may also occur. Deafness, tinnitus and a history of ear infection will suggest Ménière's disease. Cerebellar stroke is the most common central cause of vertigo.

Hyperekplexia ('startle disease'). This refers to a rare group of disorders characterised by an exaggerated involuntary motor response to startle stimuli. Major and minor forms of the disorder have been distinguished (Bakker *et al.* 2006). The major form presents in the neonate with generalised stiffness that resolves in the first few years of life; an exaggerated startle response, especially to auditory stimuli, that persists throughout life; and a generalised stiffness that follows the startle response and lasts for a few seconds. The minor form of the disorder, which involves only an exaggerated startle response, is less common and less clearly delineated. In particular, minor forms of the disorder have not been as consistently linked to genetic abnormalities as have the major forms (Tijssen *et al.* 2002). Hyperekplexia usually has a genetic basis and over 70 pedigrees have now been reported. Most have mutations in the *GLRA1* gene encoding the α_1 subunit of the glycine receptor and show an autosomal dominant pattern of inheritance. The overwhelming majority of affected individuals have the major form of hyperekplexia but there are reports of the minor form of the disorder in some family members, with or without the mutation. Thus, family history is an important pointer to the diagnosis. The startle response is dramatic, may involve myoclonic movements and be associated with a fall but there is no alteration of consciousness. Non-familial hyperekplexia is rare and may have a sporadic genetic cause (Gaitatzis *et al*. 2004). Exaggerated startle is also seen in the stiff man syndrome and in association with brainstem or severe diffuse cerebral pathology. Hyperekplexia must be differentiated from *startle-induced epilepsy*. In the latter condition, epileptic seizures are triggered by sudden stimuli, most commonly auditory. Seizures typically arise in childhood and are often not exclusively related to startle, in which case startle-induced seizures may occur as a transient phase. Assymetric tonic posturing is a common semiological feature of the seizures. Some patients have diffuse cerebral pathology and learning difficulties but around half are of normal intelligence without neurological signs. Dysplastic lesions in premotor and perisylvian cortices may account for many of the latter group (Manford *et al*. 1996b).

Paroxysmal movement disorders. Paroxysmal kinesogenic dyskinesia (or choreoathetosis) is the most common paroxysmal movement disorder (Vidailhet 2000). Patients develop sudden brief (usually less than 1 minute) attacks of dystonia or chorea triggered by voluntary movement (Bruno *et al*. 2004); 80% of patients report a brief 'aura' which may have an epigastric quality. Consciousness is not impaired. Exacerbation by stress and alcohol are common. Idiopathic cases, two-thirds of whom have a family history, begin before 20 years of age and may be associated with a history of nonfebrile infantile convulsions. Treatment with low-dose antiepileptic medication is highly effective. Later-onset cases secondary to vascular, demyelinating and traumatic lesions have also been described (Blakeley & Jankovic 2002). Genetic linkage to chromosome 16 has been reported in a number of pedigrees. In paroxysmal non-kinesogenic dyskinesia, episodes are triggered by anxiety, caffeine and alcohol but not by movement. Episodes may be of longer duration (several minutes) and onset may be at any age, often in adulthood. Treatment with clonazepam is usually effective. Most cases are familial and the pattern of inheritance is typically autosomal dominant with incomplete penetrance. Mutations affecting the myofibrillogenesis 1 (*MR1*) gene on chromosome 2 have recently been reported, and appear to be associated with a phenotype characterised by early onset and precipitation by caffeine and alcohol (Bruno *et al*. 2007). A pedigree without these specific features was found to have linkage to a site on chromosome 2 not involving the *MR1* locus (Spacey *et al*. 2006).

Episodes of spontaneous paresis with preserved consciousness lasting for hours are seen in periodic paralysis (Venance *et al*. 2006), which may present to seizure clinics. The primary periodic paralyses are autosomal dominant conditions caused by mutations in genes encoding three specific ion channels. Secondary hypokalaemic periodic paralysis may occur in thyrotoxicosis. The periodic ataxias are also dominantly inherited channelopathies that present with brief (seconds to minutes) episodes of ataxia, sometimes associated with myokymia.

Sleep disorders are quite commonly considered in the differential diagnosis of epilepsy (see Chapter 13). In narcolepsy, daytime episodes of somnolence typically occur in settings where attentional demands are reduced but they may seem precipitous, a good example being attacks during a telephone conversation. However, the episodes are usually clearly described as being preceded by an irresistible urge to sleep and are seldom mistaken for epilepsy. Afterwards, the patient wakes feeling refreshed. Emotionally triggered loss of muscle tone in cataplexy may be associated with a fall. Consciousness is not impaired and recovery almost immediate (rarely taking longer than 1 minute). Cataplexy seldom if ever occurs other than in association with narcolepsy, but it may be the presenting feature of the syndrome. The other features of narcolepsy (hypnogogic/hypnopompic hallucinations and sleep paralysis) are found in around one-third and one-quarter of patients, respectively. The distinction between epilepsy and sleep disorders associated with paroxysmal motor and behaviour disturbance may be more difficult (see Derry *et al*. 2006 for a comprehensive review). In particular, FLE, which may occur exclusively in sleep and is often characterised by bizarre semiological features, is easily mistaken for sleep disorder and vice versa. Non-REM arousal disorders (confusional arousals, somnambulism and sleep terrors) may be relatively stereotyped, and their duration (minutes) does not clearly differentiate them from epileptic automatisms. However, they tend to occur less frequently and are less likely to show clustering than epileptic seizures, especially frontal seizures. They occur during stage 3 and 4 sleep, typically 90 minutes to 2 hours after sleep onset, whereas epileptic seizures tend to occur in stage 2 sleep, usually within 30 minutes of sleep onset. *REM sleep behaviour disorder* involves complex, sometimes violent, behaviour in which dreams are enacted during a sleep automatism. After the event, patients will usually, but not invariably, remember the dream that led to their actions but have no recall of their behaviour. Older age at onset, associated degenerative neurological disease, a history of vivid dreams and rousability during the episode are useful distinguishing features. Overall, it is the lack of epileptiform features that distinguishes these parasomnias from epilepsy. However, a clear eyewitness account of the episodes is often not available and video-EEG monitoring will often be required.

Transient global amnesia

Transient global amnesia (TGA) is a striking clinical syndrome. Patients present in an alert, perplexed, often agitated state, having abruptly become aware that they are unable to remember recent events. They are also unable to retain new information. Cognitive function is otherwise remarkably preserved. Episodes last for an average of 4 hours and resolve gradually. On recovery, the patient has no memory for the episode. In most cases the episode is an isolated one and TGA is regarded as a benign condition that requires no treatment. Aetiology is uncertain. Ischaemia, cerebral venous congestion, and migraine have all been put forward as possible mechanisms (Quinette *et al.* 2006). Patients with epilepsy are specifically excluded in diagnostic criteria for TGA. However, there may be some overlap with transient epileptic amnesia. Recent descriptions of transient epileptic amnesia emphasise that clinical evidence of epilepsy is often subtle and indeed may be absent in 30% of patients (see Transient epileptic amnesia, earlier in chapter). The pattern of amnesia in the two syndromes may overlap but retrograde amnesia is the conspicuous feature in transient epileptic amnesia and may extend back in time for years. Anterograde amnesia is also present in transient epileptic amnesia but patients may have some memory of the episode on recovery, unlike those with TGA in whom the main feature is a dense anterograde memory deficit.

Endocrine and metabolic disorders

Among endocrine and metabolic disorders with paroxysmal presentations, hypoglycaemia is the most common. Symptoms may include blurred vision, diaphoresis, and behavioural changes with delirium, anxiety and agitation. Hypoglycaemia occurs most commonly in the context of insulin therapy. Other causes include alcohol, renal or hepatic disease, insulin-producing tumours and hereditary fructose intolerance. Paroxysmal symptoms may also be seen with hypocalcaemia secondary to hypoparathyroidism, phaeochromocytoma and carcinoid syndrome.

What is the aetiology?

If seizures are judged to be epileptic, it is important to determine whether they may have been provoked by some extrinsic or non-recurrent factor. Some 40% of incident seizures fall into this category (Annegers *et al.* 1995). In children, a febrile illness is the most common provoking factor. In adults, traumatic brain injury, cerebrovascular disease, alcohol withdrawal and CNS infection are the most common causes. A combination of sleep deprivation and alcohol are the most likely factors in a young adult. Where seizures seem to have occurred without obvious provoking factors, the history may point to a likely aetiology. Age at onset of seizures provides the most important clue. Epilepsy due to congenital

disorders and perinatal insults is likely to present in infancy. From early childhood through to adolescence, febrile convulsions, CNS infection and then the idiopathic generalised epilepsy syndromes predominate. Most cases of cryptogenic and symptomatic localisation-related epilepsy will have presented by early adulthood. With increasing age, trauma, malignancy and then cerebrovascular and degenerative disorders become the most likely causes. Specific enquiry should accordingly be made about perinatal history, developmental delay, febrile convulsions, head injury (with loss of consciousness), history of CNS infection and family history of epilepsy. It should be noted that patients with psychogenic non-epileptic seizures frequently report a history of neurological problems and a family history of seizures may be more common in this group than in people with epilepsy (Wilkus *et al.* 1984; Moore & Baker 1997). A recent history of progressive neurological symptoms, and systemic symptoms of malignancy, will suggest a primary or metastatic tumour. Physical examination is often not rewarding but may reveal dermatological stigmata of the neurocutaneous syndromes or signs of neurological or systemic illness.

Investigation

Electroencephalography

Most EEG recordings in patients with seizures are obtained interictally when the patient is asymptomatic. If the interictal EEG is abnormal, then it may provide support for a diagnosis of epilepsy. Conversely, if the interictal recording is normal, this may make a diagnosis of epilepsy less likely. However, the interictal EEG can never be relied on to exclude a diagnosis of epilepsy, or indeed to prove it. To appreciate the role an interictal EEG may have in 'supporting' a clinical diagnosis of epilepsy it is important to understand the specificity and sensitivity of EEG. How often is the EEG abnormal in healthy individuals? How often is it normal in people with epilepsy? What factors make a false-negative or false-positive result more likely, and how can these misleading results be avoided, or at least minimised?

There is a relative paucity of information about EEG findings in healthy individuals. The most frequently quoted evidence comes from studies of military aircrew candidates who are routinely screened with EEG. The largest of these involved over 13 000 young men with no significant past medical history and normal physical examinations (Gregory *et al.* 1993). Clearly defined epileptiform abnormalities (spikes, certain spike-and-wave discharges, and/or a spike-and-wave photoparoxysmal response) were present in 0.5%. Follow-up information on those individuals with abnormal EEG was limited in this and other studies but the results have been broadly similar, suggesting that the risk of developing epilepsy after such an EEG finding is approximately twice that in the normal population. Overall, these studies have therefore suggested that epileptiform abnormalities will be found in about 0.3–0.5% of healthy adults who are at no discernible increased risk of epilepsy. By any standards such figures for specificity seem reasonably high. If an otherwise healthy person has a blackout and the EEG shows epileptiform abnormalities, it is highly likely that epilepsy is present. Why is it then that one authority in the field (Chadwick 1994) was moved to comment that 'routine interictal EEG recording is one of the most abused investigations in clinical medicine and is unquestionably responsible for great human suffering'? The problem concerns two particular sources of false positives. The first involves 'over-reporting' and 'over-interpretation' of EEG findings: non-specific changes in the EEG, and certain normal variants, are all too easily misreported as epileptiform; or reported as 'non-specific abnormalities', which is then misinterpreted as suggesting epilepsy (Benbadis & Tatum 2003). The second problem relates to the fact that in clinical populations the prevalence of false-positive epileptiform findings may be much higher. The incidence of epileptiform abnormalities rises to 10–30% in patients with congenital or acquired CNS disorders such as head trauma, tumours and perinatal injury (Zivin & Ajmone Marsan 1968). Both souces of false-positive error are of particular relevance to patients with dissociative seizures. A proportion of such patients have learning difficulties and consequently demonstrate a higher incidence of epileptiform abnormalities than healthy controls. However, potentially more problematic is the finding that, even after excluding such patients, *non-specific* abnormalities are over-represented in patients with dissociative seizures (Reuber *et al.* 2002). The significance of this finding is uncertain, but it may relate to an association between personality disturbance and non-specific EEG findings that does not seem to be accounted for by overt neurological disorder (De la Fuente *et al.* 1998).

Approximately 50% of patients with epilepsy will demonstrate an epileptiform abnormality during their first routine EEG recording (Fowle & Binnie 2000; Smith 2005). Repeated recordings will increase the yield of significant findings, but around one-third of patients are likely never to show an abnormality during an EEG obtained in the alert state. A recording obtained during sleep (either spontaneous or drug induced) will increase the rate of positive findings to around 80%. Overall, interictal epileptiform discharges are most likely in patients with frequent seizures (Sundaram *et al.* 1990) and, in a patient with daily seizures, an entirely normal interictal EEG will raise strong suspicion of non-epileptic seizures. The sensitivity of interictal EEG is higher in children than in adults, and higher in TLE than in patients with mesial or basal (especially frontal) epileptogenic foci. Hyperventilation and photic stimulation should be included as part of routine EEG protocols. Hyperventilation will trigger a seizure in most children with juvenile absence epilepsy, which is associated with a characteristic 3-Hz discharge (thus affording a reliable and simple method of obtaining an ictal EEG in this situation). A generalised spike-and-wave photoparoxysmal response to photic stimulation is strongly correlated with clinical generalised epilepsy. Photosensitivity is rare in localisation-related epilepsy.

An ictal EEG, especially when accompanied by video recording (video-EEG telemetry) of clinical semiology, is the gold standard for diagnosis. Telemetry should always be considered when there is doubt about diagnosis, the threshold for referral being determined primarily by practical considerations concerning availability and cost, as well as how frequently the person is having seizures. The diagnostic findings in epilepsy are an ictal discharge, clear evidence of postictal slowing and/or a preserved alpha rhythm in an unresponsive patient (Meierkord *et al.* 1991). Quite large areas of cortex (a few square centimetres) need to be involved in synchronous discharges before an abnormality is seen on the scalp EEG. Simple partial seizures and frontal seizures arising in medial or basal regions are therefore often not accompanied by any scalp EEG change. An ictal EEG may still be useful in distinguishing frontal lobe seizures from dissociative episodes when seizures occur during sleep: frontal lobe seizures will be seen to arise directly from electrographically documented sleep; in patients with dissociative seizures, the EEG will reveal a period of arousal from sleep (typically inconspicuous to an observer, so-called pseudosleep) that precedes seizure onset (Duncan *et al.* 2004). Movement artefacts may obscure the EEG and, if rhythmic, may even be mistaken for epileptic discharges. The evaluation of patients with multiple seizure types requires special diligence. Because dissociative seizures often coexist with epilepsy, care must be taken to ensure that each type of seizure has been documented before concluding that the patient has, or does not have, epilepsy. It is important to verify, with the patient and with informants, that the episodes captured are indeed examples of the patient's habitual seizures. Occasionally, a patient is encountered who has a first, and last, dissociative seizure during an admission for telemetry. A further problem concerns patients who have epileptic partial seizures that trigger a dissociative non-epileptic elaboration (Kapur *et al.* 1995). Provocation techniques, for both epilepsy and non-epileptic seizures, may be used. In certain circumstances, withdrawal of antiepileptic drugs may be considered in evaluating seizures thought likely to be epileptic in order to increase the chances of capturing a seizure or possibly to unmask epileptic discharges that might be suppressed by medication. Between 50% and 90% of patients with dissociative seizures will have attacks induced by suggestion. Techniques involving placebo (e.g. intravenous saline, alcohol skin patches) are effective but raise significant ethical issues. More recently, McGonigal *et al.* (2002) were able to provoke dissociative seizures in two-thirds of patients using simple suggestion with routine photic and hyperventilation stimuli, fully disclosing the aims of the procedure to patients. These authors estimate they were able to reduce the need for prolonged telemetry admission in 47% of patients. Provocation may be of particular value in patients who have infrequent seizures and would otherwise be unsuitable for telemetry. There is a small risk of false-positive results with these provocation techniques and it is therefore critical that an informant who has witnessed the patient's seizures is available to confirm that the provoked seizure resembles the habitual ones.

The EEG has a valuable role in determining seizure type and epilepsy syndrome (Fowle & Binnie 2000; Smith 2005). Two clinical situations are particulary important in this context. The first concerns the differentiation of complex partial and absence seizures, which may sometimes be difficult based on history alone. The second concerns partial seizures with rapid secondary generalisation, which may be mistaken for primary generalised epilepsy. In addition, a number of infantile and childhood syndromes are characterised by specific EEG appearances, for example West syndrome, benign childhood epilepsy syndromes and Landau–Kleffner syndrome. Other than helping establish seizure type and identifying the syndrome, the EEG has a limited role in guiding treatment decisions. An abnormal EEG following a first seizure may influence the decision to start treatment. The risk of seizure recurrence following a first unprovoked seizure rises from 27% when the EEG is normal to 58% when epileptiform abnormalities are present (Berg & Shinnar 1994). The decision to withdraw antiepileptic drugs after seizure remission is discussed in Management of epilepsy in remission, later in chapter. A normal EEG is one factor that may be taken into account but it has a relatively low predictive value.

The EEG plays an important role in the diagnosis of nonconvulsive status epilepticus and in the management of status epilepticus in intensive care settings. In the latter situation, EEG is essential for monitoring treatment response when anaesthesia and paralysing agents may conceal overt seizure activity. Along with MRI, the EEG has a central role in the assessment of patients for surgery (see Surgical treatment of epilepsy, later in chapter).

Neuroimaging

Magnetic resonance imaging is the structural imaging method of choice in epilepsy (see Duncan 1997b; Connor & Jarosz 2001). CT has a much lower sensitivity but will be used when MRI is contraindicated or in acute settings where CT allows better access to a medically unstable patient during scanning. In addition, CT has advantages over MRI in the detection of acute intracranial haemorrhage and skull fracture and is a useful supplement to MRI in the identification of small areas of intracranial calcification. The Commission on Neuroimaging of the International League Against Epilepsy (1997) have recommended that MRI be obtained in all patients with epilepsy, with the exception of those with a definite diagnosis of idiopathic generalised epilepsy or benign rolandic epilepsy of childhood. MRI is particularly indicated

in the following situations: (i) onset of partial seizures at any age; (ii) onset of unclassified or generalised seizures in the first years of life or adulthood; (iii) where there is evidence of a focal neurological or neuropsychological deficit; (iv) when seizures are poorly controlled with first-line treatment; and (v) where there is loss of seizure control or a changing pattern of seizures. Where access to MRI is restricted, priority should be given to patients whose seizures are not controlled with medical treatment or who have progressive neurological or neuropsychological deficits.

Magnetic resonance imaging will detect a lesion in over 80% of patients with chronic epilepsy. Hippocampal sclerosis is the most commonly identified pathology. Other abnormalities include disorders of neuronal migration and cortical development, tumours, vascular malformations and acquired cortical injury. A typical MRI protocol should include oblique coronal images obtained orthogonal to the long axis of the hippocampal structures. T1- and T2-weighted datasets should be obtained. The main findings in hippocampal sclerosis are hippocampal atrophy and increased T2-weighted signal within the hippocampus. Visual inspection will detect a 20% or greater degree of hippocampal asymmetry. Quantitative methods for assessing both hippocampal volume and T2 signal abnormality have been described. The resource implications of these methods have meant that their clinical use has been restricted to the presurgical evaluation of patients with equivocal findings on qualitative review of scans. Hippocampal atrophy may be bilateral in up to 15% of cases (Margerison & Corsellis 1966; King et al. 1995) and not uncommonly occurs in association with other pathologies. Careful inspection for hippocampal sclerosis is therefore essential even if other pathology is identified, and vice versa. Subtle abnormalities of cortical development are found in up to 7% of patients with chronic partial epilepsy and are likely to account for a substantial proportion of those who are currently 'MRI-negative'. Advances in MRI hardware, including higher magnetic field strength (3 T), will improve anatomical resolution and may further improve the sensitivity of structural MRI in epilepsy.

Functional imaging has a growing role in the presurgical evaluation of localisation-related epilepsy (see Duncan 1997b, 2003; Richardson 2001). Images of cerebral blood flow obtained with SPECT demonstrate focal interictal hypoperfusion and ictal hyperperfusion. The interictal findings have a relatively poor correlation with seizure localisation but ictal hyperperfusion on SPECT is a more reliable marker of seizure onset and has an established place in presurgical assessment in some centres. PET may similarly be used to demonstrate regional metabolic changes in association with seizures. However, PET ligand studies of the distribution of benzodiazepine, opioid and other receptors seem to offer greater potential for seizure localisation. For example, benzodiazepine receptor studies with the ligand ^{11}C-flumazenil demonstrate focal reductions in receptor density that correlate well with MRI findings in hippocampal sclerosis and in malformations of cortical development. In the latter situation, ligand studies may prove helpful in locating seizure foci in MRI-negative patients. Functional MRI is being developed to delineate motor and speech cortex as part of surgical planning. Techniques linking EEG, functional MRI and structural MRI have the potential for allowing anatomical mapping of the source of interictal epileptiform discharges.

Cardiological investigations

Most cases of vasovagal syncope are readily identified on history alone and do not require further investigation. In uncertain cases, when episodes are frequent, or where underlying cardiac disorder is suggested by history or examination, cardiological assessment is required. The important alarm signals in the history are a personal or family history of heart disease, a lack of presyncopal symptoms, and a history of syncope occurring with exercise, when lying or in association with palpitations or chest pain (Brignole 2007). A routine ECG, echocardiography and a 24-hour ECG recording are usually the first steps. These are relatively inexpensive and will identify structural cardiac disease but will miss some causes of paroxysmal arrhythmia. Tilt table testing will help confirm a syncopal tendency, and will identify most cases of orthostatic syncope and many cases of vasovagal syncope. However, the sensitivity (50%) is relatively low and false-positive results are seen in up to 15% of normal individuals (Gould et al. 2006). Sensitivity may be increased with various pharmacological provoking agents but at the expense of lower specificity. In the elderly, carotid-sinus massage with ECG monitoring may be used to investigate carotid sinus hypersensitivity. This procedure also has poor specificity, with around one-third of asymptomatic individuals over the age of 65 demonstrating a false-positive result (Kerr et al. 2006). If a strong suspicion of vasovagal syncope or arrhythmia remains despite normal preliminary investigations, longer-term ECG monitoring should be considered. This can be performed using either an external or an implanted 'loop' ECG monitor. An implanted device is invasive and relatively expensive but provides high-quality recordings for up to 18 months and does not suffer from the problems of compliance encountered with external devices. Loop monitors record the ECG continuously. After an episode the patient triggers an event-switch on the device, which then stores the preceding epoch of ECG for later analysis. The device can also be programmed to save recordings automatically in association with episodes of bradycardia or tachycardia. Internal loop recorders will lead to an ECG-based diagnosis and treatment in around one-third of patients and appear to be cost-effective (Brignole et al. 2006; Farwell et al. 2006). There is growing evidence that dual-chamber cardiac pacemakers are an effective treatment for recurrent vasovagal syncope (Morgan 2006).

The occurrence of sinus bradycardia and syncope during epileptic seizures has been mentioned in the preceding section on clinical evaluation. However, the real importance of ictal bradycardia lies in its relationship to ictal asystole which, along with ictal apnoea, is likely to be an important mechanism in sudden seizure-related deaths (Nashef et al. 2007). The wider implications of ictal bradycardia in terms of management, including indications for cardiological investigations and monitoring, have not yet been established. However, in one highly selected series of 19 patients with intractable localisation-related epilepsy, monitoring with implanted ECG loop recorders over 18 months revealed ictal bradyarrhythmias in seven patients, four of whom subsequently received permanent pacemaker insertion (Rugg-Gunn et al. 2004). An important finding was that serious arrhythmias occurred only intermittently in the affected patients; between episodes of ictal bradycardia there were typically many seizures without any significant cardiac effects. Thus, an isolated normal ictal ECG recording, obtained for example during presurgical work-up, provides little or no reassurance that the patient is not at risk.

Serum prolactin

Serum prolactin rises after tonic–clonic epileptic seizures, peaking 10–20 minutes after the seizure and returning to baseline after about 6 hours (Chen et al. 2005). A rise in prolactin is less reliable following complex partial seizures, may be absent following serial epileptic seizures or in status epilepticus, and is not seen following simple partial seizures. Syncope may also be associated with elevated prolactin levels and, potentially more problematically, modest rises in prolactin have been described in patients with psychogenic non-epileptic seizures (Alving 1998; Willert et al. 2004). As a result, and because video-EEG monitoring is now more widely available, the test has fallen out of favour. However, a negative finding after an apparent tonic–clonic seizure is still helpful. Blood samples should be taken 10–20 minutes after a seizure and compared with a baseline sample taken at approximately the same time of day and at least 6 hours after a seizure. Criteria for a positive result have varied between studies but a twofold rise above baseline is widely regarded as significant. The American Academy of Neurology (Chen et al. 2005) have concluded that the postictal prolactin test is a useful adjunct for differentiating generalised and complex partial seizures from psychogenic events and recommended further studies to establish the sensitivity and specificity of the procedure.

Treatment

The aim of treatment is to achieve seizure control with a minimum of adverse effects. Complete remission is a realistic target for most patients who can then expect a quality of life comparable to that of the general population. When this is not possible, a secondary aim is reduction in seizure frequency or severity. However, this is very much a 'second best' outcome. Continuing seizures, no matter how infrequent, have a significant impact on overall quality of life, social functioning and psychiatric status (Leidy *et al.* 1999; Birbeck *et al.* 2002; Gilliam 2002). In addition, epilepsy is associated with significant mortality and a risk of accidental injury. Patients whose seizures are not fully controlled therefore constitute a special clinical group requiring careful reappraisal and a clearly defined, active management plan. Seizure freedom should not, of course, be pursued at any cost. Treatment will always represent a compromise between reducing seizure frequency or severity and keeping side effects to an acceptable minimum. Shorvon (2004) has commented that 'there is often a strange inertia in much of the treatment of chronic epilepsy'. The phrase 'well-controlled epilepsy with infrequent seizures' should always strike a note of alarm. Epilepsy that is not in remission is poorly controlled.

The higher mortality rate and risk of injury associated with epilepsy are important factors underlying the rationale for treatment. Overall, patients with epilepsy have a standardised mortality ratio of 2–3 (O'Donoghue & Sander 1997). Causes of this excess mortality include death due to the underlying cause of epilepsy, accidental injury, suicide, status epilepticus and sudden unexplained death. The risk of sudden unexplained death in epilepsy (SUDEP; see Sudden death in epilepsy) is probably small in most cases of recent-onset epilepsy but may be as high as 1 in 100 patients per year in those with medically intractable epilepsy awaiting surgery (Dasheiff 1991). Most accidental injuries in people with epilepsy are seizure related (Wirrell 2006). Children and patients with generalised tonic–clonic seizures are at greatest risk. Retrospective studies have suggested a threefold to sixfold increased risk of submersion injury, with incidents during bathing being more common than those related to swimming. Burns, fractures and head injuries are also more common. However, the overall incidence of these problems is relatively low. There has been only one prospective controlled study of accidental injury in epilepsy (Beghi & Cornaggia 2002). Over 12 months, accidental injuries occurred in 17% of 952 people with epilepsy and 12% of 909 controls. After 2 years the corresponding figures were 27% and 17%. Most injuries were minor but patients with epilepsy reported a higher rate of injuries requiring hospitalisation (3% vs 1%) or medical treatment (16% vs 10%). At each stage in treatment, these risks, together with the psychosocial burden of ongoing seizures, must be weighed against the likelihood that a proposed treatment will be successful and without significant side effects. As previously mentioned, the risks of untreated epilepsy in the early stages are probably insignificant compared with the dire consequences of a mistaken diagnosis of epilepsy. Treatment should only be instituted when diagnosis is certain.

When to start treatment

Treatment is indicated if a patient has had two or more unprovoked seizures occurring within a relatively short interval. Most would consider recurrence within 6 months or 1 year as falling into this category. In practice, seizures usually occur at shorter intervals and the decision to begin treatment is straightforward. This is especially so when a syndromic diagnosis, for example JME, has been made. A more difficult, but not uncommon, problem arises when a patient presents following a single, apparently unprovoked, tonic–clonic seizure. In this situation further investigations will help inform treatment decisions. Overall, the risk of recurrence over a 2-year period following a single unprovoked seizure is approximately 30–40%. The lowest risk (24%) is in patients with no identifiable cause and a normal EEG. Where a cause is found and the EEG is abnormal, the chance of a second seizure is as high as 65% (Berg & Shinnar 1991).

Some patients with mild forms of epilepsy may decide not to pursue treatment. The question of whether delaying treatment has an adverse effect on long-term prognosis then arises: do seizures beget seizures? Elwes *et al.* (1988) studied patients presenting with untreated tonic–clonic seizures and found the median interval between seizures showed a progressive decline, from 12 weeks between the first and second seizures to 3 weeks between the fourth and fifth. This seemed compatible with an accelerating underlying disease process. Other evidence, however, suggests that epilepsy is generally a non-progressive disorder and there is little if any harm in delaying treatment. For example, studies of untreated epilepsy have found that it may run a relatively benign course with spontaneous seizure-free periods of a year or more occurring in nearly 50% of patients (Placencia *et al.* 1994). There is also evidence that treatment begun many years after the onset of epilepsy achieves similar results to that initiated soon after seizure onset (Feksi *et al.* 1991).

Prophylactic treatment after brain injury or supratentorial neurosurgery should be avoided. Such treatment may decrease the incidence of acute symptomatic seizures in the first week, but confers no protection against seizures in the longer term (Schierhout & Roberts 1998). The needless prescription of antiepileptic drugs undoubtedly contributes to the cognitive and behavioural difficulties in many such patients. One of the most rewarding medical interventions in a neurorehabilitation setting is the withdrawal of unnecessary antiepileptic drugs, an action that is often followed by remarkable improvements in alertness, communication and overall neurological function.

Choice of treatment

The choice of initial drug treatment is dictated by type of seizure and syndrome, patient characteristics, side effects and practical considerations such as availability and cost.

Seizure type/syndrome

Carbamazepine has long been regarded as the drug of first choice for localisation-related epilepsy. Most recently, this view has been challenged by the results of a large multicentre trial in the UK, the Standard and New Antepileptic Drugs (SANAD) trial (Marson *et al.* 2007a); 1721 patients for whom carbamazepine was deemed the standard treatment were randomly allocated to receive carbamazepine, lamotrigine, oxcarbazepine, gabapentin or topiramate. In terms of efficacy, carbamazepine showed an advantage in relation to time to 12-months seizure remission, but this was statistically significant only in comparison with gabapentin. However, time to treatment failure (failure to control seizures or the advent of intolerable side effects) was longer for lamotrigine, and this difference was statistically significant in relation to all drugs except oxcarbazepine. The authors concluded that lamotrigine was a cost-effective and well-tolerated alternative to carbamazepine.

Valproate remains the drug of choice for generalised epilepsy (Marson *et al.* 2007b). As valproate is associated with adverse cosmetic and teratogenic effects (see below), young women with generalised epilepsy present a particularly difficult treatment dilemma. Ethosuxamide is an alternative treatment for absence seizures but is ineffective for generalised tonic–clonic seizures.

The spectrum of efficacy of antiepileptic drugs is listed in Table 6.15. The table is based on recent reviews (McCorry *et al.* 2004; Perucca 2005) and guidelines published by the American Acadamy of Neurology (French *et al.* 2004a,b) and the ILAE (Glauser *et al.* 2006). Felbamate and vigabatrin have been omitted from the table as their use is now restricted because of toxicity. Efficacy has been established for a number of the newer drugs as add-on treatment only.

Drug toxicity

Antiepileptic drugs are associated with four categories of adverse effects (Smith & Chadwick 2001): (i) acute dose-related toxicity; (ii) acute idiosyncratic reactions; (iii) chronic toxicity; and (iv) teratogenicity.

Acute dose-related toxicity is common. The most frequent symptoms are referable to the CNS and include drowsiness, cognitive disturbance, headache, ataxia and visual disturbance. Nausea and other gastric symptoms are also common. These symptoms are usually mild and transient. They improve as tolerance to the drug develops, usually within a week or two at any given dose, and can be relieved by lowering the dose and subsequently slowing the rate of dose titration. Nevertheless, these side effects are a common reason for treatment failure.

Acute idiosyncratic reactions are rare but potentially life-threatening and require immediate drug withdrawal. Allergic reactions with a rash occur in 2–4% of patients taking carbamazepine, phenytoin, phenobarbital and, perhaps more commonly, lamotrigine. These reactions typically occur in the first 4 weeks of treatment and may be accompanied by symptoms of systemic illness. The same drugs are also associated with Stevens–Johnson syndrome and Lyell's syndrome, rare but potentially fatal cutaneous reactions. Severe haematological complications are reported with felbamate, acetazolamide, carbamazepine, phenytoin, lamotrigine and zonisamide. Such reactions are rare with the exception of felbamate, use of which is now restricted because of its association with aplastic anaemia and liver toxicity. Acute hepatotoxicity is a rare complication of valproate and occurs almost exclusively in children with complex

Table 6.15 Effectiveness of antiepileptic drugs against different seizure types.

	Partial-onset seizures	Generalised onset: tonic–clonic seizures	Generalised onset: absence seizures
First line	Carbamazepine Lamotrigine	Valproate	Ethosuxamide
Alternatives First generation	Valproate Phenobarbital Phenytoin Benzodiazepines	Carbamazepine* Phenobarbital Phenytoin* Benzodiazepines	Valproate
Second generation	Gabapentin Levetiracetam Oxcarbazepine Tiagabine Topiramate Zonisamide Pregabalin	Lamotrigine Topiramate Levetiracetam?	Lamotrigine

* May exacerbate myoclonic and absence seizures.

neurological disorders on polytherapy. Acute liver failure is also rarely reported with phenytoin and carbamazepine.

Chronic toxicity. These effects are usually not directly life-threatening but may be irreversible. Important examples include cosmetic effects with phenytoin (hirsutism, coarsening of facial appearance, gum hyperplasia) and valproate (weight gain, alopecia and tremor), hyponatraemia with carbamazepine and oxcarbazepine, folate deficiency with phenytoin, phenobarbital, valproate and carbamazepine, weight loss and renal calculi with topiramate, visual field defects with vigabatrin (which severely restrict its use), and endocrine and bone effects with many drugs, particularly those that induce hepatic enzymes (phenytoin, carbamazepine and phenobarbital).

Teratogenicity. The risk of major congenital malformations in children born to women taking antiepileptic drugs is about 5–9%, approximately twice the rate observed in the general population (Samren *et al*. 1997; Kaneko *et al*. 1999; Holmes *et al*. 2001). The most commonly reported malformations include neural tube defects, cardiac malformations and skeletal abnormalities. Minor anomalies, including certain dysmophic facial characteristics, have also been described but their prevalence is less certain. Patients taking more than one antiepileptic drug are at greatest risk and there is evidence that the risk is related to higher doses for some drugs. Overall, the risk of major malformations is highest with valproate, especially at doses above 1000 mg daily, but phenytoin, phenobarbital, lamotrigine and carbamazepine are all implicated. However, more recently introduced drugs must not be regarded as safe. They have not been in use long enough to allow even preliminary judgements to be made. Registers of pregnancies in women with epilepsy have been established in a number of centres and are the subject of ongoing investigation. Morrow *et al*. (2006) have reported outcome in 3607 pregnancies from the UK register, the largest study so far. The analysis focused on outcome for women taking carbamazepine (900 women), valproate (715) or lamotrigine (647), as well as a small group (239) of women with epilepsy who had not taken medication during pregnancy. Overall, major congenital malformations were seen in 4.2% of births to women who had taken antiepileptic drugs during pregnancy, and in 3.5% of those who were not taking medication. The risk of malformations was 6% in women on polytherapy compared with 3.7% in those taking a single drug. The rate of malformations was greater in those exposed to valproate (6.2%) than to lamotrigine (3.2%) or carbamazepine (2.2%), but the difference was statistically significant only for the comparison between valproate and carbamazepine. The highest risk (9%) was seen in patients receiving polytherapy combinations that included valproate. Interestingly, a significant relationship between dose and risk was observed for lamotrigine, but was discernible as a trend only for valproate. These results confirm previous impressions that valproate is associated with the highest risk of major congenital malformations but also suggest that lamotrigine is not as safe as had previously been hoped. Finally, there is emerging evidence that children exposed to antiepileptic drugs *in utero* are at increased risk of developmental delay, learning and behavioural difficulties, and possibly autistic spectrum disorder (Eriksson *et al*. 2005; Rasalam *et al*. 2005; Vinten *et al*. 2005). Valproate has again been implicated in most of these studies but further prospective investigations are required.

Drug interactions are an important further complication in the treatment of epilepsy (Perucca 2006). This is mainly because antiepileptic drugs are often prescribed on a long-term basis and also because polytherapy is, unfortunately, quite common. An important category of interactions concerns drugs that induce the cytochrome P450 enzymes, the main examples being carbamazepine, phenytoin and barbiturates. Through this mechanism these drugs effectively shorten the half-lives of many other compounds, resulting in reduced serum levels and increased dosage requirements. This may affect other antiepileptic medication, oral contraceptives, anticoagulant treatment, analgesics, psychotropics and many other drugs. Enzyme inhibition may also occur, the most noteworthy example being the inhibition of lamotrigine metabolism by valproate, an action which effectively halves the dose requirements of lamotrigine. This is particularly important when prescribing lamotrigine for a patient already taking valproate, as the incidence of hypersensitivity reactions to lamotrigine seems to be related to the rate at which its serum levels rise. Accordingly, the starting dose of lamotrigine should be halved in this situation and dose increments made more slowly. In relation to psychotropics, interactions are seldom clinically significant (Spina & Perucca 2002). Reduced concentrations of tricyclic antidepressants, conventional neuroleptics (haloperidol, chlorpromazine) and atypical neuroleptics (clozapine, olanzapine, respiridone) have been reported in association with enzyme-inducing drugs. Fluoxetine and sertraline may increase serum levels of phenytoin and carbamazepine, and sertraline may cause a rise in lamotrigine levels.

Patient characteristics

Choosing the right drug for the right patient involves consideration of potential side effects in the context of patient characteristics. Age, gender and comorbidity are the most important factors in this context (Crawford *et al*. 1999; McCorry *et al*. 2004; Brodie & Kwan, 2005). Age influences the likelihood, as well as the impact, of certain adverse reactions and is often an important consideration in drug choice. For example, the hepatotoxicity associated with valproate is seldom seen in children older than 2 years. Skin reactions with lamotrigine are also more likely in children. Sedation, cognitive difficulties and behavioural problems may be associated with many of the antiepileptic treatments in children and can have a grave impact on educational achievement and social functioning. The cosmetic effects of phenytoin and valproate may be of little concern to an older man but are highly significant considerations in children and young women. Acute dose-related CNS side effects, in particular sedation, are more likely in the elderly and in patient groups with static or progressive neurological disorders affecting cognitive functioning. Whereas in younger patients these effects are usually transient, this is often not the case in the elderly or in patients with diminished cerebral reserve. In more severely impaired patients with communication difficulties, sedation may not be conspicuous and subtle behavioural changes may be the only sign of toxicity. Lamotrigine and some of the newer antiepileptic drugs with favourable cognitive profiles may be more appropriate first-line choices in these patient groups. Decreased bone mineralisation is associated particularly with enzyme-inducing drugs, presumably through effects on vitamin D metabolism, but valproate has also been implicated. Older patients and postmenopausal women are particularly at risk. Bone density scans and calcium and vitamin D supplementation need to be considered. Finally, a number of special considerations apply to women of childbearing age. In view of the high rate of unplanned pregnancies, all fertile women should be considered 'at risk', not just those who are planning pregnancy. Information must be provided about contraception, including interactions between enzyme-inducing drugs and oral contraceptive preparations, and pregnancy. Folic acid should be prescribed as a matter of routine and oral vitamin K should probably be given in the last month of pregnancy. The choice of treatment in young women with idiopathic generalised epilepsy represents a particularly difficult dilemma for which there are no straightforward solutions at present (Duncan 2007). Lamotrigine has been favoured by many in this situation but the recent demonstration of significant teratogenic risk with lamotrigine now makes the choice more difficult. The main priority must be to provide women with clear information to allow them to weigh up the various alternatives.

Individual antiepileptic drugs

The following section is intended as a guide to the principal indications and important advantages or disadvantages of the most commonly prescribed antiepileptic drugs for adults. Prescribing guidelines are provided by the *British National Formulary* (2006). A comprehensive account is given in the standard text *The Treatment of Epilepsy* (Shorvon *et al.* 2004), which includes chapters devoted to each of the drugs currently in use.

Carbamazepine

Carbamazepine is a first-line drug for partial and tonic–clonic seizures. It is ineffective for, and may exacerbate, absence and myoclonic seizures. It has well-established efficacy and is usually well tolerated: acute dose-related CNS side effects (drowsiness, dizziness, mental slowing, ataxia,

diplopia, blurred vision) are transient and can usually be avoided with a low starting dose and slow increases. Hypersensitivity reactions include rashes, seen in 10%. Severe life-threatening haematological reactions (thrombocytopenia, aplastic anaemia, agranulocytosis and pancytopenia) have an estimated incidence of around 1 in 200 000. A mild subclinical leucopenia of under 5000 cells/mm^3 is seen in around one-third of patients in the first 6 months. It may exacerbate atrioventricular conduction abnormalities and is therefore contraindicated in this situation. Carbamazepine is a hepatic enzyme inducer and has many drug interactions as a consequence.

Sodium valproate

Valproate has a wide spectrum of action. It is a drug of first choice in idiopathic generalised epilepsy and a first-line treatment for generalised seizures (of all types) and partial seizures. Acute dose-related CNS effects are mild and of a similar degree to those seen with carbamazepine. The most characteristic side effect is a dose-dependent intention tremor. Weight gain and alopecia (usually reversible on drug withdrawal) are relatively common and not infrequently lead to treatment withdrawal, especially in women. An association with polycystic ovary syndrome, presenting as menstrual disorder, obesity and hirsutism, is recognised although the incidence is uncertain. Fatal hepatotoxicity has been reported, almost exclusively in children less than 2 years old taking polytherapy in the context of complex neurological disorders. An encephalopathy associated with elevated ammonia levels has also been reported. The cosmetic, cognitive and teratogenic (see Drug toxicity, earlier) effects of valproate complicate its use in women. Valproate has a number of complex interactions with other antiepileptic drugs. The most significant relates to the addition of valproate to lamotrigine treatment, which may more than double serum concentration of the latter.

Ethosuximide

Ethosuximide is a first-line treatment for absence seizures for which it is probably equally effective as valproate. Ethosuximide is considered the drug of first choice for absence seizures in younger children (e.g. with onset before age 10) because it lacks the risk of liver toxicity associated with valproate and because generalised tonic–clonic and myoclonic seizures, for which ethosuximide is not effective, are less likely in this age group. Common side effects include gastrointestinal symptoms and non-specific CNS effects. More rarely, behavioural disturbance and psychosis have been reported.

Phenytoin

Phenytoin has a broad spectrum of action and may be considered as a first-line treatment for generalised and partial seizures. Non-linear pharmacokinetics mean that small adjustments in dosage may be accompanied by marked changes in serum levels. A therapeutic range of serum concentration is reasonably well established, although clinical experience suggests that levels at the lower end of the range may be effective for generalised seizures whereas the higher end of the range may be required in patients with partial seizures. However, clinical response and side effects, rather than serum levels, guide dose selection in individual patients. The CNS dose-related effects are often quite severe and may be less transient than with other first-line drugs. Skin hypersensitivity reactions are seen in 5–10%. There are many systemic longer-term effects. Cosmetic side effects are important and include coarsened facial features, hirsutism and gum hyperplasia. Other longer-term effects include folate and vitamin K deficiency, osteomalacia, dyskinesias and, more rarely, peripheral neuropathy and cerebellar atrophy. Phenytoin induces hepatic enzymes with consequent drug interactions. While phenytoin is effective and broad spectrum, its acute and longer term side-effect profile place it behind other first-line treatments.

Barbituates

Phenobarbital is a cheap, highly effective, broad-spectrum treatment for generalised and partial seizures. Its use has declined because of a relatively high rate of neurotoxic effects, particularly sedation, cognitive slowing, and mood and behavioural disturbance (especially in children). Other relatively common side effects include folate and vitamin K deficiency, osteomalacia and soft-tissue abnormalities. It is a potent hepatic enzyme inducer. A further disadvantage is the occurrence of dependence and a withdrawal syndrome (which may include withdrawal seizures) when the drug is discontinued. Consequently, the rate of withdrawal must be extremely slow, over many months. *Primidone* is rapidly converted to phenobarbital but may also have an independent antiepileptic action.

Benzodiazepines

Clonazepam has a broad spectrum of action and is used as adjunctive treatment for partial and generalised seizures. Its use is limited primarily by its sedative effect, which may be severe, prolonged and associated with behavioural disturbance. Tolerance is also an important disdvantage and may be associated with both a loss of efficacy in some patients and a withdrawal syndrome on discontinuation. *Clobazam* also has a broad spectrum of action but is generally better tolerated than clonazepam. It may be a very effective adjunctive treatment but tolerance leads to reduced efficacy in up to 50% of patients. It is nevertheless a very useful treatment for some patients. Clobazam also has a special place as an intermittent treatment given for seizure clusters, as prophylaxis to cover special occasions and for catamenial seizures.

Lamotrigine

Lamotrigine is a first-line drug for partial and generalised seizures and is useful as both monotherapy and adjunctive

treatment. It is well tolerated, with less marked CNS effects than some of the older agents. The most important hypersensitivity reaction is a rash, which is seen in some 10%. The rash is typically maculopapular or erythematous, associated with pruritis, and appears some 4 weeks after starting treatment. Patients must be warned about this and treatment withdrawn if a rash appears: withdrawal should be carried out over about 2 weeks, more abruptly if skin reactions are severe. While a rash is seen as a hypersensitivity reaction with other antiepileptic drugs, its importance with lamotrigine relates to an association with rare but potentially life-threatening dermatological reactions including Stevens–Johnson syndrome and toxic epidermal necrolysis, which may be relatively more common with lamotrigine than other antiepileptic drugs. These severe reactions are more often seen in children and with rapid dose escalation. Special care must therefore be taken when adding lamotrigine to a patient already taking valproate. Lamotrigine levels may be lowered by enzyme inducers but the most important interaction is with valproate, which increases lamotrigine levels.

Gabapentin

Gabapentin is a second-line agent for adjunctive treatment of partial onset seizures and secondarily generalised seizures. It is well tolerated with relatively few CNS side effects and few, if any, significant drug interactions. Its efficacy in relation to other treatments remains uncertain but its favourable side-effect profile is a strong advantage.

Topiramate

Topiramate is a second-line agent, either as adjunctive treatment or as monotherapy, for partial seizures, with or without secondary generalisation, and for generalised tonic–clonic seizures. It is associated with marked dose-related CNS side effects, which can usually be minimised by introducing the drug very slowly. Cognitive effects, including problems with attention, memory and word finding, may be present with relatively little in the way of sedation. Weight loss is also common. Renal calculi occur in up to 2%. There have been recent reports of acute myopia and closed-angle glaucoma occurring in the first month of treatment. The drug should be withdrawn as rapidly as possible if this happens.

Levetiracetam

Levetiracetam is a recently introduced treatment (adjuctive or as monotherapy) for partial seizures, with or without secondary generalisation. It is also effective adjunctive therapy for myoclonic seizures. It is generally well tolerated. Sedation and other acute CNS side effects are relatively uncommon. Insomnia, dysthymia and other psychiatric and behavioural problems have been reported. There is preliminary evidence of efficacy with doses lower than currently recommended and also of seizure exacerbation at doses in the upper end of the currently recommended range.

Vigabatrin

Approximately one-third of patients treated with vigabatrin will develop a visual field defect that is almost certainly permanent. Its use is therefore now restricted to very special circumstances in severely disabling epilepsy where all other treatment combinations have failed, e.g. West syndrome.

Recently introduced antiepileptic drugs

Oxcarbazepine, tiagabine, pregabalin and zonisamide have been introduced too recently for any clear impression to have been formed of their value and side-effect profile. They are all considered second-line choices for adjunctive treatment of partial seizures, with or without secondary generalisation. Oxcarbazepine is an analogue of carbamazepine. It appears to be better tolerated than carbamazepine, although hyponatraemia may be more common. Other reported side effects include weight gain, alopecia and gastrointestinal disturbances. Preliminary experience with tiagabine suggests that CNS side effects, including cognitive difficulties, are relatively common and a cautious approach to dosing therefore seems important.

Treatment in practice

Treatment should begin with a single drug. The starting dose should be low and increases made slowly. In most cases there is no hurry to achieve a therapeutic dose and clinicians should not hesitate to err on the cautious (slow) side of prescribing guidelines (British National Formulary 2006). There are a number of important reasons for adopting the 'start low, go slow' approach. The main aim is to avoid acute dose-related adverse effects, the most common of which is sedation. Some idiosyncratic side effects are also more likely with excessively rapid dose escalation. However, the real cost of intolerable side effects at this stage is that they may result in a potentially useful treatment being abandoned prematurely, and the first drug will often have been chosen because it has very clear advantages over the alternatives. A further important reason for slow dose increases is that many patients will achieve seizure remission at doses well below the published therapeutic range.

Patients must be informed of the most common side effects and warned to seek advice immediately should they develop symptoms of an allergic reaction (e.g. rash, flu-like symptoms). The effectiveness of treatment is, of course, judged by seizure reduction and, ultimately, cessation. This will be recognised promptly in patients who have very frequent seizures but assessing efficacy may be a more protracted affair in those whose seizures occur infrequently. Unless seizures remit quickly it is extremely helpful for patients to record seizure frequency with a diary. If there are multiple seizure types, a simple code to identify each type of seizure is useful. If seizures do not stop, the dose is gradually increased until the patient experiences dose-related side effects. Ongoing

seizures when this point is reached mean that first-line treatment has failed.

When first-line treatment fails and a second drug is chosen the aim must still be monotherapy. Whether the first drug is reduced before starting the second, or the second drug added to the first (more common), will depend on seizure frequency and the presence of side effects. One of the most important principles in the medical treatment of epilepsy is that side effects, particularly dose-related toxic effects, are far more likely with polytherapy. Thus, the chance of achieving an effective dose of the second drug without side effects is greatly improved by withdrawing the first. This often means reducing the first drug as the second is increased, ideally before side effects are encountered. If remission is achieved and the patient has remained on both drugs, it is important to withdraw the first. Unfortunately, this is often forgotten and many patients are left unnecessarily on two drugs at this stage.

Serum levels of antiepileptic drugs are useful in very limited circumstances. A 'therapeutic range' is best established for phenytoin, but even this provides a rough guide only. If a patient is seizure-free and serum levels are below the lower end of the range, there is obviously no point in increasing the dose. Equally, some patients are able to tolerate levels above the therapeutic range, without toxic effects, and may benefit. The main use of serum levels is to assess compliance. Levels obtained before and after adding a second drug can also help assess the impact of any pharmacokinetic interactions and may guide dose adjustment. In patients on polytherapy who have non-specific toxic side effects, serum levels may help identify the culprit. Antiepileptic drugs may be associated with a variety of minor haematological and biochemical disturbances. Common examples include raised transaminases caused by enzyme induction, neutropenia and hyponatraemia with carbamazepine, and thrombocytopenia with valproate. However, these are seldom of any clinical significance and routine haematological and biochemistry screening is not required. Sensible times for blood tests are at baseline and prior to commencing additional drugs. In this way, if clinically significant problems do arise, the likely agent can more easily be identified.

Management after failed monotherapy

Around 60% of patients with symptomatic or cryptogenic epilepsy will become seizure-free with monotherapy (Mattson *et al.* 1996; Sillanpaa *et al.* 1998; Kwan & Brody 2000). For idiopathic epilepsy, the figure is closer to 70%. Once initial treatment has failed, however, the chances of achieving seizure remission with medical treatment alone fall below 10%. Failed monotherapy is therefore an ominous development and requires a systematic approach. Diagnosis and aetiology must be formally reviewed. About 20% of patients with apparently intractable epilepsy will be found to have dissociative seizures. Other errors include mistaking partial-onset for generalised seizures and failing to identify a syndrome. Reassessment will also involve a thorough review of the history, in particular checking seizure semiology with the patient and informants. Video-EEG monitoring at this stage is strongly indicated if there is any doubt. Previous EEG data and neuroimaging should be reviewed. The possibility of non-compliance must be considered, together with aggravating factors (e.g. alcohol misuse) that might have been missed. A review of the medication history should address a number of questions for each drug that has been tried. Were adequate trials given? What was the maximum dose? Was there any response? Were there side effects and, if so, might these have been avoided?

Surgical treatment should be considered once no obvious problems or omissions emerge from a careful review of the treatment history. The selection of patients for surgery requires great care and is covered below. For most patients, however, resective surgery will not prove possible. Medical treatment in this group aims to optimise seizure control with the minimum of side effects. Overall, clinical trials of the newer antiepileptic drugs, given as add-on treatment, have generated remarkably similar results: around 40–50% of patients will experience a 50% reduction in seizure frequency but the chance of seizure remission is less than 5%. Reduced seizure frequency or severity may be of real benefit for some individuals, and for many the chance of remission, even if remote, is a good enough reason to give new drugs a try. However, some patients grow tired of repeated unsuccessful attempts, each one associated with side effects, and decide to remain on their 'tried and trusted' established treatment. In this situation it is important that patients are provided with information to allow them to make a balanced decision between the risks posed by ongoing seizures and the likelihood of success with new treatment. There is little evidence favouring one add-on drug from another (French *et al.* 2004b; McCorry *et al.* 2004). Combinations of drugs that have different, or at least complementary, principal modes of action are a rational choice (Table 6.16). The most commonly cited example is a combination of lamotrigine and valproate, but there is no good evidence supporting this or any other combination. A benzodiazepine, usually clobazam, prescribed over a short period can be a useful adjunct to treatment in women with perimenstrual seizure clustering (catamenial epilepsy) or to cover significant events (e.g. travel, exams, social occasions).

Management of epilepsy in remission

Once seizures have been in remission for at least 2 years, antiepileptic drug withdrawal may be considered. Overall, the risk of relapse over the 2 years following withdrawal is approximately 40%, compared with around 20% if medication had been continued (Medical Research Council Antiepileptic Drug Withdrawal Study Group 1991; Berg & Shinnar 1994; Specchio *et al.* 2002). The most important predictor of relapse is diagnosis of an epilepsy syndrome. Relapse is very rare in benign rolandic epilepsy, moderately rare (25%) in absence epilepsy (Bouma *et al.* 1996) and almost inevitable in JME (Janz 1997). For patients with symptomatic or cryptogenic partial epilepsy the risk of relapse is intermediate, somewhere between 25% and 75%. In adults (excluding patients with JME) relapse is more likely if epilepsy began in adulthood and has an identified aetiology (50% increased risk compared with cryptogenic cases) (Berg & Shinnar 1994). Additional risk factors for relapse, listed in order of decreasing importance, include shorter duration of remis-

Table 6.16 Principal modes of action of antiepileptic drugs. (From McCorry *et al.* 2004 with permission.)

Drug	GABA-mediated inhibition	Blockade of voltage-gated Na+ channels	Blockade of voltage-gated Ca2+ channels	Unknown
Phenobarbital	Yes	–	–	–
Phenytoin	–	Yes	–	–
Carbamazepine	–	Yes	–	–
Valproate	Yes	Yes	Yes	–
Ethosuxamide	–	–	Yes	–
Benzodiazepines	Yes	–	–	–
Lamotrigine	–	Yes	–	–
Gabapentin	Yes	?Yes	?Yes	–
Levetiracetam	–	–	–	Yes
Topiramate	?Yes	Yes	Yes	–
Oxcarbazepine	–	Yes	–	–
Tiagabine	Yes	–	–	–

GABA, γ-aminobutyric acid.

sion, taking two or more antiepileptic drugs, a history of myoclonic seizures, having seizures after the start of treatment, a history of tonic–clonic seizures of any type, and having an abnormal EEG (Medical Research Council Antiepileptic Drug Withdrawal Study Group 1991). These factors have been used to derive a predictive index (Medical Research Council Antiepileptic Drug Withdrawal Study Group 1993). However, probability figures may not help many patients (or their clinicians) weigh up risks and for many the chance of losing their driving licence outweighs any disadvantages of remaining on medication. It is widely presumed that if relapse occurs, then restarting previous treatment will achieve remission once again. Unfortunately, this is not so, a fact that adds a further degree of uncertainty to the decision. Up to 23% of patients who relapse after drug withdrawal may not regain freedom from seizures (Schmidt & Loscher 2005).

Surgical treatment of epilepsy

As described above, 20–30% of patients with epilepsy are unlikely to become seizure-free with medical treatment. For a proportion of this group, epilepsy surgery offers a real hope of remission. Patients with medial TLE form the largest group treated surgically. However, resections of extratemporal lesions, in particular operations involving the frontal lobe, are now more frequently performed. Additional procedures, conducted mostly in children, include hemispherectomy, multiple subpial transection and callosotomy.

The American Acadamy of Neurology has recommended that all patients with medically intractable localisation-related epilepsy be considered for surgery (Engel *et al.* 2003). Once at least two antiepileptic drugs have failed to control seizures, the chance of achieving remission with medical treatment alone is small. The point at which patients should be referred for surgical evaluation has not been defined but will depend to a large degree on the extent of disability. Given that this is likely to increase over time, and given also the risks of injury and sudden unexplained death in these patients, many believe that referral should be considered early, within 2 years of onset. It is useful to establish whether surgery is feasible at an early stage even for patients who are uncertain if they would undergo an operation. Patients will then be fully informed about the options available to them. Patients with identified lesions and those with the clinical syndrome of medial TLE are the most obvious candidates for early referral.

The aims of presurgical assessment are to identify an epileptogenic lesion and demonstrate, as far as possible, that the lesion can be removed without causing further, significant neurological or cognitive disability (Engel 1996). MRI will detect a structural lesion in over 80% of cases. If the lesion is potentially resectable, patients will usually proceed to video-EEG telemetry. Telemetry aims to establish that the seizures are indeed epileptic and also, through analysis of ictal EEG and clinical semiology, that seizures arise from the identified lesion. Invasive methods of EEG recording, including foramen ovale and subdural grid electrodes, may be required when scalp recordings are inconclusive. Ictal SPECT and interictal PET may also help localise functional abnormalities, and PET ligand studies may identify lesions not seen with MRI, thereby providing a guide for depth EEG studies in MRI-negative cases. Neuropsychological testing, particularly of verbal and non-verbal memory function, provides additional lateralising information. Studies of normal cortical function are conducted to delineate areas that must be preserved during surgery. Intracarotid amobarbital injection with language and memory testing (Wada test) is used to identify the language-dominant hemisphere and to predict the likely effect of medial temporal lobe excision on memory function. Functional MRI is likely to have a growing role in presurgical cortical mapping.

Presurgical assessment involves the evaluation of a large amount of complex information by a highly specialised multidisciplinary team. The decision to recommend operation is based on the degree of concordance between the many different findings. Psychiatric assessment prior to surgery is essential. Surgery should almost certainly not be undertaken in patients with comorbid dissociative seizures, as these are likely to persist with disastrous consequences for outcome. Overall, a history of psychiatric disorder is not a contraindication for surgery. A judgement must be made in each case about the relative contribution of psychiatric morbidity and epilepsy to the patient's quality of life. If chronic psychiatric problems are felt to be the overriding source of disability, and are viewed as largely independent of ongoing seizures, then even a successful operation may have little impact on the patient's overall well-being. The burden of a failed operation will be more profound in such patients and this will also have to be taken into consideration. Postictal psychosis might be regarded as a relative indication for surgery. However, recent evidence suggests that this, and possibly interictal psychosis, are associated with bilateral medial temporal lobe dysfunction, and this should be considered when evaluating electrophysiological and imaging data [see Postictal disorders (Psychosis)]. A higher burden of proof that disease is unilateral may be required in such cases. Presurgical psychiatric assessment will also aim to identify those patients, principally those with a past psychiatric history, who are at highest risk of developing psychiatric disorder postoperatively. The transient, but sometimes severe, depressive reactions seen after surgery have been described under Risk factors for depression, earlier. Postsurgical follow-up arrangements must be vigilant for these sequelae, which carry a risk of suicide and require prompt treatment.

Surgery involves either the resection of an epileptogenic lesion or disconnection of pathways that serve seizure propagation (Polkey 2004). Temporal lobe surgery usually involves either an anteromedial temporal lobectomy (most common) or a more selective amygdalohippocampectomy.

A recent randomised controlled trial of mesial temporal lobe surgery found that 64% of patients who received surgery were free of disabling seizures (defined as seizures involving impaired consciousness) by 1 year compared with 8% of those treated medically (Wiebe *et al.* 2001). These results are almost identical to those of earlier uncontrolled surgical series that reported seizure-free rates of 68% at 1–2 years (Engel 1996). Significant improvements in quality of life only occur in patients who become seizure-free (Birbeck *et al.* 2002). The major determinant of outcome is pathological substrate. Patients with foreign tissue lesions (low-grade tumours of astrocytic or mixed origin including DNETs and focal cortical dysplasias) have a slightly better outcome than those with medial temporal sclerosis (Berkovic *et al.* 1995). This almost certainly reflects the fact that hippocampal sclerosis is bilateral in about 13% of cases and may be difficult to detect with MRI. A normal MRI predicts a poor (20% seizure-free) outcome (Berkovic *et al.* 1995; Hennessy *et al.* 2001). Serious complications, such as stroke or large visual field defects, occur in less than 2% (Behrens *et al.* 1997). Contralateral peripheral superior quadrant visual field defects following temporal lobectomy are usually small and not noticed by the patient. Minor word-finding difficulties are relatively common, especially after dominant hemisphere operations (Hermann *et al.* 1991). Postoperative cognitive, and particularly memory, function is determined primarily by the preoperative state. Deficits are more often detected in those with high preoperative functioning, while improvements may be seen in those functioning at a low level preoperatively (Chelune *et al.* 1991). Significant new memory deficits were seen in 5% of patients in the controlled trial mentioned above. Such deficits show the expected pattern of lateralisation (Morris *et al.* 1995; Martin *et al.* 1998). Stereotactically guided radiotherapy for epilepsy is a relatively recent technique that requires further evaluation, particularly with respect to possible longer-term effects including delayed radionecrosis (Regis *et al.* 2000).

There are few data concerning outcome following neocortical (temporal and extratemporal) resections (Engel *et al.* 2003). Overall, results appear less favourable, with seizure-free rates of around 50%. As might be expected, cases with a clearly identifiable lesion have a better outcome (63% seizure-free). Hemispherectomy or multilobar resection can be a dramatically successful procedure in infants or children with extensive disease confined to one hemisphere. Seizure-free rates of 60–80% are achieved, typically with improved functioning of the affected limbs postoperatively (Devlin *et al.* 2003). Multiple subpial transection involves disruption of intracortical connections while preserving the columnar pathways necessary for normal function. It is an effective treatment in Landau–Kleffner syndrome and may produce dramatic improvements in behaviour and language function (Robinson *et al.* 2001). The technique is also performed, usually in combination with limited resection, in adults with partial onset seizures where adequate resection alone cannot be performed. A meta-analysis of over 200 such cases reported 95% seizure reduction in over two-thirds of cases, with new neurological deficits occurring in 22% (Spencer *et al.* 2002). Callosotomy, which involves resection of the corpus callosum (usually the anterior two-thirds), is a highly effective treatment for drop attacks (but not other seizure types) in children with severe symptomatic generalised epilepsy, e.g. Lennox–Gastaut syndrome. VNS may be an effective alternative in this situation (Hosain *et al.* 2000; Frost *et al.* 2001).

Vagal nerve stimulation

Vagal nerve stimulation was introduced as a treatment for epilepsy over 10 years ago (Schachter 2002). The procedure involves intermittent electrical stimulation of the vagus nerve via a stimulator inserted surgically over the anterior chest wall. The mechanism of action is unknown. Stimulation parameters are adjusted externally by means of a magnet and patients with auras can also trigger the device at seizure onset. VNS is usually considered for patients who prove unsuitable for epilepsy surgery but there is some evidence of efficacy in generalised epilepsy syndromes (Labar *et al.* 1999; Holmes *et al.* 2004; Ng & Devinsky 2004). Overall, a 50% reduction in seizure frequency is seen in approximately 30% of patients. Seizure remission rates are much lower, perhaps 5–10% (Helmers *et al.* 2003). Full benefit is often not achieved for several months. VNS is generally well tolerated: the main side effects are intermittent hoarseness of the voice and throat discomfort during stimulation but patients usually habituate to this. A reduction in antiepileptic medication is often possible. Positive effects on mood and behaviour have been reported in some studies (Elger *et al.* 2000). Further work to define which patients are most likely to benefit from VNS is required.

Psychological treatment of epilepsy

A number of observations suggest that psychological approaches to seizure control should be helpful. People with epilepsy typically report that stress is an aggravating factor and it would seem logical to expect that helping people deal better with stress might be accompanied by a reduction in seizures. A small proportion of patients describe being able to wilfully precipitate seizures by focusing on mental experiences they have as part of their aura (Fenwick & Brown 1989). If mental processes can trigger seizures, might they not also be used to inhibit them? Many patients are indeed convinced they can modify or stop seizures through voluntary acts of will (Spector *et al.* 2001). The hope that the mind might be harnessed to control the brain has also been founded on the observation that people can learn to control certain aspects of EEG recordings using biofeedback techniques (Fenwick 1992). The numerous studies in this area have been reviewed by Goldstein (1997) and are the subject of a Cochrane review (Ramaratnam *et al.* 2005). Studies have been small and poorly designed, and as yet there is no good evidence of efficacy. However, several areas deserve further investigation.

Cognitive–behaviour therapy may target background factors such as anxiety and coping skills. More specific interventions involve a variety of cognitive and relaxation techniques that patients can engage when they experience an aura or prodromal symptoms. Such cued countermeasures, conceived of as the psychological opposite of a patient's habitual experience at seizure onset, may be tailored to match individual patients' symptoms. For example, if the patient typically feels drowsy prior to a seizure, the countermeasure might aim to heighten arousal. Heightened arousal might also have a more general application in patients with epilepsy: an inverse correlation between autonomic arousal and contingent negative variation, a marker of cortical excitability, has been demonstrated and provisionally mapped to a distributed network of brain regions including thalamus, cingulate cortex, sensorimotor cortex and insula (Nagai *et al.* 2004a). In a small treatment study, the same group have reported a method of training patients to achieve heightened levels of autonomic arousal using biofeedback from (reduced) galvanic skin resistance (Nagai *et al.* 2004b). Patients were instructed to use the technique in response to seizure warnings. Six of nine patients achieved a 50% reduction in seizure frequency over a follow-up period that was limited to 3 months. These studies suggest a plausible physiological mechanism of action but, like many before them, provide only weak evidence that psychological treatment is effective.

Non-pharmacological approaches to treatment, including psychological ones, that give patients a sense of self-control and avoid toxic side effects are obviously an attractive prospect. Many clinicians would like to be able to recommend such treatment, but large well-designed clinical trials are needed to establish their efficacy.

Status epilepticus

Status epilepticus is usually defined as a condition in which epileptic activity persists for 30 minutes or more (Shorvon 2001; Walker & Shorvon 2004). Convulsive status is the term used to describe the status form of tonic–clonic seizures. The clinical features of non-convulsive status have been described under Non-convulsive status epilepticus. About 5% of adults with epilepsy will experience at least one episode of status. In children, the proportion is higher (25%). Common precipitants include drug withdrawal, intercurrent illness and metabolic disturbance. However, most status arises in people who have no prior history of epilepsy and is due to acute cerebral insult. The most common causes in this situation are CNS infection, trauma, stroke, hypoxia, metabolic disorders and alcohol withdrawal.

Convulsive status is a medical emergency. The risk of irreversible brain damage increases progressively from about 1 hour after onset and it is imperative that if seizures are not controlled by this time, anaesthesia should be instituted. For patients with established epilepsy, the duration of their habitual seizures will guide the decision about when to start treatment. As a general rule, treatment should be instituted after 5–10 minutes of continuing seizure activity. In a community setting, buccal midazolam (adult dose 10 mg) or rectal diazepam (adult dose 10–30 mg) may be given by carers or paramedics (both drugs can be repeated after 15 minutes). In medical settings, the first-line treatment is lorazepam (adult dose 4 mg) given as an intravenous bolus. An adequate airway must be secured and oxygen should always be given. The ECG should be monitored. An intravenous line is required for fluid replacement and drug administration. Blood should be taken for blood gases, glucose, renal and liver function, calcium and magnesium, full haematological screen (including platelets), clotting profile and antiepileptic drug levels. If hypoglycaemia is suspected, 50 mL of 50% glucose should be given immediately by intravenous injection. If there is suspicion of alcoholism or any other state of compromised nutrition, thiamine 250 mg should also be given. This is especially important if glucose has been administered (because of the heightened risk of Wernicke's encephalopathy). The timing of further investigations, including neuroimaging, will depend on circumstances.

If the initial bolus of lorazepam is ineffective, it may be repeated after 10 minutes, but second-line treatment should be considered at this point. Phenobarbital and phenytoin are the drugs of first choice at this stage. If the episode has been precipitated by withdrawal from antiepileptic medication, this should be restarted. If seizures continue despite these measures, the patient should be transferred to intensive care and anaesthesia instituted. Cerebral damage is caused, at least partly, by the direct effects of ongoing seizure activity. EEG monitoring is therefore critical at this stage.

Absence status is a benign condition and does not require aggressive treatment. Episodes are usually terminated quickly with benzodiazepines. There is no good evidence that aggressive treatment is warranted in complex partial status. The emphasis is instead on early recognition and treatment is with benzodiazepines. Some patients have recurrent episodes that are heralded by severe clusters of seizures. These can often be treated at home with oral benzodiazepines.

Sudden death in epilepsy

It has long been suspected that people with epilepsy are at risk of sudden unexplained death but the nature and extent of this risk were unknown until relatively recently. By 1997, Annegers was able to estimate a near 40-fold increased risk in people with epilepsy compared with the general population. Quantification of the risk is clearly of the utmost importance in counselling patients and in making treatment decisions. The overall annual incidence of SUDEP has been estimated as 0.35 per 1000 patients (Ficker *et al.* 1998), but in patients with severe intractable epilepsy it may be much higher. For example, in patients being assessed, or waiting, for epilepsy surgery an annual incidence of 1 in 100 has been reported (Dasheiff 1991). Among patients attending a tertiary care service a representative figure would be about 1 in 250 (O'Donoghue & Sander 1997; Tomson *et al.* 2005).

That the overwhelming majority of these deaths are seizure related is no longer doubted. The mechanisms are not yet clear and are the subject of intense investigation (Nashef *et al.* 2007). Progress has been made, however, and it appears that apnoea is an important mechanism in many cases. Asystole is also likely to be important, independent of respiratory arrest, and may be related to the well-documented but rare occurrence of ictal bradycardia (see Differential diagnosis of epilepsy, Syncope, earlier in chapter).

Risk factors have been investigated in observational series and case–control studies. Factors including frequent seizures, tonic–clonic seizures, taking two or more antiepileptic drugs, recent antiepileptic drug withdrawal, and never having received drug treatment have consistently emerged as important (Nashef & Langan 2004; Tomson *et al.* 2005). There is some evidence that carbamazepine may be overrepresented but this finding, and the association with polytherapy, may be surrogate markers for epilepsy severity. However, antiepileptic drugs, particularly polytherapy, are sometimes known to exacerbate seizures and this may be a factor (Perucca *et al.* 1998). Most recently, based on an analysis of antiepileptic drug levels in hair samples, Williams *et al.* (2006) have provided evidence that erratic drug compliance may also be important. Most cases of SUDEP are unwitnessed and occur at night. From this and other observations it has long been suspected that lack of supervision at night might be a risk factor (Nashef *et al.* 1995). This was confirmed by the most recent case–control study: sharing a bedroom with someone capable of giving assistance and the use of listening devices were both significant protective factors (Langan *et al.* 2005).

Several important clinical implications arise from these findings. Seizure prevention, particularly prevention of tonic–clonic seizures, must be the aim of treatment. Abrupt changes in medication should be avoided and any recently introduced drug that exacerbates seizures should be withdrawn. Patients must be warned about the dangers of not taking medication regularly. The findings also emphasise the importance of first aid advice. Patients should be attended to quickly during a seizure: simple measures such as positioning them and stimulating them if they are not breathing may be life-saving.

Table 6.17 Information for patients with epilepsy.

Nature of epilepsy
Aetiology and prognosis
Drug treatment
    Efficacy
    Side effects
    Interactions
    Compliance
Likely duration of treatment
Aggravating factors
Risks of seizures
    First aid
    Accidental injury
    Sudden unexplained death in epilepsy
Driving
Education/employment
Special issues for women

Patient education

Providing information for a patient newly diagnosed with epilepsy is a major part of treatment. The points that need to be covered are listed in Table 6.17. Information sheets published by the epilepsy societies are an invaluable resource and should be made readily available to patients and their families. Epilepsy is poorly understood by the general public and still carries the stigma of mental illness, and even of supernatural phenomena (Caveness & Gallup 1980; Jacoby *et al.* 2004; Diamantopoulos *et al.* 2006). The nature of epilepsy must therefore be carefully explained. Advice about treatment and prognosis will obviously be dictated by aetiology and syndrome diagnosis. For most patients, the good news is that medication is highly likely to stop their seizures and investigations will have ruled out any sinister, progressive underlying disease. The clinician will often have a fairly good idea from the start about the likelihood that medication will need to be continued long term. It is as well to raise this difficult issue early on. As treatment is started, discussion must cover the likely benefits and side effects of treatment. Patients need to be warned about hypersensitivity reactions but also reassured that if symptoms of dose-related toxicity develop, these can readily be dealt with by adjusting the dose and slowing the rate of dose increase. Patients need to be aware of the possibility of drug interactions. It is important to stress that medication must be taken regularly, both to be effective and because of the risks of withdrawal seizures. Advice about exacerbating factors needs to be given. Sleep deprivation should be avoided as should excessive alcohol consumption. In relation to the latter point, one or two units, once or twice a week, is probably safe (Hoppener *et al.* 1983). Patients and their carers will often be very worried about the risks of accidental injury. In general, they can be reassured that the risk is small. First aid advice (protection from injury, recovery position, when to call for help) should be provided for the patient and carers. Taking a bath unsupervised should be avoided: showers are safer and scald injuries can be prevented by thermostatic control of the hot water. Most sports are safe with a few obvious exceptions (e.g. scuba diving, rock climbing, skydiving). Swimming is generally regarded as safe if supervison is available. If seizures do not remit, patients will gradually come to conclusions about what level of risk is acceptable in trying to live as normal and independent a life as possible. How frequent seizures are and whether they are preceded by a useful warning will obviously be factored into the decision. A few patients may choose to live rather recklessly, but this may seem preferable to being overly cautious and over-protected. The issue of SUDEP needs to be discussed sensitively. A number of the special issues relating to women have already been mentioned (see Patient characteristics, earlier). These include possible drug interactions with the oral contraceptive pill, considerations relating to pregnancy, and the increased risk of bone disease in postmenopausal patients (Crawford *et al.* 1999).

Driving is an important issue that must be covered at the time of diagnosis. Driving laws vary around the world. In the UK, regulations are regularly updated. At present, an ordinary driver's licence may be granted to an individual if free of seizures for 1 year or if seizures have occurred only during sleep for at least 3 years. An additional condition is that allowing the patient to drive must not be likely to endanger the public. Thus, other factors such as neurological or psychiatric comorbidity and medication effects must be considered. Special consideration may be given following a single seizure if provoking factors are clearly identified and non-recurrent. Additional restrictions apply to a commercial drivers licence, in which case a seizure-free period of 10 years (off medication) is required, and there must be no identifiable ongoing liability to seizures. The licensing authority recommends that where medication is being withdrawn after seizure remission, the patient should not drive during the period of withdrawal and for 6 months afterwards. However, there is no requirement that the driving licence be surrendered.

Epilepsy may have far-reaching effects on education and employment prospects. Some jobs may not be possible, for example those that require a driving licence or entail sole responsibility for the safety of others, but people with epilepsy are undoubtedly subject to discrimination (Chaplin 2005). Interventions to educate employers and teachers can be extremely effective in this situation.

Treatment of psychiatric disorder in epilepsy

Patients with chronic epilepsy often represent complex and challenging management problems. Some difficulties will relate directly to ongoing seizures and their treatment. Others will be more obviously 'psychiatric': depression or psychosis for example, or social problems related to education, employment, interpersonal relationships or care provision. Yet a simple division into 'neurological' and 'psychiatric' is seldom possible or desirable. A management plan will need to consider the type of epilepsy, its underlying cause and its current and potential treatment, all of which must be set within the context of psychiatric diagnosis, cognitive function and capacity for independent living, social circumstances and support networks. The causes, treatment and outcome of each set of problems are mutually dependent. Management requires a holistic approach from a multidisciplinary team that might include nurse specialists, psychologists, occupational and speech therapists, physiotherapists, social workers and doctors. Every member of the team should have special knowledge and experience of epilepsy. The service should have links with the epilepsy societies and with support groups for patients and carers. Liaison with primary care and with other specialist services will be essential if complex management plans are to have any chance of success.

Assessment will naturally involve a review of the epilepsy history and how this relates to the psychiatric presentation. Two aspects of the neurological history are particularly important. The first concerns the temporal relationship between seizures and psychiatric disorder. The clinician must assess whether the two are related and, if so, whether psychiatric symptoms are ictal, postictal or interictal. This distinction has important implications for treatment and prognosis. Psychotic symptoms are a good example. Ictal psychotic symptoms are simply an expression of epilepsy. Their importance lies primarily in recognising them as epileptic and differentiating them from functional psychiatric disorder: seizure control will be the focus of treatment and neuroleptics have no role. If a diagnosis of postictal psychosis has been made, symptoms will be expected to resolve spontaneously in a few days. Admission and sedation with benzodiazepines may be required but neuroleptics usually will not. In the longer term, recurrence may be prevented with better control of the epilepsy. However, if the diagnosis is one of interictal psychosis, then management, including pharmacological and non-pharmacological measures, will be along lines that would be familiar to a general psychiatrist treating a patient with schizophrenia.

The second particularly important aspect of the neurological history concerns treatment history. Antiepileptic drugs are a common cause of cognitive, behavioural and psychiatric morbidity in people with epilepsy. Mood disturbance and psychosis may occur as a direct consequence of any antiepileptic drug and any changes in treatment that preceded the onset of psychiatric symptoms may implicate a specific cause. A more common problem concerns the dose-related toxic effects of drugs on the CNS, which may present with cognitive slowing, underperformance at school or work, and any number of behavioural problems. Polypharmacy is particularly associated with this clinical picture. Overly aggressive treatment of epilepsy may also sometimes cause a worsening of seizure control with further effects on psychosocial functioning. Optimising the treatment of the patient's epilepsy – achieving control of seizures with the minimum of side effects – is often one of the most important aspects of 'psychiatric' treatment.

In general, the psychiatric disorders associated with epilepsy are treated as they would be if epilepsy were not present. In the absence of any well-designed treatment trials, treatment is based on opinion and experience. This is clearly a deficiency, but it is reassuring that several decades of clinical experience have not highlighted any striking differences between the outcome of psychiatric treatment in epilepsy and that which might be expected in general psychiatric practice. As in other areas of psychiatry, treatment may involve medication, psychological treatment and social measures. The indications for each are much as they would be in the absence of epilepsy.

Psychotropic medication in epilepsy

The most frequently cited treatment problem is that most psychotropic drugs have the potential to exacerbate seizures. However, this has been overstated in the past. Useful reviews of this issue have been provided by McConnell and Duncan (1998), Alldredge (1999) and Pisani et al. (2002). Concern about the proconvulsant effect of psychotropics stems from a number of sources, including studies in animals, reports of adverse reactions to drug monitoring agencies (including reports of seizures after overdose), and data concerning the incidence of seizures in preclinical and clinical trials. It is extremely difficult to draw any clear recommendations for clinical practice from these data. Clozapine is the one drug undoubtedly associated with a significant risk of seizures. As with other psychotropic drugs the proconvulsant effect of clozapine is dose related; as a guide, seizures may be expected in 2–3% of patients (with no prior history of epilepsy) with doses in the range 300–600 mg daily (Devinsky et al. 1991). With this exception, the incidence of seizures in non-epileptic individuals treated with therapeutic doses of antidepressants and antipsychotics is very low, well below 1% (Alldredge 1999). Comparisons between individual drugs cannot be made conclusively, but there is some suggestion that the more recently introduced antidepressants are marginally less proconvulsant than tricyclics. However, none of these data reveal how significant the risk of seizures is when psychotropics are given to people with epilepsy. It is quite reasonably assumed that patients with epilepsy will be more sensitive to proconvulsant effects. However, most people with epilepsy are of course taking antiepileptic drugs and this will presumably have a moderating effect. Large well-designed trials of psychotropics in patients with epilepsy would be required to answer this question and as yet have not been done. In relation to antidepressants, small trials have reported no exacerbation of seizures with amitriptyline and nomifensine (Robertson & Trimble 1985), fluvoxamine (Harmant et al. 1990), paroxetine (Andersen et al. 1991), and citalopram, mirtazapine or reboxetine (Kuhn et al. 2003). In a report of 97 patients treated with sertraline, increased seizure frequency occurred in six patients, one definitely so, the remaining five only possibly and transiently (Kanner et al. 2000). Two studies have in fact described *improvement* in seizure control, one with fluoxetine (Favale et al. 1995) and one with citalopram (Specchio et al. 2004). While it seems improbable that antidepressants have a clinically useful antiepileptic action, these findings serve to emphasise that, in therapeutic doses, antidepressants are most unlikely to have any detrimental effect on seizure control. There are no controlled trials of neuroleptics in patients with epilepsy. Pauig et al. (1961) reported improvement in seizure frequency, or no change, in two-thirds of 100 patients with epilepsy treated with thioridazine. There are very few reports of lithium treatment in patients with epilepsy. Lithium is markedly proconvulsant in overdose but is probably not associated with any change in seizure control at therapeutic doses.

Treatment of depression and anxiety

In light of the data reviewed above, clinicians should not hesitate to prescribe antidepressants for patients with epilepsy if they would otherwise be indicated. Recommended drugs, drawn from the reviews cited above, include citalopram, escitalopram, fluoxetine, mirtazapine, moclobemide, nefazodone, paroxetine, reboxetine, sertraline, trazodone and venlafaxine. Tricyclic antidepressants (e.g. amitriptyline, clomipramine, dothiepin, lofepramine, imipramine, nortriptyline and trimipramine) are associated with a higher risk of seizure exacerbation. They should be regarded as second-line choices, but are by no means contraindicated in the presence of epilepsy. The proconvulsant effect of all these drugs is dose related. A sensible approach is therefore to start treatment at relatively low doses and to increase the dose slowly. As with antidepressant treatment outside the context of epilepsy, choice of drug and treatment failure will primarily be influenced by side effects other than any effect on seizure control. In exceptional cases, where an exacerbation of seizures does occur, it is almost always of a minor degree and an alternative drug better tolerated by that individual can usually be found. There are many potential interactions with antiepileptic drugs, especially with the hepatic enzyme-inducing drugs, and these should always be checked before prescribing. In practice there are few clinically significant interactions (i.e. interactions that involve commonly prescribed combinations or are of large effect-size). More common examples include the following: fluoxetine and sertraline may increase serum levels of phenytoin, and sertraline may cause a rise in lamotrigine levels. Electroconvulsive therapy is an effective and safe treatment for severe depression in epilepsy (Lunde *et al.* 2006). Seizure induction is usually possible without reduction of antiepileptic drugs and there is usually no discernible effect on seizure frequency.

The profound impact that epilepsy may have on almost every aspect of life has been mentioned many times in this chapter. The frustration of restricted opportunites in work and leisure, difficulties with personal relationships and the stigma, both real and perceived, attached to seizures all contribute to the development and maintenance of depression. Psychotherapeutic approaches are as important in epilepsy as they are in general psychiatry. As in other areas of psychiatry, the type of therapy is possibly not as important as the individual qualities of the therapist. In this respect, therapists with experience of epilepsy will have a number of advantages: familiarity with the practical issues likely to be involved (e.g. treatment and safety issues, work and driving restrictions) and being able to place a patient's difficulties in the context of other cases will facilitate an empathic therapeutic relationship. Epilepsy nurse specialists can play an invaluable role in providing patient and carer education, longer-term support and liaison between the different agencies often involved in caring for the most vulnerable patients (Ridsdale *et al.* 1999). Cognitive–behaviour therapy may have a special place in the management of 'seizure phobia', a term used to describe the not uncommon situation in which a patient is more disabled by fear of having seizures than by the seizures themselves (see Anxiety, earlier in chapter). Specific therapeutic strategies might include challenging negative cognitions and cognitive schema concerning epilepsy, and seeking to modify safety and avoidant behaviours (Newsom-Davis *et al.* 1998).

Treatment of psychosis

Most cases of interictal psychosis will require treatment with neuroleptic drugs. Drugs regarded as being associated with a low risk of seizure exacerbation include sulpiride, haloperidol, risperidone and trifluoperazine. Amisulpiride, olanzapine and quetiapine are regarded as having a higher risk but this is probably marginal and the choice of treatment will be dictated primarily by consideration of the more general side-effect profile of the drug. Depot neuroleptics should probably be avoided because although the risk of seizure exacerbation is low, if there is an exacerbation of seizures, the offending drug may not be quickly withdrawn. A 'start low, go slow' approach is again sensible. As with antidepressants, there are a large number of potential interactions with antiepileptic drugs but these are generally not clinically significant. The treatment of refractory psychosis poses a difficult problem because of the marked proconvulsant effect of clozapine, the only drug with established efficacy in this situation. However, Langosch and Trimble (2002) have described

six patients with refractory psychosis and epilepsy who were successfully treated with clozapine, without exacerbation of seizure frequency. Such treatment should be initiated in hospital. The most important interactions between antiepileptic drugs and clozapine are pharmacodynamic: if the patient is taking carbamazepine, this should probably be replaced because of the potential synergistic risk of agranulocytosis. Lamotrigine, or one of the newer antiepileptic drugs, may be preferable to valproate because of the likelihood of weight gain and sedation with the latter.

As already mentioned, postictal psychosis does not generally require treatment with neuroleptics. The marked agitation often seen in this disorder may necessitate hospital admission and symptomatic treatment (sedation) with benzodiazepines. If antipsychotic agents are used, it is very important that they are withdrawn promptly once symptoms have resolved. A small proportion of patients will eventually progress from postictal to chronic interictal psychosis but there is no evidence to support prophylactic use of antipsychotics to prevent this progression.

Treatment of dissociative seizures

The most important, and often the most difficult, step in managing patients with dissociative seizures is engaging them in psychiatric treatment. How the diagnosis is communicated to the patient is critical. Shen *et al.* (1990) and Mellers (2005) have discussed this issue in some detail (Table 6.18). Patients are obviously extremely sensitive to any suggestion that they are feigning their symptoms. A description of dissociation and of any likely aetiological factors to emerge in the history will help patients understand what the disorder is and why they have it (see Dissociative seizures, earlier). Dissociative seizures often reduce in frequency and may even stop after the patient is given the diagnosis (Farias *et al.*

Table 6.18 Presenting the diagnosis of dissociative seizures.

Explanation of the diagnosis
Reasons for concluding that the patient does not have epilepsy
What the patient does have (describe dissociation)

Reassurance
That patient is *not* suspected of 'putting on' the attacks
That the disorder is very common

Causes of the disorder
Triggering 'stresses' for seizures may not be immediately apparent
Any specific aetiological factors relevant
Importance of maintaining factors

Treatment
Suggest that seizures usually improve after the correct diagnosis is made
Caution that antiepileptic drug withdrawal should be gradual
Limited role of psychotropic medication
Describe psychological treatment

2003). This is especially likely when seizures are of recent onset. Many clinicians believe that suggestion may be an important adjunct to this effect. Patients should be cautioned not to stop antiepileptic drugs suddenly. Carers should be involved in these discussions, with the patient's consent, as early as possible.

Reuber *et al.* (2005) have recently provided a comprehensive review of specific approaches to treatment. Treatment should aim to control seizures but this may be achieved without any real improvement in overall outcome. Background psychosocial factors must also be addressed. Patients with dissociative seizures often have a history of depression and anxiety disorder but these symptoms are usually mild and pharmacotherapy plays a relatively minor role. The mainstay of treatment is usually some form of psychological therapy. Many approaches have been advocated but there have been no controlled treatment trials. The early literature includes several compelling reports of psychodynamic approaches, often in patients with traumatic childhood experiences. Operant behavioural programmes using simple reward systems may be very effective in patients with learning disability. Variations of therapy based on psychodynamic, insight-oriented and group-based methods are undoubtedly widely practised and require further evaluation.

The paroxysmal nature of dissociative seizures lends itself to a cognitive–behaviour approach modelled on that developed in panic disorder and post-traumatic stress disorder. Rusch *et al.* (2001) combined such approaches with psychodynamic methods in a series of 33 patients, one-third of whom had a relatively short duration of illness (less than 1 year); 63% were free of seizures at the end of treatment. In a smaller series of 20 patients with a longer history of seizures, Goldstein *et al.* (2004) reported more modest improvement in seizure control (20% seizure-free) but significant gains in work and social outcome.

The most difficult group to treat is undoubtedly those patients with coexistent epilepsy. In many cases dissociative seizures are the major source of disability but distinguishing between the different types of seizures may be very difficult. Showing patients and carers videos obtained during telemetry is invaluable but the situation often changes over time; semiology changes, new seizures appear and telemetry may have to be repeated. A significant proportion of patients continue to have seizures despite intensive treatment. A pragmatic approach in such cases, as in other somatoform disorders, is to offer long-term follow-up to provide support for the patient and family and to limit the costs and morbidity associated with further unnecessary investigations and medical interventions.

References

Acharya, V., Acharya, J. & Luders, H. (1998) Olfactory epileptic auras. *Neurology* **51**, 56–61.

Adachi, N., Matsuura, M., Okubo, Y. *et al.* (2000) Predictive variables of interictal psychosis in epilepsy. *Neurology* **55**, 1310–1314.

Agathonikou, A., Panayiotopoulos, C.P., Giannakodimos, S. & Koutroumanidis, M. (1998) Typical absence status in adults: diagnostic and syndromic considerations. *Epilepsia* **39**, 1265–1276.

Aicardi, J. (1986) Some epileptic syndromes in infancy and childhood and their relevance to the definition of epilepsy. In: Trimble, M.R. & Reynolds, E.H. (eds) *What is Epilepsy? The Clinical and Scientific Basis of Epilepsy*, ch. 3. Churchill Livingstone, Edinburgh.

Alarcon, G., Elwes, R.D., Polkey, C.E. & Binnie, C.D. (1998) Ictal oroalimentary automatisms with preserved consciousness: implications for the pathophysiology of automatisms and relevance to the international classification of seizures. *Epilepsia* **39**, 1119–1127.

Aldenkamp, A.P. & Arends, J. (2004) Effects of epileptiform EEG discharges on cognitive function: is the concept of 'transient cognitive impairment' still valid? *Epilepsy and Behavior* **5** (suppl. 1), S25–S34.

Aldenkamp, A.P., Alpherts, W.C., Bruine-Seeder, D. & Dekker, M.J. (1990) Test–retest variability in children with epilepsy: a comparison of WISC-R profiles. *Epilepsy Research* **7**, 165–172.

Alessio, A., Damasceno, B.P., Camargo, C.H., Kobayashi, E., Guerreiro, C.A. & Cendes, F. (2004) Differences in memory performance and other clinical characteristics in patients with mesial temporal lobe epilepsy with and without hippocampal atrophy. *Epilepsy and Behavior* **5**, 22–27.

Alldredge, B.K. (1999) Seizure risk associated with psychotropic drugs: clinical and pharmacokinetic considerations. *Neurology* **53** (5 suppl. 2), S68–S75.

Alper, K., Devinsky, O., Westbrook, L. *et al.* (2001) Premorbid psychiatric risk factors for postictal psychosis. *Journal of Neuropsychiatry and Clinical Neurosciences* **13**, 492–499.

Alstrom, C.H. (1950) A study of epilepsy in its clinical, social and genetic aspects. *Acta Psychiatrica et Neurologica Scandinavica Supplementum* **63**, 5–284.

Altay, E.E., Serdaroglu, A., Gucuyener, K., Bilir, E., Karabacak, N.I. & Thio, L.L. (2005) Rotational vestibular epilepsy from the temporo-parieto-occipital junction. *Neurology* **65**, 1675–1676.

Altshuler, L., Rausch, R., Delrahim, S., Kay, J. & Crandall, P. (1999) Temporal lobe epilepsy, temporal lobectomy, and major depression. *Journal of Neuropsychiatry and Clinical Neurosciences* **11**, 436–443.

Al Twaijri, W.A. & Shevell, M.I. (2002) Pediatric migraine equivalents: occurrence and clinical features in practice. *Pediatric Neurology* **26**, 365–368.

Alving, J. (1998) Serum prolactin levels are elevated also after pseudo-epileptic seizures. *Seizure* **7**, 85–89.

Andermann, F. & Berkovic, S.F. (2001) Idiopathic generalized epilepsy with generalized and other seizures in adolescence. *Epilepsia* **42**, 317–320.

Andersen, B.B., Mikkelsen, M., Vesterager, A. *et al.* (1991) No influence of the antidepressant paroxetine on carbamazepine, valproate and phenytoin. *Epilepsy Research* **10**, 201–204.

Andersson-Roswall, L., Engman, E., Samuelsson, H., Sjoberg-Larsson, C. & Malmgren, K. (2004) Verbal memory decline and adverse effects on cognition in adult patients with pharmacoresistant partial epilepsy: a longitudinal controlled study of 36 patients. *Epilepsy and Behavior* **5**, 677–686.

Annegers, J.F., Hauser, W.A., Shirts, S.B. & Kurland, L.T. (1987) Factors prognostic of unprovoked seizures after febrile convulsions. *New England Journal of Medicine* **316**, 493–498.

Annegers, J.F., Hauser, W.A., Beghi, E., Nicolosi, A. & Kurland, L.T. (1988) The risk of unprovoked seizures after encephalitis and meningitis. *Neurology* **38**, 1407–1410.

Annegers, J.F., Hauser, W.A., Lee, J.R. & Rocca, W.A. (1995) Incidence of acute symptomatic seizures in Rochester, Minnesota, 1935–1984. *Epilepsia* **36**, 327–333.

Annegers, J.F. (1997) United States perspective on definitions and classifications. *Epilepsia* **38** (suppl. 11), S9–S14.

Annegers, J.F., Hauser, W.A., Coan, S.P. & Rocca, W.A. (1998) A population-based study of seizures after traumatic brain injuries. *New England Journal of Medicine* **338**, 20–24.

Archer, J.S., Briellmann, R.S., Syngeniotis, A., Abbott, D.F. & Jackson, G.D. (2003) Spike-triggered fMRI in reading epilepsy: involvement of left frontal cortex working memory area. *Neurology* **60**, 415–421.

Audenaert, D., Van Broeckhoven, C. & De Jonghe, P. (2006) Genes and loci involved in febrile seizures and related epilepsy syndromes. *Human Mutation* **27**, 391–401.

Avoli, M., Rogawski, M.A. & Avanzini, G. (2001) Generalized epileptic disorders: an update. *Epilepsia* **42**, 445–457.

Bakker, M.J., van Dijk, J.G., van den Maagdenberg, A.M. & Tijssen, M.A. (2006) Startle syndromes. *Lancet Neurology* **5**, 513–524.

Barker, W. & Wolf, S. (1947) Studies in epilepsy. *American Journal of the Medical Sciences* **214**, 600–604.

Barkovich, A.J., Kuzniecky, R.I., Jackson, G.D., Guerrini, R. & Dobyns, W.B. (2001) Classification system for malformations of cortical development: update 2001. *Neurology* **57**, 2168–2178.

Barraclough, B. (1981) Suicide and epilepsy. In: Reynolds, E.H. & Trimble, M.R. (eds) *Epilepsy and Psychiatry*, ch. 7. Churchill Livingstone, Edinburgh.

Barry, E., Sussman, N.M., Bosley, T.M. & Harner, R.N. (1985) Ictal blindness and status epilepticus amauroticus. *Epilepsia* **26**, 577–584.

Bartolomei, F., Suchet, L., Barrie, M. & Gastaut, J.L. (1997) Alcoholic epilepsy: a unified and dynamic classification. *European Neurology* **37**, 13–17.

Bautista, R.E., Spencer, D.D. & Spencer, S.S. (1998) EEG findings in frontal lobe epilepsies. *Neurology* **50**, 1765–1771.

Bear, D.M. & Fedio, P. (1977) Quantitative analysis of interictal behaviour in temporal lobe epilepsy. *Archives of Neurology* **34**, 454–467.

Beghi, E. (2003) Overview of studies to prevent posttraumatic epilepsy. *Epilepsia* **44** (suppl. 10), 21–26.

Beghi, E. (2004) Aetiology of epilepsy. In: Shorvon, S.D., Perucca, E., Fish, D.R. & Dodson, W.E. (eds) *The Treatment of Epilepsy*, pp. 50–63. Blackwell Science, Malden, MA.

Beghi, E. & Cornaggia, C. (2002) Morbidity and accidents in patients with epilepsy: results of a European cohort study. *Epilepsia* **43**, 1076–1083.

Beghi, E., Spagnoli, P., Airoldi, L. *et al.* (2002) Emotional and effective disturbances in patients with epilepsy. *Epilepsy and Behavior* **3**, 255–261.

Behrens, E., Schramm, J., Zentner, J. & Konig, R. (1997) Surgical and neurological complications in a series of 708 epilepsy surgery procedures. *Neurosurgery* **41**, 1–9; discussion 9–10.

Benbadis, S.R. & Tatum, W.O. (2003) Overinterpretation of EEGs and misdiagnosis of epilepsy. *Journal of Clinical Neurophysiology* **20**, 42–44.

Benson, D.F. (1991) The Geschwind syndrome. *Advances in Neurology* **55**, 411–421.

Berg, A.T. & Shinnar, S. (1991) The risk of seizure recurrence following a first unprovoked seizure: a quantitative review. *Neurology* **41**, 965–972.

Berg, A.T. & Shinnar, S. (1994) Relapse following discontinuation of antiepileptic drugs: a meta-analysis. *Neurology* **44**, 601–608.

Berkley, H.J. (1901) *A Treatise on Mental Disease*. Henry Kimpton, London.

Berkovic, S.F., McIntosh, A.M., Kalnins, R.M. *et al.* (1995) Preoperative MRI predicts outcome of temporal lobectomy: an actuarial analysis. *Neurology* **45**, 1358–1363.

Berkovic, S.F., Howell, R.A., Hay, D.A. & Hopper, J.L. (1998) Epilepsies in twins: genetics of the major epilepsy syndromes. *Annals of Neurology* **43**, 435–445.

Berkovic, S.F., Arzimanoglou, A., Kuzniecky, R., Harvey, A.S., Palmini, A. & Andermann, F. (2003) Hypothalamic hamartoma and seizures: a treatable epileptic encephalopathy. *Epilepsia* **44**, 969–973.

Berkovic, S.F., Mulley, J.C., Scheffer, I.E. & Petrou, S. (2006) Human epilepsies: interaction of genetic and acquired factors. *Trends in Neurosciences* **29**, 391–397.

Bien, C.G., Benninger, F.O., Urbach, H., Schramm, J., Kurthen, M. & Elger, C.E. (2000) Localizing value of epileptic visual auras. *Brain* **123**, 244–253.

Bien, C.G., Granata, T., Antozzi, C. *et al.* (2005) Pathogenesis, diagnosis and treatment of Rasmussen encephalitis: a European consensus statement. Brain **128**, 454–471.

Binnie, C.D. (2003) Cognitive impairment during epileptiform discharges: is it ever justifiable to treat the EEG? *Lancet Neurology* **2**, 725–730.

Binzer, M., Stone, J. & Sharpe, M. (2004) Recent onset pseudoseizures: clues to aetiology. *Seizure* **13**, 146–155.

Biraben, A., Taussig, D., Thomas, P. *et al.* (2001) Fear as the main feature of epileptic seizures. *Journal of Neurology, Neurosurgery and Psychiatry* **70**, 186–191.

Birbeck, G.L., Hays, R.D., Cui, X. & Vickrey, B.G. (2002) Seizure reduction and quality of life improvements in people with epilepsy. *Epilepsia* **43**, 535–538.

Blakeley, J. & Jankovic, J. (2002) Secondary paroxysmal dyskinesias. *Movement Disorders* **17**, 726–734.

Blanke, O., Ortigue, S., Coeytaux, A., Martory, M.D. & Landis, T. (2003) Hearing of a presence. *Neurocase* **9**, 329–339.

Blume, W.T. & Wiebe, S. (2000) Occipital lobe epilepsies. *Advances in Neurology* **84**, 173–187.

Blume, W.T., Luders, H.O., Mizrahi, E., Tassinari, C., van Emde, B.W. & Engel, J. Jr (2001) Glossary of descriptive terminology for ictal semiology: report of the ILAE task force on classification and terminology. *Epilepsia* **42**, 1212–1218.

Blumer, D. (1991) Epilepsy and disorders of mood. *Advances in Neurology* **55**, 185–195.

Blumer, D. (1999) Evidence supporting the temporal lobe epilepsy personality syndrome. *Neurology* **53** (5 suppl. 2), S9–S12.

Blumer, D., Montouris, G. & Hermann, B. (1995) Psychiatric morbidity in seizure patients on a neurodiagnostic monitoring unit. *Journal of Neuropsychiatry and Clinical Neurosciences* **7**, 445–456.

Bouma, P.A., Westendorp, R.G., van Dijk, J.G., Peters, A.C. & Brouwer, O.F. (1996) The outcome of absence epilepsy: a meta-analysis. *Neurology* **47**, 802–808.

Bourgeois, B.F., Prensky, A.L., Palkes, H.S., Talent, B.K. & Busch, S.G. (1983) Intelligence in epilepsy: a prospective study in children. *Annals of Neurology* **14**, 438–444.

Bowman, E.S. & Markand, O.N. (1996) Psychodynamics and psychiatric diagnoses of pseudoseizure subjects. *American Journal of Psychiatry* **153**, 57–63.

Boylan, L.S., Flint, L.A., Labovitz, D.L., Jackson, S.C., Starner, K. & Devinsky, O. (2004) Depression but not seizure frequency predicts quality of life in treatment-resistant epilepsy. *Neurology* **62**, 258–261.

Briellmann, R.S., Kalnins, R.M., Hopwood, M.J., Ward, C., Berkovic, S.F. & Jackson, G.D. (2000) TLE patients with postictal psychosis: mesial dysplasia and anterior hippocampal preservation. *Neurology* **55**, 1027–1030.

Briellmann, R.S., Wellard, R.M. & Jackson, G.D. (2005) Seizure-associated abnormalities in epilepsy: evidence from MR imaging. *Epilepsia* **46**, 760–766.

Brignole, M. (2007) Diagnosis and treatment of syncope. *Heart* **93**, 130–136.

Brignole, M., Alboni, P., Benditt, D.G. *et al.* (2004) Guidelines on management (diagnosis and treatment) of syncope: update 2004. Executive Summary. *European Heart Journal* **25**, 2054–2072.

Brignole, M., Sutton, R., Menozzi, C. *et al.* (2006) Early application of an implantable loop recorder allows effective specific therapy in patients with recurrent suspected neurally mediated syncope. *European Heart Journal* **27**, 1085–1092.

British National Formulary (2006) BMJ Publishing Group and RPS Publishing, London.

Brodie, M.J. & Kwan, P. (2005) Epilepsy in elderly people. *British Medical Journal* **331**, 1317–1322.

Brookes, G. & Crawford, P. (2002) The associations between epilepsy and depressive illness in secondary care. *Seizure* **11**, 523–526.

Brown, S. & Bird, J. (2001) Continuing professional development: medico-legal aspects of epilepsy. *Seizure* **10**, 68–73; quiz 73–74.

Bruno, M.K., Hallett, M., Gwinn-Hardy, K. *et al.* (2004) Clinical evaluation of idiopathic paroxysmal kinesigenic dyskinesia: new diagnostic criteria. *Neurology* **63**, 2280–2287.

Bruno, M.K., Lee, H.-Y., Auburger, G.W.J. *et al.* (2007) Genotype–phenotype correlation of paroxysmal nonkinesigenic dyskinesia. *Neurology* **68**, 1782–1789.

Bruton, C.J. (1988) *The Neuropathology of Temporal Lobe Epilepsy.* Maudsley Monograph No. 31. Oxford University Press, Oxford.

Bruton, C.J., Stevens, J.R. & Frith, C.D. (1994) Epilepsy, psychosis, and schizophrenia: clinical and neuropathologic correlations. *Neurology* **44**, 34–42.

Bureau, M. & Tassinari, C.A. (2005) Epilepsy with myoclonic absences. *Brain and Development* **27**, 178–184.

Burn, J., Dennis, M., Bamford, J., Sandercock, P., Wade, D. & Warlow, C. (1997) Epileptic seizures after a first stroke: the Oxfordshire Community Stroke Project. *British Medical Journal* **315**, 1582–1587.

Butler, C.R. (2006) Transient epileptic amnesia. *Practical Neurology* **6**, 368–371.

Cascino, G.D. (1990) Epilepsy and brain tumors: implications for treatment. *Epilepsia* **31** (suppl. 3), S37–S44.

Caveness, W.F. & Gallup, G.H. Jr (1980) A survey of public attitudes toward epilepsy in 1979 with an indication of trends over the past thirty years. *Epilepsia* **21**, 509–518.

Caveness, W.F., Meirowsky, M., Rish, B.L. *et al.* (1979) The nature of post-traumatic epilepsy. *Journal of Neurosurgery* **50**, 545–553.

Chadwick, D. (1993) Seizures, epilepsy, and other episodic disorders. In: Walton, J. (ed.) *Brain's Diseases of the Nervous System*, 10th edn, ch. 22. Oxford University Press, Oxford.

Chadwick, D. (1994) Epilepsy. *Journal of Neurology, Neurosurgery and Psychiatry* **57**, 264–277.

Chadwick, D. & Smith, D. (2002) The misdiagnosis of epilepsy. *British Medical Journal* **324**, 495–496.

Chaplin, J. (2005) Vocational assessment and intervention for people with epilepsy. *Epilepsia* **46** (suppl. 1), 55–56.

Chelune, G.J., Naugle, R.I., Luders, H. & Awad, I.A. (1991) Prediction of cognitive change as a function of preoperative ability status among temporal lobectomy patients seen at 6-month follow-up. *Neurology* **41**, 399–404.

Chen, D.K., So, Y.T. & Fisher, R.S. (2005) Use of serum prolactin in diagnosing epileptic seizures: report of the Therapeutics and Technology Assessment Subcommittee of the American Academy of Neurology. *Neurology* **65**, 668–675.

Christodoulou, C., Koutroumanidis, M., Hennessy, M.J., Elwes, R.D., Polkey, C.E. & Toone, B.K. (2002) Postictal psychosis after temporal lobectomy. *Neurology* **59**, 1432–1435.

Cockerell, O.C., Johnson, A.L., Sander, J.W., Hart, Y.M., Goodridge, D.M. & Shorvon, S.D. (1994) Mortality from epilepsy: results from a prospective population-based study. *Lancet* **344**, 918–921.

Cockerell, O.C., Rothwell, J., Thompson, P.D., Marsden, C.D. & Shorvon, S.D. (1996) Clinical and physiological features of epilepsia partialis continua. Cases ascertained in the UK. *Brain* **119**, 393–407.

Commission on Classification and Terminology of the International League Against Epilepsy (1981) Proposal for revised clinical and electroencephalographic classification of epileptic seizures. *Epilepsia* **22**, 489–501.

Commission on Classification and Terminology of the International League Against Epilepsy (1989) Proposal for revised classification of epilepsy and epileptic syndromes. *Epilepsia* **30**, 389–399.

Commission on Neuroimaging of the International League Against Epilepsy (1997) Recommendations for neuroimaging of patients with epilepsy. *Epilepsia* **38**, 1255–1256.

Connor, S.E. & Jarosz, J.M. (2001) Magnetic resonance imaging of patients with epilepsy. *Clinical Radiology* **56**, 787–801.

Couprie, W., Wijdicks, E.F.M., Rooijmans, H.G.M. & Van Gijn, J. (1995) Outcome in conversion disorder: a follow up study. *Journal of Neurology, Neurosurgery and Psychiatry* **58**, 750–752.

Crawford, P. (2005) Best practice guidelines for the management of women with epilepsy. *Epilepsia* **46** (suppl. 9), 117–124.

Crawford, P.M., West, C.R., Chadwick, D.W. & Shaw, M.D. (1986a) Arteriovenous malformations of the brain: natural history in unoperated patients. *Journal of Neurology, Neurosurgery and Psychiatry* **49**, 1–10.

Crawford, P.M., West, C.R., Shaw, M.D. & Chadwick, D.W. (1986b) Cerebral arteriovenous malformations and epilepsy: factors in the development of epilepsy. *Epilepsia* **27**, 270–275.

Crawford, P., Appleton, R., Betts, T., Duncan, J., Guthrie, E. & Morrow, J. (1999) Best practice guidelines for the management of women with epilepsy. The Women with Epilepsy Guidelines Development Group. *Seizure* **8**, 201–217.

Currie, S., Heathfield, K.W.G., Henson, R.A. & Scott, D.F. (1971) Clinical course and prognosis of temporal lobe epilepsy: a survey of 666 patients. *Brain* **92**, 173–190.

Cutting, S., Lauchheimer, A., Barr, W. & Devinsky, O. (2001) Adult-onset idiopathic generalized epilepsy: clinical and behavioral features. *Epilepsia* **42**, 1395–1398.

Daniele, A., Azzoni, A., Bizzi, A., Rossi, A., Gainotti, G. & Mazza, S. (1997) Sexual behavior and hemispheric laterality of the focus in patients with temporal lobe epilepsy. *Biological Psychiatry* **42**, 617–624.

Dasheiff, R.M. (1991) Sudden unexpected death in epilepsy: a series from an epilepsy surgery program and speculation on the relationship to sudden cardiac death. *Journal of Clinical Neurophysiology* **8**, 216–222.

Daumas-Duport, C., Scheithauer, B.W., Chodkiewicz, J.-P., Laws, E.R. & Vedrenne, C. (1988) Dysembryoplastic neuroepithelial tremor: a surgically curable tumour of young patients with intractable partial seizures. Report of thirty-nine cases. *Neurosurgery* **23**, 545–556.

De la Fuente, J.M., Tugendhaft, P. & Mavroudakis, N. (1998) Electroencephalographic abnormalities in borderline personality disorder. *Psychiatry Research* **77**, 131–138.

Delanty, N., Vaughan, C.J. & French, J.A. (1998) Medical causes of seizures. *Lancet* **352**, 383–390.

Delgado-Escueta, A.V., Mattson, R.H., King, L. *et al.* (1981) The nature of aggression during epileptic seizures. *New England Journal of Medicine* **305**, 711–716.

Derry, C.P., Duncan, J.S. & Berkovic, S.F. (2006) Paroxysmal motor disorders of sleep: the clinical spectrum and differentiation from epilepsy. *Epilepsia* **47**, 1775–1791.

Devinsky, O. & Najjar, S. (1999) Evidence against the existence of a temporal lobe epilepsy personality syndrome. *Neurology* **53** (5 suppl. 2), S13–S25.

Devinsky, O., Kelley, K., Porter, R.J. & Theodore, W.H. (1988) Clinical and electroencephalographic features of simple partial seizures. *Neurology* **38**, 1347–1352.

Devinsky, O., Honigfeld, G. & Patin, J. (1991) Clozapine-related seizures. *Neurology* **41**, 369–371.

Devinsky, O., Abramson, H., Alper, K. *et al.* (1995) Postictal psychosis: a case control series of 20 patients and 150 controls. *Epilepsy Research* **20**, 247–253.

Devinsky, O., Gershengorn, J., Brown, E., Perrine, K., Vazquez, B. & Luciano, D. (1997) Frontal functions in juvenile myoclonic epilepsy. *Neuropsychiatry, Neuropsychology and Behavioral Neurology* **10**, 243–246.

Devinsky, O., Barr, W.B., Vickrey, B.G. *et al.* (2005) Changes in depression and anxiety after resective surgery for epilepsy. *Neurology* **65**, 1744–1749.

Devlin, A.M., Cross, J.H., Harkness, W. *et al.* (2003) Clinical outcomes of hemispherectomy for epilepsy in childhood and adolescence. *Brain* **126**, 556–566.

Diamantopoulos, N., Kaleyias, J., Tzoufi, M. & Kotsalis, C. (2006) A survey of public awareness, understanding, and attitudes toward epilepsy in Greece. *Epilepsia* **47**, 2154–2164.

Dodrill, C.B. (2002) Progressive cognitive decline in adolescents and adults with epilepsy. *Progress in Brain Research* **135**, 399–407.

Dodrill, C.B. (2004) Neuropsychological effects of seizures. *Epilepsy and Behavior* **5** (suppl. 1), S21–S24.

Drislane, F.W., Blum, A.S. & Schomer, D.L. (1999) Focal status epilepticus: clinical features and significance of different EEG patterns. *Epilepsia* **40**, 1254–1260.

Duncan, J.S. (1997a) Idiopathic generalized epilepsies with typical absences. *Journal of Neurology* **244**, 403–411.

Duncan, J.S. (1997b) Imaging and epilepsy. *Brain* **120**, 339–377.

Duncan, J. (2003) The current status of neuroimaging for epilepsy: editorial review. *Current Opinion in Neurology* **16**, 163–164.

Duncan, R., Oto, M., Russell, A.J. & Conway, P. (2004) Pseudosleep events in patients with psychogenic non-epileptic seizures: prevalence and associations. *Journal of Neurology, Neurosurgery and Psychiatry* **75**, 1009–1012.

Duncan, S. (2007) Teratogenesis of sodium valproate. *Current Opinion in Neurology* **20**, 175–180.

Edeh, J. & Toone, B. (1987) Relationship between interictal psychopathology and the type of epilepsy. Results of a survey in general practice. *British Journal of Psychiatry* **151**, 95–101.

Edeh, J., Toone, B.K. & Corney, R.H. (1990) Epilepsy, psychiatric morbidity, and social dysfunction in general practice. *Neuropsychiatry, Neuropsychology and Behavioral Neurology* **3**, 180–192.

Egli, M., Mothersill, I., O'Kane, M. & O'Kane, F. (1985) The axial spasm: the predominant type of drop seizure in patients with secondary generalized epilepsy. *Epilepsia* **26**, 401–415.

Ehlers, A. & Clark, D.M. (2000) A cognitive model of posttraumatic stress disorder. *Behaviour Research and Therapy* **38**, 319–345.

Elger, C.E., Helmstaedter, C. & Kurthen, M. (2004) Chronic epilepsy and cognition. *Lancet Neurology* **3**, 663–672.

Elger, G., Hoppe, C., Falkai, P., Rush, A.J. & Elger, C.E. (2000) Vagus nerve stimulation is associated with mood improvements in epilepsy patients. *Epilepsy Research* **42**, 203–210.

Ellenberg, J.H., Hirtz, D.G. & Nelson, K.B. (1986) Do seizures in children cause intellectual deterioration? *New England Journal of Medicine* **314**, 1085–1088.

Elwes, R.D., Johnson, A.L. & Reynolds, E.H. (1988) The course of untreated epilepsy. *British Medical Journal* **297**, 948–950.

Engel, J. Jr (1996) Surgery for seizures. *New England Journal of Medicine* **334**, 647–652.

Engel, J. Jr (2001) A proposed diagnostic scheme for people with epileptic seizures and with epilepsy: report of the ILAE Task Force on Classification and Terminology. *Epilepsia* **42**, 796–803.

Engel, J. Jr, Wiebe, S., French, J. *et al.* (2003) Practice parameter: temporal lobe and localized neocortical resections for epilepsy. Report of the Quality Standards Subcommittee of the American Academy of Neurology, in association with the American Epilepsy Society and the American Association of Neurological Surgeons. *Neurology* **60**, 538–547. [Erratum appears in *Neurology* 2003, **60**, 1396.]

Eriksson, K., Viinikainen, K., Monkkonen, A. *et al.* (2005) Children exposed to valproate in utero: population based evaluation of risks and confounding factors for long-term neurocognitive development. *Epilepsy Research* **65**, 189–200.

Ettinger, A., Reed, M. & Cramer, J. (2004) Depression and comorbidity in community-based patients with epilepsy or asthma. Epilepsy Impact Project Group. *Neurology* **63**, 1008–1014.

Ettinger, A.B., Reed, M.L., Goldberg, J.F. & Hirschfeld, R.M. (2005) Prevalence of bipolar symptoms in epilepsy vs other chronic health disorders. *Neurology* **65**, 535–540.

Exner, C., Boucsein, K., Lange, C. *et al.* (2002) Neuropsychological performance in frontal lobe epilepsy. *Seizure* **11**, 20–32.

Fagan, K.J. & Lee, S.I. (1990) Prolonged confusion following convulsions due to generalized nonconvulsive status epilepticus. *Neurology* **40**, 1689–1694.

Falconer, M.A. (1973) Reversibility by temporal lobe resection of the behavioural abnormalities of temporal lobe epilepsy. *New England Journal of Medicine* **289**, 451–455.

Falconer, M.A. (1974) Mesial temporal (Ammon's horn) sclerosis as a common cause of epilepsy: aetiology, treatment, and prevention. *Lancet* **ii**, 767–770.

Falconer, M.A. & Taylor, D.C. (1968) Surgical treatment of drug-resistant epilepsy due to mesial temporal sclerosis. Etiology and significance. *Archives of Neurology* **19**, 353–361.

Farias, S.T., Thieman, C. & Alsaadi, T.M. (2003) Psychogenic nonepileptic seizures: acute change in event frequency after presentation of the diagnosis. *Epilepsy and Behavior* **4**, 424–429.

Farwell, D.J., Freemantle, N. & Sulke, N. (2006) The clinical impact of implantable loop recorders in patients with syncope. *European Heart Journal* **27**, 351–356.

Fastenau, P.S., Shen, J., Dunn, D.W., Perkins, S.M., Hermann, B.P. & Austin, J.K. (2004) Neuropsychological predictors of academic underachievement in pediatric epilepsy: moderating roles of demographic, seizure, and psychosocial variables. *Epilepsia* **45**, 1261–1272.

Favale, E., Rubino, V., Mainardi, P., Lunardi, G. & Albano, C. (1995) Anticonvulsant effect of fluoxetine in humans. *Neurology* **45**, 1926–1927.

Fejerman, N., Caraballo, R. & Tenembaum, S.N. (2000) Atypical evolutions of benign localization-related epilepsies in children: are they predictable? *Epilepsia* **41**, 380–390.

Feksi, A.T., Kaamugisha, J., Sander, J.W., Gatiti, S. & Shorvon, S.D. (1991) Comprehensive primary health care antiepileptic drug treatment programme in rural and semi-urban Kenya. ICBERG (International Community-based Epilepsy Research Group). *Lancet* **337**, 406–409.

Fenton, G.W. (1972) Epilepsy and automatism. *British Journal of Hospital Medicine* **7**, 57–64.

Fenton, G.W. (1981) Psychiatric disorders of epilepsy: classificaton and phenomenology. In: Reynolds, E.H. & Trimble, M.R. (eds) *Epilepsy and Psychiatry*, pp. 12–26. Churchill Livingstone, Edinburgh.

Fenwick, P.B. (1992) The relationship between mind, brain, and seizures. *Epilepsia* **33** (suppl. 6), S1–S6.

Fenwick, P.B. & Brown, S.W. (1989) Evoked and psychogenic epileptic seizures. I. Precipitation. *Acta Neurologica Scandinavica* **80**, 535–540.

Ferlazzo, E., Zifkin, B.G., Andermann, E. & Andermann, F. (2005) Cortical triggers in generalized reflex seizures and epilepsies. *Brain* **128**, 700–710.

Ficker, D.M., So, E.L., Shen, W.K. *et al.* (1998) Population-based study of the incidence of sudden unexplained death in epilepsy. *Neurology* **51**, 1270–1274.

Fiordelli, E., Beghi, E., Bogliun, G. & Crespi, V. (1993) Epilepsy and psychiatric disturbance. A cross-sectional study. *British Journal of Psychiatry* **163**, 446–450.

Fitzpatrick, A.P. & Cooper, P. (2006) Diagnosis and management of patients with blackouts. *Heart* **92**, 559–568.

Flor-Henry, P. (1969) Psychosis and temporal lobe epilepsy: a controlled investigation. *Epilepsia* **10**, 363–395.

Forsgren, L., Bucht, G., Eriksson, S. & Bergmark, L. (1996) Incidence and clinical characterization of unprovoked seizures in adults: a prospective population-based study. *Epilepsia* **37**, 224–229.

Fowle, A.J. & Binnie, C.D. (2000) Uses and abuses of the EEG in epilepsy. *Epilepsia* **41** (suppl. 3), S10–S18.

Fox, R.H., Wilkins, D.C., Bell, J.A. *et al.* (1973) Spontaneous periodic hypothermia: diencephalic epilepsy. *British Medical Journal* **2**, 693–695.

French, J.A., Kanner, A.M., Bautista, J. *et al.* (2004a) Efficacy and tolerability of the new antiepileptic drugs I: treatment of new onset epilepsy. Report of the Therapeutics and Technology Assessment Subcommittee and Quality Standards Subcommittee of the American Academy of Neurology and the American Epilepsy Society. *Neurology* **62**, 1252–1260.

French, J.A., Kanner, A.M., Bautista, J. *et al.* (2004b) Efficacy and tolerability of the new antiepileptic drugs II: treatment of refractory epilepsy. Report of the Therapeutics and Technology Assessment Subcommittee and Quality Standards Subcommittee of the American Academy of Neurology and the American Epilepsy Society. *Neurology* **62**, 1261–1273.

Frey, L.C. (2003) Epidemiology of posttraumatic epilepsy: a critical review. *Epilepsia* **44** (suppl. 10), 11–17.

Froscher, W., Maier, V., Laage, M. *et al.* (1995) Folate deficiency, anticonvulsant drugs, and psychiatric morbidity. *Clinical Neuropharmacology* **18**, 165–182.

Frost, M., Gates, J., Helmers, S.L. *et al.* (2001) Vagus nerve stimulation in children with refractory seizures associated with Lennox–Gastaut syndrome. *Epilepsia* **42**, 1148–1152.

Frucht, M.M., Quigg, M., Schwaner, C. & Fountain, N.B. (2000) Distribution of seizure precipitants among epilepsy syndromes. *Epilepsia* **41**, 1534–1539.

Gaitatzis, A., Kartsounis, L.D., Gacinovic, S. *et al.* (2004) Frontal lobe dysfunction in sporadic hyperekplexia: case study and literature review. *Journal of Neurology* **251**, 91–98.

Gale, J.L., Thapa, P.B., Wassilak, S.G., Bobo, J.K., Mendelman, P.M. & Foy, H.M. (1994) Risk of serious acute neurological illness after immunization with diphtheria-tetanus-pertussis vaccine. A population-based case-control study. *Journal of the American Medical Association* **271**, 37–41.

Gallhofer, B., Trimble, M.R., Frackowiak, R., Gibbs, J. & Jones, T. (1985) A study of cerebral blood flow and metabolism in epileptic psychosis using positron emission tomography and oxygen. *Journal of Neurology, Neurosurgery and Psychiatry* **48**, 201–206.

Gambardella, A., Reutens, D.C., Andermann, F. *et al.* (1994) Late-onset drop attacks in temporal lobe epilepsy: a reevaluation of the concept of temporal lobe syncope. *Neurology* **44**, 1074–1078.

Garcia, P.A. & Alldredge, B.K. (1994) Drug-induced seizures. *Neurologic Clinics* **12**, 85–99.

Gastaut, H. & Collomb, H. (1954) Étude du comportement sexuel chez les epileptiques psychomoteurs. *Annales Medicopsychologiques* **112**, 657–696.

Gates, J.R. (2002) Nonepileptic seizures: classification, coexistence with epilepsy, diagnosis, therapeutic approaches, and consensus. *Epilepsy and Behavior* **3**, 28–33.

Gedda, L. & Tatarelli, R. (1971) Essential isochronic epilepsy in MZ twin pairs. *Acta Geneticae Medicae et Gemellologiae* **20**, 380–383.

Gelisse, P., Genton, P., Samuelian, J.C., Thomas, P. & Bureau, M. (2001) [Psychiatric disorders in juvenile myoclonic epilepsy.] *Revue Neurologique (Paris)* **157**, 297–302.

Gerard, M.E., Spitz, M.C., Towbin, J.A. & Shantz, D. (1998) Subacute postictal aggression. *Neurology* **50**, 384–388.

Geyer, J.D., Payne, T.A., Faught, E. & Drury, I. (1999) Postictal nose-rubbing in the diagnosis, lateralization, and localization of seizures. *Neurology* **52**, 743–745.

Gibbs, F.A. (1951) Ictal and non-ictal psychiatric disorders in temporal lobe epilepsy. *Journal of Nervous and Mental Disease* **113**, 522–528.

Gilliam, F. (2002) Optimizing health outcomes in active epilepsy. *Neurology* **58** (8 suppl. 4), S9–S19.

Glauser, T., Ben Menachem, E., Bourgeois, B. *et al.* (2006) ILAE treatment guidelines: evidence-based analysis of antiepileptic drug efficacy and effectiveness as initial monotherapy for epileptic seizures and syndromes. *Epilepsia* **47**, 1094–1120.

Gleissner, U., Helmstaedter, C. & Elger, C.E. (1998) Right hippocampal contribution to visual memory: a presurgical and postsurgical study in patients with temporal lobe epilepsy. *Journal of Neurology, Neurosurgery and Psychiatry* **65**, 665–669.

Glosser, G., Zwil, A.S., Glosser, D.S., O'Connor, M.J. & Sperling, M.R. (2000) Psychiatric aspects of temporal lobe epilepsy before and after anterior temporal lobectomy. *Journal of Neurology, Neurosurgery and Psychiatry* **68**, 53–58.

Goldstein, L.H. (1997) Effectiveness of psychological interventions for people with poorly controlled epilepsy. *Journal of Neurology, Neurosurgery and Psychiatry* **63**, 137–142.

Goldstein, L.H. & Mellers, J.D. (2006) Ictal symptoms of anxiety, avoidance behaviour, and dissociation in patients with dissociative seizures. *Journal of Neurology, Neurosurgery and Psychiatry* **77**, 616–621.

Goldstein, L.H., Deale, A.C., Mitchell-O'Malley, S.J., Toone, B.K. & Mellers, J.D.C. (2004) An evaluation of cognitive behavioral therapy as a treatment for dissociative seizures: a pilot study. *Cognitive and Behavioral Neurology* **17**, 41–49.

Goossens, L.A., Andermann, F., Andermann, E. & Remillard, G.M. (1990) Reflex seizures induced by calculation, card or board games, and spatial tasks: a review of 25 patients and delineation of the epileptic syndrome. *Neurology* **40**, 1171–1176.

Gould, P.A., Krahn, A.D., Klein, G.J., Yee, R., Skanes, A.C. & Gula, L.J. (2006) Investigating syncope: a review. *Current Opinion in Cardiology* **21**, 34–41.

Graham, P. & Rutter, M. (1968) Organic brain dysfunction and child psychiatric disorder. *British Medical Journal* **3**, 695–700.

Gregory, R.P., Oates, T. & Merry, R.T. (1993) Electroencephalogram epileptiform abnormalities in candidates for aircrew training. *Electroencephalography and Clinical Neurophysiology* **86**, 75–77.

Gudmundsson, G. (1966) Epilepsy in Iceland. A clinical and epidemiological investigation. *Acta Neurologica Scandinavica Supplementum* **25**, 7–124.

Guerrini, R. & Aicardi, J. (2003) Epileptic encephalopathies with myoclonic seizures in infants and children (severe myoclonic epilepsy and myoclonic-astatic epilepsy). *Journal of Clinical Neurophysiology* **20**, 449–461.

Gulgonen, S., Demirbilek, V., Korkmaz, B., Dervent, A. & Townes, B.D. (2000) Neuropsychological functions in idiopathic occipital lobe epilepsy. *Epilepsia* **41**, 405–411.

Gunn, J.C. (1969) The prevalence of epilepsy among prisoners. *Proceedings of the Royal Society of Medicine* **62**, 60–63.

Gunn, J. (1978) Epileptic homicide: a case report. *British Journal of Psychiatry* **132**, 510–513.

Gunn, J. & Bonn, J. (1971) Criminality and violence in epileptic prisoners. *British Journal of Psychiatry* **118**, 337–343.

Gunn, J. & Fenton, G.W. (1971) Epilepsy, automatism and crime. *Lancet* **i**, 1173–1176.

Haerer, A.F., Anderson, D.W. & Schoenberg, B.S. (1986) Prevalence and clinical features of epilepsy in a biracial United States population. *Epilepsia* **27**, 66–75.

Halmagyi, G.M. (2005) Diagnosis and management of vertigo. *Clinical Medicine* **5**, 159–165.

Harden, C.L. (2002) The co-morbidity of depression and epilepsy: epidemiology, etiology, and treatment. *Neurology* **59** (6 suppl. 4), S48–S55.

Harden, C.L. (2005) Sexuality in women with epilepsy. *Epilepsy and Behavior* **7** (suppl. 2), S2–S6.

Harmant, J., Rijckevorsel-Harmant, K., de Barsy, T. & Hendrickx, B. (1990) Fluvoxamine: an antidepressant with low (or no) epileptogenic effect. *Lancet* **336**, 386.

Hauser, W.A., Annegers, J.F. & Elveback, L.R. (1980) Mortality in patients with epilepsy. *Epilepsia* **21**, 399–412.

Hauser, W.A., Morris, M.L., Heston, L.L. & Anderson, V.E. (1986) Seizures and myoclonus in patients with Alzheimer's disease. *Neurology* **36**, 1226–1230.

Hauser, W.A., Annegers, J.F. & Kurland, L.T. (1991) Prevalence of epilepsy in Rochester, Minnesota: 1940–1980. *Epilepsia* **32**, 429–445.

Hauser, W.A., Annegers, J.F. & Kurland, L.T. (1993) Incidence of epilepsy and unprovoked seizures in Rochester, Minnesota: 1935–1984. *Epilepsia* **34**, 453–468.

Heaney, D.C., MacDonald, B.K., Everitt, A. *et al.* (2002) Socioeconomic variation in incidence of epilepsy: prospective community based study in south east England. *British Medical Journal* **325**, 1013–1016.

Helmers, S.L., Griesemer, D.A., Dean, J.C. *et al.* (2003) Observations on the use of vagus nerve stimulation earlier in the course of pharmacoresistant epilepsy: patients with seizures for six years or less. *Neurologist* **9**, 160–164.

Helmstaedter, C., Kemper, B. & Elger, C.E. (1996) Neuropsychological aspects of frontal lobe epilepsy. *Neuropsychologia* **34**, 399–406.

Helmstaedter, C., Kurthen, M., Lux, S., Reuber, M. & Elger, C.E. (2003) Chronic epilepsy and cognition: a longitudinal study in temporal lobe epilepsy. *Annals of Neurology* **54**, 425–432.

Henkel, A., Noachtar, S., Pfander, M. & Luders, H.O. (2002) The localizing value of the abdominal aura and its evolution: a study in focal epilepsies. *Neurology* **58**, 271–276.

Hennessy, M.J., Elwes, R.D., Rabe-Hesketh, S., Binnie, C.D. & Polkey, C.E. (2001) Prognostic factors in the surgical treatment of medically intractable epilepsy associated with mesial temporal sclerosis. *Acta Neurologica Scandinavica* **103**, 344–350.

Henry, J.A. & Woodruff, G.H. (1978) A diagnostic sign in states of apparent unconsciousness. *Lancet* **ii**, 920–921.

Hermann, B., Seidenberg, M., Bell, B. *et al.* (2003) Extratemporal quantitative MR volumetrics and neuropsychological status in temporal lobe epilepsy. *Journal of the International Neuropsychological Society* **9**, 353–362.

Hermann, B., Jones, J., Sheth, R., Dow, C., Koehn, M. & Seidenberg, M. (2006) Children with new-onset epilepsy: neuropsychological status and brain structure. *Brain* **129**, 2609–2619.

Hermann, B.P. & Riel, P. (1981) Interictal personality and behavioral traits in temporal lobe and generalised epilepsy. *Cortex* **17**, 125–128.

Hermann, B.P., Whitman, S. & Arntson, P. (1983) Hypergraphia in epilepsy: is there a specificity to temporal lobe epilepsy? *Journal of Neurology, Neurosurgery and Psychiatry* **46**, 848–853.

Hermann, B.P., Whitman, S., Wyler, A.R., Richey, E.T. & Dell, J. (1988) The neurological, psychosocial and demographic correlates of hypergraphia in patients with epilepsy. *Journal of Neurology, Neurosurgery and Psychiatry* **51**, 203–208.

Hermann, B.P., Wyler, A.R. & Somes, G. (1991) Language function following anterior temporal lobectomy. *Journal of Neurosurgery* **74**, 560–566.

Hermann, B.P., Wyler, A.R., Blumer, D. & Richey, E.T. (1992) Ictal fear: lateralizing significance and implications for understanding the neurobiology of pathological fear states. *Neuropsychiatry, Neuropsychology and Behavioral Neurology* **5**, 205–210.

Hermann, B.P., Seidenberg, M., Schoenfeld, J. & Davies, K. (1997) Neuropsychological characteristics of the syndrome of mesial temporal lobe epilepsy. *Archives of Neurology* **54**, 369–376.

Herzog, A.G., Drislane, F.W., Schomer, D.L. *et al.* (1990) Abnormal pulsatile secretion of luteinizing hormone in men with epilepsy: relationship to laterality and nature of paroxysmal discharges. *Neurology* **40**, 1557–1561.

Herzog, A.G., Klein, P. & Ransil, B.J. (1997) Three patterns of catamenial epilepsy. *Epilepsia* **38**, 1082–1088.

Herzog, A.G., Coleman, A.E., Jacobs, A.R. *et al.* (2003) Relationship of sexual dysfunction to epilepsy laterality and reproductive hormone levels in women. *Epilepsy and Behavior* **4**, 407–413.

Herzog, A.G., Drislane, F.W., Schomer, D.L. *et al.* (2005) Differential effects of antiepileptic drugs on sexual function and hormones in men with epilepsy. *Neurology* **65**, 1016–1020.

Hesdorffer, D.C., Hauser, W.A., Annegers, J.F. & Rocca, W.A. (1996) Severe, uncontrolled hypertension and adult-onset seizures: a case–control study in Rochester, Minnesota. *Epilepsia* **37**, 736–741.

Hinchey, J., Chaves, C., Appignani, B. *et al.* (1996) A reversible posterior leukoencephalopathy syndrome. *New England Journal of Medicine* **334**, 494–500.

Holmes, E.A., Brown, R.J., Mansell, W. *et al.* (2005) Are there two qualitatively distinct forms of dissociation? A review and some clinical implications. *Clinical Psychology Review* **25**, 1–23.

Holmes, G.L., McKeever, M. & Adamson, M. (1987) Absence seizures in children: clinical and electroencephalic features. *Annals of Neurology* **21**, 268–273.

Holmes, L.B., Harvey, E.A., Coull, B.A. *et al.* (2001) The teratogenicity of anticonvulsant drugs. *New England Journal of Medicine* **344**, 1132–1138.

Holmes, M.D., Silbergeld, D.L., Drouhard, D., Wilensky, A.J. & Ojemann, L.M. (2004) Effect of vagus nerve stimulation on adults with pharmacoresistant generalized epilepsy syndromes. *Seizure* **13**, 340–345.

Holtkamp, M., Schuchmann, S., Gottschalk, S. & Meierkord, H. (2004) Recurrent seizures do not cause hippocampal damage. *Journal of Neurology* **251**, 458–463.

Hommet, C., Sauerwein, H.C., De Toffol, B. & Lassonde, M. (2006) Idiopathic epileptic syndromes and cognition. *Neuroscience and Biobehavioral Reviews* **30**, 85–96.

Hoppener, R.J., Kuyer, A. & van der Lugt, P.J. (1983) Epilepsy and alcohol: the influence of social alcohol intake on seizures and treatment in epilepsy. *Epilepsia* **24**, 459–471.

Hosain, S., Nikalov, B., Harden, C., Li, M., Fraser, R. & Labar, D. (2000) Vagus nerve stimulation treatment for Lennox–Gastaut syndrome. *Journal of Child Neurology* **15**, 509–512.

Hrachovy, R.A. & Frost, J.D. Jr (2003) Infantile epileptic encephalopathy with hypsarrhythmia (infantile spasms/West syndrome). *Journal of Clinical Neurophysiology* **20**, 408–425.

Hughes, J., Devinsky, O., Feldmann, E. & Bromfield, E. (1993) Premonitory symptoms in epilepsy. *Seizure* **2**, 201–203.

Humm, A.M. & Matthias C.J. (2006) Unexplained syncope – is screening for carotid sinus hypersensitivity indicated in all patients aged >40 years? *Journal of Neurology, Neurosurgery & Psychiatry* **77**, 1267–1270.

Isojarvi, J.I., Repo, M., Pakarinen, A.J., Lukkarinen, O. & Myllyla, V.V. (1995) Carbamazepine, phenytoin, sex hormones, and sexual function in men with epilepsy. *Epilepsia* **36**, 366–370.

Jackson, J.H. (1889) On a particular variety of epilepsy ('intellectual aura'): one case with symptoms of organic brain disease. *Brain* **11**, 179–207.

Jacoby, A., Baker, G.A., Steen, N., Potts, P. & Chadwick, D.W. (1996) The clinical course of epilepsy and its psychosocial correlates: findings from a U.K. Community study. *Epilepsia* **37**, 148–161.

Jacoby, A., Gorry, J., Gamble, C. & Baker, G.A. (2004) Public knowledge, private grief: a study of public attitudes to epilepsy in the United Kingdom and implications for stigma. *Epilepsia* **45**, 1405–1415.

Jallon, P., Loiseau, P. & Loiseau, J. (2001) Newly diagnosed unprovoked epileptic seizures: presentation at diagnosis in CAROLE study. Coordination Active du Reseau Observatoire Longitudinal de l'Epilepsie. *Epilepsia* **42**, 464–475.

Janszky, J., Schulz, R. & Ebner, A. (2004a) Simple partial seizures (isolated auras) in medial temporal lobe epilepsy. *Seizure* **13**, 247–249.

Janszky, J., Ebner, A., Szupera, Z. *et al.* (2004b) Orgasmic aura: a report of seven cases. *Seizure* **13**, 441–444.

Janz, D. (1969) *Die Epilepsien*. Georg Thieme, Stuttgart.

Janz, D. (1997) The idiopathic generalized epilepsies of adolescence with childhood and juvenile age of onset. *Epilepsia* **38**, 4–11.

Jasper, H.H. (1964) Some physiological mechanisms involved in epileptic automatisms. *Epilepsia* **5**, 1–20.

Jennett, B. (1975) *Epilepsy After Non-missile Head Injuries*, 2nd edn. Heinemann, London.

Jennett, W.B. (1969) Early traumatic epilepsy. Definition and identity. *Lancet* **i**, 1023–1025.

Jensen, I. & Larsen, J.K. (1979a) Psychoses in drug-resistant temporal lobe epilepsy. *Journal of Neurology, Neurosurgery and Psychiatry* **42**, 948–954.

Jensen, I. & Larsen, J.K. (1979b) Mental aspects of temporal lobe epilepsy: follow-up of 74 patients after resection of a temporal lobe. *Journal of Neurology, Neurosurgery and Psychiatry* **42**, 256–265.

Jobst, B.C., Siegel, A.M., Thadani, V.M., Roberts, D.W., Rhodes, H.C. & Williamson, P.D. (2000) Intractable seizures of frontal lobe origin: clinical characteristics, localizing signs, and results of surgery. *Epilepsia* **41**, 1139–1152.

Johnson, M.R. & Sander, J.W. (2001) The clinical impact of epilepsy genetics. *Journal of Neurology, Neurosurgery and Psychiatry* **70**, 428–430. [Erratum appears in *Journal of Neurology, Neurosurgery and Psychiatry* 2001, **71**, 567.]

Jokeit, H. & Ebner, A. (1999) Long term effects of refractory temporal lobe epilepsy on cognitive abilities: a cross sectional study. *Journal of Neurology, Neurosurgery and Psychiatry* **67**, 44–50.

Jones, J.E., Hermann, B.P., Barry, J.J., Gilliam, F., Kanner, A.M. & Meador, K.J. (2005) Clinical assessment of Axis I psychiatric morbidity in chronic epilepsy: a multicenter investigation. *Journal of Neuropsychiatry and Clinical Neurosciences* **17**, 172–179.

Juul-Jensen, P. (1964) Epilepsy: a clinical and social analysis of 1020 adult patients with epileptic seizures. *Acta Neurologica Scandinavica Supplementum* **5**, 1–148.

Kaneko, S., Battino, D., Andermann, E. *et al.* (1999) Congenital malformations due to antiepileptic drugs. *Epilepsy Research* **33**, 145–158.

Kanner, A.M. (2003) Depression in epilepsy: prevalence, clinical semiology, pathogenic mechanisms, and treatment. *Biological Psychiatry* **54**, 388–398.

Kanner, A.M., Stagno, S., Kotagal, P. & Morris, H.H. (1996) Postictal psychiatric events during prolonged video-electroencephalographic monitoring studies. *Archives of Neurology* **53**, 258–263.

Kanner, A.M., Kozak, A.M. & Frey, M. (2000) The use of sertraline in patients with epilepsy: is it safe? *Epilepsy and Behavior* **1**, 100–105.

Kapur, J., Pillai, A. & Henry, T.R. (1995) Psychogenic elaboration of simple partial seizures. *Epilepsia* **36**, 1126–1130.

Keranen, T., Riekkinen, P.J. & Sillanpaa, M. (1989) Incidence and prevalence of epilepsy in adults in eastern Finland. *Epilepsia* **30**, 413–421.

Kerr, S.R., Pearce, M.S., Brayne, C., Davis, R.J. & Kenny, R.A. (2006) Carotid sinus hypersensitivity in asymptomatic older persons: implications for diagnosis of syncope and falls. *Archives of Internal Medicine* **166**, 515–520.

Kim, H., Yi, S., Son, E.I. & Kim, J. (2003) Differential effects of left versus right mesial temporal lobe epilepsy on Wechsler intelligence factors. *Neuropsychology* **17**, 556–565.

King, D., Spencer, S.S., McCarthy, G., Luby, M. & Spencer, D.D. (1995) Bilateral hippocampal atrophy in medial temporal lobe epilepsy. *Epilepsia* **36**, 905–910.

King, D.W. & Ajmone Marsan, C. (1977) Clinical features and ictal patterns in epileptic patients with temporal lobe foci. *Annals of Neurology* **2**, 138–147.

Kirshner, H.S., Hughes, T., Fakhoury, T. & Abou-Khalil, B. (1995) Aphasia secondary to partial status epilepticus of the basal temporal language area. *Neurology* **45**, 1616–1618.

Kitchen, N.D., Belli, A. & Sen, J.A. (2004) Resective surgery of vascular and infective lesions. In: Shorvon, S.D., Perucca, E., Fish,

D.R. & Dodson, W.E. (eds) *The Treatment of Epilepsy*, pp. 742–763. Blackwell Science, Malden, MA.

Knox, S.J. (1968) Epileptic automatism and violence. *Medicine, Science and the Law* **8**, 96–104.

Kogeorgos, J., Fonagy, P. & Scott, D.F. (1982) Psychiatric symptom patterns of chronic epileptics attending a neurological clinic: a controlled investigation. *British Journal of Psychiatry* **140**, 236–243.

Kondziolka, D., Lunsford, L.D. & Kestle, J.R. (1995) The natural history of cerebral cavernous malformations. *Journal of Neurosurgery* **83**, 820–824.

Koszewski, W. (1991) Epilepsy following brain abscess. The evaluation of possible risk factors with emphasis on new concept of epileptic focus formation. *Acta Neurochirurgica* **113**, 110–117.

Kotagal, P., Arunkumar, G., Hammel, J. & Mascha, E. (2003) Complex partial seizures of frontal lobe onset statistical analysis of ictal semiology. *Seizure* **12**, 268–281.

Kotsopoulos, I.A.W., De Krom, M.C.T.F., Kessels, F.G.H. *et al.* (2003) The diagnosis of epileptic and non-epileptic seizures. *Epilepsy Research* **57**, 59–67.

Koutroumanidis, M., Koepp, M.J., Richardson, M.P. *et al.* (1998) The variants of reading epilepsy. A clinical and video-EEG study of 17 patients with reading-induced seizures. *Brain* **121**, 1409–1427.

Krishnamoorthy, E.S. & Trimble, M.R. (1999) Forced normalization: clinical and therapeutic relevance. *Epilepsia* **40** (suppl. 10), S57–S64.

Kristensen, O. & Sindrup, E.H. (1978a) Psychomotor epilepsy and psychosis. I. Physical aspects. *Acta Neurologica Scandinavica* **57**, 361–369.

Kristensen, O. & Sindrup, E.H. (1978b) Psychomotor epilepsy and psychosis. II. Electroencephalographic findings (sphenoidal electrode recordings). *Acta Neurologica Scandinavica* **57**, 370–379.

Kristensen, O. & Sindrup, E.H. (1979) Psychomotor epilepsy and psychosis. III. Social and psychological correlates. *Acta Neurologica Scandinavica* **59**, 1–9.

Krumholz, A. (1999) Nonepileptic seizures: diagnosis and management. *Neurology* **53** (suppl. 2), S76–S83.

Kuhn, K.U., Quednow, B.B., Thiel, M., Falkai, P., Maier, W. & Elger, C.E. (2003) Antidepressive treatment in patients with temporal lobe epilepsy and major depression: a prospective study with three different antidepressants. *Epilepsy & Behaviour* **4**, 674–679.

Kuks, J.B.M., Cook, M.J., Fish, D.R., Stevens, J.M. & Shorvon, S.D. (1993) Hippocampal sclerosis in epilepsy and childhood febrile seizures. *Lancet* **342**, 1391–1394.

Kwan, P. & Brodie, M.J. (2000) Early identification of refractory epilepsy. *New England Journal of Medicine* **342**, 314–319.

Kwan, P. & Brodie, M.J. (2001) Neuropsychological effects of epilepsy and antiepileptic drugs. *Lancet* **357**, 216–222.

Labar, D., Murphy, J. & Tecoma, E. (1999) Vagus nerve stimulation for medication-resistant generalized epilepsy. E04 VNS Study Group. *Neurology* **52**, 1510–1512.

Lambert, M.V. (2001) Seizures, hormones and sexuality. *Seizure* **10**, 319–340.

Lambert, M.V. & Robertson, M.M. (1999) Depression in epilepsy: etiology, phenomenology, and treatment. *Epilepsia* **40** (suppl. 10), S21–S47.

Lancman, M. (1999) Psychosis and peri-ictal confusional states. *Neurology* **53** (5 suppl. 2), S33–S38.

Landolt, H. (1958) Serial electroencephalographic investigations during psychotic episodes in epileptic patients and during schizophrenic attacks. In: Lorentz de Haas, A.M. (ed.) *Lectures on Epilepsy*, ch. 3. Elsevier, Amsterdam.

Langan, Y., Nashef, L. & Sander, J.W. (2005) Case–control study of SUDEP. *Neurology* **64**, 1131–1133.

Langosch, J.M. & Trimble, M.R. (2002) Epilepsy, psychosis and clozapine. *Human Psychopharmacology* **17**, 115–119.

Lee, W.-L. & Ong, H.-T. (2004) Management of epilepsy in children. In: Shorvon, S.D., Perucca, E., Fish, D.R. & Dodson, W.E. (eds) *The Treatment of Epilepsy*, pp. 190–200. Blackwell Science, Malden, MA.

Leidy, N.K., Elixhauser, A., Vickrey, B., Means, E. & Willian, M.K. (1999) Seizure frequency and the health-related quality of life of adults with epilepsy. *Neurology* **53**, 162–166.

Lempert, T., Bauer, M. & Schmidt, D. (1994) Syncope: a videometric analysis of 56 episodes of transient cerebral hypoxia. *Annals of Neurology* **36**, 233–237.

Lennox, W.G. (1960) *Epilepsy and Related Disorders*, vols 1 and 2. Churchill, London.

Leone, M., Bottacchi, E., Beghi, E. *et al.* (1997) Alcohol use is a risk factor for a first generalized tonic–clonic seizure. The ALCE (Alcohol and Epilepsy) Study Group. *Neurology* **48**, 614–620.

Lerman, P. & Kivity, S. (1975) Benign focal epilepsy of childhood. A follow-up study of 100 recovered patients. *Archives of Neurology* **32**, 261–264.

Li, L.M., Fish, D.R., Sisodiya, S.M., Shorvon, S.D., Alsanjari, N. & Stevens, J.M. (1995) High resolution magnetic resonance imaging in adults with partial or secondary generalised epilepsy attending a tertiary referral unit. *Journal of Neurology, Neurosurgery and Psychiatry* **59**, 384–387.

Lim, J., Yagnik, P., Schraeder, P. & Wheeler, S. (1986) Ictal catatonia as a manifestation of nonconvulsive status epilepticus. *Journal of Neurology, Neurosurgery and Psychiatry* **49**, 833–836.

Logsdail, S.J. & Toone, B.K. (1988) Post-ictal psychoses. A clinical and phenomenological description. *British Journal of Psychiatry* **152**, 246–252.

Lombroso, C. (1911) *Crime: Its Causes and Remedies*. Translated by Horton, H.P. (1918). Little, Brown & Co., Boston.

Lopez-Rodriguez, F., Altshuler, L., Kay, J., Delarhim, S., Mendez, M. & Engel, J. Jr (1999) Personality disorders among medically refractory epileptic patients. *Journal of Neuropsychiatry and Clinical Neurosciences* **11**, 464–469.

Lunde, M.E., Lee, E.K. & Rasmussen, K.G. (2006) Electroconvulsive therapy in patients with epilepsy. *Epilepsy and Behavior* **9**, 355–359.

McAreavey, M.J., Ballinger, B.R. & Fenton, G.W. (1992) Epileptic seizures in elderly patients with dementia. *Epilepsia* **33**, 657–660.

McConnell, H. & Duncan, D. (1998) Treatment of psychiatric comorbidity in epilepsy. In: McConnell, H. & Snyder, P. (eds) *Psychiatric Comorbidity in Epilepsy*, pp. 245–362. American Psychiatric Press, Washington, DC.

McCorry, D., Chadwick, D. & Marson, A. (2004) Current drug treatment of epilepsy in adults. *Lancet Neurology* **3**, 729–735.

MacDonald, B.K., Cockerell, O.C., Sander, J.W. & Shorvon, S.D. (2000) The incidence and lifetime prevalence of neurological disorders in a prospective community-based study in the UK. *Brain* **123**, 665–676.

MacDonald, J.M. (1969) *Psychiatry and the Criminal*, 2nd edn. Thomas, Springfield, IL.

McGonigal, A. & Chauvel, P. (2004) Frontal lobe epilepsy: seizure semiology and presurgical evaluation. *Practical Neurology* **4**, 260–273.

McGonigal, A., Oto, M., Russell, A.J., Greene, J. & Duncan, R. (2002) Outpatient video EEG recording in the diagnosis of non-epileptic seizures: a randomised controlled trial of simple suggestion techniques. *Journal of Neurology, Neurosurgery and Psychiatry* **72**, 549–551.

McLachlan, R.S. & Blume, W.T. (1980) Isolated fear in complex partial status epilepticus. *Annals of Neurology* **8**, 639–641.

Macphee, G.J., Larkin, J.G., Butler, E., Beastall, G.H. & Brodie, M.J. (1988) Circulating hormones and pituitary responsiveness in young epileptic men receiving long-term antiepileptic medication. *Epilepsia* **29**, 468–475.

Maier, M., Mellers, J., Toone, B., Trimble, M. & Ron, M.A. (2000) Schizophrenia, temporal lobe epilepsy and psychosis: an in vivo magnetic resonance spectroscopy and imaging study of the hippocampus/amygdala complex. *Psychological Medicine* **30**, 571–581.

Manchanda, R., Miller, H. & McLachlan, R.S. (1993) Post-ictal psychosis after right temporal lobectomy. *Journal of Neurology, Neurosurgery and Psychiatry* **56**, 277–279.

Manchanda, R., Schaefer, B., McLachlan, R.S. *et al.* (1996) Psychiatric disorders in candidates for surgery for epilepsy. *Journal of Neurology, Neurosurgery and Psychiatry* **61**, 82–89.

Manford, M. (2001) Assessment and investigation of possible epileptic seizures. *Journal of Neurology, Neurosurgery and Psychiatry* **70** (suppl. 2), II3–II8.

Manford, M. & Shorvon, S.D. (1992) Prolonged sensory or visceral symptoms: an under-diagnosed form of non-convulsive focal (simple partial) status epilepticus. *Journal of Neurology, Neurosurgery and Psychiatry* **55**, 714–716. [Erratum appears in *Journal of Neurology, Neurosurgery and Psychiatry* 1992, **55**, 1223.]

Manford, M., Hart, Y.M., Sander, J.W.A.S. & Shorvon, S.D. (1992) National General Practice Study of Epilepsy (NGPSE): partial seizure patterns in a general population. *Neurology* **42**, 1911–1917.

Manford, M., Fish, D.R. & Shorvon, S.D. (1996a) An analysis of clinical seizure patterns and their localizing value in frontal and temporal lobe epilepsies. *Brain* **119**, 17–40.

Manford, M.R., Fish, D.R. & Shorvon, S.D. (1996b) Startle provoked epileptic seizures: features in 19 patients. *Journal of Neurology, Neurosurgery and Psychiatry* **61**, 151–156.

Marchetti, R.L., Azevedo, D. Jr, Campos Bottino, C.M. *et al.* (2003) Volumetric evidence of a left laterality effect in epileptic psychosis. *Epilepsy and Behavior* **4**, 234–240.

Margerison, J.H. & Corsellis, J.A. (1966) Epilepsy and the temporal lobes. A clinical, electroencephalographic and neuropathological study of the brain in epilepsy, with particular reference to the temporal lobes. *Brain* **89**, 499–530.

Markand, O.N. (2003) Lennox–Gastaut syndrome (childhood epileptic encephalopathy). *Journal of Clinical Neurophysiology* **20**, 426–441.

Marks, W.J. Jr & Laxer, K.D. (1998) Semiology of temporal lobe seizures: value in lateralizing the seizure focus. *Epilepsia* **39**, 721–726.

Marsden, C.D. & Reynolds, E.H. (1982) Neurology. In: Laidlaw, J. & Richens, A. (eds) *A Textbook of Epilepsy*, 2nd edn, Part 1, ch. 4. Churchill Livingstone, Edinburgh and London.

Marsh, L. & Krauss, G.L. (2000) Aggression and violence in patients with epilepsy. *Epilepsy and Behavior* **1**, 160–168.

Marsh, L., Sullivan, E.V., Morrell, M., Lim, K.O. & Pfefferbaum, A. (2001) Structural brain abnormalities in patients with schizophrenia, epilepsy, and epilepsy with chronic interictal psychosis. *Psychiatry Research* **108**, 1–15.

Marshall, E.J., Syed, G.M.S., Fenwick, P.B.C. & Lishman, W.A. (1993) A pilot study of schizophrenia-like psychosis in epilepsy using single photon emission computerised tomography. *British Journal of Psychiatry* **163**, 32–36.

Marson, A.G., Al Kharusi, A.M., Alwaidh, M. *et al.* (2007a) The SANAD study of effectiveness of carbamazepine, gabapentin, lamotrigine, oxcarbazepine, or topiramate for treatment of partial epilepsy: an unblinded randomised controlled trial. *Lancet* **369**, 1000–1015.

Marson, A.G., Al Kharusi, A.M., Alwaidh, M. *et al.* (2007b) The SANAD study of effectiveness of valproate, lamotrigine, or topiramate for generalised and unclassifiable epilepsy: an unblinded randomised controlled trial. *Lancet* **369**, 1016–1026.

Martin, R.C., Sawrie, S.M., Roth, D.L. *et al.* (1998) Individual memory change after anterior temporal lobectomy: a base rate analysis using regression-based outcome methodology. *Epilepsia* **39**, 1075–1082.

Master, D.R., Toone, B.K. & Scott, D.F. (1984) Interictal behaviour in temporal lobe epilepsy. In: Porter, R.J., Mattson, R.H., Ward, A.A. & Dam, M. (eds) *Advances in Epileptology: XVth Epilepsy International Symposium*, pp. 557–565. Raven Press, New York.

Mathias, C.J., Deguchi, K. & Schatz, I. (2001) Observations on recurrent syncope and presyncope in 641 patients. *Lancet* **357**, 348–353.

Matsuura, M. (1999) Epileptic psychoses and anticonvulsant drug treatment. *Journal of Neurology, Neurosurgery and Psychiatry* **67**, 231–233.

Mattson, R.H., Cramer, J.A. & Collins, J.F. (1996) Prognosis for total control of complex partial and secondarily generalized tonic clonic seizures. Department of Veterans Affairs Epilepsy Cooperative Studies No. 118 and No. 264 Group. *Neurology* **47**, 68–76.

Maudsley, H. (1873) *Body and Mind*. Macmillan & Co., London.

Maudsley, H. (1906) *Responsibility in Mental Disease*. Kegan Paul, Trench, Trübner & Co., London.

Meador, K.J. (2002) Cognitive outcomes and predictive factors in epilepsy. *Neurology* **58** (8 suppl. 5), S21–S26.

Medical Research Council Antiepileptic Drug Withdrawal Study Group (1991) Randomised study of antiepileptic drug withdrawal in patients in remission. *Lancet* **337**, 1175–1180.

Medical Research Council Antiepileptic Drug Withdrawal Study Group (1993) Prognostic index for recurrence of seizures after remission of epilepsy. *British Medical Journal* **306**, 1374–1378.

Meierkord, H., Will, B., Fish, D. & Shorvon, S. (1991) The clinical features and prognosis of pseudoseizures diagnosed using video-EEG telemetry. *Neurology* **41**, 1643–1646.

Meldrum, B.S., Vigouroux, R.A. & Brierley, J.B. (1973) Systemic factors and epileptic brain damage: prolonged seizures in para-lyzed artificially ventilated baboons. *Archives of Neurology* **29**, 82–87.

Meldrum, B.S., Horton, R.W. & Brierley, J.B. (1974) Epileptic brain damage in adolescent baboons following seizures induced by allylglycine. *Brain* **97**, 407–418.

Mellers, J.D. (2005) The approach to patients with 'non-epileptic seizures'. *Postgraduate Medical Journal* **81**, 498–504.

Mellers, J.D.C., Adachi, N., Takei, N., Cluck, A., Toone, B.K. & Lishman, W.A. (1998) SPET study of verbal fluency in schizophrenia and epilepsy. *British Journal of Psychiatry* **173**, 69–74.

Mellers, J.D., Toone, B.K. & Lishman, W.A. (2000) A neuropsychological comparison of schizophrenia and schizophrenia-like psychosis of epilepsy. *Psychological Medicine* **30**, 325–335.

Mendez, M.F., Cummings, J.L. & Benson, D.F. (1986) Depression in epilepsy. Significance and phenomenology. *Archives of Neurology* **43**, 766–770.

Mendez, M.F., Grau, R., Doss, R.C. & Taylor, J.L. (1993a) Schizophrenia in epilepsy: seizure and psychosis variables. *Neurology* **43**, 1073–1077.

Mendez, M.F., Doss, R.C. & Taylor, J.L. (1993b) Interictal violence in epilepsy. Relationship to behavior and seizure variables. *Journal of Nervous and Mental Disease* **181**, 566–569.

Mendez, M.F., Cherrier, M.M. & Perryman, K.M. (1996) Epileptic forced thinking from left frontal lesions. *Neurology* **47**, 79–83.

Messing, R.O., Closson, R.G. & Simon, R.P. (1984) Drug-induced seizures: a 10-year experience. *Neurology* **34**, 1582–1586.

Metz-Lutz, M.N., Kleitz, C., de Saint, M.A., Massa, R., Hirsch, E. & Marescaux, C. (1999) Cognitive development in benign focal epilepsies of childhood. *Developmental Neuroscience* **21**, 182–190.

Montouris, G. & Morris, G.L. III (2005) Reproductive and sexual dysfunction in men with epilepsy. *Epilepsy and Behavior* **7** (suppl. 2), S7–S14.

Moore, P.M. & Baker, G.A. (1997) Non-epileptic attack disorder: a psychological perspective. *Seizure* **6**, 429–434.

Morgan, C.L., Ahmed, Z. & Kerr, M.P. (2000) Social deprivation and prevalence of epilepsy and associated health usage. *Journal of Neurology, Neurosurgery and Psychiatry* **69**, 13–17.

Morgan, J.M. (2006) Basics of cardiac pacing: selection and mode choice. *Heart* **92**, 850–854.

Morris, H.H. III, Dinner, D.S., Luders, H., Wyllie, E. & Kramer, R. (1988) Supplementary motor seizures: clinical and electroencephalographic findings. *Neurology* **38**, 1075–1082.

Morris, R.G., Abrahams, S. & Polkey, C.E. (1995) Recognition memory for words and faces following unilateral temporal lobectomy. *British Journal of Clinical Psychology* **34**, 571–576.

Morrow, J., Russell, A., Guthrie, E. *et al.* (2006) Malformation risks of antiepileptic drugs in pregnancy: a prospective study from the UK Epilepsy and Pregnancy Register. *Journal of Neurology, Neurosurgery and Psychiatry* **77**, 193–198.

Motamedi, G. & Meador, K. (2003) Epilepsy and cognition. *Epilepsy and Behavior* **4** (suppl. 2), S25–S38.

Mullatti, N., Selway, R., Nashef, L. *et al.* (2003) The clinical spectrum of epilepsy in children and adults with hypothalamic hamartoma. *Epilepsia* **44**, 1310–1319.

Mungas, D. (1982) Interictal behavior abnormality in temporal lobe epilepsy. *Archives of General Psychiatry* **39**, 108–111.

Nagai, Y., Critchley, H.D., Featherstone, E., Fenwick, P.B., Trimble, M.R. & Dolan, R.J. (2004a) Brain activity relating to the contingent negative variation: an fMRI investigation. *Neuroimage* **21**, 1232–1241.

Nagai, Y., Goldstein, L.H., Fenwick, P.B. & Trimble, M.R. (2004b) Clinical efficacy of galvanic skin response biofeedback training in reducing seizures in adult epilepsy: a preliminary randomized controlled study. *Epilepsy and Behavior* **5**, 216–223.

Nashef, L. & Langan, Y. (2004) Sudden death in epilepsy. In: Shorvon, S.D., Perucca, E., Fish, D.R. & Dodson, W.E. (eds) *The Treatment of Epilepsy*, pp. 43–49. Blackwell Science, Malden, MA.

Nashef, L., Fish, D.R., Garner, S., Sander, J.W.A.S. & Shorvon, S.D. (1995) Sudden death in epilepsy: a study of incidence in a young cohort with epilepsy and learning difficulty. *Epilepsia* **36**, 1187–1194.

Nashef, L., Hindocha, N. & Makoff, A. (2007) Risk factors in sudden death in epilepsy (SUDEP): the quest for mechanisms. *Epilepsia* **48**, 859–871.

Nelson, K.B. & Ellenberg, J.H. (1986) Antecedents of seizure disorders in early childhood. *American Journal of Diseases of Children* **140**, 1053–1061.

Newsom-Davis, I., Goldstein, L.H. & Fitzpatrick, D. (1998) Fear of seizures: an investigation and treatment. *Seizure* **7**, 101–106.

Neyens, L.G., Aldenkamp, A.P. & Meinardi, H.M. (1999) Prospective follow-up of intellectual development in children with a recent onset of epilepsy. *Epilepsy Research* **34**, 85–90.

Ng, B.Y. (2002) Psychiatric aspects of self-induced epileptic seizures. *Australian and New Zealand Journal of Psychiatry* **36**, 534–543.

Ng, M. & Devinsky, O. (2004) Vagus nerve stimulation for refractory idiopathic generalised epilepsy. *Seizure* **13**, 176–178.

Ng, S.K., Hauser, W.A., Brust, J.C. & Susser, M. (1988) Alcohol consumption and withdrawal in new-onset seizures. *New England Journal of Medicine* **319**, 666–673.

Ng, S.K., Brust, J.C., Hauser, W.A. & Susser, M. (1990) Illicit drug use and the risk of new-onset seizures. *American Journal of Epidemiology* **132**, 47–57.

Nilsson, L., Tomson, T., Farahmand, B.Y., Diwan, V. & Persson, P.G. (1997) Cause-specific mortality in epilepsy: a cohort study of more than 9,000 patients once hospitalized for epilepsy. *Epilepsia* **38**, 1062–1068.

Nilsson, L., Ahlbom, A., Farahmand, B.Y., Asberg, M. & Tomson, T. (2002) Risk factors for suicide in epilepsy: a case control study. *Epilepsia* **43**, 644–651.

Northcott, E., Connolly, A.M., McIntyre, J. *et al.* (2006) Longitudinal assessment of neuropsychologic and language function in children with benign rolandic epilepsy. *Journal of Child Neurology* **21**, 518–522.

O'Donoghue, M.F. & Sander, J.W.A.S. (1997) The mortality associated with epilepsy, with particular reference to sudden unexpected death: a review. *Epilepsia* **38** (suppl. 11), S15–S19.

O'Donoghue, M.F., Goodridge, D.M., Redhead, K., Sander, J.W. & Duncan, J.S. (1999) Assessing the psychosocial consequences of epilepsy: a community-based study. *British Journal of General Practice* **49**, 211–214.

Okamura, T., Fukai, M., Yamadori, A., Hidari, M., Asaba, H. & Sakai, T. (1993) A clinical study of hypergraphia in epilepsy. *Journal of Neurology, Neurosurgery and Psychiatry* **56**, 556–559.

Olafsson, E., Hauser, W.A., Ludvigsson, P. & Gudmundsson, G. (1996) Incidence of epilepsy in rural Iceland: a population-based study. *Epilepsia* **37**, 951–955.

Olafsson, E., Benedikz, J. & Hauser, W.A. (1999) Risk of epilepsy in patients with multiple sclerosis: a population-based study in Iceland. *Epilepsia* **40**, 745–747.

Onuma, T., Adachi, N., Hisano, T. & Uesugi, S. (1991) 10-year follow-up study of epilepsy with psychosis. *Japanese Journal of Psychiatry and Neurology* **45**, 360–361.

Oostrom, K.J., van Teeseling, H., Smeets-Schouten, A., Peters, A.C. & Jennekens-Schinkel, A. (2005) Three to four years after diagnosis: cognition and behaviour in children with 'epilepsy only'. A prospective controlled study. Dutch Study of Epilepsy in Childhood (DuSECh). *Brain* **128**, 1546–1555.

Ottman, R., Annegers, J.F., Risch, N., Hauser, W.A. & Susser, M. (1996) Relations of genetic and environmental factors in the etiology of epilepsy. *Annals of Neurology* **39**, 442–449.

Ounsted, C., Lindsay, J. & Norman, R. (1966) *Biological Factors in Temporal Lobe Epilepsy*. Heinemann, London.

Oyebode, F. & Davison, K. (1990) Handedness and epileptic schizophrenia. *British Journal of Psychiatry* **156**, 228–230.

Palmini, A. & Gloor, P. (1992) The localizing value of auras in partial seizures: a prospective and retrospective study. *Neurology* **42**, 801–808.

Panayiotopoulos, C.P. (1999a) Early-onset benign childhood occipital seizure susceptibility syndrome: a syndrome to recognize. *Epilepsia* **40**, 621–630.

Panayiotopoulos, C.P. (1999b) Elementary visual hallucinations, blindness, and headache in idiopathic occipital epilepsy: differentiation from migraine. *Journal of Neurology, Neurosurgery and Psychiatry* **66**, 536–540.

Panayiotopoulos, C.P. (2005) Syndromes of idiopathic generalized epilepsies not recognized by the International League Against Epilepsy. *Epilepsia* **46** (suppl. 9), 57–66.

Pauig, P.M., Deluca, M.A. & Osterheld, R.G. (1961) Thioridazine hydrochloride in the treatment of behavior disorders in epileptics. *American Journal of Psychiatry* **117**, 832–833.

Perez, M.M. & Trimble, M.R. (1980) Epileptic psychosis: diagnostic comparison with process schizophrenia. *British Journal of Psychiatry* **137**, 245–249.

Perez, M.M., Trimble, M.R., Murray, N.N.F. & Reider, I. (1985) Epileptic psychosis: an evaluation of PSE profiles. *British Journal of Psychiatry* **146**, 155–163.

Perini, G.I., Tosin, C., Carraro, C. *et al.* (1996) Interictal mood and personality disorders in temporal lobe epilepsy and juvenile myoclonic epilepsy. *Journal of Neurology, Neurosurgery and Psychiatry* **61**, 601–605.

Perucca, E. (2005) An introduction to antiepileptic drugs. *Epilepsia* **46** (suppl. 4), 31–37.

Perucca, E. (2006) Clinically relevant drug interactions with antiepileptic drugs. *British Journal of Clinical Pharmacology* **61**, 246–255.

Perucca, E., Gram, L., Avanzini, G. & Dulac, O. (1998) Antiepileptic drugs as a cause of worsening seizures. *Epilepsia* **39**, 5–17.

Phillips, H.A., Favre, I., Kirkpatrick, M. *et al.* (2001) CHRNB2 is the second acetylcholine receptor subunit associated with autosomal dominant nocturnal frontal lobe epilepsy. *American Journal of Human Genetics* **68**, 225–231.

Piazzini, A. & Canger, R. (2001) Depression and anxiety in patients with epilepsy. *Epilepsia* **42** (suppl. 1), 29–31; discussion 35–36.

Pisani, F., Oteri, G., Costa, C., Di Raimondo, G. & Di Perri, R. (2002) Effects of psychotropic drugs on seizure threshold. *Drug Safety* **25**, 91–110.

Placencia, M., Sander, J.W., Roman, M. *et al.* (1994) The characteristics of epilepsy in a largely untreated population in rural Ecuador. *Journal of Neurology, Neurosurgery and Psychiatry* **57**, 320–325.

Placidi, F., Floris, R., Bozzao, A. *et al.* (2001) Ketotic hyperglycemia and epilepsia partialis continua. *Neurology* **57**, 534–537.

Polkey, C.E. (2004) Clinical outcome of epilepsy surgery. *Current Opinion in Neurology* **17**, 173–178.

Pond, D.A. (1962) Discussion following 'The schizophrenia-like psychoses of epilepsy'. *Proceedings of the Royal Society of Medicine* **55**, 316.

Pond, D.A. & Bidwell, B.H. (1960) A survey of epilepsy in fourteen general practices. II: Social and psychological aspects. *Epilepsia* **1**, 285–299.

Porter, B.E., Judkins, A.R., Clancy, R.R., Duhaime, A., Dlugos, D.J. & Golden, J.A. (2003) Dysplasia: a common finding in intractable pediatric temporal lobe epilepsy. *Neurology* **61**, 365–368.

Pulliainen, V., Kuikka, P. & Jokelainen, M. (2000) Motor and cognitive functions in newly diagnosed adult seizure patients before antiepileptic medication. *Acta Neurologica Scandinavica* **101**, 73–78.

Qin, P., Xu, H., Laursen, T.M., Vestergaard, M. & Mortensen, P.B. (2005) Risk for schizophrenia and schizophrenia-like psychosis among patients with epilepsy: population based cohort study. *British Medical Journal* **331**, 23.

Quigg, M., Broshek, D.K., Heidal-Schiltz, S., Maedgen, J.W. & Bertram, E.H. III (2003) Depression in intractable partial epilepsy varies by laterality of focus and surgery. *Epilepsia* **44**, 419–424.

Quinette, P., Guillery-Girard, B., Dayan, J. *et al.* (2006) What does transient global amnesia really mean? Review of the literature and thorough study of 142 cases. *Brain* **129**, 1640–1658.

Ramani, V. (1998) Reading epilepsy. *Advances in Neurology* **75**, 241–262.

Ramaratnam, S., Baker, G.A. & Goldstein, L.H. (2005) Psychological treatments for epilepsy. *Cochrane Database of Systematic Reviews* 4, CD002029.

Rasalam, A.D., Hailey, H., Williams, J.H. *et al.* (2005) Characteristics of fetal anticonvulsant syndrome associated autistic disorder. *Developmental Medicine and Child Neurology* **47**, 551–555.

Raymond, A.A., Halpin, S.F.S., Alsanjari, N. *et al.* (1994) Dysembryoplastic neuroepithelial tumour. Features in 16 patients. *Brain* **117**, 461–475.

Raymond, A.A., Fish, D.R., Sisodiya, S.M., Alsanjari, N., Stevens, J.M. & Shorvon, S.D. (1995) Abnormalities of gyration, heterotopias, tuberous sclerosis, focal cortical dysplasia, microdysgenesis, dysembryoplastic neuroepithelial tumour and dysgenesis of the archicortex in epilepsy. Clinical, EEG and neuroimaging features in 100 adult patients. *Brain* **118**, 629–660.

Regis, J., Bartolomei, F., Rey, M., Hayashi, M., Chauvel, P. & Peragut, J.C. (2000) Gamma knife surgery for mesial temporal lobe epilepsy. *Journal of Neurosurgery* **93** (suppl. 3), 141–146.

Reuber, M. & Elger, C.E. (2003) Psychogenic nonepileptic seizures: review and update. *Epilepsy and Behavior* **4**, 205–216.

Reuber, M., Fernandez, G., Bauer, J., Singh, D.D. & Elger, C.E. (2002) Interictal EEG abnormalities in patients with psychogenic nonepileptic seizures. *Epilepsia* **43**, 1013–1020.

Reuber, M., Andersen, B., Elger, C.E. & Helmstaedter, C. (2004) Depression and anxiety before and after temporal lobe epilepsy surgery. *Seizure* **13**, 129–135.

Reuber, M., Howlett, S. & Kemp, S. (2005) Psychologic treatment of patients with psychogenic nonepileptic seizures. *Expert Review of Neurotherapeutics* **5**, 737–752.

Richardson, M.P. (2001) CPD education and self-assessment: functional imaging in epilepsy. *Seizure* **10**, 139–156.

Ridsdale, L., Kwan, I. & Cryer, C. (1999) The effect of a special nurse on patients' knowledge of epilepsy and their emotional state. Epilepsy Evaluation Care Group. *British Journal of General Practice* **49**, 285–289.

Ring, H.A., Moriarty, J. & Trimble, M.R. (1998) A prospective study of the early postsurgical psychiatric associations of epilepsy surgery. *Journal of Neurology, Neurosurgery and Psychiatry* **64**, 601–604.

Roberts, G.W., Done, D.J., Bruton, C.J. & Crow, T.J. (1990) A 'mock-up' of schizophrenia: temporal lobe epilepsy and schizophrenia-like psychosis. *Biological Psychiatry* **28**, 127–143.

Roberts, J.K.A., Robertson, M.M. & Trimble, M.R. (1982) The lateralising significance of hypergraphia in temporal lobe, epilepsy. *Journal of Neurology, Neurosurgery and Psychiatry* **45**, 131–138.

Robertson, M.M. & Trimble, M.R. (1985) The treatment of depression in patients with epilepsy. A double-blind trial. *Journal of Affective Disorders* **9**, 127–136.

Robertson, M.M., Trimble, M.R. & Townsend, H.R. (1987) Phenomenology of depression in epilepsy. *Epilepsia* **28**, 364–372.

Robinson, R.O., Baird, G., Robinson, G. & Simonoff, E. (2001) Landau–Kleffner syndrome: course and correlates with outcome. *Developmental Medicine and Child Neurology* **43**, 243–247.

Romanelli, M.F., Morris, J.C., Ashkin, K. & Coben, L.A. (1990) Advanced Alzheimer's disease is a risk factor for late-onset seizures. *Archives of Neurology* **47**, 847–850.

Rossetti, A.O., Dworetzky, B.A., Madsen, J.R., Golub, O., Beckman, J.A. & Bromfield, E.B. (2005) Ictal asystole with convulsive syncope mimicking secondary generalisation: a depth electrode study. *Journal of Neurology, Neurosurgery and Psychiatry* **76**, 885–887.

Rugg-Gunn, F.J., Simister, R.J., Squirrell, M., Holdright, D.R. & Duncan, J.S. (2004) Cardiac arrhythmias in focal epilepsy: a prospective long-term study. *Lancet* **364**, 2212–2219.

Rusch, M.D., Morris, G.L., Allen, L. & Lathrop, L. (2001) Psychological treatment of non-epileptic events. *Epilepsy and Behavior* **2**, 277–283.

Russell, W.R. & Whitty, C.W.M. (1952) Studies in traumatic epilepsy. 1: Factors influencing the incidence of epilepsy after brain wounds. *Journal of Neurology, Neurosurgery and Psychiatry* **15**, 93–98.

Sachdev, H.S. & Waxman, S.G. (1981) Frequency of hypergraphia in temporal lobe epilepsy: an index of interictal behaviour syndrome. *Journal of Neurology, Neurosurgery and Psychiatry* **44**, 358–360.

Sachdev, P. (1998) Schizophrenia-like psychosis and epilepsy: the status of the association. *American Journal of Psychiatry* **155**, 325–336.

Sadleir, L.G. & Scheffer, I.E. (2007) Febrile seizures. *British Medical Journal* **334**, 307–311.

Sadler, R.M. & Rahey, S. (2004) Prescience as an aura of temporal lobe epilepsy. *Epilepsia* **45**, 982–984.

Salanova, V., Andermann, F., Rasmussen, T., Olivier, A. & Quesney, L.F. (1995) Parietal lobe epilepsy. Clinical manifestations and outcome in 82 patients treated surgically between 1929 and 1988. *Brain* **118**, 607–627.

Salazar, A.M., Jabbari, B., Vance, S.C., Grafman, J., Amin, D. & Dillon, J.D. (1985) Epilepsy after penetrating head injury. I. Clinical correlates: a report of the Vietnam Head Injury Study. *Neurology* **35**, 1406–1414.

Samren, E.B., van Duijn, C.M., Koch, S. *et al.* (1997) Maternal use of antiepileptic drugs and the risk of major congenital malformations: a joint European prospective study of human teratogenesis associated with maternal epilepsy. *Epilepsia* **38**, 981–990.

Sander, J.W., Hart, Y.M., Johnson, A.L. & Shorvon, S.D. (1990) National General Practice Study of Epilepsy: newly diagnosed epileptic seizures in a general population. *Lancet* **336**, 1267–1271.

Savard, G., Andermann, F., Olivier, A. & Remillard, G.M. (1991) Postictal psychosis after partial complex seizures: a multiple case study. *Epilepsia* **32**, 225–231.

Sazgar, M., Carlen, P.L. & Wennberg, R. (2003) Panic attack semiology in right temporal lobe epilepsy. *Epileptic Disorders* **5**, 93–100.

Schachter, S.C. (2002) Vagus nerve stimulation therapy summary: five years after FDA approval. *Neurology* **59** (6 suppl. 4), S15–S20.

Scheffer, I.E., Bhatia, K.P., Lopes-Cendes, I. *et al.* (1995) Autosomal dominant nocturnal frontal lobe epilepsy. A distinctive clinical disorder. *Brain* **118**, 61–73.

Scheffer, I.E., Harkin, L.A., Grinton, B.E. *et al.* (2007) Temporal lobe epilepsy and GEFS+ phenotypes associated with SCN1B mutations. *Brain* **130**, 100–109.

Schierhout, G. & Roberts, I. (1998) Prophylactic antiepileptic agents after head injury: a systematic review. *Journal of Neurology, Neurosurgery and Psychiatry* **64**, 108–112.

Schmidt, D. & Loscher, W. (2005) Uncontrolled epilepsy following discontinuation of antiepileptic drugs in seizure-free patients: a review of current clinical experience. *Acta Neurologica Scandinavica* **111**, 291–300.

Schmitz, B. (1999) Psychiatric syndromes related to antiepileptic drugs. *Epilepsia* **40** (suppl. 10), S65–S70.

Schmitz, E.B., Robertson, M.M. & Trimble, M.R. (1999) Depression and schizophrenia in epilepsy: social and biological risk factors. *Epilepsy Research* **35**, 59–68.

Schomer, D.L. (1993) Focal status epilepticus and epilepsia partialis continua in adults and children. *Epilepsia* **34** (suppl. 1), S29–S36.

Schulze-Bonhage, A., Kurth, C., Carius, A., Steinhoff, B.J. & Mayer, T. (2006) Seizure anticipation by patients with focal and generalized epilepsy: a multicentre assessment of premonitory symptoms. *Epilepsy Research* **70**, 83–88.

Scott, R.C., King, M.D., Gadian, D.G., Neville, B.G. & Connelly, A. (2003) Hippocampal abnormalities after prolonged febrile convulsion: a longitudinal MRI study. *Brain* **126**, 2551–2557.

Selway, R. & Dardis, R. (2004) Multiple subpial transection for epilepsy. In: Shorvon, S.D., Perucca, E., Fish, D.R. & Dodson, W.E. (eds) *The Treatment of Epilepsy*, pp. 812–823. Blackwell Science, Malden, MA.

Seshia, S.S. & McLachlan, R.S. (2005) Aura continua. *Epilepsia* **46**, 454–455.

Shafrir, Y. & Prensky, A.L. (1995) Acquired epileptiform opercular syndrome: a second case report, review of the literature, and comparison to the Landau–Kleffner syndrome. *Epilepsia* **36**, 1050–1057.

Shahwan, A., Farrell, M. & Delanty, N. (2005) Progressive myoclonic epilepsies: a review of genetic and therapeutic aspects. *Lancet Neurology* **4**, 239–248.

Shaw, P., Mellers, J., Henderson, M., Polkey, C., David, A.S. & Toone, B.K. (2004) Schizophrenia-like psychosis arising de novo following a temporal lobectomy: timing and risk factors. *Journal of Neurology, Neurosurgery and Psychiatry* **75**, 1003–1008.

Sheldon, R., Rose, S., Ritchie, D. *et al.* (2002) Historical criteria that distinguish syncope from seizures. *Journal of the American College of Cardiology* **40**, 142–148.

Sheldon, R., Rose, S., Connolly, S., Ritchie, D., Koshman, M.L. & Frenneaux, M. (2006) Diagnostic criteria for vasovagal syncope based on a quantitative history. *European Heart Journal* **27**, 344–350.

Shen, W., Bowman, E.S. & Markand, O.N. (1990) Presenting the diagnosis of pseudoseizure. *Neurology* **40**, 756–759.

Sherwin, I. (1981) Psychosis associated with epilepsy: significance of the laterality of the epileptogenic lesion. *Journal of Neurology, Neurosurgery and Psychiatry* **44**, 83–85.

Shorvon, S. (1994) *Status Epilepticus. Its Clinical Features and Treatment in Children and Adults*. Cambridge University Press, Cambridge.

Shorvon, S. (2001) The management of status epilepticus. *Journal of Neurology, Neurosurgery and Psychiatry* **70** (suppl. 2), II22–II27.

Shorvon, S.D. (2004) The choice of drugs and approach to drug treatments in partial epilepsy. In: Shorvon, S.D., Perucca, E., Fish, D.R. & Dodson, W.E. (eds) *The Treatment of Epilepsy*, pp. 317–333. Blackwell Science, Malden, MA.

Shorvon, S. & Walker, M. (2005) Status epilepticus in idiopathic generalized epilepsy. *Epilepsia* **46** (suppl. 9), 73–79.

Shorvon, S.D., Perucca, E., Fish, D.R. & Dodson, W.E. (eds) (2004) *The Treatment of Epilepsy*. Blackwell Science, Malden, MA.

Shukla, G.D., Srivastava, O.N. & Katiyar, B.C. (1979) Sexual disturbances in temporal lobe epilepsy: a controlled study. *British Journal of Psychiatry* **134**, 288–292.

Siegel, A.M. & Williamson, P.D. (2000) Parietal lobe epilepsy. *Advances in Neurology* **84**, 189–199.

Sillanpaa, M., Jalava, M., Kaleva, O. & Shinnar, S. (1998) Long-term prognosis of seizures with onset in childhood. *New England Journal of Medicine* **338**, 1715–1722.

Sisodiya, S.M. (2004) Malformations of cortical development: burdens and insights from important causes of human epilepsy. *Lancet Neurology* **3**, 29–38.

Sisodiya, S.M. (2005) Genetics of drug resistance in epilepsy. *Current Neurology and Neuroscience Reports* **5**, 307–311.

Slater, E., Beard, A.W. & Glithero, E. (1963) The schizophrenia-like psychoses of epilepsy. *British Journal of Psychiatry* **109**, 95–150.

Slavney, P.R. (1994) In defense of pseudoseizure. *General Hospital Psychiatry* **16**, 243–245.

Smith, D. & Chadwick, D. (2001) The management of epilepsy. *Journal of Neurology, Neurosurgery and Psychiatry* **70** (suppl. 2), 15–21.

Smith, D., Defalla, B.A. & Chadwick, D.W. (1999) The misdiagnosis of epilepsy and the management of refractory epilepsy in a specialist clinic. *Quarterly Journal of Medicine* **92**, 15–23.

Smith, S.J. (2005) EEG in the diagnosis, classification, and management of patients with epilepsy. *Journal of Neurology, Neurosurgery and Psychiatry* **76** (suppl. 2), ii2–ii7.

So, E.L., Annegers, J.F., Hauser, W.A., O'Brien, P.C. & Whisnant, J.P. (1996) Population-based study of seizure disorders after cerebral infarction. *Neurology* **46**, 350–355.

So, N.K. (1998) Mesial frontal epilepsy. *Epilepsia* **39** (6 suppl. 4), S49–S61.

So, N.K., Savard, G., Andermann, F., Olivier, A. & Quesney, L.F. (1990) Acute postictal psychosis: a stereo EEG study. *Epilepsia* **31**, 188–193.

Soteriades, E.S., Evans, J.C., Larson, M.G. *et al.* (2002) Incidence and prognosis of syncope. *New England Journal of Medicine* **347**, 878–885.

Sowa, M.V. & Pituck, S. (1989) Prolonged spontaneous complex visual hallucinations and illusions as ictal phenomena. *Epilepsia* **30**, 524–526.

Spacey, S.D., Adams, P.J., Lam, P.C. *et al.* (2006) Genetic heterogeneity in paroxysmal nonkinesigenic dyskinesia. *Neurology* **66**, 1588–1590.

Spatt, J., Langbauer, G. & Mamoli, B. (1998) Subjective perception of seizure precipitants: results of a questionnaire study. *Seizure* **7**, 391–395.

Specchio, L.M., Tramacere, L., La Neve, A. & Beghi, E. (2002) Discontinuing antiepileptic drugs in patients who are seizure free on monotherapy. *Journal of Neurology, Neurosurgery and Psychiatry* **72**, 22–25.

Specchio, L.M., Iudice, A., Specchio, N. *et al.* (2004) Citalopram as treatment of depression in patients with epilepsy. *Clinical Neuropharmacology* **27**, 133–136.

Spector, S., Cull, C. & Goldstein, L.H. (2001) High and low perceived self-control of epileptic seizures. *Epilepsia* **42**, 556–564.

Spencer, S.S., Schramm, J., Wyler, A. *et al.* (2002) Multiple subpial transection for intractable partial epilepsy: an international meta-analysis. *Epilepsia* **43**, 141–145.

Sperli, F., Spinelli, L., Pollo, C. & Seeck, M. (2006) Contralateral smile and laughter, but no mirth, induced by electrical stimulation of the cingulate cortex. *Epilepsia* **47**, 440–443.

Spina, E. & Perucca, E. (2002) Clinical significance of pharmacokinetic interactions between antiepileptic and psychotropic drugs. *Epilepsia* **43** (suppl. 2), 37–44.

Stefan, H., Schulze-Bonhage, A., Pauli, E. *et al.* (2004) Ictal pleasant sensations: cerebral localization and lateralization. *Epilepsia* **45**, 35–40.

Stefansson, S.B., Olafsson, E. & Hauser, W.A. (1998) Psychiatric morbidity in epilepsy: a case controlled study of adults receiving disability benefits. *Journal of Neurology, Neurosurgery and Psychiatry* **64**, 238–241.

Steinlein, O.K. (2004) Genes and mutations in human idiopathic epilepsy. *Brain and Development* **26**, 213–218.

Stevens, J.R. (1959) Emotional activation of the electro-encephalogram in patients with convulsive disorders. *Journal of Nervous and Mental Disease* **128**, 339–351.

Stevens, J.R. (1992) Abnormal reinnervation as a basis for schizophrenia: a hypothesis. *Archives of General Psychiatry* **49**, 238–243.

Stevens, J.R. & Hermann, B.P. (1981) Temporal lobe epilepsy, psychopathology, and violence: the state of the evidence. *Neurology* **31**, 1127–1132.

Stone, J., Campbell, K., Sharma, N., Carson, A., Warlow, C.P. & Sharpe, M. (2003) What should we call pseudoseizures? The patient's perspective. *Seizure* **12**, 568–572.

Sturm, J.W., Andermann, F. & Berkovic, S.F. (2000) 'Pressure to laugh': an unusual epileptic symptom associated with small hypothalamic hamartomas. *Neurology* **54**, 971–973.

Sundaram, M., Hogan, T., Hiscock, M. & Pillay, N. (1990) Factors affecting interictal spike discharges in adults with epilepsy. *Electroencephalography and Clinical Neurophysiology* **75**, 358–360.

Sveinbjornsdottir, S. & Duncan, J.S. (1993) Parietal and occipital lobe epilepsy: a review. *Epilepsia* **34**, 493–521. [Erratum appears in *Epilepsia* 1994, **35**, 467.]

Swartz, B.E., Simpkins, F., Halgren, E. *et al.* (1996) Visual working memory in primary generalized epilepsy: an [18]FDG-PET study. *Neurology* **47**, 1203–1212.

Symonds, C.P. (1962) Discussion following 'The schizophrenia-like psychoses of epilepsy'. *Proceedings of the Royal Society of Medicine* **55**, 314–315.

Tarkka, R., Paakko, E., Pyhtinen, J., Uhari, M. & Rantala, H. (2003) Febrile seizures and mesial temporal sclerosis: no association in a long-term follow-up study. *Neurology* **60**, 215–218.

Tarulli, A., Devinsky, O. & Alper, K. (2001) Progression of postictal to interictal psychosis. *Epilepsia* **42**, 1468–1471.

Taylor, D.C. (1972) Mental state and temporal lobe epilepsy: a correlative account of 100 patients treated surgically. *Epilepsia* **13**, 727–765.

Taylor, D.C. (1975) Factors influencing the occurrence of schizophrenia-like psychosis in patients with temporal lobe epilepsy. *Psychological Medicine* **5**, 249–254.

Taylor, D.C. & Lochery, M. (1987) Temporal lobe epilepsy: origin and significance of simple and complex auras. *Journal of Neurology, Neurosurgery and Psychiatry* **50**, 673–681.

Taylor, I., Scheffer, I.E. & Berkovic, S.F. (2003) Occipital epilepsies: identification of specific and newly recognized syndromes. *Brain* **126**, 753–769.

Tebartz van Elst, L., Baeumer, D., Lemieux, L. *et al.* (2002) Amygdala pathology in psychosis of epilepsy: a magnetic resonance imaging study in patients with temporal lobe epilepsy. *Brain* **125**, 140–149.

Thomas, P., Beaumanoir, A., Genton, P., Dolisi, C. & Chatel, M. (1992) 'De novo' absence status of late onset: report of 11 cases. *Neurology* **42**, 104–110.

Tijssen, M.A., Vergouwe, M.N., van Dijk, J.G., Rees, M., Frants, R.R. & Brown, P. (2002) Major and minor form of hereditary hyperekplexia. *Movement Disorders* **17**, 826–830.

Tinuper, P., Bisulli, F., Cerullo, A. *et al.* (2001) Ictal bradycardia in partial epileptic seizures: autonomic investigation in three cases and literature review. *Brain* **124**, 2361–2371.

Tomson, T., Walczak, T., Sillanpaa, M. & Sander, J.W.A.S. (2005) Sudden unexpected death in epilepsy: a review of incidence and risk factors. *Epilepsia* **46** (suppl. 11), 54–61.

Toone, B.K. (1981) Psychoses of epilepsy. In: Reynolds, E.H. & Trimble, M.R. (eds) *Epilepsy and Psychiatry*, ch. 10. Churchill Livingstone, Edinburgh & London.

Toone, B.K., Garralda, M.E. & Ron, M.A. (1982) The psychoses of epilepsy and the functional psychoses: a clinical and phenomenological comparison. *British Journal of Psychiatry* **141**, 256–261.

Toone, B.K., Wheeler, M., Nanjee, M., Fenwick, P. & Grant, R. (1983) Sex hormones, sexual activity and plasma anticonvulsant levels in male epileptics. *Journal of Neurology, Neurosurgery and Psychiatry* **46**, 824–826.

Toone, B.K., Edeh, J., Nanjee, M.N. & Wheeler, M. (1989) Hyposexuality and epilepsy: a community survey of hormonal and behavioural changes in male epileptics. *Psychological Medicine* **19**, 937–943.

Treiman, D.M. (1986) Epilepsy and violence: medical and legal issues. *Epilepsia* **27** (suppl. 2), S77–S104.

Treiman, D.M. (1999) Violence and the epilepsy defense. *Neurologic Clinics* **17**, 245–255.

Trimble, M.R. (1983) Personality disturbances in epilepsy. *Neurology* **33**, 1332–1334.

Trinka, E., Unterrainer, J., Haberlandt, E. *et al.* (2002) Childhood febrile convulsions: which factors determine the subsequent epilepsy syndrome? A retrospective study. *Epilepsy Research* **50**, 283–292.

Umbricht, D., Degreef, G., Barr, W.B., Lieberman, J.A., Pollack, S. & Schaul, N. (1995) Postictal and chronic psychoses in patients with temporal lobe epilepsy. *American Journal of Psychiatry* **152**, 224–231.

Upton, D. & Thompson, P.J. (1996) General neuropsychological characteristics of frontal lobe epilepsy. *Epilepsy Research* **23**, 169–177.

Vadlamudi, L., Andermann, E., Lombroso, C.T. *et al.* (2004) Epilepsy in twins: insights from unique historical data of William Lennox. *Neurology* **62**, 1127–1133.

Venance, S.L., Cannon, S.C., Fialho, D. *et al.* (2006) The primary periodic paralyses: diagnosis, pathogenesis and treatment. *Brain* **129**, 8–17.

Vermeulen, J. & Aldenkamp, A.P. (1995) Cognitive side-effects of chronic antiepileptic drug treatment: a review of 25 years of research. *Epilepsy Research* **22**, 65–95.

Verrotti, A., Greco, R., Altobelli, E. *et al.* (1999) Centro-temporal spikes in non-epileptic children: a long-term follow up. *Journal of Paediatrics and Child Health* **35**, 60–62.

Victor, M. & Brausch C. (1967) The role of abstinence in the genesis of alcoholic epilepsy. *Epilepsia* **8**, 1–20.

Victoroff, J.I., Benson, F., Grafton, S.T., Engel, J. Jr & Mazziotta, J.C. (1994) Depression in complex partial seizures. Electroencephalography and cerebral metabolic correlates. *Archives of Neurology* **51**, 155–163.

Vidailhet, M. (2000) Paroxysmal dyskinesias as a paradigm of paroxysmal movement disorders. *Current Opinion in Neurology* **13**, 457–462.

Vignal, J.P., Maillard, L., McGonigal, A. & Chauvel, P. (2007) The dreamy state: hallucinations of autobiographic memory evoked by temporal lobe stimulations and seizures. *Brain* **130**, 88–99.

Vingerhoets, G. (2006) Cognitive effects of seizures. *Seizure* **15**, 221–226.

Vinten, J., Adab, N., Kini, U. *et al.* (2005) Neuropsychological effects of exposure to anticonvulsant medication in utero. *Neurology* **64**, 949–954.

Walker, A.E. (1961) Murder or epilepsy? *Journal of Nervous and Mental Disease* **133**, 430–437.

Walker, A.E. & Jablon, S. (1961) *A Follow-up Study of Head Wounds in World War II.* Veterans Administration Medical Monograph No. 5, Washington, DC.

Walker, M., Cross, H., Smith, S. *et al.* (2005) Nonconvulsive status epilepticus: Epilepsy Research Foundation workshop reports. *Epileptic Disorders* **7**, 253–296.

Walker, M.C. & Shorvon, S.D. (2004) Emergency treatment of seizures and status. In: Shorvon, S.D., Perucca, E., Fish, D.R. & Dodson, W.E. (eds) *The Treatment of Epilepsy*, pp. 227–243. Blackwell Science, Malden, MA.

Wallace, S.J. (2001) Epilepsy in cerebral palsy. *Developmental Medicine and Child Neurology* **43**, 713–717.

Waruiru, C. & Appleton, R. (2004) Febrile seizures: an update. *Archives of Disease in Childhood* **89**, 751–756.

Waterman, K., Purves, S.J., Kosaka, B., Strauss, E. & Wada, J.A. (1987) An epileptic syndrome caused by mesial frontal lobe seizure foci. *Neurology* **37**, 577–582.

Waxman, S.G. & Geschwind, N. (1975) The interictal behavior syndrome of temporal lobe epilepsy. *Archives of General Psychiatry* **32**, 1580–1586.

Weglage, J., Demsky, A., Pietsch, M. & Kurlemann, G. (1997) Neuropsychological, intellectual, and behavioral findings in patients with centrotemporal spikes with and without seizures. *Developmental Medicine and Child Neurology* **39**, 646–651.

Whitman, S., Coleman, T.E., Patmon, C., Desai, B.T., Cohen, R. & King, L.N. (1984) Epilepsy in prison: elevated prevalence and no relationship to violence. *Neurology* **34**, 775–782.

Wiebe, S., Blume, W.T., Girvin, J.P. & Eliasziw, M. (2001) A randomized, controlled trial of surgery for temporal-lobe epilepsy. Effectiveness and Efficiency of Surgery for Temporal Lobe Epilepsy Study Group. *New England Journal of Medicine* **345**, 311–318.

Wieser, H.G. (1980) Temporal lobe or psychomotor status epilepticus. A case report. *Electroencephalography and Clinical Neurophysiology* **48**, 558–572.

Wieser, H.G. (2000) Semiology of neocortical temporal lobe epilepsy. *Advances in Neurology* **84**, 201–214.

Wieser, H.G., Hailemariam, S., Regard, M. & Landis, T. (1985) Unilateral limbic epileptic status activity: stereo EEG, behavioral, and cognitive data. *Epilepsia* **26**, 19–29.

Wilkus, R.J., Dodrill, C.B. & Thompson, P.M. (1984) Intensive EEG monitoring and psychological studies of patients with pseudoepileptic seizures. *Epilepsia* **25**, 100–107.

Willert, C., Spitzer, C., Kusserow, S. & Runge, U. (2004) Serum neuron-specific enolase, prolactin, and creatine kinase after epileptic and psychogenic non-epileptic seizures. *Acta Neurologica Scandinavica* **109**, 318–323.

Williams, D. (1966) Temporal lobe epilepsy. *British Medical Journal* **1**, 1439–1442.

Williams, J., Lawthom, C., Dunstan, F.D. *et al.* (2006) Variability of antiepileptic medication taking behaviour in sudden unexplained death in epilepsy: hair analysis at autopsy. *Journal of Neurology, Neurosurgery and Psychiatry* **77**, 481–484.

Williamson, P.D. & Jobst, B.C. (2000) Frontal lobe epilepsy. *Advances in Neurology* **84**, 215–242.

Williamson, P.D., Spencer, D.D., Spencer, S.S., Novelly, R.A. & Mattson, R.H. (1985) Complex partial seizures of frontal lobe origin. *Annals of Neurology* **18**, 497–504.

Williamson, P.D., Thadani, V.M., French, J.A. *et al.* (1998) Medial temporal lobe epilepsy: videotape analysis of objective clinical seizure characteristics. *Epilepsia* **39**, 1182–1188.

Wirrell, E.C. (2006) Epilepsy-related injuries. *Epilepsia* **47** (suppl. 1), 79–86.

Wirrell, E.C., Camfield, C.S., Camfield, P.R., Dooley, J.M., Gordon, K.E. & Smith, B. (1997) Long-term psychosocial outcome in typical absence epilepsy. Sometimes a wolf in sheeps' clothing. *Archives of Pediatrics and Adolescent Medicine* **151**, 152–158.

Wrench, J., Wilson, S.J. & Bladin, P.F. (2004) Mood disturbance before and after seizure surgery: a comparison of temporal and extratemporal resections. *Epilepsia* **45**, 534–543.

Young, W.B. & Silberstein, S.D. (2006) Migraine: spectrum of symptoms and diagnosis. *Continuum: Lifelong Learning in Neurology* **12**, 67–86.

Zeman, A.Z., Boniface, S.J. & Hodges, J.R. (1998) Transient epileptic amnesia: a description of the clinical and neuropsychological features in 10 cases and a review of the literature. *Journal of Neurology, Neurosurgery and Psychiatry* **64**, 435–443.

Zifkin, B.G. & Zatorre, R.J. (1998) Musicogenic epilepsy. *Advances in Neurology* **75**, 273–281.

Zijlmans, M., Flanagan, D. & Gotman, J. (2002) Heart rate changes and ECG abnormalities during epileptic seizures: prevalence and definition of an objective clinical sign. *Epilepsia* **43**, 847–854.

Zivin, L. & Ajmone Marsan, C. (1968) Incidence and prognostic significance of 'epileptiform' activity in the EEG of non-epileptic subjects. *Brain* **91**, 751–778.

CHAPTER 7

Intracranial Infections

Michael D. Dilley[1] and Simon Fleminger[2]

[1] Soho Centre for Health and Care, London
[2] Maudsley Hospital, London

Intracranial infections are usually the province of the neurologist or general physician but must occasionally be considered in the differential diagnosis of psychiatric patients. HIV/AIDS is of particular importance, likewise cerebral syphilis which, though rare, has shown an increasing incidence recently and has crucial treatment implications. These are dealt with in some detail, also certain encephalitic illnesses in which diagnostic confusion can arise. More space is devoted to encephalitis lethargica than its present-day incidence warrants, because of the important lessons that were learned for psychiatry during outbreaks of the disease. Meningitis, cerebral abscess and other nervous system infections are dealt with very briefly.

Acquired immunodeficiency syndrome

The appearance of AIDS on the medical and social scene, over 25 years ago in the early 1980s, has been followed by worldwide spread of the disease and escalating numbers of persons affected. Significant impact has been made on the prevalence of the disease, particularly through the use of highly active antiretroviral treatment (HAART), and knowledge about the effects of the virus as well as investigative methods to assess this have progressed significantly since the first recognised cases. Nonetheless, the virus is still rife in the USA and Europe, although its impact is far greater in sub-Saharan Africa and other developing countries. Worldwide, over 40 million adults and children are living with HIV or AIDS. There are an estimated 8500 deaths from the disease daily – two-thirds of these are in sub-Saharan Africa – and greater than 20 million have already succumbed to the disease (UNAIDS 2006).

In Western and Central Europe in 2006, there were up to 970 000 people living with the virus. During the period 1998–2005, the rate of new diagnoses nearly doubled, from 42 to 74 cases per million. The most rapid increase was seen in the UK, where in 2005 there were 7700 new diagnoses (Health Protection Agency 2005). Figures from the USA are many times in excess of this, with only seven countries worldwide estimated to have more cases. A cumulative total of some 1 150 000 HIV or AIDS cases had been reported in the USA from the start of the pandemic to 2004 (Centers for Disease Control 2006a). Altogether in 2006 reports suggest 25 million infected adults in sub-Saharan Africa, 7.8 million in South and South-east Asia, and 2 million in Latin America and the Caribbean (UNAIDS 2006).

Problems associated with the disease include not only its devastating clinical manifestations and their economic cost, but also the cultural and social problems that must be tackled in attempts to limit its spread. For the first time in a worldwide epidemic it has been necessary to try to change fundamental aspects of human behaviour by education and the dissemination of information. Moreover, this centres on topics as sensitive as sexual practices and the control of risk-taking behaviour among persons addicted to drugs. A particularly disturbing aspect concerns the risk of transmission to children born to infected women; the proportion of females has slowly risen and is particularly high, approaching 60%, in Africa, some 13.3 million people. Added difficulties arise from the stigma attached to the disease and the fear engendered among populations at special risk, particularly men who have sex with men. This is fuelled by the ever-present risk of transmission from infected but asymptomatic individuals.

Epidemiology and groups at risk

The disease was first recognised in 1981 when cases of *Pneumocystis carinii* pneumonia (PCP) and Kaposi's sarcoma were reported from California and New York in previously healthy men who were both homosexual and immunocompromised. The first UK cases were recognised soon afterwards. With

Lishman's Organic Psychiatry: A Textbook of Neuropsychiatry, 4th edition.
© 2009 Blackwell Publishing.   ISBN 978-1-4051-1860-1

hindsight, however, the disease had existed in the USA since at least 1978, and analysis of stored serum samples has indicated that the virus was entering the drug-injecting population in the mid-1970s (Des Jarlais *et al.* 1989). The origins of HIV have been the subject of intense debate. It has been reported that lentiviruses most closely related to HIV-1 have been isolated in chimpanzees, particularly the subspecies *Pan troglodytes troglodytes*, native to western equatorial Africa. Interspecies transmission is hypothesised to have occurred prior to 1940 (Sharp *et al.* 2001).

The subgroups of the population mainly affected differ with geographical location. In Western Europe, North America and Australasia, men who have sex with men are predominantly affected, followed by injecting drug users and heterosexual contacts with infected persons. On the west coast of America, the majority of HIV-infected persons are men who have sex with men, whereas on the east coast there is a higher prevalence among intravenous drug users. More than half of the estimated 200 000 drug injectors in New York in the late 1980s were infected with HIV, and appeared to be the principal source of heterosexual and perinatal transmission (Des Jarlais *et al.* 1989). In the UK, the prevalence varies among drug users, from around 7% in London to 20% in Edinburgh (Stimson 1995), a significant decrease from the previously reported 55% Edinburgh (Adler 1987). In Italy and Spain drug injection accounts for over two-thirds of the cases of AIDS, whereas in sub-Saharan Africa the commonest mode of transmission is heterosexual intercourse (UNAIDS 2006).

Figures on cases reported between 2001 and 2004 in the USA and the UK show that male homosexual transmission is clearly the commonest route. In the UK, a large proportion of infections through heterosexual intercourse are thought to derive from infections acquired abroad, particularly from African countries. Transmission via contaminated blood products was recognised from 1983, largely stemming from contaminated pooled factors VIII and IX given to haemophiliac patients. Mother-to-infant transmission in the UK may be due in large part to mothers who acquired the infection in Africa.

The virus disproportionately affects racial and ethnic minorities. In the USA, for example, during the period 2001–2004, some 50% of AIDS diagnoses were in the African-American population and 20% among the Hispanic community. In 2004, the rate of new diagnoses was seven times higher in African-American men and a startling 21 times higher among African-American women compared with their white counterparts (Centers for Disease Control 2006a).

The largest concentration of infection in the UK is in London and the South-east (Health Protection Agency 2006), accounting for 56% of all cases reported in 2005. However, there has been a gradual increase in diagnoses in other regions, including areas where HIV infection had been pre-

viously rare (Health Protection Agency 2006). While transmission between men who have sex with men remains the commonest group infected (around one-third of new diagnoses), persons infected in sub-Saharan Africa are now the group most affected by HIV in the UK. Research reported from the South-east and the Midlands suggests that the fear of discrimination and stigma associated with diagnosis are significant factors that preclude UK Africans from seeking serum testing (Elam *et al.* 2006). In the UK, levels of HIV and other sexually transmitted infections remain high in the population of men who have sex with men and new diagnoses have increased by 50% since 2000 (Health Protection Agency 2006). This has provoked fresh calls for prevention and education strategies targeting this risk group (Elford *et al.* 2005). Indeed, it is concerning that knowledge regarding HIV is deteriorating in general. In 2005, only 70% of surveyed Londoners were aware that HIV was transmitted by unprotected sexual intercourse compared with 91% in 2000 (National AIDS Trust 2006). Furthermore, in the UK the number of individuals living with HIV who have not been tested and are unaware of their status has been estimated as around one-third. This obviously not only impacts on the risk of transmission but also the potential benefits of treatment for this group (British Medical Association 2006).

The virus

The virus responsible for AIDS was isolated in 1983. It was first named lymphadenopathy-associated virus (LAV) in France and human T-cell lymphotropic virus type III (HTLV-III) in the USA, but by common consent is now termed human immunodeficiency virus (HIV). The overwhelming majority of cases worldwide are caused by HIV-1, although the related HIV-2 (LAV-2, HTLV-IV) has proved to be responsible for a similar AIDS presentation, principally among West Africans. HTLV-I is responsible for epidemics of tropical spastic paraparesis that may be transmitted sexually.

Related viruses in animals include visna virus in sheep and caprine arthritis encephalitis virus in goats, which lead to neurodegenerative disorders. Of particular interest are the simian immunodeficiency viruses (SIVs). Strains of SIV (SIVsm) most closely resembling HIV-2 and likely to be related viruses have been found in the wild in sooty mangabeys (*Cercocebus atys*) native to West Africa and also in several macaque monkeys in captivity in North America. HIV-2 is only endemic in West Africa and it seems likely that transmission between monkeys and humans has occurred there. Strains of SIV from chimpanzees (SIVcpz) resemble HIV-1, and despite initial uncertainty it is now clear that this is the likely origin of HIV-1. Cross-species transmission is hypothesised to have occurred through exposure to chimpanzee (and sooty mangabey) blood and mucosal secretions during hunting or when eating raw contaminated 'bush meat' (Robinson 1999; Sharp *et al.* 2001). These viruses are lentiviruses (i.e. slow to replicate and produce pathological effects) in the general class of retroviruses. Retroviruses have the unique characteristic of replicating by entering host cells, then using the enzyme reverse transcriptase to integrate their own genetic material into the DNA of the host cell nucleus. This continues to manufacture the virus until the cell dies, resulting in persistent infection. HIV-1 and HIV-2 resemble each other under the electron microscope but differ in the molecular weight of their constituent proteins. HIV infects cells that bear the CD4 surface receptor, using a glycoprotein on its surface (gp120) for the initial interaction. CD4 is the primary receptor for HIV and is found on monocytes, macrophages, eosinophils, dendritic cells and microglial cells in the central nervous system (CNS) as well as a subset of T-helper lymphocytes (T4 cells). Experiments have shown that CD4 receptors on the cell surface of non-human cell lines are insufficient to allow entry of HIV; subsequently, the existence of coreceptors was hypothesised and investigated. In 1995–1996, it was reported that members of the chemokine receptor family, specifically CCR5 and CXCR4, could co-facilitate the entry of HIV-1 into CD4$^+$ cells (Rowland-Jones 1999).

Once inside the cell, reverse transcriptase carried in the genome of the virus catalyses the production of a DNA copy of the single-stranded viral RNA. This migrates to the nucleus of the cell and becomes integrated into its genome. The integrated DNA copy is called a 'provirus'. Thereafter it may exist in latent form without pathogenic effect, reproducing along with the cell, or it may change to become productive and cytopathic. Such change involves the production of new viral RNA, the assembly of viral proteins that are toxic to the cell, and the budding of new virus from the surface of the cell to infect others. In individuals treated with HAART, reservoirs of latent provirus in quiescent CD4 cells have taken on new importance, as they are instrumental in preventing eradication of the virus.

Retrovirus replication is prone to errors and subsequently mutations; on average, 1–10 errors per genome per round of replication occur. This results in either replication-incompetent virions or mutations that cause drug resistance. The hallmark of active HIV infection is the gradual depletion of T4-helper lymphocytes in the blood, with correspondingly disastrous impairment of the body's immunological competence. Infection of macrophages and microglia leads to a further range of complications involving the nervous system directly as described below.

Natural history and clinical signs of HIV infection

Infection with HIV-1 follows a characteristic course, but with wide variation in the timing of the various stages.

Acute 'seroconversion' illness. This affects 50–90% of people, setting in 2–6 weeks after exposure and probably reflecting direct invasion by the virus. Symptoms often take the form of a mild glandular fever-like illness, with fever, myalgia, sore throat, lymphadenopathy and a maculopapular rash, generally subsiding within 1–2 weeks. A longer duration of seroconversion illness with more severe symptoms may predict more rapid progression to AIDS (Vanhems *et al.* 2000). More severe manifestations include mucocutaneous ulceration, or in 10% reflect nervous system invasion with aseptic meningitis accompanied by cranial nerve palsies particularly of the fifth, seventh and eighth nerves; myelopathy or neuropathy; encephalitis with delirium (McArthur 1987; Malouf *et al.* 1990), acute disseminated encephalomyelitis, transverse myelitis, polymyositis or a transient acute confusional state sometimes with seizures (Carne *et al.* 1985). Fever and malaise have been shown to have the highest sensitivity for clinical diagnosis of acute HIV-1 infection, while weight loss and oral ulceration have the highest specificity (Hecht *et al.* 2002).

Early during this period, viral nucleic acid can be detected in the blood, cerebrospinal fluid (CSF) and most organs of the body. A transient lymphopenia affects both CD4 and CD8 lymphocyte subsets (T-helper and cytotoxic cells, respectively), followed a week or two later by lymphocytosis. Viral replication is of the order of 100 million copies of HIV-1 RNA per millilitre during this acute infection stage and virus seeds to tissue reservoirs alongside destruction of CD4$^+$ T lymphocytes in gut lymphoid tissue. Towards the end of this stage HIV-1 antibodies begin to appear in the serum, conventional antibody tests becoming positive after 2–6 weeks or occasionally after a delay of several months. Prior to this, detection of plasma HIV-1 RNA may aid diagnosis.

After the initial high numbers of copies, viraemia declines significantly to a level referred to as the viral setpoint, a reliable predictor of disease progression (Mellors *et al.* 1995). Other factors that may have an effect on longer-term progression at this stage include the appearance of HIV-1-specific CD8$^+$ T cells, whose absence in macaques leads to an accelerated clinical course. Host genetic factors and, most significantly, being homozygous for a deletion in the chemokine coreceptor CCR5 can result in resistance to HIV-1 infection (Samson *et al.* 1996). Individuals expressing the HLA-B57 haplotype also show more controlled viral replication following acute infection (Altfeld *et al.* 2003).

Asymptomatic phase. This follows the acute illness and may last for many years, during which the person is nonetheless infective. Viral levels remain low in the blood, but high levels of activity are maintained in the lymphoid system. The semen, blood and possibly cervical secretions are particularly infective. There is no clear evidence of spread by saliva, ingestion or droplet inhalation, nor by casual or social contact. However, health-care workers must beware needle-stick injuries.

Generalised lymphadenopathy persists in up to one-third of patients after seroconversion, and minor skin complaints may be troublesome, including seborrhoeic dermatitis, but otherwise the person remains well. Thrombocytopenia of severe degree occasionally occurs. Throughout this period CD4 counts remain in the normal range (450–1500/μL in women; 350–1440/μL in men), but tend to decline slowly with time. The duration of the asymptomatic phase varies widely, most persons progressing to further stages within 2–10 years but some remaining well for considerably longer. Cohort studies of men who have sex with men have shown that up to half remain free from AIDS 10 years after initial infection and that 8% can remain clinically normal after 10–15 years (Buchbinder *et al.* 1994; Rutherford 1994). Moreover, some 5% appear to have non-progressive infection in that they do not show declining CD4 counts. Estimates of survival in a cohort of haemophiliac men, based on extrapolations of changes in CD4 counts, suggest that as many as one-quarter may remain free from AIDS for 20 years (Phillips *et al.* 1994). HAART has had a significant impact on survival and particularly progression of the disease (Torres & Barr 1997) and is briefly reviewed later.

Early symptomatic infection. This begins to appear as the proportion of infected lymphocytes increases. Cell-mediated immunity falls, and recurrent viral infections such as herpes or warts make an appearance. Infections may also result from common bacterial pathogens such as pneumococcus, *Haemophilus* and *Salmonella*. Recurrent vaginal candidiasis may occur in women.

Late symptomatic infection. This includes a constellation of symptoms that predict progression to AIDS. Oral candidiasis and hairy leucoplakia of the tongue and cheek are usually of serious import. Constitutional symptoms include low-grade pyrexia, night sweats, weight loss, fatigue and diarrhoea. The most valuable laboratory marker of disease progression is the declining trend in CD4 count, which correlates with progression to AIDS and HIV RNA viral load. Serum markers reflecting immune activation (β_2-microglobulin and neopterin) may yield additional information for assessing prognosis, but are less valuable. In developed countries, laboratory markers are the most reliable in terms of measuring disease progression and avoid the difficulties associated with identifying clinical signs (Mellors *et al.* 1997; Vlahov *et al.* 1998). Oral candidiasis, once seen as an excellent predictor of disease progression, may not be reliable enough unless the clinical history is also taken into account (Hilton 2000). In a cohort from New York, oral lesions were not predictive of progression in subjects with a CD4 count ≥200/μL (Begg *et al.* 1997). The value of oral lesions in predicting progression to AIDS needs further investigation in the developing world, where it may well be more useful in the absence of access to laboratory investigations (Birnbaum *et al.* 2002).

AIDS-defining illnesses. These finally make their appearance as definitive indications of severely compromised immunological function. By this stage viral replication is increasing rapidly and the CD4 count has generally fallen below 200/μL. The three principal groups of illnesses are opportunistic infections, certain neoplastic conditions and the results of direct involvement of the nervous system by HIV. This last may antedate evidence of immunodeficiency.

In the untreated, opportunistic infections are legion, affecting the lungs, gastrointestinal tract and nervous system as low-grade organisms that have previously been tolerated gain hold. Pneumonia results from *Pneumocystis carinii*, cytomegalovirus (CMV), herpes simplex virus (HSV), *Cryptococcus* and atypical mycobacteria. Tuberculosis has increased substantially in HIV-infected patients in Africa where it is a common opportunistic problem (Lucas *et al.* 1993). Severe diarrhoea may be caused by the protozoan organisms *Cryptosporidium*, *Isospora belli* and microsporidia; also *Candida*, CMV and *Mycobacterium avium intracellulare*. The range of infections affecting the CNS is discussed in detail in Opportunistic infection of the CNS, later in chapter.

Neoplasias characteristically consist of Kaposi's sarcoma of the skin or other organs, lymphomas, or more rarely squamous carcinoma of the mouth or anorectum. Direct HIV infection of the nervous system is described in Primary HIV infection of the CNS, later in this chapter. Other conditions may mark the later stages of infection, including lymphoid interstitial pneumonitis, granulomatous hepatitis and recurrent salmonella septicaemia.

Petruckevitch *et al.* (1998) conducted a retrospective cohort study between 1982 and 1995 of 2048 HIV-infected individuals in London from different ethnic and racial backgrounds to identify disease progression and survival following specific AIDS-defining conditions. PCP accounted for one-quarter of AIDS presentations and tuberculosis for 16%. High-grade lymphoma carried the highest risk of death in HIV-infected individuals, whereas tuberculosis carried the lowest risk.

Classification of HIV-related illness

Historically, three categories of disorder were recognised following the asymptomatic stage: persistent generalised lymphadenopathy (PGL), AIDS-related complex (ARC) and acquired immunodeficiency syndrome (AIDS).

PGL is identified by enlargement of lymph nodes (1 cm or more in diameter) in at least two extrainguinal sites and persisting for at least 3 months. One-third of such cases show associated splenomegaly. PGL is largely symptomless, and is often thought to carry a relatively good prognosis with respect to early further progression. However, a proportion of such patients show peripheral nerve disorder, and subjective memory difficulty and affective disorder appear to be commoner than in controls (Janssen *et al.* 1988). Neuropsychological evaluation may confirm mild cognitive impairment.

The definition of ARC is a category of chronic disease that fails to fulfill the criteria for AIDS in that there is no clear evidence of opportunistic infection or neoplasia. The diagnosis usually requires two or more of the following persisting for at least 3 months: low-grade pyrexia, weight loss exceeding 10% of body weight, PGL as defined above, oral candidiasis, diarrhoea, night sweats or fatigue interfering with work. One or more laboratory abnormalities such as decreased CD4 lymphocyte counts are sometimes required in addition.

The original diagnosis of AIDS came about only when there was reliable evidence of a disease at least moderately indicative of underlying cellular immune deficiency, for example Kaposi's sarcoma (in a person under 60) or some opportunistic infection. Other causes of cellular immune deficiency or of reduced resistance to infection had also to be excluded. In the era of antiretroviral therapy, effective prophylaxis against opportunistic infections and routine laboratory surveillance of CD4 and viral load, the case definition of AIDS has been somewhat revised. The most accepted classification system of HIV infection remains that revised by the Centers for Disease Control and Prevention (CDC) in 1993, after its initial publication in 1986. The system classifies individuals on the basis of CD4 count and three clinical categories, forming a matrix of nine mutually exclusive categories (Table 7.1).

The diagnosis of AIDS is confined to patients infected with HIV when they develop certain defined opportunistic infections or malignancies for the first time, for example PCP,

Table 7.1 Case definition of AIDS as revised by the Centers for Disease Control and Prevention in 1993.

CD4 cell count	Clinical categories		
	A	B	C
≥500/µL	A1	B1	C1
200–499/µL	A2	B2	C2
<200/µL	A3	B3	C3

Category A (asymptomatic, acute HIV infection or PGL): transient symptoms at the time of or shortly after seroconversion or no symptoms or PGL, as defined above.
Category B (symptomatic conditions): for example oropharyngeal candidiasis, oral hairy leucoplakia or constitutional symptoms such as fever >38.5°C or diarrhoea lasting >1 month.
Category C (AIDS-indicator conditions): neurological conditions such as HIV encephalopathy, PML and cerebral toxoplasmosis.

Kaposi's sarcoma or other specified conditions including HIV-related encephalopathy. In addition, the USA surveillance case definition of AIDS has been expanded to include HIV-positive persons whose CD4 lymphocyte count is less than 200/µL (or CD4 percentage <14%). As clearly seen in the matrix, categories A3, B3 and C1–C3 would fulfill the CDC definition of AIDS. An analogous classification system has been revised for HIV infection in children less than 13 years of age (Centers for Disease Control 1994).

The World Health Organization (WHO) published its clinical staging and case definition for HIV, particularly for use in resource-constrained settings, in 1990 and this was revised in 2005. The major difference between this system and the CDC system is that a CD4 count is not required, the focus being on clinical findings. The definition is divided into primary HIV infection and four clinical categories (World Health Organization 2005).

Neuropsychiatric manifestations

The HIV disease has proved to be of immense importance to neurology and psychiatry, not least in terms of the considerable economic burden that neuropsychiatric disorders add to treating patients with HIV (Yeung *et al.* 2006). Early reports by Snider *et al.* (1983) and Levy *et al.* (1985) drew attention to the range of neurological problems encountered and set the stage for their elaboration. It was also soon evident that the psychosocial consequences of infection could lead to profound emotional disturbance, even among those who were physically well or had sustained no more than a risk of exposure to the virus. Vulnerable persons, in groups at special risk, could display neurotic and sometimes psychotic symptomatology that needed to be distinguished from the effects of brain pathology. In this manner neurology and psychiatry have been drawn closer together in seeking to disentangle the impact of the disorder. In the sections that follow those disorders reflecting identifiable pathology are considered first, where possible comparing the pre- and post-HAART eras, then those that may be viewed as 'reactions' to knowledge of being infected. Estimates of the prevalence of neurological involvement in pre-HAART HIV-seropositive patients has been reported to be in the range 40–70% (Levy *et al.* 1985; Simpson & Berger 1996; Janssen 1997; Sacktor 2002). A similar prevalence rate is seen in developing countries where HAART may not be available (Grant *et al.* 1997; Satishchandra *et al.* 2000).

Special importance attaches to the resulting manifestations of CNS involvement in that they can be the presenting feature in some 10–20% of symptomatic HIV-1 infection (Levy *et al.* 1988). The nervous system is an early target in HIV disease (Resnick *et al.* 1988; Davis *et al.* 1992), with abnormalities developing in the CSF in a large proportion of asymptomatic HIV-positive individuals (Marshall *et al.*

1988). In a prospective study of homosexual men, McArthur *et al.* (1988) were able to demonstrate CSF abnormalities, and sometimes to isolate the virus from the fluid, within 6–24 months of seroconversion. Ho *et al.* (1985) detected the virus in the CSF of a patient suffering from aseptic meningitis at the actual time of seroconversion and Morris *et al.* (1998) identified a high HIV RNA viral load in the CSF from other patients with lymphocytic meningitis. There have also been reports of acute encephalopathy (Carne *et al.* 1985) and myelopathy (Denning *et al.* 1987) associated with primary HIV infection or at seroconversion. Post-mortem studies have revealed subtle polymerase chain reaction (PCR) positivity in the brains of some late symptomatic HIV-positive cases (Bell *et al.* 1993; Sinclair *et al.* 1994) and Davis *et al.* (1992) identified this finding in a case of iatrogenic HIV infection 15 days prior to death. There is, understandably, a scarcity of post-mortem studies of HIV-positive individuals who have died accidentally during the asymptomatic period. Of those that exist, they are predominantly from haemophiliacs who have died from other associations with their blood disorder or drug users who have died as a result of drug-related accidents (Gray *et al.* 1996; Esiri *et al.* 1989; Bell *et al.* 1993). The neurohistological features reported in these cases are of a predominantly CD8 lymphocytic infiltrate present in the leptomeninges and perivascular spaces of the central white matter. There is neuronal loss (An *et al.* 1996) and evidence of axonal injury is also suggested by the presence of β-amyloid precursor protein in some reports (An & Scaravilli 1997) together with microgliosis and astrocytosis. HIV DNA in the brain tissue of asymptomatic individuals has also been isolated and immune activation together with the presence of toxic cytokines has been reported.

By the time patients with AIDS, in the pretreatment era, had come to post-mortem, neuropathological changes were demonstrated in over 90% of cases, even in patients who had shown no relevant neurological symptomatology during life (Budka *et al.* 1987). Multiple pathologies were reported in about one-third of cases (Levy *et al.* 1988). The pictures observed were therefore pleomorphic and can still present considerable problems for diagnosis. Three main forms of involvement were recognised: opportunistic infections, neoplastic change and direct invasion of the nervous system by HIV. Indeed, before HAART, HIV encephalitis (HIVE) and opportunistic infections were reported in up to 50% of individuals with AIDS. A similar percentage of pretreatment cases of AIDS have been noted to show vacuolar myelopathy, myelin pallor and accumulation of macrophages in the spinal cord. Thus neurological involvement can span the entire spectrum of HIV infection, from the time of seroconversion to its most advanced manifestations. In 1991, Budka developed standard nomenclature for HIV neuropathology, which continues to be used. Additional pathology in the CNS results from vascular disorders, such

as vessel calcification, infarction, haemorrhage and vasculitis; such features have been noted where there is no evidence of opportunistic infection or HIVE, prior to the development of effective treatment strategies. The brain is also vulnerable to hypoxia and metabolic derangements due to pulmonary, hepatic and renal failure, and to the toxic effects of systemic infections or drugs, including HAART and other treatments used in the prophylaxis of opportunistic infection.

Since the introduction of HAART, there have been a number of cohort studies reporting a change in the prevalence of neuropathological manifestations of the virus, with data extending across pretreatment and treatment periods (Jellinger *et al.* 2000; Masliah *et al.* 2000; Sacktor *et al.* 2001; Morgello *et al.* 2002; Vago *et al.* 2002; Gray *et al.* 2003; Langford *et al.* 2003). While the prevalence of opportunistic infections is consistently reported as having declined, HIVE remains a more common finding than might be expected and there is the suggestion in some studies that a significant decrease in incidence has not been evident. Furthermore, Gray and colleagues have reported 'burnt-out' lesions of opportunistic infections and HIVE where neither inflammatory infiltrates nor the causal agent could be identified, representing variants of neuropathology in the context of HAART. Interest has also more recently focused on clinical deterioration after immune reconstitution as a result of HAART (Riedel *et al.* 2006).

A very approximate guide to the relative frequency of the different forms of pathology seen in the era before HAART is given by Petito *et al.*'s (1986) review of neuropathological findings in 153 patients dying from HIV disease; 28% showed evidence of HIVE, 26% encephalomyelitis due to CMV, 10% toxoplasmosis, 6% CNS lymphoma and 29% vacuomyelopathy of the cord. However, different risk groups of patients may be differently affected. Lantos *et al.* (1989) showed that haemophiliacs were less likely to develop HIVE while vascular lesions were common. Children are unlikely to develop opportunistic infections or lymphomas, but mainly show the picture of HIVE.

The frequency of CNS pathology before antiretroviral drugs (1984–1987) during monotherapy with zidovudine (1988–1994), dual therapy (1995–1996) and HAART (1997–2000) is reported by Vago *et al.*'s (2002) review of neuropathological findings in 1597 consecutive post-mortems of patients performed between 1984 and 2000; 76% were affected by opportunistic infections, HIV-related disease (encephalitis/leucoencephalopathy) or both. The prevalence of HIVE or leucoencephalopathy in each of the four periods was 54%, 32%, 18% and 15% respectively, a highly statistically significant reduction over time. Indeed, there are a number of excellent cohort studies of the neuropathology of HIV before and after HAART. On the whole these report general decreases in the prevalence of opportunistic infections, although HIVE would appear to be more common (Sacktor *et al.* 2002; Gray *et al.* 2003; Bell 2004).

Opportunistic infections of the CNS

Viral, fungal and parasitic infections of the CNS are common, while bacterial invasion is rare. The manifestations are broadly similar to those occurring in other settings except that they are more florid in the immunocompromised state. This may also be due in some instances to coinfection with HIV, which serves to exacerbate the tissue destruction.

Such infections occur in about one-third of untreated patients (De la Monte *et al.* 1987) and multiple infections are common (Gray *et al.* 1988). The incidence of the different organisms varies geographically (Everall & Lantos 1991). The principal infections encountered are toxoplasmosis and viral infection with CMV, HSV and varicella-zoster virus (VZV), also the polyomavirus leading to progressive multifocal leucoencephalopathy (PML). Fungal infections include *Cryptococcus*, *Candida albicans* or more rarely aspergillosis and coccidioidomycosis. The tubercle bacillus is occasionally involved, also other mycobacteria, *Escherichia coli*, *Listeria*, *Histoplasma* and *Treponema pallidum*. The detailed pictures are described by Levy *et al.* (1988) and the imaging appearances by Offiah and Turnbull (2006) and are presented here in summary form.

Toxoplasmosis. This is the result of reactivation of latent infection with the obligate intracellular protozoon *Toxoplasma gondii*. Primary infection is asymptomatic in 90% of immunocompetent individuals, although cervical or generalised lymphadenopathy has been seen in some. IgG antibodies to *T. gondii* are found in 20% of British and around 90% of French adults. These variations in immunocompetent prevalence are mirrored in HIV-seropositive cases. Toxoplasmosis appears to be especially frequent among patients from Haiti and Florida and also from France. The infection leads to an acute focal or diffuse meningoencephalitis, presenting usually with headache (45–65%), fever (10–75%) and altered consciousness, and focal neurological signs (50–60%) such as hemiparesis, aphasia or cerebellar ataxia. These may be preceded for several days or weeks by lethargy, confusion (40–50%) or weakness. Koppel *et al.* (1985) found that patients with focal neurological features usually proved to have toxoplasmosis and any neurological signs that may suggest CNS involvement should indicate neuroimaging, as toxoplasmosis is the most common and easily treated opportunistic infection in HIV-infected patients. Computed tomography (CT) or magnetic resonance imaging (MRI) reveal multiple ring or nodular, enhancing, isodense or hypodense white matter, corticomedullary or basal ganglia lesions (Fig. 7.1). Seizures occur in some 15% of cases. Raised intracranial pressure is rare.

The pathology consists of scattered focal areas of abscess formation, varying in size according to the patient's immunological response. Each has a necrotic core surrounded by granuloma formation consisting of an intense mononuclear

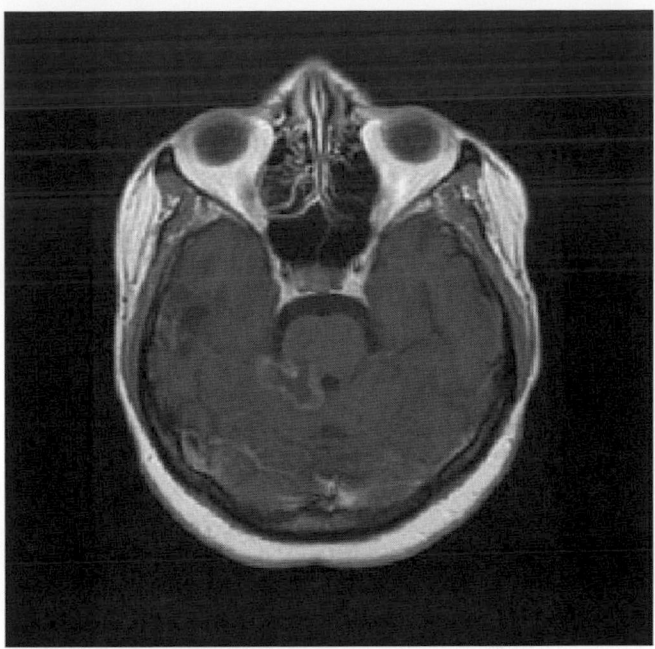

Fig. 7.1 Postcontrast MRI showing an enhancing ring lesion due to cerebral toxoplasmosis affecting the right superior cerebellar peduncle in an HIV-positive woman presenting with acute neurological and cognitive deterioration. (Courtesy of Dr John Moriarty.)

reaction. Encysted *T. gondii* and tachyzoites can usually be detected. Thrombosis of blood vessels may lead to large areas of necrosis, producing mass lesions in the brain. Early diagnosis can lead to a dramatic response to combination treatment with pyrimethamine and sulfadiazine (see Treatment of opportunistic infections, neoplasms and neuropsychiatric complications, later in chapter). Lumbar puncture often reveals a pleocytosis and elevation of protein. The incidence of toxoplasmosis has markedly decreased since the introduction of HAART (Gray *et al.* 2003; Anthony *et al.* 2005).

Cytomegalovirus. CMV is most common in patients with advanced infection and typically leads to subacute encephalitis with fever, memory and attention impairment, apathy, headache and ataxia. The pathology varies in severity from isolated cytomegalic cells to multiple necrotising lesions, the most common feature being diffuse, microglial, nodular encephalitis in the deep grey matter (Everall & Lantos 1991). The ventricular lining is frequently involved, likewise the choroid plexus. Microglia and macrophages contain intranuclear inclusions indicative of the presence of the virus. Clinical examination reveals cognitive impairment that can be similar to Korsakoff's psychosis with psychomotor retardation or dementia. MRI can be normal or reveal nonspecific abnormalities with atrophy or ventricular enlargement in 40% (Clifford *et al.* 1996). Concurrent retinitis is common and is the most frequent cause of loss of vision in

AIDS. Treatment with ganciclovir and foscarnet has been found useful in CMV retinitis and encephalitis.

Herpes simplex. This produces a severe haemorrhagic encephalitis, typically limited to the temporofrontal regions (see Non-geographically restricted sporadic encephalitides, later), presenting with headache, fever, seizures, aphasia and other focal neurological deficits (Grover *et al.* 2004). Necrosis and softening affect both the grey and white matter, and eosinophilic nuclear inclusions are seen in neurones and glial cells. Occasional cases present as an ascending myelitis.

The VZV may involve the peripheral or central nervous system, the latter leading to diffuse encephalitis with multiple necrotic lesions similar to those of PML. Small eosinophilic inclusions in neurones and glial cells contain the virus.

Progressive multifocal leucoencephalopathy. PML results from infection with the JC polyomavirus. The virus is usually acquired in childhood and remains dormant. It has not been isolated in the brains of immunocompetent patients. It usually presents with the subacute development of mental impairment accompanied by varied neurological deficits. Dementia, blindness, dysphasia, hemiparesis and ataxia are among the classic features. CT may be normal or show characteristic low-density lesions in the white matter with a 'scalloped' appearance to their margins, without mass effect, enhancement or associated oedema. MRI may show that the grey matter is involved as well, possibly reflecting a more aggressive form of the disease in the presence of AIDS (Mark & Atlas 1989). The virus can be detected in the CSF by PCR in patients with and without PML.

The lesions consist essentially of areas of demyelination with sparing of axis cylinders and often with necrosis. Polyomavirus can be detected around the margins of the bizarre glial cells that are the hallmark of the disorder: enlarged astrocytes with distorted nuclei and oligodendrocytes containing eosinophilic inclusions. The condition carries a grave prognosis, with a median survival of 4 months (Fong & Toma 1995). Ante-mortem diagnosis can be made by biopsy. No treatment has proven efficacy, although anecdotal evidence suggests benefit from high-dose acyclovir, cytosine and adenosine arabinoside, interferons and steroids. Survival may be increased with HAART (Clifford 1998), although there has been no change in the incidence of PML since the introduction of HAART (Anthony *et al.* 2005).

Cryptococcus neoformans. This is the commonest fungal infection of the CNS, typically leading to a subacute granulomatous meningitis producing a gelatinous exudate at the base of the brain. Headache and malaise may be the sole complaints, perhaps because of the minimal inflammatory response. In other patients progressive headache, photophobia and nuchal rigidity are accompanied by confused and altered behaviour. Sometimes there is additional cyst and granuloma formation within the brain, such patients presenting with focal neurological signs. Raised intracranial pressure may develop in consequence of hydrocephalus. The diagnosis is confirmed by lumbar puncture. Cells may be absent and the protein and glucose normal, but India ink staining reveals the fungus in a high proportion of cases. Detection of cryptococcal antigen in the CSF is a more reliable procedure. Treatment includes amphotericin B, flucytosine and fluconazole. Sacktor *et al.* (2001) identified that the incidence of *Cryptococcus* decreased in the Multicenter AIDS Cohort Study between 1990 and 1998, when antiretroviral treatments became available.

Candida albicans. This rarely involves the brain despite the frequency of this infection elsewhere in the body in HIV disease. When it does invade the CNS this takes the form of meningitis or multiple brain abscesses with focal neurological signs.

Coccidioidomycosis. This may produce a chronic relapsing meningitis, which is occasionally fulminant with microabscess formation in the brain.

Tuberculous infection. This can present either with a mass lesion or as tuberculous meningitis (described under Tuberculous meningitis, later).

Treponema pallidum. This may lead to neurosyphilis after an unusually brief latent interval, and sometimes despite previous adequate therapy for the initial syphilitic infection (Nieman 1991). In the immunocompromised state the manifestations of meningovascular syphilis may be especially florid, leading to unusual acute neurological syndromes, although there is controversy as to whether coinfection does result in more aggressive syphilis. Serological tests for syphilis may also be altered, becoming positive in the CSF only after repeated serial testing (Lynn & Lightman 2004). Further discussion of HIV and syphilis coinfection can be found under Neurosyphilis and HIV coinfection, later.

Neoplasia of the CNS

The commonest CNS neoplasm is a primary non-Hodgkin's malignant lymphoma; in the pre-HAART era this occurred in some 4–7% of patients with neurological complaints. Some studies suggest that the prevalence of non-Hodgkin's lymphoma has not decreased to the same extent as other sequelae of AIDS, despite antiretroviral therapy (Grulich 1999; Conti *et al.* 2000).

This is a B-cell lymphoma, unifocal in 33–50% of cases (Ciacci *et al.* 1999) but sometimes multifocal and extensive, involving the cerebral hemispheres, cerebellum and brainstem. The presentation is usually with focal neurological deficits, similar to those seen with toxoplasmosis or PML, but with more gradual onset (Stern & Marder 1991). Sometimes, however, the picture can be surprisingly non-specific with lethargy, confusion and memory impairment (Rosenblum *et al.* 1988) in as many as 60% of cases. Headache and evidence of raised intracranial pressure may be lacking and unexplained fever may occur. Seizures develop in 15–44% of cases (Chamberlain & Kormanik 1999).

The pictures on brain imaging may also be hard to distinguish from toxoplasmosis or PML. The space-occupying lesions show ill-defined margins with surrounding oedema, and may enhance irregularly (Sze *et al.* 1987). They lie mainly in the basal ganglia, thalamus, corpus callosum and cerebellum and, occasionally, brainstem. Analysis of CSF for Epstein–Barr virus (EBV) using PCR has high sensitivity and positive and negative predictive value (Cinque *et al.* 1996) and is now the investigation of choice. Biopsy may be needed for definitive diagnosis, or the distinction may ultimately be made by the rapid initial response to radiation. The long-term effects of treatment are poor, with a median length of survival of 1–3 months, even with whole-brain irradiation. Limited evidence suggests that there may be some benefit on survival for those receiving protease inhibitors as well as chemotherapy for lymphoma (Jacomet *et al.* 1997).

Pathological examination shows lymphoid cells invading vascular walls and brain tissue, along with a marked astrocytic response. EBV is found in lymphoma cells in nearly 100% of cases and may be identified by *in situ* hybridisation (Hamilton-Dutoit *et al.* 1991). Secondary brain involvement from lymphoma elsewhere in the body occurs more rarely, also metastatic deposits from Kaposi's sarcoma. Plasmocytomas and lymphoid granulomatosis may also occur.

Primary HIV infection of the CNS

As described above, it has become clear that the nervous system is a prime target for HIV in addition to its predilection for the immune system. This was not at first apparent, but has now been fully proven by electron microscopy, immunocytochemistry and *in situ* hybridisation and PCR. Shaw *et al.* (1985) were the first to identify the virus in 5 of 15 brains from AIDS patients with dementia, and Koenig *et al.* (1986) showed that the cell type harbouring the virus was the macrophage and the multinucleated giant cells deriving from it (Figs 7.2 and 7.3: see also Plates 7.1 and 7.2). Such cells often contain enormous quantities of the virus. The microglia are also involved and, like macrophages, are the only cells in the CNS to possess both CD4 and chemokine receptors. Oligodendrocytes and vascular endothelial cells may be infected, as well as astrocytes (Saito *et al.* 1994) and neurones (Torres-Munoz *et al.* 2001). The mechanism whereby HIV attaches to astrocytes and neurones, neither of which have CD4 receptors, is not clear and while the virus has been detected in some studies, the findings are not consistent. The evidence for HIV infection of cells in the CNS is summarised by Bell (2004). As has been discussed, evidence has accumulated to suggest that the nervous system is infected at an early stage of the disease, even though pronounced clinical sequelae may take a considerable time to appear.

The 'Trojan horse' hypothesis proposes that activated CD14[+]/CD16[+] or HIV-infected monocytes carry the virus through the blood–brain barrier (Fischer-Smith *et al.* 2004). There is also evidence that activated T lymphocytes can enter the CNS. Alternatively, the virus may enter and replicate in the vascular endothelium, or via the choroid plexus and CSF. Entrance by way of peripheral nerves has also been considered.

The consequences of such invasion have been clarified to some extent at the level of tissue pathology, with the delineation of several more or less distinct patterns of neuropathogenesis. However, their clinical counterparts are as yet unclear, and classification in terms of presenting clinical

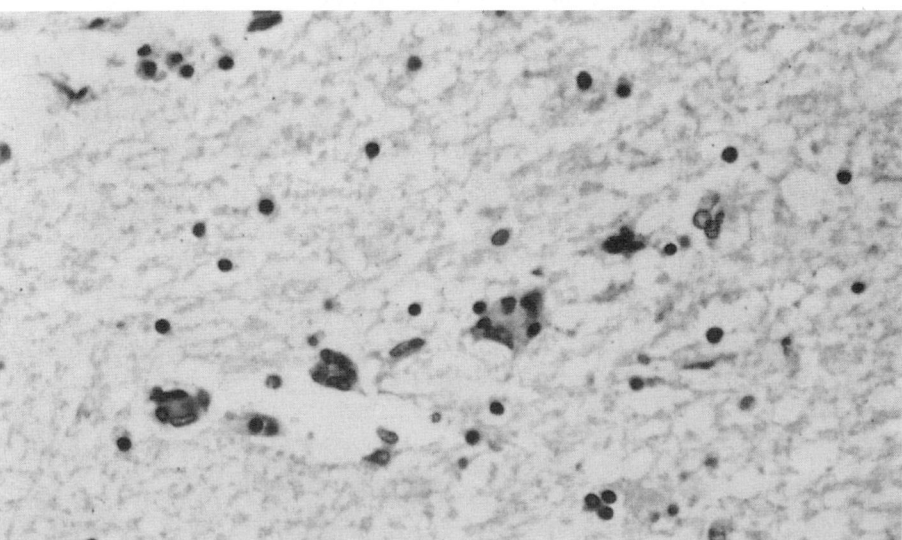

Fig. 7.2 Large multinucleated giant cells in cerebral white matter of a patient with HIV encephalitis and dementia (see also Plate 7.1). Haematoxylin and eosin, magnification ×250. (Courtesy of Dr Ian Everall.)

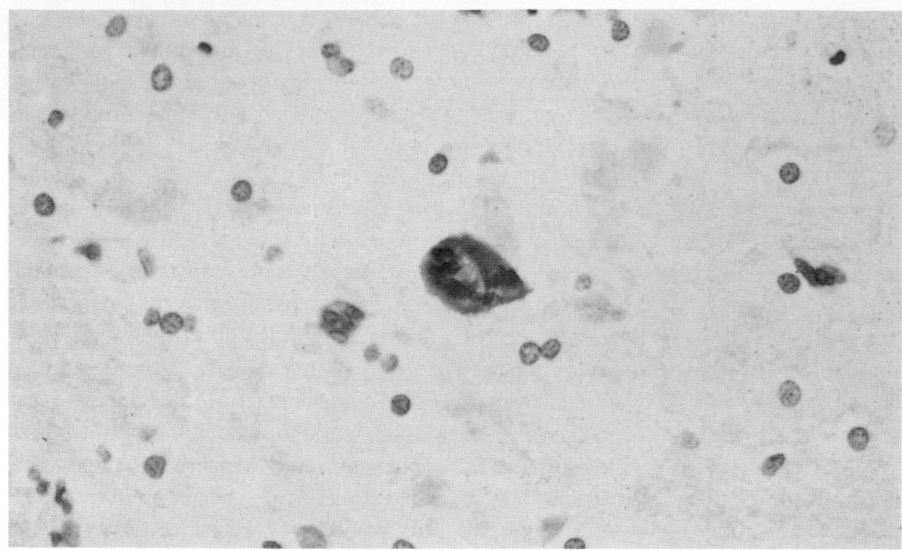

Fig. 7.3 A multinucleated giant cell from a patient with HIV encephalitis immunostained for the glycoprotein gp41 revealing viral particles (see also Plate 7.2). Magnification ×400. (Courtesy of Dr Ian Everall.)

features remains sometimes confusing in its historical nomenclature. The major clinical syndromes that appear to be due to primary brain infection are the so-called 'HIV-associated dementia' and 'HIV-associated minor cognitive and motor disorder' that had previously been called 'AIDS–dementia complex' as well as the progressive encephalopathy that occurs in children. Aseptic meningitis is almost certainly so caused. Vacuolar myelopathy of the spinal cord, distal sensory polyneuropathy (DSPN) and HIV polymyositis are also seen.

The clinical uncertainties are due to a lack of long-term prospective studies from which clinicopathological correlations may be drawn, also to the coincident operation of opportunistic infections and other pathologies in many pretreatment cases and the effects of immune reconstitution in those receiving HAART (Landay *et al.* 2002). The pathological changes associated with HIV infection are therefore briefly reviewed before consideration of the clinical pictures encountered.

HIV-associated pathology of the CNS

Budka *et al.* (1991) have produced a consensus report for the classification of HIV-associated neuropathologies as listed below. Everall and Lantos (1991) provide a concise description of the several categories. By far the most common are HIVE, HIV leucoencephalopathy and vacuolar myelopathy. With some pathologies, namely HIVE and HIV leucoencephalopathy, there is clear evidence that the lesion is caused by HIV itself, these forms not occurring in other settings of immunosuppression. In the others, the pathogenic role of direct HIV infection is less completely established.

HIV encephalitis. This term refers to the picture of multiple foci of inflammatory change throughout the cortex and white matter, also involving the basal ganglia and brainstem. The neocortex may be spared relative to deeper parts of the brain, and the globus pallidus is often particularly severely affected. The foci consist of aggregations of macrophages, microglia and multinucleated giant cells (Bell 1998), these last being the hallmark of the condition and probably deriving from macrophages (see Figs 7.2 and 7.3: see also Plates 7.1 and 7.2). The glycoprotein gp41 on the surface of HIV mediates cell fusion and may be responsible for the formation of these characteristic cell syncytia. HIV can be detected in all three types of cell. In addition, there may be foci of microglial nodules in white and grey matter together with damage to myelinated fibres. Myelin damage ranges from pallor to breakdown and loss, often with axonal injury, the latter being confirmed by the presence of β-amyloid precursor protein in the white matter varicosities and axon bulbs.

HIV leucoencephalopathy. This is the term given to such cases of HIVE with significant white matter injury. It is characterised by diffuse and usually symmetrical white matter damage, particularly in deep areas of the centrum semiovale, involving loss of myelin, reactive astrocytosis and the accumulation of macrophages and multinucleated giant cells. Such indications of inflammatory change are accompanied by alterations in small blood vessel walls and possible damage to the blood–brain barrier. A degree of overlap with HIVE is sometimes obvious and the validity of the distinction between the two is not firmly established. It is possible that they represent the same pathological process, but with accent on the white matter in HIV leucoencephalopathy.

It must be distinguished from the so-called 'myelin pallor' frequently observed in the deep white matter with myelin stains. This is an extremely common finding in patients with HIV disease and may be the sole brain abnormality at post-mortem. The myelin sheaths are preserved, and the appearances may be mainly due to increased interstitial water or represent an artefact of staining techniques.

Vacuolar myelopathy is a distinctive finding confined to the spinal cord, chiefly in the cervical and high thoracic regions and mainly affecting the dorsal and lateral white matter tracts. It is often a late development. Multiple areas show vacuolar myelin swellings, similar to the lesions seen in subacute combined degeneration due to vitamin B_{12} deficiency. Decreased CSF *S*-adenosylmethionine concentrations suggest that abnormal B_{12}-dependent transmethylation may be an important part of pathogenesis (Di Rocco *et al.* 2002). The early lesions show scattered vacuoles due to swellings within the myelin sheaths and occasional lipid-laden macrophages; with severe cases there is secondary axonal degeneration (Petito *et al.* 1985; Petito 1988; Shepherd *et al.* 1999).

Virological studies have not implicated HIV conclusively, with pathological evidence of active HIV infection being found in only 6% of cases (Petito *et al.* 1994). The virus can be cultured from the cord, but has not been demonstrated in the areas with vacuolar change. Other viruses could be responsible, or nutritional and metabolic factors could play a part.

Vacuolar leucoencephalopathy shows a not dissimilar picture affecting the white matter of the cerebral hemispheres, cerebellum, basal ganglia and brainstem. It may accompany HIV leucoencephalopathy.

Distal sensory polyneuropathy is characterised by the infiltration of lymphocytes and activated macrophages, decreased numbers of neurones and high numbers of nodules of Nageotte in the dorsal root ganglion. HIV infection of the dorsal root ganglion has been shown by PCR hybridisation *in situ* (Brannagan *et al.* 1997) but there is more evidence for the virus to be harboured in the nodules of Nageotte and perivascular inflammatory cells (Yoshioka *et al.* 1994).

Diffuse poliodystrophy consists of diffuse astrocytosis, gliosis and microglial activation in the grey matter of the cerebral cortex, basal ganglia and brainstem nuclei. This is the only category in Budka *et al.*'s (1991) classification that recognises the possibility of the neuronal loss (discussed below). The validity of diffuse poliodystrophy as a separate entity is uncertain, since gliosis is so commonly found in patients dying from HIV disease.

Cerebral vasculitis including granulomatous angiitis consists of infiltration of the walls of cerebral blood vessels with lymphocytes and multinucleated giant cells. There may be accompanying areas of necrosis.

Lymphocytic meningitis usually occurs soon after HIV infection as a self-limiting condition, but may recur or appear for the first time later in the asymptomatic or early symptomatic phases. The usual pathogens responsible for meningitis cannot be isolated, but in many cases HIV can be identified in the CSF.

Neuronal loss and cerebral atrophy with HIV infection

An important development has been the demonstration of substantial neuronal loss in the cerebral cortex of patients with HIV disease. Indeed, this is a common finding and somewhat surprising when it is considered that neurones are rarely infected by HIV (Torres-Munoz *et al.* 2001).

Everall *et al.* (1991) made counts in the frontal cortex of 11 patients with HIV disease, all without opportunistic brain infection or neoplastic change, and demonstrated a 38% depletion of neurones. Such loss was equivalently severe in the five with obvious HIVE and the six who showed only minimal pathology by way of slight astrocytosis and perivascular accumulations of mononuclear cells. Neuronal loss has since been established more widely in the occipital, parietal and superior temporal areas (Wiley *et al.* 1991; Everall *et al.* 1993a), also in the substantia nigra, putamen and cerebellar nuclei (Reyes *et al.* 1991; Abe *et al.* 1993; Everall *et al.* 1993b). However, the frontal losses have emerged as the most severe. A significant association has been observed between such losses and the presence of dementia in some studies (Achim *et al.* 1994; Wiley & Achim 1994; Asare *et al.* 1995). It is unclear as to whether cerebral atrophy is a marker of HIV dementia or of HIV infection alone (Subbiah *et al.* 1996). The presence of particularly subcortical atrophy and white matter changes on neuroimaging is remarkable in HIV-seropositive patients even in the absence of clinical deficits and has been found to be especially marked in the caudate for example on MRI (Dal Pan *et al.* 1992). Radiological changes are not necessarily associated with dementia scores.

The mechanisms responsible for HIV-associated neuronal death are unclear. It seems that the presence of HIVE with multinucleated giant cells is not an accurate marker for neuronal loss, which can occur in the presence of minimal or absent inflammatory change (Everall *et al.* 1993b). Thus dual pathogenic processes may be at work. Since neurones are only very rarely infected directly by HIV, one must postulate some 'toxic' effect on neuronal viability and it has been suggested that neuronal injury may occur through direct or indirect mechanisms. There is evidence for neuronal damage by numerous HIV proteins including env, Tat, Vpr and gp120. In studies of serum-free primary neuronal and neuroblastoma cell lines, where the confounding impact of excitatory amino acids and cytokines are absent, envelope proteins have been shown to be directly toxic. Blocking chemokine receptor signalling has been shown to prevent neuronal apoptosis induced by HIV gp120, suggesting that the envelope glycoprotein interactions with these receptors may mediate injury. gp120 has also been shown to interact with the glycine-binding site of *N*-methyl-D-aspartate (NMDA) receptors, providing another mechanism. Indirectly, it is hypothesised that effects on the NMDA receptor by phagocytic inflammatory mediators results in excessive intracellular calcium and the activation of a complex apoptotic cascade that includes initiation of capsases, free radical formation, lipid peroxidation and chromatin condensation. Apoptotic neurones have been isolated in HIV-seropositive patients by the identification of terminal deoxynucleotidyl transferase biotin-dUTP nick end labelling (TUNEL)-positive cells, DNA laddering and electron microscopic changes *post mortem*. Both microglial activation and axonal damage correlate with apoptosis, supporting the indirect inflammatory-mediated injury hypothesis (Adle-Biassette *et al.* 1999).

Dendritic morphology is also altered in the HIV-infected brain, with shortened, vacuolated and tortuous dendrites and a marked decrease in the number of dendritic spines (Wiley *et al.* 1994; Masliah *et al.* 1997). Synaptic density is reduced in the frontal cortex. These observations have been made in brains with concurrent evidence of HIVE, so they, at least, may be a product of the inflammatory process.

HIV-associated cognitive disorders

There is a wide range of cognitive impairment reported in the literature, with a bewildering nomenclature. Generally, three categories are acknowledged at present: HIV-associated dementia (HAD), minor cognitive–motor disorder (MCMD) and neuropsychological impairment. Delirium is also recognised.

HIV-associated dementia (also called AIDS–dementia complex, HIV-related encephalopathy, AIDS encephalopathy, HIV-associated cognitive/motor complex, HIV encephalitis, subacute encephalitis)

Clinical pictures of CNS impairment occur against the pathological backgrounds described above and take a variety of forms. Prominent among them is a syndrome of progressive cognitive impairment, referred to by the bewildering variety of labels listed above, and generally carrying a poor prognosis. HIV-1 infection is recognised as the most common, preventable and treatable cause of cognitive impairment in those aged under 50. Evidence increasingly suggests that cognitive impairment results in large part from direct brain invasion by HIV, but beyond that it has continued to prove complicated to relate to defined aspects of brain pathology.

Terminology and definition

In early descriptions the condition was labelled 'subacute encephalitis' and thought to be due to opportunistic brain infection, probably with CMV (Snider *et al.* 1983; Levy *et al.* 1985). It was rechristened 'AIDS–dementia complex' by Navia *et al.* (1986a,b), 'complex' being added because motor and behavioural components were often prominent in addition to the cognitive failure. This latter term has since been abandoned, as patients presenting with dementia may not have AIDS-defining illness. The Working Group of the American Academy of Neurology (1991) proposed the terms 'HIV-1-associated minor cognitive–motor complex' and 'HIV-associated dementia' to designate the minor and major forms of cognitive impairment in HIV infection, the former not involving impairment in activities of daily living.

Diagnostic criteria have been recommended by the WHO Consultation Committee (World Health Organization 1990a) and, more recently, by the Working Group of the American Academy of Neurology AIDS Task Force, both of which are essentially modifications of the ICD-10 research criteria for dementia generally (Box 7.1) (see Chapter 9). These firm definitions have allowed for a refinement of the understanding of these disorders and aid their demarcation from other clinical syndromes. Such definitions will hopefully avoid what Catalan (1991) identifies, in many surveys of HIV-positive patients, that dementia has been used as an umbrella term,

---

Box 7.1 Diagnostic criteria for cognitive impairment in HIV infection

I   Acquired abnormality in at least two of the following cognitive abilities, present for at least 1 month and causing impairment in work or activities of daily living:
  (a) Attention or concentration
  (b) Speed of information processing
  (c) Abstraction or reasoning
  (d) Visuospatial skills
  (e) Memory or learning
  (f) Speech or language
II At least one of the following:
  (a) Acquired abnormality in motor functioning
  (b) Decline in motivation or emotional control or change in social behaviour
III Absence of clouding of consciousness during a period long enough to establish presence of I, above
IV Absence of another cause of the above cognitive, motor or behavioural symptoms or signs (active CNS opportunistic infection or malignancy, psychiatric disorders, substance abuse)

---

encompassing syndromes of cognitive decline, sometimes without impairment of memory, also acute brain syndromes, motor syndromes and possibly conditions characterised chiefly by depression and other psychiatric disorders.

Epidemiology

The commonest CNS manifestation in patients with HIV disease has emerged as HIV-associated dementia. Before the development of antiretrovirals, Brew *et al.* (1988) reported that over 60% of patients dying of HIV disease in New York exhibited some degree of dementia prior to death. Catalan (1991) has reviewed various estimates of its prevalence, identifying a range from 8% to almost 40%, much probably depending on matters of patient selection and the criteria adopted for diagnosis. Prospective surveys in the UK have shown prevalence rates of 7–16% when other causes of chronic organic reactions, such as opportunistic infections, have been excluded. Grant *et al.* (2005) summarise the estimated prevalence of HAD at different stages of HIV infection: 1% in the asymptomatic phase, 3% at initial AIDS condition, 5–10% with symptomatic HIV disease and 10–20% with advanced disease. Treatment with zidovudine monotherapy was associated with a decrease in the incidence of HAD (Portegies *et al.* 1989; Chiesi *et al.* 1990; Catalan & Thornton 1993) and a decline in prevalence was initially suggested with the use of HAART, to as low as 10% in some cohorts. Nonetheless, it has been suggested in some studies that the initial improvements in prevalence figures have not been sustained. The prolongation of survival times with effective treatments obviously plays a significant role in this (Graham *et al.* 1996). Furthermore, the poor penetration into the CNS by most antiretrovirals has also been proposed as an explanation (Maschke *et al.* 2000; Clifford 2002). McArthur (2004) reports that the prevalence of HAD and MCMD remain very high at 37% in one large North American cohort and that this is not significantly different from the pre-HAART comparison group. Further exploration of the changes in both incidence and prevalence is required.

Day *et al.* (1992) identified an annual incidence of HAD in symptomatic patients of 14% and McArthur *et al.* (1993) an annual rate of 7.1%. In intravenous drug users in Edinburgh, an incidence of 9% has been reported. This study also delineated the mean time from seroconversion to HAD as 9 years (Goodwin *et al.* 1996). The decreased incidence already noted with monotherapy, unlike prevalence rates, has been largely borne out with combination antiretroviral treatment, although some groups have continued to identify increases. In the Multicenter AIDS Cohort Study for example, the incidence of HAD has dropped by 50% since the introduction of HAART (Sacktor *et al.* 2001). In the pretreatment era, HAD was associated with CD4 counts of less than 200/μL in 70% of cases. In contrast with this, in the Multicenter AIDS Cohort Study during the period when HAART became widely available (1996–1998), there was an equal distribution of cases across the range of CD4 counts and therefore more cases presenting with counts in excess of 200/μL. Similar incidence and CD4 count findings have been replicated in Europe (Brodt *et al.* 1997; Mocroft *et al.* 2000), Australia (Dore *et al.* 1999) and in intravenous drug users in Baltimore (Moore & Chaisson 1999).

Risk factors

A number of factors have been investigated that have an association with, or are predictive of, development of HIV-associated dementia. In the pre-HAART era, the Multicenter AIDS Cohort Study data allowed for the estimation of predictors for HAD by a proportional hazards survival regression model. These included lower haemoglobin and body mass index up to 6 months before AIDS, more constitutional symptoms 7–12 months before and older age at transition to AIDS (McArthur *et al.* 1993). Similarly, Wang *et al.* (1995) identified an association with increasing age, but also injection drug use. The association with drug use has been replicated in several studies (Bouwman *et al.* 1998; Maschke *et al.* 2000; Becker *et al.* 2004) and Zhang *et al.* (1998) have reported that cocaine can affect HIV entry through the blood–brain barrier, which may explain this apparent association.

Plasma viral load and CD4 cell count have been identified as positive predictors of HAD (Childs *et al.* 1999). In the Multicenter AIDS Cohort Study, an HIV RNA count in excess of 30 000 copies/mL inferred a hazard 9.1 times that of a count below 500 copies/mL; similarly, a CD4 count below

200/μL predicted a 3.4-fold increased risk compared with a CD4 count in excess of 500/μL (McArthur *et al.* 1993). While demographic factors were not reliable predictors of dementia in the Multicenter AIDS Cohort Study, female sex (Chiesi *et al.* 1996) and low educational level (De Ronchi *et al.* 2002) have been suggested as possible associations. Several studies have proposed neuropsychological risk factors, most prominent being psychomotor slowing (Sacktor *et al.* 1996). Stern *et al.* (2001) further identified abnormal scores on measures of psychomotor and executive function as well as a diagnosis of minor cognitive–motor disorder, extrapyramidal signs and systemic HIV symptoms as significantly associated. Interestingly, this study also found a strong association with depressive disorder and later developing HAD that has been supported elsewhere.

In the era of HAART, serum viral load and CD4 count are perhaps less useful factors in identifying risk of HAD. Interest has turned to CSF markers, with Ellis *et al.* (1997) showing that CSF viral load and Letendre *et al.* (1999) that CSF chemokine concentration are associated with cognitive impairment. It would appear that HAART-related improvements in cognition are associated with improvements of these CSF markers in some studies, although Cysique *et al.* (2005) advocate caution when interpreting inactive CSF markers, as they are not necessarily indicative of inactivity of cognitive impairment. Positive associations between plasma tumour necrosis factor (TNF)-α and CSF macrophage chemoattractant protein (MCP)-1 levels and developing HAD have been proposed (Sevigny *et al.* 2004).

Further investigation of the genetic susceptibility to HAD is required. Corder *et al.*'s (1998) small study was the first to investigate this intriguing hypothesis, in which an association was found between the apolipoprotein E (APOE) ε4 allele and excess dementia.

Clinical features

The principal features of HIV-associated dementia are of disabling cognitive impairment, accompanied by behavioural change and often motor deficits (Snider *et al.* 1983; Levy *et al.* 1985). Behavioural manifestations include lethargy, social withdrawal, loss of spontaneity and also marked psychomotor slowing, which could at first be mistaken for depression. A confusional state can mark the outset and malaise is frequently profound.

Navia *et al.* (1986a,b) gave the first full description of the syndrome and its pathological background. They found it in 38% of 121 patients coming to post-mortem, or almost two-thirds in the absence of opportunistic brain infection or neoplasia. In one-quarter it appeared to antedate other manifestations of AIDS. Indeed, some cases failed to show systemic features of AIDS right up to the time of death (Navia & Price 1987). However, further experience has indicated that this is rare. The onset was sometimes insidious and sometimes fairly abrupt in Navia *et al.*'s cases. Impairment of memory and loss of concentration were the commonest early symptoms. Mental slowing was prominent, and confusion often present. Approximately half presented with cognitive change, while in the remainder motor or behavioural changes predominated.

Motor dysfunction took the form of imbalance, ataxia or leg weakness, sometimes for several months before cognitive deficits appeared. Loss of fine hand coordination and deterioration of handwriting was frequently observed, together with clumsiness and tremor. Of the behavioural changes, apathy and social withdrawal were most frequent, irritability and emotional lability less so. Such changes were the opening feature in almost one-quarter of patients. The typical picture was of becoming subdued, with loss of interest and loss of emotional responsiveness.

Less common symptoms included headache, seizures and episodes of speech disturbance. Some patients showed psychotic episodes with delusions and hallucinations. Perry and Jacobsen (1986) described several patients who presented with acute psychoses resembling schizophrenia, acute paranoid disorder, mania or psychotic depression.

This clinical picture has been broadly confirmed in subsequent reports. On examination there may be little to find neurologically in the early stages, although rapid eye and limb movements may be impaired along with diffuse hyperreflexia. Later there is often ataxia of gait, leg weakness and clonus. Frontal release signs may be prominent, especially the snout reflex. Some patients show tremors and dysarthria, and evidence of peripheral neuropathy is common.

Course

The course is typically steadily progressive though punctuated at times by abrupt accelerations. Half of Navia et al.'s patients progressed to severe global impairment within 2 months, but some 20% followed a more protracted course. McArthur (1987) found that of 20 patients seen initially in the early stages, nine progressed to advanced dementia within a few months, while six remained stable and failed to deteriorate over 3–13 months. Once severely demented the mean survival time was less than 3 months. In 18 patients who died with dementia, the average interval from the first symptom of cognitive dysfunction to death was 5.5 months. McArthur et al. (1993) further reported a similar median survival of 6 months after diagnosis in the Multicenter AIDS Cohort Study. As has already been discussed, HAART has changed the course of this disorder. However, Sevigny et al. (2007) have recently reported that HAD remains a significant risk factor for death despite HAART and suggest that this may be associated with poor treatment adherence in the demented group.

Insight is often relatively preserved until late in the disorder. The delayed appearance of focal cognitive symptoms such as apraxia or agnosia is in keeping with the predominantly subcortical nature of the dementia. The final stages are marked by severe global dementia, akinetic mutism, incontinence, paraplegia and sometimes myoclonus. Even in the terminal stages, however, the level of consciousness is unimpaired.

Investigations

Electroencephalography (EEG) is often normal initially, with diffuse slowing later. Neuroimaging usually shows variable cortical atrophy and ventricular dilatation, but the absence of atrophy does not countermand the diagnosis. White matter rarefaction is common, and MRI may show areas of increased T2 signal in the white matter that becomes more diffuse as the dementia progresses (Levy et al. 1986; Olsen et al. 1988). However, the essential role of neuroimaging is to exclude features indicative of treatable conditions such as opportunistic infections or lymphomas. Numerous neuroimaging studies reported during the course of HIV infection have been summarised by Tucker et al. (2004). In brief, positron emission tomography (PET) has demonstrated subcortical hypermetabolism in the thalamus and basal ganglia in the early stages, with progression to cortical and subcortical hypometabolism later (Rottenberg et al. 1987; von Giesen et al. 2000). Single-photon emission computed tomography (SPECT) may show perfusion deficits despite the absence of gross brain lesions (Costa et al. 1988). Maini et al. (1990) found that frontoparietal hypoperfusion correlated with HAD severity and Sacktor et al. (1995a,b) identified that perfusion abnormalities could be correlated with severity of cognitive deficit but particularly motor functioning in HAD. Volumetric MRI has substantiated the association between volume loss in specific structures and declining cognition. Magnetic resonance spectroscopy (MRS) has shown reduced levels of N-acetylaspartate indicative of neuronal loss, even in areas apparently normal on structural scans (Menon et al. 1990). More recent MRS studies have supported this finding and additionally revealed increases in glial markers, myoinositol and choline/creatinine ratios with progressing dementia (Paley et al. 1996; Yiannoutsos et al. 2000). Functional MRI studies have shown reduced activation in motor paradigms in HAD and MCMD as well as differences between patients and controls in working memory tasks (Tucker et al. 2004). Diffusion tensor imaging has revealed diffuse white matter disease across the spectrum of HIV-associated cognitive impairment (Hall et al. 2004).

Examination of the CSF is essential to exclude opportunistic infections. It may be normal, but elevation of protein and a mild lymphocytic pleocytosis can occur. However, this is non-specific and can be found in asymptomatic persons. Oligoclonal bands are sometimes detected and HIV may be isolated from the fluid. Levels of β_2-microglobulin appear to correlate with the severity of the dementia (Brew et al. 1992) and reports have consistently suggested similar claims for neopterin, quinolinic acid and MCP (Perelson et al. 1997; Martin et al. 1998). The latter may be a predictive marker of

HAD when considered as a ratio of its serum concentration (Kelder *et al.* 1998). Unfortunately, as all these CSF markers are non-specific, they have not entered mainstream clinical use in the diagnosis of HAD. HIV RNA or viral load in the CSF has proven to be less clinically useful than was originally hoped (McArthur & Letendre 2006).

Differential diagnosis

The diagnosis of HIV-associated dementia during life is essentially one of exclusion. In mild examples differentiation will be required from anxiety or depression, also from fatigue and the effects of systemic illness. Metabolic causes of encephalopathy should be excluded, also the toxic effects of CNS-active medication, whether prescribed or abused, to which AIDS patients may be sensitive. When psychotic features are present it is important to consider the possibility of an independent schizophrenia or paranoid state.

With more severe dementia the essential differentiation is from opportunistic brain infections or neoplasia. Infections such as CMV, toxoplasmosis, neurosyphilis and cryptococcal or tuberculous meningitis must be carefully excluded since they lead to therapeutic options. Distinguishing features characteristic of CMV encephalitis include coexisting retinitis or colitis, electrolyte abnormalities reflecting adrenalitis, or periventricular abnormalities on MRI indicative of periventriculitis (McArthur *et al.* 1994). Other causes of dementia must clearly be considered, particularly in the middle aged or elderly.

Pathology

The pathological substrate of HIV-associated dementia remains unclear. Price (1994), and more recently in a historical review Scaravilli *et al.* (2007), summarise the attempts made to relate the severity of cognitive impairment to the extent and nature of brain pathology, but such correlations have proved far from exact.

At first it was identified that severe dementia was often associated with the prominent development of multinucleated HIVE, while mild forms tended to show little more than white matter pallor and gliosis (Wiley & Achim 1994). On the whole, this correlation has not been replicated in the majority of cohorts (Navia *et al.* 1986b; Gray *et al.* 1991; Brew *et al.* 1995; Adle-Biassette *et al.* 1999). The suggestion that cortical neuronal loss may be a clinicopathological correlate, a plausible hypothesis in view of it being consistently reported in association with HIVE, has not been supported (Giometto *et al.* 1997). Attempts to identify localised changes have revealed a range of different areas affected, including cell loss in the putamen (Everall *et al.* 1995), preferential frontal productive infection (Bell *et al.* 1998) and reactive hippocampal gliosis (Petito *et al.* 2001). Associations between dementia and leucoencephalopathy (Glass *et al.* 1993; Adle-Biassette *et al.* 1999) or poliodystrophy (Glass *et al.* 1993; Weis *et al.* 1993) have not been substantiated. A promising association

between dementia and microglial activation has been reported on a number of occasions, although this is a non-specific finding reported in other clinical scenarios. Successive stages of severity of dementia tend to arise in the context of increasing levels of systemic immunosuppression, raising the possibility that the virus both creates the opportunity for infection and then exploits it by infecting the CNS (Price 1994). However, there is much variability here as well, some patients failing to develop dementia despite repeated episodes of systemic opportunistic infection, while occasional patients develop severe dementia as the sole feature of the illness.

In an attempt to bring together the conflicting neuropathological picture, Scaravilli *et al.* (2007) propose a 'combined effects' model in the pathogenesis of HIV-associated dementia that allows for the range of conflicting evidence. They propose the concept that HAD results from the combined effects of HIV protein, glial and microglial activation mediated through oxidative stress and glutamatergic excitotoxicity.

Minor cognitive–motor disorder and neuropsychological impairment

The epidemiology of milder cognitive disorders has not been described as fully as for HAD, largely as a result of the reliability and acceptance of criteria and definitions for diagnosis. The definition of HIV-associated MCMD as proposed by the American Academy of Neurology AIDS Taskforce (1991) is shown in Box 7.2. It has been estimated

---

Box 7.2 Criteria for minor cognitive–motor disorder and neuropsychological impairment in HIV infection

I Acquired cognitive, motor or behavioural abnormalities (must have both A and B)

  A At least two of the following symptoms present for at least 1 month, verified by a reliable history:

    (1) Impaired attention or concentration

    (2) Mental slowing

    (3) Impaired memory

    (4) Slowed movements

    (5) Incoordination

    (6) Personality change, or irritability or emotional lability

  B Acquired cognitive or motor abnormality, verified by clinical neurological examination or neuropsychological testing

II Cognitive, motor or behavioural abnormalities causing mild impairment of work or activites of daily living (objectively verifiable or by report of key informant)

III Does not meet criteria for HIV-associated dementia

IV Absence of another cause of the above cognitive, motor or behavioural abnormalities (e.g. active CNS opportunistic infection or malignancy, psychiatric disorders, substance abuse)

that the prevalence is in the region of 5% in asymptomatic seropositive individuals and 18% during the symptomatic stage (Grant *et al.* 2005), although others have identified a much higher estimate of overall prevalence of 50–60%, even when treated with HAART (Sacktor *et al.* 2002). There is some suggestion that women may be at a higher risk of HIV-associated cognitive impairment (Janssen *et al.* 1992; Wojna *et al.* 2004). The transition from neuropsychological impairment to MCMD has not been clearly evaluated. Neuropsychological deficits in asymptomatic presentations are discussed in more detail under Impairment in asymptomatic HIV-positive subjects, later.

Vacuolar myelopathy of the spinal cord

Vacuolar myelopathy has been estimated to affect up to 55% of patients (Artigas *et al.* 1990) in advanced HIV infection and commonly in the context of HIV-associated dementia. Dementia had been present in 70% of the cases identified at post-mortem by Petito *et al.* (1985). Moreover, the severity of the pathological lesions correlates not only with clinical evidence of cord damage but also with the presence of dementia (Petito 1988). Sometimes, however, the motor deficit predominates over evidence of cognitive dysfunction, and worsens progressively while mentation is relatively preserved. The similarity with subacute degeneration of the cord had led to the hypothesis of a vitamin B_{12}-deficient aetiology, which has not been substantiated. Nonetheless, abnormalities in B_{12}-dependent transmethylation pathways may be important and CSF *S*-adenosylmethionine concentrations have been shown to be decreased (Di Rocco *et al.* 2002).

The picture typically evolves over weeks or months as a spastic–ataxic paraparesis, with slowness of gait, clumsiness of leg movements, sensory ataxia and eventual weakness. It may be accompanied by incontinence of the bladder and bowels and by complaints of paraesthesiae or vague discomfort in the legs. Sensation is relatively spared except for loss of vibratory and position sense unless peripheral neuropathy is also present. However, the frequent co-occurrence of the latter may render precise attribution of symptoms difficult.

Spine MRI is typically normal but can reveal non-specific tract hyperintensities. Examination of the CSF may show non-specific abnormalities, including raised protein and a mononuclear pleocytosis. Somatosensory-evoked potentials are useful in tracking the changes in myelopathy. Differential diagnoses must include cord damage due to HSV, VZV and CMV as well as lymphoma in the epidural space.

HIV-associated progressive encephalopathy of childhood

Many children born to HIV-infected mothers develop cognitive and motor disabilities, usually presenting during the first 2 years of life but with wide variability from 2 months to 5 years. Exhenry and Nadal (1996) review the manifestations of vertical HIV transmission in the CNS; 75% of children with HIV-associated progressive encephalopathy are diagnosed before 3 years (early onset) and 8% after 5 years (late onset). The diagnosis is associated with lower CD4 cell counts in the first year of life and the mean estimated length of survival after diagnosis is 22 months (Lobato *et al.* 1995). The infection is usually acquired *in utero* or possibly during birth. In occasional cases it may have been transmitted postnatally through breast-feeding. Exposure to contaminated blood products accounts for a small proportion of cases, especially those in older children.

Belman (1994) describes the heterogeneous clinical pictures that can result. Common manifestations are developmental delays, cognitive impairment, poor brain growth leading to acquired microcephaly, and corticospinal tract signs. Progressive cognitive impairment is sometimes in the forefront of the picture, whereas other children develop disabling motor involvement while cognitive function remains relatively stable. It has been suggested that cognitive deficits are more frequent than motor deficits in the late-onset group and that CD4 cell count in the first years of life predicts future school adaptation or cognitive ability (Tardieu *et al.* 1987).

The most severe syndrome takes the form of increasing spasticity, impaired brain growth and loss of previously acquired milestones. The progression of decline is usually slow but can be rapid over several weeks. Plateau periods occasionally occur, lasting for several months. The typical result is spastic quadriparesis, sometimes with rigidity, dystonia and tremor, along with progressive apathy and loss of interest in the environment. The characteristic facial appearance is of an alert, wide-eyed child with diminished blinking and a mask-like face.

Most children show a more indolent course, which can be mild with long periods during which progression is halted. Cognitive impairment becomes manifest as a decline in the rate of mental development, but previously acquired milestones are preserved. Motor involvement is again common, with paraparesis or disturbance of gait.

A stable/static form is also recognised in children with histories of developmental delay or non-progressive motor deficits. Intelligence is low but remains relatively stable and neurological deficits do not worsen. Motor dysfunction shows as poor coordination, hyperreflexia and increased tone in the legs. The role of HIV infection is less clear in these cases, but has probably served to compromise normal development.

Neuroimaging in the more severe varieties shows cerebral atrophy that can be observed to progress. White matter hypodensity is often apparent, but the characteristic finding is calcification in the basal ganglia and sometimes also in the frontal white matter. Angelini *et al.* (2000) report that late-onset presentations, after the age of 2 years, were more likely to present polymorphically and less likely to have cortical atrophy on neuroimaging.

Pathology

Post-mortem reveals atrophy on gross examination and may show the characteristic features of adult HIVE, with foci of microglia, macrophages and multinucleated giant cells. However, this is found less frequently than in adults. Characteristically the basal ganglia show calcification, chiefly in relation to blood vessels and the adjacent neuropil, and sometimes in the absence of inflammatory change elsewhere. CSF viral load has been associated with atrophy but not intracerebral calcification (Brouwers *et al.* 2000). White matter leucoencephalopathy may be present in the cerebral hemispheres. The spinal cord shows myelin pallor, often restricted in distribution to the corticospinal tracts. Vacuolar myelopathy is infrequent and usually found only in older children. Opportunistic infections and neoplasms of the brain occasionally occur in childhood but less commonly than in adulthood.

Aseptic meningitis

HIV-positive subjects who are not infrequently show a lymphocytic pleocytosis in the CSF during the asymptomatic stage (Marshall *et al.* 1988). Some, however, present with symptoms of meningitis, usually early after infection and while still relatively immunocompetent. Obvious pathogens cannot be isolated, hence the term 'aseptic', but in several cases HIV has been recovered directly from the fluid.

The condition appears to be clinically heterogeneous. In an important group the meningitis develops acutely after infection at the time of seroconversion, presenting with fever, headache, photophobia and meningism (Ho *et al.* 1985). This is typically a mild and self-limiting disorder, lasting for 1–4 weeks, although cranial nerve palsies are occasionally seen. Similar examples may occur later in the asymptomatic phase, or shortly after defining features of AIDS have appeared. Hollander and Stringari (1987) describe two patterns of presentation. One resembles the above, sometimes with recurrent bouts of acute meningeal infection. The other presents with chronic headache in the absence of meningeal signs and may run a protracted course over several months. This appears to represent a more indolent infection, with less marked abnormalities in cell count and protein in the CSF.

A number of case reports have noted the association between oral antibiotic therapy, especially with trimethoprim, and the onset of aseptic meningitis in this setting (Harrison *et al.* 1994).

Peripheral nerve and muscle disorders

Peripheral nerve disorders can complicate all stages of HIV infection and appear to be attributable to a variety of mechanisms (Hoke & Keswani 2005; McArthur *et al.* 2005; Ferrari *et al.* 2006). Evidence of direct infection by HIV is very rare (Pardo *et al.* 2001). As with CNS toxicity, it is likely that HIV proteins indirectly cause injury and loss. For example, there is evidence that upregulation of TNF-α acts as the end-point of a gp120-activated cascade resulting in apoptosis of sensory neurones (Keswani & Hoke 2003).

Acute and chronic inflammatory demyelinating polyneuropathies. These are commonest early in the disease and can be the presenting manifestation. The acute form (Guillain–Barré syndrome) can occur at the time of seroconversion. There is profound motor impairment, with loss of tendon reflexes, variable degrees of sensory loss and often radicular pains in the back and legs. The CSF protein is characteristically elevated. The pathogenesis almost certainly reflects a disorder of immune regulation. Treatment by plasmapheresis (Kiprov & Hofmann 2003) or intravenous immunoglobulin can be of benefit. Steroids must only be used with caution and with close monitoring of immune function because they may reduce resistance to opportunistic infections.

Sensory ganglioneuritis and acute cranial nerve palsies. These may also occur in the early asymptomatic phase of infection.

Distal sensory polyneuropathy. DSPN is the main form in the later stages of HIV disease, rivalling HIV dementia in prevalence, with around 30% of hospitalised patients with AIDS being identified as having DSPN. The two frequently occur together. DSPN may develop acutely or gradually, presenting usually with bilateral burning pain and hyperalgesia particularly in the soles of the feet, worse at night or after walking. Intense neuropathic pain may lead to considerable disablement. Mild distal motor involvement can often be found when carefully sought, by way of muscle atrophy or weakness. Tendon reflexes are diminished or absent at the ankles and vibratory thresholds are elevated. Nerve conduction tests show an axonal, length-dependent, sensory polyneuropathy. Occasionally the dysaesthesiae may begin in the hands. The pathogenic factors at work are unclear, and may involve infectious, toxic or nutritional processes.

Distal sensory polyneuropathy is clinically indistinguishable from antiretroviral toxic neuropathy. Some investigators have asserted that antiretrovirals may unmask a silent DSPN. A careful history of treatment and the timings of changes in preparations and doses may help to distinguish aetiological factors. Other causes of neuropathy, such as diabetes, should be excluded.

Other neuropathies. These take the form of polyradiculopathies, consisting of rapidly evolving flaccid paralysis and pain in the back and legs, or sometimes present as a cauda equina lesion. Multiple mononeuropathy (mononeuritis multiplex) appears often to be due to CMV infections, and partial response may be obtained with ganciclovir. HSV is sometimes implicated. The role of direct infection with HIV is suspected, and the virus can sometimes be isolated from the peripheral nerves.

Myopathy. This may present at any stage with slowly progressive proximal muscle weakness of the limbs, myalgia and excessive fatiguability. Serum creatine phosphokinase levels are elevated, and cautious treatment with steroids can be beneficial. The relative roles of immunological factors and infection with HIV are uncertain. Other affections of muscle include necrotising myopathy, necrotising vasculitis, nemaline rod myopathy and mitochondrial myopathy. An acute self-limiting myopathic process may also be observed at the time of seroconversion.

Impairment in asymptomatic HIV-positive subjects

In view of the known early invasion of the nervous system by HIV, the question arises whether impairments of a subtle nature may be detectable during the asymptomatic phase. The issue is important for both theoretical and practical reasons. If impairments commonly exist while asymptomatic persons are active at work and in social life, this could be relevant to their competence and reliability. In particular, impairment of judgement, risky decision-making (Hardy *et al.* 2006) or behavioural change could increase their risks of spreading the infection. Early therapeutic intervention might be indicated.

Some reports have identified a higher rate of cross-sectional neuropsychological deficit in asymptomatic individuals compared with those who are seronegative, but there are few studies that reveal that this impairment is progressive or that it precedes MCMD or HAD. In some cases abnormalities in neuropsychological function may not have clinical meaning in the sense that they are not readily associated with functional impact and may improve on retesting. To some extent problems in the sampling of persons to be tested, the selection of appropriate neuropsychological tests (Woods *et al.* 2006), variability in definitions of impairment and disorder between studies, and the need to allow for variables such as past head injury, alcohol or drug abuse, age, premorbid neurological disorders and educational background confound investigations. White, D.A. *et al.* (1995) reviewed the findings of neuropsychological studies between 1987 and 1994. They found that the median rate of impairment was 35% in asymptomatic cases and 12% in controls without the virus. Studies where large batteries of tests were performed were more likely to report impairment.

There has been a search for associations between neuropsychological impairment in asymptomatic HIV infection and various markers. Reports have not found correlations with serum HIV RNA (Dal Pan *et al.* 1998) or CD4 cell count (Podraza *et al.* 1994). CSF viral load has been a more promising indicator (McArthur *et al.* 1997). However, this has not been substantiated in another cohort taking HAART, where there were no differences in serum or CSF viral load or immune activation markers compared with those with

normal neuropsychological tests (J.C. McArthur *et al.*, unpublished results, 2002). It may be that early post-infection viral load and CD4 cell counts are of greater importance in predicting progression to neuropsychological impairment and necessitate early aggressive treatment (Ellis *et al.* 2002; Marcotte *et al.* 2003).

Despite the inherent challenges that have been encountered in establishing the neuropathological correlate of HAD, more encouragingly cognitive impairment does appear to predict histological evidence of HIVE at post-mortem, even when this impairment is mild (Cherner *et al.* 2002). Again, as in dementia, authors have suggested the importance of combining information from several markers of neuronal injury in order to identify the strongest associations with cognitive impairment before death (Moore *et al.* 2006).

Illicit substance and alcohol misuse may be special risk factors for cognitive impairment (Justice *et al.* 2004; Durvasula *et al.* 2006). In one recent study of HIV-positive methamphetamine users, cognitive impairment was associated with severe loss of frontal interneurones (Chana *et al.* 2006). Similarly, viral coinfection, for example with hepatitis C, may worsen neuropsychological performance (Letendre *et al.* 2006; Parsons *et al.* 2006).

With regard to degrees of functional cognitive impairment, it was originally suggested that this is greater in symptomatic cases when compared with asymptomatic controls (Maj *et al.* 1994). However, Heaton *et al.* (1994) identified that, among asymptomatic individuals, the level of unemployment was statistically significantly higher in the cognitively impaired group, in contrast to those unaffected. Albert *et al.* (1995) have replicated this, finding an eightfold increase in work disability, and Heaton *et al.* (2004) have provided further support utilising standardised functional measures that reveal significantly worse performance in neuropsychologically impaired individuals. Memory impairment is clearly an important indicator of decreased likelihood of return to work (van Gorp *et al.* 2007) and has a negative impact on quality of life (Tozzi *et al.* 2003).

An understanding of the progression of cognitive disorders remains elusive. Grant *et al.* (2005) review neuropsychological longitudinal studies in asymptomatic infection between 1990 and 1993. They find that there is little to suggest neuropsychological deterioration in asymptomatic cases up to 36 months follow-up. Longer term, the Multicenter AIDS Cohort Study reports significant decline before AIDS only in psychomotor speed (Selnes *et al.* 1995).

Other psychiatric disorders

In addition to the neuropsychiatric disorders described above, HIV-infected patients are also vulnerable to a variety of psychiatric disturbances, many of which may owe little or nothing to the primary effects of the virus on the CNS. The range is wide, from states of acute distress on becoming aware of HIV status to profound depression/psychotic illnesses. The latter may sometimes show an admixture of organic psychiatric symptoms, since mood disorder and psychoses can be early manifestations of brain disease. A separate group of patients consists of the 'worried well', i.e. individuals who are not infected but develop an intense fear or even a protracted conviction of harbouring the disease.

Patients with primary mental disorder are also disproportionately represented in those who have contracted the virus. In their retrospective analysis of a psychiatric cohort, Beyer *et al.* (2007) identified that the prevalence of HIV was some four times higher than that of the general population and other studies have supported this finding. The interplay between pre-existing mental illness, HIV-related factors and the effects or interactions of both psychotropic medications and HAART can make psychiatric presentations and management extremely complex. As a result comorbid mental ill health is often poorly recognised in those with the virus (Evans *et al.* 1999).

Other factors have been noted as contributing to psychiatric morbidity over and above the threats inherent in a long-term life-threatening, condition. Surveys have stressed the vulnerability of the populations from which HIV-infected persons tend to be drawn, and the powerful role of psychosocial influences in determining adverse reactions (Dilley *et al.* 1985; Faulstich 1987). The acquisition of infection can increase feelings of stigma or guilt, and provoke intense concern about others to whom the disease may have been transmitted. An additional stress is the uncertainty, extending sometimes over many years, about the course the disease will take, occurring often against a background of illness and losses among close friends and partners. In consequence it is scarcely surprising that a high prevalence of psychiatric disorder is reported in both physically asymptomatic and symptomatic persons.

An increasing number of studies have recently focused on the relationship between mental ill health and psychosocial stress on the progression of HIV infection, seeking to find associations between variability in the course of the illness between those affected and the impact of both stressors and mood disorder on cellular immunity and mortality (Ickovics *et al.* 2001; Leserman 2008). Similarly, interest has been directed at the relationship between behavioural manifestations of psychosocial factors and disease progression including the impact of treatment compliance, illicit substance misuse, sexual risk behaviours and physical exercise (for a review see Gore-Felton & Koopman 2008).

Acute psychological reactions
Acute stress reactions are most commonly observed at the time of notification of a positive serological test result. Confirmation of the diagnosis brings the realisation of fears that may have long been present, also the need to tell others, including sexual partners. Lifestyles which have previously been concealed may be exposed to parents and colleagues for the first time. The principal manifestations are acute shock, bewilderment and anxiety, typically lasting for several weeks. Major depression may be precipitated, with depersonalisation, insomnia and suicidal ideation. A preoccupation may develop with bodily symptoms thought to be indicative of commencing disease. Other reactions include anger, despair, guilt, increased use of alcohol or drugs, social withdrawal or denial. Denial may lead to a dangerous disregard of medical advice and failure to take precautions against infecting others. The incidence of acute psychological reactions at the time of testing has varied widely in different reports, perhaps reflecting the adequacy of pre- and post-test counselling. Perry *et al.* (1990a) found that psychological distress had diminished in most cases by 10 weeks after notification.

Longer-term psychiatric disorder
Longer-lasting psychiatric disorders may emerge during the asymptomatic or symptomatic stages of infection, but it is uncertain whether this is more common than in patients with other serious medical conditions (King 1989, 1993).

Anxiety presents in 4–19% of patients (Justice *et al.* 2004; Pence *et al.* 2006), predominantly in the context of adjustment disorder (Fernandez 2002) and focused on the uncertainties surrounding long-term outcome, the availability of care in the future and the loss of physical and financial independence. The risk of infecting others, or of being identified as homosexual or a drug abuser, may be at the forefront of concerns. Somatic symptoms of anxiety are sometimes interpreted as evidence of progression to further stages of the disorder, giving rise to an escalating vicious circle. Alcohol or drugs may be abused in attempts to self-medicate the symptoms of anxiety.

Depression has a varied reported prevalence, ranging from 2% to 48% of patients in different surveys, depending on those studied (Perkins *et al.* 1994; Fernandez 2002; Chander *et al.* 2006). A moderately high incidence of 15% has been reported in HAART-naive patients (Starace *et al.* 2002). The risk of depression in seropositive individuals is double that seen in an uninfected control group, independent of sexual orientation (Ciesla & Roberts 2001). In the HAART era, by way of comparison, over 30% of HIV-positive individuals in one large multicentre study met operational criteria for depression (Bing *et al.* 2001). Depression is likely to be underdiagnosed (Asch *et al.* 2003) and has been associated with the presence of personality disorder and low perceived social support (Lyketsos *et al.* 1996). A 2-year prospective cohort study of major depressive disorder in men reported a higher risk of depression in those with more advanced HIV disease at baseline, lifetime presence of multiple psychiatric illness and particularly a past history of depression as the most significant predictors of depressive illness (Atkinson *et al.* 2008). Interestingly, the presence of baseline cognitive impairment, pathology identified on neuroimaging and adverse life events did not predict a depressive episode in this study, although it is acknowledged that this may be a feature of the cohort and needs further confirmation.

Depression and withdrawal can significantly interfere with the ability to cope with the procedures required for management of the illness (Ostrow 1990; Cruess *et al.* 2003; Antoni *et al.* 2005) and particularly with adherence to antiretroviral treatment regimens (Avants *et al.* 2001; Starace *et al.* 2002; Tucker *et al.* 2003). It would appear that taking antidepressant medication could improve treatment adherence in depressed subjects, although further investigation is needed to elucidate whether treatment of depression is related to HIV outcomes (Yun *et al.* 2005). There is increasing, if sometimes conflicting, evidence of the negative impact of depressive disorders on immunological, virological and clinical outcomes in HIV even when controlling for poor HAART adherence (Cruess *et al.* 2003; Hartzell *et al.* 2008). Prior to the advent of HAART, the San Francisco Men's Health Study found that depressed individuals at baseline progressed to an AIDS diagnosis roughly 1.5 years sooner than their non-depressed counterparts (Page-Shafer *et al.* 1996). This finding has been corroborated and refuted by subsequent pre-HAART studies. Notably, the Multicenter AIDS Cohort Study (Lyketsos *et al.* 1996) did not find a significant association. Similar studies in the era of HAART, conducted over longer follow-up periods and with larger numbers, have found more consistent evidence for an association between chronic depressive symptoms and less favourable outcomes (Leserman 2008). Nonetheless, it appears that HAART does have a modest impact on reducing measures of depression and hopelessness (Rabkin *et al.* 2000).

Care in identifying depression is particularly important and especially in the context of the overlap of somatic symptoms such as fatigue, pain, appetite loss and sleeplessness that may be present throughout infection with HIV. Nonetheless, severe depressive symptoms should not be assumed to be understandable and justified, and must always receive full evaluation and treatment. Anhedonia and diurnal mood variation may be useful discriminating symptoms suggestive of depression (Treisman *et al.* 2001). The problems that may arise in distinguishing depression and the early stages of HIV-associated dementia are discussed under HIV-associated cognitive disorders in this chapter.

Obsessive–compulsive disorder. This can occur with or without depressed mood, commonly involving repeated bodily scrutiny for evidence of progression of disease. Obsessive ruminations may centre on death and dying, or endeavours to recollect past sexual partners to whom the infection may have been transmitted.

Suicide. This presents a considerable risk in both the early and late stages of the disorder. Perry *et al.* (1990b) found that suicidal ideation was common, affecting almost 30% of individuals at the time of serological testing, but falling significantly within 2 months of notification. Suicide attempts tend to cluster in the first 6 months after diagnosis, underlining the importance of pre- and post-test counselling (World Health Organization 1990b). Demographic and disease-related factors associated with suicidality have been identified as white ethnicity, male gender, homosexuality, physical health complications, frequency of AIDS-related conditions and rapidity of disease progression. Psychosocial variables associated with suicidal ideation include neuroticism, hopelessness, avoidant coping, intravenous drug use, limited social support networks and a family history of suicide (Kalichman *et al.* 2000; Haller & Miles 2003; Carrico *et al.* 2007).

Later, with symptomatic AIDS, completed suicide is considerably increased. Rates among New York residents were estimated to be some 36-fold above expectation in one retrospective review, but such a very large excess has yet to be confirmed (Marzuk *et al.* 1988; Marzuk 1991). An important consideration is the extent to which suicide in the later stages may be considered to be 'rational' in view of the poor outcome to be expected. Against this is the close association between suicide and psychiatric illness, inappropriate guilt, and erroneous perceptions about the development of the illness and methods available to relieve suffering (Glass 1988; King 1993).

Marzuk (1991) discusses other AIDS-related suicides, including persons grieving for loss of friends and family members, psychotic patients who were deluded that they suffered from AIDS, and a small group of people, mainly homosexual, who had deliberately sought to contract AIDS as a means of ending their lives.

Psychoses. These appear to be not infrequent, although the scattered reports of small numbers of cases make any estimate of prevalence uncertain and it is certainly considerably less than that of depression. Many pictures have been reported, some seemingly typical of psychoses occurring in other settings, while others have shown special features.

A considerable proportion of psychoses develop in the context of AIDS-related cognitive impairment (Sewell *et al.* 1994; Evans *et al.* 2002) and in one study 15% of patients with HAD reported psychotic symptoms (Navia & Price 1987). In others, evidence of cognitive impairment emerges only later when the more florid manifestations have been brought under control. Sometimes, however, organic symptomatology remains absent throughout the illness which presents as a purely 'functional' psychosis (Halstead *et al.* 1988) and on occasion the only indicator of underlying HIV infection.

Maj (1990) reviews the mechanisms that may be responsible: chance association, reactions to the threat of the disorder, precipitation in predisposed persons or a response to drugs abused or prescribed. Alternatively, the psychosis may reflect HIV brain infection, especially in patients with no previous history of psychiatric illness or drug abuse and who are unaware of their seropositivity (Buhrich *et al.* 1988). The predilection of the virus for the limbic regions of the brain could be relevant in this regard. De Ronchi *et al.* (2000) identified psychiatric history, lower cognitive performance and the absence of antiretroviral treatment as potential risk factors for first-episode psychosis in those with HIV infection compared with non-psychotic controls and suggested that HAART may be protective against psychosis. However, antiretrovirals have also been repeatedly implicated in the development of psychotic disorders in the literature. Foster *et al.* (2003, 2004) report the emergence of two cases of psychosis that they suggest were associated with abacavir in a combination regimen. Zidovudine (Maxwell *et al.* 1988; O'Dowd 1988; Schaerf *et al.* 1989), efavirenz (De la Garza *et al.* 2001; Peyriere *et al.* 2001) and nevirapine (Wise *et al.* 2002) are also identified in this review as being associated with *de novo* psychoses (Foster *et al.* 2003).

The variety of pictures encountered is illustrated by several reports and reviews (Thomas & Szabadi 1987; Buhrich *et al.* 1988; Halstead *et al.* 1988; Vogel-Scibilia *et al.* 1988; Harris *et al.* 1991). Delusions, hallucinations, bizarre behaviour, thought disorder, lability of mood and major affective disorder may feature prominently, with or without organic accompaniments in the mental state. Among the 31 cases reviewed by Harris *et al.* (1991), after excluding those due to substance abuse or delirium, the psychosis was the presenting feature in 12. CT was abnormal in half and the CSF in one-quarter, these patients tending to decline rapidly in physical and cognitive status.

It seems unlikely that a specific 'HIV psychosis' exists, but it appears that *mania* may be especially common and perhaps associated with HIV disease progression. In the early stages of HIV infection the incidence of manic episodes is likely to be similar to the seronegative general population at 1–2% (Lyketsos *et al.* 2001). This increases some fourfold at the onset of AIDS and is associated with cognitive impairment and higher CD4 counts (Lyketsos *et al.* 1993). Kieburtz *et al.* (1991) described eight such patients, all with evidence of cognitive impairment once the florid mood symptoms had subsided. Irritability was more prominent than elation, and all showed MRI abnormalities. King (1993) reported that all psychotic patients referred to his AIDS liaison psychiatry service exhibited major manic symptoms. Treisman *et al.* (1994) present data suggesting that when mania develops in patients with low genetic risk this tends to occur late in the disease and in the context of dementia, whereas in those with personal or family histories of affective disorder mania may occur at any stage and while cognitive function is well preserved.

The 'worried well' (AIDS phobia, pseudo-AIDS)

The intense public concern aroused by AIDS, and the amount of media attention devoted to it, have raised anxieties in many segments of the population. People at risk, particularly homosexual and bisexual men, may present themselves for testing in states of considerable alarm (termed 'AIDS anxiety' or 'AIDS panic'). Psychotic patients may incorporate AIDS into their delusions and become convinced that they are harbouring the disease (Mahorney & Cavenar 1988). Todd (1989) describes typical examples: patients present with anxiety or panic after casual affairs, especially in the face of mild physical symptoms, or with obsessional fears of touching people and compulsive hand washing, or with paranoid psychosis developing some time after an affair.

Distinct from these are a group of neurotic patients who focus on the condition as a vehicle for hypochondriacal concern. Such patients can absorb a great deal of attention in fruitless attempts at reassurance. These are the 'worried well'. They are remarkable not only for the persistence of their anxieties, which can fail to be allayed by repeated negative tests, but often for the remoteness of the chance that they have been exposed to risk of infection. An interesting constellation of influences appears to underlie this sometimes intractable disorder.

Miller *et al.* (1988) reported experience with 19 such patients. Of the 17 males, six were heterosexual, eight homosexual and three bisexual. The mean age was 35 years. The uniform presentation was with an unshakeable and anxiety-laden conviction that they had HIV infection or disease, as indicated by symptoms such as fatigue, dizziness, sweating, skin rashes, muscle pain, diarrhoea, sore throat, slight weight loss, minor mouth infections or slight lymphadenopathy. The misattribution of such features had often stemmed directly from media reports describing AIDS-related symptoms. Obsessional ruminations were almost universal, centring on thoughts of HIV disease and death, possible 'high-risk' sexual practices in the past and the dangers they may have presented to others. Repeated body checking for signs of the disease and palpation for enlarged lymph nodes were common, likewise questioning and scrutiny of spouses or partners for evidence of the disease. Three-quarters were depressed and over half suicidal. Two patients later progressed to a delusional conviction of supposed infection. Most of the patients had already made repeated attendances at clinics or general practice surgeries, often receiving several negative serological test results.

Background features included a fairly consistent picture of constrained and problematic sexual adaptation, including non-acceptance of homosexual tendencies, difficulties with sexual expression, or constricting religious or family influences on sexual behaviour. This had often resulted in episodes of covert sexual activity, either homosexual or heterosexual, with high levels of associated guilt. In most cases there was a history of no more than low-risk sexual experiences, and only two patients reported activities that could have led to infection within the previous 6 years. A past history of psychiatric disorder, mostly depression or anxiety, was common.

The remarkable persistence of such anxieties has been stressed in most reports. Negative test results may be attributed by the patient to laboratory error, to the appearance of a 'new form' of the virus, or to their inability to form antibodies as other people do (Maj 1990). Miller *et al.* (1988) acknowledge the futility of repeated reassurance, which appears merely to maintain the problem. They recommend a cognitive–behavioural strategy based on cue exposure and response prevention, with attempts at the reinterpretation of symptoms in terms of their origin in anxiety. In occasional patients, however, the excessive fear of infection may prove to be part of a major depressive illness and be responsive to antidepressant medication (Jenike & Pato 1986).

Factitious/fraudulent AIDS

In contrast to the above group who have an unfounded fear of infection, occasional patients present with unfounded claims of having the disease. Some state that they are HIV positive to secure financial assistance, rehousing or social support (King 1993). Drug abusers may hope to ensure a supply of maintenance medication and obviate therapeutic attempts to promote withdrawal. Falsified documents and forged reports may be presented to these ends (Zumwalt *et al.* 1987).

More remarkable are those patients who attend hospitals and clinics with a complex history of HIV-related illness, including opportunistic infections and their treatment, all of which turns out to have been fabricated. Sometimes a similar story has been repeated during visits at several hospitals. These patients represent a variant of Munchausen's syndrome, the underlying motive being apparently to secure medical attention. Zuger and O'Dowd (1992) describe such a patient who had received inpatient and outpatient treatment at AIDS facilities for almost a year before the true situation was established. They review 14 more cases from the literature. The usual presentations were with acute neurological or psychiatric complaints, and most patients were members of groups at high risk for HIV infection. Only HIV testing, and where possible confirmation of the history, can protect against a false diagnosis.

Bereavement and stressful life events

Fawzy *et al.* (1991) describe the multifaceted problems of bereavement in patients with AIDS, also in their families, friends and partners. In contrast with individuals suffering from other life-threatening diseases, the patient with AIDS will often have to deal with AIDS-related deaths among many associates and in unrelenting succession. Such an experience of loss of a partner or close friend has been associated with a more rapid decline in CD4 counts in surviving HIV-positive homosexual men (Kemeny *et al.* 1995). The immune activation marker neopterin is increased and natural killer cell cytotoxicity decreased in bereaved survivors (Kemeny *et al.* 1995; Goodkin *et al.* 1996).

There is a high risk of the development of abnormal bereavement reactions for a number of reasons. There may be constraints on the public display of grief when homosexuality has previously been concealed, and in the case of drug abuse there is likely to be disapproval or even a punitive response from those around. The patient's ambivalent feelings about homosexuality or drug abuse may be brought to the surface, and may conspire against the development of new supportive relationships. Family members may need to contend with the first awareness of their relative's sexual orientation or drug abuse, and may find themselves lying about the cause of death. Health-care workers who treat patients with AIDS also carry a heavy burden in adjusting to the loss of their patients.

In general, stressful life events have been repeatedly shown to have significant effects on disease progression (Leserman 2008). In one study of young people, two or more stressful events were associated with three times the risk of decline in CD4 counts over the period of follow-up (Howland *et al.* 2000). Similarly, in adult homosexual men, higher cumulative stressful event scores predicted an accelerated transition to AIDS (Leserman 2000). Since the more widespread use of HAART, negative effects of stress on immunological, virological and clinical outcomes have continued to be reported (Ironson *et al.* 2005a,b,c; Leserman *et al.* 2007).

Investigation and treatment

The attention of physicians, psychiatrists, psychologists, social workers and specially trained counsellors may be required in HIV-related disease. The problems that arise are frequently complex, in terms of both medical diagnosis and psychosocial impact. Investigations during the symptomatic stages will often involve extensive laboratory and radiographic procedures. Some of the principal findings in patients with opportunistic infections and tumours of the nervous system have been mentioned above, also findings in relation to HAD.

Serological testing and pretest discussion

The Clinical Effectiveness Group of the British Association of Sexual Health and HIV produced UK National Guidelines on HIV testing in 2006 (Rogstad *et al.* 2006) and these should be referred to with regard to all matters relating to serological testing.

The technique routinely employed for detecting HIV infection relies on assessment of antibodies to the virus using fourth-generation enzyme immunoassay (EIA) that detects all three main immunoglobulins and p24 antigen. When a positive result is obtained the test is first repeated, then checked with a more specific approach such as immunofluorescence, radioimmune precipitation or Western blotting and laboratories should have a confirmatory algorithm for such testing (Parry *et al.* 2003). Testing using PCR can be utilised during this period and may identify infection 7–10 days earlier than EIA screening. Lymphocyte culture for isolation of the virus can be useful in paediatric practice, since HIV antibody testing can remain positive through passive maternal transfer for up to 18 months. Minute amounts of HIV nucleic acid can be detected by PCR, and this can yield a measurement of viral load. Oral fluid samples can also be tested, although antibodies may take longer to become positive.

Testing should only be carried out with the patient's *informed and explicit* verbal consent, except in very rare instances, and this should be carefully documented following a pretest discussion with a professional who has specific training and expertise in HIV counselling. A positive result carries not only implications for the patient's future health but also far-reaching social, financial and often legal consequences. The specific points to be covered in the pretest discussion have been set out in the UK National Guidelines (Box 7.3).

However, there are very exceptional circumstances in which testing may need to be performed without explicit consent, namely where a test is imperative in order to secure the safety of persons other than the patient and where it is not possible for the prior consent of the patient to be obtained, for example if the patient is unconscious (General Medical Council 1988, 1993, 1997). Patients should be informed that they have been tested and why the test was performed once they regain consciousness. The result should not be disclosed to anyone (including relatives) who is not involved in their health care without the patient's permission. In psychiatric practice other situations may also arise, for example when a patient is unable or unwilling to give consent by reason of psychiatric disorder such as severe affective illness, mental handicap or an organic brain syndrome. It is then necessary before proceeding to be clear that the result would be of both real diagnostic value and likely of benefit to the patient. In many instances there is no immediate and pressing need for a definitive diagnosis, and it may be possible to defer testing until the patient becomes well enough to reconsider giving consent in the normal way. The need to know urgently for the protection of staff or other patients is likely to apply only in patients showing aggressive or seriously disinhibited behaviour.

When performed without consent, it is important to record reasons for taking such action in the patient's notes, to discuss it with the psychiatric team and to obtain a second opinion from a psychiatrist or physician. It is wise also to inform the health authority's solicitor and the relevant medical defence body. In essence the test should be carried out with awareness that the decision may have to be defended in court.

Matters of confidentiality surrounding the test result can also be problematic (General Medical Council 1988, 1993, 1997; Catalan *et al.* 1989; Rogstad *et al.* 2006). Only those team members who need to know should be informed. The importance of telling the patient's general practitioner, who is likely to be involved in future care, should be discussed with the patient and consent obtained for this. However, if after full discussion the patient refuses, his request for privacy should normally be respected. The exception is when failure of disclosure could put the health of any carer at serious risk although this needs to be considered in the context of the legal framework of the jurisdiction of the test. This is particularly so when the patient is incapacitated and cannot give consent. A careful multidisciplinary discussion and consultation with both an occupational health consultant and legal advice should be sought when making complex testing decisions. Similarly, disclosure to a spouse or partner without consent is warranted only when there is a serious and identifiable risk to a specific individual who, if not informed, would be exposed to infection.

Treatment
General aspects
General aspects of management include the need for support and counselling, not only for the infected person but often also for the family, partners and friends. Even in the asymptomatic stage it is important to allow full discussion of the disease and its significance, including the likelihood that there may be considerable delay before symptoms make an appearance. It is essential to provide detailed information about methods to minimise the risk of infecting others, including 'safe' sexual practices and, in addicts, the strict avoidance of needle-sharing. The patient should be advised to inform the dentist before any dental procedure.

Prophylactic drug treatment is often undertaken to ward off opportunistic infections such as *Pneumocystis carinii*,

---

Box 7.3 Specific points to be covered in the pretest discussion (Rogstad *et al.* 2006)

1 Benefits of testing:
   (a) Health benefits of current treatments
   (b) Knowing HIV status can allay anxiety
   (c) A positive test may motivate people to reduce risk activities
   (d) Opportunity to reduce the risk of transmission to others, e.g. infants, sexual partners
2 Risk assessment, including date of last risk activity
3 The 'window period'
4 The implications of testing for mortgages, insurance, occupational risks and confidentiality
5 Details of how the result will be given
6 Where appropriate to explore support and coping mechanisms
7 Obtaining informed consent for the test
8 Information about HIV transmission and risk reduction as necessary

tuberculosis and toxoplasmosis (Beiser 1997). Problems over employment and coping with negative reactions from associates will often need attention. Many patients will benefit from regular follow-up, when weight and blood counts can be checked routinely and enquiry made about general health and fitness. Referral to local self-help organisations will usually be of very considerable assistance.

Management of major psychiatric disorders

Depression and stress. Ferrando and Freyberg (2008) critically review the treatment of depression and identify the confounding factors in appraising the literature. Both open label and randomised controlled trials disproportionately represent homosexual and bisexual men, have variable inclusion and outcome criteria, focus on different stages of HIV disease and fail to focus on medication interactions. They found fairly consistent evidence (based on randomised clinical trials) that selective serotonin reuptake inhibitors (SSRIs), particularly fluoxetine, and the tricyclics imipramine and desipramine (Zisook *et al.* 1998; Rabkin *et al.* 1999), are effective, with a preference for SSRIs based on their favourable side-effect profile and lack of any demonstrable effect on immune status (Fernando & Freyberg 2008). Other antidepressants, including mirtazapine, have also shown promise in open label studies. Rabkin *et al.* (2004) have identified the effectiveness of testosterone, particularly for fatigue, in depressed HIV-positive men. Dexamfetamine (Wagner & Rabkin 2000), modafinil (Rabkin *et al.* 2004) and methylphenidate (Fernandez *et al.* 1995) have also shown benefit in depression and particularly in improving fatigue and demotivation.

When prescribing antidepressants it is always important to consider interactions with antiretrovirals. Protease inhibitors and nucleoside reverse transcriptase inhibitors can affect cytochrome P450 activity, resulting in altered metabolism of some antidepressant medications. Fluoxetine has been shown to cause increases in ritonavir levels. Venlafaxine, which has a more negligible effect on P450, has a potentially smaller effect on HAART (Ereshefsky & Dugan 2000) but can lower plasma levels of indinavir.

The study by Markowitz *et al.* (1998) compared combined psychological and pharmacological treatments with different modalities of psychotherapy for depression comorbid with HIV. This found that the group on combination treatment and that receiving interpersonal therapy had significant improvements in depression scores compared with supportive and cognitive–behaviour therapies. Group psychological interventions have been more extensively investigated, both alone and in combination with antidepressants, and have suggested an effect of psychotherapies alone, at least in mild to moderate depressive episodes (Targ *et al.* 1994; Zisook *et al.* 1998; Laperriere *et al.* 2005).

A meta-analysis of stress management interventions in HIV-positive adults, conducted by the National Institutes of Health (Scott-Sheldon *et al.* 2008) found that such interventions significantly improve mental health indices and quality of life but do not impact on immunological outcomes or hormonal processes, a finding echoed by Brown and Vanable (2008).

Psychosis. The evidence base for treating psychotic disorders in HIV-positive individuals is poor in comparison with mood disorders. It is likely that patients with HIV infection are considerably more sensitive to extrapyramidal effects which, alongside the subcortical psychomotor retardation associated with the virus, may be considerably disabling. For this reason, low doses and slow titrations of antipsychotics are advised, with careful monitoring for metabolic syndrome (Repetto & Petitto 2008). Interactions between HAART and antipsychotics should again be carefully considered. Ritonavir has been shown to decrease plasma concentrations of olanzapine (Penzak *et al.* 2002).

Mania. Mood stabilisers have been investigated in the management of manic symptoms associated with HIV. Sodium valproate has been suggested to increase HIV replication in some studies (Moog *et al.* 1996), although this has not been duplicated in studies looking at the drug's effect on viral load in serum and CSF (Maggi & Halman 2001; Ances *et al.* 2006). Carbamazepine and lamotrigine are both known to have effects on the enzyme systems also utilised by antiretrovirals, resulting in altered serum concentrations of both mood stabiliser and/or antiretroviral. Careful monitoring is essential. Zidovudine has been shown to have a protective influence against mania (Mijch *et al.* 1999).

Treatment of opportunistic infections, neoplasms and neuropsychiatric complications

This is a matter for specialist attention. The differential diagnosis is often wide, infections can be multiple and investigations may need to be extensive. PCP will often respond, at least early on, to co-trimoxazole, and Kaposi's sarcoma skin lesions to local radiotherapy or intralesional injections of vinblastine. Kaposi's sarcoma occurring elsewhere, such as the lungs or gastrointestinal tract, may be treated with intravenous chemotherapy. Oral candidiasis may be kept in check with nystatin suspension or amphotericin lozenges; oesophageal and severe oral infection will require ketoconazole. Details of treatment for these and other systemic infections are given in textbooks of medicine.

Many CNS pathogens can be treated similarly; for a succinct review, see the European Guidelines compiled by Portegies *et al.* (2004). *Toxoplasma* brain infection will often respond, both clinically and radiologically, to pyrimethamine and sulfadiazine, occasionally with complete resolution of symptoms and control of the disease. Improvement can be seen within 1–2 weeks, this sometimes being used empirically as a diagnostic test. If there is no response, biopsy is required to investigate for other treatable conditions such as lymphoma, tuberculosis or CMV infection. Cryptococcal infection is usually treated with amphotericin, with or without 5-flucytosine, followed by maintenance therapy with fluconazole (Manji & Connolly 1992). HSV requires acyclovir, and CMV infection foscarnet or ganciclovir; the latter should not be combined with zidovudine because of severe myelosuppression. Cerebral lymphoma often responds initially to radiotherapy.

Inflammatory neuropathies are sometimes considered best treated with plasmapheresis because of the risks of steroid therapy in the immunocompromised patient. Others, however, use steroids on the basis that autoimmune mechanisms are at work. Distal sensory neuropathy may respond to zidovudine.

Highly active antiretroviral treatment

There are four classes of antiretrovirals that are in current use: nucleoside/nucleotide analogue reverse transcriptase inhibitors (NRTIs), non-nucleoside analogue reverse transcriptase inhibitors (NNRTIs), protease inhibitors and fusion inhibitors. A full review of their mechanisms of action and the evidence that supports their use can be found in Warnke *et al.* (2007) and is only discussed briefly here.

The NRTIs are similar to the nucleoside building blocks of DNA and RNA and act by affecting reverse transcriptase activity through direct competition with nucleosides to be incorporated into viral DNA. The first NRTI, zidovudine (3-azido-2,3-diethoxythymidine, AZT, Retrovir, ZDV), has been used in treatment since 1987. It is a thymidine analogue. It is highly active against HIV *in vitro*, but is effective only against virus in the process of replication, after it has been phosphorylated. Resistant strains may accordingly develop after several months of use. It is of particular interest as it is one of the antiretrovirals that crosses the blood–brain barrier. The most frequent adverse effect of zidovudine is bone marrow suppression, resulting in anaemia or neutropenia, which may dictate dose reduction or cessation of treatment. Regular monitoring of the blood picture is therefore essential during treatment. Other side effects include nausea, anorexia, abdominal pain, rashes, headache and insomnia, largely restricted to the early weeks of treatment. A reversible myopathy occasionally develops after long-continued use.

Other NRTIs that penetrate the CNS include abacavir, didanosine and stavudine. One study of HAART combinations in HAD found that adding abacavir did not result in improved clinical or virological outcomes, although this may have been confounded by the short duration of HAART, which arguably would have not stabilised prior to the addition of abacavir (Lanier 2001). Stavudine has been shown to further ameliorate neurological symptoms in patients previously treated with zidovudine (Arendt *et al.* 1998). CSF viral load has been shown to be decreased to undetectable levels with stavudine (Gisolf *et al.* 2000).

The NNRTIs include nevirapine, delavirdine and efavirenz. These antiretrovirals act by directly binding to reverse transcriptase and subsequently block DNA polymerase activity. They do not require phosphorylation to become viricidal unlike the NRTIs. All three penetrate the blood–brain barrier, although clear evidence about their benefits in HAD remains to be established. Efavirenz has been shown to decrease CSF viral load (Tashima *et al.* 1999) and cognitive improvements have been noted with nevirapine/efavirenz combinations (von Giesen *et al.* 2002). However, efavirenz has also been associated with a number of neuropsychiatric side effects including dizziness, agitation, hallucinations, amnesia, insomnia, nightmares and deterioration in existing psychiatric illness. Of interest to the psychiatrist, it has also been shown to produce false-positive results in testing for cannabinoids.

The protease inhibitors inhibit HIV-1 protease, an enzyme responsible for cleavage of the virus into smaller functional units. Indinavir crosses the blood–brain barrier.

Several new classes of antiretroviral have been, or are in the process of being, developed. Of these, the fusion inhibitor enfuvirtide acts by altering the conformation of the helical protein that allows virus–host cell fusion. Integrase inhibitors, CCR5 receptor antagonists and maturation inhibitors are all under development.

It remains unclear whether using antiretrovirals with CNS penetration is necessary to effect improvements in neuropsychiatric symptoms. Letendre *et al.* (2004) found a correlation between the suppression of CSF viral load and the number of blood–brain barrier-penetrating antiretrovirals in the combination used. This correlation was not substantiated in another study (Antinori *et al.* 2004). Robertson *et al.* (2004) identified that a change of HAART regimen alone had an impact on neurological symptoms, regardless of whether CNS-penetrating drugs were included in the combination.

Syphilis of the CNS

Syphilitic infections of the nervous system have decreased tremendously during the last century and particularly since the introduction of penicillin. Despite the mandatory surveillance of sexually transmitted diseases in many countries, very little detailed information is available regarding the epidemiology of neurosyphilis. In the UK between 1936 and 1939 there were 1629 deaths registered as due to general paresis or tabes, but by 1966–1969 these had fallen to 224 (Wilkinson 1972).

Primary (infectious) syphilis had already shown a gradual decline from the time of the First World War onwards. A new peak arose during the Second World War but this subsided rapidly in the years that followed. However, it was feared that late manifestations would ultimately rise again, due to unwitting partial treatment in the early stages when penicillin was given for other conditions, but this did not occur.

What does seem to have happened is that partial but incomplete suppression of infection led to neurosyphilis appearing later in atypical and attenuated forms, with consequent difficulty in diagnosis in many instances. There has also been a pronounced shift away from parenchymatous neurosyphilis (general paresis and tabes dorsalis) towards meningovascular syphilis, which now accounts for most of the new cases encountered (Nieman 1991). Cases of infectious syphilis declined during the 1980s in association with the behavioural changes associated with the HIV pandemic. By the early 1990s case numbers had stabilised and although both low incidence and prevalence were evident, syphilis had not been altogether eliminated. In 1997, there were reports of an outbreak of syphilis among heterosexuals in Bristol and a subsequent increase in incidence (Simms *et al.* 2005). This coincided with similar outbreaks in Europe, North America and Australia. In the UK, London and the north-west of England had the highest incidence, from data reported up to the end of 2005 (Health Protection Agency 2006). In England and Wales, the highest number of cases are reported in men who have sex with men, where white ethnicity and HIV coinfection are the most common associations (see Neurosyphilis and HIV coinfection, later).

Paradoxically, the success of treatment brings its own particular risks, since as the disease becomes increasingly rare it runs the hazard of being more often overlooked. The psychiatrist must continue to bear it in mind, to check regularly with serological tests and look carefully for cardinal signs in the pupillary reactions and tendon reflexes. The 'classic presentation' of general paresis is nowadays rare, and syphilis of the CNS can present with virtually any form of psychiatric complaint.

Traditionally, the effects of syphilis are divided into four stages: the primary stage with the appearance of an ulcer or chancre at the site of inoculation; the secondary stage with early generalised lesions, chiefly manifest as a variety of skin and mucous membrane lesions that appear within 4–10 weeks; the tertiary stage with the appearance of late destructive lesions such as gummata, gummatous ulcers, glossitis and bone changes; and the quaternary stage of parenchymatous changes in the CNS leading to tabes dorsalis and general paresis. These divisions are empirical, and with the exception of the last not easily applied to the spectrum of changes that occur in the CNS. Whether the existing nomenclature for classifying cases of neurosyphilis is adequate has been questioned by Timmermans and Carr (2004) in their discussion of a recently reported case series. They propose a clinically based, syndromic classification whereby cases would be identified by their associated clinical presentations, i.e. 'neurosyphilis with seizures . . . with stroke . . . with cranial nerve involvement'. For practical purposes the clinical presentations of neurosyphilis can also be divided into early and late (Marra *et al.* 2000). Early neurosyphilis refers to CNS involvement during the early manifestations of the disease and largely reflects involvement of meningeal and vascular structures. Meningovascular syphilis can appear in the secondary or tertiary stages, and even with primary infections the nervous system is sometimes involved without overt signs of disorder. In more recent cohorts neuropsychiatric presentations have been identified as the most frequently reported cluster, with 50% of cases presenting symptoms such as psychosis, delirium or dementia (Timmermans & Carr 2004). The effects of syphilis on the spinal cord (myelitis, cervical pachymeningitis and syphilitic amyotrophy) are the province of neurology and are not dealt with here.

After infection, around 25% of cases result in treponemal invasion of the CSF. The majority of patients, including those coinfected with HIV, show spontaneous resolution of CNS involvement, even in the absence of treatment (Marra *et al.* 1996).

Early asymptomatic neurosyphilis

This term is used for cases with abnormalities in the CSF but no symptoms or signs of CNS disorder. The cells or protein may be raised, the pressure increased or CSF immunological tests may give a positive result. Such findings emerge in approximately 10% of cases of primary syphilis and 30% of cases of secondary syphilis when the CSF is examined routinely (Hahn & Clark 1946a). Such CSF findings are more complicated to interpret in the presence of HIV coinfection (Zetola & Klausner 2007).

Thus it appears that a meningeal reaction can set in very early in a surprising number of cases and without producing overt disorder. When adequate treatment is given the disturbance dies out within a year or two and proves to have been benign. In some cases the prognosis is favourable even when treatment has been inadequate (Hahn & Clark 1946b), though in others the changes probably have implications for the later development of quaternary neurosyphilis.

Acute syphilitic meningitis

In rare cases infection of the nervous system may be overwhelming, with the production of an acute meningitis. This usually develops within the first 2 years, and can even accompany the secondary rash within a month or two of the primary infection. The illness is indistinguishable from other forms of acute meningitis until specific tests are performed.

There is a pyrexia of approximately 39°C (102°F), with headache, delirium, neck stiffness and somnolence. Lumbar puncture reveals fluid under pressure, containing upwards of 1000 cells/mm^3, of which a considerable proportion may be polymorphs. Specific tests for syphilis may be negative in the CSF but are invariably positive in the blood. With prompt treatment there is usually good recovery, although some permanent intellectual impairment may result.

Subacute and chronic meningovascular syphilis

A variety of clinical pictures are subsumed under this heading and are most easily understood in terms of the underlying pathology. The disorders, which represent 10–35% of cases of neurosyphilis, usually declare themselves 4–10 years after the primary infection. Although peak occurrence is at 7 years, the range may extend from the first few months to 30 years or more (Lukehart *et al.* 1988).

Pathology

Changes affect the meninges, cerebral vasculature and spinal cord resulting in transient or permanent ischaemic events (Tramont 2005). In the meninges there is a diffuse inflammatory process with thickening, areas of necrosis and the formation of exudate, which may become gelatinous and adherent (gummatous leptomeningitis). Changes are often most in evidence at the base of the brain, resulting in cranial nerve lesions or hydrocephalus due to obstruction of flow of CSF. Less commonly they are localised over the convexity, or extend to envelop the whole of a hemisphere in a thickened sheath. Similar changes may extend along the perivascular channels, with the formation of localised gummata within the brain or in relation to the overlying bones of the skull.

Vascular pathology forms an integral part of the reaction in the meninges but can also involve the cerebral vessels directly. The vessels at the base of the brain are chiefly affected, first the small and then the larger branches of the circle of Willis. There is both a periarteritis and an endarteritis, the latter producing great hypertrophy of the intimal layer and leading to thrombosis. Around affected vessels there is fibroblastic proliferation and necrosis, again sometimes proceeding to scattered gummata. The large isolated gumma leading to tumour-like symptoms is extremely rare.

Clinical features

Subacute forms of meningitis may progress rapidly once they are declared, though chronic forms are often insidious and intermittent, with periods of several months between exacerbations of disease; hence the delay which may be encountered in diagnosis.

Prodromal symptoms consist of intermittent headache, lethargy and malaise. The patient is usually slow and forgetful, with difficulty in attention and concentration and impaired judgement. Emotional instability and irritability are common together with changes in personality. Mental deterioration may progress to definite evidence of dementia, sometimes with fleeting delusions or episodes of excited overactivity. Alternatively, there may be periods of clouding of consciousness or florid delirium separated by intervals of relative normality. The vague quality of the complaints, and the fleeting nature of the early disabilities, can lead to the organic nature of the disturbance being overlooked for some considerable time.

The focal evidence of basal meningitis consists chiefly of cranial nerve disturbances. The facial and auditory nerves are frequently affected and sensorineural deafness occurs in up to 20% (Singh & Romanowski 1999). Optic neuritis and iritis can present as features (Margo & Hamed 1992). Paresis of external ocular movements and abnormalities of pupil size and reaction are common, but the fully developed Argyll Robertson pupil is rarely seen. Papilloedema, optic atrophy and visual field defects from chiasmatic lesions also occur. Hypothalamic involvement may produce polyuria, obesity and somnolence. Convexity meningitis can result in focal fits, aphasia or hemiparesis. Headache is often sharply localised and the overlying skull may be tender.

When vascular pathology is predominant, minor arterial occlusions lead to episodes of transient neurological disorder: hemiparesis, hemianopia, aphasia or amnesia. Asdaghi *et al.* (2007) report two cases, both lacking a history of symptoms of systemic syphilis, of meningovascular syphilis presenting with headache and multiple cerebrovascular attacks. Occlusion of major vessels, predominantly the middle cerebral artery but also the basilar circulation, can result in a completed stroke (Flint *et al.* 2005). The picture of pseudobulbar palsy may also develop, with bilateral spasticity and emotional lability. Unusual presentations include isolated ocular palsy and trigeminal neuralgia as well as meningitic symptoms (Nieman 1991). Meningovascular syphilis may also mimic encephalitis and even multiple sclerosis. It should be considered in any acute encephalopathy, and in any acute stroke in younger patients, regardless of whether there is a clear history of systemic syphilis.

The CSF shows a moderate cellular reaction with up to 200 cells/mm^3, mostly mononuclear leucocytes, and a moderate increase in protein. The pressure is usually normal. Serological tests are usually positive in the blood but may be negative in the CSF.

With adequate treatment the prognosis is generally good provided extensive cerebral infarction has not occurred. Serial transcranial Doppler studies have identified improved vascular flow after antibiotic treatment (Flint *et al.* 2005), with one case showing little resolution of stenotic vascular change at 4 months (Kelley *et al.* 2003). Sometimes the patient is left with fits, hydrocephalus or permanent intellectual impairment.

Tabes dorsalis

Tabes dorsalis is seen in conjunction with approximately 20% of cases of general paresis. Its highly characteristic signs and symptoms may therefore alert the psychiatrist to the latter disease. It is now an extremely rare presentation in the post-antibiotic era (Kinghorn 2000), with reported evidence of a clear decline from pre-antibiotic cohorts (Wolters 1987).

Onset is usually 8–12 years after primary infection, although a range of 3–25 years is seen (Singh & Romanowski 1999). Males are affected much more frequently than females, with a peak age of onset in the fifth decade (Orban 1957). The essential pathology consists of degeneration of the ascending fibres from the dorsal root ganglia, resulting in atrophy of the dorsal roots and shrinkage and demyelination in the posterior columns of the cord together with dystrophic changes of optic nerve fibres and decreased neuronal numbers in brain, spinal cord and spinal ganglia.

Characteristic symptoms include pain, paraesthesiae and a marked disturbance of gait. These usually develop insidiously. The lightning pains of tabes are extraordinarily severe, can occur in 75–90% of patients and are typically brief and stabbing in nature and sharply localised in the legs. Burning and tearing pains may also occur, or girdle pains around the trunk. Paraesthesiae are also most common in the legs and feet; the skin may be hyperaesthetic to touch or the patient may feel he is walking on cotton wool. The ataxia is sensory in origin and due to loss of proprioceptive sensibility. The patient walks with a wide base or a typical 'high stepping' gait, and finds more difficulty in the dark when visual control is reduced. Romberg's test is positive from an early stage.

Tabetic crises consist of episodic pain in the viscera. The gastric crisis is most common, with attacks of epigastric pain and vomiting. Laryngeal crises consist of dyspnoea, cough and stridor, rectal crises of tenesmus, and vesical crises of pain in the bladder and penis. Other manifestations are impotence and sphincter disturbances.

On examination, sensory changes are found earliest in the legs. Loss of postural sense and vibration sense are marked, and compression of the Achilles tendon may fail to produce pain. Other characteristic sites of sensory loss, involving both touch and pain, are the side of the nose, the ulnar aspect of the arms, patchy loss over the trunk and the dorsum of the feet. The musculature is hypotonic and the tendon reflexes diminished or absent, particularly at the ankles. The pupils are abnormal in 90% of cases, although the full spectrum of Argyll Robertson pupil (see General paresis/Abnormalities on examination, later) tends to be a late development. Ptosis and optic atrophy are frequently seen (Simon 1985). Painless disorganisation of joints may result in gross deformity (Charcot's joints), most frequently at the knee or the hip. Perforating ulcers and other trophic skin changes may appear.

The CSF is usually under increased pressure, with a moderate number of mononuclear cells and a slightly raised protein. The Venereal Disease Research Laboratory (VDRL) test may be negative in both the blood and CSF in 20% of cases, and the fluorescent treponemal antibody absorption (FTA-ABS) test may be negative in the CSF despite an excess of cells and protein (Wiles 1993a).

Without treatment the disease is slowly progressive. General paresis may appear after a lapse of many years; even if it does not, long-standing cases may develop psychotic illnesses of a paranoid or depressive nature (Wilson 1940).

General paresis (dementia paralytica, general paralysis of the insane)

Hare (1959) has traced the fascinating history of this disease. It was first clearly described in the early nineteenth century by physicians working in the mental hospitals of Paris. It appears to have assumed epidemic proportions in France soon after the Napoleonic wars, and thereafter the spread by venereal infection can be traced along the trade routes of Europe and to the New World. Hare adduces detailed evidence to suggest that general paresis may have arisen as a new disease by mutation of the syphilitic spirochaete.

The disease occupies a unique place in several respects in the history of psychiatry. The final proof of its aetiology was an important landmark, likewise the discovery of its response to treatment. A relationship between syphilis and insanity had long been recognised, but there was much controversy before a syphilitic aetiology became accepted for general paresis. Hereditary taint, alcohol consumption, mental strain and even sexual excess were all championed as causes by various authorities despite the increasing epidemiological evidence that syphilis was responsible. The development of the Wassermann test in 1906 did not end the disputes, which persisted until Noguchi and Moore (1913) finally demonstrated *Treponema pallidum* in the brain itself. Thus a clear aetiology was eventually established for a mental disorder that was then extremely common.

Pathology

General paresis is the only syphilitic disease in which spirochaetes can be demonstrated in the tissues of the brain, and the pathology is thought to be the direct result of their action there. Macroscopically, the dura mater is thickened and opaque, and chronic subdural haemorrhage may contribute to the formation of a thick membrane over the brain (pachymeningitis haemorrhagica). The pia mater is firmly adherent to the underlying cortex. The brain itself is small and atrophied, with widening of the cerebral sulci and dilatation of the ventricles.

Microscopically, there are inflammatory lesions throughout the cortex, consisting of dense perivascular collections of lymphocytes and plasma cells and attributable to the irritation produced by the spirochaetes. Equally prominent are degenerative changes, with cortical thinning and outfall of neurones, especially in the frontal and parietal regions. Neuroglial proliferation is marked, forming a dense feltwork below the meninges and beneath the ventricular walls, the latter giving a 'frosted' granular appearance to the naked eye. Enlarged microglial cells (rod cells) are characteristically arranged in rows, and stain with Prussian blue to show iron-containing pigments in their cytoplasm. This reaction is held to be pathognomonic for general paresis.

The spinal cord may show secondary degeneration of the pyramidal tracts, or a combination of paretic and tabetic pathology with degeneration of the posterior columns.

Clinical features

In essence general paresis is a dementing process of insidious onset, but often coloured at first by other features that tend to obscure the intellectual impairment. Changes in affect or personality are frequently the presenting abnormalities as with Pick's disease (see Chapter 9); alternatively the dementing process may be concealed until some unexplained lapse of conduct brings the true situation abruptly to light. Thereafter the progress of the disorder is marked by certain characteristic features and by neurological disabilities that give the disease its name.

It is usual to describe several forms of general paresis according to salient aspects of the mental state. This remains useful in serving to underline the varied manifestations of the disease, although as indicated below the frequency of the different varieties has changed considerably, the disorder is rare and many atypical forms are now seen.

The disease affects males much more commonly than females, with a peak age of onset between 30 and 50 though the latitude is wide. Congenital general paresis can be declared in early childhood and cases are also seen in extreme old age. The time from infection is difficult to determine, but is usually quoted as being 5–25 years, with an average of 10–15 years.

Presenting features

In retrospect it is often discovered that the patient has experienced minor ill-defined symptoms such as headache, insomnia and lethargy for several months before more definite manifestations appear. Relatives commonly report an insidious change of temperament – moodiness, apathy or decreased emotional control. Other common early changes may suggest frontal lobe involvement by way of coarsening of behaviour and loss of refinement in the personality.

Episodic forgetfulness is usually the first cognitive change, followed by defective concentration, reduction of interests and mental and physical slowing in the manner typical of a dementing process. Difficulty with calculation is stressed as an early feature, also disturbances of speech and writing. Insight is impaired from an early stage.

In approximately 50% of patients the presentation is abrupt, with some striking incident that first brings the patient to medical attention (Dewhurst 1969). Sometimes it is a lapse of social conduct that reveals the true state of affairs: law-breaking, an outburst of violence or an episode of indecent exposure (Roberts & Emsley 1992). Foolish, eccentric or reckless behaviour may be the opening sign, as seen in the following examples from Wilson (1940).

> In one case the first whim was the purchase of a quantity of old silver for which payment could not be made; another patient rose in his stall at the theatre and threw sovereigns at a comedienne on the stage; a third ordered 700 hymn books for a hospital ward of 16 beds, and a ton of guano for the ward plants. Another wrote to the War Office demanding three Victoria Crosses which he considered he had won in fighting some 10 years before. At the outbreak of hostilities in August 1914, an incipient paralytic sent telegrams to all the crowned heads and rulers, proffering his services as peacemaker.

Alternatively, some organic feature may be abruptly declared, such as an episode of amnesia, a single epileptic fit or status epilepticus (Ances *et al.* 2004), or an acute delirious episode. In Dewhurst's (1969) series, 5 of 91 cases presented with attempted suicide.

Grandiose or expansive form

This was by far the most frequent type of general paresis when the condition was first described, and it has tended to remain the prototype of the disorder in medical teaching. However, there is evidence that it had already become less common in Europe during the latter half of the nineteenth century and perhaps somewhat later in England (Hare 1959). Nowadays it is comparatively rare. In large series of cases from England, America and Norway it has represented only 10%, 18% and 7% of cases, respectively (Fröshaug & Ytrehus 1956; Hahn *et al.* 1959; Dewhurst 1969). How far the change over time has depended on alterations in the host, the infecting organism or cultural factors is unknown. In some countries the proportion apparently continued to be high, for example in India (Varma 1952) and China (Liu 1960), when it had already become rare elsewhere.

Florid examples are certainly impressive and share symptoms of mania (Hoffman 1982), which may lead to their being highlighted in reports of the disease. The hallmark is the patient's bombastic and expansive demeanour, with delusions of power, wealth or social position. The patient boasts of fantastic riches, exploits in battle, or tells of his athletic and sexual prowess. He may believe he is some eminent person from the past or present, yet at the same time accepts his stay in hospital without complaint.

The mood is euphoric and frequently condescending. The patient's recital may be amusing but his jocularity is rarely infectious, the underlying dementia imparting a shallowness to the prevailing affect. If his beliefs are questioned, the mood may readily turn to petulance or anger.

With arrest of the disease the clinical picture can remain remarkably static over many years. Formerly the delusions tended to die out with progression of the disease, and expansiveness gave way to apathy, lethargy and indifference.

Simple dementing form

This appears over time to have gradually replaced the grandiose form and is now a great deal more common. It represented 20% in Dewhurst's (1969) series, 60% in Hahn et al.'s (1959) series and 48% in Fröshaug and Ytrehus' (1956) series. The usual symptoms of generalised dementia are in evidence, with impairment of memory, slowed and laboured thinking and early loss of insight. Progress may be punctuated by transient episodes of impairment of consciousness during which behaviour becomes even more confused. The affect is shallow; a mild euphoria is common, although many patients are dull and apathetic from the start. As with other dementing illnesses the patient may develop fleeting and ill-systematised delusions, mostly of a persecutory nature. Generally, however, such patients are quiet, lethargic and amenable throughout the course of the disease.

Depressive form

This important variety appears also to have increased considerably at the expense of the grandiose form. It emerged as the commonest variety (27%) in Dewhurst's (1969) series. The patient presents with classic symptoms of a depressive illness. If dementia is already advanced, it may be noted that the affect is somewhat shallow and that the patient is more readily lifted from his gloom than in primary affective disorders. Sometimes, however, no such distinction can be made. Delusions are of a typically melancholic kind; nihilistic and hypochondriacal delusions may be grotesque in degree, though again the mood may be noted to be disproportionately shallow.

Taboparetic form

In perhaps 20% of patients the picture of general paresis and tabes dorsalis are combined. Along with dementia the classic tabetic symptoms and signs (see Tabes dorsalis in this chapter) are observed. The mental symptoms are then often rather mild. True Argyll Robertson pupils and optic atrophy are seen more commonly in this variety than with general paresis alone.

Other forms

Other forms of the disorder are much less common. There may occasionally be a picture of true manic elation accompanied by flight of ideas, or a presentation with schizophrenic features that mask the true diagnosis. Paranoid delusions are then common, together with ideas of influence, passivity phenomena and auditory hallucinations of an abusing or threatening nature ('paranoid' or 'paraphrenic' form). In the 'neurasthenic' form the outstanding features are weakness, fatigue, irritability and complaints of general ill health. Presentation with an acute organic reaction represents an active and rapidly progressive form of the disease. Very occasionally this follows a fulminating course with fever, fits and a picture simulating encephalitis. Cases have been reported which for some time preserve the appearance of Korsakoff's psychosis (Wilson 1940). An epileptic or apoplectic presentation occurred in 15% of Fröshaug and Ytrehus' (1956) series and in 8.7% of Timmermans and Carrs' (2004) series. In Lissauer's type, the patient presents with hemiparesis, aphasia or other evidence of focal brain disease as a result of massive localised brain destruction. The common presentation nowadays, with a markedly attenuated picture.

Juvenile general paresis

This has always been extremely rare and is now hardly ever seen. Infection is transmitted via the placenta and the disease is declared in childhood or adolescence. The usual age of onset is between 6 and 21 years. Onset in childhood leads to learning difficulties at school and results in symptoms of mental impairment. Epileptic fits are common. Onset in adolescence leads usually to the simple dementing type of general paresis. The same neurological and CSF abnormalities are seen as in the adult form of the disease.

Abnormalities on examination

The patient frequently shows evidence of poor physical health. In the mental state there will usually be evidence of some degree of dementia if full attention is paid to the assessment of recent memory and other cognitive functions. However, this may require considerable persistence in the face of facile excuses and evasive behaviour. Confirmatory signs may be found on neurological examination even in the absence of definite organic features in the mental state. Pupillary abnormalities, tremor and dysarthria head the list of abnormal findings.

The pupils show abnormalities in about two-thirds of cases. A variety of changes is seen: inequality, irregularity and sluggishness of reactions. The full syndrome of Argyll Robertson pupil may be present but not so commonly: a small pupil, irregular in outline and with atrophy of the iris, which reacts normally to convergence but not at all to light, and does not dilate fully under the influence of a mydriatic. Optic atrophy may be in evidence even when the patient has no complaint of visual impairment.

Tremor also occurs in about two-thirds of patients when first seen. It typically involves the face and hands particularly. Close attention may be required to detect it in the lips and around the mouth. Tremor of the hands and fingers contributes to the clumsiness seen on manual tasks.

Dysarthria is partly due to the tremor of the lips and tongue. Speech becomes slurred, hesitant and jerky, and the voice feeble and lacking in intonation. Dysphasic difficulties may also be found.

Reflex abnormalities consist of exaggeration of the knee and ankle jerks, with clonus and spasticity in the lower limbs. With progression of the disease the plantar responses become extensor, and there is increasing weakness of the limbs leading eventually to severe spastic paralysis. In contrast, tendon reflexes may be absent when tabes dorsalis is combined with general paresis.

Incoordination is seen in the clumsiness of the hands and the characteristic slouching, unsteady gait. In taboparesis it becomes a marked feature, with Rombergism and the classic high-stepping gait.

Further progress

In the absence of treatment the dementia increases steadily along with marked physical deterioration. Periods of arrest or even complete remission were occasionally seen, but usually only for a few weeks or months at a time. Incontinence of urine appears early. Delusions gradually fade away with the other more florid mental features, and the patient becomes quiet, incoherent and apathetic. The characteristic picture in the later stages was of a childish gentle personality, seldom aggressive and with much of the dementia concealed beneath good-tempered polite behaviour (Storm-Mathisen 1969). Spastic paralysis and ataxia increased until the patient was enfeebled and confined to bed. Epileptic attacks, both grand mal and psychomotor, occurred in approximately half of the cases, and the progression of neurological disabilities was often speeded by the appearance of 'congestive attacks'. These consist of sudden episodes of loss of consciousness, hemiplegia, monoplegia, aphasia or hemianopia, lasting a few days or weeks at a time but eventually leaving enduring deficits in their wake. The mechanism responsible remains uncertain but a vascular basis is probable. Death usually occurred within 4–5 years of presentation. This uniformly disastrous prognosis has, of course, been dramatically altered by present methods of treatment as described below.

Atypical present-day forms of neurosyphilis

In addition to the risk of overlooking the disease on account of its rarity, we nowadays face the additional problem that neurosyphilis can occur in atypical or attenuated forms in the post-antibiotic era, as well as comorbidly with HIV. Thus while fully developed examples of general paresis and tabes dorsalis have become less often reported, modified forms of neurosyphilis with atypical presentations and relatively minor symptomatology are increasingly encountered (Anon.

1978). In Hooshmand *et al.*'s (1972) series of 241 patients in the USA, almost half presented with unrelated symptoms, the diagnosis being made by routine investigation after suspicion had been aroused by neurological or ocular findings. In one-quarter the presentation was with focal or generalised seizures (see also Luxon *et al.* 1979). Wolters (1987) compared cases from the pre- and post-antibiotic era and did not identify any significant between-group difference, other than a decline in diagnoses of tabes dorsalis. This finding was corroborated in a 1990–1999 cohort of 161 South African patients where the clinical presentations were identical to those seen prior to antibiotics (Timmermans & Carr 2004). However, the authors noted that the cohort population had poor access to health care and had likely been less exposed to equivalent quantities of antibiotics than their counterparts in Western societies (Timmermans & Carr 2004). Similar conclusions have been reached in other studies (Conde-Sendin *et al.* 2004; Delli *et al.* 2007).

In atypical cases little may appear to be pathognomonic, either in the clinical picture or on CSF examination. Hooshmand *et al.*'s (1972) criteria for the diagnosis of neurosyphilis are therefore important. They recommend a firm diagnosis when (i) the blood FTA-ABS test (see below) is positive and there are ocular or neurological findings suggestive of neurosyphilis; (ii) the FTA-ABS test is positive in both blood and CSF and the latter contains over 5 leucocytes/mm^3 in the absence of bacterial or viral meningitis; or (iii) when blood and CSF FTA-ABS tests are positive in the presence of progressive neurological symptoms not otherwise explained. In the last category there must also be either a transient leucocytosis in the CSF after administering penicillin, or the patient must improve clinically on penicillin. A positive FTA-ABS test in the blood and CSF as the sole abnormal finding may not necessarily imply active neurosyphilis, since this can have persisted as a serological finding after adequate antibiotic treatment. Subsequently, case definition criteria have also been established for the diagnosis of neurosyphilis by the CDC in 1996 (Box 7.4).

Neurosyphilis and HIV coinfection

The risk factors for acquiring syphilis are similar to those for the transmission of HIV (Zellan & Augenbraun 2004). After an initial decline in the incidence of syphilis, associated with the beginning of the HIV pandemic in the 1980s and contingent changes in sexual practice, there has been an increasing number of reported coinfections that, alarmingly, may be associated with increasingly unsafe behaviours (Buchacz *et al.* 2005). Another important factor affecting the prevalence of coinfection is the increased life expectancy associated with HAART (Fenton & Imrie 2005). The transmission of both HIV and syphilis is reciprocally potentiated, particularly through genital ulceration (Douglas *et al.* 2005) and the effects on HIV viral load and CD4 counts by syphilis (see Buchacz *et al.* 2004).

The hypothesis that atypical and attenuated presentations of neurosyphilis in immunocompetent individuals are likely associated with incomplete or ineffective antibiotic therapy has already been suggested. Similarly, changes in the presentation and natural history of neurosyphilis, despite usually adequate treatment, are associated with comorbid disorders that affect the patient's immune response, particularly HIV.

More recent epidemics of infectious syphilis have particularly involved the population of men who have sex with men (see Acquired immunodeficiency syndrome, later). Not surprisingly, presentations of neurosyphilis have similarly been increasingly reported in this group and particularly in those who are HIV seropositive (Musher 1991) some of whom have a rapid progression to neurosyphilis, with or without treatment (Johns *et al.* 1987). The CDC conducted a review of such cases across four cities in the USA in order to describe the clinical course of early symptomatic neurosyphilis in men who have sex with men, particularly HIV-positive individuals (Centers for Disease Control 2007). This found that the estimated risk of having symptomatic early neurosyphilis in this group was 1.7%, with 0.5% having persistent symptoms 6 months after treatment. Of the cases, 75% had presented with visual disturbance or new-onset headache, 12% with acute meningitis and 50% with no other signs or symptoms of syphilis whatsoever. Of concern, 25% had been undiagnosed with HIV.

Investigations

The UK Public Health Laboratory has produced guidelines that identify the most appropriate investigations for syphilis

(Egglestone & Turner 2000). They indicate that serological tests for syphilis can be divided into two groups.
1 Non-treponemal tests: the VDRL test and rapid plasma reagin (RPR) test detect non-specific treponemal antigens utilising a modified Wassermann reaction.
2 Treponemal tests: *Treponema pallidum* haemagglutination assay (TPHA), FTA-ABS and most enzyme immunoassay (EIAs).

Investigations such as the Wassermann reaction and other non-treponemal tests such as the VDRL are positive in the blood in 90% or more of untreated cases of general paresis, but this figure may be considerably lower if antibiotics have been given for some other infection or if a previous course of treatment has been carried out. They may also be negative in patients with HIV. False positives may be obtained in certain diseases, notably leprosy, systemic lupus erythematosus, thyroiditis, haemolytic anaemia and some cases of rheumatoid arthritis. The tests may also be positive for a while after some viral infections, after vaccination, during pregnancy and in an appreciable proportion of drug addicts. The cardiolipin Wassermann reaction uses a purer antigen and gives fewer false positives in these situations. The Reiter protein complement fixation (RPCF) test operates on spirochaetal material from non-pathogenic treponemes, and is therefore negative in the above diseases but may be positive in other spirochaetal infections such as yaws.

Positive results from the Wassermann reaction or VDRL, along with a positive RPCF test, means that the possibility of syphilitic infection is high. More certainty will be given in marginal cases by treponemal tests such as *Treponema* immobilisation (TPI), TPHA or FTA-ABS. The TPI test is reasonably specific to *T. pallidum* but is technically difficult to perform and not recommended in the guidelines. The TPHA test uses an indirect haemagglutination technique, yielding a high degree of specificity and lending itself to automated methods. Development of the FTA test marked an important advance, particularly in the form of an absorption test (FTA-ABS). This is generally very reliable, although false positives occasionally occur with sera containing antinuclear/rheumatoid factor or possibly because of passive diffusion of treponemal antibodies from the blood into CSF. True positive results are obtained with yaws. Negative results are occasionally seen in patients who are HIV positive. The FTA-ABS test is fortunately almost invariably positive, in both the CSF and the blood, in the modified forms of neurosyphilis encountered in present-day practice (Oates 1979). For many years the combination of VDRL and TPHA was favoured in UK laboratories. However, difficulties with automating these investigations has resulted in increasing use of EIAs that detect treponemal IgG or IgG and IgM. Treponemal IgM remains detectable in treated late disease for up to 18 months, but is usually undetectable after 3–9 months in early treated cases. Confirmatory testing with TPHA is recommended after a reactive EIA.

The possibility of negative results with certain serological tests in the blood means that the CSF must be examined in every case when the presence of neurosyphilis is even remotely suspected. Such tests are positive in the CSF in almost every untreated case of general paresis, although the VDRL may be negative in a considerable proportion (Davis & Schmitt 1989; Lee & Chen 2005). CSF FTA-ABS is a highly sensitive but poorly specific treponemal test. At lumbar puncture the pressure is often raised, there is a moderate lymphocytosis of 5–50 cells/mm^3, and the protein is also usually elevated (50–100 mg/dL). The globulin ratio is greatly increased and oligoclonal bands may be present. There is generally little correlation between the initial CSF cell or protein level and the severity of the clinical picture. A CSF without raised cells or protein may be seen if there has been previous treatment. A recent study reported that those with increased CSF tau protein were statistically more likely to have CNS involvement and therefore the measurement of CSF tau protein might be used in discriminating between syphilis with and without CNS involvement (Paraskevas *et al.* 2007).

In the great majority of patients with general paresis EEG is abnormal, with an excess of theta and slower wave activity.

Differential diagnosis

The forms of neurosyphilis are so variable in presentation that serological tests should be considered in all patients admitted to psychiatric units. In the outpatient clinic there must be a readiness to perform such tests when the index of suspicion is high. Roberts and Emsley (1992) reported 21 patients admitted to acute psychiatric units with neurosyphilis, in only three of whom the diagnosis had been considered before the results of routine serology were known. The initial diagnoses had encompassed schizophrenia, depression, mania and hysteria, in addition to delirium and dementia. Cleare *et al.* (1993) found a continuing low prevalence of positive serology (at almost 4%) among psychogeriatric inpatients, this not infrequently reflecting active disease. Other examples where mistakes were averted are reported by Sirota *et al.* (1989) and Sivakumar and Okocha (1992). At the very minimum the pupil reactions and tendon reflexes should be examined at every new consultation. However, clinical examination without serology is not always enough to avoid errors in diagnosis; this was illustrated by Steel (1960) in patients in a psychiatric observation ward and by Joffe *et al.* (1968) in patients seen in a neurological clinic. The present-day frequency of attenuated forms and atypical presentations, as well as the prevalence of comorbidity with HIV and the detrimental effects of this, make the application of routine serology very much more important.

Boyle *et al.* (1995) report the history of a 62-year-old man who presented with expressive dysphasia, anxiety and agitation in the context of his wife's hospitalisation with probable prion disease. There were no abnormalities on examination and initial investigations other than serum glucose were normal, including chest radiography and ECG. An initial diagnosis of dissociative disorder was made and the opinion of a psychiatrist sought. Cognitive testing later in his admission identified significant impairment, with a Mini-Mental State Examination (MMSE) score of 18/30. CT identified advanced cerebral atrophy. EEG revealed excessive temporal and anterior slow waves. Features of the mental state at this stage included confabulation, perseveration, social disinhibition and grandiosity. VDRL, TPHA and FTA tests were positive. CSF was VDRL and FTA positive. A diagnosis of neurosyphilis was made.

A history of change of personality, impaired emotional control and intellectual decline will immediately suggest general paresis, and the presence of tremor, dysarthria or pupillary or reflex abnormalities will almost suffice to confirm the diagnosis. However, such well-established cases are nowadays rare at the time of initial presentation. In Dewhurst's (1969) series only 24 of 91 cases were diagnosed as having neurosyphilis from the outset. The most common initial diagnoses were depressive illness, dementia, confusional states, schizophrenia, hypomania and epilepsy.

General paresis must obviously be considered in all patients who present with organic impairment of intellect, and no patient should be diagnosed as suffering from a primary dementia until syphilis has been excluded. Among older arteriopathic patients mistakes are particularly likely to be made, since tremor and dysarthria are then not entirely unexpected. However, pupillary abnormalities are rarely seen in cerebral arteriosclerosis or other dementing illnesses.

Affective psychoses appear to have been closely simulated in many of Dewhurst's patients. On occasion the clinical picture may also be typical of schizophrenia, to the extent that the CSF findings come as a surprise (Fröshaug & Ytrehus 1956). Where routine serological testing is not possible the principal safeguard must lie in careful and systematic examination of the nervous system, and due attention to any organic mental impairments which emerge.

There is a special risk of overlooking the diagnosis in alcohol-dependent patients. Emotional instability or expansiveness may be attributed to alcoholic deterioration, likewise social lapses, facile behaviour, tremulousness and dysarthria.

General paresis may be confused with cerebral tumour when headache is marked and the personality attributes of frontal lobe damage conspicuous. An anterior basal meningioma may mimic the disease closely when compression of the optic pathways leads to pupillary changes and optic atrophy.

General paresis must also be borne in mind in the differential diagnosis of epilepsy of late onset, and in all acute organic reactions when other causes are not immediately obvious.

Finally it is necessary to distinguish between general paresis and other neurosyphilitic diseases, in particular chronic meningovascular syphilis and asymptomatic neurosyphilis. In chronic meningovascular syphilis the prognosis is much better than in general paresis. Meningovascular syphilis tends to occur earlier than general paresis, shows a more acute development, and fluctuations in its course are usually marked. Insight is generally better preserved, the personality less deteriorated and focal neurological signs somewhat more common.

Treatment

Adequate treatment of syphilis in the primary stage prevents the development of general paresis later. Similarly, energetic treatment must be pursued, essentially as for general paresis, in those cases of 'asymptomatic neurosyphilis' where lumbar puncture reveals abnormalities in the CSF before any clinical signs or symptoms of nervous system involvement have become apparent. For this reason routine lumbar puncture is often advocated in every case of primary syphilis, and yearly examination of the CSF in those who show abnormalities in the early stages. In patients who are HIV positive it is generally agreed that treatment should be as for general paresis, even for those in the primary or secondary stages (Nieman 1991). On the whole, treatment of people infected with HIV is the same as those who are HIV seronegative.

Penicillin therapy

For the treatment of established general paresis, penicillin alone is generally agreed to be adequate and can eliminate syphilitic infection in the brain in the great majority of cases. Benzylpenicillin is the preparation of choice and must be given by intramuscular injection; as procaine benzylpenicillin it can be given by daily injections. However, benzathine benzylpenicillin, given as a single injection per week, will not suffice. This regimen appears to be effective for the treatment of primary syphilis in patients who are likely to be uncooperative over daily attendance, but there is now evidence that it yields inadequate CSF levels for the treatment of neurosyphilis (Mohr et al. 1976; Tramont 1976). The minimum effective dose has not been established with certainty, but aqueous benzylpenicillin 18–24 million units i.v. daily for 10–14 days is the current preferred guideline (Greenwood 1996; Centers for Disease Control 2006b).

A Herxheimer reaction is liable to occur in 5–10% of cases within the first few days of treatment. Because of this, these days of treatment are best undertaken in hospital. The reaction may consist of malaise and fever alone or result in exacerbation of symptoms, sometimes with seizures. Oral prednisone given the day before and during the first few days of treatment helps to prevent its occurrence. When sensitivity to penicillin precludes its use it may be necessary to substitute ceftriaxone 2 g parenterally for 10–14 days (CDC 2006). Chloramphenicol and doxycycline have been shown to achieve adequate penetration of the CSF and are options, although with limited data to support them. Where patients are penicillin sensitive, consideration should be given to penicillin desensitisation procedures (Arroliga & Pien 2003). Fortunately, spirochaetal resistance to penicillin does not appear to have developed; all early syphilis continues to respond and it is unlikely that other antibiotics confer extra benefit.

Other treatment

Antipsychotic drugs are indicated for the control of excitement, agitation or florid delusions or hallucinations as in any other psychotic illness and there are case reports of the use of atypicals being effective (Taycan et al. 2006), similarly antidepressant drugs for severe depressive symptoms. Anticonvulsants are required for the symptomatic treatment of epilepsy. It must be borne in mind that a small proportion of cases may represent a coincidence between asymptomatic neurosyphilis and an independent psychotic illness, and the latter will then warrant full psychiatric management in its own right.

There is some evidence to contraindicate the use of electroconvulsive therapy in general paresis, particularly in the presence of active disease as mirrored in the CSF. Sudden worsening with focal signs of neurological defect has been reported to follow electroconvulsive therapy in such cases, and Dewhurst (1969) provides data that suggest the possibility of an impaired overall prognosis.

The complete care of the patient will include planned rehabilitation when deficits persist, in the knowledge that they may show continued slow improvement for up to 2 years following arrest of the disease. From the outset it is necessary to make every effort to test the blood serology of the patient's partner and any children.

Follow-up and retreatment

Patients should be followed up both clinically and serologically after treatment, depending on disease stage and HIV status. It has been recommended that in neurosyphilis, CSF analysis should be repeated every 6 months until the cell count is normal. Inadequate treatment has been defined as failure of the CSF to normalise within a 2-year period or cell count not having decreased within 6 months. Follow-up in those who are coinfected with HIV should be aggressive. If abnormalities in cells or protein persist, a second course should be given immediately. Failure to show clinical

Intracranial Infections | **431**

improvement does not automatically warrant retreatment if the CSF has shown an entirely satisfactory response. In this situation the essential step is re-evaluation of the diagnosis, since syphilitic infection may have been coincidental with other disease.

The first sign of relapse is seen in the CSF cell count; if this rises above 5 cells/mm³ at any follow-up examination, retreatment is strongly indicated. A persistently elevated protein is not of the same significance, and can usually be disregarded if cell counts remain low and there is no clinical evidence of progression. Serological tests may remain positive in the blood and the CSF for several years after resolution of all active infection. However, rising titres in the blood serology should cause concern and may point to continuing activity or reinfection. This will always indicate the need for re-examination of the CSF at any point during the follow-up period.

Clinical evidence of progression of the disease will always raise the possibility of the need for retreatment, especially when the initial response was good. However, routine retreatment confers no additional benefit.

Outcome of treatment

The outcome that can be expected was comprehensively described by Hahn *et al.* (1959) from a multicentre follow-up study of 1086 patients in the USA. Their general conclusion is of great importance, namely that success depends essentially on early diagnosis and prompt administration of a fully adequate course of treatment.

Of mild or early cases, 80% obtained clinical remission and proved capable of resuming work. In this group there were hardly any deaths from paresis. The prognosis for ability to work and to live in the community was directly proportional to the severity of the illness and the duration of decreased work capacity at the time of treatment. However, even severely affected institutionalised patients were still capable of considerable benefit, and stood a one in three chance of improving sufficiently for rehabilitation and ultimate return to work. Certain symptoms were associated with a poor overall prognosis, including incontinence, inability to dress and neglect of personal hygiene. In patients over 60 years old, remission or improvement became much less frequent, probably because of the presence of cerebrovascular changes.

Interesting correlations were found in relation to the CSF abnormalities at the time of treatment. The more active the fluid in terms of cell count, the greater the chance of a good clinical response; at the same time, however, the likelihood of clinical progression was then also increased in certain cases. This apparent paradox is explained by the fact that pleocytosis in the CSF reflects an active and labile process, whereas an inactive fluid indicates a relatively static pathology. The latter is less susceptible to treatment but also less likely to result in clinical progression.

The quality of recovery extended to a wide range of organic mental symptoms and florid psychotic phenomena. At 5-year follow-up, the following symptoms and signs had resolved completely in over half of the patients who showed them: disorientation, convulsions, tremors, incontinence, euphoria and depression. In over one-quarter there was resolution of impaired memory, judgement, insight, speech, calculation, delusions and hallucinations. Clearly there is considerable leeway for restoration of function in favourable cases, although with long-established disease one can hope merely to halt progression of the disorder. The overall death rate 10 years after treatment was 31%, 9% being attributable to general paresis and a further 22% to other causes. Altogether this was almost four times the death rate to be expected for non-syphilitic patients of a similar age.

Currie *et al.* (1988) also identified that clinical improvement was associated with decreasing CSF pleocytosis rather than with a decline in protein levels. Wilner and Brody (1968), in a prolonged follow-up of 100 patients, showed that new neurological manifestations were liable to develop in some 30% of cases, consisting of grand mal epilepsy, paraplegia, hemiparesis, optic atrophy or oculomotor palsies. These occurred even among patients who had been treated with penicillin, the average interval between treatment and such developments being 12 years. However, it was uncertain whether this always represented progression of the neurosyphilis rather than increased susceptibility to other neurological disease, and penicillin may often have been given in inadequate dosage. Roberts and Emsley (1995) in a case series of 12 patients identified a negative correlation between 1-year improvements in MMSE scores and CSF VDRL titres and suggested that this may be an early indicator of continued disease activity, even in the absence of declared neurosyphilitic symptoms.

Encephalitis

Encephalitis refers to a primary disease in which viral agents cause inflammation of the brain. Meningoencephalitis is the more appropriate term when a marked element of meningeal irritation exists as well. Virological studies have gone some way towards isolating and demonstrating the responsible organisms, especially in large epidemics, but a large number of cases remain in which a viral aetiology is merely presumed to operate on account of the general features of the illness. This applies particularly to sporadic cases where opportunities for extensive virological investigations may not be available, but is also true of some large epidemics, notably of encephalitis lethargica in which a specific agent was never conclusively demonstrated.

In some cases of known viral infection it is uncertain whether the virus actually gains access to the CNS or whether the central nervous changes represent an autoimmune or hypersensitivity reaction to the presence of viral infection

Table 7.2 Causes of acute viral encephalitis (rarer or suspected arboviral causes are shown in parentheses). (From Solomon *et al.* 2007.)

Non-geographically restricted sporadic causes

Herpesviruses: herpes simplex virus types 1 and 2, varicella-zoster virus, Epstein–Barr virus, cytomegalovirus, human herpesvirus types 6 and 7

Enteroviruses: coxsackieviruses, echoviruses, enteroviruses 70 and 71, parechovirus, poliovirus

Paramyxoviruses: measles virus, mumps virus

Others (rarer causes): influenza viruses, adenovirus, parvovirus, lymphocytic choriomeningitis virus, rubella virus

Geographically restricted causes (mostly arthropod-borne*)

The Americas: West Nile, La Cross, St Louis, Rocio and Powassan encephalitis; Venezuelan, eastern and western equine encephalitis; Colorado tick fever virus, dengue virus and rabies virus

Europe/Middle East: tick-borne encephalitis, West Nile, Tosana, rabies (dengue virus, louping ill virus)

Africa: West Nile (Rift Valley fever virus, Crimean-Congo haemorrhagic fever, dengue, chikungunya), rabies

Asia: Japanese encephalitis, West Nile, dengue, Murray Valley encephalitis, rabies (chikungunya virus, Nipah)

Australasia: Murray Valley encephalitis, Japanese encephalitis (kunjin, dengue)

* All are arthropod-borne, except for rabies and Nipah virus.

elsewhere in the body. The latter is thought to be the principal mechanism in many of the forms of encephalitis that follow childhood infectious diseases.

It is now also apparent that viruses play a part in some subacute degenerative diseases of the brain, for example the measles virus in subacute sclerosing panencephalitis (see Encephalitis, later) and the JC polyomavirus in PML (see Acquired immunodeficiency syndrome, earlier). Direct infection of the brain with HIV-1 appears to be central to the development of HAD (see HIV-associated cognitive disorders, earlier). A comprehensive classification of encephalitis is difficult, but Table 7.2 delineates the main categories for discussion (Solomon *et al.* 2007).

The relative incidence of the different forms has been demonstrated in a study from Finland that employed PCR to identify the virus present in CSF in some 3000 cases of CNS infection (Koskiniemi *et al.* 2001). Surprisingly, and against conventional wisdom, VZV was most frequently detected (29%). HSV and enteroviruses each accounted for the aetiology in 11% and influenza A virus in 7%. However, the cause remained uncertain in the remainder. This is a common finding, with between 50% and as many as 85% of cases remaining with an unknown cause in a variety of studies.

The worldwide incidence of acute encephalitis is variable but is thought to be 3.5–7.4 per 100 000 patient-years. HSV is generally reported as the most common sporadic cause in the Western world, with an annual incidence between 1 in 250 000 and 1 in 1 000 000 persons (Granerod & Crowcroft

2007), although this may be an underestimate (Kennedy 2005).

Sejvar (2006) has identified the evolving epidemiology of viral encephalitis with particular attention to the spread of the arbovirus West Nile virus in North America. This, along with Japanese encephalitis virus, is notably thriving in new areas (Solomon & Winter 2004). There have been West Nile outbreaks in the Americas and southern Europe and the virus has also been identified in the UK, although there have not been human cases reported as yet (Buckley *et al.* 2006; Morgan 2006).

Human immunodeficiency virus and other causes of immunocompromise including transplant surgery and chemotherapy have also changed the epidemiology of encephalitis, with CMV, EBV and human herpesvirus 6 presenting more commonly in this context (Solomon *et al.* 2007).

Clinical presentation

The characteristic clinical presentation in most forms of acute encephalitis is of a flu-like prodrome rapidly developing into an illness with headache, fever, nausea and vomiting, irritability and photophobia. Virus-specific clinical features that may present are highlighted later in the discussion. Some degree of neck stiffness is often detectable, and papilloedema may develop due to cerebral oedema. The pyrexia can be variable, low grade and easily overlooked. Equally, in a study by Raschilas *et al.* (2002), 91% of adults, later diagnosed with HSV-1 encephalitis, presented with high fever on admission.

The principal feature of cerebral involvement is disturbance of consciousness, ranging from mild somnolence to coma. Delirium features prominently in some varieties and disorientation (76%) and behavioural change (41%) were prominent in Raschilas *et al.*'s cohort. Seizures are common, especially in children, and can be the opening presentation of the illness. Focal neurological signs vary greatly according to the site of major impact of the inflammatory process, and are sometimes remarkably slight or even totally absent. Among the most common are pupillary changes, ocular palsies, nystagmus, ataxia, or disturbance of the long tracts with alteration of tendon reflexes, upgoing plantar responses and pareses of the limbs. Symptoms of temporal lobe involvement such as aphasia and dysphasia strongly suggest HSV infection. Sometimes the spinal cord is involved, with retention of urine or paraparesis.

Special interest attaches to cases that present with psychiatric disorder and cases have been included to illustrate this where possible. Mental disorder was recognised in the early epidemics of encephalitis lethargica (see Encephalitis lethargica, later), which will be discussed in detail, but examples still occur with other varieties. It has been suggested that the long-term psychiatric sequelae are considerable, but there is a need for further standardised clinical investigation (Arciniegas & Anderson 2004). As an indicator of psychiatric morbidity, Dowell *et al.* (2000) report that respondents to an Encephalitis Society questionnaire on their current state of functioning identified frustration and anger (68%), anxiety (67%), mood swings (59%) and depression (58%).

Caroff *et al.* (2001) reviewed 62 cases of encephalitis and identified the initial presenting symptoms to be delusions (54%, predominantly persecutory and nihilistic), hallucinations (auditory 44%, visual 13%, olfactory 3%, gustatory 1%) and affective disorder (depression 21%, euphoria 6%). Sometimes impairment of consciousness and neurological signs are absent at the time of presentation, as in the three patients reported by Misra and Hay (1971) who were admitted to a psychiatric unit with a provisional diagnosis of schizophrenia. Virological studies were apparently not performed.

A boy of 18 was admitted with a 2-day history of odd behaviour. He was excited, overactive and aggressive, with thought disorder and catatonic features. Two days after admission one plantar response was equivocal, and 2 days later both plantars were extensor and the left abdominal reflexes diminished. Lumbar puncture revealed no abnormality. He became pyrexial and developed subacute delirium. EEG showed a reduction in alpha rhythm and generalised slow activity. He was treated with corticotrophin. Subsequently he developed postencephalitic parkinsonism.

A woman of 45 was admitted with a 3-week history of depression and irritability and a 2-week history of paranoid delusions. On examination she admitted to thought withdrawal and auditory hallucinations. Three days after admission she became pyrexial and an extensor plantar response was elicited. Lumbar puncture was normal but EEG showed a general excess of symmetrical fast activity. She developed atrial fibrillation and congestive heart failure. She was treated for encephalitis and myocarditis and eventually made a complete recovery.

Wilson (1976) presented further striking cases of this nature, showing abrupt onset of psychological disturbance and little by way of neurological dysfunction in the early stages. Crow (1978) reviews other scattered examples that illustrate the potential overlap with schizophrenia. The majority probably represent cases of HSV encephalitis (see Non-geographically restricted sporadic encephalitides in this chapter).

The course of illness can vary greatly from one patient to another, and from time to time in a single patient, no matter what the causative organism. Profound coma may improve dramatically after some days or weeks, or unexpected relapse may follow steady recovery. When the acute phase is over there is generally a long period of physical and mental recuperation that may continue for several months. Occasionally, the acute phase is succeeded by a prolonged phase of disturbed behaviour, which may outlast all evidence of active infection and closely simulate a psychogenic reaction.

Geographically restricted encephalitides

This group contains illnesses that occur in epidemics in different parts of the world and are transmitted to humans through animal or insect vectors. The majority of viruses are arthropod-borne, i.e. the vector is an infected insect, chiefly the mosquito, although in some cases ticks and mites are involved. In the Americas the main varieties are West Nile, La Crosse, Rocio and Powassan encephalitis; Venezuelan, eastern and western equine encephalitis; and Colorado tick fever, dengue and St Louis encephalitis, distinguished mainly by their geographical locations (Solomon *et al.* 2007). Louping ill is the only member of the group seen in England in humans and this is very rare. It is derived from sheep via sheep ticks. There are more reports of this virus in Europe, alongside presentations with tick-borne encephalitis (Charrel *et al.* 2004). Japanese B encephalitis virus is the main cause of viral encephalitis in Asia (Diagana *et al.* 2007) and became well known to the Western world by affecting troops in the Far East during the Second World War. It can present with acute flaccid paralysis in contrast to the usual encephalitic presentation (Chung *et al.* 2007) and is associated with psychiatric presentations including social inappropriateness, aggression, emotional lability, and affective and paranoid symptoms (Monnet 2003).

Transmission patterns of arthropod-borne viruses are often linked to the migration of birds, although changes in geographical distributions may also be seen with future climate change, potentially allowing agents such as West Nile virus, whose mosquito vector is present in the UK but dormant because of the colder climate (Morgan 2006), to flourish. West Nile virus like Japanese B encephalitis virus can also present with flaccid paralysis, as well as parkinsonism and myoclonus (Davis *et al.* 2006; DeBiasi & Tyler 2006).

Recurrent epidemics are a feature of all the diseases listed, often with a seasonal incidence in the warm summer months, and varying somewhat in virulence from one epidemic to another. In some epidemics overt disease is rare in comparison to the number of abortive cases who are found to harbour the viruses without showing signs of illness. This naturally leads to considerable difficulty in reaching a satisfactory laboratory confirmation of the disease when sporadic cases arise, although rising titres of antibodies on repeat examination may help.

Rabies

Rabies is transmitted by infected animal saliva from dogs, bats or wolves. There is a long and variable incubation period, commonly 1–2 months, but with a wide latitude extending sometimes up to a year. The onset is then sudden, with a pyrexial illness, excitement, hydrophobia and violent muscular spasms involving the oesophagus and respiratory muscles. Crises are characterised by intense fury or profound terror, and in the intervals between the mind is clear. An ascending paralysis may occur. Death occurs during paroxysms, or in coma if the patient survives sufficiently long. Rabies must be distinguished from tetanus and from hysteria when a supposedly rabid dog has bitten a patient. In hysteria true pharyngeal spasm does not occur, and the mental disturbance is amenable to sedatives and suggestion.

Nipah virus

Nipah virus is a paramyxovirus that was first identified in Malayasia in 1998–1999. It is transmitted from pigs and was initially limited to farm workers (Goh *et al.* 2000). In comparison with other encephalitides, MRI may reveal multiple white matter lesions, which have been proposed to represent vasculitic lesions causing infarction (Lim *et al.* 2003). Ng *et al.* (2004) have reported the long-term neuropsychiatric sequelae of infection; eight of nine of their cohort presented with psychiatric symptoms, with depressive disorder both immediately after recovery and up to 1 year later being the most prominent. Cognitive deficits were also identified in attention, verbal and visual memory (Ng *et al.* 2004).

Non-geographically restricted sporadic encephalitides

Herpes simplex virus

The disease is severe, with mortality in untreated cases as high as 70% (Whitley *et al.* 1998) and long-term neurological impairments prominent in survivors. HSV shows certain special features including marked psychological disturbance in the acute phase and as a major sequel. Unlike the arboviruses, there are no seasonal or gender associations. The incidence has a bimodal spread, with one-third of cases occurring in the youngest age group up to 20 years and 50% of cases in those over 50 years (Tyler 2004). In a PCR investigation, HSV was responsible for 37% of all cases of encephalitis in subjects aged 60–65 years. The second bimodal peak may represent reactivation of latent virus in the elderly (Koskiniemi *et al.* 1996).

HSV encephalitis was controversial for many years because HSV infection is very widely distributed, with antibodies detectable in 80–90% of adults. It was also known that the virus could occasionally be cultured from random samples of CSF. However, the evidence that it truly caused encephalitis came from the finding of Cowdry type A inclusion bodies in the brains of affected persons, identical with those seen in cutaneous and visceral forms of the disease. Smith *et al.* (1941) were finally able to show a convincing association with acute encephalitis by isolating the virus

from the brain of a case which showed this specific pathological feature.

It is now recognised that HSV is responsible not only for cases of ordinary acute encephalitis but also for many of the cases of 'acute inclusion body', 'acute necrotising' and 'haemorrhagic' encephalitis that had formerly been regarded as distinct entities (Drachman & Adams 1962).

Pathology

Changes characteristic of other forms of encephalitis are seen: perivascular infiltration of lymphocytes and histiocytes in the cortex and adjacent white matter, proliferation of microglia and the formation of glial nodules. The cerebral cortex is mainly affected in adults, with less involvement of subcortical structures. A distinctive feature is the severity of the process. In areas of maximal involvement there is necrosis with softening, haemorrhage and loss of all nervous and glial elements. Such lesions tend to be asymmetrical between the hemispheres, and involve the medial temporal and orbital regions especially. In biopsy material obtained early in the disease it may be possible to demonstrate herpes viral antigen by immunofluorescence or immunoperoxidase techniques, thus confirming the diagnosis (Booss & Esiri 1986).

Clinical features

Only a small proportion of patients give a history of recurrent herpes labialis (Leider *et al.* 1965; Gostling 1967). Typically, there is rapid onset with a severe illness in the acute stage. There are no characteristic features that can distinguish HSV from other causes of encephalitis (Davis 2000). Pyrexia may be up to 39.5°C (103°F) and seizures may present in all age groups. In one study of symptom clusters in encephalitis and their PCR-identified virus correlations, HSV was more commonly associated with focal encephalitis (weakness, sensory abnormalities, aphasia, visual field defects and cranial nerve palsies) than diffuse disease (neurobehavioural change and alteration of consciousness) (Domingues *et al.* 1997).

Nonetheless, a high index of suspicion should remain even in atypical cases. Sometimes the clinical picture can at first be misleading and this is the position in perhaps as many as 20% of cases (Fodor *et al.* 1998). In five of six cases reported by Drachman and Adams (1962), psychological symptoms were the most striking initial feature. At first these patients appeared only mildly unwell and it was aberrations of behaviour that called attention to the seriousness of the illness. One patient packed a case a week in advance of a short journey, one dressed at night to go to an imagined funeral, one failed to recognise his wife and another slept until four o'clock in the afternoon then suddenly rushed from the house without explanation.

Once the illness is declared, a delirious phase is often prominent before the patient sinks into coma. Hallucinations can resemble those of delirium tremens in being vivid and colourful, and in provoking a marked emotional reaction. On recovery from coma, behavioural disturbance may again be marked, with a phase of restless hyperactivity.

The prominence of psychiatric disturbance no doubt owes much to the characteristic accent of pathology on the temporal lobes and orbitofrontal structures (Greenwood *et al.* 1983). This may bring added focal symptoms such as anosmia, olfactory and gustatory hallucinations, or marked memory disturbance out of proportion to the impairment of intellect. Sometimes an area of focal necrosis becomes swollen to such a degree that the illness presents with features indicative of an acute intracranial mass, usually in the temporal lobe.

Much more rarely cases present with aseptic meningitis and run a benign course (Leider *et al.* 1965; Olson *et al.* 1967; Tyler 2004). Very occasionally there may be recurrent episodes of organic psychosis, as in the interesting patient reported by Shearer and Finch (1964): a 9-year-old boy had 17 episodes in a 3-year period, lasting a little over a week at a time, and consisting of fever, headache, drowsiness, disorientation and grossly irrational behaviour. Each episode was accompanied by EEG abnormalities and an outbreak of herpes labialis.

Investigations

Examination of the CSF should be carried out only if this is judged safe after performing CT (Solomon *et al.* 2007). Other infectious conditions can be excluded, and it may be possible to retrospectively demonstrate intrathecal synthesis of antibody to the virus, although this is not useful acutely as it takes weeks to develop (Boivin 2004).

Polymerase chain reaction is particularly useful for the detection of viral DNA in the CSF (Kleinschmidt-DeMasters *et al.* 2001), has high sensitivity (98%) and specificity (99%) (Puchhammer-Stockl *et al.* 1993) and allows the differentiation of recurrent viral infection and postinfectious immune-mediated disease (Boivin 2004). EEG shows non-specific slowing early on, and later periodic lateralising epileptiform discharges with a temporal focus (Steiner *et al.* 2005). EEG may need to be repeated, as these findings may only be temporary (Lai & Gragasin 1988).

Computed tomography can aid materially in excluding an abscess or tumour (Kaufman *et al.* 1979). The scan may be normal in the early stages, but later reveals characteristic low-density areas in one or both temporal lobes, or evidence of mass effects along with contrast enhancement (Zimmerman *et al.* 1980). MRI is more sensitive in revealing early changes at a time when therapy is most likely to be useful (Chaudhuri & Kennedy 2002). Cingulate gyrus and contralateral temporal involvement is extremely suggestive of HSV encephalitis.

Before the development of PCR techniques, brain biopsy was considered the gold standard for confirming the diagnosis. Type A inclusion bodies may be detected and the virus demonstrated in the tissue obtained. However, the procedure is not without risk and a negative result does not exclude the condition. Rising titres of antibodies in the blood may give supportive evidence, but can be useful only in retrospect. Stereotactic-guided needle aspiration is now only rarely performed.

Tyler (2004) has discussed the discrepancies between different clinical presentations when confirmatory investigations by PCR or biopsy are considered. This appraisal identifies the variable presentations of encephalitis and the danger of assuming that what may have been considered atypical features, are not actually quiescent HSV encephalitis. PCR is considerably more sensitive, and cases with subtle changes in consciousness are much more readily identified by PCR than biopsy. Comparatively, personality change is slightly less common in PCR-identified cases.

Differential diagnosis

The disease is not infrequently puzzling. In addition to cases that present as possible tumours or abscesses, other conditions can be simulated. When pyrexia is low and neurological signs markedly asymmetrical, the picture may suggest subdural haematoma or head injury. Acute and fulminating examples may resemble meningitis. The prominence of mental confusion with vivid hallucinations may lead to a diagnosis of delirium tremens, or an acute onset with drowsiness, confabulation and fits may suggest Wernicke's encephalopathy. The residual end-state can closely resemble Korsakoff's psychosis or raise the possibility of neurosyphilis.

Treatment and outcome

Treatment is often a matter of urgency. Seizures should be controlled. Corticosteroids and mannitol may be required to reduce cerebral oedema, although their use requires further investigation (Openshaw & Cantin 2005). The nucleoside analogue acyclovir should be started as soon as possible in immunocompetent patients where there is strong suspicion based on the clinical history, neuroimaging and initial CSF findings (Solomon *et al.* 2007). Acyclovir resistance has been reported in immunocompromised patients and here foscarnet can be an effective alternative (Whitley *et al.* 1998). Decompression of the brain is a useful adjunct in appropriate cases.

Factors affecting treatment outcome include age, level of consciousness at presentation, viral load and duration of encephalitis (Tyler 2004). Kaplan and Bain (1999) identify time to treatment as the best indicator of outcome, although cognitive outcomes may be best predicted by the period of transient encephalitic amnesia, which is an equivalent concept to post-traumatic amnesia in head injury (Hokkanen & Launes 1997).

Before the advent of acyclovir, approximately 70% of patients died and half of the survivors were left with sequelae that could be severe (Illis & Merry 1972). With acyclovir the prognosis has improved considerably, with fatal outcomes dropping to 20% (Sköldenberg et al. 1984; Whitley et al. 1986). However, when the temporal lobes have been damaged severely the consequences can still be grave. Mental retardation can ensue in children, or dementia in adults. Seizures, dysphasia, personality change and severe amnesic states have also been described (Oxbury & MacCallum 1973). Hierons et al. (1978) reported pictures ranging from relatively pure amnesic syndromes to severe dementia, often accompanied by bizarre behaviour reminiscent of Klüver–Bucy syndrome. The patients reported by Rose and Symonds (1960), in whom encephalitis was followed by a Korsakoff-like syndrome, were probably examples of HSV encephalitis.

The risk of cognitive impairment has been shown to be two to four times higher than that of patients with other causes of viral encephalitis (Warrington & Shallice 1984; Hokkanen et al. 1996; Pewter et al. 2007). Cognitive outcomes include dense anterograde amnesia in 25–75% (Hokkanen & Launes 2000) with variable retrograde memory impairment, which may also present in isolation (Baur et al. 2000; Harlam et al. 2001; Tsukiura et al. 2003). Dysexecutive features may also present in some 40% (Kapur et al. 1994), with impaired performance on frontal testing (Del Grosso Destreri et al. 2002; Shoqeirat et al. 1990; Hokkanen & Launes 1997). Category-specific anomia or more widespread semantic impairments are a frequently reported sequel (Barbarotto et al. 1996; Moss & Tyler 2000; Schweizer et al. 2001). Even among patients who apparently make excellent recoveries after treatment with acyclovir, neuropsychological testing may reveal evidence of cognitive deficits. Gordon et al. (1990) followed four such patients for several years, and all showed deficits on language and memory tests. Some showed additional impairments in calculation, visuoconstructive ability and facial recognition, and none were able to function at their prior level of achievement. Such results underline the importance of careful follow-up evaluation and counselling in patients who have had the disease.

Long-term psychiatric outcomes are also prominent. McGrath et al. (1997) identified a prevalence of personality and behavioural disturbance of 45%, taken from the medical records of survivors of HSV encephalitis at between 6 months and 11 years. Schizophreniform psychoses and emotional lability are rare but have also been reported (Vallini & Burns 1987; Gaber & Eshiett 2003), sometimes a considerable time after treatment and discharge.

Type B HSV encephalitis
The monkey form of HSV produces an almost invariably fatal disease in humans, and is a hazard to workers in animal laboratories. It is transmitted by the bite of an infected monkey. A vesicle is produced at the site of entry, and along with encephalitis of severe degree there is often an ascending

paraplegia. Widespread necrotic lesions are found in other organs as well as the brain.

Epstein–Barr virus
The neurological complications of infectious mononucleosis rarely include an encephalitic picture. When this does occur it may be due to direct viral invasion of the nervous system, but sometimes it appears to represent an allergic encephalomyelitis similar to that following the acute exanthemata. A benign lymphocytic meningitis (see Meningitis in this chapter) can also occur. The incidence of neurological sequelae in infectious mononucleosis is 0.4–7.3% (Silverstein et al. 1972).

Headache and meningism often accompany glandular fever. Diffuse EEG abnormalities have been reported in up to 30% of cases. However, frank neurological complications are rare. Gautier-Smith (1965) and Boughton (1970) have described patients with acute confusion progressing to stupor or coma, usually setting in abruptly within 5–9 days of the illness. Other cases present with seizures or focal cerebral disturbances such as hemiplegia. Pommer et al. (1983) reported the case of a 43-year-old patient who presented with transient global amnesia and seizures after EBV infection. Siversten and Christensen (1996) identified the onset of a severe dementia in one case from their cohort. Syndromes of brainstem, cerebellar or cord dysfunction may also be seen. The CSF shows a moderate rise in cells and protein. Complete recovery appears to be the rule.

Of considerable interest are patients who develop acute psychiatric disturbances in clear consciousness during the course of glandular fever. Raymond and Williams (1948) described a patient who became acutely psychotic within a few days of onset, settling over 3 weeks as the illness improved. Klaber and Lacey (1968) reported 5 of 76 cases presenting with severe psychiatric disorder during the course of an epidemic, only subsequently being diagnosed as suffering from glandular fever. Two showed pictures of acute schizophrenia and three acute depression. Here it seems likely that the patients were responding to the nonspecific stress of the physical illness rather than to direct nervous system involvement.

More recently, Behr et al. (2006) reported the psychiatric presentation of an immunocompromised post-transplant patient.

A 58-year-old man presented with emotional lability, depressed mood, anhedonia and loss of appetite 2 months after a bone marrow transplant for myelodysplastic syndrome. Three months later he presented with cognitive dysfunction. MRI demonstrated a frontal lesion consistent with a vascular malformation and, later in the presentation, non-enhancing periventricular hyperintensities. His cognitive state deteriorated with disorientation, poor attention and concentration, as well as impaired short-term memory. Mental state examination revealed a dysphoric mood, blunted affect and psychomotor retardation and no alteration of consciousness. On physical examination, he was afebrile and there were no focal neurological signs or meningism. EBV genome copies in peripheral blood leucocytes revealed reactivation of EBV. CSF examination identified a pleocytosis, raised protein and oligiclonal banding restricted to the CSF. Intrathecal syntheses of IgM antibodies and intrathecal production of IgG anti-EBV antibodies indicated a reactivated cerebral EBV infection. PCR for EBV DNA in CSF was positive.

EBV and fatigue

A depressive aftermath has also been widely reported following EBV, very occasional patients showing depression of psychotic intensity (White & Lewis 1987). Careful prospective studies by White, P.D. et al. (1995a,b) have shown that a persistent fatigue syndrome may develop in the 6 months following glandular fever, and that to a large extent it could be differentiated from depression. Whereas social adversity correlated significantly with the development of depression, this had little association with the development of a fatigue syndrome or delayed physical recovery (Bruce-Jones et al. 1994). An investigation by Hamblin et al. (1983) could be relevant in pointing to immunological dysfunction. However, a prospective study of 71 patients with infectious mononucleosis from primary care revealed that predictors of fatigue over 1 year had no clear immune or neuroendocrine predictors but that psychosocial factors and illness perceptions were predictive at various stages (Candy et al. 2004). Early mobilisation may have a protective effect.

In these and other cases of chronic fatigue that appears to follow a viral infection, general rehabilitative principles apply with attention paid to treating manifest or masked psychiatric disorder. Wessely et al. (1989, 1991) and Sharpe et al. (1996) give detailed descriptions of a cognitive–behavioural approach which aims, inter alia, to break the vicious cycle of exercise avoidance leading to diminished exercise tolerance and the production of further symptoms. Encouragement of the patient to engage in graded activity by planned stages requires careful assessment of the capacities in each individual and full explanation of the aims of treatment.

Enterovirus encephalitis

The enteroviruses are more likely to produce the picture of aseptic meningitis than encephalitis (see Meningitis, later). The poliomyelitis virus is distinguished by its effects on the

spinal cord and the accompanying encephalitis is usually very slight in degree, but the related coxsackieviruses and echoviruses can occasionally produce definite encephalitic manifestations.

Outbreaks are commonest in summer and autumn. The illnesses caused by coxsackieviruses and echoviruses usually run a benign course, accompanied by other systemic symptoms characteristic of the virus concerned: maculopapular rashes, muscular pains or pleurodynia. The changes in the CSF resemble those of poliomyelitis, with a moderate elevation in protein, normal sugar and 50–100 cells/mm^3 (polymorphs early and mononuclear cells later). The virus may be isolated from throat swabs or stool specimens, but is of more significance if found in the CSF. A rise in serum antibodies may be demonstrated during the course of the disease by neutralisation or complement fixation tests, although many asymptomatic infections evoke the same response. Serological testing is also made difficult by the large number of antigenically distinct viruses in this group.

Children affected before 1 year of age may occasionally be left with neurological impairment and seizures (Sells et al. 1975). Otherwise serious sequelae are uncommon with coxsackievirus and echovirus infections. Muscular weakness may persist for some time during convalescence, but true paralysis is rare. Poser et al. (1969) have reported the occasional development of postencephalitic parkinsonism after such infections, but this is usually a transient and mild disability unlike that following encephalitis lethargica (see Encephalitis lethargica, later).

Other sporadic viral encephalitides

In a great number of cases of sporadic encephalitis the cause is never identified, and the yield even with extensive virological studies remains rather low. The following known varieties are all relatively infrequent.

Varicella-zoster virus

Varicella-zoster virus is the cause of either chickenpox or shingles, depending on the immunocompetence of the patient. Some degree of meningeal reaction is common in herpes zoster, with elevation of the protein and an excess of mononuclear cells in the CSF. Features of meningitis are observed very occasionally and encephalitis occurs in up to 5% of those hospitalised with shingles and in less than 0.05% of those hospitalised with chickenpox (Mazur & Dolin 1978; Guess et al. 1986). Hall (1963) has reported a clear example of encephalitis following ophthalmic zoster and resulting in a chronic amnesic syndrome.

Hokkanen and Launes (2007) have reviewed the neuropsychiatric sequelae of herpes zoster encephalitis. They note that the acute-stage cognitive profile has not been adequately studied but that deterioration in verbal and visual reasoning, perseveration, poor recent and remote memory, attention, concentration, planning and impulse control have all been reported. Hallucinations have been reported in a number of case studies in the acute stage, but are likely a non-specific feature of delirium (Jemsek *et al*. 1983). Psychosis, irritability and mood change have been reported both acute-ly and after recovery (Hokkanen *et al*. 1997; Hokkanen & Launes 2007). Cognitive characteristics after treatment have equally received only limited attention, with the suggestion that outcomes are more favourable than in HSV encephalitis, with perhaps a subcortical picture being evident in some cases (Hokkanen *et al*. 1997).

Mumps encephalitis

It appears that the mumps virus affects the nervous system more commonly than was previously supposed, even in the absence of parotitis or other typical evidence of the disease. This is probably the only common childhood infectious disease in which the virus itself can invade the CNS. Prior to the development of routine vaccination, an aseptic men-ingitis (see Meningitis, later) was most commonly seen, although an encephalitic illness is also reported. When it occurs there is usually some degree of coincident meningitis and sometimes myelitis. Mumps encephalitis in adults is nowadays extremely rare.

Symptoms appear some 2–10 days after the onset of paro-titis, but can precede it or occur without any overt evidence of mumps elsewhere in the body. Meningeal symptoms are usually prominent, with headache, vomiting, fever, neck stiffness and irritability. Drowsiness and delirium occur, sometimes with cranial nerve palsies, ataxia or pareses in the limbs. Fits are uncommon. In the acute myelitic form there is profound paresis and sensory changes in the limbs. The varied psychiatric and neurological pictures that may be seen are reviewed by Keddie (1965).

The CSF shows a moderate pleocytosis, usually of mono-nuclear cells, from the outset. Serological tests are useful if a rise in titre of complement fixation or haemagglutination-inhibition antibodies can be demonstrated during convales-cence. Permanent sequelae are common enough to suggest that the prognosis should be guarded (Lees 1970; Johnstone *et al*. 1972).

Other para-infectious encephalitides

The forms of encephalitis that occasionally follow the acute exanthemata account for a large proportion of the cases seen in childhood. The chief causes are measles, rubella, pertussis and scarlet fever, although similar developments may be seen after viral pneumonias and infectious mononucleosis. The incidence of encephalitis in measles has been estimated as 0.1%, varying by age, with only 10% of cases occurring in adults (Gibbons *et al*. 1956) and mortality being 15–25% in the 1950s to 1960s. Encephalitis associated with rubella infection has a reported incidence of 0.2 per 1000 rubella cases, with mortality around 20% (Miller *et al*. 1956).

In Kennard and Swash's (1981) series, the predominant antecedent of many of these illnesses was an upper respira-tory tract infection of influenzal type. All share a common pathology and possibly a common pathogenesis. Closely similar illnesses may follow vaccination against smallpox or injections of serum, or sometimes they arise for no apparent reason. The brain may be involved alone or there may be more widespread effect throughout the neuraxis with brain-stem or cord involvement. In such cases the term 'acute dis-seminated encephalomyelitis' is usually employed.

The pathological changes differ from those of the virus infections already described in certain definite respects, though some degree of overlap can be seen. The brain and cord show congestion, often with petechial haemorrhages. However, the most striking changes are seen in the white matter, with discrete areas of acute perivenous demyelina-tion, mononuclear perivascular infiltration and neuroglial proliferation. There is no evidence of a direct attack on the nerve cells themselves, and the cortical neurones are charac-teristically spared completely unless there has been a com-plicating factor such as hypoxia (Booss & Esiri 1986). In acute haemorrhagic leucoencephalitis, the changes are particu-larly severely developed, along with brain congestion and swelling and foci of perivascular necrosis. There is little to suggest direct invasion of the CNS by the viruses concerned. Allergic or autoimmune mechanisms are generally held to be the cause as the picture closely resembles that of experi-mental allergic encephalomyelitis.

The clinical picture consists of headache, drowsiness, pho-tophobia and irritability, setting in some 3–14 days after the onset of the specific illness but with wide latitude of timing. There is commonly an interval of normal health between the acute viral illness and the encephalopathic development. Convulsions are common and meningism is often promi-nent. Cranial nerve palsies may appear, or myoclonic and choreiform movements may be seen. Loss of abdominal reflexes and extensor plantar responses are usual findings. The brainstem may be principally involved, with vertigo, vomiting, nystagmus and dysarthria; alternatively, in mye-litic forms there may be paraparesis with retention of urine. Peripheral nerve involvement is common. The CSF may be normal, but is often under increased pressure with a mild lymphocytic pleocytosis and moderate elevation of protein. CT or MRI may show multiple white matter abnormalities similar to those of multiple sclerosis, or more extensive sym-metrical changes in the cerebral and cerebellar white matter and basal ganglia (Kesselring *et al*. 1990). Serial MRI can be useful in contributing to the distinction from multiple sclero-sis in uncertain cases. Textbooks of neurology should be con-sulted for further details of the pictures seen with different infections.

If the patient does not succumb during the first week or two a remarkably complete recovery may be seen. The mor-tality is much higher in infants than in older children or adults. In some survivors there may be severe neurological sequelae, with hemiparesis, paraparesis, epilepsy and impairment of intellect. In children, behaviour disorders similar to those that follow encephalitis lethargica may occur. In adult survivors, varied neuropsychiatric sequelae have been reported after measles and rubella encephalitis, including schizophreniform psychosis (Stoler *et al.* 1987) and widespread impairments of memory, executive function, language and perception in some cases, similar to those seen after cases of HSV encephalitis (Pewter *et al.* 2007).

Subacute sclerosing panencephalitis

Subacute sclerosing panencephalitis (SSPE) is a rare disease in the developed world, with just 10 cases reported annually in the USA (Garg 2002). It remains rare in developing countries, but higher incidences are reported, for example 21 cases per million in India. The majority of cases have a history of measles infection. The initial features of the illness include more subtle cognitive impairment deteriorating into behavioural disturbance and clear-cut dementia. It is in this context that problems of differential diagnosis usually arise. Sometimes, however, the possibility of other psychiatric illness is raised in the early stages. Myoclonic jerks involving the head, trunk and limbs may be seen in later stages. Visual changes are reported in 10–50%, including cortical blindness, chorioretinitis and optic atrophy. In the most advanced stages the patient becomes quadriparetic with gradual decline into coma.

Cases were first described by Dawson in 1933 (subacute inclusion body encephalitis), van Bogaert in 1945 (subacute sclerosing leucoencephalitis) and Brain *et al.* in 1943 and 1948. These now appear to be essentially variants of the same disease process (Adams 1976).

Pathology

Adams (1976) described the typical pathological picture. The brain may be normal macroscopically, or firm and shrunken with areas of focal necrosis. Microscopy shows evidence of subacute inflammation, usually in both the grey and the white matter. There is perivascular infiltration with lymphocytes and plasma cells, and proliferation of astrocytes and microglia. Slight meningeal infiltration may also occur. The white matter lesions are of particular interest in that they are closely similar to those seen in para-infectious encephalomyelitis and HAD (Poser 1990). In the grey matter neuronal degeneration is apparent, often with characteristic intranuclear inclusions, and in the white matter areas of demyelination are seen with fibrous gliosis. Considerable variation is encountered from case to case.

The typical 'type A' intranuclear inclusions are strongly acidophilic homogeneous bodies with a sharp outline, separated from the nuclear membrane by a clear halo. They are the feature that originally suggested a viral aetiology, and are similar to those which occur in HSV encephalitis (see Nongeographically restricted sporadic encephalitides, later). In severely degenerated cells the inclusions may fill the nucleus so that the surrounding cytoplasm is reduced to a vestige. Sometimes they are found in the cytoplasm itself, or in glial cells as well as neurones; such changes may be focal in distribution (see Kennedy 1968).

Evidence has accumulated to suggest that the measles paramyxovirus is responsible. Almost all patients have a history of measles, usually at an early age, or of measles immunisation. Very high antibody titres to the virus are found in the serum and CSF, and specific immunofluorescence with measles antibody has been demonstrated in brain biopsy material (Connolly *et al.* 1967; Legg 1967). Electron microscopy has shown particles indistinguishable from paramyxovirus budding from cytoplasmic inclusions, and measles virus has been isolated from brain cell tissue cultures derived from patients with the disease (Horta-Barbosa *et al.* 1969). Finally, the disease has been transmitted to animals by intracerebral inoculation of brain tissue from patients with the disorder (Lehrich *et al.* 1970).

It remains unclear why such an illness should develop in a minute proportion of those who have suffered a primary measles infection. The virus probably gains access to the brain at the time of initial infection and develops into a less invasive and more persistent form that evades immune destruction (Anderson 1993). The original infection may have been with an unusual strain of virus. At some stage the latent infection then triggers an immune-mediated response that results in the widespread pathological changes in the brain. Possibilities of reactivation by subsequent infection, even by a different organism, have not been discounted.

Clinical features

The great majority of cases occur in children or adolescents, although occasional examples have been reported in middle age (Brierley *et al.* 1960; Himmelhoch *et al.* 1970) and are probably to be regarded as variants of the disease.

Classic examples present with insidious deterioration of intellect, such that the child begins to fail at school, becomes forgetful and inattentive, slowed and slovenly. Other early symptoms are nocturnal delirium with hallucinations, marked lethargy and difficult uncontrollable behaviour. The prodromal manifestations may occasionally occur alone for a period of several months, but neurological abnormalities generally develop early. Characteristically the patient develops marked involuntary movements, including myoclonic jerks of the face, fingers and limbs, athetosis or rapid torsion spasms of the trunk that lead to sudden stumbles and falls. Myoclonia may be regularly periodic, occurring at fixed intervals of 5–10 seconds for hours or days at a time. The limbs develop bilateral extrapyramidal rigidity or progressive spasticity. Epileptic fits are common, and aphasia, apraxia or akinetic mutism may appear. A low-grade pyrexia may accompany the prodromal or later stages of the disorder, but this is not invariable.

Atypical presentations sometimes raise the possibility of non-organic psychiatric illness in the early stages. For example, Koehler and Jakumeit (1976) reported a woman of 20 who presented with an apparently hysterical blindness and gave Ganser responses of a classic nature. She showed a profound lack of initiative and spent much of the time asleep. Within a week of admission, however, the true disease was declared. In the 21-year-old patient described by Salib (1988), who presented with dysmorphophobic features, the diagnosis was delayed for several months and schizophrenia was suspected initially.

Electroencephalography often shows highly characteristic features, though many variants occur. Typically there are high-voltage slow-wave complexes, synchronous in all leads, and occurring at fixed intervals of 5–10 seconds along with the myoclonic jerks. They may also appear in the absence of motor abnormalities and can sometimes be focal in the frontal or occipital regions. The CSF may show a slight increase in cells, but the total protein is often normal. A feature of diagnostic importance is that the majority of cases show a raised IgG in the CSF and a paretic curve on Lange's colloidal gold test. The complement fixation titres for measles are high in serum and CSF. CT or MRI may show white matter abnormalities and later atrophy of the cerebrum, cerebellum and brainstem (Jayakumar *et al.* 1988).

The first descriptions stressed that the disease had a hopeless prognosis, with rapidly progressive dementia over 6 weeks to 6 months and death after a period of coma and Decerebrate rigidity. However, cases have since been reported with temporary arrest for months or even years in the middle stage of the disorder, and very few have been described with partial recovery. Of Kennedy's (1968) five cases in children, two achieved remission and one returned to school after regaining much coherent speech and a diminution of myoclonic jerks. Resnick *et al.* (1968) followed a patient for 5 years who showed considerable sustained improvement despite the continued elevation of measles antibody in serum and CSF. Cobb and Morgan-Hughes (1968) mention other scattered examples in the literature and suggest that the following patient may have had the disease in a mild form.

A 21-year-old chemistry student was admitted with a 5-month history of falling attacks, momentary blank spells and recent difficulty with concentration. Neurological examination was normal apart from brisk reflexes, EEG showed persistent slow waves in the left occipitotemporal region, and CSF showed a paretic Lange curve. He was readmitted 8 months later with impairment of memory and difficulty with reading, writing and calculation, which had come on over the preceding 2 months. He showed a severe

global dementia, with loss of recent memory, disorientation in time, agraphia, acalculia and profound constructional apraxia. The Wechsler Adult Intelligence Scale (WAIS) showed a verbal IQ of 79 and a performance IQ of less than 35. Affect was flattened and inappropriate. Neurological examination was still negative, but EEG showed bilateral recurrent monophasic and biphasic slow-wave complexes.

He was treated with prednisone in addition to anticonvulsants and slowly improved. By the following year he was working, although he had been dismissed from several jobs on account of general slowness and difficulty with reading and writing. Seven years later he was working as a gardener and had recently married. He was still mildly dysgraphic, with reading difficulties and profound constructional apraxia, but he was orientated in time and place and able to do simple calculations. Psychological testing showed a verbal IQ of 82 and a performance IQ of 40.

Risk *et al.* (1978) estimated that improvement could be expected in about 5% of cases, even after severe illnesses. However, relapse may subsequently occur after remissions lasting for several years. Their experience with 118 patients showed substantial long-term improvement in six. Two of these were still improving 4–5 years later, two were stable 4–6 years later, and two relapsed after 8 and 11 years respectively. Remittent cases tended to have shown milder variants of the disease and to have been somewhat older than usual at onset.

Progressive rubella panencephalitis

A variant of SSPE has been described in which rubella rather than measles virus appears to be responsible (Townsend *et al.* 1975, 1976; Weil *et al.* 1975). This sets in, usually during the second decade, in children who have been affected by rubella *in utero*. Mental and motor deterioration develop as with SSPE, and the pathological changes in the brain are similar. The serum and CSF show elevated titres of antibodies to the rubella virus and normal titres to measles. The rubella virus has been isolated from the brain in such cases.

Other varieties of subacute encephalitis

Himmelhoch *et al.* (1970) reported an interesting group of eight cases, mostly in adults, some apparently representing variants of SSPE. Symptoms characteristic of functional psychiatric disorder were prominent in all, and seven had originally been diagnosed as suffering from depression, schizophrenia or hysteria. In some the onset was acute, with sudden withdrawal and seclusiveness following a period of coryza, malaise and headache. Retardation was prominent and a psychogenic reaction was usually diagnosed at this stage. The patients then quickly developed disorientation and visual hallucinations and showed intellectual deterioration. In others the development was more protracted, with irritability, depression, phobias and ruminations over a period of several months. They then became mute and retarded and showed progressive intellectual impairment.

The bizarreness of behaviour had strongly biased the initial diagnoses, and neurological signs had often been ignored even when they were noted. Evidence of mild confusion, disorientation or visual hallucinations had sometimes been disregarded, changes of sleep and appetite had been ascribed to depression, and fugue-like states to catatonia or hysteria.

Characteristically there were rapid fluctuations, with impaired awareness and disorientation one day followed by complete lucidity the next. Periods of aggressiveness and sexual provocativeness were often followed by profuse apology, and patients seemed bewildered by their behaviour. Bizarre behaviour became increasingly frequent as time went on. It was markedly unresponsive to pharmacotherapy. Hallucinations were mainly visual but occurred in other modalities, and clear-cut paranoid delusions were common. At times an isolated episode was hard to distinguish from schizophrenia.

There were no consistently helpful laboratory findings, but all patients showed abnormal EEG changes at some point in the disease. Some died within several weeks or months, some ran a protracted course with remissions, but three recovered to premorbid levels of intellectual functioning (Himmelhoch *et al.* 1970).

A housewife of 38 became deluded after a period of fever, coryza and headache. She was committed to hospital with a diagnosis of paranoid schizophrenia. She alternated between a delusional state, when she was boisterous, abusive and combative, and periods of complete lucidity. Neurological examination revealed nothing abnormal, and her behaviour was unresponsive to phenothiazines or electroconvulsive therapy. Her later course was stormy, with grand mal seizures and periods of coma. EEG showed episodic, synchronous, high-voltage slow waves alternating with periods of relative electrical suppression. Biopsy of the right temporal lobe showed the features of encephalitis but no inclusion bodies were found.

Over the next 3 months the patient made a partial recovery, but 6 months later she still had severe impairment of memory, with disorientation for time and place and occasional nocturnal seizures. Five years later her memory deficit had cleared markedly, but the seizures continued and she had developed progressive paraplegia. The measles antibody titre remained elevated in the serum.

A 35-year-old woman graduate with a stable previous history became abruptly combative, confused and 'animalistic'. EEG was diffusely slowed, and the CSF showed a mild pleocytosis. She became unkempt, cachectic and totally uncommunicative, and showed aggressive and sexually provocative behaviour. She was incontinent of urine and faeces and required tube feeding. Even so she had intermittent periods of complete lucidity.

One month later she began to improve, with lessening of memory deficit and improvement of intellectual functions. At the same time, however, her behaviour became increasingly difficult to control. She refused to attend group meetings, with biting, kicking or pulling up her dress when she was urged to attend. With her family she behaved rather better and ultimately she was discharged. Two further admissions were required in the next few months on account of disturbed behaviour, but thereafter she unexpectedly began to improve. At first she had to carry a notebook to help with her memory, but after 18 months this became unnecessary. After 2 years she had recovered completely and continued to function normally.

Brierley *et al.* (1960) reported another group of three patients, all with onset in the fifties and all of whom were diagnostic problems during life. One had been regarded as having dementia, but in the others a low-grade pyrexia early in the illness had raised the possibility of a viral encephalitis. One presented as a severe depressive illness coloured by bizarre behaviour and later developed minor epileptic attacks, another began with depression following a respiratory infection, and the third began with pains in the shoulders and arms then progressed to tiredness and depression over the course of several weeks. At post-mortem all showed severe encephalitic changes concentrated to a notable degree on the medial temporal lobe structures. Inclusion bodies were not present.

Differential diagnosis
Subacute encephalitis clearly gives rise to diagnostic confusion during life. It is a rare condition, so that the clinician is unlikely to see more than the very occasional case. Difficulties with diagnosis are especially likely to arise in the prodromal period. In children the picture may suggest behaviour disorder or autism, and in adults other psychiatric disorder may be simulated as described above. Careful attention must be directed towards minor neurological abnormalities, sudden involuntary jerks, evidence of nocturnal delirium or intermittent low-grade pyrexia.

Alzheimer's disease is probably the commonest misdiagnosis in the later stages in adults. Multiple sclerosis may be suggested by the combination of early neurological disability with a paretic Lange curve and negative reactions for syphilis in the CSF. HSV encephalitis can show identical inclusion bodies in biopsy material, but the course is acute, and progressive dementia and myoclonic jerking are not seen.

Classic examples of SSPE usually declare themselves eventually when involuntary movements and typical EEG features appear. Diagnostic brain biopsy may be required as a last resort.

Adenovirus encephalitis

Adenovirus infections are discussed by Booss and Esiri (1986). The several varieties are associated with acute respiratory infections, conjunctivitis and pharyngitis. Adenovirus type 7 may lead to encephalitis in children with respiratory disease, sometimes in the form of small outbreaks. Adult adenovirus encephalitis is rare and often comorbid with other conditions. The outcome is often complete recovery, although residual ataxia (Zagardo *et al.* 1998), language and visual construction impairment (Hokkanen *et al.* 1996), irritability, mood change and amnesia (West *et al.* 1985; Hokkanen *et al.* 1996) have been reported.

Influenza encephalitis

The neurological manifestations of influenza virus have been reviewed by Studahl (2003). It appears that the influenza virus itself may be responsible for occasional cases of encephalitis, perhaps with a greater incidence in children (Morishima *et al.* 2002). Small groups of cases have been reported during influenza outbreaks in many parts of the world, including the large epidemic of 'Asian' influenza (influenza type A) that affected the British Isles in 1957–1958.

A variety of pictures is seen, some setting in at the height of the upper respiratory tract infection, others beginning towards the end of the attack, and others following some days later after a brief afebrile episode. The usual picture is of headache, vomiting, delirium and coma, with transient reflex abnormalities or weakness of the limbs. The CSF may be normal or show a slight pleocytosis. EEG is often diffusely abnormal. The illness usually resolves after several days and excellent recovery is said to be the rule. Sulkava *et al.* (1981) reported four cases of encephalitis after type A influenza, with transient changes in memory, fatigue and mental 'sluggishness' that resolved within a month of recovery.

In other varieties the patient shows no more than a period of mental confusion and headache, accompanied by EEG abnormalities and succeeded by complete amnesia for the episode (Bental 1958). Cases have been reported from Barbados with an unusual hallucinatory syndrome in which bizarre smells were experienced (Lloyd-Still 1958). Other forms include spinal and radicular syndromes, transverse myelopathy and ascending motor and sensory disturbances

of the Guillain–Barré type (Flewett & Hoult 1958; Wells 1971). Severe, non-specific, transient, neurological sequelae have been reported after the influenza type B epidemic in Chicago in 1971 (Hochberg *et al.* 1975) and in Dallas in 1977 (Baine *et al.* 1980). Neuroimaging has identified widespread involvement of the cerebral cortices, subcortical white matter or thalamus, lesions in the brainstem, basal ganglia and cerebellar white matter after influenza encephalitis (Studahl 2003).

The nature of the causal relationship between these illnesses and the influenza virus remains uncertain. They are rare, even during extensive epidemics, and it is hard to exclude the possibility of coincident infection with another sporadic virus. Dunbar *et al.* (1958) estimated that their cases represented only 1 in 10 000 of the persons affected by the influenza epidemic in the area. Other possibilities are the activation of some associated neurotropic virus or the occasional development by mutation of a neurotropic strain of influenza virus. Kapila *et al.* (1958) were able to isolate influenza type A virus from the brain substance of one fatal case, but such reports are few. Examples that occur at the height of an attack may sometimes be merely attributable to the cerebral anoxia and metabolic derangements consequent on pneumonia. However, the evidence increasingly favours the view that the great majority represent an autoimmune or hypersensitivity response on the part of the brain, similar to that which occurs after other infective illnesses (see below), and precipitated by the presence of virus in the body but not necessarily within the brain (Anon. 1971). The pathology in fatal cases often supports this view by showing perivascular demyelination similar to that of postinfectious encephalitis generally.

The broader question arises of the relationship between influenza and other psychiatric disturbances that follow it. Depression appears to be common and may sometimes be unusually refractory to treatment; this has been ascribed to invasion of the brain by the influenza virus but there is no direct evidence to support the view (Anon. 1971). Psychological reactions may also be seen, and are usually ascribed to the non-specific stress of the illness and the physically weakening effects of its aftermath.

Steinberg *et al.* (1972) reopened this question by presenting a case that suggested a more direct pathophysiological relationship between the infection and a manic psychosis that followed.

The illness, in a woman of 21, began with a typical attack of influenza. After a brief remission she again became febrile, with headache, sore throat and an unproductive cough. She complained of paraesthesiae in the limbs and experienced a transient episode of blindness lasting for less than a minute. Over the next 2 weeks a typical manic illness developed, with evidence of confusion and disorientation during the first few days. The affective disturbance gradually subsided with treatment over the next few months.

Antibody titres to influenza A were abnormally high at the onset, and showed an unusually slow decline in comparison with other influenza patients while the manic illness was resolving. Despite normal findings in CSF and EEG, the authors postulated that a mild attack of influenza encephalitis had probably occurred, producing minimal brain damage which acted as an intervening factor and contributed to the subsequent affective disorder.

The evidence is clearly tenuous, but combined virological and psychiatric studies on a larger number of patients might illuminate the relationship further as Steinberg *et al.* suggest. Neuropsychological impact has been reported by Hokkanen *et al.* (1996) in a small case series of influenza type B encephalitis. The outcomes are largely favourable but further evaluation of cognitive effects is needed.

Encephalitis lethargica

An earlier generation of neurologists and psychiatrists were much concerned with this disease on account of the devastating epidemics of 1918–1920 and the chronic sequelae that occurred. From the 1930s onwards it largely disappeared, at least in its original form. Sporadic cases continue to appear in the literature with a degree of regularity (Shill & Stacy 2000; Kiley & Esiri 2001; Dale *et al.* 2004, 2007; Gonul *et al.* 2007; Raghav *et al.* 2007) but there have been no further epidemics. Strangely, no causative organism was isolated despite extensive research, and laboratory proof has never been available to uphold the diagnosis in disputed cases. This remains the case in sporadic reports of the disorder, where it has been impossible to identify viral particles in the CNS. Von Economo's assertion that influenza virus was not implicated has been borne out by examination of the archived encephalitis lethargica brain material, which has failed to reveal 1918 influenza RNA (Taubenberger *et al.* 1997; McCall *et al.* 2001). Recent interest has been directed to an autoimmune cause in light of the presence of CSF oligoclonal bands in a number of cases (Dale *et al.* 2004) and a treatment response to steroids (Blunt *et al.* 1997).

Historically, the thousands of cases available for observation displayed a wealth of psychopathological phenomena that could be clearly ascribed to pathological changes in the brain. This had an important influence on psychiatric thinking at a time when psychodynamic explanations for mental pathology were gaining significant ground. Certainly it focused attention on the relation between mental symptoms and brain structure in a way few affections of the nervous system had done before. The sequelae of the disease demonstrated that an organic basis could sometimes exist for 'functional' disturbances, including tics, psychosis, far-reaching disturbances of personality and, particularly, compulsions and other profound disturbances of will. Hendrick (1928) reviews the attempts that were made by psychiatrists of every school to capitalise on the lessons to be learned from encephalitis lethargica for understanding the neuroses and psychoses, and von Economo (1929) wrote

. . . just as we find it hard today to follow up the trend of thought of our scientific predecessors for whom bacteriology and the lore of brain localisation did not exist, future generations will hardly be able to appreciate our pre-encephalitic neurological and psychiatric conceptions, particularly with regard to so-called functional disturbances.

There is, of course, a danger that these important lessons will be forgotten with the passage of time. The clinical features of the disease are therefore described in some detail.

Encephalitis lethargica was first reported by von Economo in 1917, after a small local epidemic had led to numerous patients being seen in the Vienna Psychiatric Clinic with strange symptoms that did not fit into any known diagnostic category. The shared features were slight influenza-like prodromata followed by a variety of nervous manifestations, marked lethargy, disturbance of sleep and disturbance of ocular movement. At post-mortem the picture of microscopic foci of inflammation, particularly in the grey matter of the midbrain and basal ganglia, was sufficiently constant to suggest a common cause despite the variety of phenomena that occurred. Complete recognition followed in the great pandemic that started in London in 1918 and spread throughout Europe during the next 2 years, approximately coincident with the influenza pandemic of that time. The polymorphic forms of the disease continued to be a striking feature, fresh epidemics often running close to type and differing from those nearby both in the acute phases and in the incidence of sequelae.

There was a seasonal pattern, with most epidemics beginning in early winter. The peak incidence was in early adult life, from age 15 to 45 years, though no age group was spared. At one time a toxic agent was suspected, but the general pattern combined to suggest an airborne infective agent, gaining access via the nasopharynx and transferred by carriers or those in the presymptomatic stages of infection. The agent was shown to be filterable and the disease was transmissible to monkeys by injection of brain tissue from infected patients, but the cause itself continued to elude attempts to isolate it. It was a matter of controversy whether the coincident influenza epidemics had predisposed the host to react abnormally to some relatively innocuous organism, and some evidence suggested that the herpes virus might itself be responsible. These questions were not decisively settled, but the great majority of contemporary epidemiological evidence suggested that an independent virus was responsible.

In retrospect it appeared that this was not entirely a new disease, and similar widespread epidemics could be traced in history. von Economo was at least somewhat aware of this in that his mother recalled an epidemic of a similar stuporose disorder in Italy, the nona, in 1890–1891 and contemporary writing reported a similar illness described as the *Schlafkrankheit* in Tubingen in 1712. In England a second peak of encephalitis lethargica occurred in 1924, but thereafter there was a striking fall-off of new cases throughout the 1930s, although sporadic cases continued to be seen and small local epidemics appeared from time to time.

The following description is largely taken from von Economo's (1929) classic account.

Acute clinical picture

A prodromal stage lasting several days consisted of malaise, mild pharyngitis, headache, lassitude and low pyrexia, all symptoms being slight and resembling the prodomata of influenza. A great variety of nervous symptoms then appeared, depending on the localisation of the virus within the CNS.

The 'basic' form, and that most usual in sporadic cases, was the *somnolent–ophthalmoplegic* variety. Somnolence developed after the prodromal phase, with slight signs of meningeal irritation. Initially there was merely a tendency to drowsiness from which the patient could easily be roused, sometimes with evidence of confusion or mild delirium. If recovery did not occur at this stage, the disorder progressed further to more or less permanent sleep for weeks or sometimes months, often deepening to coma. On recovery, disturbances of sleep function might persist for many months during convalescence. Pareses of the cranial nerves set in early, especially of the third and sixth, with ptosis, paralysis of ocular movements and less commonly pupillary abnormalities or nystagmus. Such signs were usually persistent, but sometimes fugitive and fleeting. Facial palsy or bulbar palsy occasionally developed. In the limbs isolated pareses and reflex abnormalities were seen, with spasticity, hypotonia or ataxia.

In other cases the picture was dominated after the prodromal stage by signs of motor unrest. This was the *hyperkinetic form*, with myoclonic twitches, severe jerking chorea, wild jactitations and anxious excited behaviour. Sometimes compulsive tic-like movements, torticollis and torsion spasm appeared. Oculomotor signs and epileptic fits were common. Delirium could be marked, with constant unrest by day and night, sometimes closely resembling delirium tremens with anxiety amounting to terror in response to vivid hallucinations. Typically the acute disturbance lasted only a few days, but insomnia or reversal of sleep rhythm then usually persisted for weeks or months after recovery.

The *parkinsonian form* was characterised by rigidity and akinesis from the outset. Movements were remarkably slowed and sparse, the patient lying still for hours at a time or responding with profound psychomotor retardation. Speech, like motor movements, was greatly delayed, yet the patient could be shown to be mentally intact despite the appearance of dementia. The limbs showed increased tone and often a coarse tremor. The gait was festinant, and salivation occurred as in paralysis agitans. Catatonic phenomena could be seen, including classic flexibilitas cerea. Along with these features somnolence, sleep inversion and oculomotor signs might be in evidence. Many progressed thereafter to the chronic parkinsonian phase of the disease.

The *psychotic forms* were rare, but presented with acute psychiatric disturbance as the initial feature. Here mistakes in diagnosis frequently occurred until neurological signs declared themselves. The usual picture was of an acute organic reaction, but stupor, depression, hypomania and catatonia were also reported. Sometimes impulsive and bizarre behaviour was the sole manifestation for several days, accompanied by bewildered and fearful affect. Alternatively, mental conflicts were brought to the fore, adding a psychogenic colouring to the presenting symptoms. Several examples were reported by Sands (1928).

A woman of 28 developed a sore throat lasting a week. A few days later she became excited, rambling and impulsive and was diagnosed as suffering from manic–depressive psychosis. No neurological abnormalities were found. She became extremely fearful, asking whether she was about to die or if something terrible was going to happen to her family. She spoke irrelevantly and was very tense. The pupils were later found to be irregular with sluggish reactions, and the tendon reflexes were diminished. In the following week she developed choreiform and athetoid movements and a left facial weakness. She died a few days later after a period of disorientation, high pyrexia and noisy disturbed behaviour.

A woman of 32 suddenly became restless and noisy, sang and screamed, and claimed to be the daughter of Christ and impregnated by him. She lay in bed in a strained attitude, and was markedly deluded and uncooperative. The pupils were widely dilated and reacted sluggishly to light, and the tendon reflexes were diminished. She continued in a state of excitement for 3 days then became drowsy, with diplopia and irregularity of the pupils. Three weeks later she recovered completely.

A woman of 30 developed headache for 2 days, then became excitable, restless and uncooperative. She was admitted to hospital with a diagnosis of manic-depressive psychosis. She proved to be deluded and occasionally hallucinated, and claimed at times to be a physician or a great singer. Her temperature was found to be 38.9°C (102°F), and the CSF was under increased pressure with 6 cells/mm³. Many weeks later she developed ocular palsies and other neurological signs typical of encephalitis lethargica.

It was disputed whether some cases might run their course as a psychotic illness alone without somatic symptoms at any stage. This could neither be proved nor disproved owing to the lack of specific tests for the disease. However, in 1924 the Board of Control in the UK reported that many patients had been admitted to mental hospitals with diagnoses of non-specific confusional, delusional and hallucinatory states, yet in later years proved to show the classic sequelae of encephalitis lethargica (Anon. 1966). The psychiatric literature abounded with case reports, and arguments centred on whether the cases had been missed because the neurological signs had been mild and fleeting, or whether the disease could present as a 'cerebral' form without localised manifestations.

Other forms presented with acute bulbar palsy, or monosymptomatically with intense chorea, persistent hiccough or neuritis. Abortive types were common in most epidemics, with symptoms capable of arousing suspicion during the epidemic but easily overlooked at other times. During the acute phase there was usually rapid debility and loss of weight. Fever might accompany the prodromal phase or persist throughout, while other cases ran their whole course without pyrexia. A moderate leucocytosis was often present but was not invariable. Examination of the CSF was not in any way decisive, although most cases showed some abnormalities. Many abortive cases developed only the prodrome, while others recovered early after definite symptoms and signs had appeared. Some ran a fulminating course with death after a few days or weeks. Usually, however, the acute disturbances lasted for several weeks, with some months more before ocular palsies, lethargy and sleep disturbances resolved.

A protracted convalescence was not uncommon, with repeated relapses and fresh exacerbations. Convalescence also brought prolonged asthenic states, incapacitating depressive illness and a variety of sleep disturbances: insomnia, sleep inversion and narcoleptic phenomena.

On recovery, focal neurological abnormalities might persist. Paralysis of external ocular movements or of isolated eye muscles was frequently permanent, also pupillary abnormalities, difficulty with accommodation and inability to converge the eyes. Hemiparesis, aphasia or other focal cerebral symptoms might remain, likewise chorea, tics, torticollis or epilepsy. Hypothalamic damage was seen in adiposity, menstrual disturbance, impotence or precocious puberty. However, the outstanding sequelae were parkinsonism and changes of personality as considered below.

Altogether in clinically well-marked acute cases, some 40% ended fatally, 40% were left with residual deficits and 20% recovered completely. Approximately half of those with residual deficits were permanently disabled from working, mostly on account of progressive parkinsonian symptoms (von Economo 1929).

Chronic sequelae

The most seriously disabling sequelae consisted of parkinsonian developments, change of personality and mental defect. Severe psychiatric illnesses were also seen. The incidence of each varied in different epidemics, but a definite relationship emerged with regard to the age at which the acute infection had occurred. Adults tended to develop parkinsonism, children personality disturbances, and infants were left with mental defect. Generalised dementia did not appear to occur when the mature brain had been affected.

Parkinsonism sometimes developed gradually out of the acute stage, or could set in unexpectedly after full recovery. In the interval the patient may have shown persistent symptoms such as headache, irritability and sleep disturbance but this was by no means invariable. Indeed as time went by it became apparent that sequelae could develop after many months or years of completely normal health. In contrast, personality change and mental defect were usually evident immediately after the acute infection. The severity of sequelae was unrelated to the severity of the original attack.

Postencephalitic parkinsonism

This was the most common sequel and could develop even when parkinsonian symptoms had been absent during the acute phase. Its development was usually insidious, with weakness and slowing of movements or the gradual development of a stiff and unnatural posture. The ensuing picture closely resembled other forms of parkinsonism, with masklike face, stooping posture, festinant gait and excessive salivation. Tremor was less common than in paralysis agitans; the typical pill-rolling tremor was rarely seen, but coarser tremor and violent shaking of the limbs occasionally occurred.

Paucity of movement was sometimes a striking sign even in the absence of paresis or marked rigidity. It appeared that in large degree this represented a *primary disturbance of willed movement*, such that the patient was unable to supply the volitional impulse despite a wish to perform. There might be much difficulty in passing from rest to activity, the patient remaining for minutes on end in a state of trance-like immobility. Or a movement once started might freeze halfway, as when raising a spoon to the mouth. Later typical rigidity developed, with extrapyramidal increase of tone that was obvious on examination. Characteristically, the akinesis and the rigidity could vary markedly, improving at some stage during the day, or allowing some activities while preventing others that required exactly the same musculature. Speech became slurred, jerky and monotonous, and writing was often strikingly small and cramped (micrographia).

Other distinctive features were *repetitive motor phenomena* in the form of tics, blepharospasm, torticollis, spells of sighing and yawning, or complex respiratory spasms. Complicated motor stereotypies developed in advanced cases, for example stamping of the feet accompanied by writhing movements of the head and neck. Speech might show marked repetitive phenomena: of a phrase (echolalia), word (pallilalia) or syllable (logoclonia).

A *compulsive element* was often very prominent indeed, and emerged in speech and thought as well as in motor behaviour. A repeated phrase or question might accompany the motor movements, or the latter might be 'subjectivated' in a characteristic fashion; the patient would state 'I have got to move my hand that way' rather than 'I have a twitch in my hand' as would be the case with ordinary tics. Compulsive thoughts and urges also appeared independently of the motor phenomena, with the patient ruminating endlessly on restricted themes or being driven to complex rituals. Compulsive urges sometimes led to trouble with the law, for example with repeated episodes of indecent exposure. Claude *et al.* (1927) reported patients with compulsions to tear their clothes, pull out teeth, tie themselves with bonds and to strangle cats; they stressed the abrupt appearance of the obsessions, their fixity over time and the patient's clear awareness of the absurdity of the acts. It is of considerable theoretical interest that motor and psychological features of compulsion should so regularly have occurred together and in intimate association. Schilder (1938) considered that the compulsive phenomena could often be directly traced to motor sources. The encephalitic process liberated motor impulses, with a tendency towards impulsive actions of a sadistic nature, and when checked these led in turn to the compulsions.

Oculogyric crises were another characteristic feature, again often intimately associated with compulsive phenomena. For a few minutes, or rarely hours, the eyes would deviate upwards or to the side, perhaps with contortions of the head, neck and extremities. Flushing and other autonomic disturbances were common accompaniments. At the onset the patient might be beset by some obsessive thought or enact some complex compulsive ritual. The crisis was sometimes accompanied by a fugue-like mental state, with inability to speak and lack of response to commands, or by marked affective disturbance: surges of depression, anxiety or fear, ideas of reference or feelings of persecution. Schwab *et al.* (1951) mention a patient whose episodes of paranoia were localised

to one side of her body during oculogyric crises: she felt that everything and everybody on her left were hostile and unfriendly, whereas the environment on her right was normal. When the attack was over her thinking returned to normal. Suggestibility was sometimes found to be an important factor, oculogyric attacks being provoked by talking about them or terminating in response to a sharp command. Attacks could also be precipitated by annoyance, shock or grief, and could be contagious in a ward of patients similarly affected. Thus again we see the complex admixture of motor and psychological phenomena that characterised the disease.

The typical mental state in postencephalitic parkinsonism was of marked slowing (bradyphrenia) and lack of the normal fluidity of thought, though otherwise with good preservation of mental clarity. Depression was common, in the early stages at least, and suicide was frequent. Torpor, irritability and disinclination for activity usually accompanied the compulsive elements of the disease (psychasthenia). Later, apathy became the striking emotional feature, with marked difficulty in arousing an affective reaction and little evidence of subjective distress. The parkinsonism itself usually advanced steadily, sometimes with intermittent progressions, but sometimes came to a halt with fixed residual defect. The combination of physical and mental disabilities inevitably meant that a large number of victims were permanently incapacitated for work, and such patients came to form a substantial proportion of the chronic mental hospital population. Oliver Sacks (1973) has provided a striking account of the remarkable motor and behavioural abnormalities encountered in a group of very long-term institutionalised survivors in the USA, and of the effects of attempted treatment with levodopa.

Postencephalitic personality change

Children and young adolescents were mostly the victims of this serious development, but adults were not completely immune. It was estimated that approximately one-third of patients below the age of 16 developed some form of mental change after encephalitis lethargica. Frequently it was accompanied by other sequelae such as parkinsonism, sleep disturbance, obesity or other evidence of hypothalamic damage.

The common change was towards overactivity and impulsive antisocial behaviour, as though the child now had lessened control over his instinctual drives. He became excited and restless, with inability to settle at school or remain occupied at any task for long. He was talkative, importunate and disinhibited, often indulging in stealing or sexual misbehaviour. Emotional lability was marked, with cheerful affectionate behaviour one moment and outbursts of anger the next. Moral and social senses were undermined, so that the child became destructive, abusive and hard to control. There was usually no primary intellectual deficit, although as time went by education suffered severely or became impossible. Frequently the child appeared to be aware of the change in himself, to apologise repeatedly, yet immediately afterwards be compelled to err again. The subsequent course was often unfavourable, with worsening over the years leading eventually to institutionalisation. Fairweather's (1947) account of postencephalitic patients admitted to Rampton State Institution for patients with violent and dangerous propensities gives a vivid illustration of the pictures that could ensue, with repeated serious aggression, sexual perversions and self-mutilation. At puberty improvement occurred in perhaps one-third of cases. In later years some 50% developed parkinsonian changes, with ultimate benefit where the behaviour disorder was concerned (Slater & Roth 1969).

Postencephalitic psychoses

A variety of psychotic illnesses supervened in other patients on recovery from the acute stages. Depression and hypomania were relatively common, also paranoid–hallucinatory states and a variety of illnesses resembling schizophrenia. Severe hypochondriasis of 'psychotic' severity was often reported.

Hall (1929) described 18 patients from among 113 cases of encephalitis lethargica, mostly with manic–depressive psychoses or schizophrenia. They differed from the generality of psychoses in that delusions were more transient and variable, and even relatively mild depression was accompanied by profound retardation and immobility. Fairweather (1947) noted that 25% of men and 12% of women admitted to Rampton after encephalitis lethargica were deluded, mainly in a paranoid fashion.

Davison and Bagley (1969) review the evidence concerning schizophrenia. Paranoid–hallucinatory psychoses were estimated to occur in 15–30% of postencephalitics, and psychoses indistinguishable from paraphrenia or dementia praecox in 10% of those admitted to mental hospitals. All reported patients were selected for psychiatric disorder so the true frequency is unknown, but clearly such developments were not uncommon. Davison and Bagley's analysis of 40 cases from the literature revealed only one with a schizoid premorbid personality and two with family histories of schizophrenia, discounting the view that there was usually a predisposition towards the disorder.

Present-day encephalitis lethargica

It would be a matter of some importance if sporadic cases of the disease were common and indeed some authors have suggested that the disease continues at a low endemic rate (Dale *et al.* 2007). This raises the possibility that there may be a substantial chance that the diagnosis could be overlooked, especially with mild affections, yet the sequelae might still dictate considerable psychiatric disability. The problem is difficult to resolve: the laboratory findings were variable when the disease was epidemic, and specific confirmatory tests were not achieved.

Recently, however, the suggestion that the present-day encephalitis lethargica phenotype may be immune-mediated has gathered momentum. Dale *et al.* (2004) reported 20 cases, including two adults, with a classical neuropsychiatric presentation. Over half of these cases had suffered pharyngitis or tonsillitis prior to developing the illness, with an associated positive anti-streptolysin-O titre in two-thirds. None had evidence of viral encephalitis. The CSF showed elevated protein and oligoclonal IgG bands, previously also noted by Howard and Lees (1987), Blunt *et al.* (1997) and Kiley and Esiri (2001). Neuroimaging in 40% revealed inflammatory changes in basal ganglia and midbrain tegmentum. These changes were shown to resolve on recovery. Perhaps most interestingly, anti-basal ganglia antibodies were identified on Western blot in 95% of cases, with similar immunohistochemistry to Sydenham's chorea. Giovannoni and Martino (2004) have suggested that encephalitis lethargica is likely part of the spectrum of immune-mediated neuropsychiatric sequelae of streptococcal infections that also includes PANDAS (paediatric autoimmune neuropsychiatric disorders associated with *Streptococcus*) (Swedo *et al.* 1998).

Most recently, Dale *et al.* (2007) identified two hyperkinetic cases with impulsive and compulsive behaviours, rabbit-like orofacial dyskinesia and sensitivity to neuroleptics as well as dopamimetic drugs. They suggest dopamine depletion followed by dopamine-receptor hypersensitivity as a neurochemical model for encephalitis lethargica.

Dewar and Wilson (2005), in reporting a further case, review the cognitive outcomes of contemporary reports of encephalitis lethargica. They identify the limited formal evaluation of neuropsychological outcomes in the majority of case reports and go on to identify impaired executive function, concept formation, complex mental flexibility, verbal abstraction and non-verbal recall in their patient. They advocate the importance of cognitive rehabilitation.

Blunt *et al.* (1997) identified the benefit of steroids and levodopa in two cases.

One patient had a psychosis and a mute–akinetic syndrome associated with myoclonus. The second patient presented with a psychosis and fever, developing severe dyskinesias involving the mouth, trunk and limbs, together with respiratory irregularities and presumed hypothalamic disturbance and disturbance of consciousness. In both cases, initial CSF examination revealed an elevated white cell count (predominantly lymphocytes), elevated protein in case 2, and oligoclonal bands in both cases. CT of the brain was normal but in both cases EEG revealed diffuse slow-wave activity. ^{18}F-dopa PET in case 2 was normal. In case 1, levodopa improved the akinesia, while the myoclonus responded to clonazepam. In case 2, the severe dyskinesias failed to respond to a number of drugs, and she ultimately required paralysis to relieve her almost continuous movements. Both patients responded rapidly and dramatically to intravenous methylprednisolone.

Rail *et al.* (1981) reviewed eight further examples occurring during the preceding two decades, some presenting with prominent psychiatric features. Pathological examination of the brain in two patients showed extensive loss of neurones from the substantia nigra and locus coeruleus, along with widespread neurofibrillary changes elsewhere in the brainstem, dentate nuclei and corpus striatum. They stressed that the diagnosis still rested essentially on the clinical features, and suggested that the following criteria be applied: an encephalitic illness, parkinsonism developing acutely or after a delay of months or years, alteration in the sleep cycle, oculogyric crises that are not drug induced, ocular or pupillary changes, respiratory disturbances, involuntary movements, corticospinal tract signs and mental abnormalities. While these represent the specific features of encephalitis lethargica, it is clear that not all will be present in every case.

Johnson and Lucey (1987) have reported two suspected examples in young men, both presenting with severe catatonic stupor in the setting of depressive psychosis. One had a low-grade pyrexia and the other showed blepharospasm and complex compulsive rituals.

The debate concerning latter-day examples was extended by Hunter and Jones (1966), who argued that sporadic cases might be appearing in mild or attenuated form and with clinical pictures increasingly dominated by psychiatric manifestations. Consequently, the neurological signs on which the diagnosis depends could readily be overshadowed. They reported six possible cases seen during a 3-month period in a psychiatric hospital. All had presented with psychiatric syndromes, and all had initially been seen at general hospitals where diagnoses of hypomania, depression and anxiety neurosis had been applied.

Two were admitted in a state of excitement and confusion, two after overdoses of sleeping pills, one in a catatonic state and one at his own request on account of feeling ill and 'nervous'. Most had a history of progressive personality change over the course of several months, with irritability, emotionality, perplexed–paranoid developments and impaired memory and concentration. They complained of malaise, headache, lethargy, hypersomnia, insomnia, giddiness, blurred and double vision, and altered taste and smell. All had worsened in the week or two before admission, with increasing agitation and depression, paranoid and bizarre bodily delusions, and nocturnal excitement and hallucinosis.

On examination all showed some degree of mental confusion, three had mild pyrexia and all had some ocular abnormality. A variety of other neurological signs were present, often fluctuating from day to day. The authors suggested that the range of symptoms and presumed cerebral localisation was strongly reminiscent of encephalitis lethargica.

It is extremely difficult to evaluate these examples, but perhaps encephalitic antecedents should more often be considered in the differential diagnosis of psychiatric patients. Hunter *et al.* (1969) pursued the question further by examining the CSF in 256 patients admitted to a psychiatric unit. More than one-quarter showed minor biochemical abnormalities and some who underwent serial measures showed a return to normality when the clinical condition improved.

Leigh (1946) and Espir and Spalding (1956) reported other cases in the context of acute influenza.

A police cadet of 16 developed headache and later that afternoon was found unconscious in bed. An hour later he was confused and talked nonsense. In the evening he lost consciousness again and was admitted to the Radcliffe Infirmary, Oxford. On examination he responded to painful stimulation but did not speak. There was a pyrexia of 37.8°C (100°F) and some nasal discharge. Myoclonic twitching was observed around the mouth and in the limbs. The pupils were unresponsive to light and the right eye was deviated laterally. All limbs were flaccid with normal tendon reflexes but with bilateral extensor plantar responses. The CSF was under pressure (240 mmHg) but showed normal constituents. The white blood count was normal. EEG showed a generalised disturbance but no focal abnormalities. The fever subsided next day but the level of consciousness fluctuated over the next 3 weeks. There were almost continuous involuntary movements of chewing, swallowing, yawning and writhing of the limbs. He was occasionally incontinent of urine. The pupils became unequally dilated, conjugate movements of the eyes were defective in vertical directions, and slight left facial weakness appeared.

Thereafter he slowly recovered and was discharged 2 months after the onset. He was still almost completely mute and apt to have crying spells, but within the next few weeks he was speaking normally and returned to work a month or two later. During the next 18 months he complained of undue sleepiness by day and was treated with dexamfetamine sulphate. In other respects he seemed to have recovered completely. Subsequently, however, he committed a series of crimes, mainly of a violent and unpremeditated nature and with little attempt at concealment. Previously he had been of exemplary character. The legal proceedings which followed brought him under medical supervision some 4 years after the initial illness. He then described episodes lasting 15–20 minutes during which his eyes involuntarily turned upwards and to the right in a manner strongly suggestive of oculogyric crises. There was occasional titubation of the head, his facial expression was stiff and there was slight cogwheel rigidity of the upper limbs.

Espir and Spalding support their diagnosis of encephalitis lethargica by pointing out that such a picture is rarely produced by the many known types of present-day viral encephalitis. Ophthalmoplegia is rare with other varieties, and parkinsonism a distinctly uncommon complication. The prolonged sleep disturbance during convalescence was also typical.

It is also worth considering whether encephalitic processes may have contributed to the prevalence of 'catatonia' in earlier psychiatric practice. Mahendra (1981) reviews the decline of 'catatonic schizophrenia' over the past 40 years, and suggests that many examples in the earlier literature may have owed much to a viral, and possibly an encephalitic, origin. Present-day catatonia, when it occurs, may be seen in association with an impressive range of physical conditions, ranging from brain lesions and infections to toxic and metabolic disorders (Gelenberg 1976). In the absence of clearly organic determinants it appears now to be associated with affective disorder very much more commonly than with schizophrenia (Abrams & Taylor 1976).

Meningitis

Meningeal infection is less liable to lead to diagnostic problems than encephalitis. In most varieties pyrexia and neck stiffness are soon in evidence, headache is marked and lumbar puncture rapidly confirms the diagnosis. Tuberculous meningitis is the important exception, sometimes presenting with insidious and ill-defined mental changes as described below. Enduring sequelae are also less common after meningitis than encephalitis provided full and effective treatment has been instituted early. Three varieties are discussed: bacterial meningitis, aseptic meningitis and tuberculous meningitis.

Bacterial meningitis

The principal organisms responsible are *Neisseria meningitidis*, *Streptococcus pneumoniae*, *Staphylococcus aureus*,

Haemophilus influenzae and *E. coli*. In a nationwide study of community-acquired meningitis in the Netherlands, van de Beek *et al.* (2004) identified that among adults *N. meningitidis* accounted for 37% of cases and *Strep. pneumoniae* 51%. The introduction of a conjugated vaccine for *Haemophilus* has had a significant impact on the number of such cases in the developed world (Schuchat *et al.* 1997).

Headache is usually the presenting feature, with pyrexia and rapidly increasing evidence of general ill health. Vomiting, photophobia and irritability are common from an early stage. Fits are frequent in children but rare in adults. Mental disturbance takes the form of an acute organic reaction, with drowsiness extending to coma and sometimes hallucinations, excitement and other features of delirium.

Neck stiffness and a positive Kernig's sign are important confirmatory features. Pupillary abnormalities and oculomotor palsies are common, slight incoordination or tremor may appear in the limbs, and the tendon reflexes are sluggish. The plantar reflexes are sometimes upgoing. Van de Beek *et al.* (2004) found that 95% of their cohort presented with at least two of the four cardinal symptoms: headache, fever, neck stiffness and altered mental status.

The CSF is under increased pressure and is often cloudy or frankly purulent. Polymorphonuclear cells may number thousands per cubic millimetre, and the protein is raised. The causative organisms may be cultured or demonstrated on films.

Bacterial meningitis can result in damage to both cortical and subcortical areas and neurological outcomes are obviously dependent on the degree and location of injury. In a study in England and Wales, Bedford *et al.* (2001) described outcomes in 1584 children who had meningitis at age 5 and who had been treated for the disease and survived. In this group 1.8% had died within 5 years and there was a 10-fold increased risk of having moderate to severe disability: 7.5% had learning disability, 8.1% motor disability, 7.3% seizures, 25.8% hearing impairment and 12% behavioural disturbance. Those with pneumococcal infection had higher rates of significant disability than those infected with *Haemophilus* or *N. meningitidis*. Impairments have been shown to persist into adolescence, 7 years after early meningitis. Grimwood *et al.* (2000) reported that of their cohort of 109 children, 9% continued to have major neurological, hearing or learning disability and 30% had less severe impairments compared with 11% of controls.

In adults, Hoogman *et al.* (2007) conducted a large, prospective, multicentre investigation of cognitive outcome in adult survivors of meningitis. Thirty-two per cent had cognitive impairment, with those who had survived pneumococcal infection performing poorly on memory tasks and psychomotor speed compared with those who had been treated for meningococcal meningitis. Cognitive slowness was stable over time after acute infection, and male sex and cranial nerve involvement were predictors of poor cognitive outcomes. The prevalence of cognitive disturbance was similar for both pneumococcal and meningococcal infection.

In another study, over 70% of adult survivors had neurological and mental symptoms at 3 years after acute infection, with poorer outcomes in those infected by *Strep. pneumoniae* (Merkelbach *et al.* 2000). There were again reductions in psychomotor speed as well as concentration, visuoconstructive capacity and visual memory and generally lower psychometric performance scores compared with verbal subscales. The pattern was consistent with that observed in subcortical cognitive disorders. Interestingly, Beck Depression Inventory scores in this group were significantly higher than in the controls and did not correlate with neuropsychological test results. Similarly, increased risk of cognitive slowness or cognitive disorder has been corroborated in other studies and many report that *Strep. pneumoniae* may be particularly implicated (van de Beek *et al.* 2002; Weisfelt *et al.* 2006a,b), although the most recent and statistically powerful sample does not support such a difference (Hoogman *et al.* 2007).

In adults, mild but prolonged depression is common during convalescence, no doubt partly as a reaction to the stress of the illness. A period of fatigue and inefficiency may precede full recovery, and loss of libido may last for several months. Pai (1945) investigated 51 adults after meningococcal meningitis, all of whom were seen in a neuropsychiatric unit. Sulphonamides had been used in the treatment of some but not all cases. Sixteen patients showed intellectual deterioration or organic change of personality, and these were the ones who had had severe meningitis with marked delirium. In the other 35 patients psychogenic factors seemed to predominate. Disorders of gait and hysterical paresis had often set in after complete recovery and could be related to external stress. Depression was almost universal. Evidence of premorbid instability could often be discerned, but not in every case. Four patients had developed obsessional disorders for the first time. Other symptoms such as headache, blackouts and temporary loss of memory were occasionally hard to apportion to psychogenic or physiogenic causes.

Aseptic meningitis (acute benign lymphocytic meningitis)

Broadly speaking, aseptic meningitis can be defined as any type of meningitis where CSF bacterial cultures are negative. Viral meningitis is by far the most common aetiology, with the enteroviruses (including poliomyelitis, coxsackievirus and echovirus) being most frequently incriminated in some 80% of cases (Rotbart *et al.* 2004; Lee & Davies 2007). In their study of the causes of aseptic meningitis and encephalitis in an adult population, Kupila *et al.* (2006) reported confirmed diagnoses in only 50% of cases, highlighting often inconclusive investigations. Enterovirus infection accounted for 46% of cases, HSV-2 31%, and VZV 8%. Other viral causes include

acute lymphocytic choriomeningitis virus, EBV and other herpes viruses. HIV infection must also be borne in mind (see Acquired immunodeficiency syndrome, earlier). Non-viral causes must also be considered, including the early stages of tuberculous meningitis, brain abscess, neurosyphilis, leptospirosis and particularly incomplete treatment of bacterial meningitis. There are a number of non-infectious causes to consider as well: iatrogenic (including post vaccination and medication-related cases), collagen vascular disorders, sarcoid and neoplastic disease (Kumar 2005).

Viral meningitis occurs across the lifespan but is particularly common in younger children. The incidence in those aged over 16 in the large 1966 birth cohort from Finland was 7.6 per 100 000 (Kupila *et al.* 2006). Cases occur in small epidemics and also arise sporadically. Epidemics are commoner in the summer and autumn when the circulation of enteroviruses among the population reaches a peak.

The onset is abrupt with symptoms similar to those of bacterial meningitis, but most illnesses are mild, running a course of 2–10 days then subsiding spontaneously. General malaise may persist for several weeks thereafter. Occasionally, the meningitic symptoms and the CSF abnormalities persist much longer and tuberculous meningitis may then be diagnosed in error.

The CSF is under increased pressure and contains 50–1000 cells/mm^3, of which most are lymphocytes. The protein is elevated but the chloride and glucose content are usually normal. CSF cell count does not reliably differentiate bacterial and viral aseptic meningitis. Dubos *et al.* (2006) suggest that the combination of CSF protein and serum procalcitonin may be helpful discriminators between bacterial and aseptic causes in children up to 16 years old. Testing of the CSF with PCR is commonly undertaken for enteroviruses, herpesviruses and VZV. Positive identification of a viral cause has an impact on antibiotic prescribing and length of hospital stay (Ramers *et al.* 2000).

Enduring sequelae are distinctly rare, except for the paralysis that follows poliomyelitis and some infections with coxsackievirus type A7. On the other hand, minor temporary debilities are fairly common during convalescence. Muller *et al.* (1958) carried out a long-term follow-up of a large group of cases of aseptic meningitis and 'meningoencephalitis of unknown cause', and compared them with controls from the normal population. No major differences could be found with regard to mental symptoms, occupation, school performance or social adjustment. Of 238 patients, only four were definitely mentally disordered with impaired capacity for work, two had epilepsy, two had tonic pupils and two had endocrine disorder. There appears to be no increase in chronic fatigue following viral meningitis as opposed to other viral infections and it seems to be predicted by psychiatric morbidity and prolonged convalescence rather than by the severity of the viral illness itself (Hotopf *et al.* 1996).

Tuberculous meningitis

In 1998, the WHO reported that some 2000 million people across the world were infected with tuberculosis, although only 10% presented with clinical manifestations. Tuberculous meningitis, in contrast to its pulmonary and other extrapulmonary counterparts, had predominantly been a disease of the young. However, in HIV-positive subjects, the risk of infection with tuberculosis increases to one in three (Selwyn *et al.* 1989) and there is also a contingent increase in cases of tuberculous meningitis (Bishburg *et al.* 1986) that correlate with decreasing CD4 counts (DeCock 1997).

The macroscopic cerebral pathology is characteristic. A yellowish, gelatinous, inflammatory exudate forms mainly at the base of the brain in the anterior basal cisterns, brainstem and cerebellum and extending along the lateral sulci. The basal exudate is often organised and adherent, obstructing the flow of CSF and leading to hydrocephalus and also damage to efferent cranial nerves. Arteritis is prominent in large and small vessels and areas of infarction may occur. Miliary tubercles are visible on the leptomeninges and along the principal cerebral arteries. Microscopically, the inflammatory reaction can be seen to involve the floor of the third ventricle but is usually nowhere pronounced. The neurones show degenerative changes and old caseous foci can often be found in the substance of the brain.

This more than any other form of meningitis is liable to lead to diagnostic error. Thwaites and Hien (2005) have reviewed the diagnostic and treatment dilemmas at length. The onset is insidious, fever is low grade and often considerably delayed, and neck stiffness can be very slight. Meningism is not characteristically reported, with only 2% presenting these symptoms initially. Many of the clinical features are non-specific, making it difficult to arrive at the diagnosis on history and examination alone (Kent *et al.* 1993; Hosoglu *et al.* 1998). Recent exposure and extrameningeal tuberculosis are features that may increase suspicion (Karstaedt *et al.* 1998).

A prodromal phase of vague ill health is usual, lasting for 2–3 weeks or longer. Anorexia is marked (60–80%), but headache may be transient or even absent at this stage. Mental changes form an integral part of the picture, typically apathy, irritability and insidious change of personality. As long ago as 1868, Trousseau stressed that 'sadness setting in unaccountably is a premonitory sign of great value in a child'. Williams and Smith (1954) found that the earliest mental changes in their cases were often so gradual that they were imperceptible except to those who knew the patient well beforehand. A change towards clouded awareness was usually the first definite sign, the patient lying quietly and without apprehension. In one case the presenting symptom was of subjective impairment of memory.

As the disease progresses, headache (50–80%) intensifies and low-grade pyrexia develops. Focal signs appear in the form of palsies of cranial nerves III (5–15%), VI (30–40%) and VII (10–20%), coarse tremor of the limbs and reflex abnormalities. Hemiplegia (10–20%) or other gross neurological defects may occur, and seizures present in around 50% of children and 5% of adults. Papilloedema is a late development, but choroidal tubercles are seen in the retina in up to 20% of cases (Wiles 1993b). These are rounded or oval yellow patches, approximately half the size of the optic disc.

The CSF is under increased pressure, with a lymphocytosis of 100–1000 cells/mm^3. The protein is increased in the majority of cases, the sugar is reduced in around 70% and the chloride also much reduced. Atypical CSF findings are not uncommon in those who have HIV and sometimes also in the elderly. The diagnosis is confirmed when tubercle bacilli can be identified or cultured from the fluid, but this is not achieved in every case: if there is strong diagnostic suspicion, analysis should be repeated. Large volumes of CSF may be required (10 mL is recommended). CSF culture of mycobacteria is the gold standard investigation but takes up to 8 weeks.

Computed tomography and MRI may show hydrocephalus, oedema, tuberculomata, focal infarcts and exudate in basal brain cisterns. The latter two are highlighted by gadolinium-enhanced T1-weighted images, making MRI preferable (Rovira *et al.* 1980; Bhargava *et al.* 1982; Bullock & Welchman 1982; Tartaglione *et al.* 1998). Nonetheless, it is unclear whether neuroimaging is effective in discriminating between tuberculous meningitis and other cerebral pathology. MRI is considered to be preferential to CT in identifying brainstem and cerebellar pathology.

The mental abnormalities increase, with drowsiness, confusion, disorientation and inability to sustain a rational conversation. Characteristically, the patient sleeps when alone but becomes disturbed when roused, in contrast to the perpetual 'silent struggling delirium' of purulent meningitis. Occasionally the patient is hallucinated and wildly delirious. The terror may resemble that of delirium tremens, or Wernicke's encephalopathy may be simulated when the onset is abrupt and oculomotor palsies are present. Formerly, typhoid was often suggested by the combination of headache, fever and delirium.

Without treatment progressive hydrocephalus develops, coma (30–60%) supervenes and the patient dies in a state of decerebrate rigidity. The 'confusional' stage has been reported to evolve during treatment to an 'amnesic' stage which may last for many weeks. Williams and Smith (1954) have described this picture in detail. Throughout the amnesic phase the patient is usually euphoric and shows little concern about his memory difficulties (neurosyphilis is important in the differential diagnosis; see Syphilis of the CNS in this chapter). Some, however, are withdrawn, negativistic, paranoid or acutely depressed. During recovery, memory continues to lag behind improvement in other intellectual faculties. Retention of current events improves gradually, or occasionally returns with dramatic suddenness. The period of retrograde amnesia meanwhile steadily contracts towards the time of onset of the illness.

With cure of the infection, as judged by the return of the CSF to normal, there is usually a complete restitution of normal memory functions, although a persistent amnesic gap remains for the period of overt confusion and disorientation. Williams and Smith followed 19 cases for periods of up to 4 years; none showed measurable defects of intellect, personality or memorising ability, although four complained of subjective forgetfulness for minor day-to-day events. Three others complained of slight impairment of concentration or were said by their relatives to show a lessened sense of responsibility. However, all were amnesic for the early weeks or months of the illness, even those who had seemed alert and rational throughout. Six had a persistent retrograde amnesia, sometimes extending for periods of months or years prior to the illness, with haziness for details, some complete gaps and inability to organise past events into the correct temporal sequence.

A young man of 22 developed severe tuberculous meningitis. He had a long and difficult illness requiring some 9 months of treatment. Three years later he was doing well in clerical work and had recently been promoted. His memorising of current experience was normal. However, he still had a substantial retrograde amnesia for events some 6 months before the clinical onset of his illness, and had entirely lost some specific skills such as typing acquired during this period. The amnesia extended also to the first 4 months of the illness itself.

With present-day management a full physical and mental recovery can usually be secured when diagnosis has been prompt. Williams and Smith (1954) found that the majority of patients returned gradually to their former efficiency. Headache or neurotic developments were conspicuous by their absence. However, when neurological complications have been grave at the height of the illness there may be residual hemiparesis, paraparesis, epilepsy or intellectual impairment in association with hydrocephalus. Blindness or visual defects may result from optic atrophy, and deafness occurs in a minority. Hypothalamic damage occasionally leads to diabetes insipidus, disturbance of sleep rhythm or precocious puberty in children.

Lorber (1961) followed the long-term results in 100 children who survived the acute illness. A large variety of sequelae were seen but the number of children seriously affected was surprisingly small. Of this group, 77 had made a complete recovery, including some with very severe neurological abnormalities during the active phase of the illness; 23 showed defects in the form of paresis, fits, deafness or blindness, sometimes with gratifying improvement over time.

Fits persisted in only eight children despite their frequency in the acute stages. Six of the 23 were profoundly mentally retarded; all of these had been under 2 years of age and severely affected when first seen, and all had major neurological sequelae. Details of treatment are fully described in an excellent review by Thwaites and Hien (2005).

Cerebral abscess

Cerebral abscesses can present with remarkably few definite signs and symptoms. Headache may be slight and intermittent but is the most common reported symptom in those able to provide a history, papilloedema is often late, focal cerebral signs can be minimal and pyrexia tends to be absent in the chronic stage. It is essential therefore to consider the diagnosis when change of temperament or mild confusion is accompanied by evidence of ill health for which no immediate cause is obvious. In a retrospective series of patients seen at Atkinson Morley Hospital for neurosurgical interventions for brain abscess, Carpenter *et al.* (2007) found that psychiatric symptoms, and particularly confusion with or without alteration of conscious level, was present from the start in 51% of cases, only closely followed by headache in 49%.

Cerebral abscess is rarely seen without a focus of infection elsewhere, although this may be well concealed. Important sources near the brain include infection of the middle ear and mastoid cells, dental infections and extension from the frontal and sphenoidal sinuses. Head injury may convey infection by direct penetration or may open up pathways from the sinuses or ear when the base of the skull is fractured. The principal extracranial source is chronic suppurative disease of the lungs and pleura: bronchiectasis, lung abscess and empyema. Less commonly the abscess results from a general pyaemic infection caused by pelvic or abdominal suppuration, osteomyelitis, boils, cellulitis or subacute bacterial endocarditis. Paradoxical embolism of infected material may occur via septal defects in patients with congenital heart disease. With extracranial sources the abscesses are often multiple. In some 20–30% of cases the extracerebral source of the abscess remains unclear (Mathiesen & Johnson 1997).

The organisms chiefly responsible are streptococci, staphylococci or *E. coli*. The developing abscess arises from an area of suppurating encephalitis that becomes progressively walled off from the surrounding brain by a fibrous and glial reaction. Inflammation of the overlying meninges varies in severity with the activity of the lesion. The abscess may grow large, with distortion and compression of surrounding brain structures, but intracranial pressure may be little disturbed because the process is so gradual.

Classic, though rarely demonstrated, symptoms are headache, vomiting and mild delirium, but these may often be submerged in the symptoms of the predisposing infection. Alternatively, the abscess may remain quiescent at the time of the original infection, and a latent interval of many months may follow before symptoms are declared. In the interim the patient shows evidence of chronic ill health: intermittent headache, malaise, loss of appetite and weight, constipation, occasional chills, depression and irritability. Ultimately, more definite signs appear, sometimes closely simulating cerebral tumour. Headache intensifies and may be paroxysmal, evidence of toxaemia increases, fits may occur and focal neurological signs are declared.

The common temporal lobe abscess is usually derived from middle ear infection. Motor signs are often very slight, and careful testing of the visual fields may be needed to display the quadrantic hemianopia. Dysphasic symptoms may be detected with abscesses of the dominant lobe. The alternative route from the middle ear is to the cerebellum. Signs can again be slight, with nystagmus, hypotonia and incoordination of the ipsilateral limbs, or cranial nerve pareses from involvement of the nearby brainstem. Frontal lobe abscesses arise from sinus infection or frontal fracture, and may lack all focal signs apart from unilateral anosmia. Concentration and memory may be markedly impaired and personality change much in evidence. In all such cases signs of raised intracranial pressure can be slight or absent, even with very large abscesses, and papilloedema may be late.

Some degree of aseptic meningitis may produce obvious neck stiffness on examination. Examination of the CSF rarely helps diagnosis and can be fatal if intracranial pressure is increased. CT has revolutionised the diagnosis of cerebral abscess, locating the abscess and allowing determination of its size and mass effect and whether the ventricles have been breached by the lesion (Moorthy & Rajshekhar 2008). The abscess is revealed after scan enhancement and has a characteristic appearance: the capsule shows as a ring-shaped area of increased density surrounded by cerebral oedema. MRI appearances are often specific enough for exact diagnosis – the capsule forming a discrete isointense or hyperintense ring surrounding a central cavity (Sze & Zimmerman 1988). Nonetheless, MRI is rarely necessary for diagnosis in preference to CT, other than in identifying the early cerebritis stages of abscess formation.

Treatment of cerebral abscess involves aspiration and excision followed by antibiotic therapy (Bernardini 2004; Moorthy & Rajshekhar 2008). With modern management the mortality has fallen progressively and the success rate for treatment is around 90%. Some degree of permanent incapacity may nonetheless persist, and epilepsy is liable to develop in up to 70% of cases. Intraventricular rupture and low initial Glasgow Coma Scale score are associated with poor outcomes (Takeshita *et al.* 1992).

Other infective processes

Acute organic reactions may accompany many systemic infections, especially at the extremes of life. An obvious example is the delirium sometimes seen with the acute exanthemata of childhood, likewise the impairment of consciousness or delirium that occurs with pneumonia in the elderly. Slater and Roth (1969) discuss the various causes which may be operative. Cerebral anoxia often appears to be responsible, or the influence of toxins derived from the infecting microorganisms. More complex metabolic disturbances or the accumulation of toxic intermediate products must sometimes be postulated. Fever itself may play a direct part.

However, in the infections considered below, there is more definite evidence of cerebral involvement by the disease process itself. The conditions are dealt with briefly, and textbooks of general medicine should be consulted for further details.

Lyme disease

Lyme disease is caused by the spirochaete *Borrelia burgdorferi*, which is transmitted to humans through tick bites. It occurs in several regions of the USA and Europe, and cases have recently been reported from the UK, especially the New Forest area. It can lead to cutaneous, neurological, arthritic and cardiac manifestations, although the course is usually benign and self-limiting. The clinical pictures encountered are described by Burgdorfer (1987), and British experience of the disease is summarised by Bateman and White (1990) and O'Connell (1995).

The tick bite is followed by a characteristic rash (erythema migrans), which develops after some days or weeks and is often the pointer to the diagnosis. This consists of a spreading annular erythema that extends slowly outwards, usually on the trunk or limbs. It may be accompanied by systemic disturbances such as fever, headache or backache.

Neurological manifestations develop in some 15% of cases during the ensuing weeks or months, or can be the presenting feature. Eight cases from the New Forest region were described by Bateman *et al.* (1988). Some show a chronic low-grade meningitis with persistent headache and dizziness, others intense burning radicular pains and/or lower motor neurone facial palsies (Bannwarth's syndrome). Focal neurological signs and seizures may indicate brain parenchymal involvement. Complete recovery is the rule, though cases of chronic progressive encephalomyelitis have been reported in Europe and a syndrome resembling multiple sclerosis in the USA. Occasional patients are left with chronic fatigue and sometimes mild neuropsychological impairments. Recurrent attacks of arthritis may affect both large and small joints, and a transient myocarditis may occur, but these have been rare in the UK.

When the diagnosis is suspected, serological tests for antibodies to *B. burgdorferi* should be carried out (O'Connell 1995). False negatives and false positives can occur, but rising titres over several weeks may give definitive evidence of the infection. The results may be positive in the CSF when the serum is negative, so lumbar puncture should be performed when there are neurological manifestations. The CSF shows pleocytosis with raised protein levels and often oligoclonal bands. The presence of borrelial DNA may be detected by PCR.

Treatment consists of penicillin or tetracycline and should be given promptly once the skin rash is detected. In the presence of neurological complications penicillin must be given parenterally, and cefotaxime may be required (Muhlemann 1992).

Typhus fever

Of the several varieties of typhus, that due to *Rickettsia prowazekii* is the most common. Epidemics are intimately associated with famines and wars and the infection is transmitted by the body louse. Mental and neurological manifestations are usually prominent, and there is abundant evidence that the causative organism invades the nervous system directly. The rickettsiae invade the endothelial cells of small blood vessels, producing foci of thrombosis and necrosis in various organs including the brain. Characteristic 'typhus nodules' consist of perivascular accumulations of glial, endothelial and phagocytic cells.

Symptoms consist of pyrexia, delirium, malaise, severe headache, cough and generalised aching. A characteristic rash appears on the fifth day of fever. More definite nervous system manifestations appear towards the end of the febrile period and are of serious import. Headache becomes continuous and periods of delirium alternate with stupor or coma. Focal signs appear in the form of hemiplegia, ataxia, bulbar dysfunction, deafness or optic neuritis. Meningeal irritation is common and the CSF shows a lymphocytosis and increased globulin. Among survivors evidence of cerebral damage frequently persists.

Trypanosomiasis (sleeping sickness)

The South African forms of trypanosomiasis are due to the protozoans *Trypanosoma brucei gambiense* and *T. brucei rhodesiense*. They are transmitted by the bite of the tsetse fly. An initial febrile stage consists of bouts of pyrexia, asthenia, adenitis, rashes and hepatosplenomegaly. This merges into the sleeping sickness stage, which is essentially a chronic meningoencephalitis with the organisms appearing in the CSF. The patient develops tremors, fits, incoordination or hemiplegia. Mental disturbances are prominent, with somnolence, apathy and eventually coma. Death usually occurs within a year if the disease is untreated.

Cerebral malaria

Delirium may be marked at the peaks of fever in any variety of malaria, but sometimes there is more acute and dramatic evidence of cerebral involvement. This is most common with infections due to *Plasmodium falciparum* (malignant tertian malaria). In fatal cases the brain is seen to be congested and oedematous, with numerous areas of haemorrhage and softening around vessels.

The cerebral capillaries are filled with parasites in various stages of development. The cerebral symptoms usually appear in the second or third week of the illness, but they may sometimes be the initial manifestation. They can be cataclysmic in onset. Severe delirium is accompanied by bursting headache and high pyrexia. The patient is often combative and excitable before coma supervenes. Fits can be the presenting feature and focal signs are common: hemiplegia, dysphasia, hemianopia or cerebellar ataxia. Retinal haemorrhages and papilloedema may occur.

The picture can simulate encephalitis, meningitis, cerebral tumour, epilepsy, cerebrovascular lesions or a variety of acute psychiatric disorders (Boshes 1947). Mistakes are particularly likely to be made in the rare examples when the patient is afebrile. Nadeem and Younis (1977) also stressed that clouding of consciousness may be absent initially. Of 39 patients admitted to a Sudanese psychiatric hospital with mental illness precipitated by physical disease, 17 proved to have malaria. Half of these showed psychiatric disturbances in clear consciousness. Thus where malaria is endemic it must be borne in mind in all patients with psychoses of acute onset, whether or not organic features are evident in the mental state.

Rapid treatment is vital, so examination of blood smears must not be delayed in suspected cases. Care must be taken to enquire about countries in which the patient may have lived or travelled whenever an acute organic reaction occurs without obvious cause. The number of cases reported in the UK has increased substantially over the years as a result of visits by businessmen and back-packers to heavily infected regions (Wyatt 1992).

Cerebral cysticercosis

The cysticercus stage of the tapeworm, usually *Taenia solium*, may occur in humans. Common sites include the skeletal muscles and the brain. The infestation is extremely common in Mexico. McCormick *et al.* (1982) and Grisolia and Wiederholt (1982) describe the typical clinical pictures.

Multiple cysts are usually present within the brain and the main damage appears to occur when the larvae begin to die. There is then an intense inflammatory reaction in an attempt to wall off the irritating process. The circulation of the CSF is often obstructed.

The usual presentation is with focal seizures, or with symptoms of raised intracranial pressure due to internal hydrocephalus. Localising signs are relatively uncommon, though sudden neurological deficits can result from infarcts. Very occasionally dementia is the presenting feature. Retinal involvement may accompany the CNS disturbance.

The CSF shows a pleocytosis including eosinophils, an increase in protein and a positive reaction to serological tests for cysticercosis. However, the latter may be negative in up to 40% of patients (McCormick *et al.* 1982). Calcification of the cysts may be seen on radiography, both within the skull and in the skeletal muscles. Neuroimaging is valuable in revealing the lesions or the resulting hydrocephalus when skull radiography is negative.

References

Abe, H., Weis, S. & Mehraein, P. (1993) Degeneration of the cerebellar dentate nucleus and the inferior olivary nucleus in HIV-1 infection: a morphometric study. *Clinical Neuropathology* **12** (suppl.), S7.

Abrams, R. & Taylor, M.A. (1976) Catatonia: a prospective clinical study. *Archives of General Psychiatry* **33**, 579–581.

Achim, C.L., Wang, R., Miners, D.K. & Wiley, C.A. (1994) Brain viral burden in HIV infection. *Journal of Neuropathology and Experimental Neurology* **53**, 284–294.

Adams, J.H. (1976) Parasitic and fungal infections of the nervous system. In: Blackwood, W. & Corsellis, J.A.N. (eds) *Greenfield's Neuropathology*, 3rd edn, ch. 7. Edward Arnold, London.

Adle-Biassette, H., Chretien, F., Wingertsmann, L. *et al.* (1999) Neuronal apoptosis does not correlate with dementia in HIV infection but is related to microglial activation and axonal damage. *Neuropathology and Applied Neurobiology* **25**, 123–133.

Adler, M.W. (1987) ABC of AIDS. Development of the epidemic. *British Medical Journal* **294**, 1083–1085.

Albert, S.M., Marder, K., Dooneief, G. *et al.* (1995) Neuropsychological impairment in early HIV infection: a risk factor for work disability. *Archives of Neurology* **52**, 525–530.

Altfeld, M., Addo, M.M., Rosenberg, E.S. *et al.* (2003) Influence of HLA-B57 on clinical presentation and viral control during acute HIV-1 infection. *AIDS* **17**, 2581–2591.

An, S.F. & Scaravilli, F. (1997) Early HIV-1 infection of the central nervous system. *Archives d'Anatomie et de Cytologie Pathologiques* **45**, 94–105.

An, S.F., Giometto, B. & Scaravilli, F. (1996) HIV-1 DNA in brains in AIDS and pre-AIDS: correlation with the stage of disease. *Annals of Neurology* **40**, 611–617.

Ances, B.M., Shellhaus, R., Brown, M.J., Rios, O.V., Herman, S.T. & French, J.A. (2004) Neurosyphilis and status epilepticus: case report and literature review. *Epilepsy Research* **59**, 67–70.

Ances, B.M., Letendre, S., Buzzell, M. *et al.* (2006) Valproic acid does not affect markers of human immunodeficiency virus disease progression. *Journal of Neurovirology* **12**, 403–406.

Anderson, M. (1993) Virus infections of the nervous system. In: *Brain's Diseases of the Nervous System*, 10th edn, ch. 9. Oxford University Press, Oxford.

Angelini, L., Zibordi, F., Triulzi, F. *et al.* (2000) Age-dependent neurologic manifestations of HIV infection in childhood. *Neurological Sciences* **21**, 135–142.

Anon. (1966) Leading article: Encephalitis of lethargica type in a mental hospital. *Lancet* **ii**, 1014–1015.

Anon. (1971) Leading article: Influenza and the nervous system. *British Medical Journal* **1**, 357–358.

Anon. (1978) Modified neurosyphilis. *British Medical Journal* **2**, 647–648.

Anthony, I.C., Ramage, S.N., Carnie, F.W., Simmonds, P. & Bell, J. E. (2005) Influence of HAART on HIV-related CNS disease and neuroinflammation. *Journal of Neuropathology and Experimental Neurology* **64**, 529–536.

Antinori, A., Cozzi-Lepri, A., Ammassari, A. *et al.* (2004) Relative prognostic value of self-reported adherence and plasma NNRTI/PI concentrations to predict virological rebound in patients initially responding to HAART. *Antiviral Therapy* **9**, 291–296.

Antoni, M.H., Cruess, D.G., Klimas, N. *et al.* (2005) Increases in a marker of immune system reconstitution are predated by decreases in 24-h urinary cortisol output and depressed mood during a 10-week stress management intervention in symptomatic HIV-infected men. *Journal of Psychosomatic Research* **58**, 3–13.

Arciniegas, D.B. & Anderson, C.A. (2004) Viral encephalitis: neuropsychiatric and neurobehavioral aspects. *Current Psychiatry Reports* **6**, 372–379.

Arendt, G., Giesch, H.J. & Jablonowski, H. (1998) Stavudine stops neuro-AIDS in AZT non-responders. Abstract 564/32207 presented at the XII World Conference on AIDS, Geneva, Switzerland, 1998.

Arroliga, M.E. & Pien, L. (2003) Penicillin allergy: consider trying penicillin again. *Cleveland Clinic Journal of Medicine* **70**, 313–314, 317–318, 320–321 passim.

Artigas, J., Grosse, G., Habedank, S., Heise, W. & Niedobitek, F. (1990) [Morphology of vacuolar changes in the spinal cord of AIDS patients (vacuolar myelopathy).] *Pathologe* **11**, 260–267.

Asare, E.K., Glass, J.D., Luthert, P.J. *et al.* (1995) Neuronal pattern differences in HIV-associated dementia. *Neuropathology and Applied Neurobiology* **21**, 151.

Asch, S.M., Kilbourne, A.M., Gifford, A.L. *et al.* (2003) Underdiagnosis of depression in HIV: who are we missing? *Journal of General Internal Medicine* **18**, 450–460.

Asdaghi, N., Muayqil, T., Scozzafava, J., Jassal, R., Saqqur, M. & Jeerakathil, T.J. (2007) The re-emergence in Canada of meningovascular syphilis: 2 patients with headache and stroke. *Canadian Medical Association Journal* **176**, 1699–1700.

Atkinson, J.H., Heaton, K.K., Patterson, T.L. *et al.* (2008) Two-year prospective study of major depressive disorder in HIV-infected men. *Journal of Affective Disorders* **108**, 225–234.

Avants, S.K., Margolin, A., Warburton, L.A., Hawkins, K.A. & Shi, J. (2001) Predictors of nonadherence to HIV-related medication regimens during methadone stabilization. *American Journal on Addictions* **10**, 69–78.

Baine, W.B., Luby, J.P. & Martin, S.M. (1980) Severe illness with influenza B. *American Journal of Medicine* **68**, 181–189.

Barbarotto, R., Capitani, E. & Laiacona, M. (1996) Naming deficit in herpes simplex encephalitis. *Acta Neurologica Scandinavica* **93**, 272–280.

Bateman, D.E. & White, J.E. (1990) Lyme disease. *Hospital Update* August, 677–681.

Bateman, D.E., Lawton, N.F., White, J.E., Greenwood, R.J. & Wright, D.J.M. (1988) The neurological complications of *Borrelia burgdorferi* in the New Forest area of Hampshire. *Journal of Neurology, Neurosurgery and Psychiatry* **51**, 699–703.

Baur, B., Ullner, I., Iimbinger, J., Fesl, G. & Mai, N. (2000) Music memory provides access to verbal knowledge in a patient with global amnesia. *Neurocase* **6**, 415–421.

Becker, J.T., Lopez, O.L., Dew, M.A. & Aizenstein, H.J. (2004) Prevalence of cognitive disorders as a function of age in HIV virus function. *AIDS* **18** (suppl. 1), 511–518.

Bedford, H., De Louvois, J., Halket, S., Peckham, C., Hurley, R. & Harvey, D. (2001) Meningitis in infancy in England and Wales: follow up at age 5 years. *British Medical Journal* **323**, 533–536.

Begg, M.D., Lamster, I.B., Panageas, K.S., Mitchell-Lewis, D., Phelan, J.A. & Grbic, J.T. (1997) A prospective study of oral lesions and their predictive value for progression of HIV disease. *Oral Diseases* **3**, 176–183.

Behr, J., Schaefer, M., Littmann, E., Klingebiel, R. & Heinz, A. (2006) Psychiatric symptoms and cognitive dysfunction caused by Epstein–Barr virus-induced encephalitis. *European Psychiatry* **21**, 521–522.

Beiser, C. (1997) Recent advances. HIV infection: II. *British Medical Journal* **314**, 579–583.

Bell, J.E. (1998) The neuropathology of adult HIV infection. *Revue Neurologique (Paris)* **154**, 816–829.

Bell, J.E. (2004) An update on the neuropathology of HIV in the HAART era. *Histopathology* **45**, 549–559.

Bell, J.E., Busuttil, A., Ironside, J.W. *et al.* (1993) Human immunodeficiency virus and the brain: investigation of virus load and neuropathologic changes in pre-AIDS subjects. *Journal of Infectious Diseases* **168**, 818–824.

Bell, J.E., Brettle, R.P., Chiswick, A. & Simmonds, P. (1998) HIV encephalitis, proviral load and dementia in drug users and homosexuals with AIDS. Effect on neocortical involvement. *Brain* **121**, 2043–2052.

Belman, A.L. (1994) HIV-1 associated central nervous system disease in infants and children. In: Price, R.W. & Perry, S.W. (eds) *HIV, AIDS and the Brain*, ch. 16. Association for Research in Nervous and Mental Disease, vol. 72. Raven Press, New York.

Bental, E. (1958) Acute psychoses due to encephalitis following Asian influenza. *Lancet* **ii**, 18–20.

Bernardini, G.L. (2004) Diagnosis and management of brain abscess and subdural empyema. *Current Neurology and Neuroscience Reports* **4**, 448–456.

Beyer, J.L., Taylor, L., Gersing, K.R. & Krishnan, K.R. (2007) Prevalence of HIV infection in a general psychiatric outpatient population. *Psychosomatics* **48**, 31–37.

Bhargava, S., Gupta, A.K. & Tandon, P.N. (1982) Tuberculous meningitis: a CT study. *British Journal of Radiology* **55**, 189–196.

Bing, E.G., Burnam, M.A., Longshore, D. *et al.* (2001) Psychiatric disorders and drug use among human immunodeficiency virus-infected adults in the United States. *Archives of General Psychiatry* **58**, 721–728.

Birnbaum, W., Hodgson, T.A., Reichart, P.A., Sherson, W., Nittayannanta, S.W. & Axell, T.E. (2002) Prognostic significance of HIV-associated oral lesions and their relation to therapy. *Oral Diseases* **8** (suppl. 2), 110–114.

Bishburg, E., Sunderam, G., Reichman, L.B. & Kapila, R. (1986) Central nervous system tuberculosis with the acquired immunodeficiency syndrome and its related complex. *Annals of Internal Medicine* **105**, 210–213.

Blunt, S.B., Lane, R.J., Turjanski, N. & Perkin, G.D. (1997) Clinical features and management of two cases of encephalitis lethargica. *Movement Disorders* **12**, 354–359.

Boivin, G. (2004) Diagnosis of herpesvirus infections of the central nervous system. *Herpes* **11** (suppl. 2), 48A–56A.

Booss, J. & Esiri, M.M. (1986) *Viral Encephalitis. Pathology, Diagnosis and Management*. Blackwell Scientific Publications, Oxford.

Boshes, B. (1947) Neuropsychiatric manifestations during the course of malaria: experiences in the Mediterranean theater in World War II. *Archives of Neurology and Psychiatry* **58**, 14–27.

Boughton, C.R. (1970) Neurological complications of glandular fever. *Medical Journal of Australia* **2**, 573–575.

Bouwman, F.H., Skolasky, R.L., Hes, D. *et al.* (1998) Variable progression of HIV-associated dementia. *Neurology* **50**, 1814–1820.

Boyle, A., Zafar, R., Riley, V. & Lindesay, J. (1995) Neurosyphilis presenting with dissociative symptoms. *Journal of Neurology, Neurosurgery and Psychiatry* **59**, 452–453.

Brain, W.R., Greenfield, J.G. & Russell, D.S. (1943) Discussion on recent experiences of acute encephalomyelitis and allied conditions. *Proceedings of the Royal Society of Medicine* **36**, 319–322.

Brain, W.R., Greenfield, J.G. & Russell, D.S. (1948) Subacute inclusion encephalitis (Dawson type). *Brain* **71**, 365–385.

Brannagan, T.H. III, Nuovo, G.J., Hays, A.P. & Latov, N. (1997) Human immunodeficiency virus infection of dorsal root ganglion neurons detected by polymerase chain reaction in situ hybridization. *Annals of Neurology* **42**, 368–372.

Brew, B.J., Sidtis, J.J., Rosenblum, M. & Price, R.W. (1988) AIDS dementia complex. *Journal of the Royal College of Physicians of London* **22**, 140–144.

Brew, B.J., Bhalla, R.B., Paul, M. *et al.* (1992) Cerebrospinal fluid β2-microglobulin in patients with AIDS dementia complex: an expanded series including response to zidovudine treatment. *AIDS* **6**, 461–465.

Brew, B.J., Rosenbaum, M., Cronin, K. & Price, R.W. (1995) AIDS dementia complex and HIV-1 brain infection: clinical–virological correlations. *Annals of Neurology* **38**, 559–560.

Brierley, J.B., Corsellis, J.A.N., Hierons, R. & Nevin, S. (1960) Subacute encephalitis of later adult life: mainly affecting the limbic areas. *Brain* **83**, 357–368.

British Medical Association (2006) Sexually transmitted infection update. Available at http//www.web.bma.org.uk/ap.nsf/content/stiupd06

Brodt, H.R., Kamps, B.S., Gute, P., Knupp, B., Staszewski, S. & Helm, E.B. (1997) Changing incidence of AIDS-defining illnesses in the era of antiretroviral combination therapy. *AIDS* **11**, 1731–1738.

Brouwers, P., Civitello, L., Decarli, C., Wolters, P. & Sei, S. (2000) Cerebrospinal fluid viral load is related to cortical atrophy and not to intracerebral calcifications in children with symptomatic HIV disease. *Journal of Neurovirology* **6**, 390–397.

Brown, J.L. & Vanable, P.A. (2008) Cognitive-behavioral stress management interventions for persons living with HIV: a review and critique of the literature. *Annals of Behavioral Medicine* **35**, 26–40.

Bruce-Jones, W.D.A., White, P.D., Thomas, J.M. & Clare, A.W. (1994) The effect of social adversity on the fatigue syndrome, psychiatric disorders and physical recovery, following glandular fever. *Psychological Medicine* **24**, 651–659.

Buchacz, K., Patel, P., Taylor, M. *et al.* (2004) Syphilis increases HIV viral load and decreases CD4 cell counts in HIV-infected patients with new syphilis infections. *AIDS* **18**, 2075–2079.

Buchacz, K., Greenberg, A., Onorato, I. & Janssen, K.J. (2005) Syphilis epidemic and human immunodeficiency virus (HIV) incidence among men who have sex with men in the United

States: implication for HIV prevention. *Sexually Transmitted Diseases* **32** (10 suppl.), 573–579.

Buchbinder, S.P., Katz, M.H., Hessol, N.A., O'Malley, P.M. & Holmberg, S.D. (1994) Long-term HIV-1 infection without immunological progression. *AIDS* **8**, 1123–1128.

Buckley, A., Dawson, A. & Gould, E.A. (2006) Detection of seroconversion to West Nile virus, Usutu virus and Sindbis virus in UK sentinel chickens. *Virology Journal* **3**, 71.

Budka, H. (1991) Neuropathology of human immunodeficiency virus infection. *Brain Pathology* **1**, 163–175.

Budka, H., Costanzi, G., Cristina, S. *et al.* (1987) Brain pathology induced by infection with the human immunodeficiency virus (HIV). A histological, immunocytochemical and electron microscopal study of 100 autopsy cases. *Acta Neuropathologica* **75**, 185–198.

Budka, H., Wiley, C.A., Kleihues, P. *et al.* (1991) HIV-associated disease of the nervous system: review of nomenclature and proposal for neuropathology-based terminology. *Brain Pathology* **1**, 143–152.

Buhrich, N., Cooper, D.A. & Freed, E. (1988) HIV infection associated with symptoms indistinguishable from functional psychosis. *British Journal of Psychiatry* **152**, 649–653.

Bullock, M.R. & Welchman, J.M. (1982) Diagnostic and prognostic features of tuberculous meningitis on CT scanning. *Journal of Neurology, Neurosurgery and Psychiatry* **45**, 1098–1101.

Burgdorfer, W. (1987) Lyme disease. In: Weatherall, D.J., Ledingham, J.G.G. & Warrell, D.A. (eds) *Oxford Textbook of Medicine*, 2nd edn, pp. 324–327. Oxford University Press, Oxford.

Candy, B., Chalder, T., Cleare, A.J., Wessely, S. & Hotopf, M. (2004) A randomised controlled trial of a psycho-educational intervention to aid recovery in infectious mononucleosis. *Journal of Psychosomatic Research* **57**, 89–94,

Carne, C.A., Tedder, R.S. & Smith, A. (1985) Acute encephalopathy coincident with seroconversion for anti-HTLV-III. *Lancet* **ii**, 1206–1208.

Caroff, S.N., Mann, S.C., McCarthy, M., Naser, J., Rynn, M. & Morrison, M. (1998) Acute infectious encephalitis complicated by neuroleptic malignant syndrome. *Journal of Clinical Psychopharmacology* **18**, 349–351.

Caroff, S.N., Mann, S.C., Gliatto, M.F., Sullivan, K.A. & Campbell, E.C. (2001) Psychiatric manifestation of acute viral encephalitis. *Psychiatric Annals* **31**, 193–204.

Carpenter, J., Stapleton, S. & Holliman, R. (2007) Retrospective analysis of 49 cases of brain abscess and review of the literature. *European Journal of Clinical Microbiology and Infectious Diseases* **26**, 1–11.

Carrico, A.W., Johnson, M.O., Morin, S.F. *et al.* (2007) Correlates of suicidal ideation among HIV-positive persons. *AIDS* **21**, 1199–1203.

Catalan, J. (1991) HIV-associated dementia: review of some conceptual and terminological problems. *International Review of Psychiatry* **3**, 321–330.

Catalan, J. & Thornton, S. (1993) Whatever happened to HIV dementia? *International Journal of STD and AIDS* **4**, 1–4.

Catalan, J., Riccio, M. & Thompson, C. (1989) HIV disease and psychiatric practice. *Psychiatric Bulletin* **13**, 316–332.

Centers for Disease Control (1986) Classification system for human T-lymphotropic virus type III/lymphadenopathy-associated virus infections. *Morbidity and Mortality Weekly Report* **35**, 334–339.

Centers For Disease Control (1992) 1993 revised classification system for HIV infection and expanded surveillance case definition for AIDS among adolescents and adults. *Morbidity and Mortality Weekly Report* **41** (RR-17), 1–19.

Centers for Disease Control (1994) Revised classification system for human immunodeficiency virus infection in children less than 13 years of age, official authorised addenda: human immunodeficiency virus infection codes and official guidelines for coding and reporting ICD-9-CH. *Morbidity and Mortality Weekly Report* **43** (RR-12).

Centers for Disease Control (2006) HIV and STI surveillance: mapping the issues. *Morbidity and Mortality Weekly Report* **55**, 589–592.

Centers for Disease Control (2006b) Sexually transmitted disease treatment guidelines. *Morbidity and Mortality Weekly Report* **55** (KR11), 1–94.

Centers for Disease Control (2007) Symptomatic early neurosyphilis among HIV-positive men who have sex with men – four cities, United States, January 2002–June 2004. *Morbidity and Mortality Weekly Report* **56**, 625–628.

Chamberlain, M.C. & Kormanik, P.A. (1999) AIDS-related central nervous system lymphomas. *Journal of Neuro-oncology* **43**, 269–276.

Chana, G., Everall, I.P., Crews, L. *et al.* (2006) Cognitive deficits and degeneration of interneurons in HIV+ methamphetamine users. *Neurology* **67**, 1486–1489.

Chander, G., Himelhoch, S. & Moore, R.D. (2006) Substance abuse and psychiatric disorders in HIV-positive patients: epidemiology and impact on antiretroviral therapy. *Drugs* **66**, 769–789.

Charrel, R.N., Attoui, H., Butenko, A.M. *et al.* (2004) Tick-borne virus diseases of human interest in Europe. *Clinical Microbiology and Infection* **10**, 1040–55.

Chaudhuri, A. & Kennedy, P.G. (2002) Diagnosis and treatment of viral encephalitis. *Postgraduate Medical Journal* **78**, 575–583.

Cherner, M., Masliah, E., Ellis, R.J. *et al.* (2002) Neurocognitive dysfunction predicts postmortem findings of HIV encephalitis. *Neurology* **59**, 1563–1567.

Chiesi, A., Agresti, M.G., Dally, L.G. *et al.* (1990) [Decrease in notifications of AIDS dementia complex in 1989–1990 in Italy: possible role of the early treatment with zidovudine.] *Medicina (Firenze)* **10**, 415–416.

Chiesi, A., Vella, S., Dally, L.G. *et al.* (1996) Epidemiology of AIDS dementia complex in Europe. *Journal of Acquired Immune Deficiency Syndromes and Human Retrovirology* **11**, 39–44.

Childs, E.A., Lyles, R.H., Selnes, O.A. *et al.* (1999) Plasma viral load and CD4 lymphocytes predict HIV-associated dementia and sensory neuropathy. *Neurology* **52**, 607–613.

Chung, C.C., Lee, S.S., Chen, Y.S. *et al.* (2007) Acute flaccid paralysis as an unusual presenting symptom of Japanese encephalitis: a case report and review of the literature. *Infection* **35**, 30–32.

Ciacci, J.D., Tellez, C., Vonroenn, J. & Levy, R.M. (1999) Lymphoma of the central nervous system in AIDS. *Seminars in Neurology* **19**, 213–221.

Ciesla, J.A. & Roberts, J.E. (2001) Meta-analysis of the relationship between HIV infection and risk for depressive disorders. *American Journal of Psychiatry* **158**, 725–730.

Cinque, P., Vago, L., Dahl, H. *et al.* (1996) Polymerase chain reaction on cerebrospinal fluid for diagnosis of virus-associated opportunistic diseases of the central nervous system in HIV-infected patients. *AIDS* **10**, 951–958.

Claude, H., Baruk, H. & Lamache, A. (1927) Obsessions-impulsions consécutives à l'encéphalite épidémique. *Encéphale* **22**, 716–720.

Cleare, A.J., Jacoby, R., Tovey, S.J. & Bergmann, K. (1993) Syphilis, neither dead nor buried: a survey of psychogeriatric inpatients. *International Journal of Geriatric Psychiatry* **8**, 661–664.

Clifford, D.B. (2002) AIDS dementia. *Medical Clinics of North America* **86**, 537–550, vi.

Clifford, D.B., Arribas, J.R., Storch, G.A., Tourtellote, W. & Wippold, F.J. (1996) Magnetic resonance brain imaging lacks sensitivity for AIDS associated cytomegalovirus encephalitis. *Journal of Neurovirology* **2**, 397–403.

Cobb, W.A. & Morgan-Hughes, J.A. (1968) Non-fatal subacute sclerosing leucoencephalitis. *Journal of Neurology, Neurosurgery and Psychiatry* **31**, 115–123.

Conde-Sendin, M.A., Amela-Peris, R., Aladro-Benito, Y. & Maroto, A.A. (2004) Current clinical spectrum of neurosyphilis in immunocompetent patients. *European Neurology* **52**, 29–35.

Connolly, J.H., Allen, I.V., Hurwitz, L.J. & Miller, J.H.D. (1967) Measles-virus antibody and antigen in subacute sclerosing panencephalitis. *Lancet* **i**, 542–544.

Conti, S., Masocco, M., Pezzotti, P. *et al.* (2000) Differential impact of combined antiretroviral therapy on the survival of italian patients with specific AIDS-defining illnesses. *Journal of Acquired Immune Deficiency Syndromes* **25**, 451–458.

Corder, E.H., Robertson, K., Lannfelt, L. *et al.* (1998) HIV-infected subjects with the E4 allele for APOE have excess dementia and peripheral neuropathy. *Nature Medicine* **4**, 1182–1184.

Costa, D.C., Ell, P.J., Burns, A., Philpot, M. & Levy, R. (1988) CBF tomograms with ^{99m}Tc-HMPAO in patients with dementia (Alzheimer type and HIV) and Parkinson's disease: initial results. *Journal of Cerebral Blood Flow and Metabolism* **8**, S109–S115.

Crow, T.J. (1978) Viral causes of psychiatric disease. *Postgraduate Medical Journal* **54**, 763–767.

Cruess, D.G., Petitto, J.M., Leserman, J. *et al.* (2003) Depression and HIV infection: impact on immune function and disease progression. *CNS Spectrums* **8**, 52–58.

Currie, J.N., Coppeto, J.R. & Lessell, S. (1988) Chronic syphilitic meningitis resulting in superior orbital fissure syndrome and posterior fossa gumma. A report of two cases followed for 20 years. *Journal of Clinical Neuro-ophthalmology* **8**, 145–159.

Cysique, L.A., Brew, B.J., Halman, M. *et al.* (2005) Undetectable cerebrospinal fluid HIV RNA and beta-2 microglobulin do not indicate inactive AIDS dementia complex in highly active antiretroviral therapy-treated patients. *Journal of Acquired Immune Deficiency Syndromes* **39**, 426–429.

Dale, R.C., Church, A.J., Surtees, R.A. *et al.* (2004) Encephalitis lethargica syndrome: 20 new cases and evidence of basal ganglia autoimmunity. *Brain* **127**, 21–33.

Dale, R.C., Webster, R. & Gill, D. (2007) Contemporary encephalitis lethargica presenting with agitated catatonia, stereotypy, and dystonia-parkinsonism. *Movement Disorders* **22**, 2281–2284.

Dal Pan, G.J., McArthur, J.H., Aylward, E. *et al.* (1992) Patterns of cerebral atrophy in HIV-1-infected individuals: results of a quantitative MRI analysis. *Neurology* **42**, 2125–2130.

Dal Pan, G.J., Fazadegan, H., Selner, O. *et al.* (1998) Sustained cognitive decline in HIV infection: relationship to CD4$^+$ cell count, plasma viraemia and p24 antigenemia. *Journal of Neurovirology* **4**, 95–99.

Davis, L.E. (2000) Diagnosis and treatment of acute encephalitis. *Neurologist* **6**, 145–159.

Davis, L.E. & Schmitt, J.W. (1989) Clinical significance of cerebrospinal fluid tests for neurosyphilis. *Annals of Neurology* **25**, 50–55.

Davis, L.E., Hjelle, B.L., Miller, V.E. *et al.* (1992) Early viral brain invasion in iatrogenic human immunodeficiency virus infection. *Neurology* **42**, 1736–1739.

Davis, L.E., Debiasi, R., Goade, D.E. *et al.* (2006) West Nile virus neuroinvasive disease. *Annals of Neurology* **60**, 286–300.

Davison, K. & Bagley, C.R. (1969) Schizophrenia-like psychoses associated with organic disorders of the central nervous system: a review of the literature. In: Herrington, R.N. (ed.) *Current Problems in Neuropsychiatry*, Part II, pp. 113–183. British Journal of Psychiatry Special Publication No. 4. Headley Brothers, Ashford, Kent.

Dawson, J.R. (1933) Cellular inclusions in cerebral lesions of lethargic encephalitis. *American Journal of Pathology* **9**, 7–15.

Day, J.J., Grant, L., Atkinson, J.H. *et al.* (1992) Incidence of AIDS dementia complex in a two year follow-up of AIDS and ARC patients on an initial phase II AZT placebo-controlled study: San Diego Cohort. *Journal of Neuropsychiatry and Clinical Neurosciences* **4**, 15.

DeBiasi, R.L. & Tyler, K.L. (2006) West Nile virus meningoencephalitis. *Nature Clinical Practice Neurology* **2**, 264–275.

DeCock, K.M. (1997) HIV drug strategies in the West, and AIDS everywhere else. An interview with Kevin M. DeCock, MD, FRCP, DTM&H. Interview by Mark Mascolini. *Journal of the International Association of Physicians in AIDS Care* **3**, 23–26, 28–31.

De la Garza, C.L., Paoletti-Duarte, S., Garcia-Martin, C. & Gutierrez-Casares, J.R. (2001) Efavirenz-induced psychosis. *AIDS* **15**, 1911–1912.

De la Monte, S.M., Schooley, R.T., Hirsch, M.S. & Richardson, E.P. (1987) Subacute encephalomyelitis of AIDS and its relation to HTLV-III infection. *Neurology* **37**, 562–569.

Del Grosso Destreri, N., Farina, E., Calabrese, E., Pinardi, G., Imbornone, E. & Mariani, C. (2002) Frontal impairment and confabulation after herpes simplex encephalitis: a case report. *Archives of Physical Medicine and Rehabilitation* **83**, 423–426.

Delli, F.S., Mourellou, O., Chaidemenos, G., Anagnostou, E. & Amaxopoulos, K. (2007) Neurosyphilis a reality again. *Journal of the European Academy of Dermatology and Venereology* **21**, 398–399.

Denning, D.W., Anderson, J., Rudge, P. & Smith, H. (1987) Acute myelopathy associated with primary infection with human immunodeficiency virus. *British Medical Journal* **294**, 143–144.

De Ronchi, D., Faranca, I., Forti, P. *et al.* (2000) Development of acute psychotic disorders and HIV-1 infection. *International Journal of Psychiatry in Medicine* **30**, 173–183.

De Ronchi, D., Faranca, I., Berardi, D. *et al.* (2002) Risk factors for cognitive impairment in HIV-1-infected persons with different risk behaviors. *Archives of Neurology* **59**, 812–818.

Des Jarlais, D.C., Friedman, S.R., Novick, D.M. *et al.* (1989) HIV-1 infection among intravenous drug users in Manhattan, New York City, from 1977 through 1987. *Journal of the American Medical Association* **261**, 1008–1012.

Dewar, B.K. & Wilson, B.A. (2005) Cognitive recovery from encephalitis lethargica. *Brain Injury* **19**, 1285–1291.

Dewhurst, K. (1969) The neurosyphilitic psychoses today: a survey of 91 cases. *British Journal of Psychiatry* **115**, 31–38.

Diagana, M., Preux, P.M. & Dumas, M. (2007) Japanese encephalitis revisited. *Journal of the Neurological Sciences* **262**, 165–170.

Dilley, J.W., Ochitill, H.N., Perl, M. & Volberding, P.A. (1985) Findings in psychiatric consultations with patients with acquired immune deficiency syndrome. *American Journal of Psychiatry* **142**, 82–86.

Di Rocco, A., Bottiglieri, T., Werner, P. *et al.* (2002) Abnormal cobalamin-dependent transmethylation in AIDS-associated myelopathy. *Neurology* **58**, 730–735.

Domingues, R.B., Tsanaclis, A.M., Pannuti, C.S., Mayo, M.S. & Lakeman, F.D. (1997) Evaluation of the range of clinical presentations of herpes simplex encephalitis by using polymerase chain reaction assay of cerebrospinal fluid samples. *Clinical Infectious Diseases* **25**, 86–91.

Dore, G.J., Correll, P.K., Li, Y., Kaldor, J.M., Cooper, D.A. & Brew, B.J. (1999) Changes to AIDS dementia complex in the era of highly active antiretroviral therapy. *AIDS* **13**, 1249–1253.

Douglas, J.M. Jr, Peterman, T.A. & Fenton, K.A. (2005) Syphilis among men who have sex with men: challenges to syphilis elimination in the United States. *Sexually Transmitted Diseases* **32**, S80–S83.

Dowell E., Easton, A. & Solomon, T. (2000) *The Consequences of Encephalitis. Report of a Postal Survey*. The Encephalitis Society, Malton, UK.

Drachman, D.A. & Adams, R.D. (1962) Herpes simplex and acute inclusion-body encephalitis. *Archives of Neurology* **7**, 45–63.

Dubos, F., Moulin, F., Gajdos, V. *et al.* (2006) Serum procalcitonin and other biologic markers to distinguish between bacterial and aseptic meningitis. *Journal of Pediatrics* **149**, 72–76.

Dunbar, J.M., Jamieson, W.M., Langlands, J.H.H. & Smith, G.H. (1958) Encephalitis and influenza. *British Medical Journal* **1**, 913–915.

Durvasula, R.S., Myers, H.F., Mason, K. & Hinkin, C. (2006) Relationship between alcohol use/abuse, HIV infection and neuropsychological performance in African American men. *Journal of Clinical and Experimental Neuropsychology* **28**, 383–404.

Egglestone, S.I. & Turner, A.J. (2000) Serological diagnosis of syphilis. *Communicable Disease and Public Health* **3**, 158–162.

Elam, G., De Souza-Thomas, L. & Ward, H. (2006) HIV and AIDS in the United Kingdom African communities: guidelines produced for prevention and care. *Euro Surveillance* **11**, E060126 5.

Elford, J., Bolding, G., Sherr, L. & Hart, G. (2005) High-risk sexual behaviour among London gay men: no longer increasing. *AIDS* **19**, 2171–2174.

Ellis, R.J., Hsia, K., Spector, S.A. *et al.* (1997) Cerebrospinal fluid human immunodeficiency virus type 1 RNA levels are elevated in neurocognitively impaired individuals with acquired immunodeficiency syndrome. *Annals of Neurology* **42**, 679–688.

Ellis, R.J., Moore, D.J., Childers, M.E. *et al.* (2002) Progression to neuropsychological impairment in human immunodeficiency virus infection predicted by elevated cerebrospinal fluid levels of human immunodeficiency virus RNA. *Archives of Neurology* **59**, 923–928.

Ereshefsky, L. & Dugan, D. (2000) Review of the pharmacokinetics, pharmacogenetics, and drug interaction potential of antidepressants: focus on venlafaxine. *Depression and Anxiety* **12** (suppl. 1), 30–44.

Esiri, M.M., Scaravilli, F., Millard, P.R. & Harcourt-Webster, J.N. (1989) Neuropathology of HIV infection in haemophiliacs: comparative necropsy study. *British Medical Journal* **299**, 1312–1315.

Espir, M.L.E. & Spalding, J.M.K. (1956) Three recent cases of encephalitis lethargica. *British Medical Journal* **1**, 1141–1144.

Evans, D.L., Staab, J.P., Petitto, J.M. *et al.* (1999) Depression in the medical setting: biopsychosocial interaction and treatment consideration. *Journal of Clinical Psychiatry* **60** (suppl. 4), 40–55; discussion 56.

Evans, D.L., Ten Have, T.R., Douglas, S.D. *et al.* (2002) Association of depression with viral load, CD8 T lymphocytes, and natural killer cells in women with HIV infection. *American Journal of Psychiatry* **159**, 1752–1759.

Everall, I.P. & Lantos, P.L. (1991) The neuropathology of HIV: a review of the first 10 years. *International Review of Psychiatry* **3**, 307–320.

Everall, I.P., Luthert, P.J. & Lantos, P.L. (1991) Neuronal loss in the frontal cortex in HIV infection. *Lancet* **337**, 1119–1121.

Everall, I.P., Luthert, P.J. & Lantos, P.L. (1993a) Neuronal number and volume alterations in the neocortex of HIV infected individuals. *Journal of Neurology, Neurosurgery and Psychiatry* **56**, 481–486.

Everall, I., Luthert, P. & Lantos, P. (1993b) A review of neuronal damage in human immunodeficiency virus infection: its assessment, possible mechanism and relationship to dementia. *Journal of Neuropathology and Experimental Neurology* **52**, 561–566.

Everall, I., Barnes, H., Spargo, E. & Lantos, P. (1995) Assessment of neuronal density in the putamen in human immunodeficiency virus (HIV) infection. Application of stereology and spatial analysis of quadrats. *Journal of Neurovirology* **1**, 126–129.

Exhenry, C. & Nadal, D. (1996) Vertical human immunodeficiency virus-1 infection: involvement of the central nervous system and treatment. *European Journal of Pediatrics* **155**, 839–850.

Fairweather, D.S. (1947) Psychiatric aspects of the post-encephalitic syndrome. *Journal of Mental Science* **93**, 201–254.

Faulstich, M.E. (1987) Psychiatric aspects of AIDS. *American Journal of Psychiatry* **144**, 551–556.

Fawzy, F.I., Fawzy, N.W. & Pasnau, R.O. (1991) Bereavement in AIDS. *Psychiatric Medicine* **9**, 469–481.

Fenton, K.A. & Imrie, J. (2005) Increasing rates of sexually transmitted diseases in homosexual men in Western Europe and the United States: why? *Infectious Disease Clinics of North America* **19**, 311–331.

Fernandez, F. (2002) Neuropsychiatric aspects of human immunodeficiency virus (HIV) infection. *Current Psychiatry Reports* **4**, 228–231.

Fernandez, F., Levy, J.K., Samley, H.R. *et al.* (1995) Effects of methylphenidate in HIV-related depression: a comparative trial with desipramine. *International Journal of Psychiatry in Medicine* **25**, 53–67.

Fernando, S.J. & Freyberg, Z. (2008) Treatment of depression in HIV positive individuals: a critical review. *International Review of Psychiatry* **20**, 61–71.

Ferrando, S.J. & Freyberg, Z. (2008) Treatment of depression in HIV positive individuals: a critical review. *International Review of Psychiatry* **20**, 61–71.

Ferrari, S., Vento, S., Monaco, S. *et al.* (2006) Human immunodeficiency virus-associated peripheral neuropathies. *Mayo Clinic Proceedings* **81**, 213–219.

Fischer-Smith, T., Croul, S., Adeniyi, A. *et al.* (2004) Macrophage/microglial accumulation and proliferating cell nuclear antigen expression in the central nervous system in human immunodeficiency virus encephalopathy. *American Journal of Pathology* **164**, 2089–2099.

Flewett, T.H. & Hoult, J.G. (1958) Influenzal encephalopathy and postinfluenzal encephalitis. *Lancet* **ii**, 11–15.

Flint, A.C., Liberato, B.B., Anziska, Y., Schantz-Dunn, J. & Wright, C.B. (2005) Meningovascular syphilis as a cause of basilar artery stenosis. *Neurology* **64**, 391–392.

Fodor, P.A., Levin, M.S., Weinberg, A., Sandberg, E., Sylman, J. & Tyler, K.L. (1988) Atypical herpes simplex virus encephalitis diagnosed by PCR amplification of viral DNA from CSF. *Neurology* **51**, 554–559.

Fong, I.W. & Toma, E. (1995) The natural history of progressive multifocal leukoencephalopathy in patients with AIDS. *Clinical Infectious Diseases* **20**, 1305–1310.

Foster, R., Olajide, D. & Everall, I.P. (2003) Antiretroviral therapy-induced psychosis: case report and brief review of the literature. *HIV Medicine* **4**, 139–144.

Foster, R., Taylor, C. & Everall, I.P. (2004) More on abacavir-induced neuropsychiatric reactions. *AIDS* **18**, 2449.

Fröshaug, H. & Ytrehus, A. (1956) A study of general paresis with special reference to the reasons for the admission of these patients to hospital. *Acta Psychiatrica et Neurologica Scandinavica* **31**, 35–60.

Gaber, T.A. & Eshiett, M. (2003) Resolution of psychiatric symptoms secondary to herpes simplex encephalitis. *Journal of Neurology, Neurosurgery and Psychiatry* **74**, 1164; author reply 1164.

Garg, R.K. (2002) Subacute sclerosing panencephalitis. *Postgraduate Medical Journal* **78**, 63–70.

Gautier-Smith, P.C. (1965) Neurological complications of glandular fever (infectious mononucleosis). *Brain* **88**, 323–334.

Gelenberg, A.J. (1976) The catatonic syndrome. *Lancet* **i**, 1339–1341.

General Medical Council (1988) *HIV Infection and AIDS: The Ethical Considerations.* General Medical Council, London.

General Medical Council (1993) *HIV Infection and AIDS: The Ethical Considerations.* General Medical Council, London.

General Medical Council (2006) Serious communicable diseases, October 1997, withdrawn September.

Gibbons, J.L., Miller, H.G. & Stanton, J.B. (1956) Para-infectious encephalomyelitis and related syndromes: a critical review of the neurological complication of certain specific fevers. *Quarterly Journal of Medicine* **25**, 427–505.

Giometto, B., An, S.F., Groves, M. *et al.* (1997) Accumulation of beta-amyloid precursor protein in HIV encephalitis: relationship with neuropsychological abnormalities. *Annals of Neurology* **42**, 34–40.

Giovannoni, G. & Martino, D. (2004) Antibasal ganglia antibodies and their relevance to movement disorders. *Current Opinion in Neurology* **17**, 425–432.

Gisolf, E.H., Enting, R.H., Jurriaans, S. *et al.* (2000) Cerebrospinal fluid HIV-1 RNA during treatment with ritonavir/saquinavir or ritonavir/saquinavir/stavudine. *AIDS* **14**, 1583–1589.

Glass, J.D., Wesselingh, S.L., Selnes, O.A. & McArthur, J.C. (1993) Clinical–neuropathologic correlation in HIV-associated dementia. *Neurology* **43**, 2230–2237.

Glass, R.M. (1988) AIDS and suicide. *Journal of the American Medical Association* **259**, 1369–1370.

Goh, K.J., Tan, C.T., Chew, N.K. *et al.* (2000) Clinical features of Nipah virus encephalitis among pig farmers in Malaysia. *New England Journal of Medicine* **342**, 1229–1235.

Goodkin, K., Feaster, D.J., Tuttle, R. *et al.* (1996) Bereavement is associated with time-dependent decrements in cellular immune function in asymptomatic human immunodeficiency virus type 1-seropositive homosexual men. *Clinical and Diagnostic Laboratory Immunology* **3**, 107–118.

Goodwin, G., Pretsell, B., Chiswick, A., Egan, V. & Brettle, R. (1996) The Edinburgh cohort of HIV positive injecting drug users at 10 years after infection: a case–control study of the evolution of dementia. *AIDS* **10**, 431–440.

Gordon, B., Selnes, O.A., Hart, J. Jr, Hanley, D.F. & Whitley, R.J. (1990) Long-term cognitive sequelae of acyclovir-treated herpes simplex encephalitis. *Archives of Neurology* **47**, 646–647.

Gore-Felton, C. & Koopman, C. (2008) Behavioral mediation of the relationship between psychosocial factors and HIV disease progression. *Psychosomatic Medicine* **70**, 569–574.

Gostling, J.V.T. (1967) Herpetic encephalitis. *Proceedings of the Royal Society of Medicine* **60**, 693–696.

Graham, N.M., Hoover, D.R., Park, L.P. *et al.* (1996) Survival in HIV-infected patients who have received zidovudine: comparison of combination therapy with sequential monotherapy and continued zidovudine monotherapy. *Annals of Internal Medicine* **124**, 1031–1038.

Granerod, J. & Crowcroft, N.S. (2007) The epidemiology of acute encephalitis. *Neuropsychological Rehabilitation* **17**, 406–428.

Grant, A.D., Djomand, G. & DeCock, K.M. (1997) Natural history and spectrum of disease in adults with HIV/AIDS in Africa. *AIDS* **11** (suppl. B), S43–S54.

Grant, I., Sacktor, H. & McArthur, J. (2005) HIV neurocognitive disorders. In: Gendelman, H.E., Grant, I., Everall, I., Lipton, S.A. & Swindells, S. (eds) *The Neurology of AIDS*, 2nd edn, pp. 357–373. Oxford University Press, London.

Gray, F., Gherardi, R., Keohane, C., Favolini, M., Sobel, A. & Poirier, J. (1988) Pathology of the central nervous system in 40 cases of acquired immune deficiency syndrome (AIDS). *Neuropathology and Applied Neurobiology* **14**, 365–380.

Gray, F., Geny, C., Dournon, E., Fenelon, G., Lionnet, F. & Gherardi, R. (1991) Neuropathological evidence that zidovudine reduces incidence of HIV infection of brain. *Lancet* **337**, 852–853.

Gray, F., Scaravilli, F., Everall, I. *et al.* (1996) Neuropathology of early HIV-1 infection. *Brain Pathology* **6**, 1–15.

Gray, F., Chretien, F., Vallat-Decouvelaere, A.V. & Scaravilli, F. (2003) The changing pattern of HIV neuropathology in the HAART era. *Journal of Neuropathology and Experimental Neurology* **62**, 429–440.

Greenwood, R.J. (1996) Neurosyphilis. In: Weatherall, D.J., Ledingham, J.G.G. & Warrell, D.A. (eds) *Oxford Textbook of*

Medicine, 3rd edn, section 24.15.5. Oxford University Press, Oxford.

Greenwood, R., Bhalla, A., Gordon, A. & Roberts, J. (1983) Behaviour disturbances during recovery from herpes simplex encephalitis. *Journal of Neurology, Neurosurgery and Psychiatry* **46**, 809–817.

Grimwood, K., Anderson, P., Anderson, V., Tan, L. & Nolan, T. (2000) Twelve year outcomes following bacterial meningitis: further evidence for persisting effects. *Archives of Disease in Childhood* **83**, 111–116.

Grisolia, J.S. & Wiederholt, W.C. (1982) CNS cysticercosis. *Archives of Neurology* **39**, 540–544.

Grover, D., Newsholme, W., Brink, N., Manji, H. & Miller, R. (2004) Herpes simplex virus infection of the central nervous system in human immunodeficiency virus-type 1-infected patients. *International Journal of STD and AIDS* **15**, 597–600.

Grulich, A.E. (1999) AIDS-associated non-Hodgkin's lymphoma in the era of highly active antiretroviral therapy. *Journal of Acquired Immune Deficiency Syndromes* **21** (suppl. 1), S27–S30.

Guess, H.A., Broughton, D.D., Melton, L.J. & Kirland, L.T. (1986) Population-based studies of varicella complications. *Pediatrics* **78**, 723–727.

Hahn, R.D. & Clark, E.G. (1946a) Asymptomatic neurosyphilis: a review of the literature. *American Journal of Syphilis, Gonorrhoea and Venereal Diseases* **30**, 305–316.

Hahn, R.D. & Clark, E.G. (1946b) Asymptomatic neurosyphilis: prognosis. *American Journal of Syphilis, Gonorrhoea and Venereal Diseases* **30**, 513–548.

Hahn, R.D., Webster, B., Weickhardt, G. *et al.* (1959) Penicillin treatment of general paresis (dementia paralytica). *Archives of Neurology and Psychiatry* **81**, 557–590.

Hall, P. (1963) Korsakov's syndrome following herpes-zoster encephalitis. *Lancet* **i**, 752.

Hall, S.B. (1929) Mental aspect of epidemic encephalitis. *British Medical Journal* **1**, 444–446.

Haller, D.L. & Miles, D.R. (2003) Suicidal ideation among psychiatric patients with HIV: psychiatric morbidity and quality of life. *AIDS and Behavior* **7**, 101–108.

Halstead, S., Riccio, M., Harlow, P., Oretti, R. & Thompson, C. (1988) Psychosis associated with HIV infection. *British Journal of Psychiatry* **153**, 618–623.

Hamblin, T.J., Hussain, J., Akbar, A.N., Tang, Y.C., Smith, J.L. & Jones, D.B. (1983) Immunological reason for chronic ill health after infectious mononucleosis. *British Medical Journal* **287**, 85–88.

Hamilton-Dutoit, S.J., Pallesen, G., Franzmann, M.B. *et al.* (1991) AIDS-related lymphoma. Histopathology, immunophenotype, and association with Epstein–Barr virus as demonstrated by in-situ nucleic acid hybridization. *American Journal of Pathology* **138**, 149–163.

Hardy, D.J., Hinkin, C.H., Levine, A.J., Castellon, S.A. & Lam, M.N. (2006) Risky decision making assessed with the gambling task in adults with HIV. *Neuropsychology* **20**, 355–360.

Hare, E.H. (1959) The origin and spread of dementia paralytica. *Journal of Mental Sciences* **105**, 594–626.

Harlam, C., Cook, M. & Coltheart, M. (2001) 'I know your name but not your face'. Explaining modality based differences in access to biographical knowledge in a patient with retrograde amnesia. *Neurocase* **7**, 189–199.

Harris, M.J., Jeste, D.V., Gleghorn, A. & Sewell, D.D. (1991) New-onset psychosis in HIV-infected patients. *Journal of Clinical Psychiatry* **52**, 369–376.

Harrison, M.S., Simonte, S.J. & Kauffman, C.A. (1994) Trimethoprim-induced aseptic meningitis in a patient with AIDS: case report and review. *Clinical Infectious Diseases* **19**, 431–434.

Hartzell, J.D., Janke, I.E. & Weintrob, A.C. (2008) Impact of depression on HIV outcomes in the HAART era. *Journal of Antimicrobial Chemotherapy* **62**, 246–255.

Health Protection Agency (2005) UK Collaborative Group for HIV and other Sexually Transmitted Infections in the UK. Health Protection Agency Centre for Infection, London.

Health Protection Agency (2006) HIV/STIs. *Communicable Disease Report Weekly* **16** (4).

Heaton, R.K., Velin, R.A., McCutchan, J.A. *et al.* (1994) Neuropsychological impairment in human immunodeficiency virus-infection: implications for employment. *Psychosomatic Medicine* **56**, 8–17.

Heaton, R.K., Marcotte, T.D., Mindt, M.R. *et al.* (2004) The impact of HIV-associated neuropsychological impairment on everyday functioning. *Journal of the International Neuropsychological Society* **10**, 317–331.

Hecht, F.M., Busch, M.P., Rawal, B. *et al.* (2002) Use of laboratory tests and clinical symptoms for identification of primary HIV infection. *AIDS* **16**, 1119–1129.

Hendrick, I. (1928) Encephalitis lethargica and the interpretation of mental disease. *American Journal of Psychiatry* **7**, 989–1014.

Hierons, R., Janota, I. & Corsellis, J.A.N. (1978) The late effects of necrotising encephalitis of the temporal lobes and limbic areas: a clinico-pathological study of 10 cases. *Psychological Medicine* **8**, 21–42.

Hilton, J.F. (2000) Functions of oral candidiasis episodes that are highly prognostic for AIDS. *Statistics in Medicine* **19**, 989–1004.

Himmelhoch, J., Pincus, J., Tucker, G. & Detre, T. (1970) Sub-acute encephalitis: behavioural and neurological aspects. *British Journal of Psychiatry* **116**, 531–538.

Ho, D.D., Rota, T.R., Schooley, R.T. *et al.* (1985) Isolation of HTLV-III from cerebrospinal fluid and neural tissues of patients with neurologic syndromes related to the acquired immunodeficiency syndrome. *New England Journal of Medicine* **313**, 1493–1497.

Hochberg, F.H., Nelson, K. & Janzen, W. (1975) Influenza type B-related encephalopathy. The 1971 outbreak of Reye Syndrome in Chicago. *Journal of the American Medical Association* **231**, 817–821.

Hoffman, B.F. (1982) Reversible neurosyphilis presenting as chronic mania. *Journal of Clinical Psychiatry* **43**, 338–339.

Hoke, A. & Keswani, S.C. (2005) Neuroprotection in the PNS: erythropoietin and immunophilin ligands. *Annals of the New York Academy of Sciences* **1053**, 491–501.

Hokkanen, L. & Launes, J. (1997) Duration of transient amnesia correlates with cognitive outcome in acute encephalitis. *Neuroreport* **8**, 2721–2725.

Hokkanen, L. & Launes, J. (2000) Cognitive outcome in acute sporadic encephalitis. *Neuropsychology Review* **10**, 151–167.

Hokkanen, L. & Launes, J. (2007) Neuropsychological sequelae of acute-onset sporadic viral encephalitis. *Neuropsychological Rehabilitation* **17**, 450–477.

Hokkanen, L., Poutiainen, E., Valanne, L., Salonen, O., Iivanainen, M. & Launes, J. (1996) Cognitive impairment after acute encephalitis: comparison of herpes simplex and other aetiologies. *Journal of Neurology, Neurosurgery and Psychiatry* **61**, 478–484.

Hokkanen, L., Launes, J., Poutiainen, E. *et al.* (1997) Subcortical type cognitive impairment in herpes zoster encephalitis. *Journal of Neurology* **244**, 239–245.

Hollander, H. & Stringari, S. (1987) Human immunodeficiency virus-associated meningitis. Clinical course and correlations. *American Journal of Medicine* **83**, 813–816.

Hoogman, M., van de Beek, D., Weisfelt, M., de Gans, J. & Schmand, B. (2007) Cognitive outcome in adults after bacterial meningitis. *Journal of Neurology, Neurosurgery and Psychiatry* **78**, 1092–1096.

Hooshmand, H., Escobar, M.R. & Kopf, S.W. (1972) Neurosyphilis. A study of 241 patients. *Journal of the American Medical Association* **219**, 726–729.

Horta-Barbosa, L., Fuccillo, D.A., London, W.T., Jabbour, J.T., Zeman, W. & Sever, J.L. (1969) Isolation of measles virus from brain cell cultures of two patients with subacute sclerosing panencephalitis. *Proceedings of the Society for Experimental Biology and Medicine* **132**, 272–277.

Hosoglu, S., Ayaz, C., Geyik, M.F., Kokoglu, O.F. & Ceviz, A. (1998) Tuberculous meningitis in adults: an eleven-year review. *International Journal of Tuberculosis and Lung Disease* **2**, 553–557.

Hotopf, M., Noah, N. & Wessely, S. (1996) Chronic fatigue and minor psychiatric morbidity after viral meningitis: a controlled study. *Journal of Neurology, Neurosurgery and Psychiatry* **60**, 504–509.

Howard, R.S. & Lees, A.J. (1987) Encephalitis lethargica. A report of four recent cases. *Brain* **110**, 19–33.

Howland, L.C., Gortmaker, S.L., Mofenson, L.M. *et al.* (2000) Effects of negative life events on immune suppression in children and youth infected with human immunodeficiency virus type 1. *Pediatrics* **106**, 540–546.

Hunter, R. & Jones, M. (1966) Acute lethargica-type encephalitis. *Lancet* **ii**, 1023–1024.

Hunter, R., Jones, M. & Malleson, A. (1969) Abnormal cerebrospinal fluid total protein and gamma-globulin levels in 256 patients admitted to a psychiatric unit. *Journal of the Neurological Sciences* **9**, 11–38.

Ickovics, J.R., Hamburger, M.E., Vlahov, D. *et al.* (2001) Mortality, CD4 cell count decline, and depressive symptoms among HIV-seropositive women: longitudinal analysis from the HIV Epidemiology Research Study. *Journal of the American Medical Association* **285**, 1466–1474.

Illis, L.S. & Merry, R.T. (1972) Treatment of herpes simplex encephalitis. *Journal of the Royal College of Physicians of London* **7**, 34–44.

Ironson, G., Balbin, E., Stuetzle, R. *et al.* (2005a) Dispositional optimism and the mechanisms by which it predicts slower disease progression in HIV: proactive behavior, avoidant coping, and depression. *International Journal of Behavioral Medicine* **12**, 86–97.

Ironson, G., O'Cleirigh, C., Fletcher, M.A. *et al.* (2005b) Psychosocial factors predict CD4 and viral load change in men and women with human immunodeficiency virus in the era of highly active antiretroviral treatment. *Psychosomatic Medicine* **67**, 1013–1021.

Ironson, G., Weiss, S., Lydston, D. *et al.* (2005c) The impact of improved self-efficacy on HIV viral load and distress in culturally diverse women living with AIDS: the SMART/EST Women's Project. *AIDS Care* **17**, 222–236.

Jacomet, C., Girard, P.M., Lebrette, M.G., Farese, V.L., Monfort, L. & Rozenbaum, W. (1997) Intravenous methotrexate for primary central nervous system non-Hodgkin's lymphoma in AIDS. *AIDS* **11**, 1725–1730.

Janssen, R.S. (1997) Epidemiology and neuroepidemiology of human immunodeficiency virus infection. In: Berger, J.R. & Levy, R.M. (eds) *AIDS and the Nervous System*, 2nd edn, pp. 13–37. Lippincott-Raven, Philadelphia.

Janssen, R.S., Saykin, A.J., Kaplan, J.E. *et al.* (1988) Neurological symptoms and neuropsychological abnormalities in lymphadenopathy syndrome. *Annals of Neurology* **23** (suppl.), S17–S18.

Janssen, R.S., Nwanyanwu, O.C., Selik, R.M. & Stehr-Green, J.K. (1992) Epidemiology of human immunodeficiency virus encephalopathy in the United States. *Neurology* **42**, 1472–1476.

Jayakumar, P.N., Taly, A.B., Arya, B.Y.T. & Nagaraj, D. (1988) Computed tomography in subacute sclerosing panencephalitis: report of 15 cases. *Acta Neurologica Scandinavica* **77**, 328–330.

Jellinger, K.A., Setinek, U., Drlicek, M., Bohm, G., Steurer, A. & Lintner, F. (2000) Neuropathology and general autopsy findings in AIDS during the last 15 years. *Acta Neuropathologica* **100**, 213–220.

Jemsek, J., Greenberg, S.B., Taber, L., Harvey, D., Gershon, A. & Couch, R.B. (1983) Herpes zoster-associated encephalitis: clinicopathologic report of 12 cases and review of the literature. *Medicine (Baltimore)* **62**, 81–97.

Jenike, M.A. & Pato, C. (1986) Disabling fear of AIDS responsive to imipramine. *Psychosomatics* **27**, 143–144.

Joffe, R., Black, M.M. & Floyd, M. (1968) Changing clinical picture of neurosyphilis: report of seven unusual cases. *British Medical Journal* **1**, 211–212.

Johns, D.R., Tierney, M. & Felsenstein, D. (1987) Alteration in the natural history of neurosyphilis by concurrent infection with the human immunodeficiency virus. *New England Journal of Medicine* **316**, 1569–1572.

Johnson, J. & Lucey, P.A. (1987) Encephalitis lethargica, a contemporary cause of catatonic stupor. A report of two cases. *British Journal of Psychiatry* **151**, 550–552.

Johnstone, J.A., Ross, C.A.C. & Dunn, M. (1972) Meningitis and encephalitis associated with mumps infection. A 10 year survey. *Archives of Disease in Childhood* **47**, 647–651.

Justice, A.C., McGinnis, K.A., Atkinson, J.H. *et al.* (2004) Psychiatric and neurocognitive disorders among HIV-positive and negative veterans in care: Veterans Aging Cohort Five-Site Study. *AIDS* **18** (suppl. 1), S49–S59.

Kalichman, S.C., Heckman, T., Kochman, A., Sikkema, K. & Bergholte, J. (2000) Depression and thoughts of suicide among middle-aged and older persons living with HIV-AIDS. *Psychiatric Services (Washington, DC)* **51**, 903–907.

Kapila, C.C., Kaul, S., Kapur, S.C., Kalayanam, T.S. & Banerjee, D. (1958) Neurological and hepatic disorders associated with influenza. *British Medical Journal* **2**, 1311–1314.

Kaplan, C.P. & Bain, K.P. (1999) Cognitive outcome after emergent treatment of acute herpes simplex encephalitis with acyclovir. *Brain Injury* **13**, 935–941.

Kapur, N., Barker, S., Burrows, E.H. *et al.* (1994) Herpes simplex encephalitis: long term magnetic resonance imaging and neuropsychological profile. *Journal of Neurology, Neurosurgery and Psychiatry* 57, 1334–1342.

Karstaedt, A.S., Valtchanova, S., Barriere, R. & Crewe-Brown, H.H. (1998) Tuberculous meningitis in South African urban adults. *Quarterly Journal of Medicine* 91, 743–747.

Kaufman, D.M., Zimmerman, R.D. & Leeds, N.E. (1979) Computed tomography in herpes simplex encephalitis. *Neurology* 29, 1392–1396.

Keddie, K.M.G. (1965) Toxic psychosis following mumps. *British Journal of Psychiatry* 111, 691–696.

Kelder, W., McArthur, J.C., Nance-Sproson, T., McClernon, D. & Griffin, D.E. (1998) Beta-chemokines MCP-1 and RANTES are selectively increased in cerebrospinal fluid of patients with human immunodeficiency virus-associated dementia. *Annals of Neurology* 44, 831–835.

Kelley, R.E., Minagar, A., Kelley, B.J. & Brunson, R. (2003) Trancranial Doppler monitoring of response to therapy for meningovascular syphilis. *Journal of Neuroimaging* 13, 85–87.

Kemeny, M.E., Weiner, H., Duran, R., Taylor, S.E., Visscher, B. & Fahey, J.L. (1995) Immune system changes after the death of a partner in HIV-positive gay men. *Psychosomatic Medicine* 57, 547–554.

Kennard, C. & Swash, M. (1981) Acute viral encephalitis: its diagnosis and outcome. *Brain* 104, 129–148.

Kennedy, C. (1968) A ten-year experience with subacute sclerosing panencephalitis. *Neurology* 18 (suppl.), 58–59.

Kennedy, P.G. (2005) Viral encephalitis. *Journal of Neurology* 252, 268–272.

Kent, S.J., Crowe, S.M., Yung, A., Lucas, C.R. & Mijch, A.M. (1993) Tuberculous meningitis: a 30-year review. *Clinical Infectious Diseases* 17, 987–994.

Kesselring, J., Miller, D.H., Robb, S.A. *et al.* (1990) Acute disseminated encephalomyelitis. MRI findings and the distinction from multiple sclerosis. *Brain* 113, 291–302.

Keswani, S.C. & Hoke, A. (2003) Incidence of and risk factors for HIV-associated distal sensory polyneuropathy. *Neurology* 61, 279; author reply 279–280.

Kieburtz, K., Zettelmaier, A.E., Ketonen, L., Tuite, M. & Caine, E.D. (1991) Manic syndrome in AIDS. *American Journal of Psychiatry* 148, 1068–1070.

Kiley, M. & Esiri, M.M. (2001) A contemporary case of encephalitis lethargica. *Clinical Neuropathology* 20, 2–7.

King, M.B. (1989) Psychological status of 192 out-patients with HIV infection and AIDS. *British Journal of Psychiatry* 154, 237–242.

King, M.B. (1993) *AIDS, HIV and Mental Health.* Cambridge University Press, Cambridge.

Kinghorn, G. (2000) Re-emergence of syphilis. *Hospital Medicine* 61, 675.

Kiprov, D.D. & Hofmann, J.C. (2003) Plasmapheresis in immunologically mediated polyneuropathies. *Therapeutic Apheresis and Dialysis* 7, 189–196.

Klaber, M. & Lacey, J. (1968) Epidemic of glandular fever. *British Medical Journal* 3, 124.

Kleinschmidt-DeMasters, B.K., Debiasi, R.L. & Tyler, K.L. (2001) Polymerase chain reaction as a diagnostic adjunct in herpesvirus infections of the nervous system. *Brain Pathology* 11, 452–464.

Koehler, K. & Jakumeit, U. (1976) Subacute sclerosing panencephalitis presenting as Leonhard's speech-prompt catatonia. *British Journal of Psychiatry* 129, 29–31.

Koenig, S., Gendelman, H.E., Orenstein, J.M. *et al.* (1986) Detection of AIDS virus in macrophages in brain tissue from AIDS patients with encephalopathy. *Science* 233, 1089–1093.

Koppel, B.S., Wormser, G.P., Tuchman, A.J., Maayan, S., Hewlett, D. Jr & Daras, M. (1985) Central nervous system involvement in patients with acquired immune deficiency syndrome (AIDS). *Acta Neurologica Scandinavica* 71, 337–353.

Koskiniemi, M., Piiparinen, H., Mannonen, L., Rantalaiho, T. & Vaheri, A. (1996) Herpes encephalitis is a disease of middle aged and elderly people: polymerase chain reaction for detection of herpes simplex virus in the CSF of 516 patients with encephalitis. *Journal of Neurology, Neurosurgery and Psychiatry* 60, 174–178.

Koskiniemi, M., Rantalaiho, T., Piiparinen, H. *et al.* (2001) Infections of the central nervous system of suspected viral origin: a collaborative study from Finland. *Journal of Neurovirology* 7, 400–408.

Kumar, R. (2005) Aseptic meningitis: diagnosis and management. *Indian Journal of Pediatrics* 72, 57–63.

Kupila, L., Vuorinen, T., Vainionpaa, R., Hukkanen, V., Marttila, R.J. & Kotilainen, P. (2006) Etiology of aseptic meningitis and encephalitis in an adult population. *Neurology* 66, 75–80.

Lai, C.W. & Gragasin, M.E. (1988) Electroencephalography in herpes simplex encephalitis. *Journal of Clinical Neurophysiology* 5, 87–103.

Landay, A.L., Bettendorf, D., Chan, E. *et al.* (2002) Evidence of immune reconstitution in antiretroviral drug-experienced patients with advanced HIV disease. *AIDS Research and Human Retroviruses* 18, 95–102.

Langford, T.D., Letendre, S.L., Larrea, G.J. & Masliah, E. (2003) Changing patterns in the neuropathogenesis of HIV during the HAART era. *Brain Pathology* 13, 195–210.

Lanier, E.R., Sturge, G., McClernon, D. *et al.* (2001) HIV-1 reverse transcriptase sequence in plasma and cerebrospinal fluid of patients with AIDS dementia complex treated with Abacavir. *AIDS* 15, 747–751.

Lantos, P.L., McLaughlin, J.E., Scholtz, C.L., Berry, C.L. & Tighe, J.R. (1989) Neuropathology of the brain in HIV infection. *Lancet* i, 309–310.

Laperriere, A., Ironson, G.H., Antoni, M.H. *et al.* (2005) Decreased depression up to one year following CBSM+ intervention in depressed women with AIDS: the smart/EST women's project. *Journal of Health Psychology* 10, 223–231.

Lee, B.E. & Davies, H.D. (2007) Aseptic meningitis. *Current Opinion in Infectious Diseases* 20, 272–277.

Lee, D.M. & Chen, M.Y. (2005) The re-emergence of syphilis among homosexually active men in Melbourne. *Australian and New Zealand Journal of Public Health* 29, 390–391.

Lees, F. (1970) *The Diagnosis and Treatment of Diseases Affecting the Nervous System*, vols 1 and 2. Staples Press, London.

Legg, N.J. (1967) Virus antibodies in subacute sclerosing panencephalitis: a study of 22 patients. *British Medical Journal* 3, 350–352.

Lehrich, J.R., Katz, M., Rorke, L.B., Barbanti-Brodano, G. & Koprowski, H. (1970) Subacute sclerosing panencephalitis. Encephalitis in hamsters produced by viral agents isolated from human brain cells. *Archives of Neurology* **23**, 97–102.

Leider, W., Magoffin, R.L., Lennette, E.H. & Leonards, L.N.R. (1965) Herpes-simplex-virus encephalitis: its possible association with reactivated latent infection. *New England Journal of Medicine* **273**, 341–347.

Leigh, A.D. (1946) Infections of the nervous system occurring during an epidemic of influenza B. *British Medical Journal* **2**, 936–938.

Leserman, J. (2000) The effects of depression, stressful life events, social support, and coping on the progression of HIV infection. *Current Psychiatry Reports* **2**, 495–502.

Leserman, J. (2008) Role of depression, stress, and trauma in HIV disease progression. *Psychosomatic Medicine* **70**, 539–545.

Leserman, J., Pence, B.W., Whetten, K. *et al.* (2007) Relation of lifetime trauma and depressive symptoms to mortality in HIV. *American Journal of Psychiatry* **164**, 1707–1713.

Letendre, S.L., Lanier, E.R. & McCutchan, J.A. (1999) Cerebrospinal fluid beta chemokine concentrations in neurocognitively impaired individuals infected with human immunodeficiency virus type 1. *Journal of Infectious Diseases* **180**, 310–319.

Letendre, S.L., McCutchan, J.A., Childers, M.E. *et al.* (2004) Enhancing antiretroviral therapy for human immunodeficiency virus cognitive disorders. *Annals of Neurology* **56**, 416–423.

Letendre, S.L., Woods, S.P., Ellis, R.J. *et al.* (2006) Lithium improves HIV-associated neurocognitive impairment. *AIDS* **20**, 1885–1888.

Levy, R.M., Bredesen, D.E. & Rosenblum, M.L. (1985) Neurological manifestations of the acquired immunodeficiency syndrome (AIDS): experience at UCSF and review of the literature. *Journal of Neurosurgery* **62**, 475–495.

Levy, R.M., Rosenbloom, S. & Perrett, L.V. (1986) Neuroradiologic findings in AIDS: a review of 200 cases. *American Journal of Radiology* **147**, 977–983.

Levy, R.M., Bredesen, D.E. & Rosenblum, M.L. (1988) Opportunistic central nervous system pathology in patients with AIDS. *Annals of Neurology* **23** (suppl.), S7–S12.

Lim, C.C., Lee, W.L., Leo, Y.S. *et al.* (2003) Late clinical and magnetic resonance imaging follow up of Nipah virus infection. *Journal of Neurology, Neurosurgery and Psychiatry* **74**, 131–133.

Liu, M.C. (1960) General paralysis of the insane in Peking between 1933 and 1943. *Journal of Mental Science* **106**, 1082–1092.

Lloyd-Still, R.M. (1958) Psychosis following Asian influenza in Barbados. *Lancet* **ii**, 20–21.

Lobato, M.N., Spira, T.J. & Rogers, M.F. (1995) CD4+ T lymphocytopenia in children: lack of evidence for a new acquired immunodeficiency syndrome agent. *Pediatric Infectious Disease Journal* **14**, 527–535.

Lorber, J. (1961) Long-term follow-up of 100 children who recovered from tuberculous meningitis. *Pediatrics* **28**, 778–791.

Lucas, S.B., Hounnou, A., Peacock, C. *et al.* (1993) The mortality and pathology of HIV infection in a West African city. *AIDS* **7**, 1569–1579.

Lukehart, S.A., Hook, E.W. III, Baker-Zander, S.A., Collier, A.C., Critchlow, C.W. & Handsfield, H.H. (1988) Invasion of the central nervous system by *Treponema pallidum*: implications for diagnosis and treatment. *Annals of Internal Medicine* **109**, 855–862.

Luxon, L., Lees, A.J. & Greenwood, R.J. (1979) Neurosyphilis today. *Lancet* **i**, 90–93.

Lyketsos, C.G., Hanson, A.L., Fishman, M., Rosenblatt, A., McHugh, P.R. & Treisman, G.J. (1993) Manic syndrome early and late in the course of HIV. *American Journal of Psychiatry* **150**, 326–327.

Lyketsos, C.G., Hoover, D.R., Guccione, M. *et al.* (1996) Changes in depressive symptoms as AIDS develops. The Multicenter AIDS Cohort Study. *American Journal of Psychiatry* **153**, 1430–1437.

Lyketsos, C.G., Breitner, J.C. & Rabins, P.V. (2001) An evidence-based proposal for the classification of neuropsychiatric disturbance in Alzheimer's disease. *International Journal of Geriatric Psychiatry* **16**, 1037–1042.

Lynn, W.A. & Lightman, S. (2004) Syphilis and HIV: a dangerous combination. *Lancet Infectious Diseases* **4**, 456–466.

McArthur, J.C. (1987) Update on HIV infection. Neurological aspects. *Maryland Medical Journal* **36**, 32–34.

McArthur, J.C. (2004) HIV dementia: an evolving disease. *Journal of Neuroimmunology* **157**, 3–10.

McArthur, J.C. & Letendre, S.L. (2006) Is the glass three-quarters full or one-quarter empty? *Journal of Infectious Diseases* **194**, 1628–1631.

McArthur, J.C., Cohen, B.A., Farzedegan, H. *et al.* (1988) Cerebrospinal fluid abnormalities in homosexual men with and without neuropsychiatric findings. *Annals of Neurology* **23** (suppl.), S34–S37.

McArthur, J.C., Hoover, D.R., Bacellar, H. *et al.* (1993) Dementia in AIDS patients: incidence and risk factors. Multicenter AIDS Cohort Study. *Neurology* **43**, 2245–2252.

McArthur, J.C., Selnes, O.A., Glass, J.D., Hoover, D.R. & Bacellar, H. (1994) HIV dementia: incidence and risk factors. In: Price, R.W. & Perry, S.W. (eds) *HIV, AIDS, and the Brain*, ch. 14. Association for Research in Nervous and Mental Disease vol. 72. Raven Press, New York.

McArthur, J.C., McClernon, D.R., Cronin, M.F. *et al.* (1997) Relationship between human immunodeficiency virus-associated dementia and viral load in cerebrospinal fluid and brain. *Annals of Neurology* **42**, 689–698.

McArthur, J.C., Brew, B.J. & Nath, A. (2005) Neurological complications of HIV infection. *Lancet Neurology* **4**, 543–555.

McCall, S., Henry, J.M., Reid, A.H. & Taubenberger, J.K. (2001) Influenza DNA not detected in archival brain tissues from acute encephalitis lethargica cases or in postencephalitis Parkinson cases. *Journal of Neuropathology and Experimental Neurology* **60**, 696–704.

McCormick, G.F., Zee, C.-S. & Heiden, J. (1982) Cysticercosis cerebri. *Archives of Neurology* **39**, 534–539.

McGrath, N., Anderson, N.E., Croxson, M.C. & Powell, K.F. (1997) Herpes simplex encephalitis treated with acyclovir: diagnosis and long term outcome. *Journal of Neurology, Neurosurgery and Psychiatry* **63**, 321–326.

Maggi, J.D. & Halman, M.H. (2001) The effect of divalproex sodium on viral load: a retrospective review of HIV-positive patients with manic syndromes. *Canadian Journal of Psychiatry* **46**, 359–362.

Mahendra, B. (1981) Where have all the catatonics gone? *Psychological Medicine* **11**, 669–671.

Mahorney, S.L. & Cavenar, J.O. (1988) A new and timely delusion: the complaint of having AIDS. *American Journal of Psychiatry* **145**, 1130–1132.

Maini, C.L., Piogorini, F., Pan Fu *et al.* (1990) Cortical cerebral blood flow in HIV-1 related dementia complex. *Nuclear Medicine Communications* **11**, 639–648.

Maj, M. (1990) Psychiatric aspects of HIV-1 infection and AIDS. *Psychological Medicine* **20**, 547–563.

Maj, M., Satz, P., Janssen, R. *et al.* (1994) WHO Neuropsychiatric AIDS study, cross-sectional phase II. Neuropsychological and neurological findings. *Archives of General Psychiatry* **51**, 51–61.

Malouf, R., Jacquette, G., Dobkin, J. & Brust, J.C. (1990) Neurologic disease in human immunodeficiency virus-infected drug abusers. *Archives of Neurology* **47**, 1002–1007.

Manji, H. & Connolly, S. (1992) AIDS and the central nervous system: part 2. *Hospital Update* January, 28–38.

Marcotte, T.D., Deutsch, R., McCutchan, J.A. *et al.* (2003) Prediction of incident neurocognitive impairment by plasma HIV RNA and CD4 levels early after HIV seroconversion. *Archives of Neurology* **60**, 1406–1412.

Margo, C.E. & Hamed, L.M. (1992) Ocular syphilis. *Survey of Ophthalmology* **37**, 203–220.

Mark, A.S. & Atlas, S.W. (1989) Progressive multifocal leukoencephalopathy in patients with AIDS: appearance on MR images. *Radiology* **173**, 517–520.

Markowitz, J.C., Kocsis, J.H., Fishman, B. *et al.* (1998) Treatment of depressive symptoms in human immunodeficiency virus-positive patients. *Archives of General Psychiatry* **55**, 452–457.

Marra, C.M., Gary, D.W., Kuypers, J. & Jacobson, M.A. (1996) Diagnosis of neurosyphilis in patients infected with human immunodeficiency virus type 1. *Journal of Infectious Diseases* **174**, 219–221.

Marra, C.M., Boutin, P., McArthur, J.C. *et al.* (2000) A pilot study evaluating ceftriaxone and penicillin G as treatment agents for neurosyphilis in human immunodeficiency virus-infected individuals. *Clinical Infectious Diseases* **30**, 540–544.

Marshall, D.W., Brey, R.L., Cahill, W.T., Houk, R.W., Zajac, R.A. & Boswell, R.N. (1988) Spectrum of cerebrospinal fluid findings in various stages of human immunodeficiency virus infection. *Archives of Neurology* **45**, 954–958.

Martin, C., Albert, J., Hansson, P., Pehrsson, P., Link, H. & Sonnerborg, A. (1998) Cerebrospinal fluid mononuclear cell counts influence CSF HIV-1 RNA levels. *Journal of Acquired Immune Deficiency Syndromes and Human Retrovirology* **17**, 214–219.

Marzuk, P.M. (1991) Suicidal behavior and HIV illness. *International Review of Psychiatry* **3**, 365–371.

Marzuk, P.M., Tierney, H., Tardiff, K. *et al.* (1988) Increased risk of suicide in persons with AIDS. *Journal of the American Medical Association* **259**, 1333–1337.

Maschke, M., Kastrup, O., Esser, S., Ross, B., Hengge, U. & Hufnagel, A. (2000) Incidence and prevalence of neurological disorders associated with HIV since the introduction of highly active antiretroviral therapy (HAART). *Journal of Neurology, Neurosurgery and Psychiatry* **69**, 376–380.

Masliah, E., Heaton, R.K., Marcotte, T.D. *et al.* (1997) Dendritic injury is a pathological substrate for human immunodeficiency virus-related cognitive disorders. *Annals of Neurology* **42**, 963–972.

Masliah, E., Deteresa, R.M., Mallory, M.E. & Hansen, L.A. (2000) Changes in pathological findings at autopsy in AIDS cases for the last 15 years. *AIDS* **14**, 69–74.

Mathiesen, G.E. & Johnson, J.P. (1997) Brain abscess. *Clinical Infectious Diseases* **25**, 763–781.

Maxwell, S., Scheftner, W.A., Kessler, H.A. & Busch, K. (1988) Manic syndrome associated with zidovudine treatment. *Journal of the American Medical Association* **259**, 3406–3407.

Mazur, M.H. & Dolin, R. (1978) Herpes zoster at the NIH: a 20 year experience. *American Journal of Medicine* **65**, 738–744.

Mellors, J.W., Kingsley, L.A., Rinaldo, C.R. Jr *et al.* (1995) Quantitation of HIV-1 RNA in plasma predicts outcome after seroconversion. *Annals of Internal Medicine* **122**, 573–579.

Mellors, J.W., Munoz, A., Giorgi, J.V. *et al.* (1997) Plasma viral load and CD4+ lymphocytes as prognostic markers of HIV-1 infection. *Annals of Internal Medicine* **126**, 946–954.

Menon, D.K., Baudouin, C.J., Tomlinson, D. & Hoyle, C. (1990) Proton MR spectroscopy and imaging of the brain in AIDS: evidence of neuronal loss in regions that appear normal with imaging. *Journal of Computer Assisted Tomography* **14**, 882–885.

Merkelbach, S., Sittinger, H., Schweizer, I. & Muller, M. (2000) Cognitive outcome after bacterial meningitis. *Acta Neurologica Scandinavica* **102**, 118–123.

Mijch, A.M., Judd, F.K., Lyketsos, C.G., Ellen, S. & Cockram, A. (1999) Secondary mania in patients with HIV infection: are antiretrovirals protective? *Journal of Neuropsychiatry and Clinical Neuroscience* **11**, 475–480.

Miller, D., Acton, T.M.G. & Hedge, B. (1988) The worried well: their identification and management. *Journal of the Royal College of Physicians of London* **22**, 158–165.

Misra, P.C. & Hay, G.G. (1971) Encephalitis presenting as acute schizophrenia. *British Medical Journal* **1**, 532–533.

Mocroft, A., Katlama, C., Johnson, A.M. *et al.* (2000) AIDS across Europe, 1994–98: the EuroSIDA study. *Lancet* **356**, 291–296.

Mohr, J.A., Griffiths, W., Jackson, R., Saadah, H., Bird, P. & Riddle, J. (1976) Neurosyphilis and penicillin levels in cerebrospinal fluid. *Journal of the American Medical Association* **236**, 2208–2209.

Monnet, F.P. (2003) Behavioural disturbances following Japanese B encephalitis. *European Psychiatry* **18**, 269–273.

Moog, C., Kuntz-Simon, G., Caussin-Schwemling, C. & Obert, G. (1996) Sodium valproate, an anticonvulsant drug, stimulates human immunodeficiency virus type 1 replication independently of glutathione levels. *Journal of General Virology* **77**, 1993–1999.

Moore, D.J., Masliah, E., Rippeth, J.D. *et al.* (2006) Cortical and subcortical neurodegeneration is associated with HIV neurocognitive impairment. *AIDS* **20**, 879–887.

Moore, R.D. & Chaisson, R.E. (1999) Natural history of HIV infection in the era of combination antiretroviral therapy. *AIDS* **13**, 1933–1942.

Moorthy, R.K. & Rajshekhar, V. (2008) Management of brain abscess: an overview. *Neurosurgical Focus* **24**, E3.

Morgan, D. (2006) Control of arbovirus infections by a coordinated response: West Nile Virus in England and Wales. *FEMS Immunology and Medical Microbiology* **48**, 305–312.

Morgello, S., Mahboob, R., Yakoushina, T., Khan, S. & Hague, K. (2002) Autopsy findings in a human immunodeficiency virus-infected population over 2 decades: influences of gender, ethnicity, risk factors, and time. *Archives of Pathology and Laboratory Medicine* **126**, 182–190.

Morishima, T., Togashi, T., Yokota, S. *et al.* (2002) Encephalitis and encephalopathy associated with an influenza epidemic in Japan. *Clinical Infectious Diseases* **35**, 512–517.

Morris, L., Silber, E., Sonnenberg, P. *et al.* (1998) High human immunodeficiency virus type 1 RNA load in the cerebrospinal fluid from patients with lymphocytic meningitis. *Journal of Infectious Diseases* **177**, 473–476.

Moss, H.E. & Tyler, L.K. (2000) A progressive category-specific semantic deficit for non-living things. *Neuropsychologia* **38**, 60–82.

Muhlemann, M.F. (1992) Uncommon infections: 3. Lyme disease. *Prescribers Journal* **32**, 77–82.

Muller, R., Nylander, I., Larsson, L.-E., Widen, L. & Frankenhaeuser, M. (1958) Sequelae of primary aseptic meningoencephalitis. *Acta Psychiatrica et Neurologica Scandinavica Supplementum* **126**, 1–115.

Musher, D.M. (1991) Syphilis, neurosyphilis, penicillin, and AIDS. *Journal of Infectious Diseases* **163**, 1201–1206.

Nadeem, A.A. & Younis, Y.O. (1977) Physical illness and psychiatric disorders in Tigani El-Mahi Psychiatric Hospital (Sudan). *East African Medical Journal* **54**, 207–210.

National AIDS Trust (2006) Public attitudes towards HIV. Available at http//www.nat.org.uk

Navia, B.A. & Price, R.W. (1987) The acquired immunodeficiency syndrome dementia complex as the presenting or sole manifestation of human immunodeficiency virus infection. *Archives of Neurology* **44**, 65–69.

Navia, B.A., Jordan, B.D. & Price, R.W. (1986a) The AIDS dementia complex: I. Clinical features. *Annals of Neurology* **19**, 517–524.

Navia, B.A., Cho, E.-S., Petito, C.K. & Price, R.W. (1986b) The AIDS dementia complex: II. Neuropathology. *Annals of Neurology* **19**, 525–535.

Ng, B.Y., Lim, C.C., Yeoh, A. & Lee, W.L. (2004) Neuropsychiatric sequelae of Nipah virus encephalitis. *Journal of Neuropsychiatry and Clinical Neuroscience* **16**, 500–504.

Nieman, E.A. (1991) Neurosyphilis yesterday and today. *Journal of the Royal College of Physicians of London* **25**, 321–324.

Noguchi, H. & Moore, J.W. (1913) A demonstration of treponema pallidum in the brain in cases of general paralysis. *Journal of Experimental Medicine* **17**, 232–238.

Oates, J.K. (1979) Serological tests for syphilis and their clinical use. *British Journal of Hospital Medicine* **21**, 612–617.

O'Connell, S. (1995) Lyme disease in the United Kingdom. *British Medical Journal* **310**, 303–308.

O'Dowd, M.A. (1988) Psychosocial issues in HIV infection. *AIDS* **2** (suppl. 1), S201–S205.

Offiah, C.E. & Turnbull, I.W. (2006) The imaging appearances of intracranial CNS infections in adult HIV and AIDS patients. *Clinical Radiology* **61**, 393–401.

Olsen, W.L., Longo, F.M., Mills, C.M. & Norman, D. (1988) White matter disease in AIDS: findings at MR imaging. *Radiology* **169**, 445–448.

Olson, L.C., Buescher, E.L., Artenstein, M.S. & Parkman, P.D. (1967) Herpes virus infections of the human central nervous system. *New England Journal of Medicine* **277**, 1271–1277.

Openshaw, H. & Cantin, E.M. (2005) Corticosteroids in herpes simplex virus encephalitis. *Journal of Neurology, Neurosurgery and Psychiatry* **76**, 1469.

Orban, T. (1957) Experiences with a follow-up of 200 tabetic patients. *Acta Psychiatrica et Neurologica Scandinavica* **32**, 89–102.

Ostrow, D.G. (1990) *Psychiatric Aspects of Human Immunodeficiency Virus Infection.* Upjohn Company, Kalamazoo, MI.

Oxbury, J.M. & MacCallum, F.O. (1973) Herpes simplex virus encephalitis: clinical features and residual damage. *Postgraduate Medical Journal* **49**, 387–389.

Page-Shafer, K., Delorenze, G.N., Satariano, W.A. & Winkelstein, W. Jr (1996) Comorbidity and survival in HIV-infected men in the San Francisco Men's Health Survey. *Annals of Epidemiology* **6**, 420–430.

Pai, M.N. (1945) Change in personality after cerebrospinal fever. *British Medical Journal* **1**, 289–293.

Paley, M., Cozzone, P.J., Alonso, J. *et al.* (1996) A multicenter proton magnetic resonance spectroscopy study of neurological complications of AIDS. *AIDS Research and Human Retroviruses* **12**, 213–222.

Paraskevas, G.P., Kapaki, E., Kararizou, E., Mitsonis, C., Sfagos, C. & Vassilopoulos, D. (2007) Cerebrospinal fluid tau protein is increased in neurosyphilis: a discrimination from syphilis without nervous system involvement? *Sexually Transmitted Diseases* **34**, 220–223.

Pardo, C.A., McArthur, J.C. & Griffin, J.W. (2001) HIV neuropathy: insights in the pathology of HIV peripheral nerve disease. *Journal of the Peripheral Nervous System* **6**, 21–27.

Parry, J.V., Mortimer, P.P., Perry, K.R., Pillay, D. & Zuckerman, M. (2003) Towards error-free HIV diagnosis: guidelines on laboratory practice. *Communicable Disease and Public Health* **6**, 334–350.

Parsons, T.D., Tucker, K.A., Hall, C.D. *et al.* (2006) Neurocognitive functioning and HAART in HIV and hepatitis C virus co-infection. *AIDS* **20**, 1591–1595.

Pence, B.W., Miller, W.C., Whetten, K., Eron, J.J. & Gaynes, B.N. (2006) Prevalence of DSM-IV-defined mood, anxiety, and substance use disorders in an HIV clinic in the Southeastern United States. *Journal of Acquired Immune Deficiency Syndromes* **42**, 298–306.

Penzak, S.R., Hon, Y.Y., Lawhorn, W.D., Shirley, K.L., Spratlin, V. & Jann, M.W. (2002) Influence of ritonavir on olanzapine pharmacokinetics in healthy volunteers. *Journal of Clinical Psychopharmacology* **22**, 366–370.

Perelson, A.S., Essunger, P. & Ho, D.D. (1997) Dynamics of HIV-1 and CD4+ lymphocytes in vivo. *AIDS* **11** (suppl. A), S17–S24.

Perkins, D.O., Stern, R.A., Golden, R.N., Murphy, C., Naftolowitz, D. & Evans, D.L. (1994) Mood disorders in HIV infection: prevalence and risk factors in a nonepicenter of the AIDS epidemic. *American Journal of Psychiatry* **151**, 233–236.

Perry, S. & Jacobsen, P. (1986) Neuropsychiatric manifestations of AIDS-spectrum disorders. *Hospital and Community Psychiatry* **37**, 135–142.

Perry, S.W., Jacobsberg, L.B., Fishman, B., Weiler, P.H., Gold, J.W.M. & Frances, A.J. (1990a) Psychological responses to serological testing for HIV. *AIDS* **4**, 145–152.

Perry, S., Jacobsberg, L. & Fishman, B. (1990b) Suicidal ideation and HIV testing. *Journal of the American Medical Association* **263**, 679–682.

Petito, C.K. (1988) Review of central nervous system pathology in human immunodeficiency virus infection. *Annals of Neurology* **23** (suppl.), S54–S57.

Petito, C.K., Navia, B.A., Cho, E.-S., Jordan, B.D., George, D.C. & Price, R.W. (1985) Vacuolar myelopathy pathologically resembling subacute combined degeneration in patients with the acquired immunodeficiency syndrome. *New England Journal of Medicine* **312**, 874–879.

Petito, C.K., Cho, E.-S., Lemann, W., Navia, B.A. & Price, R.W. (1986) Neuropathology of acquired immunodeficiency syndrome (AIDS): an autopsy review. *Journal of Neuropathology and Experimental Neurology* **45**, 635–646.

Petito, C.K., Vecchio, D. & Chen, Y.T. (1994) HIV antigen and DNA in AIDS spinal cords correlates with macrophage infiltration and not with vacuolar myelopathy. *Journal of Neuropathology and Experimental Neurology* **53**, 86–94.

Petito, C.K., Roberts, B., Cantando, J.D., Rabinstein, A. & Duncan, R. (2001) Hippocampal injury and alterations in neuronal chemokine co-receptor expression in patients with AIDS. *Journal of Neuropathology and Experimental Neurology* **60**, 377–385.

Petruckevitch, A., Del Amo, J., Phillips, A.N. *et al.* (1998) Disease progression and survival following specific AIDS-defining conditions: a retrospective cohort study of 2048 HIV-infected persons in London. *AIDS* **12**, 1007–1013.

Pewter, S.M., Williams, W.H., Haslam, C. & Kay, J.M. (2007) Neuropsychological and psychiatric profiles in acute encephalitis in adults. *Neuropsychological Rehabilitation* **17**, 478–505.

Peyriere, H., Mauboussin, J.M., Rouanet, I., Fabre, J., Reynes, J. & Hillaire-Buys, D. (2001) Management of sudden psychiatric disorders related to efavirenz. *AIDS* **15**, 1323–1324.

Phillips, A.N., Sabin, C.A., Elford, J., Bofill, M., Janossy, G. & Lee, C.A. (1994) Use of CD4 lymphocyte count to predict long-term survival free of AIDS after HIV infection. *British Medical Journal* **309**, 309–313.

Podraza, A.M., Bornstein, R.A., Whitacre, C.C. *et al.* (1994) Neuropsychological performance and CD4 levels in HIV-1 asymptomatic infection. *Journal of Clinical and Experimental Neuropsychology* **16**, 777–783.

Pommer, B., Pilz, P. & Harrer, G. (1983) Transient global amnesia as a manifestation of Epstein–Barr virus encephalitis. *Journal of Neurology* **229**, 125–127.

Portegies, P., De Gans, J., Lange, J.M. *et al.* (1989) Declining incidence of AIDS dementia complex after introduction of zidovudine treatment. *British Medical Journal* **299**, 819–821.

Portegies, P., Solod, L., Cinque, P. *et al.* (2004) Guidelines for the diagnosis and management of neurological complications of HIV infection. *European Journal of Neurology* **11**, 297–304.

Poser, C.M. (1990) Notes on the pathogenesis of subacute sclerosing panencephalitis. *Journal of the Neurological Sciences* **95**, 219–224.

Poser, C.M., Huntley, C.J. & Poland, J.D. (1969) Para-encephalitic parkinsonism. Report of an acute case due to coxsackie virus type B2 and re-examination of the etiologic concepts of post-encephalitic parkinsonism. *Acta Neurologica Scandinavica* **45**, 199–215.

Price, R.W. (1994) Understanding the AIDS dementia complex: the challenge of HIV and its effects on the central nervous system. In: Price, R.W. & Perry, S.W. (eds) *HIV, AIDS, and the Brain*, ch. 1. Association for Research in Nervous and Mental Disease vol. 72. Raven Press, New York.

Puchhammer-Stockl, E., Heinz, F.X., Kundi, M. *et al.* (1993) Evaluation of the polymerase chain reaction for diagnosis of herpes simplex virus encephalitis. *Journal of Clinical Microbiology* **31**, 146–148.

Rabkin, J.G., Wagner, G. & Rabkin, R. (1999) Fluoxetine treatment for depression in patients with HIV and AIDS: a randomized, placebo-controlled trial. *American Journal of Psychiatry* **156**, 101–107.

Rabkin, J.G., Ferrando, S.J., Lin, S.H., Sewell, M. & McElhiney, M. (2000) Psychological effects of HAART: a 2-year study. *Psychosomatic Medicine* **62**, 413–422.

Rabkin, J.G., Wagner, G.J., McElhiney, M.C., Rabkin, R. & Lin, S.H. (2004) Testosterone versus fluoxetine for depression and fatigue in HIV/AIDS: a placebo-controlled trial. *Journal of Clinical Psychopharmacology* **24**, 379–385.

Raghav, S., Seneviratne, J., McKelvie, P.A., Chapman, C., Talman, P.S. & Kempster, P.A. (2007) Sporadic encephalitis lethargica. *Journal of Clinical Neuroscience* **14**, 696–700.

Rail, D., Scholtz, C. & Swash, M. (1981) Post-encephalitic parkinsonism: current experience. *Journal of Neurology, Neurosurgery and Psychiatry* **44**, 670–676.

Ramers, C., Billman, G., Hartin, M., Ho, S. & Sawyer, M.H. (2000) Impact of a diagnostic cerebrospinal fluid enterovirus polymerase chain reaction test on patient management. *Journal of the American Medical Association* **283**, 2680–2685.

Raschilas, F., Wolff, M., Delatour, F. *et al.* (2002) Outcome of and prognostic factors for herpes simplex encephalitis in adult patients: results of a multicenter study. *Clinical Infectious Diseases* **35**, 254–260.

Raymond, R.W. & Williams, R.L. (1948) Infectious mononucleosis with psychosis: report of case. *New England Journal of Medicine* **239**, 542–544.

Repetto, M.J. & Petitto, J.M. (2008) Psychopharmacology in HIV-infected patients. *Psychosomatic Medicine* **70**, 585–592.

Resnick, J.S., Engel, W.K. & Sever, J.L. (1968) Subacute sclerosing panencephalitis. *New England Journal of Medicine* **279**, 126–129.

Resnick, L., Berger, J.R., Shapshak, P. & Tourtellotte, W.W. (1988) Early penetration of the blood–brain barrier by HIV. *Neurology* **38**, 9–14.

Reyes, M.G., Faraldi, F., Senseng, C.S., Flowers, C. & Fariello, R. (1991) Nigral degeneration in acquired immune deficiency syndrome (AIDS). *Acta Neuropathologica* **82**, 39–44.

Riedel, D.J., Pardo, C.A., McArthur, J. & Nath, A. (2006) Therapy Insight: CNS manifestations of HIV-associated immune reconstitution inflammatory syndrome. *Nature Clinical Practice Neurology* **2**, 557–565.

Risk, W.S., Haddad, F.S. & Chemali, P. (1978) Substantial spontaneous long-term improvement in subacute sclerosing panencephalitis. Six cases from the Middle East and a review of the literature. *Archives of Neurology* **35**, 494–502.

Roberts, M.C. & Emsley, R.A. (1992) Psychiatric manifestations of neurosyphilis. *South African Medical Journal* **82**, 335–337.

Roberts, M.C. & Emsley, R.A. (1995) Cognitive change after treatment for neurosyphilis. Correlation with CSF laboratory measures. *General Hospital Psychiatry* **17**, 305–309.

Robertson, K.R., Robertson, W.T., Ford, S. *et al.* (2004) Highly active antiretroviral therapy improves neurocognitive functioning. *Journal of Acquired Immune Deficiency Syndromes* **36**, 562–566.

Robinson, J.G. (1999) Wildlife harvest in logged tropical forests. *Science* **284**, 595–596.

Rogstad, K., Palfreeman, A., Rooney, G. *et al.* (2006) UK National Guidelines on HIV Testing 2006. *International Journal of STD and AIDS* **17**, 668–676.

Rose, F.C. & Symonds, C.P. (1960) Persistent memory defect following encephalitis. *Brain* **83**, 195–212.

Rosenblum, M.L., Levy, R.M., Bredesen, D.E., So, Y.T., Wara, W. & Ziegler, J.L. (1988) Primary central nervous system lymphomas in patients with AIDS. *Annals of Neurology* **23** (suppl.), S13–S16.

Rotbart, H.A., Sawyer, M.H., Fast, S. *et al.* (1994) Diagnosis of enteroviral meningitis by using PCR with a colorimetric microwell detection assay. *Journal of Clinical Microbiology* **32**, 2590–2592.

Rottenberg, D.A., Moeller, J.R., Strother, S.C. *et al.* (1987) The metabolic pathology of the AIDS dementia complex. *Annals of Neurology* **22**, 700–706.

Rovira, M., Romero, F., Torrent, O. & Ibarra, B. (1980) Study of tuberculous meningitis by CT. *Neuroradiology* **19**, 137–141.

Rowland-Jones, S. (1999) The role of chemokine receptors in HIV infection. *Sexually Transmitted Infections* **75**, 148–151.

Rutherford, G. (1994) Long term survival in HIV-1 infection. *British Medical Journal* **309**, 283–284.

Sacks, O. (1973) *Awakenings*. Duckworth, London.

Sacktor, N. (2002) The epidemiology of human immunodeficiency virus-associated neurological disease in the era of highly active antiretroviral therapy. *Journal of Neurovirology* **8** (suppl. 2), 115–121.

Sacktor, N., Van Heertum, K.L., Dooneief, G. *et al.* (1995a) A comparison of cerebral SPECT abnormalities in HIV-positive homosexual men with and without cognitive impairment. *Archives of Neurology* **52**, 1170–1173.

Sacktor, N., Prohovnik, I., Van Heertum, K.L. *et al.* (1995b) Cerebral single-photon emission computed tomography abnormalities in human immunodeficiency virus type 1 infected gay men without cognitive impairment. *Archives of Neurology* **52**, 607–611.

Sacktor, N.P., Bacellar, H., Hoover, D.R. *et al.* (1996) Psychomotor slowing in HIV infection: a predictor of dementia, AIDS and death. *Journal of Neurovirology* **2**, 404–410.

Sacktor, N., Lyles, R.H., Skolasky, R. *et al.* (2001) HIV-associated neurologic disease incidence changes: Multicenter AIDS Cohort Study, 1990–1998. *Neurology* **56**, 257–260.

Sacktor, N., McDermott, M.P., Marder, K. *et al.* (2002) HIV-associated cognitive impairment before and after the advent of combination therapy. *Journal of Neurovirology* **8**, 136–142.

Saito, Y., Sharer, L.R., Epstein, L.G. *et al.* (1994) Overexpression of nef as a marker for restricted HIV-1 infection of astrocytes in postmortem pediatric central nervous tissues. *Neurology* **44**, 474–481.

Salib, E.A. (1988) Subacute sclerosing panencephalitis (SSPE) presenting at the age of 21 as a schizophrenia-like state with bizarre dysmorphophobic features. *British Journal of Psychiatry* **152**, 709–710.

Samson, M., Libert, F., Doranz, B.J. *et al.* (1996) Resistance to HIV-1 infection in caucasian individuals bearing mutant alleles of the CCR-5 chemokine receptor gene. *Nature* **382**, 722–725.

Sands, I.J. (1928) The acute psychiatric type of epidemic encephalitis. *American Journal of Psychiatry* **7**, 975–987.

Satishchandra, P., Nalini, A., Gourie-Devi, M. *et al.* (2000) Profile of neurologic disorders associated with HIV/AIDS from Bangalore, south India (1989–96). *Indian Journal of Medical Research* **111**, 14–23.

Scaravilli, F., Bazille, C. & Gray, F. (2007) Neuropathologic contributions to understanding AIDS and the central nervous system. *Brain Pathology* **17**, 197–208.

Schaerf, F.W., Miller, R.R., Lipsey, J.R. & McPherson, R.W. (1989) ECT for major depression in four patients infected with human immunodeficiency virus. *American Journal of Psychiatry* **146**, 782–784.

Schilder, P. (1938) The organic background of obsessions and compulsions. *American Journal of Psychiatry* **94**, 1397–1413.

Schuchat, A., Robinson, K., Wenger, J.D. *et al.* (1997) Bacterial meningitis in the United States in 1995. Active Surveillance Team. *New England Journal of Medicine* **337**, 970–976.

Schwab, R.S., Fabing, H.D. & Prichard, J.S. (1951) Psychiatric symptoms and syndromes in Parkinson's disease. *American Journal of Psychiatry* **107**, 901–907.

Schweizer, T.A., Dixon, M.J., Westwood, D. & Piskopos, M. (2001) Contribution of visual and semantic proximity to identification performance in a viral encephalitis patient. *Brain and Cognition* **46**, 260–264.

Scott-Sheldon, L.A., Kalichman, S.C., Carey, M.P. & Fielder, R.L. (2008) Stress management intervention for HIV-positive adults: a meta-analysis of randomized controlled trials, 1989–2006. *Health Psychology* **27**, 129–139.

Sejvar, J.J. (2006) The evolving epidemiology of viral encephalitis. *Current Opinion in Neurology* **19**, 350–357.

Sells, C.J., Carpenter, R.L. & Ray, C.G. (1975) Sequelae of central-nervous-system enterovirus infections. *New England Journal of Medicine* **293**, 1–4.

Selnes, O.A., Galai, N., Bacellar, H. *et al.* (1995) Cognitive performance after progression to AIDS: a longitudinal study from the Multicenter AIDS Cohort Study. *Neurology* **45**, 267–275.

Selwyn, P.A., Hartel, D., Wasserman, W. & Drucker, E. (1989) Impact of the AIDS epidemic on morbidity and mortality among intravenous drug users in a New York City methadone maintenance program. *American Journal of Public Health* **79**, 1358–1362.

Sevigny, J.J., Albert, S.M., McDermott, M.P. *et al.* (2004) Evaluation of HIV RNA and markers of immune activation as predictors of HIV-associated dementia. *Neurology* **63**, 2084–2090.

Sevigny, J.J., Albert, S.M., McDermott, M.P. *et al.* (2007) An evaluation of neurocognitive status and markers of immune activation as predictors of time to death in advanced HIV infection. *Archives of Neurology* **64**, 97–102.

Sewell, D.D., Jeste, D.V., Atkinson, J.H. *et al.* (1994) HIV-associated psychosis: a study of 20 cases. San Diego HIV Neurobehavioral Research Center Group. *American Journal of Psychiatry* **151**, 237–242.

Sharp, P.M., Bailes, E., Chaudhuri, R.R., Rodenburg, C.M., Santiago, M.O. & Hahn, B.H. (2001) The origins of acquired

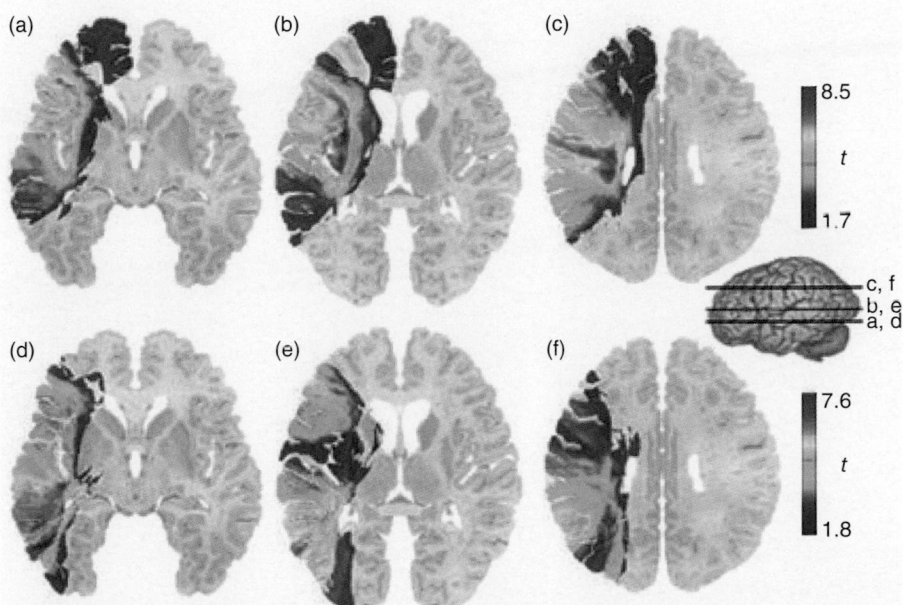

Plate 2.1 Representative slices from VLSM maps computed for fluency and auditory comprehension performance of 101 aphasic stroke patients.

These maps are coloured depictions of *t*-test results evaluating patients' performance on a voxel-by-voxel basis, for fluency (a–c) or auditory comprehension (d–f). High scores (red) indicate that lesions to these voxels have a highly significant effect on behaviour. Dark blue voxels indicate that the lesions had relatively little impact on behaviour. From Bates *et al.* (2003), *Nature Neuroscience* **6**, 448–450. See also Fig. 2.1.

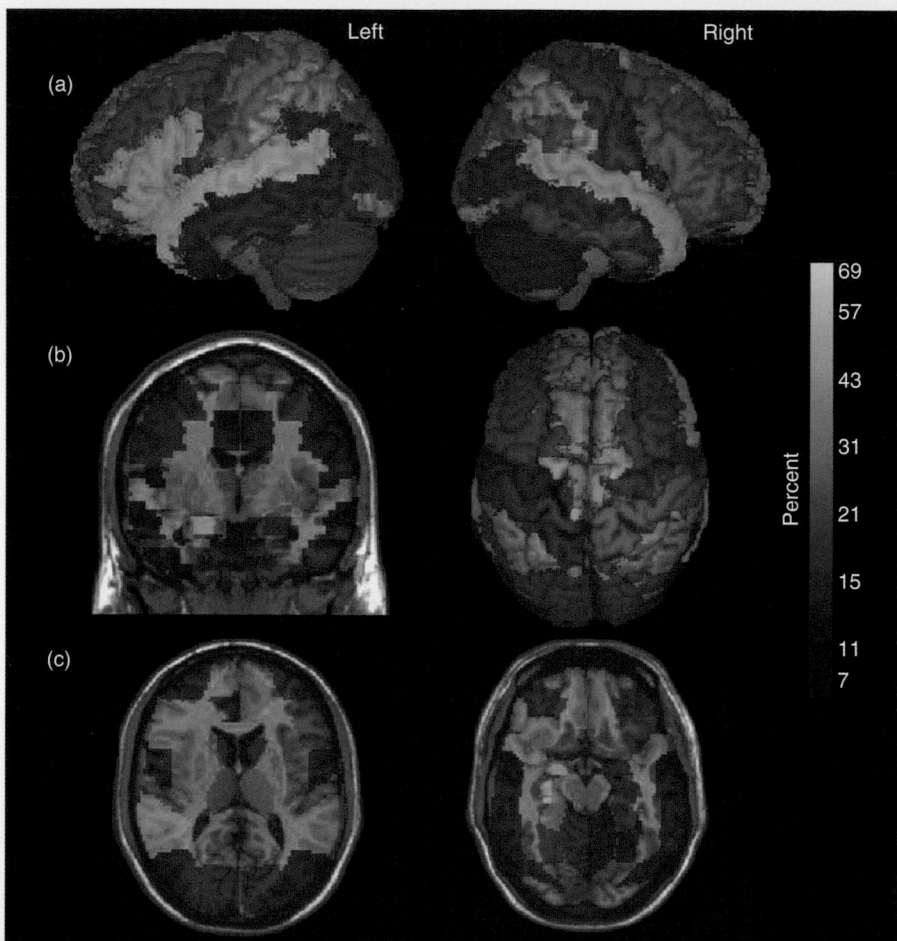

Plate 2.2 Brain regions in which significant volume deficits in patients with schizophrenia were reported in voxel-based morphometry studies (*N*=15), by percentage of studies reporting the deficit. In row (a), left and right whole-brain three-dimensional images are overlaid with all regions in which significant volume deficits in patients with schizophrenia were reported. In row (b), a coronal view and an axial three-dimensional image are shown. In row (c), axial views are shown. From Honea *et al.* (2005), *Am J Psychiatry* **162**, 2233–2245. © 2005 American Psychiatric Association. See also Fig. 2.2.

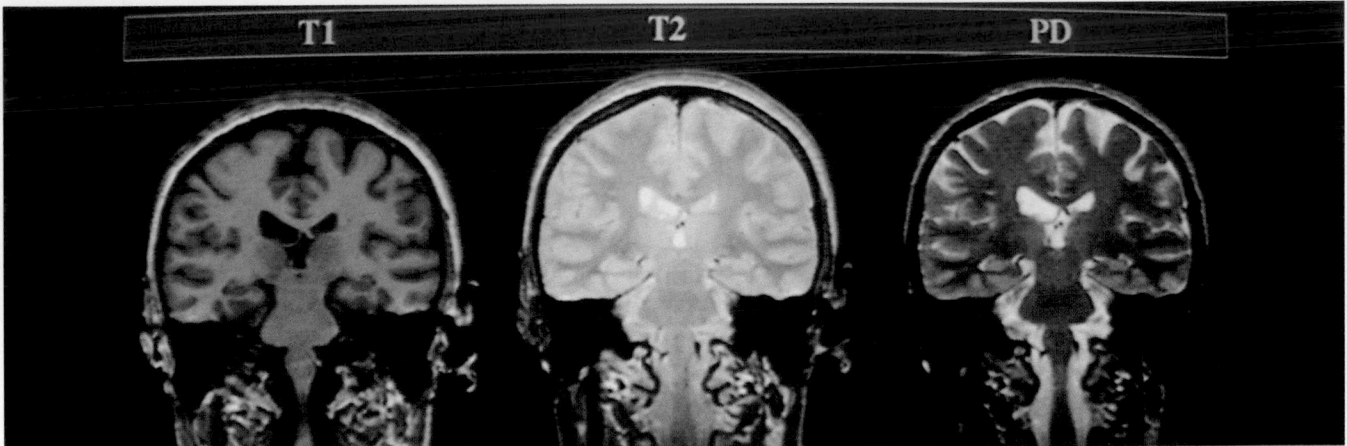

Plate 3.1 Coronal magnetic resonance brain images illustrating different scanning sequences (see also Fig. 3.5). T1, inversion recovery; T2, spin-echo; PD, proton density. (Courtesy of Dr Nancy Andreasen.)

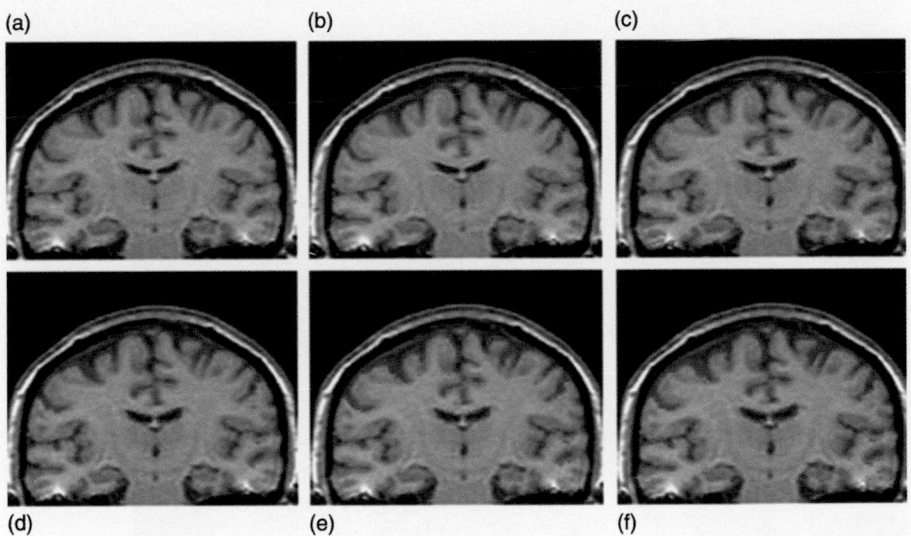

Plate 3.2 Serially acquired T1-weighted MRI scans from an initially asymptomatic patient destined to develop familial Alzheimer's disease. Scans were acquired over 4 years before criteria for dementia were met; the first symptoms were reported between scans (d) and (e). Each scan has been positionally registered to the baseline scan; red overlay represents tissue loss compared with baseline. See also Fig. 3.10. (From Fox & Schott 2004 with permission.)

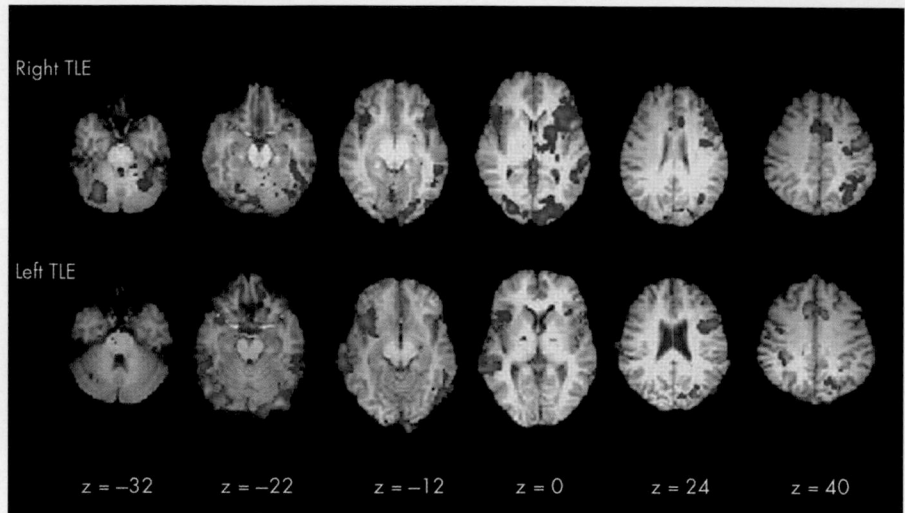

Plate 3.3 Functional magnetic resonance imaging: differences in relative language lateralisation for a verbal fluency task can be found between patients with right or left temporal lobe epilepsy (TLE). Illustrative activation maps are shown here, co-registered with individual high-resolution structural MRI. Cluster detection was done on all voxels above $z = 2.3$ to determine clusters significantly activated (corrected $P < 0.01$) in the experimental task condition. The patient with right TLE has predominantly left hemisphere activation. In contrast, the activation map for the patient with left TLE shows bihemispheric activations. See also Fig. 3.15. (From Matthews & Jezzard 2004 with permission.)

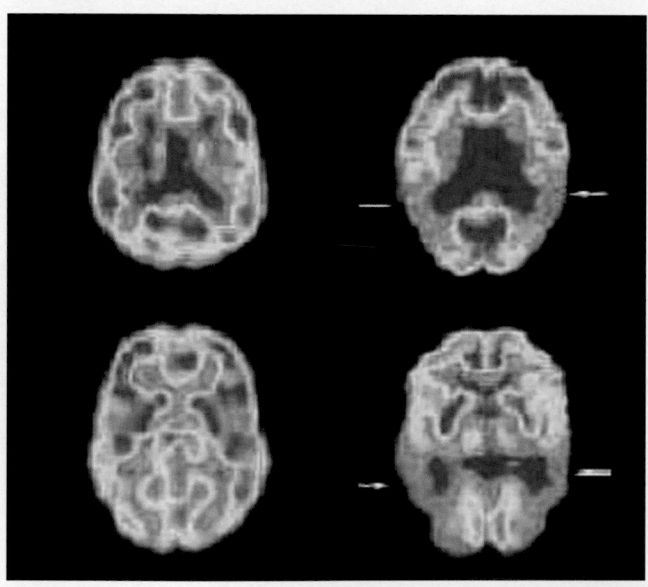

Plate 3.4 Fluorodeoxyglucose positron emission tomography images in Alzheimer's disease: (left) normal brain; (right) Alzheimer's brain. Arrows point to area of posterior hypometabolism. See also Fig. 3.16. Available at http://www.uhseastpetscan.com/zportal/portals/pat/brain/Alzheimers_Disease/pet_scans

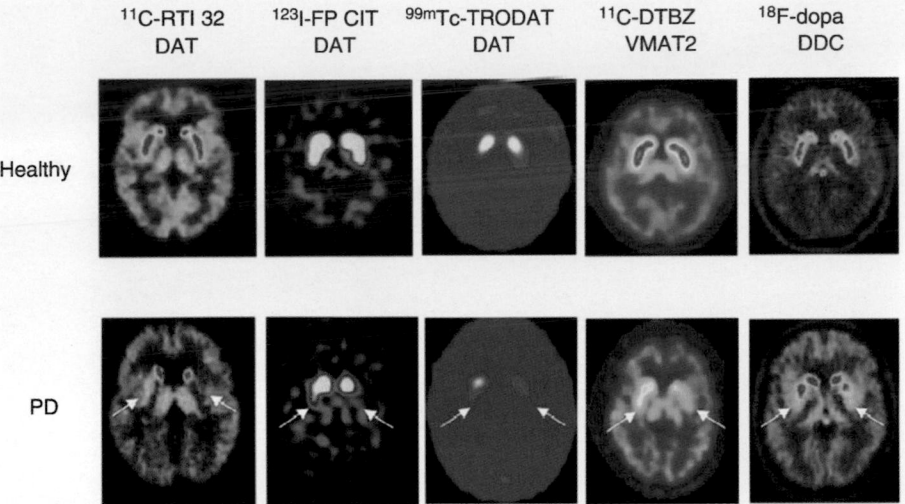

Plate 3.5 Striatal uptake of dopamine transporter (DAT) ^{11}C-RTI-32, ^{123}I-β-CIT, ^{99m}Tc-TRODAT, vesicular monoamine transporter (VMAT2) ^{11}C-DTBZ, and dopa decarboxylase (DDC) ^{18}F-dopa in a healthy control subject and a patient with early Parkinson's disease (PD). In PD the putamens are targeted asymmetrically. See also Fig. 3.17. (From Brooks & Piccini 2006 with permission.)

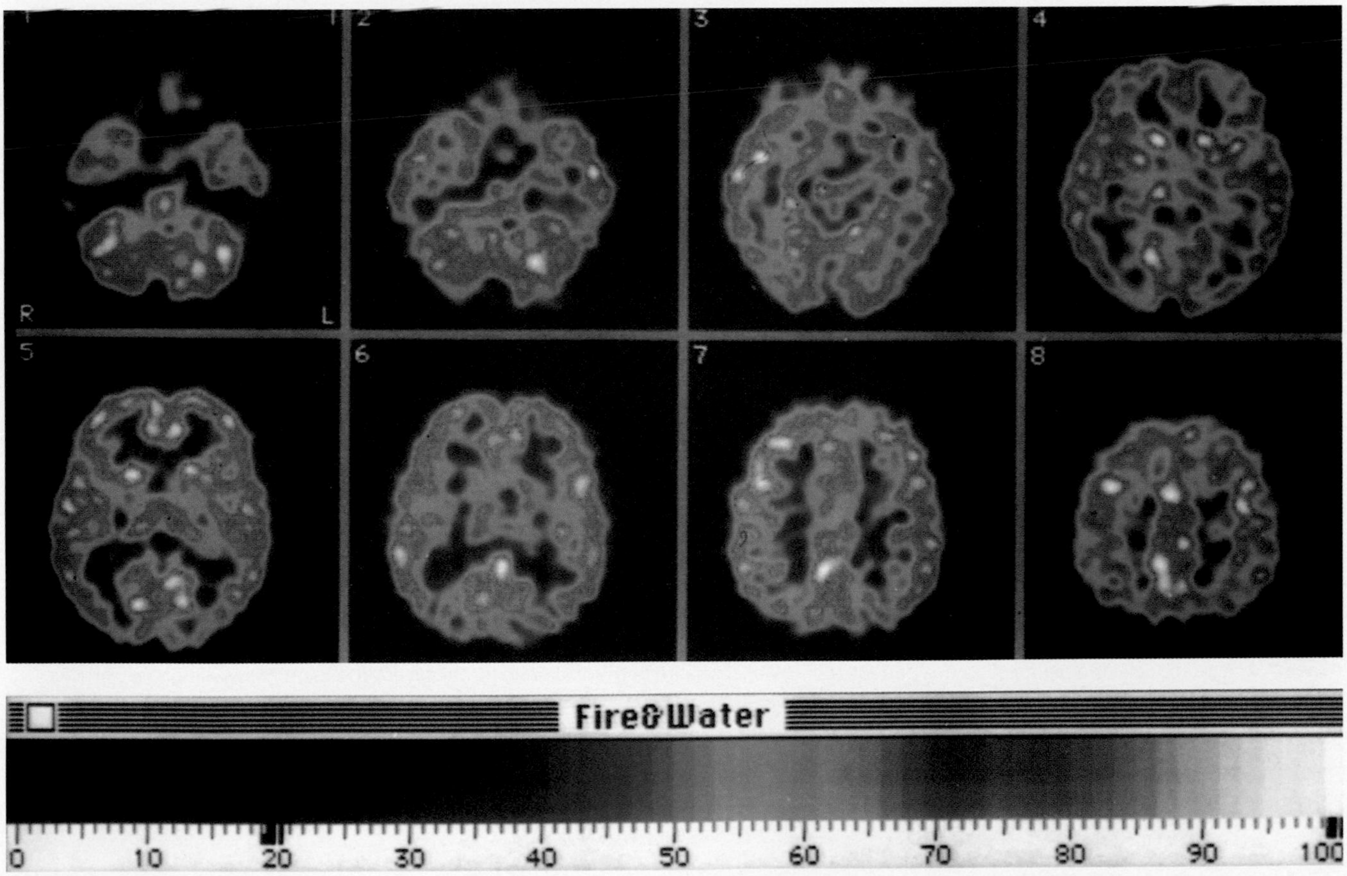

Plate 3.6 An HMPAO-SPECT scan from a normal subject, using a Strichman Medical Equipment multislice, head-dedicated scanner. The slices are orientated parallel to the orbitomeatal plane. See also Fig. 3.18. (Courtesy of the Department of Nuclear Medicine, King's College Hospital, London.)

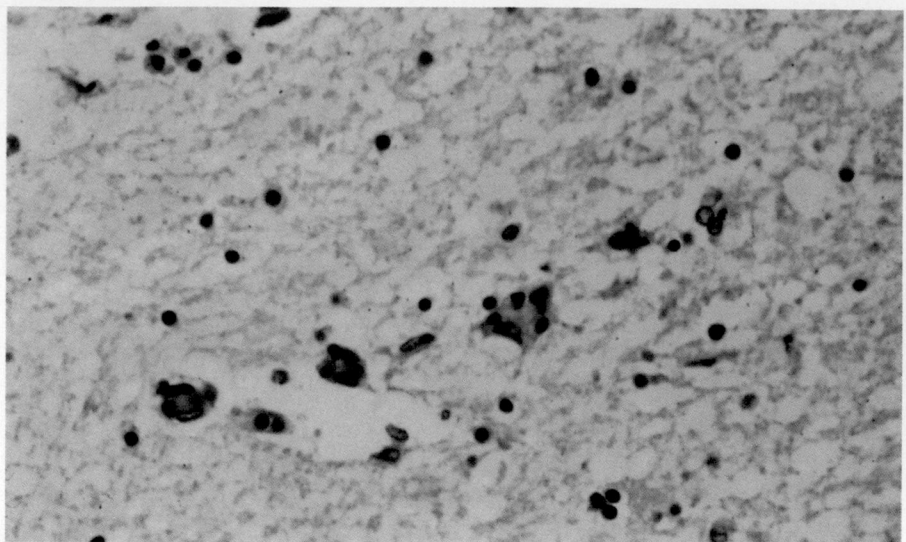

Plate 7.1 Large multinucleated giant cells in cerebral white matter of a patient with HIV encephalitis and dementia (see also Fig. 7.2). Haematoxylin and eosin, magnification ×250. (Courtesy of Dr Ian Everall.)

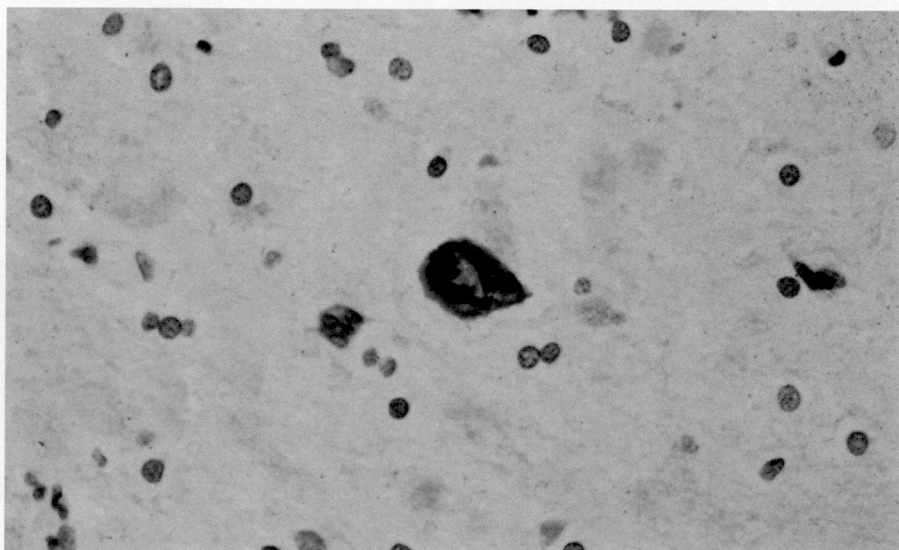

Plate 7.2 A multinucleated giant cell from a patient with HIV encephalitis immunostained for the glycoprotein gp41 revealing viral particles (see also Fig. 7.3). Magnification ×400. (Courtesy of Dr Ian Everall.)

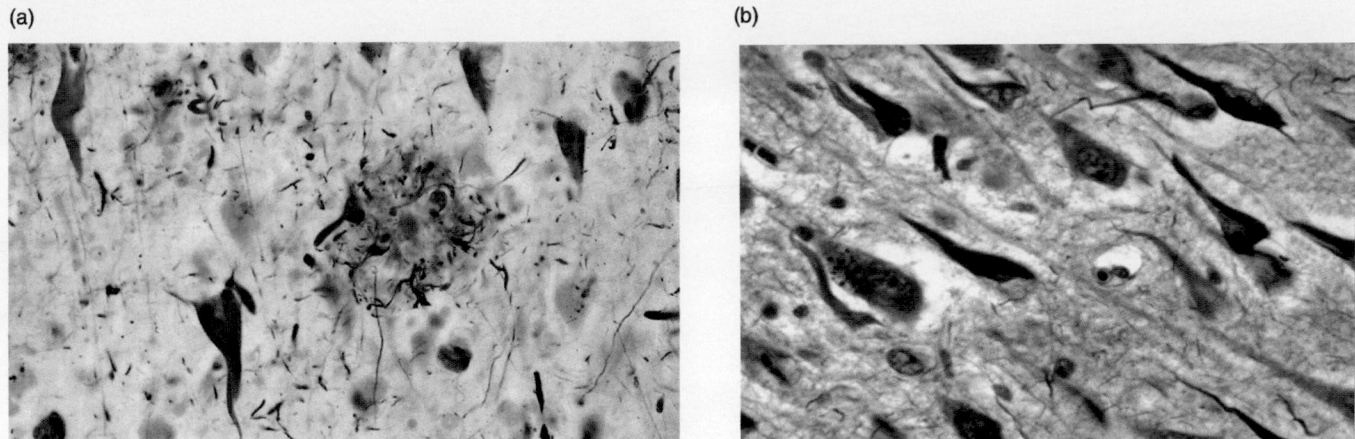

Plate 9.1 (a) Neuritic plaque and (b) neurofibrillary tangles (see also Fig. 9.1).

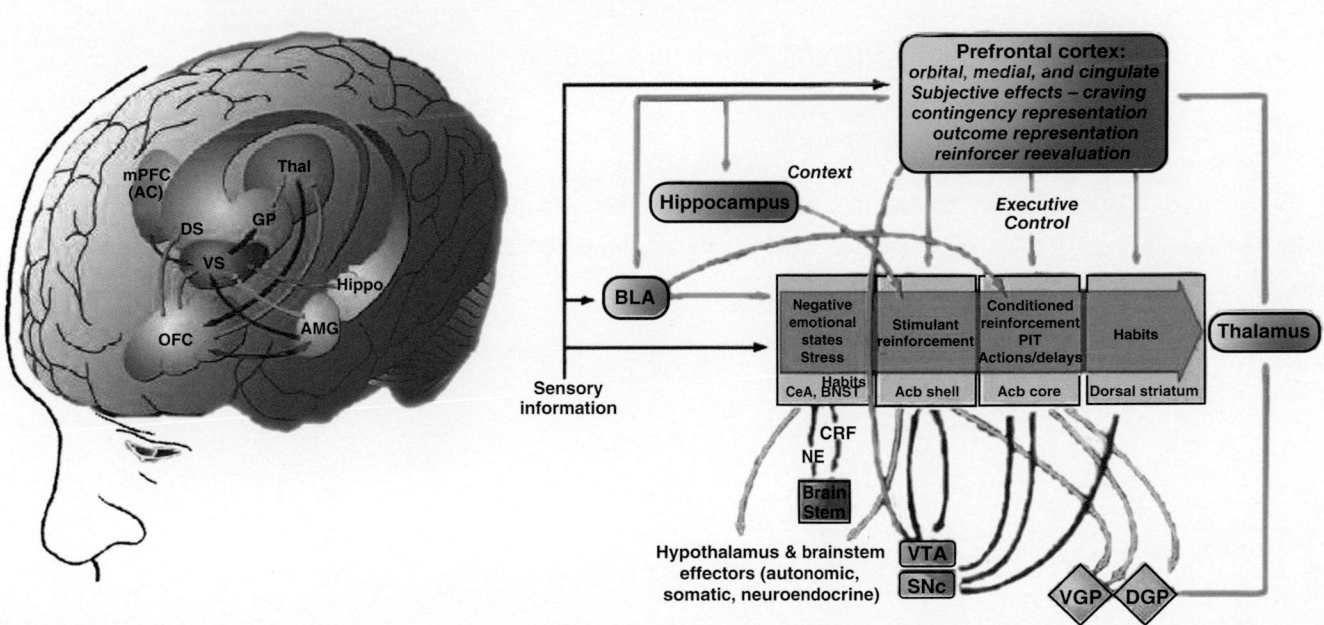

Plate 11.1 Key elements of the neurocircuitry of addiction (see also Fig. 11.1). (From Koob *et al.* 2008 with permission.)

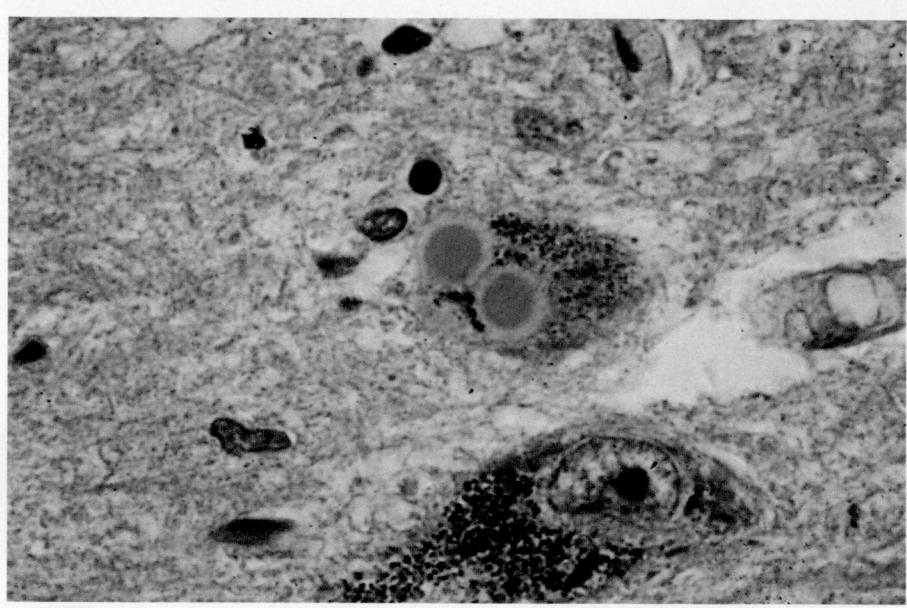

Plate 12.1 Lewy bodies in the substantia nigra (haematoxylin and eosin). Magnification ×600. (Courtesy of Professor Peter Lantos.) See also Fig. 12.1.

immune deficiency syndrome viruses: where and when? *Philosophical Transactions of the Royal Society of London B* **356**, 867–876.

Sharpe, M., Hawton, K., Simkin, S. *et al.* (1996) Cognitive behaviour therapy for the chronic fatigue syndrome: a randomised controlled trial. *British Medical Journal* **312**, 22–26.

Shaw, G.M., Harper, M.E., Hahn, B.H. *et al.* (1985) HTLV-III infection in brains of children and adults with AIDS encephalopathy. *Science* **227**, 177–182.

Shearer, M.L. & Finch, S.M. (1964) Periodic organic psychosis associated with recurrent herpes simplex. *New England Journal of Medicine* **271**, 494–497.

Shepherd, E.J., Brettle, R.P., Liberski, P.P. *et al.* (1999) Spinal cord pathology and viral burden in homosexuals and drug users with AIDS. *Neuropathology and Applied Neurobiology* **25**, 2–10.

Shill, H.A. & Stacy, M.A. (2000) Malignant catatonia secondary to sporadic encephalitis lethargica. *Journal of Neurology, Neurosurgery and Psychiatry* **69**, 402–403.

Shoqeirat, M.A., Mayes, A., MacDonald, C., Meudell, P. & Pickering, A. (1990) Performance on tests sensitive to frontal lobe lesions by patients with organic amnesia: Leng & Parkin revisited. *British Journal of Clinical Psychology* **29**, 401–408.

Silverstein, A., Steinberg, G. & Nathanson, M. (1972) Nervous system involvement in infectious mononucleosis. The heralding and/or major manifestation. *Archives of Neurology* **26**, 353–358.

Simms, I., Fenton, K.A., Ashton, M. *et al.* (2005) The re emergence of syphilis in the United Kingdom: the new epidemic phases. *Sexually Transmitted Diseases* **32**, 220–226.

Simon, R.P. (1985) Neurosyphilis. *Archives of Neurology* **42**, 606–613.

Simpson, D.M. & Berger, J.R. (1996) Neurologic manifestations of HIV infection. *Medical Clinics of North America* **80**, 1363–1394.

Sinclair, E., Gray, F., Ciardi, A. & Scaravilli, F. (1994) Immunohistochemical changes and PCR detection of HIV provirus DNA in brains of asymptomatic HIV-positive patients. *Journal of Neuropathology and Experimental Neurology* **53**, 43–50.

Singh, A.E. & Romanowski, B. (1999) Syphilis: review with emphasis on clinical, epidemiologic, and some biologic features. *Clinical Microbiology Reviews* **12**, 187–209.

Sirota, P., Eviatar, J. & Spivak, B. (1989) Neurosyphilis presenting as psychiatric disorders. *British Journal of Psychiatry* **155**, 559–561.

Sivakumar, K. & Okocha, C.I. (1992) Neurosyphilis and schizophrenia. *British Journal of Psychiatry* **161**, 251–254.

Siversten, B. & Christensen, P.B. (1996) Acute encephalitis. *Acta Neurologica Scandinavica* **93**, 156–159.

Sköldenberg, B., Forsgren, M., Alestig, K. *et al.* (1984) Acyclovir versus vidarabine in herpes simplex encephalitis. Randomised multicentre study in consecutive Swedish patients. *Lancet* **ii**, 707–711.

Slater, E. & Roth, M. (1969) *Clinical Psychiatry*, 3rd edn. Baillière, Tindall & Cassell, London.

Smith, M.G., Lennette, E.M. & Reames, H.R. (1941) Isolation of the virus of herpes simplex and the demonstration of intranuclear inclusions in a case of acute encephalitis. *American Journal of Pathology* **17**, 55–68.

Snider, W.D., Simpson, D.M., Nielsen, S., Gold, W.M., Metroka, C.E. & Posner, J.B. (1983) Neurological complications of acquired

immune deficiency syndrome: analysis of 50 patients. *Annals of Neurology* **14**, 403–418.

Solomon, T. & Winter, P.M. (2004) Neurovirulence and host factors in flavivirus encephalitis: evidence from clinical epidemiology. *Archives of Virology* Suppl. **18**, 161–170.

Solomon, T., Hart, I.J. & Beeching, N.J. (2007) Viral encephalitis: a clinician's guide. *Practical Neurology* **7**, 288–305.

Starace, F., Bartoli, L., Aloisi, M.S. *et al.* (2002) Cognitive and affective disorders associated to HIV infection in the HAART era: findings from the NeuroICONA study. Cognitive impairment and depression in HIV/AIDS. *Acta Psychiatrica Scandinavica* **106**, 20–26.

Steel, R. (1960) GPI in an observation ward. *Lancet* **i**, 121–123.

Steinberg, D., Hirsch, S.R., Marston, S.D., Reynolds, K. & Sutton, R.N.P. (1972) Influenza infection causing manic psychosis. *British Journal of Psychiatry* **120**, 531–535.

Steiner, I., Budka, H., Chaudhuri, A. *et al.* (2005) Viral encephalitis: a review of diagnostic methods and guidelines for management. *European Journal of Neurology* **12**, 331–343.

Stern, Y. & Marder, K. (1991) The neurology and neuropsychology of HIV infection. In: Boller, F. & Grafman, J. (eds) *Handbook of Neuropsychology*, vol. 5, ch. 12. Elsevier Science Publications, Holland.

Stern, Y., McDermott, M.P., Albert, S. *et al.* (2001) Factors associated with incident human immunodeficiency virus-dementia. *Archives of Neurology* **58**, 473–479.

Stimson, G.V. (1995) AIDS and injecting drug use in the United Kingdom, 1987–1993: the policy response and the prevention of the epidemic. *Social Science and Medicine* **41**, 699–716.

Stoler, M., Meshulam, B., Zoldan, J. & Sirota, P. (1987) Schizophreniform episode following measles infection. *British Journal of Psychiatry* **150**, 861–862.

Storm-Mathisen, A. (1969) General paresis. A follow up study of 203 patients. *Acta Psychiatrica Scandinavica* **45**, 118–132.

Studahl, M. (2003) Influenza virus and CNS manifestations. *Journal of Clinical Virology* **28**, 225–232.

Subbiah, P., Mouton, P., Fedor, H., McArthur, J.C. & Glass, J.D. (1996) Stereological analysis of cerebral atrophy in human immunodeficiency virus-associated dementia. *Journal of Neuropathology and Experimental Neurology* **55**, 1032–1037.

Sulkava, R., Rissanen, A. & Pyhala, R. (1981) Post-influenzal encephalitis during the influenza A outbreak in 1979/1980. *Journal of Neurology, Neurosurgery and Psychiatry* **44**, 161–163.

Swedo, S.E., Leonard, H.L., Garvey, M. *et al.* (1998) Pediatric autoimmune neuropsychiatric disorders associated with streptococcal infections: clinical description of the first 50 cases. *American Journal of Psychiatry* **155**, 264–271.

Sze, G. & Zimmerman, R.D. (1988) The magnetic resonance imaging of infections and inflammatory diseases. *Radiologic Clinics of North America* **26**, 839–859.

Sze, G., Brant-Zawadzki, N., Norman, D. & Newton, T.H. (1987) The neuroradiology of AIDS. *Seminars in Roentgenology* **22**, 42–53.

Takeshita, M., Kagawa, M., Yonetani, H. *et al.* (1992) Risk factors for brain abscess in patients with congenital cyanotic heart disease. *Neurologia Medico-Chirurgica (Tokyo)* **32**, 667–670.

Taubenberger, J.K., Reid, A.H., Krafft, A.E., Bijwaard, K.E. & Fanning, T.G. (1997) Initial genetic characterization of the 1918 'Spanish' influenza virus. *Science* **275**, 1793–1796.

Tardieu, M., Blanche, S., Rouzioux, C., Veber, F., Fischer, A. & Griscelli, C. (1987) [Nervous system involvement in HIV1 infections in infants.] *Archives Francaises de Pediatrie* **44**, 495–499.

Targ, E.F., Karasic, D.H., Diefenbach, P.N., Anderson, D.A., Bystritsky, A. & Fawzy, F.I. (1994) Structured group therapy and fluoxetine to treat depression in HIV-positive persons. *Psychosomatics* **35**, 132–137.

Tartaglione, T., Di Lella, G.M., Cerase, A., Leone, A., Moschini, M. & Colosimo, C. (1998) Diagnostic imaging of neurotuberculosis. *Rays* **23**, 164–180.

Tashima, K.T., Caliendo, A.M., Ahmad, M. *et al.* (1999) Cerebrospinal fluid human immunodeficiency virus type 1 (HIV-1) suppression and efavirenz drug concentrations in HIV-1-infected patients receiving combination therapy. *Journal of Infectious Diseases* **180**, 862–864.

Taycan, O., Ugur, M. & Ozmen, M. (2006) Quetiapine vs. risperidone in treating psychosis in neurosyphilis: a case report. *General Hospital Psychiatry* **28**, 359–361.

Thomas, C.S. & Szabadi, E. (1987) Paranoid psychosis as the first presentation of a fulminating lethal case of AIDS. *British Journal of Psychiatry* **151**, 693–695.

Thwaites, G. & Hien, T.T. (2005) TB meningitis: too many questions, too few answers. *Lancet Neurology* **4**, 139.

Timmermans, M. & Carr, J. (2004) Neurosyphilis in the modern era. *Journal of Neurology, Neurosurgery and Psychiatry* **75**, 1727–1730.

Todd, J. (1989) AIDS as a current psychopathological theme: a report on five heterosexual patients. *British Journal of Psychiatry* **154**, 253–255.

Torres, R.A. & Barr, M. (1997) Impact of combination therapy for HIV infection on inpatient census. *New England Journal of Medicine* **336**, 1531–1532.

Torres-Munoz, J., Stockton, P., Tacoronte, N., Roberts, B., Maronpot, R.R. & Petito, C.K. (2001) Detection of HIV-1 gene sequences in hippocampal neurons isolated from postmortem AIDS brains by laser capture microdissection. *Journal of Neuropathology and Experimental Neurology* **60**, 885–892.

Townsend, J.J., Baringer, J.R., Wolinsky, J.S. *et al.* (1975) Progressive rubella panencephalitis. Late onset after congenital rubella. *New England Journal of Medicine* **292**, 990–993.

Townsend, J.J., Wolinsky, J.S. & Baringer, J.R. (1976) The neuropathology of progressive rubella panencephalitis of late onset. *Brain* **99**, 81–90.

Tozzi, V., Balestra, P., Galgani, S. *et al.* (2003) Neurocognitive performance and quality of life in patients with HIV infection. *AIDS Research and Human Retroviruses* **19**, 643–652.

Tramont, E.C. (1976) Persistence of *Treponema pallidum* following penicillin G therapy. *Journal of the American Medical Association* **236**, 2206–2207.

Tramont, E.C. (2005) *Treponema pallidum (syphilis)*. Elsevier, Philadelphia.

Treisman, G., Fishman, M., Lyketsos, C. & McHugh, P.R. (1994) Evaluation and treatment of psychiatric disorders associated with HIV infection. In: Price, R.W. & Perry, S.W. (eds) *HIV, AIDS, and the Brain*, ch. 13. Association for Research in Nervous and Mental Disease vol. 72. Raven Press, New York.

Treisman, G.J., Angelino, A.F. & Hutton, H.E. (2001) Psychiatric issues in the management of patients with HIV infection. *Journal of the American Medical Association* **286**, 2857–2864.

Trousseau, A. (1868) *Lectures on Clinical Medicine*, vol. 35, p. 453. New Sydenham Society, London. Quoted by Williams, M. & Smith, H.V. (1954) *Journal of Neurology, Neurosurgery and Psychiatry* **17**, 173–182.

Tsukiura, T., Ohtake, H., Fujii, T., Miura, R., Ogawa, T. & Yamadori, A. (2003) Presumed ability to recognise keywords related to remote events in the absence of retrieval of relevant knowledge: a case of postencephalitic amnesia. *Brain and Cognition* **51**, 1–11.

Tucker, J.S., Burnam, M.A., Sherbourne, C.D., Kung, F.Y. & Gifford, A.L. (2003) Substance use and mental health correlates of non-adherence to antiretroviral medications in a sample of patients with human immunodeficiency virus infection. *American Journal of Medicine* **114**, 573–580.

Tucker, K.A., Robertson, K.R., Lin, W. *et al.* (2004) Neuroimaging in human immunodeficiency virus infection. *Journal of Neuroimmunology* **157**, 153–162.

Tyler, K.L. (2004) Update on herpes simplex encephalitis. *Reviews in Neurological Diseases* **1**, 169–178.

UNAIDS (2006) *AIDS Epidemic Update: special report on HIV/AIDS*. Joint United Nations Programme on HIV/AIDS.

Vago, L., Bonetto, S., Nebuloni, M. *et al.* (2002) Pathological findings in the central nervous system of AIDS patients on assumed antiretroviral therapeutic regimens: retrospective study of 1597 autopsies. *AIDS* **16**, 1925–1928.

Vallini, A.D. & Burns, R.L. (1987) Carbamazepine as therapy for psychiatric sequelae of herpes simplex encephalitis. *Southern Medical Journal* **80**, 1590–1592.

Van Bogaert, L. (1945) Une leuco-encéphalite sclérosante subaigue. *Journal of Neurology, Neurosurgery and Psychiatry* **8**, 101–120.

Van de Beek, D., Schmand, B., de Gans, J. *et al.* (2002) Cognitive impairment in adults with good recovery after bacterial meningitis. *Journal of Infectious Diseases* **186**, 1047–1052.

Van de Beek, D., De Gans, J., Spanjaard, L., Weisfelt, M., Reitsma, J.B. & Vermeulen, M. (2004) Clinical features and prognostic factors in adults with bacterial meningitis. *New England Journal of Medicine* **351**, 1849–1859.

Van Gorp, W.G., Rabkin, J.G., Ferrando, S.J. *et al.* (2007) Neuropsychiatric predictors of return to work in HIV/AIDS. *Journal of the International Neuropsychological Society* **13**, 80–89.

Vanhems, P., Hirschel, B., Phillips, A.N. *et al.* (2000) Incubation time of acute human immunodeficiency virus (HIV) infection and duration of acute HIV infection are independent prognostic factors of progression to AIDS. *Journal of Infectious Diseases* **182**, 334–337.

Varma, L.P. (1952) The incidence and clinical features of general paresis. *Indian Journal of Neurology and Psychiatry* **3**, 141–163.

Vlahov, D., Graham, N., Hoover, D. *et al.* (1998) Prognostic indicators for AIDS and infectious disease death in HIV-infected injection drug users: plasma viral load and CD4+ cell count. *Journal of the American Medical Association* **279**, 35–40.

Vogel-Scibilia, S.E., Mulsant, B.H. & Keshavan, M.S. (1988) HIV infection presenting as psychosis: a critique. *Acta Psychiatrica Scandinavica* **78**, 652–656.

Von Economo, C. (1929) *Encephalitis Lethargica: Its Sequelae and Treatment*. Translated by Newman, K.O. (1931). Oxford University Press, London.

Von Giesen, H.J., Antke, C., Hefter, H., Wenserski, F., Seitz, R.J. & Arendt, G. (2000) Potential time course of human immunodeficiency virus type 1-associated minor motor deficits: electrophysiologic and positron emission tomography findings. *Archives of Neurology* **57**, 1601–1607.

Von Giesen, H.J., Koller, H., Theisen, A. & Arendt, G. (2002) Therapeutic effects of nonnucleoside reverse transcriptase inhibitors on the central nervous system in HIV-1-infected patients. *Journal of Acquired Immune Deficiency Syndromes* **29**, 363–367.

Wagner, G.J. & Rabkin, R. (2000) Effects of dextroamphetamine on depression and fatigue in men with HIV: a double-blind, placebo-controlled trial. *Journal of Clinical Psychiatry* **61**, 436–440.

Wang, F., So, Y., Vittinghof, E. *et al.* (1995) Incidence, proportion of and risk factors for AIDS patients diagnosed with HIV dementia, central nervous system toxoplasmosis and cryptococcal meningitis. *Journal of Acquired Immune Deficiency Syndrome and Human Retrovirology* **8**, 75–82.

Warnke, D., Barreto, J. & Temesgen, Z. (2007) Antiretroviral drugs. *Journal of Clinical Pharmacology* **47**, 1570–1579.

Warrington, E.K. & Shallice, T. (1984) Category specific semantic impairments. *Brain* **107**, 829–854.

Weil, M.L., Itabashi, H.H., Cremer, N.E., Oshiro, L.S., Lennette, E.H. & Carnay, L. (1975) Chronic progressive panencephalitis due to rubella virus simulating subacute sclerosing panencephalitis. *New England Journal of Medicine* **292**, 994–998.

Weis, S., Haug, H. & Budka, H. (1993) Neuronal damage in the cerebral cortex of AIDS brains: a morphometric study. *Acta Neuropathologica* **85**, 185–189.

Weisfelt, M., van de Beek, D., Hoogman, M., Hardeman, C., de Gans, J. & Schmand, B. (2006a) Cognitive outcome in adults with moderate disability after pneumococcal meningitis. *Journal of Infection* **52**, 433–439.

Weisfelt, M., van de Beek, D., Spanjaard, L., Reitsma, J.B. & de Gans, J. (2006b) Clinical features, complications, and outcome in adults with pneumococcal meningitis: a prospective case series. *Lancet Neurology* **5**, 123–129.

Wells, C.E.C. (1971) Neurological complications of so-called influenza. A winter study in South-east Wales. *British Medical Journal* **1**, 369–373.

Wessely, S., David, A., Butler, S. & Chalder, T. (1989) Management of chronic (post-viral) fatigue syndrome. *Journal of the Royal College of General Practitioners* **39**, 26–29.

Wessely, S., Butler, S., Chalder, T. & David, A. (1991) The cognitive behavioural management of the post-viral fatigue syndrome. In: Jenkins, R. & Mowbray, J.F. (eds) *Post-viral Fatigue Syndrome*, ch. 22. John Wiley & Sons, Chichester.

West, T.E., Papasian, C.J., Park, B.H. & Parker, S.W. (1985) Adenovirus type 2 encephalitis and concurrent Epstein–Barr virus infection in the adult man. *Archives of Neurology* **42**, 815–817.

White, D.A., Heaton, R.K. & Monsch, A.U. (1995) Neuropsychological studies of asymptomatic human immunodeficiency virus-type-1 infected individuals. *Journal of the International Neuropsychological Society* **1**, 304–315.

White, P.D. & Lewis, S.W. (1987) Delusional depression after infectious mononucleosis. *British Medical Journal* **295**, 97–98.

White, P.D., Thomas, J.M., Amess, J., Grover, S.A., Kangro, H.O. & Clare, A.W. (1995a) The existence of a fatigue syndrome after glandular fever. *Psychological Medicine* **25**, 907–916.

White, P.D., Grover, S.A., Kangro, H.O., Thomas, J.M., Amess, J. & Clare, A.W. (1995b) The validity and reliability of the fatigue syndrome that follows glandular fever. *Psychological Medicine* **25**, 917–924.

Whitley, R.J., Alford, C.A., Hirsch, M.S. *et al.* (1986) Vidarabine versus acyclovir therapy in herpes simplex encephalitis. *New England Journal of Medicine* **314**, 144–149.

Whitley, R.J., Kimberlin, D.W. & Roizman, B. (1998) Herpes simplex viruses. *Clinical Infectious Diseases* **26**, 541–553; quiz 554–555.

Wiles, C.M. (1993a) Spirochaetal diseases, some other specific infections and intoxications and their neurological complications. In: Walton, J. (ed.) *Brain's Diseases of the Nervous System*, 10th edn, ch. 8. Oxford University Press, Oxford.

Wiles, C.M. (1993b) The meninges: bacterial (excluding spirochaetal disease) and fungal meningitis; intracranial abscess. In: Walton, J. (ed.) *Brain's Diseases of the Nervous System*, 10th edn, ch. 7. Oxford University Press, Oxford.

Wiley, C.A. & Achim, C. (1994) Human immunodeficiency virus encephalitis is the pathological correlate of dementia in acquired immunodeficiency syndrome. *Annals of Neurology* **36**, 673–676.

Wiley, C.A., Masliah, E., Morey, M. *et al.* (1991) Neocortical damage during HIV infection. *Annals of Neurology* **29**, 651–657.

Wilkinson, A.E. (1972) Problems in the treatment of venereal disease: bacterial resistance: treatment. *Journal of the Royal College of Physicians of London* **6**, 175–180.

Williams, M. & Smith, H.V. (1954) Mental disturbances in tuberculous meningitis. *Journal of Neurology, Neurosurgery and Psychiatry* **17**, 173–182.

Wilner, E. & Brody, J.A. (1968) Prognosis of general paresis after treatment. *Lancet* **ii**, 1370–1371.

Wilson, L.G. (1976) Viral encephalopathy mimicking functional psychosis. *American Journal of Psychiatry* **133**, 165–170.

Wilson, S.A.K. (1940) *Neurology*. Edward Arnold, London.

Wise, M.E., Mistry, K. & Reid, S. (2002) Drug points: Neuropsychiatric complications of nevirapine treatment. *British Medical Journal* **324**, 879.

Wojna, V., Carlson, K.A., Luo, X. *et al.* (2004) Proteomic fingerprinting of human immunodeficiency virus type 1-associated dementia from patient monocyte-derived macrophages: a case study. *Journal of Neurovirology* **10** (suppl. 1), 74–81.

Wolters, E.C. (1987) Neurosyphilis: a changing diagnostic problem? *European Neurology* **26**, 23–28.

Woods, S.P., Morgan, E.E., Marquie-Beck, J., Carey, C.L., Grant, I. & Letendre, S.L. (2006) Markers of macrophage activation and axonal injury are associated with prospective memory in HIV-1 disease. *Cognitive and Behavioral Neurology* **19**, 217–221.

Working Group of the American Academy of Neurology AIDS Task Force (1991) Nomenclature and research case definitions for neurologic manifestations of human immunodeficiency virus type 1 (HIV-1) infection. *Neurology* **41**, 778–785.

World Health Organization (1990a) *Report of the second consultation on the neuropsychiatric aspects of HIV-1 infection*, Global Programme on AIDS, Geneva, Annex 3. Ref. No. WHO/GPA/MNH 90.1. World Health Organization, Geneva.

World Health Organization (1990b) *Suicidal Behaviour Among People with HIV and AIDS*. Report on a WHO consultation. WHO Regional Office for Europe, Copenhagen.

World Health Organization (2005) *Interim WHO Clinical Staging of HIV/AIDS and HIV/AIDS Case Definition for Surveillance*. World Health Organization, Geneva.

Wyatt, G.B. (1992) Malaria, the mimic. *Journal of the Medical Defence Union* **3**, 54–55.

Yeung, H., Krentz, H.B., Gill, M.J. & Power, C. (2006) Neuropsychiatric disorders in HIV infection: impact of diagnosis on economic costs of care. *AIDS* **20**, 2005–2009.

Yiannoutsos, C.T., Ernst, T., Chang, L. *et al.* (2004) Regional patterns of brain metabolites in AIDS dementia complex. *Neuroimage* **23**, 928–935.

Yoshioka, M., Shapshak, P., Srivastava, A.K. *et al.* (1994) Expression of HIV-1 and interleukin-6 in lumbosacral dorsal root ganglia of patients with AIDS. *Neurology* **44**, 1120–1130.

Yun, L.W., Maravi, M., Kobayashi, J.S., Barton, P.L. & Davidson, A.J. (2005) Antidepressant treatment improves adherence to antiretroviral therapy among depressed HIV-infected patients. *Journal of Acquired Immune Deficiency Syndromes* **38**, 432–438.

Zagardo, M.T., Shanholtz, C.B., Zoarski, G.H. & Rothman, M.I. (1998) Rhombencephalitis caused by adenovirus: MR imaging appearance. *American Journal of Neuroradiology* **19**, 1901–1903.

Zellan, J. & Augenbraun, M. (2004) Syphilis in the HIV-infected patient: an update on epidemiology, diagnosis, and management. *Current HIV/AIDS Reports* **1**, 142–147.

Zetola, N.M. & Klausner, J.D. (2007) Syphilis and HIV infection: an update. *Clinical Infectious Diseases* **44**, 1222–1228.

Zhang, L., Looney, D., Taub, D. *et al.* (1998) Cocaine opens the blood-brain barrier to HIV-1 invasion. *Journal of Neurovirology* **4**, 619–626.

Zimmerman, R.D., Russell, E.J., Leeds, N.E. & Kaufman, D. (1980) CT in the early diagnosis of herpes simplex encephalitis. *American Journal of Roentgenology* **134**, 61–66.

Zisook, S., Peterkin, J., Goggin, K.J., Sledge, P., Atkinson, J.H. & Grant, I. (1998) Treatment of major depression in HIV-seropositive men. *Journal of Clinical Psychiatry* **59**, 217–224.

Zuger, A. & O'Dowd, M.A. (1992) The Baron has AIDS: a case of factitious human immunodeficiency virus infection and review. *Clinical Infectious Diseases* **14**, 211–216.

Zumwalt, R.E., McFeeley, P.J. & Maito, J. (1987) Fraudulent AIDS. *Journal of the American Medical Association* **257**, 3231.

CHAPTER 8

Cerebrovascular Disorders

Simon Fleminger

Maudsley Hospital, London

Diseases of the vascular system contribute greatly to the sum total of psychiatric disability, chiefly in the elderly population and mainly as a result of stroke. Strokes, cerebrovascular accidents and subarachnoid haemorrhage are therefore considered first, with emphasis on their psychiatric sequelae and the problems encountered in rehabilitation. Over recent years much has been learnt about the biological basis of migraine and this important common condition is considered next. Finally, certain diseases of rather obscure aetiology, such as systemic lupus erythematosus and other forms of vasculitis, are described. The psychiatric components of such illnesses have gained increasing recognition and appear to be attributable in part to involvement of the cerebral vasculature.

Stroke

Strokes are the third commonest cause of death after heart disease and cancer in the Western world. The incidence of a first stroke is about 2 per 1000 per year (Bamford *et al.* 1988) and it has been estimated that almost one in four men and one in five women aged 45 can expect to have a stroke if they live to 85 (Bonita 1992). Therefore, in a population of 250 000 (the basis for a district general hospital) more than 500 strokes will occur per annum, of which about 150 will be added to the accumulating number needing continuing care (Hurwitz & Adams 1972). As a result, stroke is probably the most frequent cause of severe disability in the community (Harris *et al.* 1971). Moreover, approximately one-quarter of victims affected are under 65 years of age and are thus disabled during the productive years of their lives.

The principal causes of stroke are atherosclerosis and hypertension. Among predisposing causes, factors susceptible to modification include hypertension, heart disease, diabetes, raised serum lipids and smoking. Severely threatening life events may be commoner in stroke victims than controls throughout the year preceding the stroke (House *et al.* 1990).

There is new interest and vigour in solving the problems of rehabilitating survivors, although psychiatrists are often little involved in the process. This is disappointing, in that much of the disability resulting from strokes is mental rather than physical, and psychological influences can be paramount in determining what progress is made. In what follows, the general background to cerebrovascular accidents is briefly sketched before reviewing what is known of the psychological and psychiatric aftermaths.

Classification of stroke

Older definitions of stroke have tended to demand that symptoms should have lasted more than 24 hours, partly in order to distinguish stroke from transient ischaemic attacks. However, such definitions are less valuable now that very early interventions, within the first 3 hours of onset, may need to be implemented in patients who are nevertheless probably going to develop permanent symptoms. In practice any recent disturbance of cerebral function meeting the criteria described in Box 8.1, and with no apparent cause other than a vascular origin, should be regarded as a stroke.

There are two essential pathological processes underlying stroke: infarction (ischaemia) and haemorrhage. Infarction is commoner than haemorrhage by a ratio of approximately 4 : 1. It is not only more frequent as an acute development but very much more so as a source of enduring disability. Thus approximately three-quarters of patients with infarctions survive, whereas almost two-thirds of patients with cerebral haemorrhage die within a year (Bamford *et al.* 1990). Infarction may result from thrombosis of vessels or from emboli which come to lodge within them. Haemorrhage may be primarily into the substance of the brain or into the subarachnoid space. Hypertension is a risk factor for both cerebral infarct and haemorrhage, although the strength of the association is greater for haemorrhage (Song *et al.* 2004).

Lishman's Organic Psychiatry: A Textbook of Neuropsychiatry, 4th edition.
© 2009 Blackwell Publishing.   ISBN 978-1-4051-1860-1

Cerebral haemorrhage

Intracranial haemorrhage, representing some 15% of all strokes, may be divided into subarachnoid haemorrhage from a ruptured cerebral artery aneurysm and primary intracerebral haemorrhage. The differentiation is not always absolute, since bleeding may occur into brain tissue in the neighbourhood of a ruptured aneurysm, and blood may gain access to the ventricular system and subarachnoid space after primary intracerebral haemorrhage. Subarachnoid haemorrhage is dealt with later in this chapter.

Primary intracerebral haemorrhage is most common in patients between the ages of 60 and 80 and is usually associated with hypertension, particularly in younger patients, for example in their forties or fifties. The precise mechanism whereby haemorrhage develops continues to be the subject of controversy. Deep haemorrhages, into basal ganglia, thalamus, pons and cerebellum, are regarded as more closely associated with hypertension than are lobar haemorrhages into temporal, frontal, parietal or occipital lobes. It is has been proposed that lipohyalinosis of the small penetrating arteries due to hypertension may result in deep intracerebral haemorrhage or lacunar infarcts (Jackson & Sudlow 2006). On the other hand, in lobar haemorrhage, particularly in the elderly, cerebral amyloid angiopathy, with deposition of congophilic amyloid-B protein in cerebral cortical and leptomeningeal vessels, may be the main pathological process (Labovitz & Sacco 2001).

Comparing groups of patients it is possible to demonstrate differences between the clinical presentation of those with cerebral haemorrhage compared with those with cerebral infarct. For example, in intracerebral haemorrhage the onset is often during exertion and rarely during sleep as with cerebral infarct. Headache, vomiting and loss of consciousness are more common with haemorrhage. However, these differ-

ences are not specific enough to allow a diagnosis at the individual level. For this purpose it is essential to perform computed tomography (CT) of the brain, or magnetic resonance imaging (MRI) with appropriate T2* gradient echo Sequences, to identify acute haemorrhage. In practice neuroimaging is required as soon as possible after presentation to determine if the stroke is due to an infarct, which can be treated with thrombolysis, or to haemorrhage, in which case thrombolysis is contraindicated.

Deep haemorrhage into basal ganglia and adjacent internal capsule will produce a dense contralateral hemiplegia and may be accompanied by deviation of the head and eyes away from the side of the lesion. The formation of a large intracerebral haematoma can lead to secondary effects due to tentorial herniation and brainstem compression. Another site of predilection is the cerebellum, leading to a similar picture but with vertigo and ataxia during the early stages. With haemorrhage into the pons consciousness is usually lost rapidly, the pupils are unequal or pinpoint, hyperpyrexia may occur and quadriplegia is likely to be present.

Early mortality is high, and survivors are usually severely disabled. However, mild examples with only brief loss of consciousness may make a reasonably good recovery. Medical treatment during the acute stages rests primarily on excellent nursing care.

Cerebral infarction

The two most widely used classifications of cerebral infarcts are based on aetiology or on location (Box 8.2). There is some degree of overlap between the two because for some causes of stroke there are areas of particular vulnerability. This is the case for small-artery occlusions (lacunar infarcts), which are localised to subcortical structures and brainstem. It has been estimated that about 50% of ischaemic strokes (infarcts) are due to large-artery atherosclerosis, 25% to lacunar infarcts and 20% to cardiac embolism, with only 5% due to rarer causes (Davenport & Dennis 2000).

Large-artery atherosclerosis may result from cerebral thrombosis or local emboli, the two often being difficult to distinguish clinically. Lipid material accumulates beneath the intima of affected vessels and as the plaques thicken the lumen narrows and thrombus may form. The vessels chiefly involved are the aorta, carotid arteries, middle cerebral arteries and vertebrobasilar arteries. The occlusion may result from local thrombus formation within the stenotic vessel or thromboemboli from proximal arteries. In some a transient fall in blood pressure, as after myocardial infarction, further compromises flow in vessels already critically affected and precipitates the thrombosis. The size of the infarct will depend on the vessels principally involved and also on the efficiency of the collateral circulation. The result is often a total anterior circulation infarct (TACI).

Cerebral small-vessel disease of the small penetrating arteries supplying the basal ganglia, thalamus, internal capsule

Box 8.2 Classification of cerebral infarcts

By cause (Adams *et al.* 1993)

Large-artery atherosclerosis

- Thrombosis and/or embolism related to stenosis or occlusion of a major brain artery or branch cortical artery
- A history of intermittent claudication, transient ischaemic attacks (TIAs) in the same vascular territory, a carotid bruit or diminished pulses supports the diagnosis
- Need to exclude cardiac emboli

Cardioembolism

- Arterial occlusions presumed due to emboli from the heart
- Evidence of TIAs in more than one territory, or systemic emboli support the diagnosis
- High-risk sources include mitral valve stenosis, prosthetic valve, atrial fibrillation, myocardial infarct within 4 weeks, dilated cardiomyopathy and atrial myxoma

Small-artery occlusion, lacunar infarcts

- Presents with lacunar syndrome
- Normal CT/MRI or subcortical lesion less than 1.5 cm diameter
- Diagnosis supported by presence of hypertension

Stroke of other aetiology

- Non-atherosclerotic vasculopathy, hypercoagulable states, arterial dissection, haematological disorders, fat emboli

Stroke of undetermined aetiology

By location (Bamford *et al.* 1991)

Total anterior circulation infarcts

- Large anterior circulation infarcts with both cortical and subcortical involvement. Hemiplegia plus hemianopia plus aphasia or visuospatial neglect
- Worst prognosis: 60% dead and 4% independent at 1 year

Partial anterior circulation infarcts

- Predominantly cortical infarcts. More localized cerebral deficit, e.g. aphasia or visuospatial neglect or motor or sensory deficit or hemianopia
- Most likely to have early recurrent stroke

Posterior circulation infarcts

- Associated with vertebrobasilar arterial territory. Ipsilateral cranial nerve deficit plus contralateral motor or sensory deficit or cerebellar signs
- High recurrence rate throughout first year

Lacunar infarcts

- Confined to the territory of the deep perforating arteries. Pure motor hemiparesis or hemisensory deficit
- Best prognosis: 11% dead and 60% independent at 1 year

or pons causes lacunar infarcts (Fisher 1982) and/or white matter changes. As noted above, lipohyalinosis of the vessel wall may be found and hypertension is an associated finding in the majority of cases. Lacunar infarcts may be multiple and almost microscopic in size. Leucoaraiosis describes the presence of multiple lesions in the deep hemispheric and periventricular white matter seen on neuroimagining. Both lacunar infarcts and leucoaraiosis are probably due to endothelial dysfunction associated with breakdown of the blood–brain barrier, harmful leakage into the perivascular spaces, and impaired autoregulation (Hassan *et al.* 2003; Wardlaw 2005) in and around the small penetrating arteries, for example the lenticulostriate arteries. Cerebral microbleeds may be seen on gradient echo MRI (Werring *et al.* 2005).

Cardiac emboli should be suspected when there is atrial fibrillation, mitral stenosis, subacute bacterial endocarditis or a recent myocardial infarction. Rare forms include paradoxical embolism, in which a congenital cardiac malformation allows material from the veins of the legs to reach the brain by bypassing the pulmonary circulation.

The clinical picture in cerebral thrombosis usually develops abruptly, though less so than with embolism. Occasionally the development is ingravescent, with the neurological deficit increasing over hours or days and progressing in a stepwise or saltatory fashion. Onset is often during sleep. In cerebral embolism, whether cardiac or from the large vessels, the clinical picture is usually extremely acute in onset, developing within seconds or a minute and often during activity. The neurological deficit is typically maximal from the outset, often with rapid resolution over the first few hours thereafter. Regardless of the cause of the cerebral infarction, headache may be present in the early stages but is often absent throughout. Some degree of mental confusion is common, but consciousness may be little if at all impaired. However, large infarcts may be followed by swelling of the affected hemisphere, leading to coma. Coma following infarcts of the posterior circulation is due to direct effects on brainstem pathways involved in maintaining conscious level.

The prognosis for cerebral infarction is much better than for cerebral haemorrhage. Approximately 20% of patients die in the acute stage, 20% recover completely and 60% are left with residual disability. Recovery from emboli is in general much quicker and more complete than after thrombosis, since collateral channels will usually be more readily available. In both, however, much will depend on the size of the infarct produced.

Cerebral arterial syndromes

Occlusion of the proximal stem of the *middle cerebral artery* will usually lead to a TACI (see Box 8.2), with ischaemia in both the deep and superficial territories of the middle cerebral artery (Bamford *et al.* 1991). A TACI is defined by the presence of a contralateral hemiparesis or sensory deficit plus hemianopia (due to involvement of the optic radiation) plus a disorder of higher cortical function. The latter, dependent on which hemisphere is affected, may be a dysphasia, agnosic syndrome, or body image disturbance with visuospatial neglect. In some cases of TACI, the anterior cerebral artery is also involved.

Partial anterior circulation infarct may be seen if more distal parts of the middle cerebral artery are affected or with isolated occlusions of the anterior cerebral artery. More localised disturbance including weakness mainly involves the face, arm and hand, or an isolated disorder of higher cortical function is found after distal occlusion of branches of the middle cerebral artery. Infarctions in the distribution of the *anterior cerebral artery* lead to contralateral hemiparesis affecting the leg more severely than the arm. There may be a grasp reflex in the hand. Cortical sensory loss and motor dysphasia are often present as well. Mental changes may resemble those of a global dementia and incontinence may be a prominent feature. Residual personality changes of frontal lobe type may occur.

Mesulam *et al.* (1976) drew attention to the states of mental confusion that can follow middle cerebral infarctions on the right, sometimes leading to diagnostic difficulties in that focal signs may consist of little more than left-sided cortical sensory loss and visual inattention. A toxic or metabolic cause for the acute organic reaction had often been suspected in their patients. Salient features were inattentiveness to relevant stimuli and inability to maintain a coherent stream of thought or behaviour. Disorientation, anomia, incontinence, an abnormal gait and lack of concern for the illness were characteristic. An example follows.

> A 61-year-old man was discovered in an incoherent agitated state, banging on doors and shouting in the night. He was disoriented in all spheres, very distractible, and with a severely diminished span of attention. His speech contained paraphasic errors and there were difficulties in naming objects. Gait was unsteady and he was incontinent and unkempt. Over the next few days the agitation gave way to an amiable placid state, but the incoherence and impaired attention span persisted for several weeks. Angiography showed occlusion of the right angular branch of the middle cerebral artery (Mesulam *et al.* 1976).

A common tell-tale sign of occlusion of the *internal carotid artery* is monocular blindness, fleeting or permanent, in the eye contralateral to hemiplegia, due to interruption of blood flow in the ophthalmic or retinal arteries. However, internal carotid artery occlusion can be entirely asymptomatic, emerging as a chance finding at post-mortem. If the circulation should fail, infarction occurs principally in the territory of the middle cerebral artery, although the distribution of the anterior cerebral artery may be involved as well. Much depends on the efficiency of the collateral circulation and the patency of the circle of Willis.

Border-zone infarcts, otherwise known as watershed infarcts, occur at the boundary between adjacent arterial territories (Fig. 8.1). *Internal border-zone infarcts* are subcortical and occur where the territories of the deep penetrating branches (Heubner, lenticulostriate and anterior choroidal arteries) of the major cerebral arteries meet the cortical branches of the anterior, middle and posterior cerebral arteries (Donnan *et al.* 1993). *Cortical border-zone infarcts* occur at the boundary between the territory of the middle cerebral artery and the anterior and/or posterior cerebral artery; they occur in a sickle-shaped zone on the lateral surface of the hemisphere (Fisher 1968), with the junction between the parietal and occipital lobes being particularly vulnerable. The border-zone area is vulnerable because it is at the limits of perfusion of the arteries supplying the two adjacent areas. Therefore under conditions of reduced blood flow, for example due to severe systemic hypotension, these areas will be the first to suffer ischaemia. Border-zone infarcts are associated with internal carotid artery stenosis or occlusion, but emboli thrown off from behind and around the stenosis may be as important as the haemodynamic effects of the stenosis (Barnett 1997). It has been proposed that a healthy perfusion pressure can wash out emboli, particularly microemboli, and therefore 'impaired washout is an important but neglected concept that intertwines hypoperfusion, embolization, and brain infarction' (Caplan & Hennerici 1998).

The resulting clinical picture of border-zone infarcts is varied and often indistinguishable from that of middle cerebral infarction. Occasionally, an isolated agnosia, visual or auditory, is seen with an infarct in the zone between middle and posterior cerebral arteries. Sometimes mental symptoms may predominate with general slowing, decreased spontaneous activity, dyspraxia and incontinence, all pointing to a frontal lobe deficit. If the abruptness of onset and fluctuation in the symptoms is not appreciated, the nature of the lesion may not be detected, as in the following example reported by Fisher (1968).

> A man of 68 had shown a change of personality for some 4 months, consisting of selfishness, overeating and impoliteness, combined with clumsiness, falling, spilling food, episodic difficulty in speaking and urinary incontinence. On examination he stared vacantly into space, spoke in a quiet voice, forgot quickly and was clumsy in all his movements. There were elements of dysphasia, both hands were dyspraxic, and he broke spasmodically into tears. Angiography showed left carotid occlusion but this was felt to be irrelevant. He died suddenly and post-mortem revealed an extensive watershed infarct in the left hemisphere.

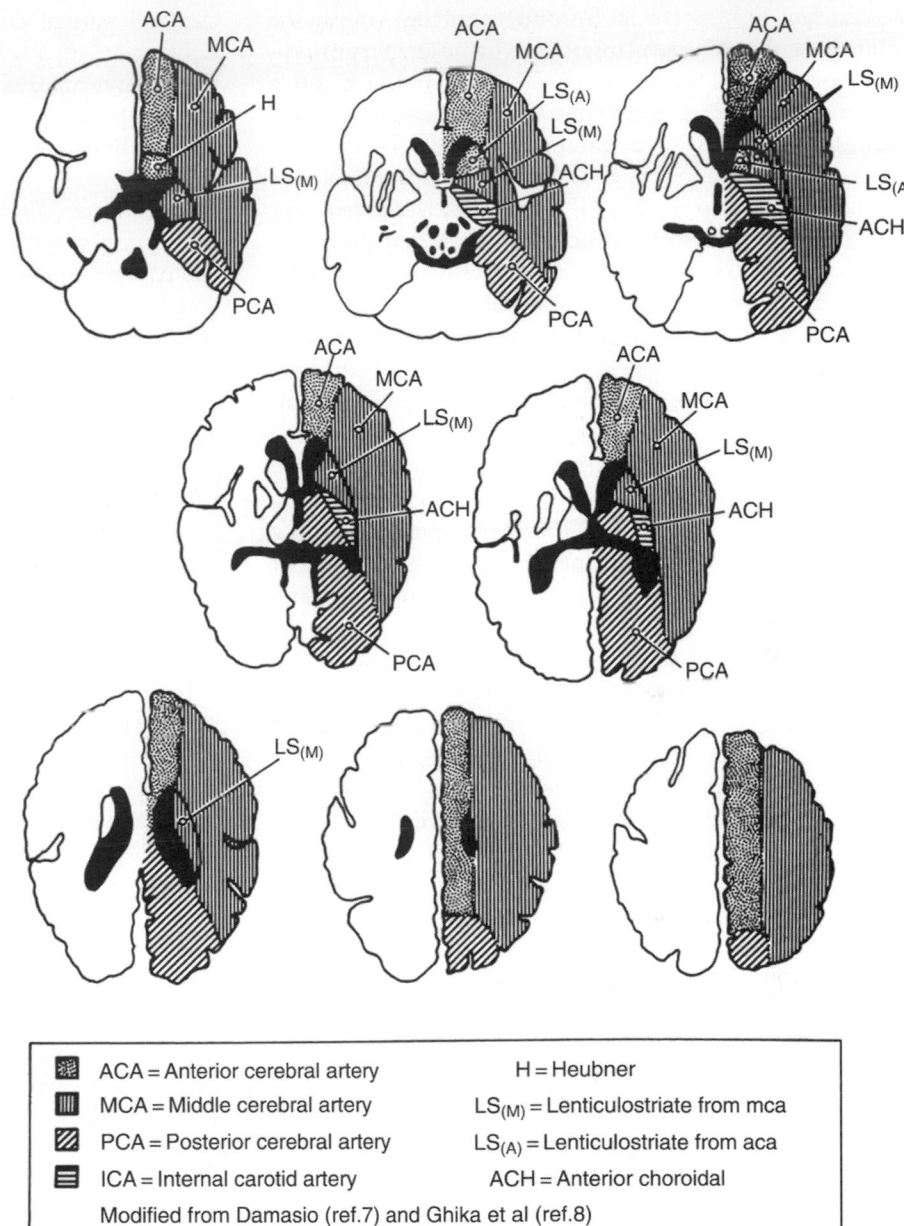

Fig. 8.1 Territories of the major cerebral arteries. (From Del Sette *et al.* 2000 with permission.)

▦	ACA = Anterior cerebral artery		H = Heubner
▥	MCA = Middle cerebral artery		LS(M) = Lenticulostriate from mca
▨	PCA = Posterior cerebral artery		LS(A) = Lenticulostriate from aca
▤	ICA = Internal carotid artery		ACH = Anterior choroidal

Modified from Damasio (ref.7) and Ghika et al (ref.8)

Almost half of *posterior cerebral artery* strokes are due to cardiac emboli (Yamamoto *et al.* 1999; Cals *et al.* 2002). The main effect of posterior cerebral artery infarction is a contralateral hemianopia, sometimes with visual hallucinations, visual agnosias or spatial disorientation. Visual perseveration may consist of a train of objects repeating within the affected field, or persistence of an image in the centre of the field after the object is removed (Caplan 1980). Alexia without agraphia occurs when damage has affected the dominant occipital lobe along with the splenium of the corpus callosum (see Chapter 2, under Pure word-blindness). Bilateral infarctions may lead to cortical blindness, sometimes with conspicuous denial of disability (Anton's syndrome). Adams

and Hurwitz (1974) stressed that psychological disturbances are frequent with posterior cerebral infarctions. Transient mental confusion and agitation has been reported in 7% (Cals *et al.* 2002) to 40% (Ng *et al.* 2005). This may be the only manifestation apart from a hemianopia which is difficult to demonstrate. Amnesic syndromes may also figure prominently when the hippocampus and other limbic structures are involved bilaterally on the inferomedial surfaces of the temporal lobes (Victor *et al.* 1961; Benson *et al.* 1974). In those with unilateral lesions amnesia may be more common if the left hemisphere is involved (Cals *et al.* 2002).

The two posterior cerebral arteries are fed by the basilar artery, which is formed by the two vertebral arteries. From the *vertebrobasilar system*, perforating branches supply the brainstem and cerebellum. Infarctions in the territory of individual branches of the vertebrobasilar system can lead to a multitude of pictures. The hallmark is brainstem involvement, with bilateral or unilateral pyramidal signs and a variety of ipsilateral cranial nerve palsies. Ipsilateral cerebellar deficits may also be present. Major obstacles to recovery include disturbances of balance and persistent dizziness. Intellectual processes may be affected. In seven patients admitted to a rehabilitation unit with isolated brainstem lesions, five of which were infarcts, impaired attention and executive function was found although disturbance of memory was unusual (Garrard *et al.* 2002). Subtle impairments of cognitive function may be seen even in those with small isolated lacunar infarcts of the brainstem (van Zandvoort *et al.* 2003). These findings have been confirmed in a large series of subtentorial strokes which found that executive impairment was common, regardless of whether the stroke involved the brainstem or cerebellum (Hoffmann & Schmitt 2004).

Total occlusion of the basilar artery is usually rapidly fatal, with loss of consciousness, a decerebrate state and quadriplegia. The various pictures of coma, decerebration and akinetic mutism that may follow brainstem infarction are described by Plum and Posner (1972). One rare but striking picture is the so-called 'locked-in' syndrome which follows a circumscribed infarction affecting the descending motor pathways in the ventral part of the pons. This is compatible with full wakefulness and alertness, despite aphonia and total paralysis of the limbs, trunk and lower cranial nerves. Such patients are responsive and sentient but may only be able to communicate using blinking and eye movements. In a survey of carers of 44 patients with locked-in syndrome, 38 due to brainstem stroke and six to trauma, the majority reported little if any problems with cognitive function, although memory problems were described in 18% (Leon-Carrion *et al.* 2002). These findings are consistent with more detailed neuropsychological testing in patients with locked-in syndrome who may (New & Thomas 2005) or may not (Allain *et al.* 1998) show evidence of impairment.

Caplan (1980) reviews further striking pictures with prominent behavioural change following occlusion of the rostral branches of the basilar artery ('top of the basilar' syndrome). The result is infarction in the midbrain, thalamus and portions of the temporal and occipital lobes, producing an array of visual, oculomotor and behavioural abnormalities often with changes in alertness and sleep–wake cycle. Motor dysfunction can be minimal, leading to difficulties with diagnosis. The remarkable syndrome of *peduncular hallucinosis* consists of vivid well-formed hallucinations, sometimes confined to a half-field of vision and occurring with or without visual field defects. The hallucinations are recognised by the patient as unreal despite their dramatic nature.

Caplan's patient saw a parrot in beautiful plumage to the right, and pictures of a relative flashed on the wall to the left. Others have reported vivid hallucinations of animals, of children at play with toys, fleeting images of the head of a dog or intricate lines and colours lasting for an hour or two at a time. States of *bizarre disorientation* accompanied by somnolence may likewise reflect disturbance in the rostral portions of the brainstem reticular formation. In response to questions one patient said she was lying on a beach at Nice, another that she was speaking to friends on the telephone. Such answers, entirely divorced from the current reality, may appear as an extraordinary form of confabulation. Other patients may dream excessively, with inability to distinguish the dreams from reality. Oculomotor disturbances and pupillary abnormalities will usually betray the origins of such abnormal mental states.

The diverse cognitive and behavioural effects of thalamic infarcts, which can partly be explained by which thalamic nuclei are involved, have recently been reviewed (Carrera & Bogousslavsky 2006). Confusion and altered conscious level are often early manifestations. Personality change, particularly disinhibition and apathy, executive difficulties often with perseveration, and occasionally psychotic mood change may follow. Amnesic syndromes may be seen as well as aphasia or visuospatial neglect. Central pain may be more common after right-sided thalamic lesions (Nasreddine & Saver 1997). Quite often both paramedian thalamic nuclei are supplied by a single paramedian artery, which partly explains why bilateral thalamic infarcts are not all that uncommon (Schmahmann 2003).

Very small lacunar infarcts may be asymptomatic, but those 0.5–1.5 cm in diameter are likely to produce deficits (Fisher 1982; Gautier 1983). Lacunar infarcts do not result in any disturbance of higher cortical function or visual field deficit. Pure motor hemiparesis, due to lacunes in the posterior limb of the internal capsule or pons, hemisensory stroke, often with lacunes in the posterolateral thalamus, and ataxic hemiparesis (dysarthria clumsy hand syndrome or ipsilateral ataxia with crural hemiparesis) are seen. The deficits resulting from lacunar infarcts are usually slight and recover rapidly and the risk of death early after the stroke is relatively small. However, after several years 10% or more, particularly those with leucoaraiosis, will develop a vascular dementia (Norrving 2003) (described in Chapter 9), sometimes accompanied by a pseudobulbar palsy.

Transient ischaemic attacks

The classic definition of a transient ischaemic attack (TIA) is acute loss of focal cerebral or monocular function that resolves completely within 24 hours, and with no other explanation for the symptoms than inadequate blood supply. This definition was introduced in an attempt to distinguish episodes that resulted in no permanent brain infarction from stroke. Most TIAs only last a few minutes and leave no permanent infarct. However, for episodes lasting between 4 and 24 hours the majority of patients will have evidence of brain infarction on diffusion-weighted MRI (Engelter *et al.* 1999). And, given that thrombolysis for stroke has to be given within about 3 hours of the onset of symptoms to be effective, the classical definition of TIA is no longer useful. TIAs are therefore now more usually defined as 'a brief episode of neurologic dysfunction caused by focal brain or retinal ischemia, with clinical symptoms typically lasting less than one hour, and without evidence of acute infarction' (Albers *et al.* 2002).

The feature common to all TIAs is temporary reduction of the blood supply to a small area of the brain, long enough to cause manifest but transient loss of function. Both stroke and TIAs can be considered as lying on a spectrum of outcomes from brain ischaemia (Albers *et al.* 2002), with atherothromboembolism, cardiogenic embolism and intracranial small-vessel disease probably accounting for 95% of cases (Bamford 2001). Many TIAs are probably caused by small emboli that temporarily occlude blood flow before breaking up (del Zoppo 2004). The emboli may consist of platelet aggregates, cholesterol or small fragments of thrombus. Emboli passing up the major vessels have been detected as high-intensity transient signals (HITS) on Doppler sonography (Markus *et al.* 1995), although in almost all cases such HITS are asymptomatic. Nevertheless, the presence of HITS may indicate an increased risk for TIA or stroke.

In occasional cases haemodynamic factors may be responsible. Thus a sudden fall in cardiac output, or systemic hypotension due to any cause, may compromise flow in vessels already critically narrowed by atherosclerosis. Anaemia or polycythaemia may be background factors facilitating the development of attacks.

TIAs in the carotid territory typically show contralateral pareses, paraesthesiae, hemianopias or dysphasia, sometimes with transient blurring or even episodes of total blindness in the ipsilateral eye (amaurosis fugax). Microemboli may actually be observed in the retinal arteries on ophthalmoscopy in such cases. Motor impairments may take the form of a brief monoparesis involving only part of a limb. Transient numbness of the face or arm is a common variety. Mental confusion may occasionally be marked but in general non-focal symptoms are absent. Vertebrobasilar TIAs present with a multitude of pictures. Spells of vertigo, tinnitus or diplopia are typical. Episodes of paresis or numbness may involve different sides of the body in successive attacks. Drop attacks are commonly attributable to such a cause in the elderly–the person falls abruptly to the ground without loss of consciousness, then can rise immediately – as a result of acute and transient failure of the antigravity muscles. Sometimes a staggering ataxia may be combined with dysarthria and drowsiness, leading to an impression of drunkenness. Visual phenomena include blurred vision, altitudinal or homonymous hemianopias, or scintillation scotomata.

Box 8.3 Differential diagnosis of transient ischaemic attack

- Migraine aura
- Structural brain lesion (subdural, intracranial tumour, aneurysm, intracranial haemorrhage, sinus thrombosis)
- Postictal deficit (e.g. Todd's paresis)
- Epilepsy
- Hypoglycaemia
- Simple faint
- Labyrinthine disease
- Multiple sclerosis
- Transient global amnesia
- Cerebral infection
- Panic attack

Transient bilateral blindness may occur where both posterior cerebral arteries are implicated.

Because TIAs are associated with significant morbidity in the days and months that follow, accurate identification is important, several differential diagnoses need to be considered (Box 8.3). One-tenth of patients will have a stroke within 90 days and one-quarter within 5 years; 20% will have had a stroke or myocardial infarct or be dead by 1 year. Those at greatest risk of later stroke have longer-lasting TIAs, repeated TIAs while receiving antiplatelet therapy, or have crescendo TIAs (more than three events in 3 days of increasing severity, duration or frequency). Other high-risk factors for subsequent stroke include having a cardioembolic source, being over 60 years of age, and having diabetes mellitus or hypertension. Weakness or speech impairment during the episode also increases the risk (Shah & Edlow 2004). Investigations will therefore be aimed at identifying risk factors for subsequent stroke, and the cause of the TIA. Investigations are likely to include a full blood screen, ECG, echocardiography and, depending on the territory involved, carotid Doppler sonography. MRI with diffusion-weighted imaging is the best way of determining if there is any evidence of brain infarction.

Once neuroimaging has excluded the possibility of an intracerebral bleed, antiplatelet agents (e.g. aspirin or clopidogrel) are the mainstay of medical management. Anticoagulation has no value unless there is clear indication of a cardiac source of emboli, for example atrial fibrillation, prosthetic heart valve or recent myocardial infarct. Carotid endarterectomy has an important role in the prevention of later infarction in patients with greater than 70% stenosis of the carotid artery (Barnett *et al.* 1998).

Neuroimaging of stroke

The acute management of stroke, within the first few hours of onset, goes hand in hand with neuroimaging protocols, developed over the last few years, designed to help the clinician decide whether intravenous thrombolysis is indicated (Masdeu *et al.* 2006). Having confirmed that the neuroimaging findings are indeed those of a vascular lesion, the first priority is then to separate haemorrhagic stroke, in which case thrombolysis is contraindicated, from ischaemic stroke. Subsequently, assessment of the extent of ischaemic but salvageable brain (the penumbra) around the core of non-viable tissue may improve selection of those most likely to benefit from thrombolysis. Neuroimaging may also help identify the cause of the stroke, for example picking up multiple cortical infarcts suggestive of cardiac emboli.

In the acute stage, infarcts of the major cerebral arteries are considered to produce three zones of hypoperfused tissue (Muir *et al.* 2006). The *core* of the infarct, where the opportunity for anastomotic perfusion is least, is defined as the zone where cells will inevitably die. Within the core there may be a zone where only neurones die, surrounding a zone where the ischaemia is so severe that no cell, including glial elements, has a chance of survival. The *penumbra* is the ischaemic zone surrounding the core and is defined as the zone where tissue may either die or survive in the long term. Here the blood flow is about 10–20 mL/min per 100 g. The consequent ischaemia impairs neuronal function, giving rise to neurological symptoms over and above those arising from neuronal death in the core. Finally, surrounding the penumbra is a zone of *oligaemia*, with blood flow greater than 20 mL/min per 100 g but less than the normal value of about 50 mL/min per 100 g, where oxygen extraction is increased, neuronal function is maintained and cell death in the long term is unlikely.

In the acute stage the size of the core determines the extent to which there will be inevitable permanent damage, whereas the size of the penumbra indicates the potential for recovery and for thrombolysis to salvage brain tissue. Therefore identifying the extent of these zones, using neuroimaging, is clinically useful. CT of the brain is quick, generally more accessible than MRI, and detects any early significant intracerebral haemorrhage; by about 10 days any haemorrhage loses its high signal on CT and becomes isodense with brain and is therefore more easily missed. Within the first 3 hours of onset of the stroke, CT brain scan is generally used as part of the protocol to determine if a patient is suitable for thrombolysis (Masdeu *et al.* 2006). However, CT is not as sensitive as MRI for the detection of stroke. In the acute stages a severe stroke can be surprisingly difficult to detect on CT, although detection rates can be improved when the image is systematically examined for early signs of stroke (Barber *et al.* 2000). CT perfusion, which involves tracking an intravenous bolus of contrast media as it passes through the brain, may be used as an alternative to MRI (see below) for identifying the penumbra.

MRI has greater sensitivity for ischaemic changes, and can detect haemorrhage using gradient echo sequences. Because it takes longer than CT imaging and because there are more contraindications to its use, it may not be so useful in the emergency room. Diffusion-weighted imaging (DWI) is an MRI sequence that measures the degree to which water molecules are free to diffuse. Cells dying from ischaemia develop intracellular oedema as sodium ions enter the cell; water is thus removed from the extracellular compartment, resulting in reduced free diffusion of water. The consequent reduction in the apparent diffusion coefficient is detected as a signal on DWI. DWI therefore detects the extent of the core of the infarct. In perfusion-weighted imaging (PWI) a bolus of gadolinium is injected intravenously and its passage through the brain is then tracked, enabling areas of reduced perfusion to be identified, as measured for example by delays in the time-to-peak. What is of interest is the extent to which the area of reduced perfusion, identified on PWI, is larger than the core of dying tissue, identified on DWI. This area of DWI/PWI mismatch is thought to represent the penumbra. However, there may be situations when the DWI/PWI mismatch does not match the penumbra, for example because the DWI lesion includes some tissue that is in fact salvageable (Guadagno *et al.* 2004). Nevertheless, there are two clinical situations where DWI/PWI findings are useful. Patients with a middle cerebral artery stroke and a large extensive DWI lesion (i.e. the core) and little mismatch are very likely to do badly. The stroke may become 'malignant', with severe raised intracranial pressure and cerebral herniation; decompressive hemicraniectomy, to relieve the raised intracranial pressure, may reduce mortality in these patients. On the other hand, even as late as 3–6 hours after stroke onset, if there is a large area of mismatch (suggesting a large penumbra), then thrombolysis may improve outcome.

Any advantage in identifying DWI/PWI mismatch is largely limited to anterior circulation strokes. On the other hand, routine MRI combined with DWI is particularly useful for detecting posterior fossa or lacuna strokes. MRI gradient echo sequences can visualise intracerebral haemorrhages including microbleeds or petechial haemorrhages below the 5-mm-diameter threshold necessary for detection using CT. There is uncertainty as to whether such microbleeds should be regarded as a contraindication to thrombolysis. MRI can also identify occluded arteries, which lose the normal flow void within the lumen, or those with dissection of the wall. These observations may be complemented by visualisation of the occluded arterial tree by magnetic resonance angiography (MRA). MRI plus MRA is the method of choice for the diagnosis and follow-up of cerebral venous thrombosis as a cause of stroke (Masdeu *et al.* 2006). Other neuroimaging techniques that may have a role in the investigation of stroke include cerebral angiography and Doppler studies of the cerebral vessels.

Positron emission tomography (PET) and single-photon emission computed tomography (SPECT) may demonstrate remote effects (*diaschisis*) at a distance from the point of infarction (Baron 1987; Costa & Ell 1991). This is best observed in ipsilateral cortex, particularly frontal, after thalamic infarcts, in contralateral cerebellum after large supratentorial infarcts (crossed cerebellar diaschisis) (Sobesky *et al.* 2005), and in contralateral areas of cortex after unilateral cerebral ischaemia (transhemispheric diaschisis). The diaschisis may be accompanied by neuropsychological (Caselli *et al.* 1991) or neurological (Seitz *et al.* 1999) deficits that may recover quickly.

In the hours and days after stroke, neurological recovery is due to reperfusion. With improvement in blood flow the penumbra shrinks as neurones that were previously unable to function return to activity. This may be followed by a period of improvement over several weeks due to the spontaneous regression of brain oedema and other acute histopathological processes in and around the stroke. Over this same period the remote effects of the stroke, particularly diaschisis, improve. Any later recovery is probably, at least in part, due to reorganisation of function (Butefisch *et al.* 2006).

Frackowiak and colleagues used PET to investigate patterns of adaptation and reorganisation in patients who had recovered from hemiplegic stroke (Chollet *et al.* 1991). Finger movements on the unaffected side activated regional blood flow in the contralateral sensorimotor and premotor cortex and the ipsilateral cerebellar hemisphere. The same movements in the recovered hand produced more widespread activations, including significant increases bilaterally in sensorimotor and premotor cortex and both cerebellar hemispheres. Thus bilateral involvement of motor systems was seen when the recovered fingers were employed, indicating significant reorganisation and recruitment of ipsilateral motor pathways. In a further study, Weiller *et al.* (1992) obtained evidence of the recruitment of additional motor systems involving inferior parietal and anterior insular regions. Activations were also observed in cingulate and prefrontal areas that are not normally involved in finger movement but are known to be involved in selective attentional and intentional mechanisms, suggesting that these too may play an important part in the recovery process. Rather similar patterns of reorganisation, with activation of motor and premotor cortex contralateral to the lesioned side, have been identified using functional (f)MRI to study a finger-tracking task in patients several years after stroke (Carey *et al.* 2002). This reorganisation was only seen in those who were exposed to a motor training programme, compared with those who were not, an observation that has important implications for stroke rehabilitation.

Investigation and medical management of TIA and stroke

The management of stroke within 3 hours of onset is dominated by the need to determine whether there is any evidence of cerebral haemorrhage on neuroimaging. If there is no haemorrhage, it may be possible to start thrombolytic treatment with recombinant tissue plasminogen activator (rt-PA). The sooner rt-PA is started, the greater the benefit. It will also be necessary to evaluate the patient's cardiovascular status; possible sources of emboli must be sought with care. Anticoagulant therapy may be indicated where embolism is suspected, or operative intervention may be needed on a stenosed or atheromatous carotid artery, but these are matters for neurological assessment. More recently it has been proposed that in some cases with a large lesion on DWI in the middle cerebral artery territory early decompressive hemicraniectomy may reduce mortality. There is no evidence that neuroprotection helps.

Patients with intracerebral haemorrhage are at risk of further bleeding and of developing hydrocephalus. In the acute stage, expert nursing and physiotherapy are essential. Patients admitted to a stroke unit are less likely to die than those admitted to routine medical admission wards (Stroke Unit Trialists' Collaboration 2001). Particularly in the younger patient or those with recurrent stroke, specific causes of stroke should be considered (Box 8.4).

Sequelae of stroke

The disablement resulting from strokes is frequently a mixture of physical and mental problems. The latter may be attributable directly to the brain damage sustained, or largely represent the individual's reaction to the handicaps imposed on him. In either event the patient's personality and life situation can have a profound effect on overall adjustment to the disability, and the mental components of the picture will often be decisive in determining the level of success achieved in rehabilitation.

In what follows an attempt is made to review the principal components of psychiatric disability after stroke, but first the

---

Box 8.4 Additional investigations in young or recurrent stroke (Brown 2001)

- MRI
- Autoantibody screen
- Anticardiolipin antibodies
- Thrombophilia screen
- Sickle cell
- Serum homocysteine
- Serum lactate (CADASIL)
- Syphilis serology
- Drug screen
- 24-hour ECG recording
- Transthoracic echocardiography
- Transoesophageal echocardiography
- Cerebral angiography

question of overall prognosis is considered. The general picture of the incidence of defects and quality of survival provides the framework against which to view the range and extent of the problems encountered.

Overall prognosis

On average, after a stroke about one-quarter of patients die within 1 month (Wolfe 2000). The wide variation in mortality rates across studies, from 18 to over 50%, presumably reflects the differing age and health status of the populations studied. The highest mortality is associated with primary intracerebral haemorrhage and subarachnoid haemorrhage; 1-year case fatality is about 34–40%. In terms of impairment it has been estimated that at 6 months after the stroke (Wolfe 2000) about half continue to have partial or complete motor loss, one-quarter are not orientated and about 15% have a significant aphasia. As a result more than 20% of patients are at least moderately dependent. A population-based survey 5 years after stroke (Wilkinson *et al.* 1997) found one-third to be moderately or severely disabled, and two-fifths were more disabled than they had been at 3 months after the stroke. Presumably intervening vascular events and other effects of ageing explained some of the deterioration. Perhaps the high rates of depression also contributed to the deterioration; almost one-quarter were depressed. In a study of 286 survivors of stroke at 3 and 15 months (Pohjasvaara *et al.* 2002), both deteriorating depression and deteriorating cognition were associated with an increase in dependence at 15 months.

Early epileptic seizures, within the first week, are seen in about 3–6% of patients after ischaemic stroke (Camilo & Goldstein 2004; Ryvlin *et al.* 2006), but the risk is perhaps fourfold greater with intracerebral haemorrhage (Vespa *et al.* 2003). Other risk factors include a cortical lesion and severe stroke. Although only about 2–4% of patients will develop epilepsy in the longer term, stroke is the commonest single cause of late-onset epilepsy (Ryvlin *et al.* 2006). Those stroke patients who develop epilepsy probably have a worse outcome and may have greater risk of psychosis (see below). Early epileptic seizures may be a risk factor for cognitive impairment after stroke (Cordonnier *et al.* 2007).

Cognitive impairment and dementia

The mental impairment that may follow a single stroke usually proves to be focal in nature once the initial clouding of consciousness has cleared. For some time, however, global confusion and disorientation may be much in evidence, and can be slow to clear when cerebral damage has been extensive. It may be aggravated by anoxia from congestive cardiac failure or respiratory infection, or be attributable in part to the patient's difficulty in coping with new-found barriers to communication with his environment. As the situation improves the true extent of cognitive dysfunction is revealed. The longer clouding of consciousness has persisted, the more likely that residual mental deficits are severe and extensive.

Considerable difficulty may be encountered in assessing the extent of global intellectual impairment, particularly if the patient is dysphasic or with marked constructional difficulties. Agitation, depression or apathy in the early stages may give a false impression of dementia, as may visual disorientation or agnosic difficulties. A circumscribed amnesic syndrome due to posterior cerebral infarction may not at first be appreciated as such.

Much of our understanding of the classic focal cortical syndromes (the dysphasias, apraxias and body image disturbances) has come from studies of stroke survivors. The essentials of such disorders have been outlined in Chapter 1 and are not repeated here. Such disorders have important impacts on rehabilitation. Disturbances of language contribute a large added handicap and source of frustration, frequently outlasting recovery of motor function. Patients with expressive loss but good comprehension will in general make much better adjustment than when understanding is faulty. Apraxic disturbances may persist as a barrier to rehabilitation when motor paralysis has cleared, particularly an apraxia of gait. Disorders of attention, including neglect, often improve spontaneously but otherwise may prove difficult to treat particularly as they are often accompanied by lack of insight.

The concepts of vascular dementia and multi-infarct dementia are discussed alongside the other dementias in Chapter 9. The focus here is on *poststroke dementia*, a term introduced to describe those patients found to suffer global cognitive impairment after stroke (Leys *et al.* 2005). Thus the index event in studies of poststroke dementia is the stroke, and all types of dementia irrespective of their cause are included. The most common are vascular dementia and Alzheimer's disease. In some cases the dementia will have been present before the stroke, in others the stroke will have caused the dementia, and in others the dementia will have had its onset at some time between the stroke and the assessment.

Estimates of the prevalence of poststroke dementia vary widely, from 6 to 32%. Much of this variance may be because of the different classification criteria that have been used. The age of the cohort studied and the interval between assessment and stroke will affect prevalence rates. Stroke doubles the risk of new-onset cases of dementia (i.e. not present when assessed shortly after the stroke) over the years after the stroke (Kokmen *et al.* 1996), and this includes a doubling of the risk of Alzheimer's disease. Risk factors for poststroke dementia include lower educational level, prestroke cognitive decline (but not sufficient for dementia diagnosis), and more severe stroke. Left hemisphere strokes are more likely to be associated with dementia. Dementia after stroke is more common in those who, on CT or MRI, have silent infarcts (i.e. infarcts not associated with any corresponding neurological defect), global atrophy or white matter disease (leucoaraiosis) (Leys *et al.* 2005).

Very occasionally dementia may follow a single strategically situated stroke. The syndrome of cognitive impairment after strokes of the left angular gyrus, with a receptive aphasia and constructional deficits, may easily be mistaken for the clinical picture found in Alzheimer's disease (Benson & Cummings 1982). Bilateral strokes involving the basal forebrain can produce a dementia as a result of severe impairment of executive function and memory. Bilateral thalamic strokes may produce dementia. De Boucaud *et al.* (1968) reported an example with post-mortem findings of old haemorrhagic softenings in both thalami and no pathological changes in the cortex. The dementia was accompanied by disturbance of gait. Bilateral medial thalamic infarctions typically lead to a hypersomnolent apathetic state and vertical gaze disturbance, with dementia of the 'subcortical' type (Kumral *et al.* 2001). Such lesions are seen with occlusion of the paramedian arteries of the thalamus. Indeed because the thalamus is supplied by four arteries, each with a very distinct origin and territory, thalamic strokes may be quite localised and offer unique insights into brain–behaviour relationships. It has been suggested that distinct patterns of behavioural change, even following unilateral lesions, can be seen depending on which of the four main thalamic arterial territories is affected (Carrera & Bogousslavsky 2006). Infarcts of the anterior thalamic territory may produce apathy, amnesia and a behavioural syndrome (still to be validated by other research groups and which perhaps bears some semblance to confabulation) of perseveration and 'superimposition of unrelated information'; amnesia, loss of self-activation and disinhibition with personality change follow paramedian infarcts; executive dysfunction follows inferolateral lesions, and neglect and aphasia after posterior lesions.

Poststroke dementia has a serious adverse effect on both the mortality (Desmond *et al.* 2002) and morbidity of stroke. It also increases the risk of stroke recurrence. Deficits in cognitive function are therefore among the more serious of the sequelae of stroke, delaying and often gravely compromising attempts at rehabilitation. Such elements in the clinical picture may be less immediately obvious than the hemiplegia or other physical handicap, yet often prove to be the factors responsible for failure to regain independence. Thus among patients who become long-stay invalids, permanently confined to chair or bed, paralysis by itself rather seldom accounts for their incapacity and may even contribute little towards it (Adams & Hurwitz 1963, 1974).

Personality change

Personality changes after stroke are among the most troublesome of the sequelae of stroke, and may overshadow the intellectual deficits. It may be difficult to determine if the change in personality is directly attributable to brain damage. When this is the case, widespread vascular changes are probably responsible and the personality change may progress even though the focal sequelae of the stroke improve. The changes usually prove to be the prelude to a progressive dementing illness.

> A woman of 69 had a very mild stroke affecting the left arm transiently. She seemed well for a while thereafter, but gradually changed, becoming irritable, hard to please and with vague complaints of headache and giddiness. She became anxious and did not want to be left alone. Loss of interests and slowing were accompanied by episodes of confusion and disorientation. On examination 15 months after the stroke she was not grossly demented, but showed some difficulty in understanding questions and had only a vague idea of the date. There was a residual left hemiparesis, a left homonymous hemianopia, some dyscalculia and a mild nominal dysphasia. However, her affective state was worse than her intellect: she was mostly apathetic and dull, though cheerful in a facile way at times. Eventually she needed long-term hospitalisation (Slater 1962).

In such cases the pattern of problems encountered is not dissimilar to those found in any dementing illness. Typically one sees a 'reduction of margins'. The patient cannot adjust to new circumstances, and small matters make him anxious, irritable or depressed. He avoids new experiences and restricts himself to an unvarying routine. Confrontation with a task or with social demands carries the risk of provoking a catastrophic reaction. The patient may become abusive and uncooperative if asked to make any effort, yet be affable and obliging when left in peace. Hypochondriacal concerns may become evident and constitutional predispositions may also be revealed or accentuated. A previously lonely person may become suspicious or frankly paranoid. It may be only at a later stage, when for example the emotional state is recognisably abnormal with dulled and flattened responsiveness, that it becomes evident that the patient has a dementia.

When the carers of unselected cohorts of patients with stroke are asked to describe the personality changes, several attributes are typically endorsed. At 1 year after stroke over half of 84 patients were rated by their carers as being slowed down, excessively worried, miserable or complaining of aches and pains, and over one-third as withdrawn, irritable, fearful or unpredictable (Anderson *et al.* 1995). At 9 months after the stroke, patients were rated as being more bored, frustrated, unhappy, worried, irritable and unreasonable, and less active, independent, patient, confident and enthusiastic compared with the retrospective assessment of the pre-stroke state (Stone *et al.* 2004). Greater changes in personality were reported in patients who were diagnosed as depressed, who had worse scores on an extended activities of daily living scale, and for whom the carer had more emotional distress as rated by the carer's score on the Hospital Anxiety and Depression Scale (HADS). Patients with total anterior circulation strokes were most at risk.

Caregiver burden

Much of the burden of care of stroke comes to fall on carers, often the spouse of the patient and themselves no longer young. Early in the course of adopting this responsibility carers will express their concerns about the challenge. When this was examined during rehabilitation on average 12 weeks after injury (Belciug 2006), carers were worried about making sure that the patient would be safe at all times and dealing with the emotional aspects of the patient's care. Carers also wanted to know what the future needs would be and what to do in specific situations when the patient could not do something for himself. These anticipatory worries may partly explain why carers rate the patient as more impaired than patients rate themselves (Knapp & Hewison 1999). However, at 3 years carers remain burdened by feelings of heavy responsibility, uncertainty about patients' care needs, constant worries, restraints in social life, and feelings that patients rely on them alone (Scholte op Reimer *et al*. 1998).

A review of 20 studies of caregivers of stroke patients found that about 40% of carers are depressed (Han & Haley 1999). When non-caregiver controls had been studied they showed much lower rates of depression. How much of the effect is specific to looking after patients with stroke, as opposed to other disabled patients, is uncertain. Carers with worse social networks and worse physical health report more depressive symptoms. The carers of patients who were depressed or had more abnormal behaviour were also more likely to be depressed. Nevertheless, carers of patients who were more physically dependent did not seem to be at increased risk. Some studies suggest that carer ill health may deteriorate over time after the injury (Schlote *et al*. 2006). However, one 2-year follow-up found relatively low levels of carer stress and depression, and these remained fairly constant over time (Wade *et al*. 1986). Associations between patient characteristics and carer depression, including being less independent or more depressed, present in the first year after stroke were no longer present at 2 years.

Does stress in the caregiver result in worse outcome for the patient? The best test of this is to demonstrate that interventions, directed at the carer to reduce carer burden, improve patient outcome. As yet there is little evidence to support this. Indeed it may not be easy to relieve caregiver burden. A review of studies designed to improve well-being in carers using problem-solving interventions found some effects in some studies (Lui *et al*. 2005). For example, in a randomised study of patients and their families a few weeks after stroke, one-third of caregivers were visited at home to be taught problem-solving skills using a systematic four-step approach (Grant *et al*. 2002). Telephone contact, initially weekly, was then used to consolidate the intervention. After 3 months the intervention group, compared with a sham intervention and a control treatment-as-usual group, showed better problem-solving and were less depressed. However, they did not

show less carer burden. The study did not attempt to examine any impact the intervention might have had on the patients themselves. In a study of 240 stroke patients randomised to receive visits from a specialist outreach nurse to provide information, advice and support over the first 12 months compared with treatment as usual, there was no reduction in stress in carers (Forster & Young 1996). Mildly disabled patients showed small gains in activity. In a randomised controlled trial (RCT) of a family support organiser, aimed at both patient and carer, those who received the intervention did obtain more social services support and felt better informed, but there was no significant improvement in a measure of reintegration into normal living (Tilling *et al*. 2005). Therefore it is not yet possible to give firm advice as to what technique to use to reduce carer stress, and whether in fact it will make much difference anyway.

Depression and other mood disorders

It is scarcely surprising that depressive reactions should be common in survivors of strokes. Ullman (1962) vividly describes the subjective impact which the experience may have. The patient finds himself abruptly in the grip of something novel, frightening and ill understood. Even slight interference in free communication with those around will greatly intensify feelings of isolation, threat or loss. When the acute stage is over there is a variety of factors around which depression may come to be organised: the frustrations of physical handicaps, uncertainty about the prospects of their resolution, the enforced dependency and imposition of the invalid role. In the longer term the patient may face loss of job and status, financial insecurity, a sense of uselessness or the prospect of permanent loss of independence.

At what stage should such depressive reactions be regarded as a case of depression? It could be argued that there is a danger of overestimating depression after stroke if physical symptoms of stroke are interpreted as evidence of depression (Box 8.5). Patients diagnosed with depression after stroke, compared with primary depression (depression that is not secondary to brain disease or other factors), have more physical symptoms and less evidence of melancholia (Beblo & Driessen 2002). However, somatic symptoms are not necessarily a confounder. Depressed stroke patients are much more likely to endorse symptoms like fatigue and sleep disturbance than stroke patients who are not depressed (Williams *et al*. 2005). Nevertheless, depression in patients who are aphasic after stroke may be missed.

Most studies find that survivors of stroke, when compared with age-matched controls, are more depressed. Indeed stroke patients have been found to show a higher incidence of depression than orthopaedic controls or patients suffering from traumatic brain injuries, despite equivalent levels of disability in terms of activities of daily living or cognitive dysfunction (Folstein *et al*. 1977; Robinson & Szetela 1981). However, one study comparing survivors of stroke with survivors of myocardial infarction found no difference (Aben *et al.* 2003).

A systematic review of studies of depression after stroke found that the estimates of the prevalence of depression vary according to which rating scales have been used (Hackett & Anderson 2005), but that even using clinical assessments, e.g. based on *Diagnostic and Statistical Manual of Mental Disorders* (DSM)-IV criteria, there is considerable variation in reported frequencies across individual studies. Nevertheless, when the findings across studies were collated the pooled estimates were fairly consistent, indicating that about one-third of patients had significant depressive symptoms, regardless of whether the cases were ascertained from the community, from hospital or from rehabilitation settings. The pooled estimates of the time course of depression were largely based on different cross-sectional studies, each study assessing depression at a different time after stroke; only a small minority of studies had longitudinally assessed depression. Whether the study was early, in the first few weeks and months after stroke, or late, on average the rate of depression did not change. However, even though the rate of depression at each time point remains fairly constant, depression early after stroke has a good chance of remitting over the course of the first year; this is counterbalanced by the finding that other patients become depressed for the first time many months after stroke. Nevertheless, some longitudinal studies show a trend for rates of depression to decline over the first

1–2 years (Morris *et al.* 1990; House *et al.* 1991; Astrom *et al.* 1993; Verdelho *et al.* 2004), but not all studies (Wade *et al.* 1987; Herrmann *et al.* 1998).

Based on the same systematic review of papers, Hackett and Anderson (2005) found that the best predictor of depression was stroke severity, including the extent of physical disability and cognitive impairment. One matter of interest is whether the laterality of the stroke is related to depression. Early studies suggested that left hemisphere infarcts, particularly if located anteriorly, were more likely to produce depression (Robinson & Price 1982; Robinson *et al.* 1984), although a systematic review of studies reporting rates of depression related to laterality of stroke found no effect (Carson *et al.* 2000). However, this conclusion has been rebutted (Narushima *et al.* 2003) and one systematic review (Bhogal *et al.* 2004) found that left-sided stroke is associated with depression if the study examines patients early after stroke, or in hospital. More recent studies have failed to demonstrate an effect of laterality (Verdelho *et al.* 2004; Nys *et al.* 2005; Aben *et al.* 2006; Paolucci *et al.* 2006).

It seems likely that biological factors will be especially important in the early weeks following the infarct (Nys *et al.* 2005), but that with the passage of time, social and interpersonal factors will become increasingly important in determining the affective state. Clinical wisdom suggests that depression will be strongly determined by aspects of the premorbid personality. Patients of striving and self-sufficient disposition may react more adversely to handicap and those who have experienced anxiety and depressive reactions under previous stress will be at increased risk. Neuroticism, as assessed by self-rating 1 month after stroke on the NEO Five Factor Inventory (Costa & McCrae 1985), has been found to be associated with depression (Aben *et al.* 2006). Much will also depend on the family setting and relationships with which the patient is surrounded. Quite frequently, at the era of life where most strokes occur, the patient is relatively unsupported: the spouse may have died or be infirm, and children will have moved away. In their systematic review Hackett and Anderson (2005) found that adverse social factors, particularly those related to social isolation, are associated with depression. However, it was less easy to demonstrate, consistently across studies, effects of age, personal history of depression or stroke subtype. Possible reasons for the discrepancies among the different investigations are likely to include differing levels of physical and cognitive impairment, pre-existing brain damage as well as the time elapsed since the stroke occurred. A host of psychosocial variables in the samples studied may be important, including the proportion of patients having religious beliefs, which may protect against the development of depression (Giaquinto *et al.* 2007).

On occasion it may be difficult to recognise depression, especially when the development has been insidious. Sometimes it is masked by stoical attitudes, or absorbed into habitual or automatic patterns of behaviour. The importance of recognising depression need scarcely be stressed. Stroke is associated with suicidal thoughts in perhaps 10% of patients (Kishi *et al.* 1996; Pohjasvaara *et al.* 2001; Williams 2005) and probably doubles the risk of suicide (Stenager *et al.* 1998; Teasdale & Engberg 2001). Depression may lead to lack of cooperation or poor motivation for rehabilitation, and is associated with generally worse outcomes (Williams 2005) and greater use of health care (Jia *et al.* 2006). It is associated with greater depression in carers (Dennis *et al.* 1998). Depression early after stroke increases mortality over the subsequent years (Morris *et al.* 1993; House *et al.* 2001; Williams *et al.* 2004). Indeed depression probably increases the risk of having a stroke in the first place (Williams 2005).

Emotionalism after stroke
A heightened tendency to cry, often uncontrollably and with little warning, has traditionally been attributed to pseudobulbar palsy resulting from bilateral lesions of the corticobulbar tracts. In such a setting, crying may occur with little or no provocation. However, the disorder has broader connotations, and is not uncommon as an embarrassing and disabling aftermath of strokes.

House *et al.* (1989) followed up 128 patients who had suffered a first-ever stroke and examined them specifically for heightened emotionalism. The criteria were that the patient should experience an increase in episodes of crying (or more rarely laughing), with little or no warning, and with an inability to control them. At 6 months, 21% of patients reported such symptoms, and at 12 months 11%. All showed crying as the principal problem, but two had episodes of pathological laughter in addition. In most the disorder had set in during the 4–6 weeks following the stroke, with a tendency to ameliorate over the following year. In virtually all patients the episodes were provoked by emotional stimuli of a sad or sentimental nature.

The patients as a group scored higher on indices of depression than the remainder, but they were also more intellectually impaired and showed more extensive lesions on CT. A special relationship appeared to obtain with lesions in the anterior left hemisphere, patients with such lesions showing longer-lasting disorder. Stroke survivors with emotionalism, compared to those without, exhibit more irritability and ideas of reference (Calvert *et al.* 1998) and intrusive thoughts about their stroke (Eccles *et al.* 1999).

Prevention and treatment of poststroke depression and emotionalism
Though it is be hoped that appropriate treatment can be quickly rewarding, it is important to distinguish depressive disorder from simple loss of confidence, or from the emotional lability associated with intellectual impairment. It is also necessary to remain sensitively aware that sometimes,

in severely disabled patients, feelings of resignation and futility are realistically based; some elderly patients really are so frail, and the odds so genuinely against them, that their wish 'not to bother' deserves to be treated with proper respect. Needless to say this is an aspect of differential diagnosis that requires the utmost care.

Given that probably one-third to half of patients go on to suffer depression in the year after stroke, and that depression is associated with adverse sequelae (see above), several studies have attempted to prevent depression after stroke. Most have used antidepressants prescribed prophylactically to all patients, whether depressed or not, to see if patients on drug treatment are less likely to become depressed over subsequent months. For example, 137 patients were randomised to receive sertraline or placebo within 4 weeks of stroke (Rasmussen *et al.* 2003). Significantly fewer scored above cut-off on the Hamilton Depression Rating Scale at 1 year, although this finding was jeopardised by the fact that half had dropped out of the study by then. In fact a rigorous systematic review (most recently updated in August 2005) concluded that there was insufficient evidence to support the clinical argument that antidepressants should be used to prevent depression after stroke (Hackett *et al.* 2005). In only five of nine studies was it possible to estimate whether rates of diagnosable depression were reduced. There was a significant finding in favour of antidepressants, but this relied heavily on one study that used indolaxine, a drug not generally available, as well as the study using sertraline just described. Nevertheless, no adverse effects were found related to antidepressant use. The review concluded that if it were possible to identify patients at high risk of depression, there might be a role for prophylactic antidepressants for these patients. A more recent review found in favour of antidepressants for preventing depression, although the review included studies with only 4-week treatment trials (Chen *et al.* 2006). There have been two more recent studies with reasonable durations of treatment, in both cases started within 2 weeks of stroke. Almeida *et al.* (2006) compared 24 weeks of sertraline with placebo; there was no significant reduction in rates of depression in patients on sertraline. The other study by Niedermaier *et al.* (2004) compared 1 year of mirtazapine with treatment as usual (no placebo so the study was not blinded); fewer on mirtazapine suffered depression. Given these ambivalent findings, at present the evidence probably does not justify the routine use of antidepressants in all patients who have suffered a stroke.

The review by Hackett *et al.* (2004) also found three studies of psychotherapeutic techniques aimed at preventing depression. Using the General Health Questionnaire (GHQ) as a measure of psychological distress, there was a small effect in favour of psychotherapy (weighted mean difference –1.41; CI –2.64 to –0.18). However, this result relied heavily on the positive results of one study and there was no significant effect on reducing rates of depression. More recently, a study of a 3-month exercise programme after stroke, designed to investigate general improvements in outcome, found that at 3 months significantly fewer of the exercise group were depressed (14% vs. 35%), although by 9 months the effect was no longer statistically significant (Lai *et al.* 2006).

Turning now to the effectiveness of antidepressants in relieving poststroke depression, several studies have been published since this was first documented by Lipsey *et al.* (1984). On the basis of a systematic review of these studies, Hackett *et al.* (2004) concluded that there was no strong evidence that antidepressants were able to increase rates of remission of depression after stroke. However, there was evidence of a reduction (improvement) in scores on depression rating scales. Even though the findings of the review have been disputed (Chen *et al.* 2006), it seems reasonable to conclude that while antidepressants do improve mood in patients who are depressed after stroke, the effect is not as great as in primary depression, i.e. in patients without brain disease. Given that antidepressants may increase anxiety when used to treat poststroke depression (Hackett *et al.* 2004), some would argue that they should only be used if there is good evidence of major depression. On the other hand, because selective serotonin reuptake inhibitors (SSRIs) are unlikely to produce side effects, perhaps all patients with possible depression (e.g. those with poor motivation) should be treated; not to do so may mean that patients who might benefit are not given the opportunity. However, any such therapeutic trial needs to be closely monitored for evidence of benefit, and if none is found there should be a clear protocol for stopping the antidepressant.

In the absence of powerful effects of antidepressant medication, it is all the more important to consider psychological treatments of poststroke depression. These were evaluated in an RCT of patients with depression 1–6 months after stroke (Lincoln & Flannaghan 2003). They were offered 10 sessions of cognitive–behaviour therapy, delivered by a community psychiatric nurse, over 3 months or an equivalent level of contact but with no formal cognitive–behaviour therapy (attentional placebo) or treatment as usual; there were about 40 patients in each arm. There was no effect on depression. On the other hand, a study of care management of depression, with patients recruited 1–2 months after stroke, found lower rates of depression after 12 weeks in the treatment group compared with treatment as usual (Williams *et al.* 2007). However, the care management intervention ('Activate–Initiate–Monitor') was essentially aimed at improving compliance with antidepressant medication. Therefore far higher rates of antidepressant use were seen in the treatment group. As such it is difficult to be sure how much of the effect

was due to any psychological support the patients received, and how much was due to antidepressants. Nevertheless, the findings support clinical wisdom; if antidepressants are going to be prescribed this is best done in the setting of a clear management plan (see for example the guidance for prescribing antidepressants following acquired brain injury; Royal College of Physicians 2005).

Given such ambivalent findings in terms of the treatment effects of antidepressants, it is too early to be convinced by suggestions that antidepressants may improve cognition or reduce mortality after stroke. However, tricyclic antidepressants have also been shown to be remarkably effective in patients who develop 'emotional incontinence' with pathological laughing and crying, whether or not this is associated with other features of pseudobulbar palsy (Lawson & MacLeod 1969). Even in the absence of subjective depression, such medication can apparently alleviate the disruptive and socially embarrassing effects of the disorder. A systematic review of the evidence was less optimistic. It concluded that large effect sizes could be seen, but noted that the confidence intervals were wide and that there was no consistency across studies in terms of the measure of emotionalism or the antidepressant that had been used (House *et al.* 2004). Despite these cautions most clinicians would recommend a trial of an SSRI in somebody with disabling emotionalism after stroke.

Other mood disorders

A generalised anxiety disorder is found in about 25% of stroke patients (Castillo *et al.* 1995; Leppavuori *et al.* 2003) usually in association with depression. In a careful follow-up of patients, House *et al.* (1991) stressed the importance of persistent agoraphobia and social withdrawal in a small proportion of cases. Such developments were often associated with fear of looking conspicuous on account of disabilities, or fear of recurrence provoked by physical activity. Tension, worry and lack of energy were common complaints.

Mania occurs after stroke, but not sufficiently frequently to reliably estimate its prevalence. Mania may be associated with right temporal lesions (Starkstein *et al.* 1990). Hypomanic pictures have also been reported (Van der Lugt & De Visser 1967), and from the data presented by Starkstein *et al.* (1988) may be expected to be commoner after right hemisphere strokes than left. They reported 12 cases of mania after a variety of brain lesions, seven being restricted to the right hemisphere, one to the left, and four with bilateral or midline damage. Of the four strokes in this series, two were in the right hemisphere, one in the left and one was a right thalamocapsular bleed. The episodes of mania often followed the strokes within days or weeks.

A remarkable example of bipolar affective disorder following thalamic infarction was described by McGilchrist *et al.* (1993).

A 43-year-old man with mild hypercholesterolaemia and indications of autoimmune dysfunction experienced an episode of transient loss of consciousness, followed by drowsiness and left-sided pyramidal signs for 24 hours. Thereafter he appeared to have undergone a marked change of personality, becoming apathetic, dulled and fatuous, and eating and sleeping excessively. At intervals of 3 weeks or so he would suddenly become alert, excitable and elated for about 36 hours, then relapse to his former condition. The picture was sufficiently bizarre to suggest at one time that he might be malingering.

When referred for a second opinion 18 months later he was histrionic and tearful, smiled incongruously and had poor self-esteem. He was profoundly apathetic and self-care was poor. He complained that he was like 'an engine that won't tick over'. CT revealed bilateral thalamic infarcts, and SPECT showed severe hypoperfusion of both frontal lobes. Psychological testing showed poor performance on a visual memory task and impaired frontal functioning on the Trail Making and the Cognitive Estimates tests. While in hospital he showed two episodes of elation lasting for several days, the second being frankly manic with pressure of speech, flight of ideas and possibly auditory hallucinations.

It was concluded that the thalamic infarctions had led, via diaschisis, to metabolic hypofunction in the frontal lobes, resulting in the abrupt onset of cyclical mood disorder accompanied by features of frontal lobe dysfunction.

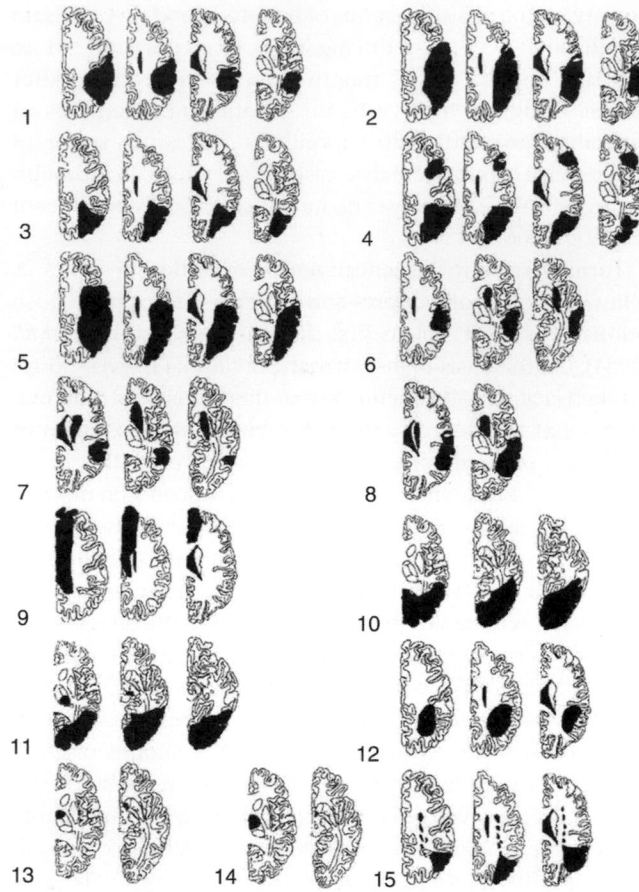

Fig. 8.2 Location of strokes in 15 patients with delusional ideation in the days following stroke. (From Kumral & Ozturk 2004 with permission.)

Attention has been drawn to another aspect of differential diagnosis by Förstl and Sahakian (1991). Three patients were described who were admitted to hospital with supposed major depression, exhibiting severe psychomotor retardation, weight loss, exhaustion and self-reproach. All had evidence of infarcts or atrophy in the left frontal lobe, and SPECT scanning in two showed left frontal hypoperfusion. The shared clinical feature was abrupt improvement under hospital care, with relapse to extreme lack of initiative and energy on discharge to the home environment. Such cycles were followed repeatedly, with the patients neglecting to eat or drink and spending most of their time at home in bed. It was suggested that this may represent a specific syndrome of extreme abulia (i.e. lack of will) consequent on left frontal pathology. Milder forms of apathy are quite common after stroke, and though they are usually observed in patients who are also depressed, may be seen in isolation (Starkstein *et al.* 1993).

Psychoses

There are few figures against which to gauge the incidence of non-affective psychotic illness after cerebrovascular accidents; it has been estimated at about 1–2% (Rabins *et al.* 1991), although follow-up series will fail to find any cases at 1 year (Tang *et al.* 2002). The most thorough study of the incidence of delusional ideas rated 360 patients admitted within 1 day

of stroke every day while they were in hospital (Kumral & Ozturk 2004). Delusional ideation was found in 15 patients (4%), with onset within a few days of stroke. It was often associated with other behavioural problems, for example agitation. All patients were treated with haloperidol or quetiapine and the delusions lasted on average 13 days, tending to ameliorate alongside the other behavioural problems. All patients with delusional ideas had right hemisphere stroke (Fig. 8.2), particularly posterior temporoparietal, and they also tended to show mild evidence of generalised cerebral atrophy. It was therefore not surprising to find that in four cases there was Capgras delusion, and one other case of delusional misidentification. These findings are very much in line with Price and Mesulam (1985), who described five cases of delusions occurring in the acute phase after stroke, all with right hemisphere lesions.

Levine and Finklestein (1982) have also noted an apparent relationship between cerebrovascular lesions of the right hemisphere, specifically of the right temporoparieto-occipital areas, and the development of psychotic illnesses some time later. Eight patients were described, with the psychoses appearing some weeks or years after the stroke. All but one had developed seizures in the interim, which may have been a connecting factor. The psychoses developed acutely, with formed auditory and visual hallucinations; the majority of patients showed agitation, persecutory delusions and confusion, but in some the hallucinatory phenomena were relatively pure. All had constructional apraxia, and most showed a variety of other neurological residua. The right-sided location in every case may have reflected the freedom from dysphasia, allowing the psychoses to be revealed, or alternatively may have reflected the predisposing effects of spatial disabilities in leading to environmental misinterpretations. The combination of right hemisphere infarcts with poststroke seizures as a risk for psychosis has been found in a further five cases (Rabins *et al.* 1991). Pre-existing subcortical atrophy appeared to be an additional risk factor.

Hallucinosis, in which the patient retains insight into the unreal nature of the hallucinated material, has traditionally been related to lesions in the midbrain and pons, the peduncular hallucinosis of Lhermitte (1922, 1932) described in Chapter 1 (Basic concepts and terminology/Organic hallucinosis). Such hallucinosis can occur in the visual or auditory modalities, is typically complex and vivid, and usually resolves within days or weeks. The midbrain lesion responsible has been demonstrated on MRI (Geller & Bellur 1987). On the other hand, hallucinations may be seen after cortical strokes; 4 of 641 patients had auditory hallucinations in the early poststroke period and in all cases the lesion was in the right temporal lobe (Lampl *et al.* 2005).

Given the concern that antipsychotics, when used to treat psychosis in the elderly, may be associated with an increased risk of stroke, care is required when prescribing these agents to patients who have suffered a stroke. Psychosis in the early days after stroke may well resolve spontaneously. If antipsychotics are to be prescribed, any potential risks should be discussed with the patient and the family.

Rehabilitation after stroke

The processes of recovery after stroke are largely spontaneous. Early recovery involves resolution of the histochemical effects of the stroke. As noted above, targeted treatments during this period are aimed at promoting survival of cells in the penumbra. However, numerous less specific matters need to be addressed that can all be considered under the rubric of rehabilitation. Good guidance on what should be available has been published (Bates *et al.* 2005) (Box 8.6).

Patients who receive organised inpatient care, as generally provided on a stroke unit, over the early days and weeks are more likely to be alive and independent at 1 year (Stroke Unit Trialists' Collaboration 2001). The care will optimise the systemic management of the patient, e.g. by paying close attention to hydration, blood pressure and assessment of swallowing function. Nursing and therapy will minimise

---

Box 8.6 Management of rehabilitation after stroke
(from Bates *et al.* 2005)

- The primary goal of rehabilitation is to prevent complications, minimise impairments and maximise function
- Secondary prevention is fundamental to preventing stroke recurrence
- Early assessment and intervention are critical to optimise rehabilitation
- Standardised evaluations and valid assessment tools are essential to the development of a comprehensive treatment plan
- Evidence-based interventions should be based on functional goals
- Every candidate for rehabilitation should have access to an experienced and coordinated rehabilitation team to ensure optimal outcome
- The patient and family and/or caregiver are essential members of the rehabilitation team
- Patient and family education improves the likelihood of informed decision-making, social adjustment and maintenance of rehabilitation gains
- The rehabilitation team should utilise community resources for community reintegration
- Ongoing medical management of risk factors and comorbidities is essential to ensure survival

---

secondary complications such as bed sores, contractures and subluxation of joints. As soon as feasible more specific rehabilitation will be available, early on relying heavily on physiotherapy (Young & Forster 2007). It is possible that such early rehabilitation interventions can influence neuroplastic change such that there is transfer of lost functions to unaffected brain areas, and reorganisation within the brain to allow other areas to contribute more. There is good evidence that physiotherapy is helpful, particularly in terms of exercise training to improve balance and gait. However, attempts to demonstrate the value of physiotherapy in improving limb function, as in hemiparetic stroke, have been less successful. Likewise there is little good evidence to demonstrate that speech and language therapy can improve dysphasia, though the speech and language therapist is likely to have an important role in assessment of swallowing function and helping to improve communication.

Later rehabilitation is likely to concentrate on adaptive responses and coping strategies. It may proceed in the hospital, the home or specialised rehabilitation units, depending on circumstances and the severity of the problems involved. Proper liaison among the different members of the team is essential for success, also adequate continuing care when the patient returns home. Therapy targeted at patients who have returned home can improve outcome, a review of the evidence suggesting that for every 100 patients treated, seven will be spared a poor outcome (Outpatient Service Trialists 2003). Ongoing physiotherapy may be required but there is likely to be greater input from the occupational therapist who will concentrate on matters of fine motor control, particularly in the upper limbs. Retraining may be needed for activities of daily living: how to dress, feed, wash and cook despite the handicaps that persist. The provision of simple mechanical aids can be of immense help in restoring capabilities that would otherwise be lost. Community occupational therapy is effective at improving activities of daily living including mobility and use of public transport (Walker *et al.* 2004).

Sensory handicaps gravely complicate rehabilitation, particularly sensory impairments in paralysed limbs. Loss of position sense that persists after the early weeks carries a bad prognosis in hemiplegic patients, and may need special training under visual and tactile control. Cortical sensory loss, with defective discrimination, adds to difficulties with fine manipulation of the fingers. Hemianopic or quadrantic field defects tend to resolve with time, or the alert patient learns to compensate for them. However, in the early stages or when there is mental impairment, care must be taken to approach the patient from the sound side, and to arrange the disposition of belongings and work materials accordingly. Refractive errors or defective hearing must not be overlooked as remediable sources of additional difficulty.

Rehabilitation for cognitive impairments has received much interest and more detailed guidance on what should be offered, based on evidence of efficacy, has been produced by a European Federation of Neurological Sciences Task Force (Cappa *et al.* 2005). Even though this was a review of therapy for all causes of acquired brain injury, including traumatic brain injury and stroke, the principles are nevertheless by and large relevant to stroke.

Disturbed body awareness and sensory inattention can provide a serious obstacle to progress. A tendency to ignore the left half of space may be a greater barrier, contributing to falls and mishaps and hindering mastery of a new environment. Persistent denial or disowning of hemiplegic limbs carries an especially poor prognosis for recovery of independence, and is often accompanied by prolonged incontinence. Unilateral neglect is more common with right hemisphere stroke. One study found 43% of right hemisphere stroke as opposed of 20% of left-sided stroke had neglect at the time of presentation, falling to 17% and 5% respectively at 3 months (Ringman *et al.* 2004). Most cases therefore resolve spontaneously within weeks and there is no good evidence that stimulation and exercises improve on this (Lincoln & Bowen 2006).

Communication disorders warrant close and early attention. The dysphasic patient has lost not only the ability to speak but also his primary means of relating with those around. Once communication is re-established, however small in degree, the patient's frustration and fear begin to diminish. A first aim must be to establish emotional contact with the patient, using whatever channels of communication are most intact. Pictures may be used with which he can indicate requests, even though he cannot read or speak. Cards with words or short phrases may be useful later on. Gestures or visual signs may be employed when verbal understanding is very poor, coupled with one or two concrete words but avoiding a confusing flow of speech. Later in recovery instructions must be carefully spaced, given slowly, and as far as possible in the same manner on each occasion. Thus a special approach is needed from all the staff. Every attempt must be made to avoid withdrawal after early failures, to keep the patient involved and active, and to stimulate a continuing desire to communicate.

Formal speech therapy has rarely been rigorously tested, which is surprising in view of the magnitude of the problem. A Cochrane systematic review of the evidence concluded that 'speech and language therapy treatment for people with aphasia after a stroke has not been shown either to be clearly effective or clearly ineffective within a RCT' (Greener *et al.* 2000). Nevertheless, although it is uncertain whether the final level achieved exceeds that which would have occurred spontaneously, few doubt the effects of retraining programmes on emotional adjustment and morale.

Impairment of memory must be specially catered for with a more gradual programme, frequent rehearsals and the provision of props and supports by way of notes and written instructions. The relative preservation of old memories may initially produce a misleading impression until ability to acquire new knowledge is specifically tested. Strategies for rehabilitation of memory impairments rest largely on the premise that it will not be possible to affect the degree of impairment, but that by using compensatory strategies it may be possible to reduce the consequent disability and handicap that the memory impairment produces. More general techniques concentrate on organising the study of material to be learned, chunking information into subsets and breaking down new skills into a series of steps. More specific methods include the use of mnemonic devices such as first-letter cueing, rhyming strategies, visual imagery, or 'motor coding' whereby a movement is associated with a name to be remembered. Where multiple items are to be remembered these may be 'pegged' to a standard list of words, or to standard loci such as body parts or rooms within a house. Embedding the items in a brief manufactured story can be particularly effective. A review of memory rehabilitation across patients with different acquired brain injuries, including stroke, found errorless learning to be effective, whereas the case for the method of vanishing cues was not so robust (Kessels & de Haan 2003). However, there have been rather few attempts to demonstrate in stroke patients alone that rehabilitation can improve memory (Majid *et al.* 2000).

Other intellectual impairments are a serious barrier to progress when at all extensive. Ill-sustained attention, perseveration, fatiguability and failure to grasp instructions may combine to render attempts at rehabilitation fruitless. To maximise the chances of success, verbal instructions must be presented in simple language with deliberate methodical repetition. Practical demonstrations of what is expected may get the ideas across when other methods have failed. The pace will necessarily be slow, and allowance must be made for variability in performance from day to day.

Motivation is among the most crucial determinants of progress and every means must be taken to optimise and maintain it. The day-to-day enthusiasm and encouragement of the therapeutic team is an essential ingredient, and the patient's own awareness of progress then plays back to reinforce it. All through the programme, proper communication must be maintained so that he is aware of the plans and goals at every stage. Motivational interviewing is a specific technique that was originally designed to help patients with addictions, but more recently has been used in a variety of setting where poor motivation may jeopardise improvements in health. In an RCT, weekly sessions of motivational interviewing over 4 weeks on a rehabilitation unit after stroke were found to improve mood at 3 months, but not to have any impact on disability scores (Watkins *et al.* 2007).

A watch must be kept for evidence of depression, which may well respond to appropriate medication or psychological therapy. Tactful handling may be required in the face of discouragement, withdrawal or obstinacy. Clear guidelines must sometimes be drawn up, especially for patients with intellectual impairment who will benefit from a structured environment. In contrast, flexibility must be built into the programme to allow for patients with differing needs and personalities. Rigid conformity to set standards cannot always be expected, and in some persons will be counterproductive.

Attention must also be devoted to the relatives of the patient. They too will need full discussion of aims and procedures, and help in adjusting to the disabilities that are likely to remain. Careful physical rehabilitation may be doomed to failure if insufficient attention has been given to the family situation and to the impact of the problem on family members. Here the social worker has a vital part to play, and should be brought into the picture at an early stage. Much time may be needed to allay unrealistic expectations or needless anxieties and fears. The stroke and its repercussions may have had a far-reaching effect on many members of the household, disturbing the family equilibrium and requiring a reorganisation of roles. Preparations for discharge must be made well in advance, on a practical as well as an emotional level. The patient's assets and liabilities must be carefully assessed, likewise the family and community resources available to help. Physical adaptations may be needed in the home by way of ramps or simple supports. Proper liaison will be required with local authority and voluntary services. Where work is being considered, extended evaluation and retraining will often be indicated. Sheltered employment may need

to be found when the patient is too disabled to cope on the open market.

In older patients, and those severely disabled, attendance at a day centre or social centre may need to be organised. Transport problems in particular will need attention. For those who remain at home every effort must be made to combat feelings of loneliness and isolation, by building new contacts, encouraging a return to hobbies and mobilising community resources.

Sadly, some patients will need to remain in institutions, usually by virtue of extensive mental impairments in addition to their neurological defects. Others will have complicating pathologies, such as heart disease or arthritis, which have conspired to make effective rehabilitation impossible. Here nursing care and occupational therapy will be required long term in order to maintain a reasonable quality of life. Adequate stimulation must be ensured, with routines that are as varied and congenial as possible. Psychotropic medication will occasionally be required to combat anxiety and depression.

Subarachnoid haemorrhage

It is estimated that subarachnoid haemorrhage, with an incidence of about 6–7 per 100 000 per year in most populations, makes up some 5% of cerebrovascular accidents (van Gijn *et al.* 2007). It is particularly important because, even though the incidence increases with age, it affects a younger age group than other strokes; half of patients with subarachnoid haemorrhage are less than 55 years old. Reduced level of consciousness on admission is one of the best predictors of poor outcome. The World Federation of Neurosurgical Societies (WFNS) scale for grading subarachnoid haemorrhage is therefore based heavily on the Glasgow Coma Scale (GCS), starting at grade I, defined by a GCS score of 15 and no motor deficit, and ending at grade V, defined by a GCS score of 3–6 with or without motor deficit (Teasdale *et al.* 1988). The mortality rate is high; about half of cases die. Nevertheless, correct management can substantially reduce mortality. In about 80% of cases subarachnoid haemorrhage is the result of rupture of an intracranial aneurysm.

Non-aneurysmal perimesencephalic haemorrhage came to be recognised as a cause of subarachnoid haemorrhage when CT imaging allowed visualisation of the location of the subarachnoid blood. In non-aneurysmal perimesencephalic haemorrhage, which accounts for about 10% of subarachnoid haemorrhage, the blood is usually restricted to the cisterns around the midbrain (van Gijn *et al.* 1985). The headache is not as dramatic in onset as in aneurysmal rupture, clinical signs are generally mild at most and the outcome is good. The angiogram is negative and it seems likely that venous, rather than arterial, bleeding is responsible. Non-aneurysmal perimesencephalic haemorrhage has no impact on quality of life (Brilstra *et al.* 1997) and is not discussed further.

Other causes of subarachnoid haemorrhage include ruptured angiomas, bleeds from intracranial and spinal tumours, blood dyscrasias or inflammatory conditions of the brain and meninges. Some represent primary intracerebral or cerebellar haemorrhages that have bled into the ventricular system and thereby reached the subarachnoid space. A table of rare causes of subarachnoid haemorrhage can be found in the review by van Gijn *et al.* (2007).

Aneurysms arise from defects in the media, usually at the forks of the cerebral arteries. The great majority arise close to the circle of Willis at the base of the brain. Common sites are on the anterior cerebral or anterior communicating arteries, at the point of division of the middle cerebral arteries, or where the posterior communicating artery arises from the upper end of the internal carotid artery. Rupture occurs spontaneously and suddenly, with bleeding directly into the subarachnoid space and often into the adjacent brain substance as well. Most ruptured aneurysms are less than 1 cm in diameter. Another common site for intracranial aneurysms is the intracavernous part of the internal carotid, but aneurysms here more often lead to local pressure effects than to subarachnoid haemorrhage (see below).

Intracranial aneurysms steadily become more common with age such that they are present in about 2% of adults. In the vast majority of cases these aneurysms will never rupture. It may therefore be difficult to estimate whether the risks of preventive treatment of an aneurysm found incidentally, during cerebral imaging for some other purpose, outweigh the benefits of any reduced risk of rupture; useful guidance is to be found in a recent meta-analysis of the risk (Wermer *et al.* 2007a). In a study of patients with previously treated aneurysm, those who were subsequently found to have a further silent aneurysm that was then left untreated did not seem to suffer adverse psychological effects (van der Schaaf *et al.* 2006). There is therefore an argument for the importance of doing nothing for silent aneurysms (Brainin 2006). On the other hand, when subjects with a strong familial history of aneurysmal subarachnoid haemorrhage are screened, those found to have a silent aneurysm then have worse psychosocial outcome than those who screen negative (Wermer *et al.* 2005a). A recent study found that elective surgery improved quality of life in patients in whom an unruptured intracranial aneurysm had been found incidentally (Yamashiro *et al.* 2007).

Risk factors for subarachnoid haemorrhage include smoking, hypertension and drinking alcohol to excess, as well as having a larger aneurysm. In about 20% of cases activity, including physical exertion or sexual intercourse, seems to have precipitated rupture of the aneurysm. In about 10% of cases the subarachnoid haemorrhage is familial, in which case large and multiple aneurysms are more frequent. Genetic factors have not been identified, although those with autosomal dominant polycystic kidney disease are at high risk.

Acute clinical picture and management

The onset is abrupt with intense, often catastrophic pain in the head, mainly in the occipital region but radiating into the neck and later becoming generalised. Vomiting, photophobia and fits may occur and onset may be complicated by cardiac arrest in a small minority. Consciousness may be lost from the outset and about one-third of cases present in coma, although some patients retain full awareness throughout. Others are drowsy, confused and irritable. Sometimes the mental symptoms overshadow the headache to such an extent that the diagnosis is not immediately apparent. From a case series of over 700, nine cases were identified who presented with delirium (Reijneveld *et al.* 2000). Only three cases had headache and only three had witnessed loss of consciousness. Although four of the cases had an anterior communicating artery (ACoA) aneurysm and five had hydrocephalus, it was not possible to identify any definite predictors of delirium. One study of 66 patient within 4 days of subarachnoid haemorrhage found that 11 (16%) fulfilled criteria for delirium (Caeiro *et al.* 2005). These 11 patients with delirium were more likely to have intraventricular bleeding and hydrocephalus, and to be older; two of them had bifrontal haematoma. There have been several case reports over the years of subarachnoid haemorrhage presenting with behavioural change including akinetic mutism, delusional misidentification or an amnesic–confabulatory syndrome (Mobbs *et al.* 2001). In some cases the patients were accused of drunkenness at the onset or of being hysterical (Walton 1956). Very occasionally a patient will present with amnesic symptoms akin to transient global amnesia.

A man in his early fifties presented with headache and vomiting which started in the morning. During the course of the day he developed a state, lasting several hours, during which he repetitively asked what has happening, saying that he could not remember anything. There was no loss of personal identity. Subsequently a diagnosis of subarachnoid haemorrhage from an ACoA aneurysm was made, and the angiogram showed spasm of the anterior cerebral arteries. He later underwent surgery but his postoperative recovery was complicated by hydrocephalus. He was left with a severely disabling Korsakoff syndrome (see below), which was associated with numerous bizarre confabulations and delusions, for example the belief that surgically implanted small metal arrows were in his brain and were coming out through his ear. These confabulatory delusions gradually resolved over many months. He was left with a severe amnesic state, but was nevertheless by 2 years after the haemorrhage, perhaps aided by treatment with donepezil, able to live by himself with a little support from his family.

Neck stiffness generally becomes intense but is not always present. Papilloedema may develop immediately or within a few days, and subhyaloid haemorrhages may be observed spreading from the edges of the optic discs. Focal ophthalmoplegias are common, and aphasia or hemiplegia may result from arterial spasm or intracerebral extension. Rupture of ACoA aneurysms may damage basal forebrain, which lies immediately above the aneurysm. Localising signs are often absent but ischaemia can be extensive in one or both frontal lobes, presumably due to occlusion or spasm of the anterior cerebral arteries. Middle cerebral artery aneurysms lie in the sylvian fissure or embedded in the frontal or temporal lobes nearby. Rupture is often accompanied by hemiparesis due to vascular spasm in the territory of the middle cerebral artery or haematoma formation. Posterior communicating aneurysms lie medial to the uncus of the temporal lobe. They often bleed directly into the subarachnoid space, but infarction can be widespread in the territory of the middle cerebral arteries, and there may also be interference with the fine perforating vessels to the basal ganglia and hypothalamus.

During the first few days, subarachnoid blood is generally visible as high signal on routine brain CT, which is therefore the critical initial investigation. Lumbar puncture is now restricted to those cases, about 3%, with a typical clinical picture but no evidence of subarachnoid blood on CT. Conventional cerebral angiography is the definitive investigation; however, using this as the gold standard, CT angiography can now achieve about 95% sensitivity for identification of aneurysms and has the advantage of being much less invasive and with less likelihood of complications.

Immediate bed rest is mandatory, with sedation, analgesics and good general nursing and medical care. Even at this early stage psychological support for the family and patient is helpful. One study has looked at the value of a specialist liaison nurse on the neurosurgical unit (Pritchard *et al.* 2004). The nurse was a senior neurosurgical ward nurse whose role was to support and counsel patients with subarachnoid haemorrhage and their families. Once the liaison nurse was in place, the progress of a cohort of patients admitted over a 2-year period was compared with a cohort of patients admitted over the previous 18 months. At 6 months after discharge the patients who had access to the specialist liaison nurse showed better emotional adjustment and confidence, and greater satisfaction with their inpatient treatment.

In the early days after subarachnoid haemorrhage, once the diagnosis has been established, there are three main considerations: (i) minimise the risk of rebleeding, (ii) try to prevent delayed cerebral ischaemia, and (iii) manage any hydrocephalus. Rebleeding is the major cause of poor outcome; without intervention more than one-third of patients will rebleed within the first few weeks. This risk can be reduced by surgical intervention, but in the past this necessarily involved a craniotomy and surgical clipping of the aneurysm and the threat of aggravating cerebral ischaemia.

Over the last few years clipping has largely been replaced by coiling of the aneurysm using an intra-arterial catheter. Once the end of the catheter is in place in the aneurysm, small platinum coils are detached to rest in the aneurysm which then becomes occluded by reactive thrombosis. There is a chance of the aneurysm subsequently reopening and some clinicians regard long-term follow-up angiography as mandatory (Feigin & Findlay 2006). In a large RCT comparing coiling to clipping, largely restricted to patients in good clinical condition with small aneurysms of the anterior circulation, coiling was significantly less likely to be associated with poor outcome at 1 year (van der Schaaf *et al.* 2005); compared with clipping, the number needed to treat to prevent one poor outcome was 15. The advantage of coiling, in terms of survival, was maintained at 7-year follow-up (Molyneux *et al.* 2005). Platinum coils also have the advantage over many neurosurgical aneurysmal clips in that they are non-magnetic and patients can therefore undergo MRI subsequently. However, some aneurysms will be unsuitable for coiling because of their anatomical configuration.

Cerebral ischaemia, sometimes involving vessels at a distance from the aneurysm, is a considerable problem for many patients over the hours and days after subarachnoid haemorrhage, reaching a peak after 1–2 weeks. Infarcts, usually involving the cortex, may be found in almost 40% of patients (Rabinstein *et al.* 2005). In some they are single infarcts often near the aneurysm but in others multiple infarcts at a distance from the site of rupture are seen. Patients with a large amount of subarachnoid blood or with loss of consciousness are at increased risk. Vasospasm may be partly to blame, but global ischaemia and hypotension are contributory factors. Treatment with calcium antagonists, in particular nimodipine for 3 weeks, reduces the risk of poor outcome (Rinkel *et al.* 2005) and is now standard practice.

Hydrocephalus may develop at any time after subarachnoid haemorrhage. Usually it develops in the acute phase, in the hours after the haemorrhage. However, not all patients with ventriculomegaly on the acute CT scan will need shunting because in about half there will be spontaneous improvement (Hasan *et al.* 1989). Shunting should be restricted to those with good clinical evidence of need and be for as short as possible, because of the risk of ventriculitis. Nevertheless, the clinician needs to remember that hydrocephalus may be a cause of deterioration in mental state, months or years after haemorrhage.

In the long term perhaps 2–3% of patients will rebleed over the 10 years after surgical clipping for subarachnoid haemorrhage (Wermer *et al.* 2005b) and the figure is not much different for coiling (Sluzewski *et al.* 2005). Epilepsy is seen in about 5% of cases in the first year, being more common in those with worse WFNS grading and worse outcome. Coma persisting for more than 24 hours is a bad prognostic sign. Axonal damage, assessed using neurofilament levels in ventricular cerebrospinal fluid (CSF) over the first few days, may contribute to poor outcome (Petzold *et al.* 2006). With modern management some two-thirds of patients may be expected to survive a first bleed, although one-third of survivors will be left with major neurological disability. In patients with no aneurysm demonstrable on angiography the mortality and morbidity rates are considerably lower. High levels of pituitary deficiency have been found after subarachnoid haemorrhage and it has been suggested that this may contribute to chronic symptoms in a proportion of cases (Kreitschmann-Andermahr *et al.* 2004).

Psychiatric sequelae of subarachnoid haemorrhage

Severe, but usually transient, confusion and states of akinetic mutism can be seen in the early stages of recovery. The later sequelae, after 2–11 years, were described by Walton (1952, 1956) among 120 survivors. Important residua included persistent headache in 23%, organic mental symptoms in 9% and anxiety symptoms in 27%. The anxiety was occasionally severely disabling, resulting in chronic psychiatric invalidism.

Subsequently, two large series of patients were reported with attention directed primarily at the psychiatric sequelae. Storey (1967, 1970, 1972) studied 261 patients who had suffered a subarachnoid haemorrhage 6 months to 6 years earlier, noting the site of the responsible aneurysm and correlating this with the psychiatric aftermaths; 81 patients had bled from ACoA aneurysms, 71 from middle cerebral aneurysms, 72 from posterior communicating aneurysms and seven from multiple aneurysms, while in the remaining 30 no aneurysm could be detected. Logue *et al.* (1968) confined attention to 79 survivors of haemorrhages from anterior cerebral aneurysms, studied 6 months to 8.5 years later. Both studies confirmed the high incidence of mental disablement among survivors, especially as a result of organic mental impairments and personality change attributable to brain damage. Rather surprisingly both also stressed that, compared with how the survivor had been before the haemorrhage, improvement in personality could occasionally occur, mainly evident to relatives but sometimes also to the patients themselves.

Cognitive impairments including amnesia and confabulation

Storey (1967) found persistent intellectual difficulties in about 40% of patients as judged by simple clinical criteria. They were rated as moderate to severe in some 10% of cases, and occasional patients remained grossly demented and bedridden. Those with middle cerebral aneurysms fared considerably worse than other groups, while patients with no demonstrable aneurysms had the lowest morbidity of all. In the study by Logue *et al.* (1968), patients with anterior cerebral aneurysms showed 10% with global dementia but many

more with minor persistent deficits; 40% showed dysphasic errors on detailed testing. Memory was often more impaired than intelligence. Further studies have demonstrated cognitive impairments even in survivors of subarachnoid haemorrhage who have had good outcome (Hutter & Gilsbach 1993; Mayer *et al.* 2002), although not all studies find evidence of impairment (McKenna *et al.* 1989). Predictors of worse cognitive outcome include lower GCS score on admission and ventricular enlargement (see table 4 of Haug *et al.* 2007) and the presence of large amounts of subarachnoid blood; those with left-sided infarction may be most affected (Hutter *et al.* 2001; Kreiter *et al.* 2002).

Executive function, memory and speed of information processing seem to be most vulnerable. For example, when 20 patients with ACoA aneurysms were compared with 17 with aneurysms of other branches of the internal carotid artery on a neuropsychological test battery at least 6 months after subarachnoid haemorrhage, no differences between the two groups could be found (Tidswell *et al.* 1995). However, in both groups, compared with controls, there were deficits on executive function and in memory. Cognitive impairment improves over the first year (Samra *et al.* 2007). Nevertheless, long-term cognitive deficits are found, for example as late as 7 years (Stenhouse *et al.* 1991). However, subjective complaints of memory problems or absent-mindedness may have more to do with patients' dissatisfaction with their situation, in particular social support, than with objective evidence of cognitive impairment (Toomela *et al.* 2004).

Most of the patients studied in the papers reviewed above underwent surgical clipping of the ruptured aneurysm. It is therefore reasonable to ask how much of any cognitive impairment present months and years after haemorrhage is due to the immediate effects of the aneurysm and how much to the surgery to clip the aneurysm. This was assessed by testing 27 patients in good condition while on the neurosurgical unit after the haemorrhage but before surgery, and then again after they had recovered from surgery and many months later (Maurice-Williams *et al.* 1991). In the majority of patients there was no evidence of an adverse effect of surgery on cognitive performance, with the exception of two patients with definite surgical complications.

More recent studies have considered whether clipping or coiling produces less cognitive impairment. Four non-randomised studies have looked at outcomes over the first year following treatment of patients with either clipping or coiling. In the largest study (*N* = 40 in each arm matched for severity of the haemorrhage), there was a trend for greater impairment in the group treated surgically with clipping (Hadjivassiliou *et al.* 2001). This seemed to be confirmed by two smaller studies which found that those treated with coiling had less impairment of executive function and memory (Chan *et al.* 2002; Fontanella *et al.* 2003). However, another small non-randomised study found in favour of clipping, although this effect disappeared once National Adult Reading Test (NART) estimates of premorbid IQ were taken into account, leaving both groups showing equivalent impairment (Frazer *et al.* 2007). Furthermore, in none of these studies were patients randomised to receive coiling or clipping, and therefore the findings could have more to do with factors that governed whether an aneurysm was clipped or coiled rather than which procedure was in fact used. The most rigorous study is therefore an RCT of 109 patients randomly assigned to either surgical treatment (clipping) or endovascular treatment (coiling) (Koivisto *et al.* 2000). No differences between the two groups on neuropsychological testing at 3 or 12 months were found.

In conclusion, when it comes to neuropsychological outcome the evidence that clipping is worse than coiling is not very strong, but there is certainly very little to suggest that clipping is better. However, there is good evidence that patients treated with coils have less evidence of damage on MRI; 45% of clipped patients showed lesions consistent with superficial brain retraction on MRI, whereas only 10% of coiled patients did, and surgically treated patients also had more ischaemic lesions in the territory of the parent artery (Koivisto *et al.* 2000). Likewise, in one of the non-randomised studies referred to above, it was only in the clipped group that there was evidence of focal encephalomalacia, presumably due to the effects of the surgery itself (Hadjivassiliou *et al.* 2001).

Although some studies have found that those with ACoA aneurysms do worse (Bornstein *et al.* 1987; Kreiter *et al.* 2002), in general it has been surprisingly difficult to demonstrate that the site of the aneurysm has a bearing on neuropsychological outcome (Desantis *et al.* 1989; Richardson 1991; Ogden *et al.* 1993; Tidswell *et al.* 1995). For example, in a recent RCT of the effects of hypothermia on outcome after surgical clipping of subarachnoid haemorrhage, over 150 patients with good outcome (good outcome or moderate disability on the Glasgow Outcome Scale) were tested at 9 and 15 months across a range of cognitive tests (Samra *et al.* 2007); 25% of patients showed cognitive impairment, defined as two standard deviations below the mean of the control population on a composite cognitive test score, with a trend toward a smaller proportion being impaired at 15 months. However, the location of the aneurysm did not affect the proportion demonstrating cognitive impairment, nor did treatment with hypothermia.

However, these findings contrast with the literature, and anecdotal experience, which suggests that ACoA aneurysms are particularly associated with severe executive and memory impairment in some cases, producing a Korsakoff syndrome of amnesia, disorientation, poor insight and confabulation (DeLuca & Diamond 1995). This evidence is based heavily on case studies (Volpe & Hirst 1983; Parkin *et al.* 1988) and case series showing that memory impairment is common in patients with ACoA aneurysms (Gade 1982; Alexander &

Freedman 1984; Laiacona *et al.* 1989; Stenhouse *et al.* 1991). For example, Lindqvist and Norlén (1966) reported amnesic syndromes in 17 of 33 patients after operations on ACoA aneurysms. Eleven improved markedly within 6 months, but five appeared destined to be permanent. Transient confabulation was noted in almost one-quarter of Logue *et al.*'s (1968) cases and two striking examples of enduring memory difficulties have been reported after operative intervention on ACoA aneurysms (Sweet *et al.* 1966; Talland *et al.* 1967).

Preoperatively both patients had been confused and apathetic, but immediately postoperatively they showed severe disorientation, nonsensical confabulation, and some retrograde and virtually complete anterograde amnesia. The disorientation improved considerably within a few weeks, and at the same time their confabulation changed from fantastic fabrications to temporal misplacement of actual incidents. Over the next 3 years the memory disorder became chronic, together with impotence and lack of initiative. The lesions seen at operation had involved the posteromedial aspects of the orbital surface of both frontal lobes and the adjoining medial surface of the hemispheres, the so-called septal region in front of the lamina terminalis and anterior commissure. The crucial region was thought to lie in the septal region bilaterally.

Others have also suggested that damage to basal forebrain (septal nuclei, substantia innominata, nucleus accumbens, anterior hypothalamus) is responsible for the amnesia (Damasio *et al.* 1985). This is consistent with the CT findings of Vilkki *et al.* (1989); patients with medial frontal infarcts, which were usually due to ACoA aneurysms, were more likely to have memory impairments than those with infarcts in other locations.

Why is it that the rigorous cases series described above so often fail to demonstrate a particular relationship of ACoA aneurysm to amnesic disorder? It is probably because Korsakoff's syndrome is a relatively uncommon, though specific, outcome of ACoA aneurysm rupture. If only one in ten patients with an ACoA aneurysm develops an 'ACoA syndrome' with confabulation and severe amnesia, then in any small case series this effect may easily be swamped by other cases with ACoA aneurysm with non-specific heterogeneous outcomes similar to those with aneurysms in other locations. The problem is nicely demonstrated in the study of Bottger *et al.* (1998). In this consecutive series of 30 patients tested some months after ACoA aneurysm, the full Korsakoff syndrome of disorientation, confabulation, amnesia and lack of insight was only seen in three cases. The other cases showed various degrees of executive and memory and attentional problems, probably rather similar to the impairments seen with other aneurysm locations. It is also worth noting that the three Korsakoff cases all had Glasgow Outcome Scale ratings of 3 (severe disability). These cases would therefore never have appeared in several of the studies described above, which only studied patients with good outcome or moderate disability. It may also be the case that now coiling is replacing clipping, the ACoA syndrome will be less frequently seen.

There are probably several pathogenic factors that cause disruption of basal forebrain after ACoA aneurysm rupture, producing the amnesic syndrome: hydrocephalus (Theander & Granholm 1967), cerebral vasospasm (Volpe & Hirst 1983; Weidauer *et al.* 2007), interference with the small perforating arteries at operation (Gade 1982), and haemorrhage directly from the aneurysm into the brain tissue immediately above. The observation that in some cases there is a latent interval of several days before the syndrome appears, followed by spontaneous recovery usually over a few weeks (Tarachow 1939; Walton 1953), is compatible with the effects of either hydrocephalus or cerebral vasospasm.

Donepezil may improve memory function in patients with basal forebrain damage due to subarachnoid haemorrhage. Eleven such patients, mostly with ACoA aneurysms, with a chronic amnesic syndrome lasting at least 1 year and tested on average over 6 years after the haemorrhage, were offered donepezil in an open study over a period of 12 weeks (Benke *et al.* 2005). Compared with their performance on tests of memory at baseline, improvements were seen after 12 weeks of donepezil whereas there were no significant effects on tests of attention or executive function. Four weeks after drug discontinuation there was a significant drop in memory performance. No measurements of disability were made, to see if these changes on tests of memory impairment translated into reductions in disability.

Personality changes

Personality deterioration after subarachnoid haemorrhage usually has an obvious organic stamp and occurs in a setting of intellectual impairment. Prominent changes include loss of drive and vitality, decreased interest and initiative, withdrawal, irritability and easily provoked anxiety. Emotional lability and catastrophic tendencies may be marked. Storey (1970) described a picture of 'organic moodiness' with chronic shallow depression, often lifting in response to some new stimulus but rapidly falling back again with boredom, loss of interest and easy fatigue. Changes reminiscent of the frontal lobe syndrome may occur, with uninhibited selfish behaviour, tactlessness, elevation of mood and a decreased tendency to worry. Some of these latter aspects can be construed as improvements in personality, as discussed below.

Personality impairment was rated as moderate or severe in 19% of Storey's patients, and mild in 22% more. It was most common after rupture of middle cerebral aneurysms, and in general the incidence paralleled that of intellectual impairment and neurological disability. The exception was a significant tendency for patients with ACoA aneurysms to show relatively less intellectual impairment in the presence of personality deterioration. Descriptions of disinhibited behaviour, lessened worry and lessened irritability were commoner in those with anterior aneurysms than other

groups, lending support to the classic idea of a frontal lobe syndrome. In an attempt to define any decision-making deficits that might be responsible for the personality change, patients with ACoA aneurysms have been tested on a gambling task. As a group they showed increased risk-taking behaviour (Mavaddat *et al.* 2000), possibly due to disruption of orbital prefrontal cortex. On the other hand, using the same task a rather different pattern of responding was found in survivors of middle cerebral or posterior communicating artery aneurysms. They showed altered sensitivity to both reward and punishment, and impulsive responding (Salmond *et al.* 2006). However, neither study measured whether there was in fact any personality change in the individuals tested.

Improvement in personality was noted by relatives in 13 of Storey's patients, eight after bleeds from anterior aneurysms. The same was seen in nine of Logue *et al.*'s (1968) patients. In both series, therefore, approximately 10% of patients with anterior bleeds showed a favourable outcome of this nature. Storey's patients were described as being more pleasant to live with, less sarcastic and irritable, less anxious and fussy, and often more affectionate and tolerant. Most were aware of increased well-being subjectively. The majority had previously been tense, perfectionistic or inhibited. Two who had been gloomy and readily fatigued became cheerful, vigorous and lost their tension headaches. Another lost compulsive rituals of long standing. Two of the 13 showed minor forgetfulness, but in the remainder there was no detectable intellectual impairment. None showed loss of drive or fall-off in work ability. A more recent study found that 13% of patients reported a positive personality change, although the paper gives no further description of what was meant by this (Wermer *et al.* 2007b).

However, Logue *et al.* (1968) found that a price was usually paid for the improvements, in terms of memory impairment or an increase in irritability or outspokenness. The improvements consisted mainly of a decreased tendency to worry or get depressed. In three patients there was relief of preexisting endogenous depression, and another showed virtual relief of an obsessional neurosis. Both Storey and Logue attributed the improvements to a 'leucotomy effect' consequent on frontal lobe damage or ischaemia.

Anxiety and depression

Walton (1952) emphasised anxiety symptoms in 27% of his cases, half with premorbid neurotic tendencies and half without. The anxiety was often severe and incapacitating, centring largely on fear of recurrence of the haemorrhage. Some patients were afraid for months afterwards to leave the house, or retired to bed immediately they had a headache. In some instances the situation had been worsened by medical advice to avoid exertion.

Storey (1972) found symptoms of anxiety or depression in one-quarter of patients, being moderate or severe in 14%.

Such symptoms showed an association with indices of brain damage, but depression could also be severe when there was no evidence of brain damage whatever. The depressives without neurological signs had been more neurotic and prone to depression in their premorbid personalities, while those with brain damage had more often been energetic and were therefore perhaps reacting to their loss of function. The patients in whom aneurysms had not been detected appeared to form a special group, with a similar incidence of depression to the remainder despite considerably less evidence of intellectual impairment or neurological disability. Depression was commonest of all, and more liable to be severe and persistent, in patients with posterior communicating aneurysms, where rupture is known to interfere with the fine perforating vessels to the hypothalamus.

More recently, three studies have relied on the HADS to determine symptoms of depression and anxiety. Using a score of greater than 10 on the HADS as a cut-off, indicating that the patient was at least 'probably depressed', 8.5% (9 months after haemorrhage, good to fair outcome patients only) (Powell *et al.* 2002), 17% (on average at 16 months) (Morris *et al.* 2004) and 9% (2–19 years) (Wermer *et al.* 2007b) were identified as probably depressed. Almost twice as many scored above 10 on the anxiety scale of HADS, the figures being 17%, 38% and 11% respectively. However, using the Beck Depression Inventory (BDI) and the State Trait Anxiety Inventory (STAI), Fontanella *et al.* (2003) failed to find significantly elevated scores for depression or anxiety compared with controls in patients with good outcome assessed 6 months after subarachnoid haemorrhage.

It has been suggested that post-traumatic stress disorder (PTSD) is quite a common sequelae. In a survey of 28 patients referred to a neuropsychology clinic after subarachnoid haemorrhage, almost one-third of patients were assessed as meeting diagnostic criteria for PTSD (Berry 1998). This finding receives some support from Powell *et al.* (2002). Patients were recruited consecutively at the time of haemorrhage and rated themselves on the Revised Impact of Events Scale at 3 and 9 months; 30% of patients scored in the clinical range on both subscales (intrusive thoughts and avoidance) at 3 months, falling to 15% at 9 months. At 18 months, three of the patients seemed to be cases of PTSD (Powell *et al.* 2004). However, none of the 63 patients studied by Rodholm *et al.* (2002) (see next section) were found to fulfil criteria for PTSD.

Other disturbances

Psychotic developments appear to be rare. Storey (1972) found no examples of psychosis among 261 patients who were studied closely from the psychiatric point of view. One of his patients developed schizophrenia a year later, but the illness seemed unrelated to the haemorrhage.

'Neurasthenic' symptoms can occasionally be marked, with fatigue, headache, dizziness and sensitivity to noise.

These were persistent and incapacitating in 7 of 56 patients followed by Theander and Granholm (1967), and present in mild degree in many more. Their origin was obscure and showed no relation to the duration of loss of consciousness. Walton (1952) commented on the general similarity between such symptoms after subarachnoid haemorrhage and after head injury, an observation that others have made (Hellawell & Pentland 2001).

At this point it is worth reviewing the studies of Rodholm *et al.* (2001, 2002) who prospectively studied a cohort of 63 patients over the first year after haemorrhage. At 3, 6 and 12 months every patient was assessed by psychiatric interview and classified according to a somewhat idiosyncratic classification of organic mental disorders developed in Sweden (Lindqvist & Malmgren 1993). So, for example, at 6 months three were found to have an emotional–motivational blunting disorder (EMD), 11 had Korsakoff's amnestic disorder (KAD) and 29 (49%) had astheno-emotional disorder (AED). The authors demonstrated that EMD and KAD were related to injury severity, as measured by conscious level on admission at the time of the haemorrhage, whereas AED was not. Of those with either EMD or KAD at 1 year, two-thirds were at least very drowsy or very confused on admission. In contrast, four-fifths of those with AED were alert or at most drowsy or confused on admission, a proportion that was not very different from the whole cohort. Patients with AED were likely to improve over the first year, the proportions at 3, 6 and 12 months being 60%, 49% and 38% respectively. However, in almost all those who had EMD or KAD at 3 months, it was still present at 1 year.

Rodholm *et al.* (2001) went on to describe AED in more detail in those who did not have evidence of either EMD or KAD or 'non-organic psychiatric disorder'. Thus the excluded patients included six who were diagnosed as suffering a non-organic psychiatric disorder usually on the basis of depressive symptoms that were either present before the haemorrhage or only appeared during the course of the first year, not having been present at 3 months. In this select sample studied at 1 year, of whom one-third were diagnosed as AED, common symptoms included fatigue, concentration impairment, memory difficulties, sound sensitivity, emotional instability and irritability. This constellation is very similar to that found in post-concussion syndrome.

Therefore a picture emerges which is reminiscent of that seen in traumatic brain injury. Some neuropsychiatric sequelae, for example personality change with disinhibition or poor motivation, and the amnesic syndrome, are tightly determined by the severity of brain injury. In contrast, patients also suffer a range of symptoms, of which fatigue, headache, dizziness and emotional changes are the commonest, that are less easy to understand simply as a consequence of brain injury, more likely to improve over the early months, and probably more related to psychological factors.

Psychosocial and long-term outcome

One year after subarachnoid haemorrhage almost 50% of survivors report incomplete recovery. This was the finding in a population-based study of over 200 patients, comprising 95% of the target cohort, who were available for telephone interview between 12 and 18 months after haemorrhage; 50% reported memory problems, 40% mood problems and 10% reported being dependent in terms of everyday activities (Hackett & Anderson 2000). On the SF-36 assessment of quality of life, patients reported significant restrictions in work and other activities.

Even when studies are restricted to patients with good neurosurgical outcome, many are found to have disabling psychosocial problems that relate to cognitive, emotional and behavioural sequelae. Three studies have restricted their ascertainment to patients rated good or fair outcome on the Glasgow Outcome Scale. In one study the majority of patients, examined at 1–5 years, nevertheless reported restrictions in the domains of motivation and/or mental capacity and/or social relationships (Hutter *et al.* 1995). They tended to suffer worse headaches than before the haemorrhage, almost one-third were depressed, and almost one-third reported that they had lost their job or been demoted or retired. In a second study, only 3 of 20 patients fully employed at the time of the haemorrhage were still employed at that level 19 months later (Buchanan *et al.* 2000). Common symptoms were high levels of fatigue and intolerance of noise and social contact. Reduced libido was seen in over half. Very few reported positive effects of the injury and family members reported that they themselves had high levels of distress and burden. Finally, in their study of 52 patients recruited consecutively and compared with controls matched carefully for age, sex and psychosocial status, Powell *et al.* (2002) demonstrated the lowered levels of social participation 9 months after subarachnoid haemorrhage. On measures of self-organisation and productive employment, over half the patients scored above the 90th centile of the control population scores (i.e. were less active). There was subtle evidence of cognitive impairment, with greater impairment evident at 3 months than 9 months, by which time only prose recall was impaired. Elevated levels of depressed mood, intrusive thoughts and avoidance were reported (described above).

Most of the improvement in disability takes place over the first year. Using the 8-point extended Glasgow Outcome Scale to measure disability on several occasions over the first 5 years, it was possible to demonstrate significant improvements in outcome (e.g. from severe disability to moderate disability) in the first 6 months (Svensson & Starmark 2002). However, after 12 months and over the next 4 years patients were as likely to deteriorate one point as they were to improve one point, with the vast majority of patients remaining unchanged.

It is therefore not surprising to find that symptoms remain in the long term. A postal survey of relatives of patients with subarachnoid haemorrhage or traumatic brain injury who had been admitted to a neurosurgical unit 5–7 years before found that they frequently reported that the patient had symptoms of impatience, passivity or tiredness (Hellawell & Pentland 2001). There was a considerable degree of overlap in the symptoms described by the two groups. Another study examined outcome 4–7 years after haemorrhage and found similar problems, but gained the impression that the cohort had improved over the years and many had a positive attitude to life (Ogden *et al.* 1997). For example, more than 75% of subjects reported that though they had for several months or years after the haemorrhage suffered fatigue or sleepiness, these had now resolved. The largest study is of over 600 patients most of whom had at most slight disability after a subarachnoid haemorrhage between 2 and 19 years (average 9 years) previously (Wermer *et al.* 2007b). At interview patients were asked about symptoms and handicap. One-quarter of patients who had been working before the haemorrhage were no longer working, and a further one-quarter were working reduced hours or in a less demanding position. Almost 60% reported personality change, the commonest changes being increased agitation/irritability, increased emotionality and apathy. Overall 35% reported memory problems, although the proportion lessened as time since haemorrhage increased. The most frequent symptoms were fatigue, headaches, concentration problems and dizziness, with only one-quarter of patients saying that they had made a complete symptomatic recovery. Thus the pattern and extent of problems, compared to what has been described above in the first months and years after haemorrhage, does not seem to change much in the very long term.

Emotional precipitation of subarachnoid haemorrhage

Occasional examples are reported of cerebrovascular accidents that show a striking temporal relationship to emotionally stressful events. However, the most dramatic instances appear to involve patients with subarachnoid haemorrhage. Particularly striking examples have been recorded by Storey (1969, 1972), in which the haemorrhage followed immediately upon some emotionally traumatic event, presumably by virtue of the rise of blood pressure engendered. Thus a woman answered the door to a policeman who told her that the woman next door, her closest friend, had hanged herself: she said 'Oh, my God' and forthwith had her haemorrhage. Another woman was watching television when an aeroplane on a test flight was shown exploding in the air; she believed (erroneously as it turned out) that her son was on it, put her hands to her head and had the haemorrhage within seconds of the disaster. Another had a subarachnoid haemorrhage within a minute of being told by her husband that he knew of her adultery and was going to divorce her.

Altogether Storey found evidence of a striking emotional precipitant in four of his original 261 patients, and two further less dramatic examples. All were in women, although 43% of the series were male. Such precipitation appeared to be markedly more common in patients with no obvious source for the haemorrhage than in patients with aneurysms demonstrable on angiography. On the other hand, Powell *et al.* (2002) found no evidence of higher stress levels, from self-report after the event, in patients with subarachnoid haemorrhage compared with controls.

Giant cerebral aneurysms

The great majority of aneurysms giving rise to subarachnoid haemorrhage are small, rarely exceeding 1 or 2 cm in diameter. Massive aneurysms are distinctly uncommon, but when present can give rise to much diagnostic confusion and are often not even considered in differential diagnosis.

Best known is aneurysm of the intracavernous portion of the internal carotid artery, which may compress surrounding nerves leading to ophthalmoplegias and sensory loss of trigeminal distribution. They most commonly present with diplopia and pain in the face, eye or head (Stiebel-Kalish *et al.* 2005). Occasionally, they rupture to give rise to a carotid–cavernous fistula that may produce pulsating exophthalmos and a bruit.

Those situated on the circle of Willis at the base of the brain rarely rupture, but can produce local pressure effects simulating basal space-occupying lesions. Bull (1969) reported 22 such cases collected over a similar number of years. Common complaints were of visual disturbance or headache. However, in six patients mental changes predominated; dementia was the presenting feature, usually but not invariably accompanied by neurological signs such as cranial nerve deficits or hemiparesis.

Morley (1967) reviewed the literature concerning unruptured vertebrobasilar aneurysms, which can lead to a variety of pictures simulating multiple sclerosis, posterior fossa tumours or vertebrobasilar ischaemia. Three of his own five cases had at first been diagnosed as psychiatrically unwell; vague symptoms of headache, nondescript dizziness, slowed speech and a muted facial expression had led to an impression of depressive illness. Mental impairment was also sometimes evident.

Hypertensive encephalopathy

This was never a common condition, with less than one in six patients with malignant hypertension suffering encephalopathy (Healton *et al.* 1982), and is even rarer now that better management of hypertension prevents the malignant phase. Nevertheless, it is still very occasionally seen, particularly in patients with eclampsia (Becker 2006). When it does arise it is always a serious medical emergency. Very occasionally it may be the presenting manifestation of the hypertension.

Onset is acute with headache, drowsiness, apprehension and mental confusion. Epileptic fits frequently occur. Sometimes focal neurological signs, including cortical blindness and hemiplegia, may be found but are not usually part of the picture. Vomiting may occur and papilloedema frequently develops. The disorder evolves rapidly, often within the space of 24 hours, and if untreated progresses to coma with fatal outcome in a high proportion of cases. The diastolic blood pressure is extremely high, often exceeding 140 mmHg. Patients generally make a full recovery although three cases have been described in which hypertensive episodes in childhood appear to have been followed by temporal lobe epilepsy and hippocampal sclerosis (Solinas *et al.* 2003).

Serial images are required to differentiate the acute effects of hypertensive encephalopathy from the ischaemic demyelination of white matter, characteristically in a periventricular distribution, that is associated with chronic hypertension. One long-term sequela of hypertensive encephalopathy, found on gradient echo MRI, is evidence of numerous punctate haemorrhages (Weingarten *et al.* 1994).

Cerebral oedema, particularly involving the basal ganglia and brainstem, may be found on MRI as an acute reversible effect of hypertensive encephalophathy. Another reversible finding is high signal on T2 sequences in white matter, particularly posteriorly in the cerebral hemispheres. A single case report using diffusion- and perfusion-weighted MRI suggests that vasogenic oedema is responsible for this reversible posterior leucoencephalopathy (Sundgren *et al.* 2002). The syndrome of reversible posterior leucoencephalopathy (Hinchey *et al.* 1996) may also be associated with immunosuppressive drugs and with renal failure.

Pathological examination may reveal a normal brain, but usually there is marked oedema or petechial haemorrhages and microinfarcts. Byrom (1954) showed in the rat that with hypertension of advanced degree there was intense segmental constriction of cerebral arterioles, attributable to attempts at autoregulation that fail when the pressure exceeds a certain limit. Dilatation occurs between the constricted segments and the vessel wall is damaged, leading to hyperperfusion and cerebral oedema, which may be the essential factors underlying hypertensive encephalopathy (Skinhoj & Strandgaard 1973).

Migraine

Migraine is a common and sometimes severely incapacitating disorder. Neuropsychiatric phenomena may feature prominently in the course of the attacks. Good reviews are to be found in Goadsby (2006) and Silberstein (2004). Silberstein *et al.* (2002) provide a more detailed review of neuropsychiatric sequelae.

The syndrome of migraine is hard to delineate precisely since to some extent boundaries are blurred between this and other forms of headache, particularly tension-type headache. Migraine is a familial disorder, characterised by recurrent attacks of headache widely variable in intensity, frequency and duration, commonly unilateral, usually associated with anorexia, nausea and vomiting, and sometimes preceded by or associated with neurological and mood disturbances (Critchley 1969). Comprehensive criteria for both diagnosis and classification of migraine have been proposed by the International Headache Society (IHS) (Subcommittee IHSC 2004) (Box 8.7). The IHS classification distinguishes several types of migraine, of which the most common are migraine without aura and migraine with aura. In the presence of aura the diagnosis of migraine headache is usually unmistakable, but headache in the absence of aura may be less easy to diagnose. For headache without aura, a meta-analysis recently identified the five criteria that best predict the diagnosis of migraine, using the IHS criteria as the gold standard (Detsky *et al.* 2006):

- *P*ulsating;
- duration of 4–72 h*O*urs;
- *U*nilateral;
- *N*ausea;
- *D*isabling.

If a patient's headache is found to meet four or five of these '*POUND*ing' criteria, then it is very likely that migraine is present. Although estimates vary quite widely, it is reasonable to conclude that over the previous year about 12% of adults will have had at least one attack of migraine. The male to female ratio is about 1 : 3 and the lifetime prevalence about 16% (Hirtz *et al.* 2007).

Clinical features

Onset is usually in childhood or early adult life, some 25% of cases beginning before the age of 10 and very few after 50. A childhood history of cyclical vomiting with abdominal pain can sometimes be traced as a precursor. Affected individuals show an increased frequency of epilepsy, Raynaud's phenomenon, stroke and affective disorders (Silberstein 2004). A family history of migraine is reported in some two-thirds of cases.

A proportion of patients report premonitory symptoms. This has been studied prospectively in 76 patients who reported having non-headache symptoms that predicted an attack (Giffin *et al.* 2003). Using patient hand-held electronic diaries that were adjusted so that entries could not be retrospectively altered or deleted, patients recorded these symptoms and whether they were in fact followed by migraine. When such symptoms were recorded in the diaries they were followed by migraine within 72 hours on 72% of occasions. The most common premonitory symptoms were tiredness, difficulty concentrating, stiff neck and irritability. Such symptoms were also very common during the attack and after. In other words, there was not a specific constellation of symptoms that only occurred during the premonitory phase, although yawning, hunger or food cravings, and increased energy were more common before than during the attack. The authors suggested that the presence of non-headache symptoms before, during and after a migraine attack were consistent with a model of migraine as an episodic dysfunction of trigeminovascular regulation, probably mediated at the level of the brainstem (see below).

Headache is the most constant element, lasting usually for 8–24 hours but occasionally several days, and varying from mild discomfort to pain of incapacitating violence. It is mostly unilateral at onset, though tending to become diffuse later in the attack. Throbbing is common, at least initially, with aggravation on coughing or jolting. Anorexia, nausea and vomiting usually develop, also photophobia and intolerance of noise. Autonomic changes may include pallor, facial oedema, conjunctival injection, abdominal distension or the passing of one or more loose stools. In attacks of any

---

Box 8.7 Diagnosis and classification of migraine proposed by the International Headache Society (Subcommittee IHSC 2004)

Diagnostic criteria

A At least five attacks fulfilling criteria B–D

B Headache attacks lasting 4–72 hours (untreated or unsuccessfully treated)

C Headache has at least two of the following characteristics:
1 Unilateral location
2 Pulsating quality
3 Moderate or severe pain intensity
4 Aggravation by, or causing avoidance of, routine physical activity

D During headache at least one of the following:
1 Nausea and/or vomiting
2 Photophobia and phonophobia

E Not attributed to another disorder

Classification

1 Migraine
1.1 Migraine without aura
1.2 Migraine with aura (with and without headache and including familial hemiplegic migraine and basilar-type migraine)
1.3 Childhood periodic syndromes that are commonly precursors of migraine (cyclical vomiting, abdominal migraine and benign paroxysmal vertigo of childhood)
1.4 Retinal migraine
1.5 Complications of migraine (including migrainous infarction and migraine-triggered seizure)

severity the patient is usually obliged to lie down until the episode has passed.

This variety is designated *migraine without aura* (previously 'common migraine'). Difficulty will be encountered in distinguishing it from tension-type headache in certain cases. In perhaps one-third of cases (Launer *et al.* 1999) the headache is preceded by an aura, the syndrome then being known as *migraine with aura* (previously 'classic migraine') (Kirchmann 2006). Various dramatic neurological symptoms may be seen but the commonest is visual disturbance as the first indication of an impending attack. The aura usually builds up over 5–20 minutes, lasts some 10–60 minutes and subsides as the headache sets in, usually within the hour. Occasionally no headache follows. Most typical are the well-known 'fortification spectra' (teichopsia), starting near the fixation point in one half-field and expanding to the periphery as a semicircle of shimmering highly coloured zig-zag lights. Other forms consist of moving coils, curving lights or rippling sensations in the visual field. Not all are confined to one half-field of vision. A negative scotoma may follow in their wake, or constitute the whole of the aura in itself. Monocular scotoma can occur due to involvement of retinal vessels. Other disturbances include micropsia, macropsia, distortions of shape and position, 'zoom vision' and 'mosaic vision'. Occasionally there are hallucinations and distortion of taste, smell and hearing. Tactile paraesthesiae may coexist with the visual disturbances or occur alone. Problems with language may take the form of anomia or difficulty with speaking (Ardila & Sanchez 1988). Body image disturbances, though rare, can take fascinating forms, as discussed in Psychiatric features associated with attacks (later in chapter). After the attack there is often a period of resolution lasting a few hours. The person may feel tired or washed out or have difficulties concentrating. Sometimes scalp tenderness is present. Mood changes include irritability and depression, but the occasional person feels refreshed or euphoric after the attack.

A not uncommon variant, seen in about 10% of cases, is *basilar-type migraine* or *basilar artery migraine* (Bickerstaff 1961a; Kirchmann *et al.* 2006). The attacks begin with a visual aura, sometimes extending to both half-fields and obscuring vision, then proceeding to symptoms of brainstem dysfunction such as vertigo, dysarthria, ataxia, tinnitus, and sensory symptoms distally in the limbs and around the lips and tongue. Symptoms are often bilateral. After several minutes to three-quarters of an hour these give way to throbbing headache usually of occipital distribution. Loss of consciousness may be interposed between the brainstem symptoms and headache, lasting sometimes for up to half an hour and presumably due to ischaemia of the reticular formation. The impairment is gradual in onset, resembling deep sleep rather than syncope. Attacks of basilar migraine appear to be especially common in women. The episodes are usually interspersed among classic attacks.

Familial hemiplegic migraine (Thomsen *et al.* 2002) is an autosomal dominant condition characterised by attacks of transient hemiplegia that are followed by headache (Ducros *et al.* 2001). The hemiparesis is always associated with sensory, language or visual disturbances and in one-fifth of cases the attacks are accompanied by confusion or drowsiness. The aura symptoms tend to be of longer duration than in other types of migraine. In a proportion, particularly in younger patients and sometimes following a mild head injury, prolonged episodes of an encephalopathic-like illness, lasting days and weeks, may be seen (Ducros *et al.* 2001). The majority of cases have symptoms of basilar migraine, and in 20% of families patients have permanent cerebellar signs. Familial hemiplegic migraine is rare and is largely of interest in view of the genetic findings (see below), which are generally not found in sporadic hemiplegic migraine.

Other varieties of migraine include attacks in which components other than headache dominate the clinical picture (previously known as 'migraine equivalents'). The headache may be mild or even totally absent, leading to considerable diagnostic difficulty if a history of more typical attacks is not forthcoming. Thus the visual aura or other neurological disturbance may occur alone, or there may be episodes of nausea and vomiting, abdominal pain or drowsiness. Some of the mental phenomena that may constitute equivalents are discussed below. Migraine aura can occasionally mimic TIA, and some TIAs, particularly in the basilar artery territory, can be associated with headache. Slow progression of symptoms may be a helpful distinction, generally present in migraine aura and absent in TIAs.

Cluster headaches, previously called 'migrainous neuralgia', consist of severe unilateral head or face pain, usually periorbital, typically occurring in bouts over a period of several weeks and often appearing at exactly the same time each day. Attacks are accompanied by lacrimation and nasal blockage on the ipsilateral side, and sometimes by Horner's syndrome. Cluster headaches are no longer considered to be a migraine variant, and are classified by the IHS as one of the trigeminal autonomic cephalalgias. Activation of hypothalamic, rather than brainstem, blood flow is found (May *et al.* 1998).

Retinal migraine is probably at best exceedingly rare. A review of the literature of case reports of retinal migraine found that the vast majority failed to meet, for one reason or other, the IHS criteria of at least two attacks of fully reversible monocular visual symptoms followed by migraine headache (Hill *et al.* 2007). The accompanying editorial described retinal migraine as an oxymoron (Winterkorn 2007) because it is highly unlikely that the pathophysiology underlying migraine aura, involving spreading depression over the cortex (see below), could apply to the retina. 'Ophthalmoplegic migraine', with attacks of headache accompanied by paresis of external ocular movement, again often outlasting the headache, is no longer considered a migraine variant and is classified by the IHS as a cranial neuralgia (Subcommittee IHSC 2004).

Course and outcome

Once established, migraine is commonly a lifelong complaint, although spells of relief may occur for years at a time. The frequency and severity of attacks vary greatly from one patient to another. Some are affected at fairly regular intervals, and a small number of women are especially susceptible around the time of their menstrual periods. Temporary relief during pregnancy is well attested in approximately 60% of cases. The prevalence declines beyond the age of 50 years in both men and women (Steiner *et al.* 2003). Nevertheless, in some patients headaches become more frequent over time and the illness is considered to have 'transformed' into chronic migraine, defined as headaches without aura on at least 15 days a month for at least 6 months. Precipitating factors, for example fatigue or sleep, stress, particular foods or drinks, menstruation, weather (Prince *et al.* 2004) and infections, are probably not particular to migraine headache, being almost as common before episodes of non-migraine headache (Chabriat *et al.* 1999).

Migraine is associated with strokes. Dorfman *et al.* (1979) demonstrated infarctions by angiography or CT in four young adults with migraine, one representing a posterior cerebral artery occlusion and three infarctions in the middle cerebral territory. However, Broderick and Swanson (1987) were able to find only 20 examples of stroke occurring with an attack among almost 5000 patients at the Mayo Clinic. Good recovery was usual, only two being left with moderate disability and 14 with mild or minimal disability. Bogousslavski *et al.* (1988) made a careful comparison between 22 patients who suffered a stroke during an attack and matched migraine patients who had suffered strokes remote from attacks. A second control group consisted of non-migraineurs with stroke. Those with stroke during an attack were less likely to have cardiovascular abnormalities as potential sources of emboli, and more likely to have a prolonged duration of attack. Such features suggested that strokes which occur during the course of attacks were intimately related to the pathophysiology of the migraine process, i.e. probably attributable to prolonged oligaemia in the territory responsible for the auras. The conclusion from a review of the relation between stroke and migraine is that the risk of suffering ischaemic stroke is increased in patients with migraine, particularly in young women (Bousser & Welch 2005). However, the absolute risk is nevertheless very low, i.e. the vast majority of young patients with migraine with aura will not suffer a stroke.

Findings of possible relevance have come from brain imaging. Hungerford *et al.* (1976) found evidence of infarction in 6 of 53 patients with very severe migraine, three of the infarctions corresponding in site to aspects of the clinical history. Of the 13 patients with permanent neurological sequelae, 11 showed some abnormality on the scan. MRI has also revealed abnormalities, chiefly scattered areas of high T2 signal intensity in the subcortical white matter, sometimes with larger cortical changes resembling infarcts. In a meta-analysis of seven studies, white matter abnormalities were found to be almost four times as common in migraine patients as controls (Swartz & Kern 2004); the increased risk was seen even in those studies restricted to patients less than 55 years old. One large study of subclinical brain lesions found that the risk of deep white matter abnormalities, as opposed to periventricular abnormalities, was raised by migraine, particularly in those with aura and frequent attacks and particularly in women (Kruit *et al.* 2004). In those with extensive periventricular lesions or large lacunar infarcts in deep white matter, it is important to rule out other conditions, including CADASIL (cerebral autosomal dominant arteriopathy with subcortical infarcts and leucoencephalopathy) and small-vessel disease. Small silent infarcts are found in about 10% of migraine, almost all in the posterior circulation particularly involving cerebellum (Kruit *et al.* 2005).

The mechanism underlying the increased risk of ischaemic stroke in migraine is unknown. Migrainous infarcts, i.e. infarcts during a migraine attack, only account for a small proportion of the risk at most; most ischaemic strokes in patients with migraine occur between migraine attacks (Bousser & Welch 2005). It may be the case that ischaemia-induced migraine is more common than migraine-induced ischaemia (Olesen *et al.* 1993); in a significant proportion of cases with both migraine and cerebral infarct, a definite cause for the infarct (e.g. cardioembolic source or carotid stenosis) was found. Various vascular disorders, including patent foramen ovale (Domitrz *et al.* 2007), mitral valve prolapse, thrombocythaemia and systemic lupus erythematosus, may be associated with increased rates of migraine, in addition to their increased risk of stroke. Finally, it must be remembered that MELAS (mitochondrial myopathy, encephalopathy, lactic acidosis and stroke), CADASIL (Gladstone & Dodick 2005) and a condition of autosomal dominant vascular retinopathy, migraine and Raynaud's phenomenon are three rare conditions that may produce both ischaemic stroke and migraine with aura (Bousser & Welch 2005).

Epilepsy and migraine occur together more frequently in the same person than would be predicted by a chance association. About 6% of patients with migraine have epilepsy, much higher than the rate in the general population (Haut *et al.* 2006). Furthermore, in a study of 1948 patients with epilepsy and 1411 of their parents and siblings, 24% of those with epilepsy had migraine compared with 12% of relatives without epilepsy. There was no convincing relationship between type of epilepsy and risk of migraine (Ottman & Lipton 1994). Both epilepsy and migraine may be related to the menstrual cycle, and the same drugs may be effective in both conditions. It has been suggested that both may be disorders of neuronal hyperexcitability (Aurora *et al.* 1999; Haut *et al.* 2006); two studies have found that migraineurs are more likely to experience phosphenes during transcranial magnetic stimulation of the occipital cortex, though one study has failed to replicate this.

Pathophysiology

The hypothesis that migraine should be understood as a disorder of neuronal hyperexcitability has gained support from the finding that many patients with familial hemiplegic migraine have genetic mutations. In all cases these mutations involve polymorphisms of genes regulating ion translocation. The first to be identified was a mutation in the gene, on chromosome 19, for the voltage-gated calcium channel (Ducros *et al.* 2001). Since then families have been found where the mutation is either in the gene coding for the Na^+/K^+ pump or in the gene for the neuronal voltage-gated sodium channel. It has been suggested that in each case, whether the abnormality is in the voltage-gated calcium or sodium channel or the Na^+/K^+ pump, the final common pathway to the migraine aura is excessive potassium or glutamate release which facilitates cortical spreading depression (see below) (Sanchez-Del-Rio *et al.* 2006). However, these changes in ionic regulation may also affect neuronal activity in brainstem nuclei (see below).

Previous hypotheses suggesting that migraine aura was caused by vasoconstriction, with the headache produced by the subsequent vasodilation, have now been discarded. Instead, migraine is now conceived as being related to events in the cortex and adjacent meninges on the one hand and in the brainstem on the other. These events are linked by sensory fibres of the trigeminal nerve conveying signals from meningeal nociceptors to the brainstem, and efferent fibres of the parasympathetic system controlling meningeal blood vessels, this afferent and efferent loop being part of the trigeminovascular system (Pietrobon & Striessnig 2003). The events of interest comprise:

- cortical spreading depression over the cerebral cortex, which is relevant to the aura of migraine but perhaps not to migraine without aura;
- effects of neuropeptides and other neurotransmitters, particularly 5-hydroxytryptamine (5HT), on meningeal vasculature and nociceptors;
- altered function of aminergic brainstem nuclei and their parasympathetic outflow.

Cortical spreading depression, a wave of neuronal and glial depolarisation with reduced neuronal activity and reduced blood flow that spreads across the cortex at a rate of about 2–3 mm/min, is very probably the cause of migraine aura (Sanchez-Del-Rio *et al.* 2006). In animals, spreading depression can be triggered by local application of high concentration of potassium, which then causes a wave of depolarisation to spread outwards. The extracellular concentrations of potassium, nitric oxide and glutamate are raised. In patients with migraine aura the studies of Lauritzen (1994) and colleagues have shown a wave of oligaemia travelling across the cortex, usually starting posteriorly and spreading anteriorly over the course of 15–45 minutes to involve parietal and temporal regions. The spread of oligaemia is independent of the territories supplied by the larger cerebral vessels, but like cortical spreading depression may fail to cross prominent cortical sulci (e.g. parieto-occipital sulcus) (Hadjikhani *et al.* 2001). The reduction in blood flow, of the order of 20–30%, is coupled to the reduced metabolic demand (Olesen *et al.* 1981; Lauritzen 1994), an observation which tallies with the absence of ischaemic change on diffusion-weighted MRI (Cutrer *et al.* 1998). A short phase of hyperaemia on the leading edge of the oligaemia may be responsible for the flashing jagged lights of the visual aura; using fMRI in three patients with visual aura it was possible to link the increase in BOLD signal, indicating greater blood oxygenation, to the patient's experience of scintillations moving across the visual field (Hadjikhani *et al.* 2001). Nitric oxide and inflammatory cytokines released from cortex affected by spreading depression may sensitise overlying meninges and trigger the migraine headache.

Activation of nociceptors in the meninges and meningeal vessels is responsible for the headache of migraine, whether or not preceded by aura. Neuropeptides, especially calcitonin gene-related peptide (CGRP), released by nerve terminals of the trigeminal sensory nerves act as vasodilators and contribute to what is effectively an inflammatory response with plasma extravasation and mast cell degranulation in the dura (neurogenic inflammation). 5HT is also involved because ergotamine and triptans both work by blocking 5HT receptors at various levels of the pathway, including those on meningeal blood vessels and trigeminal nerve endings. Sensitisation of the trigeminal nerve and its sensory nuclei explains why a proportion of patients complain of cutaneous allodynia in the trigeminal distribution (Burstein *et al.* 2000). The trigeminal nerve carries the sensory nociceptive signals to the brainstem.

In the rostral brainstem (dorsolateral pons), increased blood flow on PET is found during acute migraine headache (Bahra *et al.* 2001) and in those with chronic migraine (Matharu *et al.* 2004). In those with unilateral headache this effect is lateralised, although one group studying nine patients all with right-sided headache found contralateral brainstem activation (Weiller *et al.* 1995), whereas another group studying glyceryl trinitrate-triggered attacks found ipsilateral brainstem activation (Afridi *et al.* 2005). The activation continues after the headache is controlled by sumatriptan, suggesting that it is not simply a response to painful stimuli coming from the meninges and other intracranial vessels but may play an active role in the pathogenesis of the headache. The lateralised nature of the activation may explain why the headache is lateralised in many patients.

These findings are consistent with the hypothesis that migraine headache (Goadsby 2006) is explained by abnormal behaviour of aminergic brainstem nuclei that take part in the trigeminovascular loop (Pietrobon & Striessnig 2003). These nuclei, which include the trigeminal nucleus pars caudalis on the afferent side and the superior salivary nucleus on the efferent side, modulate sensory input from the meninges and, via their parasympathetic afferents, influence cranial vasculature. The consequent vasodilation enhances the inflammatory response described above.

The site of the changes responsible for auras must differ widely from one form to another. Teichopsia and homonymous field defects almost certainly originate in the occipital lobes, illusions of altered size, shape and position in the optic radiations, and bitemporal hemianopias from disturbance of chiasmatic vessels. The middle cerebral or internal carotids are likely to be involved in hemiplegic migraine, and the vertebrobasilar system in patients with brainstem manifestations. In fact it is probable that in many attacks a large part of the cerebral vasculature is affected diffusely, the focal symptoms merely reflecting ischaemia in the territory most severely involved, hence the vague but definite symptoms of slowed cerebration and somnolence common in attacks.

In the case of prolonged neurological phenomena, as in hemiplegic migraine, local oedema or hypoxia consequent on the spasm may be responsible for the symptoms.

Psychiatric aspects

Virtually all observers, neurologists and psychiatrists alike, stress the influence that psychological factors may have in migraine and the importance attaching to them in treatment. A considerable literature has accumulated concerning the personality of migraine sufferers and the role of emotions and conflicts in precipitating attacks. Early reports suggested that it was possible to identify a personality type that was particularly prone to suffering migraine. However, the anecdotal observations on which such conclusions were based are vulnerable, not least to ascertainment effects. It has for example been shown that personality type may predict who attends clinic for help rather than who in fact has headache (see below). With more rigorous methods, avoiding ascertainment bias and using reliable measures of personality and other psychopathology, the story is found to be a little more complicated. Mental phenomena are also recognised as common accompaniments of the migraine ictus, and may sometimes assume bizarre expression leading to diagnostic difficulty. These aspects are briefly reviewed.

Anxiety and depression

Patients with migraine are at increased risk of anxiety and depression. Population surveys consistently show that the risk of a person with migraine suffering depression or anxiety is at least twofold to threefold that of somebody without headache (Table 8.1). For example, a study of 1007 adults in Detroit found a lifetime prevalence of migraine of 12.8% and a 1-year prevalence of 9.2% (Breslau *et al.* 1991). Approximately half had migraine with aura; 26.5% of migraineurs had major depression compared with 9% of the non-migraine subjects, giving an odds ratio (OR) of about 3. The rates of any anxiety disorder were 53% and 27% respectively (OR 2.6).

In a prospective study of a cohort of 27- and 28-year-olds in Zurich, 61 of the 457 subjects were deemed to suffer from migraine, and these showed a significant excess of major depression, bipolar spectrum disorder (i.e. cyclothymia and hypomania), generalised anxiety and social phobia (Merikangas *et al.* 1990). For example, 14.7% of the migraineurs compared with 7.3% of controls had major depression (OR 2.2). The association with anxiety disorders was particularly strong, the corresponding figures being 31.2% versus 14.1% (OR 2.7). Retrospective data suggested a characteristic time course, with anxiety often manifested in childhood, followed by the development of migraine some years later, and then by discrete episodes of depression in early adult life. Similar figures were found by Swartz *et al.* (2000); of 1729 adults, those with migraine compared with controls had elevated risks for major depression (OR 2.2), panic disorder (OR 3.4) and phobias (OR 1.4). In a combined USA/UK study of over 300 adults with migraine and 300 controls, using PRIME-MD (Primary Care Evaluation of Mental Disorders) to identify depression, 47% of migraineurs compared with 17% of controls were depressed (Lipton *et al.* 2000). There were independent contributions of depression and of migraine to the Reduction in quality of life seen in the patients with migraine.

In general these studies (Table 8.1) find that the increased risk of having an anxiety disorder is greater than that for having depression. In those studies that have looked at the overlap, many cases are found to have mixed anxiety and depression. The risk of suicide attempt is also increased in migraine, and it is of interest that not all this excess risk is explained by the presence of depression (Breslau 1992).

It is a mathematical necessity that when people in a cohort must belong to only one of four categories (i.e. both depressed and suffering migraine, depressed but not suffering migraine, suffering migraine but not depressed, neither depressed nor suffering migraine), then the OR for depression if you suffer migraine is the same as the OR for migraine if you suffer depression. Therefore these studies also tell us that those who are depressed, and those with anxiety disorders, are at increased risk of suffering migraine. Thus in studies of patients presenting with major depression (Hung *et al.* 2005; Oedegaard & Fasmer 2005), about half are found to have migraine.

Various studies have looked at the specificity of the effect. Is the excess risk of emotional disorder restricted to migraine headache, or is it also seen in non-migraine headache? For those with migraine is the risk greater for those with or

Table 8.1 Rates and odds ratio (OR) for anxiety and depression in people with migraine and people without headache defined in population-based surveys.

Reference	Country	Method	Major depression (%)			Anxiety disorder (%)		
			With migraine	Without migraine	OR	With migraine	Without migraine	OR
Stewart *et al.* (1989) Data calculated from figures Migraine *N* = 235 Control *N* = 9757	USA	Telephone interview, migraine in previous week, lifetime risk of panic attack				39.6	6.8	8.9
Merikangas *et al.* (1990) Migraine *N* = 61 Control *N* = 396	Switzerland	Psychiatric interview, DSM-III	14.7	7.3	2.2	31.2	14.1	2.7
Breslau *et al.* (1991) *N* = 1007	USA	Interview, IHS 1988 classification for migraine, DSM-IIIR	26.5	9	3	53	27	2.6
Swartz *et al.* (2000) Migraine *N* = 118 Control *N* = 1225	USA	Interview, IHS 1988 classification for migraine, DSM-IIIR			2.2			3.4
Lipton *et al.* (2000) Migraine *N* = 389 Control *N* = 379	USA/UK	Telephone interview, IHS 1988 classification for migraine, PRIME-MD diagnosis for depression (Hahn *et al.* 1999)	47	17	4.4			
Breslau *et al.* (2003) Migraine *N* = 536 Control *N* = 586	USA	Interview, IHS 1988 classification for migraine, CIDI diagnosis for DSM-IV depression	40.7	16	3.5			
Zwart *et al.* (2003) Migraine *N* ≈ 5600 Control *N* ≈ 27 000	Norway	Questionnaire survey, IHS 1988 migraine within last year, HADS ≥11	4.3	2.3	2.7	9.2	3.1	3.2
McWilliam *et al.* (2004) Migraine *N* = 340 Control *N* = 2692	USA	Telephone interview and questionnaire: 'Have you experienced or been treated for migraine over last 12 months'. CIDI short form for DSM-IV depression and anxiety disorder	28.5	12.3	2.8	17.4	5.5	3.6
Patel *et al.* (2004) Migraine *N* = 1265 Control *N* = 6062	USA	Telephone interview, IHS 1988 classification for migraine, PRIME-MD diagnosis for depression	28.1	10.3	3.4			

CIDI, Composite International Diagnostic Interview; HADS, Hospital Anxiety and Depression Scale; IHS, International Headache Society.

without aura? The first study to examine this found that patients with migraine were more likely to be depressed than patients with tension-type headache, but did not check that this was not simply related to greater severity of headaches (Merikangas *et al.* 1994). A subsequent study comparing 536 people with migraine with 162 with severe headache and 586 controls found no significant difference between rates of depression in migraine and non-migraine headache, although there was a trend for the former to suffer worse depression (Breslau *et al.* 2000). Lifetime prevalence of major depression was 40.7% in migraine, 35.8% in severe non-migraine headache and 16% in controls, giving adjusted ORs

of 3.5 and 3.2 respectively. If anything, migraine patients with aura were more likely to suffer depression than patients with migraine without aura, the rates of major depression being 49% (OR 4.9) and 37% (OR 3.0) respectively.

A similar picture emerges from Norway based on a population survey of over 90 000 residents aged over 20 years. From this survey full questionnaire returns were available for 49 000, allowing the presence of migraine or other headache to be compared with the presence of anxiety and depression, the latter measured using HADS. Although the study had the advantage of being large, it relied on questionnaire assessment for the diagnosis of migraine with aura, migraine without aura, and other headache. This probably had the effect of making the study less powerful at detecting any differences between these three conditions because of cross-contamination across the three cohorts. In other words, because of misclassification some of the migraine with aura cohort will contain patients with migraine without aura, and so on. Nevertheless, a previous study had shown that the questionnaire methods had reasonable reliability compared with interview diagnoses. It was also reassuring that their figure of 12% with migraine headache within the previous 12 months is consistent with other prevalence studies; more than twice as many, 26%, had non-migraine headache. In the first paper (Zwart *et al.* 2003), rates of anxiety and depression were compared in those with migraine headache, non-migraine headache and controls. The risk of both depression and anxiety was increased in both migraine and non-migraine headache, with ORs between 2 and 3. The risk was slightly, but not significantly, higher in migraine, and was higher for anxiety than for depression in both types of headache. In both cases, i.e. regardless of headache type, there was a strong dose–response relationship: those with more frequent headache were more likely to be depressed. The second paper (Oedegaard *et al.* 2006) considered whether those with migraine with aura were more at risk of anxiety and depression than patients with migraine without aura. No significant difference was found between these two groups, although there was a trend for migraine with aura to have higher rates of anxiety and depression, and this was significant for the risk of depression in women with aura.

Therefore patients with migraine are not very different from patients with non-migraine headache in terms of their vulnerability to emotional disorders, although if anything the risk is greatest in those with migraine with aura and least in those with non-migraine headache. In fact the risk of depression and anxiety in migraine may not be very different from that found in arthritis or back pain (McWilliams *et al.* 2004). This suggests that it is the pain of migraine headache that results in depression and anxiety. However, one longitudinal study of the relation between depression and migraine suggests that depression may increase a person's vulnerability to migraine. At baseline both migraineurs and non-migraine headache sufferers had similar rates of lifetime major depression (42% vs. 36%) (Breslau *et al.* 2003). The authors then looked at those people who did not have headache at baseline to find out if they developed a first migraine attack over the 2-year follow-up. Being depressed at baseline markedly increased the risk of developing migraine compared with not being depressed (OR 3). This effect was specific for new-onset migraine headache; being depressed did not raise the risk of developing non-migraine headache over the next 2 years. The study did not report antidepressant usage, so it is possible that being on an antidepressant, rather than being depressed, was causing the increased risk of migraine. However, another study found the presence of phobia, not depression, to predict who would develop migraine. In this study participants were identified by community sampling in 1981 and followed up 12–15 years later (Swartz *et al.* 2000). Full psychiatric assessments were made at both time points. A total of 1343 patients who had not been suffering headaches in 1981 were followed up; of these, 118 (8.8%) had developed migraine (incident migraine). Those with an affective disorder in 1981 were not at greater risk of developing migraine, neither was there any effect of antidepressant usage. Only a phobia diagnosis in 1981 was associated with increased risk of developing migraine (OR 1.7).

Personality and stress in migraine

Many accounts stress the driving conscientious personality of migraine sufferers, often with marked obsessional traits and above-average intelligence. Such a picture originated with the work of Wolff (1937, 1963). Wolff's migraineurs were described as overtly obedient but with traits of stubbornness and inflexibility. Most were ambitious and preoccupied with achievement and success, attempted to dominate their environments, and were exacting and meticulous. Many harboured strong resentments that were linked to their intolerance and superabundance of drive. Sexual dissatisfaction was common. Such features, when present, appeared to furnish optimal conditions for the precipitation of attacks. Psychoanalysts have highlighted certain other constellations in the personality, for example repressed hostility and unresolved ambivalence resulting in compulsive behaviour and rigidity (Fromm-Reichmann 1937; Sperling 1964) or the role of sexual conflicts.

However, it is unlikely that generalisations can be made about the personality make-up of migraine patients. Sacks (1970) illustrated the variety of emotional needs that attacks appeared to fulfil, and found it impossible to fit his material into stereotypes of obsessive personality or chronically repressed hostility. Selby and Lance (1960) made a rough categorisation of their patients and considered that the personality range differed little from what occurs in the population generally: 23% showed obsessional trends, 22% were hyperactive and found it hard to relax, 13% showed overt anxiety symptoms and 42% were considered 'normal'. However, these studies used somewhat idiosyncratic methods of personality assessment. It is possible that more sensitive and better-validated methods of personality assessment might yield positive results.

Studies using standard measure of personality, for example the Minnesota Multiphasic Personality Inventory (MMPI) or Cloninger's seven-factor Temperament and Character Inventory (TCI), do find evidence of increased rates of neuroticism, or traits consistent with neuroticism such as harm avoidance or social introversion. In China a study of 80 patients with migraine found them to have elevated scores on the paranoia and social introversion scales of the MMPI compared with non-headache controls (Fan & Zhou 1999).

Elevated scores on hysteria and hypochondriasis improved with treatment of the migraine (Fan *et al.* 1999). Nylander *et al.* (1996) found that 26 migraine patients from a large Swedish family were no different from controls on the TCI, except that the subjects with migraine had slightly higher scores on novelty seeking (i.e. less likely to seek novelty); the authors suggested this was because they had high levels of somatic anxiety symptoms. Another study using the TCI obtained a slightly different result; patients with migraine without aura had higher scores than controls on problems with anger management and harm avoidance (Abbate-Daga *et al.* 2007). Psychasthenia and social introversion may be higher in those with chronic as opposed to episodic migraine (Karakurum *et al.* 2004). Comparing migraine with or without aura, only the migraine without aura group were found to have increased scores on a measure of aggression–hostility judged against healthy controls; no abnormal personality traits were found in migraine with aura patients (Cao *et al.* 2002). Patients who responded to sumatriptan have been compared to those who did not respond (Meckling *et al.* 2001); the former, if women, had headache that was more influenced by menstrual factors, whereas the non-responders had higher rates of anxiety and neuroticism.

However, increased rates of neuroticism may not be specific for migraine headache; studies have found elevated scores on measures of anxiety, neuroticism and harm avoidance that are equivalent in patients with migraine and those with tension-type headache (Di Piero *et al.* 2001; Cao *et al.* 2002; Mongini *et al.* 2005). Indeed, in one study only tension-type headache, not migraine, was associated with high neuroticism scores on the Eysenck Personality Inventory (EPI) (Rasmussen 1992). These observations are in line with a study that examined the effect of undertaking a mental arithmetic task as a mental stressor in patients with migraine or tension-type headache; in both headache groups symptoms of fatigue took longer to recover compared with controls (Stronks *et al.* 1999).

The studies that have just been described were by and large performed on clinic populations, with the danger that special selection may have been at work. Waters' (1971) survey of a community-based sample is informative. No evidence was found to support the contention that migraine is especially common among persons of higher intelligence, although it was noted that a higher proportion of the more intelligent sufferers had consulted doctors about their headaches. Similarly, there was no indication that migraine was especially frequent among persons in social classes I and II, a finding that has been replicated (Rasmussen 1992). However, Waters did find a tendency for a higher proportion of migraineurs in social classes I and II to have consulted their doctors. More recently, the characteristics of headache suffers who sought medical advice and treatment over the previous 2 years was compared with those, with approximately the

same headache severity, who did not (Ziegler & Paolo 1995). The proportion of migraine sufferers in each group was about the same but the clinic attenders had higher rates of psychasthenia, hysteria, hypochondriasis, social introversion and depression. This selection bias might well explain some of the findings described in the previous paragraphs.

Henryk-Gutt and Rees (1973) surveyed a large population of government employees and matched the migraine sufferers with carefully chosen controls, thus overcoming the selective processes involved in medical referral. Semi-structured interviews and personality inventories were used to explore psychological aspects of the disorder. They obtained no evidence of increased ambitiousness, striving or obsessionality among the migraine subjects, nor was there any relation to hostility and guilt. However, 'neuroticism', as measured by the EPI, was significantly higher than among controls, likewise indices of emotionality as manifest in current nervous symptoms, current emotional difficulties, liability to mood swings and tendencies to bottle up anger and resentments. Another study based on a community sample also found elevated scores on the neuroticism scale of the EPI, but this time only in women (Breslau *et al.* 1996). However, in a study of 728 women aged between 40 and 72 years attending a population-based mammography screening service, overall there was no association between lifetime migraine headache and personality traits (Mattsson & Ekselius 2002).

Therefore the evidence that a particular personality type predisposes a person to suffering migraine is not very strong. Nevertheless, it seems quite likely that people with migraine do have higher scores on neuroticism traits, including harm avoidance, psychasthenia and social introversion, particularly if they attend a migraine clinic. Migraine subjects may therefore be constitutionally predisposed towards increased emotional reactivity, and this increased reactivity of the autonomic nervous system could conceivably provide the predisposing factor for the development of attacks. Such factors probably also increase the risk of being treatment unresponsive and developing chronic migraine. However, such character traits are not very specific for migraine headache, and may be common to all patients with headache. Furthermore, there seems no evidence that patients with migraine with aura are at particularly high risk of increased neuroticism, indeed the opposite.

Psychological precipitants

Many observers place psychological factors high on the list of features that may provoke episodes of migraine. It is common to find that periods of stress, or the anticipation of stress, are associated with attacks. Sustained emotional tension seems to be more important than acute emotional disturbance, the crucial factor being the degree to which feelings are sustained, bottled up and inadequately expressed (Rees 1971). Frustrations and resentments may operate powerfully in this way. Another well-documented finding is the tendency for some patients to develop attacks during the 'let down period' after intense activity and striving. Consequently, some have attacks quite regularly when a harassing day is over, at weekends or on the first day of a holiday. However, many patients insist that the majority of their attacks are entirely without discernible precipitants. Emotional disturbance therefore appears to be a common but by no means universal factor. Migraine subjects attending a headache clinic report higher levels of stress on the Perceived Stress Questionnaire than do controls (Wacogne *et al.* 2003), including more 'intrusive thoughts about work' and 'feeling under pressure'.

Some two-thirds of clinic-based samples report that emotional precipitants are important, though rarely as the sole invariant factor (Selby & Lance 1960; Dalsgaard-Nielsen 1965). In their community survey, Henryk-Gutt and Rees (1973) found about 60% in whom problems at work or problems with interpersonal relationships were regarded as direct precipitants. Relief from strain was noted as a factor in about one-third. In controls with non-migrainous headaches such features were less commonly blamed. In almost half of the migraine subjects the disorder had had its onset during a period of emotional stress. The subjects were then asked to keep records of their attacks for a 2-month period, noting any special events or emotions coinciding with the attacks. Over half of the episodes recorded proved to be related to emotionally stressful events. Other precipitants such as alcohol, food or hunger were by comparison very rare. In approximately one-third of attacks no cause whatever could be discerned. A more recent study used very similar methods in 20 women with migraine, again over a 2-month period (Holm *et al.* 1997); 14 (70%) showed at least some relation between the amount of stress they experienced and their headache, and in four women there was a strong correlation between daily stress and headache severity. From a review of three previous studies, not including that of Henryk-Gutt and Rees (1973), the authors confirmed that on average about half of migraine subjects showed an effect of stress on likelihood of migraine headache. In general the effect was seen on the day of the stressor, but in one study stress preceded migraine headache by 1–3 days.

Psychiatric features associated with attacks

As noted above, feelings of irritability and anxiety may last for several hours as a prelude to attacks. More rarely patients may experience unusual health and vigour, sometimes amounting to elation. A rebound of energy is also described in the wake of attacks, with feelings of buoyancy and increased drive. Others by contrast remain listless and fatigued for several days. Such features may sometimes occur with sufficient regularity to suggest that they are an essential part of the pathophysiology of the disorder.

Mental changes are almost universal during the attack itself. Anxiety and irritability are common early on, with drowsiness and lethargy as the headache continues. Depression can be severe. Cerebration is typically slowed, with poor concentration and poor ability to think coherently. Klee (1968) made a detailed analysis of patients with migraine severe enough to warrant hospitalisation, and found that attacks were accompanied by marked impairment of memory in 10%, clouding of consciousness or delirium in 8%, pronounced anxiety in 8%, complex visual and auditory hallucinations in 6%, changes of body image in 6% and severe depression in 4%. Altogether 22% of patients experienced at least one mental symptom severely enough to affect them greatly in the course of their attacks.

Alterations of consciousness range from blunting of alertness, through states of marked lethargy and drowsiness to frank loss of consciousness. The latter is the so-called 'migrainous syncope', sometimes occurring during the aura and sometimes later in the attack. Typically the patient lapses into unconsciousness over a period of several minutes, appears as though sleeping deeply, then emerges from the episode in the same gradual fashion. Such attacks have been described as characteristic of basilar artery migraine (Bickerstaff 1961b) but can also be seen with hemiplegic migraine and other varieties. On rare occasions there may be short-lived periods of coma with incontinence or even epileptic fits at the height of attacks.

Mental 'confusion' can be marked. Sometimes it represents a focal disturbance of cerebral function with dysphasic, apraxic or agnosic manifestations. Disturbance of memory can be the main component, as described below by Sacks (1970), or there may be elaborate 'dreamy states', probably reflecting temporal lobe dysfunction, with feelings of *déjà vu*, timelessness, depersonalisation or forced reminiscence.

A 44-year-old man suffered very occasional attacks of migraine from adolescence, ushered in by scintillation scotomata. In one attack a profound dream-like state followed the visual phenomena.

First I couldn't think where I was, and then I suddenly realised that I was back in California . . . It was a hot summer day. I saw my wife moving about on the verandah, and I called her to bring me a Coke. She turned to me with an odd look on her face, and said 'Are you sick or something?' I suddenly seemed to wake up, and realised that it was a winter's day in New York, and there was no verandah and that it wasn't my wife but my secretary who was standing in the office looking strangely at me.

Other examples clearly represent acute organic reactions due to generalised cerebral dysfunction, with disorientation and clouding of consciousness. Medicaments administered for treatment of the attack may sometimes be partly responsible. Such states may be coloured by anxiety, restlessness and complex visual and auditory hallucinations. A paranoid element may be marked. The condition may amount to a frank delirium, lasting throughout the headache for several hours or days. Very occasionally the headache fails to materialise and the mental disturbance then appears as a psychotic episode in itself ('mental migraine equivalent'). Psychosis is very rare as a fully developed manifestation, and is usually seen as an elaboration of an acute organic reaction.

> A 37-year-old housewife had suffered attacks of migraine from 19, increasing in severity since the age of 32. Attacks began with headache, later proceeding to paraesthesiae in the right hand and leg with weakness of the limbs and a variety of visual phenomena. They often lasted for 3 or 4 days. During a particularly severe attack which lasted for a week she had to be admitted to a mental hospital. On the preceding day she had become increasingly restless with clouding of consciousness, had heard neighbours making unpleasant comments about her and believed she had been stuck with knives. For the first few days in hospital she was disorientated, restless and appeared hallucinated both visually and aurally. She heard children's voices and the voice of her general practitioner, and believed her legs had been amputated. This psychotic episode disappeared within a few days and she was amnesic for it afterwards. Her last clear memory was of lying down to sleep at home, and the next of waking in hospital (Klee 1968).

However, Bhatia (1990) has described a patient with Capgras syndrome, setting in during the headache despite normal orientation and memory and persisting for several weeks. Fuller *et al.* (1993) described a case in which psychotic features were in the forefront of the picture, four episodes occurring over a 17-year period and each setting in within 24 hours of migraine attacks, and only one being associated with disorientation.

Hallucinatory elements may sometimes dominate the picture, as in one of Klee's (1968) patients who saw greyish-coloured Red Indians, 20 cm high, crowding round in the room in which he lay. On another occasion he picked up hallucinatory musical instruments from the floor. Another patient saw 'white living creatures', stationary and rather indistinct, apparently unaccompanied by clouding of consciousness or disorientation.

Florid examples of confusion are probably rare, at least in adults. However, in children it seems not uncommon for migraine to present in this fashion. Gascon and Barlow (1970) observed four children who showed acute organic reactions lasting from 6 to 24 hours. Although headache developed in every case it was usually not detected until the mental disturbance had receded. Ehyai and Fenichel (1978) found five similar examples among 100 consecutive cases of childhood migraine, with episodes of agitated confusion lasting from several minutes to hours, and succeeded by diffuse EEG changes indicative of cerebral ischaemia. Such attacks tended to recur on follow-up but were eventually replaced by typical migraine.

Amnesia may feature prominently in some episodes, either alongside the visual aura or as a variant of classic attacks.

> A 37-year-old doctor complained of episodes of mental disturbance lasting 3–6 hours at a time, and occurring once or twice per year from the age of 18. They began with a feeling of mild depression, then strangeness, then mental confusion. Throughout the attack he remained perfectly orientated, yet was unable to organise his thinking and had large defects in his memory. Facts and events seemed isolated and devoid of normal associations. He was unable to remember things for more than half a minute and found it difficult to converse as a result, repeating questions and appearing absent-minded to onlookers. Close questioning revealed migraine attacks with scotomata and fortification spectra occurring between such episodes. The more typical attacks were also associated with very mild confusion (Nielsen 1930).

Caplan *et al.* (1981) have reported an association between the syndrome of transient global amnesia and migraine, describing 12 migraineurs who experienced a typical amnesic episode. Six were cases of common migraine and six of classic migraine. Of the latter, three experienced their classic aura accompanying the attack and headache followed it; two more had pounding headache during the attack. Altogether 9 of 12 experienced headache in the course of the amnesic episode. Pathophysiological mechanisms similar to those of migraine may be present in a substantial proportion of patients with transient global amnesia.

Body image disturbances may occur just before, during or after attacks of headache. Parts of the body are felt to be magnified, diminished, distorted, reduplicated or absent. Lippman (1952) reported several examples, all in classic migraine, including patients in whom the abnormal sensations could constitute the entire attack without headache developing. One patient felt as though the neck or hip were extending out on one side, another that the left ear was ballooning out for 15 cm or more, another that the head had grown to tremendous proportions and had become light, floating up to the ceiling. One patient felt alternating enlargements and diminutions in the size of the right half of the body, coming and going throughout the headache period. Patients who feel exceedingly tall or extremely minute during attacks are suggestive of *Alice in Wonderland* and Lewis Carroll was known to have suffered from migraine.

Lippman (1952) also described experiences of physical duality associated with migraine. During attacks such patients felt a conviction of having two bodies, usually for several seconds at a time, before, during or after the headache. Qualities such as observation, judgement and perception were typically transferred to the 'other' body which for the moment seemed the more real of the two, but throughout the experience the patient remained aware of the actual body and its position in space. Feelings of fear, mild wonder or amazement were common accompaniments. This striking phenomenon is best illustrated by one of Lippman's (1952) examples.

A woman of 37 wrote:

'Until . . . 5 years ago, I felt the queer sensation of being two persons. This sensation came just before a violent headache attack and at no other time. Very often it came as I was serving breakfast. There would be my husband and children, just as usual, and in a flash they didn't seem to be quite the same. They were my husband and children all right – but they certainly weren't the same . . . There was something queer about it all. I felt as if I were standing on an inclined plane, looking down on them from a height of a few feet watching myself serve breakfast. It was as if I were in another dimension, looking at myself and them. I was not afraid, just amazed. I always knew that I was really with them. Yet there was 'I' and there was 'me' – and in a moment I was one again!

Cognitive impairment and migraine

Progressive mental impairment has occasionally been noted in sufferers from severe migraine, although a causal connection has not been clearly established and any association would certainly appear to be rare. Symonds (1951) considered it probable that in some cases there might be slight but cumulative brain damage as a result of successive small infarctions and this is consistent with the observation that MRI studies find an increased risk of small infarcts in the white matter. An example is reported by Bradshaw and Parsons (1965):

A 39-year-old nursing sister had suffered migraine from the age of 7, increasing after a period of worry some years before. After injecting herself with ergotamine tartrate during one attack she developed a right hemiplegic episode with dysphasia. This improved slowly over 5 weeks but left a slight residual deficit. Angiography and other investigations showed no abnormalities. Follow-up showed unequivocal evidence of progressive impairment of mental faculties, leading to memory impairment, falling standards of work, lack of insight and emotional instability. Further migraine attacks had continued, some with right-sided paraesthesiae. Her mother had suffered right hemiplegic migraine, and from the age of 52 had shown mental changes that progressed to gross dementia over the course of several years.

Pedersen (1980) has described three patients with cortical atrophy and marked signs of reduced intellect. No other causes could be found to account for this, and two of the patients had shown a marked increase in frequency of attacks prior to the onset of the dementia.

With regard to psychometry, Klee and Willanger (1966) found evidence of slight impairment in six of eight patients, and Zeitlin and Oddy (1984) reported impairments in comparison to a carefully matched control group. In the latter study, 19 patients with histories of migraine extending over 10 years were matched to controls in terms of age, sex, social class, verbal IQ and education. All were under 50 with a mean age of 36 years. Significant impairments were revealed on choice reaction time tests, Trail Making Test and Paced Auditory Serial Addition Test (PASAT), and on recognition memory for words. However, no associations emerged with measures of the severity of migraine or the use of ergotamine. A review of 12 studies of interictal neuropsychological testing in adult migraineurs found surprisingly little evidence of neuropsychological impairment (O'Bryant *et al.* 2005); the evidence suggested 'some subtle but possibly significant changes in cognition'. Psychomotor slowing was the commonest finding. Indeed, migraine with aura patients had more evidence of impairments. However, there was no evidence that migraine results in greater cognitive decline with ageing (and see also Kalaydjian *et al.* 2007) or is a risk factor for Alzheimer's disease.

Chronic migraine or transformed migraine

Occasional sufferers from migraine may enter a phase in which very frequent, severe and unremitting headaches develop. Typically this is coupled with malaise, anorexia, sleeplessness and loss of weight. Depression of considerable severity is usually an integral part of the picture. Over-medication may prove to be partly responsible, but in many cases psychological influences are clearly at work in initiating or perpetuating the disorder.

The deterioration may be decisively linked to the development of a depressive illness, the migraine and the affective disorder thereafter reinforcing each other. In other patients it may be difficult to discern which components have been primary in initiating the vicious circle once the condition has become entrenched. *Transformed migraine* is the term now used to describe the situation when headache occurs on at least 15 days of the month for on average, if untreated, more than 4 hours a day.

Differential diagnosis

Migraine headaches must first be differentiated from other causes of pain in the head and face: chronic sinus disease, glaucoma, hypertension and raised intracranial pressure. In the majority of cases the history will be sufficient to allow such a distinction, aided by physical examination or simple investigations. More difficulty may be encountered in making a firm distinction between migraine and tension headaches, both of which are common, chronic and frequently incapacitating.

Problems with neurological diagnosis are likely to arise in cases of 'complicated migraine', where marked neurological deficits accompany or follow attacks. Here a neurological opinion is essential, even though a basis in structural cerebral pathology will emerge in only a minute proportion of cases. An angioma must be considered when the deficits well outlast the headache, and especially when attacks of hemiplegic migraine involve one side of the body exclusively. Ophthalmoplegic attacks limited to one side will raise the possibility of an aneurysm of the internal carotid or posterior communicating arteries. In basilar migraine the prominence of brainstem deficits may suggest the possibility of some brainstem lesion. And even classic migraine attacks may warrant investigation if they first declare themselves in adult life, particularly if the auras tend to occur alone without much by way of headache.

Occasionally, difficulty can arise in distinguishing migraine from epilepsy, and indeed the two may occur together. When loss of consciousness occurs with migraine it is usually gradual in onset and a good deal less profound than in epilepsy. Even when sudden, it is usually succeeded by headache far exceeding that which follows an epileptic attack. Doubt can also arise over the complex auras of migraine, especially when these occur as isolated events. However, visual phenomena are far commoner in migraine than in epilepsy and often assume their highly specific form. Paraesthesiae are rarely bilateral in epilepsy, and proceed with much greater rapidity than in migraine.

Patients presenting with episodes of confusion may be suspected of delirium due to toxic or metabolic factors. Long-lasting acute organic reactions may be diagnosed as transient paranoid reactions. Episodes coloured by marked mood disturbance may resemble the swings of manic–depressive disorder, especially when preceded or followed by a rebound of elation and hyperactivity. Episodes of syncope in migraine may be regarded as hysterical dissociation, particularly when the impairment of consciousness is not profound and is preceded by a dramatic train of symptoms. In all such variants the true situation is usually revealed by the development of headache later in the attack or by a history of more typical migraine attacks in the past.

Treatment

Details of medical treatment are dealt with in the reviews by Goadsby (2006) and Silberstein (2004). Triptans, selective $5HT_{1B/1D}$ receptor agonists, have markedly improved control of migraine for many sufferers. They are used in the treatment of the acute attack, and can work even if given several hours after the onset of headache. In addition to relieving headache they have beneficial effects on nausea and photophobia. They are usually given orally, but alternative routes of administration, including nasal spray and suppositories, may be needed when nausea and vomiting are present. Sumatriptan has been followed by a range of newer agents. Triptans may be contraindicated in patients with ischaemic heart disease, uncontrolled hypertension and in pregnancy. A recent evidence-based review suggested that alternative treatments for acute migraine included aspirin in combination with metoclopramide, and ergotamine either by nasal spray or rectally (Tfelt-Hansen 2006). An exciting new class of drugs, developed from translation of laboratory work into clinical practice, are the CGRP antagonists; one clinical trial demonstrated that these agents may be effective in treating acute migraine (Olesen *et al.* 2004).

Prophylactic drug therapy may be indicated when two or more attacks are regularly experienced per month (Bigal & Lipton 2006). Those preventive drugs that receive an evidence-based stamp of approval, both in terms of efficacy and with relative lack of side effects, include valproate, amitriptyline, propranolol and timolol (Tfelt-Hansen 2006). Propranolol is widely regarded as the drug of first choice for prophylactic treatment, and has been shown to be effective in a high proportion of patients. Other drugs with good evidence of efficacy but with problematic side effects include methysergide and pizotifen.

However, pharmacological aspects are merely a part of the total management required in patients with migraine of disabling severity. Attention may need to be directed towards a host of factors specific to the individual: regularisation of sleep and meal times, judicious avoidance of stress where this is possible, and perhaps attention to provocative substances in the diet. In addition, social and psychological factors will usually warrant close consideration when attacks have become frequent and incapacitating.

It is important to detect and treat depressive or anxiety states that are aggravating the situation (Griffith & Razavi

2006). A recent study suggests that buspirone, a $5HT_{1A}$ agonist, may be effective in reducing headache in migraine patients suffering anxiety (Lee *et al.* 2005). One must similarly be alert to sources of emotional turmoil that have arisen, especially conflicts at work or in interpersonal relationships. When the patient's personality and life situation are well understood, the attacks may be seen as providing oblique expression for various feelings and moods that are denied expression in other ways: imposing a halt after prolonged activity, allowing temporary respite for the working through of stresses and conflicts, providing an outlet for repressed anger, or fulfilling a self-punitive role in chronically depressed individuals (Sacks 1970). Mitchell (1971) has indicated the value which may be obtained from behaviourally orientated techniques in reducing the frequency and severity of attacks. Training in relaxation has been shown to produce enduring improvement, likewise hypnosis aimed at reducing tension or apprehension (Lance 1993). Occipital nerve stimulation may prove to be useful for patients with chronic migraine (Matharu *et al.* 2004).

Subdural haematoma

The majority of subdural haematomas follow head injury. Subdural haematomas are regarded as acute if less than 1 week old or chronic if more than 1 month old. Chronic subdural haematomas have a prevalence of about 1 in 10 000; in 25–50% of cases no history of head trauma is found (El-Kadi *et al.* 2000). Predisposing factors include alcohol, blood dyscrasias or anticoagulant treatment, ventriculoperitoneal shunt and epilepsy. Blood accumulates in the subdural space from rupture of veins running between the cortex and the dural venous sinuses. It becomes encysted between the dura and arachnoid and may swell by osmosis to reach a very large size. Localising signs often remain minimal, however, since the brain is compressed from without. The collections usually lie over the frontal or parietal lobes and are bilateral in one-third to half of cases.

Those which declare themselves acutely after head injury present either with failure to regain consciousness or with fluctuating confusion and torpor often lapsing into coma. Hemiparesis and ocular changes are usually evident, but neurological deficits can be surprisingly slight and overshadowed by the mental disturbance. Quite often the haematoma is suspected only because the patient's recovery from the injury is slower than expected.

However, it is chronic subdural haematoma that is notorious for leading to mistakes in diagnosis, particularly among the elderly. The antecedent head injury may be trivial and go unrecognised, and there may be few clear pointers to the presence of a space-occupying lesion within the skull. Sometimes there is a latent interval of days, weeks or months after injury before the declaration of symptoms. Very occasionally a year or more may elapse. This picture, with a long interval between injury and presentation, is more typically seen in older patients. Younger patients tend to present earlier and with symptoms and signs of raised intracranial pressure such as vomiting, headache and papilloedema (Machulda & Haut 2000).

In classic examples there is vague headache that sets in gradually and may or may not be localised. It may be present only intermittently or occasionally be entirely absent. Dullness, sluggishness and difficulty with concentration slowly increase in severity. Lapses of memory and episodes of mental aberration occur. The level of consciousness fluctuates widely, with periods of apparent normality alternating with periods of drowsiness, changing from day to day or even from hour to hour. The variability in the mental state is often the most important indicator of the condition. Physical signs may be few, with inequality of the pupils, transient ocular paralyses or upgoing plantar responses. Pyramidal tract involvement may progress to hemiparesis, and a grasp reflex may be present. Papilloedema remains absent in a large proportion of cases. Epileptic fits may occur but are rare (Ohno *et al.* 1993). Ultimately the patient lapses into intermittent mutism or semicoma, but even at this stage evidence of neurological involvement can be surprisingly slight.

In a study of patients before and after surgery, reductions in thalamic blood flow were associated with impairment of conscious level and alertness, and consequently mentation (Tanaka *et al.* 1992). Reductions in cerebral blood flow (CBF) were most pronounced in thalamus and putamen before surgery. After surgery the biggest improvement in blood flow was seen in thalamus, and this improvement correlated with improvements in cognition. Patients with chronic subdural haematoma with altered conscious level or dementia, compared with those presenting with headache or motor symptoms, may have greater reductions in blood flow bilaterally in thalamus and ipsilaterally in frontal cortex (Inao *et al.* 2001). Reduced thalamic blood flow was related to the degree of midline shift.

Wide variation may be seen from the typical picture. Occasional patients present with severe headache but no physical signs, others with episodes of confusion and restlessness. In long-standing cases there may be insidious failure of intellect progressing to generalised dementia. In a retrospective survey, Black (1984) analysed the mental changes recorded in 79 patients discharged from hospital with subdural haematomas. In 20% mental symptoms had been the initial manifestation, and 58% had developed them by the time of admission. Delirium occurred in 24 patients, with lethargy and fluctuating clouding of consciousness. Dementia was present in seven, coma in six and three patients showed depression with minimal changes in consciousness or intellect.

Problems with diagnosis are particularly severe among the elderly, where the classic picture has been found to be the exception rather than the rule, occurring in only 5 of 52 examples reported by Bedford (1958). The typical story was of an aged person, already somewhat enfeebled, recently becoming mentally confused. Drowsiness was not always present, and concomitant disease such as pneumonia, uraemia or cardiac failure provided further diagnostic distractions. The diagnosis may therefore be overlooked until the patient declines and becomes somnolent or comatose. Despite the utmost vigilance, only 40% of Bedford's cases were diagnosed during life.

In a psychiatric hospital post-mortem study, Cole (1978) found subdural haematomas to be the commonest form of space-occupying lesion. Six acute and eight chronic haematomas were discovered among 200 routine post-mortems, yet the diagnosis had been made before death only once. In the chronic cases particularly, signs were often minimal and fluctuation of consciousness had rarely been conspicuous. A terminal seizure or sudden death had sometimes been the first indication of a change in the patient's condition. In the elderly a cerebrovascular accident had often been held responsible when neurological deficits were present.

Apart from dementia, differentiation must be made from cerebral infarction, cerebral tumour and alcoholism. Important features distinguishing subdural haematomas from strokes are the slow steady increase in neurological deficit, the presence of some lack of responsiveness, and lack of improvement mentally despite comparatively slight physical disability (Carter 1972). Sometimes the two occur together when cerebral infarction has led to a fall with striking of the head. Cerebral tumour may be closely simulated when there is evidence of raised intracranial pressure. The fluctuating course of the drowsiness and mental confusion can then be an important differentiating feature. Chronic alcoholism may lead to similar drowsiness and intermittent mental aberration, and alcoholics are liable to head injuries which are then forgotten. Thus 7 of 14 examples of subdural haematoma discovered by Selecki (1965) among patients admitted to a psychiatric hospital were in deteriorated chronic alcoholics.

CT will usually provide definitive evidence, showing displacement of midline structures, obliteration of the ventricle on the ipsilateral side and a low-density area underlying the skull. However, care must be taken, particularly with bilateral haematomas, which can sometimes be missed by CT (Davenport *et al.* 1994). The clotted blood is initially more dense than brain, becoming hypodense as it liquefies; it therefore passes through an isodense phase during the transitional period. Clues may lie in the generalised absence of sulci and a small ventricular system, but such signs are often equivocal. MRI has been shown to be greatly superior to CT, particularly in the demonstration of small subdural collections (Williams & Hogg 2000). In general, acute subdural haematomas are low signal and hypointense compared with brain on T2 MRI sequences, and isointense or hyperintense on T1 sequences; conversely, most chronic subdural haematomas are hyperintense on T2 sequences. Subdural haematomas with high signal on T1 sequences may be less likely to rebleed after surgery.

Evacuation of the haematoma can lead to excellent results, particularly in early cases. However, much depends on the presence of complicating pathologies, and the prognosis often proves to be poor in the elderly. Other factors that predict worse outcome are greater depth of coma at presentation and longer interval between the head injury and detection of the haematoma (El-Kadi *et al.* 2000). Mehta (1965) stressed the high morbidity among survivors, particularly by way of organic mental impairments. However, more recent follow-up studies find that the majority of cases treated for chronic subdural haematoma emerge with little if any disability, and only 10–20% have moderate or severe disability. These better outcomes probably reflect earlier detection and better surgical techniques. One small follow-up study of patients treated for chronic subdural haematoma only found retrieval-based memory deficits compared with controls (Machulda & Haut 2000). Another study of 26 patients requiring surgery for chronic subdural haematoma found that half of the 18 patients who had scores in the dementia range on MMSE preoperatively made a full psychological recovery after surgery (Ishikawa *et al.* 2002).

Systemic lupus erythematosus

Systemic lupus erythematosus (SLE) is a multiorgan autoimmune connective tissue disorder. The helpful review by D'Cruz (2006) describes the various clinical presentations and gives a broad overview of the condition, whereas that by D'Cruz *et al.* (2007) is valuable for those who need more detail about pathogenesis and treatment. SLE and antiphospholipid syndrome overlap both clinically and immunologically, and therefore some of what follows should be read alongside the discussion of antiphospholipid syndrome (see below).

Identification of anti-DNA antibodies is critical to diagnosis and alows SLE to be distinguished from other disorders such as rheumatoid arthritis and scleroderma. Cerebral involvement is prominent in a high proportion of cases. Moreover, it is evident that very occasionally neuropsychiatric complications can set in early, before the involvement of other systems is clinically obvious. Hence it has become important to include appropriate screening tests in the detailed evaluation of certain neurological and psychiatric patients as described below.

The disease is markedly more common in females, with a female to male ratio of 9 : 1. It mainly occurs in young adult life, with a mean age of onset of 30 years, but the range is wide. There is marked variation in rates across ethnic groups, so that for example the prevalence in white Americans is less than 10 per 100 000, whereas for Afro-Caribbean people it is over 100 per 100 000.

Pathogenesis

Antibodies against intracellular components are probably involved in the development of tissue lesions. An interesting study of US military personnel was able to identify the point at which people who were later to develop SLE turned autoantibody positive (Arbuckle *et al.* 2003). Thousands of healthy men and women had their blood taken and stored every 2 years over several years; 130 developed SLE. In 72 of these patients antibodies to DNA appeared on average 2.7 years before they developed clinical symptoms of the disease, and in some cases up to 9 years before. There seemed to be a surge of autoantibody activity just before illness onset, but it was also evidence that disease onset could not be predicted by antibody activity alone, and that other factors must be at play. Environmental factors include sunlight, silica and mercury, and numerous drugs (Sarzi-Puttini *et al.* 2005). Some cases seem to be precipitated by infection with Epstein–Barr virus. This may be because of molecular mimicry by the Epstein–Barr virus of Ro, a small intracellular RNA–protein complex. Ro autoantibodies are very common in SLE and among the first to be produced. They are also found in Sjögren's syndrome and are thus otherwise known as SS-A (Sjögren's syndrome A) antibodies. Using the database just described, the researchers were able to identify patients in whom the very first autoantibody produced, years before disease onset, was against Ro (McClain *et al.* 2005). Antibodies against this Ro epitope directly cross-reacted with a peptide from the Epstein–Barr virus nuclear antigen (EBNA). Thus Epstein–Barr virus infection might elicit antibodies against EBNA, which then cross-react with Ro and trigger an autoimmune reaction against Ro, and thus SLE.

One hypothesis suggests that disease arises because of a failure of the systems within the body to deal with the products of dead and dying cells (Munoz *et al.* 2005). Normally these products are rapidly phagocytosed and removed. However, in those with SLE the products of cell death are not properly cleared and instead become autoantigens that provoke an immune response, and this is particularly the case for intracellular components not normally visible to the immune system. For example, cells that are dying from apoptosis are understood to signal this fact by changes on their cell surface that indicate 'eat me' to local phagocytes. They are then silently removed without stimulating any inflammatory process. However, if the system is too slow, intracellular products of the dying cell will leak out and trigger autoantibody production. C-reactive protein (CRP) may be one of the pentraxin glycoproteins that activates the complement pathway and opsonises the dying cell for phagocytosis. CRP levels are relatively low in SLE, and an allele of one of the CRP genes has been found to be associated with the disorder. Another genetic link is with a polymorphism of the programmed cell death 1 gene (*PDCD1*).

The autoimmune hallmarks of SLE are autoantibodies against DNA, nucleus and other intracellular elements, activation of T and B cells, circulating immune complexes, and complement activation (Kyttaris *et al.* 2005). Cytokines, in particular interferon, are also involved. Some autoantibod-

ies may be associated with particular clinical presentations (Egner 2000; Sawalha & Harley 2004). As will be seen, it is the antiphospholipid antibodies, characteristic of antiphospholipid syndrome, that are particularly associated with neuropsychiatric SLE.

General clinical features

The onset is usually insidious with the development of fatigue, malaise and low-grade intermittent fever. A migratory arthritis or arthralgia ultimately develops in the majority of cases, closely resembling that of rheumatoid arthritis or rheumatic fever. Diffuse muscle aching is a common accompaniment as are painless mouth ulcers. Skin changes are frequent, although the classic butterfly eruption over the nose and cheeks is by no means always seen. Other skin manifestations include purpura, Raynaud's phenomenon and alopecia. Photosensitivity of the skin may be pronounced.

Lymphadenopathy, oedema and anaemia are often disclosed. Of the viscera, the kidneys are probably most frequently involved, also the pleura, lungs, heart and pericardium. Patients may present acutely with organ failure. Liver involvement is exceptional and gross splenomegaly rare. Anorexia, nausea, abdominal pain and vomiting are common. Hypertension is often considerable in degree and retinopathy may develop. A proportion of patients will develop antiphospholipid syndrome (see later in chapter).

The course of the disease may be acute, subacute or chronic and is generally difficult to predict. Chronic progression with repeated exacerbations and remissions appears to be a frequent pattern. It can be a recurrent mild illness with prolonged asymptomatic intervals. Worse prognosis is seen in those with multisystem involvement or multiple autoantibodies. The 5-year survival rates have improved from 50% reported in the 1950s to greater than 90% in the 1990s, with 15-year survival rates in excess of 80% in some series (Gladman 1992). This is probably attributable to earlier diagnosis, better treatment and the more frequent recognition of mild forms of the disease. Nevertheless, central nervous system (CNS) involvement still ranks with renal failure and accelerated atherosclerosis among the commoner causes of death.

Haemolytic anaemia is often accompanied by leucopenia, especially lymphopenia, and occasionally by thrombocytopenia. The erythrocyte sedimentation rate (ESR) is raised in about 90% of cases, showing an approximate correlation with the current stage of activity of the disease. Yet the CRP is often normal, giving a characteristic pattern of raised ESR and normal CRP. The detection of antinuclear antibodies by indirect immunofluorescence is the most sensitive screening test, identifying over 95% of cases (Venables 1993). In practice almost all patients with SLE have positive antinuclear antibodies at a dilution of 1:80 (Egner 2000). Antibodies to double-stranded DNA are more specific to the disorder, being virtually restricted to SLE. Other antibodies against ribosomes, histones, ribonucleoprotien, Ro and phospholipids including cardiolipin, some of which are not specific for SLE, may be found. Biopsy of skin lesions, or occasionally renal biopsy, may give valuable confirmation of the diagnosis.

SLE carries a significant risk of accelerated atherosclerosis. Antiphospholipid antibodies, renal disease and steroid treatment may play a part in this process (Jennekens & Kater 2002), but for many it is not fully explained. Although SLE as an attributable risk for stroke is low (i.e. of all patients with stroke, only very few have SLE), nevertheless young people with stroke should be screened for SLE and antiphospholipid syndrome.

Neuropsychiatric problems in SLE

Neuropsychiatric manifestations are now being reported in up to 60% of patients with SLE, when comprehensively studied and followed for reasonably long periods of time. Indeed Hughes (1974) suggests that CNS involvement may overtake renal disease as the major clinical problem in the disorder, in that it carries a high mortality and the response to treatment is uncertain.

The neurological and psychiatric features of SLE lack any characteristic form or pattern but are as varied as other manifestations of the disease. Table 8.2 summarises six recent studies that have assessed the prevalence of various neuropsychiatric symptoms and signs in SLE. The data in the table are not based on any assessment that the symptom or sign is attributable to SLE; it is simply an assessment of whether the symptom or sign is present. As can be seen many of the neuropsychiatric accompaniments are non-specific, with high rates for example of headache and mood disorders. Indeed some authors (Denburg et al. 1997) highlight the rather non-specific nature of neuropsychiatric SLE and suggest that the rates of some psychiatric symptoms are similar to those seen for example in general medical outpatients. When authors attempt to define the neuropsychiatric morbidity found in patients with SLE that is definitely attributable to the SLE, seizure disorder, cerebrovascular disease, neuropathy and acute confusional states feature most strongly (Hanly et al. 2007).

Anxiety, depression and sleep disturbance are common, but may not be very different from the rates found in other rheumatology patients (Pincus et al. 1999). However, Ganz et al. (1972) showed that depression was chiefly responsible for the increased incidence of psychiatric disorder in SLE compared with rheumatoid arthritis. In patients with SLE, depressive symptoms were twice as common as organic mental symptoms, occurring in 51% and 22% respectively. In a more recent study of 52 patients with SLE but without overt neuropsychiatric symptoms compared with 29 patients with rheumatoid arthritis, those with SLE were more depressed

and more distressed (Kozora et al. 2005a). At least some of the sleep disturbance found in SLE is probably due to pain (Gudbjornsson & Hetta 2001) or depression (Costa et al. 2005). Fatigue is a common symptom in SLE (Wysenbeek et al. 1993) and is associated with reduced aerobic fitness and muscle strength (Tench et al. 2002).

Some authors suggest that neuropsychiatric symptoms may appear several years before the diagnosis of SLE, but here again the matter of attribution has to be taken into account; many of those symptoms might have been present even if the patient had never developed SLE. Nevertheless, in some cases there is good anecdotal evidence for psychiatric disturbance as the presenting feature. Lim et al. (1988) reported a patient who presented with acute behavioural change, paranoid ideas and a degree of impairment of consciousness, and who was soon afterwards found to have SLE with renal involvement. Three further psychotic episodes coincided with recrudescences of physical symptoms. Hopkinson et al. (1992) discovered three cases of SLE on routine screening of 296 admissions to acute psychiatric units. In the series of Lim et al. (1988), 12% of patients with SLE had a psychotic illness at some stage. The point prevalence of psychosis is much lower, of the order of 2–5%, and in many of these cases occurs in the context of a delirious state (Ovsiew & Utset 2002).

In the past delirium was probably the most frequent of the mental abnormalities. For example, it was present at some time or another in approximately 30% of patients in Heine's (1969) series. Often referred to as 'lupus psychosis' it would last for hours or days, then subside completely. The picture may be of quiet confusion and clouding of consciousness, or more florid delirium with visual and auditory hallucinations and excessive motor activity (Johnson & Richardson 1968). The degree of disorientation and memory impairment may fluctuate markedly from time to time. However, more recent studies (see Table 8.2) find only about 3% with acute confusional states. This presumably reflects earlier diagnosis of SLE, such that much milder cases are now forming the majority. In this setting mood disorders become the most common of the mental disorders to be found (Table 8.2).

Cognitive impairment is usually mild, often evanescent, and similar to that seen in subcortical disease. Attention and concentration, memory and processing speed are most vulnerable, followed by executive and visuospatial problems. For example, in cases that show cognitive impairment only 5% of patients are found to have 'cortical' deficits on MMSE (Leritz et al. 2000). Of patients with evidence of CNS involvement, 75% will have some degree of cognitive impairment compared with about 25% of those without other evidence of neuropsychiatric SLE (Carbotte et al. 1986; Kozora et al. 1996). The degree of impairment is also related to overall disease activity, so that patients with severe disease, whether or not it involves the CNS, are more likely to show impairment (Sweet et al. 2004). There is no consistent evidence that steroid use

Table 8.2 Prevalence (%) of neuropsychiatric symptoms and signs in systemic lupus erythematosus. (Based on Mok *et al.* 2006.)

	Ainiala *et al.* (2001) (Finland)	Brey *et al.* (2002) (Hispanic 56%)	Sanna *et al.* (2003) (London)	Afeltra *et al.* (2003) (Italy)	Mok *et al.* (2006) (Chinese)	Hanly *et al.* (2007) (White 52%)	Mean
No. of patients	46	128	323	61	282	572	
Mean age (years)	45	43	42	40	39	35	
Duration of illness (years)	14	8	11	10	7	5 months	
Per cent female	85	94	95	87	91	88	
Per cent on steroids	54	60	—	100	66	68	
Cerebrovascular disease	15	2	18	24	7	8	12
Headache	54	57	24	21	3	39	28
Movement disorder*	2	1	1	0	0.7	0.8	1
Seizure disorder	9	16	8	11	6	8	10
Polyneuropathy	28	22	3	13	0	4	12
Cranial neuropathy	7	2	2	4	2	2	3
Cognitive dysfunction	80†	79†	11†	52†	3.5	5	38
Acute confusional state	7	0	4	0	3.5	5	3
Anxiety disorder	13	24	7	6	1.1	7	10
Mood disorder	44	51	17	27	3.5	12	26
Psychosis	0	5	8	0	5.3	3	4

* When defined, chorea is most common.
† Assessed using battery of neuropsychological tests.

plays much of a role, although the occasional study does find greater cognitive impairment in those taking steroids (McLaurin *et al.* 2005); however this may simply be because use of steroids is a surrogate marker of more severe disease. In those without clinically manifest CNS disease it may be difficult to link cognitive impairment to findings on cerebral imaging. In this setting one study found 35% to have enlarged ventricles or white matter hyperintensities, and 35% to have neuropsycholgical impairment, but the two were not closely related (Kozora *et al.* 1998).

Cognitive impairment is often found to be associated with the presence of psychiatric problems, particularly depression. In one study, as the psychiatric illness improved over time so did the cognitive impairment (Hay *et al.* 1994). Perhaps this is why other follow-up studies have also found a good proportion of those with cognitive impairment when first seen to be performing in the normal range a year or two later (Hanly *et al.* 1994). In another study, 123 patients were assessed every 4 months over at least 3 years on a battery of computerised neuropsychological tests particularly involving psychomotor speed (McLaurin *et al.* 2005). Over time there was a marked improvement in test scores, presumably at least partly due to practice effects. Stable scores were found in a follow-up of 51 stable patients, seen for their second evaluation on average 20 months after the first (Carlomagno *et al.* 2000). Of the 51 patients, 15 had cognitive impairment and in 14 this was still present at 20 months. Not one of the 15 cases deteriorated, although four patients had developed cognitive impairment in the mean time. Even after 5 years there is no evidence for progressive deterioration (Waterloo *et al.* 2002); as a group, 28 patients showed no change in the majority of neuropsychological test results, and in fact on two of the nine tests they showed improved performance at 5 years.

It seems likely that mild cognitive impairment is more vulnerable to psychological state and more likely to remit compared with more severe impairment that tends to be constant over time, and is better explained by the severity of SLE, particular if it affects the CNS, and its treatment. This divergence may explain the apparently contradictory findings of studies which have looked at psychiatric predictors of cognitive impairment in patients with SLE (Harrison & Ravdin 2002). As many studies find an association, particularly with depression or psychological distress, as fail to find an effect. For example, in a small study of 11 depressed SLE patients compared with seven non-depressed patients, no differences were found on neuropsychological test performance (Denburg *et al.* 1997). Moreover, in 20 patients assessed during a flare-up of their SLE, eight had a psychiatric diagnosis, largely anxiety disorder with or without panic disorder (Segui *et al.* 2000). A year later when the disease was no longer active, only two remained psychiatrically unwell. However, cognitive impairment, assessed using the rather crude MMSE, showed no change over the year despite the improvement in mental health. This finding is in contrast to that of Hay *et al.* (1994) (see earlier). Furthermore, in a careful study comparing 52 patients with SLE but without neurological involvement with 27 patients with neuropsychiatric SLE and with controls, depression was found to be the best predictor of cognitive impairment (Monastero *et al.* 2001). The neuropsychiatric SLE patients had higher scores on both depression and anxiety measured using the Hamilton Depression Rating Scale and the Hamilton Anxiety Rating Scale. However, no significant differences were found between the two SLE groups on the neuropsychological test battery, although the neuropsychiatric patients tended to be worse on all measures. In a multivariate analysis the patient's score on the Hamilton Depression Rating Scale was the only clinical variable to predict severity of cognitive impairment. More recently, Kozora *et al.* (2006) compared 22 patients with neuropsychiatric SLE with 31 non-neuropsychiatric SLE and healthy controls and found that symptoms of depression, fatigue, pain and complaints of cognitive dysfunction were more common in SLE, although only objective cognitive impairment was greater in the neuropsychiatric SLE cases. Within the cases with neuropsychiatric SLE the four symptoms of depression, fatigue, pain and objective cognitive impairment were all associated with one another, an association not seen in the other SLE cases nor in controls. The authors suggested a single common aetiology might explain this symptom cluster.

Headache is perhaps the most common of all neurological problems encountered in the disease, often with features typical of migraine (McCune & Golbus 1988), with about half of migraine patients having aura. However, it may be difficult to be confident that the headache is due to SLE (Hanly *et al.* 2007). A review of headache in SLE concluded that although 32% of SLE patients reported migraine and 23% tension-type headache, there was little evidence that these rates are different from those in controls (Mitsikostas *et al.* 2004).

Seizures, ischaemic strokes and TIAs, and neuropathies are the common neurological manifestations of SLE (see Table 8.2). In contrast, in antiphospholipid syndrome the neurological picture is dominated by ischaemic strokes and TIAs (Table 8.3). The conditions overlap. Strokes are more likely in antiphospholipid antibody-positive SLE than antiphospholipid antibody-negative SLE. Some of this increased risk may be because patients with SLE who are antiphospholipid antibody positive are more likely to have heart valve disease (Khamashta *et al.* 1990). Furthermore, patients with antiphospholipid syndrome are most likely to have epilepsy if they also have SLE; in primary antiphospholipid syndrome 6% of patients have epilepsy, whereas when antiphospholipid syndrome is secondary to SLE the rate is 13% (Shoenfeld *et al.* 2004). In fact it seems likely that patients with both SLE and antiphospholipid syndrome are at greatest risk of neuropsychiatric sequelae. For example, in

Table 8.3 Neurological disorders occurring at some stage in 1000 patients during the course of antiphospholipid syndrome. (From Cervera *et al.* 2002.)

	Number of patients
Migraine	202
Stroke	198
Transient ischaemic attack	111
Epilepsy	70
Multi-infarct dementia	25
Chorea	13
Acute encephalopathy	11
Transient amnesia	7
Cerebral venous thrombosis	7

667 patients with SLE neuropsychiatric problems were more common in the 15% with a comorbid diagnosis of antiphospholipid syndrome (Alarcon-Segovia *et al.* 1997). There was no good evidence that any particular neurological manifestation was selectively affected, although cerebrovascular disease was the only condition that was statistically more common in antiphospholipid syndrome-positive SLE.

In SLE, cranial nerve palsies are among the commoner neurological signs. Usually they set in suddenly without prodromes and most are transient. Disorders of external ocular movement, pupillary abnormalities and vertigo are the most frequent, more rarely disorders of the fifth, seventh and bulbar nerves. Visual field defects are often partly due to retinal changes. Papilloedema may result from a local retinal lesion and optic atrophy may follow. Peripheral neuropathy is usually symmetrical and distal, with both sensory and motor deficits. Chorea is probably the most common of the movement disorders, but these also include tremors, parkinsonian rigidity and ataxia due to brainstem lesions. All are relatively rare. Choreiform movements in association with SLE may at first be diagnosed as Sydenham's chorea. Paraparesis due to transverse myelitis of the cord occurs infrequently. The neurological symptoms and signs of SLE may therefore sometimes resemble those found in multiple sclerosis, so for example optic neuropathy and internuclear ophthalmoplegia are common to both, as are CSF oligoclonal bands.

In SLE and antiphospholipid syndrome, seizures, generalised or partial, are not uncommon and often unexplained by a brain lesion visible on neuroimaging (Cimaz *et al.* 2006). In patients with SLE, those who are anticardiolipin antibody positive are more likely to have seizures. In patients with antiphospholipid syndrome, part of the increased risk of epilepsy is explained by the extent of cerebrovascular disease and, to a lesser extent, valvular heart disease. However, much of the increased risk is not related to ischaemic events, and it seems quite likely that antibodies acting on neurones may be responsible (Shoenfeld *et al.* 2004). As already noted, patients with both SLE and antiphospholipid syndrome are at greatest risk of epilepsy, compared with SLE alone (Appenzeller *et al.* 2004) or antiphospholipid syndrome alone (Shoenfeld *et al.* 2004).

These findings have led to research into antiphospholipid antibodies in patients with epilepsy (Cimaz *et al.* 2006). However, several studies have found that antiphospholipid antibodies, anticardiolipin antibodies and lupus anticoagulant seem to be as common in control populations as they are in epilepsy. Subgroup analyses have found that higher frequency of seizures may be associated with antibody-positive status. In children there may be a better case for the association between being antiphospholipid antibody positive and having epilepsy. All such studies are complicated by the observation that some of the anticonvulsants may be associated with autoantibody production.

Hinchey *et al.* (1996) have described a posterior reversible encephalopathy syndrome in which white matter changes are found on T2-weighted MRI posteriorly in the brain (see also section on hypertensive encephalopathy earlier in chapter). Patients often present with headache, seizures and visual or mental disturbance, and the condition is associated with hypertension, renal disease and rheumatoid conditions. Diffusion-weighted MRI suggests that the high signal in white matter is due to oedema, probably vasogenic, and this is consistent with the observation that the MRI findings often improve as the condition remits. The condition is rare, but several of the cases have been in patients with SLE (Kur & Esdaile 2006; Magnano *et al.* 2006). In these patients visual loss and seizures are characteristic, severe hypertension and headaches almost always present along with renal disease, and the condition is often related to treatment with immunosuppressive drugs. The majority made a full recovery once the hypertension was treated.

Neuroimaging in SLE

Neuroimaging may be useful in the assessment of a patient with SLE by identifying lesions that are clinically silent, or clarifying the extent to which the brain has been affected when neuropsychiatric symptoms are present. Sometimes it may help to indicate the cause of the neurological disorder, for example showing that a large-vessel stroke as opposed to deterioration of diffuse periventricular white matter disease is responsible for a recent-onset confusional state. However, much of what follows is of more theoretical interest. How easy is it to demonstrate abnormalities on neuroimaging in patients with SLE, and in particular neuropsychiatric SLE? And does the picture that is found tell us about causation of symptoms?

Earlier studies suggested that MRI is not very good at distinguishing cases with neuropsychiatric SLE from those without: in both cases a good proportion, perhaps as many as

50%, have normal MRI (Tanabe & Weiner 1997). Although MRI generally could distinguish between patients with focal signs and those without, those with clinically 'diffuse' neuropsychiatric syndromes, including for example headache, seemed to have as many abnormalities as those without. In those with clinically diffuse syndromes, the non-focal lesions that were found were said to be frequently reversible with steroid treatment, suggesting they were due to oedema. However, more recent studies, reviewed by Govoni *et al.* (2004), have found MRI abnormalities to be more frequent in neuropsychiatric SLE (Sanna *et al.* 2000; Bosma *et al.* 2002). So, for example, in patients without neuropsychiatric involvement, 25–50% of patients show abnormalities; this rises to 75% in patients with neuropsychiatric SLE. Perhaps the study with the least risk of ascertainment bias is that from Finland where they were careful to ensure that all cases of SLE within the 440 000 catchment were identified (Ainiala *et al.* 2005); 43 patients with SLE, 19 of whom had neuropsychiatric SLE, were carefully matched to 43 controls from the same population database and assessed for SLE illness severity and evidence of neuropsychiatric problems. MRI scan data were blindly rated for evidence of lesions on T1 and T2 sequences and were analysed using computer software to determine CSF volume as a proportion of intracranial volume, a measure of cerebral atrophy. Patients with SLE were different from controls on all three counts; they had greater cerebral atrophy and more evidence of both T1 and T2 lesions. Furthermore, within the SLE group greater MRI abnormalities were associated with presence of neuropsychiatric SLE. In particular, patients with cognitive impairment had more severe cerebral atrophy and T2 lesions, those with cerebrovascular disease were more severely affected on all three measures, and those with seizures had worse cerebral atrophy. No other single neuropsychiatric problem was associated with MRI change. Cerebral atrophy and T1 lesions also correlated with cumulative steroid usage.

The commonest MRI finding, seen in 15–60% (Govoni *et al.* 2004), is small punctate lesions in subcortical white matter, mainly periventricular or subcortical. In the past these were sometimes regarded as evidence of vasculitis, but in fact probably represent small areas of infarction or ischaemia due to a localised vasculopathy. Other relatively common abnormalities are cortical atrophy and ventricular dilatation, periventricular white matter changes, and major infarcts. Occasionally there will be evidence of cerebral venous thrombosis. T1 lesions are more likely to represent the gliosis of infarcts and demyelinating lesions that are well established. Lesions on T2-weighted imaging are more likely to resolve, sometimes as a result of steroid therapy, and this may be because they are at least partly due to cerebral oedema. Gadolinium-enhancing lesions on MRI, suggesting a breakdown of the blood–brain barrier, are not common, but when seen also tend to disappear with treatment (Miller *et al.* 1992). It has been suggested that T2-weighted small punctate lesions, mainly localised to white matter, represent small-vessel vasculopathy (see later).

More sophisticated MRI techniques include measures of DWI and magnetisation transfer imaging (MTI). The former relies on the signal change associated with alterations in the ability of water molecules to diffuse in the extracellular or intracellular space. In particular, early signal change on DWI may be found when intracellular oedema occurs, for example due to cerebral ischaemia. Intracellular water has a more restricted ability to diffuse and the consequent reduction in the apparent diffusion coefficient (ADC) can be seen as high signal on DWI. On the other hand, a breakdown in tissue integrity can be manifest as an increase in ADC. This is what was found in a study of 11 patients with neuropsychiatric SLE but without MRI evidence of infarcts, only allowing white matter lesions of less than 5 mm. The findings were not striking and could not be seen by direct visualisation of DWI images, but instead relied on inspection of the histogram of ADC activity across all brain pixels, showing that patients with SLE had more pixels with high ADC values (Bosma *et al.* 2003). On the other hand, in a less sophisticated study of 20 unselected cases of neuropsychiatric SLE, high signal (reduced ADC) was found on DWI, largely in association with infarcts or vasogenic oedema (Moritani *et al.* 2001).

By detecting macromolecues that have been diluted or destroyed, MTI may be more sensitive to brain damage than standard MRI measures. It is for example affected by the concentration of phospholipids and myelin. In healthy brain the signal, as expressed by the magnetisation transfer ratio (MTR), is relatively homogeneous across brain voxels. Brain damage tends to a cause a decrease in and flattening of the peak of the histogram of number of voxels against activity, as found for example in normal-appearing white matter in multiple sclerosis. In SLE there is preliminary evidence that MTI may be able to detect abnormalities not otherwise evident on MRI. Rovaris *et al.* (2000) studied nine patients with neuropsychiatric SLE and 15 with SLE without neuropsychiatric involvement and were able to compare the findings with controls and patients with multiple sclerosis. The analysis was restricted to normal-appearing brain tissue by removing from the analysis pixels affected by macroscopic lesions on MRI. Normal-appearing brain tissue in patients with neuropsychiatric SLE or multiple sclerosis was similar with significantly lower peaks than those found in both controls and SLE patients without neuropsychiatric involvement. However, the authors do not take account of the fact that the neuropsychiatric SLE patients were on average about 10–14 years older than the other groups. Another study of neuropsychiatric SLE patients who did not have infarcts, probably based at least partly on the same cohort described above showing higher ADC values, found that MTI changes correlated with clinical measures of neurological, cognitive and psychiatric functioning. More recently the same group has found that these changes in the MTR histogram peak height over time are in line with the patients' clinical condition (Emmer *et al.* 2006), and that changes in MTI appear to be related to the presence of IgM anticardiolipin antibodies (Steens *et al.* 2006).

Further support for disturbance of cerebral cellular function in SLE comes from magnetic resonance spectroscopy (MRS), which can measure the signal from several chemicals found in cerebral tissue. The neurochemical signal from *N*-acetylaspartic acid (NAA) is found almost exclusively in neurones, with lower signal suggesting neuronal dysfunction. Choline-related metabolites contribute to the Cho peak of MRS and this tends to be raised in the presence of brain injury. On the other hand, the creatine (Cr) signal is regarded as being relatively constant regardless of disease status, so is used as an internal reference. The NAA/Cr and Cho/Cr ratios are therefore regarded as measuring NAA and Cho activity respectively. In SLE there is reduced NAA signal not only in injured areas but also in normal-appearing white matter (Govoni *et al.* 2004; Appenzeller *et al.* 2006). However, within normal-appearing brain tissue it was only areas defined as hypoperfused using ^{99}Tc-labelled hexamethyl-propyleneamine oxine (HMPAO)-SPECT that showed altered NAA/Cho and Cho/Cr ratios, lower and higher respectively, compared with areas with normal perfusion (Castellino *et al.* 2005). A lowered NAA/Cho ratio may be a particularly sensitive marker of disease activity and in 12 patients with SLE the ratio correlated with scores on cognitive testing (Brooks *et al.* 1999). However, in a small study of seven cases of SLE without neuropsychiatric involvement compared with seven controls, no differences were found between the groups on NAA/Cr despite the SLE patients having significant cognitive impairment (Kozora *et al.* 2005b). Furthermore, in a study of 90 patients with SLE, with 50 having repeat scanning after 12 months, the NAA/Cr ratio mapped more closely to SLE disease activity than clinical evidence of CNS involvement (Appenzeller *et al.* 2005).

SPECT is one of the most sensitive techniques for detecting cerebral changes in SLE (Govoni *et al.* 2004). The typical picture is of widespread multifocal areas of reduced uptake suggesting patchy perfusion, most frequently in the distribution of the middle cerebral artery. Abnormalities are found in 86–100% of patients with major symptoms of neuropsychiatric SLE, and even in patients without neuropsychiatric involvement 10–50% will show abnormalities on SPECT. Of particular interest is the ability of SPECT to reveal changes in brain tissue that appears normal on conventional MRI. Moreover, as noted above these SPECT abnormalities tally with metabolic changes, identified using MRS, in the hypoperfused but normal MRI-appearing tissue. Using ^{99}Tc-labelled ethylcysteinate dimer (ECD)-SPECT, global hypoperfusion particularly involving frontal and temporal lobes has been found to distinguish patients with and without CNS involvement (Appenzeller *et al.* 2007). In a study of 56 patients with SLE, mostly with mild or stable disease, HMPAO-SPECT was compared with the results of a battery of neuropsychological tests (Waterloo *et al.* 2001). Psychomotor slowing correlated with regional CBF as measured by SPECT in parietal lobe, but could also be explained by evidence of cerebral infarcts on MRI. In fact the SPECT findings did not add to what was already known using conventional MRI. This finding runs counter to others which suggest that evidence of hypoperfusion on SPECT does explain some of the cognitive impairment of SLE that cannot be explained by manifest brain injury using conventional MRI. In support of this failure to find added value of SPECT, the authors cite studies finding poor correlation between SPECT and PET, and one study using PET which failed to demonstrate glucose hypometabolism in patients with cognitive impairment. However, one study did find changes in glucose hypometabolism using PET in patients with SLE and neuropsychiatric involvement compared to those without (Weiner *et al.* 2000). Almost all patients with significant cognitive impairment also had reduced metabolism in parieto-occipital regions regardless of findings on MRI. Another study measured regional CBF in 20 SLE patients with no history of stroke, movement disorder or dementia, and no major (i.e. >2 mm) lesions on MRI using ^{99}Tc-ECD-SPECT (Oda *et al.* 2005). Compared with controls reduced regional CBF was found in posterior cingulate and thalamus, but only in the seven patients with either psychosis (*N* = 3) or mood disorder (*N* = 4). This may in part reflect the changes in blood flow produced by mental symptoms.

Aetiology and pathogenesis of neuropsychiatric manifestations in SLE and antiphospholipid syndrome

Pathological changes in the brain have been abundantly described in SLE, chiefly in the form of disease of small blood vessels leading to scattered infarctions and haemorrhages. The smaller arterioles and capillaries are principally affected, with evidence of inflammatory, destructive and proliferative changes. The commonest finding at post-mortem is a small-vessel non-inflammatory proliferative vasculopathy consisting of intimal proliferation with fibrinoid degeneration in the vessel walls or hyalinisation with necrosis (Johnson & Richardson 1968; Jennekens & Kater 2002). This may be associated with microglial proliferation around the capillaries or with microhaemorrhages due to extravasation of erythrocytes and fibrin. The vascular changes are especially prevalent in the cortex and brainstem. Small vessels may show 'beading', with alternating stenosis and dilatation on angiography (Tanabe & Weiner 1997), similar to that seen in cerebral vasculitis. On the other hand, a true 'vasculitis' is only present in about 10% of cases (Belmont *et al.* 1996). Cerebral SLE can therefore be understood as a diffuse but patchy microvascular disorder, and this explains why multiple fairly localised perfusion defects are seen on SPECT (see earlier). This small-vessel cerebral angiopathy probably explains the cognitive impairment of patients who otherwise have no neuropsychiatric involvement (Jennckens & Kater 2002). Infarcted areas are usually small and multiple, although extensive areas of softening and large intracerebral haemorrhages occasionally occur. Serum S-100B levels are raised in SLE, particularly in those with neuropsychiatric involvement, probably because of ongoing neuronal damage (Schenatto *et al.* 2006).

Clinicopathological correlations at post-mortem are far from exact. O'Connor and Musher (1966) found that gross impairment of CNS function could exist with no demonstrable lesions at post-mortem; conversely, patients without neuropsychiatric manifestations could show widespread cerebral pathology. Other factors such as uraemia, electrolyte disturbance and hypertension may therefore make their own contributions to mental disturbance.

An additional mechanism may depend on immunological reactions that implicate brain tissue. Thus a review of cerebral inflammation and degeneration in neuropsychiatric SLE suggests that brain-specific autoantibody production, immune complex deposition, and intrathecal production of proinflammatory cytokines are likely to be involved (Trysberg & Tarkowski 2004). The best evidence is for the role of antiphospholipid and anticardiolipin antibodies and lupus anticoagulant (Sanna *et al.* 2003). Antiphospholipid antibodies increase the likelihood of large-vessel cerebrovascular disease, and also probably contribute to the small-vessel vasculopathy. Whether in addition they have direct effects on neuronal tissue is uncertain, although this is a case frequently made for anticardiolipin antibodies. For example, antiphospholipid antibodies have been shown to bind to neuronal tissue, causing membrane depolarisation of synaptosomes (Chapman *et al.* 1999). Moreover, anticardiolipin antibodies may interact with the GABA receptor-mediated chloride channel of snail neurones (Liou *et al.* 1994).

Other immunological markers that have been associated with neuropsychiatric SLE include the proinflammatory cytokine interleukin (IL)-6. A recent review found that 20 autoantibodies had been studied in SLE and antiphospholipid syndrome, 11 being specific for brain and nine systemic (Zandman-Goddard *et al.* 2007). The review suggests that cognitive impairment, psychosis and depression could often be linked to one or other of these antibodies. However, the review did not take account of the many studies with negative findings. For example, early suggestions that antiribosomal P antibodies are particularly associated with neuropsychiatric disorder have not been confirmed (Gerli *et al.* 2002).

There has been recent interest in antibodies to N-methyl-D-aspartate (NMDA) receptors. Antibodies to double-stranded DNA are one of the hallmarks of SLE, and in some patients a subset of these antibodies may cross-react with the ligand-binding domain of the NMDA receptor (Kowal *et al.* 2006). In mice these anti-NMDA receptor antibodies cause neuronal apoptosis. In a clinical study, although there was no effect of anti-NMDA antibody activity on cognitive impairment, high titres were associated with depression; 6 of 11 patients with depression had high titres, whereas only 10 of 48 non-depressed patients did (Lapteva *et al.* 2006).

Considerable attention has been given to the possible role of steroids in precipitating confusional episodes, with a consensus of opinion that they can only rarely be held responsible. Thus similar episodes were often reported before steroids were introduced, they continue to be reported in patients not having such treatment, lowering of the dose has an inconsistent effect, and episodes do not necessarily recur when steroids are given again during later relapses. Nevertheless, the possibility must be borne in mind that steroids may occasionally have an aggravating or precipitating effect.

Neuropsychiatric SLE may produce changes in the cortical organisation of psychomotor processing. Patients without any neurological involvement of their right arm, and with no lesion on MRI affecting the left pyramidal tract, were studied using fMRI. When asked to move their right arm under test conditions they showed a larger area of activation of contralateral sensorimotor cortex than did normal controls (Rocca *et al.* 2006).

Treatment

The treatment of SLE is best undertaken by experts, particularly as there is now a variety of new immunosuppressant agents available. Current practice is outlined by D'Cruz *et al.* (2007). In addition to specific treatment, patients should be warned to avoid undue exposure to the sun, and intercurrent infections should be treated promptly since they can lead to exacerbations. Preparations containing estrogen, such as the contraceptive pill, are best avoided partly because they may cause the disease to flare up and partly because of the increased risk of thrombotic events.

Steroids remain one of the mainstays of treatment for the systemic effects of the disease and are also important in managing certain neuropsychiatric developments. Prednisolone is used most commonly. Cyclophosphamide can be very successful, for example in those with renal disease, but has worrying side effects. Mycophenolate mofetil, a drug that inhibits B and T cell proliferation as well as having other immunosuppressive actions, has been introduced and will probably replace cyclophosphamide for the treatment of renal SLE because it is far better tolerated and probably more effective. Rituximab, a monoclonal antibody directed against B cells and used in lymphoma, has the potential to produce remissions, perhaps when other treatments have failed.

The management of neuropsychiatric manifestations can prove difficult, though fortunately most episodes are transient and self-limiting. Special attention must be paid to clouding of consciousness or mild intellectual impairment in what appear at first sight to be non-organic disturbances. EEG and MRI can be helpful in deciding the likelihood of an organic cerebral cause, but are not an accurate guide in every case. Other causes must be carefully considered: uraemia, electrolyte disturbance, hypertension, infection or steroid administration. In a prospective survey of 36 episodes of cerebral disturbance, Wong *et al.* (1991) considered that active SLE was responsible in less than one-quarter of cases, with infection, steroids or hypertensive encephalopathy accounting for the remainder. When confusion or delirium appear with fresh relapses of the disorder, steroids may help considerably in their resolution. On other occasions, however, they may stand to aggravate rather than help the clinical picture, some psychotic episodes responding to a reduction in current dosage.

For patients who are reasonably stable, physical exercise appears to be helpful. Tench *et al.* (2003) studied 93 reasonably stable but largely sedentary patients who were randomised to receive an exercise programme, a relaxation programme or treatment as usual. Those in the exercise programme were asked to exercise, for example by going for a walk, for at least 30–50 minutes at least three times a week. After the 12-week treatment, significantly more patients in the exercise group rated themselves as having less fatigue and at least 'much improved' on the Clinical Global Impression Scale, compared with either the relaxation or treatment as usual group. It is therefore important to consider opportunities for exercise alongside other psychosocial issues. Matters such as the home environment and financial responsibilities have to be considered, as do the needs of the family. The attitudes of clinicians may have large impacts on quality of life, and good communication between doctor and patient, as in any condition particularly when long-lasting, is crucial (Seawell & Danoff-Burg 2004).

Vasculitis of the central nervous system

Vasculitis is inflammation of the blood vessel wall and is synonymous with angiitis. The classification of vasculitis has changed over the years. Recent insights into the pathogenesis of these conditions have led to a reappraisal of the best way to classify vasculitis, in particular as it affects the nervous system. Even though there is no universal agreement on the terms to be used, most authorities now agree on the value of a classification that acknowledges the size of the vessels preferentially affected, the presence or absence of autoantibodies, and whether the condition affects the CNS in isolation or is accompanied by systemic disease (Carolei & Sacco 2003; Younger 2004) (Table 8.4). It is accepted that regardless of which system is used the categories will overlap to some extent with one another.

Systemic vasculitis is usually referred to as primary when no cause for the condition in terms of infection, drugs or malignancy is found (Zandi & Coles 2007). Some authors

Table 8.4 Vasculitis involving the CNS.

Systemic vasculitis (generally involves multiple organs including the CNS)
Small vessels (arterioles, capillaries and venules) (generally ANCA
    positive)
    Wegener's granulomatosis*
    Microscopic polyangiitis*
    Churg–Strauss syndrome*
    Henoch–Schönlein purpura[†]

Medium-sized vessels (medium and small arteries)
    Polyarteritis nodosa

Large vessels (arteries) (ANCA negative)
    Giant-cell (temporal) arteritis
    Takayasu's arteritis

Vasculitis confined to the CNS[‡]
Primary angiitis of the CNS
    Granulomatous angiitis of the CNS
    Benign angiitis of the CNS

Note that there are more patients with vasculitis involving the CNS as a result of a systemic vasculitis than there are patients with a vasculitis confined to the CNS.
* One of the primary small-vessel vasculitides (Pavone *et al.* 2006).
[†] Often regarded as a hypersensitiviy vasculitis, e.g. following drug administration, ANCA negative, IgA complex positive.
[‡] In some cases of systemic vasculitis, the vasculitis is found only in the CNS.
ANCA, antineutrophil cytoplasmic antibody.

suggest that vasculitis associated with the connective tissue disorders, for example when occasionally seen in SLE or rheumatoid arthritis, should also be regarded as secondary. Conditions that mimic vasculitis, such as infective endocarditis or mitochondrial disease, need to be excluded.

The vasculitides that affect the CNS can also be regarded as primary and secondary. However, in this case, 'primary' means there is no systemic vasculitis to explain the CNS involvement (Table 8.4). Vasculitis of the CNS, in the absence of systemic involvement, is usually called primary angiitis of the CNS, although others refer to it as idiopathic or isolated angiitis of the CNS. Certain principles are generally common to all the cerebral vasculitides.

• There is a very pleomorphic clinical picture: acute or insidious onset; diffuse, focal or multifocal signs and symptoms; single incident or relapsing/remitting. Presentations may include headache, delirium, seizures, subarachnoid haemorrhage, strokes/TIAs, focal neurological symptoms and signs, cranial neuropathies, cord lesions, peripheral neuropathy (particularly mononeuritis multiplex), or psychosis or mood disorder.

• Psychiatric sequelae are related to encephalopathy, focal cortical lesions and psychological reaction to illness.

• It is necessary to have a high index of suspicion; the vasculitides are rare but treatable.

- They are often accompanied by general systemic symptoms, malaise, fever and weight loss. In systemic vasculitis, any organ may be affected but particularly kidney. Systemic vasculitis with secondary involvement of CNS is more common that primary vasculitis (angiitis) of the CNS.
- Acute-phase markers, ESR and CRP, are often raised. Antineutrophil cytoplasmic antibodies (ANCAs) are sometimes present.
- MRI shows diffuse cortical and deep white matter ischaemic lesions, strokes or subarachnoid haemorrhage, or gadolinium meningeal enhancement.
- CSF shows increased protein and moderate pleocytosis; there may be oligoclonal bands.
- There is a need to exclude other diseases, particularly those that closely mimic vasculitis.
- Angiography shows characteristic beading of arteries, and sequential stenosis and ectasia (dilatation), but this is non-specific unless it involves multiple vessels in multiple vascular territories.
- Biopsy is the definitive diagnosis, but there may be false negatives when vasculitis is focal. Cerebral, meningeal, nerve or arterial biopsy should be taken. Diagnosis may be based on biopsy of another organ, e.g. renal biopsy.
- The vasculitides generally respond to treatment with steroids with or without cyclophosphamide or other immunosuppressive agents.
- Without treatment there is high morbidity and mortality. Therefore there is a high potential for avoidable mortality and morbidity.

Vasculitis, both systemic and involving the CNS, may be secondary to infection, malignancy or drugs (Siva 2001). Viral infections that commonly cause a vasculitis include human immunodeficiency virus (HIV), cytomegalovirus (CMV), varicella-zoster, herpes simplex, and hepatitis B and C. Various bacterial infections may be responsible and include of course *Treponema pallidum* and *Mycobacterium tuberculosis*, but also *Haemophilus influenzae* and *Borrelia burgdorferi* (the cause of Lyme disease). Fungi, such as *Aspergillus*, and protozoa, such as malaria and *Toxoplasma*, should also enter the differential diagnosis.

CNS vasculitis has also been reported in patients with lymphoma and Hodgkin's disease as well as leukaemia. It may occur as a hypersensitivity reaction to drugs. Cerebral vasculitis has been reported in amphetamine abusers and there are anecdotal reports of vasculitis in cocaine and other drug users. However, the evidence that drugs of abuse cause a vasculitis is not strong. Firstly, it is unusual to have confirmation that any vascular event or angiopathy is in fact due to a vasculitis. Secondly, even if it is a vasculitis, it is necessary to rule out other causes of vasculitis such as endocarditis, HIV, hepatitis B or syphilis. The best evidence for drug-induced vasculitis is probably for cocaine, amphetamine and related drugs that produce vasoconstriction (Siva 2001).

Although less than 5% of strokes are due to vasculitis, in the young patient with stroke vasculitis should be considered. Vasculitis should also be a differential diagnosis in any neuropsychiatric case in which steadily accumulating evidence of organicity is found in a patient who originally presented with unremarkable psychiatric symptoms. The following case vignette is typical of the uncertainty that surrounds many such cases.

A 28-year-old man presented with a year's history of treatment-resistant atypical depression, with boredom and finding life meaningless. Increasing euphoria, personality change with disinhibition, accompanied by fleeting diplopia and headaches, developed over the course of several months. An early CT brain scan was negative. He then presented with a sudden onset of dysarthria, left hemiplegia, right cerebellar ataxia and ophthalmoplegia. MRI showed a large T2 high-signal lesion in the right basal ganglia. Brain biopsy excluded a lymphoma but failed to confirm a vasculitis because no vessels were to be found in the small fragments of biopsy material. All other investigations were also negative, although an angiogram was not performed. Five months later he deteriorated with a similar lesion in the right pons extending into the midbrain and temporal lobes. This appeared to respond to treatment with steroids, as did a subsequent relapse a few months later. The presumed diagnosis was a primacy angiitis of the CNS (Hocaoglu & Tan 2005).

Primary angiitis of the nervous system

Primary angiitis of the CNS (PACNS) has evolved as a diagnostic entity over the last 50 years since the original descriptions of a granulomatous angiitis restricted to the nervous system (Calabrese 2001). These conditions are exceedingly rare but are important to neurology and psychiatry in that they can affect the nervous system alone without evidence of vasculitis elsewhere. As cases have accumulated, and with MRI allowing enhanced case ascertainment, the initial gloomy prognosis has been modified. Cases have been described that lead a relatively benign course, even without treatment. Some authors separate PACNS into benign angiitis of the CNS and the more typical granulomatous angiitis of the CNS (Calabrese 2001). However, these two entities overlap considerably, with more features in common than set them apart. PACNS should be considered when after extensive investigation a patient has unexplained neurological problems. There then needs to be evidence of a cerebral arteritis, and evidence that this is confined to the CNS. Disorders capable of mimicking a cerebral vasculitis need to be excluded.

Sigal (1987) reviewed the 61 cases in the literature to that date. Men were affected slightly more often than women, although recent studies show an equal male–female ratio. The mean age of onset was 46 years, but the range is wide with cases reported in childhood and old age. Presentation is often remarkably non-specific, with the acute or subacute onset of headache, confusion and memory disturbance. The most common presentation is headache with encephalopathy plus multifocal signs (Siva 2001). Cognitive impairment, which may progress to a dementia, and alterations of personality and other psychiatric symptoms can be to the fore. Other neurological sequelae include cranial neuropathies, intracerebral or subarachnoid haemorrhage (Kumar *et al.* 1997), seizures and less commonly strokes or spinal cord disease. Meningeal involvement may be prominent. Non-specific symptoms of malaise, nausea and low-grade fever occurred in a significant proportion of cases. The onset is often insidious, and followed by a relapsing/remitting course. The picture may initially suggest encephalitis, cerebral tumour, meningovascular syphilis, multiple sclerosis or sarcoid of the nervous system. The vasculitis may be secondary to infection, particularly with varicella-zoster virus, HIV, CMV and hepatitis B or C.

The ESR may be normal and is more likely to be raised if there is small-vessel involvement. The CSF typically shows increased protein and a lymphocytic pleocytosis; it is abnormal in 80–90% of cases and in some cases shows oligoclonal bands. The EEG shows diffuse or focal slowing in some 80% of patients. MRI may demonstrate infarcts or foci of oedema or ischaemia. MRI may also show gadolinium enhancement of the meninges. In a small proportion of cases findings on MRI resemble demyelinating disease. SPECT or PET may show focal areas of hypoperfusion.

Clearly, however, such investigations are insufficient for diagnosis or for excluding the condition, and when suspected angiography will always be required. This shows diffuse or localised changes in large and small arteries, with irregularities, beading and aneurysmal formation. If findings on cerebral angiography are to be relied on as evidence of vasculitis, then they need to be reasonably secure. There are many causes of localised changes on angiography that mimic arteritis. Without biopsy-proven histological evidence of a vasculitis, it is probably unwise to rely on anything less than multiple-vessel involvement in multiple vascular territories as the standard for angiographic evidence of cerebral vasculitis. It has been suggested that cases diagnosed solely on angiographic findings may have a more benign course than those in whom there is biopsy-proven angiitis, but this has not been confirmed (Woolfenden *et al.* 1998). A case series of 16 such cases found 12 to have headache, seven seizures, and stroke or TIA in eight (Abu-Shakra *et al.* 1994); two presented with impairment of consciousness, and a further three had cognitive impairment. One patient presented with psychosis, but it is not possible to determine if

this patient also had cognitive impairment or seizures; two patients were left with cognitive impairment at follow-up, on average a little over 2 years later. In both cases it was a multi-infarct dementia.

A wedge biopsy of cerebral cortex with overlying meninges is essential for the definitive diagnosis. If possible an area that shows changes on MRI is selected. Histology reveals an inflammatory process in the small and medium-sized arteries and arterioles of the brain parenchyma and leptomeninges; to a lesser extent venules and veins may be affected. Intimal thickening and fibrosis are accompanied by multinucleated giant cells and granuloma formation. Surrounding brain may show ischaemic changes including infarction, demyelination and axonal degeneration.

The diagnosis needs to be almost certain before embarking on the aggressive immunosuppressive treatment that is required, with its significant morbidity. Most authorities would therefore recommend a cerebral biopsy before starting treatment, even though this may be negative in one-quarter of cases, partly in order to rule out other conditions (Moore 1994). The prognosis was extremely poor before the advent of steroid medication. This, with cytotoxic agents such as cyclophosphamide and azathioprine, now brings hopeful prospects of treatment. In a series of 41 cases, followed up for on average 4 years, only 10% had died, and 80% were left with no, or only mild, disability (Calabrese 2001).

Polyarteritis nodosa

Polyarteritis nodosa, recently the subject of a useful review (Segelmark & Selga 2007), is characterised by involvement of many systems of the body and not infrequently the nervous system. It is quite rare, with a prevalence of about 30 per million. Many cases are associated with hepatitis B infection, and occasionally HIV or CMV or other virus infections. A hypersensitivity reaction is suspected in some cases. There may be a preceding history of streptococcal infection, and on rare occasions it may follow the administration of phenytoin, sulphonamides or other drugs.

A 1992 consensus conference on the nomenclature of vasculitic conditions restricted the definition of polyarteritis nodosa to a disease of small and medium-sized arteries (Jennette *et al.* 1994). Vasculitis involving smaller vessels, arterioles, capillaries and venules, often associated with glomerulonephritis and with positive ANCA antibodies and which would previously have been placed within the polyarteritis nodosa rubric, was now to be called microscopic polyangiitis.

The underlying pathology is a focal arteritis of small and medium-sized vessels. The larger arteries may also suffer due to involvement of their nutrient vessels. Highly characteristic focal dilatations are seen along affected vessels and whitish-grey nodules may be apparent macroscopically. A cellular reaction occurs at the site of the changes in and around the vessel walls. Necrosis of the artery wall leads to rupture, and intimal proliferation causes thrombosis. Polyarteritis nodosa, along with Wegener's granulomatosis and microscopic polyangiitis, is one of the systemic necrotising vasculitides.

The onset is usually in middle age but the range is wide. Males and females are equally affected. The disorder may declare itself abruptly or insidiously, and tends to run a subacute or chronic course with relapses and remissions. Most patients have symptoms such as headache, malaise, weakness and a low-grade intermittent fever at onset. Weight loss may be profound and multisystem involvement is usually soon apparent. Renal insufficiency leads to severe hypertension in a high proportion of cases, and crises of abdominal pain result from infarctions in the mesenteric vessels and their tributaries. Gastrointestinal and renal involvement has a significant deleterious effect on prognosis. Arthritis and myositis are common. Pleuritic pain and pneumonitis may develop, and cardiac involvement leads to myocardial infarction, congestive cardiac failure and pericarditis. Skin lesions include livedo reticularis, purpura, ecchymoses, subcutaneous nodules, necrotic ulcers and superficial gangrene. In addition to hypertensive retinopathy, the eyes may show evidence of scleritis, keratitis, choroiditis, retinal artery occlusion or optic atrophy.

Laboratory investigations usually disclose anaemia, raised ESR, and reversal of the albumin–globulin ratio. However, there are no specific laboratory tests for the disorder. Leucocytosis is common, sometimes with eosinophilia. Most cases show uraemia, albuminuria and abnormal sediment in the urine. Chest radiography may show pulmonary infiltration or a pleural reaction. The CSF is sometimes under increased pressure, with elevation of protein, pleocytosis or xanthochromia. Arteriography via the aorta may reveal a diagnostic picture by way of multiple small aneurysms, focal dilatations, or infarcted areas in the kidneys or other abdominal organs. Biopsies from skin, liver, kidney or small nerves serve to confirm the diagnosis.

The disease formerly carried an extremely poor prognosis, death usually being attributable to renal failure or to coronary, mesenteric or cerebral infarction. Treatment with steroids and immunosuppressive drugs, usually in combination with one another, now offers hope of delaying or even halting progression. Hypertension warrants vigorous management and anticoagulants may be indicated.

Nervous system involvement

Peripheral neuropathy is the most frequent neurological finding and will be found in 70% of cases. The nerves suffer via their nutrient arteries, leading to multiple infarctions along their course. The result is usually a mononeuropathy or mononeuritis multiplex, with paraesthesiae, weakness and wasting. A symmetrical polyneuropathy is less common.

Cerebral manifestations appear in up to half of cases eventually, but usually in the later part of the illness (Moore 1994). A diffuse encephalopathic-like illness with cognitive impairment or seizures may be seen, perhaps more frequently in those with small artery involvement. In contrast, disease affecting the medium-sized arteries is more likely to present with intracerebral haemorrhage or subarachnoid haemorrhage or stroke-like episodes. Cranial nerve lesions are common, causing blurring of vision, vertigo, tinnitus and disorders of external ocular movement. Occasionally, a local mass of brain necrosis may simulate a tumour. Headache is common, sometimes attributable to hypertension and sometimes to arachnoiditis at the base of the brain. Epileptic seizures may result from uraemia, hypertension, diffuse encephalopathy or focal lesions in the brain.

Mental changes can figure prominently and occurred in 26 of 114 cases from the Mayo Clinic (Ford & Siekert 1965). The usual picture was of confusion and disorientation, sometimes with visual hallucinations and delusions. Delirium, 'mania' and paranoia were seen occasionally. Forgetfulness was noted in many patients, and seven showed marked intellectual deterioration. Eight showed a fluctuating impairment of consciousness varying from somnolence to coma.

Occasional cases are reported in which polyarteritis nodosa appears to be largely confined to the nervous system. MacKay et al. (1950) described a patient who for 2 years showed intermittent diplopia, hemiparesis and cranial nerve disorders accompanied by a low pyrexia, then developed depression and progressive dementia leading to death over several months. At post-mortem the typical changes of polyarteritis nodosa were largely confined to the brain and cord.

Primary small-vessel vasculitides

Wegener's granulomatosis, microscopic polyangiitis and Churg–Strauss syndrome all affect small vessels and are all associated with ANCAs. Inflammation and fibrinoid necrosis of small-vessel walls (arterioles, capillaries or venules), with few or no immune deposits, is characteristic of each of these conditions. They are all relatively rare. The majority of patients will have general constitutional symptoms at presentation, for example a flu-like illness or generalised malaise. Involvement of the upper and lower respiratory tract is common. The granulomas of Wegener's granulomatosis commonly affect the ear, nose and throat, whereas Churg–Strauss syndrome typically presents with asthma; an eosinophilic vasculitis particularly involving the lungs is characteristic. On the other hand, renal involvement is also frequently seen and this is particularly common in microscopic polyangiitis, which may be associated with a rapidly progressive glomerulonephritis (Guillevin et al. 1999). Other organs that may be affected include skin, liver and heart.

ANCAs may be detected using indirect immunofluorescence with ethanol-fixed human neutrophils as substrate.

Using this method it is possible to distinguish two patterns of immunofluorescence as ANCAs bind to their target: a granular cytoplasmic pattern (c-ANCA) and a perinuclear pattern (p-ANCA). The c-ANCA pattern tends to be associated with antibodies directed against proteinase 3, and this is what is generally found in Wegener's granulomatosis. However, there are reports of ANCAs against myeloperoxidase also producing the c-ANCA pattern, and this is found in Churg–Strauss syndrome. ANCAs against myeloperoxidase usually produce the p-ANCA pattern, and this is typically seen in microscopic polyangiitis. Patients with small-vessel vasculitis who are p-ANCA positive have the lowest risk of relapse (Pavone *et al.* 2006). There is reasonably good evidence that ANCAs have a pathogenic role in these conditions by activating neutrophils and by binding to a target antigen in the endothelium of the vessel to cause cell damage (Preston *et al.* 2002). In Wegener's granulomatosis, a rise in ANCA has shown to predict relapse of the disease (Slot & Tervaert 2004).

About one-quarter of cases, particularly those with Churg–Strauss syndrome, will have a neuropathy. Cerebral involvement is relatively uncommon, with perhaps only 1 in 20 affected (Pavone *et al.* 2006), although the figures may be higher for Wegener's granulomatosis.

Wegener's granulomatosis is characterised by necrotising granulomas in the upper and lower respiratory tract with a systemic necrotising vasculitis (Slot & Tervaert 2004). ANCAs are detected in the majority of patients (see above). Damage to the nasal septum may cause a saddle deformity of the nose when the cartilage supporting the bridge of the nose collapses. Between 10% and 20% of cases develop a neuropathy, the commonest being mononeuritis multiplex followed by a symmetrical distal neuropathy. Neurological involvement may also be a consequence of invasion of the base of the skull by large granulomas arising from nasal or paranasal sites. These may for example directly penetrate the orbits or intracranial cavity, or involve major arteries supplying the brain or cranial nerves. Less than 10% of cases will have a cerebral vasculitis, often with intracerebral or subarachnoid haemorrhage (Siva 2001).

A recent case series describes six cases with CNS involvement from a database of 80 cases of Wegener's granulomatosis (Seror *et al.* 2006). Two had a pachymeningitis, presenting with headaches: in one case the meningitis affected the falx causing an obstructive hydrocephalus, and in the other a diffuse meningitis was associated with seizures and behavioural change. In three cases the pituitary was affected; in one of these there had been a previous central retinal artery occlusion and a TIA involving the middle cerebral artery some years before, suggestive of cerebral vasculitis. One case had a typical picture of cerebral vasculitis with an intracerebellar haemorrhage followed by T2-enhancing lesions in the cerebrum. The subsequent review of the literature suggests

three clinical patterns of cerebral Wegener's granulomatosis: a chronic hypertrophic pachymeningitis (Jinnah *et al.* 1997), pituitary gland involvement, and cerebral vasculitis.

Untreated the prognosis for Wegener's granulomatosis is poor, with 1-year mortality of 80%, but with treatment three-quarters of patients will survive 5 years. Treatment generally relies on achieving remission with a combination of steroids and cyclophosphamide. Because cyclophosphamide is so toxic, RCTs have explored the consequences of replacing cyclophosphamide, once remission has been achieved, with a less toxic immunosuppressant. These have shown that it is safe to change to azathioprine or methotrexate for long-term maintenance therapy (Hellmich *et al.* 2006).

Giant-cell arteritis (temporal arteritis)

Giant-cell arteritis is a disease of large arteries and a disease of later years, rarely appearing before 60 years of age and being commonest in those aged 75–85 years (Weyand & Goronzy 2003). In North America and Europe it is the most common of the systemic vasculitides, with an incidence of the order of 100 per million per year (Siva 2001); it is much less common in east Asia. It is a disease of the aorta and its branches, but is particularly likely to affect the extracranial branches of the carotid artery. Of these the temporal arteries are most commonly affected, hence the alternative name temporal arteritis. Arteries show a subacute inflammatory reaction with necrosis, granulation and giant-cell formation. CD4+ T cells play a primary role in the pathogenesis. They penetrate the endothelium of the vasa vasorum, not the main vessel wall, and with the help of antigen-presenting cells then cause inflammation across the width of the arterial wall. Intimal proliferation may lead to thrombosis and occlusion. The ciliary arteries, which supply the optic nerve and disc, are involved in about 30% of cases. The aorta and its major branches are too large to occlude and instead damage to the vessel wall may produce dissection, rupture or aneurysmal dilatation. The disease is related to polymyalgia rheumatica and the two may occur together.

Clinically, there is often a prodromal phase of vague malaise with muscle and joint pains lasting for several weeks or months. A low pyrexia may develop and weight loss and depression may be marked. Characteristic headache then appears, sometimes abruptly, situated principally over the affected vessels in the temporal region. The temporal arteries may be palpable and exquisitely tender. Suffering is usually intense, with throbbing or lancinating pain and severe insomnia. Jaw claudication, with pain on chewing, is also characteristic.

The acute stage lasts for a week or two but tenderness may persist rather longer. At any time in the early days or weeks the serious complication of ciliary artery obstruction may follow, leading to impairment or loss of vision in one or both eyes, hence the importance of prompt diagnosis and treatment. Ophthalmoplegias may also occur. The systemic disturbance continues throughout the stage of headache and visual complications, and may last for many months more. Peripheral neuropathy and muscle pain and wasting may occur. Infarctions can follow from involvement of the carotid or vertebral vessels. McCormick and Neuberger (1958) describe the brain lesions that may be observed at post-mortem, including involvement of small intracerebral vessels by giant-cell arteritis.

Mental disturbances sometimes feature prominently during the illness, with confusion, delirium, memory impairment and drowsiness proceeding to coma (Cloake 1951). Vereker (1952) described examples in the literature with restlessness, disorientation, severe memory difficulties and episodes of delirium, often with abrupt resolution after several weeks. Coma is a serious development, but patients can recover after several days. Vereker also stressed the frequency of severe depression in the disease, and considered that in many examples it was attributable to cerebral arterial disease rather than being secondary to the headache. Russell (1959) found that 7 of 35 patients were depressed and four were confused during the stage of headache.

The ESR is greatly raised and there may be a leucocytosis. However, in about 10% of cases the ESR may be normal in the early stages (Russell & Grahm 1988). Biopsy of an inflamed artery serves to confirm the diagnosis. Steroids meet with dramatic success in treatment and must not be delayed. They are given in high dosage initially then reduced after 1–2 weeks to maintenance levels, which are continued for 6–12 months or sometimes indefinitely. Mason and Walport (1992) discuss the regimens involved. Anticoagulants may also be indicated in the acute stages. Giant-cell arteritis is a self-limiting disease so that once the acute phase is treated the illness usually becomes inactive within a few months to a year or two.

Takayasu's arteritis, pulseless disease, is also a disease of large vessels, particularly the aorta and its main branches and is found mainly in young women. Distal pulses are commonly absent. The disease may lead a fairly chronic course. Being much more common in Japan and eastern Asia, it has the opposite geographical distribution to giant-cell arteritis. Neurological sequelae, stroke or TIA, are not very common though headache is found in about half of cases.

Other conditions associated with vasculitis

Susac's syndrome consists of a triad of microangiopathy of the brain and retina with hearing loss; it is predominantly found in young women (Susac 1994) and is of uncertain aetiology. Headache is a common presenting symptom. The encephalopathy may be acute or insidious and several cases show insidious development of personality change associated with cognitive impairment. There is therefore the potential for such cases to present to a psychiatrist.

Thromboangiitis obliterans is virtually confined to male smokers, presenting usually between 25 and 40 years of age. The pathology is characterised by highly cellular and inflammatory occlusive thrombus with relative sparing of the blood vessel wall (Olin & Shih 2006). The medium-sized vessels of the legs are predominantly affected. Anti-endothelial cell antibodies may be pathogenic. A relapsing/remitting course is characteristic, affecting short segments of the vessels at a time so that lesions in all stages of activity are found at different sites. The common presentation is with intermittent claudication, leading eventually to gangrene of the toes. Superficial venous thromboses frequently occur. The affected limb is pulseless, cyanosed and cold. Nocturnal pain is typically relieved by hanging the leg downwards out of bed.

Cerebral involvement is rare but well attested, usually only when the peripheral disease is well established, though in occasional cases is the presenting feature. The possibility of the disease should therefore be borne in mind when young adult males develop cerebrovascular symptoms, especially in the absence of hypertension. The vessels principally affected are the internal carotid and anterior and middle cerebral arteries (Cloake 1951). Infarctions follow in the corresponding territories. In the early stages the deficits may be slight and transient, suggesting that they are due to episodes of spasm or emboli. Epileptic seizures are common and headache of migrainous type may occur. Later dementia can be profound with an end-state similar to that of multi-infarct dementia.

Polycythaemia rubra vera

Polycythaemia, one of the myeloproliferative disorders, exhibits an increase in red cell mass and usually an excess of white blood corpuscles and platelets as well. It presents mainly in middle or later life, and with a slight male preponderance. Sometimes it declares itself insidiously, or it may present with acute complications such as cerebrovascular accident or major thrombotic episode (Weatherall 1996). Patients may experience angina or claudication, or suffer recurrent emboli or venous thromboses. Complaints of pruritus are common. The facies is typically plethoric with injected conjunctivae, and splenomegaly and hepatomegaly are often present.

Neuropsychiatric features can be prominent and have been reported in half to three-quarters of cases (Silverstein *et al.* 1962). Impairment of the cerebral circulation leads to headache, impaired concentration, dizziness, vertigo and visual blurring. Episodes of confusion may progress to dementia. The increased blood viscosity predisposes to TIAs and cerebral infarctions. Murray and Hodgson (1991) reported a patient who developed a severe depressive illness with psychotic features after a series of TIAs, ultimately with good resolution after electroconvulsive treatment. Mania after an episode of delirium has also been reported (Chawla

& Lindesay 1993). Other cerebral symptoms occasionally include chorea, narcolepsy and seizures.

Willison *et al.* (1980) showed that patients with high-normal or above-normal haematocrit (range 0.46–0.77) were impaired on tests of alertness (tests of digit copying, counting backwards, letter cancellation and coding) compared with controls matched for age and occupation. After vene-section the haematocrit fell from a mean of 0.54 to 0.45 and the test scores improved. The extent of improvement correlated significantly with increases in CBF as measured by ^{133}Xe inhalation. More recently, there has been a report of a 65-year-old man with a haematocrit of 60% who presented with confusional episodes and abulia, and severe executive impairments and moderate deficits in constructional praxis. There was a marked improvement in the confusional episodes following treatment of the polycythaemia, with some improvement on neuropsychological test performance (Di Pollina *et al.* 2000).

Cerebral venous sinus thrombosis

Largely because of CT and MRI, cerebral venous sinus thrombosis has changed in status from a rare fatal diagnosis only made at post-mortem to an illness that explains 1–2% of strokes (Renowden 2004). The outcome is very diverse and in general probably better than for arterial strokes. The onset is also more variable, with subacute or fluctuating presentations seen in two-thirds of cases (Masuhr *et al.* 2004). The commonest symptom is headache (80–90%), followed by focal neurological deficits, seizures or papilloedema (each in about 50%) (Bousser 2000). A good proportion, from 10% to 60% in different series, will show alteration of consciousness.

Four main patterns of presentation have been described (Bousser 2000):
• One pattern is typical of any stroke, with focal deficits, although epileptic seizures are very much more common than in arterial stroke.
• An isolated syndrome of raised intracranial pressure, with headaches, papilloedema and sometimes a sixth nerve palsy, often mimicking benign intracranial hypertension.
• Of most interest to the neuropsychiatrist is a subacute encephalopathy without localising signs but with delirium often accompanied by seizures.
• In the case of cavernous sinus thrombosis, a progressive, often painful, third or sixth nerve palsy.

Young women are at greatest risk, particularly if taking oral contraceptives or in the perinatal period. Other risk factors include head injury and infection, particularly of the middle ear. Cerebral venous sinus thrombosis has been reported as a rare complication of lumbar puncture. Systemic illness with cachexia, malignancies, heart failure or pulmonary embolism, and coagulation disorders are also on the long list of potential causes (Stam 2005). The commonest

sites of thrombosis are the superior sagittal sinus and the transverse sinus with more than one site usually affected (Stam 2005). The clinical picture depends somewhat on the site of thrombosis. Thrombosis of the cerebral veins tends to produce localised infarction, which is often haemorrhagic. Thrombosis of the major sinuses results in raised intracranial pressure, but without hydrocephalus.

CT and MRI are crucial for diagnosis (Masuhr *et al.* 2004). The first clue may be the pattern of ischaemia and infarction, which is often multifocal, haemorrhagic and does not match arterial territories. Evidence of thrombus in the sinuses may be easily missed; depending on the state of maturation it may hypointense, isointense or hyperintense on CT or MRI. Over the first few days it may be isointense on T1 MRI sequences and hypointense on T2 sequences; then over the next few weeks hyperintense, firstly on T1 and then on T2 sequences. The pictures after a month can be quite variable depending on whether there has been recanalisation; in most cases the sinuses are isointense on T1 and hyperintense on T2 sequences. MRA allows the visualisation of the blocked veins and sinuses.

Treatment consists of the management of any precipitating factors and anticoagulation in selected cases. The mortality is of the order of 10–20%, and is worse in those presenting with a reduced conscious level. However, many make a full recovery and seem to be left with no sequelae.

There has been relatively little written about the long-term outcome in terms of cognitive and behavioural sequelae. In one study, based on an RCT of anticoagulant treatment in 59 patients, eight had died and four could not be followed up (de Bruijn *et al.* 2000); 47 patients were available for follow-up on average 18 months after the thrombosis. About one-third of patients showed impairments on cognitive testing. Nevertheless, all bar three scored above 23 out of 30 on the MMSE. Worst performance was on the visuospatial maze test, with 15 of 46 patients scoring less than the 10th centile. In about 40–50% of patients their employment potential had been adversely affected by the thrombosis. In a cases series of 38 patients with thrombosis, 34 were available for assessment on average 3.5 years later (Buccino *et al.* 2003). Cognitive performance, as assessed using the MMSE, was normal in all except one who scored 21 and one 26 out of 30. Working memory impairments could be identified in six (18%). Depression, with a BDI of greater or equal to 10 was also found in six patients, but in no case did the BDI exceed 13. These two studies suggest that most patients make a good recovery after cerebral venous sinus thrombosis.

References

Abbate-Daga, G., Fassino, S. *et al.* (2007) Anger, depression and personality dimensions in patients with migraine without aura. *Psychotherapy and Psychosomatics* **76**, 122–128.

Aben, I., Verhey, F. *et al.* (2003) A comparative study into the one year cumulative incidence of depression after stroke and myocardial infarction. *Journal of Neurology, Neurosurgery and Psychiatry* **74**, 581–585.

Aben, I., Lodder, J. *et al.* (2006) Focal or generalized vascular brain damage and vulnerability to depression after stroke: a 1-year prospective follow-up study. *International Psychogeriatrics* **18**, 19–35.

Abu-Shakra, M., Khraishi, M. *et al.* (1994) Primary angiitis of the CNS diagnosed by angiography. *Quarterly Journal of Medicine* **87**, 351–358.

Adams, G.F. & Hurwitz, L.J. (1963) Mental barriers to recovery from strokes. *Lancet* **ii**, 533–537.

Adams, G.F. & Hurwitz, L.J. (1974) *Cerebrovascular Disability and the Ageing Brain*. Churchill Livingstone, Edinburgh & London.

Adams, H.P., Bendixen, B.H. Jr *et al.* (1993) Classification of subtype of acute ischemic stroke. Definitions for use in a multicenter clinical trial. TOAST. Trial of Org 10172 in Acute Stroke Treatment. *Stroke* **24**, 35–41.

Afeltra, A., Garzia, P. *et al.* (2003) Neuropsychiatric lupus syndromes: relationship with antiphospholipid antibodies. *Neurology* **61**, 108–110.

Afridi, S.K., Matharu, M.S. *et al.* (2005) A PET study exploring the laterality of brainstem activation in migraine using glyceryl trinitrate. *Brain* **128**, 932–939.

Ainiala, H., Loukkola, J. *et al.* (2001) The prevalence of neuropsychiatric syndromes in systemic lupus erythematosus. *Neurology* **57**, 496–500.

Ainiala, H., Dastidar, P. *et al.* (2005) Cerebral MRI abnormalities and their association with neuropsychiatric manifestations in SLE: a population-based study. *Scandinavian Journal of Rheumatology* **34**, 376–382.

Alarcon-Segovia, D., Estanol, B. *et al.* (1997) Antiphospholipid antibodies and the antiphospholipid syndrome. Clinical relevance in neuropsychiatric systemic lupus erythematosus. *Annals of the New York Academy of Sciences* **823**, 279–288.

Albers, G.W., Caplan, L.R. *et al.* (2002) Transient ischemic attack: proposal for a new definition. *New England Journal of Medicine* **347**, 1713–1716.

Alexander, M.P. & Freedman, M. (1984) Amnesia after anterior communicating artery aneurysm rupture. *Neurology* **34**, 752–757.

Allain, P., Joseph, P.A. *et al.* (1998) Cognitive functions in chronic locked-in syndrome: a report of two cases. *Cortex* **34**, 629–634.

Almeida, O.P., Waterreus, A. *et al.* (2006) Preventing depression after stroke: results from a randomized placebo-controlled trial. *Journal of Clinical Psychiatry* **67**, 1104–1109.

Anderson, C.S., Linto, J. *et al.* (1995) A population-based assessment of the impact and burden of caregiving for long-term stroke survivors. *Stroke* **26**, 843–849.

Appenzeller, S., Cendes, F. *et al.* (2004) Epileptic seizures in systemic lupus erythematosus. *Neurology* **63**, 1808–1812.

Appenzeller, S., Li, L.M. *et al.* (2005) Evidence of reversible axonal dysfunction in systemic lupus erythematosus: a proton MRS study. *Brain* **128**, 2933–2940.

Appenzeller, S., Costallat, L.T. *et al.* (2006) Magnetic resonance spectroscopy in the evaluation of central nervous system manifestations of systemic lupus erythematosus. *Arthritis and Rheumatism* **55**, 807–811.

Appenzeller, S., Amorim, B.J. *et al.* (2007) Voxel-based morphometry of brain SPECT can detect the presence of active central nervous system involvement in systemic lupus erythematosus. *Rheumatology (Oxford)* **46**, 467–472.

Arbuckle, M.R., McClain, M.T. *et al.* (2003) Development of autoantibodies before the clinical onset of systemic lupus erythematosus. *New England Journal of Medicine* **349**, 1526–1533.

Ardila, A. & Sanchez, E. (1988) Neuropsychologic symptoms in the migraine syndrome. *Cephalalgia* **8**, 67–70.

Astrom, M., Adolfsson, R. *et al.* (1993) Major depression in stroke patients. A 3-year longitudinal study. *Stroke* **24**, 976–982.

Aurora, S.K., Cao, Y. *et al.* (1999) The occipital cortex is hyperexcitable in migraine: experimental evidence. *Headache* **39**, 469–476.

Bahra, A., Matharu, M.S. *et al.* (2001) Brainstem activation specific to migraine headache. *Lancet* **357**, 1016–1017.

Bamford, J. (2001) Assessment and investigation of stroke and transient ischaemic attack. *Journal of Neurology, Neurosurgery and Psychiatry* **70** (suppl. 1), I3–I6.

Bamford, J., Sandercock, P. *et al.* (1988) A prospective study of acute cerebrovascular disease in the community: the Oxfordshire Community Stroke Project 1981–86. 1. Methodology, demography and incident cases of first-ever stroke. *Journal of Neurology, Neurosurgery and Psychiatry* **51**, 1373–1380.

Bamford, J., Sandercock, P. *et al.* (1990) A prospective study of acute cerebrovascular disease in the community: the Oxfordshire Community Stroke Project 1981–86. 2. Incidence, case fatality rates and overall outcome at one year of cerebral infarction, primary intracerebral and subarachnoid haemorrhage. *Journal of Neurology, Neurosurgery and Psychiatry* **53**, 16–22.

Bamford, J., Sandercock, P. *et al.* (1991) Classification and natural history of clinically identifiable subtypes of cerebral infarction. *Lancet* **337**, 1521–1526.

Barber, P.A., Demchuk, A.M. *et al.* (2000) Validity and reliability of a quantitative computed tomography score in predicting outcome of hyperacute stroke before thrombolytic therapy. ASPECTS Study Group. Alberta Stroke Programme Early CT Score. *Lancet* **355**, 1670–1674.

Barnett, H.J. (1997) Hemodynamic cerebral ischemia. An appeal for systematic data gathering prior to a new EC/IC trial. *Stroke* **28**, 1857–1860.

Barnett, H.J., Taylor, D.W. *et al.* (1998) Benefit of carotid endarterectomy in patients with symptomatic moderate or severe stenosis. North American Symptomatic Carotid Endarterectomy Trial Collaborators. *New England Journal of Medicine* **339**, 1415–1425.

Baron, J.C. (1987) Remote metabolic effects of stroke. In: Wade, J., Knežević, S., Maximilian, V.A., Mubrin, Z. & Prohovnik, I. (eds) *Impact of Functional Imaging in Neurology and Psychiatry*, ch. 8. Current Problems in Neurology vol. 5, pp. 91–100.

Bates, B., Choi, J.Y. *et al.* (2005) Veterans Affairs/Department of Defense Clinical Practice Guideline for the Management of Adult Stroke Rehabilitation Care: executive summary. *Stroke* **36**, 2049–2056.

Beblo, T. & Driessen, M. (2002) No melancholia in poststroke depression? A phenomenologic comparison of primary and poststroke depression. *Journal of Geriatric Psychiatry and Neurology* **15**, 44–49.

Becker, K. (2006) Hypertensive encephalopathy, eclampsia, and reversible posterior leukoencephalopathy. *Critical Care Neurology* **12**, 30–45.

Bedford, P.D. (1958) Discussion: intracranial haemorrhage: diagnosis and treatment. *Proceedings of the Royal Society of Medicine* **51**, 209–213.

Belciug, M.P. (2006) Concerns and anticipated challenges of family caregivers following participation in the neuropsychological feedback of stroke patients. *International Journal of Rehabilitation Research* **29**, 77–80.

Belmont, H.M., Abramson, S.B. *et al.* (1996) Pathology and pathogenesis of vascular injury in systemic lupus erythematosus. Interactions of inflammatory cells and activated endothelium. *Arthritis and Rheumatism* **39**, 9–22.

Benke, T., Koylu, B. *et al.* (2005) Cholinergic treatment of amnesia following basal forebrain lesion due to aneurysm rupture: an open-label pilot study. *European Journal of Neurology* **12**, 791–796.

Benson, D.F. & Cummings, J.L. (1982) Angular gyrus syndrome simulating Alzheimer's disease. *Archives of Neurology* **39**, 616–620.

Benson, D.F., Marsden, C.D. & Meadows, J.C. (1974) The amnesic syndrome of posterior cerebral artery occlusion. *Acta Neurologica Scandinavica* **50**, 133–145.

Berry, E. (1998) Post-traumatic stress disorder after subarachnoid haemorrhage. *British Journal of Clinical Psychology* **37**, 365–367.

Bhatia, M.S. (1990) Capgras syndrome in a patient with migraine. *British Journal of Psychiatry* **157**, 917–918.

Bhogal, S.K., Teasell, R. *et al.* (2004) Lesion location and poststroke depression: systematic review of the methodological limitations in the literature. *Stroke* **35**, 794–802.

Bickerstaff, E.R. (1961a) Basilar artery migraine. *Lancet* **i**, 15–17.

Bickerstaff, E.R. (1961b) Impairment of consciousness in migraine. *Lancet* **ii**, 1057–1059.

Bigal, M.E. & Lipton, R.B. (2006) The preventive treatment of migraine. *Neurologist* **12**, 204–213.

Black, D.W. (1984) Mental changes resulting from subdural haematoma. *British Journal of Psychiatry* **145**, 200–203.

Bogousslavski, J., Regli, F. *et al.* (1988) Migraine stroke. *Neurology* **38**, 223–227.

Bonita, R. (1992) Epidemiology of stroke. *Lancet* **339**, 342–344.

Bornstein, R.A., Weir, B.K. *et al.* (1987) Neuropsychological function in patients after subarachnoid hemorrhage. *Neurosurgery* **21**, 651–654.

Bosma, G.P., Middelkoop, H.A. *et al.* (2002) Association of global brain damage and clinical functioning in neuropsychiatric systemic lupus erythematosus. *Arthritis and Rheumatism* **46**, 2665–2672.

Bosma, G.P., Huizinga, T.W. *et al.* (2003) Abnormal brain diffusivity in patients with neuropsychiatric systemic lupus erythematosus. *American Journal of Neuroradiology* **24**, 850–854.

Bottger, S., Prosiegel, M. *et al.* (1998) Neurobehavioural disturbances, rehabilitation outcome, and lesion site in patients after rupture and repair of anterior communicating artery aneurysm. *Journal of Neurology, Neurosurgery and Psychiatry* **65**, 93–102.

Bousser, M.G. (2000) Cerebral venous thrombosis: diagnosis and management. *Journal of Neurology* **247**, 252–258.

Bousser, M.G. & Welch, K.M. (2005) Relation between migraine and stroke. *Lancet Neurology* **4**, 533–542.

Bradshaw, P. & Parsons, M. (1965) Hemiplegic migraine: a clinical study. *Quarterly Journal of Medicine* **34**, 65–85.

Brainin, M. (2006) Finding silent cerebral aneurysms: the importance of doing nothing. *Journal of Neurology, Neurosurgery and Psychiatry* **77**, 713.

Breslau, N. (1992) Migraine, suicidal ideation, and suicide attempts. *Neurology* **42**, 392–395.

Breslau, N., Davis, G.C. *et al.* (1991) Migraine, psychiatric disorders, and suicide attempts: an epidemiologic study of young adults. *Psychiatry Research* **37**, 11–23.

Breslau, N., Chilcoat, H.D. *et al.* (1996) Further evidence on the link between migraine and neuroticism. *Neurology* **47**, 663–667.

Breslau, N., Schultz, L.R. *et al.* (2000) Headache and major depression: is the association specific to migraine? *Neurology* **54**, 308–313.

Breslau, N., Lipton, R.B. *et al.* (2003) Comorbidity of migraine and depression: investigating potential etiology and prognosis. *Neurology* **60**, 1308–1312.

Brey, R.L., Holliday, S.L. *et al.* (2002) Neuropsychiatric syndromes in lupus: prevalence using standardized definitions. *Neurology* **58**, 1214–1220.

Brilstra, E.H., Hop, J.W. *et al.* (1997) Quality of life after perimesencephalic haemorrhage. *Journal of Neurology, Neurosurgery and Psychiatry* **63**, 382–384.

Broderick, J.P. & Swanson, J.W. (1987) Migraine-related strokes. Clinical profile and prognosis in 20 patients. *Archives of Neurology* **44**, 868–887.

Brooks, W.M., Jung, R.E. *et al.* (1999) Relationship between neurometabolite derangement and neurocognitive dysfunction in systemic lupus erythematosus. *Journal of Rheumatology* **26**, 81–5.

Brown, M.M. (2001) Identification and management of difficult stroke and TIA syndromes. *Journal of Neurology, Neurosurgery and Psychiatry* **70** (suppl. 1), 17–22.

Buccino, G., Scoditti, U. *et al.* (2003) Neurological and cognitive long-term outcome in patients with cerebral venous sinus thrombosis. *Acta Neurologica Scandinavica* **107**, 330–335.

Buchanan, K.M., Elias, L.J. *et al.* (2000) Differing perspectives on outcome after subarachnoid hemorrhage: the patient, the relative, the neurosurgeon. *Neurosurgery* **46**, 831–838; discussion 838–840.

Bull, J. (1969) Massive aneurysms at the base of the brain. *Brain* **92**, 535–570.

Burstein, R., Cutrer, M.F. *et al.* (2000) The development of cutaneous allodynia during a migraine attack: clinical evidence for the sequential recruitment of spinal and supraspinal nociceptive neurons in migraine. *Brain* **123**, 1703–1709.

Butefisch, C.M., Kleiser, R. *et al.* (2006) Post-lesional cerebral reorganisation: evidence from functional neuroimaging and transcranial magnetic stimulation. *Journal de Physiologie (Paris)* **99**, 437–454.

Byrom, F.B. (1954) The pathogenesis of hypertensive encephalopathy and its relation to the malignant phase of hypertension. Experimental evidence from the hypertensive rat. *Lancet* **ii**, 201–211.

Caeiro, L., Menger, C., Ferro, J.M., Albuquerque, R. & Fiqueira, M.L. (2005) Delirium in acute subarachnoid haemorrhage. *Cerebrovascular Diseases* **19**, 31–38.

Calabrese, L. (2001) Primary angiitis of the central nervous system: the penumbra of vasculitis. *Journal of Rheumatology* **28**, 465–466.

Cals, N., Devuyst, G. *et al.* (2002) Pure superficial posterior cerebral artery territory infarction in The Lausanne Stroke Registry. *Journal of Neurology* **249**, 855–861.

Calvert, T., Knapp, P. *et al.* (1998) Psychological associations with emotionalism after stroke. *Journal of Neurology, Neurosurgery and Psychiatry* **65**, 928–929.

Camilo, O. & Goldstein, L.B. (2004) Seizures and epilepsy after ischemic stroke. *Stroke* **35**, 1769–1775.

Cao, M., Zhang, S. *et al.* (2002) Personality traits in migraine and tension-type headaches: a five-factor model study. *Psychopathology* **35**, 254–258.

Caplan, F., Chedru, F. *et al.* (1981) Transient global amnesia and migraine. *Neurology* **31**, 1167–1170.

Caplan, L.R. (1980) 'Top of the basilar' syndrome. *Neurology* **30**, 72–79.

Caplan, L.R. & Hennerici, M. (1998) Impaired clearance of emboli (washout) is an important link between hypoperfusion, embolism, and ischemic stroke. *Archives of Neurology* **55**, 1475–1482.

Cappa, S.F., Benke, T. *et al.* (2005) EFNS guidelines on cognitive rehabilitation: report of an EFNS task force. *European Journal of Neurology* **12**, 665–680.

Carbotte, R.M., Denburg, S.D. *et al.* (1986) Prevalence of cognitive impairment in systemic lupus erythematosus. *Journal of Nervous and Mental Disease* **174**, 357–364.

Carey, J.R., Kimberley, T.J. *et al.* (2002) Analysis of fMRI and finger tracking training in subjects with chronic stroke. *Brain* **125**, 773–788.

Carlomagno, S., Migliaresi, S. *et al.* (2000) Cognitive impairment in systemic lupus erythematosus: a follow-up study. *Journal of Neurology* **247**, 273–279.

Carolei, A. & Sacco, S. (2003) Central nervous system vasculitis. *Neurological Sciences* **24** (suppl. 1), S8–S10.

Carrera, E. & Bogousslavsky, J. (2006) The thalamus and behavior: effects of anatomically distinct strokes. *Neurology* **66**, 1817–1823.

Carson, A.J., MacHale, S. *et al.* (2000) Depression after stroke and lesion location: a systematic review. *Lancet* **356**, 122–126.

Carter, A.B. (1972) Clinical aspects of cerebral infarction. In: Vinken, P.J. & Bruyn, G.W. (eds) *Handbook of Clinical Neurology*, ch. 12. North-Holland Publishing Co., Amsterdam.

Caselli, R.J., Graff-Radford, N.R. *et al.* (1991) Thalamocortical diaschisis: single photon emission tomographic study of cortical blood flow changes after focal thalamic infarction. *Neuropsychiatry, Neuropsychology and Behavioral Neurology* **4**, 193–214.

Castellino, G., Govoni, M. *et al.* (2005) Proton magnetic resonance spectroscopy may predict future brain lesions in SLE patients: a functional multi-imaging approach and follow up. *Annals of the Rheumatic Diseases* **64**, 1022–1027.

Castillo, C.S., Schultz, S.K. *et al.* (1995) Clinical correlates of early-onset and late-onset poststroke generalized anxiety. *American Journal of Psychiatry* **152**, 1174–1179.

Cervera, R., Piette, J.C. *et al.* (2002) Antiphospholipid syndrome: clinical and immunologic manifestations and patterns of disease expression in a cohort of 1,000 patients. *Arthritis and Rheumatism* **46**, 1019–1027.

Chabriat, H., Danchot, J. *et al.* (1999) Precipitating factors of headache. A prospective study in a national control-matched survey in migraineurs and nonmigraineurs. *Headache* **39**, 335–338.

Chan, A., Ho, S. *et al.* (2002) Neuropsychological sequelae of patients treated with microsurgical clipping or endovascular embolization for anterior communicating artery aneurysm. *European Neurology* **47**, 37–44.

Chapman, J., Cohen-Armon, M. *et al.* (1999) Antiphospholipid antibodies permeabilize and depolarize brain synaptoneurosomes. *Lupus* **8**, 127–133.

Chawla, M. & Lindesay, J. (1993) Polycythaemia, delirium and mania. *British Journal of Psychiatry* **162**, 833–835.

Chen, Y., Guo, J.J., Zhan, S. & Patel, N.C. (2006) Treatment effects of antidepressants in patients with post-stroke depression: a meta-analysis. *Annals of Pharmacotherapy* **40**, 2115–2122.

Chollet, F., V. Di Piero, *et al.* (1991) The functional anatomy of motor recovery after stroke in humans: a study with positron emission tomography. *Annals of Neurology* **29**, 63–71.

Cimaz, R., Meroni, P.L. *et al.* (2006) Epilepsy as part of systemic lupus erythematosus and systemic antiphospholipid syndrome (Hughes syndrome). *Lupus* **15**, 191–197.

Cloake, P.C.P. (1951) Certain vascular diseases of the nervous system. In: Feiling, A. (ed.) *Modern Trends in Neurology*, ch. 14. Butterworths, London.

Cole, G. (1978) Intracranial space-occupying masses in mental hospital patients: necropsy study. *Journal of Neurology, Neurosurgery and Psychiatry* **41**, 730–736.

Cordonnier, C., Henon, H. *et al.* (2007) Early epileptic seizures after stroke are associated with increased risk of new-onset dementia. *Journal of Neurology, Neurosurgery and Psychiatry* **78**, 514–516.

Costa, D.C. & Ell, P.J. (1991) *Brain Blood Flow in Neurology and Psychiatry*. Churchill Livingstone, Edinburgh & London.

Costa, D.D., Bernatsky, S. *et al.* (2005) Determinants of sleep quality in women with systemic lupus erythematosus. *Arthritis and Rheumatism* **53**, 272–278.

Costa, P.T. Jr & McCrae, R.R. (1985) *The NEO Personality Inventory Manual*. Psychological Assessment Resources Inc., Odessa, FL.

Critchley, M. (1969) Definition of migraine. In: Cochrane, A.L. (ed.) *Background to Migraine. Third Migraine Symposium*, ch. 18. Heinemann, London.

Cutrer, F.M., Sorensen, A.G. *et al.* (1998) Perfusion-weighted imaging defects during spontaneous migrainous aura. *Annals of Neurology* **43**, 25–31.

Dalsgaard-Nielsen, T. (1965) Migraine and heredity. *Acta Neurologica Scandinavica* **41**, 287–300.

Damasio, A.R., Graff-Radford, N.R. *et al.* (1985) Amnesia following basal forebrain lesions. *Archives of Neurology* **42**, 263–271.

Davenport, R. & Dennis, M. (2000) Neurological emergencies: acute stroke. *Journal of Neurology, Neurosurgery and Psychiatry* **68**, 277–288.

Davenport, R.J., Statham, P.F.X. *et al.* (1994) Detection of bilateral isodense subdural haematomas. *British Medical Journal* **309**, 792–794.

D'Cruz, D.P. (2006) Systemic lupus erythematosus. *British Medical Journal* **332**, 890–894.

D'Cruz, D.P., Khamashta, M.A. *et al.* (2007) Systemic lupus erythematosus. *Lancet* **369**, 587–596.

De Boucaud, P., Vital, C.I. *et al.* (1968) Thalamic dementia of vascular origin. *Revue Neurologique* **119**, 461–468.

de Bruijn, S.F., Budde, M. *et al.* (2000) Long-term outcome of cognition and functional health after cerebral venous sinus thrombosis. *Neurology* **54**, 1687–1689.

Del Sette, M., Eliasziw, M. *et al.* (2000) Internal borderzone infarction: a marker for severe stenosis in patients with symptomatic internal carotid artery disease. For the North American Symptomatic Carotid Endarterectomy (NASCET) Group. *Stroke* **31**, 631–636.

DeLuca, J. & Diamond, B.J. (1995) Aneurysm of the anterior communicating artery: a review of neuroanatomical and neuropsychological sequelae. *Journal of Clinical and Experimental Neuropsychology* **17**, 100–121.

del Zoppo, G.J. (2004) TIAs and the pathology of cerebral ischemia. *Neurology* **62** (8 suppl. 6), S15–S19.

Denburg, S.D., Carbotte, R.M. *et al.* (1997) Cognition and mood in systemic lupus erythematosus. Evaluation and pathogenesis. *Annals of the New York Academy of Sciences* **823**, 44–59.

Dennis, M., O'Rourke, S. *et al.* (1998) A quantitative study of the emotional outcome of people caring for stroke survivors. *Stroke* **29**, 1867–1872.

Desantis, A., Laiacona, M. *et al.* (1989) Neuropsychological outcome of patients operated upon for an intracranial aneurysm: analysis of general prognostic factors and of the effects of the location of the aneurysm. *Journal of Neurology, Neurosurgery and Psychiatry* **52**, 1135–1140.

Desmond, D.W., Moroney, J.T. *et al.* (2002) Mortality in patients with dementia after ischemic stroke. *Neurology* **59**, 537–543.

Detsky, M.E., McDonald, D.R. *et al.* (2006) Does this patient with headache have a migraine or need neuroimaging? *Journal of the American Medical Association* **296**, 1274–1283.

Di Piero, V., Bruti, G. *et al.* (2001) Aminergic tone correlates of migraine and tension-type headache: a study using the tridimensional personality questionnaire. *Headache* **41**, 63–71.

Di Pollina, L., Mulligan, R. *et al.* (2000) Cognitive impairment in polycythemia vera: partial reversibility upon lowering of the hematocrit. *European Neurology* **44**, 57–59.

Domitrz, I., Mieszkowski, J. & Kaminska, A. (2007) Relationship between migraine and patent foramen ovale: a study of 121 patients with migraine. *Headache* **47**, 1311–1318.

Donnan, G., Norrving, B. *et al.* (1993) Subcortical infarction: classification and terminology. *Cerebrovascular Disease* **3**, 248–251.

Dorfman, L.J., Marshall, W.H. *et al.* (1979) Cerebral infarction and migraine: clinical and radiologic correlations. *Neurology* **29**, 317–322.

Ducros, A., Denier, C. *et al.* (2001) The clinical spectrum of familial hemiplegic migraine associated with mutations in a neuronal calcium channel. *New England Journal of Medicine* **345**, 17–24.

Eccles, S., House, A. *et al.* (1999) Psychological adjustment and self reported coping in stroke survivors with and without emotionalism. *Journal of Neurology, Neurosurgery and Psychiatry* **67**, 125–126.

Egner, W. (2000) The use of laboratory tests in the diagnosis of SLE. *Journal of Clinical Pathology* **53**, 424–432.

Ehyai, A. & Fenichel, G.M. (1978) The natural history of acute confusional migraine. *Archives of Neurology* **35**, 368–370.

El-Kadi, H., Miele, V.J. & Kaufman, H.H. (2000) Prognosis of chronic subdural hematomas. *Neurosurgical Clinics of North America* **11**, 553–567.

Emmer, B.J., Steens, S.C. *et al.* (2006) Detection of change in CNS involvement in neuropsychiatric SLE: a magnetization transfer study. *Journal of Magnetic Resonance Imaging* **24**, 812–816.

Engelter, S.T., Provenzale, J.M. *et al.* (1999) Diffusion MR imaging and transient ischemic attacks. *Stroke* **30**, 2762–2763.

Fan, A.Y. & Zhou, A.N. (1999) MMPI manifestations of Chinese migraine syndromes: a control study. *American Journal of Chinese Medicine* **27**, 37–42.

Fan, A.Y., Gu, R.J. *et al.* (1999) MMPI changes associated with therapeutic intervention: a migraine control study. *Headache* **39**, 581–585.

Feigin, V.L. & Findlay, M. (2006) Advances in subarachnoid hemorrhage. *Stroke* **37**, 305–308.

Fisher, C.M. (1968) Dementia in cerebral vascular disease. In: Toole, J.F., Siekert, R. & Whisnant, J. (eds) *Transactions of the Sixth Conference on Cerebral Vascular Diseases*. Grune & Stratton, New York.

Fisher, C.M. (1982) Lacunar strokes and infarcts: a review. *Neurology* **32**, 871–876.

Folstein, M.F., Maiberger, R. *et al.* (1977) Mood disorder as a specific complication of stroke. *Journal of Neurology, Neurosurgery and Psychiatry* **40**, 1018–1020.

Fontanella, M., Perozzo, P. *et al.* (2003) Neuropsychological assessment after microsurgical clipping or endovascular treatment for anterior communicating artery aneurysm. *Acta Neurochirurgica (Wien)* **145**, 867–872.

Ford, R.G. & Siekert, R.G. (1965) Central nervous system manifestations of periarteritis nodosa. *Neurology* **15**, 114–122.

Forster, A. & Young, J. (1996) Specialist nurse support for patients with stroke in the community: a randomised controlled trial. *British Medical Journal* **312**, 1642–1646.

Förstl, H. & Sahakian, B. (1991) A psychiatric presentation of abulia: three cases of left frontal lobe ischaemia and atrophy. *Journal of the Royal Society of Medicine* **84**, 89–91.

Frazer, D., Ahuja, A. *et al.* (2007) Coiling versus clipping for the treatment of aneurysmal subarachnoid hemorrhage: a longitudinal investigation into cognitive outcome. *Neurosurgery* **60**, 434–441; discussion 441–442.

Fromm-Reichmann, F. (1937) Contribution to the psychogenesis of migraine. *Psychoanalytic Review* **24**, 26–33.

Fuller, G.N., Marshall, A. *et al.* (1993) Migraine madness: recurrent psychosis following migraine. *Journal of Neurology, Neurosurgery and Psychiatry* **56**, 416–418.

Gade, A. (1982) Amnesia after operations on aneurysms of the anterior communicating artery. *Surgical Neurology* **18**, 46–49.

Ganz, V.H., Gurland, B.J. *et al.* (1972) The study of the psychiatric symptoms of systemic lupus erythematosus: a biometric study. *Psychosomatic Medicine* **34**, 207–220.

Garrard, P., Bradshaw, D. *et al.* (2002) Cognitive dysfunction after isolated brain stem insult. An underdiagnosed cause of long term morbidity. *Journal of Neurology, Neurosurgery and Psychiatry* **73**, 191–194.

Gascon, G. & Barlow, C. (1970) Juvenile migraine, presenting as an acute confusional state. *Pediatrics* **45**, 628–635.

Gautier, J.C. (1983) Cerebral ischaemia in hypertension. In: Russell, R.W.R. (ed.) *Vascular Disease of the Central Nervous System*, ch. 12. Churchill Livingstone, Edinburgh & London.

Geller, T.J. & Bellur, S.N. (1987) Peduncular hallucinosis: magnetic resonance imaging confirmation of mesencephalic infarction during life. *Annals of Neurology* **21**, 602–604.

Gerli, R., Caponi, L. *et al.* (2002) Clinical and serological associations of ribosomal P autoantibodies in systemic lupus erythematosus: prospective evaluation in a large cohort of Italian patients. *Rheumatology (Oxford)* **41**, 1357–1366.

Giaquinto, S., Spiridigliozzi, C. *et al.* (2007) Can faith protect from emotional distress after stroke? *Stroke* **38**, 993–997.

Giffin, N.J., Ruggiero, L. *et al.* (2003) Premonitory symptoms in migraine: an electronic diary study. *Neurology* **60**, 935–940.

Gladman, D.D. (1992) Prognosis of systemic lupus erythematosus and factors that affect it. *Current Opinion in Rheumatology* **4**, 681–687.

Gladstone, J.P. & Dodick, D.W. (2005) Migraine and cerebral white matter lesions: when to suspect cerebral autosomal dominant arteriopathy with subcortical infarcts and leukoencephalopathy (CADASIL). *Neurologist* **11**, 19–29.

Goadsby, P.J. (2006) Recent advances in the diagnosis and management of migraine. *British Medical Journal* **332**, 25–29.

Govoni, M., Castellino, G. *et al.* (2004) Recent advances and future perspective in neuroimaging in neuropsychiatric systemic lupus erythematosus. *Lupus* **13**, 149–158.

Grant, J.S., Elliott, T.R. *et al.* (2002) Telephone intervention with family caregivers of stroke survivors after rehabilitation. *Stroke* **33**, 2060–2065.

Greener, J., Enderby, P. *et al.* (2000) Speech and language therapy for aphasia following stroke. *Cochrane Database of Systematic Reviews* 2, CD000425.

Griffith, J.L. & Razavi, M. (2006) Pharmacological management of mood and anxiety disorders in headache patients. *Headache* **46** (suppl. 3), S133–S141.

Guadagno, J.V., Warburton, E.A. *et al.* (2004) Does the acute diffusion-weighted imaging lesion represent penumbra as well as core? A combined quantitative PET/MRI voxel-based study. *Journal of Cerebral Blood Flow and Metabolism* **24**, 1249–1254.

Gudbjornsson, B. & Hetta, J. (2001) Sleep disturbances in patients with systemic lupus erythematosus: a questionnaire-based study. *Clinical and Experimental Rheumatology* **19**, 509–514.

Guillevin, L., Durand-Gasselin, B. *et al.* (1999) Microscopic polyangiitis: clinical and laboratory findings in eighty-five patients. *Arthritis and Rheumatism* **42**, 421–430.

Hackett, M.L. & Anderson, C.S. (2000) Health outcomes 1 year after subarachnoid hemorrhage: an international population-based study. The Australian Cooperative Research on Subarachnoid Hemorrhage Study Group. *Neurology* **55**, 658–662.

Hackett, M.L. & Anderson, C.S. (2005) Predictors of depression after stroke: a systematic review of observational studies. *Stroke* **36**, 2296–2301.

Hackett, M.L., Anderson, C.S. *et al.* (2004) Interventions for treating depression after stroke. *Cochrane Database of Systematic Reviews* 3, CD003437.

Hackett, M.L., Anderson, C.S. *et al.* (2005) Management of depression after stroke: a systematic review of pharmacological therapies. *Stroke* **36**, 1098–1103.

Hadjikhani, N., Sanchez-Del-Rio, M. *et al.* (2001) Mechanisms of migraine aura revealed by functional MRI in human visual cortex. *Proceedings of the National Academy of Sciences USA* **98**, 4687–4692.

Hadjivassiliou, M., Tooth, C.L. *et al.* (2001) Aneurysmal SAH: cognitive outcome and structural damage after clipping or coiling. *Neurology* **56**, 1672–1677.

Hahn, S., Kroenke, K. *et al.* (1999) Primary Care Evaluation of Mental Disorders: PRIME-MD. In: Maruish, M. (ed.) *The Use of Psychological Testing for Treatment Planning and Outcome Assessment*, pp. 871–920. Lawrence Earlbaum Associates, Mahwah, NJ.

Han, B. & Haley, W.E. (1999) Family caregiving for patients with stroke. Review and analysis. *Stroke* **30**, 1478–1485.

Hanly, J.G., Fisk, J.D. *et al.* (1994) Clinical course of cognitive dysfunction in systemic lupus erythematosus. *Journal of Rheumatology* **21**, 1825–1831.

Hanly, J.G., Urowitz, M.B. *et al.* (2007) Neuropsychiatric events at the time of diagnosis of systemic lupus erythematosus: an international inception cohort study. *Arthritis and Rheumatism* **56**, 265–273.

Harris, A.I., Cox, E. *et al.* (1971) *Handicapped and Impaired in Great Britain*, Part 1, p. 375. Office of Population Censuses and Surveys, London.

Harrison, M.J. & Ravdin, L.D. (2002) Cognitive dysfunction in neuropsychiatric systemic lupus erythematosus. *Current Opinion in Rheumatology* **14**, 510–514.

Hasan, D., Vermeulen, M. *et al.* (1989) Management problems in acute hydrocephalus after subarachnoid hemorrhage. *Stroke* **20**, 747–753.

Hassan, A., Hunt, B.J. *et al.* (2003) Markers of endothelial dysfunction in lacunar infarction and ischaemic leukoaraiosis. *Brain* **126**, 424–432.

Haug, T., Sorteberg, A. *et al.* (2007) Cognitive outcome after aneurysmal subarachnoid hemorrhage: time course of recovery and relationship to clinical, radiological, and management parameters. *Neurosurgery* **60**, 649–656; discussion 656–657.

Haut, S.R., Bigal, M.E. *et al.* (2006) Chronic disorders with episodic manifestations: focus on epilepsy and migraine. *Lancet Neurology* **5**, 148–157.

Hay, E.M., Huddy, A. *et al.* (1994) A prospective study of psychiatric disorder and cognitive function in systemic lupus erythematosus. *Annals of the Rheumatic Diseases* **53**, 298–303.

Healton, E.B., Brust, J.C. *et al.* (1982) Hypertensive encephalopathy and the neurologic manifestations of malignant hypertension. *Neurology* **32**, 127–132.

Heine, B.E. (1969) Psychiatric aspects of systemic lupus erythematosus. *Acta Psychiatrica Scandinavica* **45**, 307–326.

Hellawell, D.J. & Pentland, B. (2001) Relatives' reports of long term problems following traumatic brain injury or subarachnoid haemorrhage. *Disability and Rehabilitation* **23**, 300–5.

Hellmich, B., Lamprecht, P. *et al.* (2006) Advances in the therapy of Wegener's granulomatosis. *Current Opinion in Rheumatology* **18**, 25–32.

Henryk-Gutt, R. & Rees, W.L. (1973) Psychological aspects of migraine. *Journal of Psychosomatic Research* **17**, 141–153.

Herrmann, N., Black, S.E. *et al.* (1998) The Sunnybrook Stroke Study: a prospective study of depressive symptoms and functional outcome. *Stroke* **29**, 618–624.

Hill, D.L., Daroff, R.B. *et al.* (2007) Most cases labeled as retinal migraine are not migraine. *Journal of Neuro-ophthalmology* **27**, 3–8.

Hinchey, J., Chaves, C. *et al.* (1996) A reversible posterior leukoencephalopathy syndrome. *New England Journal of Medicine* **334**, 494–500.

Hirtz, D., Thurman, D.J. *et al.* (2007) How common are the common neurologic disorders? *Neurology* **68**, 326–337.

Hocaoglu, C. & Tan, M. (2005) Isolated angiitis of the central nervous system: a case presented with atypical psychiatric symptoms. *Progress in Neuropsychopharmacology and Biological Psychiatry* **29**, 627–631.

Hoffmann, M. & Schmitt, F. (2004) Cognitive impairment in isolated subtentorial stroke. *Acta Neurologica Scandinavica* **109**, 14–24.

Holm, J.E., Lokken, C. *et al.* (1997) Migraine and stress: a daily examination of temporal relationships in women migraineurs. *Headache* **37**, 553–558.

Hopkinson, N.D., Bendall, P. *et al.* (1992) Screening of acute psychiatric admissions for previously misdiagnosed systemic lupus erythematosus. *British Journal of Psychiatry* **161**, 107–110.

House, A., Dennis, M. *et al.* (1989) Emotionalism after stroke. *British Medical Journal* **298**, 991–994.

House, A., Dennis, M. *et al.* (1990) Life events and difficulties preceding stroke. *Journal of Neurology, Neurosurgery and Psychiatry* **53**, 1024–1028.

House, A., Dennis, M. *et al.* (1991) Mood disorders in the year after first stroke. *British Journal of Psychiatry* **158**, 83–92.

House, A., Knapp, P. *et al.* (2001) Mortality at 12 and 24 months after stroke may be associated with depressive symptoms at 1 month. *Stroke* **32**, 696–701.

House, A.O., Hackett, M.L. *et al.* (2004) Pharmaceutical interventions for emotionalism after stroke. *Cochrane Database of Systematic Reviews* **2**, CD003690.

Hughes, G.V. (1974) Systemic lupus erythematosus. *British Journal of Hospital Medicine* **12**, 309–319.

Hung, C.I., Wang, S.J. *et al.* (2005) Risk factors associated with migraine or chronic daily headache in out-patients with major depressive disorder. *Acta Psychiatrica Scandinavica* **111**, 310–315.

Hungerford, G.D., Du Boulay, G.H. *et al.* (1976) Computerised axial tomography in patients with severe migraine: a preliminary report. *Journal of Neurology, Neurosurgery and Psychiatry* **39**, 990–994.

Hurwitz, L.J. & Adams, G.F. (1972) Rehabilitation of hemiplegia: indices of assessment and prognosis. *British Medical Journal* **1**, 94–98.

Hutter, B.O. & Gilsbach, J.M. (1993) Which neuropsychological deficits are hidden behind a good outcome (Glasgow = I) after aneurysmal subarachnoid hemorrhage? *Neurosurgery* **33**, 999–1005; discussion 1005–1006.

Hutter, B.O., Gilsbach, J.M. *et al.* (1995) Quality of life and cognitive deficits after subarachnoid haemorrhage. *British Journal of Neurosurgery* **9**, 465–475.

Hutter, B.O., Kreitschmann-Andermahr, I. *et al.* (2001) Health-related quality of life after aneurysmal subarachnoid hemorrhage: impacts of bleeding severity, computerized tomography findings, surgery, vasospasm, and neurological grade. *Journal of Neurosurgery* **94**, 241–251.

Inao, S., Kawai, T. *et al.* (2001) Relation between brain displacement and local cerebral blood flow in patients with chronic subdural haematoma. *Journal of Neurology, Neurosurgery and Psychiatry* **71**, 741–746.

Ishikawa, E., Yanaka, K. *et al.* (2002) Reversible dementia in patients with chronic subdural hematomas. *Journal of Neurosurgery* **96**, 680–683.

Jackson, C.A. & Sudlow, C.L. (2006) Is hypertension a more frequent risk factor for deep than for lobar supratentorial intracerebral haemorrhage? *Journal of Neurology, Neurosurgery and Psychiatry* **77**, 1244–1252.

Jennekens, F.G. & Kater, L. (2002) The central nervous system in systemic lupus erythematosus. Part 2. Pathogenetic mechanisms of clinical syndromes: a literature investigation. *Rheumatology (Oxford)* **41**, 619–630.

Jennette, J.C., Falk, R.J. *et al.* (1994) Nomenclature of systemic vasculitides. Proposal of an international consensus conference. *Arthritis and Rheumatism* **37**, 187–192.

Jia, H., Damush, T.M. *et al.* (2006) The impact of poststroke depression on healthcare use by veterans with acute stroke. *Stroke* **37**, 2796–2801.

Jinnah, H.A., Dixon, A. *et al.* (1997) Chronic meningitis with cranial neuropathies in Wegener's granulomatosis. Case report and review of the literature. *Arthritis and Rheumatism* **40**, 573–577.

Johnson, R.T. & Richardson, E.P. (1968) The neurological manifestations of systemic lupus erythematosus: a clinical-pathological study of 24 cases and review of the literature. *Medicine (Baltimore)* **47**, 337–369.

Kalaydjian, A., Zandi, P.P. *et al.* (2007) How migraines impact cognitive function: findings from the Baltimore ECA. *Neurology* **68**, 1417–1424.

Karakurum, B., Soylu, O. *et al.* (2004) Personality, depression, and anxiety as risk factors for chronic migraine. *International Journal of Neuroscience* **114**, 1391–1399.

Kessels, R.P. & de Haan, E.H. (2003) Implicit learning in memory rehabilitation: a meta-analysis on errorless learning and vanishing cues methods. *Journal of Clinical and Experimental Neuropsychology* **25**, 805–814.

Khamashta, M.A., Cervera, R. *et al.* (1990) Association of antibodies against phospholipids with heart valve disease in systemic lupus erythematosus. *Lancet* **335**, 1541–1544.

Kirchmann, M. (2006) Migraine with aura: new understanding from clinical epidemiologic studies. *Current Opinion in Neurology* **19**, 286–293.

Kirchmann, M., Thomsen, L.L. *et al.* (2006) Basilar-type migraine: clinical, epidemiologic, and genetic features. *Neurology* **66**, 880–886.

Kishi, Y., Robinson, R.G. *et al.* (1996) Suicidal plans in patients with stroke: comparison between acute-onset and delayed-onset suicidal plans. *International Psychogeriatrics* **8**, 623–634.

Klee, A. (1968) *A Clinical Study of Migraine with Particular Reference to the Most Severe Cases.* Munksgaard, Copenhagen.

Klee, A. & Willanger, R. (1966) Disturbances of visual perception in migraine. *Acta Neurologica Scandinavica* **42**, 400–414.

Knapp, P. & Hewison, J. (1999) Disagreement in patient and carer assessment of functional abilities after stroke. *Stroke* **30**, 934–938.

Koivisto, T., Vanninen, R. *et al.* (2000) Outcomes of early endovascular versus surgical treatment of ruptured cerebral aneurysms. A prospective randomized study. *Stroke* **31**, 2369–2377.

Kokmen, E., Whisnant, J.P. *et al.* (1996) Dementia after ischemic stroke: a population-based study in Rochester, Minnesota (1960–1984). *Neurology* **46**, 154–159.

Kowal, C., Degiorgio, L.A. *et al.* (2006) Human lupus autoantibodies against NMDA receptors mediate cognitive impairment. *Proceedings of the National Academy of Sciences USA* **103**, 19854–19859.

Kozora, E., Thompson, L.L. *et al.* (1996) Analysis of cognitive and psychological deficits in systemic lupus erythematosus patients without overt central nervous system disease. *Arthritis and Rheumatism* **39**, 2035–2045.

Kozora, E., West, S.G. *et al.* (1998) Magnetic resonance imaging abnormalities and cognitive deficits in systemic lupus erythematosus patients without overt central nervous system disease. *Arthritis and Rheumatism* **41**, 41–47.

Kozora, E., Ellison, M.C. *et al.* (2005a) Major life stress, coping styles, and social support in relation to psychological distress in patients with systemic lupus erythematosus. *Lupus* **14**, 363–372.

Kozora, E., Arciniegas, D.B. *et al.* (2005b) Cognition, MRS neurometabolites, and MRI volumetrics in non-neuropsychiatric systemic lupus erythematosus: preliminary data. *Cognitive and Behavioral Neurology* **18**, 159–162.

Kozora, E., Ellison, M.C. *et al.* (2006) Depression, fatigue, and pain in systemic lupus erythematosus (SLE): relationship to the American College of Rheumatology SLE neuropsychological battery. *Arthritis and Rheumatism* **55**, 628–635.

Kreiter, K.T., Copeland, D. *et al.* (2002) Predictors of cognitive dysfunction after subarachnoid hemorrhage. *Stroke* **33**, 200–208.

Kreitschmann-Andermahr, I., Hoff, C. *et al.* (2004) Prevalence of pituitary deficiency in patients after aneurysmal subarachnoid hemorrhage. *Journal of Clinical Endocrinology and Metabolism* **89**, 4986–4992.

Kruit, M.C., van Buchem, M.A. *et al.* (2004) Migraine as a risk factor for subclinical brain lesions. *Journal of the American Medical Association* **291**, 427–434.

Kruit, M.C., Launer, L.J. *et al.* (2005) Infarcts in the posterior circulation territory in migraine. The population-based MRI CAMERA study. *Brain* **128**, 2068–2077.

Kumar, R., Wijdicks, E.F. *et al.* (1997) Isolated angiitis of the CNS presenting as subarachnoid haemorrhage. *Journal of Neurology, Neurosurgery and Psychiatry* **62**, 649–651.

Kumral, E. & Ozturk, O. (2004) Delusional state following acute stroke. *Neurology* **62**, 110–113.

Kumral, E., Evyapan, D. *et al.* (2001) Bilateral thalamic infarction. Clinical, etiological and MRI correlates. *Acta Neurologica Scandinavica* **103**, 35–42.

Kur, J.K. & Esdaile, J.M. (2006) Posterior reversible encephalopathy syndrome: an underrecognized manifestation of systemic lupus erythematosus. *Journal of Rheumatology* **33**, 2178–2183.

Kyttaris, V.C., Katsiari, C.G. *et al.* (2005) New insights into the pathogenesis of systemic lupus erythematosus. *Current Rheumatology Reports* **7**, 469–475.

Labovitz, D.L. & Sacco, R.L. (2001) Intracerebral hemorrhage: update. *Current Opinion in Neurology* **14**, 103–108.

Lai, S.M., Studenski, S. *et al.* (2006) Therapeutic exercise and depressive symptoms after stroke. *Journal of the American Geriatric Society* **54**, 240–247.

Laiacona, M., DeSantis, A. *et al.* (1989) Neuropsychological follow-up of patients operated for aneurysms of anterior communicating artery. *Cortex* **25**, 261–273.

Lampl, Y., Lorberboym, M. *et al.* (2005) Auditory hallucinations in acute stroke. *Behavioral Neurology* **16**, 211–216.

Lance, J.W. (1993) *Mechanism and Management of Headache.* Butterworth Heinemann, Oxford.

Lapteva, L., Nowak, M. *et al.* (2006) Anti-N-methyl-D-aspartate receptor antibodies, cognitive dysfunction, and depression in systemic lupus erythematosus. *Arthritis and Rheumatism* **54**, 2505–2514.

Launer, L.J., Terwindt, G.M. *et al.* (1999) The prevalence and characteristics of migraine in a population-based cohort: the GEM study. *Neurology* **53**, 537–542.

Lauritzen, M. (1994) Pathophysiology of the migraine aura. The spreading depression theory. *Brain* **117**, 199–210.

Lawson, I.R. & MacLeod, R.D.M. (1969) The use of imipramine ('Tofranil') and other psychotrophic drugs in organic emotionalism. *British Journal of Psychiatry* **115**, 281–285.

Lee, S.T., Park, J.H. *et al.* (2005) Efficacy of the 5-HT1A agonist, buspirone hydrochloride, in migraineurs with anxiety: a randomized, prospective, parallel group, double-blind, placebo-controlled study. *Headache* **45**, 1004–1011.

Leon-Carrion, J., van Eeckhout, P. *et al.* (2002) The locked-in syndrome: a syndrome looking for a therapy. *Brain Injury* **16**, 571–582.

Leppavuori, A., Pohjasvaara, T. *et al.* (2003) Generalized anxiety disorders three to four months after ischemic stroke. *Cerebrovascular Disease* **16**, 257–264.

Leritz, E., Brandt, J. *et al.* (2000) Subcortical cognitive impairment in patients with systemic lupus erythematosus. *Journal of the International Neuropsychological Society* **6**, 821–825.

Levine, D.N. & Finklestein, S. (1982) Delayed psychosis after right temporoparietal stroke or trauma: relation to epilepsy. *Neurology* **32**, 267–273.

Leys, D., Henon, H. *et al.* (2005) Poststroke dementia. *Lancet Neurology* **4**, 752–759.

Lhermitte, J. (1922) Syndrome de la calotte du pédoncule cérébral. Les troubles psycho-sensoriels dans les lésions du mésocéphale. *Revue Neurologique* **38**, 1359–1365.

Lhermitte, J. (1932) L'hallucinose pédonculaire. *Encéphale* **27**, 422–435.

Lim, L., Ron, M.A. *et al.* (1988) Psychiatric and neurological manifestations in systemic lupus erythematosus. *Quarterly Journal of Medicine* **66**, 27–38.

Lincoln, N.B. & Bowen, A. (2006) The need for randomised treatment studies in neglect research. *Restorative Neurology and Neuroscience* **24**, 401–408.

Lincoln, N.B. & Flannaghan, T. (2003) Cognitive behavioral psychotherapy for depression following stroke: a randomized controlled trial. *Stroke* **34**, 111–115.

Lindqvist, G. & Malmgren, H. (1993) Organic mental disorders as hypothetical pathogenetic processes. *Acta Psychiatrica Scandinavica Supplementum* **373**, 5–17.

Lindqvist, G. & Norlén, G. (1966) Korsakoff's syndrome after operation on ruptured aneurysm of the anterior communicating artery. *Acta Psychiatrica Scandinavica* **42**, 24–34.

Liou, H.H., Wang, C.R. *et al.* (1994) Anticardiolipin antisera from lupus patients with seizures reduce a GABA receptor-mediated chloride current in snail neurons. *Life Sciences* **54**, 1119–1125.

Lippman, C.W. (1952) Certain hallucinations peculiar to migraine. *Journal of Nervous and Mental Disease* **116**, 346–351.

Lipsey, J.R., Robinson, R.G. *et al.* (1984) Nortriptyline treatment of post-stroke depression: a double-blind study. *Lancet* **i**, 297–300.

Lipton, R.B., Hamelsky, S.W. *et al.* (2000) Migraine, quality of life, and depression: a population-based case–control study. *Neurology* **55**, 629–635.

Logue, V., Durward, M. *et al.* (1968) The quality of survival after rupture of an anterior cerebral aneurysm. *British Journal of Psychiatry* **114**, 137–160.

Lui, M.H., Ross, F.M. *et al.* (2005) Supporting family caregivers in stroke care: a review of the evidence for problem solving. *Stroke* **36**, 2514–2522.

McClain, M.T., Heinlen, L.D. *et al.* (2005) Early events in lupus humoral autoimmunity suggest initiation through molecular mimicry. *Nature Medicine* **11**, 85–89.

McCormick, H.M. & Neuberger, K.T. (1958) Giant-cell arteritis involving small meningeal and intracerebral vessels. *Journal of Neuropathology and Experimental Neurology* **17**, 471–478.

McCune, W.J. & Golbus, J. (1988) Neuropsychiatric lupus. *Rheumatic Disease Clinics of North America* **14**, 149–167.

McGilchrist, I., Goldstein, L.H. *et al.* (1993) Thalamo-frontal psychosis: a case report. *British Journal of Psychiatry* **163**, 113–115.

Machulda, M.M. & Haut, M.W. (2000) Clinical features of chronic subdural hematoma: neuropsychiatric and neuropsychologic changes in patients with chronic subdural hematoma. *Neurosurgical Clinics of North America* **11**, 473–477.

MacKay, M.E., McLardy, T. *et al.* (1950) A case of periarteritis nodosa of the central nervous system. *Journal of Mental Science* **96**, 470–475.

McKenna, P., Willison, J.R. *et al.* (1989) Cognitive outcome and quality of life one year after subarachnoid haemorrhage. *Neurosurgery* **24**, 361–367.

McLaurin, E.Y., Holliday, S.L. *et al.* (2005) Predictors of cognitive dysfunction in patients with systemic lupus erythematosus. *Neurology* **64**, 297–303.

McWilliams, L.A., Goodwin, R.D. *et al.* (2004) Depression and anxiety associated with three pain conditions: results from a nationally representative sample. *Pain* **111**, 77–83.

Magnano, M.D., Bush, T.M. *et al.* (2006) Reversible posterior leukoencephalopathy in patients with systemic lupus erythematosus. *Seminars in Arthritis and Rheumatism* **35**, 396–402.

Majid, M.J., Lincoln, N.B. *et al.* (2000) Cognitive rehabilitation for memory deficits following stroke. *Cochrane Database of Systematic Reviews* **3**, CD002293.

Markus, H.S., Thomson, N.D. *et al.* (1995) Asymptomatic cerebral embolic signals in symptomatic and asymptomatic carotid artery disease. *Brain* **118**, 1005–1011.

Masdeu, J.C., Irimia, P. *et al.* (2006) EFNS guideline on neuroimaging in acute stroke. Report of an EFNS task force. *European Journal of Neurology* **13**, 1271–1283.

Mason, J.C. & Walport, M.J. (1992) Giant cell arteritis. Probably underdiagnosed and overtreated. *British Medical Journal* **305**, 68–69.

Masuhr, F., Mehraein, S. *et al.* (2004) Cerebral venous and sinus thrombosis. *Journal of Neurology* **251**, 11–23.

Matharu, M.S., Bartsch, T. *et al.* (2004) Central neuromodulation in chronic migraine patients with suboccipital stimulators: a PET study. *Brain* **127**, 220–230.

Mattsson, P. & Ekselius, L. (2002) Migraine, major depression, panic disorder, and personality traits in women aged 40–74 years: a population-based study. *Cephalalgia* **22**, 543–551.

Maurice-Williams, R.S., Willison, J.R. *et al.* (1991) The cognitive and psychological sequelae of uncomplicated aneurysm surgery. *Journal of Neurology, Neurosurgery and Psychiatry* **54**, 335–340.

Mavaddat, N., Kirkpatrick, P.J. *et al.* (2000) Deficits in decision-making in patients with aneurysms of the anterior communicating artery. *Brain* **123**, 2109–2117.

May, A., Bahra, A. *et al.* (1998) Hypothalamic activation in cluster headache attacks. *Lancet* **352**, 275–278.

Mayer, S.A., Kreiter, K.T. *et al.* (2002) Global and domain-specific cognitive impairment and outcome after subarachnoid hemorrhage. *Neurology* **59**, 1750–1758.

Meckling, S.K., Becker, W.J. *et al.* (2001) Sumatriptan responsiveness and clinical, psychiatric and psychologic features in migraine patients. *Canadian Journal of Neurological Sciences* **28**, 313–318.

Mehta, T. (1965) Subdural haematoma. *Journal of the Indian Medical Association* **44**, 635–641.

Merikangas, K.R., Angst, J. *et al.* (1990) Migraine and psychopathology. Results of the Zurich cohort study of young adults. *Archives of General Psychiatry* **47**, 849–853.

Merikangas, K., Stevens, D. *et al.* (1994) Psychopathology and headache syndromes in the community. *Headache* **34**, S17–S26.

Mesulam, M.-M., Waxman, S.G. *et al.* (1976) Acute confusional states with right middle cerebral artery infarctions. *Journal of Neurology, Neurosurgery and Psychiatry* **39**, 84–89.

Miller, D.H., Buchanan, N. *et al.* (1992) Gadolinium-enhanced magnetic resonance imaging of the central nervous system in systemic lupus erythematosus. *Journal of Neurology* **239**, 460–464.

Mitchell, K.R. (1971) A psychological approach to the treatment of migraine. *British Journal of Psychiatry* **119**, 533–534.

Mitsikostas, D.D., Sfikakis, P.P. *et al.* (2004) A meta-analysis for headache in systemic lupus erythematosus: the evidence and the myth. *Brain* **127**, 1200–1209.

Mobbs, R.J., Chandran, K.N. *et al.* (2001) Psychiatric presentation of aneurysmal subarachnoid haemorrhage. *Australian and New Zealand Journal of Surgery* **71**, 69–70.

Mok, C.C., To, C.H. *et al.* (2006) Neuropsychiatric damage in Southern Chinese patients with systemic lupus erythematosus. *Medicine (Baltimore)* **85**, 221–228.

Molyneux, A.J., Kerr, R.S. *et al.* (2005) International subarachnoid aneurysm trial (ISAT) of neurosurgical clipping versus endovascular coiling in 2143 patients with ruptured intracranial aneurysms: a randomised comparison of effects on survival, dependency, seizures, rebleeding, subgroups, and aneurysm occlusion. *Lancet* **366**, 809–817.

Monastero, R., Bettini, P. *et al.* (2001) Prevalence and pattern of cognitive impairment in systemic lupus erythematosus patients with and without overt neuropsychiatric manifestations. *Journal of the Neurological Sciences* **184**, 33–39.

Mongini, F., Rota, E. *et al.* (2005) A comparative analysis of personality profile and muscle tenderness between chronic migraine and chronic tension-type headache. *Neurological Sciences* **26**, 203–7.

Moore, P.M. (1994) Vasculitis of the central nervous system. *Seminars in Neurology* **14**, 307–312.

Moritani, T., Shrier, D.A. *et al.* (2001) Diffusion-weighted echoplanar MR imaging of CNS involvement in systemic lupus erythematosus. *Academic Radiology* **8**, 741–53.

Morley, J.B. (1967) Unruptured vertebro-basilar aneurysms. *Medical Journal of Australia* **2**, 1024–1027.

Morris, P.G., Wilson, J.T. *et al.* (2004) Anxiety and depression after spontaneous subarachnoid hemorrhage. *Neurosurgery* **54**, 47–52; discussion 52–54.

Morris, P.L., Robinson, R.G. *et al.* (1990) Prevalence and course of depressive disorders in hospitalized stroke patients. *International Journal of Psychiatry in Medicine* **20**, 349–364.

Morris, P.L., Robinson, R.G. *et al.* (1993) Association of depression with 10-year poststroke mortality. *American Journal of Psychiatry* **150**, 124–129.

Muir, K.W., Buchan, A. *et al.* (2006) Imaging of acute stroke. *Lancet Neurology* **5**, 755–768.

Munoz, L.E., Gaipl, U.S. *et al.* (2005) SLE: a disease of clearance deficiency? *Rheumatology (Oxford)* **44**, 1101–1107.

Murray, D. & Hodgson, R. (1991) Polycythaemia rubra vera, cerebral ischaemia and depression. *British Journal of Psychiatry* **158**, 842–844.

Narushima, K., Kosier, J.T. *et al.* (2003) A reappraisal of poststroke depression, intra- and inter-hemispheric lesion location using meta-analysis. *Journal of Neuropsychiatry and Clinical Neuroscience* **15**, 422–430.

Nasreddine, Z.S. & Saver, J.L. (1997) Pain after thalamic stroke: right diencephalic predominance and clinical features in 180 patients. *Neurology* **48**, 1196–1199.

New, P.W. & Thomas, S.J. (2005) Cognitive impairments in the locked-in syndrome: a case report. *Archives of Physical Medicine and Rehabilitation* **86**, 338–343.

Ng, Y.S., Stein, J. *et al.* (2005) Clinical characteristics and rehabilitation outcomes of patients with posterior cerebral artery stroke. *Archives of Physical Medicine and Rehabilitation* **86**, 2138–2143.

Niedermaier, N., Bohrer, E. *et al.* (2004) Prevention and treatment of poststroke depression with mirtazapine in patients with acute stroke. *Journal of Clinical Psychiatry* **65**, 1619–1623.

Nielsen, J.M. (1930) Migraine equivalent. *American Journal of Psychiatry* **9**, 637–641.

Norrving, B. (2003) Long-term prognosis after lacunar infarction. *Lancet Neurology* **2**, 238–245.

Nylander, P.O., Schlette, P. *et al.* (1996) Migraine: temperament and character. *Journal of Psychiatric Research* **30**, 359–368.

Nys, G.M., van Zandvoort, M.J. *et al.* (2005) Early depressive symptoms after stroke: neuropsychological correlates and lesion characteristics. *Journal of the Neurological Sciences* **228**, 27–33.

O'Bryant, S.E., Marcus, D.A. *et al.* (2005) Neuropsychology of migraine: present status and future directions. *Expert Review of Neurotherapeutics* **5**, 363–70.

O'Connor, J.F. & Musher, D.M. (1966) Central nervous system involvement in systemic lupus erythematosus. *Archives of Neurology* **14**, 157–164.

Oda, K., Matsushima, E. *et al.* (2005) Abnormal regional cerebral blood flow in systemic lupus erythematosus patients with psychiatric symptoms. *Journal of Clinical Psychiatry* **66**, 907–913.

Oedegaard, K.J. & Fasmer, O.B. (2005) Is migraine in unipolar depressed patients a bipolar spectrum trait? *Journal of Affective Disorders* **84**, 233–242.

Oedegaard, K.J., Neckelmann, D. *et al.* (2006) Migraine with and without aura: association with depression and anxiety disorder in a population-based study. The HUNT Study. *Cephalalgia* **26**, 1–6.

Ogden, J.A., Mee, E.W. *et al.* (1993) A prospective study of impairment of cognition and memory and recovery after subarachnoid hemorrhage. *Neurosurgery* **33**, 572–586; discussion 586–587.

Ogden, J.A., Utley, T. *et al.* (1997) Neurological and psychosocial outcome 4 to 7 years after subarachnoid hemorrhage. *Neurosurgery* **41**, 25–34.

Ohno, K., Maehara, T. *et al.* (1993) Low incidence of seizures in patients with chronic subdural haematoma. *Journal of Neurology, Neurosurgery and Psychiatry* **56**, 1231–1233.

Olesen, J., Larsen, B. *et al.* (1981) Focal hyperemia followed by spreading oligemia and impaired activation of rCBF in classic migraine. *Annals of Neurology* **9**, 344–352.

Olesen, J., Friberg, L. *et al.* (1993) Ischaemia-induced (symptomatic) migraine attacks may be more frequent than migraine-induced ischaemic insults. *Brain* **116**, 187–202.

Olesen, J., Diener, H.C. *et al.* (2004) Calcitonin gene-related peptide receptor antagonist BIBN 4096 BS for the acute treatment of migraine. *New England Journal of Medicine* **350**, 1104–1110.

Olin, J.W. & Shih, A. (2006) Thromboangiitis obliterans (Buerger's disease). *Current Opinion in Rheumatology* **18**, 18–24.

Ottman, R. & Lipton, R.B. (1994) Comorbidity of migraine and epilepsy. *Neurology* **44**, 2105–2110.

Outpatient Service Trialists (2003) Therapy-based rehabilitation services for stroke patients at home. *Cochrane Database of Systematic Reviews* 1, CD002925.

Ovsiew, F. & Utset, T. (2002) Neuropsychiatric aspects of rheumatic disease. In: Yudofsky, S.C. & Hales, R.E. (eds) *Textbook of Neuropsychiatry and Clinical Neurosciences,* pp. 813–850 American Psychiatric Publishing, Washington, DC.

Paolucci, S., Gandolfo, C. *et al.* (2006) The Italian multicenter observational study on post-stroke depression (DESTRO). *Journal of Neurology* **253**, 556–562.

Parkin, A.J., Leng, N.R. *et al.* (1988) Memory impairment following ruptured aneurysm of the anterior communicating artery. *Brain and Cognition* **7**, 231–243.

Patel, N.V., Bigal, M.E. *et al.* (2004) Prevalence and impact of migraine and probable migraine in a health plan. *Neurology* **63**, 1432–1438.

Pavone, L., Grasselli, C. *et al.* (2006) Outcome and prognostic factors during the course of primary small-vessel vasculitides. *Journal of Rheumatology* **33**, 1299–1306.

Pedersen, K.K. (1980) Migraene og demens. *Ugeskrift for Laeger* **142**, 1346–1347.

Petzold, A., Keir, G. *et al.* (2006) Axonal damage and outcome in subarachnoid haemorrhage. *Journal of Neurology, Neurosurgery and Psychiatry* **77**, 753–759.

Pietrobon, D. & Striessnig, J. (2003) Neurobiology of migraine. *Nature Reviews Neuroscience* **4**, 386–398.

Pincus, T., Swearingen, C. *et al.* (1999) Toward a multidimensional Health Assessment Questionnaire (MDHAQ): assessment of advanced activities of daily living and psychological status in the patient-friendly health assessment questionnaire format. *Arthritis and Rheumatism* **42**, 2220–2230.

Plum, F. & Posner, J.B. (1972) *Diagnosis of Stupor and Coma.* Davis, Philadelphia.

Pohjasvaara, T., Vataja, R. *et al.* (2001) Suicidal ideas in stroke patients 3 and 15 months after stroke. *Cerebrovascular Disease* **12**, 21–26.

Pohjasvaara, T., Vataja, R. *et al.* (2002) Cognitive functions and depression as predictors of poor outcome 15 months after stroke. *Cerebrovascular Disease* **14**, 228–233.

Powell, J., Kitchen, N. *et al.* (2002) Psychosocial outcomes at three and nine months after good neurological recovery from aneurysmal subarachnoid haemorrhage: predictors and prognosis. *Journal of Neurology, Neurosurgery and Psychiatry* **72**, 772–781.

Powell, J., Kitchen, N. *et al.* (2004) Psychosocial outcomes at 18 months after good neurological recovery from aneurysmal subarachnoid haemorrhage. *Journal of Neurology, Neurosurgery and Psychiatry* **75**, 1119–1124.

Preston, G.A., Yang, J.J. *et al.* (2002) Understanding the pathogenesis of ANCA: where are we today? *Cleveland Clinic Journal of Medicine* **69** (suppl. 2), SII51–SII54.

Price, B.H. & Mesulam, M. (1985) Psychiatric manifestations of right hemisphere infarctions. *Journal of Nervous and Mental Disease* **173**, 610–614.

Prince, P.B., Rapoport, A.M. *et al.* (2004) The effect of weather on headache. *Headache* **44**, 596–602.

Pritchard, C., Foulkes, L. *et al.* (2004) Cost–benefit analysis of an integrated approach to reduce psychosocial trauma following neurosurgery compared with standard care: two-year prospective comparative study of enhanced specialist liaison nurse service for aneurysmal subarachnoid hemorrhage (ASAH) patients and carers. *Surgical Neurology* **62**, 17–27.

Rabins, P.V., Starkstein, S.E. *et al.* (1991) Risk factors for developing atypical (schizophreniform) psychosis following stroke. *Journal of Neuropsychiatry and Clinical Neurosciences* **3**, 6–9.

Rabinstein, A.A., Weigand, S. *et al.* (2005) Patterns of cerebral infarction in aneurysmal subarachnoid hemorrhage. *Stroke* **36**, 992–997.

Rasmussen, A., Lunde, M. *et al.* (2003) A double-blind, placebo-controlled study of sertraline in the prevention of depression in stroke patients. *Psychosomatics* **44**, 216–221.

Rasmussen, B.K. (1992) Migraine and tension-type headache in a general population: psychosocial factors. *International Journal of Epidemiology* **21**, 1138–1143.

Rees, W.L. (1971) Psychiatric and psychological factors in migraine. In: Cumings, J.N. (ed.) *Background to Migraine. Fourth Migraine Symposium*, ch. 6. Heinemann, London.

Reijneveld, J.C., Wermer, M. *et al.* (2000) Acute confusional state as presenting feature in aneurysmal subarachnoid hemorrhage: frequency and characteristics. *Journal of Neurology* **247**, 112–116.

Renowden, S. (2004) Cerebral venous sinus thrombosis. *European Radiology* **14**, 215–226.

Richardson, J.T. (1991) Cognitive performance following rupture and repair of intracranial aneurysm. *Acta Neurologica Scandinavica* **83**, 110–122.

Ringman, J.M., Saver, J.L. *et al.* (2004) Frequency, risk factors, anatomy, and course of unilateral neglect in an acute stroke cohort. *Neurology* **63**, 468–474.

Rinkel, G.J., Feigin, V.L. *et al.* (2005) Calcium antagonists for aneurysmal subarachnoid haemorrhage. *Cochrane Database of Systematic Reviews* 1, CD000277.

Robinson, R.G. & Price, T.R. (1982) Post-stroke depressive disorders: a follow-up study of 103 patients. *Stroke* **13**, 635–641.

Robinson, R.G. & Szetela, B. (1981) Mood change following left hemisphere brain injury. *Annals of Neurology* **9**, 447–453.

Robinson, R.G., Kubos, K.L. *et al.* (1984) Mood disorders in stroke patients. Importance of location of lesion. *Brain* **107**, 81–93.

Rocca, M.A., Agosta, F. *et al.* (2006) An fMRI study of the motor system in patients with neuropsychiatric systemic lupus erythematosus. *Neuroimage* **30**, 478–484.

Rodholm, M., Starmark, J.E. *et al.* (2001) Astheno-emotional disorder after aneurysmal SAH: reliability, symptomatology and relation to outcome. *Acta Neurologica Scandinavica* **103**, 379–385.

Rodholm, M., Starmark, J.E. *et al.* (2002) Organic psychiatric disorders after aneurysmal SAH: outcome and associations with age, bleeding severity, and arterial hypertension. *Acta Neurologica Scandinavica* **106**, 8–18.

Rovaris, M., Viti, B. *et al.* (2000) Brain involvement in systemic immune mediated diseases: magnetic resonance and magnetisation transfer imaging study. *Journal of Neurology, Neurosurgery and Psychiatry* **68**, 170–177.

Royal College of Physicians (2005) Use of antidepressant medication in adults undergoing recovery and rehabilitation following acquired brain injury. Clinical effectiveness and evaluation unit. Royal College of Physicians, British Society of Rehabilitation Medicine, and British Geriatrics Society. Concise Guidance to Good Practice 4. Royal College of Physicians, London.

Russell, R.W.R. (1959) Giant cell arteritis. A review of 35 cases. *Quarterly Journal of Medicine* **28**, 471–489.

Russell, R.W.R. & Grahm, E.M. (1988) Giant cell arteritis. In: Hopkins, A. (ed.) *Headache. Problems in Diagnosis and Management*, ch. 8. W.B. Saunders, London.

Ryvlin, P., Montavont, A. *et al.* (2006) Optimizing therapy of seizures in stroke patients. *Neurology* **67** (12 suppl. 4), S3–S9.

Sacks, O.W. (1970) *Migraine: The Evolution of a Common Disorder.* Faber, London.

Salmond, C.H., DeVito, E.E. *et al.* (2006) Impulsivity, reward sensitivity, and decision-making in subarachnoid hemorrhage survivors. *Journal of the International Neuropsychological Society* **12**, 697–706.

Samra, S.K., Giordani, B. *et al.* (2007) Recovery of cognitive function after surgery for aneurysmal subarachnoid hemorrhage. *Stroke* **38**, 1864–1872.

Sanchez-Del-Rio, M., Reuter, U. *et al.* (2006) New insights into migraine pathophysiology. *Current Opinion in Neurology* **19**, 294–298.

Sanna, G., Piga, M. *et al.* (2000) Central nervous system involvement in systemic lupus erythematosus: cerebral imaging and serological profile in patients with and without overt neuropsychiatric manifestations. *Lupus* **9**, 573–583.

Sanna, G., Bertolaccini, M.L. *et al.* (2003) Neuropsychiatric manifestations in systemic lupus erythematosus: prevalence and association with antiphospholipid antibodies. *Journal of Rheumatology* **30**, 985–992.

Sarzi-Puttini, P., Atzeni, F. *et al.* (2005) Environment and systemic lupus erythematosus: an overview. *Autoimmunity* **38**, 465–472.

Sawalha, A.H. & Harley, J.B. (2004) Antinuclear autoantibodies in systemic lupus erythematosus. *Current Opinion in Rheumatology* **16**, 534–540.

Schenatto, C.B., Xavier, R.M. *et al.* (2006) Raised serum S100B protein levels in neuropsychiatric lupus. *Annals of the Rheumatic Diseases* **65**, 829–31.

Schlote, A., Richter, M. *et al.* (2006) A longitudinal study of health-related quality of life of first stroke survivors' close relatives. *Cerebrovascular Disease* **22**, 137–142.

Schmahmann, J.D. (2003) Vascular syndromes of the thalamus. *Stroke* **34**, 2264–2278.

Scholte op Reimer, W.J., de Haan, R.J. *et al.* (1998) The burden of caregiving in partners of long-term stroke survivors. *Stroke* **29**, 1605–1611.

Seawell, A.H. & Danoff-Burg, S. (2004) Psychosocial research on systemic lupus erythematosus: a literature review. *Lupus* **13**, 891–899.

Segelmark, M. & Selga, D. (2007) The challenge of managing patients with polyarteritis nodosa. *Current Opinion in Rheumatology* **19**, 33–38.

Segui, J., Ramos-Casals, M. *et al.* (2000) Psychiatric and psychosocial disorders in patients with systemic lupus erythematosus: a longitudinal study of active and inactive stages of the disease. *Lupus* **9**, 584–588.

Seitz, R.J., Azari, N.P. *et al.* (1999) The role of diaschisis in stroke recovery. *Stroke* **30**, 1844–1850.

Selby, G. & Lance, J.W. (1960) Observations on 500 cases of migraine and allied vascular headache. *Journal of Neurology, Neurosurgery and Psychiatry* **23**, 23–32.

Selecki, B.R. (1965) Intracranial space-occupying lesions among patients admitted to mental hospitals. *Medical Journal of Australia* **1**, 383–390.

Seror, R., Mahr, A. *et al.* (2006) Central nervous system involvement in Wegener granulomatosis. *Medicine (Baltimore)* **85**, 54–65.

Shah, K.H. & Edlow, J.A. (2004) Transient ischemic attack: review for the emergency physician. *Annals of Emergency Medicine* **43**, 592–604.

Shoenfeld, Y., Lev, S. *et al.* (2004) Features associated with epilepsy in the antiphospholipid syndrome. *Journal of Rheumatology* **31**, 1344–8.

Sigal, L.H. (1987) The neurologic presentation of vasculitic and rheumatologic syndromes. *Medicine* **66**, 157–180.

Silberstein, S.D. (2004) Migraine. *Lancet* **363**, 381–391.

Silberstein, S.D., Lipton, R.B. *et al.* (2002) Neuropsychiatric aspects of primary headache disorders. In: Yudofsky, S.D. & Hales, R.E. (eds) *Textbook of Neuropyschiatry and Clinical Neurosciences*, pp. 451–488. American Psychiatric Publishing, Washington, DC.

Silverstein, A., Gilbert, H. *et al.* (1962) Neurologic complications of polycythaemia. *Annals of Internal Medicine* **57**, 909–916.

Siva, A. (2001) Vasculitis of the nervous system. *Journal of Neurology* **248**, 451–468.

Skinhoj, E. & Strandgaard, S. (1973) Pathogenesis of hypertensive encephalopathy. *Lancet* **i**, 461–462.

Slater, E.T.O. (1962) Psychological aspects. In: *Modern Views on 'Stroke' Illness*. The Chest and Heart Association, London.

Slot, M.C. & Tervaert, J.W. (2004) Wegener's granulomatosis. *Autoimmunity* **37**, 313–315.

Sluzewski, M., van Rooij, W.J. *et al.* (2005) Late rebleeding of ruptured intracranial aneurysms treated with detachable coils. *American Journal of Neuroradiology* **26**, 2542–2549.

Sobesky, J., Thiel, A. *et al.* (2005) Crossed cerebellar diaschisis in acute human stroke: a PET study of serial changes and response to supratentorial reperfusion. *Journal of Cerebral Blood Flow and Metabolism* **25**, 1685–1691.

Solinas, C., Briellmann, R.S. *et al.* (2003) Hypertensive encephalopathy: antecedent to hippocampal sclerosis and temporal lobe epilepsy? *Neurology* **60**, 1534–1536.

Song, Y.M., Sung, J. *et al.* (2004) Blood pressure, haemorrhagic stroke, and ischaemic stroke: the Korean national prospective occupational cohort study. *British Medical Journal* **328**, 324–325.

Sperling, M. (1964) A further contribution to the psychoanalytic study of migraine and psychogenic headaches. *International Journal of Psychoanalysis* **45**, 549–557.

Stam, J. (2005) Thrombosis of the cerebral veins and sinuses. *New England Journal of Medicine* **352**, 1791–1798.

Starkstein, S.E., Boston, J.D. *et al.* (1988) Mechanisms of mania after brain injury. 12 case reports and review of the literature. *Journal of Nervous and Mental Disease* **176**, 87–100.

Starkstein, S.E., Mayberg, H.S. *et al.* (1990) Mania after brain injury: neuroradiological and metabolic findings. *Annals of Neurology* **27**, 652–659.

Starkstein, S.E., Fedoroff, J.P. *et al.* (1993) Apathy following cerebrovascular lesions. *Stroke* **24**, 1625–1630.

Steens, S.C., Bosma, G.P. *et al.* (2006) Association between microscopic brain damage as indicated by magnetization transfer imaging and anticardiolipin antibodies in neuropsychiatric lupus. *Arthritis Research and Therapy* **8**, R38.

Steiner, T.J., Scher, A.I. *et al.* (2003) The prevalence and disability burden of adult migraine in England and their relationships to age, gender and ethnicity. *Cephalalgia* **23**, 519–527.

Stenager, E.N., Madsen, C. *et al.* (1998) Suicide in patients with stroke: epidemiological study. *British Medical Journal* **316**, 1206.

Stenhouse, L.M., Knight, R.G. *et al.* (1991) Long-term cognitive deficits in patients after surgery on aneurysms of the anterior communicating artery. *Journal of Neurology, Neurosurgery and Psychiatry* **54**, 909–914.

Stewart, W.F., Linet, M.S. *et al.* (1989) Migraine headaches and panic attacks. *Psychosomatic Medicine* **51**, 559–569.

Stiebel-Kalish, H., Kalish, Y. *et al.* (2005) Presentation, natural history, and management of carotid cavernous aneurysms. *Neurosurgery* **57**, 850–857.

Stone, J., Townend, E. *et al.* (2004) Personality change after stroke: some preliminary observations. *Journal of Neurology, Neurosurgery and Psychiatry* **75**, 1708–1713.

Storey, P.B. (1967) Psychiatric sequelae of subarachnoid haemorrhage. *British Medical Journal* **3**, 261–266.

Storey, P.B. (1969) The precipitation of subarachnoid haemorrhage. *Journal of Psychosomatic Research* **13**, 175–182.

Storey, P.B. (1970) Brain damage and personality change after subarachnoid heamorrhage. *British Journal of Psychiatry* **117**, 129–142.

Storey, P.B. (1972) Emotional disturbances before and after subarachnoid haemorrhage. In: Porter, R. & Knight, J. (eds) *Physiology, Emotion and Psychosomatic Illness*, pp. 337–343. Ciba Foundation Symposium No. 8 (new series). Associated Scientific Publishers, Amsterdam.

Stroke Unit Trialists' Collaboration (2001) Organised inpatient (stroke unit) care for stroke. *Cochrane Database of Systematic Reviews* **3**, CD000197.

Stronks, D.L., Tulen, J.H. *et al.* (1999) Personality traits and psychological reactions to mental stress of female migraine patients. *Cephalalgia* **19**, 566–574.

Subcommittee IHSC (2004) International classification of headache disorders. *Cephalalgia* **24** (suppl. 1), 1–160.

Sundgren, P.C., Edvardsson, B. *et al.* (2002) Serial investigation of perfusion disturbances and vasogenic oedema in hypertensive encephalopathy by diffusion and perfusion weighted imaging. *Neuroradiology* **44**, 299–304.

Susac, J.O. (1994) Susac's syndrome: the triad of microangiopathy of the brain and retina with hearing loss in young women. *Neurology* **44**, 591–593.

Svensson, E. & Starmark, J.E. (2002) Evaluation of individual and group changes in social outcome after aneurysmal subarachnoid haemorrhage: a long-term follow-up study. *Journal of Rehabilitation Medicine* **34**, 251–259.

Swartz, K.L., Pratt, L.A. *et al.* (2000) Mental disorders and the incidence of migraine headaches in a community sample: results from the Baltimore Epidemiologic Catchment area follow-up study. *Archives of General Psychiatry* **57**, 945–950.

Swartz, R.H. & Kern, R.Z. (2004) Migraine is associated with magnetic resonance imaging white matter abnormalities: a meta-analysis. *Archives of Neurology* **61**, 1366–1368.

Sweet, J.J., Doninger, N.A. *et al.* (2004) Factors influencing cognitive function, sleep, and quality of life in individuals with systemic lupus erythematosus: a review of the literature. *Clinical Neuropsychologist* **18**, 132–147.

Sweet, W.H., Talland, G.A. *et al.* (1966) A memory and mood disorder associated with ruptured anterior communicating aneurysm. *Transactions of the American Neurological Association* **91**, 346–348.

Symonds, C. (1951) Migrainous variants. *Transactions of the Medical Society of London* **67**, 237–250.

Talland, G.A., Sweet, W.H. *et al.* (1967) Amnesic syndrome with anterior communicating artery aneurysm. *Journal of Nervous and Mental Disease* **145**, 179–192.

Tanabe, J. & Weiner, M.W. (1997) MRI-MRS of the brain in systemic lupus erythematosus. How do we use it to understand causes of clinical signs? *Annals of the New York Academy of Sciences* **823**, 169–184.

Tanaka, A., Kimura, M. *et al.* (1992) Computed tomography and cerebral blood flow correlations of mental changes in chronic subdural hematoma. *Neurosurgery* **30**, 370–377; discussion 377–378.

Tang, W.K., Ungvari, G.S. *et al.* (2002) Psychiatric morbidity in first time stroke patients in Hong Kong: a pilot study in a rehabilitation unit. *Australian and New Zealand Journal of Psychiatry* **36**, 544–549.

Tarachow, S. (1939) The Korsakoff psychosis in spontaneous subarachnoid haemorrhage. *American Journal of Psychiatry* **95**, 887–899.

Teasdale, G.M., Drake, C.G. *et al.* (1988) A universal subarachnoid hemorrhage scale: report of a committee of the World Federation of Neurosurgical Societies. *Journal of Neurology, Neurosurgery and Psychiatry* **51**, 1457.

Teasdale, T.W. & Engberg, A.W. (2001) Suicide after a stroke: a population study. *Journal of Epidemiology and Community Health* **55**, 863–866.

Tench, C., Bentley, D. *et al.* (2002) Aerobic fitness, fatigue, and physical disability in systemic lupus erythematosus. *Journal of Rheumatology* **29**, 474–481.

Tench, C.M., McCarthy, J. *et al.* (2003) Fatigue in systemic lupus erythematosus: a randomized controlled trial of exercise. *Rheumatology (Oxford)* **42**, 1050–1054.

Tfelt-Hansen, P. (2006) A review of evidence-based medicine and meta-analytic reviews in migraine. *Cephalalgia* **26**, 1265–1274.

Theander, S. & Granholm, L. (1967) Sequelae after spontaneous subarachnoid haemorrhage, with special reference to hydrocephalus and Korsakoff's syndrome. *Acta Neurologica Scandinavica* **43**, 479–488.

Thomsen, L.L., Eriksen, M.K. *et al.* (2002) A population-based study of familial hemiplegic migraine suggests revised diagnostic criteria. *Brain* **125**, 1379–1391.

Tidswell, P., Dias, P.S. *et al.* (1995) Cognitive outcome after aneurysm rupture: relationship to aneurysm site and perioperative complications. *Neurology* **45**, 875–882.

Tilling, K., Coshall, C. *et al.* (2005) A family support organiser for stroke patients and their carers: a randomised controlled trial. *Cerebrovascular Disease* **20**, 85–91.

Toomela, A., Pulver, A. *et al.* (2004) Possible interpretation of subjective complaints in patients with spontaneous subarachnoid haemorrhage. *Journal of Rehabilitation Medicine* **36**, 63–69.

Trysberg, E. & Tarkowski, A. (2004) Cerebral inflammation and degeneration in systemic lupus erythematosus. *Current Opinion in Rheumatology* **16**, 527–533.

Ullman, M. (1962) *Behavioural Changes in Patients Following Strokes*. Thomas, Springfield, IL.

Van der Lugt, P.J.M. & De Visser, A.P. (1967) Two patients with a vital expansive syndrome following a cerebrovascular accident. *Psychiatria, Neurologia, Neurochirurgia* **70**, 349–359.

van der Schaaf, I., Algra, A. *et al.* (2005) Endovascular coiling versus neurosurgical clipping for patients with aneurysmal subarachnoid haemorrhage. *Cochrane Database of Systematic Rev* **4**, CD003085.

van der Schaaf, I.C., Wermer, M.J. *et al.* (2006) Psychosocial impact of finding small aneurysms that are left untreated in patients previously operated on for ruptured aneurysms. *Journal of Neurology, Neurosurgery and Psychiatry* **77**, 748–752.

van Gijn, J., van Dongen, K.J. *et al.* (1985) Perimesencephalic hemorrhage: a nonaneurysmal and benign form of subarachnoid hemorrhage. *Neurology* **35**, 493–497.

van Gijn, J., Kerr, R.S. *et al.* (2007) Subarachnoid haemorrhage. *Lancet* **369**, 306–318.

van Zandvoort, M., de Haan, E. *et al.* (2003) Cognitive functioning in patients with a small infarct in the brainstem. *Journal of the International Neuropsychological Society* **9**, 490–494.

Venables, P.J.W. (1993) Diagnosis and treatment of systemic lupus erythematosus. *British Medical Journal* **307**, 663–666.

Verdelho, A., Henon, H. *et al.* (2004) Depressive symptoms after stroke and relationship with dementia: a three-year follow-up study. *Neurology* **62**, 905–911.

Vereker, R. (1952) The psychiatric aspects of temporal arteritis. *Journal of Mental Science* **98**, 280–286.

Vespa, P.M., O'Phelan, K. *et al.* (2003) Acute seizures after intracerebral hemorrhage: a factor in progressive midline shift and outcome. *Neurology* **60**, 1441–1446.

Victor, M., Angevine, J.B., Mancall, E.L. & Fisher, C.M. (1961) Memory loss with lesions of hippocampal formation. *Archives of Neurology* **5**, 244–263.

Vilkki, J., Holst, P. *et al.* (1989) Cognitive deficits related to computed tomographic findings after surgery for a ruptured intracranial aneurysm. *Neurosurgery* **25**, 166–172.

Volpe, B.T. & Hirst, W. (1983) Amnesia following the rupture and repair of an anterior communicating artery aneurysm. *Journal of Neurology, Neurosurgery and Psychiatry* **46**, 704–709.

Wacogne, C., Lacoste, J.P. *et al.* (2003) Stress, anxiety, depression and migraine. *Cephalalgia* **23**, 451–455.

Wade, D.T., Legh-Smith, J. *et al.* (1986) Effects of living with and looking after survivors of a stroke. *British Medical Journal* **293**, 418–420.

Wade, D.T., Legh-Smith, J. & Hewer, R.A. (1987) Depressed mood after stroke. A community study of its frequency. *British Journal of Psychiatry* **151**, 200–205.

Walker, M.F., Leonardi-Bee, J. *et al.* (2004) Individual patient data meta-analysis of randomized controlled trials of community occupational therapy for stroke patients. *Stroke* **35**, 2226–2232.

Walton, J.N. (1952) The late prognosis of subarachnoid haemorrhage. *British Medical Journal* **2**, 802–808.

Walton, J.N. (1953) The Korsakoff syndrome in spontaneous subarachnoid haemorrhage. *Journal of Mental Science* **99**, 521–530.

Walton, J.N. (1956) *Subarachnoid Haemorrhage.* Livingstone, Edinburgh and London.

Wardlaw, J.M. (2005) What causes lacunar stroke? *Journal of Neurology, Neurosurgery and Psychiatry* **76**, 617–619.

Warlow, C., Dennis, M., van Gijn, J. *et al.* (eds) (1996) *Stroke. A Practical Guide to Management.* Blackwell Science, Oxford.

Waterloo, K., Omdal, R. *et al.* (2001) Neuropsychological dysfunction in systemic lupus erythematosus is not associated with changes in cerebral blood flow. *Journal of Neurology* **248**, 595–602.

Waterloo, K., Omdal, R. *et al.* (2002) Neuropsychological function in systemic lupus erythematosus: a five-year longitudinal study. *Rheumatology (Oxford)* **41**, 411–415.

Waters, W.E. (1971) Migraine: intelligence, social class and familial prevalence. *British Medical Journal* **2**, 77–81.

Watkins, C.L., Auton, M.F. *et al.* (2007) Motivational interviewing early after acute stroke: a randomized, controlled trial. *Stroke* **38**, 1004–1009.

Weatherall, D.J. (1996) Polycythaemia vera. In: Weatherall, D.J., Ledingham, J.G.G. & Warrell, D.A. (eds) *Oxford Textbook of Medicine*, section 22.3.8. Oxford University Press, Oxford.

Weidauer, S., Lanfermann, H. *et al.* (2007) Impairment of cerebral perfusion and infarct patterns attributable to vasospasm after aneurysmal subarachnoid hemorrhage: a prospective MRI and DSA study. *Stroke* **38**, 1831–1836.

Weiller, C., Chollet, F., Friston, K., Wise, R.J.S. & Frackowiak, R.S.J. (1992) Functional reorganization of the brain in recovery striatocapsular infarction in man. *Annals of Neurology* **31**, 463–472.

Weiller, C., May, A. *et al.* (1995) Brain stem activation in spontaneous human migraine attacks. *Nature Medicine* **1**, 658–660.

Weiner, S.M., Otte, A. *et al.* (2000) Diagnosis and monitoring of central nervous system involvement in systemic lupus erythematosus: value of F-18 fluorodeoxyglucose PET. *Annals of the Rheumatic Diseases* **59**, 377–385.

Weingarten, K., Barbut, D. *et al.* (1994) Acute hypertensive encephalopathy: findings on spin-echo and gradient-echo MR imaging. *American Journal of Roentgenology* **162**, 665–670.

Wermer, M.J., van der Schaaf, I.C. *et al.* (2005a) Psychosocial impact of screening for intracranial aneurysms in relatives with familial subarachnoid hemorrhage. *Stroke* **36**, 836–840.

Wermer, M.J., Greebe, P. *et al.* (2005b) Incidence of recurrent subarachnoid hemorrhage after clipping for ruptured intracranial aneurysms. *Stroke* **36**, 2394–2399.

Wermer, M.J., van der Schaaf, I.C. *et al.* (2007a) Risk of rupture of unruptured intracranial aneurysms in relation to patient and aneurysm characteristics: an updated meta-analysis. *Stroke* **38**, 1404–1410.

Wermer, M.J., Kool, H. *et al.* (2007b) Subarachnoid hemorrhage treated with clipping: long-term effects on employment, relationships, personality, and mood. *Neurosurgery* **60**, 91–97; discussion 97–98.

Werring, D.J., Coward, L.J. *et al.* (2005) Cerebral microbleeds are common in ischemic stroke but rare in TIA. *Neurology* **65**, 1914–1918.

Weyand, C.M. & Goronzy, J.J. (2003) Medium- and large-vessel vasculitis. *New England Journal of Medicine* **349**, 160–169.

Wilkinson, P.R., Wolfe, C.D. *et al.* (1997) A long-term follow-up of stroke patients. *Stroke* **28**, 507–512.

Williams, L.S. (2005) Depression and stroke: cause or consequence? *Seminars in Neurology* **25**, 396–409.

Williams, L.S., Ghose, S.S. *et al.* (2004) Depression and other mental health diagnoses increase mortality risk after ischemic stroke. *American Journal of Psychiatry* **161**, 1090–1095.

Williams, L.S., Brizendine, E.J. *et al.* (2005) Performance of the PHQ-9 as a screening tool for depression after stroke. *Stroke* **36**, 635–638.

Williams, L.S., Kroenke, K. *et al.* (2007) Care management of post-stroke depression: a randomized, controlled trial. *Stroke* **38**, 998–1003.

Williams, V.L. & Hogg, J.P. (2000) Magnetic resonance imaging of chronic subdural hematoma. *Neurosurgical Clinics of North America* **11**, 491–498.

Willison, J.R., Du Boulay, G.H. *et al.* (1980) Effects of high haematocrit on alertness. *Lancet* **i**, 846–848.

Winterkorn, J.M. (2007) Retinal migraine is an oxymoron. *Journal of Neuro-ophthalmology* **27**, 1–2.

Wolfe, C.D. (2000) The impact of stroke. *British Medical Bulletin* **56**, 275–286.

Wolff, H.G. (1937) Personality features and reactions of subjects with migraine. *Archives of Neurology and Psychiatry* **37**, 895–921.

Wolff, H.G. (1963) The relation of life situations, personality features, and reactions to the migraine syndrome. In: *Headache and Other Head Pain*, ch. 11, 2nd edn. Oxford University Press, New York.

Wong, K.L., Woo, E.K.W. *et al.* (1991) Neurologic manifestations of systemic lupus erythematosus: a prospective study. *Quarterly Journal of Medicine* **81**, 857–870.

Woolfenden, A.R., Tong, D.C. *et al.* (1998) Angiographically defined primary angiitis of the CNS: is it really benign? *Neurology* **51**, 183–188.

Wysenbeek, A.J., Leibovici, L. *et al.* (1993) Fatigue in systemic lupus erythematosus. Prevalence and relation to disease expression. *British Journal of Rheumatology* **32**, 633–635.

Yamamoto, Y., Georgiadis, A.L. *et al.* (1999) Posterior cerebral artery territory infarcts in the New England Medical Center Posterior Circulation Registry. *Archives of Neurology* **56**, 824–832.

Yamashiro, S., Nishi, T. *et al.* (2007) Improvement of quality of life in patients surgically treated for asymptomatic unruptured intracranial aneurysms. *Journal of Neurology, Neurosurgery and Psychiatry* **78**, 497–500.

Young, J. & Forster, A. (2007) Review of stroke rehabilitation. *British Medical Journal* **34**, 86–90.

Younger, D.S. (2004) Vasculitis of the nervous system. *Current Opinion in Neurology* **17**, 317–336.

Zandi, M.S. & Coles, A.J. (2007) Notes on the kidney and its diseases for the neurologist. *Journal of Neurology, Neurosurgery and Psychiatry* **78**, 444–449.

Zandman-Goddard, G., Chapman, J. *et al.* (2007) Autoantibodies involved in neuropsychiatric SLE and antiphospholipid syndrome. *Seminars in Arthritis and Rheumatism* **36**, 297–315.

Zeitlin, C. & Oddy, M. (1984) Cognitive impairment in patients with severe migraine. *British Journal of Clinical Psychology* **23**, 27–35.

Ziegler, D.K. & Paolo, A.M. (1995) Headache symptoms and psychological profile of headache-prone individuals. A comparison of clinic patients and controls. *Archives of Neurology* **52**, 602–606.

Zwart, J.A., Dyb, G. *et al.* (2003) Depression and anxiety disorders associated with headache frequency. The Nord-Trondelag Health Study. *European Journal of Neurology* **10**, 147–152.

CHAPTER 9

Alzheimer's Disease and Other Dementias (Including Pseudodementias)

Simon Lovestone

Institute of Psychiatry, King's College, London

Dementia is described in the *Diagnostic and Statistical Manual of Mental Disorders* (DSM)-IV as a disorder with memory impairment and at least one other symptom from aphasia, apraxia, agnosia or disturbances in executive functioning accompanied by impairment in social and occupational function. The decline must represent a decline from a previously higher level of functioning. The causes are many and may be both cerebral and extracerebral, but must be distinguished from delirium. Prominent among them are certain intrinsic degenerative diseases of the brain occurring in middle or late life. These, the so-called primary dementias, are the subject of this chapter. Later in the chapter the concept of mild cognitive impairment, an intermediate state and in some people, but not all, a prodrome of dementia, is discussed.

By far the commonest of the primary dementias of late life is Alzheimer's disease (AD), chiefly by virtue of its sharply rising incidence with age. However, it is also true that AD is the commonest of the early-onset (previously called presenile) dementias, namely those with onset before age 65 years, although the relative proportions are less marked. Next in frequency are the vascular dementias, previously called 'multi-infarct' or 'arteriosclerotic' dementia, both in the late and early-onset age ranges. An interesting question is whether vascular dementia is strictly speaking a secondary rather than a primary degenerative brain process: in other words, does all the neurodegeneration of vascular dementia arise from simple loss of vascular supply to neurones (strictly a secondary dementia) or does a local and relative anoxia induce or enhance a complex neurodegenerative process (making it a primary dementia)? While this of some considerable interest in terms of pathophysiology, vascular dementia has traditionally been considered with the primary dementias. Dementia with Lewy bodies (DLB) is in most series of post-mortem and clinical prevalence studies the third most common dementia. Pick's disease, other frontal dementias, Huntington's disease and the prion disorders, including Creutzfeldt–Jakob disease (CJD), constitute the best known of the remaining primary dementias and are all much less common. When the distinctive pathologies of the above conditions fail to be revealed at post-mortem in a patient with a primary dementing illness, it is usual to speak of a 'simple' or 'non-specific' primary dementia, although in the context of detailed neuropathology this is a vanishing and rare event. Rather more common is the presence of large amounts of AD pathology in people without dementia (MRC CFAS 2001).

An alternative approach to classification is emerging from neuropathological studies. As discussed below, one of the key neuropathological lesions of AD is the neurofibrillary tangle, which is composed of aggregates of tau protein, a protein that normally functions to stabilise microtubules in axons. Other conditions also have aggregates of tau protein, including progressive supranuclear palsy (PSP), corticobasal degeneration and some of the frontotemporal dementias (FTDs). As these disorders have some common pathologies and presumably therefore common mechanisms, it has been proposed that they be considered together as the 'tauopathies' (Lee *et al.* 2001). In contrast, other disorders, including DLB, Parkinson's disease and multisystem atrophy, feature aggregations of a protein, synuclein, in Lewy bodies and other lesions. These disorders have been called the 'synucleinopathies' (Duda *et al.* 2000), in contrast again to the 'amyloidopathies' that encompass the prion disorders such as CJD, some of the rarer dementias such as familial British or Danish dementia and AD. Herein lies one of the flaws of such a classification, as AD is both a tauopathy and an amyloidopathy, and some cases, including early-onset autosomal dominant AD, have Lewy bodies also and are therefore synucleinopathies. There is probably more overlap than clear distinction between these different pathologies. Nonetheless, the classification is important, as it is the first attempt

Lishman's Organic Psychiatry: A Textbook of Neuropsychiatry, 4th edition.
© 2009 Blackwell Publishing.   ISBN 978-1-4051-1860-1

to classify the primary dementias according to mechanism and pathology rather than by clinical features. It draws attention to the fact that very different clinical pictures can emerge as a consequence of very similar pathological processes, the different clinical picture reflecting less pathology than the neuroanatomical locations of the lesions (compare, for example, the synucleinopathies Parkinson's disease and DLB and the tauopathies PSP and FTD) and possibly the relative admixture of lesions. Even more importantly, if there are common mechanisms, then it suggests the possibilities of common therapies. For example, a disease-modifying therapy reducing the formation of tau aggregates might conceivably be as useful in PSP as in AD. For the time being, however, this neuropathological and putative mechanistic formulation of classification remains to be proven and the conventional symptom-based classification has more clinical utility, not least in predicting outcome.

The general clinical picture is similar in all common dementias: a progressive disintegration of intellect, memory and personality accompanied by loss of functional abilities and behavioural disturbances. The different conditions are distinguished to some extent by the rapidity of their course or by associated symptoms and signs, as described when the individual disorders are considered in turn. Differential diagnosis has improved and in most cases the disorders can be distinguished with some considerable degree of accuracy in life, although a definitive diagnosis is revealed only by careful post-mortem examination of the brain, and even then a measure of uncertainty can remain in some cases. The relationship between the three commonest dementias, particularly AD, vascular dementias and DLB, is complex and these forms frequently coexist (Holmes *et al.* 1999; MRC CFAS 2001). The contribution of the various pathological events associated with these diagnoses to the actual symptoms of dementia is often unclear in a single case or indeed overall.

It is as true today as it was in the previous editions of this book that in terms of overall outcome these diseases share a uniformly poor long-term prognosis although symptomatic treatments have improved. Given the huge advances in understanding the pathophysiology of the conditions and the strides being taken to develop disease-modifying drugs, it is to be hoped that this will, in the foreseeable future, no longer be the case. However, even without disease-modifying or primary preventive strategies, it is no longer the chief aim in diagnostic practice to distinguish them from the secondary dementias, i.e. to search for the other causes of chronic organic reactions that may have some therapeutic issue. Indeed the frequency of these 'reversible' dementias, previously thought to be a major diagnostic dilemma, is very low. In a meta-analysis of studies including nearly 6000 patients with dementia, only 9% were found to be potentially reversible and only 0.6% actually reversed (Clarfield 2003). Although detection of this "less than 1% of all dementias" is important, the main aim of diagnostic practice now is to determine if it is appropriate to prescribe one of the growing

numbers of symptomatic treatments; to consider, in the case of vascular dementia, the role of secondary preventive measures; and in all the dementias to offer sufferers and families advice, support and, where appropriate, prognostic information. Diagnosis or detection of behavioural disturbance is also a task of immense importance for the clinician and in many but not all cases a combination of behavioural, environmental and pharmacological approaches can manage even the most disturbed of patients.

Alzheimer's disease

Dementia setting in after the age of 65 (late-onset, previously called senile, dementia) has usually been considered separately from that occurring in younger patients. The organisation of clinical services for the elderly, and the development of the specialities of geriatrics and psychogeriatrics or old age psychiatry, has served to reinforce the practice. While this has had undoubted benefits in terms of development of clinical services for the elderly and indeed for professional consolidation of the various clinical disciplines, it has had the unfortunate consequence that late-onset dementia has tended to acquire nosological status as a separate and distinct entity in clinical and even in some research writing. In fact the dementias of the elderly can have several causes, as at any other age, and with advancing age multiple causes will often be operative together.

The most common pathology displayed at post-mortem in elderly demented patients is closely similar to, if not identical with, that of AD in younger persons. Historically, this was labelled 'parenchymatous senile dementia' and then 'senile dementia of the Alzheimer type' (SDAT) but now simply AD. The change in terminology reflects the increasing body of evidence that the conditions are likely to be identical whether setting in before or after age 65 years. The distinction between early onset and late onset, with age 65 as the cut-off, has more relevance to social factors such as retirement than to biology. In many respects it has added confusion to an already complicated field. A more meaningful distinction might be between very early-onset AD occurring before age 50–55, very late-onset AD occurring after age 80–85 and the majority of AD occurring between these age ranges. There is very good evidence of a genetic distinction between these categories, with almost all autosomal dominant AD occurring before age 55 and with apolipoprotein E gene (*APOE*) variation being a susceptibility factor for later-onset AD but with this gene having less importance in the very elderly. Despite this clear evidence of genetic aetiological differences between very early-onset, late-onset and very late-onset AD, the neuropathological features are very similar and there is no evidence to suggest differences in the pathological mechanisms leading to neurodegeneration. Therefore we consider all forms of AD together and do not adhere to the convention of distinguishing 'presenile' from 'senile' AD despite the precedents of both Alzheimer and Lishman.

Community, clinic-based and neuropathological studies all concur that AD is the commonest of the dementias, occurring in up to two-thirds of all dementias (Polvikoski *et al.* 2001; Stevens *et al.* 2002). A second large group consists of the vascular dementias, whereas an admixture of these two common forms of pathology determines a third. Considerable evidence suggests that these mixed dementia may in fact be the predominant neuropathological presentation, with increasing acknowledgement that this may not be only a chance occurrence of two common conditions. DLB occurs more frequently in some series than others, perhaps reflecting post-mortem diagnostic practices as well as clinical factors, but in any case is an important category of patients coming to post-mortem with dementia. The relatively small remainder of cases is likely to show a range of other causative pathologies, or the brain may be normal apart from the changes expected with age.

In this chapter, the sections on AD, vascular dementia and DLB describe the clinical picture and underlying pathology of these conditions in some detail.

Prevalence and incidence

As a consequence of increasing longevity in the population, the prevalence of dementia has risen and continues to rise alarmingly. It was estimated that in 1997 there were approximately 2.3 million persons with dementia in the USA, with a further 360 000 new cases arising annually (Brookmeyer *et al.* 1998). It is estimated that in 2008 there were approximately 5.2 million persons with dementia in the USA, with over 410 000 new cases arising annually (Alzheimer's Association 2008, Alzheimer's Disease Facts and figures www.alz.org/national/documents/report_alzfactsfigures2008.pdf). In the UK there are an estimated 750 000 people with dementia and, globally, over 24 million people, with these prevalence figures forecast to rise to over 80 million by 2040 (Ferri *et al.* 2005). Altogether dementia now ranks as the third most common cause of death in the USA, on a par with cardiovascular disease (Ewbank 1999).

The implications of a problem on such a scale for the cost and provision of care are clearly enormous. Kay *et al.* (1970) were able to show that admission rates to hospital in 1970 for the elderly demented exceeded the rates for all other psychoses combined, likewise that their demands on hospital and residential facilities outstripped those due to all other forms of disability in old age. Not surprisingly the costs, in particular to health services but also to carers and families, is simply huge, being estimated at between £7 billion and £14 billion in the UK, compared with costs of £3 billion for stroke, £4 billion for heart disease and £1.6 billion for cancer (Lowin *et al.* 2001). These estimates include family and other non-service caregiving costs but even the direct costs to health services are considerable in AD, one estimate of direct Medicaid costs in the USA being $14 492 per AD recipient (Martin *et al.* 2000). The costs of dementia rise with severity, one study from

Denmark for example showing that the costs of mild dementia were DKK93 000 rising to DKK206 000 for severe dementia (Andersen, C.K. *et al.* 1999). Most of the change in costs with severity result from decline in function rather than specifically cognition (Wolstenholme *et al.* 2002) as it is functional loss above all else that demands intervention both in the community and even more so in residential and nursing homes.

Yet even these statistics from diagnosed patients underestimate the size of the problem. The Newcastle upon Tyne survey of a random sample of people living at home, coupled with a census of institutions in the same area, disclosed that fewer than one-fifth of even the more severe cases were in hospitals or homes for the elderly (Kay *et al.* 1964). Only a proportion of dementia in the community is recognised by services, with general practitioners being aware of perhaps half to two-thirds of all dementia among their patients (O'Connor *et al.* 1988). Neuropathological studies of elderly people concur with these findings with, for example, the prevalence of neuropathological features sufficient to cause AD being twice as common as a clinical diagnosis of AD in a large prospectively examined community-based cohort (Polvikoski *et al.* 2001).

All epidemiological studies have shown that of the dementias, AD is the most common, although increasingly the contribution of multiple pathologies to the manifestation of dementia is recognised. The European Community Concerted Action on the Epidemiology and Prevention of Dementia Group (EURODEM) initiative is a collaboration between multiple epidemiological studies of dementia across Europe; in an analysis of six such studies, Rocca *et al.* (1991) found similar prevalence rates of AD in the different participating countries. Overall, European prevalence was 2% for the age group 30–59, rising exponentially with age to 11% in people aged 80–89 years. Some studies have found even higher prevalence rates: in a study of nearly 4000 persons in the USA, the prevalence was 3% in those aged 65–74 years, rising to 47% in those over 85 years old (Evans *et al.* 1989). Some of the differences reported between studies almost certainly reflect methodological differences (Jorm *et al.* 1987) but overall the rates are of the order of 5% for all those aged 65 years and older, doubling thereafter every 5 years to a total of 20–30% of all those aged over 85 years. Incidence figures reflect these high rates. In a UK study the incidence of AD in a community-based sample over the age of 75 years was 2.7 per 1000 person-years at risk, with the rates for men being twice those of women (Brayne *et al.* 1995).

Neuropathological studies concur with clinical studies that AD is the commonest of all dementias, occurring in approximately 60% of cases with dementia (MRC CFAS 2001). These figures are not substantially different from the seminal studies of Blessed, Tomlinson and Roth that mapped the late-onset dementias (Blessed *et al.* 1968; Tomlinson *et al.* 1970). However, in the MRC Cognitive Function in Ageing Study, a longitudinal examination of cognitive change in the elderly in the community, it was clear that not only AD but cerebrovascular changes were common and the admixture of both pathologies was very frequent (MRC CFAS 2001). It is also clear that presence of pathology itself is not enough to induce dementia as one-third of people without dementia had similar amounts of pathology as those with dementia. This disparity between pathological load and cognition has been observed in other studies (Leaper *et al.* 2001; Meguro *et al.* 2001; Bigio *et al.* 2002; Riley *et al.* 2002). This remains something of a puzzle: perhaps some people are more vulnerable to a given amount of pathological insult because they have less of a quantity, loosely termed 'reserve'. What reserve might be is open to question. It might be that reserve is a physical attribute of the brain such as numbers of neurones or synapses or a functional, cognitive, attribute such as connectivity or plasticity. It might be inherited or arise as a consequence of environment. There is some evidence for both. Stern (2002) conceptualised these two components, cognition and brain, as active and passive elements of reserve. Alternatively, it might be that the neuropathological features of AD are only the tip of the iceberg and that cognitive impairment and dementia result from loss of neuronal function that is not apparent on post-mortem where only the insoluble, stable, gross pathological defects are present. This is not unlikely as there is some evidence that the earliest effects of pathological change in AD is loss of axonal transport, a process that would not necessarily be apparent at post-mortem.

Clinical features

The onset of AD is usually after the age of 40, although rare cases have been reported at younger ages. Given the exponential increase in incidence after age 75, the vast majority of people with AD are elderly, although early-onset AD remains an important condition both in terms of providing dementia services and in understanding the pathogenesis of the condition. At all ages females outnumber males by a ratio of 2 or 3:1, with the exception of the early-onset familial forms of the condition, which as an autosomal dominant inherited condition occurs equally in males and females.

For both early-onset and late-onset and familial and non-familial forms, the onset is usually insidious and can be dated only imprecisely. The slow development of the intellectual deterioration often allows the patient to preserve considerable social competence until the disease is well advanced. Insight is lost relatively early in the condition, something relatives sometimes consider a fortunate occurrence, but it is important to remember that often partial insight is retained in the early stages.

It remains true that the early stages are commonly overlooked by relatives and even by medical attendants, although this is more likely to be the case in late-onset than early-onset AD. Partly this is due to low expectations of the elderly but

partly also to a genuinely less intellectually challenging life for many people post retirement. Failing memory and lack of initiative and interest tend to be regarded by many, including family and friends, as no more than an accentuation of the normal processes of ageing and this shows little signs of changing. An exaggeration of such traits as obstinacy, egocentricity and rigid adherence to old habits may be viewed likewise. Moreover, old people may already have adopted a circumscribed routine within which cognitive failure is slow to be exposed.

While the onset of dementia is insidious, it not infrequently comes to attention as a result of some acute disturbance. An intercurrent illness may have taxed the reserves of the failing brain beyond their limit or resulted in an acute episode of delirium. Or a sudden change of environment or the loss of a partner may have abruptly revealed the inroads made by the disorder. Other cases come to notice as a result of the social disorganisation produced by the dementing process: the patient may wander away and get lost, become suddenly abusive on account of paranoid delusions or harm himself due to some clumsiness or accident.

Three main phases to the disease are commonly distinguished. The first, often lasting for 2 or 3 years, is characterised by failing memory, muddled inefficiency over the tasks of everyday life and spatial disorientation. The second stage brings more rapid progress of intellectual and personality deterioration and focal symptoms appear. An accent on the parietal lobes is common, with dysphasia, apraxia, agnosia and acalculia. The third or terminal stage consists of profound apathetic dementia in which the patient becomes bedridden and doubly incontinent. Gross neurological disability may sometimes develop, such as spastic hemiparesis or severe striatal rigidity and tremor. Forced grasping and groping may be seen, along with sucking reflexes. The frequency of epilepsy has sometimes been quoted as a distinctive feature of AD and a history of seizures was reported in 3% of one series (Burns *et al.* 1991a) and more than 20% in another (Volicer *et al.* 1995). Minor seizures may occur early in the disease, although grand mal fits appear to be mainly a late development. In the terminal phase of the disease, bodily wasting may be rapid despite adequate preservation of appetite. In a systematically assessed cohort of largely advanced dementia, the commonest neurological sign was a snout reflex, present in 41%, extrapyramidal signs were observed in 12% and myoclonus in 5% (Burns *et al.* 1991a).

Differences between early-onset and late-onset AD
There are few well-documented and consistent differences between early- and late-onset AD. This is complicated by the fact that true early-onset (i.e. before age 55 years) AD is not infrequently familial and there is some evidence for particular neuropathological patterns in some families and possibly clinical patterns too. However, the general clinical picture for early- and late-onset AD follows the same pattern of decline

except that the onset may be particularly hard to discern and parietal lobe symptomatology is less regularly conspicuous in the elderly. Among older patients it is possible that the disorder can sometimes follow a relatively protracted course as a result of more 'benign' development of pathological changes, and physical frailty and concomitant systemic illnesses are more likely to complicate late-onset than early-onset AD. Patients with early-onset AD are more likely to decline quicker (Lucca *et al.* 1993; O'Hara *et al.* 2002) and more likely to have difficulties with word comprehension and naming ability (Imamura *et al.* 1998), although clinically apparent speech impairments occur in both early- and late-onset AD (Cummings *et al.* 1985). There may be greater visuospatial deficits in people with early-onset AD (Fujimori *et al.* 1998). There are no neuropathological or neurochemical features exclusive to either early- or late-onset AD. For example, cerebrospinal fluid (CSF) measures of cholinesterase activity and choline showed no difference between early- and late-onset AD (Kumar *et al.* 1989). On balance, therefore, while there may be subtle neurocognitive differences and the general frailty of some people with late-onset AD may be reflected in the clinical presentation, the pattern of decline and the neuropathological substrates of that decline are remarkably similar no matter what the age of onset.

Symptoms in Alzheimer's disease

Cognitive impairment

The cognitive changes of dementia differ in kind and quantity from those experienced as a consequence of ageing. They are often considered as the four As: amnesia, aphasia (more correctly dysphasia in AD), apraxia (or dyspraxia) and agnosia.

Amnesia

Memory impairment is an invariable and early symptom of AD. Typically the loss is for recent events, with relative sparing of working memory in the very early stages and of remote memories even to moderate stages of disease. Recent memory function or recall is tested as part of the Mini-Mental State Examination (MMSE) (Folstein *et al.* 1975), and in the very early stages of disease the patient might typically be able to repeat three items (working memory) but fail to recall all three after only a few minutes. The rate of forgetting of new memories is greater in AD than in other groups with amnesias (Moss *et al.* 1986) as is the rate of storage into long-term memory (Petersen *et al.* 1994). However the rate of forgetting of fully stored memories may not be any lower than similarly aged people (Becker *et al.* 1987), suggesting that the primary neuropsychological deficit in AD is one of encoding and storing memories rather than failure to retrieve or to primary loss of memories.

As the disease process progresses, even more remote memories are lost and amnesia is manifested as episodic,

semantic and visuospatial deficits. Episodic memory is that for events and there is, as expected, a gradient for loss with more recent events being lost before more remote events. This may represent a combination both of greater rehearsal of older events and of a failure to store recent events effectively. Semantic memory is inexorably connected to, but distinct from, language: it is the knowledge and understanding of words, facts and concepts and in AD is relatively preserved early in the disease process but becomes compromised as the disease progresses. Semantic memory can be tested by word fluency (e.g. 'Name all the animals you can in one minute'). Visuospatial skills are addressed in the MMSE by copying of pentagons and are manifested clinically by becoming disorientated in strange environments, perhaps by wandering and by becoming lost even in a familiar environment.

Aphasias

Early in the disease process language loss may be hard to detect as the patient uses a variety of strategies to conceal this. However, carers and others in close contact with the patient will often comment upon it and many patients themselves find it a frustrating and difficult symptom. Nevertheless, the loss of speech often does not progress or not progress as profoundly or rapidly as in FTDs, which can proceed to mutism relatively early in the condition. Aphasias early in the disease process may be associated with more rapid decline (O'Hara *et al.* 2002). The earliest changes are word-finding difficulties and this can be tested for by asking the patient to name an increasingly complex set of items (e.g. jacket, sleeve, cuff, seam). The patient may try to compensate with circumlocutions and generic or indefinite terms. At this stage syntax may appear superficially intact but close analyses may reveal unfinished sentences, inappropriate usage of tense and other relatively minor errors. As the disease progresses, receptive difficulties become increasingly apparent and in the final stages of the disease speech becomes increasingly degraded with perseverations, echolalias, decreased fluency and non-speech verbalisations.

Apraxias

Difficulties with complex motor tasks not due to a primary motor deficit are a major determinant of the care needs of a person with dementia because they result in increasingly poor self-care and increasing risk of harm. In the early stages this may be elicited by asking the patient to enact a command (ideomotor apraxia) and in a more detailed and goal-orientated manner by a dressing or kitchen assessment often conducted by an occupational therapist.

Agnosia

The failure to correctly interpret a sensory input, or agnosia, is common in AD and particular attention is drawn to prosopagnosia and especially autoprosopagnosia. This failure to recognise one's own face can be particularly disturbing and can cause diagnostic confusion to the unwary.

An elderly lady was referred as suffering from visual hallucinations. She reported seeing faces when out shopping leering at her from shop windows. A visit to her house revealed bathroom mirrors that had been taped up and covered in newspapers. On questioning she commented that the face she saw was always wearing the same hat as she commonly wore and it was easy to demonstrate the symptom by showing her a mirror. Interestingly she recognised that the face bore many similarities to her own but commented that it looked older than she did.

This symptom results, as in the case above, in the 'mirror sign' where patients interpret their reflection in the mirror as a stranger and may even be observed to converse with it.

Executive function

The ability to plan, to organise and to maintain attention are lost early and consistently in AD. However, of the various cognitive deficits it is probably the most taxing to assess, especially in someone showing amnestic and aphasics difficulties. The serial 7s of the MMSE is probably the most commonly assessed executive function, with the Stroop test or card-sorting test being used in more detailed assessments. Executive functioning is considered to be a primary frontal lobe function and relative sparing of memory with a predominance of executive function loss and speech deficits suggests a frontal lobe predominant dementia. Other tests of frontal lobe function can be usefully employed, including bedside tests of perseveration (e.g. copying hand sequences).

Sourander and Sjögren (1970) drew attention to the frequency of behavioural abnormalities suggestive of temporal lobe dysfunction in early-onset AD, particularly phenomena reminiscent of Klüver–Bucy syndrome in animals after bilateral temporal lobe excision. Late phenomena included strong tendencies to examine and touch objects with the mouth (hyperorality), and tendencies to be stimulus-bound to contact and touch every object in sight (hypermetamorphosis). Hyperphagia was often a terminal phenomenon, with indiscriminate eating of any material available. The emotional changes of apathy and dullness were similarly reminiscent of the pathological tameness of monkeys with Klüver–Bucy syndrome. Such manifestations were observed in over three-quarters of patients with AD, and in some of them the full gamut of phenomena was displayed. The human counterpart of Klüver–Bucy syndrome has been occasionally observed with other cerebral disorders such as arteriosclerosis, Pick's disease and cerebral tumours, but Sourander and Sjögren considered that in most cases it formed an essential part of the symptomatology of AD. To some extent this was confirmed in late-onset AD by Burns *et al.* (1990a), who found features of Klüver–Bucy syndrome frequently in late-onset AD although the full syndrome only

rarely. The association with temporal lobe loss was also confirmed.

Functional impairment

Declining ability to perform everyday tasks (activities of daily living, ADL) is an invariable accompaniment to the cognitive loss in AD. Indeed deficits in ADL are an essential component of the DSM-IV diagnostic process for AD. ADL is often considered as basic (self-care) and instrumental and it is the latter that are lost first. Assessing ADL loss is important not only as this represents a core component of severity assessments but also because loss of function is an important predictor of institutionalisation (Riter & Fries 1992). Reisberg *et al.* (1986, 1989) have done much to describe the pattern of decline in function in AD and this has been encompassed in the Functional Assessment Staging (FAST) and Global Deterioration Scale (GDS) both of which use descriptions of functional loss to grade severity in AD (Reisberg *et al.* 1982; Reisberg 1988). Thus FAST stage 1 is a normal adult with no functional loss; stage 2, the patient might have some difficulty in finding personal belongings; stage 3, compatible with very early AD, the patient will have functional difficulties apparent only in demanding circumstances such as at work; stage 4, representing mild AD, the patient might need assistance with handling finances; stage 5, the patient could have difficulty in dressing as in moderate AD; stage 6, the patient would have loss of most basic ADL ability; and stage 7, the patient would be at the end stage of dementia where the patient would become bedbound. These seven broad stages have been expanded into substages in updates of FAST (Reisberg 1986).

Perhaps surprisingly there is only a modest correlation between the loss in cognition and the loss in function, and the MMSE is not a reliable predictor of the functional ability of any one individual, especially in the less impaired (Reed *et al.* 1989). Thus Teri *et al.* (1989) showed that age was a better predictor of functional loss than cognitive state. Functional loss must therefore be evaluated on an individual basis but in practice this can be difficult in the mildly affected. Instrumental functional abilities are highly gender, class and age-cohort specific. One patient reports making an error when using a power drill, another finds switching programs on the computer difficult and a third reports using a hot wash cycle for delicate woollens in the washing machine. All are real examples and your guesses as to patient characteristics are likely to be both correct and not prejudicial. While scales have been developed (see Burns *et al.* 2002) these tend to be most useful in the moderate stages of the condition. In practice in the clinic the question 'Is there anything you used to do that you find difficult now?' to both patient and informant is a good start. As the subject deteriorates, loss of function dictates much of the care needs and has important safety considerations and an occupational therapy assessment is invaluable in assessing function both in staged environments such as a mock-up kitchen and importantly in the patient's own home.

Behavioural and psychological symptoms

Alzheimer recognised the importance of non-cognitive symptoms, noting in his seminal case study that 'the first noticeable symptom of illness shown by this 51-year-old woman was suspiciousness of her husband. [At times] believing that people were out to murder her, [she] started to scream loudly. At times she . . . seems to have auditory hallucinations' (Alzheimer 1907; Jarvik & Greenson 1987). The many symptoms of AD, other than cognitive changes and functional losses, are now brought together under the rubric 'behavioural and psychological symptoms of dementia' (BPSD). These symptoms are common and core features of AD and not secondary or rare features. Broadly speaking, BPSD can be grouped together as psychotic, mood and activity related (Table 9.1). The prevalence is high but, as can be seen in the table, highly variable in different studies. Much of this variability results from different criteria adopted for symptoms, some studies counting symptoms of depression and others only major depression meeting DSM-IV criteria. Also the frequency varies according to the stage of the disease and few studies are truly prospective. Disease-lifetime prevalence of BPSD is very high indeed and few patients escape some symptoms. Some evidence suggests that certain behavioural symptoms occur together: Hope et al. (1997) found three distinct syndromes, overactivity, aggressive behaviour and psychosis, whereas in the Cache County study patients were grouped into those with psychotic symptoms, those with affective symptoms and those with no or only one symptom (Lyketsos et al. 2001).

Looking after people with dementia is difficult and looking after people with behavioural disturbance is harder. A considerable body of work suggests that it is BPSD that impacts most on carers (Coen et al. 1997; Donaldson et al. 1998). Sleep disturbance is particularly difficult for carers: it saps energy and is difficult to manage. BPSD are also a major determinant of entry into institutional care (Cohen et al. 1993; Vernooij-Dassen et al. 1997). As this has become increasingly recognised, BPSD have become a target for therapy, both pharmacological and behavioural.

Psychotic symptoms

Depending partly on how it is defined, some form of psychosis occurs in up to one-third of people with AD. There is some evidence that those with psychotic features tend to decline quicker than those without (Drevets & Rubin 1989; Rosen & Zubenko 1991) but are not at greater risk of early mortality (Stern et al. 1994; Samson et al. 1996). There is no consistency in the literature regarding whether psychoses occur most frequently early or late in the condition but there is an inherent confounder in these studies in that it is easier to ascertain psychosis in the early stages where individuals retain language and can make their experiences understood. Psychosis must be a supremely distressing symptom and it is no surprise to find a number of studies showing an association between psychosis and aggression (Deutsch et al. 1991; Aarsland et al. 1996; Gormley et al. 1998). However, psychotic features are also associated with depression, suggesting that perhaps there is a common mechanism to behavioural disturbance in AD (Bassiony et al. 2002).

Delusions are the most common symptom and have a distinct flavour distinguishing them from the delusions of mood disorders or schizophrenia. Most common of all are delusions of theft, sometimes accompanied by a relatively complex explanation as to how the object was stolen.

Table 9.1 Frequency of behavioural and psychological symptoms in Alzheimer's disease.

Symptoms	Prevalence (%) (approximate)	Example references
Psychotic		
Hallucinations	20–30	Teri et al. (1988), Deutsch et al. (1991)
Paranoid or delusional ideation	20–30	Drevets & Rubin (1989), Deutsch et al. (1991)
Misidentification syndromes	10–20	Reisberg et al. (1987), Deutsch et al. (1991)
Mood		
Depression	10–25	Greenwald et al. (1989), Rovner et al. (1989), Sultzer et al. (1992)
Mania	<5	Burns et al. (1990b), Lyketsos et al. (1995)
Anxiety	>50	Jost & Grossberg (1996), Teri et al. (1999)
Activity		
Apathy	15–40	Starkstein et al. (2001), Lyketsos et al. (2002)
Agitation	30–70	Tractenberg et al. (2003b), McCurry et al. (2004)
Wandering	15–40	Klein et al. (1999), Holtzer et al. (2003)
Aggression	20–40	Deutsch et al. (1991), Eastley & Wilcock (1997)
Circadian rhythm disturbance	30–80	Tractenberg et al. (2003a), McCurry et al. (2004)

An elderly woman with AD became increasingly in need of social services as she no longer allowed her daughter into her flat. When her daughter visited she was treated with suspicion and at times shouted at and on one occasion had a stick raised to her. Needless to say this was distressing to the daughter and made caring for the patient difficult. Eventually the patient confessed to a community nurse that she believed that the daughter was systematically robbing her of her life savings and as evidence demonstrated that she did not know where her purse was. She claimed her daughter had taken it and when it was pointed out that the daughter had not been allowed to visit said the daughter came into the flat at night, climbing through the windows.

Although true delusions, the delusions of AD are usually secondary in that often the primary psychopathological event is amnesia. In the case above the primary event appeared to be mislaying a purse, which led to the secondary delusion of theft, a belief which was held with unusual conviction, was not amenable to reason and was manifestly erroneous (Sims 1988).

Hallucinations in AD are also distinct from those in other, primary, psychoses. Visual are the most common followed by auditory and then olfactory and tactile. Visual hallucinations may be complex, often of small animals or people and may be unaccompanied by fear or anxiety. Typically they are silent and sometimes the person with dementia has some insight, recognising that these experiences are in some way different from normal perceptions. Visual hallucinations form the most distinct of the clinical triad that make the diagnosis of DLB but are not in themselves pathognomonic, since visual hallucinations also occur in people with classical AD pathology.

Misidentification syndromes are distinct from prosopagnosias: in a true misidentification syndrome the person with AD is able to identify the face correctly (in person or from a photograph) but believes that an impostor has 'taken over' or replaced the other. One very common manifestation of a misidentification syndrome is where family members are mistaken for one another. Many children of people with AD become accustomed to being addressed as if they were a sibling or spouse of the patient. It can be difficult to distinguish a true misidentification event from a word-finding difficulty for names.

There have been considerable attempts to understand the underlying pathophysiology of psychosis in AD, partly for its own sake but also partly because it might contribute to the search for understanding of primary psychoses. Functional neuroimaging suggests relative hypoperfusion of dorsolateral frontal and dorsolateral parietal regions in AD with psychosis compared with AD without psychosis (Kotrla et al. 1995; Mega et al. 2000) and this may be in line with Cummings

(1985) who postulated disruptions to the corticolimbic systems as being common to many 'organic' delusions. It may be the relative activity of cholinergic and dopaminergic pathways in this system that is important and using receptor binding a moderate increase in D_3 binding in AD with psychosis was found in one post-mortem study (Sweet et al. 2001), although others failed to find a change in dopamine activity (Bierer et al. 1993) or a relative decrease in serotonergic activity (Zubenko et al. 1991).

Surprisingly, perhaps, as it is the exception rather than the rule, it is genetic studies that have been most replicable. Thus sib-pairs have been shown to share non-cognitive features more often than expected by chance alone in replicated studies (Tunstall et al. 2000; Sweet et al. 2002), and using a linkage approach susceptibility regions for AD plus psychosis have been found on regions of the genome also associated with schizophrenia (Bacanu et al. 2002). Given the neurophysiological evidence for dopamine and serotonin alterations in AD with psychosis, this was the obvious starting point for candidate association studies and it seems that variation in serotonin receptors is associated with risk of hallucinations (Holmes et al. 1998; Nacmias et al. 2001; Rocchi et al. 2003) and variation in dopamine receptors with risk of delusions (Sweet et al. 1998; Holmes et al. 2001).

Affective symptoms

Depression in particular has a complicated relationship with AD. Depression is a common non-cognitive feature, can be a precursor or prodromal syndrome (Schweitzer et al. 2002) and can be confused with dementia (pseudodementia). Of these, perhaps the most important is the first in that it is treatable and yet too often not treated. The prevalence of depression in AD differs widely according to the research methodology used and depends to a large degree on what is meant by depression. Major depressive episodes occur in approximately 10% or less of patients but minor depressive episodes occur in up to 30% and perhaps a majority of patients suffer some symptoms of depression (Reifler et al. 1986; Weiner et al. 1994, 2002; Migliorelli et al. 1995; Ballard et al. 1996; Brodaty & Luscombe 1996; Jost & Grossberg 1996; Li et al. 2001). Another difficulty is determining depression in different stages of dementia. Although scales for assessing depression in dementia are available (e.g. Cornell Scale for Depression in Dementia; Alexopoulos et al. 1988), assessing more subtle signs of depression becomes harder as the primary condition progresses.

It has been reported that there is a preferential loss of neurones in the *locus coeruleus* and possibly the dorsal raphe nucleus in AD with depression (Zweig et al. 1988; Förstl et al. 1992), suggesting that loss of noradrenergic or serotonergic function may be important. However, most neuropathological association studies are fraught with difficulties: the time between assessment and post-mortem may be considerable, the assessment of clinical features may have been only at one time point, and the numbers are frequently small. Although the association of loss of particular monoaminergic neurotransmitter neurones and depression in AD is intellectually satisfying, it remains to be fully replicated and some studies fail to find such an association (Hoogendijk *et al.* 1999).

Family studies show little linkage between late-onset depression (LOD) and AD, suggesting that there are no common genetic factors between the conditions (Heun *et al.* 2001). This is important as the finding that LOD is associated with AD could be explained by LOD inducing AD, LOD being a prodrome for AD, or LOD and AD having common risk factors. Common environmental factors cannot be excluded but common genetic factors seem to have been. It seems unlikely that LOD might induce AD but disruption of the hypothalamic–pituitary axis has been suggested and some internal mediator of biological stress increasing the pathology of AD cannot be entirely discounted. However, it seems much more likely that LOD occurring in people in their sixth or seventh decades is in many cases an early manifestation of the AD process (Steffens *et al.* 1997; Schweitzer *et al.* 2002). However, depression as a symptom of dementia does seem to have some genetic factors, since siblings tend to share AD plus depression (Tunstall *et al.* 2000).

Differences between AD and normal ageing

Cognitive deficits of AD and normal ageing

There has been much controversy regarding the question as to whether AD is simply an extreme form of, or is qualitatively different from, normal ageing. The debate has raged on the grounds of cognition and brain changes. Part of the problem with regard to cognitive neuroscience is that the symptoms of normal ageing and AD are superficially similar in that memory begins to fail in both. However, the evidence is increasingly clear that if memory declines in late life, it is a secondary effect of processing ability in contrast to a primary failure of memory systems in AD. In late life, fluid intelligence, or problem-solving ability, is almost certainly affected (Denney 1985), although learnt skills and crystallised intelligence is not. Memory tasks involving processing of information are affected whereas the tasks that minimise working memory are relatively unaffected (Babcock & Salthouse 1990). Older people encode information poorly and are less effective in utilising strategies and instruction for retrieval (Verhaeghen & Marcoen 1996; Nyberg *et al.* 2002; West *et al.* 2002). All this amounts to some loss of effective memory together with a slowing of processing speed and changes in spatial cognition and language when they involve processing functions. In contrast, in AD there is primary loss of memory, language and spatial cognitive abilities. Milwain and Iversen (2002) argue that this difference between normal cognitive ageing and AD reflects the known anatomical location and spread of AD pathology. Thus AD commences in the limbic system, the seat of episodic memory, and it is this func-

tion that is lost first in AD but which is relatively unaffected in ageing. The pathology then spreads to the frontal and parietal association cortices in line with the primary semantic and spatial deficits of AD but not ageing. This raises the prospect of increasingly refined cognitive tests that might distinguish between normal ageing and the very early onset of AD (Nestor *et al.* 2004).

Brain changes of late-onset AD and normal ageing

All components of the cerebral pathology of AD may also be found in aged persons who have appeared to be mentally intact up to the time of death. Thus it has been argued that cerebral atrophy and its attendant histological changes are so common in later life that the structural state of the brain, as at present revealed, is of doubtful significance in relation to the disease process (Rothschild 1956). Some other qualitative differences might be waiting to be discovered, although this now seems unlikely, or alternatively it might be the mode of the patient's reaction to the ageing processes within the brain which holds the key to dementia.

It was the careful mapping of the neuropathology of the brains of elderly people combined with attention to their clinical features prior to death that really established late-onset AD as a disease entity, separate from normal ageing and akin to early-onset AD. The importance of the comprehensive studies of Corsellis (1962) and the series of reports from Newcastle upon Tyne (Roth *et al.* 1967; Blessed *et al.* 1968; Tomlinson *et al.* 1968, 1970; summarised by Roth 1971) cannot be overstated in this respect.

Corsellis (1962) examined the brains of a large group of aged patients who had died in a psychiatric hospital, and found a high level of agreement between the clinical diagnosis during life and the severity of the neuropathological changes. Both parenchymatous and vascular changes tended to become more common with advancing age, but the great majority of those diagnosed as suffering from dementia showed cerebral pathology of at least moderate severity compared with only one-quarter of those who had suffered from 'functional' mental disorders.

The Newcastle workers undertook prospective studies, beginning with clinical and psychometric observations during life, and compared these with quantitative measures of neuropathological changes after death. The subjects included elderly demented patients, patients with 'functional' psychiatric illness, and mentally well-preserved persons who had died from accidents or other acute illnesses. The non-demented elderly subjects frequently showed senile plaques (now often called neuritic plaques) in the cortex and neurofibrillary changes in the hippocampi. Outfall of cells and granulovacuolar degeneration were also seen in some degree in the absence of dementia. However, quantitative estimates of the number of plaques, or of the severity of neurofibrillary changes, proved to correlate very highly indeed with scores of intellectual and personality impairment. In fact the relationship between impairment and mean plaque count was broadly linear. Moreover, plaques were present in all layers of the cortex in demented subjects, but often restricted to the superficial layers in those who had shown no intellectual decline. Very large conglomerate plaques were far commoner in demented than in normal subjects.

Wilcock and Esiri (1982) confirmed the Newcastle findings and focused particular attention on the significance of neurofibrillary change. Ball (1976) had already demonstrated an enormous increase in the number of tangle-bearing neurones in the hippocampi when AD patients were compared with age-matched controls, and Wilcock and Esiri sought to relate this to the severity of the dementia. Counts of both plaques and tangles were made in the cortex and hippocampi in patients with AD and in controls of equivalent age. Tangle formation proved to be highly correlated with the severity of dementia prior to death in the majority of areas sampled, in addition to distinguishing reliably between demented and non-demented subjects. Plaque counts showed significant associations of a similar nature but less impressively so. Moreover, tangle counts correlated with the severity of choline acetyltransferase reductions in the brain (Wilcock et al. 1982). It would appear therefore that the extensive development of neurofibrillary tangles may be of particular significance as a histological marker of AD. Tomlinson (1982) concludes from his considerable experience that while tangles can be found in the hippocampal pyramidal layer and occasionally in the hippocampal gyrus in healthy aged subjects, it is extremely rare to find them in the neocortex at any age in the absence of dementia. It might be added that the absence of neurofibrillary tangle pathology from the cerebellum, even in the context of heavy plaque load, is even more striking. Other more recent studies have confirmed that it is tangles rather than plaques that correlate best with severity of dementia (Nagy et al. 1995) but caution is warranted before over-interpreting these data: it may be, indeed some evidence suggests is likely to be, that tangles are relatively stable structures whereas plaques are more dynamic and can be removed by glia and possibly other processes. Furthermore, neither plaques nor tangles may be the 'cause' of dementia. Both may be the end-stage of the biochemical process that is actually the root cause of loss of neuronal function. Thus it may be oligomeric forms of amyloid invisible to the neuropathologist, or highly phosphorylated tau occurring years or decades before death, that results in dementia symptoms.

However, it does appear that AD arises clinically when the pathological changes of senescence develop beyond a certain degree of severity. In addition to these pathological lesions there is increasingly clear evidence of profound cell loss from the cortex when AD patients are compared with age-matched controls (Terry et al. 1981; Terry & Katzman 1983). Changes in the morphology of dendrites (Scheibel 1978) and reductions in their fields of arborisation (Buell & Coleman 1979, 1981)

have been reported. However, in contrast to this, in neurones containing tangles arborisation is actually increased (Gertz et al. 1991; McKee et al. 1989), perhaps as an attempt at compensation for loss of function.

A refinement of the distinction between AD and ageing comes with the argument as to whether AD is an age-related disorder or a disorder of ageing. The former suggests a disease state that is more common in a given age range (in this case age 75 to end of life) and the latter suggests a gradual and inevitable accumulation of brain damage with time. If the former, an age-related disorder, were the case, then it might be expected that incidence rates would fall at the upper end of the age range whereas they would continue to rise exponentially if AD were simply a function of age. The epidemiological evidence is not clear on this point for the obvious reason that it is very difficult to perform sufficiently large prospective studies of people at the very upper limits of the human lifespan. In an analysis of studies with approaching 30 000 pooled person life-years, the incidence in women continued to rise after the age of 90 whereas that in men started to fall (Andersen, K. et al. 1999). Even with studies of this size it cannot be concluded whether AD is an age-related disease or a disorder of ageing.

Investigations

Neuroimaging

Historically, neuroimaging has been used most in dementia to exclude other pathologies, some of which may be treatable. However, the cost-effectiveness of such a screening policy is highly dubious: in sequential series few if any potentially reversible conditions were identified by imaging that were not already suspected (Scheltens et al. 2002). Increasingly, however, the case is being made for neuroimaging to be used in the diagnostic work-up to enhance or refine diagnosis and not just to exclude other conditions (Knopman et al. 2001; Frisoni et al. 2003).

Cerebral atrophy, shown by widened sulci and enlarged ventricles on computed tomography (CT) or magnetic resonance imaging (MRI), is obvious in many patients, although overlap with age-matched controls prevents this from being used as a firm diagnostic criterion. Longitudinal studies have demonstrated that atrophy tends to worsen albeit with wide variability (Burns et al. 1991b; DeCarli et al. 1992). A more focused examination of the medial temporal lobe structures improves the diagnostic and prognostic value of structural imaging (Jobst et al. 1992; Horn et al. 1996; De Leon et al. 1997).

Hippocampal volume has most consistently been shown to be reduced early in AD and to be a marker of progression. Many studies have found evidence that medial temporal lobe structures, in particular hippocampal volume, are reduced early in AD and can be used to distinguish early AD from normal individuals (Convit et al. 2000; Jack et al. 2000;

Mizuno *et al.* 2000; Wahlund *et al.* 2000; Wolf *et al.* 2001). Some studies have shown a single MRI examination to provide a measure of atrophy that correlates with subsequent progression (Mungas *et al.* 2002). Scheltens *et al.* (2002) reviewed a series of studies that reported diagnostic sensitivity and specificity values ranging from 70% to 100% depending partly on the measures of hippocampal volume used and partly on the comparator groups in the studies. Overall, the sensitivity and specificity for detection of mild to moderate AD compared with controls was 85% and 88%.

Increasing attention is being paid to the possibility of using structural neuroimaging as a biomarker to measure change in AD. In particular, the studies of Fox and Rossor have shown that coregistration of serial MRI scans allows detection and quantitation of relatively subtle atrophic change (Fox *et al.* 2000). They find an annual change of 2.4% in AD compared with 0.4% in normal controls. Based on changes of this magnitude they are able to produce power calculations for the use of serial MRI as a biomarker of change in clinical trials of putative disease-modifying therapies, showing that for a year-long trial approximately 200 people in each arm of a trial would need to be assessed in order to have 90% power to detect a 20% effect-size of the drug (Fox *et al.* 2000). These figures compare very favourably with the numbers needed and the length of trial required were the sole outcome to be clinical change. De Santi *et al.* (2001) have suggested that although detecting change, coregistration of MRI is less sensitive than serial positron emission tomography (PET). Others have reviewed the evidence for the use of neuroimaging in measuring progression of AD (Kantarci & Jack 2003; Matthews *et al.* 2003).

Changes in cerebral blood flow and metabolism have been clearly demonstrated by functional imaging techniques. Early studies by Frackowiak *et al.* (1981), using PET, demonstrated substantial decreases in both cerebral blood flow and oxygen utilisation in SDAT, affecting both grey and white matter and implicating the parietal and temporal regions most severely. Sequential studies showed further decline with clinical deterioration, frontal hypometabolism appearing when deterioration was advanced. In contrast, the visual cortex and the primary sensorimotor cortex were relatively spared.

Mirroring blood flow, metabolism is also depressed in dementia (Pakrasi & O'Brien 2005). Using ^{18}F-fluorodeoxyglucose (FDG)-PET, Chase *et al.* (1984) observed relationships between hypometabolism in the left perisylvian region and language impairment, right posterior parietal region and visuospatial impairment, left angular gyrus and dyscalculia, and frontal hypometabolism in relation to personality change and attentional deficits. Haxby *et al.* (1988) found that frontal hypometabolism correlated with poor verbal fluency and attentional skills, whereas parietal hypometabolism was associated with impairment in verbal comprehension, arithmetical ability and visuospatial func-

tioning. Hypometabolism of brain in AD has been extensively confirmed using FDG-PET (De Leon *et al.* 2004; Mosconi 2005) and correlates with amyloid burden (Mega *et al.* 1999). In one systematic review the sensitivity and specificity of FDG-PET in the diagnosis of AD relative to controls was found to be 86% and 86%, respectively, (Patwardhan *et al.* 2004).

One interesting development has been the demonstration that these changes in metabolism are present in very young people at genetic risk of dementia (Bookheimer *et al.* 2000; Burggren *et al.* 2002; Reiman *et al.* 2004). It has been suggested that this marks the very early stages of dementia but an alternative possibility is that people carrying the *APOE* ε4 allele have instead a mild developmental difference in their brains and it is this that is related to increased risk of dementia in late life.

Proton magnetic resonance spectroscopy (^{1}H-MRS) has been used to examine the metabolic changes in the brain of a patient with AD, particularly *N*-acetylaspartate (NAA), a marker of neuronal integrity; creatine and phosphocreatine, markers of systemic energy use and storage; choline-containing compounds, markers of cell density and proliferation; and myoinositol, a possible marker of glial cells. The pattern of MRS changes in AD has been well established (Valenzuela & Sachdev 2001), showing reduced NAA and increased myoinositol. Concentrations of NAA correlate with plaque density and neurofibrillary tangles (Klunk *et al.* 1996) and reductions in NAA/creatine and phosphocreatine correlate with disease severity (Jessen *et al.* 2000).

Increasingly, functional MRI studies are being used to identify lesions in networks in AD and to search for evidence of plasticity and compensatory activity (Demetriades 2002; Devous 2002; Salmon 2002). However, possibly the most exciting prospect for the future is to develop molecular-based markers of AD processes. The first of these was a marker of amyloid formation used in PET studies (Cai *et al.* 2004; Klunk *et al.* 2004) but it is likely that other molecular markers will be developed and translated to more accessible imaging technologies including MRI.

Electroencephalography

Electroencephalography (EEG) shows abnormalities more frequently in AD than in any other form of dementia (Boutros & Struve 2002; Jeong 2004). The early stage consists of reduction of alpha activity, which may sometimes disappear entirely. This is particularly characteristic of AD and is perhaps of some value in distinguishing it from other varieties, in particular FTD where the EEG remains normal even relatively late in the disorder (Förstl *et al.* 1996). Later in the disease course in AD, diffuse slow waves appear, typically irregular theta activity with superimposed runs of delta. Focal or paroxysmal features are rare, even in patients with epileptic fits. Quantitative EEG may be useful in diagnosis in certain cases (Nuwer 1997).

Operational diagnostic criteria for AD

The diagnostic criteria for AD put forward by a working group established by the National Institute of Neurological and Communicative Disorders and Stroke and the Alzheimer's Disease and Related Disorders Association (NINCDS-ADRDA criteria) (McKhann *et al.* 1984) have become firmly established as a research, and to a large extent clinical, tool for diagnosing AD (Box 9.1). These criteria define probable and possible AD in life and definite AD as a post-mortem diagnosis (importantly accompanied by clinical features and not an exclusively neuropathological process).

In a prospective study of 50 elderly patients followed to post-mortem, Burns *et al.* (1990c) have shown the value of the NINCDS-ADRDA criteria. Of 32 patients diagnosed as 'probable' AD this was correct in 28, and of 18 'possible' cases the diagnosis was confirmed in 14 (i.e. sensitivities of 88%

and 78%, respectively). Mistakes mainly involved DLB in the former and vascular dementia in the latter. Jobst *et al.* (1998) found a specificity of 61% and a sensitivity of 96%. Lopez *et al.* (1999) found a similarly high sensitivity for AD but note that this condition is overdiagnosed. In a prospective study of over 2000 people coming to post-mortem, sensitivity was 93% and specificity 55% (Mayeux *et al.* 1998). These are remarkably consistent results and an American consensus group has expressed confidence in the use of both DSM and NINCDS-ADRDA criteria for clinical diagnosis of dementia (Knopman *et al.* 2001).

Course and outcome

The disease runs a progressive course, with death following some 2–8 years after onset. In Heston *et al.*'s (1981) material a trend could be seen for survival to increase a little from a mean of 7 years in those under 49 to 8.5 years for those aged

---

Box 9.1 NINCDS-ADRDA diagnostic criteria

I Diagnosis of probable AD

- Dementia established by clinical examination and documented by the MMSE, Blessed Dementia Scale or similar examination and confirmed by neuropsychological tests
- Deficits in two or more areas of cognition
- Progressive worsening of memory and other cognitive functions
- No disturbance of consciousness
- Onset between 40 and 90 years of age
- Absence of systemic disorders or other brain diseases to account for the progressive deficits in memory and cognition

II Such diagnosis is supported by:

- Progressive deterioration of specific cognitive functions such as language, motor skills and perception
- Impaired ADL and altered patterns of behaviour
- Family history of similar disorder, particularly if confirmed neuropathologically
- Laboratory results of normal lumbar puncture, normal EEG pattern or non-specific EEG changes, evidence of atrophy on CT with progression on serial observations

III Other features consistent with such diagnosis, after excluding other causes of dementia

- Plateaus in the course of progression
- Associated symptoms of depression, insomnia, incontinence, delusions, illusions, hallucinations, catastrophic outbursts, sexual disorders, weight loss and other neurological abnormalities (especially with more advanced disease) including increased muscle tone, myoclonus and gait disorder
- Seizures in advanced disease
- CT normal for age

IV Features that make such a diagnosis unlikely

- Sudden apoplectic onset
- Focal neurological signs such as hemiparesis, sensory loss, visual field deficits and incoordination early in the course
- Seizures or gait disturbances at the onset or very early in the course

V Diagnosis of possible AD

- May be made on the basis of the dementia syndrome, in the absence of other neurological, psychiatric or systemic disorders sufficient to cause dementia, and in the presence of variations in the onset, presentation or clinical course
- May be made in the presence of a second systemic or brain disorder sufficient to produce dementia, which is not considered to be the cause of the dementia
- Should be used in research studies when a single, gradually progressive severe cognitive deficit is identified in the absence of other identifiable cause

VI Diagnosis of definite AD

- The clinical criteria for probable AD and histopathological evidence obtained from biopsy or post-mortem

VII Classification of AD for research purposes

- Should specify features that may differentiate subtypes of the disorder, such as familial occurrence, onset before 65 years, presence of trisomy 21 and coexistence of other relevant conditions such as Parkinson's disease

55–74. In more elderly groups the survival was on average shorter, presumably due to deaths from competing causes, but even so the span could sometimes exceed 20 years. Seltzer and Sherwin (1983) made direct comparisons of 'relative survival time' between patients with onset before and after the age of 65 (by comparing observed length of survival for each individual with his expected survival from actuarial tables), and found significantly shorter survival for those in the presenile category. Rare cases are described in which the disorder becomes arrested for a time, but these must be regarded as exceptional. Neither remissions nor fluctuations characterise the disease.

A number of studies have attempted to use clinical features to try to define a subtype of aggressive AD or characteristics of more rapid decline. In a study of over 1000 patients, retrospective analysis found age at onset, MMSE, years of education, gender, ethnicity, living arrangement, presence of aphasia, delusions, hallucinations, and extrapyramidal signs to be independent variables associated with more rapid decline based on annual MMSE change (O'Hara *et al.* 2002). In line with this, in the Rotterdam study, age at onset and MMSE at presentation both predict decline (Ruitenberg *et al.* 2001a). The most consistent finding of many studies is that the worse the cognitive state at presentation, the worse the rate of subsequent decline and this holds true even in the very early stages of AD and prodromal AD (Lucca *et al.* 1993; Marra *et al.* 2000; Storandt *et al.* 2002). Aphasia and apraxia have been found by others to be predictors of rapid decline and mortality (Burns *et al.* 1991c; Yesavage *et al.* 1993). Loss of function is a predictor of mortality, and behavioural disturbance, perhaps unsurprisingly, a predictor of entry into nursing homes (Bianchetti *et al.* 1995). Once in a nursing home increased age, male sex, limitation in physical function, evidence of malnutrition, pressure sores, diabetes mellitus and cardiovascular disease predicts a more rapid decline to death (Gambassi *et al.* 1999).

Neuropathology

In a paper in 1907, Alzheimer described the clinical features and neuropathology of one of his patients, Auguste D. The lesions he described were subsequently shown by Corsellis and the Newcastle group to also occur in the brains of older people with dementia, thus suggesting that the two conditions were essentially the same, although there may be differences in aetiology and possibly in pathogenesis. The two key lesions are the amyloid or neuritic (previously senile) plaque and the neurofibrillary tangle.

Neuritic plaques (Fig. 9.1a)

These lesions are extracellular deposits of an amyloid, defined as an aggregated protein that has a high proportion of β-pleated sheet and shows birefringence when stained with Congo red. All amyloid deposits share this biochemical property but the parent molecules from which they are derived are different. In the case of AD the parent molecule is amyloid precursor protein (APP), the metabolism and genetics of which are discussed below. The neuritic plaque has a dense amyloid core surrounded by neuritic change and is visible on various silver staining techniques as pioneered by Nissl and utilised by Alzheimer, in addition to being readily visible with Congo red staining. When the amyloid peptide and its parent molecule were discovered, antibodies were developed that allowed the more subtle techniques of immunocytochemistry to be used on brain material. This revealed that the amyloid peptide was also deposited in diffuse aggregates that were not Congo-red positive. Strictly speaking these are therefore not amyloid deposits but this distinction is often lost. It is likely though that these diffuse plaques are precursors of the mature, neuritic plaque as seen by Alzheimer. The plaque is found in all cortical areas of brain and also occurs in striatum and the cerebellum (Braak *et al.* 1989; Braak and Braak 1990, 1991). There appears to be

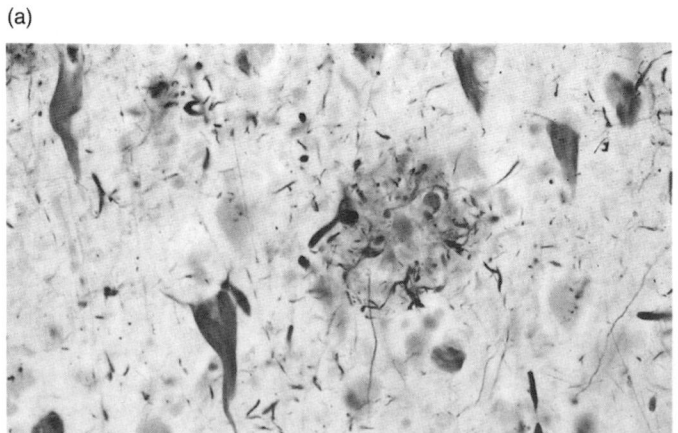
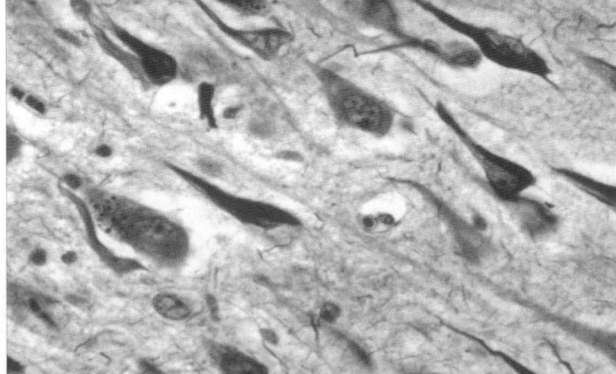

Fig. 9.1 (a) Neuritic plaque and (b) neurofibrillary tangles (see also Plate 9.1).

relatively little correlation between overall plaque density and cognitive state (Nagy *et al.* 1995; Green *et al.* 2000), and plaque counts are not sensitive to differentiation between normal ageing and AD, although this may suggest simply that they are among the earliest changes of AD rather than indicating they are not pathological (Gold *et al.* 2001; Haroutunian *et al.* 1998). It is important to distinguish neuritic plaques from diffuse or non-neuritic plaques as the latter do correlate reasonably well with cognitive state (Dickson 1997). However, it is true that both plaques and tangles occur in people not known to have dementia (Davis *et al.* 1999; MRC CFAS 2001).

Neurofibrillary tangles (Fig. 9.1b)

Tangles are intraneuronal aggregates of a protein, tau, normally found in the axon. They are readily visible with silver staining techniques such as Bielschowsky: initially they appear as aggregates in the cell body, and then as they increasingly fill the cell body, particularly in pyramidal neurones, they appear as flame-shaped accumulations extending into the axonal hillock. Also seen with Bielschowsky staining are fine hair-like structures in the brain substance known as neuropil threads. Most probably these are tangles accumulating in the axons and dendrites of affected neurones. Under the electron microscope neurofibrillary tangles can be shown to be composed of many separate filaments, most appearing to be paired structures with a periodicity suggesting two twisted ropes. These are paired helical filaments and are abnormal and not to be confused with other normal filamentous structures in neurones such as neurofilaments and microtubules, of which more details will be given later. Paired helical filaments (and also straight filaments) occur not only in tangles but also in neuropil threads and in the neuritis surrounding neuritic plaques.

Tangles occur first in the entorhinal cortex and spread in a systematic fashion through hippocampus to wider cortical structures but always sparing the cerebellum (Braak *et al.* 1994; Braak & Braak 1998). In fact the important studies of Braak have shown that the earliest changes in neurones are an increase in tau phosphorylation and a redistribution of tau from the axon to the cell body. This appears to occur some years, possibly decades, before the clinical onset of dementia and both changes in tau phosphorylation and changes in tau expression and/or redistribution may be necessary precursors of the tau aggregation that results in tangle formation. It is not known, but is the subject of much interest and speculation, why some areas of brain are exquisitely sensitive and others apparently completely resistant to tangle formation. In advanced AD the distribution of tangles is very extensive and neurones in many areas become sparse. Tangles are insoluble and remain after the neurone dies, at which point the tangle is known as a 'ghost' or 'tombstone' tangle.

Other pathological changes in the AD brain

The steady accumulation of plaques and tangles is accompanied by synaptic loss (Adams 1991; DeKosky & Scheff 1990;

Terry *et al.* 1991) and this, together with actual neuronal loss, is likely responsible for most of the clinical features of AD. However, an effect of altered tau phosphorylation and redistribution, as observed by Braak as the earliest sign of AD pathology, on neuronal function cannot be excluded. Another lesion occurring in AD, the significance of which is unknown, is the granulovacuolar body, an intraneuronal change occurring often in pyramidal neurones. Amyloid material also occurs in amyloid angiopathy, in the walls of small vessels. As noted above, many studies have shown extensive non-amyloid atherosclerotic change in AD as well and it is becoming clear that this likely contributes to the disease process, possibly by accelerating plaque or tangle formation, possibly by affecting neuronal function or stability directly.

Neurochemistry

One of the most important breakthroughs in understanding AD was the realisation that it is, at least partially, predominantly a disorder of cholinergic neurones. The cholinergic hypothesis of AD rests on two main strands: evidence that cholinergic neurones are lost first and foremost in AD, and evidence from animal studies that cholinergic neurones are essential for memory. The evidence that cholinergic markers are lost most in AD came from the groups of Peter Whitehouse, Gordon Wilcock, Elaine and Robert Perry and others and demonstrated reductions in cholinergic neurones in the nucleus basalis of Meynert and reductions in markers of cholinergic activity there and elsewhere in the brain (reviewed in Francis *et al.* 1999). From animal work it was known that lesions of the cholinergic system, either surgical or chemical with the cholinergic antagonist scopolamine, induced cognitive defects in rodents. *In vivo* but indirect evidence in humans that lesions of the cholinergic system hasten decline in dementia comes from retrospective studies of those taking antidepressants or antipsychotics with anticholinergic actions (Holmes *et al.* 1997; McShane *et al.* 1997). The cholinergic hypothesis led to an intense effort to design compounds to increase cholinergic function including precursor therapies such as lecithin, receptor agonist approaches and the cholinesterase inhibitors. It was this latter approach that proved the first successful drug therapy in AD.

Despite this outstanding success, the cholinergic hypothesis is only part of the story as far as neurochemical attrition in AD goes. Lyness *et al.* (2003) reviewed all the studies on regional cell loss in AD published between 1966 and 2000 and performed a meta-analysis of relative cell loss. Compared with the dopaminergic substantia nigra, where there is relatively little cell loss, the attrition was greatest in the cholinergic nucleus basalis and the noradrenergic locus coeruleus, closely followed by the serotonergic dorsal raphe nucelus. This huge analysis of a considerable body of work stretching two decades demonstrates that there is extensive loss of noradrenergic and serotonergic neurones, with loss of the former being as extensive as loss of cholinergic tracts and suggests that there may be some merit in replacing these functions in addition to replacing cholinergic function.

There is less convincing evidence for glutametergic deficits in AD (Cowburn *et al.* 1990), although there is some evidence of decreased glutamate *in vivo* from MRS studies (Antuono *et al.* 2001; Hattori *et al.* 2002).

Molecular biology

Formation of amyloid

Research in AD entered a new phase when David Allsop, then separately Glenner and Wong, and Beyreuther and Masters, discovered the nature of the amyloid protein core of the plaque first observed by Alzheimer (Allsop *et al.* 1983; Glenner & Wong 1984; Masters *et al.* 1985). Glenner and Wong noted that 'This protein may be derived from a unique serum precursor which may provide a diagnostic test for Alzheimer's disease and a means to understand its pathogenesis'. These predictions have largely been borne out. The peptide is indeed derived from a larger precursor, fragments of which can be detected in serum although the whole protein itself is cell-bound. Using these fragments as biomarkers has not proved possible but certainly the pathogenesis of the plaque has become understood and 20 years after this seminal study compounds designed to reduce amyloid formation are entering clinical trials.

The precursor from which the amyloid peptide (known as Aβ) is derived is APP, a nearly ubiquitous protein present in all cell types and showing a large degree of cross-species homology (Kang *et al.* 1987). The role of this protein is not fully understood but it is becoming increasingly clear that it is a complex molecule that serves not a single but many functions. One role is to act as a cellular receptor (specifically as a G protein-coupled receptor, where binding to APP would be expected to induce signalling events, the nature of which are as yet unknown) (Nishimoto *et al.* 1993). Another suggestion is that as a molecule with a large extracellular region, APP

might function in cell–cell contact or adhesion events, possibly at the synapse. The metabolic products of APP have functions quite distinct from those of the intact molecule. The APP fragment released by cleavage at the cell membrane (sAPPα) functions as a complement factor inhibitor and the intracellular fragment released by cleavage of APP within the cell membrane translocates to the cell nucleus and is involved in gene transcription events (Cao & Sudhof 2001). These are just two of many actions and sAPPα, Aβ and the other metabolic products of APP have many binding partners, all of which suggest a complex biology. It is widely assumed that the critical events in AD are not so much loss of this rich biology but a toxic gain of function, a neurotoxicity due to the Aβ fragment. However, it is worth bearing in mind that APP and its fragments have important roles to play in memory and cognition (Turner *et al.* 2003). This is most apparent in relation to long-term potentiation, the process whereby neurones, most often in hippocampus, can be shown to 'remember' a rapid and strong electrical stimulus. The excitatory postsynaptic potential increases in response to such a tetanic stimulus and this increased response is then replicated even for milder subsequent stimuli: the neurones have been potentiated (Bear & Malenka 1994). This protein synthesis-dependent process is the best available cellular correlate of memory and is consistently inhibited by Aβ (Turner *et al.* 2003).

Amyloid precursor protein is metabolised by three secretase activities: α-secretase, β-secretase or β-amyloid cleaving enzyme (BACE), and γ-secretase (this has been extensively reviewed; see for example Haass & De Strooper 1999; Wilson *et al.* 1999; Allinson *et al.* 2003) (Fig. 9.2). The site for α-secretase is within the moiety itself and so cleavage by this route cannot yield intact Aβ and hence this pathway is known as non-amyloidogenic. On the other hand, sequential cleavage by BACE and then γ-secretase yields fragments of 40–42 amino acids in length. Aβ-42 is more likely to form fibrils *in vitro* (as occurs in the plaque in the AD brain) and is therefore

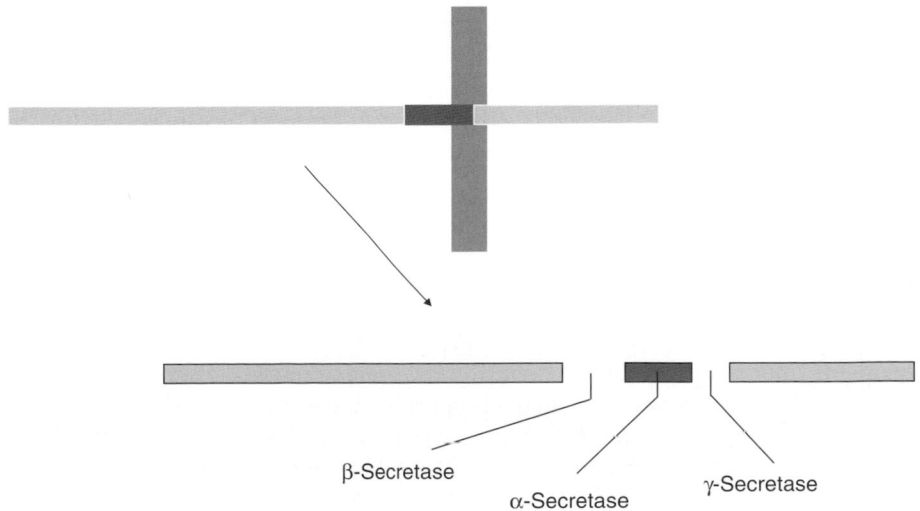

Fig. 9.2 Metabolism of amyloid precursor protein.

β-Secretase

α-Secretase

γ-Secretase

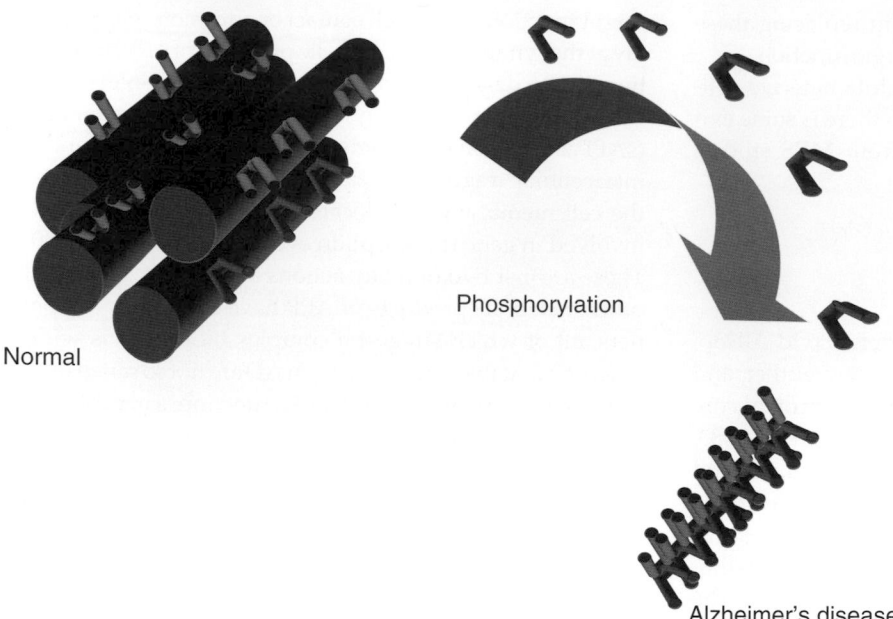

Normal

Phosphorylation

Alzheimer's disease

Fig. 9.3 Tau phosphorylation and aggregation.

thought to be more pathogenic than Aβ-40. The identity of these various enzymes has been sought with vigour as these are obvious sites for therapeutic intervention. BACE and its homologue BACE2 has been identified and cloned (Saunders *et al.* 1999) and inhibitors have been produced that might have potential as therapies to prevent amyloid formation (Potter & Dressler 2000). For various reasons, not least the fact that loss of the gene is fatal to mice, targeting γ-secretase for therapy is harder. However, the identity of this interesting enzyme has been shown to reside within a complex of proteins that includes presenilin-1 (see below), nicastrin, APH-1 and PEN-2 (De Strooper 2003). This γ-secretase complex is of fundamental importance to the brain as in addition to cleaving APP it also cleaves a protein Notch responsible for lateral inhibition, the process whereby one precursor cell adopts a neuronal cell fate and signals to its neighbours to choose other destinations (Beatus & Lendahl 1998). One Notch gene is involved in the disorder CADASIL (cerebral autosomal dominant arteriopathy with subcortical infarcts and leucoencephalopathy), an inherited condition with migraine, stroke, neuropsychiatric symptoms and dementia (Davous 1998). It would not be surprising to find Notch and its related genes involved in other neuropsychiatric conditions.

Formation of tangles

Neurofibrillary tangles are composed of the microtubule-associated protein tau, present in tangles in a highly phosphorylated form and aggregated into paired helical filaments. Normally, tau binds to and stabilises microtubules, which are essential for axonal transport (reviewed in Goedert 1993; Paglini *et al.* 2000). Much of psychiatry and neurology concentrates on synaptic events but this is mere

expediency secondary to the availability of drugs that happen to work at the synapse. However, the synapse has little or no protein-generating capability and all the functional proteins, or their subunits or precursors, at the synapse have been generated in the cell body and then transported down axons. This fast axonal transport is microtubule dependent and in turn tau dependent, as tau and other microtubule-binding proteins are responsible for maintaining the integrity and function of the microtubules. In AD, tau is highly phosphorylated and the microtubule-binding properties of tau are regulated by phosphorylation (Fig. 9.3). The highly phosphorylated tau of the AD brain fails to effectively bind to microtubules and in cells fails to stabilise them. It is noteworthy that in the AD brain, neurones affected by tangle formation lack a normal microtubule cytoskeleton. This suggests that the regulation of tau phosphorylation is critical in AD (Lovestone & Reynolds 1997). A considerable body of work now suggests glycogen synthase kinase (GSK)-3 as a predominant but probably not exclusive tau kinase. GSK-3 is an interesting enzyme as it is effectively inhibited by lithium, although whether this is responsible for lithium's therapeutic or toxic actions is unclear (Eldar-Finkelman 2002).

Amyloid cascade hypothesis

The finding of mutations in the *APP* gene associated with familial early-onset AD (FAD; see Genetic factors, later) demonstrated that APP was fundamental in the pathogenesis. Mutations in the gene tend to occur at or close to the sites of amyloidogenic cleavage by BACE and γ-secretase and this very strongly suggests that dysregulation of APP metabolism is an early event in AD pathology. This is the basis of the amyloid cascade hypothesis (Fig. 9.4), in which altered regu-

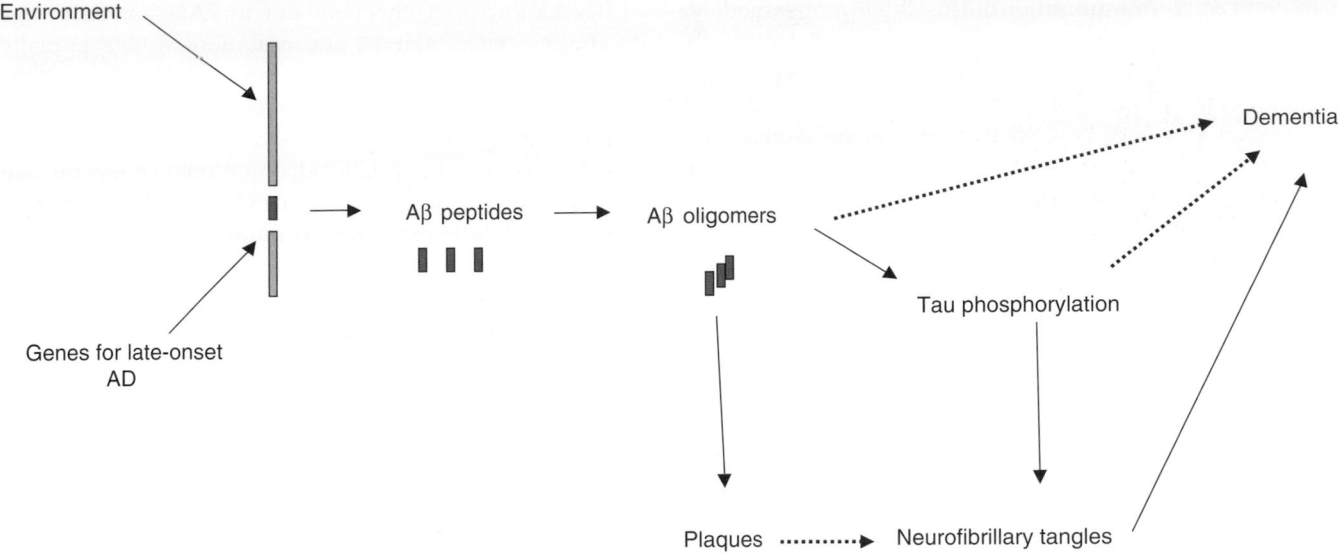

Fig. 9.4 Amyloid cascade hypothesis.

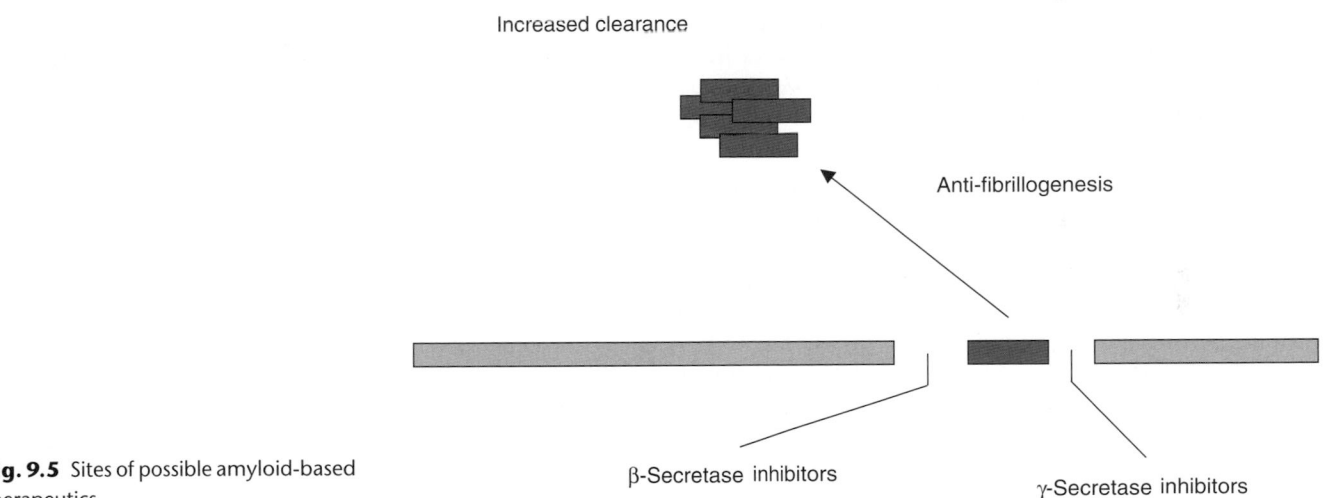

Fig. 9.5 Sites of possible amyloid-based therapeutics.

lation of APP would yield increased Aβ and this in turn would induce tau phosphorylation, aggregation into tangles, neuronal death and hence dementia (Hardy & Higgins 1992). One and a half decades later, this hypothesis has not been seriously challenged, although it has been extensively refined in its detail (Mudher & Lovestone 2002). Remarkably, all the fundamental predictions of the model have been confirmed; most importantly the observation that all the known mutations causing FAD increase either total Aβ or the more fibrillogenic Aβ-42. The gap in the hypothesis is most obvious between amyloid and tau: in neurones in culture Aβ-42 is toxic and induces tau phosphorylation, most likely by inducing GSK-3 activity (Takashima *et al.* 1998; Alvarez *et al.* 1999). However, in transgenic mice massive deposition of amyloid in animals carrying the FAD mutations does not result in

extensive tau phosphorylation, no tangles and little or no evidence of a dementia. This fact suggests a critique of animal modelling of human disease rather than a serious objection to the amyloid cascade hypothesis.

Disease-modifying therapy and the amyloid cascade hypothesis

The huge accumulation of evidence in favour of the cascade starting with amyloid and ending with tau suggests therapies for AD many of which are in development (Fig. 9.5). Drugs to reduce Aβ formation such as BACE inhibitors have been developed, as have small-molecule inhibitors of Aβ aggregation. An alternative approach would be to increase clearance of amyloid deposits from the brain and one of the most promising developments was the demonstration that passive or active immunisation did just this in mouse models. Unfortunately, the same in humans proved toxic, although there was evidence that plaque load was reduced (Nicoll *et al.* 2003). The immunisation approach is being modified in an attempt to reduce the toxicity while retaining amyloid-clearance efficacy. Breaking the link between amyloid and tau is being pursued, not least with GSK-3 inhibitors. Determining whether any of these approaches actually reduces the pathology in brain given that there are few biomarkers and no actual markers of pathology is a challenge.

Genetic factors

Early-onset autosomal dominant FAD

The only subclassification of AD that has biological justification is between familial forms and non-familial forms. However, even this is complicated by the fact that there is a considerable genetic component even to the apparently non-familial forms. Individual families with pedigrees suggestive of autosomal dominant inheritance had long been recognised and when linkage in some of these families was mapped to a region on chromosome 21, attention turned to the obvious candidate in this region, APP. After some initial confusion caused by genetic heterogeneity between families, a mutation in the *APP* gene resulting in a valine/isoleucine change at position 717 of the APP protein was found in a family from London by the group led by John Hardy, then working at St Mary's Hospital. Subsequently, other mutations were found in the same region of the gene. This region is at the γ-secretase site and it is likely that coding changes in the amino acid sequence alter the activity of γ-secretase on the APP protein. In cells and in transgenic animals, overexpression of human APP with these mutations results in increased Aβ-41 formation and plaques. Subsequently, a double mutation in the region of the gene coding for the sequence recognised by BACE was found in a Swedish family (*APPswe*) and, as for other mutations in APP, this change (at position 670/671) results in Aβ formation and plaque formation in animal models. All this is powerful evidence in favour of the amyloid cascade hypothesis, but even more compelling evidence for the hypothesis comes from the fact that mutations within the Aβ moiety of APP do not result in increased Aβ formation in model systems and do not cause classical AD but instead hereditary cerebral haemorrhage with amyloidosis (Dutch type) or variants of this condition. In 2005, there were 16 known pathogenic mutations in the *APP* gene, with new mutations being posted at http://www.alzforum.org/res/com/mut/default.asp as they are reported. However, there are some families with apparent linkage to chromosome 21 that do not have *APP* mutations and it may be that there are other disease loci on this chromosome. It is likely that the reason why AD neuropathology is an invariable accompaniment of Down's syndrome (Mann 1988) is trisomy *APP*.

It was known that other families with FAD showed linkage to chromosomes 14 and 1 and mutations were eventually found in a novel gene named presenilin 1 (PS-1 for protein, *PSEN1* for gene) on chromosome 14. A swift hunt through the human genome database found a homologous gene on chromosome 1 and, as predicted, mutations in this gene in an ethnic group showing chromosome 1 linkage (Volga German people). To date there are over 70 mutations in *PSEN1* known to cause AD, with new mutations still being reported. It is still not known whether these mutations result in a toxic gain in function or a loss of normal function but it is clear that the end-result is a change in APP processing. Transgenic animals have been generated harbouring both *PSEN1* and *APP* mutations with consequent increased amyloid pathology (but surprisingly little tau pathology).

The age of onset in families carrying *PSEN1* mutations tends to be earlier, and those carrying *PSEN2* mutations later, than those with *APP* mutations. However, there is considerable variation between families and even to a degree within families. Non-penetrance of a *PSEN1* mutation has been reported but not (yet) for *PSEN2* or *APP* (Rossor *et al.* 1996). Based on linkage, to chromosome 3 for example, there are likely to be one or two other genes causing FAD. Mutations in the *TAU* gene have been found in FTD and there are reports of familial motor neurone disease with dementia, the genes for which have not yet been reported (although linkage results suggests a gene on chromosome 9). It will be important to determine the biological relationship between these genes, and disorders with few clinical similarities may turn out to have considerable mechanistic and pathological overlap.

The genetics of FAD has been extensively reviewed (Clark & Goate 1993; Hardy 1996; Price *et al.* 1998; Selkoe 2000). It has undoubtedly been the most important spur to understanding the molecular pathogenesis. However, it is important to recall that FAD is an extremely rare condition, occurring in perhaps 5 per 100 000 population at risk (Campion *et al.* 1999), a figure that equates to approximately 600 people in the entire UK (Liddell *et al.* 2001). Nonetheless, for these families precise diagnosis of AD can be made in life and predictive testing can be offered (Liddell *et al.* 2001). This should only be performed in the context of a clinical genetics department and there is international agreement that protocols developed for Huntington's disease should be followed (Lovestone 1999). These include first determining a mutation in an affected family member (and for AD determining that a mutation is indeed pathogenic – not a trivial task). Counselling should be offered and would normally take place over 3–6 months; people at 25% a priori risk (i.e. grandchildren) should not be tested as this would provide a de facto prediction on the intermediary generation, and caution should be exercised in those with serious affective or other psychiatric features (Lovestone & Lashwood 2001).

Late-onset AD

Previously, late-onset AD was thought to be largely a sporadic condition, although a family history is found in up to one-third of patients. However, the most important reason for lack of family history is attrition due to other diseases: relatively few of the currently aged cohort have sufficiently large and aged pedigrees to be informative. Clearly if both parents die before the age of onset of AD (say before 75–80), then one cannot infer anything from a lack of family history. A series of studies instead examined age-related incidence of AD in family members, finding a cumulative incidence by the age of 90 years of up to 50% (Breitner *et al.* 1988; Huff *et al.* 1988; Farrer *et al.* 1989; Korten *et al.* 1993). This demonstrates the importance of susceptibility genes that do not cause but increase risk of AD. From twin studies, it has been estimated that the heritability of late-onset AD is 60–70% (Bergem *et al.* 1997; Gatz *et al.* 1997; Pedersen *et al.* 2001), of which one gene (*APOE*) accounts for less than half of the genetic variance (Owen *et al.* 1994) and with an estimated four or more genes waiting to be discovered (Daw *et al.* 2000). In very late-onset AD the importance of genetic factors appears to diminish (Silverman *et al.* 2003).

One unequivocal genetic susceptibility locus for AD has been discovered, the *APOE* gene. There are three common variants or alleles of the gene, *APOEε2*, *APOEε3* and *APOEε4*, differing by only two single-nucleotide polymorphisms (SNPs) that result in two different amino acid changes. The *APOEε4* variant increases risk, by perhaps threefold to fourfold in the heterozygote state and up to 10-fold in the homozygote state. At the age of 65 this has the effect of a threefold difference in life expectancy between *APOEε4* carriers and non-carriers (Seshadri *et al.* 1995), but at earlier ages the effect on life expectancy is negligible (even though *APOEε4* also increases risk of cardiovascular disease in men). *APOE* only modulates risk and does not 'cause' the disease; as *APOEε4* is not the commonest variant, the majority of people with AD do not carry this risk gene. In fact, it may be that *APOE* only alters risk at all by altering the age of onset of AD, with *APOEε4* carriers acquiring the disease earliest and *APOEε2* carriers the latest (Meyer *et al.* 1998). This has been characterised as *APOE* affecting 'when and not if' AD occurs.

The means by which *APOE* alters risk are not known. The *APOEε2/3/4* variant is a major mediator of cholesterol levels and so the risk may not be directly on the brain at all. Alternatively, *APOE* has been shown in different studies to affect Aβ aggregation and clearance, tau phosphorylation, synaptic plasticity and numerous other processes that could plausibly be important in AD. Given the robust association between *APOEε4* and AD, considerable thought has been given to whether genetic testing for this gene could contribute to diagnosis or prognosis or whether there are pharmacogenetic uses for testing. This has been the subject of a number of consensus groups (see for example Brodaty *et al.* 1995; Farrer *et al.* 1995; Alzheimers Association and National Institute for

Aging 1998), which have concluded that there are no clinical roles for testing as *APOE* genotype does not improve diagnostic accuracy enough to warrant its use, confers too little risk to be of value in prediction and does not have any replicated effects on response to cholinesterase inhibitors. However, it is likely that at some point there may be some use for genetic testing in late-onset AD, perhaps with a combination of genes or to predict conversion from mild cognitive impairment. This is a prospect anticipated with some trepidation by many. It is sobering that the decade from 1993 to 2003 of accumulated research on the genetics of late-onset AD yielded one gene of uncertain function and no clinical utility and has led to no significant insights into the pathophysiology of AD. Although almost certainly an essential and inevitable research strategy, it demonstrates that the genetics of complex common conditions is no rapid route to therapy.

A huge number (more than 100 in 2003) of other genes have been reported to be associated with late-onset AD in case–control association studies. However, none of these have yet been reliably replicated, emphasising the difficulty currently facing attempts to find genetic susceptibility factors for many common and complex diseases. It is something of a puzzle and a huge concern as to why it has proved so difficult to replicate findings. It might be that all these 100 or so putative associations are false positives or it might be that due to study population stratification, associations that are true for a subgroup (by gender, age, ethnicity or any one of a myriad of other factors) appear in one study but not another. It is likely that this difficult and frustrating situation will only be resolved by studying very much larger groups (thousands rather than the hundreds typical of most studies). An alternative approach is to perform linkage on related individuals and a series of such studies concur that there is a region on chromosome 10 associated with AD, although the actual genomic regions in these various studies do not completely overlap (Bertram *et al.* 2000; Ertekin-Taner *et al.* 2000; Myers *et al.* 2000; Li *et al.* 2002; Blacker *et al.* 2003).

Genotype–phenotype correlations

There is a considerable amount of evidence that individual variation in the phenotype of AD (the manifestation of the illness in a particular individual) may have a genetic component. In siblings with AD, depression and agitation are shared traits and depression may be more frequent in first-degree relatives of probands with AD and depression (Pearlson *et al.* 1990; Tunstall *et al.* 2000). Some of the genetic component responsible for this variation in the pattern of non-cognitive symptoms has been shown, in replicated studies, to lie in 5-hydroxytryptamine and dopaminergic receptor polymorphisms (Holmes *et al.* 1998, 2001; Sweet *et al.* 1998; Nacmias *et al.* 2001). Age of onset of AD is also inheritable, most obviously in the autosomal dominant families where age of onset has some constancy within families (Mullan & Crawford 1994) but also due to *APOE* variation (Meyer *et al.* 1998) and a locus on chromosome 10 (Li *et al.* 2002). The relationship between genetic factors and BPSD has also been examined through linkage studies, with some evidence for genetic loci on chromosomes 2, 6 and 21 influencing the occurrence of psychosis in AD (Bacanu *et al.* 2002).

Environmental risk factors

Of all the risk factors for AD, age is overwhelmingly the most important, doubling the risk every year after the age of 65. So important is this that it has led some to speculate that AD is an invariable accompaniment of ageing (Ritchie & Kildea 1995). In line with this are studies showing accumulation of AD pathology in the elderly without apparent dementia (MRC CFAS 2001) and epidemiological studies showing no decrease in incidence in very elderly women (Andersen, K. *et al.* 1999), although the finding that incidence falls in very elderly men would counter this somewhat. However, even this most apparently obvious environmental risk factor may have an inherited component as there is an interesting interaction between age and genetic factors, with the only confirmed risk factor for AD altering age of onset rather than having absolute risk of suffering the condition (Breitner *et al.* 1999; Meyer *et al.* 1998). Family-based studies confirm that age of onset tends to be shared by siblings and that not all of this sharing is accounted for by *APOE*, suggesting that other genetic loci are involved (Tunstall *et al.* 2000) and a linkage study shows a region on chromosome 10 associated with earlier age of onset not only of AD but also Parkinson's disease (Li *et al.* 2002). These findings serve to emphasise that the distinction between gene and environment is an entirely false one and that it is interaction between the gene and environment that is critical.

Head injury: effects on amyloid and tau related pathology

A reasonably large number of case–control studies have suggested that closed head injury resulting in some loss of consciousness is commoner in people with AD. A meta-analysis of these studies confirmed an increased risk of head injury with a relative risk of 1.8 (Mortimer *et al.* 1991). However, in a later meta-analysis, subsequent studies showed no increase in risk. Overall, including all 15 studies examining the association, a modest increase of risk with an odds ratio (OR) of 1.6 was found, although this was entirely due to an increased risk in males exposed to head injury (Fleminger *et al.* 2003). Although the risk due to head injury is only modest and not entirely replicable, there is a clear mechanism to explain such an association as studies of brains of people dying of head injury show increased amounts of amyloid peptide deposition (Roberts *et al.* 1994). It is likely that this is a neuroprotective response, but one that can in some people who survive

the head injury go on to induce the changes of AD. In addition, repetitive head injury not resulting in loss of consciousness is a associated with dementia, for example the dementia pugilistica syndrome of boxers. The shearing action on axons that accompanies such blows to the head induces extensive damage, including tau aggregations similar to those of AD and also deposition of amyloid peptide (Roberts *et al.* 1990). Some studies have been able to demonstrate that this deposition of amyloid is increased in people carrying at least one *APOEε4* allele and that clinical response to brain injury is *APOE* dependent (Horsburgh *et al.* 2000), suggesting another gene–environment interaction although evidence for such an interaction in clinical studies of head injury and AD is lacking (Mortimer *et al.* 1991).

Vascular factors

Vascular dementia is partly defined by the presence of vascular risk factors but it is probably true that these same factors also increase risk of AD itself. Thus hypertension, smoking and peripheral artery disease are all associated with AD (reviewed in Prince 1995; Fujishima & Tsuchihashi 1999; Skoog *et al.* 1999). The clearest association between AD and vascular risk factors (as distinct from those studies examining all dementias and vascular risk where the association may obviously be confounded by vascular dementia) is between hypertension and AD. However, even here, some cautionary notes are warranted. Thus, for example, Qiu *et al.* (2003) find an association between hypertension and AD with an OR of 1.5 but also find an association with low blood pressure. In contrast, Posner *et al.* (2002) show that hypertension is not associated with increased risk of AD demonstrating, if nothing else, that epidemiological associations can be as hard to replicate as genetic ones. However, the importance of this risk factor is the straightforward means of preventing it, and one study has demonstrated that treating hypertension can reduce the risk of AD (Forette *et al.* 2002). There is a possible gene–environment interaction between hypertension and AD in that the gene encoding angiotensin-converting enzyme (ACE) is associated with both, although it has to be said that the association is not consistently replicated in either condition (Kehoe *et al.* 1999; Schunkert 1997). In addition, an interaction between *APOE* and vascular risk is reported in some studies (Hofman *et al.* 1997; Stewart *et al.* 2001) but not all (Prince *et al.* 2000). Neuropathological studies have consistently shown a high degree of overlap between vascular and AD pathologies (Holmes *et al.* 1999; MRC CFAS 2001) but it is also true that minor amounts of vascular damage are common in the population, for example 34% in controls compared with 43% in neuropathologically confirmed AD cases in one study (Jellinger & Attems 2003).

A raised homocysteine level is a highly reproducible risk factor for vascular disease and has been consistently shown to be associated with AD (Clarke *et al.* 1998; McIlroy *et al.* 2002; Shea *et al.* 2002; Miller *et al.* 2003; Nagga *et al.* 2003;

Religa *et al.* 2003; Selley 2003). Whether this association is mediated through vascular damage inducing AD, through an association with vascular dementia *per se* or some other neuronal effect altering the AD pathogenic process is not known. However, it does raise the possibility of preventive measures to reduce homocysteine levels using dietary folate supplementation. Early trials have not shown any benefits on cognition in healthy elderly or in people with dementia, although long-term preventive trials have not yet been performed (Malouf *et al.* 2003; Sommer *et al.* 2003).

Inflammation and non-steroidal anti-inflammatory drugs

Following the important observation that AD appeared rare in conditions such as leprosy and arthritis, a series of studies examined the effects of non-steroidal anti-inflammatory drugs (NSAIDs) on the incidence of AD. Reviewing the literature, McGeer *et al.* (1996) noted the apparent protection offered by both steroids (OR 0.7) and NSAIDs (OR 0.5). Subsequent studies have all confirmed this finding but it seems to be that long-term use of these drugs is necessary to confer protection (Stewart *et al.* 1997; in't Veld *et al.* 2001; Zandi *et al.* 2002a). The clear finding from epidemiology that NSAIDs and other anti-inflammatory drugs are protective chimes with findings from neuropathology that there is extensive inflammatory change in the AD brain (reviewed in Akiyama *et al.* 2000). There is an excess of microglia, many associated with neuritic plaques, and extensive evidence of upregulation and secretion of inflammatory response proteins such as complement and its constituents, the cytokines and acute-phase proteins. A gene–environment interaction has been sought and a number of genetic factors relevant to inflammation have been associated with AD but none reliably replicated.

It is tempting to speculate that the inflammatory process in AD is initiated by plaque formation and, as in other inflammatory diseases, progresses to the point where it causes local damage thus creating a spiral of disease. However, more recent evidence suggests that some but not all NSAIDs alter the processing of APP, possibly by activating either, or both, BACE and γ-secretase (Weggen *et al.* 2001, 2003; Sastre *et al.* 2003). It is interesting that not all NSAIDs are equal in this respect, and noteworthy that ibuprofen, one of the drugs that alters APP metabolism, reduced pathology in the brains of mice overexpressing APP, with evidence of a reduction in the formation of the soluble amyloid peptides that form plaques (Lim *et al.* 2001). If the action of NSAIDs on APP were the mechanism of effect in offering protection against AD then only some compounds would be expected to be protective, whereas if the mechanism were directly on inflammation then all anti-inflammatories should be efficacious. A series of trials have reported no protection with a variety of NSAIDs and cyclooxygenase (COX)-2 inhibitors (NSAIDs are joint COX-1 and COX-2 inhibitors) without any success. However,

it is too early to conclude whether this is because non-APP-altering drugs have been used or whether the failure to demonstrate an effect is due to trial design – too late in the disease process, too short or too small.

Diabetes: insulin signalling defect or vascular insult?

A series of epidemiological studies have demonstrated that diabetes increases risk of dementia (reviewed in Stewart & Liolitsa 1999; Gasparini *et al.* 2002), with only one study showing no association (MacKnight *et al.* 2002). An obvious explanation for this association would be that diabetes causes vascular disease and that it is this that in turn causes the dementia. If this were the case, then diabetes should be associated with vascular dementia and not AD. Both case–control and cohort studies have attempted to determine whether this association is due to vascular dementia or AD or both, with mixed results: some suggest that both are increased in those with diabetes (Peila *et al.* 2002), some that diabetes increases the risk of vascular dementias (Katzman *et al.* 1989; Boston *et al.* 1999; Hébert *et al.* 2000) but not AD (Nielson *et al.* 1996; Curb *et al.* 1999; Hassing *et al.* 2002), one that diabetes increases risk of AD but not vascular dementia (Brayne *et al.* 1998), and three large longitudinal cohort studies show that diabetes is a risk factor for AD independently of whether or not it is a risk factor for vascular dementia (OR 1.3–1.9) (Ott *et al.* 1996, 1999; Luchsinger *et al.* 2001).

Other evidence points to a specific defect in insulin signalling (i.e. insulin resistance) in AD (Winograd *et al.* 1991; Meneilly & Hill 1993) and insulin resistance itself appears to be a risk factor for AD (Kuusisto *et al.* 1997). Thus it has been shown that there is increased plasma and CSF insulin both at baseline (Craft *et al.* 1998) and after oral glucose load in AD compared with controls (Fujisawa *et al.* 1991) and that impaired serum insulin response to hyperglycaemia correlates with cognitive impairment even after controlling for vascular factors (Stolk *et al.* 1997) and also with dementia progression (Craft *et al.* 1993). This is in line with post-mortem evidence that brain insulin receptors are increased in AD (Hoyer *et al.* 1998), suggesting upregulation in response to resistance, and tyrosine phosphorylation, an insulin signalling event, is reduced in AD (Frolich *et al.* 1999). Insulin has been shown to regulate both the metabolism of APP (Solano *et al.* 2000) and the phosphorylation of tau (Hong & Lee 1997), in both instances reducing the processing of these proteins that leads to pathological lesions in AD. Mice with disrupted insulin signalling, induced by either diet or targeted genetic lesions, have increased tau phosphorylation (Yanagisawa *et al.* 1999; Planel *et al.* 2001; Schubert *et al.* 2003).

Given that insulin resistance and diabetes increase the risk of AD, it follows that susceptibility loci associated with insulin resistance/diabetes might also be risk factors for AD. Three studies provide tentative evidence that this may the case. In Pima Indian women, polymorphic variation in a phosphatidylinositol 3-kinase subunit, P85α, is associated with insulin resistance and diabetes and the same SNP increased AD risk in women but not men, analogous to the pattern of risk in relation to diabetes, with an OR of 2 (Liolitsa *et al.* 2002). Others have shown variation in the insulin receptor gene to be associated with earlier onset of AD (Majores *et al.* 2002), and variation in PPARα (peroxisome proliferator-activated receptor), also involved with glucose metabolism, to be associated with dementia (Brune *et al.* 2003). The usual caveat, that none of these studies have yet had replications published, remains.

Education: 'use it or lose it' and the brain reserve hypothesis

Case–control studies have tended to suggest that remaining in education for longer offers some protection against dementia (Schmand *et al.* 1997). In some studies this was due to an effect of education on non-Alzheimer dementia (Fratiglioni *et al.* 1991; Cobb *et al.* 1995) and education may be a confounder in that it independently affects scores on dementia screening instruments (O'Carroll & Ebmeier 1995), possibly resulting in lower rates of detection in the highly educated. However, a series of large epidemiological studies do suggest a direct interaction between education and AD (Evans *et al.* 1997; Launer *et al.* 1999; Letenneur *et al.* 1999; Qiu *et al.* 2001). Most convincing has been the Nun study where a protective effect of education was suggested by the association of complex language use in young adults with decreased AD pathology many decades later (Butler *et al.* 1996; Mortimer *et al.* 2003).

Explaining the apparent association between education and protection against AD has proved difficult. That longitudinal studies confirm the case–control studies does tend to negate the parsimonious explanation that people with high levels of education are simply not detected as having dementia. There is an interaction between gender and education in that it is only in women that an effect is seen (Letenneur *et al.* 2000), but this does not provide an explanation of why there is an effect. Interestingly, in a study of African-Americans there was an interaction between education and place of residence, suggesting that living in an urban environment increases risk of AD and that low education might just be a marker of a protective, rural lifestyle (Hall *et al.* 2000). Others have found early-life factors to alter the risk of AD but that education does not modify this effect (Moceri *et al.* 2000). Alternatively, it may be that education is a marker of mid-life protective factors and there is reasonably consistent evidence that increased physical and mental activity offers some protection against AD (Friedland *et al.* 2001; Laurin *et al.* 2001; Lindsay *et al.* 2002; Wilson *et al.* 2002). Maybe the highly educated stay active longer. This might be considered the 'use it or lose it' hypothesis. An alternative possible explanation of the protection offered by education is the 'cognitive reserve' hypothesis, which broadly stated postulates that those with more education have more function and can therefore sustain

a greater neurodegenerative 'hit' than those with fewer reserves. Quite what cognitive reserve equates to in the brain is pure conjecture, presumably networks, neurones or synapses. In this context it is both intriguing and perhaps surprising that head circumference is also associated with risk of dementia, a larger head offering some measure of protection (Schofield *et al.* 1997; Borenstein *et al.* 2001), although small neuroimaging studies are less supportive of this finding (Jenkins *et al.* 2000; Edland *et al.* 2002). The combination of small head and low education is particularly risky as far as AD is concerned (Mortimer *et al.* 2003). Perhaps big heads mean big brains, which in turn means more brain to lose before dementia becomes apparent. Most interestingly in this context, animals that overexpress the tau-kinase GSK-3 have very small brains (Spittaels *et al.* 2002).

Gender and the role of estrogen

Women are over-represented in all cohorts of the elderly and especially so in those with dementia and AD in particular. However, this is not just due to the increased longevity of women as the incidence of AD is greater in women than in men and the risk of vascular dementia is not increased (Andersen, K. *et al.* 1999). Nevertheless, the increase in incidence was only apparent in the very elderly in at least one large prospective study (Ruitenberg *et al.* 2001b). Assuming that there is a true increase in incidence for women, what might this be due to? The most obvious mechanism is the loss of protection of estrogen and related hormones after the menopause and there is ample evidence that estrogen has some neuroprotective properties, particularly against amyloid-induced neurotoxicity (Green *et al.* 1996; Mook-Jung *et al.* 1997; Svensson & Nordberg 1999). Then it was found that hormone-replacement therapy (HRT) offers protection against AD and might even mitigate against some of the cognitive loss once the disease has started (Ohkura *et al.* 1995; Paganini-Hill & Henderson 1996). This led to huge optimism that HRT might be used as a disease-modifying therapy, although enthusiasm was tempered by some epidemiological studies failing to find an association (Seshadri *et al.* 2001) or finding association only with very long-term use (Zandi *et al.* 2002b). Trials of HRT, both naturalistic and randomised and controlled, have proved negative (Mulnard *et al.* 2000; Thal *et al.* 2003).

Other risk factors: ethnicity, depression and diet

Historically, although AD is common in many different ethnic groups, it was always said to be rare in black African peoples. Hendrie's group have made careful studies of prevalence and incidence of AD in African-Americans and Nigerians, showing a much lower incidence in those living in Africa. It must be said that genetic, cultural and environmental diversity is at least as large between African nations as between black and white people and so there are likely to be many differences between African-American and Nigerian people that go beyond the environmental differences (Hendrie *et al.* 2001). Nonetheless, this suggests that a low incidence of dementia in Africa may be due to some protective factor.

Prior depression has also been found to be a risk factor for AD (Jorm *et al.* 1991; Speck *et al.* 1995; Steffens *et al.* 1997; Jorm 2000). Jorm and colleagues identify six possible mechanisms for this association (Jorm 2000), none of which can be confidently excluded. Perhaps the explanation needing fewest radical speculations is the one that depression represents a very early prodromal symptom.

Aluminium was once thought to be associated with dementia but, with the exception of the very high aluminium load in early kidney dialysis (before the use of chelating agents), this association has largely been excluded, although not before a great deal of anxiety was caused to relatives and people worried about AD. Dietary intake of vitamin C or vitamin E has been raised as possible risk factors but the results from epidemiology are inconsistent (Engelhart *et al.* 2002; Luchsinger *et al.* 2003). It may well be that only trials will determine whether these antioxidants offer any protection. Fish oils are suggested to be protective (Kalmijn *et al.* 1997; Morris *et al.* 2003a), whereas polyunsaturated fats increase risk (Morris *et al.* 2003b). In animals a diet rich in cholesterol induces amyloid plaque formation, cholesterol levels alter the processing of the APP protein, and lowering cholesterol levels using statins may be a useful approach to AD therapy in humans for the future (Crisby *et al.* 2002; Petanceska *et al.* 2002; Morris *et al.* 2003a).

Mild cognitive impairment

Mild cognitive impairment (MCI) is a term that has achieved considerable prominence and attention. It has long been clear that there is a group of individuals who are somewhat impaired but who do not have a full dementia syndrome. The difficulty with nosology has been what impairment means: impaired in relation to all adults, young adults, age-matched controls? And for any of these, how much impairment does there need to be for an individual to be considered 'not normal for age'? Attempts have been made to group these people in various categories, including benign senescent forgetfulness, age-associated memory impairment, and others. However, it has been the formulation of MCI by Petersen *et al.* (2001a) that has become widely accepted. Criteria for MCI vary somewhat and are not as established as criteria for the various dementia conditions. However, common to all criteria are (i) that the patient should not meet criteria for dementia; (ii) that there should be some report of cognitive impairment by either the patient or an informant; (iii) that there should be objective evidence of cognitive impairment or decline; and (iv) that there should be no substantial evidence of functional impairment. Some criteria refine these elements, suggesting for example that objective

evidence for cognitive impairment should be a score more than 1.5 standard deviations away from age-adjusted norms. Other refinements include the distinction between amnestic (memory only) and other MCI and between single- and multi-dimensional MCI (Winblad *et al.* 2004). However, one of the difficulties common to all criteria relates to the upper-level criteria that the patient should not have dementia. Oftentimes this will be a question of clinical judgement and it is readily apparent that whether a patient receives a label of MCI or mild AD depends to a large degree on the inclinations of the clinician and specifically how diligently functional impairments are sought and what weight the clinician places on these. While there are excellent scales and measures for assessing function in more advanced dementia, doing the same in very early dementia is difficult and rests entirely on a careful, detailed and sometimes lengthy history. Often functional impairment is specific to an individual and is both culture and gender bound. While one person's functional impairment may be manifested in restricted use of the full capability of a washing machine, another's may be inability to rewire the machine. At least for currently elderly cohorts this example illustrates a probable gender bias and neither functional impairment is detectable without considerable effort. When combined with very mild cognitive impairment and other features, some clinicians would give a diagnosis of dementia; others would not.

This difficulty with diagnostic categories possibly explains some of the discrepancies in the literature on outcomes of MCI. In a systematic review we found rates of conversion to dementia ranged from 2% to 30% per year (Bruscoli & Lovestone 2004). However, diagnostic differences did not seem to account for all this substantial variability. When considering a variety of variables that might account for these different conversion rates, the one that stood out was the origin of the subjects of the study. Where subjects were recruited from a community-based study annual conversion rate was 7.5%, but where subjects were recruited from clinics the conversion rate was significantly different at 15%, despite apparently identical diagnostic criteria. It seems that there is something about people who manage to negotiate the care pathway to a memory clinic that is different from those people identified with the same symptoms in the community. It is likely that the care pathway acts as a selective filter, favouring people with early dementia because they, their carers or their primary physicians recognise the seriousness of the condition in a large proportion of individuals. The task, not yet completed, for researchers is to identify what this factor is.

Various attempts have been made to identify biological factors that might help to predict which people with MCI are more likely to convert to dementia. *APOE* status does predict a higher conversion rate in some but not all studies and promising data have been produced for CSF measures of AD-related proteins and a variety of imaging techniques

(Blennow 2004; Bruscoli & Lovestone 2004; De Leon *et al.* 2004; Maccioni *et al.* 2004; Chong *et al.* 2006). However, none of these findings are yet fully replicated and suitable for use in the clinic.

Nonetheless, despite problems with nosology and with the difficulty in distinguishing people with MCI who progress compared with those who do not, MCI is now a widely used concept in both clinical and research settings. Guidelines recommend that patients should be screened for MCI and monitored for conversion to dementia (Petersen *et al.* 2001b). In the research arena MCI has become the focus for some clinical trials, as preventing conversion from MCI to dementia might indicate that a drug had not only symptomatic effects but disease-modifying or preventive benefits.

Pseudodementia

While some patients in the memory clinic have clear and unarguable cognitive impairment but do not quite meet the criteria for dementia, others have questionable cognitive impairment and yet have sometimes received the diagnosis of dementia. A concept used only rarely today is that of pseudodementia, indicating a patient who appears demented but is not, perhaps because of depression or some other condition. Careful clinical examination is usually sufficient to make a distinction.

Vascular dementia and vascular cognitive impairment

Concepts of vascular dementia have undergone considerable revision in the last two to three decades. The recent history of this revision and the various consensus groups that have attempted to refine our understanding of vascular dementia is reviewed by Román *et al.* (2004). It is now widely understood that vascular pathology coexists with other forms of pathology in many, if not most, cases of dementia. The coexistence of vascular pathology and AD pathology in particular is common and, to complicate matters, both occur to a substantial degree in elderly people without known dementia (Fernando & Ince 2004). There is an inherent problem in disentangling these relationships. Alzheimer's pathology, vascular pathology and cognitive impairment are all common in the elderly and all are likely to coexist as a consequence, quite apart from any mechanistic relationship between pathological processes. Trying to understand which process is important in individual patients in life is extremely problematical. Even with the power of modern imaging, determining the vascular damage to the brain at a sub-stroke level is difficult in life and so researchers are left with post-mortem studies that attempt to extrapolate backwards to determine the relationship between pathology and early symptoms. These difficulties go some way to explaining the currently somewhat confused understanding of vascular dementia.

Nonetheless, it is clear that vascular disease does impact on cognition and four broad categories are emerging: multi-infarct dementia, small-vessel disease, post-stroke dementia and specific vascular dementia syndromes (e.g. CADASIL). These are discussed in turn but it should be understood that there is considerable overlap and that a categorical distinction between types of vascular dementia is inherently problematical. In an attempt to move on from the preconceptions and confusions associated with the term 'vascular dementia', O'Brien *et al.* (2003) have introduced the concept of *vascular cognitive impairment* (VCI), a term that encompasses all forms of cognitive impairment related to vascular disease in the brain. It remains to be seen whether this term will replace 'vascular dementia' in either clinical or research uses.

Multi-infarct dementia

Multi-infarct dementia is perhaps the most widely used category of vascular dementia and to a large degree the category on which diagnostic criteria are built. Clinically it is found with almost equal frequency in males and females, with perhaps a slight excess in males. It usually begins during the late sixties and seventies, although well-confirmed examples are occasionally seen in patients in their forties.

Arteriosclerosis may be obvious in the peripheral and retinal vessels and hypertension will frequently be present, be long-standing and may be severe. Attempts have been made to define the clinical characteristics of multi-infarct dementia but the evidence linking these symptoms with a specific pathological pattern is not overwhelming. The onset is frequently more acute than in AD, and a substantial number of cases only come to medical attention after a frank cerebrovascular accident has occurred. When the onset is gradual, emotional or personality changes may antedate definite evidence of memory and intellectual impairment. Other common early features include somatic symptoms such as headache, dizziness, tinnitus and syncope, which may be the main complaints for some considerable time. Once established the cognitive impairments characteristically fluctuate in severity and progression is said to be stepwise. Apoplectiform features punctuate the progress of the disorder and are due to episodes of cerebral infarction. Commonly they consist of abrupt episodes of hemiparesis, sensory change, dysphasia or visual disturbances. At first they are transient and followed by gradual restitution of function, but later each leaves more permanent neurological deficits in its wake. Each episode may be followed by an abrupt increase in the severity of the dementia. Lacunar infarcts may lead to a variety of neurological defects, including ataxia, dysarthria and motor and sensory disturbances, culminating in the picture of pseudobulbar palsy (dysarthria, dysphagia and emotional incontinence) together with bradykinesia and *marche à petit pas*.

Other features that suggest multi-infarct dementia include the patchy nature of the psychological deficits that result. Thus the basic personality may be well preserved until late in the disease, whereas in other dementing illnesses this is undermined from an early stage. Capacity for judgement may persist for a surprisingly long time, and a remarkable degree of insight is sometimes retained. As a result the patient often reacts to awareness of his decline by severe anxiety and depression. Other emotional changes include lability, no doubt due to lesions in the basal parts of the brain, and a tendency towards explosive emotional outbursts. Episodes of noisy weeping or laughing may occur on minor provocation, often without accompanying subjective distress or elation.

Perhaps the most reliable distinguishing characteristic of multi-infarct dementia is the course it pursues. This is rarely smoothly progressive as in AD, but typically punctuated by abrupt step-like progressions. Acute exacerbations are sometimes followed by improvement for a time, and in the early stages at least, periods of remission may last for months at a time. These features depend on the pathogenesis of the disorder in terms of repeated cerebral infarctions.

Birkett (1972) found that neurological abnormalities predicted arteriosclerosis more accurately than any mental feature. Even in the absence of gross defects, such as dysphasia or hemiparesis, there will often be minor focal signs. The tendon reflexes are often unequal, the plantars extensor or pupil reactions impaired. Parkinsonian features may be conspicuous, likewise evidence of pseudobulbar palsy as described above. Epileptic seizures are found in about 20% of cases, and attacks of syncope are common.

The EEG shows a picture similar to that of AD but the changes tend to be more severe. However, advanced examples can sometimes show normal records. A distinctive feature may be the appearance of focal abnormalities in the region of local cerebral thromboses: a low-amplitude delta focus may emerge if the infarction is sufficiently extensive, and some asymmetry may persist for several weeks thereafter. Frontal delta activity may appear when there are episodes of delirium. Harrison *et al.* (1979) found that the EEG more often showed focal or lateralising abnormalities in patients diagnosed as having multi-infarct dementia than in equivalently impaired patients with AD. The occurrence of paroxysmal activity or of a normal EEG is also commoner in the former than the latter (Erkinjuntti & Sulkava 1991).

Neuroimaging will usually show evidence of cerebral atrophy, sometimes marked in degree. Both old and recent infarctions may be revealed. Multiple small lacunar infarcts will often escape direct detection on CT and the suspicion of vascular dementia should direct the clinician to MRI rather than CT.

The clinical picture of multi-infarct dementia has to a large degree driven the categorical distinctions drawn up to differentiate 'vascular dementia' from AD and other dementias. The 'ischaemic index' proposed by Hachinski *et al.* (1975) has been one of the most widely employed as a guide to distinguishing multi-infarct dementia from AD. Features in the clinical history and on examination are given a weighted score as follows: abrupt onset (2), stepwise deterioration (1), fluctuating course (2), nocturnal confusion (1), relative preservation of personality (1), depression (1), somatic complaints (1), emotional incontinence (1), history of hypertension (1), history of strokes (2), evidence of associated atherosclerosis (1), focal neurological symptoms (2) and focal neurological signs (2). Patients scoring 7 or above are classified as having multi-infarct dementia and those scoring 4 or below as having non-vascular dementia, typically AD. The separation of patients on such a basis can be valuable in refining groups for research purposes, and when used with caution can give some guidance to diagnosis in the individual case. However, the index was drawn up on relatively young and mildly affected patients; a very considerable degree of overlap may be expected in the elderly especially when the dementia is more advanced.

The Hachinski index is still often used, although it has largely been superseded in the research context by the semi-operationalised diagnostic criteria drafted by the neuroepidemiology branch of the National Institute of Neurological Disorders and Stroke in association with the Association Internationale pour la Recherche et l'Enseignement en Neurosciences (NINDS-AIREN) (Román *et al.* 1993). These are summarised in Box 9.2. The NINDS-AIREN criteria sidestep any attempt to define 'mixed' cases of AD and vascular dementia and patients or subjects in research can fulfill both these criteria and the NINCDS-ADRDA criteria for AD simultaneously. These criteria have relatively high specificity but very low sensitivity (Holmes *et al.* 1999).

Small-vessel disease

Evidence of pathology to the vasculature of the brain, falling short of infarct, is common in the elderly and thought to be a major cause of cognitive impairment and indeed dementia. This small-vessel disease is found accompanying AD pathology in one-third or more of those with dementia in the community (Holmes *et al.* 1999) and is probably the major cause of VCI. In small-vessel disease there is evidence of damage to the microvasculature in the brain, demyelination, axonal loss and gliosis (Pantoni & Simoni 2003; Ringelstein & Nabavi 2005).

There are two cardinal features of small-vessel disease: (i) white matter lesions (WMLs), which may be apparent as periventricular lucency (also known as leucoaraiosis) or as deep white matter hyperintensities; and (ii) central grey matter lacunae (Schmidtke & Hull 2005). When first detected on CT, leucoaraiosis was thought to be rare, occurring in some 2% of routine scans on patients with cerebral

---

Box 9.2 NINDS-AIREN clinical criteria

I Criteria for probable vascular dementia

1 Dementia diagnosed according to defined operational criteria and documented by neuropsychological testing. Among the exclusion criteria are aphasia or major sensorimotor impairments which preclude such testing. Dementia in this context implies cognitive decline from a previously higher level of functioning, whether it has a stable, ameliorating or progressive course. The decline must be manifest in impairment of memory and in two or more other cognitive domains. The resulting deficits must be severe enough to interfere with ADL which are *not* due to the physical effects of stroke alone

2 The presence of cerebrovascular disease as detected by focal deficits on neurological examination consistent with stroke (whether or not there is a history of stroke), together with evidence of relevant cerebrovascular disease on brain imaging (CT or MRI). The latter includes multiple large-vessel infarcts, a single strategically placed infarct, multiple basal ganglia or white matter lacunes, or extensive periventricular WMLs. Severity standards are set for excluding trivial infarcts, occasional lacunes or minor periventricular lucencies

3 A relationship between **1** and **2** must be manifest, either by onset of dementia within 3 months of a recognised stroke, or by abrupt deterioration or stepwise progression in cognitive function in the absence of a history of stroke

II Clinical features consistent with probable vascular dementia

1 Early presence of gait disturbance (*marche à petit pas*, magnetic, apraxic–ataxic or parkinsonian gait)

2 A history of unsteadiness and frequent unprovoked falls

3 Early frequency or urinary incontinence

4 Pseudobulbar palsy

5 Personality and mood changes

6 Psychomotor retardation, perseveration and difficulty in shifting and maintaining sets

III Features that make a diagnosis of vascular dementia uncertain

1 Early onset of memory deficit and progressive worsening of memory and other cognitive functions in the absence of corresponding focal lesions on brain imaging

2 Absence of focal neurological signs other than cognitive disturbance

3 Absence of cerebrovascular lesions on CT or MRI

IV Clinical criteria for possible vascular dementia

1 Dementia with focal neurological signs, but absence of confirmation of cerebrovascular disease on brain imaging

2 Absence of clear temporal relationship between dementia and stroke

3 Subtle onset and variable course (plateau or improvement) of cognitive deficits and evidence of relevant cerebrovascular disease

V Criteria for definite vascular dementia

1 Clinical criteria for probable vascular dementia

2 Histopathological evidence of cerebrovascular disease obtained from biopsy or post-mortem

3 Absence of neurofibrillary tangles and neuritic plaques exceeding those expected for age

4 Absence of other disorder capable of producing dementia

---

atrophy (Valentine *et al.* 1980). Most of those affected were hypertensive and two-thirds showed evidence of dementia. Zeumer *et al.* (1980) found similar changes in 15 patients, all with progressive dementia and histories of transient, usually recurrent, neurological deficits. All but one were hypertensive and two showed pseudobulbar palsy. Microinfarcts were visible in the basal ganglia in one-third of cases. One of the patients came to post-mortem and showed the histological features of Binswanger's disease. It therefore seemed likely at the time that this might be a neuroradiological marker of the condition. However, with time, growing awareness and the increased use of MRI it became apparent that WMLs are a frequent observation in patients with dementia and in elderly people with memory complaints (Minett *et al.* 2005). They probably represent areas of demyelination resulting from ischaemia. However, their relationship to dementia is disputed. In one community study only 8% of the population were free of WMLs (de Leeuw *et al.*

2001) and the presence of WMLs was predicted largely by mid-life hypertension (de Leeuw *et al.* 2000; van Dijk *et al.* 2004). Not all WMLs are equal and periventricular lucencies in particular appear to be more significantly associated with disease or pathology: periventricular, but not deep white matter, changes are more common in patients diagnosed with AD (Burns *et al.* 2005), and periventricular lesions are more predictive of dementia (Prins *et al.* 2004) and cerebral atrophy than deep white matter hyperintensities (Barber *et al.* 2000). It might be that deep white matter hyperintensities are the result of lifelong vascular damage to the brain – end-organ damage – but it is periventricular lucency that is a marker of VCI. Some evidence in favour of this comes from a study showing that diabetes with and without accompanying hypertension is strongly associated with deep white matter hyperintensities but not periventricular lesions (van Harten *et al.* 2007). Deep white matter lesions may have consequences on the brain beyond dementia and are associated with depression and motor deficits (O'Brien *et al.* 2003).

The distinction between small-vessel disease and other forms of VCI is as difficult as the distinction between VCI and AD. However, small-vessel disease is most likely to present as a subcortical disorder with a slowly evolving dementia associated with focal neurological deficits, often in hypertensive patients and frequently accompanied by motor signs or other focal neurological deficits. Semi-operational criteria for neuroimaging features (WMLs and lacunae) have been proposed but agreement between raters has been poor and there are no widely accepted imaging criteria in routine clinical use. Schmidtke and Hull (2005) have reviewed neuropsychological deficits in small-vessel disease compared with AD; word fluency and clock-reading appear to have some value in discriminating the disorders.

Binswanger's disease is a subtype of small-vessel disease, previously thought to be rare and first described by Binswanger (1894) under the title 'encephalitis subcorticalis chronica progressiva'. The condition derives from pathological changes affecting the long perforating vessels to the deep white matter and subcortical nuclear masses, resulting in multiple small areas of infarction (lacunes) together with the cardinal feature of diffuse demyelination of the white matter. The arcuate fibres beneath the sulci are by contrast spared, and the cortex itself is substantially intact. The white matter changes are usually extensive, demyelination being associated with pronounced fibrillary gliosis. Possible pathogenic mechanisms include diffuse ischaemia consequent on subacute hypertensive encephalopathy (Caplan & Schoene 1978), or chronic hypoperfusion in the watershed area between the territories of the cortical medullary arteries and the long perforating branches to the white matter (Loizou *et al.* 1981).

Clinical features stressed from the outset were of a slowly evolving dementia associated with focal neurological deficits, usually in hypertensive patients in their fifties or sixties. Caplan and Schoene (1978) clarified the picture from a description of cases proven at post-mortem. They noted persistent hypertension, a history of acute strokes, a lengthy course, and dementia accompanied by prominent motor signs and usually by pseudobulbar palsy. However, the distinctive clinical manifestation was the subacute progression of focal neurological deficits. Such deficits commonly developed in a gradual fashion over some weeks or months, the picture then stabilising with long plateau periods lasting for months or occasionally years. This feature appeared to separate the patients with Binswanger's disease from those whose dementia rested on large-vessel occlusions or on a lacunar state without accompanying white matter demyelination. The dementia varied considerably in its manifestations: some patients showed a phase of ebullience and lack of inhibition, others progressive loss of spontaneity. Memory disorder was not invariably prominent.

Poststroke dementia

The risk of dementia increases substantially after stroke, especially in the elderly. Prevalence studies show up to one-third of those aged above 55 years to have dementia in the 5-year period after stroke compared with a little over 5% of the general population; in a population-based study, the incidence of dementia after stroke was nearly nine times greater than predicted (Mackowiak-Cordoliani *et al.* 2005). The mechanism of poststroke dementia is not understood but is likely to be complex, some patients having strategic infarcts, others multiple infarcts and others with continuing small-vessel disease. Although there is some evidence that hemispheric lesions increase risk of poststroke dementia, overall the relationship between site of lesion and risk of dementia is not at all clear. In addition to a direct effect of the stroke on brain function, in some patients incipient AD will become apparent after stroke either because cognitive or brain reserve is diminished or because the effects of the stroke make cognitive or functional deficits apparent to the patients themselves or, more likely, to carers.

Specific vascular syndromes

A small number of specific syndromes give rise to a vascular dementia. These include CADASIL, a rare familial disorder that presents with migraine, usually but not always accompanied by aura, recurrent small subcortical infarcts leading to dementia, transient ischaemic attacks and sometimes severe affective disturbance. Neuroimaging reveals white matter abnormalities in subcortical white matter and basal ganglia (Chabriat *et al.* 1995). Onset is typically in the forties, the pedigree will reveal autosomal dominant inheritance and the patient will be free from the typical vascular risk factors (Davous 1998). The disorder is caused by mutations in the *NOTCH3* gene (Joutel *et al.* 1997), which codes for a transmembrane protein involved in complex intracellular signalling and, interestingly, both neuronal development and memory (Louvi *et al.* 2006). Whether either of these functions of Notch proteins are relevant to CADASIL remains to be seen. Identifying families with CADASIL allows presymptomatic counselling and testing.

Other genetic disorders also give rise to vascular lesions in the brain. One of the most intriguing of these is hereditary cerebral haemorrhage with amyloidosis (Dutch type), which presents with haemorrhagic strokes and dementia (Maat-Schieman *et al.* 2005). This autosomal dominant disorder results from mutations in the *APP* gene just as in some early-onset FAD. However, the mutation results in decreased Aβ-42 in contrast to the increase seen in AD and with the AD mutations in the same gene (Bornebroek *et al.* 2003). The primary pathology is cerebral amyloid angiopathy and this is just one of the inherited angiopathies; others include hereditary cerebral haemorrhage with amyloidosis (Icelandic type) and chromosome 13 familial dementia in British and Danish kindreds (Frangione *et al.* 2001).

Relationship between AD and vascular dementia

Alzheimer's disease pathology and vascular pathology frequently coincide in people with dementia. What is the nature of this relationship? Is it simply common things occurring commonly together or is there a more complex interrelationship between pathologies in the brain that result in dementia? It is unlikely that there is a simple answer to this question that intrigues many researchers in the field. It is possible that there are common risk factors, that AD exacerbates vascular disease, that vascular pathology exacerbates AD or that the two pathological processes are additive in their effects on cognition and function.

There is some evidence for common risk factors. For example, hypertension and diabetes are both de facto risk factors for vascular dementia but both are also apparently independent risk factors for AD (Biessels *et al.* 2006; Skoog & Gustafson 2006). The difficulty in disentangling risk factors for AD and vascular dementia in life will be immediately obvious, and there is a certain tautology involved as the presence of vascular risk factors makes a diagnosis in life of vascular dementia more likely and so an association of vascular risk factors with vascular disease is not unexpected. Other common risk factors have been sought including genetic factors. *APOE* variation is strongly associated with both AD and cardiac disease, although there is only conflicting evidence of an association with vascular dementia (Frank *et al.* 2002; Bang *et al.* 2003; Baum *et al.* 2006; Davidson *et al.* 2006) and probably no association with stroke (Sudlow *et al.* 2006). Variation in the gene encoding ACE is probably weakly associated with hypertension and AD, although again there is no reported association with vascular dementia as would be expected if it were a common risk factor (Zuliani *et al.* 2001; Kolsch *et al.* 2005).

The possibility that AD pathological processes might exacerbate vascular disease has not been explored thoroughly but is plausible. As well as amyloid deposition in plaques, congophilic angiopathy representing amyloid deposition in blood vessel walls is a near-universal finding in AD and is the predominant pathology in some families with *APP* mutations (Castellani *et al.* 2004a). In these families haemorrhage is the predominant pathological finding but it is plausible that the thickening of the endothelial wall that accompanies the angiopathy of AD might contribute to ischaemic events and small-vessel disease resulting in a vascular dementia-type pathology. Alternatively, vascular disease may itself initiate or propagate Alzheimer's pathology (Kalback *et al.* 2004; Humpel & Marksteiner 2005) through diverse possible mechanisms all centring on the increased vulnerability of neurones in ischaemic conditions.

Box 9.3 Subtypes of vascular dementia

I Large or several infarcts (>50 mL loss of tissue): multi-infarct dementia

II Multiple small infarcts (>3 mm, with minimum diameter 5 mm): small-vessel disease, involving greater than three coronal levels, with hyalinisation, cerebral amyloid angiopathy, lacunar infarcts, perivascular changes

III Strategic infarcts, e.g. thalamus, hippocampus

IV Cerebral hypoperfusion, e.g. hippocampal sclerosis, ischaemic anoxic damage

V Cerebral haemorrhages

VI Cerebrovascular changes with AD pathology

However, the most parsimonious explanation is that vascular damage to the brain and Alzheimer's pathology are independent processes that have synergistic effects on cognition. Post-mortem studies tend to support this idea, with evidence that the cognitive impairment for a given AD load is greater than expected if vascular disease is also present (Nagy *et al.* 1997; Snowdon *et al.* 1997). Such effects might arise from the addition of pathologies in the same brain areas or may be synergistic if they result in dysfunction of different, but interacting, systems.

Neuropathology in vascular dementia

Kalaria *et al.* (2004) have reviewed the various pathological lesions found in vascular dementia and have proposed a set of key variables to be collected at post-mortem and a pathological classification system for subtyping vascular dementia (Box 9.3). These authors note that the commonest lesions are complete infarctions, found in 75% of cases, followed by lacunar infarcts and small infarcts in 50% of cases, cystic infarcts in 25% of cases, cerebral amyloid angiopathy in 10% and haemorrhages in only 2% of cases. Large infarcts, visible to the naked eye, often occur in the watersheds supplied by the major arteries and consist of a core of complete infarction surrounded by a penumbra of ischaemic tissue. A gliosis accompanies infarction and results in scar formation. Lacunae usually result from cavitating infarcts, occurring most frequently in the white matter but may result from haemorrhage. Small-vessel disease takes various forms but all involve damage to the end-arterial wall with hyalinisation, degeneration of the vascular smooth muscle and other changes indicative of arteriosclerosis. Cerebral amyloid angiopathy is the consequence of deposition of aggregated amyloid protein in or near the vessel wall, resulting in thickening and, almost certainly, loss of function.

Epidemiology of vascular dementia

Vascular dementia is common but given the comments above about the difficulties of diagnosis in life and the pitfalls of mixed disease, estimating how common is difficult. Clinically, 15–20% of patients in many series are diagnosed as having vascular dementia, although this is higher (up to 40–50%) in some studies (Kuller *et al.* 2005; Román 2002). However, patients often meet criteria for both AD and vascular dementia, suggesting that pathological studies are necessary. In post-mortem studies of series with dementia also, co-occurrence of pathologies is common and so in order to estimate true prevalence figures population-based pathological studies are needed. A recent meta-analysis found six such studies but these only reinforce the problems in correlating specific pathological findings with clinical syndromes (Zaccai *et al.* 2006). Thus one study found that one-third of subjects had neuropathologically defined AD although the prevalence of clinically diagnosed AD was only 16%. Half of those with AD pathology at post-mortem were not diagnosed with any dementia in life or had vascular dementia and, conversely, one-third of those with clinical AD had insufficient evidence at post-mortem for a definitive diagnosis of AD. All the studies find a high degree of co-occurrence of AD and vascular dementia as do pathological cohorts of people with dementia. At present, the best that can be said is that vascular dementia in all its forms is common, is probably the second most prevalent pathology affecting the elderly with dementia and occurs very frequently together with AD pathology.

The risk factors for vascular dementia are, not surprisingly, evidence of vascular disease, especially in the brain. Past history of stroke, evidence of white matter damage on neuroimaging, hypertension, elevated cholesterol and adverse lipid profile, diabetes and some genetic variants are all risk factors in most studies (Schmidt *et al.* 2002; Kuller *et al.* 2005; Rea *et al.* 2005; Hayden *et al.* 2006; Panza *et al.* 2006). However, it should be noted that in some studies high cholesterol (Mielke *et al.* 2005) and hypertension (Ruitenberg *et al.* 2001c) in late life appears to be protective.

The natural history of dementia is classically described as stepwise or intermittent, especially in multi-infarct dementia. However, the clinicopathological correlation is not strong and slowly progressive dementia also occurs in people with pathological evidence of vascular dementia. A review of the literature suggested that progression of vascular dementia was not distinguishable from that of AD (Chui & Gonthier 1999).

Summary

Vascular dementia is a concept in transition. The concept of vascular dementia as a separate disorder with different clinical profile, different set of risk factors and different pathology is no longer sustainable. An attempt has been made to replace the term 'vascular dementia' with 'vascular cognitive impairment', although this seems to sidestep the fundamental problem rather than addressing it. What is clear is that vascular damage to the brain contributes significantly to impairment and to dementia specifically. Vascular damage frequently coincides with AD pathology and trying to disentangle the relative contribution of the two pathologies to functional and cognitive impairment in groups of subjects or in individual patients is exceedingly difficult and may ultimately prove impossible.

However, some concepts have remained valid and useful despite these challenges. It is clear that the separation of vascular damage into small-vessel and multi-infarct types together with cerebral amyloid angiopathy represents a true distinction, although it remains to be seen whether there are many clinicopathological correlations. The concept of vascular risk factors has received a great deal of support and it is clear that vascular risk factors are also, by and large, dementia risk factors although in most cases they are risk factors for both AD and vascular dementia. As the contribution of vascular damage to dementia and as the importance of vascular risk factors becomes increasingly recognised, vascular dementia becomes an ever more important target for therapy.

Dementia with Lewy bodies

Lewy bodies, which are the hallmark of the brainstem pathology of Parkinson's disease, were found relatively recently to occur diffusely in the cerebral cortex and to be accompanied by a dementia syndrome with characteristic clinical features. The nosological status of DLB (previously variously called diffuse Lewy body disease, cortical Lewy body dementia or senile dementia of the Lewy body type) remains a subject of some controversy and its relationship to its allied disorders, AD and Parkinson's disease, is not yet fully understood. DLB is the second or third most common dementia after AD. The frequency in different series varies somewhat from 10% to 20% and whether it is more common than vascular disease depends partly on probable selection biases in post-mortem series and partly on the definitions used for vascular dementia. In any case it is an important cause of dementia.

Clinical features

Males have outnumbered females in some but not all series, with onset typically in the sixties or seventies. Disease duration is on average approximately 10 years but with a wide range (Ransmayr 2000). The classical triad of symptoms of DLB comprises fluctuating cognitive impairment, parkinsonism and visual hallucinations (Byrne *et al.* 1990; Kalra *et al.* 1996; Brown 1999). The fluctuation may be day to day or even hour to hour and may be difficult to distinguish from delirium. Not infrequently patients have had episodes of admission to medical units for acute confusional states from which they apparently spontaneously recovered before the diagnosis was made. Attention and EEG variability correlate with systematic assessment of fluctuation and although informants sometimes report all dementia patients as showing some variability, the clinical fluctuation is greater in DLB than in other dementia syndromes (Walker *et al.* 2000). The exception is the dementia that occurs in Parkinson's disease which, like DLB, also shows considerable fluctuation in attention (Ballard *et al.* 2002a). A review of studies comparing DLB with AD showed that visuoperceptual and attentional–executive impairments were more severe in DLB (Collerton *et al.* 2003).

Visual hallucinations in DLB are complex, often of people or animals, usually undersized and silent, and may not be distressing to the patient. Similar symptoms occur, albeit with less frequency, in Parkinson's disease dementia (Aarsland *et al.* 2001). Psychosis is a common feature of AD also but visual hallucinations are less common in AD than in DLB. Functional neuroimaging suggests that visual hallucinations are particularly associated with hypometabolism in the primary visual cortex together with relatively preserved metabolism in the right temporoparietal association cortex (Imamura *et al.* 1999). The Newcastle group has made a strong case for the fluctuation and psychotic symptoms of DLB to have their origin in a relatively more profound cholinergic deficit relative to AD (Perry *et al.* 1993, 1994; Perry & Perry 1995).

Importantly, hallucinations and delusions occurring early in a dementia syndrome strongly suggest a diagnosis of DLB (Ballard *et al.* 1999a). In fact all the symptoms of DLB are more discriminative relative to AD when found to occur early in the course of the dementia (Del Ser *et al.* 2001). With time, many AD patients become psychotic, have motor symptoms and fluctuation, making clinical distinction from DLB increasingly difficult. In addition, the presence of extrapyramidal symptoms at presentation is highly predictive of Lewy body pathology (Haan *et al.* 2002). Although the presence of symptoms of DLB at presentation is highly predictive of Lewy body pathology, the reverse is not true. In patients with a clinical diagnosis of AD in life but with Lewy bodies found at post-mortem, retrospective assessment of their symptom complex did not show any particular clinical pattern, whether the type of symptoms experienced or indeed the rate of progression (Stern *et al.* 2001).

Parkinsonism occurring after or anteceding dementia by no more than a year is part of the diagnostic criteria for DLB. Rigidity and gait abnormalities are more prominent than tremor, although this can occur. Falls are common (Ballard *et al.* 1999b) The motor manifestations show the typical features of Parkinson's disease, with bradykinesia, rigidity, tremor, mask-like facies and stooped posture. Involuntary movements are sometimes reported, also myoclonus, quadriparesis, dysarthria and dysphagia (Burkhardt *et al.* 1988). Orthostatic hypotension may occur and unexplained losses of consciousness are often seen.

Diagnostic guidelines for DLB, based on the core triad of symptoms (of which two are necessary) and a set of common supportive features, were reached by consensus and then updated (McKeith *et al.* 1996, 1999, 2005). Supportive features include falls, syncope, neuroleptic sensitivity, delusions, non-visual hallucinations, depression and rapid eye movement (REM) sleep disturbance. Notice is especially drawn to the neuroleptic sensitivity. Patients with DLB are highly sensitive to severe extrapyramidal and other adverse effects of these drugs and considerable caution should be exercised in treating psychosis in DLB. Early indications suggested that the accuracy of the consensus diagnostic criteria in relation to post-mortem confirmation was at best modest (Lopez *et al.* 1999), with acceptable levels of specificity but poor sensitivity (McKeith *et al.* 2003).

McKeith *et al.* (1992) described the spectrum of clinical features in detail, making a retrospective case note comparison between 21 cases of DLB and 37 cases of AD proven histologically. The DLB patients tended to show milder cognitive impairment at presentation, and more often showed marked fluctuations at any stage. Episodes of clouding of consciousness occurred in 80% of patients. Visual hallucinations were commoner than in AD, and were often complex, vivid and rapidly moving. One patient saw an express train going through his room, another gypsies climbing through the window. Auditory hallucinations and persecutory delusions were also frequent. The fluctuating nature of such symptoms and their tendency to worsen at night suggested an acute confusional state superimposed on the dementia. Fluctuation was also observed in memory, language and visuospatial abilities; lucid periods with near-normal memory capacity were sometimes recorded until late in the disease. Almost half of the patients with DLB had falls or transient and unexplained losses of consciousness, which were rare in those with AD. Depression was significantly more common in DLB and was sometimes the reason for the initial referral.

Extrapyramidal features in this series were no commoner at presentation than in the AD group, but developed more frequently and more severely later on. An important observation was that they almost always appeared to be directly related to the prescription of antipsyhcotic medication. Moreover, the patients with DLB appeared to be unusually susceptible to severe reactions to antipsychotics such as chlorpromazine or haloperidol, developing first sedation and then acute onset of rigidity accompanied by postural instability and falls. Rapid deterioration led to death in many cases. There were no such acute reactions in those patients with AD.

Course and outcome

On present evidence it would seem that the clinical course, though widely variable, is shorter than with AD (Olichney *et al*. 1998). In McKeith *et al*.'s (1992) series, the time from onset of symptoms to death was a mean of 1.8 years in the group with DLB and 4.8 years in the group with AD, although others typically find a longer survival time after diagnosis. Those who suffered adverse reactions to antipsychotic treatment fared particularly badly, surviving a mean of less than 1 year. In patients with AD the presence of Lewy bodies and extrapyramidal symptoms predicts a faster decline (Haan *et al*. 2002).

Pathology

At post-mortem the brain usually shows mild cortical atrophy and ventricular enlargement. Pallor is detected in the substantia nigra and locus coeruleus. The distinctive pathological finding is the occurrence of numerous Lewy bodies in the cortex. They are also found in the substantia nigra, other brainstem nuclei and basal forebrain regions, although often less in number than in Parkinson's disease. In Parkinson's disease, occasional Lewy bodies can sometimes be detected in the cortex, but not in anything approaching the numbers seen in DLB.

Lewy bodies consist of rounded eosinophilic inclusions within neurones. They are easily detected in the brainstem, where they stain deeply with haematoxylin and eosin, and where the pale halo around the filamentous core is highlighted by the surrounding neuromelanin. In the cortex, however, they are less eosinophilic and less clearly circumscribed, making their detection less straightforward. The use of anti-ubiquitin antibodies has been an important advance, permitting reliable estimates of Lewy body frequency and proving to be twice as sensitive as conventional stains in revealing them in cortical areas (Lennox *et al*. 1989).

In rare cases Lewy bodies have been found without any accompanying Alzheimer-type pathology (Gurd *et al*. 2000) but this is uncommon (so-called pure Lewy body dementia). The severity of Alzheimer pathology is usually described as well below what would be expected in AD and insufficient to make such a diagnosis on its own. Moreover, the relative distribution of Lewy bodies and Alzheimer pathology do not mirror one another closely. Lewy bodies also occur in AD (Arai *et al*. 2001), even in autosomal dominant AD with known mutations (Rosenberg *et al*. 2000; Lippa *et al*. 2001; Yokota *et al*. 2002). Cortical Lewy bodies in Parkinson's disease are associated with cognitive impairment (Mattila *et al*. 2000).

Varying degrees of cell loss are reported in the cortex, although less severely than in AD. Cell loss is also seen in the substantia nigra and other subcortical nuclei, but less than in Parkinson's disease. Severe reductions in choline acetyl transferase activity have been found in the temporal neocortex, exceeding even that found in AD (Perry *et al*. 1990, 1993, 1994). Caudate dopamine levels are also depleted, paralleling the neuronal loss in the substantia nigra.

The Lewy body core is composed of aggregates of a protein α-synuclein (Spillantini *et al*. 1997; Hashimoto *et al*. 2004), making DLB one of the synucleinopathies, also including multiple system atrophy, pure autonomic failure and Parkinson's disease itself (Marti *et al*. 2003). α-Synuclein is normally found in the presynaptic compartment and may be important in learning and memory. Mutations in the coding gene have been found to be a very rare cause of familial Parkinson's disease.

Frontotemporal dementia

The term 'frontal' or 'frontotemporal' dementia is used to signify those dementias which depend principally on degeneration within the anterior parts of the brain, as detected by mode of presentation, neuroimaging procedures or post-mortem examination. Some confusion has arisen between Pick's disease, which is properly a neuropathological diagnosis, and FTD, which is a clinical diagnosis. As discussed below, the nosological status of FTD is being clarified by a growing understanding of molecular pathogenesis and the FTDs are best considered as a set of clinical syndromes that show some common features but which have a variety of neuropathological substrates. Pick's disease is one pathological variant of FTD but does not have a typical clinical presentation allowing the pathology to be predicted in life. FTDs are of special importance to psychiatry because of their tendency to present with behavioural disorder and change of personality. In the age range 45–65 years, FTD is an important disorder with an estimated prevalence of 3–15 per 100 000, not very different from that of AD (Bird *et al*. 2003). In some series males predominate and a significant proportion, probably in the range 20–40%, is familial.

Clinical features

The features of FTD are relatively distinct from the other major dementia syndromes and are characterised by change in personality and behaviour accompanied by emotional blunting and apathy and in many cases speech and language deficits (Snowden *et al*. 2002). These symptoms occur in the context of relatively preserved memory, especially visual memory. Features of Klüver–Bucy syndrome are frequently present.

Hodges (2001) describes three distinctive forms of FTD: frontal variant FTD, semantic dementia and progressive nonfluent aphasia. In the Cambridge series, the first two syndromes accounted for 40% each and the progressive aphasias approximately 20%. Others find frontal variant FTD to be the majority of cases of FTD (Snowden *et al.* 2002). A few cases present as mixed or a very rare clinical variant. Frontal variant FTD presents with classical features of loss of frontal lobe function, specifically orbitobasal structures, namely disinhibition, stereotypy, lack of impulse control and antisocial behaviour. Apathy and loss of executive function resulting in inability to plan are universal but also common in AD and are less useful in differential diagnosis. Compulsive repetitive behaviours or speech patterns are common and Snowden *et al.* (2002) suggest that these behaviours occur more in those with striatal-predominant as opposed to neocortical-predominant pathology; this is in contrast to those with apathy as a dominant syndrome, where the pathology is predominantly frontal. On neuropsychological testing memory is relatively spared but tests of frontal lobe function usually reveal considerable impairment. Hodges (2001) makes the point that many of these tests are particularly sensitive to dorsolateral and not orbitobasal function; nonetheless commonly used neuropsychological tests such as the Wisconsin Card Sorting Test and the Stroop and bedside tests of verbal fluency are useful. Amnesia develops with time but even in relatively advanced dementia, spatial memory can be preserved.

Semantic dementia is, in effect, the temporal variant of FTD and presents with complaints of loss of memory for words but is usually accompanied by a receptive dysfunction that the patient may be completely unaware of. Especially in predominant right-sided atrophy, the semantic loss is frequently accompanied by prosopagnosia. i.e. loss of recognition and naming of faces. Orientation is preserved and, interestingly, where there is memory impairment it is predominantly remote rather than recent memories that are most affected. As might be expected, all tests of verbal cognition are affected but categorical naming tests (naming of defined lists, e.g. animals, in a given time period) are especially so. At least in the mild to moderate stages, patients will perform normally on tests of executive function and non-verbal problem-solving tasks such as Raven's Progressive Matrices.

Non-fluent progressive aphasia presents with speech dysfluency and word-finding difficulties often accompanied by deterioration in spelling (Mesulam 2001). Comprehension is relatively preserved but patients eventually develop global cognitive decline accompanied by profound language difficulty and early autism. This progression may be very protracted. Patients can have only primary verbal defects for 10–15 years (Mesulam 2001). In contrast to semantic dementia and frontal variant FTD, the pathological findings in non-fluent progressive aphasia are very variable and in some instances this is a variant presentation of AD while in others the various FTD pathologies are present. The left temporal lobe is typically preferentially atrophied.

In all FTD variants the onset is usually in the presenile period, with a range from 45 to 70 years (Gustafson *et al.* 1992). There was a small preponderance of males in the series of Neary *et al.* (1988).

A woman of 42 gradually lost her interests and became inefficient at work. She complained of stomach pains for which no cause could be found. Some months later she began repetitive checking behaviour and counting rituals and became progressively untidy and withdrawn. The following year it was apparent that her memory was impaired and her verbal fluency was poor, although she still remained fully orientated. Two years later she was withdrawn, incontinent and mostly mute. She sat swaying and rocking, often singing in a fatuous manner. Marked frontal atrophy and ventricular enlargement were apparent on CT. The EEG remained normal.

An accountant of 40 showed a 2-year decline in efficiency at work and self-care, and developed severe compulsive behaviour. He would check that the front door was closed up to 10 times per hour. A diagnosis of obsessional neurosis was made, although it was noted that insight was lacking. His mood tended to be jovial. During the following year he developed child-like behaviour with yelps and shouts, and became gluttonous, often stealing from other people's plates. When seen 4 years from onset new learning was poor but he gave the dates of past events correctly. He was orientated for place and year but was wrong for the month. He performed very poorly on proverb interpretation. The EEG was normal, but CT showed severe frontal atrophy.

Neurological examination typically shows no abnormalities, other than the emergence of primitive reflexes such as grasping, pouting or sucking. The plantar reflexes may be extensor. Fascicular twitchings are sometimes observed, and some patients develop dysarthria and dysphagia. Late in the disease the patient may become immobile through akinesia and rigidity.

The EEG is usually normal, even late into the disease, in marked contrast to all other forms of dementia and this can be a useful and relatively specific diagnostic marker. Brain imaging may show atrophy largely confined to the fronto-temporal regions, usually with ventricular enlargement. Functional brain imaging, particularly hexamethylpropyleneamine oxine single-photon emission computed tomography (HMPAO-SPECT), can have special importance in revealing diminished blood flow or metabolism selectively affecting the anterior brain regions, even when structural scans show little abnormality.

A professional man of 44 had been suspended from work because of poor performance and certain errors of judgement over the preceding year. A neurologist suspected early dementia, but other consultant neurologists and psychiatrists considered him to be normal. It was thought that the problem might lie with over-critical colleagues rather than with himself. His wife, however, described a gradual change of personality, with rigidity of habits and a tendency towards irritability and agitation. On occasion he had been embarrassing in social situations, making insensitive comments of a personal nature to casual acquaintances. She described marked lacunae in his distant memory, for example for a holiday they had taken some years ago. He admitted to memory problems but in other respects considered that he was well.

Examination showed normal mood and he made good rapport. He was fully orientated and well informed about recent events, but seemed totally amnesic for significant episodes from his past life. He made occasional paraphasic errors and his verbal fluency was poor. Physical examination showed no abnormalities. The EEG was normal, and CT showed only marginal abnormalities over the left sylvian fissure and possible dilatation of the left anterior horn. These were considered to be of doubtful significance. However, SPECT showed clear evidence of hypoperfusion over both frontal lobes.

Follow-up over the next 2 years showed very gradual deterioration, with increasing lack of initiative, disinhibition and obsessionality. Psychometric testing revealed increasing naming difficulties and problems with card sorting. His mother had suffered from a slowly progressive dementing illness of a similar nature.

FTD-related conditions

Progressive supranuclear palsy and corticobasal degeneration (CBD) are both now considered to be related to FTD (Boeve *et al.* 2003). This change in their nosological status came about because of findings from pathology: all are tauopathies. However, CBD in particular also shows some clinical overlap with common if not universal cognitive difficulties, particularly frontal lobe deficits and the difficulties of speech and language typical of FTD (Graham *et al.* 2003). The assessment of speech can be difficult because of complicating dysarthria but it is clear that there is commonly a cognitive aphasia in this condition.

Differential diagnosis

The subtle nature of the behavioural change in the early stages, and the lack of conspicuous cognitive defects, may lead to long delays before the correct diagnosis is made. A personality disorder may be suspected, especially when some life event appears to have provoked the change in demeanour. Other patients are suspected of alcoholism, or of hypomania when there is elevated mood and disinhibition. Agitation and hypochondria may give the impression of an anxiety or depressive state, and compulsive features may lead to the diagnosis of obsessive–compulsive neurosis. It is not uncommon for the patient to have received treatment for such disorders before the organic nature of the illness becomes evident through progressive lack of self-care and the advent of clear cognitive deficits.

Huntington's disease may be suspected when personality change and psychotic features are prominent, and especially when other family members are affected. Differentiation from AD will rarely be difficult, though occasional patients with AD present with behavioural change and with anterior rather than posterior hypoperfusion on SPECT. Some cases of FTD are accompanied by motor neurone disease.

Pathology

The gross appearance of the brain at post-mortem is of generalised atrophy combined with striking circumscribed shrinkage of certain lobes, most commonly the frontal and temporal lobes. In the frontal lobes the orbital surface may be affected alone, and in the temporal lobes the posterior half of the superior temporal gyrus may stand out as relatively spared. The distribution of atrophy varies considerably from case to case, but major involvement of the parietal lobes is unusual and occipital atrophy extremely rare. The gyri are roughened and brownish, often with a characteristic 'knife-blade' appearance. The ventricles are dilated, often with great enlargement of the horn of the lateral ventricle beneath the site of maximal cortical atrophy. The basal ganglia and thalamus also show atrophy, sometimes pronounced in the caudate nucleus, but the cerebellum is usually spared.

There has been considerable reassessment and revision of the pathological features of FTD and associated diseases in recent years following the discovery of mutations in the *TAU* gene in one variant, frontotemporal dementia with parkinsonism linked to chromosome 17 (FTDP-17). It is now recognised that many (but not all) cases of FTD, Pick's disease, PSP and CBD share tau-positive pathology (Neary *et al.* 1998; Neary 1999; Munoz *et al.* 2003; Kertesz & Munoz 2004). The critical pathological distinctions are between the presence and absence of inclusions and the type of tau pathology where present. Three main pathological subtypes constitute the majority of cases. Microvacuolar is the commonest and features a superficial layer spongiform change (extracellular in contrast to the intraneuronal spongiform changes of the transmissible encephalopathies) caused by neuronal loss, a relative absence of gliosis and absence of intraneuronal distinctive lesions. In contrast, in the Pick's type of pathology there is profound gliosis, an absence of spongiform change and there are swollen neurones with tau- and ubiquitin-positive inclusions. Pick bodies are specific inclusions. In the third and least common pathological presentation, microvacuolar change is accompanied by features of motor neurone disease. In all cases the gross pathology is of atrophied temporal and frontal lobes.

Tau is a microtubule-associated protein normally expressed in axons (Avila *et al.* 2004). In AD, the distribution of tau within the neurone changes. Early in the disease, in fact in the prodromal phase before the onset of clinical dementia, tau is apparent in a soluble and hyperphosphorylated state in cell bodies in neurones and then, as the disease progresses, in neurofibrillary tangles. In the FTDs, tau-positive inclusions are found in neurones and glia, although these inclusions do not have the same morphological appearance as neurofibrillary tangles in AD. However, as in AD, tau is aggregated, relatively insoluble and highly phosphorylated relative to normal adult tau. There are six isoforms of tau in human adult central nervous system, all expressed by differential splicing of a single gene (D'Souza & Schellenberg 2005). The isoforms differ by having three or four microtubule-binding domains (3R or 4R) and none, one or two N-terminal inserts of unknown function. The relative predominance of the different isoforms differs in the various FTDs and associated disorders. Thus 3R tau predominates in Pick's disease and 4R tau in CBD and PSP. Some cases have no tau lesions but do have lesions that stain with antibodies to ubiquitin. Ubiquitin is a protein that is tagged to proteins to target them for degradation.

Some cases of FTD are inherited in an autosomal dominant fashion whereas others are apparently sporadic. Familial cases of not only FTDP-17 but also more common variants of FTD have been found to have mutations in the *TAU* gene (Heutink 2000; Pickering-Brown 2004; Goedert & Jakes 2005). Broadly speaking these mutations fall into two classes: (i) those that occur in or near the microtubule-binding domains are likely to affect the normal function of tau; and (ii) those that are in the exon 10 splice site alter the relative expression of 3R and 4R tau (Rademakers *et al.* 2004). As some of the FTDs have an excess of 3R tau and others an excess of 4R tau, it can be assumed that the relative expression of both classes of isoform is more important than the absolute expression. If the normal ratio of 3R to 4R tau is disrupted, or if the tau has a mutation in or close to the microtubule-binding domains, then tau appears to no longer properly bind microtubules but instead aggregates, becomes highly phosphorylated and thereby disrupts neuronal function leading to neuronal loss. The neuronal dysfunction

caused by abnormalities in tau remains to be fully elucidated but evidence from cell and animal studies suggests one important function that is disrupted is axonal transport. Other families with FTD or variants have been linked to chromosomes 3 and 9 and it is likely that the responsible genes will be identified soon.

Distinction between FTD and AD

In FTD changes of character and disposition are often noted from the onset, whereas memory disturbance is almost invariably the presenting feature in AD. Incontinence occurring early in the course of the dementia has also been regarded as indicative of FTD, and may similarly be due to the accent of pathology on the frontal lobes.

Parietal lobe symptomatology in the form of dysphasia, apraxia and agnosia is said to be much less common in FTD than AD, likewise disturbances of gait and other extrapyramidal features. Aspects of Klüver–Bucy syndrome may be detected early in FTD but are generally a late development in AD.

The facile hilarity and aspontaneity of Pick's disease has been contrasted with the depressed anxious mood and overactivity of patients with AD, though aspontaneity occurs in the latter condition also. The disturbance of circadian rhythms with nocturnal activity that occurs so often in AD is relatively lacking in FTD (Harper *et al.* 2001).

The preservation of a normal EEG, even in the presence of moderately advanced dementia, will suggest FTD, likewise atrophy restricted to the anterior half of the brain as revealed by CT or MRI. However, intermediate pictures will quite often be encountered. SPECT holds the promise of more reliable differential diagnosis.

It appears therefore to be chiefly in the mode of onset of the disorder and in the neurological concomitants that a clinical differentiation is to be sought. The differentiation is more easily made in the earlier than the later stages, since ultimately any differences become submerged.

Huntington's disease

Huntington's disease has attracted a great deal of interest and attention. Choreiform movements are combined with dementia, serving as a clinical marker that has allowed its genetic background to be studied with care. Since Huntington's original account in 1872, cases have been reported from all over the world and no race appears to be immune. Prevalence varies markedly from one investigation to another. Very high figures have been reported from Tasmania, while in parts of Japan the disease appears to be extremely rare. Overall, in Europe, the prevalence is about 4–8 per 100 000 population (Harper 1992), although there are foci of higher prevalence. An astonishingly dense focus is known to have existed for a long time in the Moray Firth area of Scotland, with the equivalent of 560 cases per 100 000 in a small fishing community on the east coast of Ross-shire (Lyon 1962).

Aetiology

The disease is an autosomal dominant disorder and as a consequence half of the offspring of an affected person can be expected to develop the disorder, with equal incidence in males and females. Cases in Massachusetts and Connecticut have been traced back to emigrants from England, principally to three men and their wives who left from Bures in Suffolk in 1630 and thereafter produced 11 generations of choreics (Vessie 1932). However, subsequent work has cast doubt on some of the genealogies in Vessie's study (Harper & Morris 1991). A family history is not always forthcoming, even among classic examples. This may be the result of several factors: the early death of a parent, illegitimacy, lack of an adequate history, or concealed and circumscribed knowledge within the immediate family circle.

Huntington's disease results from an expansion in the CAG repeat within exon 1 of the gene encoding huntingtin (htt). As CAG is the codon for glutamine, this results in a string of glutamines being incorporated into the protein and Huntington's disease is one of a series of polyglutamine disorders, themselves a subset of the triplet repeat disorders (Koshy & Zoghbi 1997). Myotonic dystrophy and fragile X are examples of triplet repeat disorders caused by non-glutamine triplet repeat expansions; dentatorubral-pallidoluysian atrophy is an example of another polyglutamine disorder. The normal repeat length in the *HTT* gene is 36 or less. An expansion of 40 or more codons causes Huntington's disease, with a correlation between size of expansion and virulence of the disease. Large expansions tend to result in earlier onset of disease (Stine *et al.* 1993) and in some, but not all, studies with more severe neurodegeneration as measured by imaging (Culjkovic *et al.* 1999; Roth *et al.* 2005) or at post-mortem (Rosenblatt *et al.* 2003) or with more rapid clinical decline (Ward *et al.* 2006).

There are a number of features common to diseases resulting from this type of genetic variability, most characteristic of which is the phenomenon of anticipation, whereby there is a tendency for the triplet to expand during meiosis thus resulting in a predisposition to longer repeats in offspring. As the severity of the disorder, as evidenced by its age of onset, is related to the size of the repeat, this translates to a propensity for the disorder to be of earlier onset in children. As the triplet instability is greater in the generation of male gametes, there is also a tendency for the disorder to show increased anticipation in the children of male sufferers (Nance 1997). Juvenile onset is associated with larger expansions, often secondary to paternal transmission. Onset in infants can be a

consequence of massive expansion of the triplet repeat (Seneca *et al.* 2004).

The mechanism whereby an expansion in the triplet repeat causes Huntington's disease is not fully understood. In animal models expression of the expansion region alone is sufficient to cause disease, suggesting a predominant toxic gain-of-function effect rather than a loss of normal function (Bates & Gonitel 2006; Borrell-Pages *et al.* 2006). These mouse and cellular models have added considerably to the understanding of Huntington's disease and have provided models on which to develop therapeutic strategies. The Huntington's disease repeats tend to aggregate and when these aggregates occur in nuclei this appears to mediate toxicity (Yang *et al.* 2002). Inhibiting the formation of these aggregates *in vivo* reverses toxicity (Kazantsev *et al.* 2002), as does increasing turnover of aggregates by stimulating autophagy (Berger *et al.* 2006). Clearly this is promising, but this is a rapidly advancing field and it is by no means certain that a toxic effect of Huntington's disease aggregates in nucleus, possibly affecting gene transcription events, is the only pathogenic mechanism.

Genetic counselling and presymptomatic testing

Huntington's disease provides an archetypal example of best practice when it comes to the use of genetics in clinical practice. This has been reviewed extensively elsewhere (Simpson & Harding 1993; Scourfield *et al.* 1997; Ensenauer *et al.* 2005). Prior to the availaibilty of direct gene testing, a large proportion of unaffected family members indicated that they would welcome a predictive test but only a small proportion went on to have one (Tyler & Harper 1983; Meissen & Berchek 1987). Persons who do go on to be tested generally do well and psychological well-being measures improve after testing, whatever the result (Bloch *et al.* 1992; Huggins *et al.* 1992; Simpson *et al.* 1992; Wiggins *et al.* 1992; Adam *et al.* 1993). Surprisingly, some of those receiving 'good news' have the worst outcomes (Almqvist *et al.* 2003). This matches with clinical experience: living with a family with Huntington's disease, growing up with a 50% risk, is an experience that dominates individuals' lives. People having presymptomatic testing talk about their lives having been 'put on hold'. For some, having this threat of disease removed or having uncertainty removed is liberating. For others the readjustment to a life of health and removal from the world of disease can be difficult and all people undergoing presymptomatic counselling require extensive support. International consensus has laid out the ground rules for this support: counselling by two professionals, sessions separated by a minimum of 3 months, and results only given in person and only after the parent of the counselee has received a diagnosis and/or genetic confirmation. Pitfalls in counselling are common and it is essential that such counselling takes place in the context of clinical genetics units.

Clinical features

The onset is usually in the fourth and fifth decades, with an average in the mid-forties. Variation is wide, however, and onset may occur in childhood and in extreme old age. In general the age of onset among sibs tends to be closer than among members of different families, but the correlation is not sufficiently close to be of much value in genetic counselling. There is evidence that the disease follows a more severe course when onset is early rather than late, also that emotional disturbance is more prominent as a premonitory feature. There is some suggestion of other changes in manifestation with age of onset, striate rigidity predominating in the early twenties, choreic symptoms in middle age and intention tremor after the age of 60. Special features of the disease in childhood are considered below.

Considerable variation may be seen in the relationship between the neurological and psychiatric features. In the typical case involuntary movements precede dementia, although the reverse can also be seen. Occasionally, several years may separate the appearance of the two components, or the two may begin and proceed throughout together. Certainly once both are well established each tends to worsen in conformity with the other.

Very occasionally chorea may be the sole manifestation. Dementia without chorea has similarly been recorded, even when chorea was prominent in previous generations of the family. Other variations include the form the neurological abnormalities take, progressive rigidity with parkinsonism replacing the typical choreic movements in up to 10% of cases. All such variations usually appear sporadically; despite some indications in the literature, it is not well established that in different families the form of the disease tends to breed true.

Presenting symptoms

The presenting symptoms were almost equally divided between neurological and psychiatric features in Heathfield's (1967) survey. Neurological presentations were usually with choreiform movements, or less often with unsteadiness of gait, a tendency to fall or general clumsiness. Psychiatric presentations could be with symptoms of incipient dementia, but even more commonly with change of disposition, emotional disturbance and paranoia. Families with predominant psychiatric symptoms have been reported (Lovestone *et al.* 1996; Tsuang *et al.* 2000; Correa *et al.* 2006), suggesting that there may be risk factors for psychosis in these families independent of the *HTT* gene mutation.

Most observers agree that psychiatric changes are often present for some considerable time before chorea or intellectual impairment develops. A change in personality may be marked, the patient becoming morose and quarrelsome, or slowed, apathetic and neglectful. These are well recognised as premonitory symptoms by those who have practical dealings with communities in which the disease is relatively common. Paranoid developments may be the earliest change, with marked sensitivity and ideas of reference. Sometimes a florid schizophrenic illness may be present for several years before the true diagnosis becomes apparent. Depression and anxiety may be marked from the outset.

Neurological features

The neurological features often go unrecognised at their first appearance. The typical early choreic movements consist of randomly distributed and irregularly timed muscle jerks, brief in duration and unpredictable in their appearance. At first the patient is merely thought to be clumsy or fidgety. Early movements may be no more than the twitching of a finger, or fleeting facial grimaces that pass for mannerisms. The movements usually start in the muscles of the face, hands or shoulders, or are first manifest in subtle changes of gait. Speech is often affected early with slight dysarthria. For some time the patient may conceal the involuntary nature of the movements by exploiting them to perform some habitual activity such as smoothing the hair or the clothes.

With worsening of the disease the pathological nature of the motor disturbance becomes abundantly obvious. The movements are abrupt, jerky, rapid and repetitive but variable from one muscle group to another. They may be aggravated by voluntary movement but may also occur spontaneously. The face shows fleeting changes of expression and constant writhing contortions that bestow a grotesque appearance. The fingers twitch, the arms develop athetoid twisting movements and the proximal musculature is affected with shrugging of the shoulders. However, it is characteristic that even late into the disease the movements largely cease during sleep.

The gait is sometimes affected by a curious dance-like ataxia that results from the variable choreic influences on the lower limbs: the weight tends to be carried on the heels while the toes are dorsiflexed, and often a foot will remain suspended off the ground for longer than usual. Eventually the patient walks with a wide base, exaggerated lumbar lordosis, wide arm abduction and zig-zag progression due to lurching of the trunk. Progress is interrupted by pauses and even backward steps, and accompanied by a great increase in choreiform movements of the upper limbs. Hemichorea, massively affecting one half of the body, may be seen. Involvement of the diaphragm and bulbar muscles may lead to jerky breathing, explosive or staccato speech, dysphagia and difficulty in protruding the tongue.

In addition to such involuntary movements, Folstein *et al.* (1986) emphasise a characteristic disorder of voluntary activity that can be an important aid to diagnosis. The rhythm and speed of fine motor movements is disturbed, with conspicuous slowness in the performance of tasks. Disturbances of eye movement have also been reported, often from early in the disease and with gradual worsening over time. Patients have difficulty in initiating fast saccades when asked to glance quickly at objects in the periphery, also impairments of smooth pursuit and gaze fixation (Quarrell & Harper 1991).

In some patients extrapyramidal rigidity may be present, or spasticity with pyramidal signs. As mentioned above, some cases develop striate rigidity rather than chorea, perhaps especially when the onset is at an early age (the so-called Westphal variant). This is commonly associated with akinesia, tremor and cogwheel rigidity, and occasionally progresses to torsion dystonia. Fits are more frequent in this variety than in the generality of cases (16% compared with 3%) (Myrianthopoulos 1966).

Dementia

The cognitive impairment is commonly insidious in development. Brandt and Butters (1986) and Folstein (1989) summarise the studies that have sought to characterise the dementia in detail. General inefficiency at work and in the management of daily affairs is usually the presenting feature, rather than obvious memory impairment. A prevailing apathy, setting in early and impeding cognitive functioning, has been stressed as characteristic (McHugh & Folstein 1975). In consequence the patient's performance on everyday tasks is usually more slipshod than psychological testing would predict during the early stages of the disorder. Executive dysfunction is present and correlates with caudate atrophy (Peinemann *et al.* 2005). Overall, in early disease, the pattern is of decreased attention, executive dysfunction, and deficits in immediate memory with relatively preserved general cognition, semantic memory and delayed recall memory (Ho *et al.* 2003). Executive dysfunction is interesting in that patients show deficits in planning but not execution of tasks (Watkins *et al.* 2000).

Slowing of cognitive responses is usually marked from an early stage. Rigidity is observed in thinking and behaviour, with difficulty in changing easily from one activity to another. Memory impairment can usually be demonstrated when carefully sought, even in patients examined within a year of onset of the chorea (Butters *et al.* 1978). However, it is rarely conspicuous as in AD, and it gradually becomes submerged in general difficulties with attention, concentration and organisation of thought. The relative sparing of memory as the disease progresses is consonant with the pathological finding that the limbic areas of the brain are often less affected than in other dementing processes. Disorientation in time and place tends similarly to be a late development.

Detailed investigation into the nature of the memory deficits shows certain distinctive features as outlined by Brandt and Rich (1995). Thus the predominant difficulty appears to lie with deficient retrieval strategies rather than acquisition deficits, in that free recall can be markedly impaired in the presence of near-normal multiple-choice recognition. The retrograde amnesia is usually severe and generalised, being equally impaired across the decades and not showing the temporal gradient of Korsakoff's syndrome. This again reflects impaired retrieval processes. However, recognition as well as recall deficits are observed and a meta-analysis of the literature suggests that both make substantial contributions to the episodic memory deficits in the disease (Montoya *et al.* 2006a).

With regard to implicit (procedural) memory, there is an interesting difference from the deficits seen with AD; lexical priming is well preserved (e.g. on word-stem completion tasks) while the acquisition of motor and perceptual skills is impaired. This pattern is the reverse of that seen in AD, probably reflecting the accent of neuronal loss in the basal ganglia.

Focal psychological features are also rare in comparison with other primary dementias (Bruyn 1968; McHugh & Folstein 1975). Word-finding difficulties can occur, and verbal fluency is severely affected from the early stages, but dysphasia, dyslexia, apraxia and agnosia are seldom detected. However, tests of visuospatial functioning are typically poorly performed. Judgement is often severely impaired as part of the widespread intellectual decline, but insight is commonly retained for a considerable length of time. The patient may thus be aware of his mental changes, complaining that he feels dulled, slow and forgetful and that his thinking is muddled.

These clinical impressions were confirmed by Aminoff *et al.* (1975), who examined 11 patients with the disease an average of 6 years after onset, and when all were sufficiently impaired to have warranted premature retirement from work. The intellectual deterioration was found to be global, with a pattern of results on psychometric testing which approximated to that of the decline normally occurring in old age. Memory was not selectively impaired, and no patient showed focal symptoms such as dysphasia or dyspraxia. Of the 11, seven were fully orientated for time, place and person, and nine retained full insight into their condition.

Distractibility is a marked and characteristic feature, and can be seen as the counterpart of the disturbed motor patterns. Depression may be severe, especially while insight is retained, and suicide is a considerable risk in the early stages. Eventually, however, the mood is of apathy or fatuous euphoria, and inertia and self-neglect become pronounced. Episodes of restlessness and irritability or outbursts of excitement may occur from time to time, and some patients become difficult to manage on account of spiteful, quarrelsome or violent behaviour. A picture resembling akinetic mutism may mark the terminal stages.

The special features of the dementia in Huntington's disease – poor cognitive ability generally but a lack of language disorder or other focal cortical deficits – has suggested that it owes much to subcortical rather than cortical pathology. The pronounced apathy that accompanies and develops along with it is also typical of subcortical dementia. In line with this, apathy but not depression accounts for some of the variance in episodic memory and other cognitive deficits in early Huntington's disease (Baudic *et al*. 2006). Dementia is usually a relatively late symptom but exceptions are recorded where it is the predominant presenting symptom (Cooper, D.B. *et al*. 2006).

Affective and psychotic disturbance

Affective and psychotic features become obtrusive in many cases, often early in the course or even preceding the onset of chorea or dementia. Most common symptoms are dysphoria, agitation, irritability, apathy and anxiety (Paulsen *et al*. 2001a). Major depressive illness is frequent, sometimes recurrent and can be responsive to drugs or electroconvulsive therapy. A schizophrenic or paraphrenic picture may also be seen. Delusions of persecution can be pronounced, with religiosity and sometimes grandiosity. Ideas of reference are perhaps accentuated by the attention attracted by the involuntary movements and bizarre facial expressions.

Folstein *et al*. (1983) surveyed the incidence of affective disorder among 88 patients (from 63 kindreds) drawn from a defined geographical area in Maryland; 41% showed major affective disorder, 32% being depressive and 9% bipolar. This development had antedated the Huntington's disease by 2–20 years in almost two-thirds of cases. Moreover, it appeared to be confined to certain families, suggesting that the association may represent genetic heterogeneity within Huntington's disease. Five probands with affective disorder and five without were subjected to detailed family studies; affective disorder accompanied the Huntington's disease significantly more often in the families of the former than the latter, and was also somewhat commoner among unaffected family members. Suicide had already been stressed by Huntington (1910), and has been found to account for 7% of deaths among non-hospitalised patients (Reed & Chandler 1958).

The schizophrenia-like pictures can also be an early development. McHugh and Folstein (1975) prefer the term 'delusional–hallucinatory states', noting the emergence of psychotic symptoms from a pervasive delusional mood. They describe the typical progression as follows: the patient is overwhelmed by a vague impression of an uncanny change in reality which becomes laden with meaning of an uncertain nature. Delusions and hallucinations distil from this, often welling up suddenly and usually lasting several months. Treatment with neuroleptics can lead to considerable improvement. McHugh and Folstein suggest that the admixture of dementia with such a picture may account for many of the reports of severe personality change and paranoid features among patients with Huntington's disease.

Behavioural change

Change of behaviour and/or personality was noted in 42% of 65 patients identified in the Oxfordshire region (Watt &

Seller 1993). Aggression and violence, usually against the spouse, was the most common change, followed by suspiciousness and outbursts of temper. Aggression was particularly common among men and quarrelsomeness among women.

Preclinical changes

Autosomal dominant conditions offer the opportunity to unambiguously study the very earliest symptoms, as family members carrying the mutation can be identified and studied in detail prior to obvious manifestation of disease. For Huntington's disease the relatively preserved age of onset within families and correlation with expansion length allows particularly detailed phenotypic studies at around the time of expected onset. In one very large study, preclinical symptoms included anxiety, paranoid ideation and psychoticism in one cluster of subjects and depression in another (Marshall *et al*. 2007). Neuropsychometric testing shows deficits in memory prior to executive dysfunction and motor speed in preclinical mutation carriers (Robins Wahlin *et al*. 2007). Berrios *et al*. (2002) found evidence for cognitive deficits but not personality or mood changes when comparing carriers with non-carriers in families with Huntington's disease and make the case that being part of a family with such a disease is itself highly stressful. They conclude that cognitive dysfunction is likely to be due to biological effects and personality or mood changes to psychological mechanisms. Some of these cognitive impairments are detectable more than 2 years before disease onset (Paulsen *et al*. 2001b); in line with this, functional imaging shows changes, notably diminished activation of the left anterior cingulate cortex, in presymptomatic subjects (Reading *et al*. 2004).

Investigations

Electroencephalography characteristically shows poorly developed or complete loss of alpha rhythms. There may be generalised low-voltage fast activity or random slow activity, but this too may disappear as the disease progresses. In consequence the record may become entirely flat. Occasionally, however, a normal record may be obtained even in the presence of advanced dementia.

Computed tomography and MRI show dilated ventricles, often particularly affecting the frontal regions. Atrophy of the heads of the caudate nuclei may be clearly apparent, with loss of the normal convex bulging into the lateral walls of the frontal horns. Various linear measures have been proposed for establishing this feature as an aid to diagnosis, but they are not sufficiently specific to be of value in the individual case (Shoulson & Plassche 1980). In addition MRI studies have shown significant reductions in the thalamus and the medial temporal lobe structures (Jernigan *et al*. 1991).

Functional imaging techniques can be of particular value by revealing marked hypometabolism in the caudate and putamen. Using PET, Kuhl *et al.* (1982, 1985) showed that this developed early in the disease and before tissue loss was evident on CT. In contrast, metabolic values were often normal in other brain regions despite severe disability and CT evidence of atrophy. Caudate hypometabolism was also observed in occasional subjects at risk of Huntington's disease, even while they were asymptomatic. Mazziotta *et al.* (1987) confirmed this in a large group of at-risk persons; 31% showed bilateral reductions in caudate glucose metabolism, which was close to the 34% estimate for the likelihood of developing the disease when age and other factors were taken into account. Smith *et al.* (1988) and Gemmell *et al.* (1989) showed that reductions of cerebral blood flow may be detected with SPECT in the caudate nuclei in a large proportion of patients. This, being more widely available, is likely to find clinical application in uncertain cases.

A recent systematic review of imaging studies in Huntington's disease showed that both structural and functional imaging has demonstrated striatal and cortical atrophy that correlates well with cognitive deficits (Montoya *et al.* 2006b), suggesting that the complex cognitive deficits in Huntington's disease that accompany the motor disorder result from abnormal connectivity between the basal ganglia and the cortex.

The value of PET in remedying a false diagnosis of Huntington's disease was illustrated in a woman of 55. For the past 10 years she had shown a slowly progressive dementia, along with increasing motor disorder by way of a stiff unsteady gait, writhing of the hands and choreiform movements of the face. The antecedent family history was at that time uncertain, but her sister in New Zealand was known to suffer from an entirely similar illness. The motor disorder in both cases had been judged to be typical of Huntington's disease. The EEG showed moderate diffuse theta and occasional delta waves.

However, CT showed well-preserved caudate nuclei, despite very pronounced cortical atrophy and ventricular dilatation. Her sister's scan was remarkably similar. Doubts about the diagnosis were further reinforced when vigorous efforts to trace the family history revealed longevity in the parents and their many siblings, with no evidence of dementia or movement disorder in any of them. The parents proved to be first cousins.

It was therefore concluded likely that the illness represented a recessively inherited dementing disorder, with adventitious movements attributable to the neuroleptics that had been administered for many years. In confirmation that Huntington's disease was unlikely, PET showed excellently preserved metabolism in the caudate nuclei, but with poor metabolism in both frontal lobes and both thalami.

Course and outcome

The course after the first definitive manifestations is generally much longer than with other primary dementing illnesses. The average duration is reported as 15–20 years, but with wide variation, some cases showing very slow progression over several decades.

Special features in childhood

Huntington's disease may occasionally set in during childhood or adolescence, although the true diagnosis will sometimes only be made at post-mortem. In several respects the disease tends to differ from the adult form, yet the pathological changes at post-mortem are the same (Hayden 1981; O'Shea & Falvey 1991). Muscular rigidity and tremor are commoner than choreiform movements, the mental deterioration tends to be rapid, and epileptic fits occur in more than half of the cases. The time to death is generally much shorter than with adult cases.

After developing normally the child begins to fail at school and shows difficulties with concentration. Change of personality and anxiety are common. He may become clumsy, ataxic and dysarthric. The absence of chorea readily leads to other diagnoses even in families known to harbour the disease. Friedreich's ataxia may be suspected, or Wilson's disease or postencephalitic parkinsonism. When a change of personality is the predominant manifestation, this may all too easily be ascribed to external factors, especially when the onset is at the approach of adolescence.

A 25-year-old man was admitted to hospital for the mentally handicapped. He was judged to have low intellect and to suffer from a personality disorder. He showed ataxia, tremor, dysarthria and muscular rigidity, but these were thought to be due to the neuroleptics he had been given. He was illegitimate and the fate of his father was unknown. His mother insisted that he had been a bright and inquisitive child, and that until the age of 11 he had progressed well at school. From then on he had shown unwillingness to work and increasingly aggressive behaviour. On leaving school he obtained simple labouring jobs, and was repeatedly arrested for thefts and other misdemeanours. From 18 he became increasingly withdrawn and developed dysarthria. During several hospital admissions thereafter he had been variously regarded as psychopathic or mentally subnormal, and was treated with a variety of neuroleptics. At 22 he was arrested for indecent exposure and other sexual offences.

Psychometric assessment was difficult, but he obtained an IQ equivalent of 67 on the coloured progressive matrices, compared with a verbal reasoning score of 103 recorded when he was 11. Detailed review 2 years later showed a parkinsonian gait, dysarthria and markedly increased tone in the limbs. There were jerking tremors around the mouth and in the fingers of the left hand. He spoke only monosyllabically, but proved to be fully orientated in time and place.

EEG revealed the absence of alpha rhythm and a very low amplitude tracing. CT showed flattening of the heads of the caudate nuclei (Fig 9.6). Over the next few weeks he declined abruptly, and post-mortem brain examination showed the typical pathology of Huntington's disease (Brooks *et al.* 1987).

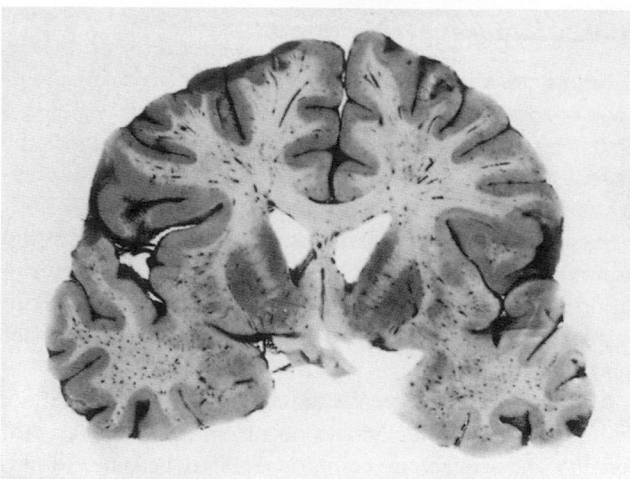

Fig. 9.6 Autopsy appearances of a patient with Huntington's disease, confirming shrinking of the heads of the caudate nuclei. Reproduced from Brooks, D.S., Murphy, D., Janota, I. & Lishman, W.A. (1987), *British Journal of Psychiatry* **151**, 850–852.

It has been known for some time that 'juvenile-onset' cases, i.e. those setting in before the age of 20, are more likely to demonstrate paternal than maternal transmission. For example, Osborne *et al.* (1982) found that children with onset before the age of 10 had an affected father approximately four times as frequently as an affected mother. This puzzling feature now finds an explanation from recent discoveries in molecular genetics.

The death rate of children in the first decade is known to be high in families with Huntington's disease, and has often been vaguely ascribed to 'mental deficiency' or 'spinal paralysis' (Oliver & Dewhurst 1969). The infant mortality is also high, and Oliver and Dewhurst suggest that this may be partially due to undiagnosed cases occurring even in infancy. Such deaths are often attributed to birth injury, spasticity or quadriplegia. However, social factors are also likely to be important in contributing to the infant mortality, since families with Huntington's disease are often disadvantaged and sometimes severely disorganised (see below).

Other psychiatric associations

The frequent occurrence of change of personality and emotional disturbance as premonitory symptoms of the disease has already been mentioned, also the marked psychotic features which may accompany the dementia. The association with severe depressive illness may have special genetic determinants. In addition, certain other psychiatric associations deserve emphasis.

A large number of psychiatric abnormalities, sometimes severe in degree, are reported when detailed studies of families with Huntington's disease are undertaken. Some fami-

lies are severely disorganised on account of a multitude of pathologies, involving both the patients themselves and their relatives. Epilepsy, schizophrenia, mental defect and a variety of other degenerative brain diseases have been reported. How far these may represent common genetic determinants remains to be established. It is possible that to some extent assortative mating between patients from Huntington families and those with other physical and psychiatric handicaps may contribute to the frequency of such disabilities.

Minski and Guttmann (1938) noted a variety of psychopathological features in the relatives of cases, particularly a personality characterised by explosive irritability and readiness to take offence. Suicide has been reported to be frequent even among members unaffected directly by the disease (Bickford & Ellison 1953). It is unclear how far this may be due to endogenous mental illness or the result of knowledge of the consequences of the condition. Watt and Seller (1993) found that one-third of first-degree relatives of patients gave a history of depression, mainly reactive to stresses within the family or to the onset of definitive illness in a family member. No support was obtained for a direct pathogenic effect of the Huntington gene in leading to depression or to personality disturbance in as yet unaffected persons.

In a study of 102 patients, Dewhurst *et al.* (1970) vividly illustrate the psychosocial consequences of the disorder: 10 attempted suicide and 13 self-mutilation; 19 were alcoholics and 18 had had convictions for serious criminal offences. Of those who had married, 38% subsequently divorced or separated, usually because of social or intellectual deterioration in the patient. Sexual disturbances were common: excessive demands, sexual assault, sexual deviation, impotence and frigidity. Notably there was often a history of promiscuity with the production of illegitimate offspring. The children were sometimes found to be at risk from their parents, with examples of serious neglect.

Oliver (1970) showed that unaffected siblings from Huntington families could also become victims of their disturbed environment. Ninety-three out of 150 either died young, became psychotic or suffered such disturbance as psychopathy, chronic alcoholism, criminality or divorce.

Mistakes in diagnosis

Huntington's disease may be mistaken for many other psychiatric and neurological illnesses, certainly in the early stages. Surveys have shown that over one-third of cases may be wrongly diagnosed initially (Bolt 1970; Dewhurst *et al.* 1970).

In a systematic study of patients in Maryland, Folstein *et al.* (1986) found that 11% had been given some other diagnosis, mainly because the existence of a diagnosed family member was not known to their doctor. Systematic interviewing of relatives revealed 47 cases additional to the 212 already known, and in half of these there had been some other false diagnosis. Moreover, 15% of the 212 cases reported by community physicians proved on review not to have Huntington's disease but to be suffering from other neurological and psychiatric conditions. Sometimes tardive dyskinesia consequent on medication had led to the mistake.

Psychiatric misdiagnoses are the most common, especially a label of schizophrenia or paranoid psychosis. When schizophrenic features are obtrusive, the chorea may readily be ascribed to 'schizophrenic mannerisms' or to the medications given. Affective psychosis, anxiety state and personality disorder may be the initial diagnosis. Other forms of dementia will often be suspected when a family history is not forthcoming, and the motor abnormalities which develop may then be ascribed to dyskinesia induced by phenothiazines.

Bolt (1970) found that diagnoses of neurosis or affective psychosis were almost invariably revised before the patient's death, but sometimes a diagnosis of schizophrenia or paranoid psychosis was not. A diagnosis of some other form of dementia or of neurological disease was much less likely to be corrected.

Neurological mistakes include multiple sclerosis, Wilson's disease, Parkinson's disease, neurosyphilis, cerebellar disorders and ataxia due to drug abuse. Arteriosclerotic or senile chorea may be misleading in the elderly: distinguishing features include the absence of a family history, and mental changes that are less conspicuous or progressive; moreover, these are often vascular in origin and can therefore be abrupt in onset and with a tendency towards resolution. The rare syndrome of *hereditary chorea without dementia* (benign familial chorea) may also be misleading (Quarrell & Harper 1991). This autosomal dominant disorder usually presents in childhood and mainly affects the head, face and upper limbs. In most families there is little progression beyond childhood, although worsening has occasionally been seen throughout adult life (Schady & Meara 1988). Intellect remains unimpaired.

The childhood form of Huntington's disease is liable to be mistaken for mental subnormality, Friedreich's ataxia, Wilson's disease, epilepsy, spasticity or birth injury. Sydenham's chorea may be simulated, but is usually sudden in onset and associated with other rheumatic manifestations.

Whenever the picture of Huntington's disease is atypical, and particularly when seizures, areflexia or muscle wasting are present, neuroacanthocytosis should be suspected. The examination of fresh blood films may then immediately clarify the diagnosis.

Pathology

The brain is usually small and atrophic although this varies greatly in degree. It is generally difficult to correlate the intensity of pathological changes with the severity of mental symptoms. The frontal lobes are often the site of maximal cortical change. Marked dilatation of the ventricular system is characteristic, especially of the frontal horns, along with striking atrophy of the caudate nuclei. Instead of bulging into the lateral ventricles these may be represented by a mere rim of tissue along the ventrolateral edge of the dilated anterior horns. The putamen is also atrophic, although the globus pallidus usually escapes in large degree.

Microscopic examination shows cell loss accompanied by gliosis. This can usually be detected in the cortex even when atrophy is not severe. It is particularly marked in the frontal lobes. Severe cell loss is invariably present in the caudate and putamen together with much astrocytic proliferation. The loss of small nerve cells is particularly striking. Similar changes of less degree are sometimes found in the globus pallidus, substantia nigra or cerebellar nuclei.

The white matter shows diffuse loss of nerve fibres, often with consequent narrowing of the corpus callosum. Vascular changes are not marked and cannot be incriminated in the pathogenesis of the disorder. The presence of neuronal nuclear inclusions was first highlighted by transgenic animal models and subsequently revealed in the human disease. Formal assessment of intranuclear inclusions using immunocytochemistry can contribute to the accuracy of post-mortem diagnosis (Maat-Schieman *et al.* 2007).

Biochemical studies

Although the genetic mechanisms causing Huntington's disease have been fully explained, the biochemical mechanisms have not and it is far from clear how expansions in the *HTT* gene give rise to neurodegeneration. In post-mortem studies, Perry *et al.* (1973) and others have shown reduced levels of γ-aminobutyric acid (GABA) in the basal ganglia and substantia nigra of brains from patients with Huntington's disease compared with brains from neurologically normal persons. GABA is an inhibitory synaptic transmitter, so its lack could be significant in relation to the movement disorder. Subsequently, a marked reduction in the enzyme responsible for the synthesis of GABA (glutamic acid decarboxylase, GAD) in the putamen and globus pallidus was demonstrated (Bird *et al.* 1973; Bird & Iverson 1974). Levels were normal in the frontal cortex, thus indicating a selective loss of GABA-containing neurones from the basal ganglia. It is now known that GABA receptors are depleted in the striatum from early in the disease, and before there is extensive cell loss and atrophy (Walker *et al.* 1984).

Cholinergic neurones are also severely deficient in the striatum, as reflected in low levels of choline acetyltransferase and of cholinergic receptors. In contrast, the dopaminergic system is spared (Spokes 1980). Indeed dopamine (and noradrenaline) have proved to be elevated in the striatum and substantia nigra, perhaps as a consequence of the low

GABA levels since GABA inhibits the release of dopamine in the nigrostriatal system.

A model was therefore proposed whereby the intact nigrostriatal pathway in Huntington's disease releases approximately normal quantities of dopamine onto a considerably reduced population of striatal neurones, leading to net dopamine overstimulation of those that remain (Spokes 1980; Marsden 1982). Dopamine overactivity in the striatum is known to provoke chorea. This could therefore be the key neuropharmacological feature of Huntington's disease, at least where the movement disorder is concerned; a similar excess of dopamine in the mesolimbic system may underlie the behavioural manifestations and psychoses seen with the disease.

In addition to neurochemical abnormalities and possible excitotoxic insults, there is evidence for oxidative stress and mitochondrial abnormalities in Huntington's disease (Browne & Beal 2006; Trushina & McMurray 2007). The mitochondrial toxin 3-nitropropionic acid (3NP) induces a Huntington's disease-like disorder in experimental animal studies, and both neurochemical and imaging investigations in these animals suggest that mitochondrial toxicity might combine with N-methyl-D-aspartate (NMDA)-induced excitotoxicty to induce neuronal cell damage (Lee & Chang 2004; Brouillet et al. 2005; Perez-De la Cruz & Santamaria 2007). In people with Huntington's disease, neurones bearing NMDA receptors are lost early and NMDA agonists, like 3NP, recapitulates some aspects of the disease in animal models, adding weight to this combined excitotoxicity/mitochondrial abnormality hypothesis (Fan & Raymond 2007).

Finally, it is remarkable how many neurological disorders have aggregated, relatively insoluble, protein inclusions. Huntington's disease joins AD, DLB, CJD, Parkinson's disease and others in this respect (Lovestone & McLoughlin 2002). Two protein machineries are responsible for clearing 'unwanted' proteins in both the aggregated and non-aggregated state: the ubiquitin–proteosome system and the process of autophagy. A defect in either or both has been postulated as an 'upstream' or primary cause in various of these diseases. For Huntington's disease, the evidence from model organisms and cells that there might be a defect in autophagy is strong (Ravikumar & Rubinsztein 2006; Rubinsztein et al. 2005) and might suggest novel therapeutic possibilities.

Prion diseases

The prion diseases, also known as the transmissible spongiform encephalopathies (TSEs), comprise a group of disorders of humans and other mammals, some of which are important causes of primary neurodegenerative dementias including CJD, Gerstmann–Sträussler–Scheinker disease (GSS) and fatal familial insomnia (FFI). These disorders are characterised neuropathologically by vacuolation, astrocytosis, neuronal loss and aggregation of a proteinaceous infectious particle or *prion*. Aguzzi and Polymenidou (2004) review the history of research of these disorders, noting that scrapie (a TSE in sheep) was described in the nineteenth century and that the transmissible nature of the condition was demonstrated in the 1930s. The first disease in humans to be described as a TSE was Kuru, a disorder of indigenous peoples in Papua New Guinea resulting from ritualistic cannibalism. This was the lifework of Gajdusek who was also the first to demonstrate that CJD was also transmissible to non-human primates. The prion disorders became an urgent and pressing public health concern when in the late 1980s there was an epidemic of a TSE in cattle in the UK (bovine spongiform encephalopathy, BSE) and then in the late 1990s when a variant of CJD in humans was first described and then shown to have arisen from BSE (Ironside 2003). These concerns are receding as an epidemic in humans has not occurred, although the risk has not disappeared (Manson et al. 2006). Nonetheless, two decades of intense research has yielded the most extraordinary body of work that has described a novel aetiology of disease and one that, for a time, challenged the very bedrock of biological understanding (Glatzel et al. 2005).

Prion biology

Arguably, the central dogma proposed by Watson and Crick (DNA to RNA to protein) has had two major challenges: the discovery of reverse transcriptase (RNA to DNA) by Temin, Dulbecco and Baltimore in 1970 and the demonstration by Prusiner in the early 1980s that characteristics, in this case disease, can be passed from one organism to another by proteins alone (Prusiner 1982). Placed in this context it is easy to see why the prion-only hypothesis of the TSEs has been subjected to such a thorough critique. Nonetheless, it has withstood this and is accepted, almost unanimously, by those in the field although there remain many unanswered questions.

The endogenous prion protein (PrPc) is a normal protein, highly abundant in neurones and believed to be involved in copper metabolism, oxidative balance and neuroprotection (Cui et al. 2003; Roucou et al. 2004; Leach et al. 2006). PrPc contains a high proportion of α-helices but can undergo conversion to a tertiary structure with more than 40% β-pleated sheets. This form, known as PrPSc, tends to form insoluble aggregates as do other β-pleated peptides (e.g. Aβ of AD). However, in this case, the β-pleated PrPSc has two apparently unique characteristics: it is almost completely resistant to degradation by proteases and can interact with native PrPc and promote its conversion to PrPSc. It is this second characteristic that confers the infectious property on prions.

However, the process whereby PrPSc initiates pathogenesis *in vivo* remains controversial. One view is that the pathogenic process can be initiated by a single pathogenic molecule that converts a normal endogenous molecule to a pathogenic form, which in turn converts further endogenous molecules, thus setting off a train of events resulting in massive conversion of endogenous PrPc and thus disease. The initiating event might be exogenous protein (iatrogenic TSE or variant CJD in humans; probably BSE in cattle), a random event in a genetically prone animal (scrapie in sheep, sporadic CJD in humans), or a mutation massively increasing conversion to PrPSc (GSS, FFI or familial CJD). An alternative view is that a balance normally exists between a pool of PrPSc and PrPc, albeit heavily weighted to PrPc. A small shift in this balance, it is suggested, might lead to a nucleation event with the formation of small amounts of aggregated PrPSc and this nucleus would act as a seed for further conversion of PrPc to aggregated PrPSc. A further view is that PrPc is in equilibrium with an intermediate state that interacts with a chaperone before aggregating with PrPSc (Fasano et al. 2006). All these ideas are variants of the prion-only hypothesis but determining the precise mechanism of pathogenesis is obviously important for therapeutics.

The prion-only hypothesis generates a number of predictions all of which have turned out to be true. Thus, for example, it was predicted that as infectivity was dependent on protein–protein interactions, then as PrP is not identical in all species there would be some species specificity in infectivity and this seems to be true: infectivity is far more virulent within a species than between species (Baron 2002; Moore et al. 2005). Similarly, as infection is postulated to result from an interaction between exogenous and endogenous protein, then it was predicted that animals lacking the endogenous protein would be resistant and this too turns out to be the case (Bueler et al. 1993; Weissmann & Flechsig 2003). Most strikingly, altering the host gene confers a different pattern of disease. Thus normal mice show much longer incubation times when infected with hamster scrapie than when infected with mouse scrapie. However, the situation is altered when transgenic mice are artificially created by the introduction of the hamster prion gene (Prusiner et al. 1990; Prusiner 1991; Prusiner & DeArmond 1991). Incubation times for hamster scrapie are then dramatically reduced. In elegant experiments the converse has also been shown to occur. In other words, the relative species barrier can be broken by genetic manipulation of the host prior to infection.

Surprisingly, however, given the wealth of research and the huge advances that have been made in understanding infectivity, little is known about the mechanism whereby PrPSc accumulation induces neurodegeneration. It is not depletion of PrPc because animals lacking the protein show little or no ill effects (Bueler et al. 1993). Nor is it simply accumulation of PrPSc, as chronic accumulation of this protein in the absence of PrPc is also harmless (Brandner et al. 1996). It seems most likely that the intracellular location of PrP is critical and that translocation from the endoplasmic reticulum to the cytosol or perhaps a transmembrane location underlies neurotoxicity (Aguzzi & Polymenidou 2004; Harris 2003).

The prion gene

Further molecular genetic studies have concentrated on the prion gene (PRNP) itself. This has emerged as abnormal in many patients suffering from CJD or GSS. In a family with CJD, Owen et al. (1989) found a mutation consisting of a 144-bp insertion in the prion gene, and Hsiao et al. (1989) found a point mutation at codon 102 in two families with GSS. The potential pathogenicity of such mutations was clearly demonstrated by Hsiao et al. (1990); transgenic mice created to carry the codon 102 mutation spontaneously developed spongiform degeneration some 5–6 months later.

The PRNP gene is highly conserved between species and has a simple structure, consisting of three exons only, with the open reading frame contained entirely within the second of these. An N-terminal repeat region of a nonapeptide followed by four octapeptides is the site of variation in the number of repeats but not a site for normal or pathogenic point variation. There are such variants elsewhere in the gene, including those mutations causing familial TSEs (Mead 2006). These autosomal dominant disorders (CJD, GSS and FFI) have been associated with more than 30 different mutations in PRNP, resulting in a premature stop codon, an amino acid substitution or the insertion of an octapeptide repeat. There is a degree of genotype–phenotype correlation in these familial TSEs (discussed below). In addition to variants or mutations causing autosomal dominant TSEs, there are a number of common polymorphic variants, mostly SNPs in the gene, some of which alter susceptibility to the disease. Most notable of these is that at codon 129, which might code for either methionine or valine (M129V). This variant has a strong influence on susceptibility, with homozygosity to the 129V variant conferring increased risk of both sporadic and iatrogenic CJD (Collinge et al. 1991; Palmer et al. 1991). To date all variant (v)CJD cases have been homozygous for 129M, although there has been one heterozygous patient reported as having preclinical vCJD; this individual had received blood from a donor with CJD and had extensive evidence of prion protein accumulation in the peripheral lymphoreticular system but died of unrelated causes (Zeidler et al. 1997a; Peden et al. 2004). The phenotype of the disease is also affected by the genotype, with homozygous 129M individuals showing classical clinical presentation of sporadic CJD whereas presentation with slower progression, absence of myoclonus and absence of the typical EEG findings were associated with other genotypes (Parchi et al. 1999).

The finding of susceptibility variants raises the possibility that different populations may have intrinsically different risk of CJD as the variant frequencies show marked differences across ethnic groups. Thus the 129M allele frequency is approximately 0.65 in the UK, higher in Africa and higher still in Japan where 129V is rare (Mead 2006). This is an example of a gene–environment interaction, oft searched for but rarely found; another SNP in PRNP (E219K) shows a similar effect in influencing susceptibility (Shibuya *et al.* 1998). Other susceptibility loci may exist and are being actively sought in both humans and in animal models.

Epidemiology of CJD

A relatively short time ago CJD was held to be a rare disorder with even rarer familial forms and the occasional clustering. A review of cases in France over a 15-year period to 1982 found a frequency of less than one case per million, of which 6% were familial (Brown *et al.* 1987). Clusters of CJD have been reported worldwide but in some instances are likely to be due to chance occurrence of more than one case in the same area (Cousens *et al.* 1999; Beaudry *et al.* 2002), in other instances to be due to familial disease (Chapman & Korczyn 1991), and in yet other cases remain unexplained and might be due to an environmental effect, possibly exogenous prion exposure (Arakawa *et al.* 1991; Cousens *et al.* 2001; Mad'ar *et al.* 2003).

However, the epidemic of BSE in the UK has raised the possibility of a substantial change in the frequency of TSEs. The epidemic in cattle peaked in 1992 and over 180 000 animals have developed the disease, with very many more likely to have been slaughtered in the preclinical phase (Anderson *et al.* 1996). Dairy farmers claim to readily identify cattle in the early phases of disease with subtle changes in behaviour, especially in the milking parlour (Anon, personal communication). Strict control was introduced on the feeding of cattle, with ruminant protein being banned as feed first for ruminants and then any farmed animal. Peaks in BSE also occurred in other countries in Europe and North America and controls were also introduced outside the UK. These control measures have almost eliminated TSEs from the UK cattle herd, although occasional cases still do occur. Scrapie is of course endemic but sheep to human transmission is not thought to have occurred. Chronic wasting disease is a TSE disorder of deer and is also common, occurring in up to 10% of the farmed population, but it too has not been shown to have crossed the species barrier although concerns remain.

Variant CJD was first described in 1996 and then shown to be linked to BSE by strain typing in mice and by biochemical approaches (Manson *et al.* 2006). In March 2007 there were 165 cases of vCJD known to the national CJD surveillance unit (http://www.cjd.ed.ac.uk/). All reported cases are homozygous for 129M. This raises the possibility that 129VV homozygotes or 129MV heterozygotes may have carrier status and may succumb or be themselves capable of transmitting disease. Evidence in favour of this concerning scenario came from studies of appendices which showed two 129VV individuals who were asymptomatic but who had extensive PrP accumulation (Ironside *et al.* 2006), as well as from the individual referred to above who had evidence of PrP accumulation following infected blood transfusion and

who was 129MV (Peden *et al.* 2004). Given these concerns, the long-term impact of BSE and other TSEs in farmed animals on the population remains to be seen.

Iatrogenic TSEs result from the accidental transfer of PrP from one individual to another during a medical procedure. Originally this was thought to occur only with the direct transfer of neuronal material, either through tissue use or a neurosurgical procedure. There was an outbreak of CJD following the use of pituitary-derived growth hormone and gonadotrophins (Brown 1988), and transmission was also shown to occur with corneal and dural transplants (Lang *et al.* 1998), resulting in disease with a slightly different clinical presentation. More recently, concern has been raised regarding blood and other non-neural tissue transfer as it has become increasingly realised that PrP deposits occur extensively in the lymphoreticular system, even though pathological expression is limited to the nervous system (Aguzzi & Glatzel 2006; Ironside 2006).

Clinical features of CJD

The clinical features of sporadic CJD are very diverse. Both sexes appear to be equally affected, although a female preponderance has sometimes been reported. The onset is usually in the fifth or sixth decade but cases are reported with onset at any adult age. A prodromal stage is usually described, lasting weeks or months and characterised by neurasthenic symptoms. The patient complains of fatigue, insomnia, anxiety and depression, and shows a gradual change towards mental slowness and unpredictability of behaviour. Occasionally the mood is mildly elevated with loquacity and inappropriate laughter. Already at this stage there may be evidence of impaired memory and concentration, the limbs may appear to be weak and the gait unsteady. Frequently, however, objective findings are lacking and a 'functional' psychiatric disorder is suspected. This is especially likely in patients in whom the early symptoms remit for several weeks at a time. In a review of sporadic CJD cases sleep disturbance, anxiety and psychosis were the commonest symptoms and psychiatric symptoms in general occurred in 80% of patients in the first 3–4 months of illness (Wall *et al.* 2005).

An instructive example was reported by Keshavan *et al.* (1987).

A 38-year-old man became forgetful and disorientated from Christmas 1983, but this was attributed to heavy alcohol consumption and depression. His marital situation and business affairs had become chaotic. When admitted to a psychiatric hospital 6 months later his mental state showed marked fluctuations, with disorientation and bizarre memory disturbances alternating with periods of lucidity. He was emotionally labile and gave approximate answers to questions, and the presumptive diagnosis was of hysterical pseudodementia.

In August 1984, EEG showed mixed theta and delta activity, attributed to possible alcoholic encephalopathy, but CT was normal. No abnormal neurological signs could be detected apart from a pout reflex and a shuffling gait. During the following month he deteriorated markedly and became regressed in his behaviour. In October he was referred for a further opinion, at which stage it was impossible to test cognitive functions because of extreme distractibility. He was perplexed, gazed vacantly and spoke in a slurred incoherent babble. At this stage neurological examination revealed gross apraxia, generalised myoclonic jerks and choreoathetoid movements. He was incontinent of urine and faeces. CT now showed some evidence of atrophy, and EEG showed prominent slow waves maximal over the left frontotemporal region. He then followed a downhill course until his death in March 1985, when post-mortem confirmed the diagnosis of CJD.

Intellectual deterioration or neurological defects soon become prominent. The latter are extremely variable but are liable to involve motor functions, speech or vision. Myoclonic jerks are almost invariably seen. There may be ataxia of cerebellar type, spasticity of limbs with progressive paralysis, extrapyramidal rigidity, tremor or choreoathetoid movements, depending on the brain regions principally involved. Involvement of the anterior horn cells of the cord may lead to muscular fibrillation and atrophy, especially of the small hand muscles, resembling amyotrophic lateral sclerosis. Speech disturbances are common with dysphasia and dysarthria, likewise parietal lobe symptoms such as right–left disorientation, dyscalculia and finger agnosia. Vision may be severely affected with rapidly progressive cortical blindness. Apart from this, sensory changes are usually absent. Brainstem involvement may lead to nystagmus, dysphagia or bouts of uncontrollable laughing and crying. Epileptic fits may occur.

Attempts have been made to classify this bewildering variety of phenomena but with little success. A given case may show a succession of different neurological features as the disease progresses. A broad classification into those which begin with cerebellar symptoms and those with parietal lobe symptoms has been suggested, similarly into cases with and without spinal cord or visual cortex involvement.

Intellectual deterioration follows or appears along with the neurological defects and evolves with great rapidity. An acute organic picture may be present initially, with clouding of consciousness or frank delirium. Auditory hallucinations and delusions may be marked, and confabulation is often seen. Ultimately a state of profound dementia is reached,

accompanied by gross rigidity or spastic paralysis and often a decorticate or decerebrate posture. Repetitive myoclonic jerking of muscle groups is often still evident late in the disease. Emaciation is usually profound by the time death occurs.

Considerable effort has been expended in identifying a diagnostic test for CJD with most attention being paid to markers in CSF. Both 14-3-3 protein and tau are elevated and show modest sensitivity and specificity in diagnosis (Geschwind *et al.* 2003; Van Everbroeck *et al.* 2003; Castellani *et al.* 2004b). CT may show cortical atrophy and ventricular enlargement but this is rarely gross in degree. Indeed, CT can be essentially normal when the dementia is well advanced, a feature that was suggested to be of some importance in differential diagnosis (Galvez & Cartier 1984). The use of MRI has been of more value in diagnosis and prognosis of CJD. Increased grey matter signal in sporadic CJD is associated with shorter survival (Urbach *et al.* 1998) and diffusion-weighted imaging shows high specificity and sensitivity for both diagnosis and prediction of clinical course (Shiga *et al.* 2004; Young *et al.* 2005). Most notably, however, the MRI finding of a bilateral pulvinar signal (the 'pulvinar sign') is very highly sensitive and specific for vCJD (Zeidler *et al.* 2000; Collie *et al.* 2001).

Electroencephalography is almost always markedly abnormal (Wieser *et al.* 2006). A variety of changes have been reported and different findings may emerge at different stages of the illness. Initially there is some diffuse or focal slowing. Later, paroxysmal sharp waves or slow spike-and-wave discharges appear; these are bilaterally synchronous and may accompany the myoclonic jerks. Ultimately, a characteristic pattern emerges of synchronous triphasic sharp wave complexes at 1–2 Hz, superimposed on progressive suppression of cortical background activity. The triphasic discharges are at first intermittent, but evolve to a periodic picture at rates of 1–2 Hz. The latter changes may be helpful in diagnosis, though usually only late in the course of the disease.

The course is much more rapid than with most other primary dementing illnesses, the great majority of patients dying within 2 years. Death is usually preceded by a period of deepening coma that lasts for several weeks.

Pathology

The brain may appear to be somewhat atrophied but often there is little abnormal to detect macroscopically. Histological examination shows great variability from case to case, but the essential features consist of neuronal degeneration, great proliferation of astrocytes and a characteristic spongy appearance of the grey matter. In some varieties the latter may be so pronounced that it is visible to the naked eye. The degenerated neurones often show an accumulation of lipid material.

The accent of the pathology may fall on different regions, accounting for the various clinical pictures that are seen. The cortex is nearly always involved, although often with relative sparing of the parietal and occipital lobes. The hippocampi may also escape. In different cases there may be a marked emphasis on the corpus striatum, thalamus, cerebellum, substantia nigra, brainstem and spinal cord. The corticospinal tracts and also the extrapyramidal pathways are often severely degenerated.

The 'status spongiosus' of the cortex is highly characteristic, showing as finely meshed vacuolation under the microscope. The vacuoles then enlarge and coalesce to form microcysts (Lantos *et al.* 1992; Bell & Ironside 1993). Severely affected areas have the appearance of being riddled with tiny cavities. In some varieties this is widely disseminated. Electron microscopy shows the presence of vacuoles within the cytoplasm of neurones and astrocytes, particularly within dendrites, and the accumulation of abnormal cytoskeletal protein. Status spongiosus is not entirely pathognomonic for CJD, having occasionally been reported in SDAT, Pick's disease, Wilson's disease and other degenerative conditions.

There are usually no senile plaques or neurofibrillary tangles as in AD, no massive circumscribed atrophy as in Pick's disease, and no evidence of an inflammatory reaction. However, some cases show extracellular amyloid plaques especially in the cerebellum. The cerebral vessels appear healthy, or if cerebrovascular disease is present this appears to be incidental. Immunocytochemistry using antibodies to prion protein gives a positive reaction, which can be useful diagnostically in uncertain cases.

Variant and familial forms of CJD

Variant CJD was first described in 1996 by Will *et al.* and shows both clinical and pathological differences from sporadic CJD (Stewart & Ironside 1998; Collinge 1999). The onset is much earlier, typically in young adults, and course is more rapid. The onset is usually with neuropsychiatric symptoms including depression, anxiety and behavioural changes (Zeidler *et al.* 1997b). This is followed rapidly by cerebellar ataxia and myoclonus, followed later by cognitive deterioration and ending in a prolonged period of akinetic mutism. A small proportion of patients (<10%) may present with cerebellar ataxia at outset (Cooper, S.A. *et al.* 2006). The neuropathology is also distinct, showing florid amyloid plaques surrounded by vacuolation (Will *et al.* 1996).

Familial CJD is rare but shows some genotype–phenotype correlations. Thus families with the octapeptide repeat and those with G114V and H187R mutations show notably early neuropsychiatric symptoms and/or personality problems (Mead 2006). Mead (2006) reviews this phenotypic variability and correlation with mutation and notes that families with the E200K mutation present with rapidly progressive dementia with myoclonus in their late fifties, with those also having 129M homozygosity showing a unique PrP deposit

in the cerebellum. On the other hand, families with the octapeptide repeat show a high degree of phenotypic variability, with age of onset from 21 to 82 years and a very highly variable clinical presentation, disease course and neuropathological findings.

Other TSEs

Gerstmann–Sträussler–Scheinker disease is an inherited TSE also resulting from mutations in the *PRNP* gene. It is rare, with a frequency of 1–10 per 10 million population (Liberski & Budka 2004). It typically presents with progressive ataxia, extrapyramidal symptoms, dysarthria and dementia and has an early age of onset, usually in the fourth or fifth decade (Collins *et al.* 2001). The average disease duration is 7 years and the neuropathology includes elements of the TSEs such as spongiform change and astrocytosis, as well as features of AD as there are, in many cases, neurofibrillary tangles (Ghetti *et al.* 1994) and amyloid plaques. The tangles are composed of the same protein (tau) as in AD, but the plaques are predominantly PrP.

Fatal familial insomnia is also a *PRNP* mutation disorder. Interestingly, the mutation D178N in the gene results in FFI when codon 129 codes for methionine but results in CJD when codon 129 codes for valine. The clinical picture is of disruption in circadian cycles resulting in insomnia, dysautonomia and motor dysfunction (Benarroch & Stotz-Potter 1998). On examination there may be chronic hypertension and loss of nocturnal decrease in blood pressure. Laboratory studies show hypercortisolism together with elevated catecholamine levels and abnormal rhythms of growth hormone, prolactin and melatonin. Neuropathological findings include severe thalamic degeneration.

Assessment and differential diagnosis

Every patient suspected of a primary dementia requires comprehensive evaluation. This will in all cases require certain investigatory procedures in addition to the routines of history-taking and clinical examination. It is commonly held that the principal aim must be to exclude a remediable cause for the patient's symptoms and that the diagnosis of AD is one of exclusion. However, truly reversible causes of dementia are rare, vanishingly so in the elderly, and although important to be alert to the possibility, a specialist in old age psychiatry may never see such a case. Nor is it true that the diagnosis is one of exclusion: AD, the commonest dementia, has a characteristic presentation and can be confidently diagnosed following a careful clinical evaluation. Diagnosis is important because it carries with it prognostic information, treatment options and is highly valued by families and carers. A full evaluation is important not only to assess the primary disorder but also other concomitant disorders that may still be aggravating the situation and will sometimes have caused the patient to present at this particular time. Indeed cognition is profoundly affected by physical illness even in those without dementia, and treating systemic illness improves cognition even to the point of changing patients below the threshold for dementia on screening scales to the normal range (Inouye *et al.* 2006; Milosevic *et al.* 2007). This is important but in most cases a thorough evaluation would readily distinguish between the physically ill with cognitive symptoms and those with a primary dementia.

Conditions amenable to treatment include pathologies within the skull such as cerebral tumour, subdural haematoma, normal-pressure hydrocephalus and general paresis, also certain systemic disorders that may be impairing cerebral function indirectly. These indirect impairments include the several causes of cerebral anoxia, myxoedema, hypoglycaemia, metabolic derangements due to renal or hepatic disease, vitamin deficiencies, alcoholism, and intoxication due to various drugs and chemicals. The tendency, especially in the elderly, for a depressive illness to masquerade as dementia or to aggravate its manifestations must also be remembered. However, depression presenting in late life can be prodromal for dementia and even apparent dementia reversing with resolution of depression (pseudodementia) turns out not to be a benign condition as 5 years later the majority will have an established dementia (Saez-Fonseca *et al.* 2007).

The proportion of patients that appear not to have dementia at all has been reported as relatively high in an early series of reports of consecutive series of suspected dementia cases, largely early onset and mostly admitted to neurological units (Marsden & Harrison 1972; Victoratos *et al.* 1977; Smith & Kiloh 1981). In these series some 15% of the patients were judged not to be demented after full evaluation, but to be suffering from some other organic psychosyndrome or from non-organic psychiatric disorder. Tumours and normal-pressure hydrocephalus were not infrequent in these series. Among the eight tumours in Marsden and Harrison's series three were benign, three had no abnormal neurological signs and seven showed global impairment of intellect without focal psychological deficits. Non-organic psychiatric disorder masquerading as dementia was common in the UK and Australian series, and amounts to 8% of cases overall. Depression is most often responsible. In discussing such results, Wells (1978) concludes that potentially correctable disorders (depression, drug toxicity, hydrocephalus, benign intracranial masses) may be expected in some 15% of patients, with an additional 20–25% in whom some useful intervention will be possible (control of hypertension, withdrawal of alcohol or genetic counselling).

More recent reports confirm a substantially different rate of non-degenerative and non-vascular dementia in early-onset versus late-onset cases. In a large study from the Rochester Epidemiology Project, of all incident dementia cases, 30% of early-onset but only 8% of late-onset cases were due to non-degenerative and non-vascular dementia, with the commonest causes being cancer, chronic mental illness and alcoholism (Knopman *et al.* 2006). Interestingly, two commonly held views are dispelled by this report: (i) none of the causes of 'reversible dementia' commonly sought, including normal-pressure hydrocephalus, subdural hematoma, hypothyroidism, vitamin B_{12} deficiency or neurosyphilis, were found and (ii) not a single case of dementia was found to be reversible after treatment. The prevalence of non-degenerative and non-vascular apparent dementia appears to be declining, possibly as a consequence of improved diagnostic practice or possibly because the numbers of people with uncomplicated dementia coming to the attention of specialists is increasing. A review in 1988 of nearly 3000 subjects with dementia found 13% to have a potentially reversible dementia and a follow-up meta-analysis to 2002 including over 5500 patients with dementia showed only 9% to have a potentially reversible dementia and only 0.6% to actually reverse (Clarfield 1988, 2003). These results may not hold true everywhere: in one report from India, a relatively high proportion of neuroinfections and vitamin B_{12} deficiency was found and in many cases the dementia was indeed reversible (Srikanth & Nagaraja 2005).

A broad attitude to the question of differential diagnosis must be maintained throughout all stages of the clinical enquiry. The history provides important clues, similarly the physical and mental state examinations. Psychometric assessment can be very helpful, especially in borderline cases and in confirming or refuting the global nature of the patient's intellectual difficulties. Certain ancillary investigations will always be needed, as set out below. In the majority of cases the definitive diagnosis will soon become apparent, but occasionally the picture will be perplexing and the search may need to be far ranging. Occasionally, complete investigation will leave one with probabilities rather than certainties, and it will then be necessary to see what course the disorder takes with time. Lack of clear confirmation of the diagnosis will mean that it is essential to keep the patient under regular review, with readiness to investigate anew if later developments are in any way unusual.

History

Family history can be of prime importance in early-onset cases and when the presentation is atypical. Differential diagnosis of a familial dementia includes AD, FTDs, Huntington's disease or familial spongiform encephalopathies. A marked family history of affective disorder may occasionally help towards the identification of depressive pseudodementia.

Antecedent history may contain clues of great significance. Even slight head injury can lead to a subdural haematoma, especially in elderly, arteriosclerotic or alcoholic subjects. This may declare itself only after a considerable latent interval. Normal-pressure hydrocephalus may likewise be traceable to prior head injury, subarachnoid haemorrhage or meningitis.

Recent fits, faints or episodes of collapse will indicate the possibility of a cerebral tumour, cerebral infarction, episodic hypoglycaemia or an undiagnosed myocardial infarction that has led to cerebral anoxia. Previous episodes of transient neurological disturbance will raise the question of vascular dementia or multiple sclerosis.

Special care must be taken whenever there is a previous history of anaemia, heart disease or chronic pulmonary disorder which may now be leading to cerebral anoxia. The recent administration of an anaesthetic may be significant, or any episode of carbon monoxide poisoning or prolonged coma due to drug overdosage.

Recent illnesses must be viewed in relation to their effects on cerebral function, in particular hepatic or renal disease which may have led to metabolic disturbance, or infective processes that may have resulted in a cerebral abscess.

Dietary neglect may have produced vitamin B or folic acid deficiency, either as a primary aetiological factor or as a complication of the dementing process. A history of gastrectomy may be especially significant in relation to vitamin B_{12} deficiency. Some patients with dementia and vitamin B_{12} deficiency do improve after correction of the deficit and those that do may have a somewhat different neuropsychological presentation (Osimani *et al.* 2005).

Alcoholism deserves careful and sometimes pressing enquiry. The progressive inefficiency and deterioration of habits in alcoholic subjects can present as a possible dementing process, and Korsakoff's syndrome can at first sight be mistaken for global intellectual impairment. Drug abuse should be suspected when the picture fluctuates from time to time or when there is a history of similar episodes in the past. A history of relevant behaviours will bring the possibility of HIV infection to mind. Medication recently prescribed should also always be determined. In obscure cases the patient's occupation warrants consideration, with enquiry about the possibility of chronic poisoning from lead, manganese or other chemicals.

Certain symptoms are of importance. Headache, visual disturbance or vomiting will raise the possibility of a space-occupying lesion. Epileptic fits, especially with focal onset, must similarly be noted with care. Other complaints that may indicate focal rather than diffuse cerebral disease include special difficulty with language, trouble in recognising people or objects, or inability to carry out habitual acts and manipulations.

Benson and Cummings (1982) have drawn attention to the 'angular gyrus syndrome' which may easily be confused with AD on account of the number of features they have in common. Such patients present with posterior aphasia, alexia with agraphia, Gerstmann's syndrome and constructional deficits, usually as a consequence of cerebral inf-

arction. The abrupt onset, if known, will give the clue, likewise the preservation of memory and topographical orientation. Malaise, loss of energy and anorexia will suggest anaemia, uraemia or occult malignant disease. A cough of recent onset and severe loss of weight will suggest carcinoma of the lung, which can sometimes present with dementia in the absence of secondary cerebral deposits. Sensitivity to cold will immediately raise the possibility of myxoedema, and excessive thirst or bone pain may suggest parathyroid disorder.

Mode of evolution of the illness is of great diagnostic importance. Separate note must be taken of the nature of the principal early difficulties, the duration up to the time of presentation, the certainty or uncertainty of onset, and the steadiness or otherwise of progression.

Onset with memory disturbance is characteristic of most primary dementias, especially AD, which is the commonest form. In the elderly this may for a time be difficult to distinguish from the 'normal' memory difficulties of old age; the dysmnesia of senescence typically progresses very slowly, and occurs in a setting of relative preservation of other cognitive processes, whereas in dementia other aspects of intellect usually soon come to be implicated. Any onset with symptoms other than memory disturbance should always raise suspicion. Marked affective disturbance or change of personality may be seen with Pick's disease, other frontal dementias or Huntington's disease, but may equally be indicative of a frontal lobe tumour or general paresis.

A short duration immediately raises the possibility of a secondary dementia due to cerebral tumour, covert cerebral infarction, AIDS or some extracranial cause. In most primary dementing illnesses the symptoms are of long duration, usually of many months by the time the patient presents for attention.

Caution should be paid when interpreting apparently sudden onset as the suddenness may simply represent infrequency of contact between the patient and the informant, especially in the elderly. Anecdotally, onset is not infrequently at national holidays, Christmas and Easter for example, when the elderly person with an early but as yet unrecognised dementia may have more contact with family members, may have more cognitive and functional tasks to perform (e.g. cooking, shopping) and may find themselves in an unfamiliar environment (staying with a relative, being taken on holiday). All these may 'reveal' the dementia, which may then present to the clinician as sudden onset.

A definite date for the onset is also rarely obtained in the primary dementias, which tend to begin so insidiously that neither the patient nor family can give a precise timing to the earliest manifestations. In contrast, with cerebral tumours there is usually some episode or symptom that can later be recalled as the first indication of the illness. This information can be important in tumours that are unaccompanied by headache or other evidence of raised intracranial pressure, or for example in frontal meningiomas which can present with global dementia and lack all focal signs.

Steady progression without remission is typical of all the primary dementias with the exception of multi infarct dementia. Marked fluctuations from time to time must therefore immediately suggest that one may be dealing not with a chronic but an acute organic reaction, or at least with an acute component superimposed on the basic dementing process. Considerable difficulty can sometimes be encountered in differentiating between a subacute organic reaction and dementia, especially multi-infarct dementia. The elderly are unusually vulnerable to the effects of anoxia or metabolic derangements, and the responsible somatic disease may not be very obvious. A markedly intermittent course, with periods of possible clouding of consciousness or delirium, should therefore be noted with care, and will indicate the need for survey of the cardiac, pulmonary, renal, hepatic and endocrine systems. Fluctuations and periods of remission will also raise the possibility of a subdural haematoma or drug abuse. An intermittent course with discrete episodes of abnormal behaviour may suggest hypoglycaemia, and when severe this can leave enduring dementia in its wake.

Examination

Physical examination is important in suggesting remediable causes of dementia but more so in revealing systemic disorders that may be aggravating the situation, especially in the elderly. The general appearance may suggest myxoedema or malnutrition. Inspection of the skin and tongue may indicate dehydration, vitamin depletion or anaemia. A patient who looks unwell will be suspected of metabolic disorder, malignant disease or some infective process. Common foci of infection in the elderly include low-grade pneumonia or bronchitis, and in women cystitis. A low-grade intermittent pyrexia may raise the possibility of subacute encephalitis, cerebral abscess, collagen vascular disorder or, on rare occasions, multiple embolisation in association with subacute bacterial endocarditis. The cardiovascular state always requires appraisal with regard to hypertension, arteriosclerosis, congestive cardiac failure and the patency of the carotid arteries in the neck.

Neurological examination will rarely reveal marked localising signs in the primary dementias, with the exception of some cases of vascular and poststroke dementia and the rare cases of CJD. Evidence of focal paresis or sensory loss in association with a slowly progressive dementia therefore immediately raises the possibility of a space-occupying lesion. Considerable care must sometimes be taken to exclude visual field defects or unilateral anosmia, which can be difficult in patients who are less than fully cooperative.

Examination of the optic fundi may reveal evidence of raised intracranial pressure. The pupil reactions may betray general paresis, and nystagmus will suggest barbiturate intoxication. A Kayser–Fleischer ring at the corneal margins will indicate Wilson's disease. Pronounced ataxia in association with memory disturbance will suggest the residue of Wernicke's encephalopathy, and peripheral neuropathy will raise the possibility of alcoholism or heavy metal poisoning. Evidence of dysarthria, minor dysphagia or a brisk jaw jerk may indicate early pseudobulbar palsy, and should be carefully assessed when cerebral arteriosclerosis is suspected.

Early incontinence and unsteadiness of gait are important pointers towards normal-pressure hydrocephalus. Close observation may sometimes be required for the detection of the early choreiform movements of Huntington's disease, and myoclonic jerking in association with dementia will raise the possibility of CJD. Evidence of Parkinson's disease or multiple sclerosis must not be overlooked. The prominent development of parkinsonian features, either early or late in the course, will suggest DLB. Rigidity, tremor or dystonia in the younger patient will raise suspicion of Wilson's disease.

Mental state evaluation is principally directed at establishing the global nature of the intellectual disorder. Care must be taken to avoid mistaking dysphasia, circumscribed amnesic difficulties or parietal lobe symptomatology for global dementia. Somnolence, in the absence of uraemia or other metabolic disorder, will suggest hypothalamic damage. A marked degree of emotional lability with pathological laughing and crying will suggest a vascular process, with an accent on the basal regions of the brain. Any suspicion of clouding of consciousness will immediately raise the possibility that one is dealing with an acute organic reaction rather than dementia, or that there is some complicating toxic, infective or metabolic disorder present.

The mental state evaluation is equally important for the detection of depression presenting as dementia (i.e. pseudodementia). Inconsistencies in the patient's performance may raise the question of a Ganser state, hysterical pseudodementia or even, on rare occasions, simulation. The patient's attitude to his symptoms and the degree to which his purported disabilities interfere with daily life can be observations of crucial importance. Affective changes sometimes need to be sought with care. A marked depressive component may indicate depressive pseudodementia, or concurrent depression may be aggravating the situation in a patient with organic cerebral disease.

Assessment of non-cognitive symptoms in established dementia is critical and should be an ongoing task. These include behavioural change, depression, anxiety, psychosis and personality changes and may be achieved in the clinical context by interview of the informant, assessment of the patient and in many cases with the addition of one of the many excellent scales used widely in research.

Psychometric testing will often be of value. Bedside cognitive testing will be performed in all instances and will include assessment of multiple domains of cognition; it has become routine to incorporate a standard assessment measure such as the MMSE as a measure of severity, although it should be remembered that this scale was developed as a screening scale. Tests of frontal and parietal function help in the differential diagnosis. Further detailed psychometry, usually by a psychologist, is often helpful but rarely mandatory. It may help in the distinction between organic and non-organic psychiatric illness and with the question of diffuse versus focal cerebral disorder. In very early cases psychometry provides a measured baseline against which future progress can be assessed.

Assessment of function is critical to the full evaluation of the patient. A wide variety of scales are available for research but in clinical practice a very careful history from the patient and the informant is usually sufficient. It can be difficult to assess loss of function in the very early stages and careful and patient assessment of complex tasks that might be expected of the patient and were once easily accomplished is necessary. The assessment of an occupational therapist is often essential to both aid diagnosis and help plan management.

Diogenes' syndrome, squalor and self-neglect
(Cooney & Hamid 1995)

Patients are occasionally found to be living in a state of extreme squalor and gross physical neglect, yet prove to be free from any psychiatric disorder sufficient to account for it. In particular, their cognitive functions may emerge as relatively or completely intact. This has been designated Diogenes' syndrome or 'senile self-neglect', although the nosological status of the condition remains uncertain (Pavlou & Lachs 2006). Some may be in the early stages of a dementing illness while others appear to be suffering essentially from personality disorder. Quite often such patients prove to be solitary and reclusive individuals who are reacting to stress, bereavement or loneliness. Hoarding rituals may have become entrenched, and serious medical illness or disability is not uncommon. Orrell *et al.* (1989) have reported marked frontal lobe dysfunction on neuropsychological examination in some instances, raising the possibility that frontal lobe dementia may occasionally be responsible. Reports of such patients underline the need for careful assessment of elderly patients even when first appearances are strongly suggestive of advanced AD. A cross-sectional survey showed 70% of people with self-neglect had a mental health problem, although only half of those had had any contact with mental health services (Halliday 2000).

Investigations

In the primary dementias there are no specific abnormalities in the blood, urine, CSF or neuroimaging. However, there are some indicators that help in differential diagnosis and some promising developments in biomarker research. For the most part investigations are directed at detecting remediable conditions or uncovering systemic disorders that may be worsening the clinical picture.

It is widely accepted that a minimum investigation screen for every patient with dementia includes full blood count, blood urea, serum electrolytes and liver function tests. Tests of thyroid function and vitamin B_{12} and folate, and in some patients syphilis serology, are appropriate. If delirium is suspected, urine examination should be supplemented by microscopy and where necessary culture. Chest radiography may be performed for the evaluation of cardiac and pulmonary status and as a screen for primary or secondary carcinoma.

Electroencephalography is oft-neglected but can be useful. Non-specific changes occur early in AD and yet the EEG remains entirely normal relatively late in FTD. Specific changes are seen in CJD. The ECG is an important investigation if the patient is being considered for acetylcholinesterase therapy.

Neuroimaging of some sort is considered mandatory by most European and American specialist groups (Beck *et al.* 2000; Knopman *et al.* 2001; Frisoni *et al.* 2003; Kantarci & Jack 2003; Waldemar *et al.* 2007). CT can be used to identify vascular lesions and treatable masses but MRI adds greatly to specificity. Special indications for scanning will include any remote suspicion of a cerebral tumour or subdural haematoma, the presence of focal neurological signs, a history suggestive of cerebral infarction or head injury, or clinical pointers towards normal-pressure hydrocephalus. Imaging shows cerebral atrophy with ventricular dilatation and prominence of cortical sulci but without distortion or displacement of the ventricular system. The distribution of atrophy may point towards a diagnosis of Pick's disease or other frontal dementia, or marked shrinkage of the heads of the caudate nuclei may indicate Huntington's disease. Evidence of old and recent cerebral infarctions may suggest a vascular basis for the dementia. However, these changes are neither sensitive nor specific markers of dementia and questions have been raised regarding its utility in assessment. SPECT and even PET can be used to identify a characteristic pattern of regional brain hypometabolism. Posterior parietotemporal deficits in regional blood flow or metabolism, though not pathognomonic, may add to a suspicion of Alzheimer's dementia while sharply circumscribed frontal deficits may indicate FTD for example.

A raft of neuroimaging techniques are being developed that might be of use in diagnosing or monitoring progression in AD. These include the use of diffusion tension imaging, functional MRI or PET-based molecular markers of amyloid (Jagust 2004; Masdeu *et al.* 2005; Walker & Walker 2005; Catani 2006). None of these techniques have yet escaped the research context into the clinic but do show promise in doing so.

Lumbar puncture is rarely of value in the routine assessment of people with dementia and is not recommended in typical cases (Waldemar *et al.* 2007). However, it may be undertaken if the cause for the dementia remains uncertain and when there is no reason to suspect a cerebral tumour or raised intracranial pressure. Examination of the CSF can be decisive in the diagnosis of general paresis in cases when blood serology has been negative. Dementia can also occur with syphilitic arteritis which has produced scattered cerebral infarcts. The first indication of a subdural haematoma may come from an elevated CSF pressure, increased protein or xanthochromia. Subacute and chronic forms of encephalitis may likewise be detected only after examination of the fluid. The assessment of 14-3-3 protein may be useful as it has good sensitivity and specificity for CJD. Biomarkers in CSF are being actively sought and the most promising of these are tau and amyloid (Fagan *et al.* 2005; Sunderland *et al.* 2005). Whether these tests will become part of recommended clinical practice remains to be seen.

Very occasionally it will be deemed advisable to exclude other rare conditions that can give rise to dementia. Wilson's disease is detected by the estimation of serum caeruloplasmin and confirmed by liver biopsy. Neuroacanthocytosis requires examination of fresh blood films and metachromatic leucodystrophy the estimation of arylsulphatase-A in the blood or urine, or biopsies of the peripheral nerve or rectal wall. Kufs disease is detectable by skeletal muscle or rectal biopsy, Whipple's disease by lymph node or jejunal biopsy, and mitochondrial myopathies by a search for 'ragged red fibres' in skeletal muscle biopsy. A search for sarcoid may involve radiography of the phalanges, biopsy of the lymph nodes or skin lesions, and the Kveim intradermal test. Most familial dementias can be categorised by genetic testing, although it is important to bear in mind that this is not a diagnostic test as the mutation will have been present for life. Even in these cases where an absolute molecular categorisation can be made, the diagnosis of whether the patient is affected relies on the clinician's skill and sensitivity in establishing the very early symptoms.

Management of dementia

The reader would be well advised to consult recent guidelines on management of dementia for current treatment strategies, especially when it comes to pharmacotherapy of both the dementia and the behavioural symptoms in dementia. Here the general principles of management are discussed. The first step in management is always full medical evaluation along the lines already discussed. This is necessary for firm establishment of the diagnosis, the exclusion of remediable conditions masquerading as primary dementia, and to check on any concurrent disease that may be aggravating the symptoms. In cases where the first evaluation has given equivocal results, this must be borne in mind during follow-up, with readiness to reopen investigations if the course is in any way unusual.

Diagnosis and information

After establishing the diagnosis, both the disease and the person suffering from it together with their carers and wider family must be kept in mind. Difficult decisions will often have to be made over such questions as continuation with work in early-onset cases and how fully to explain about prognosis. The clinician will need to consider, with the patient and his or her family, whether the patient should continue to drive and later perhaps whether to continue to live at home. On all these issues much will depend on factors specific to the individual and his family.

Attitudes to sharing the diagnosis with the patient are changing and now almost all patients with mild dementia wish to be told (Pinner & Bouman 2003). Family members may be less sure and indeed may request the clinician not to disclose the diagnosis, placing him or her in a difficult situation (Hughes *et al.* 2002). Disclosing diagnosis and discussing prognosis is a sensitive task and needs to be approached with skill and with care. Reassurance is not, in the end, reassuring when inappropriate and yet it is true that an unnecessarily pessimistic attitude concentrating on only negative consequences and a hopeless outlook is not helpful to either the patient or the carer. General counselling principles apply here as much as elsewhere in medicine and the most thoughtful clinicians will convey an attitude of care and attention, will share the facts and information they have, will have time to address fears and concerns and will above all be guided and led by the recipient of the information, be that the patient or the family.

Many families and patients benefit from contact with a carer or lay organisation. There are many such including the Alzheimer's Society in the UK and the Alzheimer's Association in the USA. An umbrella body, Alzheimer's Disease International, encourages the growth of similar societies throughout the world. These groups provide a wealth of information through local groups, through their websites and with pamphlets, books and leaflets. No carer should remain ignorant of their existence. Carer groups are immensely valuable for many families and may be organised by clinical services or the lay societies.

One issue that should be addressed as early as possible concerns the long-term financial and legal standing of the patient. In the UK the establishment of a lasting power of attorney, whereby the patient's financial affairs are placed in the hands of another, is the main mechanism for this. There are similar arrangements in many other countries. Most countries, including the UK, have separate legal frameworks for establishing decision-making on behalf of a person already rendered incapable of making complex decisions and for setting out advance directives for future health care and for passing over decision-making to a responsible other person before capacity is lost. Clearly, where possible, the latter is preferable.

Community and residential care

The vast majority of people with dementia remain at home for an extensive period and many remain at home throughout their illness. A comprehensive service for people with dementia will integrate medical and other clinical care providers with social care providers. A case or key worker can help to integrate these elements with services provided by the voluntary sector. The care of a person with dementia is complex and changes as the illness progresses. The patient's needs will differ over time and the family will have needs as well that should be considered.

In the early stages all that may be required is information and possibly the support of a care worker or a support group. As the patient becomes more impaired then home care might include the provision of meals, cleaning services, shopping, supervision or other services. Carers can be provided with support and respite. A day unit, usually a day-centre, sometimes a day-hospital, might be needed to provide respite and also more detailed ongoing assessment and activites. In some services home care can be provided multiple times a day, seven days a week; in other areas such requirements point to the need for residential care.

When the patient can no longer be managed at home, optimal placement must be arranged. Much will depend on local facilities and the extent to which social, psychiatric and geriatric services have become organised. Families may resist residential care at first, feeling guilty or considering this a slight on their provision of care. Sensitive handling is needed. Care does not stop at the door of a residential home and the best homes are well supported by local service providers. Preparation should ideally be made well in advance of the time when this is likely to be required, although this is not always possible. The needs of different patients are widely variable, and should ideally be matched by a similarly broad range of resources.

The stress experienced by families caring for a demented relative, sometimes called burden, has been extensively studied (Burns 2000). Up to one-quarter of all carers experience significant stress or anxiety and the rates of carer burden are higher when caring for a patient with more severe behavioural symptoms (Sorensen *et al.* 2006), although there are other determinants of carer stress including younger carers, financial difficulties and perceived stigma (Freyne *et al.* 1999; Schneider *et al.* 1999; Cooper *et al.* 2007).

The range of therapies for people with dementia is wide, although the evidence base for many is variable (Bates *et al.* 2004; Robinson *et al.* 2006). The reader is directed towards recent studies of validation therapy (Neal & Briggs 2003; Tondi *et al.* 2007), reality orientation therapy (Onder *et al.* 2005), cognitive stimulation therapy (Spector *et al.* 2003) and

aromatherapy (Ballard *et al.* 2002b; Thorgrimsen *et al.* 2003) for example. While awaiting a more complete evidence base the pragmatic clinician combines the possible with the appreciated and hopes for the best.

Medical management

The medical management of dementia is undergoing rapid developments, with the availability of new drugs for both the disease itself and treatment of behavioural symptoms. Optimal physical health must be maintained if the patient's deterioration is to be slowed and the best use made of residual functions at any given stage. Attention to adequate nutrition, hydration and vitamin replacement can sometimes meet with gratifying improvement. The elimination of infection is a matter for repeated checks, particularly chronic infection within the lungs or urinary tract. Any tendency towards congestive cardiac failure, cardiac dysrhythmia or anaemia must be treated energetically. Hypertension, when severe, will warrant appropriate management. Special care must be taken to guard against iatrogenic disorders, particularly electrolyte imbalance due to diuretics and toxicity from other drugs. A recent study showed a very substantial effect of drugs on rates of progression, with some prescribed drugs accelerating and some slowing progression (Ellul *et al.* 2007).

In vascular dementia there will often be a special case for strict control of hypertension, and sometimes for treatment with anticoagulants or aspirin. However, management decisions should be made on the basis of cardiac disease because there is insufficient evidence to currently recommend any treatment for the dementia itself (Waldemar *et al.* 2007). Other vascular risk factors such as hypercholesterolaemia or diabetes will need special attention. Vasculitis may require treatment with corticosteroids.

Adequate physical exercise must be encouraged, sometimes with the aid of physiotherapy. Orthopaedic complications may need attention in the elderly. Adequate daily activity will induce normal fatigue and lessen the incidence of disturbed and restless nights. It will also help defer the time when nursing in bed, and hence the terminal stages, are reached. There is some evidence that exercise may even delay decline (Rolland *et al.* 2007).

Psychotropic medication will often be needed to allay agitation and depression. In general, however, one will wish to avoid using drugs with strong anticholinergic effects for prolonged periods, in view of the known cholinergic deficits in AD. Treatment of depression should be vigorous and pharmacotherapy should avoid antidepressants with significant anticholinergic action; arguably this makes one of the best cases for using a selective serotonin reuptake inhibitor (SSRI). Disappointingly, few trials have been conducted but those that have show a beneficial effect of SSRIs (Lyketsos *et al.* 2003; Rao *et al.* 2006). Pharmacotherapy must be combined with non-pharmacological management.

Treatment of other BPSD also requires a combined pharmacological and non-pharmacological approach, with the emphasis on the latter not only because it is most efficacious but because it is safest (Ayalon *et al.* 2006; Angelini *et al.* 2007; Bird *et al.* 2007). Pharmacological treatment of BPSD is difficult and the general approach of 'start low, go slow' should be adopted. Atypical antipsychotics have been most studied and a meta-analysis finds some evidence of efficacy in BPSD (Schneider *et al.* 2006a). However, antipsychotic medication is most efficacious for psychosis and rarely has any effects on generalised behavioural disturbance other than general sedation. The evidence that atypical antipsychotics have an increased rate of serious adverse effects and indeed increased mortality in this group of patients is growing and these drugs should be used only under very strict scrutiny, by engaged clinicians reviewing the need for the medication regularly and only in extremis when all other approaches have failed. It may be that the lack of evidence for adverse effects of typical antipsychotics simply represents absence of evidence rather than evidence of safety. In general, the results from one large multicentre trial match the views of many clinicans who have come to the conclusion that for many patients the benefits of antipsychotics in dementia is outweighed by their side effects (Schneider *et al.* 2006b).

Alzheimer's disease

In the late 1990s the first specific drugs for AD received a licence. The acetylcholinesterase inhibitors, currently donepezil, rivastigmine and galanthamine, have been shown to be efficacious and safe in AD (Francis *et al.* 1999; Birks 2006; Burns *et al.* 2006). Their use is widely recommended, although reimbursement and support for their prescription is variable, not least as there is little evidence that they are cost-effective. In the UK an extensive set of reviews by the National Institute for Clinical Excellence (NICE) has currently concluded that they should be prescribed for patients with moderate AD only. A second class of drug, currently represented only by memantine, was shown to be efficacious in severe dementia and is licensed and widely prescribed in the USA and in Europe but is not recommended by NICE (Robinson & Keating 2006; Cosman *et al.* 2007).

In general terms, treatment with cholinesterase inhibitors has followed guidelines established for a decade or so (Lovestone *et al.* 1997). Patients should be monitored throughout: early and frequently for titration and for assessment of side effects and less often but continuously for efficacy. Expectations of patients and carers should be managed: these drugs have a modest effect, at best, and decline continues regardless. When a patient progresses to the point that the drug is unlikely to be having a benefit, then it should be stopped and carers should have been warned that this will occur at the outset. A drug holiday can be useful in establishing whether the drug is still having an effect, although precipitous falls in cognition can occur and carers should be primed to urgently restart medication.

Other disorders

There is no evidence for a specific indication of any therapeutic approach in a non-AD dementia. However, there is some limited evidence that patients with DLB respond to cholinesterase inhibitors and to levodopa (McKeith *et al.* 2005; Liepelt *et al.* 2007) and excellent evidence that these patients can have a severe and sometimes fatal response to antipsychotic medication. The evidence base for the use of cholinesterase inhibitors in vascular dementia is not as strong as that for AD and the drugs are not licensed for that condition. However, given that most patients with 'vascular dementia' also have changes of AD and vice versa, it is not surprising that many patients respond to cholinesterase inhibitors in much the same way as patients with AD (Erkinjuntti *et al.* 2004). There is little or no evidence that lowering blood pressure is beneficial to the dementia condition (McGuinness *et al.* 2006). Specific treatment may help in Huntington's disease for the control of choreic movements. Phenothiazines are widely employed for this purpose and have been shown to be effective, especially haloperidol. However, a meta-analysis and systematic review failed to make any robust clinically relevant reccomendations (Bonelli & Wenning 2006).

References

Aarsland, D., Cummings, J.L., Yenner, G. & Miller, B. (1996) Relationship of aggressive behavior to other neuropsychiatric symptoms in patients with Alzheimer's disease. *American Journal of Psychiatry* **153**, 243–247.

Aarsland, D., Ballard, C., Larsen, J.P. & McKeith, I. (2001) A comparative study of psychiatric symptoms in dementia with Lewy bodies and Parkinson's disease with and without dementia. *International Journal of Geriatric Psychiatry* **16**, 528–536.

Adam, S., Wiggins, S., Whyte, P. *et al.* (1993) Five year study of prenatal testing for Huntington's disease: demand, attitudes, and psychological assessment. *Journal of Medical Genetics* **30**, 549–556.

Adams, I.M. (1991) Structural plasticity of synapses in Alzheimer's disease. *Molecular Neurobiology* **5**, 411–419.

Aguzzi, A. & Glatzel, M. (2006) Prion infections, blood and transfusions. *Nature Clinical Practice Neurology* **2**, 321–329.

Aguzzi, A. & Polymenidou, M. (2004) Mammalian prion biology: one century of evolving concepts. *Cell* **116**, 313–327.

Akiyama, H., Barger, S., Barnum, S. *et al.* (2000) Inflammation and Alzheimer's disease. *Neurobiology of Aging* **21**, 383–421.

Alexopoulos, G.S., Abrams, R.C., Young, R.C. & Shamoian, C.A. (1988) Cornell Scale for Depression in Dementia. *Biological Psychiatry* **23**, 271–284.

Allinson, T.M., Parkin, E.T., Turner, A.J. & Hooper, N.M. (2003) ADAMs family members as amyloid precursor protein alpha-secretases. *Journal of Neuroscience Research* **74**, 342–352.

Allsop, D., Landon, M. & Kidd, M. (1983) The isolation and amino acid composition of senile plaque core protein. *Brain Research* **259**, 348–352.

Almqvist, E.W., Brinkman, R.R., Wiggins, S. & Hayden, M.R. (2003) Psychological consequences and predictors of adverse events in the first 5 years after predictive testing for Huntington's disease. *Clinical Genetics* **64**, 300–309.

Alvarez, G., Muñoz-Montaño, J.R., Satrústegui, J., Avila, J., Bogónez, E. & Díaz-Nido, J. (1999) Lithium protects cultured neurons against β-amyloid-induced neurodegeneration. *FEBS Letters* **453**, 260–264.

Alzheimer, A. (1907) Über eine eigenartige Erkrankung der Hirnrinde. *Allgemeine Zeitschrift für Psychiatrie* **64**, 146–148.

Alzheimers Association and National Institute for Aging (1998) Consensus report of the Working Group on Molecular and Biochemical Markers of Alzheimer's Disease. *Neurobiology of Aging* **19**, 109–116.

Aminoff, M.J., Marshall, J., Smith, E.M. & Wyke, M.A. (1975) Pattern of intellectual impairment in Huntington's chorea. *Psychological Medicine* **5**, 169–172.

Andersen, C.K., Sogaard, J., Hansen, E. *et al.* (1999) The cost of dementia in Denmark: the Odense study. *Dementia* **10**, 295–304.

Andersen, K., Launer, L.J., Dewey, M.E. *et al.* (1999) Gender differences in the incidence of AD and vascular dementia: the EURODEM Studies. *Neurology* **53**, 1992–1997.

Anderson, R.M., Donnelly, C.A., Ferguson, N.M. *et al.* (1996) Transmission dynamics and epidemiology of BSE in British cattle. *Nature* **382**, 779–788.

Angelini, A., Bendini, C., Neviani, F. & Neri, M. (2007) Behavioral and psychological symptoms of dementia (BPSD) in elderly demented subjects: is the long lasting use of atypical antipsychotic drugs useful and safe? *Archives of Gerontology and Geriatrics* **44** (suppl.), 35–43.

Antuono, P.G., Jones, J.L., Wang, Y. & Li, S.J. (2001) Decreased glutamate + glutamine in Alzheimer's disease detected in vivo with (1)H-MRS at 0.5 T. *Neurology* **56**, 737–742.

Arai, Y., Yamazaki, M., Mori, O., Muramatsu, H., Asano, G. & Katayama, Y. (2001) α-Synuclein-positive structures in cases with sporadic Alzheimer's disease: morphology and its relationship to tau aggregation. *Brain Research* **888**, 287–296.

Arakawa, K., Nagara, H., Itoyama, Y. *et al.* (1991) Clustering of three cases of Creutzfeldt–Jakob disease near Fukuoka City, Japan. *Acta Neurologica Scandinavica* **84**, 445–447.

Avila, J., Lucas, J.J., Perez, M. & Hernandez, F. (2004) Role of tau protein in both physiological and pathological conditions. *Physiological Reviews* **84**, 361–384.

Ayalon, L., Gum, A.M., Feliciano, L. & Arean, P.A. (2006) Effectiveness of nonpharmacological interventions for the management of neuropsychiatric symptoms in patients with dementia: a systematic review. *Archives of Internal Medicine* **166**, 2182–2188.

Babcock, R.L. & Salthouse, T.A. (1990) Effects of increased processing demands on age differences in working memory. *Psychology and Aging* **5**, 421–428.

Bacanu, S.A., Devlin, B., Chowdari, K.V., DeKosky, S.T., Nimgaonkar, V.L. & Sweet, R.A. (2002) Linkage analysis of Alzheimer disease with psychosis. *Neurology* **59**, 118–120.

Ball, M.J. (1976) Neurofibrillary tangles and the pathogenesis of dementia: a quantitative study. *Neuropathology and Applied Neurobiology* **2**, 395–410.

Ballard, C., Bannister, C., Solis, M., Oyebode, F. & Wilcock, G. (1996) The prevalence, associations and symptoms of depression amongst dementia sufferers. *Journal of Affective Disorders* **36**, 135–144.

Ballard, C., Holmes, C., McKeith, I. *et al.* (1999a) Psychiatric morbidity in dementia with Lewy bodies: a prospective clinical and neuropathological comparative study with Alzheimer's disease. *American Journal of Psychiatry* **156**, 1039–1045.

Ballard, C.G., Shaw, F., Lowery, K., McKeith, I. & Kenny, R. (1999b) The prevalence, assessment and associations of falls in dementia with Lewy bodies and Alzheimer's disease. *Dementia* **10**, 97–103.

Ballard, C.G., Aarsland, D., McKeith, I. *et al.* (2002a) Fluctuations in attention: PD dementia vs DLB with parkinsonism. *Neurology* **59**, 1714–1720.

Ballard, C.G., O'Brien, J.T., Reichelt, K. & Perry, E.K. (2002b) Aromatherapy as a safe and effective treatment for the management of agitation in severe dementia: the results of a double-blind, placebo-controlled trial with Melissa. *Journal of Clinical Psychiatry* **63**, 553–558.

Bang, O.Y., Kwak, Y.T., Joo, I.S. & Huh, K. (2003) Important link between dementia subtype and apolipoprotein E: a meta-analysis. *Yonsei Medical Journal* **44**, 401–413.

Barber, R., Gholkar, A., Scheltens, P., Ballard, C., McKeith, I.G. & O'Brien, J.T. (2000) MRI volumetric correlates of white matter lesions in dementia with Lewy bodies and Alzheimer's disease. *International Journal of Geriatric Psychiatry* **15**, 911–916.

Baron, T. (2002) Identification of inter-species transmission of prion strains. *Journal of Neuropathology and Experimental Neurology* **61**, 377–383.

Bassiony, M.M., Warren, A., Rosenblatt, A. *et al.* (2002) The relationship between delusions and depression in Alzheimer's disease. *International Journal of Geriatric Psychiatry* **17**, 549–556.

Bates, G.P. & Gonitel, R. (2006) Mouse models of triplet repeat diseases. *Molecular Biotechnology* **32**, 147–158.

Bates, J., Boote, J. & Beverley, C. (2004) Psychosocial interventions for people with a milder dementing illness: a systematic review. *Journal of Advanced Nursing* **45**, 644–658.

Baudic, S., Maison, P., Dolbeau, G. *et al.* (2006) Cognitive impairment related to apathy in early Huntington's disease. *Dementia and Geriatric Cognitive Disorders* **21**, 316–321.

Baum, L., Lam, L.C., Kwok, T. *et al.* (2006) Apolipoprotein E epsilon4 allele is associated with vascular dementia. *Dementia and Geriatric Cognitive Disorders* **22**, 301–305.

Bear, M.F. & Malenka, R.C. (1994) Synaptic plasticity: LTP and LTD. *Current Opinion in Neurobiology* **4**, 389–399.

Beatus, P. & Lendahl, U. (1998) Notch and neurogenesis. *Journal of Neuroscience Research* **54**, 125–136.

Beaudry, P., Parchi, P., Peoc'h, K. *et al.* (2002) A French cluster of Creutzfeldt–Jakob disease: a molecular analysis. *European Journal of Neurology* **9**, 457–462.

Beck, C., Cody, M., Souder, E., Zhang, M. & Small, G.W. (2000) Dementia diagnostic guidelines: methodologies, results, and implementation costs. *Journal of the American Geriatric Society* **48**, 1195–1203.

Becker, J.T., Boller, F., Saxton, J. & McGonigle-Gibson, K.L. (1987) Normal rates of forgetting of verbal and non-verbal material in Alzheimer's disease. *Cortex* **23**, 59–72.

Bell, J.E. & Ironside, J.W. (1993) Neuropathology of spongiform encephalopathies in humans. *British Medical Bulletin* **49**, 738–777.

Benarroch, E.E. & Stotz-Potter, E.H. (1998) Dysautonomia in fatal familial insomnia as an indicator of the potential role of the thalamus in autonomic control. *Brain Pathology* **8**, 527–530.

Benson, D.F. & Cummings, J.L. (1982) Angular gyrus syndrome simulating Alzheimer's disease. *Archives of Neurology* **39**, 616–620.

Bergem, A.L.M., Engedal, K. & Kringlen, E. (1997) The role of heredity in late-onset Alzheimer disease and vascular dementia: a twin study. *Archives of General Psychiatry* **54**, 264–270.

Berger, Z., Ravikumar, B., Menzies, F.M. *et al.* (2006) Rapamycin alleviates toxicity of different aggregate-prone proteins. *Human Molecular Genetics* **15**, 433–442.

Berrios, G.E., Wagle, A.C., Markova, I.S., Wagle, S.A., Rosser, A. & Hodges, J.R. (2002) Psychiatric symptoms in neurologically asymptomatic Huntington's disease gene carriers: a comparison with gene negative at risk subjects. *Acta Psychiatrica Scandinavica* **105**, 224–230.

Bertram, L., Blacker, D., Mullin, K. *et al.* (2000) Evidence for genetic linkage of Alzheimer's disease to chromosome 10q. *Science* **290**, 2302–2303.

Bianchetti, A., Scuratti, A., Zanetti, O. *et al.* (1995) Predictors of mortality and institutionalization in Alzheimer disease patients 1 year after discharge from an Alzheimer dementia unit. *Dementia* **6**, 108–112.

Bickford, J.A.R. & Ellison, R.M. (1953) The high incidence of Huntington's chorea in the Duchy of Cornwall. *Journal of Mental Science* **99**, 291–294.

Bierer, L.M., Knott, P.J., Schmeidler, J.M. *et al.* (1993) Post-mortem examination of dopaminergic parameters in Alzheimer's disease: relationship to noncognitive symptoms. *Psychiatry Research* **49**, 211–217.

Biessels, G.J., Staekenborg, S., Brunner, E., Brayne, C. & Scheltens, P. (2006) Risk of dementia in diabetes mellitus: a systematic review. *Lancet Neurology* **5**, 64–74.

Bigio, E.H., Hynan, L.S., Sontag, E., Satumtira, S. & White, C.L. (2002) Synapse loss is greater in presenile than senile onset Alzheimer disease: implications for the cognitive reserve hypothesis. *Neuropathology and Applied Neurobiology* **28**, 218–227.

Binswanger, O. (1894) Die Abgrenzung der allgemeinen progressiven Paralyse. *Berliner klinische Wochenshrift* **31**, 1137–1139.

Bird, E.D. & Iverson, L.L. (1974) Huntington's chorea: postmortem measurement of glutamic acid decarboxylase, choline acetyl-transferase and dopamine in basal ganglia. *Brain* **97**, 457–472.

Bird, E.D., MacKay, A.V.P., Rayner, C.N. & Iversen, L.L. (1973) Reduced glutamic-acid-decarboxylase activity of post-mortem brain in Huntington's chorea. *Lancet* **i**, 1090–1092.

Bird, M., Jones, R.H., Korten, A. & Smithers, H. (2007) A controlled trial of a predominantly psychosocial approach to BPSD: treating causality. *International Psychogeriatrics* **19**, 874–891.

Bird, T., Knopman, D., VanSwieten, J. *et al.* (2003) Epidemiology and genetics of frontotemporal dementia/Pick's disease. *Annals of Neurology* **54** (suppl. 5), S29–S31.

Birkett, D.P. (1972) The psychiatric differentiation of senility and arteriosclerosis. *British Journal of Psychiatry* **120**, 321–325.

Birks, J. (2006) Cholinesterase inhibitors for Alzheimer's disease. *Cochrane Database of Systematic Reviews* CD005593.

Blacker, D., Bertram, L., Saunders, A.J. *et al.* (2003) Results of a high-resolution genome screen of 437 Alzheimer's Disease families. *Human Molecular Genetics* **12**, 23–32.

Blennow, K. (2004) CSF biomarkers for mild cognitive impairment. *Journal of Internal Medicine* **256**, 224–234.

Blessed, G., Tomlinson, B.E. & Roth, M. (1968) The association between quantitative measures of dementia and of senile change in the cerebral grey matter of elderly subjects. *British Journal of Psychiatry* **114**, 797–811.

Bloch, M., Adam, S., Wiggins, S., Huggins, M. & Hayden, M.R. (1992) Predictive testing for Huntington disease in Canada: the experience of those receiving an increased risk. *American Journal of Medical Genetics* **42**, 499–507.

Boeve, B.F., Lang, A.E. & Litvan, I. (2003) Corticobasal degeneration and its relationship to progressive supranuclear palsy and frontotemporal dementia. *Annals of Neurology* **54** (suppl. 5), S15–S19.

Bolt, J.M.W. (1970) Huntington's chorea in the West of Scotland. *British Journal of Psychiatry* **116**, 259–270.

Bonelli, R.M. & Wenning, G.K. (2006) Pharmacological management of Huntington's disease: an evidence-based review. *Current Pharmaceutical Design* **12**, 2701–2720.

Bookheimer, S.Y., Strojwas, M.H., Cohen, M.S. *et al.* (2000) Patterns of brain activation in people at risk for Alzheimer's disease. *New England Journal of Medicine* **343**, 450–456.

Borenstein, G.A., Mortimer, J.A., Bowen, J.D. *et al.* (2001) Head circumference and incident Alzheimer's disease: modification by apolipoprotein E. *Neurology* **57**, 1453–1460.

Bornebroek, M., De, J.C., Haan, J., Kumar-Singh, S., Younkin, S., Roos, R. & Van, B.C. (2003) Hereditary cerebral hemorrhage with amyloidosis Dutch type (AbetaPP 693): decreased plasma amyloid-beta 42 concentration. *Neurobiology of Disease* **14**, 619–623.

Borrell-Pages, M., Zala, D., Humbert, S. & Saudou, F. (2006) Huntington's disease: from huntingtin function and dysfunction to therapeutic strategies. *Cellular and Molecular Life Sciences* **63**, 2642–2660.

Boston, P.F., Dennis, M.S. & Jagger, C. (1999) Factors associated with vascular dementia in an elderly community population. *International Journal of Geriatric Psychiatry* **14**, 761–766.

Boutros, N.N. & Struve, F. (2002) Electrophysiological assessment of neuropsychiatric disorders. *Seminars in Clinical Neuropsychiatry* **7**, 30–41.

Braak, E., Braak, H. & Mandelkow, E.-M. (1994) A sequence of cytoskeleton changes related to the formation of neurofibrillary tangles and neuropil threads. *Acta Neuropathologica* **87**, 554–567.

Braak, H. & Braak, E. (1990) Alzheimer's disease: striatal amyloid deposits and neurofibrillary changes. *Journal of Neuropathology and Experimental Neurology* **49**, 215–224.

Braak, H. & Braak, E. (1991) Neuropathological stageing of Alzheimer-related changes. *Acta Neuropathologica* **82**, 239–259.

Braak, H. & Braak, E. (1998) Evolution of neuronal changes in the course of Alzheimer's disease. *Journal of Neural Transmission* **105** (suppl. 53), 127–140.

Braak, H., Braak, E., Bohl, J. & Lang, W. (1989) Alzheimer's disease: amyloid plaques in the cerebellum. *Journal of the Neurological Sciences* **93**, 277–287.

Brandner, S., Isenmann, S., Raeber, A. *et al.* (1996) Normal host prion protein necessary for scrapie-induced neurotoxicity. *Nature* **379**, 339–343.

Brandt, J. & Butters, N. (1986) The neuropsychology of Huntington's disease. *Trends in Neurosciences* **9**, 118–120.

Brandt, J. & Rich, J.B. (1995) Memory disorders in the dementias. In: Baddeley, A.D., Wilson, B.A. & Watts, F.N. (eds) *Handbook of Memory Disorders*, ch. 10. John Wiley & Sons, Chichester.

Brayne, C., Gill, C., Huppert, F.A. *et al.* (1995) Incidence of clinically diagnosed subtypes of dementia in an elderly population. Cambridge Project for Later Life. *British Journal of Psychiatry* **167**, 255–262.

Brayne, C., Gill, C., Huppert, F.A. *et al.* (1998) Vascular risks and incident dementia: results from a cohort study of the very old. *Dementia* **9**, 175–180.

Breitner, J.C., Silverman, J.M., Mohs, R.C. & Davis, K.L. (1988) Familial aggregation in Alzheimer's disease: comparison of risk among relatives of early-and late-onset cases, and among male and female relatives in successive generations. *Neurology* **38**, 207–212.

Breitner, J.C., Wyse, B.W., Anthony, J.C. *et al.* (1999) APOE-epsilon4 count predicts age when prevalence of AD increases, then declines: the Cache County Study. *Neurology* **53**, 321–331.

Brodaty, H. & Luscombe, G. (1996) Depression in persons with dementia. *International Psychogeriatrics* **8**, 609–622.

Brodaty, H., Conneally, M., Gauthier, S., Jennings, C., Lennox, A. & Lovestone, S. (1995) Consensus statement on predictive testing. *Alzheimer Disease and Associated Disorders* **9**, 182–187.

Brookmeyer, R., Gray, S. & Kawas, C. (1998) Projections of Alzheimer's disease in the United States and the public health impact of delaying disease onset. *American Journal of Public Health* **88**, 1337–1342.

Brooks, D.S., Murphy, D., Janota, I. & Lishman, W.A. (1987) Early-onset Huntington's chorea: diagnostic clues. *British Journal of Psychiatry* **151**, 850–852.

Brouillet, E., Jacquard, C., Bizat, N. & Blum, D. (2005) 3-Nitropropionic acid: a mitochondrial toxin to uncover physiopathological mechanisms underlying striatal degeneration in Huntington's disease. *Journal of Neurochemistry* **95**, 1521–1540.

Brown, D.F. (1999) Lewy body dementia. *Annals of Medicine* **31**, 188–196.

Brown, P. (1988) The clinical neurology and epidemiology of Creutzfeldt–Jakob disease, with special reference to iatrogenic cases. *Ciba Foundation Symposia* **135**, 3–23.

Brown, P., Cathala, F., Raubertas, R.F., Gajdusek, D.C. & Castaigne, P. (1987) The epidemiology of Creutzfeldt–Jakob disease: conclusion of a 15-year investigation in France and review of the world literature. *Neurology* **37**, 895–904.

Browne, S.E. & Beal, M.F. (2006) Oxidative damage in Huntington's disease pathogenesis. *Antioxidants and Redox Signaling* **8**, 2061–2073.

Brune, S., Kolsch, H., Ptok, U. *et al.* (2003) Polymorphism in the peroxisome proliferator-activated receptor alpha gene influences the risk for Alzheimer's disease. *Journal of Neural Transmission* **110**, 1041–1050.

Bruscoli, M. & Lovestone, S. (2004) Is MCI really just early dementia? A systematic review of conversion studies. *International Psychogeriatrics* **16**, 129–140.

Bruyn, G.W. (1968) Huntington's chorea: historical, clinical and laboratory synopsis. In: Vinken, P.J. & Bruyn, G.W. (eds) *Handbook of Clinical Neurology*, vol. 6, ch. 13. North-Holland Publishing Co., Amsterdam.

Bueler, H., Aguzzi, A., Sailer, A. *et al.* (1993) Mice devoid of PrP are resistant to scrapie. *Cell* **73**, 1339–1347.

Buell, S.J. & Coleman, P.D. (1979) Dendritic growth in the aged human brain and failure of growth in senile dementia. *Science* **206**, 854–856.

Buell, S.J. & Coleman, P.D. (1981) Quantitative evidence for selective dendritic growth in normal human ageing but not in senile dementia. *Brain Research* **214**, 23–41.

Burggren, A.C., Small, G.W., Sabb, F.W. & Bookheimer, S.Y. (2002) Specificity of brain activation patterns in people at genetic risk for Alzheimer disease. *American Journal of Geriatric Psychiatry* **10**, 44–51.

Burkhardt, C.R., Filley, C.M., Kleinschmidt-DeMasters, B.K., de la Monte, S., Norenberg, M.D. & Schneck, S.A. (1988) Diffuse Lewy body disease and progressive dementia. *Neurology* **38**, 1520–1528.

Burns, A. (2000) The burden of Alzheimer's disease. *International Journal of Neuropsychopharmacology* **3**, 31–38.

Burns, A., Jacoby, R. & Levy, R. (1990a) Psychiatric phenomena in Alzheimer's disease. IV: Disorders of behaviour. *British Journal of Psychiatry* **157**, 86–94.

Burns, A., Jacoby, R. & Levy, R. (1990b) Psychiatric phenomena in Alzheimer's disease. III: Disorders of mood. *British Journal of Psychiatry* **157**, 81–86.

Burns, A., Luthert, P., Levy, R., Jacoby, R. & Lantos, P. (1990) Accuracy of clinical diagnosis of Alzheimer's disease. *BMJ* **301**, 1026.

Burns, A., Jacoby, R. & Levy, R. (1991a) Neurological signs in Alzheimer's disease. *Age and Ageing* **20**, 45–51.

Burns, A., Jacoby, R. & Levy, R. (1991b) Computed tomography in Alzheimer's disease: a longitudinal study. *Biological Psychiatry* **29**, 383–390.

Burns, A., Lewis, G., Jacoby, R. & Levy, R. (1991c) Factors affecting survival in Alzheimer's disease. *Psychological Medicine* **21**, 363–370.

Burns, A., Lawlor, B. & Craig, S. (2002) Rating scales in old age psychiatry. *British Journal of Psychiatry* **180**, 161–167.

Burns, A., O'Brien, J., Auriacombe, S. *et al.* (2006) Clinical practice with anti-dementia drugs: a consensus statement from British Association for Psychopharmacology. *Journal of Psychopharmacology* **20**, 732–755.

Burns, J.M., Church, J.A., Johnson, D.K. *et al.* (2005) White matter lesions are prevalent but differentially related with cognition in aging and early Alzheimer disease. *Archives of Neurology* **62**, 1870–1876.

Butler, S.M., Ashford, J.W. & Snowdon, D.A. (1996) Age, education, and changes in the Mini-Mental State Exam scores of older women: findings from the Nun Study. *Journal of the American Geriatric Society* **44**, 675–681.

Butters, N., Sax, D., Montgomery, K. & Tarlow, S. (1978) Comparison of the neuropsychological deficits associated with early and advanced Huntington's disease. *Archives of Neurology* **35**, 585–589.

Byrne, E.J., Lennox, G., Lowe, J. & Reynolds, G. (1990) Diffuse Lewy body disease: the clinical features. *Advances in Neurology* **53**, 283–286.

Cai, L., Chin, F.T., Pike, V.W. *et al.* (2004) Synthesis and evaluation of two ^{18}F-labeled 6-iodo-2-(4′-*N,N*-dimethylamino)phenylimi dazo[1,2-a]pyridine derivatives as prospective radioligands for beta-amyloid in Alzheimer's disease. *Journal of Medicinal Chemistry* **47**, 2208–2218.

Campion, D., Dumanchin, C., Hannequin, D. *et al.* (1999) Early-onset autosomal dominant Alzheimer disease: prevalence, genetic heterogeneity, and mutation spectrum. *American Journal of Human Genetics* **65**, 664–670.

Cao, X. & Sudhof, T.C. (2001) A transcriptionally active complex of APP with Fe65 and histone acetyltransferase Tip60. *Science* **293**, 115–120.

Caplan, L.R. & Schoene, W.C. (1978) Clinical features of subcortical arteriosclerotic encephalopathy (Binswanger disease). *Neurology* **28**, 1206–1215.

Castellani, R.J., Smith, M.A., Perry, G. & Friedland, R.P. (2004a) Cerebral amyloid angiopathy: major contributor or decorative response to Alzheimer's disease pathogenesis. *Neurobiology of Aging* **25**, 599–602.

Castellani, R.J., Colucci, M., Xie, Z. *et al.* (2004b) Sensitivity of 14-3-3 protein test varies in subtypes of sporadic Creutzfeldt–Jakob disease. *Neurology* **63**, 436–442.

Catani, M. (2006) Diffusion tensor magnetic resonance imaging tractography in cognitive disorders. *Current Opinion in Neurology* **19**, 599–606.

Chabriat, H., Vahedi, K., Iba Zizen, M.T. *et al.* (1995) Clinical spectrum of CADASIL: a study of 7 families. Cerebral autosomal dominant arteriopathy with subcortical infarcts and leukoencephalopathy. *Lancet* **346**, 934–939.

Chapman, J. & Korczyn, A.D. (1991) Genetic and environmental factors determining the development of Creutzfeldt–Jakob disease in Libyan Jews. *Neuroepidemiology* **10**, 228–231.

Chase, T.N., Foster, N.L., Fedio, P., Brooks, R., Mansi, L. & Di Chiro, G. (1984) Regional cortical dysfunction in Alzheimer's disease as determined by positron emission tomography. *Annals of Neurology* **15** (suppl.), S170–S174.

Chong, M.S., Lim, W.S. & Sahadevan, S. (2006) Biomarkers in preclinical Alzheimer's disease. *Current Opinion in Investigative Drugs* **7**, 600–607.

Chui, H. & Gonthier, R. (1999) Natural history of vascular dementia. *Alzheimer Disease and Associated Disorders* **13** (suppl. 3), S124–S130.

Clarfield, A.M. (1988) The reversible dementias: do they reverse? *Annals of Internal Medicine* **109**, 476–486.

Clarfield, A.M. (2003) The decreasing prevalence of reversible dementias: an updated meta-analysis. *Archives of Internal Medicine* **163**, 2219–2229.

Clark, R.F. & Goate, A.M. (1993) Molecular genetics of Alzheimer's disease. *Archives of Neurology* **50**, 1164–1172.

Clarke, R., Smith, A.D., Jobst, K.A., Refsum, H., Sutton, L. & Ueland, P.M. (1998) Folate, vitamin B$_{12}$, and serum total homocysteine levels in confirmed Alzheimer disease. *Archives of Neurology* **55**, 1449–1455.

Cobb, J.L., Wolf, P.A., Au, R., White, R. & D'Agostino, R.B. (1995) The effect of education on the incidence of dementia and Alzheimer's disease in the Framingham Study. *Neurology* **45**, 1707–1712.

Coen, R.F., Swanwick, G.R., O'Boyle, C.A. & Coakley, D. (1997) Behaviour disturbance and other predictors of carer burden in Alzheimer's disease. *International Journal of Geriatric Psychiatry* **12**, 331–336.

Cohen, C.A., Gold, D.P., Shulman, K.I., Wortley, J.T., McDonald, G. & Wargon, M. (1993) Factors determining the decision to institutionalize dementing individuals: a prospective study. *Gerontologist* **33**, 714–720.

Collerton, D., Burn, D., McKeith, I. & O'Brien, J. (2003) Systematic review and meta-analysis show that dementia with Lewy bodies is a visual–perceptual and attentional–executive dementia. *Dementia and Geriatric Cognitive Disorders* **16**, 229–237.

Collie, D.A., Sellar, R.J., Zeidler, M., Colchester, A.C., Knight, R. & Will, R.G. (2001) MRI of Creutzfeldt–Jakob disease: imaging features and recommended MRI protocol. *Clinical Radiology* **56**, 726–739.

Collinge, J. (1999) Variant Creutzfeldt–Jakob disease. *Lancet* **354**, 317–323.

Collinge, J., Palmer, M.S. & Dryden, A.J. (1991) Genetic predisposition to iatrogenic Creutzfeldt–Jakob disease. *Lancet* **337**, 1441–1442.

Collins, S., McLean, C.A. & Masters, C.L. (2001) Gerstmann–Straussler–Scheinker syndrome, fatal familial insomnia, and kuru: a review of these less common human transmissible spongiform encephalopathies. *Journal of Clinical Neuroscience* **8**, 387–397.

Convit, A., de Asis, J., De Leon, M.J., Tarshish, C.Y., De Santi, S. & Rusinek, H. (2000) Atrophy of the medial occipitotemporal, inferior, and middle temporal gyri in non-demented elderly predict decline to Alzheimer's disease. *Neurobiology of Aging* **21**, 19–26.

Cooney, C. & Hamid, W. (1995) Review: Diogenes syndrome. *Age and Ageing* **24**, 451–453.

Cooper, C., Balamurali, T.B. & Livingston, G. (2007) A systematic review of the prevalence and covariates of anxiety in caregivers of people with dementia. *International Psychogeriatrics* **19**, 175–195.

Cooper, D.B., Ales, G., Lange, C. & Clement, P. (2006) Atypical onset of symptoms in Huntington disease: severe cognitive decline preceding chorea or other motor manifestations. *Cognitive and Behavioral Neurology* **19**, 222–224.

Cooper, S.A., Murray, K.L., Heath, C.A., Will, R.G. & Knight, R.S. (2006) Sporadic Creutzfeldt–Jakob disease with cerebellar ataxia at onset in the UK. *Journal of Neurology, Neurosurgery and Psychiatry* **77**, 1273–1275.

Correa, B., Xavier, M. & Guimaraes, J. (2006) Association of Huntington's disease and schizophrenia-like psychosis in a Huntington's disease pedigree. *Clinical Practice and Epidemiology in Mental Health* **2**, 1.

Corsellis, J.A.N. (1962) *Mental Illness and the Ageing Brain*. Maudsley Monograph No. 9. Oxford University Press, Oxford.

Cosman, K.M., Boyle, L.L. & Porsteinsson, A.P. (2007) Memantine in the treatment of mild-to-moderate Alzheimer's disease. *Expert Opinion on Pharmacotherapy* **8**, 203–214.

Cousens, S.N., Linsell, L., Smith, P.G. *et al.* (1999) Geographical distribution of variant CJD in the UK (excluding Northern Ireland). *Lancet* **353**, 18–21.

Cousens, S., Smith, P.G., Ward, H. *et al.* (2001) Geographical distribution of variant Creutzfeldt–Jakob disease in Great Britain, 1994–2000. *Lancet* **357**, 1002–1007.

Cowburn, R.F., Hardy, J.A. & Roberts, P.J. (1990) Glutamatergic neurotransmission in Alzheimer's disease. *Biochemical Society Transactions* **18**, 390–392.

Craft, S., Dagogo-Jack, S.E., Wiethop, B.V. *et al.* (1993) Effects of hyperglycemia on memory and hormone levels in dementia of the Alzheimer type: a longitudinal study. *Behavioral Neuroscience* **107**, 926–940.

Craft, S., Peskind, E., Schwartz, M.W., Schellenberg, G.D., Raskind, M. & Porte, D. Jr (1998) Cerebrospinal fluid and plasma insulin levels in Alzheimer's disease: relationship to severity of dementia and apolipoprotein E genotype. *Neurology* **50**, 164–168.

Crisby, M., Carlson, L.A. & Winblad, B. (2002) Statins in the prevention and treatment of Alzheimer disease. *Alzheimer Disease and Associated Disorders* **16**, 131–136.

Cui, T., Daniels, M., Wong, B.S. *et al.* (2003) Mapping the functional domain of the prion protein. *European Journal of Biochemistry* **270**, 3368–3376.

Culjkovic, B., Stojkovic, O., Vojvodic, N. *et al.* (1999) Correlation between triplet repeat expansion and computed tomography measures of caudate nuclei atrophy in Huntington's disease. *Journal of Neurology* **246**, 1090–1093.

Cummings, J.L. (1985) Organic delusions: phenomenology, anatomical correlations, and review. *British Journal of Psychiatry* **146**, 184–197.

Cummings, J.L., Benson, F., Hill, M.A. & Read, S. (1985) Aphasia in dementia of the Alzheimer type. *Neurology* **35**, 394–397.

Curb, J.D., Rodriguez, B.L., Abbott, R.D. *et al.* (1999) Longitudinal association of vascular and Alzheimer's dementias, diabetes, and glucose tolerance. *Neurology* **52**, 971–975.

Davidson, Y., Gibbons, L., Purandare, N. *et al.* (2006) Apolipoprotein E epsilon4 allele frequency in vascular dementia. *Dementia and Geriatric Cognitive Disorders* **22**, 15–19.

Davis, D.G., Schmitt, F.A., Wekstein, D.R. & Markesbery, W.R. (1999) Alzheimer neuropathologic alterations in aged cognitively normal subjects. *Journal of Neuropathology and Experimental Neurology* **58**, 376–388.

Davous, P. (1998) CADASIL: a review with proposed diagnostic criteria. *European Journal of Neurology* **5**, 219–233.

Daw, E.W., Payami, H., Nemens, E.J. *et al.* (2000) The number of trait loci in late-onset Alzheimer disease. *American Journal of Human Genetics* **66**, 196–204.

DeCarli, C., Haxby, J.V., Gillette, J.A., Teichberg, D., Rapoport, S.I. & Schapiro, M.B. (1992) Longitudinal changes in lateral ventricular volume in patients with dementia of the Alzheimer type. *Neurology* **42**, 2029–2036.

DeKosky, S.T. & Scheff, S.W. (1990) Synapse loss in frontal cortex biopsies in Alzheimer's disease: correlation with cognitive severity. *Annals of Neurology* **27**, 457–464.

de Leeuw, F.E., De Groot, J.C., Oudkerk, M. *et al.* (2000) Aortic atherosclerosis at middle age predicts cerebral white matter lesions in the elderly. *Stroke* **31**, 425–429.

de Leeuw, F.E., De Groot, J.C., Achten, E. *et al.* (2001) Prevalence of cerebral white matter lesions in elderly people: a population based magnetic resonance imaging study. The Rotterdam Scan Study. *Journal of Neurology, Neurosurgery and Psychiatry* **70**, 9–14.

De Leon, M.J., George, A.E., Golomb, J. *et al.* (1997) Frequency of hippocampal formation atrophy in normal aging and Alzheimer's disease. *Neurobiology of Aging* **18**, 1–11.

De Leon, M.J., Desanti, S., Zinkowski, R. *et al.* (2004) MRI and CSF studies in the early diagnosis of Alzheimer's disease. *Journal of Internal Medicine* **256**, 205–223.

Del Ser, T., Hachinski, V., Merskey, H. & Munoz, D.G. (2001) Clinical and pathologic features of two groups of patients with dementia with Lewy bodies: effect of coexisting Alzheimer-type lesion load. *Alzheimer Disease and Associated Disorders* **15**, 31–44.

Demetriades, A.K. (2002) Functional neuroimaging in Alzheimer's type dementia. *Journal of the Neurological Sciences* **203–204**, 247–251.

Denney, N.W. (1985) A review of life span research with the Twenty Questions Task: a study of problem-solving ability. *International Journal of Aging and Human Development* **21**, 161–173.

De Santi, S., De Leon, M.J., Rusinek, H. *et al.* (2001) Hippocampal formation glucose metabolism and volume losses in MCI and AD. *Neurobiology of Aging* **22**, 529–539.

De Strooper, B. (2003) Aph-1, Pen-2, and Nicastrin with Presenilin generate an active gamma-Secretase complex. *Neuron* **38**, 9–12.

Deutsch, L.H., Bylsma, F.W., Rovner, B.W., Steele, C. & Folstein, M.F. (1991) Psychosis and physical aggression in probable Alzheimer's disease. *American Journal of Psychiatry* **148**, 1159–1163.

Devous, M.D. Sr (2002) Functional brain imaging in the dementias: role in early detection, differential diagnosis, and longitudinal studies. *European Journal of Nuclear Medicine and Molecular Imaging* **29**, 1685–1696.

Dewhurst, K., Oliver, J.E. & McKnight, A.L. (1970) Sociopsychiatric consequences of Huntington's disease. *British Journal of Psychiatry* **116**, 255–258.

Dickson, D.W. (1997) Neuropathological diagnosis of Alzheimer's disease: a perspective from longitudinal clinico-pathological studies. *Neurobiology of Aging* **18** (suppl.), S21–S26.

Donaldson, C., Tarrier, N. & Burns, A. (1998) Determinants of carer stress in Alzheimer's disease. *International Journal of Geriatric Psychiatry* **13**, 248–256.

Drevets, W.C. & Rubin, E.H. (1989) Psychotic symptoms and the longitudinal course of senile dementia of the Alzheimer type. *Biological Psychiatry* **25**, 39–48.

D'Souza, I. & Schellenberg, G.D. (2005) Regulation of tau isoform expression and dementia. *Biochimica et Biophysica Acta* **1739**, 104–115.

Duda, J.E., Lee, V.M. & Trojanowski, J.Q. (2000) Neuropathology of synuclein aggregates. *Journal of Neuroscience Research* **61**, 121–127.

Eastley, R. & Wilcock, G.K. (1997) Prevalence and correlates of aggressive behaviours occurring in patients with Alzheimer's disease. *International Journal of Geriatric Psychiatry* **12**, 484–487.

Edland, S.D., Xu, Y., Plevak, M. *et al.* (2002) Total intracranial volume: normative values and lack of association with Alzheimer's disease. *Neurology* **59**, 272–274.

Eldar-Finkelman, H. (2002) Glycogen synthase kinase 3: an emerging therapeutic target. *Trends in Molecular Medicine* **8**, 126–132.

Ellul, J., Archer, N., Foy, C.M. *et al.* (2007) The effects of commonly prescribed drugs in patients with Alzheimer's disease on the rate of deterioration. *Journal of Neurology, Neurosurgery and Psychiatry* **78**, 233–239.

Engelhart, M.J., Geerlings, M.I., Ruitenberg, A. *et al.* (2002) Dietary intake of antioxidants and risk of Alzheimer disease. *Journal of the American Medical Association* **287**, 3223–3229.

Ensenauer, R.E., Michels, V.V. & Reinke, S.S. (2005) Genetic testing: practical, ethical, and counseling considerations. *Mayo Clinic Proceedings* **80**, 63–73.

Erkinjuntti, T. & Sulkava, R. (1991) Diagnosis of multi-infarct dementia. *Alzheimer Disease and Associated Disorders* **5**, 112–121.

Erkinjuntti, T., Roman, G. & Gauthier, S. (2004) Treatment of vascular dementia: evidence from clinical trials with cholinesterase inhibitors. *Journal of the Neurological Sciences* **226**, 63–66.

Ertekin-Taner, N., Graff-Radford, N., Younkin, L.H. *et al.* (2000) Linkage of plasma Aβ42 to a quantitative locus on chromosome 10 in late-onset Alzheimer's disease pedigrees. *Science* **290**, 2303–2304.

Evans, D.A., Funkenstein, H.H., Albert, M.S. *et al.* (1989) Prevalence of Alzheimer's disease in a community population of older persons. Higher than previously reported. *Journal of the American Medical Association* **262**, 2551–2556.

Evans, D.A., Hebert, L.E., Beckett, L.A. *et al.* (1997) Education and other measures of socioeconomic status and risk of incident Alzheimer disease in a defined population of older persons. *Archives of Neurology* **54**, 1399–1405.

Ewbank, D.C. (1999) Deaths attributable to Alzheimer's disease in the United States. *American Journal of Public Health* **89**, 90–92.

Fagan, A.M., Csernansky, C.A., Morris, J.C. & Holtzman, D.M. (2005) The search for antecedent biomarkers of Alzheimer's disease. *Journal of Alzheimers Disease* **8**, 347–358.

Fan, M.M. & Raymond, L.A. (2007) N-methyl-D-aspartate (NMDA) receptor function and excitotoxicity in Huntington's disease. *Progress in Neurobiology* **81**, 272–293.

Farrer, L.A., O'Sullivan, D.M., Cupples, L.A., Growdon, J.H. & Myers, R.H. (1989) Assessment of genetic risk for Alzheimer's disease among first-degree relatives. *Annals of Neurology* **25**, 485–493.

Farrer, L.A., Brin, M.F., ELsas, L. *et al.* (1995) Statement on use of apolipoprotein E testing for Alzheimer disease. *Journal of the American Medical Association* **274**, 1627–1629.

Fasano, C., Campana, V. & Zurzolo, C. (2006) Prions: protein only or something more? Overview of potential prion cofactors. *Journal of Molecular Neuroscience* **29**, 195–214.

Fernando, M.S. & Ince, P.G. (2004) Vascular pathologies and cognition in a population-based cohort of elderly people. *Journal of the Neurological Sciences* **226**, 13–17.

Ferri, C.P., Prince, M., Brayne, C. *et al.* (2005) Global prevalence of dementia: a Delphi consensus study. *Lancet* **366**, 2112–2117.

Fleminger, S., Oliver, D.L., Lovestone, S., Rabe-Hesketh, S. & Giora, A. (2003) Head injury as a risk factor for Alzheimer's disease: the evidence 10 years on; a partial replication. *Journal of Neurology, Neurosurgery and Psychiatry* **74**, 857–862.

Folstein, M.F., Folstein, S.E. & McHugh, P.R. (1975) Mini-Mental State: a practical method of grading the cognitive state of patients for the clinician. *Journal of Psychiatric Research* **12**, 189–198.

Folstein, S.E. (1989) *Huntington's Disease. A Disorder of Families*. Johns Hopkins University Press, Baltimore.

Folstein, S.E., Abbott, M.H., Chase, G.A., Jensen, B.A. & Folstein, M.F. (1983) The association of affective disorder with Huntington's disease in a case series and in families. *Psychological Medicine* **13**, 537–542.

Folstein, S.E., Leigh, R.J., Parhad, I.M. & Folstein, M.F. (1986) The diagnosis of Huntington's disease. *Neurology* **36**, 1279–1283.

Forette, F., Seux, M.L., Staessen, J.A. *et al.* (2002) The prevention of dementia with antihypertensive treatment: new evidence from the systolic hypertension in europe (SYST-EUR) study. *Archives of Internal Medicine* **162**, 2046–2052.

Förstl, H., Burns, A., Luthert, P., Cairns, N., Lantos, P. & Levy, R. (1992) Clinical and neuropathological correlates of depression in Alzheimer's disease. *Psychological Medicine* **22**, 877–884.

Förstl, H., Besthorn, C., Hentschel, F., Geiger-Kabisch, C., Sattel, H. & Schreiter-Gasser, U. (1996) Frontal lobe degeneration and Alzheimer's disease: a controlled study on clinical findings, volumetric brain changes and quantitative electroencephalography data. *Dementia* **7**, 27–34.

Fox, N.C., Cousens, S., Scahill, R., Harvey, R.J. & Rossor, M.N. (2000) Using serial registered brain magnetic resonance imaging to measure disease progression in Alzheimer disease: power calculations and estimates of sample size to detect treatment effects. *Archives of Neurology* **57**, 339–344.

Frackowiak, R.S., Pozzilli, C., Legg, N.J. *et al.* (1981) Regional cerebral oxygen supply and utilization in dementia. A clinical and physiological study with oxygen-15 and positron tomography. *Brain* **104**, 753–778.

Francis, P.T., Palmer, A.M., Snape, M. & Wilcock, G.K. (1999) The cholinergic hypothesis of Alzheimer's disease: a review of progress. *Journal of Neurology, Neurosurgery and Psychiatry* **66**, 137–147.

Frangione, B., Revesz, T., Vidal, R. *et al.* (2001) Familial cerebral amyloid angiopathy related to stroke and dementia. *Amyloid* **8** (suppl. 1), 36–42.

Frank, A., ez-Tejedor, E., Bullido, M.J., Valdivieso, F. & Barreiro, P. (2002) APOE genotype in cerebrovascular disease and vascular dementia. *Journal of the Neurological Sciences* **203–204**, 173–176.

Fratiglioni, L., Grut, M., Forsell, Y. *et al.* (1991) Prevalence of Alzheimer's disease and other dementias in an elderly urban population: relationship with age, sex, and education. *Neurology* **41**, 1886–1892.

Freyne, A., Kidd, N., Coen, R. & Lawlor, B.A. (1999) Burden in carers of dementia patients: higher levels in carers of younger sufferers. *International Journal of Geriatric Psychiatry* **14**, 784–788.

Friedland, R.P., Fritsch, T., Smyth, K.A. *et al.* (2001) Patients with Alzheimer's disease have reduced activities in midlife compared with healthy control-group members. *Proceedings of the National Academy of Sciences USA* **98**, 3440–3445.

Frisoni, G.B., Scheltens, P., Galluzzi, S. *et al.* (2003) Neuroimaging tools to rate regional atrophy, subcortical cerebrovascular disease, and regional cerebral blood flow and metabolism: consensus paper of the EADC. *Journal of Neurology, Neurosurgery and Psychiatry* **74**, 1371–1381.

Frolich, L., Blum-Degen, D., Riederer, P. & Hoyer, S. (1999) A disturbance in the neuronal insulin receptor signal transduction in sporadic Alzheimer's disease. *Annals of the New York Academy of Sciences* **893**, 290–293.

Fujimori, M., Imamura, T., Yamashita, H. *et al.* (1998) Age at onset and visuocognitive disturbances in Alzheimer disease. *Alzheimer Disease and Associated Disorders* **12**, 163–166.

Fujisawa, Y., Sasaki, K. & Akiyama, K. (1991) Increased insulin levels after OGTT load in peripheral blood and cerebrospinal fluid of patients with dementia of Alzheimer type. *Biological Psychiatry* **30**, 1219–1228.

Fujishima, M. & Tsuchihashi, T. (1999) Hypertension and dementia. *Clinical and Experimental Hypertension* **21**, 927–935.

Galvez, S. & Cartier, L. (1984) Computed tomography findings in 15 cases of Creutzfeldt–Jakob disease with histological verification. *Journal of Neurology, Neurosurgery and Psychiatry* **47**, 1244–1246.

Gambassi, G., Landi, F., Lapane, K.L., Sgadari, A., Mor, V. & Bernabei, R. (1999) Predictors of mortality in patients with Alzheimer's disease living in nursing homes. *Journal of Neurology, Neurosurgery and Psychiatry* **67**, 59–65.

Gasparini, L., Netzer, W.J., Greengard, P. & Xu, H. (2002) Does insulin dysfunction play a role in Alzheimer's disease? *Trends in Pharmacological Sciences* **23**, 288–293.

Gatz, M., Pedersen, N.L., Berg, S. et al. (1997) Heritability for Alzheimer's disease: the study of dementia in Swedish twins. *Journal of Gerontology* **52A**, M117–M125.

Gemmell, H.G., Sharp, P.F., Smith, F.W. et al. (1989) Cerebral blood flow measured by SPET as a diagnostic tool in the study of dementia. *Psychiatry Research* **29**, 327–329.

Gertz, H.J., Kruger, H., Patt, S. & Cervos Navarro, J. (1991) Tangle-bearing neurons show more extensive dendritic trees than tangle-free neurons in area CA1 of the hippocampus in Alzheimer's disease. *Brain Research* **548**, 260–266.

Geschwind, M.D., Martindale, J., Miller, D. et al. (2003) Challenging the clinical utility of the 14-3-3 protein for the diagnosis of sporadic Creutzfeldt–Jakob disease. *Archives of Neurology* **60**, 813–816.

Ghetti, B., Tagliavini, F., Giaccone, G. et al. (1994) Familial Gerstmann–Straussler–Scheinker disease with neurofibrillary tangles. *Molecular Neurobiology* **8**, 41–48.

Glatzel, M., Stoeck, K., Seeger, H., Luhrs, T. & Aguzzi, A. (2005) Human prion diseases: molecular and clinical aspects. *Archives of Neurology* **62**, 545–552.

Glenner, G.G. & Wong, C.W. (1984) Alzheimer's disease: initial report of the purification and characterization of a novel cerebrovascular amyloid protein. *Biochemical and Biophysical Research Communications* **120**, 885–890.

Goedert, M. (1993) Tau protein and the neurofibrillary pathology of Alzheimer's disease. *Trends in Neuroscience* **16**, 460–465.

Goedert, M. & Jakes, R. (2005) Mutations causing neurodegenerative tauopathies. *Biochimica et Biophysica Acta* **1739**, 240–250.

Gold, G., Kovari, E., Corte, G. et al. (2001) Clinical validity of A beta-protein deposition staging in brain aging and Alzheimer disease. *Journal of Neuropathology and Experimental Neurology* **60**, 946–952.

Gormley, N., Rizwan, M.R. & Lovestone, S. (1998) Clinical predictors of aggressive behaviour in Alzheimer's disease. *International Journal of Geriatric Psychiatry* **13**, 109–115.

Graham, N.L., Bak, T.H. & Hodges, J.R. (2003) Corticobasal degeneration as a cognitive disorder. *Movement Disorders* **18**, 1224–1232.

Green, M.S., Kaye, J.A. & Ball, M.J. (2000) The Oregon brain aging study: neuropathology accompanying healthy aging in the oldest old. *Neurology* **54**, 105–113.

Green, P.S., Gridley, K.E. & Simpkins, J.W. (1996) Estradiol protects against p-amyloid (25–35)-induced toxicity in SK-N-SH human neuroblastoma cells. *Neuroscience Letters* **218**, 165–168.

Greenwald, B.S., Kramer Ginsberg, E., Marin, D.B. et al. (1989) Dementia with coexistent major depression. *American Journal of Psychiatry* **146**, 1742–1748.

Gurd, J.M., Herzberg, L., Joachim, C. et al. (2000) Dementia with Lewy bodies: a pure case. *Brain and Cognition* **44**, 307–323.

Gustafson, L., Brun, A. & Passant, U. (1992) Frontal lobe degeneration of non-Alzheimer type. *Baillieres Clinical Neurology* **1**, 559–582.

Haan, M.N., Jagust, W.J., Galasko, D. & Kaye, J. (2002) Effect of extrapyramidal signs and lewy bodies on survival in patients with Alzheimer disease. *Archives of Neurology* **59**, 588–593.

Haass, C. & De Strooper, B. (1999) Review: Neurobiology: the presenilins in Alzheimer's disease. Proteolysis holds the key. *Science* **286**, 916–919.

Hachinski, V.C., Iliff, L.D., Zilhka, E. et al. (1975) Cerebral blood flow in dementia. *Archives of Neurology* **32**, 632–637.

Hall, K.S., Gao, S.J., Unverzagt, F.W. & Hendrie, H.C. (2000) Low education and childhood rural residence: risk for Alzheimer's disease in African Americans. *Neurology* **54**, 95–99.

Halliday, S. (2000) William Farr: campaigning statistician. *Journal of Medical Biography* **8**, 220–227.

Hardy, J. (1996) New insights into the genetics of Alzheimer's disease. *Annals of Medicine* **28**, 255–258.

Hardy, J.A. & Higgins, G.A. (1992) Alzheimer's disease: the amyloid cascade hypothesis. *Science* **256**, 184–185.

Haroutunian, V., Perl, D.P., Purohit, D.P. et al. (1998) Regional distribution of neuritic plaques in the nondemented elderly and subjects with very mild Alzheimer disease. *Archives of Neurology* **55**, 1185–1191.

Harper, D.G., Stopa, E.G., McKee, A.C. et al. (2001) Differential circadian rhythm disturbances in men with Alzheimer disease and frontotemporal degeneration. *Archives of General Psychiatry* **58**, 353–360.

Harper, P.S. (1992) The epidemiology of Huntington's disease. *Human Genetics* **89**, 365–376.

Harper, P.S. & Morris, M.R. (1991) Introduction: a historical background. In: Harper, P.S. (ed.) *Huntington's Disease*, ch. 1. W.B. Saunders, London.

Harris, D.A. (2003) Trafficking, turnover and membrane topology of PrP. *British Medical Bulletin* **66**, 71–85.

Harrison, M.J.G., Thomas, D.J., Du Boulay, G.H. & Marshall, J. (1979) Multi-infarct dementia. *Journal of the Neurological Sciences* **40**, 97–103.

Hashimoto, M., Kawahara, K., Bar-On, P., Rockenstein, E., Crews, L. & Masliah, E. (2004) The role of alpha-synuclein assembly and metabolism in the pathogenesis of Lewy body disease. *Journal of Molecular Neuroscience* **24**, 343–352.

Hassing, L.B., Johansson, B., Nilsson, S.E. et al. (2002) Diabetes mellitus is a risk factor for vascular dementia, but not for Alzheimer's disease: a population-based study of the oldest old. *International Psychogeriatrics* **14**, 239–248.

Hattori, N., Abe, K., Sakoda, S. & Sawada, T. (2002) Proton MR spectroscopic study at 3 Tesla on glutamate/glutamine in Alzheimer's disease. *Neuroreport* **13**, 183–186.

Haxby, J.V., Grady, C.L., Koss, E. *et al.* (1988) Heterogeneous anterior–posterior metabolic patterns in dementia of the Alzheimer type. *Neurology* **38**, 1853–1863.

Hayden, K.M., Zandi, P.P., Lyketsos, C.G. *et al.* (2006) Vascular risk factors for incident Alzheimer disease and vascular dementia: the Cache County study. *Alzheimer Disease and Associated Disorders* **20**, 93–100.

Hayden, M.R. (1981) *Huntington's Chorea*. Springer-Verlag, New York.

Heathfield, K.W.G. (1967) Huntington's chorea. *Brain* **90**, 203–232.

Hébert, R., Lindsay, J., Verreault, R., Rockwood, K., Hill, G. & Dubois, M.F. (2000) Vascular dementia: incidence and risk factors in the Canadian Study of Health and Aging. *Stroke* **31**, 1487–1493.

Hendrie, H.C., Ogunniyi, A., Hall, K.S. *et al.* (2001) Incidence of dementia and Alzheimer disease in two communities: Yoruba residing in Ibadan, Nigeria, and African Americans residing in Indianapolis, Indiana. *Journal of the American Medical Association* **285**, 739–747.

Heston, L.L., Mastri, A.R., Anderson, E. & White, J. (1981) Dementia of the Alzheimer type. Clinical genetics, natural history and associated conditions. *Archives of General Psychiatry* **38**, 1085–1090.

Heun, R., Papassotiropoulos, A., Jessen, F., Maier, W. & Breitner, J.C.S. (2001) A family study of Alzheimer disease and early- and late-onset depression in elderly patients. *Archives of General Psychiatry* **58**, 190–196.

Heutink, P. (2000) Untangling tau-related dementia. *Human Molecular Genetics* **9**, 979–986.

Ho, A.K., Sahakian, B.J., Brown, R.G. *et al.* (2003) Profile of cognitive progression in early Huntington's disease. *Neurology* **61**, 1702–1706.

Hodges, J.R. (2001) Frontotemporal dementia (Pick's disease): clinical features and assessment. *Neurology* **56**, S6–S10.

Hofman, A., Ott, A., Breteler, M.M. *et al.* (1997) Atherosclerosis, apolipoprotein E, and prevalence of dementia and Alzheimer's disease in the Rotterdam Study. *Lancet* **349**, 151–154.

Holmes, C., Fortenza, O., Powell, J. & Lovestone, S. (1997) Do neuroleptic drugs hasten cognitive decline in dementia? Carriers of apolipoprotein E ε4 allele seem particularly susceptible to their effects. *British Medical Journal* **314**, 1411.

Holmes, C., Arranz, M.J., Powell, J.F., Collier, D.A. & Lovestone, S. (1998) 5-HT$_{2A}$ and 5-HT$_{2C}$ receptor polymorphisms and psychopathology in late onset Alzheimer's disease. *Human Molecular Genetics* **7**, 1507–1509.

Holmes, C., Cairns, N., Lantos, P. & Mann, A. (1999) Validity of current clinical criteria for Alzheimer's disease, vascular dementia and dementia with Lewy bodies. *British Journal of Psychiatry* **174**, 45–50.

Holmes, C., Smith, H., Ganderton, R. *et al.* (2001) Psychosis and aggression in Alzheimer's disease: the effect of dopamine receptor gene variation. *Journal of Neurology, Neurosurgery and Psychiatry* **71**, 777–779.

Holtzer, R., Tang, M.X., Devanand, D.P. *et al.* (2003) Psychopathological features in Alzheimer's disease: course and relationship with cognitive status. *Journal of the American Geriatric Society* **51**, 953–960.

Hong, M. & Lee, V.M.Y. (1997) Insulin and insulin-like growth factor-1 regulate tau phosphorylation in cultured human neurons. *Journal of Biological Chemistry* **272**, 19547–19553.

Hoogendijk, W.J., Sommer, I.E., Pool, C.W. *et al.* (1999) Lack of association between depression and loss of neurons in the locus coeruleus in Alzheimer disease. *Archives of General Psychiatry* **56**, 45–51.

Hope, T., Keene, J., Fairburn, C., McShane, R. & Jacoby, R. (1997) Behaviour changes in dementia. 2: Are there behavioural syndromes? *International Journal of Geriatric Psychiatry* **12**, 1074–1078.

Horn, R., Ostertun, B., Fric, M., Solymosi, L., Steudel, A. & Möller, H.J. (1996) Atrophy of hippocampus in patients with Alzheimer's disease and other diseases with memory impairment. *Dementia* **7**, 182–186.

Horsburgh, K., McCarron, M.O., White, F. & Nicoll, J.A.R. (2000) The role of apolipoprotein E in Alzheimer's disease, acute brain injury and cerebrovascular disease: evidence of common mechanisms and utility of animal models. *Neurobiology of Aging* **21**, 245–255.

Hoyer, S., Blum-Degen, D., Bernstein, H.G. *et al.* (1998) Brain insulin and insulin receptors in aging and sporadic Alzheimer's disease. *Journal of Neural Transmission* **105**, 423–438.

Hsiao, K., Baker, H.F., Crow, T.J. *et al.* (1989) Linkage of a prion protein missense variant to Gerstmann–Straussler syndrome. *Nature* **338**, 342–345.

Hsiao, K.K., Scott, M., Foster, D., Groth, D.F., DeArmond, S.J. & Prusiner, S.B. (1990) Spontaneous neurodegeneration in transgenic mice with mutant prion protein. *Science* **250**, 1587–1590.

Huff, F.J., Auerbach, J., Chakravarti, A. & Boller, F. (1988) Risk of dementia in relatives of patients with Alzheimer's disease. *Neurology* **38**, 786–790.

Huggins, M., Bloch, M., Wiggins, S. *et al.* (1992) Predictive testing for Huntington disease in Canada: adverse effects and unexpected results in those receiving a decreased risk. *American Journal of Medical Genetics* **42**, 508–515.

Hughes, J.C., Hope, T., Reader, S. & Rice, D. (2002) Dementia and ethics: the views of informal carers. *Journal of the Royal Society of Medicine* **95**, 242–246.

Humpel, C. & Marksteiner, J. (2005) Cerebrovascular damage as a cause for Alzheimer's disease. *Current Neurovascular Research* **2**, 341–347.

Huntington, G. (1910) Recollections of Huntington's chorea as I saw it at East Hampton, Long Island, during my boyhood. *Journal of Nervous and Mental Disease* **37**, 255–257.

Imamura, T., Takatsuki, Y., Fujimori, M. *et al.* (1998) Age at onset and language disturbances in Alzheimer's disease. *Neuropsychologia* **36**, 945–949.

Imamura, T., Ishii, K., Hirono, N. *et al.* (1999) Visual hallucinations and regional cerebral metabolism in dementia with Lewy bodies (DLB). *Neuroreport* **10**, 1903–1907.

Inouye, S.K., Zhang, Y., Han, L., Leo-Summers, L., Jones, R. & Marcantonio, E. (2006) Recoverable cognitive dysfunction at hospital admission in older persons during acute illness. *Journal of General Internal Medicine* **21**, 1276–1281.

in't Veld, B.A., Ruitenberg, A., Hofman, A. *et al.* (2001) Nonsteroidal antiinflammatory drugs and the risk of Alzheimer's disease. *New England Journal of Medicine* **345**, 1515–1521.

Ironside, J.W. (2003) The spectrum of safety: variant Creutzfeldt–Jakob disease in the United Kingdom. *Seminars in Hematology* **40**, 16–22.

Ironside, J.W. (2006) Variant Creutzfeldt–Jakob disease: risk of transmission by blood transfusion and blood therapies. *Haemophilia* **12** (suppl. 1), 8–15.

Ironside, J.W., Bishop, M.T., Connolly, K. *et al.* (2006) Variant Creutzfeldt–Jakob disease: prion protein genotype analysis of positive appendix tissue samples from a retrospective prevalence study. *British Medical Journal* **332**, 1186–1188.

Jack, C.R. Jr, Petersen, R.C., Xu, Y. *et al.* (2000) Rates of hippocampal atrophy correlate with change in clinical status in aging and AD. *Neurology* **55**, 484–489.

Jagust, W. (2004) Molecular neuroimaging in Alzheimer's disease. *NeuroRx* **1**, 206–212.

Jarvik, L. & Greenson, H. (1987) Translation of Alzheimer A. *Alzheimer Disease and Associated Disorders* **1**, 7–8.

Jellinger, K.A. & Attems, J. (2003) Incidence of cerebrovascular lesions in Alzheimer's disease: a postmortem study. *Acta Neuropathologica* **105**, 14–17.

Jenkins, R., Fox, N.C., Rossor, A.M., Harvey, R.J. & Rossor, M.N. (2000) Intracranial volume and Alzheimer disease: evidence against the cerebral reserve hypothesis. *Archives of Neurology* **57**, 220–224.

Jeong, J. (2004) EEG dynamics in patients with Alzheimer's disease. *Clinical Neurophysiology* **115**, 1490–1505.

Jernigan, T.L., Salmon, D.P., Butters, N. & Hesselink, J.R. (1991) Cerebral structure on MRI. Part II. Specific changes in Alzheimer's and Huntington's diseases. *Biological Psychiatry* **29**, 68–81.

Jessen, F.M., Block, W.P., Traber, F.P. *et al.* (2000) Proton MR spectroscopy detects a relative decrease of N-acetylaspartate in the medial temporal lobe of patients with AD. *Neurology* **55**, 684–688.

Jobst, K.A., Smith, A.D., Szatmari, M. *et al.* (1992) Detection in life of confirmed Alzheimer's disease using a simple measurement of medial temporal lobe atrophy by computed tomography. *Lancet* **340**, 1179–1183.

Jobst, K.A., Barnetson, L.P. & Shepstone, B.J. (1998) Accurate prediction of histologically confirmed Alzheimer's disease and the differential diagnosis of dementia: the use of NINCDS-ADRDA and DSM-III-R criteria, SPECT, X-ray CT, and Apo E4 in medial temporal lobe dementias. Oxford Project to Investigate Memory and Aging. *International Psychogeriatrics* **10**, 271–302.

Jorm, A.F. (2000) Is depression a risk factor for dementia or cognitive decline? A review. *Gerontology* **46**, 219–227.

Jorm, A.F., Korten, A.E. & Henderson, A.S. (1987) The prevalence of dementia: a quantitative integration of the literature. *Acta Psychiatrica Scandinavica* **76**, 465–479.

Jorm, A.F., van Duijn, C.M., Chandra, V. *et al.* (1991) Psychiatric history and related exposures as risk factors for Alzheimer's disease: a collaborative re-analysis of case–control studies. EURODEM Risk Factors Research Group. *International Journal of Epidemiology* **20** (suppl. 2), S43–S47.

Jost, B.C. & Grossberg, G.T. (1996) The evolution of psychiatric symptoms in Alzheimer's disease: a natural history study. *Journal of the American Geriatric Society* **44**, 1078–1081.

Joutel, A., Corpechot, C., Ducros, A. *et al.* (1997) *Notch3* mutations in cerebral autosomal dominant arteriopathy with subcortical infarcts and leukoencephalopathy (CADASIL), a mendelian condition causing stroke and vascular dementia. *Annals of the New York Academy of Sciences* **826**, 213–217.

Kalaria, R.N., Kenny, R.A., Ballard, C.G., Perry, R., Ince, P. & Polvikoski, T. (2004) Towards defining the neuropathological substrates of vascular dementia. *Journal of the Neurological Sciences* **226**, 75–80.

Kalback, W., Esh, C., Castano, E.M. *et al.* (2004) Atherosclerosis, vascular amyloidosis and brain hypoperfusion in the pathogenesis of sporadic Alzheimer's disease. *Neurological Research* **26**, 525–539.

Kalmijn, S., Launer, L.J., Ott, A., Witteman, J.C., Hofman, A. & Breteler, M.M. (1997) Dietary fat intake and the risk of incident dementia in the Rotterdam Study. *Annals of Neurology* **42**, 776–782.

Kalra, S., Bergeron, C. & Lang, A.E. (1996) Lewy body disease and dementia. A review. *Archives of Internal Medicine* **156**, 487–493.

Kang, J., Lemaire, H.G., Unterbeck, A. *et al.* (1987) The precursor of Alzheimer's disease amyloid A4 protein resembles a cell-surface receptor. *Nature* **325**, 733–736.

Kantarci, K. & Jack, C.R. Jr (2003) Neuroimaging in Alzheimer disease: an evidence-based review. *Neuroimaging Clinics of North America* **13**, 197–209.

Katzman, R., Aronson, M., Fuld, P. *et al.* (1989) Development of dementing illnesses in an 80-year-old volunteer cohort. *Annals of Neurology* **25**, 317–324.

Kay, D.W., Beamish, P. & Roth, M. (1964) Old age mental disorders in Newcastle upon Tyne. I. A study of prevalence. *British Journal of Psychiatry* **110**, 146–158.

Kay, D.W., Bergmann, K., Foster, E.M., McKechnie, A.A. & Roth, M. (1970) Mental illness and hospital usage in the elderly: a random sample followed up. *Comprehensive Psychiatry* **11**, 26–35.

Kazantsev, A., Walker, H.A., Slepko, N. *et al.* (2002) A bivalent Huntingtin binding peptide suppresses polyglutamine aggregation and pathogenesis in *Drosophila*. *Nature Genetics* **30**, 367–376.

Kehoe, P.G., Russ, C., McIlroy, S. *et al.* (1999) Variation in *DCP1*, encoding ACE, is associated with susceptibility to Alzheimer disease. *Nature Genetics* **21**, 71–72.

Kertesz, A. & Munoz, D. (2004) Relationship between frontotemporal dementia and corticobasal degeneration/progressive supranuclear palsy. *Dementia and Geriatric Cognitive Disorders* **17**, 282–286.

Keshavan, M.S., Lishman, W.A. & Hughes, J.T. (1987) Psychiatric presentation of Creutzfeldt–Jakob disease. A case report. *British Journal of Psychiatry* **151**, 260–263.

Klein, D.A., Steinberg, M., Galik, E. *et al.* (1999) Wandering behaviour in community-residing persons with dementia. *International Journal of Geriatric Psychiatry* **14**, 272–279.

Klunk, W.E., Xu, C., Panchalingram, K., McClure, R.J. & Pettegrew, J.W. (1996) Quantitative ^{1}H and ^{31}P MRS of PCA extracts of postmortem Alzheimer's disease brain. *Neurobiology of Aging* **17**, 349–357.

Klunk, W.E., Engler, H., Nordberg, A. *et al.* (2004) Imaging brain amyloid in Alzheimer's disease with Pittsburgh Compound-B. *Annals of Neurology* **55**, 306–319.

Knopman, D.S., DeKosky, S.T., Cummings, J.L. *et al.* (2001) Practice parameter: diagnosis of dementia (an evidence-based review). Report of the Quality Standards Subcommittee of the American Academy of Neurology. *Neurology* **56**, 1143–1153.

Knopman, D.S., Petersen, R.C., Cha, R.H., Edland, S.D. & Rocca, W.A. (2006) Incidence and causes of nondegenerative nonvascular dementia: a population-based study. *Archives of Neurology* **63**, 218–221.

Kolsch, H., Jessen, F., Freymann, N. *et al.* (2005) ACE I/D polymorphism is a risk factor of Alzheimer's disease but not of vascular dementia. *Neuroscience Letters* **377**, 37–39.

Korten, A.E., Jorm, A.F., Henderson, A.S., Broe, G.A., Creasey, H. & McCusker, E. (1993) Assessing the risk of Alzheimer's disease in first-degree relatives of Alzheimer's disease cases. *Psychological Medicine* **23**, 915–923.

Koshy, B.T. & Zoghbi, H.Y. (1997) The CAG/polyglutamine tract diseases: gene products and molecular pathogenesis. *Brain Pathology* **7**, 927–942.

Kotrla, K.J., Chacko, R.C., Harper, R.G., Jhingran, S. & Doody, R. (1995) SPECT findings on psychosis in Alzheimer's disease. *American Journal of Psychiatry* **152**, 1470–1475.

Kuhl, D.E., Phelps, M.E., Markham, C.H., Metter, J., Riege, W.H. & Winter, J. (1982) Cerebral metabolism and atrophy in Huntington's disease determined by ^{18}FDG and computed tomographic scan. *Annals of Neurology* **12**, 425–434.

Kuhl, D.E., Markham, C.H., Metter, E.J., Riege, W.H., Phelps, M.E. & Mazziotta, J.C. (1985) Local cerebral glucose utilization in symptomatic and presymptomatic Huntington's disease. In: Sokoloff, L. (ed.) *Brain Imaging and Brain Function*, pp. 199–209. Association for Research in Nervous and Mental Disease, vol. 63. Raven Press, New York.

Kuller, L.H., Lopez, O.L., Jagust, W.J. *et al.* (2005) Determinants of vascular dementia in the Cardiovascular Health Cognition Study. *Neurology* **64**, 1548–1552.

Kumar, V., Giacobini, E. & Markwell, S. (1989) CSF choline and acetylcholinesterase in early-onset vs. late-onset Alzheimer's disease patients. *Acta Neurologica Scandinavica* **80**, 461–466.

Kuusisto, J., Koivisto, K., Mykkänen, L. *et al.* (1997) Association between features of the insulin resistance syndrome and Alzheimer's disease independently of apolipoprotein E4 phenotype: cross sectional population based study. *British Medical Journal* **315**, 1045–1049.

Lang, C.J., Heckmann, J.G. & Neundorfer, B. (1998) Creutzfeldt–Jakob disease via dural and corneal transplants. *Journal of the Neurological Sciences* **160**, 128–139.

Lantos, P.L., McGill, I.S., Janota, I. *et al.* (1992) Prion protein immunocytochemistry helps to establish the true incidence of prion diseases. *Neuroscience Letters* **147**, 67–71.

Launer, L.J., Andersen, K., Dewey, M.E. *et al.* (1999) Rates and risk factors for dementia and Alzheimer's disease: results from EURODEM pooled analyses. *Neurology* **52**, 78–84.

Laurin, D., Verreault, R., Lindsay, J., MacPherson, K. & Rockwood, K. (2001) Physical activity and risk of cognitive impairment and dementia in elderly persons. *Archives of Neurology* **58**, 498–504.

Leach, S.P., Salman, M.D. & Hamar, D. (2006) Trace elements and prion diseases: a review of the interactions of copper, manganese and zinc with the prion protein. *Animal Health Research Reviews* **7**, 97–105.

Leaper, S.A., Murray, A.D., Lemmon, H.A. *et al.* (2001) Neuropsychologic correlates of brain white matter lesions depicted on MR images: 1921 Aberdeen Birth Cohort. *Radiology* **221**, 51–55.

Lee, V.M., Goedert, M. & Trojanowski, J.Q. (2001) Neurodegenerative tauopathies. *Annual Review of Neuroscience* **24**, 1121–1159.

Lee, W.T. & Chang, C. (2004) Magnetic resonance imaging and spectroscopy in assessing 3-nitropropionic acid-induced brain lesions: an animal model of Huntington's disease. *Progress in Neurobiology* **72**, 87–110.

Lennox, G., Lowe, J., Morrell, K., Landon, M. & Mayer, J. (1989) Anti-ubiquitin immunocytochemistry is more sensitive than conventional techniques in the detection of diffuse Lewy body disease. *Journal of Neurology, Neurosurgery and Psychiatry* **52**, 67–71.

Letenneur, L., Gilleron, V., Commenges, D., Helmer, C., Orgogozo, J.M. & Dartigues, J.F. (1999) Are sex and educational level independent predictors of dementia and Alzheimer's disease? Incidence data from the PAQUID project. *Journal of Neurology, Neurosurgery and Psychiatry* **66**, 177–183.

Letenneur, L., Launer, L.J., Andersen, K. *et al.* (2000) Education and the risk for Alzheimer's disease: sex makes a difference. *American Journal of Epidemiology* **151**, 1064–1071.

Li, Y., Meyer, J.S. & Thornby, J. (2001) Depressive symptoms among cognitively normal versus cognitively impaired elderly subjects. *International Journal of Geriatric Psychiatry* **16**, 455–461.

Li, Y.J., Scott, W.K., Hedges, D.J. *et al.* (2002) Age at onset in two common neurodegenerative diseases is genetically controlled. *American Journal of Human Genetics* **70**, 985–993.

Liberski, P.P. & Budka, H. (2004) Gerstmann–Straussler–Scheinker disease. I. Human diseases. *Folia Neuropathologica* **42** (suppl. B), 120–140.

Liddell, M.B., Lovestone, S. & Owen, M.J. (2001) Genetic risk of Alzheimer's disease: advising relatives. *British Journal of Psychiatry* **178**, 7–11.

Liepelt, I., Maetzler, W., Blaicher, H.P., Gasser, T. & Berg, D. (2007) Treatment of dementia in parkinsonian syndromes with cholinesterase inhibitors. *Dementia and Geriatric Cognitive Disorders* **23**, 251–267.

Lim, G.P., Yang, F., Chu, T. *et al.* (2001) Ibuprofen effects on Alzheimer pathology and open field activity in APPsw transgenic mice. *Neurobiology of Aging* **22**, 983–991.

Lindsay, J., Laurin, D., Verreault, R. *et al.* (2002) Risk factors for Alzheimer's disease: a prospective analysis from the Canadian Study of Health and Aging. *American Journal of Epidemiology* **156**, 445–453.

Liolitsa, D., Powell, J. & Lovestone, S. (2002) Genetic variability in the insulin signalling pathway may contribute to the risk of late onset Alzheimer's disease. *Journal of Neurology, Neurosurgery and Psychiatry* **73**, 261–266.

Lippa, C.F., Schmidt, M.L., Lee, V.M. & Trojanowski, J.Q. (2001) Alpha-synuclein in familial Alzheimer disease: epitope mapping parallels dementia with Lewy bodies and Parkinson disease. *Archives of Neurology* **58**, 1817–1820.

Loizou, L.A., Kendall, B.E. & Marshall, J. (1981) Subacute arteriosclerotic encephalopathy: a clinical and radiological investigation. *Journal of Neurology, Neurosurgery and Psychiatry* **44**, 294–304.

Lopez, O.L., Litvan, I., Catt, K.E. *et al.* (1999) Accuracy of four clinical diagnostic criteria for the diagnosis of neurodegenerative dementias. *Neurology* **53**, 1292–1299.

Louvi, A., Arboleda-Velasquez, J.F., and Artavanis-Tsakonas, S. (2006) CADASIL: a critical look at a Notch disease. *Developmental Neuroscience* **28**, 5–12.

Lovestone, S. (1999) Early diagnosis and the clinical genetics of Alzheimer's disease. *Journal of Neurology* **246**, 69–72.

Lovestone, S. & Lashwood, A. (2001) Genetic counselling. In: Tomas, P., Davison, A. & Rance, C. (eds) *Clincial Counselling in Medical Settings*, pp. 24–38. Brunner-Rotledge, East Sussex, UK.

Lovestone, S. & McLoughlin, D.M. (2002) Protein aggregates and dementia: is there a common toxicity? *Journal of Neurology, Neurosurgery and Psychiatry* **72**, 152–161.

Lovestone, S. & Reynolds, C.H. (1997) The phosphorylation of tau: a critical stage in neurodevelopmental and neurodegenerative processes. *Neuroscience* **78**, 309–324.

Lovestone, S., Hodgson, S., Sham, P., Differ, A.M. & Levy, R. (1996) Familial psychiatric presentation of Huntington's disease. *Journal of Medical Genetics* **33**, 128–131.

Lovestone, S., Graham, N. & Howard, R. (1997) Guidelines on drug treatments for Alzheimer's disease. *Lancet* **350**, 232–233.

Lowin, A., Knapp, M. & McCrone, P. (2001) Alzheimer's disease in the UK: comparative evidence on cost of illness and volume of health services research funding. *International Journal of Geriatric Psychiatry* **16**, 1143–1148.

Lucca, U., Comelli, M., Tettamanti, M., Tiraboschi, P. & Spagnoli, A. (1993) Rate of progression and prognostic factors in Alzheimer's disease: a prospective study. *Journal of the American Geriatric Society*. **41**, 45–49.

Luchsinger, J.A., Tang, M.X., Stern, Y., Shea, S. & Mayeux, R. (2001) Diabetes mellitus and risk of Alzheimer's disease and dementia with stroke in a multiethnic cohort. *American Journal of Epidemiology* **154**, 635–641.

Luchsinger, J.A., Tang, M.X., Shea, S. & Mayeux, R. (2003) Antioxidant vitamin intake and risk of Alzheimer disease. *Archives of Neurology* **60**, 203–208.

Lyketsos, C.G., Corazzini, K. & Steele, C. (1995) Mania in Alzheimer's disease. *Journal of Neuropsychiatry and Clinical Neuroscience* **7**, 350–352.

Lyketsos, C.G., Sheppard, J.M., Steinberg, M. *et al.* (2001) Neuropsychiatric disturbance in Alzheimer's disease clusters into three groups: the Cache County study. *International Journal of Geriatric Psychiatry* **16**, 1043–1053.

Lyketsos, C.G., Lopez, O., Jones, B., Fitzpatrick, A.L., Breitner, J. & DeKosky, S. (2002) Prevalence of neuropsychiatric symptoms in dementia and mild cognitive impairment: results from the cardiovascular health study. *Journal of the American Medical Association* **288**, 1475–1483.

Lyketsos, C.G., DelCampo, L., Steinberg, M. *et al.* (2003) Treating depression in Alzheimer disease: efficacy and safety of sertraline therapy, and the benefits of depression reduction: the DIADS. *Archives of General Psychiatry* **60**, 737–746.

Lyness, S.A., Zarow, C. & Chui, H.C. (2003) Neuron loss in key cholinergic and aminergic nuclei in Alzheimer disease: a metaanalysis. *Neurobiology of Aging* **24**, 1–23.

Lyon, R.L. (1962) Huntington's chorea in the Moray Firth area. *British Medical Journal* **1**, 1301–1306.

Maat-Schieman, M., Roos, R. & van Diunen, S. (2005) Hereditary cerebral hemorrhage with amyloidosis-Dutch type. *Neuropathology* **25**, 288–297.

Maat-Schieman, M., Roos, R., Losekoot, M. *et al.* (2007) Neuronal intranuclear and neuropil inclusions for pathological assessment of Huntington's disease. *Brain Pathology* **17**, 31–37.

Maccioni, R.B., Lavados, M., Maccioni, C.B. & Mendoza-Naranjo, A. (2004) Biological markers of Alzheimer's disease and mild cognitive impairment. *Current Alzheimer Research* **1**, 307–314.

McCurry, S.M., Gibbons, L.E., Logsdon, R.G. & Teri, L. (2004) Anxiety and nighttime behavioral disturbances. Awakenings in patients with Alzheimer's disease. *Journal of Gerontological Nursing* **30**, 12–20.

McGeer, P.L., Schulzer, M. & McGeer, E.G. (1996) Arthritis and anti-inflammatory agents as possible protective factors for Alzheimer's disease: a review of 17 epidemiologic studies. *Neurology* **47**, 425–432.

McGuinness, B., Todd, S., Passmore, P. & Bullock, R. (2006) The effects of blood pressure lowering on development of cognitive impairment and dementia in patients without apparent prior cerebrovascular disease. *Cochrane Database of Systematic Reviews* CD004034.

McHugh, P.R. & Folstein, M.F. (1975) Psychiatric syndromes of Huntington's chorea. In: Benson, D.F. & Blamer, D. (eds) *Psychiatric Aspects of Neurologic Disease*, ch. 13. Grune & Stratton, New York.

McIlroy, S.P., Dynan, K.B., Lawson, J.T., Patterson, C.C. & Passmore, A.P. (2002) Moderately elevated plasma homocysteine, methylenetetrahydrofolate reductase genotype, and risk for stroke, vascular dementia, and Alzheimer disease in Northern Ireland. *Stroke* **33**, 2351–2356.

McKee, A.C., Kowall, N.W. & Kosik, K.S. (1989) Microtubular reorganization and dendritic growth response in Alzheimer's disease. *Annals of Neurology* **26**, 652–659.

McKeith, I.G., Perry, R.H., Fairbairn, A.F., Jabeen, S. & Perry, E.K. (1992) Operational criteria for senile dementia of Lewy body type (SDLT). *Psychological Medicine* **22**, 911–922.

McKeith, I.G., Galasko, D., Kosaka, K. *et al.* (1996) Consensus guidelines for the clinical and pathologic diagnosis of dementia with Lewy bodies (DLB): report of the consortium on DLB international workshop. *Neurology* **47**, 1113–1124.

McKeith, I.G., Perry, E.K., Perry, R.H. & Consortium Dementia Lewy Bodies (1999) Report of the second dementia with Lewy body international workshop: diagnosis and treatment. *Neurology* **53**, 902–905.

McKeith, I.G., Burn, D.J., Ballard, C.G. *et al.* (2003) Dementia with Lewy bodies. *Seminars in Clinical Neuropsychiatry* **8**, 46–57.

McKeith, I.G., Dickson, D.W., Lowe, J. *et al.* (2005) Diagnosis and management of dementia with Lewy bodies. Third Report of the DLB Consortium. *Neurology* **65**, 1863–1872.

McKhann, G., Drachman, D., Folstein, M., Katzman, R., Price, D. & Stadlan, E.M. (1984) Clinical diagnosis of Alzheimer's disease: report of the NINCDS-ADRDA Work Group under the auspices of Department of Health and Human Services Task Force on Alzheimer's Disease. *Neurology* **34**, 939–944.

MacKnight, C., Rockwood, K., Awalt, E. & McDowell, I. (2002) Diabetes mellitus and the risk of dementia, Alzheimer's disease and vascular cognitive impairment in the Canadian Study of Health and Aging. *Dementia and Geriatric Cognitive Disorders* **14**, 77–83.

Mackowiak-Cordoliani, M.A., Bombois, S., Memin, A., Henon, H. & Pasquier, F. (2005) Poststroke dementia in the elderly. *Drugs and Aging* **22**, 483–493.

McShane, R., Keene, J., Gedling, K., Fairburn, C., Jacoby, R. & Hope, T. (1997) Do neuroleptic drugs hasten cognitive decline in dementia? Prospective study with necropsy follow up. *British Medical Journal* **314**, 266–270.

Mad'ar, R., Maslenova, D., Ranostajova, K., Straka, S. & Baska, T. (2003) Analysis of unusual accumulation of Creutzfeldt–Jakob disease cases in Orava and Liptov regions (northern Slovak focus) 1983–2000. *Central European Journal of Public Health* **11**, 19–22.

Majores, M., Kolsch, H., Bagli, M. *et al.* (2002) The insulin gene VNTR polymorphism in Alzheimer's disease: results of a pilot study. *Journal of Neural Transmission* **109**, 1029–1034.

Malouf, M., Grimley, E.J. & Areosa, S.A. (2003) Folic acid with or without vitamin B12 for cognition and dementia. *Cochrane Database of Systematic Reviews* CD004514.

Mann, D.M. (1988) Alzheimer's disease and Down's syndrome. *Histopathology* **13**, 125–137.

Manson, J.C., Cancellotti, E., Hart, P., Bishop, M.T. & Barron, R.M. (2006) The transmissible spongiform encephalopathies: emerging and declining epidemics. *Biochemical Society Transactions* **34**, 1155–1158.

Marra, C., Silveri, M.C. & Gainotti, G. (2000) Predictors of cognitive decline in the early stage of probable Alzheimer's disease. *Dementia* **11**, 212–218.

Marsden, C.D. (1982) Basal ganglia and disease. *Lancet* **ii**, 1141–1146.

Marsden, C.D. & Harrison, M.J. (1972) Outcome of investigation of patients with presenile dementia. *British Medical Journal* **2**, 249–252.

Marshall, J., White, K., Weaver, M. *et al.* (2007) Specific psychiatric manifestations among preclinical Huntington disease mutation carriers. *Archives of Neurology* **64**, 116–121.

Marti, M.J., Tolosa, E. & Campdelacreu, J. (2003) Clinical overview of the synucleinopathies. *Movement Disorders* **18** (suppl. 6), S21–S27.

Martin, B.C., Ricci, J.F., Kotzan, J.A., Lang, K. & Menzin, J. (2000) The net cost of Alzheimer disease and related dementia: a population-based study of Georgia Medicaid recipients. *Alzheimer Disease and Associated Disorders* **14**, 151–159.

Masdeu, J.C., Zubieta, J.L. & Arbizu, J. (2005) Neuroimaging as a marker of the onset and progression of Alzheimer's disease. *Journal of the Neurological Sciences* **236**, 55–64.

Masters, C.L., Simms, G., Weinman, N.A., Multhaup, G., McDonald, B.L. & Beyreuther, K. (1985) Amyloid plaque core protein in Alzheimer disease and Down syndrome. *Proceedings of the National Academy of Sciences USA* **82**, 4245–4249.

Matthews, B., Siemers, E.R. & Mozley, P.D. (2003) Imaging-based measures of disease progression in clinical trials of disease-modifying drugs for Alzheimer disease. *American Journal of Geriatric Psychiatry* **11**, 146–159.

Mattila, P.M., Rinne, J.O., Helenius, H., Dickson, D.W. & Röyttä, M. (2000) Alpha-synuclein-immunoreactive cortical Lewy bodies are associated with cognitive impairment in Parkinson's disease. *Acta Neuropathologica* **100**, 285–290.

Mayeux, R., Saunders, A.M., Shea, S. *et al.* (1998) Utility of the apolipoprotein E genotype in the diagnosis of Alzheimer's disease. *New England Journal of Medicine* **338**, 506–511.

Mazziotta, J.C., Phelps, M.E., Pahl, J.J. *et al.* (1987) Reduced cerebral glucose metabolism in asymptomatic subjects at risk for Huntington's disease. *New England Journal of Medicine* **316**, 357–362.

Mead, S. (2006) Prion disease genetics. *European Journal of Human Genetics* **14**, 273–281.

Mega, M.S., Chu, T., Mazziotta, J.C. *et al.* (1999) Mapping biochemistry to metabolism: FDG-PET and amyloid burden in Alzheimer's disease. *Neuroreport* **10**, 2911–2917.

Mega, M.S., Lee, L., Dinov, I.D., Mishkin, F., Toga, A.W. & Cummings, J.L. (2000) Cerebral correlates of psychotic symptoms in Alzheimer's disease. *Journal of Neurology, Neurosurgery and Psychiatry* **69**, 167–171.

Meguro, K., Shimada, M., Yamaguchi, S. *et al.* (2001) Cognitive function and frontal lobe atrophy in normal elderly adults: implications for dementia not as aging-related disorders and the reserve hypothesis. *Psychiatry and Clinical Neurosciences* **55**, 565–572.

Meissen, G.J. & Berchek, R.L. (1987) Intended use of predictive testing by those at risk for Huntington disease. *American Journal of Medical Genetics* **26**, 283–293.

Meneilly, G.S. & Hill, A. (1993) Alterations in glucose metabolism in patients with Alzheimer's disease. *Journal of the American Geriatric Society* **41**, 710–714.

Mesulam, M.M. (2001) Primary progressive aphasia. *Annals of Neurology* **49**, 425–432.

Meyer, M.R., Tschanz, J.T., Norton, M.C. *et al.* (1998) *APOE* genotype predicts when, not whether, one is predisposed to develop Alzheimer disease. *Nature Genetics* **19**, 321–322.

Mielke, M.M., Zandi, P.P., Sjogren, M. *et al.* (2005) High total cholesterol levels in late life associated with a reduced risk of dementia. *Neurology* **64**, 1689–1695.

Migliorelli, R., Tesón, A., Sabe, L., Petracchi, M., Leiguarda, R. & Starkstein, S.E. (1995) Prevalence and correlates of dysthymia and major depression among patients with Alzheimer's disease. *American Journal of Psychiatry* **152**, 37–44.

Miller, J.W., Green, R., Ramos, M.I. *et al.* (2003) Homocysteine and cognitive function in the Sacramento Area Latino Study on Aging. *American Journal of Clinical Nutrition* **78**, 441–447.

Milosevic, D.P., Kostic, S., Potic, B. *et al.* (2007) Is there such thing as 'Reversible Dementia' (RD)? *Archives of Gerontology and Geriatrics* **44** (suppl.), 271–277.

Milwain, E. & Iversen, S. (2002) Cognitive change in old age. In: Jacoby, R. & Oppenheimer, C. (eds) *Psychiatry in the Elderly*, pp. 43–79. Oxford University Press, Oxford.

Minett, T.S., Dean, J.L., Firbank, M., English, P. & O'Brien, J.T. (2005) Subjective memory complaints, white-matter lesions, depressive symptoms, and cognition in elderly patients. *American Journal of Geriatric Psychiatry* **13**, 665–671.

Minski, L. & Guttmann, E. (1938) Huntington's chorea: a study of thirty-four families. *Journal of Mental Science* **84**, 21–96.

Mizuno, K., Wakai, M., Takeda, A. & Sobue, G. (2000) Medial temporal atrophy and memory impairment in early stage of Alzheimer's disease: an MRI volumetric and memory assessment study. *Journal of the Neurological Sciences* **173**, 18–24.

Moceri, V.M., Kukull, W.A., Emanuel, I., van Belle, G. & Larson, E.B. (2000) Early-life risk factors and the development of Alzheimer's disease. *Neurology* **54**, 415–420.

Montoya, A., Pelletier, M., Menear, M., Duplessis, E., Richer, F. & Lepage, M. (2006a) Episodic memory impairment in Huntington's disease: a meta-analysis. *Neuropsychologia* **44**, 1984–1994.

Montoya, A., Price, B.H., Menear, M. & Lepage, M. (2006b) Brain imaging and cognitive dysfunctions in Huntington's disease. *Journal of Psychiatry and Neuroscience* **31**, 21–29.

Mook-Jung, I., Joo, I., Sohn, S., Kwon, H.J., Huh, K. & Jung, M.W. (1997) Estrogen blocks neurotoxic effects of β-amyloid (1–42) and induces neurite extension on B103 cells. *Neuroscience Letters* **235**, 101–104.

Moore, R.A., Vorberg, I. & Priola, S.A. (2005) Species barriers in prion diseases: brief review. *Archives of Virology Supplement* **19**, 187–202.

Morris, M.C., Evans, D.A., Bienias, J.L. et al. (2003a) Consumption of fish and n-3 fatty acids and risk of incident Alzheimer disease. *Archives of Neurology* **60**, 940–946.

Morris, M.C., Evans, D.A., Bienias, J.L. *et al.* (2003b) Dietary fats and the risk of incident Alzheimer disease. *Archives of Neurology* **60**, 194–200.

Mortimer, J.A., van Duijn, C.M., Chandra, V. *et al.* (1991) Head trauma as a risk factor for Alzheimer's disease: a collaborative re-analysis of case–control studies. *International Journal of Epidemiology* **20** (suppl. 2), S28–S35.

Mortimer, J.A., Snowdon, D. & Markesbery, W. (2003) Head circumference, education and risk of dementia: findings from the Nun study. *Journal of Clinical and Experimental Neuropsychology* **25**, 671–679.

Mosconi, L. (2005) Brain glucose metabolism in the early and specific diagnosis of Alzheimer's disease FDG-PET studies in MCI and AD. *European Journal of Nuclear Medicine and Molecular Imaging* **32**, 486–510

Moss, M.B., Albert, M.S., Butters, N. & Payne, M. (1986) Differential patterns of memory loss among patients with Alzheimer's disease, Huntington's disease, and alcoholic Korsakoff's syndrome. *Archives of Neurology* **43**, 239–246.

MRC CFAS (2001) Pathological correlates of late-onset dementia in a multicentre, community-based population in England and Wales. Neuropathology Group of the Medical Research Council Cognitive Function and Ageing Study (MRC CFAS). *Lancet* **357**, 169–175.

Mudher, A. & Lovestone, S. (2002) Alzheimer's disease: do tauists and baptists finally shake hands? *Trends in Neuroscience* **25**, 22–26.

Mullan, M. & Crawford, F. (1994) The molecular genetics of Alzheimer's disease. *Molecular Neurobiology* **9**, 15–22.

Mulnard, R.I., Cotman, C.W., Kawas, C. *et al.* (2000) Estrogen replacement therapy for treatment of mild to moderate Alzheimer disease: a randomized controlled trial. *Journal of the American Medical Association* **283**, 1007–1015.

Mungas, D., Reed, B.R., Jagust, W.J. *et al.* (2002) Volumetric MRI predicts rate of cognitive decline related to AD and cerebrovascular disease. *Neurology* **59**, 867–873.

Munoz, D.G., Dickson, D.W., Bergeron, C., Mackenzie, I.R., Delacourte, A. & Zhukareva, V. (2003) The neuropathology and biochemistry of frontotemporal dementia. *Annals of Neurology* **54** (suppl. 5), S24–S28.

Myers, A., Holmans, P., Marshall, H. *et al.* (2000) Susceptibility locus for Alzheimer's disease on chromosome 10. *Science* **290**, 2304–2305.

Myrianthopoulos, N.C. (1966) Huntington's chorea. *Journal of Medical Genetics* **3**, 298–314.

Nacmias, B., Tedde, A., Forleo, P. *et al.* (2001) Association between 5-HT(2A) receptor polymorphism and psychotic symptoms in Alzheimer's disease. *Biological Psychiatry* **50**, 472–475.

Nagga, K., Rajani, R., Mardh, E., Borch, K., Mardh, S. & Marcusson, J. (2003) Cobalamin, folate, methylmalonic acid, homocysteine, and gastritis markers in dementia. *Dementia and Geriatric Cognitive Disorders* **16**, 269–275.

Nagy, Z., Esiri, M.M., Jobst, K.A. *et al.* (1995) Relative roles of plaques and tangles in the dementia of Alzheimer's disease: correlations using three sets of neuropathological criteria. *Dementia* **6**, 21–31.

Nagy, Z., Esiri, M.M., Jobst, K.A. *et al.* (1997) The effects of additional pathology on the cognitive deficit in Alzheimer disease. *Journal of Neuropathology and Experimental Neurology* **56**, 165–170.

Nance, M.A. (1997) Clinical aspects of CAG repeat diseases. *Brain Pathology* **7**, 881–900.

Neal, M. & Briggs, M. (2003) Validation therapy for dementia. *Cochrane Database of Systematic Reviews* CD001394.

Neary, D. (1999) Overview of frontotemporal dementias and the consensus applied. *Dementia and Geriatric Cognitive Disorders* **10** (suppl. 1), 6–9.

Neary, D., Snowden, J.S., Northen, B. & Goulding, P. (1988) Dementia of frontal lobe type. *Journal of Neurology, Neurosurgery and Psychiatry* **51**, 353–361.

Neary, D., Snowden, J.S., Gustafson, L. *et al.* (1998) Frontotemporal lobar degeneration: a consensus on clinical diagnostic criteria. *Neurology* **51**, 1546–1554.

Nestor, P.J., Scheltens, P. & Hodges, J.R. (2004) Advances in the early detection of Alzheimer's disease. *Nature Medicine* **10** (suppl.), S34–S41.

Nicoll, J.A., Wilkinson, D., Holmes, C., Steart, P., Markham, H. & Weller, R.O. (2003) Neuropathology of human Alzheimer disease after immunization with amyloid-beta peptide: a case report. *Nature Medicine* **9**, 448–452.

Nielson, K.A., Nolan, J.H., Berchtold, N.C., Sandman, C.A., Mulnard, R.A. & Cotman, C.W. (1996) Apolipoprotein-E genotyping of diabetic dementia patients: is diabetes rare in Alzheimer's disease. *Journal of the American Geriatric Society* **44**, 897–904.

Nishimoto, I., Okamoto, T., Matsuura, Y., Takahashi, S., Murayama, Y. & Ogata, E. (1993) Alzheimer amyloid protein precursor complexes with brain GTP-binding protein G_o. *Nature* **362**, 75–79.

Nuwer, M. (1997) Assessment of digital EEG, quantitative EEG, and EEG brain mapping: report of the American Academy of Neurology and the American Clinical Neurophysiology Society. *Neurology* **49**, 277–292.

Nyberg, L., Persson, J. & Nilsson, L.G. (2002) Individual differences in memory enhancement by encoding enactment: relationships to adult age and biological factors. *Neuroscience and Biobehavioral Reviews* **26**, 835–839.

O'Brien, J.T., Erkinjuntti, T., Reisberg, B. *et al.* (2003) Vascular cognitive impairment. *Lancet Neurology* **2**, 89–98.

O'Carroll, R. & Ebmeier, K. (1995) Education and prevalence of Alzheimer's disease and vascular dementia. Premorbid ability influences measures used to identify dementia. *British Medical Journal* **311**, 125–126.

O'Connor, D.W., Pollitt, P.A., Hyde, J.B., Brook, C.P., Reiss, B.B. & Roth, M. (1988) Do general practitioners miss dementia in elderly patients? *British Medical Journal* **297**, 1107–1110.

O'Hara, R., Thompson, J.M., Kraemer, H.C. *et al.* (2002) Which Alzheimer patients are at risk for rapid cognitive decline? *Journal of Geriatric Psychiatry and Neurology* **15**, 233–238.

Ohkura, T., Isse, K., Akazawa, K., Hamamoto, M., Yaoi, Y. & Hagino, N. (1995) Long-term estrogen replacement therapy in female patients with dementia of the Alzheimer type: 7 case reports. *Dementia* **6**, 99–107.

Olichney, J.M., Galasko, D., Salmon, D.P., Hofstetter, C.R., Katzman, R. & Thal, L.J. (1998) Cognitive decline is faster in Lewy body variant than in Alzheimer's disease. *Neurology* **51**, 351–357.

Oliver, J.E. (1970) Huntington's chorea in Northamptonshire. *British Journal of Psychiatry* **116**, 241–253.

Oliver, J. & Dewhurst, K. (1969) Childhood and adolescent forms of Huntington's disease. *Journal of Neurology, Neurosurgery and Psychiatry* **32**, 455–459.

Onder, G., Zanetti, O., Giacobini, E. *et al.* (2005) Reality orientation therapy combined with cholinesterase inhibitors in Alzheimer's disease: randomised controlled trial. *British Journal of Psychiatry* **187**, 450–455.

Orrell, M.W., Sahakian, B.J. & Bergmann, K. (1989) Self-neglect and frontal lobe dysfunction. *British Journal of Psychiatry* **155**, 101–105.

Osborne, J.P., Munson, P. & Burman, D. (1982) Huntington's chorea. Report of 3 cases and review of the literature. *Archives of Disease of Childhood* **57**, 99–103.

O'Shea, B. & Falvey, J. (1991) Juvenile Huntington's disease. *Irish Journal of Psychological Medicine* **8**, 149–153.

Osimani, A., Berger, A., Friedman, J., Porat-Katz, B.S. & Abarbanel, J.M. (2005) Neuropsychology of vitamin B12 deficiency in elderly dementia patients and control subjects. *Journal of Geriatric Psychiatry and Neurology* **18**, 33–38.

Ott, A., Stolk, R.P., Hofman, A., van Harskamp, F., Grobbee, D.E. & Breteler, M.M. (1996) Association of diabetes mellitus and dementia: the Rotterdam Study. *Diabetologia* **39**, 1392–1397.

Ott, A., Stolk, R.P., van Harskamp, F., Pols, H.A.P., Hofman, A. & Breteler, M.M.B. (1999) Diabetes mellitus and the risk of dementia: the Rotterdam Study. *Neurology* **53**, 1937–1942.

Owen, F., Poulter, M., Lofthouse, R. *et al.* (1989) Insertion in prion protein gene in familial Creutzfeldt–Jakob disease. *Lancet* **i**, 51–52.

Owen, M., Liddell, M. & McGuffin, P. (1994) Alzheimer's disease. *British Medical Journal* **308**, 672–673.

Paganini-Hill, A. & Henderson, V.W. (1996) Estrogen replacement therapy and risk of Alzheimer disease. *Archives of Internal Medicine* **156**, 2213–2217.

Paglini, G., Peris, L., Mascotti, F., Quiroga, S. & Caceres, A. (2000) Tau protein function in axonal formation. *Neurochemical Research* **25**, 37–42.

Pakrasi, S. & O'Brien, J.T. (2005) Emission tomography in dementia. *Nuclear Medicine Communications* **26**, 189–196.

Palmer, M.S., Dryden, A.J., Hughes, J.T. & Collinge, J. (1991) Homozygous prion protein genotype predisposes to sporadic Creutzfeldt–Jakob disease. *Nature* **352**, 340–342.

Pantoni, L. & Simoni, M. (2003) Pathophysiology of cerebral small vessels in vascular cognitive impairment. *International Psychogeriatrics* **15** (suppl. 1), 59–65.

Panza, F., D'Introno, A., Colacicco, A.M. *et al.* (2006) Lipid metabolism in cognitive decline and dementia. *Brain Research Reviews* **51**, 275–292.

Parchi, P., Giese, A., Capellari, S. *et al.* (1999) Classification of sporadic Creutzfeldt–Jakob disease based on molecular and phenotypic analysis of 300 subjects. *Annals of Neurology* **46**, 224–233.

Patwardhan, M.B., McCrory, D.C., Matchar, D.B., Samsa, G.P. & Rutschmann, O.T. (2004) Alzheimer disease: operating characteristics of PET. A meta-analysis. *Radiology* **231**, 73–80.

Paulsen, J.S., Ready, R.E., Hamilton, J.M., Mega, M.S. & Cummings, J.L. (2001a) Neuropsychiatric aspects of Huntington's disease. *Journal of Neurology, Neurosurgery and Psychiatry* **71**, 310–314.

Paulsen, J.S., Zhao, H., Stout, J.C. *et al.* (2001b) Clinical markers of early disease in persons near onset of Huntington's disease. *Neurology* **57**, 658–662.

Pavlou, M.P. & Lachs, M.S. (2006) Could self-neglect in older adults be a geriatric syndrome? *Journal of the American Geriatric Society* **54**, 831–842.

Pearlson, G.D., Ross, C.A., Lohr, W.D., Rovner, B.W., Chase, G.A. & Folstein, M.F. (1990) Association between family history of affective disorder and the depressive syndrome of Alzheimer's disease. *American Journal of Psychiatry* **147**, 452–456.

Peden, A.H., Head, M.W., Ritchie, D.L., Bell, J.E. & Ironside, J.W. (2004) Preclinical vCJD after blood transfusion in a PRNP codon 129 heterozygous patient. *Lancet* **364**, 527–529.

Pedersen, N.L., Posner, S.F. & Gatz, M. (2001) Multiple-threshold models for genetic influences on age of onset for Alzheimer disease: findings in Swedish twins. *American Journal of Medical Genetics* **105**, 724–728.

Peila, R., Rodriguez, B.L. & Launer, L.J. (2002) Type 2 diabetes, APOE gene, and the risk for dementia and related pathologies: the Honolulu–Asia Aging Study. *Diabetes* **51**, 1256–1262.

Peinemann, A., Schuller, S., Pohl, C., Jahn, T., Weindl, A. & Kassubek, J. (2005) Executive dysfunction in early stages of Huntington's disease is associated with striatal and insular atrophy: a neuropsychological and voxel-based morphometric study. *Journal of the Neurological Sciences* **239**, 11–19.

Perez-De la Cruz, V. & Santamaria, A. (2007) Integrative hypothesis for Huntington's disease: a brief review on experimental evidence. *Physiological Research* **56**, 513–526.

Perry, E.K. & Perry, R.H. (1995) Acetylcholine and hallucinations: disease-related compared to drug-induced alterations in human consciousness. *Brain and Cognition* **28**, 240–258.

Perry, E.K., Marshall, E., Perry, R.H. *et al.* (1990) Cholinergic and dopaminergic activities in senile dementia of Lewy body type. *Alzheimer Disease and Associated Disorders* **4**, 87–95.

Perry, E.K., Irving, D., Kerwin, J.M. *et al.* (1993) Cholinergic transmitter and neurotrophic activities in Lewy body dementia: similarity to Parkinson's and distinction from Alzheimer disease. *Alzheimer Disease and Associated Disorders* **7**, 69–79.

Perry, E.K., Haroutunian, V., Davis, K.L. *et al.* (1994) Neocortical cholinergic activities differentiate Lewy body dementia from classical Alzheimer's disease. *Neuroreport* **5**, 747–749.

Perry, T.L., Hansen, S. & Kloster, M. (1973) Huntington's chorea: deficiency of γ-aminobutyric acid in brain. *New England Journal of Medicine* **288**, 337–342.

Petanceska, S.S., DeRosa, S., Olm, V. *et al.* (2002) Statin therapy for Alzheimer's disease: will it work? *Journal of Molecular Neuroscience* **19**, 155–161.

Petersen, R.C., Smith, G.E., Ivnik, R.J., Kokmen, E. & Tangalos, E.G. (1994) Memory function in very early Alzheimer's disease. *Neurology* **44**, 867–872.

Petersen, R.C., Doody, R., Kurz, A. *et al.* (2001a) Current concepts in mild cognitive impairment. *Archives of Neurology* **58**, 1985–1992.

Petersen, R.C., Stevens, J.C., Ganguli, M., Tangalos, E.G., Cummings, J.L. & DeKosky, S.T. (2001b) Early detection of dementia: mild cognitive impairment (an evidence-based review). Report of the Quality Standards Subcommittee of the American Academy of Neurology. *Neurology* **56**, 1133–1142.

Pickering-Brown, S. (2004) The tau gene locus and frontotemporal dementia. *Dementia and Geriatric Cognitive Disorders* **17**, 258–260.

Pinner, G. & Bouman, W.P. (2003) Attitudes of patients with mild dementia and their carers towards disclosure of the diagnosis. *International Psychogeriatrics* **15**, 279–288.

Planel, E., Yasutake, K., Fujita, S.C. & Ishiguro, K. (2001) Inhibition of protein phosphatase 2A overrides Tau protein kinase I/glycogen synthase kinase 3b and cyclin-dependent kinase 5 inhibition and results in tau hyperphosphorylation in the hippocampus of starved mouse. *Journal of Biological Chemistry* **276**, 34298–34306.

Polvikoski, T., Sulkava, R., Myllykangas, L. *et al.* (2001) Prevalence of Alzheimer's disease in very elderly people: a prospective neuropathological study. *Neurology* **56**, 1690–1696.

Posner, H.B., Tang, M.X., Luchsinger, J., Lantigua, R., Stern, Y. & Mayeux, R. (2002) The relationship of hypertension in the elderly to AD, vascular dementia, and cognitive function. *Neurology* **58**, 1175–1181.

Potter, H. & Dressler, D. (2000) The potential of BACE inhibitors for Alzheimer's therapy. *Nature Biotechnology* **18**, 125–126.

Price, D.L., Tanzi, R.E., Borchelt, D.R. & Sisodia, S.S. (1998) Alzheimer's disease: genetic studies and transgenic models. *Annual Review of Genetics* **32**, 461–493.

Prince, M.J. (1995) Vascular risk factors and atherosclerosis as risk factors for cognitive decline and dementia. *Journal of Psychosomatic Research* **39**, 525–530.

Prince, M., Lovestone, S., Cervilla, J. *et al.* (2000) The association between *APOE* and dementia does not seem to be mediated by vascular factors. *Neurology* **54**, 397–402.

Prins, N.D., van Dijk, E.J., den Heijer, T. *et al.* (2004) Cerebral white matter lesions and the risk of dementia. *Archives of Neurology* **61**, 1531–1534.

Prusiner, S.B. (1982) Novel proteinaceous infectious particles cause scrapie. *Science* **216**, 136–144.

Prusiner, S.B. (1991) Molecular biology of prion diseases. *Science* **252**, 1515–1522.

Prusiner, S.B. & DeArmond, S.J. (1991) Molecular biology and pathology of scrapie and the prion diseases of humans. *Brain Pathology* **1**, 297–310.

Prusiner, S.B., Scott, M., Foster, D. *et al.* (1990) Transgenetic studies implicate interactions between homologous PrP isoforms in scrapie prion replication. *Cell* **63**, 673–686.

Qiu, C., Backman, L., Winblad, B., Aguero-Torres, H. & Fratiglioni, L. (2001) The influence of education on clinically diagnosed dementia incidence and mortality data from the Kungsholmen Project. *Archives of Neurology* **58**, 2034–2039.

Qiu, C., von Strauss, E., Fastbom, J., Winblad, B. & Fratiglioni, L. (2003) Low blood pressure and risk of dementia in the Kungsholmen Project: a 6-year follow-up study. *Archives of Neurology* **60**, 223–228.

Quarrell, O.W.J. & Harper, P.S. (1991) The clinical neurology of Huntington's disease. In: Harper, P.S. (ed.) *Huntington's Disease*, ch. 2. W.B. Saunders, London.

Rademakers, R., Cruts, M. & Van Broeckhoven, C. (2004) The role of tau (MAPT) in frontotemporal dementia and related tauopathies. *Human Mutation* **24**, 277–295.

Ransmayr, G. (2000) Dementia with Lewy bodies: prevalence, clinical spectrum and natural history. *Journal of Neural Transmission Supplement* **60**, 303–314.

Rao, V., Spiro, J.R., Rosenberg, P.B., Lee, H.B., Rosenblatt, A. & Lyketsos, C.G. (2006) An open-label study of escitalopram (Lexapro) for the treatment of 'Depression of Alzheimer's disease' (dAD). *International Journal of Geriatric Psychiatry* **21**, 273–274.

Ravikumar, B. & Rubinsztein, D.C. (2006) Role of autophagy in the clearance of mutant huntingtin: a step towards therapy? *Molecular Aspects of Medicine* **27**, 520–527.

Rea, T.D., Breitner, J.C., Psaty, B.M. *et al.* (2005) Statin use and the risk of incident dementia: the Cardiovascular Health Study. *Archives of Neurology* **62**, 1047–1051.

Reading, S.A., Dziorny, A.C., Peroutka, L.A. *et al.* (2004) Functional brain changes in presymptomatic Huntington's disease. *Annals of Neurology* **55**, 879–883.

Reed, B.R., Jagust, W.J. & Seab, J.P. (1989) Mental status as a predictor of daily function in progressive dementia. *Gerontologist* **29**, 804–807.

Reed, T.E. & Chandler, J.H. (1958) Huntington's chorea in Michigan. I: Demography and genetics. *American Journal of Human Genetics* **10**, 201–225.

Reifler, B.V., Larson, E., Teri, L. & Poulsen, M. (1986) Dementia of the Alzheimer's type and depression. *Journal of the American Geriatric Society* **34**, 855–859.

Reiman, E.M., Chen, K., Alexander, G.E. *et al.* (2004) Functional brain abnormalities in young adults at genetic risk for late-onset Alzheimer's dementia. *Proceedings of the National Academy of Sciences USA* **101**, 284–289.

Reisberg, B. (1986) Dementia: a systematic approach to identifying reversible causes. *Geriatrics* **41**, 30–46.

Reisberg, B. (1988) Functional assessment staging (FAST). *Psychopharmacology Bulletin* **24**, 653–659.

Reisberg, B., Ferris, S.H., De Leon, M.J. & Crook, T. (1982) The Global Deterioration Scale for assessment of primary degenerative dementia. *American Journal of Psychiatry* **139**, 1136–1139.

Reisberg, B., Ferris, S.H., Shulman, E. *et al.* (1986) Longitudinal course of normal aging and progressive dementia of the Alzheimer's type: a prospective study of 106 subjects over a 3.6 year mean interval. *Progress in Neuropsychopharmacology and Biological Psychiatry* **10**, 571–578.

Reisberg, B., Borenstein, J., Salob, S.P., Ferris, S.H., Franssen, E. & Georgotas, A. (1987) Behavioral symptoms in Alzheimer's disease: phenomenology and treatment. *Journal of Clinical Psychiatry* **48** (suppl.), 9–15.

Reisberg, B., Ferris, S.H., De Leon, M.J. *et al.* (1989) The stage specific temporal course of Alzheimer's disease: functional and behavioral concomitants based upon cross-sectional and longitudinal observation. *Progress in Clinical and Biological Research* **317**, 23–41.

Religa, D., Styczynska, M., Peplonska, B. *et al.* (2003) Homocysteine, apolipoprotein E and methylenetetrahydrofolate reductase in Alzheimer's disease and mild cognitive impairment. *Dementia and Geriatric Cognitive Disorders* **16**, 64–70.

Riley, K.P., Snowdon, D.A. & Markesbery, W.R. (2002) Alzheimer's neurofibrillary pathology and the spectrum of cognitive function: findings from the Nun Study. *Annals of Neurology* **51**, 567–577.

Ringelstein, E.B. & Nabavi, D.G. (2005) Cerebral small vessel diseases: cerebral microangiopathies. *Current Opinion in Neurology* **18**, 179–188.

Ritchie, K. & Kildea, D. (1995) Is senile dementia 'age-related' or 'ageing-related'? Evidence from meta-analysis of dementia prevalence in the oldest old. *Lancet* **346**, 931–934.

Riter, R.N. & Fries, B.E. (1992) Predictors of the placement of cognitively impaired residents on special care units. *Gerontologist* **32**, 184–190.

Roberts, G.W., Allsop, D. & Bruton, C. (1990) The occult aftermath of boxing. *Journal of Neurology, Neurosurgery and Psychiatry* **53**, 373–378.

Roberts, G.W., Gentleman, S.M., Lynch, A., Murray, L., Landon, M. & Graham, D.I. (1994) β Amyloid protein deposition in the brain after severe head injury: implications for the pathogenesis of Alzheimer's disease. *Journal of Neurology, Neurosurgery and Psychiatry* **57**, 419–425.

Robins Wahlin, T.B., Lundin, A. & Dear, K. (2007) Early cognitive deficits in Swedish gene carriers of Huntington's disease. *Neuropsychology* **21**, 31–44.

Robinson, D.M. & Keating, G.M. (2006) Memantine: a review of its use in Alzheimer's disease. *Drugs* **66**, 1515–1534.

Robinson, L., Hutchings, D., Corner, L. *et al.* (2006) A systematic literature review of the effectiveness of non-pharmacological interventions to prevent wandering in dementia and evaluation of the ethical implications and acceptability of their use. *Health Technology Assessment* **10**, iii, ix–108.

Rocca, W.A., Hofman, A., Brayne, C. *et al.* (1991) Frequency and distribution of Alzheimer's disease in Europe: a collaborative study of 1980–1990 prevalence findings. The EURODEM Prevalence Research Group. *Annals of Neurology* **30**, 381–390.

Rocchi, A., Micheli, D., Ceravolo, R. *et al.* (2003) Serotoninergic polymorphisms (5-HTTLPR and 5-HT2A): association studies with psychosis in Alzheimer disease. *Genetic Testing* **7**, 309–314.

Rolland, Y., Pillard, F., Klapouszczak, A. *et al.* (2007) Exercise program for nursing home residents with Alzheimer's disease: a 1-year randomized, controlled trial. *Journal of the American Geriatric Society* **55**, 158–165.

Román, G.C. (2002) Vascular dementia may be the most common form of dementia in the elderly. *Journal of the Neurological Sciences* **203–204**, 7–10.

Román, G.C., Tatemichi, T.K., Erkinjuntti, T. *et al.* (1993) Vascular dementia: diagnostic criteria for research studies. Report of the NINDS-AIREN International Workshop. *Neurology* **43**, 250–260.

Román, G.C., Sachdev, P., Royall, D.R. *et al.* (2004) Vascular cognitive disorder: a new diagnostic category updating vascular cognitive impairment and vascular dementia. *Journal of the Neurological Sciences* **226**, 81–87.

Rosen, J. & Zubenko, G.S. (1991) Emergence of psychosis and depression in the longitudinal evaluation of Alzheimer's disease. *Biological Psychiatry* **29**, 224–232.

Rosenberg, C.K., Pericak-Vance, M.A., Saunders, A.M., Gilbert, J.R., Gaskell, P.C. & Hulette, C.M. (2000) Lewy body and Alzheimer pathology in a family with the amyloid-β precursor protein APP717 gene mutation. *Acta Neuropathologica* **100**, 145–152.

Rosenblatt, A., Abbott, M.H., Gourley, L.M. *et al.* (2003) Predictors of neuropathological severity in 100 patients with Huntington's disease. *Annals of Neurology* **54**, 488–493.

Rossor, M.N., Fox, N.C., Beck, J., Campbell, T.C. & Collinge, J. (1996) Incomplete penetrance of familial Alzheimer's disease in a pedigree with a novel presenilin-1 gene mutation. *Lancet* **347**, 1560.

Roth, J., Klempii, J., Jech, R. *et al.* (2005) Caudate nucleus atrophy in Huntington's disease and its relationship with clinical and genetic parameters. *Functional Neurology* **20**, 127–130.

Roth, M. (1971) Classification and aetiology in mental disorders of old age: some recent developments. In: Kay, D.W.K. & Walk, A. (eds) *Recent Developments in Psychogeriatrics*, ch. 1. British Journal of Psychiatry Special Publication No. 6. Headley Brothers, Ashford, Kent.

Roth, M., Tomlinson, B.E. & Blessed, G. (1967) The relationship between quantitative measures of dementia and of degenerative changes in the cerebral grey matter of elderly subjects. *Proceedings of the Royal Society of Medicine* **60**, 254–259.

Rothschild, D. (1956) Senile psychoses and psychoses with cerebral arteriosclerosis. In: Kaplan, O.J. (ed.) *Mental Disorders in Later Life*, p. 435. Stanford University Press, Stanford, CA.

Roucou, X., Gains, M. & LeBlanc, A.C. (2004) Neuroprotective functions of prion protein. *Journal of Neuroscience Research* **75**, 153–161.

Rovner, B.W., Broadhead, J., Spencer, M., Carson, K. & Folstein, M.F. (1989) Depression and Alzheimer's disease. *American Journal of Psychiatry* **146**, 350–353.

Rubinsztein, D.C., Ravikumar, B., Cevedo-Arozena, A., Imarisio, S., O'Kane, C.J. & Brown, S.D. (2005) Dyneins, autophagy, aggregation and neurodegeneration. *Autophagy* **1**, 177–178.

Ruitenberg, A., Kalmijn, S., de Ridder, M.A. *et al.* (2001a) Prognosis of Alzheimer's disease: the Rotterdam Study. *Neuroepidemiology* **20**, 188–195.

Ruitenberg, A., Ott, A., Van Swieten, J.C., Hofman, A. & Breteler, M.M. (2001b) Incidence of dementia: does gender make a difference? *Neurobiology of Aging* **22**, 575–580.

Ruitenberg, A., Skoog, I., Ott, A. *et al.* (2001c) Blood pressure and risk of dementia: results from the Rotterdam study and the Gothenburg H-70 Study. *Dementia and Geriatric Cognitive Disorders* **12**, 33–39.

Saez-Fonseca, J.A., Lee, L. & Walker, Z. (2007) Long-term outcome of depressive pseudodementia in the elderly. *Journal of Affective Disorders* **101**, 123–129

Salmon, E. (2002) Functional brain imaging applications to differential diagnosis in the dementias. *Current Opinion in Neurology* **15**, 439–444.

Samson, N.W., van Duijn, C.M., Hop, W.C.J. & Hofman, A. (1996) Clinical features and mortality in patients with early-onset Alzheimer's disease. *European Neurology* **36**, 103–106.

Sastre, M., Dewachter, I., Landreth, G.E. *et al.* (2003) Nonsteroidal anti-inflammatory drugs and peroxisome proliferator-activated receptor-gamma agonists modulate immunostimulated processing of amyloid precursor protein through regulation of beta-secretase. *Journal of Neuroscience* **23**, 9796–9804.

Saunders, A.J., Kim, T.-W. & Tanzi, R.E. (1999) *BACE* maps to chromosome 11 and a *BACE* homolog, *BACE2*, reside in the obligate Down syndrome region of chromosome 21. *Science* **286**, 1255a.

Schady, W. & Meara, R.J. (1988) Hereditary progressive chorea without dementia. *Journal of Neurology, Neurosurgery and Psychiatry* **51**, 295–297.

Scheibel, A.B. (1978) Structural aspects of the aging brain: spine systems and the dendritic arbor. In: Katzman, R., Terry, R.D. & Bick, K.L. (eds) *Alzheimer's Disease: Senile Dementia and Related Disorders*, pp. 353–373. Aging vol. 7. Raven Press, New York.

Scheltens, P., Fox, N., Barkhof, F. & De Carli, C. (2002) Structural magnetic resonance imaging in the practical assessment of dementia: beyond exclusion. *Lancet Neurology* **1**, 13–21.

Schmand, B., Smit, J., Lindeboom, J. *et al.* (1997) Low education is a genuine risk factor for accelerated memory decline and dementia. *Journal of Clinical Epidemiology* **50**, 1025–1033.

Schmidt, R., Fazekas, F., Enzinger, C., Ropele, S., Kapeller, P. & Schmidt, H. (2002) Risk factors and progression of small vessel disease-related cerebral abnormalities. *Journal of Neural Transmission Supplement* **62**, 47–52.

Schmidtke, K. & Hull, M. (2005) Cerebral small vessel disease: how does it progress? *Journal of the Neurological Sciences* **229–230**, 13–20.

Schneider, J., Murray, J., Banerjee, S. & Mann, A. (1999) EUROCARE: a cross-national study of co-resident spouse carers for people with Alzheimer's disease: I. Factors associated with carer burden. *International Journal of Geriatric Psychiatry* **14**, 651–661.

Schneider, L.S., Dagerman, K. & Insel, P.S. (2006a) Efficacy and adverse effects of atypical antipsychotics for dementia: meta-analysis of randomized, placebo-controlled trials. *American Journal of Geriatric Psychiatry* **14**, 191–210.

Schneider, L.S., Tariot, P.N., Dagerman, K.S. et al. (2006b) Effectiveness of atypical antipsychotic drugs in patients with Alzheimer's disease. *New England Journal of Medicine* **355**, 1525–1538.

Schofield, P.W., Logroscino, G., Andrews, H.F., Albert, S. & Stern, Y. (1997) An association between head circumference and Alzheimer's disease in a population-based study of aging and dementia. *Neurology* **49**, 30–37.

Schubert, M., Brazil, D.P., Burks, D.J. *et al.* (2003) Insulin receptor substrate-2 deficiency impairs brain growth and promotes tau phosphorylation. *Journal of Neuroscience* **23**, 7084–7092.

Schunkert, H. (1997) Polymorphism of the angiotensin-converting enzyme gene and cardiovascular disease. *Journal of Molecular Medicine* **75**, 867–875.

Schweitzer, I., Tuckwell, V., O'Brien, J. & Ames, D. (2002) Is late onset depression a prodrome to dementia? *International Journal of Geriatric Psychiatry* **17**, 997–1005.

Scourfield, J., Soldan, J., Gray, J., Houlihan, G. & Harper, P.S. (1997) Huntington's disease: psychiatric practice in molecular genetic prediction and diagnosis. *British Journal of Psychiatry* **170**, 146–149.

Selkoe, D.J. (2000) The genetics and molecular pathology of Alzheimer's disease: roles of amyloid and the presenilins. *Neurology Clinics* **18**, 903–922.

Selley, M.L. (2003) Increased concentrations of homocysteine and asymmetric dimethylarginine and decreased concentrations of nitric oxide in the plasma of patients with Alzheimer's disease. *Neurobiology of Aging* **24**, 903–907.

Seltzer, B. & Sherwin, I. (1983) A comparison of clinical features in early- and late-onset primary degenerative dementia. *Archives of Neurology* **40**, 143–146.

Seneca, S., Fagnart, D., Keymolen, K. *et al.* (2004) Early onset Huntington disease: a neuronal degeneration syndrome. *European Journal of Pediatrics* **163**, 717–721.

Seshadri, S., Drachman, D.A. & Lippa, C.F. (1995) Apolipoprotein E ε4 allele and the lifetime risk of Alzheimer's disease. What physicians know, and what they should know. *Archives of Neurology* **52**, 1074–1079.

Seshadri, S., Zornberg, G.L., Derby, L.E., Myers, M.W., Jick, H. & Drachman, D.A. (2001) Postmenopausal estrogen replacement therapy and the risk of Alzheimer disease. *Archives of Neurology* **58**, 435–440.

Shea, T.B., Lyons-Weiler, J. & Rogers, E. (2002) Homocysteine, folate deprivation and Alzheimer neuropathology. *Journal of Alzheimers Disease* **4**, 261–267.

Shibuya, S., Higuchi, J., Shin, R.W., Tateishi, J. & Kitamoto, T. (1998) Codon 219 Lys allele of PRNP is not found in sporadic Creutzfeldt–Jakob disease. *Annals of Neurology* **43**, 826–828.

Shiga, Y., Miyazawa, K., Sato, S. *et al.* (2004) Diffusion-weighted MRI abnormalities as an early diagnostic marker for Creutzfeldt–Jakob disease. *Neurology* **63**, 443–449.

Shoulson, I. & Plassche, W. (1980) Huntington disease: the specificity of computed tomography measurements. *Neurology* **30**, 382–383.

Silverman, J.M., Smith, C.J., Marin, D.B., Mohs, R.C. & Propper, C.B. (2003) Familial patterns of risk in very late-onset Alzheimer disease. *Archives of General Psychiatry* **60**, 190–197.

Simpson, S.A. & Harding, A.E. (1993) Predictive testing for Huntington's disease: after the gene. The United Kingdom Huntington's Disease Prediction Consortium. *Journal of Medical Genetics* **30**, 1036–1038.

Simpson, S.A., Besson, J., Alexander, D., Allan, K. & Johnston, A.W. (1992) One hundred requests for predictive testing for Huntington's disease. *Clinical Genetics* **41**, 326–330.

Sims, A. (1988) *Symptoms in the Mind.* Bailliere Tindall, London.

Skoog, I. & Gustafson, D. (2006) Update on hypertension and Alzheimer's disease. *Neurological Research* **28**, 605–611.

Skoog, I., Kalaria, R.N. & Breteler, M.M.B. (1999) Vascular factors and Alzheimer disease. *Alzheimer Disease and Associated Disorders* **13** (suppl. 3), S106–S114.

Smith, F.W., Besson, J.A.O., Gemmell, H.G. & Sharp, P.F. (1988) The use of technetium-99m-HMPAO in the assessment of patients with dementia and other neuropsychiatric conditions. *Journal of Cerebral Blood Flow and Metabolism* **8**, S116–S122.

Smith, J.S. & Kiloh, L.G. (1981) The investigation of dementia: results in 200 consecutive admissions. *Lancet* **i**, 824–827.

Snowden, J.S., Neary, D. & Mann, D.M. (2002) Frontotemporal dementia. *British Journal of Psychiatry* **180**, 140–143.

Snowdon, D.A., Greiner, L.H., Mortimer, J.A., Riley, K.P., Greiner, P.A. & Markesbery, W.R. (1997) Brain infarction and the clinical expression of Alzheimer disease. The Nun Study. *Journal of the American Medical Association* **277**, 813–817.

Solano, D.C., Sironi, M., Bonfini, C., Solerte, S.B., Govoni, S. & Racchi, M. (2000) Insulin regulates soluble amyloid precursor protein release via phosphatidyl inositol 3 kinase-dependent pathway. *FASEB Journal* **14**, 1015–1022.

Sommer, B.R., Hoff, A.L. & Costa, M. (2003) Folic acid supplementation in dementia: a preliminary report. *Journal of Geriatric Psychiatry and Neurology* **16**, 156–159.

Sorensen, S., Duberstein, P., Gill, D. & Pinquart, M. (2006) Dementia care: mental health effects, intervention strategies, and clinical implications. *Lancet Neurology* **5**, 961–973.

Sourander, P. & Sjögren, H. (1970) The concept of Alzheimer's disease and its clinical implications. In: Wolstenholme, G.E.W. & O'Connor, M. (eds) *Alzheimer's Disease*, pp. 433, 435, 439 and 449. Ciba Foundation Symposium. Churchill, London.

Speck, C.E., Kukull, W.A., Brenner, D.E. *et al.* (1995) History of depression as a risk factor for Alzheimer's disease. *Epidemiology* **6**, 366–369.

Spector, A., Thorgrimsen, L., Woods, B. *et al.* (2003) Efficacy of an evidence-based cognitive stimulation therapy programme for people with dementia: randomised controlled trial. *British Journal of Psychiatry* **183**, 248–254.

Spillantini, M.G., Schmidt, M.L., Lee, V.M., Trojanowski, J.Q., Jakes, R. & Goedert, M. (1997) Alpha-synuclein in Lewy bodies. *Nature* **388**, 839–840.

Spittaels, K., Van Den Haute, C., Van Dorpe, J. *et al.* (2002) Neonatal neuronal overexpression of glycogen synthase kinase-3beta reduces brain size in transgenic mice. *Neuroscience* **113**, 797–808.

Spokes, E.G.S. (1980) Neurochemical alterations in Huntington's chorea: a study of post-mortem brain tissue. *Brain* **103**, 179–210.

Srikanth, S. & Nagaraja, A.V. (2005) A prospective study of reversible dementias: frequency, causes, clinical profile and results of treatment. *Neurology India* **53**, 291–294.

Starkstein, S.E., Petracca, G., Chemerinski, E. & Kremer, J. (2001) Syndromic validity of apathy in Alzheimer's disease. *American Journal of Psychiatry* **158**, 872–877.

Steffens, D.C., Plassman, B.L., Helms, M.J., Welsh-Bohmer, K.A., Saunders, A.M. & Breitner, J.C. (1997) A twin study of late-onset depression and apolipoprotein E epsilon 4 as risk factors for Alzheimer's disease. *Biological Psychiatry* **41**, 851–856.

Stern, Y. (2002) What is cognitive reserve? Theory and research application of the reserve concept. *Journal of the International Neuropsychological Society* **8**, 448–460.

Stern, Y., Albert, M., Brandt, J. *et al.* (1994) Utility of extrapyramidal signs and psychosis as predictors of cognitive and functional decline, nursing home admission, and death in Alzheimer's disease: prospective analyses from the Predictors Study. *Neurology* **44**, 2300–2307.

Stern, Y., Jacobs, D., Goldman, J. *et al.* (2001) An investigation of clinical correlates of Lewy bodies in autopsy-proven Alzheimer disease. *Archives of Neurology* **58**, 460–465.

Stevens, T., Livingston, G., Kitchen, G., Manela, M., Walker, Z. & Katona, C. (2002) Islington study of dementia subtypes in the community. *British Journal of Psychiatry* **180**, 270–276.

Stewart, G.E. & Ironside, J.W. (1998) New variant Creutzfeldt–Jakob disease. *Current Opinion in Neurology* **11**, 259–262.

Stewart, R. & Liolitsa, D. (1999) Type 2 diabetes mellitus, cognitive impairment and dementia. *Diabetic Medicine* **16**, 93–112.

Stewart, R., Russ, C., Richards, M., Brayne, C., Lovestone, S. & Mann, A. (2001) Apolipoprotein E genotype, vascular risk and early cognitive impairment in an African Caribbean population. *Dementia and Geriatric Cognitive Disorders* **12**, 251–256.

Stewart, W.F., Kawas, C., Corrada, M. & Metter, E.J. (1997) Risk of Alzheimer's disease and duration of NSAID use. *Neurology* **48**, 626–632.

Stine, O.C., Pleasant, N., Franz, M.L., Abbott, M.H., Folstein, S.E. & Ross, C.A. (1993) Correlation between the onset age of Huntington's disease and length of the trinucleotide repeat in IT-15. *Human Molecular Genetics* **2**, 1547–1549.

Stolk, R.P., Breteler, M.M., Ott, A. *et al.* (1997) Insulin and cognitive function in an elderly population. The Rotterdam Study. *Diabetes Care* **20**, 792–795.

Storandt, M., Grant, E.A., Miller, J.P. & Morris, J.C. (2002) Rates of progression in mild cognitive impairment and early Alzheimer's disease. *Neurology* **59**, 1034–1041.

Sudlow, C., Martinez Gonzalez, N.A., Kim, J. & Clark, C. (2006) Does apolipoprotein E genotype influence the risk of ischemic stroke, intracerebral hemorrhage, or subarachnoid hemorrhage? Systematic review and meta-analyses of 31 studies among 5961 cases and 17,965 controls. *Stroke* **37**, 364–370.

Sultzer, D.L., Levin, H.S., Mahler, M.E., High, W.M. & Cummings, J.L. (1992) Assessment of cognitive, psychiatric, and behavioral disturbances in patients with dementia: the Neurobehavioral Rating Scale. *Journal of the American Geriatric Society* **40**, 549–555.

Sunderland, T., Gur, R.E. & Arnold, S.E. (2005) The use of biomarkers in the elderly: current and future challenges. *Biological Psychiatry* **58**, 272–276.

Svensson, A.L. & Nordberg, A. (1999) β-Estradiol attenuate amyloid β-peptide toxicity via nicotinic receptors. *Neuroreport* **10**, 3485–3489.

Sweet, R.A., Nimgaonkar, V.L., Kamboh, M.I., Lopez, O.L., Zhang, F. & DeKosky, S.T. (1998) Dopamine receptor genetic variation, psychosis, and aggression in Alzheimer disease. *Archives of Neurology* **55**, 1335–1340.

Sweet, R.A., Hamilton, R.L., Healy, M.T. *et al.* (2001) Alterations of striatal dopamine receptor binding in Alzheimer disease are associated with Lewy body pathology and antemortem psychosis. *Archives of Neurology* **58**, 466–472.

Sweet, R.A., Nimgaonkar, V.L., Devlin, B., Lopez, O.L. & DeKosky, S.T. (2002) Increased familial risk of the psychotic phenotype of Alzheimer disease. *Neurology* **58**, 907–911.

Takashima, A., Honda, T., Yasutake, K. *et al.* (1998) Activation of tau protein kinase I glycogen synthase kinase-3β by amyloid β peptide (25–35) enhances phosphorylation of tau in hippocampal neurons. *Neuroscience Research* **31**, 317–323.

Teri, L., Larson, E.B. & Reifler, B.V. (1988) Behavioral disturbance in dementia of the Alzheimer's type. *Journal of the American Geriatric Society* **36**, 1–6.

Teri, L., Borson, S., Kiyak, H.A. & Yamagishi, M. (1989) Behavioral disturbance, cognitive dysfunction, and functional skill. Prevalence and relationship in Alzheimer's disease. *Journal of the American Geriatric Society* **37**, 109–116.

Teri, L., Ferretti, L.E., Gibbons, L.E. *et al.* (1999) Anxiety in Alzheimer's disease: prevalence and comorbidity. *Journal of Gerontology* **54A**, M348–M352.

Terry, R.D. & Katzman, R. (1983) Senile dementia of the Alzheimer type. *Annals of Neurology* **14**, 497–506.

Terry, R.D., Peck, A., De Teresa, R., Schechter, R. & Horoupian, D.S. (1981) Some morphometric aspects of the brain in senile dementia of the Alzheimer type. *Annals of Neurology* **10**, 184–192.

Terry, R.D., Masliah, E., Salmon, D.P. *et al.* (1991) Physical basis of cognitive alterations in Alzheimer's disease: synapse loss is the major correlate of cognitive impairment. *Annals of Neurology* **30**, 572–580.

Thal, L.J., Thomas, R.G., Mulnard, R., Sano, M., Grundman, M. & Schneider, L. (2003) Estrogen levels do not correlate with improvement in cognition. *Archives of Neurology* **60**, 209–212.

Thorgrimsen, L., Spector, A., Wiles, A. & Orrell, M. (2003) Aroma therapy for dementia. *Cochrane Database of Systematic Reviews* CD003150.

Tomlinson, B.E. (1982) Plaques, tangles and Alzheimer's disease. *Psychological Medicine* **12**, 449–459.

Tomlinson, B.E., Blessed, G. & Roth, M. (1968) Observations on the brains of non-demented old people. *Journal of the Neurological Sciences* **7**, 331–356.

Tomlinson, B.E., Blessed, G. & Roth, M. (1970) Observations on the brains of demented old people. *Journal of the Neurological Sciences* **11**, 205–242.

Tondi, L., Ribani, L., Bottazzi, M., Viscomi, G. & Vulcano, V. (2007) Validation therapy (VT) in nursing home: a case–control study. *Archives of Gerontology and Geriatrics* **44** (suppl.), 407–411.

Tractenberg, R.E., Singer, C.M., Cummings, J.L. & Thal, L.J. (2003a) The Sleep Disorders Inventory: an instrument for studies of sleep disturbance in persons with Alzheimer's disease. *Journal of Sleep Research* **12**, 331–337.

Tractenberg, R.E., Weiner, M.F., Patterson, M.B., Teri, L. & Thal, L.J. (2003b) Comorbidity of psychopathological domains in community-dwelling persons with Alzheimer's disease. *Journal of Geriatric Psychiatry and Neurology* **16**, 94–99.

Trushina, E. & McMurray, C.T. (2007) Oxidative stress and mitochondrial dysfunction in neurodegenerative diseases. *Neuroscience* **145**, 1233–1248.

Tsuang, D., Almqvist, E.W., Lipe, H. *et al.* (2000) Familial aggregation of psychotic symptoms in Huntington's disease. *American Journal of Psychiatry* **157**, 1955–1959.

Tunstall, N., Owen, M.J., Williams, J. *et al.* (2000) Familial influence on variation in age of onset and behavioural phenotype in Alzheimer's disease. *British Journal of Psychiatry* **176**, 156–159.

Turner, P.R., O'Connor, K., Tate, W.P. & Abraham, W.C. (2003) Roles of amyloid precursor protein and its fragments in regulating neural activity, plasticity and memory. *Progress in Neurobiology* **70**, 1–32.

Tyler, A. & Harper, P.S. (1983) Attitudes of subjects at risk and their relatives towards genetic counselling in Huntington's chorea. *Journal of Medical Genetics* **20**, 179–188.

Urbach, H., Klisch, J., Wolf, H.K., Brechtelsbauer, D., Gass, S. & Solymosi, L. (1998) MRI in sporadic Creutzfeldt–Jakob disease: correlation with clinical and neuropathological data. *Neuroradiology* **40**, 65–70.

Valentine, A.R., Moseley, I.F. & Kendall, B.E. (1980) White matter abnormality in cerebral atrophy: clinico-radiological correla-tions. *Journal of Neurology, Neurosurgery and Psychiatry* **43**, 139–142.

Valenzuela, M.J. & Sachdev, P. (2001) Magnetic resonance spectroscopy in AD. *Neurology* **56**, 592–598.

van Dijk, E.J., Breteler, M.M., Schmidt, R. *et al.* (2004) The association between blood pressure, hypertension, and cerebral white matter lesions: cardiovascular determinants of dementia study. *Hypertension* **44**, 625–630.

Van Everbroeck, B., Quoilin, S., Boons, J., Martin, J.J. & Cras, P. (2003) A prospective study of CSF markers in 250 patients with possible Creutzfeldt–Jakob disease. *Journal of Neurology, Neurosurgery and Psychiatry* **74**, 1210–1214.

van Harten, B., Oosterman, J.M., Potter van Loon, B.J., Scheltens, P. & Weinstein, H.C. (2007) Brain lesions on MRI in elderly patients with type 2 diabetes mellitus. *European Neurology* **57**, 70–74.

Verhaeghen, P. & Marcoen, A. (1996) On the mechanisms of plasticity in young and older adults after instruction in the method of loci: evidence for an amplification model. *Psychology and Aging* **11**, 164–178.

Vernooij-Dassen, M., Felling, A. & Persoon, J. (1997) Predictors of change and continuity in home care for dementia patients. *International Journal of Geriatric Psychiatry* **12**, 671–677.

Vessie, R.P. (1932) On the transmission of Huntington's chorea for 300 years: the Bures family group. *Journal of Nervous and Mental Disease* **76**, 553–573.

Victoratos, G.C., Lenman, J.A. & Herzberg, L. (1977) Neurological investigation of dementia. *British Journal of Psychiatry* **130**, 131–133.

Volicer, L., Smith, S. & Volicer, B.J. (1995) Effect of seizures on progression of dementia of the Alzheimer type. *Dementia* **6**, 258–263.

Wahlund, L.O., Julin, P., Johansson, S.E. & Scheltens, P. (2000) Visual rating and volumetry of the medial temporal lobe on magnetic resonance imaging in dementia: a comparative study. *Journal of Neurology, Neurosurgery and Psychiatry* **69**, 630–635.

Waldemar, G., Dubois, B., Emre, M. *et al.* (2007) Recommendations for the diagnosis and management of Alzheimer's disease and other disorders associated with dementia: EFNS guideline. *European Journal of Neurology* **14**, e1–e26.

Walker, F.O., Young, A.B., Penney, J.B., Dovorini-Zis, K. & Shoulson, I. (1984) Benzodiazepine and GABA receptors in early Huntington's disease. *Neurology* **34**, 1237–1240.

Walker, M.P., Ayre, G.A., Perry, E.K. *et al.* (2000) Quantification and characterisation of fluctuating cognition in dementia with Lewy bodies and Alzheimer's disease. *Dementia* **11**, 327–335.

Walker, Z. & Walker, R.W. (2005) Imaging in neurodegenerative disorders: recent studies. *Current Opinion in Psychiatry* **18**, 640–646.

Wall, C.A., Rummans, T.A., Aksamit, A.J., Krahn, L.E. & Pankratz, V.S. (2005) Psychiatric manifestations of Creutzfeldt–Jakob disease: a 25-year analysis. *Journal of Neuropsychiatry and Clinical Neuroscience* **17**, 489–495.

Ward, J., Sheppard, J.M., Shpritz, B., Margolis, R.L., Rosenblatt, A. & Brandt, J. (2006) A four-year prospective study of cognitive functioning in Huntington's disease. *Journal of the International Neuropsychological Society* **12**, 445–454.

Watkins, L.H., Rogers, R.D., Lawrence, A.D., Sahakian, B.J., Rosser, A.E. & Robbins, T.W. (2000) Impaired planning but intact decision making in early Huntington's disease: implications for specific fronto-striatal pathology. *Neuropsychologia* **38**, 1112–1125.

Watt, D.C. & Seller, A. (1993) A clinico-genetic study of psychiatric disorder in Huntington's chorea. *Psychological Medicine Monograph Supplement* **23**, 1–43.

Weggen, S., Eriksen, J.L., Das, P. *et al.* (2001) A subset of NSAIDs lower amyloidogenic Abeta42 independently of cyclooxygenase activity. *Nature* **414**, 212–216.

Weggen, S., Eriksen, J.L., Sagi, S.A. *et al.* (2003) Evidence that nonsteroidal anti-inflammatory drugs decrease Abeta 42 production by direct modulation of gamma-secretase activity. *Journal of Biological Chemistry* **278**, 31831–31837.

Weiner, M.F., Edland, S.D. & Luszczynska, H. (1994) Prevalence and incidence of major depression in Alzheimer's disease. *American Journal of Psychiatry* **151**, 1006–1009.

Weiner, M.F., Doody, R.S., Sairam, R., Foster, B. & Liao, T. (2002) Prevalence and incidence of major depressive disorder in Alzheimer's disease: findings from two databases. *Dementia and Geriatric Cognitive Disorders* **13**, 8–12.

Weissmann, C. & Flechsig, E. (2003) PrP knock-out and PrP transgenic mice in prion research. *British Medical Bulletin* **66**, 43–60.

Wells, C.E. (1978) Chronic brain disease; an overview. *American Journal of Psychiatry* **135**, 1–12.

West, R., Jakubek, K. & Wymbs, N. (2002) Age-related declines in prospective memory: behavioral and electrophysiological evidence. *Neuroscience and Biobehavioral Reviews* **26**, 827–833.

Wieser, H.G., Schindler, K. & Zumsteg, D. (2006) EEG in Creutzfeldt–Jakob disease. *Clinical Neurophysiology* **117**, 935–951.

Wiggins, S., Whyte, P., Huggins, M. *et al.* (1992) The psychological consequences of predictive testing for Huntington's disease. Canadian Collaborative Study of Predictive Testing. *New England Journal of Medicine* **327**, 1401–1405.

Wilcock, G.K. & Esiri, M.M. (1982) Plaques, tangles, and dementia: a quantitative study. *Journal of the Neurological Sciences* **56**, 343–356.

Wilcock, G.K., Esiri, M.M., Bowen, D.M. & Smith, C.C.T. (1982) Alzheimer's disease. Correlations of cortical choline acetyltransferase activity with the severity of dementia and histological abnormalities. *Journal of the Neurological Sciences* **57**, 407–417.

Will, R.G., Ironside, J.W., Zeidler, M. *et al.* (1996) A new variant of Creutzfeldt–Jakob disease in the UK. *Lancet* **347**, 921–925.

Wilson, C.A., Doms, R.W. & Lee, V.M.Y. (1999) Intracellular APP processing and Aβ production in Alzheimer disease. *Journal of Neuropathology and Experimental Neurology* **58**, 787–794.

Wilson, R.S., Bennett, D.A., Bienias, J.L. *et al.* (2002) Cognitive activity and incident AD in a population-based sample of older persons. *Neurology* **59**, 1910–1914.

Winblad, B., Palmer, K., Kivipelto, M. *et al.* (2004) Mild cognitive impairment: beyond controversies, towards a consensus. Report of the International Working Group on Mild Cognitive Impairment. *Journal of Internal Medicine* **256**, 240–246.

Winograd, C.H., Jacobson, D.H., Minkoff, J.R. *et al.* (1991) Blood glucose and insulin response in patients with senile dementia of the Alzheimer's type. *Biological Psychiatry* **30**, 507–511.

Wolf, H., Grunwald, M., Kruggel, F. *et al.* (2001) Hippocampal volume discriminates between normal cognition: questionable and mild dementia in the elderly. *Neurobiology of Aging* **22**, 177–186.

Wolstenholme, J.L., Fenn, P., Gray, A.M., Keene, J., Jacoby, R. & Hope, T. (2002) Estimating the relationship between disease progression and cost of care in dementia. *British Journal of Psychiatry* **181**, 36–42.

Yanagisawa, M., Planel, E., Ishiguro, K. & Fujita, S.C. (1999) Starvation induces tau hyperphosphorylation in mouse brain: implications for Alzheimer's disease. *FEBS Letters* **461**, 329–333.

Yang, W., Dunlap, J.R., Andrews, R.B. & Wetzel, R. (2002) Aggregated polyglutamine peptides delivered to nuclei are toxic to mammalian cells. *Human Molecular Genetics* **11**, 2905–2917.

Yesavage, J.A., Brooks, J.O., Taylor, J. & Tinklenberg, J. (1993) Development of aphasia, apraxia, and agnosia and decline in Alzheimer's disease. *American Journal of Psychiatry* **150**, 742–747.

Yokota, O., Terada, S., Ishizu, H. *et al.* (2002) NACP/alpha-Synuclein, NAC, and beta-amyloid pathology of familial Alzheimer's disease with the E184D presenilin-1 mutation: a clinicopathological study of two autopsy cases. *Acta Neuropathologica* **104**, 637–648.

Young, G.S., Geschwind, M.D., Fischbein, N.J. *et al.* (2005) Diffusion-weighted and fluid-attenuated inversion recovery imaging in Creutzfeldt–Jakob disease: high sensitivity and specificity for diagnosis. *American Journal of Neuroradiology* **26**, 1551–1562.

Zaccai, J., Ince, P. & Brayne, C. (2006) Population-based neuropathological studies of dementia: design, methods and areas of investigation: a systematic review. *BMC Neurology* **6**, 2.

Zandi, P.P., Anthony, J.C., Hayden, K.M., Mehta, K., Mayer, L. & Breitner, J.C. (2002a) Reduced incidence of AD with NSAID but not H2 receptor antagonists: the Cache County Study. *Neurology* **59**, 880–886.

Zandi, P.P., Carlson, M.C., Plassman, B.L. *et al.* (2002b) Hormone replacement therapy and incidence of Alzheimer disease in older women: the Cache County Study. *Journal of the American Medical Association* **288**, 2123–2129.

Zeidler, M., Stewart, G., Cousens, S.N., Estibeiro, K. & Will, R.G. (1997a) Codon 129 genotype and new variant CJD. *Lancet* **350**, 668.

Zeidler, M., Johnstone, E.C., Bamber, R.W. *et al.* (1997b) New variant Creutzfeldt–Jakob disease: psychiatric features. *Lancet* **350**, 908–910.

Zeidler, M., Sellar, R.J., Collie, D.A. *et al.* (2000) The pulvinar sign on magnetic resonance imaging in variant Creutzfeldt–Jakob disease. *Lancet* **355**, 1412–1418.

Zeumer, H., Schonsky, B. & Sturm, K.W. (1980) Predominent white matter involvement in subcortical arteriosclerotic encephalopathy (Binswanger's disease). *Journal of Computer Assisted Tomography* **4**, 14–19.

Zubenko, G.S., Moossy, J., Martinez, A.J. *et al.* (1991) Neuropathologic and neurochemical correlates of psychosis in primary dementia. *Archives of Neurology* **48**, 619–624.

Zuliani, G., Ble', A., Zanca, R. *et al.* (2001) Genetic polymorphisms in older subjects with vascular or Alzheimer's dementia. *Acta Neurologica Scandinavica* **103**, 304–308.

Zweig, R.M., Ross, C.A., Hedreen, J.C. *et al.* (1988) The neuropathology of aminergic nuclei in Alzheimer's disease. *Annals of Neurology* **24**, 233–242.

10

Endocrine Diseases and Metabolic Disorders

Neil A. Harrison[1] **and Michael D. Kopelman**[2]

[1] Institute of Cognitive Neuroscience, University College, London
[2] Institute of Psychiatry, King's College, London

The relationship between endocrinology and psychiatry continues to attract considerable attention. Endocrine disorders can be accompanied by prominent abnormalities of the mental state, as for example in hypothyroidism and hyperthyroidism, and epochs of life such as after childbirth that are associated with rapid changes in hormonal levels appear to be associated with special liability to mental disturbance. Conversely, it is now clear that primary emotional disorders are accompanied by changes in neuroendocrine regulatory functions and may even predispose to the development of endocrine disorders such as diabetes mellitus.

Historically, treatment by means of hormones has often been viewed as a possibility in psychiatry. Kraepelin (1896) once proposed that dementia praecox was basically an endocrine disorder. Others have speculated on the role of hormones in regulating the 'biological background of psychic life', noting their influence on characteristics such as impulsivity, attention, arousal and motivational drive (Bleuler 1967). More recently, studies of patients treated for hypopituitarism have revealed that hormones such as growth hormone, previously thought to play a role only in childhood and adolescence, continue to be important to mental well-being and metabolic function throughout adult life. On the other hand, exogenous administration of hormones, most notably corticosteroids, may lead to the development of cognitive, psychotic or affective disorder.

Recent research has continued to pursue the question of how hormones influence fundamental aspects of brain development and human behaviour during both early childhood development and later adult life. Experimental work in animals has clarified the morphological basis by which lack of thyroxine during early development impairs the maturation of behaviour (Eayers 1968). Prenatal steroid hormones have a decisive influence in animals on sexual differentiation and on a wide range of sexual and social behaviours (McCarthy 1994; Signoret & Balthazart 1994). Elegant experimental design coupled with functional neuroimaging technologies are also beginning to provide exciting new insights into the mechanisms through which hormones such as vasopressin and oxytocin influence social recognition and the expression of appropriate social responses in adult life (Kosfeld *et al.* 2005; Storm & Tecott 2005). Findings such as these illustrate the important interactions between endocrine systems and psychological function and in the words of William James 'make us realise more deeply than ever how much our mental life is knit up with our corporeal frame' (James 1890).

This chapter includes sections on Turner's and Klinefelter's syndromes and the metabolic disorders of hypoglycaemia, malnutrition, vitamin B deficiencies, uraemia and electrolyte disturbance. Research into Turner's syndrome continues to illuminate the differential roles of imprinted genes on the X chromosome and hormonal deficiencies on the specific cognitive deficits and difficulties in social functioning seen in girls with the condition. The metabolic disorders illustrate the importance of a stable biochemical and metabolic milieu for the proper functioning of the central nervous system (CNS). They are a group of disorders seen quite frequently in unwell patients admitted to medical or surgical wards and are encountered quite commonly by liaison psychiatrists in general hospitals. Porphyria is included as a rare but striking example of an inborn error of metabolism with important psychiatric features.

The chapter focuses on the clinical psychiatric manifestations of the primary endocrine disorders, discussed together with the results of relevant research literature. Whilst a significant majority of patients with the conditions discussed will present either to a general physician or general practitioner, occasional individuals will present in such a way that psychiatric manifestations dominate the clinical picture and the endocrine disturbance may go unnoticed. With some conditions, for example hypothyroidism and Addison's disease, the psychiatric abnormalities may be so marked that there is a constant risk of mistaken diagnosis.

Lishman's Organic Psychiatry: A Textbook of Neuropsychiatry, 4th edition.
© 2009 Blackwell Publishing.   ISBN 978-1-4051-1860-1

Diabetes mellitus

Diabetes mellitus is a group of metabolic diseases characterized by hyperglycaemia resulting from defects in insulin production, insulin action or both. Recent consensus opinion has advised a change to an aetiopathologically based classificatory system (Expert Committee on the Diagnosis and Classification of Diabetes Mellitus 2003), with the vast majority of cases fitting into one of two broad categories. In type 1 diabetes the associated abnormalities of protein, carbohydrate and fat metabolism are the result of insufficient insulin action on peripheral target tissues as a result of reduced insulin secretion, whereas in type 2 diabetes these metabolic abnormalities are the result of diminished tissue response to insulin with or without an associated deficiency in insulin secretion. Type 1 diabetes is associated with pancreatic islet β-cell loss that results in proneness to ketosis. Most cases typically present by age 20 and appear to be the result of an autoimmune reaction, possibly triggered by an environmental insult, on a background of raised genetic susceptibility. Type 2 diabetes likely results from a combination of inadequate insulin secretion and peripheral insulin resistance. Insulin levels may be higher than seen in normals but are insufficient to overcome resistance in liver, muscle and adipose tissue. Published prevalences of type 2 diabetes depend on the diagnostic criteria used and the age and racial composition of the population studied, being higher in older populations and in certain ethnic groups such as Pima Indians living in the USA. In the UK, the prevalence of diabetes mellitus is 3–5% (Forrest *et al.* 1986; Yudkin *et al.* 1993), with type 2 diabetes seven to eight times more common than type 1.

It is well established that genetic mechanisms contribute to the development of both forms of the disease, and interesting progress has been made in relation to type 1 diabetes (Bennett *et al.* 1995; Kennedy *et al.* 1995). Multiple loci are clearly involved, including loci on chromosome 6 in the human leucocyte antigen (HLA) region, and on chromosome 11 in close relation to the insulin gene itself. The insulin gene is flanked upstream by multiple repeats of a 14-bp sequence, variations in length of the sequence correlating with disease susceptibility, perhaps through a direct effect on transcription of the insulin gene. Genetic influences in type 2 diabetes are especially apparent in patients who are not overweight, including, it seems, changes in mitochondrial DNA. Textbooks of medicine should be consulted for the general clinical associations of the disorder and the principles of management by diet, insulin and oral hypoglycaemic agents.

Diagnosis of diabetes is of importance to psychiatry for a number of reasons. Psychiatric disorders, particularly emotional disorders, are more prevalent in the diabetic population, whilst the development of depression in diabetic patients is associated with poorer glycaemic control, higher

Table 10.1 Criteria for the diagnosis of diabetes mellitus. (From American Diabetes Association 2004.)

Normoglycaemia
Fasting plasma glucose (FPG) <5.6 mmol/L
2-hour post-load glucose (PG)* <7.8 mmol/L

Impaired fasting glucose or impaired glucose tolerance
Impaired fasting glucose: FPG ≥5.6 and <7.0 mmol/L
Impaired glucose tolerance: 2-hour PG ≥7.8 and <11.1 mmol/L

Diabetes[†]
FPG ≥7.0 mmol/L
2-hour PG ≥11.1 mmol/L
Symptoms of diabetes and casual plasma glucose concentration ≥11.1 mmol/L

---

* This test requires the use of a glucose load containing the equivalent of 75 g anhydrous glucose dissolved in water.
[†] In the absence of unequivocal hyperglycaemia, a diagnosis of diabetes must be confirmed, on a subsequent day, by measurement of FPG, 2-hour PG or random plasma glucose (if symptoms are present). The FPG test is greatly preferred because of ease of administration, convenience, acceptability to patients and lower cost. Fasting is defined as no caloric intake for at least 8 hours.

prevalence of multiple diabetic complications and greater functional impairment. Furthermore, mood disorder appears to be an independent risk factor for the development of type 2 diabetes. A number of medications commonly used by psychiatrists, including all the antipsychotic drugs, are associated with an increased incidence of diabetes. It is therefore important that all practising psychiatrists should be familiar with current diagnostic criteria for diabetes mellitus, enabling any patient developing diabetes to be rapidly identified and referred for appropriate treatment. Failure to do so will unnecessarily expose patients seen by psychiatrists to increased risk of developing cardiovascular disease and diabetic microvascular complications. Diagnostic criteria are shown in Table 10.1. These issues are discussed below, along with the question of brain damage in diabetic patients. When evidence of brain damage emerges this may be attributable to episodes of hypoglycaemia or diabetic coma or, alternatively, to the high incidence of atherosclerosis that exists in patients with diabetes. The picture of diabetic coma, and certain common neurological complications, are also briefly described.

In several ways the situation imposed by diabetes is unusual in comparison with other chronic diseases. Patients with diabetes are required to comply with strict dietary restrictions and daily self-administered injections. This incurs a responsibility that is rare in other illnesses. Adherence to dietary regimens may be particularly difficult during periods of loneliness, depression or tension, whilst rebellion in adolescents may be associated with wilful neglect of treatment. Pruritis and decreased sexual interest may contribute to emotional complications, and impotence and amenorrhoea can be early complaints even in undiagnosed diabetics. Physical handicaps resulting from ocular and other complications further increase the burden of the disease. A major fear among many who inject insulin is the occurrence of a hypoglycaemic attack, especially those that lack the adrenergic warning in which loss of self-control or bizarre behaviour may occur. Tighter glycaemic control has led to more frequent hypoglycaemic episodes, which may themselves be associated with chronic long-term disability (Diabetes Control and Complications Trial Group 1997).

Depression as a risk factor for diabetes

Recent longitudinal studies suggest that depression is an important independent risk factor for the development of type 2 diabetes. Individuals with psychiatric illnesses often also have a number of risk factors for the development of diabetes, including physical inactivity and obesity (Hayward 1995). However, even after controlling for potential confounders such as age, race, gender, socioeconomic class, education, health service use, other psychiatric disorders and body weight, depression remains a significant risk factor for the development of diabetes (Musselman et al. 2003).

Eaton et al. (1996) in a follow-up study of 3481 participants in the Epidemiological Catchment Area study showed that subjects who had experienced an episode of major depressive disorder had a 2.2 times higher risk of developing type 2 diabetes in the following 13 years. Controlling for age, race, sex, socioeconomic status, education, use of health services, other psychiatric disorders and body weight did not weaken the association. In a second large prospective cohort, Kawakami et al. (1999) followed 2764 male employees of a Japanese electrical company for 8 years. Participants were screened at study entry for depression using the Zung self-rating depression scale and yearly for development of diabetes. Over the 8-year follow-up 43 subjects developed type 2 diabetes, of whom nine had moderate or severe levels of depression at study onset. After controlling for eleven other risk factors (age, education, occupation, work shift, obesity, leisure-time, physical activity, smoking, alcohol consumption, chronic medical conditions and family history), subjects with moderate to severe levels of depressive symptoms at baseline had a 2.3 times higher risk of type 2 diabetes at follow-up compared with those who were not depressed or had low levels of depressive symptoms at study onset.

Prevalence of depression in diabetic patients

Debate continues to surround the issue of whether depression is more prevalent in patients with diabetes mellitus, particularly with respect to patients with other chronic diseases. Studies using self-report measures tend to produce much higher prevalences than those that determine the presence of psychiatric comorbidities using structured or semi-structured diagnostic interview (Anderson et al. 2001). Many studies were also very small and exposed to selection bias, studies were non-randomised and, in some, subjects had volunteered.

Two meta-analyses have reviewed the literature in this area. Gavard et al. (1993) found a mean prevalence of depression in individuals with diabetes of 14% by diagnostic interview and 32% using self-report symptom scales in controlled studies and 15.4% and 19.6% in uncontrolled. The meta-analysis by Anderson et al. (2001) included studies of 'clinically relevant' depression in diabetes. Within this definition they included studies of both major and minor (or subsyndromal) depression, both of which have been shown to be associated with increased medical morbidity and mortality even after adjustment for health status and health behaviours. They included 42 studies, 48% of which were controlled. Of the controlled studies, 10 reported depression estimates separately by type of diabetes, giving an odds ratio of 2.9 in both the type 1 and type 2 groups compared with non-diabetic controls. Analysis yielded similar odds ratios for men and women, for community versus clinical groups, and for self-report measures versus clinician assessment. They concluded that although the prevalence of depression varied considerably across trials, the odds ratio comparing diabetic with non-diabetic groups was more consistent, with patients with diabetes twice as likely to be suffering from depression as non-diabetic controls (95% CI 1.8–2.2).

However, a subsequent large cross-sectional community study using a modified version of the Composite International Diagnostic Interview found that people with diabetes were no more likely than the non-diabetic population to have a mental disorder as defined by the Diagnostic and Statistical Manual of Mental Disorders (DSM)-IV (Kruse et al. 2003), although a higher prevalence of anxiety disorders was found. The odds ratio for an anxiety disorder was 1.93 (95% CI 1.19–3.14). A higher prevalence of affective disorders was found in the diabetic group, though this did not survive correction for age, sex, marital status and socioeconomic status. A further study comparing patients who had previously been hospitalised with either diabetes or osteoarthritis found no difference in rates of subsequent hospitalisation for moderate or severe depression between these groups (Kessing et al. 2003). Due to the specific nature of this group, generalisation to the wider diabetic population is difficult though the authors argue that these results suggest that older patients with diabetes do not have an increased risk of developing severe depression compared to patients with other chronic diseases.

Impact of depression on the course of diabetes

Patients with diabetes may sometimes show a close relationship between distressing life events and periods of poor diabetic control, which may even lead to the development of ketotic coma.

Increased levels of depressive symptoms are associated with poorer adherence to a diabetic diet, poorer compliance with oral hypoglycaemic medication and greater functional impairment (Ciechanowski 2000) and meta-analyses link depression in diabetes with hyperglycaemia and an increased risk of complications (de Groot *et al.* 2000; Lustman *et al.* 2000). Three randomised controlled trials have shown that treatment with either antidepressant medication or cognitive behavioural therapy that results in improvement in mood is also associated with an improvement in glycaemic control (Lustman *et al.* 1997, 1998, 2000). In patients with pre-existing diabetes, depression is also an independent risk factor for coronary heart disease and appears to accelerate the presentation of coronary heart disease (Forrest *et al.* 2000).

Whether direct metabolic consequences of depression are responsible for the increased prevalence of diabetes in depression and for the increase in diabetic complications, or whether these result from the secondary effects due to poor dietary and medication compliance, remains uncertain. When under stress or depressed some people may overeat and neglect their diet or increase their alcohol consumption. Occasionally, patients may also deliberately neglect their medication to precipitate hospital admission at times of crisis.

Depression is also associated with abnormalities in a number of metabolically significant pathways. Early experimental observations showed that emotionally stressful experiences can produce fluctuations in levels of blood glucose and ketone bodies in both normal people and those with diabetes (Hinkle & Wolf 1952a,b). Psychologically stressful conditions are accompanied by release of hormones that counter the action of insulin (i.e. catecholamines, glucocorticoids, growth hormone and glucagons) and are correlated with higher blood glucose levels in non-diabetics (Wing 1985). Numerous studies have reported that depressive disorders are associated with activation of these counter-regulatory hormones (Musselman *et al.* 2003). The initial acute increase in blood glucose in response to stress is associated with increased activity of the sympathoadrenal and hypothalamic–pituitary–adrenal axis with release of adrenaline (epinephrine) and glucagon. This is followed by the combined actions of growth hormone and glucocorticoids, which prolong the increase in blood glucose over hours (Surwit *et al.* 1992).

Some authors have suggested that chronic depressive symptoms may be conceptualised as a stress response gone awry, with the increased release of counter-regulatory hormones and cortisol, activated sympathetic nervous system activity and/or other endocrine disturbances impairing the body's ability to handle a carbohydrate load (Musselman *et al.* 2003). A further consequence of this increased counter-regulatory hormone release may be the impaired insulin and glucose tolerances seen in insulin and glucose tolerance tests respectively in patients with major depression.

Whatever the mechanisms, mild and more severe depression may have an important bearing on the course of diabetes, leading to worsening of diabetic control and increased diabetic complications. Effective treatment facilitates adherence to diet and exercise and results in improved glycaemic control.

Brain damage in diabetes

Diabetes is associated with both microvascular and macrovascular disease and in type 1 diabetes the risk of additional exposure to intermittent severe hypoglycaemia, all of which may play a part in the development of brain damage in patients with diabetes. Prospective epidemiological studies have shown that diabetes is associated with a greater than twofold increase in the risk of deterioration in cognitive function test scores over 4 years of follow-up (Fontbonne *et al.* 2001). In women the risk of cognitive decline was greatest in those with diabetes of the longest duration (Knopman *et al.* 2001). Stroke is more frequent in diabetes and the risk of vascular dementia is increased 1.5–2.8 fold (Strachan *et al.* 2003). Conflicting data exist on the association of type 2 diabetes and Alzheimer's disease, with some authors arguing for a direct relation and others suggesting that any increased incidence is due to an increase in misclassified cerebrovascular disease. To date studies have lacked sufficiently detailed clinical assessments to allow the differential contribution of macrovascular disease, hypertension, chronic hyperglycaemia, hyperinsulinaemia and other factors to be determined and future detailed prospective studies are required to determine the relative contributions of each of these mechanisms.

Severe protracted hypoglycaemia associated with type 1 diabetes is rare but may lead to permanent neurological and cognitive deficits. Occasional reports have also described localised neuroimaging changes predominantly affecting the frontal lobes and deep grey matter, which appear more susceptible to hypoglycaemia-induced damage (Auer & Siesjo 1993). Acute hypoglycaemia is associated with symptoms of neuroglycopenia (see Acute and subacute neuroglycopenia, later) and may, if left uncorrected, proceed to coma. Cognitive function following acute mild hypoglycaemic episodes recovers within an hour though mood disturbances may take longer to recover (Strachan *et al.* 2000). In more severe hypoglycaemic episodes cognitive function has usually recovered within a day and a half, although mood disturbance and energy levels may be recovered more slowly (Strachan *et al.* 2000). The role of recurrent severe hypoglycaemic episodes in inducing persistent cognitive impairment and brain damage has been the subject of many recent trials, perhaps triggered by the recognition that subjects on intensive insulin therapy are at a threefold higher risk of severe hypoglycaemic episodes (Diabetes Control and Complications Trial Research Group 1997).

An early study (Bale 1973) that compared individuals with diabetes for 15 years or more with age- and sex-matched controls showed an association between diabetes and impaired scores on a test of new learning and suggested an association between low scores and apparent severity of past hypoglycaemic episodes. However, subsequent prospective studies have reported no association between the frequency of previous severe hypoglycaemic attacks and long-term cognitive impairment (Diabetes Control and Complications Trial Research Group 1996; Reichard *et al.* 1996; Austin & Deary 1999). Austin & Deary (1999) re-analysed the data from the Diabetes Control and Complications Trial and found that repeated episodes of hypoglycaemia were not associated with a decline in spatial ability, processing speed, memory or verbal ability. Ferguson *et al.* (2003) assessed whether a history of previous hypoglycaemia and the presence of background retinopathy was related to cognitive function and brain structure in 74 young people with type 1 diabetes. Severe hypoglycaemia did not influence cognitive ability or brain structure, whilst diabetic retinopathy was associated with small focal lesions in the basal ganglia and worse scores in terms of performance IQ, verbal fluency, and attention and concentration. Taken together these results suggest that at least in younger people with diabetes, episodes of hypoglycaemia are not generally associated with significant long-term cognitive impairment.

However, cross-sectional and case–control studies of older adults with a longer duration of disease have demonstrated a modest but significant decrement in cognitive function associated with the frequency of preceding severe hypoglycaemia. Wredling *et al.* (1990) compared 17 patients with insulin-dependent diabetes and histories of recurrent severe hypoglycaemic episodes with 17 diabetic patients without. The groups were matched for sex, age, duration of diabetes, injection frequency, dose of insulin and socioeconomic factors. On neuropsychological assessment, the group who had experienced hypoglycaemic episodes performed significantly less well on tests of finger tapping, digit span, Necker cube reversals and maze learning. Langan *et al.* (1991) tested 100 insulin-dependent patients on an extensive psychometric battery, after excluding those who had evidence of other causes of brain damage including cerebrovascular disease. Using a questionnaire to assess the number, frequency and severity of previous hypoglycaemic episodes, the authors found significant correlations between the frequency of severe hypoglycaemia and an index of intellectual decline (discrepancy between NART and WAIS IQ), all of the WAIS performance subtests and a forced choice reaction time test. Speed of information processing as measured by the Paced Auditory Serial Addition Task correlated with the estimated number of hypoglycaemic episodes sustained during the patient's lifetime.

> A patient reported by Mace (1987) raised the possibility of memory impairment secondary to self-induced hypoglycaemias. A 29-year-old computer manager had abused many drugs and had drunk excessively from his teens; diabetes was diagnosed at 25. He developed severe hypoglycaemic episodes, some with convulsions and automatisms and prolonged bouts of disinhibited behaviour. In hospital it was noted that such episodes were frequent when he was left to measure and administer his own insulin, but stopped when it was given under nursing supervision. He denied deliberate abuse of insulin, but phials and syringes were found concealed among his possessions along with other drugs. His memory was clearly faulty for events of the previous year, and testing confirmed the presence of severe verbal memory deficits. It was difficult to know how far the insulin hypoglycaemias had contributed to this rather than the abuse of alcohol and other drugs.

Diabetic coma

In addition to the complications discussed above, patients with diabetes are susceptible to two metabolic emergencies: diabetic ketoacidosis and hyperosmolar non-ketotic coma. Diabetic ketoacidosis is a complication of type 1 diabetes and usually occurs on cessation of insulin or in the face of markedly increased requirements, such as during infection or at times of increased emotional stress; very occasionally, patients may present in this way without being known diabetics. Hyperosmolar non-ketotic coma usually occurs in type 2 diabetes.

Prodromal symptoms of diabetic ketoacidosis consist of weakness, thirst, dull headache, abdominal pain, nausea, vomiting and drowsiness. The onset may be abrupt or insidious. It is sometimes very gradual over several hours, so that a patient with a dangerous ketosis may still be fully ambulant. Air hunger and heavy laboured breathing develop. The patient becomes increasingly listless and in about 10% becomes comatose, sometimes after a period of restlessness, irritability and confusion. The pulse is weak and rapid and the blood pressure low. Dehydration is marked, the face flushed, and acetone may be smelled on the breath. Investigations will reveal large amounts of glucose and ketones in the urine, and blood glucose with ketosis. Acidosis is marked and the blood urea may be raised. Cerebral oedema and disseminated intravascular coagulation are serious complications. On initial examination the picture may be hard to distinguish from hypoglycaemic coma or from advanced renal failure. Overdosage with salicylates can also give a closely similar picture. In older subjects the differential diagnosis must sometimes include a cerebrovascular accident, since glycosuria may also occur in such a situation.

Hyperosmolar non-ketotic coma is a condition of profound dehydration. There is no associated ketoacidosis, but serum osmolality and glucose are both extremely high. It typically occurs in elderly patients who become hyperglycaemic due to an infection or other complication; they are unable to drink sufficiently to make up for urinary losses resulting from a hyperglycaemic diuresis. Onset may be gradual, sometimes developing over several days or weeks. The presenting picture may be of gradually increasing lethargy and impairment of consciousness but, unlike ketotic coma, seizures and focal neurological signs are common. The patient may at first be thought to be suffering from an acute stroke, presenting with hemiparesis, aphasia or simple or complex hallucinations (Guisado & Arieff 1975). The condition is usually reversible with correction of the metabolic abnormalities. Autonomic changes can include hyperpnoea and hypertension.

Neurological complications

Neurological complications of diabetes are common. Peripheral neuropathy may affect 10–50% of diabetic patients (Chaudhuri 1997) and can be a severe and distressing complication. Newly diagnosed patients sometimes complain of pain, paraesthesiae and restlessness of limbs, usually distally, symptoms that generally resolve with treatment of the hyperglycaemia. Other reversible neuropathies may be due to individual nerve or nerve root damage or due to cranial neuropathies. Diabetic amyotrophy (femoral neuropathy) is an unpleasant and often extremely painful condition that frequently develops over several weeks and is associated with wasting in one or both anterior thigh muscles. Most patients recover completely but may require strong analgesia for many months. Acute or subacute cranial nerve lesions, usually affecting cranial nerves III or VI or more rarely IV or VII, may also occur. If the third cranial nerve is affected, the pupil is usually spared. Recovery is usually complete within 6–8 weeks. In the elderly irreversible pupillary changes include meiosis, irregular pupils with sluggish light reflex, and sometimes the classic Argyll Robertson pupil (pseudotabes).

A symmetrical somatic polyneuropathy often develops over many years and is related to the duration of diabetes and other microvascular complications. Unfortnately no treatment has been shown to satisfactorily treat this. A painful neuropathy may occur in association. These may present with painful feet, the pain often being severe and unremitting with a burning type sensation and frequently accompanied by allodynia and hyperpathia. Patients may also complain of restless legs or of a sensation of swollen feet. Autonomic dysfunction, usually of the parasympathetic nervous system with preserved sympathetic function, is also common. Impotence is the commonest symptom, and sildenafil and related agents are now widely prescribed in diabetic clinics. Other symptoms such as postural hypotension, gustatory sweating and gastrointestinal complications may

occur. Diabetes is also a risk factor for carotid or vertebrobasilar circulation territory strokes and transient ischaemic attacks and is associated with a relative risk of 1.5–3 (Marshall 1993).

Hypoglycaemic disorders including insulinomas

Spontaneous hypoglycaemia is associated with a number of diseases but is seen most frequently clinically following overjudicious use of insulin in diabetes mellitus. Its importance in psychiatry lies in the range of predominantly cerebral symptoms associated with hypoglycaemic disorders and because accurate identification of hypoglycaemic episodes, which may mimic many psychiatric conditions, may lead to diagnosis of the underlying disorder and curative treatment.

The definition of hypoglycaemia is broadly accepted as a blood glucose concentration below 3 mmol/L (Marks & Teale 2001). There is considerable interindividual variability in both the symptoms experienced during hypoglycaemic episodes (Hepburn et al. 1991) and the blood glucose levels at which they occur. In experimentally induced hypoglycaemia, symptoms are not usually present until the arterial blood glucose falls below 3.5 mmol/L, equivalent to a venous blood glucose level of 3.3 mmol/L, just below the level at which homeostatic mechanisms opposing the action of insulin become active. The symptoms are caused by neuroglycopenia, literally a shortage of glucose in neurones, and have been classified into three distinct syndromes (Marks & Teale 2001; Marks 1981a).

Acute and subacute neuroglycopenia

This is the commonest picture associated with experimental hypoglycaemia and with iatrogenic hypoglycaemia associated with excess insulin or oral hypoglycaemic agents. It is characterised by profuse sweating, anxiety and panic, or an unnatural detached feeling similar to depersonalisation, together with feelings of hunger, tachycardia, tremor and paraesthesia. All are attenuated by adrenergic and cholinergic blockade. Speech and visual disturbances, confusion, fatigue and an ataxic gait are also found. The first group of symptoms is ascribed to the autonomic nervous system, though with the exception of tachycardia all occur with hypoglycaemia in totally sympathectomised patients. Angina may be precipitated if coronary artery disease exists.

When seen in insulin-treated diabetes mellitus, subacute neuroglycopenia is referred to as hypoglycaemic unawareness (see under Brain damage in diabetes). It is characterised by a reduction in spontaneous movements and speech, somnolence, poor performance at habitual tasks, memory impairments and behaviour that is out of character. Patients may become disinhibited, foolhardy or aggressive in manner, closely resembling alcoholic intoxication. Others become apathetic and withdrawn, with slurred speech and somnolence. The degree of functional impairment is out of proportion to subjective discomfort, and the person typically lacks realisation of the changes within himself. In rare instances, insulin-induced hypoglycaemia results in offending, in which case it constitutes grounds in UK law for a 'sane' (or 'non-insane') automatism (Fenwick 1990).

Brief episodes of unconsciousness and provocation of seizure activity with automatisms may occur in both acute and subacute neuroglycopenic syndromes. Occasionally focal neurological disturbances such as diplopia, hemiparesis or dysphasia may be seen without obvious diffuse cerebral disturbance. If normoglycaemia is not restored, progression to stupor, coma or death from cerebral oedema may occur.

Chronic neuroglycopenia

Chronic neuroglycopenia is rare and virtually confined to patients with insulinomas and patients with diabetes mellitus treated overzealously with insulin. It is characterised by the insidious development of personality change, poor memory and intellectual deterioration resembling dementia or psychosis with paranoid features. Emotional changes may be prominent, with irritability, apathy or emotional lability. The course may be punctuated by episodes of acute or subacute neuroglycopenia. The symptoms and signs are unaltered on the temporary restoration of normoglycaemia but permanent removal of the cause may lead to long-term improvement over a year or more (Marks 1981a).

Glucose passes through the blood–brain barrier via a facilitated transport system using specific glucose transporter proteins. Blood glucose is an important factor in determining the rate of glucose transport and adaptation develops in the face of prolonged hyperglycaemia or hypoglycaemia. This explains in part why diabetic patients experience neuroglycopenic symptoms at higher blood glucose levels, and habitually hypoglycaemic patients at lower levels, than normal subjects. It may also explain why apparently healthy people with no discernible abnormality of glucose homeostasis suffer postprandial symptoms at blood glucose levels tolerated without difficulty by most.

Hypoglycaemic episodes are associated with a wide range of underlying disorders, including severe liver, renal, cardiac and respiratory failure, sepsis, starvation including anorexia nervosa, hypopituitarism, Addison's disease and hypothyroidism. Important to psychiatry are the toxic and drug-induced causes. Alcohol may provoke a reactive hypoglycaemia and salicylates, quinine, haloperidol, beta-blockers, the sulphonylureas and insulins, and many others have been associated with drug-induced hypoglycaemia. Insulinomas are a rare but important cause of hypoglycae-

mia because they may produce a wide range of clinical pictures that are usually intermittent and because there may be normal health between attacks, making diagnosis often very challenging. Other causes, less likely to be seen by psychiatrists, include glycogen storage disease, hereditary fructose intolerance, galactosaemia, carnitine deficiency and disorders of gluconeogenesis.

Alcohol-induced hypoglycaemia

Hypoglycaemia may occur in response to various drugs and poisons of which alcohol is the most important. Alcohol exerts its hypoglycaemic effect mainly by inhibiting gluconeogenesis. It specifically inhibits gluconeogenesis from lactate but not from pyruvate, alanine or glycerol and it does not affect glycogenolysis. Hepatic glycogen stores are rarely sufficient to replace glucose used by insulin-independent tissues such as the brain for more than 8 hours. Consequently, hypoglycaemia most commonly occurs after this time, typically in the chronically alcohol dependent, 6–36 hours after a large intake, and it may first show itself by inducing coma. Sometimes it develops sooner, when it may be overlooked in the face of obvious intoxication. Recovery is usually prompt after the administration of glucose. It is possible that the condition accounts for a considerable number of deaths in alcoholic subjects.

Recurrent attacks are rare but have been reported (Fredericks & Lazor 1963; de Moura *et al.* 1967), usually in those with a long history of alcohol dependency. Arky *et al.* (1968) drew attention to the severe alcohol-induced hypoglycaemia liable to occur in insulin-dependent diabetics. They reported five patients who had repeatedly been admitted to hospital following alcohol-induced hypoglycaemic episodes; two died without recovery from coma and three were left with permanent memory impairments or dementia.

Meal-induced hypoglycaemia

Mild hypoglycaemia with symptoms resembling acute neuroglycopenia occurring after ingestion of food, but not provoked by fasting, are common. These symptoms occur more often in asthenic and emotionally labile persons, and may be associated with minor psychiatric instability in a manner which initiates a vicious circle. Exercise may provoke or aggravate the symptoms, but food or glucose do not bring decisive relief. Between attacks the patient often reports that he feels run down and is functioning below his optimum. The now-discredited oral glucose test, which has a high false-positive rate (>50%), was previously widely used in the assessment of postprandial hypoglycaemia and led to an epidemic of non-hypoglycaemia across the developed world from the 1950s to the 1980s (Jager & Young 1974). However, the failure of this classification to either aid diagnosis or provide a better understanding of the underlying pathophysiology has led to its demise (Service 1995). No specific treatment is indicated for individuals with symptoms occurring after food ingestion other than advice to avoid provocating foods. Some individuals who are susceptible to even mild lowering of their blood glucose may have a defect in blood–brain glucose transport or neurotic personality traits (Genter *et al.* 1994; Jager & Young 1974) but do not have detectable abnormality of glucose homeostasis (Marks & Teale 2001).

Factitious hypoglycaemia

Surreptitious use of insulin or sulphonylureas to induce hypoglycaemic symptoms can pose a difficult diagnostic problem. It is seen predominantly among those working in health-related occupations, more often in women, and in close relatives of diabetics who have access to their medications. It has also been noted among teenage female diabetics who misuse their insulin (Anon. 1978). Hypoglycaemia may be induced for the benefit of the symptoms experienced or as part of attention-seeking behaviour. Sometimes it may occur in association with Munchausen's syndrome, with patients submitting to laparotomy and even subtotal pancreatectomy.

Presentation is with erratically occurring neuroglycopenic symptoms suggestive of insulinoma. Many patients are admitted in coma. Scarlett *et al.* (1977) described seven subjects with factitious hypoglycaemia in whom symptoms had been present for 2 months to 6 years. Two had had subtotal pancreatectomies before the true cause was discovered; one had been diagnosed with diabetes 17 years previously, probably erroneously; and two had given insulin to their children, one with a fatal result. Another described the exquisite pleasure of going to sleep not knowing whether she would regain consciousness, after injecting insulin.

Jordan *et al.* (1977) described patients abusing sulphonylurea who presented in a similar manner. They estimated that factitious hypoglycaemia was at least as common as insulinomas. Inappropriately raised plasma insulin during hypoglycaemic episodes occurs in both insulin and sulphonylurea abuse, although low C-peptide levels occur only with insulin use. After oral hypoglycaemic agents, C-peptide levels are likely to be raised as a result of β-cell stimulation, a picture that can be virtually indistinguishable from insulinoma. Diagnosis must then be made by demonstrating the drugs in the blood or urine (see Table 10.2).

Marks (1981a) describes a separate group of patients, also paramedical workers or relatives of diabetics, who present with attacks simulating acute neuroglycopenia, sometimes gradually proceeding to coma. However, blood glucose and electroencephalography (EEG) remain normal throughout the episodes. Recovery occurs spontaneously or may be provoked by saline injection. The situation is considered to represent a conversion disorder.

Insulinomas

Insulinomas are rare, occurring in 4 per million person-years (Service 1991). Benign adenomas of the pancreatic islet cells are the most common cause, occurring in the body and tail of the pancreas in two-thirds. Occasionally ectopic insulinomas occur in the vicinity of the duodenum or porta hepatis. Less than 10% are malignant. Approximately 6% occur as part of multiple endocrine neoplasia (MEN) syndrome type 1, a familial disorder associated with adenomas of the parathyroid, pituitary or other endocrine glands (see under Hyperparathyroidism, later in chapter). They are slightly more common in women and may occur at any age.

Episodes of odd behaviour and disturbances of consciousness are the main reasons for referral. Symptoms have commonly been present for months or years by the time the diagnosis is made, sometimes for as long as 30 years. Very occasionally, long remissions may be detected in the histories. Almost any psychiatric syndrome may be simulated, depending quite probably on the individual's constitution. The detailed content of attacks may differ from one occasion to another and diagnostic confusion is common. The essential clue usually lies in the episodic and recurrent nature of the attacks. An added difficulty is that organic features are not always evident, the change of consciousness sometimes being so slight that it passes unnoticed except to those familiar with the patient.

Typically attacks of subacute, or less often, acute neuroglycopenia occur. They gradually increase in frequency, initially occurring at intervals of several weeks or months but by presentation are often occurring several times per week. Attacks may commence abruptly, or with slowly worsening weakness, ataxia and confusion. Sweating, nystagmus, incoordination or focal neurological signs such as hemiparesis or positive Babinski responses may be seen during an attack. Coma is rare except in the most severe episodes. Initially attacks are commonest at midday, though later they occur more characteristically before breakfast and during the night. Only one-quarter of patients give a clear history of a relationship to fasting and only 10% to exercise, while relief by eating is even more rarely noticed by the patient (Marks 1981b). Typically the patient has complete amnesia for the content of the attacks, and occasionally for additional periods during which behaviour was seemingly normal. Between attacks he usually feels quite well. In a small proportion, chronic neuroglycopenia may occur with progressive mental or physical disability and little or no history of episodic disturbance.

Cases from the literature illustrate some of the diagnostic difficulties.

A 44-year-old man suffered from attacks of confusion with bizarre behaviour over a 5-year period. Each lasted from a few minutes to several hours and increased in frequency until they were occurring four to five times per week. He had partial or complete amnesia for the attacks, which were initially interpreted as fugue states. On one occasion whilst driving he started driving recklessly with complete disregard for his passenger. On another he wandered semi-confused at work for 2 hours, conducting coherent conversations with some people but ultimately removed his shirt and stared foolishly at people who tried talking to him. An episode when he clenched an axe in a menacing manner, after chopping wood, and wandered around his neighbourhood with a dazed expression led to his admission. In other episodes he was described as being pale, sweating, appearing limp and unsteady with drunken behaviour and double vision. During prolonged starvation it was possible to demonstrate intermittent disturbances of awareness that became progressively more marked even though the blood sugar values were essentially unchanged. Periods of acute motor excitement with confusion and aggressive behaviour could similarly begin and end without significant changes in the blood sugar (Romano & Coon 1942).

A 27-year-old man was referred as a psychiatric emergency with bouts of aggressive and destructive behaviour. During attacks he was disorientated with inappropriate behaviour, sweating and a violent tremor. Following them he had no recollection of what had occurred. He had a history of learning difficulties and of head injury at the age of 18 years. His father had a history of similar bouts of violent behaviour. The initial differential diagnosis included aggressive psychopathy, mental impairment with behaviour disturbance, and post-traumatic epilepsy. Prolonged fasting provoked a typical attack at 16 hours, associated with hypoglycaemia and relieved by glucose. At laparotomy multiple islet-cell tumours were found. A diagnosis of multiple endocrine adenomatosis (pluriglandular syndrome) was made as hyperparathyroidism was also present. His father had died with 'islet-cell-secreting tumour of the pancreas and calcification of the kidneys' (Carney et al. 1971).

Differential diagnosis of insulinomas

The following psychiatric and neurological conditions may often be suspected before the diagnosis of an insulinoma is made.
- Anxiety disorders may be suggested by episodes of anxiety, panic and depersonalisation.
- Personality disorder may be suggested by a history of episodes of aggressive or antisocial conduct, for which the patient claims amnesia or only a hazy recollection.
- Manic–depressive or schizophrenic psychoses may very occasionally be diagnosed. Rare cases of insulinoma have been reported to present with acute depressive psychoses, no doubt as a result of individual predisposition.

- Dementia may be closely simulated in cases with chronic deterioration of intellect and personality. Superimposed episodes of acute and transient disturbance may resemble the step-like course of multi-infarct dementia.
- A space-occupying lesion may be suspected when attacks provoke epilepsy, or when headache and focal neurological symptoms accompany clouding of consciousness. Carotid artery stenosis may be suggested by attacks of dysphasia or hemiplegia, or vertebrobasilar insufficiency when vertigo and diplopia are prominent features.
- Epilepsy is a relatively rare form of presentation of hypoglycaemia except in childhood. However, any episodic and recurrent neurological disorder is likely to raise the question of epilepsy, and the content of attacks may closely resemble the automatisms of complex partial seizures.
- Intoxication with other metabolic disorders such as uraemia or liver failure may be closely simulated, or endocrine disorders such as thyrotoxicosis, hypoparathyroidism or phaeochromocytoma.

Rare cases may present with peripheral neuropathy. Narcolepsy may sometimes be considered, or attacks of somnolence may suggest Kleine–Levin syndrome. Angina, vasovagal attacks, orthostatic hypotension and Stokes–Adams attacks may also be considered.

Investigation of hypoglycaemia

Spontaneous hypoglycaemia should be considered in anyone who presents with an episode of subacute neuroglycopenia, even if there may be an alternative explanation for the symptoms. A blood sample should be obtained when the patient is symptomatic, a process that may require training the patient or a friend or relative in collecting a capillary blood sample (Gama et al. 2003). Most patients with episodic spontaneous hypoglycaemia will have at least one overnight (18-hour) fasting blood glucose concentration below 2 mmol/L, when measured on three separate occasions.

The prolonged fast or 72-hour fast test has been advocated as the test of choice for investigating hypoglycaemia. It should be conducted in hospital under careful supervision. During the fast the patient is allowed to drink non-calorific and caffeine-containing drinks and is encouraged to be ambulant during the day. Blood glucose, insulin, C-peptide and proinsulin are tested 6 hourly until blood glucose is less than 3.5 mmol/L, when sampling is reduced to 1–2 hourly and the patient tested regularly for signs or symptoms of neuroglycopenia. The fast should be terminated if the blood glucose falls below 2.5 mmol/L in association with symptoms or signs of neuroglycopenia or if neither symptoms of neuroglycopenia nor episodes of hypoglycaemia have occurred at 72 hours. Glucose, insulin, C-peptide, proinsulin, β-hydroxybutyrate and sulphonylurea are tested at the end of the fast and plasma glucose response to glucagon before refeeding. When a deficiency is suspected, plasma cortisol, growth hormone or glucagon should also be measured at the beginning and end of the fast.

Interpretation of the findings of the 72-hour fast is shown in Table 10.2. To complicate interpretation, healthy, young, lean women may have plasma glucose concentrations of 2.5 mmol/L or even less following prolonged fasting in the absence of symptoms (Service 1999). Other provocation tests include the exercise test; the mixed meal test, the C-peptide suppression test and tolbutamide test are also occasionally used.

Electroencephalography

Sequential EEG changes were recorded during the course of insulin coma therapy, which was previously used for the treatment of schizophrenia. The EEG response to hypoglycaemia varies considerably between individuals, though is relatively stereotyped within individuals. In general, the correlation between symptoms and EEG change is closer than between symptoms and blood sugar levels. The earliest change to be detected is the appearance of delta rhythms on overbreathing. Spontaneous theta and delta waves then occur, and later asynchronous irregular waves and a flattened tracing. The abnormalities are often most marked over the temporal lobes. In hypoglycaemic coma the EEG consists of high-voltage delta waves as in other metabolic comas. After severe hypoglycaemic episodes, abnormalities may persist in the EEG for several days before reverting to normal.

Treatment of hypoglycaemia

The aims of treatment of hypoglycaemic disorders are twofold: to relieve neuroglycopenic symptoms by restoring normal plasma glucose levels and to treat the underlying cause. Neuroglycopenic symptoms can be relieved by oral glucose tablets, which should be carried by patients awaiting investigation when hypoglycaemic attacks are known to occur; during more severe attacks glucose may be given intravenously as a 5 or 10% solution or as a bolus of 50% solution.

Treatment of the underlying cause depends on the specific causal mechanism. Causative medications should be withdrawn, patients with alcohol dependency advised on the dangers of hypoglycaemia and individuals suspected of insulinomas should be referred to centres specialising in the management. The possibility of coincident hypoadrenalism or hypopituitarism must then be borne in mind, and parenteral hydrocortisone considered.

Outcome of hypoglycaemia

The immediate outcome for most attacks is excellent. The symptoms usually resolve spontaneously even without specific treatment. Sometimes, however, neurological and psychiatric manifestations may outlast the actual period of hypoglycaemia. Dysphasia, hemiparesis and stupor have been reported to persist for hours or even weeks after restoring the blood sugar to normal, also negativism, restlessness, apathy and prolonged behaviour disorder (Markowitz et al. 1961). Such disturbances are thought to rest on a vascular basis that ultimately resolves. Recovery from hypoglycaemic coma may similarly be delayed for hours or even weeks in occasional cases. After prolonged coma recovery may be incomplete, with evidence of permanent brain damage and dementia (Arky et al. 1968).

The outcome after surgery for insulinoma is excellent in the great majority of cases. The typical patient who has presented with intermittent episodes of neuroglycopenia ceases to have such attacks, whatever form they have taken, and normal health is restored.

While this is the experience of most observers, occasional reports have indicated a less favourable picture on prolonged follow-up. Markowitz et al. (1961) followed six early cases after a lapse of 25 years, and found that five had shown either persisting or newly acquired mental disturbances in the interim. These were sometimes severe, including manic–depressive psychosis, irrational or erratic behaviour and other aberrations of personality, and were thought possibly to represent the aftermath of brain damage sustained during the hypoglycaemic episodes. A surprisingly high incidence of peptic ulceration and haemorrhage had also developed, even though ulcerogenic pancreatic tumours had not appeared to be present.

The rarer presentations in the form of chronic psychosis or intellectual deterioration may be expected to improve to some degree after operation, but here recovery is seldom complete. In these cases, as after prolonged episodes of hypoglycaemic coma, irreversible brain damage often proves to have occurred. Thus among 100 patients with psychosis or 'long-term insanity' in the detailed review by Laurent et al. (1971), 37 showed little or no improvement after removal of the hypoglycaemic tumour. The longer the duration of symptoms before the diagnosis, the greater was the risk of permanent mental disability.

Cerebral pathology of hypoglycaemia

Pathological changes in the brain following acute episodes of hypoglycaemia have mainly been studied in cases following insulin coma therapy. The brain may show oedema and vascular congestion, whilst survival after profound hypoglycaemic coma may be associated with ventricular dilatation, cortical atrophy and hippocampal atrophy. Neurones show ischaemic cell changes and associated gliosis. Cell damage may occur in scattered foci, but is more typically laminar with emphasis on the third and fifth layers (Brierley 1981). Relative sparing of the visual cortex is usual, but the corpus

Table 10.2 Diagnostic interpretation of the results of a 72-hour fast.*

Diagnosis	Symptoms or signs	Glucose† (mg/day)	Insulin‡§ (µU/ml)	C-peptide§¶ (nmol/litre)	Proinsulin§‖ (pmol/litre)	β-Hydroxy-butyrate (mmol/litre)	Change in glucose** (mg/dl)	Sulponylurea in plasma
Normal	No	≥40	<6	<0.2	<5	>2.7	<25	No
Insulinoma	Yes	≤45	≥6††	≥0.2	≥5	≤2.7	≥25	No
Factitious hypoglycaemia from insulin	Yes	≤45	≥6‡‡	<0.2	<5	≤2.7	≥25	No
Sulphonylurea-induced hypoglycaemia	Yes	≤45	≥6	≥0.2	≥5	≤2.7	≥25	Yes§§
Hypoglycaemia mediated by insulin-like growth factor	Yes	≤45	≤6	<0.2	<5	≤2.7	≥25	No
Non-insulin-mediated hypoglycaemia	Yes	≤45	<6	<0.2	<5	>2.7	<25	No
Inadvertent feeding during the fast	No	≥45	<6	<0.2	<5	≤2.7	≥25	No
Non-hypoglycaemia disorder	Yes	≥40	<6	<0.2	<5	>2.7	<25	No

* Measurements are made at the point the decision is made to end the fast.

† Sequential plasma glucose measurements in the hypoglycaemia range fluctuate. Plasma glucose levels ≤45 mg per decilitre at the time a decision is made to end the fast may rise to as much as 50 mg per decilitre when the fast is factually ended approximately one hour later. Plasma glucose levels may be as low as 40 mg per decilitre during prolonged fasting in normal women. To convert values to millimoles per litre multiply by 0.05551.

‡ Measured by double-antibody radioimmunoassay (lower limit of detection, 5 µU per millilitre). To convert values to picomoles per litre, multiply by 6.0.

§ In normal subjects plasma insulin, C-peptide, and proinsulin levels may be higher if the plasma glucose levels is ≥60 mg per decilitre.

¶ Measured by the immunochemiluminometric technique (lower limit of detection, 0.033 nmol per itre).

‖ Measured by the immunochemiluminometric technique (lower limit of detection, 0.2 pmol per litre).

** In response to intravenous glucagon (peak value minus value at the end of fast). To convert values to millimoles per litre, multiply by 0.05551.

†† Ratios of insulin to glucose are of no diagnostic value in patients with insulinomas.

‡‡ Plasma insulin levels may be very high (>100 µU per millilitre or >1000 µU per millilitre) in factitious hypoglycaemia from insulin.

§§ Unlike the first generation of sulphonylurea drugs, which were easily measured, second-generation drugs are not.

striatum and the hippocampi appear to be especially vulnerable, as in cerebral hypoxia (see Chapter 4, Neuronal death). However, in hypoglycaemia the cerebellar Purkinje cells appear to be less affected (Richardson *et al.* 1959).

Hypothyroidism

Hypothyroidism remains of great importance in psychiatric practice and is notorious for leading to mistakes in diagnosis. The prevalence, nature and clinical course of the behavioural and psychological disturbances associated with hypothyroidism (myxoedema) were first described in a report by the Clinical Society of London (1888). This described some degree of mental disturbance, ranging from irritability and agoraphobia to dementia and melancholia in almost all untreated patients with hypothyroidism. Subsequently, it has been recognised that the effect of prolonged hypothyroidism on brain function may be severe and potentially irreversible. Furthermore, on account of its insidious development with minor and often diffuse complaints at first presentation, diagnosis of hypothyroidism may be considerably delayed and isolated case reports of hypothyroid patients presenting with psychiatric manifestations continue to appear in the literature.

The widespread availability of cheap reliable laboratory tests for quantification of thyroid hormone levels has objectified diagnosis, although this has also led to the identification of a larger group of patients with biochemically borderline hypothyroidism. These patients have few if any specific symptoms with often ill-defined complaints, and ideal management currently remains unclear. Recent research has also suggested that a group of residual symptoms may remain despite 'adequate' replacement therapy with thyroxine. A number of randomised controlled trials investigating response to treatment with a more physiological combination of tri-iodothyronine and thyroxine have produced conflicting results and the issue of best treatment of residual symptoms currently remains unresolved.

Hypothyroidism is a common condition with an incidence that increases markedly with age, especially from middle age onward. Like hyperthyroidism, it is very much commoner in women than men, in a ratio of approximately 8:1. Classification based on severity subdivides hypothyroidism into mild and overt forms: in the former, serum thyroid-stimulating hormone (TSH) alone is raised; in the latter, a reduction in serum free thyroxine is also seen. The large Whickham study identified raised serum TSH (mild or overt hypothyroidism) in 7.5% of women and 2.8% of men in a UK community population (Tunbridge *et al.* 1977). Subsequent studies have found similar figures with incidences rising markedly with age, up to 21% in a female group aged over 74 years in one study, with the ratio of mild to overt hypothyroidism ranging from 5:1 to 15:1 (Roberts & Ladenson 2004).

Physical features

Overt hypothyroidism is associated with a familiar set of symptoms and signs. The appearance is characteristic, with a pale puffy complexion and baggy eyelids. The skin is dry and rough, with a non-pitting oedematous appearance over the face and limbs and in the supraclavicular fossae. Hair loss may have been noticed and hair may have become lank and dry in texture. Speech is slow, and the voice often coarse, thick and toneless. The whole disposition of the patient tends to be sluggish and inert. The pulse is usually slowed and angina, congestive heart failure or pericardial effusion may occur. Appetite is diminished, the patient is often constipated and ileus and intestinal pseudo-obstructions may occur. Hearing, taste and smell may be impaired due to deposits of mucoid material. Intolerance of cold is often a prominent early complaint. Menorrhagia is common in women and impotence in men. Vague generalised aches and pains of a rheumatic nature may occur. Very occasionally muscular weakness may be the initial manifestation.

Neuropsychiatric features

Initially psychological changes are non-specific and ill-defined. Cognitive disturbances include the inability to concentrate, poor attention, bradyphrenia, calculation difficulties and difficulty understanding complex questions. Memory is often affected from an early stage, with failure to register events and forgetfulness for day-to-day events. Memory for remote events may also deteriorate in chronic cases. Psychomotor retardation is seen and ready fatigueability is conspicuous. With chronic disease, the ability to perform everyday routine tasks is decreased and such tasks take a progressively longer time to complete. Patients become less concerned about and responsive to others, and there is marked inability to sustain mental exertion. The patient also becomes less capable of learning and performing new tasks. Speech is reduced and perseverations are frequently seen. Alterations in the accuracy of perception may also develop with a tendency to illusion formation, and later hallucinations in the visual or other modalities and may lead to the development of paranoid ideas. Historical accounts describe a progression to increasing drowsiness, with lethargy and difficulty in arousal.

In the earlier stages the patient is subjectively aware of such changes, and may complain of poor memory or difficulty concentrating. The profound loss of interest and initiative carries the risk of delaying medical attention. Because of these changes in attention and concentration, slowing of thought and actions, and reduced responsiveness to others, the diagnosis may be confused with one of depression. Indeed, as discussed below, depression develops more commonly in hypothyroidism though irritability is also a frequent feature, and some patients become markedly agitated and aggressive.

Mild hypothyroidism

Several studies have suggested that mild symptoms of hypothyroidism are commoner and scores on measures of depression and anxiety higher in patients with subclinical hypothyroidism than in age-matched controls. These findings, however, are inconsistent with other studies that have found no significant differences (Cooper 2001). A number of small studies have also examined the effect of mild hypothyroidism on memory and concluded that small improvements in function are associated with thyroxine therapy in this group. However, the strength of the evidence for these associations is small, and a recent consensus statement indicates that the data supporting the association of subclinical thyroid disease with symptoms or adverse events are few (Surks *et al.* 2004).

In this review of the literature, the subclinical hypothyroid group comprises those with TSH above or below 10 mIU/L. The authors do not recommend routine treatment of patients with TSH below 10 mIU/L unless symptoms compatible with hypothyroidism are also present. In the symptomatic condition, it is recommended that a treatment trial extending to several months should be considered at the clinician's discretion, with continuing treatment predicated by clear symptomatic benefit. Measurement of TSH levels every 6–12 months is advised to monitor for progression to overt hypothyroidism. In the group with TSH above 10 mIU/L, treatment with levothyroxine is considered reasonable in view of the higher conversion rate to overt hypothyroidism, although the evidence that such treatment leads to reduced cholesterol levels or symptoms is deemed inconclusive. The exception is pregnant women, who should be referred for expert advice.

Schizophrenic and affective psychoses

It is against the background of the neuropsychiatric changes described above that the more severe psychiatric disturbances of hypothyroidism develop. The psychoses that develop are non-specific and may mimic the psychoses seen in schizophrenia or the affective psychoses. They may develop acutely or run a subacute course over several weeks or months. Importantly, careful history and examination will often reveal a few stigmata of hypothyroidism (Whybrow & Bauer 2000) and assessment of cognitive function may aid differential diagnosis. Though confusion may occur in acute schizophrenia, visual hallucinations with marked and persistent cognitive disturbances are rare. The only unifying feature, upheld by many observers, is the frequency of a paranoid colouring whatever form the psychosis may take (Asher 1949).

In Asher's (1949) classic paper on 'myxoedematous madness' in 14 patients, five showed an organic reaction with hallucinations and persecutory ideas, five the picture of schizophrenia with a marked paranoid colouring, two presented as advanced dementia, and two with depressive features.

Organic psychoses usually show the features of delirium, with florid delusions and hallucinations, mental confusion and impairment of consciousness. Delusions of persecution may be gross and bizarre. Auditory hallucinations appear to be particularly common. Dementia develops as an extension of the mental impairment characteristic of the condition generally. Depressive and schizophrenic psychoses may or may not be accompanied by organic mental features, though the latter are usually found when sought with care. Paranoid symptoms again figure prominently. Schizophrenic psychoses will in general be coloured by mental slowing, and often include features indicative of organic cerebral impairment.

Few behavioural studies have been conducted in patients with hypothyroidism unselected for psychiatric disorder and therefore the incidence of psychosis in hypothyroidism is difficult to determine. In the early 1888 review before the availability of treatment, it was of the order of 15%. However, our ability to reliably detect early-onset cases through the widespread availability of laboratory testing has reduced current levels to considerably below this.

Depressive syndrome

Depressive affect has been reported as a frequent association with hypothyroidism (Whybrow *et al.* 1969) and a regular feature of early case series. Despite this there are few good studies describing prevalence rates.

Several of the metabolic and behavioural changes seen in hypothyroidism are common to depression, suggesting that changes in the pituitary–thyroid system may play a role in the modulation of mood. The most common abnormality in thyroid function testing among patients with depression is a mild elevation in serum thyroxine concentration, which falls with clinical response to treatment (Whybrow & Bauer 2000). Serum TSH response to thyrotropin-releasing hormone is blunted in 25% of depressed patients and the nocturnal surge of TSH is lost in depression, returning to normal with recovery (Whybrow & Bauer 2000).

Mild hypothyroidism is also more frequent in rapid cycling bipolar disorder, occurring in up to 25% of cases. Thyroxine supplementation of established treatment for bipolar disorder has been shown to reduce the number of episodes (Whybrow & Bauer 2000).

Neurological accompaniments

Ankle reflexes may be slowed with marked delay in the relaxation phase, though these are not specific and have also been described in diabetes mellitus and anorexia nervosa

(Larner 1995). Muscle weakness is a very common complaint that often does not correlate with biochemical severity and may persist despite therapy (Duyff *et al.* 2000). A predominantly sensory axonal peripheral neuropathy and proximal neuropathy and more rarely focal muscle enlargement or wasting may also occur (Askmark *et al.* 2000). Sleep apnoea may occur as a result of obesity or upper airway obstruction.

Jellinek (1962) drew attention to the occurrence of fits, faints, and cerebrovascular accidents in patients with hypothyroidism. Four patients were reported with generalised seizures that responded to thyroid replacement, others with attacks of syncope, and others with unusual confusional episodes suggesting temporal lobe dysfunction. Cerebrovascular accidents and episodes of previous transient cerebral ischaemia were found to have occurred in several of his patients, and hypothyroidism is known to be associated with a coagulopathy and raised risk of cardiovascular disease (Roberts & Ladenson 2004).

Cerebellar ataxia is an uncommon consequence of advanced hypothyroidism that does not seem to correlate with biochemical severity (Barnard *et al.* 1971). Jellinek and Kelly (1960) drew attention to the disorder in a description of six cases presenting with cerebellar disturbance in the form of ataxia, tremor, dysarthria and nystagmus that remitted promptly with replacement therapy. Though the aetiology remains unclear, the prompt response to therapy suggests a metabolic rather than structural cause in the majority of cases.

Hypothyroid coma is a grave condition which carries a high mortality. It typically develops in association with superimposed infection, surgery or trauma (Kaminski & Ruff 1989). It should be suspected in any patient with severe impairment of consciousness and hypothermia. The skin feels icy cold, and a low-reading rectal thermometer is required to confirm the hypothermia. Respiration may be sluggish, and cardiac failure or dysrhythmia is a feature of serious significance.

Investigations

As with hyperthyroidism, it is essential to confirm the diagnosis by laboratory tests before starting treatment. The total and free thyroxine levels are low, although serum triiodothyronine may be normal. Elevated plasma TSH will indicate primary thyroid failure, whereas normal basal levels will suggest a pituitary origin. The latter is confirmed by an absent, subnormal or delayed response to thyrotropin-releasing hormone. The estimation of circulating autoantibodies to thyroglobulin and thyroid peroxidase may help to establish the cause, for example Hashimoto's thyroiditis.

The serum cholesterol is elevated, the heart is usually enlarged and the ECG shows a low-voltage tracing with flattened or inverted T waves. The EEG shows lowered voltage and slowing of the dominant frequencies; occasionally it is normal despite severe hypothyroidism but this is rare. The protein in the cerebrospinal fluid may be moderately raised.

Neuropsychology

The neurocognitive deficits in hypothyroid adults are listed in Table 10.3.

Table 10.3 Neurocognitive deficits in hypothyroid adults. (From Dugbartey 1998.)

Cognitive domain	Treatment outcome	Psychometric test
General intelligence	Not generally affected	WAIS, WAIS-R, DRS
Complex attention and concentration	Improvement after 5–7 months Equivocal change 5–10 months	PASAT, SDMT TMT (Part A and B)
Memory	Improvement No change (treatment may prevent further decline)	Inglis paired associates learning test CVMT, FMT, RCFT, SRT, WMS
Perceptual and visuospatial function	Improvement No improvement	WAIS-R (Block design and Object assembly subsets) Cube copying
Language (expressive)	No improvement	Word fluency (Animals)
Language (receptive)	Not available	Word discrimination, oral reading
Executive/frontal system	Not available No change	Go-No Go, Word fluency, Luria's m's and n's Porteus mazes
General screening	No change Progressive decline	Modified MMSE MMSE
Motor function	No change	Grip strength

CVMT, Continuous Visual Memory Test; DRS, Dementia Rating Scale; FMT, Milner Facial Memory Test; PASAT, Paced Auditory Serial Addition Task; RCFT, Rey-Osterrieth Complex Figure Test; SDMT, Symbol Digit Modalities Test; SRT, Selective Reminding Test; TMT, Trailmaking Task; WAIS(-R), Wechsler Adult Intellegence Scale (-Revised); WMS, Wechsler Memory Test.

Differential diagnosis

Not uncommonly, hypothyroidism is first diagnosed only after a patient has been symptomatic for a considerable time. The suspicion of hypothyroidism is usually derived from the characteristic facial appearance or other physical symptoms and signs, but unless the disorder is specifically considered these may easily be overlooked. In the 14 cases reported by Asher (1949), all with florid mental illnesses, the hypothyroidism had been missed by the referring doctor in every case. In the more severe psychotic illnesses, organic features are usually evident in the mental state but not invariably so.

Even without overt evidence of hypothyroidism, psychiatric patients may warrant investigation if they have a history of thyroidectomy or of having required thyroid medication in the past. These were the factors that prompted investigation in 5 of 18 patients surveyed by Tonks (1964) in a psychiatric hospital. Patients on long-term lithium therapy are also at increased risk of developing hypothyroidism and require regular monitoring of serum TSH levels.

Aetiology of mental disturbances

The specific pathophysiology responsible for the behavioural and emotional disturbances seen in hypothyroidism remains unknown. Early investigations showed a 38% reduction in cerebral blood flow and 27% reduction in oxygen and glucose consumption in patients with hypothyroidism (Scheinberg et al. 1950). An associated near-twofold increase in cerebrovascular resistance led to the hypothesis that cerebral hypometabolism was a consequence of increased cerebrovascular resistance and reduced cardiac output rather than altered cerebral metabolic demands (Sokoloff 1953; O'Brien & Harris 1968), with the relative cerebral hypoxia worsened by frequently coexistent anaemia.

Smith and Ain (1995) using ^{31}P magnetic resonance spectroscopy reported a relative increase in frontal phosphocreatine/inorganic phosphate ratio in response to treatment of hypothyroidism, suggesting a treatment-related increase in frontal lobe metabolism; in contrast, Constant et al. (2001) using positron emission tomography (PET) showed globally reduced neural metabolism in hypothyroidism that they argued could not be explained by increased vascular resistance alone. Nuclear receptors for tri-iodothyronine are prominent in the brain particularly in neurones and are found in high concentrations in the amygdala and hippocampus, regions associated with modulation of mood, and in low concentrations in the brainstem and cerebellum (Ruel et al. 1985). The question of whether the cerebral hypometabolism seen in hypothyroidism is a consequence of a direct action of thyroid hormones on neurones or is secondary to altered cerebral blood flow therefore remains unanswered and will perhaps await the development of techniques to directly measure CNS thyroid metabolism in vivo. Nevertheless, the associated mental symptomatology can be largely ascribed to changes in cerebral metabolism, regardless of cause. Such changes are also reflected in the EEG findings described above, and these can also be observed to improve with substitution therapy.

Cases of major affective disorder and schizophrenia are likely to be determined by both organic factors and genetic and environmental factors. In the rare examples where organic features are entirely absent from the mental state, the cerebral metabolic defect has probably served merely as a precipitant. However, the situation is not entirely straightforward, since patients with purely depressive symptomatology with no evidence of hypothyroidism have been found to respond to thyroxine, often after other forms of treatment have failed entirely (Bauer et al. 1998).

Outcome of mental disturbances

The treatment of hypothyroidism is usually highly rewarding, with behavioural disturbances responding well to adequate thyroxine therapy, although supplementation with an antidepressant or neuroleptic is often initially helpful. The great majority of patients with serious psychiatric developments can also be expected to respond, even those with overt dementia, provided too long an interval has not elapsed. However, Jellinek (1962) stressed that several of his cases were left with measurable defects of intellect and memory after being rendered euthyroid, mostly those who had remained undiagnosed for very long periods of time or where treatment had been inadequate.

Where response to thyroxine is concerned, the frankly organic psychoses can generally be expected to do better than psychoses with predominantly 'functional' symptomatology. This was confirmed by Tonks (1964), who surveyed 18 hypothyroid patients in a psychiatric hospital during a period of treatment with thyroid preparations alone; the proportion that made complete and lasting recoveries was much higher among patients who showed evidence of disturbance of consciousness, by way of disorientation or confusion, than among those who did not. The duration of the illnesses was also important, in that no patient with a mental illness exceeding 2 years had a satisfactory response to the trial of thyroid replacement therapy alone. The only clearly organic condition that failed to respond was a patient with chronic progressive dementia and aphasia of 7 years' duration. In most patients cognitive dysfunction also improves markedly with treatment (Haggerty et al. 1990; Osterweil et al. 1992). However, studies have also suggested that residual symptoms remain in patients on 'adequate' thyroxine treatment, raising the possibility of augmenting therapy with tri-iodothyronine.

Additional measures in the form of phenothiazines, antidepressant medication or electroconvulsive therapy may be necessary in psychotic disorders, and particularly so when organic features are absent from the mental state. It must be borne in mind, however, that phenothiazines carry a small risk of precipitating hypothermic coma in hypothyroid patients, as in an early case reported by Mitchell *et al.* (1959).

It is necessary to introduce thyroxine with caution at the beginning of treatment, especially in the elderly, because of the possibility of myocardial damage. The starting dose of L-thyroxine sodium should not exceed 50 μg daily. If there is no evidence of cardiac failure or angina, this may be increased by 25–50 μg per day every 2–3 weeks until the maintenance dose of 100–150 μg daily is reached.

Very occasionally the initiation of treatment is accompanied by the emergence of psychotic disorder, which interestingly usually takes the form of mania. Josephson and Mackenzie (1980) refer to 18 examples in the literature, 12 being manic illnesses and the others mixed affective or depressive disorders. The symptoms usually began within 4–7 days of starting thyroxine treatment, resolving over 1–2 weeks irrespective of further therapeutic intervention. All recovered completely. Such patients often had a personal or family history of psychiatric disorder and had frequently been depressed or delusional prior to starting treatment.

Replacement with thyroxine and tri-iodothyronine?

Despite 'adequate' therapy with thyroxine, with TSH within the desired range, many hypothyroid patients complain of persistent lethargy and other persisting psychological symptoms. A large community-based study using the general health questionnaire (GHQ) and a validated thyroid symptom questionnaire showed that, compared with controls, 26% more hypothyroid patients with a normal TSH showed caseness, defined as a score of 3 or more on the GHQ. This significant difference persisted after correction for chronic disease, drug use, age and sex (Saruvanan *et al.* 2002). Whether this represents a failure of thyroxine replacement to accurately mimic the normal physiological milieu, is the result of being labelled with a disease, or is due to case ascertainment bias (i.e. individuals with an inclination to complain and seek medical care are more likely to be diagnosed with subclinical hypothyroidism) remains unclear.

A randomised clinical trial has suggested that combined therapy with tri-iodothyronine and thyroxine leads to improved cognitive performance, mood and physiological well-being compared with treatment with thyroxine alone (Bunevicius *et al.* 1999). However, subsequent randomised clinical trials have failed to replicate these findings, leading to suggestions that it is perhaps only patients with complete absence of thyroid function alone who may benefit from combined therapy (Clyde *et al.* 2003; Cooper 2003a; Sawka *et al.* 2003; Walsh *et al.* 2003). Optimum treatment of persistent psychological symptoms and mood disturbance therefore currently remains unclear.

Hyperthyroidism

Hyperthyroidism results from excess of the circulating thyroid hormones thyroxine and tri-iodothyronine. Thyroid hormones regulate energy and heat production, facilitate healthy development of the CNS, regulate somatic growth, puberty, and the synthesis of proteins important in cardiac, hepatic, neurological and muscular functions.

Although there is a rough correlation between levels of circulating hormones and severity of symptoms (Trzepacz *et al.* 1989), individuals, particularly the elderly, may present with widely differing sets of symptoms. Hyperthyroidism has a number of different causes where goitrous enlargement may or may not be present. Graves' disease is the most common cause, though the development of one or more autonomously functioning thyroid nodules is commonly seen in the elderly. There are a number of other rarer causes of hyperthyroidism including forms of thyroiditis and neoplasia, which will not be detailed here. For a comprehensive list see the recent review by Cooper (2003b) or a textbook of medicine.

A large British-based population survey from the 1970s identified unsuspected and undiagnosed hyperthyroidism in 0.5% of women (Tunbridge *et al.* 1977). A more recent survey in the USA found hyperthyroidism in 0.5% of randomly selected individuals, with subclinical or mild hyperthyroidism in a further 0.8% (Hollowell *et al.* 2002). Females are much more commonly affected than males in a ratio of approximately 6:1. Commonest presentation is in the second and third decades of life though the range is wide.

Attention has been directed to the role of stress and emotional disturbance in precipitating hyperthyroidism, in particular Graves' disease, and on the psychological constitution of those who develop the disorder. The onset is often abrupt and may be seen to follow directly upon some stressful event or emotional crisis. It is hard, however, to exclude the possibility that such emotional traumas may themselves have been the by-products of early and unsuspected thyroid overactivity. Gray and Hoffenberg (1985) failed to find an association between stressful life events and the onset of thyrotoxicosis or any cause when compared with a control group of non-toxic goitre. However, Matos-Santos *et al.* (2001) showed significantly more stressful life events with significantly greater impact in the 12 months preceding onset of symptoms in a Graves' disease group than a control group with toxic nodular goitre. These authors argue that Gray and Hoffenberg failed to find an association because they grouped all thyrotoxic patients together rather than looking specifically at Graves' disease, which is associated with an autoimmune aetiology.

Follow-up studies investigating premorbid personality using standardised personality measures suggest that neurotic features are transient rather than indicative of pre-existing personality traits in hyperthyroid patients (Jadresic 1990).

Common psychological accompaniments

Psychological disturbance of some degree is universal with hyperthyroidism. Patients frequently complain of nervousness and fatigue, and appear restless, overactive and irritable, sometimes with hyperacuity of perception and over-reaction to noise. Heightened tension leads to impatience and intolerance of frustration, and emotional lability may develop. Generalised anxiety has been reported in 80% and an association with panic disorder and the earlier 'atypical organic brain syndrome' and 'organic anxiety syndrome' has been described (Kathol *et al.* 1986; Jadresic 1990).

Depression can be prominent and found with symptoms of agitation rather than retardation (Woodbury 1918; Brownlie *et al.* 2000). Kathol *et al.* (1986) found that almost one-third of 29 consecutive patients seen in an endocrine clinic met criteria for major depression. In the elderly, an 'apathetic' hyperthyroidism with anergia and mental slowing occurs, classically presenting without the characteristic eye signs of hyperthyroidism (Thomas 1970). The acute confusional states described as occurring as part of thyroid crises are now rarely seen.

Heightened arousal leads to distractibility and impairment of concentration with difficulty sustaining focused attention. In addition, careful examination may reveal definite cognitive impairments, in the form of difficulty with simple arithmetic or with recent memory of which the patient may be unaware (Whybrow *et al.* 1969). In a survey of the populations of two psychiatric hospitals, comprising a total of over 1200 persons, McLarty *et al.* (1978) found just eight patients with thyrotoxicosis. In six the hyperthyroidism had been unsuspected prior to the survey, and in five it seemed to be contributing to the mental illness.

Psychoses

Psychosis is an uncommon association of hyperthyroidism, which may occasionally be the presenting feature and lead directly to psychiatric referral. A recent study of thyrotoxic psychosis from New Zealand suggested that in contemporary practice approximately 1% of thyrotoxic patients are first diagnosed with a major psychiatric illness (Brownlie *et al.* 2000).

Acute organic reactions accompany 'thyroid crises' and show the typical picture of delirium, usually accompanied by fever. They were formerly one of the commonest forms of major mental illness encountered in the disease, but are now very rare because of modern methods of treatment. They constitute a grave emergency and warrant urgent intervention.

Affective and schizophreniform psychoses are sometimes indistinguishable from their naturally occurring counterparts. A number of reports have suggested that mania is more frequent than depression (Lee *et al.* 1991), although the study by Brownlie *et al.* (2000) reported an equal incidence of manic (7/18) and depressive psychosis, with two cases presenting with a schizophreniform psychosis and one with a paranoid psychosis. Other authors have reported that schizophrenic illnesses of various types have sometimes been found to outnumber affective psychoses.

Hyperthyroidism is not associated with a specific type of psychosis, but it is generally considered that a distinctive colouring may be lent by the hyperthyroidism. Thus a manic component may accompany otherwise typical schizophrenic symptomatology, and agitation is often profound in the presence of depression. Most observers are also agreed that paranoid features are especially common whatever form the psychosis may take. The diagnostic distinctions between the affective and schizophrenic reactions are often blurred, and an admixture of organic psychiatric features is relatively common.

Johnson (1928) found only 24 examples of psychosis among over 2000 patients referred for thyroidectomy, when patients with obvious confusion or delirium were excluded. Most were depressive states with hallucinations and delusions. Checkley (1978) was unable to detect a clear time relationship in a careful survey of patients with manic–depressive psychosis who had also had thyrotoxicosis, and argued that if the hyperthyroidism had so little effect on the course of the affective disorder in patients long subject to manic–depressive episodes, it would seem unlikely to serve as a precipitant in patients without such liability. However, Brownlie *et al.* (2000) in a study of 18 patients found a family history of psychiatric illness in only two and a distant past psychiatric history in four. Even after excluding patients with a past psychiatric history, the number of cases of psychosis associated with hyperthyroidism requiring admission was still significantly greater than the 0.36 expected from analysis of community admission data.

Dunlap and Moersch (1935) reported 143 patients with mental disturbance accompanying hyperthyroidism; over 70% were organic psychosyndromes, but 26 patients showed manic–depressive psychoses (mostly depressions), two had dementia praecox and two were paranoid. Bursten (1961) found 10 patients with psychosis among 54 hyperthyroid patients seen in a general hospital during a 4-year period.

Neurological manifestations

A fine low-amplitude tremor at 8–10 Hz that resembles an exaggerated physiological tremor is common. It is most prominent in the small metacarpophalangeal joints in the fingers and in the tongue and eyelids. It is best seen when the arms and fingers are held extended and can be seen both during action and at rest. It appears to be mediated by peripheral β adrenoreceptors (Marsden *et al.* 1970). Chorea and athetosis are rare complications believed to be associated with enhanced striatal dopaminergic sensitivity (Delong

1996). Neuropathy is uncommon and upper motor neurone signs rare, occasionally presenting with muscle wasting and a clinical picture resembling amyotrophic lateral sclerosis (Logothetis 1961). Muscle weakness is common and most prominent in the shoulder girdles, and upper arms and legs. Many patients have clinical signs of myopathy, tendon reflexes are brisk and fasciculations occasionally seen. The well-known signs of lid-lag and upper lid retraction may be accompanied by exophthalmos due to swelling of the retro-orbital tissues.

Generalised seizures are occasionally precipitated by thyrotoxicosis and tend to resolve with treatment of the thyrotoxicosis. EEG changes seen in up to 50% of patients are usually reversible when euthyroidism is achieved (Abend & Tyler 1989). An association between hyperthyroidism and myasthenia gravis is well recognised. Periodic paralysis indistinguishable from familial hypokalaemic periodic paralysis may also occur. Beta-blockers tend to prevent the attacks, which resolve with restoration of normal thyroid function (Conway *et al*. 1974).

Investigations

Laboratory diagnosis of hyperthyroidism is usually straightforward. Most patients have increased unbound thyroxine and tri-iodothyronine and reduced concentrations of TSH. Free or unbound values are measured to avoid difficulties caused by changes in thyroid-binding protein. In 1%, free thyroxine levels are normal with raised free tri-iodothyronine (tri-iodothyronine toxicosis). Failure to suppress TSH in the presence of raised thyroxine raises the possibility of inappropriate thryrotropin syndrome due to a TSH-secreting pituitary tumour or thyroid hormone resistance (Cooper 2003b). In a small number of cases, however, the results may be borderline or even self-contradictory. The clinical features then require careful appraisal, and referral for specialist investigation is usually indicated.

Thyroid function tests have been found to be transiently abnormal in psychiatric patients shortly after admission to hospital. Among 480 newly admitted psychiatric patients, Cohen and Swigar (1979) found abnormalities in total thyroxine, thyroxine-binding capacity and free thyroxine in 9% of the patients, which usually returned to normal within a few weeks. They labelled this 'acute stress hyperthyroidism'. Low thyroxine levels were found in a similar proportion, also often resolving spontaneously.

Differential diagnosis

The differential diagnosis between hyperthyroidism and anxiety neurosis is a classic and often difficult exercise. Presenting symptoms can be virtually identical in both conditions; both show tachycardia, fine finger tremor, palpitations and loss of weight, and both may appear to have been precip-itated by stressful events. The presence of previous symptomatology of anxiety disorders in thyrotoxic patients can lead to further blurring of the diagnostic criteria between the two conditions.

Careful analysis of the features shown by large numbers of patients with hyperthyroidism has clarified the physical symptoms and signs that are of most importance in indicating this disorder (Wayne 1960). The symptoms, in descending order of discriminating value, are sensitivity to heat and preference for cold, increased appetite, loss of weight, sweating, palpitations, tiredness, 'nervousness' and dyspnoea on effort. In order of importance, the signs are cardiac dysrhythmia (typically atrial fibrillation), hyperkinetic movements, tachycardia exceeding 90 beats per minute, a palpable thyroid gland, a bruit audible over the thyroid, exophthalmos, lid retraction, hot hands, lid-lag and fine finger tremor. These lists show how closely anxiety disorders may be simulated.

Gurney *et al*. (1967) reviewed the features found in euthyroid patients with psychiatric disorder who were initially referred with suspected thyrotoxicosis. Higher frequency of psychological precipitants for the illness, a lower age of onset, more frequent 'hysterical' symptoms and panic attacks, and more neurotic features in the personality were found compared to patients with thyrotoxicosis.

Hyperthyroidism should therefore be strongly suspected when a patient gives a clear history of sensitivity to heat and a preference for cold, and this deserves careful specific enquiry. Similarly, the classical signs of exophthalmos, lid retraction and lid-lag will, when present, give a clear pointer to a diagnosis of hyperthyroidism. Precipitation by stress is found more commonly and impressively in the anxiety disorders. Perhaps the most decisive feature in differentiating the two conditions is the preservation or otherwise of appetite in the face of steady loss of weight; in hyperthyroidism appetite is characteristically increased, whereas in anxiety states it is reduced.

In the presence of frank psychosis, diagnostic difficulties are liable to be increased and the hyperthyroidism may sometimes go unrecognised for a considerable time. It is necessary to beware of the occasional case of hyperthyroidism in which fluctuations occur with periods of spontaneous resolution. Repeated episodes of affective disorder may be particularly misleading:

> A man of 40 was admitted to hospital with a typical attack of hypomania that responded satisfactorily to chlorpromazine during the next 3 weeks. Ten days later he was readmitted with a relapse after discontinuing the medication, but once again he responded rapidly to chlorpromazine. Three months later he developed marked weakness and depression, and for the first time appeared to be physically unwell. It was noted that he had a persistent tachycardia, a warm

moist skin and possibly an enlarged thyroid gland. Investigations confirmed hyperthyroidism, and retrospective enquiry revealed steady loss of weight and increased appetite since shortly before the first episode of hypomania. The admission notes on the two previous occasions had shown a tachycardia that had been overlooked at the time.

'Apathetic' hyperthyroidism, presenting with anergia and mental slowing, may cause particular diagnostic difficulty. The typical picture is of a middle-aged or elderly patient with considerable weight loss and apathy or depression (Lahey 1931; Thomas *et al.* 1970). Cardiovascular symptoms may overshadow other evidence of thyrotoxicosis, and eye signs in particular tend to be absent. Depression, particularly agitated, can also be the presenting feature in younger patients. Folks and Petrie (1982) describe a woman of 23 presenting with depression, insomnia and early morning waking, who after an overdose of amitriptyline was found to be thyrotoxic. The affective disorder resolved as the hyperthyroidism came under control. Alcoholism may be wrongly blamed for the tremulousness and emotional lability of hyperthyroid patients (Davis *et al.* 1971).

Aetiology of mental disturbances

The common psychological accompaniments of hyperthyroidism are probably the direct result of increased thyroxine levels and subsequent metabolic derangements within the CNS. This is supported by the uniformity of the common mental changes seen, their fluctuations with exacerbations of the disorder, and their rapid response to antithyroid treatment. In Kathol *et al.*'s (1986) investigation generalised anxiety disorder, but not depression, showed a strong relationship with measures of the free thyroxine index. Cerebral catecholamines may also be intimately involved, particularly increased sensitivity of β-adrenergic receptors. Beta-blocker medications improve psychiatric symptoms in hyperthyroidism despite unaltered levels of thyroid hormones (Trzepacz *et al.* 1988). Similarly, the acute organic reactions are also likely to have an origin in brain metabolic disturbance and usually appear only at peaks of thyrotoxicosis.

The precise aetiology of psychotic developments is incompletely understood. Constitutional predisposition has been suggested to explain severe affective or schizophrenic disorders, although a recent study has suggested that the situation may be complex (Brownlie *et al.* 2000). The psychosis may be precipitated by the metabolic derangement or by the resulting emotional turmoil. Simple coincidence may account for the two developments, but the parallel course which they sometimes pursue suggests that a causal relationship of some sort is likely to exist quite commonly. At all

events, once the processes are under way they doubtless augment one another.

Occasionally, psychoses may develop during treatment with antithyroid drugs (e.g. carbimazole) when thyroid hormone levels are falling. Some are associated with periods of transient hypothyroidism, although others occur when a patient has been rendered euthyroid (Brewer 1969; Herridge & Abey-Wickrama 1969; Bewsher *et al.* 1971; Brownlie *et al.* 2000).

Outcome of mental disturbances

The result of treatment is generally good, with resolution of emotional disorder as the patient is rendered euthyroid. Sometimes, however, emotional instability persists, and in most cases is probably attributable to premorbid tendencies. Kathol *et al.* (1986) found that depression and anxiety resolved in the great majority of cases with antithyroid treatment alone. Occasionally, however, additional psychotropic medication may be necessary. Acute organic and affective psychoses usually also respond rapidly as the thyrotoxicosis comes under control. Schizophrenic psychoses may run a more variable course, but as with other psychoses in which a precipitating cause is apparent the prognosis will usually be better than for schizophrenia that arises spontaneously.

Hyperparathyroidism

Hyperparathyroidism has increasingly gained recognition as a relatively uncommon though important cause of psychiatric morbidity. It is important because, if missed, patients may unnecessarily suffer many years of psychiatric illness that if treated would lead to prompt symptomatic relief. Most cases of primary hyperparathyroidism are due to a solitary adenoma of one of the four parathyroid glands. Hyperfunction in multiple glands (hyperplasia, multiple adenoma and polyclonal hyperfunction) occurs in up to 15%, with less than 1% due to parathyroid carcinoma. A small minority form part of the autosomal dominantly inherited MEN syndrome. MEN type 1, caused by an inactivating mutation of the tumour suppressor *MEN1* gene, is associated with hyperparathyroidism in 85%, endocrine tumours of the pancreas (Zollinger–Ellison syndrome) in 35%, and tumours of the anterior pituitary (prolactinoma) in 25%. MEN type 2a is characterised by hyperparathyroidism in 70%, phaeochromocytomas and medullary carcinoma of the thyroid. It is caused by an autosomal dominantly inherited activating mutation of the *RET* proto-oncogene.

Primary hyperparathyroidism affects women three times as commonly as men. The incidence of primary hyperparathyroidism rises sharply with age, peaking between 55 and 70 years. One study from the Mayo Clinic found a peak incidence of 188.5 per 100 000 in women aged over 60 years (Heath 1980) and it has been claimed that the prevalence in this group may be as high as 1%. Secondary hyperparathyroidism may result from any cause of hypocalcaemia though is most commonly seen in chronic renal failure due to a combination of hyperphosphataemia and decreased renal production of 1,25-dihydroxyvitamin D.

Physical features

Currently, most patients diagnosed with hyperparathyroidism appear to be asymptomatic (Silverberg *et al.* 1999), although a number of studies have recently suggested that this 'asymptomatic' group may have subtle neurobehavioural symptoms such as fatigue and generalised weakness that resolve after surgery (Burney *et al.* 1999). Prior to the widespread use of multichannel electrolyte analysers renal calculi or diffuse nephrocalcinosis was present in the majority at presentation, though they are now seen in only about 20% (Silverberg *et al.* 1999). Primary hypercalcaemia may also cause cardiac calcification and left ventricular hypertrophy, although there is currently some controversy over whether any of these changes adversely affects life expectancy.

In earlier studies physical complaints were the predominant feature in the great majority, typically presenting with pain, fracture or deformity of bones, renal colic or profound muscular weakness. Occasionally patients present with a myopathic syndrome (Patten & Pages 1984) consisting of proximal muscular weakness, wasting, hypotonia and discomfort on movement. Other common symptoms that may suggest the condition are increased thirst, polyuria, dull diffuse headache, anorexia and nausea. On examination corneal calcification may be seen close to the corneoscleral junction as linear aggregations of granular material.

Psychiatric features

Many of the studies on the psychiatric features of hyperparathyroidism reflect the clinical spectrum seen before the introduction of multichannel electrolyte analysers. In a large series, Petersen (1968) found psychiatric symptoms in two-thirds of patients even after excluding patients who had been referred specifically because of psychiatric disturbance; in one-third the mental abnormalities were severe. Watson (1968) found that a small group presented with mental symptoms alone, whilst Karpati and Frame (1964) identified 4 of 33 patients in whom psychiatric complaints dominated the clinical picture such that they had been referred initially for psychiatric or neurological consultation: a woman of 40 presented with depression that had proved resistant to drugs and psychotherapy for several years before hyperparathyroidism was diagnosed; a woman of 64 had a 2-year history of agitated depression with tremulousness, disorientation, confusion and severe headache; a man of 43 presented with increasing nervousness and obsessive–compulsive features that subsided after operation; and the fourth patient presented with a confusional state accompanied by severe headache.

The commonest mental change in these series was depression with anergia, the patient gradually becoming tired and listless with marked lack of initiative and spontaneity. In Petersen's series, 36% showed these changes, almost all of whom had been unable to work on account of lack of energy during the months preceding operation. Tension and irritability sometimes accompanied the depression, and explosive outbursts were occasionally seen.

In 12% of Petersen's cases organic mental symptoms were present, chiefly impairment of memory or general mental slowing. Acute organic psychoses occurred in 5% of cases, with spells of mental confusion, or acute delirious episodes with hallucinations, paranoia and aggressive behaviour. Stuporose states were also described as were recurrent convulsions leading to coma. Numann *et al.* (1984) showed that even those patients without specific neuropsychiatric complaints at presentation showed significant improvement on tests of verbal memory, verbal reasoning and cognition postoperatively, suggesting that the slow development of these deficits made them less likely to be identified and reported. Very occasionally the degree of intellectual impairment can give rise to a mistaken diagnosis of early-onset dementia.

Psychosis in the absence of an acute psychotic state appears to be rare, and when present is probably coincidental. However, Alarcón and Franceschini (1984) describe a clear example of paranoid psychosis without disorientation or other organic features that resolved after parathyroidectomy and Kleinfeld *et al.* (1984) refer to a case with mania as the sole clinical manifestation.

More recent studies suggest a much milder presentation (Mundy *et al.* 1980), though assessment of apparently 'asymptomatic' patients with mildly elevated parathyroid hormone (PTH) using health status questionnaires such as SCL-90 and SF-36 has shown considerable levels of psychological and functional morbidity that improve rapidly following surgery (Joborn *et al.* 1989; Burney *et al.* 1999). Decreased levels of 5-hydroxyindoleacetic acid (5-HIAA) and homovanillic acid have also been found in the cerebrospinal fluid (CSF) of patients with hyperparathyroidism associated with psychiatric symptoms, reductions that are reversed postoperatively and associated with improved mental functioning at 1 year after surgery (Joborn *et al.* 1988).

Investigations

Most patients with primary hyperparathyroidism have high serum PTH and calcium concentrations. Ionised calcium levels may be more sensitive and should be repeated if clinical suspicion remains despite normal levels. Two-site immunoassays for PTH are now used routinely to detect biologically active forms and minimise cross-reactivity with PTH-related peptide. Serum alkaline phosphatase is raised with bone involvement and renal stones or calcification may be detected on radiography. Hand radiography may occasionally be informative. Computed tomography (CT) of the brain may show calcification in the caudate nuclei and frontal lobes, although this is very much less common than in hypoparathyroidism since the calcium deposits are usually finely distributed. The EEG shows widespread slow activity, sometimes with paroxysms of frontal delta waves at high serum calcium concentrations.

Differential diagnosis

The disorder should be borne in mind in patients who show chronic affective disorder, anxiety or somatisation in association with suspicious physical symptoms. Symptoms of polydipsia and polyuria or a prolonged, insidiously developing and diagnostically unclear change of personality should trigger assessment of calcium and phosphate, and measurement of calcium and phosphate should be part of the work-up of all patients presenting with acute confusion or fluctuating conscious level.

Aetiology of mental disturbances

The aetiology of the psychiatric disturbance is uncertain, although the elevation of serum calcium appears to play a central role. In his careful review, Petersen (1968) found that the severity of the psychological disturbance appeared to relate to serum calcium levels: affective disorder and disturbances of drive corresponded to a serum calcium of 3–4 mmol/L, acute organic reactions with florid delirium appeared at 4–4.7 mmol/L, and somnolence and coma were found with levels exceeding 4.7 mmol/L. Such a series of changes could sometimes be traced in a single patient. However, subsequent studies have challenged the association between severity of symptoms and serum calcium level, and florid symptoms have been described even in patients with only mildly raised calcium levels (Alarcón 1985). Bleuler (1967) felt that the psychiatric disorders associated with hyperparathyroidism were more constant between patients than those seen with most other endocrine disorders and it has been suggested that this may be because in hyperparathyroidism they depend on a widespread ionic intermediary rather than the direct cerebral effects of a hormone (Lishman 1997). The possible role of hypomagnesaemia remains unclear. The PTH-2 receptor is expressed in various brain regions (Usdin et al. 1995), and a brain-specific ligand for this receptor, a hypothalamic neuropeptide, has also been described (Usdin et al. 1999), raising the possibility that psychiatric disturbance in hyperparathyroidism may indeed be a direct effect of PTH on the brain.

Outcome

Parathyroidectomy performed by an experienced surgeon is successful in almost 95% of cases and is usually associated with complete resolution of disorders of affect and drive and of the organic psychoses. The time to recovery has been found to be independent of the duration of the disease and of

the severity of the mental changes, and to parallel closely the fall in serum calcium. The rare psychotic states of long duration, with thought disorder and paranoia, may respond less satisfactorily but probably owe a good deal to premorbid vulnerability.

Contemporary presentation with oligosymptomatic or asymptomatic presentation has raised the debate on when patients should be referred for surgery. The natural history of hyperparathyroidism appears to be rather benign. During a 10-year follow-up only 27% of initially asymptomatic patients had evidence of disease progression, defined as the development of one or more new indications for parathyroidectomy (Silverberg et al. 1999). However, symptom checklists have shown higher morbidity in 'asymptomatic' patients compared with controls and improvements with surgery, suggesting that truly asymptomatic hyperparathyroidism may be rarer than previously thought.

Hypoparathyroidism

Like hyperparathyroidism, comprehensive reviews of the literature in the 1960s identified hypoparathyroidism as a cause of remediable psychiatric disorder and is now very well recognised. Denko and Kaelbling (1962) identified numerous cases in the literature of patients presenting to varied specialties often over many years and failing to be diagnosed, resulting in the much-delayed institution of treatment that offers an excellent chance of reversing both the physical and psychiatric changes.

Hypoparathyroidism may result from a number of diverse insults to the parathyroid glands. Surgery to the neck, typically for thyroid pathology, may damage the parathyroid glands or disrupt their blood supply, so a history of neck surgery should always be sought in the investigation of suspected hypoparathyroidism. Developmental defects such as DiGeorge's syndrome and the closely related velocardiofacial syndrome, which affect development of the third and fourth branchial arches, result in varying degrees of parathyroid and thyroid hypoplasia. Both syndromes are associated with rearrangement and microdeletions affecting the short arm of chromosome 22. Hypoparathyroidism is also a prominent component of autoimmune polyglandular syndrome type 1, also known as polyendocrinopathy–candidiasis–ectodermal dystrophy syndrome, an autosomal recessively inherited syndrome caused by mutations in the autoimmune regulator gene (AIRE) (Bjorses et al. 2000). Defects in the gene for PTH and in the regulation of PTH secretion (autosomal dominant hypercalciuric hypocalcaemia) have also been described. Occasionally, it may also present in association with Albright's hereditary osteodystrophy. The deficiency of PTH leads to a low serum calcium and a raised serum phosphate. Chronic deficiency may lead to calcium deposits in the skin, lens of the eye and brain.

Fuller Albright described a group of patients who presented with certain developmental and skeletal defects, now collectively termed Albright's hereditary osteodystrophy, and biochemical abnormalities suggesting end-organ resistance to the actions of PTH. The disorder was subsequently dubbed pseudohypoparathyroidism (PHP) and different forms are classified based on the presence or absence of Albright's hereditary osteodystrophy with or without hormone resistance. The most frequently seen variants include PHP type 1a, pseudo-pseudohypoparathyroidism (PPHP) and PHP type 1b.

• PHP-1a: affected individuals have features of Albright's hereditary osteodystrophy that typically include obesity, short stature, brachydactyly (abnormally shortened bones of the hands and feet, typically affecting the fourth and fifth metacarpals), ectopic calcification and mental retardation. They present with hypocalcaemia with hyperphosphataemia despite elevated serum PTH. Hormone resistance is not usually limited to PTH and individuals frequently show resistance to TSH and gonadotrophins; resistance to growth hormone-releasing hormone and calcitonin has also been described.

• PPHP: affected individuals have the phenotypic features of Albright's hereditary osteodystrophy as described for PHP-1a but do not show evidence of resistance to PTH or other hormones.

• PHP-1b: in contrast to PPHP, affected individuals present with signs and symptoms of PTH resistance but lack features of Albright's hereditary osteodystrophy. Hormone resistance may also be limited to a single tissue, typically the kidney.

The molecular defects responsible for each of the three main forms of PHP appear to reside in the gene encoding the α-subunit of the stimulatory GTP-binding protein ($G_{s\alpha}$). $G_{s\alpha}$ is a ubiquitously expressed signalling protein that mediates the cellular action of numerous hormones and neurotransmitters. Patients with PHP-1a have heterogeneous mutations in one of the $G_{s\alpha}$ exons, leading to reduced protein levels and cellular activity. This suggests that all the hormones affected in PHP-1a act via receptors coupled to $G_{s\alpha}$. Curiously, $G_{s\alpha}$ mutations are also seen in PPHP, where hormone resistance is not seen, and the two disorders are often seen in the same kindred. Interestingly, it has recently been shown that PPHP develops if the $G_{s\alpha}$ mutation is inherited from a male with either PPHP or PHP-1a, whereas PHP-1a results from inheritance of the $G_{s\alpha}$ mutation from a female with either PPHP or PHP-1a. Further, PHP-1b results from a deletion upstream of the $G_{s\alpha}$ gene and is transmitted only from a female, which appears to result in tissue-specific loss of methylation of this gene. A good contemporary review is by Bastepe and Juppner (2003).

Physical features

Hypoparathyroidism should be suspected in patients with symptoms of chronic tetany or when ocular cataracts develop at an unusually young age. A history of operation on the neck should always raise the possibility of hypoparathyroidism. The continued publication of case reports of untreated hypoparathyroidism and its associated morbidity should serve as a reminder that if it is not considered, symptoms may be endured for many years before diagnosis is made (Bellamy & Kendall-Taylor 1995).

Tetany occurs in the form of numbness and tingling in the hands and feet or around the mouth. With more severe degrees the patient experiences muscular cramps and stiffness in the limbs, carpopedal spasm or laryngeal stridor. In carpopedal spasm, the metacarpophalangeal joints are flexed and the interphalangeal joints of the thumb and fingers are extended to produce a characteristic posture of the hand called *main d'accoucheur*. Epilepsy can be the first and sometimes the only manifestation. In addition to cataracts the patients may have a dry coarse skin, scanty hair, trophic changes in the nails and poor dental development. Calcium deposits may be detected in the skin or appear on skull radiography as calcification in the region of the basal ganglia. Clinically useful signs include twitching of the facial muscles on tapping the facial nerve below the zygoma (Chvostek's sign) and the production of carpopedal spasm by temporarily occluding the circulation to the arm (Trousseau's sign). Very occasionally papilloedema may be observed.

Psychiatric features

Denko and Kaelbling's (1962) literature review served to highlight the high incidence and wide variety of psychiatric disturbances seen in hypoparathyroidism. They estimated that at least half of the cases attributable to surgery had psychiatric symptoms, with an even higher prevalence in hypoparathyroidism with a non-surgical aetiology. The subsequent literature on psychiatric manifestations of hypoparathyroidism is sparse and limited predominantly to case reports and case series.

Denko and Kaelbling classified their 268 cases into five categories: intellectual impairment, organic brain syndrome, psychosis 'functional', pseudoneurosis and undiagnosable. Organic psychiatric syndromes were seen most commonly in the postsurgical group where features of an acute confusional state developed in association with rapid postsurgical biochemical changes. The most common clinical picture in the idiopathic group, which included all non-surgical and non-PHP cases, was intellectual decline. These patients, who had experienced much more insidious and chronic biochemical changes, showed sustained difficulty with concentration, emotional lability and impairment of intellectual functions.

Response to treatment was variable, the majority showing some improvement in overall intellectual function especially if young, though some remained intellectually impaired. Others have shown improvement in concentration, memory, disorientation and apathy with correction of the hypocalcaemia (Hossain 1970; Illum & Dupont 1985). Kowdley *et al.* (1999) investigated the pattern of cognitive deficits in a case–control study of 11 subjects with chronic hypoparathyroidism treated with calcium and vitamin D supplementation (nine postsurgical, two idiopathic). Some degree of cognitive impairment was seen in seven (65%) of the hypoparathyroid group, of whom two were considered to be severely impaired. Greatest impairment occurred on the Trailmaking B test, forward digit span and oral fluency, which the authors argued was consistent with damage to prefrontal cortex, basal ganglia and thalamus.

'Pseudoneurosis' was described by Denko and Kaelbling as the next most common change in both surgical and idiopathic groups. Children show temper tantrums and night terrors, and adults become depressed, nervous and irritable with frequent crying spells and marked social withdrawal. The emotional disturbances may fluctuate in degree or show periods of spontaneous resolution. Fourman *et al.* (1963) showed that 50% of patients who had undergone thyroidectomy in whom the plasma calcium was merely at the lower limit of normal had mental symptoms in the form of tension and anxiety, panic attacks, depression and lassitude. Often there were no other pointers to parathyroid insufficiency and the symptoms were therefore indistinguishable from those commonly found in what are now classified as anxiety disorders. In a subsequent double-blind trial of calcium citrate tablets and placebo, the authors were able to show a significant improvement in psychiatric symptom scores with treatment (Fourman *et al.* 1967). The most consistent changes were with regard to depression and reduced appetite. Subsequent studies on the clinical efficacy of calcium/vitamin D treatment in chronic hypoparathyroidism are sparse. Though terminating life-threatening hypocalcaemia and debilitating tetanic symptoms, treatment with calcium and vitamin D does not replace the missing hormone, PTH, and may not reverse all the mental symptoms associated with hypoparathyroidism. Arlt *et al.* (2002) found significantly higher global complaint scores on the SCL-90-R, B-L Zersson and GBB-24 in a cross-sectional controlled study of 25 unselected women on standard treatment for postsurgical hypoparathyroidism compared with thyroid surgery controls. Greatest increases were seen in the subtest scores for anxiety, phobic anxiety, somatisation and depression. Twelve of the hypoparathyroidism cases compared with six thyroid surgery controls had severe impairments of well-being, results that remained significant even when those with residual low serum calcium levels were excluded.

More rarely, psychotic illnesses of manic–depressive or schizophrenic type may be seen, particularly in cases due to surgery. Again spontaneous remissions or response to other forms of treatment may delay diagnosis of the underlying condition.

In PHP and PPHP, intellectual impairment is by far the most frequent psychiatric abnormality, occurring in approximately half of reported cases. The prominence of intellectual impairment in PHP and PPHP suggests that it is unlikely to be based solely on the hypocalcaemia (Abrams & Jay 1998).

Investigations

Diagnosis is made on the basis of measurement of serum calcium, magnesium, phosphate and PTH levels. The serum calcium and magnesium are low, serum phosphate is raised, and the urinary excretion of calcium and phosphate reduced. Serum alkaline phosphatase is normal. PTH levels are low except in PHP when they may be normal or raised. Radiological studies show an association between hypoparathyroidism, PHP and basal ganglia calcification. In the study by Frame and Marel (1983), skull radiographs showed calcification in 28% of patients with idiopathic hypoparathyroidism and in 48% of those with PHP. CT studies appear to show a higher prevalence of intracranial calcification in chronic hypoparathyroidism, though caution should be exercised in interpreting these findings in view of publication biases. Illum and Dupont (1985) found calcification in 69% of patients with idiopathic hypoparathyroidism and 100% of those with PHP. Globus pallidus calcification was ubiquitous, caudate nucleus was involved in 14 of 19 cases, and calcification of the putamen, thalamus and cerebral cortex was also commonly seen. EEG abnormalities may be present even in the absence of epilepsy, usually generalised but sometimes surprisingly focal (Watson 1972) (see Table 10.4 and Figure 10.1).

Differential diagnosis

The diagnoses that may be mistakenly entertained include mental retardation, early-onset dementia, anxiety disorders, somatisation disorder, idiopathic epilepsy and cerebral tumour. Diagnosis of an anxiety or somatisation disorder may be suggested by the peculiar and intermittent nature of the symptoms, including bizarre paraesthesiae and muscular spasms. Moreover, the patient may give a vague and perplexing account with obvious difficulty in observing and describing the symptoms. Attacks may be triggered by emotional influences, since hyperventilation will readily lead to tetanic symptoms. Hypochondriasis is readily suggested by the generally heightened level of anxiety, the vagueness of the complaints and the occurrence of periods of spontaneous remission. As a result patients with hypoparathyroidism are sometimes found to have carried a label of psychogenic disorder for several years before the true diagnosis is made. In other cases well-defined mood swings have led to an initial diagnosis of manic–depressive disorder (Denko & Kaelbling 1962).

Table 10.4 Classification of bilateral calcification involving striatum, pallidum and dentate nucleus. (From Manyam 2005.)

Striatopallidodentate calcinosis

Primary
Autosomal dominant
Familial
Sporadic

Secondary
Endocrinological
   Hypoparathyroidism
   Pseudohypoparathyroidism
   Pseudo-pseudohypoparathyroidism
   Hyperparathyroidism
Developmental
   Cockayne's syndrome
   Syndrome of microcephaly, demyelination and
   striatopallidodentate calcification
Connective tissue disorders: systemic lupus erythematosus
Toxic: lead

Bilateral striopallidal ('basal ganglia') calcinosis

Physiological: ageing (over 50 years)
Developmental
   Angiomatous malformation with vein of Galen aneurysm
   Down's syndrome
   Oculocraniosomatic disease (Kearns–Sayre syndrome)
Degenerative
   Aicardi–Goutieres syndrome
   Coats' syndrome

Diffuse cerebral microangiopathy
   Hyperkinetic mutism
Genetic
   Biotinidase deficiency (AR)
   Carbonic anhydrase II deficiency (osteopetrosis, renal tubular
   acidosis and basal ganglia calcification) (AR)
   COFS syndrome with familial 1;16 translocation (AR)
   Lipomembranous polycystic osteodysplasia (AR)
   Tapetoretinal degeneration (AD)
Infectious
   AIDS
   Active Epstein–Barr virus infection
   Meningoencephalitis
   Mumps encephalitis
Metabolic
   Dihydropteridine reductase deficiency
   MELAS syndrome
   Post-hypoxic/ischaemic
Neoplastic: acute lymphocytic leukaemia
Physical agents: radiation therapy
Toxic: carbon monoxide poisoning

Bilateral cerebellar calcification

Primary
Idiopathic

Secondary
Infection: syphilis
Vascular: haematoma

AD, autosomal dominant; AR, autosomal recessive; MELAS, mitochondrial encephalomyopathy–lactic acidosis–stroke-like symptoms.

Epileptic attacks may be thought to be idiopathic in origin, and the serum calcium should be determined in every epileptic patient when the precise cause of the attacks remains uncertain. Occasionally, increased intracranial pressure and papilloedema are encountered in patients with hypoparathyroidism, this reversing with correction of the serum calcium; cerebral tumour may be closely simulated, especially when fits are present and alteration of personality has occurred.

Outcome

The response to correction of the serum biochemistry is usually gratifying. Anxiety and depressive symptoms are reported to clear in the majority of cases, although recent studies suggest that even with adequate replacement therapy with calcium and vitamin D supplementation and a serum calcium within the normal range these symptoms may be more common than in controls (Arlt *et al.* 2002). Acute confusional states, especially after surgery, resolve rapidly. Ongoing debate surrounds the issue of whether chronic cognitive impairments resolve with correction of the serum biochemistry. Denko and Kaelbling (1962) noted that when adequate details were given, about half the cases of idiopathic hypoparathyroidism with intellectual impairment improved whereas very few cases were unchanged or worse. Patients with PHP may also improve cognitively when the serum chemistry is corrected, but rarely to a spectacular extent. More recent studies have suggested that even in treated idiopathic and postsurgical hypoparathyroidism intellectual impairment can become chronic and some have suggested that the cognitive impairment is linked to the degree of basal ganglia calcification and to associated motor abnormalities (Kowdley *et al.* 1999). Other complications such as the incidence of cataracts and renal stones appear to increase with chronicity in hypoparathyroidism despite normalisation of serum calcium, suggesting that calcium homeostasis is not normalised with current therapy (Arlt *et al.* 2002). Findings such as these have triggered investigation of the use of more physiological treatments in hypoparathyroidism using subcutaneous PTH or parathyroid allotransplantation.

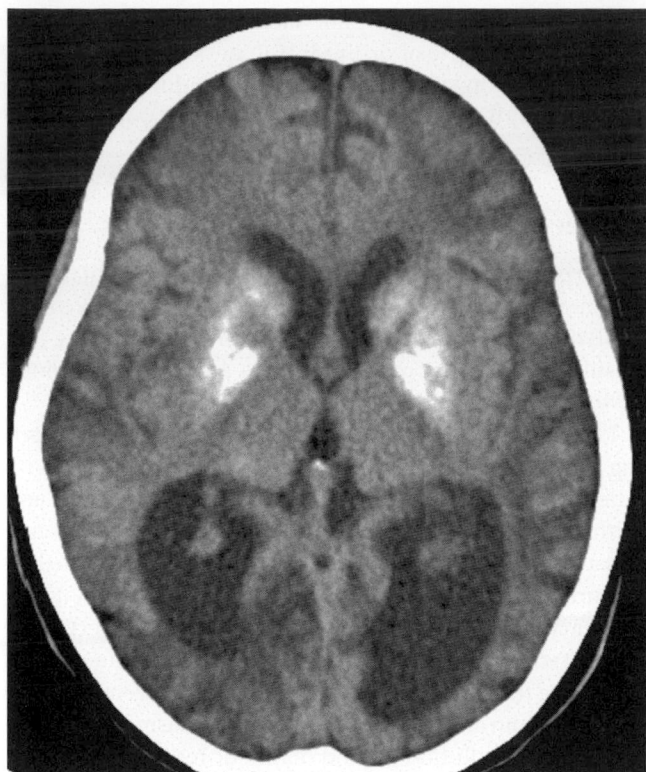

Fig. 10.1 CT scan of basal ganglia calcification from a patient with mitochondrial encephalomyelopathy with lactic acidosis (MELAS syndrome) showing extensive infarction in both cerebral hemispheres and basal ganglia calcification (caudate, lentiform).

Hypopituitarism (Simmond's disease)

Historically, the commonest cause of hypopituitarism was ischaemic necrosis of the anterior pituitary gland as a result of postpartum haemorrhage (Sheehan's syndrome). Today the commonest cause of panhypopituitarism is pituitary tumours, in particular prolactin-secreting macroadenomas in adults or craniopharyngioma in children. A rare cause of panhypopituitarism is head injury associated with fracture of the base of the skull.

Physical features

The condition is commonly of long duration, sometimes having extended over many years prior to first presentation. Leading symptoms include weakness, ready fatigue and marked sensitivity to cold. There is loss of libido, with amenorrhoea in females and impotence in males. Loss of weight is common, but despite the earlier name of 'pituitary cachexia' is not universal. Nor is it extreme until the terminal stages of the disorder (Sheehan & Summers 1949). In cases with pituitary neoplasms, weight may actually be gained if hypothalamic function is disturbed. Anorexia is common but in some cases appetite is well preserved.

Cardinal signs on examination are a thin dry skin, which fails to tan normally and may become wrinkled as in premature ageing, a flat expressionless face and loss of pubic and axillary hair. The body temperature is often subnormal, the pulse slow with a low blood pressure.

Psychiatric features

The mental picture can be equally striking. The frequency of psychiatric disorder was shown by Kind's (1958) survey of cases from the literature and from his own experience; 90% showed psychiatric symptoms and in half these were severe.

Depression may be marked, sometimes with outbursts of irritability. Drive and initiative are impaired, and the patient comes to spend progressively longer in bed. Virtually all patients show apathy, inertia and somnolence in some degree. Ultimately most are dull and drowsy, prone to self-neglect and indifferent about their state. The degree of psychological change commonly seen is greater than in other chronic debilitating diseases, and the patient's poor physical condition is therefore unlikely to be the complete explanation.

Impairment of memory may occasionally figure prominently and give rise to an impression of a dementing process. Other severe psychiatric complications include episodes of delirium in relation to impending metabolic crises, or more rarely chronic paranoid hallucinatory psychoses.

Metabolic crises may lead on from delirium to hypopituitary stupor or coma, which is always a grave complication. Such severe developments usually set in only several years after the physical disorder has made its first appearance. The following case reported by Blau and Hinton (1960) illustrates the problems that may arise.

A woman of 46 was admitted with drowsiness, neck stiffness and a moderate pyrexia of 2 days' duration. She opened her eyes to her name but would not obey commands and resisted examination. Meningitis was diagnosed at first, but scanty pubic and axillary hair soon led to the diagnosis of Simmond's disease.

Falling blood pressure required intravenous noradrenaline (norepinephrine) in addition to intravenous glucose and hydrocortisone. She emerged from the semicomatose state but remained incontinent and uncooperative and proved to be deluded about her attendants. Violent behaviour necessitated transfer to a psychiatric hospital 2 weeks later, and over the next month she fluctuated from apathy to to outbursts of restlessness with aggressive shouting. Memory and orientation were faulty and she was unable to concentrate for long. During the next few weeks she settled into a calm rather foolish euphoria and was correctly orientated for most of the time.

> She was followed up with regular treatment with corti-sone. Three months after recovery from the coma her mental state and intellectual functions were back to normal. She had recovered her libido, which had deteriorated along with her general health since the birth of her child 10 years previously.

As with Addison's disease, hypopituitarism rarely leads to functional psychoses but commonly to acute organic reactions in association with crises of metabolic disturbance. In both endocrine conditions, alterations of mood form an integral part of the clinical picture and take the form of apathy, anergia and indifference. In all these respects the psychiatric accompaniments and complications are in contrast to those of Cushing's disease, where functional psychoses are common and where the usual mood change is towards depression and emotional lability.

Differential diagnosis

Hypopituitarism must be differentiated from hypothyroidism, in which the facial appearance of the patient is very different, and from Addison's disease, in which pigmentation is a prominent feature. In questionable cases full endocrine assessment is essential before embarking on the appropriate replacement therapy.

From the psychiatric point of view, neurosis and dementia may sometimes be closely simulated, but the principal differential diagnosis is from anorexia nervosa. Many of the early reported cases of hypopituitarism seem in retrospect to have been anorexia nervosa and vice versa (Sheehan & Summers 1949). Now that the situation has been clarified, however, there is rarely clinical doubt, even though both share the cardinal feature of amenorrhoea. Severe weight loss is rare except terminally in hypopituitarism, whereas it is usually a presenting feature in anorexia nervosa. Similarly, appetite may sometimes be well preserved in hypopituitarism. Loss of pubic and axillary hair is unusual in anorexia nervosa, and the fine downy facial hair of anorexia nervosa is rare in hypopituitarism. The psychological features of the two conditions are also very different: in hypopituitarism the patient is dull, apathetic and somnolent, whereas in anorexia nervosa the patient is typically restless and surprisingly active; distinctive attitudes to food and the body image are lacking in hypopituitarism, whereas they form an important constellation of symptoms in anorexia nervosa. When serious doubt exists, full endocrine assessment will clarify the differential diagnosis.

Outcome

Response to replacement therapy is usually good. Within a few days patients experience return of interest and energy, and most lose their symptoms entirely. In cases of very long duration, however, apathy and lack of drive may persist in some degree. Cortisol or prednisolone alone may suffice, though thyroxine is sometimes given in addition. Gonadal steroids may be required to restore libido and potency in the male.

Hyperprolactinaemia

Hyperprolactinaemia is of importance to psychiatry in two regards: patients with hyperprolactinaemia have been shown to have increased rates of depression, anxiety and hostility, and hyperprolactinaemia is a common and often distressing side effect of the antipsychotic drugs.

Prolactin-secreting adenomas are the commonest secreting tumours of the pituitary. They frequently present with amenorrhoea and more rarely galactorrhoea in women and with impotence and infertility in men. Hyperprolactinaemia is usually due to a microadenoma, a small tumour less than 10 mm in diameter that comprises lactotrophs in the anterior pituitary. Less common are macroadenomas, which may present with headache or visual field disturbance due to focal erosion of the floor of the sella turcica or displacement of the infundibulum and pressure on the optic chiasm. Despite the use of high-resolution CT and magnetic resonance imaging (MRI), there remains a group of patients in whom no pituitary adenoma can be seen. This group may be associated with very small microadenomas undetectable with current imaging or may, as suggested by some investigators, be due to 'functional' hyperprolactinaemia (Sobrinho 1991).

Fava et al. (1981) used the Kellner questionnaire and semi-structured interview and identified more symptoms of depression, anxiety and hostility in patients with hyperprolactinaemia compared with amenorrhoeic controls with normal prolactin levels. Keller et al. (1985) found hyperprolactinaemic patients to be more depressed and anxious than normals and suggested that these symptoms were worse in those with normal pituitary fossa radiographs compared with those with larger tumours causing erosion of the sella turcica. These symptoms have been shown to improve with dopaminergic agents such as bromocriptine, used in the medical management of hyperprolactinaemia (Buckman & Kellner 1985), although generally they respond poorly to antidepressants. In a review of studies on the psychosomatic aspects of hyperprolactinaemia, Fava et al. (1983) suggested that women seem to be more prone to suffer from the behavioural effects of prolactin than males. Reavley et al. (1997), in a case–control study of 65 women with hyperprolactinaemia, showed an increased incidence of anxiety, measured with the HAD and SCL-90 scales, in hyperprolactinaemic women compared with a control group with nonfunctioning pituitary adenomas and normal prolactin levels. Greater psychological distress was found in the group showing no abnormality on CT compared with those with pituitary microadenomas and comparable serum prolactin levels. The authors suggested that these findings supported the concept of 'functional' hyperprolactinaemia where raised prolactin in the absence of a pituitary adenoma is an endocrine marker of primarily psychological disturbance.

In a number of recent reviews, Wieck and Haddad have drawn attention to the chronic effects of iatrogenic hyperprolactinaemia, a common side effect of antipsychotic use (Wieck & Haddad 2002; Haddad & Wieck 2004). Hypothalamic dopamine is the predominant inhibitor of prolactin release, an action mediated via binding to D_2 receptors on the surface of pituitary lactotrophs. All conventional antipsychotics and some of the atypical ones, notably risperidone and amisulpride, block D_2 receptors on lactotrophs, removing the inhibitory influence of dopamine and causing a marked and sustained increase in serum prolactin levels. In addition to the effects highlighted above, hyperprolactinaemia has adverse effects on sexual function, the breasts and, via secondary hypo-estrogenism, bone mineral density. It may lead to breast enlargement and galactorrhoea, ovarian dysfunction, infertility, reduced libido, atrophic changes in the urethra and vaginal mucosa, reduced vaginal lubrication and dyspareunia. Acne and mild hirsutism may also develop and the loss of the protective effect of estrogens on bone resorption can lead to reduced bone mineral density. Two small studies have suggested an association between chronic antipsychotic medication and reduced bone mineral density (Ataya et al. 1988; Halbreich et al. 1995). Although these findings are only preliminary and both studies suffered from a number of methodological difficulties, they suggest that the consequences of chronic hyperprolactinaemia on the skeleton secondary to antipsychotic use need to be carefully considered.

Acromegaly

Acromegaly results from overproduction of growth hormone, usually from a pituitary somatotroph adenoma though rarely from simple hyperplasia of the eosinophil cells of the anterior pituitary gland. The actions of growth hormone are effected via insulin-like growth factor (IGF)-1, a peptide with endocrine, paracrine and autocrine actions generated in many tissues. It is also responsible for the clinical features seen in acromegaly. Skeletal overgrowth develops insidiously, leading to increased hand, foot and hat size, prognathism, enlarged tongue, wide spacing of the teeth and coarsening of the facial features. Most patients also complain of neurological and musculoskeletal symptoms such as headaches, nerve entrapments, muscle weakness and joint pain. Insulin resistance occurs in the majority though clinical diabetes mellitus is seen in only 20%. Obstructive sleep apnoea, hypertension and hypogonadism are seen frequently. Life expectancy is considerably shortened, with increased rates of death from cardiovascular, cerebrovascular and respiratory disease.

The literature on psychological and psychiatric accompaniments remains sparse. The first case series was performed by Bleuler (1951) on 22 patients seen at the Burghoelzli Clinic, Zurich and an additional six cases from the clinic of the New York Hospital. He described alterations of personality, mainly a lack of initiative and spontaneity, sometimes interrupted by brief periods of impulsive behaviour and changes of mood ('frequent cheerfulness, self-satisfaction and elation occur with passivity and indifference') and regarded brief periods of moodiness with frequent mood swings as characteristic. Bradyphrenia was observed in the late stages though no intellectual impairment was seen. Social attitudes were characterised by egocentricity and lack of consideration and interest in others, leading to problems with other members of the family and at work. In contrast to earlier reports he found no evidence for an increased incidence of schizophrenic or mood-related psychosis, arguing that the previously reported association was likely due to publication bias.

Few subsequent systematic studies have sought to follow up these impressions. Anecdotal reports have emphasised depression and anxiety and loss of impulse control, coupled with loss of self-confidence and concern over body size (Avery 1973). Margo (1981) reported a patient with a chronic depressive illness with prominent psychomotor retardation beginning 12 years before the acromegaly was diagnosed. Sivakumar and Williams (1991) described a patient with insidious-onset depression and marked behavioural change characterised by pathological gambling out of keeping with his premorbid personality. However, repeated neuropsychometry including tests of frontal lobe functioning failed to show any associated cognitive impairment. Spence (1995) also described apparent loss of impulse control in a woman who presented with psychotic depression and sudden onset of impulsive shoplifting prior to diagnosis of acromegaly 3 years later.

It is hard in such examples to know how far simple coincidence or publication bias may be responsible. Abed et al. (1987) used standardised assessments (GHQ and Present State Examination) and failed to find any general increase in psychiatric morbidity, nor a specific increase in depression when compared with rates in other population studies in a survey of 51 acromegalic patients. Indeed, the scores were significantly lower than in certain other samples, and the interviewer was impressed with the optimism and even elation shown by many of the subjects. No overall relationship could be found between growth hormone levels and psychiatric morbidity; however, females showed significantly higher morbidity rates than males, and 10 of the 11 subjects who scored above the cut-off points for psychiatric illness were women. However, the instruments used in this study were unsuited to the measurement of personality change and formal neuropsychometry was not performed so these aspects remain to be elucidated. Historically, a number of reports have described patients as sometimes reserved, touchy and irritable, with emotional lability, and traits of obstinacy and impulsivity. How far such features may be understandable as reactions to disfigurement, headache and limb pain or whether they depend on metabolic changes or basal brain compression has not been clarified.

Neurological complications include mild proximal myopathy, carpal tunnel syndrome and visual field defects. Carpal tunnel syndrome has been reported in up to 64% at presentation, showing a significant improvement when circulating growth hormone levels are reduced (Baum *et al*. 1986). Using MRI, Jenkins *et al*. (2000) found oedema of the median nerve rather than a change in the volume of the contents of the carpal tunnel, as seen in idiopathic carpal tunnel syndrome, and went on to argue that appropriate management is therefore aggressive treatment of the underlying pituitary hypersecretion rather than surgical decompression. Recent studies on the association of visual field defects with acromegaly suggest that they are now less commonly seen. Studies from the 1970s suggested that they were present in up to 90% of all pituitary tumours, whereas contemporary studies suggest that this is now approximately 20% (Rivoal *et al*. 2000). Hypersomnia may be a consequence of sleep apnoea occasioned by airway obstruction due to macroglossia and hypertrophy of the pharyngeal soft tissues (Perks *et al*. 1980; Seggev *et al*. 1986). In some cases, however, the daytime somnolence remits rapidly on treatment of the acromegaly, suggesting that it is not solely due to airway obstruction.

Trans-sphenoidal removal of the responsible pituitary adenoma is the treatment of choice for most patients (Paisley & Trainer 2003). However, the presence of macroadenomas in 70% often means that tumour removal is incomplete, necessitating additional medical therapy and/or radiotherapy. Previously, dopamine agonists such as bromocriptine and cabergoline that inhibit growth hormone were the mainstay of treatment. Whilst associated with symptomatic relief in the majority of patients, they led to a normalisation of growth hormone and IGF-1 in only about 35% and were associated with a number of unpleasant side effects including headache and mood disturbance. There have also been a number of case reports of their association with schizophreniform or manic-like psychoses (Le Feuvre *et al*. 1982; Turner 1984; Boyd 1995). Long-acting somatostatin analogues such as octreotide and lanreotide, which inhibit growth hormone secretion via somatomedin receptor subtypes 2 and 5 expressed on adenomas, can induce tumour shrinkage and have been associated with a normalisation of growth hormone/IGF-1 in up to 65% of individuals (Paisley & Trainer 2003). A recently developed growth hormone receptor antagonist, pegvisomant, has been shown to achieve superior biochemical disease control in two controlled trials and has recently been licensed in the European Union.

Diabetes insipidus

Diabetes insipidus is a syndrome of polyuria with secondary polydipsia and comprises two types: inadequate production of circulating antidiuretic hormone (ADH, vasopressin) is the cause of central diabetes insipidus, whereas a lack of ADH action on the kidney causes nephrogenic diabetes insipidus. ADH is synthesised in the supraoptic and paraventricular nuclei of the hypothalamus and then transported to the posterior pituitary from where it is released into the circulation. ADH binds to V_2 receptors on the nephron collecting tubules, stimulating adenylate cyclase and ultimately the insertion of aquaporin water channels, which result in increased water reabsorption and the consequent production of a more concentrated urine.

Central diabetes insipidus develops when insufficient ADH is produced by the posterior pituitary. Causes include hypothalamic tumours, traumatic head injury, infiltration (e.g. sarcoidosis), infection (e.g. tuberculosis) and transsphenoidal surgery; 10–30% of cases are idiopathic. Occasionally, the condition is familial, inherited as an autosomal dominant condition due to mutations in the ADH signal peptide or in the neurophysins. It may present abruptly at any age without apparent cause, usually as an isolated abnormality but occasionally with other indications of hypothalamic disorder.

Nephrogenic diabetes insipidus is caused by a failure of the renal tubules to respond normally to ADH. Causes in adults include hypercalcaemia, potassium depletion and the prolonged intake of excessive amounts of water, all of which can impair the action of ADH on the nephron. A variety of drugs, including lithium, may also be responsible. Polyuria from lithium treatment can develop when plasma levels are within the therapeutic range; 40% of patients on lithium experience thirst, with perhaps 12% developing polyuria (Ledingham 1983). In most cases this resolves within several weeks of withdrawing the drug. It may also occur as a rare sex-linked recessive disorder affecting males, due to defects in the ADH receptor gene or less frequently as an autosomal recessive, due to defects in the vasopressin-sensitive aquaporin 2 channel.

Both central and nephrogenic diabetes insipidus result in the production of large volumes of dilute urine, normally accompanied by thirst. Urine osmolality is low, but plasma osmolality is usually only slightly raised provided the thirst mechanisms are intact and the patient drinks adequately. If thirst does not occur, or if fluid intake is prevented, a dangerous degree of hypernatraemia and dehydration may develop. The differential diagnosis of diabetes insipidus includes primary renal disease, diabetes mellitus, polydipsias induced by drugs such as chlorpromazine or thioridazine (which may stimulate drinking by a direct action on the hypothalamus) and primary or psychogenic polydipsia.

The treatment of choice for neurogenic diabetes insipidus is the synthetic ADH analogue desmopressin (1-deamino-8-D-arginine vasopressin, DDAVP). It has a long duration of action and may be given once or twice daily orally, by nasal spray or subcutaneously. Nephrogenic diabetes insipidus is more difficult to treat. Most are treated with thiazide diuretics to cause volume contraction and reduce glomerular filtration rate.

Primary polydipsia (psychogenic polydipsia)

Primary polydipsia may be associated with a wide range of psychopathology: psychosis, mood disorders and personality disorder. In psychotic patients it is frequently delusionally motivated. Barlow and De Wardener (1959) described nine cases in whom long-standing personality disorder was common, often with hypochondriasis and depression. Six had experienced episodes of conversion disorder and some had histories of compulsive eating. Denial and evasion were sometimes a prominent part of the picture. Mercier-Guidez and Loas (2000), in a study of all psychiatric inpatients in a defined geographical area, estimated that polydipsia and polyuria occur in 11% of all psychiatric inpatients, especially those with chronic schizophrenia.

Primary polydipsia may simulate diabetes insipidus closely. In both conditions the fluid intake and output are raised and urine osmolality is low. In primary polydipsia, however, plasma osmolality is also likely to be low and hyponatraemia may develop when water intake is so excessive that it exceeds the kidneys' ability to excrete it. Onset may be clearly related to a depressive phase or period of stress, or other evidence of psychiatric disorder may be present. The onset will often be gradual rather than abrupt, and consumption may tend to fluctuate from hour to hour or day to day in contrast to the steadily increased intake of diabetes insipidus. Nocturia is uncommon compared with diabetes insipidus when it is commonly seen (Table 10.5).

Distinguishing primary polydipsia from diabetes insipidus

Not infrequently, however, the distinction can be difficult despite water deprivation testing. In normal subjects fluid deprivation over an 8-hour period leaves plasma osmolality unchanged, while urine osmolality rises to twice that of the plasma. In diabetes insipidus the plasma osmolality rises but that of the urine remains relatively low. In primary polydipsia both the initial plasma and urine osmolality are low, and plasma osmolality rises to normal at the end of the test.

However, urine osmolality may fail to rise to twice that of the plasma because the prolonged excessive water intake may have led to a secondary nephrogenic diabetes insipidus. Prolonged water deprivation (carefully monitored) for 2–4 days may be necessary to allow the return of normal renal function, or this may be even longer delayed.

When compulsive water drinking is mistaken for diabetes insipidus and treated with ADH, hyponatraemia and symptoms of water intoxication can develop (see Hyponatraemia, later). Water intoxication also seems to be a special hazard in compulsive water drinking associated with psychosis; numerous examples of such a complication have been described in patients with schizophrenia, sometimes presenting acutely with vomiting, impairment of consciousness or fits (Jose *et al.* 1979; Khamnei 1984; Singh *et al.* 1985; Grainger 1992). Fatalities have been reported from time to time (Vieweg *et al.* 1985).

Both Jose *et al.* (1979) and Khamnei (1984) noted that a high proportion of patients with water intoxication secondary to polydipsia were psychotic, sometimes with evidence of the syndrome of inappropriate ADH secretion (SIADH). In other cases there have been indications of enhanced renal sensitivity to vasopressin (Goldman *et al.* 1988; Emsley *et al.* 1989). However, how far such features may reflect hypothalamic or other disorders intrinsic to the psychosis is uncertain. Multiple factors may often be at work, including the effects of medical illnesses or drugs (Fowler *et al.* 1977; Illowsky & Kirch 1988).

Many psychotropic medications, including all antidepressants, phenothiazines, haloperidol, thiothixine, carbamazepine and tranylcypromine, can precipitate SIADH (Sandifer 1983; Grainger 1992). In half of the cases reviewed by Sandifer, hyponatraemia, usually in association with SIADH, had developed within a week of starting medication. When hyponatraemia is found in a patient taking psychotropic medication it is important to test the response to a water load while on and off the drug, after ensuring that the serum sodium has been restored to normal.

It is important to enquire for a history of polydipsia in any psychotic patient who presents with seizures or lowering of consciousness. Similarly, the discovery of polyuria with a low urinary specific gravity should always lead to careful observation of the patient's water intake. This may on

Table 10.5 Differentiation of primary polydipsia and diabetes insipidus. (From Asbury & McKhann 2002.)

Feature	Primary polydipsia	Diabetes insipidus
Onset of polyuria	Gradual	Sudden
Nocturia	Unusual	Common
Random plasma osmolality	Sometimes <28.5 mosmol/L	Normal or elevated
Morning plasma osmolality	Normal	Elevated
Morning urine osmolality	Normal	Inappropriately low
Plasma ADH concentration	Normal relative to plasma osmolality	Low relative to plasma osmolality (in neurogenic diabetes insipidus)

occasion be skilfully concealed. Treatment must aim at restricting fluid intake, along with attempts to obtain maximal control of the patient's psychiatric disorder. Where long-term fluid restriction proves to be impractical or when an offending medication must be continued, demeclocycline may be useful in normalising serum sodium by inhibiting the action of ADH on the kidneys (Illowsky & Kirch 1988).

Cushing's syndrome

Cushing's syndrome is caused by chronic excess of glucocorticoids and has a number of different aetiologies. The most common form, accounting for 60–80% of cases in most series, is a pituitary adenoma producing excess corticotrophin (ACTH). This results in secondary bilateral hyperplasia of the adrenal cortices and is known as Cushing's disease (Mampalam et al. 1988). Typically, these pituitary tumours are microadenomas (<1 cm in diameter) and are rarely large enough to cause chiasmatic compression or raised intracranial pressure. Cushing's syndrome may also be caused by ectopic ACTH secretion (e.g. by small-cell lung carcinoma) or by ACTH-independent mechanisms, with excess cortisol production resulting from unilateral adrenocortical tumours, either benign or malignant, or by bilateral adrenal hyperplasia or dysplasia (Boscaro et al. 2001). Iatrogenic and factitious Cushing's syndrome may occasionally be associated with exogenous administration of ACTH, though is more commonly seen with long-term treatment with glucocorticoids such as prednisolone or dexamethasone.

Apart from differing levels of circulating ACTH, the endocrine abnormalities are the same whether due to adrenal or pituitary disease: a sustained excessive production of cortisol that obliterates the normal diurnal rhythm, and usually excessive production of adrenal androgens as well. Alcohol dependency may also produce clinical features identical to those seen in Cushing's syndrome in a minority of susceptible individuals. The clinical picture may be accompanied by abnormalities of cortisol secretion and in particular a loss of circadian rhythm. The mechanism through which alcohol interferes with cortisol secretion is unclear, although it has been suggested that it interferes with steroidogenic pathways by decreasing 11β-hydroxysteroid dehydrogenase activity (Groote Veldman et al. 1996). The clinical and hormonal features typically resolve within days or weeks when the alcohol intake stops and this is the simplest way of avoiding a false diagnosis (Smals et al. 1976; Morgan 1982; Boscaro et al. 2000).

Cushing's syndrome is rare: the annual incidence of Cushing's disease is 0.1–1.0 per 100 000 and is three to eight times more common in women than in men (Boscaro et al. 2001). Incidence peaks in women between the ages of 25 and 50 years though the range of ages at onset is wide. A tendency has also been noted for the disorder to start during pregnancy, at the menopause or at puberty, or while the subject is undergoing a prolonged period of psychological stress, with repeated studies showing an association between onset of the hypothalamic–pituitary form of Cushing's disease and stressful life events (Sonino et al. 1993a).

The great majority of cases present for medical attention on account of the physical disorder that develops, but psychiatric features are strikingly frequent and can be severe. Moreover, occasional cases have been reported to present with psychiatric illnesses from the outset, as discussed below, and the endocrine disorder may then be recognised only after a considerable delay.

Physical features

The physical changes most commonly seen in Cushing's syndrome are shown in Table 10.6, together with their relative frequencies in one series. However, it should be noted that the occurrence of any single feature varies so widely between series that no single finding is necessary for diagnosis. Truncal obesity is almost always present and associated with supraclavicular fat accumulation, a cervical fat pad (the well-known 'buffalo hump'), facial fullness (the moon face) and purple striae produced by rapid expansion of the trunk and abdomen. The complexion is plethoric and hirsutism may be marked. Excessive bruising or extensive ecchymoses and atrophy of the skin may also be seen. Skin pigmentation may develop from the direct action of excessive ACTH on melanocytes. Hypertension is often severe and glucose intolerance or frank diabetes mellitus may also develop. Amenorrhoea is usual in women, and impotence, testicular atrophy or gynaecomastia commonly seen in men. Other important features include proximal muscle weakness and associated muscle wasting, a liability to intercurrent infections, especially fungal, and osteoporosis leading to backache or

Table 10.6 Frequency of physical signs and symptoms in a group of 302 individuals with Cushing's syndrome. (From Boscaro et al. 2001.)

Sign/symptom	Frequency (%)
Truncal obesity	96
Facial fullness	82
Diabetes or glucose intolerance	80
Gonadal dysfunction	74
Hirsutism, acne	72
Hypertension	68
Muscle weakness	64
Skin atrophy and bruising	62
Osteoporosis	38
Oedema	18
Polydipsia/polyuria	10
Fungal infections	6

The mean age of the 302 patients (239 female and 63 male) was 38.4 years (SD 13.5 years, range 8–75 years).

vertebral collapse. However, the clinical phenotype is not always florid and suspicion should always arise with a less complete picture especially if there is concomitant recent weight gain, impaired glucose tolerance and high blood pressure (Arnaldi *et al.* 2003).

Psychiatric features

In an early series of 25 consecutive patients seen in a general hospital, Trethowan and Cobb (1952) showed that psychiatric disturbance is common and reflects the findings in more recent studies. Of their patients, four were described as severely disturbed and psychotic, six as moderately disturbed and eight mildly disturbed; three had relatively insignificant psychiatric symptoms but only four could be declared mentally normal. Jeffcoate *et al.* (1979) surveyed 40 patients of whom 22 were depressed, five severely, and four showed other psychiatric disorders (mania, chronic anxiety and an acute organic reaction). Only one-third was judged to be free from mental disorder. Whybrow and Hurwitz's (1976) literature review supported these findings and suggested that less than 4% showed euphoria, in contrast to the situation when exogenous steroids are administered for therapeutic purposes. Later prospective studies such as that by Starkman *et al.* (1981) have reported an even higher frequency of psychiatric symptoms (Table 10.7). Irritability was the earliest symptom in most cases, often antedating the physical manifestations. Patients described themselves as having become oversensitive and unable to ignore minor irritations. Verbal dyscontrol was frequent, patients noting that they were overly argumentative and unable to 'hold their tongue'. Depressed mood was reported in three-quarters. It was often of sudden onset and was usually intermittent rather than sustained, rarely lasting for longer than 3 days at a time. Social withdrawal when present was related to feelings of discomfort in large groups and seemingly due to feelings of shame at their physical appearance.

Depression is widely reported as one of the most frequent psychiatric symptoms and is often seen with paranoid features. Cohen's (1980) study was important as it reported a consecutive and unselected series of 29 patients with Cushing's syndrome examined closely from the psychiatric point of view; 25 (86%) showed a significant degree of depression, this being mild in seven, moderate in 13 and severe in five. The author also found that almost half of the series had a family history of depression or suicide, or a past history of early bereavement or separation, and six had experienced a major emotional disturbance shortly preceding the onset of the endocrine disorder. These are all factors of known importance in the genesis of depression and raised the possibility of an aetiological link between Cushing's syndrome and depressive illness. Moreover, depression was particularly common among the 21 patients with a pituitary origin for

Table 10.7 Frequency of psychiatric symptoms in a group of 35 individuals with Cushing's syndrome. (From Starkman *et al.* 1981.)

Symptom	Frequency (%)
Increased fatigue	100
Decreased energy	97
Irritability	86
Impaired memory	83
Depressed mood	74
Decreased libido	69
Middle insomnia	69
Anxiety	66
Impaired concentration	66
Crying	63
Restlessness	60
Late insomnia	57
Social withdrawal	46
Hopelessness	43
Guilt	37
Increased appetite	34
Dreams	31
Early insomnia	29
Decreased appetite	20
Thought blocking	17
Speeding thoughts	14
Elation–hyperactivity	11
Slowing thoughts	11
Perceptual distortions	11
Rapid, loud speech	9
Paranoid thoughts	9
Hyperactivity	9
Depersonalisation	3
Persistent anhedonia	3
Derealisation	3
Decreased fatigue	3
Increased energy	3

their Cushing's syndrome, and all six patients with a disturbing life event preceding it fell into this group.

More recent studies using standardised diagnostic criteria have found major depression meeting DSM criteria in 57–80% (Haskett 1985; Kelly 1996), with no significant differences in the prevalence of depression between patients with pituitary-dependent and -independent forms (Sonino *et al.* 1993b; Kelly 1996). However, the presence of major depression has been associated with older age, female gender, higher pretreatment cortisol levels and a more severe clinical condition (Sonino *et al.* 1998). Acute anxiety may also figure prominently, with one small study (Loosen *et al.* 1992) showing that 79% of the subjects with Cushing's disease fulfilled DSM-III-R criteria for generalised anxiety disorder. Apathy verging on stupor may be seen and fatigue and asthenia derived from the physical disorder often colours the psychiatric picture.

The psychoses accompanying Cushing's syndrome are mostly depressive in nature. When they occur they are typically florid illnesses with delusions and auditory hallucinations, often with paranoid symptoms. Retardation may be severe, sometimes bordering on stupor. Anxious agitation may replace the retardation in other cases, or there may be acute brief episodes of grossly disturbed behaviour. Marked fluctuations in the severity of the condition appear to be characteristic. Most recent studies using standardised diagnostic criteria have failed to identify any cases of schizophrenia or acute confusional states (Kelly 1996) or found them only in conjunction with particularly high cortisol and ACTH levels (Starkman et al. 1981). However, case reports occasionally appear in the literature and may reflect a tendency to publish unusual patients (Johnson 1975).

There has been considerable interest in defining the cognitive changes associated with Cushing's syndrome and more broadly in conditions associated with excess glucocorticoids. Typically, patients with Cushing's syndrome complain of difficulties with concentration and memory. In her study on 48 subjects with untreated Cushing's disease, Starkman (2001) showed significantly lower scores on four of five verbal IQ subtests but on only one non-verbal subtest in patients with Cushing's disease compared with healthy controls. Verbal but not visual learning and delayed recall at 30 minutes were also significantly decreased in the Cushing's disease group. This selective impairment in verbal compared with visuospatial learning appeared to be a result of impaired initial learning rather than retention or retrieval. There was no significant association between severity of depression and cognitive performance, suggesting that the behavioural domains of mood and cognition may be affected independently of each other in response to hypercortisolaemia. A similar pattern of cognitive impairment is also described in post-traumatic stress disorder (Bremner et al. 1995) that is associated with raised cortisol levels and in subjects who have received several days of stress-level exposure to corticosteroids (Newcomer et al. 1999).

Aetiology of mental disturbances

The depression so characteristic of Cushing's syndrome is doubtless partly a reaction to the physical disfigurements and discomforts produced by the disease. But a more direct connection is suggested in those cases where affective disorder is an early or even presenting feature, and by the frequency with which the depression reaches 'psychotic' intensity.

Cohen's (1980) observations are particularly interesting in this regard. The common finding of factors predisposing to depression in the histories of his patients may merely illustrate their vulnerability to depression in the face of physical illness; on the other hand, it may indicate something more – a

close pathophysiological link between the genesis of depression and the genesis of some forms of Cushing's syndrome. Thus it is noteworthy in his series that depression was significantly more common in primary pituitary than primary adrenal forms of the syndrome, a difference that had already been discerned by Carroll (1976) from cases in the literature. Disturbing life events, antecedent to the development of the endocrine disorder, were confined to this form of the disease. However, more discriminating controlled studies will be necessary before concluding that Cushing's syndrome may sometimes be induced by stress.

The depression of Cushing's syndrome has often been contrasted with the elevation of mood characteristically seen when steroids or ACTH are administered for therapeutic purposes. Whether the difference is due to differing plasma levels of biologically active steroids or to the long-continued chronic elevation of steroids in Cushing's syndrome is not known. Neither Cohen (1980) nor Kelly et al. (1983) could relate the severity of depression to the levels of circulating cortisol in their patients, yet its alleviation after surgical removal of the hyperplastic adrenal glands suggests that it must owe a good deal to some substance they produce. Hypothalamic factors may also be presumed to play a part in view of the complex neuroendocrine relationships now apparent in the control and regulation of the hypothalamic–pituitary axis. In cases of pituitary origin, additional factors could be the increased levels of β-endorphin and methionine-enkephalin that are secreted along with ACTH (Fava et al. 1987).

The discovery of glucocorticoid and mineralocorticoid receptors in the brain (McEwen et al. 1986) has stimulated interest in the pathophysiological mechanisms by which cortisol may affect cognitive and emotional functioning. Animal studies have shown that the hippocampi are especially vulnerable to excess or deficit of glucocorticoids and exposure to exogenous corticosteroids induces changes in hippocampal pyramidal cell morphology and pyramidal cell loss (Sapolsky et al. 1990). Prolonged exposure to high levels of glucocorticoids is associated with impaired long-term potentiation (Kerr et al. 1991) and impairs memory performance. Starkman et al. (1992) and subsequently others (Bourdeau et al. 2002) have shown variability in hippocampal formation volume in Cushing's syndrome on MRI, with 27% of subjects having a hippocampal volume outside the 95% confidence interval for the normal hippocampal volume quoted in the literature, the reduction in volume of the hippocampal formation correlating significantly with measures of verbal memory impairment and negatively with the levels of plasma cortisol. The hippocampal formation contains the highest proportion of corticosteroid-binding sites in the brain, particularly in the CA1, CA3 and dentate regions, which may make it particularly vulnerable in Cushing's disease. It should be noted, however, that normal hippocampal volumes quoted in the literature show fourfold variation (Colchester *et al.* 2001), so there is not yet an unequivocal reference standard.

Recent studies by Starkman *et al.* (1999) and Bourdeau *et al.* (2002, 2005) suggest that the hippocampal and general cerebral atrophy reported in Cushing's syndrome may be partially or even fully reversible following successful treatment of the underlying endocrinopathy. Furthermore, there is some evidence to suggest that this improvement in hippocampal and possibly general cerebral volume is associated with an improvement in function, particularly in learning (Starkman *et al.* 2003). In their study of 22 patients treated surgically for Cushing's disease, Starkman *et al.* showed a mean increase in hippocampal volume of $3.2 \pm 2.5\%$ at a mean of 16 months after surgery. The percentage increase in hippocampal volume significantly correlated with the magnitude of the change in urinary free cortisol levels. Bourdeau *et al.* used third ventricle diameter and bicaudate diameters as surrogate measures of cerebral atrophy and showed highly significant improvements in both in 38 patients with Cushing's syndrome treated surgically at an average of 40 months' follow-up. The mechanism for this apparent increase in cerebral volume is currently unclear. It is interesting to speculate that this may be the result of increased pyramidal cell dendritic branching or the production of new hippocampal neurones, a consequence of granule cell neurogenesis in the dentate gyrus resulting from reduced cortisol suppression. Eriksson *et al.* (1998) have also demonstrated production of new hippocampal neurones in human brain though, as cautioned by Starkman, these apparent increases in volume may simply be the result of an increase in the water content of grey and white matter resulting from the reduction in cortisol levels. In this regard it should be noted that corticosteroids are frequently used and often effective in reducing cerebral oedema associated with intracranial tumours.

Outcome

A successful psychiatric outcome can be expected when the endocrine disorder is effectively treated. The physical and mental symptoms usually improve in parallel until the patient regains his former stability. Depression is regularly observed to recede after adrenalectomy, pituitary operation or treatment with metyrapone, often starting to abate within days or weeks though sometimes taking as long as a year to clear completely (Jeffcoate *et al.* 1979; Cohen 1980; Kelly *et al.* 1983). Needless to say, when psychiatric disturbance has long antedated the Cushing's syndrome, there may be little or no change when the latter is remedied.

With florid psychotic illnesses the results can be dramatic, as in the following case vignettes.

For details of the medical management of the condition readers should consult a textbook of medicine.

A woman presented initially with physical symptoms of Cushing's syndrome, but on admission to hospital developed an acute psychotic picture with auditory and visual hallucinations and delusions about changing her sex. This was thought to have been precipitated partly by the mounting anxiety surrounding her admission to hospital. She became markedly paranoid and agitated, developed confusional episodes and showed bizarre catatonic motor phenomena. The entire condition responded well to bilateral extirpation of the hyperplastic adrenal glands and her mental state returned to normal within a few days of the operation. Follow-up 3 years later showed that she remained entirely well (Hickman *et al.* 1961).

A soldier of 23 with a good service record became abruptly confused and hallucinated, and showed severely disturbed behaviour with grandiose and religious delusions. He was diagnosed as schizophrenic and treated extensively with electroconvulsive therapy. It was not until 1 year later that Cushing's syndrome was diagnosed. He continued to be severely disturbed, but pituitary irradiation 18 months and 2 years after onset led to transitory amelioration of the psychotic symptoms. Two and a half years after onset bilateral adrenalectomy was performed, and thereafter there was steady and gradual improvement until full premorbid stability was regained (Hertz *et al.* 1955).

Addison's disease

Primary adrenal insufficiency or Addison's disease results in a deficiency of all adrenal steroids: glucocorticoids, mineralocorticoids and adrenally produced androgens. It has a prevalence of 93–140 per million (Arlt & Allolio 2003) and affects women more commonly than men. Peak onset is in the fourth decade. In developed countries the most common cause is autoimmune destruction of the adrenal glands. Autoantibodies seen in the disorder appear to be directed against the 21-hydroxylase enzyme, involved in steroidogenesis, and other endogenous adrenal cell antigens (Winqvist 1992).

Addison's disease with an autoimmune aetiology (60% of cases) occurs as part of the autoimmune polyglandular syndrome (APS), whereas in the remaining 40% of cases the disease occurs alone. APS type I is a childhood disease characterised by chronic mucocutaneous candidiasis, hypoparathyroidism, primary adrenal insufficiency and, in a minority, childhood alopecia, chronic active hepatitis and malabsorption. It is caused by mutations in the autoimmune regulator gene (*AIRE*) and is inherited in an autosomal recessive manner (Nagamine *et al.* 1997). APS type II, or Schmidt's syndrome, is a disease of adults and comprises adrenal insufficiency, hypothyroidism, primary gonadal failure and type 1 diabetes; vitiligo, chronic atrophic gastritis or celiac disease may also occasionally be seen. It is inherited as an autosomal dominant disorder with incomplete penetrance.

Tuberculous infiltration is the second most common cause of Addison's disease in developed countries and the most common cause in developing countries. Secondary adrenal insufficiency may result from suppression of the hypothalamic–pituitary–adrenal axis, typically following chronic administration of glucocorticoids though rarely may also be due to local hypothalamic or pituitary lesions. It too is seen more commonly in women than men and has a peak incidence in the sixth decade, later than that seen in primary adrenal insufficiency (Nilsson *et al.* 2000).

Physical features

The onset of symptoms is gradual and the usual presentation is with general weakness, lack of stamina and fatigue. Chronic glucocorticoid deficiency leads to weight loss, nausea and anorexia and may account for muscle, joint and abdominal pain. Orthostatic hypotension with postural dizziness is seen in 90%, and may be seen in association with salt craving resulting from mineralocorticoid deficiency. Loss of dehydroepiandrosterone (DHEA), the major precursor of the adrenally produced sex steroids, can lead to loss of libido, dry skin and loss of axillary and pubic hair and is seen predominantly in women. On examination most have hyperpigmentation in palm creases and buccal mucosa due to the increased production of pituitary ACTH and other pro-opiomelanocortin-related peptides. Resistance to stress is lowered and sensitivity to infections increased. There is often pronounced intolerance of cold and the body temperature is usually low. Symptoms of hypoglycaemia may appear at higher levels of blood sugar than is usual. There is an increased liability to convulsions, and the EEG is often abnormal with diffuse high-amplitude slow activity. Very occasionally, potassium retention may lead to hyperkalaemic periodic paralysis and may be the sole presentation (see Potassium depletion, later).

As many as half of all patients diagnosed with Addison's disease may present with a life-threatening adrenal crisis (Zellisen 1994), a medical emergency characterised by profound hypotension or hypovolaemic shock, acute abdominal pain, vomiting and often fever, that may be prevented if early diagnosis is made. It may occur spontaneously or in response to infection or drugs such as morphine or anaesthetic agents.

Psychiatric features

Psychiatric abnormalities are present in almost all patients with Addison's disease. The commonest changes are similar to those expected in chronic physical exhaustion: depression, emotional withdrawal, apathy and loss of drive and initiative. There are sometimes sudden fluctuations of mood, or episodes of marked anxiety and irritability. Cleghorn (1965) described mental symptoms of apathy and negativism in 80% of cases, depressive withdrawal and irritability in 50%, whilst suspiciousness was seen in 15%, agitated behaviour in 10% and paranoia with delusions in 5%. Memory impairment also occurs in up to three-quarters of cases (Michael & Gibbons 1963). Mild dementia may be simulated on account of the mental anergia, poverty of thought and general air of indifference. Considerable perceptual impairment may also be seen, with increased thresholds to tactile, auditory and olfactory stimuli (Leigh & Kramer 1984). Drowsiness can be conspicuous, although increased irritability, restlessness and insomnia are also seen. The severity of the changes may fluctuate over time, varying directly with the severity of the endocrine disorder.

Psychotic pictures of a depressive or schizophrenic nature are rare, in contrast to the clinical picture in Cushing's disease. However, Cleghorn (1951) reported examples of acute and chronic paranoia, hallucinatory states and schizophreniform psychoses. Such disturbances may be very short-lived and are sometimes intimately related to impending crises. McFarland (1963) reviewed reports of 10 patients with schizophrenia, six with affective psychosis and one with organic psychosis and concluded that the form of psychotic development was unpredictable. One of his patients presented with hypomania that masked the adrenal disorder until the patient lapsed into coma after electroconvulsive treatment, when severe hyponatraemia was discovered.

Investigation

Addison's disease must be differentiated from hypopituitarism and from other chronic debilitating diseases. Weight loss, hypotension and pigmentation may all be seen, for example, in carcinoma, tuberculosis, malabsorption or malnutrition. It is therefore essential to investigate adrenal function adequately before making the diagnosis.

Hyponatraemia is present in about 90% of cases of primary adrenal insufficiency, and hyperkalaemia in 65% (Kong 1994); thus normal serum sodium and potassium values do not preclude the diagnosis. The simultaneous measurement of early-morning serum cortisol and plasma ACTH separates primary adrenal insufficiency from normals or those with secondary disease (Oelkers 1992). In primary adrenal failure plasma ACTH is usually greatly increased, with a low or low-normal cortisol. Alternatively, the synthetic ACTH (tetracosactide, Synacthen) test may be used. This will show a failure of serum cortisol response at 30 or 60 minutes after injection of 250 µg of tetracosactide in primary adrenal failure whereas in secondary hypoadrenalism the response may be delayed. The insulin tolerance test is regarded as the gold standard for the assessment of suspected secondary adrenal deficiency (Arlt & Allolio 2003). Assessment of adrenal cortex autoantibodies, especially those directed against 21-hydroxylase, may also be helpful especially in suspected isolated primary adrenal insufficiency.

From the psychiatric point of view an erroneous diagnosis of a neurotic or stress-related disorder or early dementia may easily be made. The depression and generalised weakness may be attributed to neurasthenia, especially when pigmentation is slight and serum electrolytes are normal. The impression of a neurotic or stress-related disorder is strengthened by the anorexia, irritability and diminished libido, and by the fluctuation of symptoms over time. Dementia, or a chronic amnesic syndrome, is suggested when memory difficulties are prominent.

Treatment and outcome

Chronic glucocorticoid replacement with hydrocortisone is usually given in two or three daily doses, with the majority given in the morning to mimic physiological secretion patterns. Mineralocorticoid replacement in primary adrenal failure is with fludrocortisone. Adrenal androgen replacement with DHEA is not current clinical practice. Adequate replacement therapy is usually highly successful in alleviating most physical and mental disturbances. The patient's sense of well-being quickly improves, and appetite and energy gradually return to previous levels. Glucocorticoids appear to be more important than mineralocorticoids for reversing the mental symptoms and abolishing the EEG abnormalities, indicating that these do not rest entirely on disturbances of electrolyte and water balance (Reichlin 1968). Whether current therapy with glucocorticoids and mineralocorticoids abolishes all the symptoms of Addison's disease or whether a lack of androgens is associated with increased fatigue, reduced vitality perception and well-being or with subtle cognitive deficits is currently debated (Lovas *et al.* 2002; Riedel 1993). A number of randomised placebo-controlled trials of DHEA replacement have reported conflicting effects on subjective health status, mood and sexuality (Arlt *et al.* 1999; Hunt *et al.* 2000; Johannsson *et al.* 2002; Lovas *et al.* 2003). A precise definition of the clinical syndrome of DHEA deficiency would allow more sensitive and disease-specific instruments to be developed and the benefits or not of replacement to be assessed (Lovas *et al.* 2003).

Malnutrition

Severe chronic malnutrition is accompanied by well-described psychological changes: apathy, emotional lability and impairment of memory. Confusional states are not uncommon though acute psychosis is rare. Much of the early literature on the effects of chronic severe malnutrition came from studies of survivors of the Nazi concentration camps and prisoner of war camps in Germany, Russia and the Far East (Helweg-Larsen *et al.* 1952; Thygesen 1970). These suggested that neurotic symptoms did not develop and antecedent psychoneurotic and compulsive symptoms disappeared, with interest becoming focused on food alone (Thygesen *et al.* 1970).

At 23-year follow-up of Danish concentration camp survivors, Thygesen *et al.* (1970) showed that fatigue, depression, lability of affect, sleeplessness with nightmares, and reduction in learning capacity and concentration were common and suggested that with time these may fade into a state of premature senescence with intellectual reduction and associated cerebral atrophy. Others have also shown an increase in the late development of spinal cord lesions and parkinsonism that cannot be ascribed to the late effects of known tropical diseases or specific vitamin deficiencies (Gibberd & Simmonds 1980). However, the combination of severe malnutrition with chronic emotional stress in these groups makes it difficult to isolate the specific effects of malnutrition from those associated with comorbid post-traumatic stress disorder, which is now recognised to be common in these groups (Sutker *et al.* 1993) and is associated with very similar symptoms.

There has since been debate about whether chronic severe malnutrition predisposes to an increased risk of subsequent accelerated cognitive decline and dementia. Sutker *et al.* (1990, 1992) found specific deficits in tests of attention, concentration and memory as well as on abstraction and organisation in former prisoners of war that was most marked in those with weight loss of more than 35% of total body weight. These findings have been questioned by Sulway *et al.* (1996) who found no significant differences in cognitive performance on a battery of neuropsychological tests or of the prevalence of dementia in a group of Australian prisoners of war compared with Second World War veterans regardless of magnitude of weight loss. They argued that their failure to show cognitive deficits was due to more closely matched controls and suggested that previously found cognitive deficits may be due to an increased incidence of depression seen in prisoners of war that appears to decrease with age. A more recent case–control study of prisoners of war repatriated from North Vietnam also failed to show a significant difference on neuropsychometry compared with naval controls (Williams *et al.* 2002).

In infants and young children, on the other hand, there is firmer evidence that starvation is liable to damage the brain. Rodent studies showed that growth retardation induced by protein-energy malnutrition during suckling was not entirely reversed with subsequent feeding (Dobbing 1990; Levistsky & Strupp 1995) and pathology showed evidence of permanent cortical injury, with reduction in the density and arborisations of dendrites and abnormal myelination and width of cortical cells. Neurotransmitter systems were also altered permanently, for example the number of noradrenaline receptors was reduced compared with controls (Levitsky & Strupp 1995). All brain regions appear to be vulnerable. Cravioto and Delicardie (1970) showed a difference in IQ in malnourished children compared with their adequately nourished siblings, helping to confirm that the differences in cognitive function are due mainly to early malnourishment rather than differences in their psychosocial environment, and there have now been so many well-controlled studies from many countries worldwide that the severe cognitive effects of early life malnutrition are no longer in doubt (Scrimshaw 1998; O'Connor et al. 2000). Pollitt (2000) has reviewed longitudinal studies of the cognitive effects of supplementary feeding at different periods of early life and tentatively concludes that supplementary feeding during the first 18–24 months of life may help to prevent part of the cognitive delays caused by extreme poverty and malnutrition. Beyond this period the developmental benefits of supplements vary as a function of the breadth of intervention, e.g. nutrition, health, education and duration of intervention. Current studies are investigating the consequences of malnutrition on emotional and motor development and interrelation between these variables.

Under normal circumstances malnutrition of this degree is rarely encountered in Western societies. However, even in populations where the general standard of nutrition is high there are groups prone to inadequate or imbalanced food intake who may present with vitamin depletion. Those with learning disabilities or chronic mental illness and the homeless often live precariously in the community and vitamin deficiencies may add to their symptomatology. The aged population is similarly at risk, especially when depression or early dementia impairs standards of self-care. Individuals with alcohol dependency face the multiple hazards of inadequate intake, poor absorption and special demands made on vitamin reserves for the metabolism of alcohol. These are all groups that are particularly liable to come to psychiatric attention. Patients with chronic gastrointestinal disease and malabsorption are another group at risk, while any physical illness may deplete reserves. Profound deficiencies may be revealed postoperatively, especially in patients maintained for a considerable time on intravenous fluids.

Of all the vitamins it is the members of the B complex, particularly thiamine and nicotinic acid, that have proved to be of most importance in psychiatric practice. Other deficiencies will often coexist in chronic malnutrition, but specific roles for vitamins A, C and D have not been clearly identified in relation to mental disorder. Vitamin B_{12} and folic acid have been increasingly studied in relation to psychiatric illness and this evidence is also reviewed. Vitamin E has also been increasingly implicated in the aetiology of Parkinson's disease (see Chapter 12).

Vitamin B deficiency

Laboratory studies provide a firm basis for expecting functional and pathological changes in the CNS as a result of vitamin B deprivation. Many components of the B complex are known to play an essential role in metabolic processes within the brain: thiamine pyrophosphate is a coenzyme involved in carbohydrate metabolism, particularly the oxidation of pyruvate, and may also be necessary for the proper transmission of nerve impulses; nicotinic acid and its amide act as constituent parts of coenzymes necessary for glucose metabolism; riboflavin acts similarly; pantothenic acid is concerned with the formation of acetylcholine; and pyridoxine becomes converted into pyridoxal phosphate, a coenzyme fundamental to several enzyme systems concerned in brain metabolic processes.

It was not until the 1930s that the full significance of vitamin B deficiency in relation to psychiatric disorder began to be appreciated, although mental disorder had been recognised as an integral part of the syndrome of pellagra from its earliest descriptions. In the 1930s, however, the various constituents of the B complex were identified, and careful observation soon extended awareness of their functions. Experimental studies showed that deprivation could lead to psychological symptoms well before definitive manifestations were declared in other systems of the body. Acute and severe depletion of vitamin reserves also proved to be responsible for fulminating neuropsychiatric disorders that had not previously been thought to be nutritional in origin.

The wide natural dispersion of the B vitamins has made it difficult to work out precise relationships in naturally occurring disorders, and multiple deficiencies will often operate together. Sometimes, however, the evidence linking specific deficiencies to specific clinical pictures has been clarified by noting the therapeutic response to vitamins given singly. Thiamine and nicotinic acid have emerged as the vitamins of greatest importance in neuropsychiatric disorders, with others such as pyridoxine, pantothenic acid and riboflavin contributing mainly to ancillary symptoms. Moreover, with both thiamine and nicotinic acid it is clear that different syndromes of deficiency can follow, depending on the severity of depletion and the time over which it has operated.

Thiamine (B_1) deficiency classically leads to beriberi, with neuropathy, cardiac failure or peripheral oedema. This clinical picture results from chronic severe depletion. In the shorter term a neurasthenic picture may result, with fatigue, weakness and emotional disturbance, well before the physical features appear. Acute and fulminant depletion can lead to the picture of Wernicke's encephalopathy. This probably occurs through a combination of dietary insufficiency, impaired intestinal absorption and possibly a genetically determined abnormality of transketolase (Mukherjee et al.

1987) in the context of low bodily stores. The changes in Wernicke's encephalopathy may be confined to the CNS, and other evidence of vitamin lack may be entirely absent. See Chapter 4 (Wernicke's encephalopathy, Korsakoff's syndrome) for further discussion on the neuropsychiatric consequences of thiamine deficiency.

Nicotinic acid (niacin) deficiency shows a similar range of disorders. Subacute deficiency produces the syndrome of pellagra, with gastrointestinal symptoms, skin lesions and psychiatric disturbance. In the early stages a neurasthenic picture may be seen in relative isolation. Acute and sudden depletion may lead to a picture of 'encephalopathy', sometimes with few or no symptoms or signs in other systems to point to vitamin deficiency.

Pyridoxine (B$_6$) deficiency can lead to convulsions in infants on deficient diets or in those with unusually high requirements. Pronounced abnormalities appear in the EEG and mental deterioration may develop. Symptoms and the EEG changes may resolve within minutes of injection of the vitamin. Lack of pyridoxine may also contribute to the neuropathy seen with severe malnutrition. Experimental deficiency in adults, or the use of pyridoxine antagonists, leads to irritability, confusion and lethargy (Fabrykant 1960). Some authors have suggested that pyridoxine deficiency may contribute to depressive illness (Carney *et al.* 1979, 1982). Among patients admitted to a psychiatric unit, deficiencies of pyridoxine, and perhaps of riboflavin, were present in a higher proportion of those with affective disorder than with other psychiatric conditions. Pyridoxine deficiency has also been implicated in premenstrual syndrome and depression in patients taking oral contraceptives. Systematic review by Wyatt *et al.* (1999) concluded that doses of vitamin B$_6$ up to 100 mg daily are likely to be of benefit in treating premenstrual symptoms and premenstrual depression, with odds ratios compared with placebo of 2.32 and 1.69 respectively. However, these authors commented that these conclusions were limited by the low quality of most of the trials included.

Riboflavin (B$_2$) deficiency is characterised by sore throat, glossitis, angular stomatitis, lacrimation, photophobia, seborrhoeic dermatitis, and a normochromic normocytic anaemia. In study of severe and specific riboflavin restriction in healthy volunteers, Sterner and Price (1973) found personality changes on the Minnesota Multiphasic Personality Inventory (MMPI) that appeared to reflect increasing lethargy, hypersensitivity and a multitude of minor somatic complaints; however, these findings have not been replicated (Powers 2003). Subclinical riboflavin deficiency may contribute to increased concentrations of plasma homocysteine, with an associated increased risk of cardiovascular disease, and it may also be associated with impaired handling of iron and night blindness.

Pantothenic acid deficiency has been incriminated in leading to sensory neuropathy and the 'burning feet' syndrome. However, as in the case of riboflavin, a role in naturally occurring neurological or psychiatric disorder has not been clearly established.

Various aspects of vitamin B deficiency may prove to be commoner than expected among a wide range of psychiatric patients (Carney *et al.* 1982). Among 172 successive admissions to a psychiatric unit, 30% were considered to be deficient in thiamine, 27% in riboflavin and 9% in pyridoxine as assessed by red cell enzyme functions. More than half were deficient in at least one of the three, despite being drawn from a reasonably affluent community. Thiamine deficiency was mainly found in patients with alcohol dependency, drug addiction, schizophrenia and depression where poor diet may be expected. In contrast, those with pyridoxine deficiency often showed little evidence of malnutrition, and there was a significant association with depressive illness. Controlled studies examining the role of folate deficiency and hypocysteine for example will be required to determine whether such vitamin deficiencies may sometimes play an aetiological role in the genesis of depressive disorder, or whether they contribute more widely to psychiatric morbidity.

A number of studies have kept volunteer subjects on diets deficient in B vitamins in order to determine the earliest clinical features associated with deficiency. The findings are in broad agreement, particularly in emphasising the prominence of mental symptoms. Brozek and Caster (1957) confirmed the psychological effect of severe thiamine depletion using more precise dietary techniques. General weakness and extreme anorexia were associated with marked irritability and depression, and scores on the hysteria, hypochondriasis and depression scales of the MMPI deteriorated considerably. Continuation of the diet led ultimately to peripheral neuropathy and impairment on tests of manual speed, coordination and reaction time, but general intelligence was unaffected. The reintroduction of thiamine restored appetite promptly and produced a dramatic change in the attitude of the subjects, with a slower improvement in peripheral neuropathy.

Mental changes in pellagra

Multiple vitamin deficiencies or an imbalance in dietary amino acids may be operative in pellagra, although lack of nicotinic acid is by far the most important and replacement can lead to rapid relief of symptoms. Endemic pellagra disappeared with the improvement in nutritional education and widespread supplementation of grain cereals with nicotinic acid. It is now seen sporadically in patients with chronic alcoholism and poor nutritional status (Ishii & Nishihara 1981) or rarely in the malnourished homeless (Kertesz 2001). It is also a rare manifestation of the carcinoid syndrome, in which up to 60% of tryptophan is catabolised by what is usually a minor pathway, and of Hartnup disease, an inherited disorder in which several amino acids including tryptophan are poorly absorbed from the diet. In both conditions symptoms of pellagra may be cured by the administration of large amounts of niacin.

The characteristic triad of pellagra includes gastrointestinal disorder, skin lesions and psychiatric disturbance. The commonest gastrointestinal disturbances are anorexia and diarrhoea and vomiting. Skin changes are classically bilateral and symmetrical, presenting in sun-exposed areas and may include vesicles or bullae on extremities and desquamation and roughening of the skin on the dorsum of the hands. Eczema-like lesions around the mouth and nose and stomatitis are also often seen (Ishii & Nishihara 1981).

Prodromal features are similar to those seen in experimental thiamine deficiency. General deterioration of mental and physical health may predate more definite manifestations by weeks or months. Most prominent is a subjective feeling of incapacity for mental and physical effort, coupled with numerous other vague complaints: anorexia, insomnia, nervousness, apprehension, dizziness, headache, palpitations and paraesthesiae. Characteristically these fluctuate markedly from day to day. Irritability and emotional instability may dominate the picture. Depression can be severe with considerable risk of suicide. At a later stage the mental processes are obviously impaired, memory is poor and confabulation may appear. Such changes were well described in areas where pellagra was previously endemic, and patients themselves often recognised them as prodromes of the more florid manifestations of the disease. However, the rarity of pellagra today means that they are often misconstrued when sporadic cases arise.

More prolonged and severe nicotinic acid deficiency leads to the florid psychiatric manifestations of pellagra. These may sometimes develop without the above prodromes. They are often associated with gastrointestinal and skin changes but may occur alone or dominate the picture. The commonest presentation is an acute organic reaction with disorientation, confusion and impairment of memory. Excitement and outbursts of violent behaviour may occur, depression is often conspicuous, or paranoia may develop with hallucinations and delusions of persecution. Occasionally, chronic untreated pellagra may progress with a picture similar to Korsakoff's syndrome or as a slowly progressive generalised dementia. A neuropathological series by Ishii and Nishihara (1981) emphasises the importance of considering a diagnosis of pellagra in chronic alcoholism even in the absence of the classical skin changes. Of 74 patients with chronic alcoholism, 20 had neuropathologically diagnosable pellagra, of whom 19 had been diagnosed with delirium tremens at admission, presenting with confusion, hallucinations, insomnia, gait disturbance and

incontinence of urine and faeces. Only six had evidence of skin lesions.

Acute psychosis also responds to nicotinic acid, often in a dramatic fashion with calm and rational behaviour restored within a few days of vitamin replacement and occasionally within hours. It is very rare for treatment to fail in acute presentations, though the response in chronic cases with severe mental impairment may be less successful (Spies *et al.* 1938; McLester 1943). Neurological disturbances such as tremor, ataxia and sometimes dysarthria and dysphagia develop late in the course. A sensorimotor peripheral neuropathy is common, with paraesthesiae, pain and tenderness, chiefly in the distal leg muscles.

The early symptoms of pellagra are not associated with morphological changes within the brain and are presumed to depend on reversible biochemical changes within neurones. However, established pellagra is associated with a characteristic pathology: ballooning of the cell wall with loss of Nissl substance and compression of the nucleus to one side, affecting especially Betz cells in the motor cortex (Meyer 1901) and pontine, dorsal vagal and other brainstem nuclei (Leigh 1952). Symmetrical demyelination of the posterior fasciculus gracilis and cuneus, and to a lesser extent crossed pyramidal and spinocerebellar tracts, may also be seen (Spillane 1947). Degeneration of myelin in peripheral nerves has also been found (Wilson 1940).

Hartnup disease

Pellagra-like features occur as episodic attacks during childhood, then tend to subside during adult life. Increased renal clearance of neutral amino acids, including tryptophan, is accompanied by defective absorption of tryptophan from the gut. Some cases are asymptomatic and discovered only on routine screening. Other patients present with a photosensitive skin rash, often accompanied by psychiatric disturbance, cerebellar ataxia or other neurological abnormalities. Oral nicotinamide helps substantially during attacks, though these tend to subside spontaneously. Psychiatric features range from emotional lability in the milder cases to apathy, irritability, depression, confusion and delirium in the more marked examples (Hersov & Rodnight 1960). The coexistent photosensitive skin rash is an important clue to the underlying biochemical abnormality.

Acute nicotinic acid deficiency encephalopathy

Literature from the 1930s and 1940s described a syndrome of various forms of acute organic reaction that showed an excellent response to large doses of nicotinic acid. The clinical picture was of stupor or delirium, often dramatic in development and carrying a high mortality. Weakness and lethargy were common but anxiety and agitation could be marked. Extrapyramidal features, with cogwheel rigidity, and grasping and sucking reflexes were frequent accompaniments. Glossitis or stomatitis was frequently but not always present. In some the neuropsychiatric picture was the sole manifestation. Most patients had a history of malnutrition in combination with a history of chronic alcohol abuse. Thiamine replacement had no effect on the clinical picture but nicotinic acid in large dosage produced recovery usually in 3–5 days. Mortality was drastically reduced by such treatment, from 90% to 14%. Those who survived were often left with memory deficits.

The contemporary rarity of this syndrome in the UK and North America is probably associated with the routine use of high-potency vitamin therapy in the management of patients presenting with alcohol dependency (Lishman 1981). Reports from Japan and elsewhere suggest that the syndrome may still exist in the chronically malnourished and emphasise the importance of high-potency multivitamin replacement in all patients with chronic alcohol abuse or in whom chronic malnutrition may be suspected for other reasons (Ishii & Nishihara 1981; Kertesz 2001).

Ishii and Nishihara suggest that when an alcoholic patient develops neurological signs, particularly extrapyramidal rigidity, in addition to mental and gastrointestinal symptoms, nicotinic acid deficiency must be strongly suspected even in the absence of skin lesions. Gait disturbance, incontinence and hyperreflexia are further important features differentiating the syndrome from uncomplicated delirium tremens. In many cases it may be expected that thiamine deficiency will also be operative; however, only two of Ishii and Nishihara's 20 patients showed the pathology of Wernicke's encephalopathy in addition to that of pellagra. Similar findings were reported in 33 patients with chronic alcohol dependency from France (Hauw *et al.* 1988; Serdaru *et al.* 1988). Neurological features included marked oppositional hypertonus (*gegenhalten*) myoclonus, confusion and clouding of consciousness. At autopsy, chromatolysis was observed in neurones of the brainstem and cerebellar dentate nuclei, typical in all respects of nicotinic acid deficiency.

Vitamin B_{12} deficiency

Pernicious anaemia is widely recognised to be associated with subacute combined degeneration of the cord but it may also be accompanied by abnormalities of the mental state. This was probably recognised by Addison in his initial description of 'fatal idiopathic anaemia' in which he stated that 'the mind occasionally wanders' (Addison 1849). Langdon drew attention to these changes in 1905 with reports of loss of inhibition, peevishness and general mental deterioration in patients with pernicious anaemia. Of his nine patients, one was depressed, one institutionalised and another had been 'mentally peculiar' for 2 years with auditory hallucinations. It has been suggested that some of the mental symptoms, such as apathy and somnolence, may be related to the anaemia associated with vitamin B_{12} deficiency (Shulman 1967), whereas others including affective disor-

der, schizophrenia, paranoia, episodes of disorientation and delirium, and progressive dementia have been attributed directly to the B_{12} deficiency (Holmes 1956). Renewed interest in the cerebral manifestations of pernicious anaemia followed the work of Holmes (1956) and Smith (1960) which showed that they were not infrequent and responded rapidly to vitamin B_{12} replacement. These manifestations also emphasised that mental symptoms may occasionally be seen many months or even years before the development of anaemia or of peripheral neurological manifestations.

Surveys of psychiatric populations have often shown a large number of patients with low serum B_{12} levels. Recent studies have suggested that serum B_{12} levels have limited sensitivity for detecting clinically meaningful cobalamin deficiency in tissue and, as discussed below in the introduction to the section on folate, other measures may be more sensitive. Elevated serum levels of methylmalonate and total homocysteine, the accumulated substrates of two important cobalamin-dependent reactions, indicate tissue deficiency of cobalamin even in some patients with normal serum cobalamin levels (Savage *et al.* 1994). Recent studies in elderly non-hospital populations using these combined measures identified tissue deficiency of cobalamin in 5–23%, with reliance on serum B_{12} levels alone underestimating tissue deficiency by up to 50% (Hutto 97; Clarke *et al.* 2004).

An additional difficulty is that the low levels of B_{12}, or alteration in the levels of methylmalonic acid or homocysteine, may be the consequence rather than the cause of the abnormal mental state, since B_{12} deficiency can result from inadequate nutrition. However, daily requirements of B_{12} are small and it would normally take many years before simple dietary lack would become manifest in this way. Nevertheless, a low serum iron or folic acid can contribute to lowering of the serum B_{12}, which may therefore result from a mixed nutritional deficiency in patients with depression or dementia who have neglected their diet.

In an attempt to resolve this, Zucker *et al.* (1981) reviewed numerous case reports in the literature, using strictly defined criteria before accepting a causal link between B_{12} deficiency and psychiatric disturbance. They identified 15 patients where the relationship seemed well established. Among their requirements were the absence of other organic causes for the mental symptoms, a non-relapsing course, poor response to other treatments, and a positive and well-maintained response to B_{12} administration. Criteria for the diagnosis of B_{12} deficiency were also specified with care. The psychiatric pictures in the patients identified were heterogeneous, with a preponderance of organic mental symptoms, depression, paranoia, irritability and episodes of assaultative behaviour. Marked psychiatric disorder could sometimes occur in the absence of neurological abnormalities or anaemia.

Neurological symptoms have previously been considered a late manifestation of B_{12} deficiency, typically occurring after the development of anaemia. Lindenbaum *et al.* (1988) reviewed 141 consecutive patients with neuropsychiatric abnormalities due to cobalamin deficiency and found that 28% had no anaemia or macrocytosis. The haematocrit was normal in 34, mean cell volume was normal in 25, and both tests were normal in 19. Characteristic features in such patients included paraesthesiae, sensory loss, ataxia, dementia and psychiatric disorders. Methylmalonic acid and total homocysteine were also markedly elevated in these patients. Serum cobalamin levels were above 150 pmol/L in two patients, between 75 and 150 pmol/L in 16, and below 75 pmol/L in only 22. Except for one patient who died during the first week of treatment, all these patients showed an improvement in their mental state in response to vitamin B_{12} replacement. The authors concluded that neuropsychiatric disorders due to cobalamin deficiency occur commonly in the absence of anaemia or an elevated mean cell volume and that measurement of serum methylmalonic acid and total homocysteine were useful in the diagnosis of these patients.

Mood disorders

The role of vitamin B_{12} in the facilitation of monoamine transmitter release and the mechanism by which low levels may lead to depressed mood have been discussed above and have led to a renewed interest in the role of vitamin B_{12}, folate, homocysteine and other components of one-carbon metabolism in the aetiology of depression. Epidemiological studies have found that up to 31% of depressed patients have low serum vitamin B_{12} levels, though many have been criticised for lack of a consistently defined cut-off or clear or consistent control groups (Hutto 1997).

Overall the evidence supporting an association between vitamin B_{12} deficiency and depression remains quite sparse. With the exception of one study (Levitt & Joffe 1993), most studies in non-elderly groups have found no correlation between cobalamin levels and depression measured with the Hamilton Depression Scale. Studies in elderly groups have provided slightly stronger data. A community study of physically disabled women aged over 65 years found that subjects with B_{12} deficiency were twice as likely to be severely depressed as non-deficient controls (Penninx *et al.* 2000). The Rotterdam community study screened 3884 elderly people for depressive symptoms, with those positive to the screen undergoing assessment with the Present State Examination. Hyperhomocysteinaemia, vitamin B_{12} deficiency and to a lesser extent folate deficiency were all related to depressive disorders; however, only the association with B_{12} remained significant after adjustment for functional disability and cardiovascular disease (Tiemeier *et al.* 2002).

Conversely, the Hordaland homocysteine cross-sectional study failed to find an association between low vitamin B_{12} levels and depression or anxiety disorder in approximately 6000 middle-aged and elderly subjects (Bjelland *et al.* 2003). However, the study did identify a significant association of

hyperhomocysteinaemia and the T/T methylenetetrahydrofolate reductase (MTHFR) genotype (which is associated with elevated homocysteine levels under low folate conditions) with depression without comorbid anxiety. These studies and others increasingly suggest a role for components of the 1-carbon metabolic pathway in depression, although further studies will be required to dissect the contributions of individual components.

Psychosis

Case reports and case series over many years have associated psychotic symptoms with vitamin B_{12} deficiency. Early case series reported incidences of psychosis in 0–16% of patients with pernicious anaemia (Woltman 1924; Herman & Rost 1937); however, in a prospective study of 27 patients with pernicious anaemia none developed psychosis (Shulman 1967). In their review of B_{12} deficiency and psychiatric disorders, Zucker *et al.* (1981) found that 10 of 15 cases presented with psychiatric symptoms, all of whom had paranoid delusions, seven had hallucinations (one visual, three auditory and three both visual and auditory), seven were depressed and six had some organic features. One study showed that patients with psychotic depression had significantly lower mean vitamin B_{12} levels compared with patients with non-psychotic depression (Levitt & Joffe 1988). Whether vitamin B_{12} deficiency contributes to the development of psychosis, is a precipitant in predisposed individuals, is a coincidental finding or is a consequence of secondary nutritional origin remains unclear.

Other organic psychiatric disorders

In Shulman's (1967) prospective study, approximately three-quarters of the patients with pernicious anaemia showed anterograde memory deficits on a simple learning test. Retesting after treatment showed that the majority had returned to normal, sometimes within 20 hours of the first injection. Eastley *et al.* (2000) reported on 1432 patients seen at the Bristol memory clinic over a 13-year period; 125 had a low serum B_{12}, 66 presenting with a dementing illness and 22 with mild cognitive impairment. In this case–control design, none of the DSM-III diagnosed dementia group showed a significant improvement in neuropsychological function on replacement therapy; however, those presenting with cognitive impairment showed a significant improvement in verbal fluency compared with controls, with non-significant improvement on other measures.

Whilst absolute or functional B_{12} deficiency appears to be relatively common, especially in the elderly population with evidence to suggest reversal of mild cognitive deficits and other neuropsychiatric features, deficiency of B_{12} is a remarkably rare cause of a reversible dementia. Reversible dementias account for approximately 1% of all-cause dementia (Walstra *et al.* 1997), of which vitamin B_{12} deficiency has been implicated in approximately 1% (Clarfield 1988). Chiu's

(1996) review of the literature identified only 14 papers published between 1966 and 1995 reporting on cognitive impairments or dementia attributable to B_{12} deficiency and their response to treatment. She could identify only 10 patients in this literature with dementia who significantly improved or resolved with B_{12} treatment. Whether this is because changes associated with long-standing disease, as compared with milder presentations, lead to treatment resistance or simply because B_{12} deficiency was an association but not causative cannot be determined.

Neurological accompaniments
Numbness of the extremities is the commonest early symptom described in all series. Patients may also complain of tingling, pins and needles, 'feet going to sleep', burning or other dysaesthenic sensations (Victor & Lear 1956). Paraesthesiae are generally symmetrical and usually start, or are more severe in, the feet than the hands. Other more unusual symptoms, such as coldness, stiffness, band-like sensations, wetness or tightness, may also be described (Victor & Lear 1956). Motor weakness and sensory ataxia may be described as fatiguability and unsteadiness when walking.

Neurological signs were detailed by Healton et al. (1991) who reviewed 143 patients seen in two large centres over an 18-year period. Neurological signs were seen in 80%. Of these, diminished peripheral vibration sense was the most common sign, seen in nearly 90%, and best detected with a 256-Hz tuning fork (Herbert 1988). Impaired proprioception occurred only in those with diminished vibration sense. Cutaneous sensation was impaired in only four subjects where vibration sense was intact and a further two cases showed ataxia in the absence of impaired vibration sense. Weakness of the limbs, always in association with sensory deficits, and symmetrical in all but one case was seen in only 16. An extensor plantar reflex was found in 17 of 153. Deep tendon reflexes were unhelpful; increased, normal and decreased reflexes were all seen. Mental impairment, which earlier studies associated with more severe and prolonged deficiency, was seen in 18. These findings emphasise the importance of a thorough neurological examination including vibration sense testing in all patients suspected of vitamin B_{12} deficiency. The finding of these symptoms and signs without other identified cause arouse the suspicion of subacute combined degeneration of the cord in any psychiatric patient.

Pathology and other investigations
Pathological findings in the brains of patients dying with pernicious anaemia have been described since early in the twentieth century (Pfeiffer 1915). Adams and Kubik (1944) showed that the cerebral findings in patients with symptoms of suspiciousness, memory loss and confusion were similar to those seen in the spinal cord in subacute combined degen-

eration. EEG abnormalities are seen in a high proportion of cases of confirmed pernicious anaemia (Walton et al. 1954; Kunze & Leitenmaier 1976): mild abnormalities show as excessive slow activity, severe abnormalities as delta activity that is sometimes paroxysmal or focal. These abnormalities appear to bear no simple relationship to the severity of the anaemia but instead appear to reflect a specific defect of cerebral metabolism. Abnormal somatosensory-evoked potentials are frequently seen in subtle vitamin B_{12} deficiency, showing a pattern that suggests a central abnormality in at least half (Jones et al. 1987; Karnaze & Carmel 1990). The majority of EEG abnormalities are reversible with treatment, sometimes starting within 7–10 days of the first B_{12} injection. The few cases published also suggest an improvement in central and possibly peripheral somatosensory-evoked potential abnormalities with treatment. Structural T2-weighted MRI in a patient with pernicious anaemia and a 4-month history of progressive cognitive decline showed extensive areas of high-intensity signal in the periventricular white matter (Scherer 2003). A study using tensor-diffusion imaging in a similar patient showed reduced anisotropy in periventricular white matter tracts, suggesting that B_{12} deficiency was associated with white matter tract disruptions in this region (Kealey & Provenzale 2002).

Early metabolic studies also revealed impaired uptake of oxygen and glucose by the brain, especially in the presence of mental symptoms such as forgetfulness, confusion and disorientation, which again responded to replacement therapy (Scheinberg 1951). These were also unrelated to the severity of anaemia, appearing to be a specific result of B_{12} deficiency which suggests that similar disturbances of metabolism may occur in patients with low serum B_{12} even in the absence of pernicious anaemia. There appear to have been no modern studies using either functional MRI or PET that have investigated the effect of vitamin B_{12} deficiency on cerebral functioning.

These observations emphasise the importance of considering B_{12} deficiency in the differential diagnosis of all patients with unexplained acute organic reactions or cognitive impairment, and to pursue treatment vigorously at the earliest opportunity.

Routine screening
Currently there are no clear guidelines for the screening of patients presenting with psychiatric or cognitive disorders or the healthy elderly in whom high prevalences of individual or combined B_{12} and folate deficiencies have been described (Clarke et al. 2004). Chiu (1996) had suggested that all patients presenting with any degree of cognitive impairment be screened, especially if they have neurological or mild haematological signs of B_{12} deficiency. Within other psychiatric groups the situation is less clear, though it would seem sensible to consider B_{12} measurement in any patient presenting with abnormal mental state in association with

neurological signs such as unexplained impaired vibration sense or haematological changes such as anaemia, macrocytosis or neutrophil hypersegmentation. Any psychiatric patient with a history of gastric surgery or patients with regional ileitis or malabsorption syndromes such as steatorrhoea should also be screened. Low B_{12} levels are also common in vegans.

A further difficulty is determining which of the factors important in one-carbon metabolism to measure. Interactions between vitamin B_{12}, folate, homocysteine, methylmalonate, S-adenosylmethionine (SAM) and other components may lead to recommendations that multiple components be measured to obtain a clear picture of deficiency in any individual.

Treatment

Uncomplicated pernicious anaemia should be treated with intramuscular injections of hydroxocobalamin 1 mg three times a week for 2 weeks to replenish stores, then 1 mg every 3 months. With subacute combined degeneration of the cord, twice the loading dose is given in the early weeks of treatment, and this is equally advisable in patients with suspected cerebral involvement.

Folic acid deficiency

Folate, vitamins B_{12}, B_6 and B_2 and homocysteine, a sulphur-containing amino acid, are all components of the biochemical reactions involved in one-carbon metabolism. Accumulated data from the last four decades have implicated some or all of these components in abnormal development of the nervous system, in the increased risk of neurodegenerative conditions including stroke, Alzheimer's disease and Parkinson's disease, and in the pathogenesis of a number of psychiatric disorders, particularly folate in depression. A better understanding of the role of these individual components in neuronal homeostasis has led to new insights into the mechanisms through which deficiency of individual elements may disrupt these homeostatic mechanisms and lead to CNS dysfunction with consequent symptom expression.

The amino acid methionine plays a central role in one-carbon metabolism, a series of biosynthetic pathways crucial for DNA synthesis and repair and numerous other methylation reactions. Dietary methionine alone is insufficient to meet all of the body's methylation (one-carbon) requirements and additional methionine must be generated *de novo* from the one-carbon folate pool. Folate converts methionine to SAM, which is the major donor for most methyltransferase reactions. When folate levels are low, SAM is depleted. This leads to reduced DNA cytosine methylation, which results in hypomethylated DNA and enhanced gene transcription, and DNA strand breakage and may impair DNA repair mechanisms, leading to genetic mutations or the triggering of apoptosis (Mattson & Shea 2003). SAM also plays a role in the methylation of proteins, phospholipids and neurotransmitters.

Folate and vitamin B_{12} are also cofactors in the re-methylation of homocysteine to methionine and deficiency of either may lead to increased homocysteine levels. The nervous system has been shown to be particularly sensitive to extracellular homocysteine, which promotes neuronal excitotoxicity via stimulation of N-methyl-D-aspartate (NMDA) receptors and increases oxidative stress that results in neuronal DNA damage and triggering of apoptosis. For further details on the role of folate and homocysteine metabolism in neural plasticity see the review by Mattson and Shea (2003).

Deficiency of folate during pregnancy is associated with a greatly increased risk of neural tube defects whilst vitamin B_{12} deficiency is associated with elevated fetal homocysteine levels and increases the incidence of CNS developmental defects. Deficiency during infancy may result in psychomotor retardation, sensory neuropathy, severe hypotonia, seizures and apathy, which may result from impaired methylation.

Careful assessment of patients presenting to physicians or haematologists with megaloblastic anaemia due to either folate or vitamin B_{12} deficiency has shown that between half and two-thirds will have CNS complications responsive to appropriate vitamin-replacement therapy (Shorvon *et al.* 1980). These clinical manifestations have a considerable degree of overlap, although peripheral neuropathy and acute combined degeneration of the cord are seen more frequently with vitamin B_{12} deficiency and depression with deficiency of folate. In one series of 24 patients admitted medically for severe folate deficiency, an organic brain syndrome including depression was present in 71% compared with 31% of controls (Reynolds 1973). Historical reports from the beginning of the twentieth century suggest that if left untreated all patients will go on to develop similar complications (Reynolds 1979).

Numerous studies over the last 40 years have shown a high incidence of folate deficiency in psychiatric patient groups, especially those with depression and in the mentally unwell elderly. Many of the earlier studies used serum folate levels, which are known to be lowered by a number of medications and by alcohol, though more recent studies using more reliable red-cell folate measurement have shown similar findings (Reynolds 2002). Carney *et al.* (1990) surveyed 285 consecutive patients seen in a psychiatric unit and found borderline (<200 μg/L) and definite (<150 μg/L) red cell folate deficiency in 31% and 12% of patients respectively. The levels in patients with depression were significantly lower than in other groups, but patients with alcohol dependency were also severely affected. The prevalence of folate deficiency in the elderly and results of studies suggesting an association between folate deficiency and cognitive decline are discussed in the section below.

In all such surveys it is hard to assess the causal significance of the low folate found. In the majority of cases deficient nutrition may have been responsible and, as with B_{12} deficiency, this may often be secondary to the mental disorder itself. Should a causal relationship between folate deficiency and psychiatric disturbance exist it is also quite probable that this will impair food intake still further and establish a vicious circle. Regardless of direction of causality, several studies have shown that folate replacement is associated with a greater improvement in mental state (Carney & Sheffield 1970; Coppen et al. 1986). Godfrey et al. (1990) reported a double-blind placebo-controlled trial of adding methylfolate to standard psychotropic medication in 41 patients with low red cell folate, 24 with depression and 17 with schizophrenia. Methylfolate supplementation was associated with significant improvement in clinical outcome in both patient groups, which was more evident at 6 months than at 3 months. Subsequent studies have focused predominantly on the role of folate replacement in depression as discussed below.

Depression

The first reports of an association between folate deficiency and depression appeared in the 1960s with the development of reliable assays for folate (Alpert et al. 2000). Shorvon et al. (1980) examined the mental state of general medical patients presenting with megaloblastic anaemia due to either B_{12} or folate deficiency and found depression to be the commonest disturbance, occurring in 50% of the low folate group compared with 20% of those with B_{12} deficiency. Depressive symptoms have featured prominently in series of patients with folate deficiency associated with a number of different aetiologies, including malabsorption (Botez & Reynolds 1979), anticonvulsant-treated epilepsy (Edeh & Toone 1985), megaloblastic anaemia (Shorvon et al. 1980) and dietary restriction (Herbert 1961).

Conversely more than 20, mainly case–control, studies have shown low folate levels in patients with psychiatric disorders, especially those with depression (Alpert et al. 2000). Findings of the newer studies that use red blood cell folate assays, which are more indicative of intracellular stores, are generally comparable, showing that up to one-third of depressed patients have deficient or low folate levels (Carney et al. 1990; Godfrey et al. 1990; Bottiglieri et al. 2000). Bottiglieri et al. (2000) showed that this was invariably associated with evidence of functional deficiency, reflected by raised homocysteine levels. Furthermore, those with high plasma homocysteine had significantly lower concentrations of SAM and the monoamine metabolites of serotonin, dopamine and noradrenaline (i.e. 5-HIAA, homovanillic acid and 3-methoxy-4-hydroxyphenylglycol) in the CSF. There is also evidence to suggest that patients with depression who are also folate deficient may have more severe affective disorders and respond less well to conventional treatment

(Reynolds et al. 1970). Placebo-controlled trials have shown an improvement in mood at 4 months after treatment with 15 mg folic acid daily (Botez & Reynolds 1979) and double-blind placebo-controlled trials have shown improved affective morbidity after 1 year of 200 µg folic acid daily in patients with bipolar disorder treated with lithium (Coppen et al. 1986). Addition of 500 µg of folic acid to fluoxetine also significantly improved antidepressant response at 10 weeks in women in one study (Coppen & Bailey 2000).

However, population-based cross-sectional studies investigating the association between components of the one-carbon metabolic pathway and depression have found a much weaker association between depression and low folate. Bjelland et al. (2003) in a large study of nearly 6000 middle-aged and elderly subjects found no association of depression with either low folate or vitamin B_{12}, although hyperhomocysteinaemia (odds ratio 1.90) and the T/T MTHFR genotype (odds ratio 1.69) were both significantly associated. Tiemeier et al. (2002) in a large group of elderly subjects from Holland found only a mild non-significant association between depression and low serum folate, although a stronger association with vitamin B_{12} deficiency and raised homocysteine was seen. Significant associations between depression and raised methylmalonic acid and non-significant association with low vitamin B_{12} but not folate were also reported in findings from the Women's Health and Aging Study (Penninx et al. 2000). A recent Cochrane systematic review of the use of folate in depression concluded that the limited evidence suggests that folate may have a potential role as a supplement to other treatments for depression (Taylor et al. 2003).

Together these studies suggest that the association between folate and other components of the one-carbon metabolic pathway and depression are much more complicated than was previously thought. The observation that the MTHFR T/T genotype confers increased risk suggests that altered vitamin B status may be a risk factor for, rather than the result of, depression and signals the need for prospective and adequately sized double-blind studies. A causal relationship between folate deficiency and depression is also consistent with biogenic theories of affective disorder. Methylfolate is required for the synthesis of SAM which, as discussed earlier, is involved in numerous methylation reactions in the nervous system, including the synthesis of monoamines and other neurotransmitters. Moreover, SAM has been shown to have antidepressant properties of its own (Reynolds et al. 1984; Reynolds 1991).

Dementia

CSF folate levels are several times higher than in serum, suggesting that folic acid is likely to be important in cerebral metabolism. Occasional case reports have pointed to a close relationship between folic acid deficiency and organic psychiatric illness. Anand (1964) described a patient with megaloblastic anaemia, myelopathy, impairment of memory and moderate dementia of 'frontal lobe type', who showed no response to B_{12} but improved in all respects after starting folic acid. Read *et al.* (1965) similarly described an 82-year-old patient with megaloblastic anaemia due to nutritional deficiency in whom mental confusion and double incontinence improved with folic acid. Two further striking examples were provided by Strachan and Henderson (1967), both with advanced dementia. In each case the folate deficiency followed chronic malnutrition, and the dementia responded gradually to treatment with folic acid; there was a coincident megaloblastic anaemia in both cases but the blood picture returned to normal several months before the mental symptoms resolved. However, in view of the relative frequency of folate deficiency, especially in the elderly, these presentations with severe mental impairment appear to be a rare feature of folate deficiency (Melamed 1979).

Absolute or functional deficiency of folate has been shown to be quite a frequent finding in both healthy and mentally unwell elderly populations. In a case–control study in 164 patients with Alzheimer's disease, Clarke *et al.* (1998) found a significant association between raised homocysteine, low folate and vitamin B_{12} levels and cognitive decline. A prospective population-based study in 370 healthy Swedish individuals over 75 years old showed that the presence of folate or vitamin B_{12} deficiency doubled the risk of subsequently developing Alzheimer's disease (Wang *et al.* 2001). Meanwhile Reynolds *et al.* (1973) showed that among patients presenting in a general hospital with very low folate levels, cognitive abnormalities were significantly commoner than in controls, whilst a study in a community of healthy elderly subjects, many with folate levels within the normal range, folate levels correlated with measures of cognitive impairment (Goodwin *et al.* 1983). Similar considerations to those described above in non-elderly populations need to be borne in mind in the interpretation of these findings. Low folate levels have been found in association with depression, which may also be a precursor to cognitive decline; however, poor nutrition resulting from the disease process can also be found in both of these groups.

A recent UK population-based cross-sectional analysis of 3511 people over the age of 65 years showed that conventional folate deficiency (<5 nmol/L) or functional folate deficiency (serum folate <7 nmol/L and homocysteine >20 µmol/L) was present in 1 in 20 people aged between 65 and 74 years and in almost 1 in 10 of those aged over 75. Similar prevalences of vitamin B_{12} deficiency were also found (Clarke *et al.* 2004). These authors highlight the association between low folate and raised homocysteine as a risk factor in ischaemic heart disease and stroke (Homocysteine Studies Collaboration 2002).

Schizophrenia and epilepsy

A small case–control study investigated homocysteine levels in folate-deficient patients with schizophrenia and normal controls and showed that homocysteine levels were higher in schizophrenia (Susser *et al.* 1998). It has been argued that homocysteine may mediate the effects of folate and B_{12} deficiencies in schizophrenia because elevated levels in this group are not always associated with conventional folate or B_{12} deficiency. Genetic analyses have suggested that individuals with the C677T polymorphism in the gene encoding the MTHFR enzyme, which is present in 10–12% of the population and associated with a 70% reduction in enzyme activity leading to folate-resistant increase in homocysteine levels, contributes to cases of schizophrenia (Regland 1997). Clinical improvement with folate supplementation in schizophrenia has also been shown in a randomised placebo-controlled trial (Godfrey *et al.* 1990).

Laboratory work in animal models of epilepsy has shown that folates at high concentrations in the peripheral circulation or injected intraventricularly have excitatory properties and can induce seizures (Reynolds 2002). The recognition that a number of antiepileptic medications, such as phenytoin, primidone and phenobarbital, were associated with lowering of folate levels and folate-replacement therapy with reports of increased seizure frequency led to the suggestion that this antifolate effect may be responsible for their efficacy (Smith & Obbens 1979). Whilst it is now widely acknowledged that this is not the principal mechanism of action of these or other antiepileptic medications, evidence that folate may block or reverse γ-aminobutyric acid (GABA)-mediated inhibition may explain their observed excitatory properties (Reynolds 1991).

Treatment

Replacement with folic acid 5 mg three times daily should be implemented in the face of biochemically confirmed folate deficiency; lower doses (400 µg) are used for prophylaxis of neural tube defects in women wishing to become pregnant. However, replacement of folate should always be preceded by screening for B_{12} deficiency, B_{12} levels tend to fall when folic acid is started (Reynolds *et al.* 1971), and there is a risk of precipitating neurological disturbances by giving folic acid to patients with undiagnosed pernicious anaemia. There are no clear guidelines for the appropriate dose, formulation or duration of folate therapy for neuropsychiatric disorders associated with deficiency. Well-constructed, randomised, placebo-controlled trials will be needed before recommendations in this area can be made.

Electrolyte disturbances

A delicate balance must be maintained in the chemical environment, both intracellularly and extracellularly, to maintain the proper functioning of the CNS. With regard to this balance, certain relatively simple components have been identified: the correct acid–base balance, the proper gradient of sodium and potassium across the cell membrane, and the correct concentration of calcium, magnesium and phosphate. These factors may be disturbed separately or together in many disease processes and mental symptoms may follow.

The metabolic dynamics involved in the production of mental symptoms are often complex, since disturbance of one aspect of electrolyte balance can have repercussions on others. Alterations in cerebral blood flow may follow and complicate the situation further. Nevertheless, the correct appreciation of the primary disturbance is of the utmost importance if appropriate treatment is to follow.

Electrolyte disturbance plays a prominent part in certain endocrine disorders and in uraemia. It complicates respiratory disorders and can assume great importance postoperatively or in other situations when patients are maintained on intravenous fluids for long periods of time.

Hypernatraemia

Hypernatraemia may develop from either excess water loss or decreased water intake, usually in the context of impaired consciousness, when the powerful thirst drive is impaired, or immobility. As serum osmolarity rises, water shifts from the intracellular to the extracellular spaces; therefore small increases in serum sodium or osmolarity reflect a large reduction in total body water. In environments of extreme heat, in fever, burns and conditions associated with hyperventilation, insensible water loss from the skin and lungs may reach several litres a day. Hypernatraemia will only develop if water replacement is unable to match these losses. The commonest cause of hypernatraemia is water loss through the kidneys, due to diuretics, osmotic diuresis or diabetes insipidus. ADH deficiency, excessive mineralocorticoid activity and rarely excess sodium intake (e.g. in the preparation of infant formula) are other causes of hypernatraemia. Sudden development of hypernatraemia may develop in acute pituitary failure.

In the context of preserved consciousness, hypernatraemia is associated with intense thirst. Hypernatraemia presents most commonly clinically in the very young or old and in those unable to express their needs due to impaired conscious level. Clinically, hypernatraemia is associated with dryness of the mouth, a greyish complexion and weight loss. The plasma sodium, chloride and urea tend to rise. Homeostatic brain mechanisms limit neuronal shrinkage by stimulating the synthesis of intracellular organic osmolytes, especially myoinositol, that serve to limit neuronal water efflux (Pasantes-Morales 1996). As water loss outstrips homeostatic mechanisms, patients develop increasing mental confusion and lethargy that gives way to delirium and coma (Swanson 1976). There is an increase in muscle tone. Brain shrinkage may be associated with tearing of bridging veins and hypernatraemia with venous thrombosis in the sagittal or other sinuses (Luttrell & Finberg 1959). Seizures may occur as a result of these complications (Bruck et al. 1968) or during rehydration, possibly as a result

of osmotic swelling of neurones. Central pontine myelinolysis is another complication associated with over-rapid rehydration.

The elderly are especially at risk in view of their narrow limits of physiological balance, diminished capacity for renal tubular absorption, and liability to chronic debilitating disease. Jana and Romano-Jana (1973) have described four cases of 'hypernatraemic psychosis' in which elderly patients were admitted to a psychiatric hospital in a confused and disorientated state.

Hyponatraemia

Hypotonic hyponatraemia is due to either primary water gain, with secondary sodium loss, or primary sodium depletion, with secondary water gain. Causes of primary sodium loss include:
• burns;
• prolonged sweating in tropical climates;
• gastrointestinal losses due to prolonged vomiting, fistulae, obstruction with tube drainage and diarrhoea;
• renal causes such as diuretics (especially thiazides), osmotic diuresis, Addison's disease, salt-wasting nephropathy and acute non-oliguric tubular necrosis.

The classic symptoms and signs of heat exhaustion include weakness, dizziness, pallor, profuse sweating, diminution of urine, rapid pulse and respiration, low blood pressure and cramping pains in the abdomen and limbs. The onset is usually sudden, and the response to sodium chloride by mouth is dramatic. However, the picture can be misleading when it sets in very gradually.

Primary water gain in the presence of normovolaemia is most commonly caused by SIADH. Common causes of SIADH are CNS disorders such as meningitis, encephalitis, haemorrhage, stroke, tumours or head injury; pulmonary diseases such as pneumonia, empyema, tuberculosis and carcinoma; malignant tumours especially those of lung, duodenum and pancreas; and pharmacological agents including hypoglycaemics, thiazide diuretics and psychotropics (see under Distinguishing primary polydipsia from diabetes insipidus, earlier). Adrenal insufficiency and hypothyroidism may also cause hyponatraemia. An important cause of primary water gain in psychiatric patients is compulsive water drinking, when water intake may overwhelm the renal excretory capacity (see also section cited above).

The clinical manifestations of hyponatraemia are principally neuropsychiatric, related to osmotic water shifts that lead to increased intracranial fluid volume and cerebral oedema. Symptoms depend on the rate of onset and the absolute serum sodium level, with symptoms much more likely to occur if hyponatraemia develops rapidly. Nausea, vomiting, anorexia and malaise are common early symptoms with marked lassitude and change of mood. With further reduction in sodium, headache, confusion and blurring of vision may occur, then impairment of consciousness, delirium and coma. Muscle twitches and cramps are sometimes seen, and seizures, usually generalised, occur with sodium levels below 120 mmol/L (Price & Mesulam 1987).

Treatment consists of giving salt by mouth or, when necessary, intravenous saline. The administration of water alone or glucose in water can be dangerous, as the hypotonicity is aggravated further. Over-rapid correction of severe hyponatraemia risks causing central pontine myelinosis. Retrospective studies have led to the recommendation that the rate of rise in serum sodium should be limited to <12 mmol/L in the first 24 hours and 25 mmol/L in the first 48 hours (Sterns *et al.* 1986); however even at these rates myelinolysis has been described (Karp 1995).

Hypokalaemia

Hypokalaemia may result from decreased intake, shift into cells or increased loss. A common cause is inadequate replacement in patients maintained for long periods on intravenous fluids. With the exception of chronic starvation and anorexia, and possibly the elderly on poor diets, diminished intake is seldom the sole cause, with the amount of K^+ in the diet almost always exceeding that excreted in the urine. Movement of K^+ intracellularly may transiently decrease serum K^+ and may be seen after myocardial infarction, in hypokalaemic periodic paralysis, and when diabetic ketosis is treated vigorously with insulin infusions. Increased loss may occur through the gastrointestinal tract or the kidneys. Gastrointestinal causes include hyperemesis gravidarum, chronic diarrhoea due to ulcerative colitis, malabsorption syndromes such as steatorrhoea, or via long-term laxative abuse. Renal causes include K^+ wasting associated with Cushing's disease and Conn's syndrome, the massive diuresis that may arise in diabetes mellitus, the diuretic phase following acute renal failure, and the rare Liddle's syndrome, in association with renal tubular acidosis and Bartter's syndrome. It may also result from the administration of diuretics, ACTH or adrenal steroids.

The clinical manifestations of hypokalaemia vary greatly between individuals and depend on the severity of hypokalaemia. Symptoms seldom develop until K^+ is less than 3 mmol/L. Fatigue, myalgia and proximal muscle weakness are common, although cranial nerve-innervated muscles are typically spared. More severe hypokalaemia is associated with progressive weakness and eventually complete flaccid paralysis. Smooth muscle may also be affected and presents with constipation, abdominal distention or paralytic ileus. Lethargy, apathy and depression, which can be profound in degree, are common accompaniments.

Apprehension and irritability are sometimes marked and an anxiety state may be simulated. Emotionally induced hyperventilation may be thought to be responsible for paraesthesiae, vague muscle discomfort and transient visual disturbances. Very occasionally a typical acute organic reac-

tion is seen, with disorientation, confusion, impairment of memory and delirium. In familial periodic paralysis emotional stress may precipitate an attack. Mitchell and Feldman (1968) report an example of a patient with renal tubular acidosis who was first thought to show a conversion disorder.

> A woman of 30 complained of marked weakness of the arms and legs after a fall some hours earlier, and was unable to walk. There was a long previous history of anorexia, occasional vomiting, constipation and muscle spasms, and there had been several similar falls in preceding months. Marital difficulties were prominent and a conversion disorder was diagnosed. She slowly regained strength and was discharged after 4 days. One month later she was readmitted with extreme weakness of several hours' duration, and complained of sleeping excessively and frequent headaches. The serum potassium was low at 2.4 mmol/L but again spontaneous recovery occurred. Two days later there were similar complaints, the serum potassium was 1.8 mmol/L and the ECG showed typical changes. There had been no evidence of impairment of consciousness at any stage.

The ECG shows characteristic changes due to delayed ventricular repolarisation though these do not correlate well with plasma K^+ concentration. Early changes include flattening or inversion of the T wave, a prominent U wave, ST-segment depression and a prolonged QT interval.

Oral replacement with potassium chloride or bicarbonate is generally safest though nasogastric or intravenous infusion of potassium chloride may be needed if oral intake is impossible, and should be undertaken very cautiously. Normal saline is ideally used, as dextrose solutions promote insulin-mediated movement of K^+ into cells.

Hyperkalaemia

Potassium homeostasis is largely dependent on renal function and hence significant hyperkalaemia is mainly seen in renal failure. Severe Addisonian crises, acidosis, with or without insulin deficiency, and the use of drugs such as potassium-sparing diuretics and angiotensin-converting enzyme inhibitors are other associations. Cardiac toxicity precludes the appearance of nervous system manifestations in most cases, with bradycardia due to heart block, ventricular dysrhythmia or fibrillation and ultimately ventricular asystole (Riggs 1989). The most frequent neurological manifestation is diffuse muscle weakness and fatiguability akin to that seen with potassium depletion, which may rarely progress to a flaccid quadraparesis. This is most striking seen in association with Addison's disease.

Potassium channel antibody disorders

Diseases of potassium channels are caused by either autoantibodies against potassium channels or mutations in their encoding genes (Buckley 2005). Benign neonatal febrile convulsions, hereditary deafness syndromes, neuromyotonia, episodic ataxia, and intractable epilepsy have all been associated with mutations in voltage-gated potassium channels (VGKCs). The neurological syndromes associated with elevated potassium channel antibodies range from pure peripheral nerve hyperexcitability (PNH) to syndromes confined to the CNS such as limbic encephalitis. There can be varying degrees of CNS, autonomic and peripheral involvement.

The spectrum of PNH ranges from mild cramp fasciculation syndrome to more disabling neuromyotonia. In neuromyotonia there is muscle twitching and cramps, often associated with increased sweating. There may be sensory symptoms, especially dysaesthesia without numbness, which is probably a consequence of hyperexcitability of the sensory nerves (Buckley 2005). Occasionally, there is hand posturing resembling dystonia. On examination, there is visible myokymia (severe twitching) and muscle cramps often accompanied by muscle hypertrophy. Electromyography reveals fibrillations and fasciculation potentials at rest and a characteristic pattern of multiple responses to a single stimulus. The serum creatine kinase level may be elevated, and VGKC antibodies are elevated in 40% of patients. The clinical syndromes in patients with and without antibodies are indistinguishable. Hart *et al*. (2002) have classified PNH syndromes using the following characteristics:

- can be an isolated disorder or occur with CNS features;
- can be paraneoplastic, e.g. with thymomas;
- can be associated with other peripheral neuropathies or with other autoimmune diseases (e.g. myasthenia, systemic lupus erythematosus);
- can be non-immune-mediated (e.g. in motor neurone disease) or mediated by toxins or gold;
- can result from either gene mutations or other hereditary syndromes.

VGKC antibodies have also been identified in patients with non-paraneoplastic limbic encephalitis. Vincent *et al*. (2004) described 10 patients with limbic encephalitis associated with potassium channel antibodies, and Thieben *et al*. (2004) described seven such patients. These patients had a profound amnesic syndrome and were positive for potassium channel antibodies. On MRI, there was commonly signal alteration or atrophy in the medial temporal lobes bilaterally (8 of 10 cases in the Vincent *et al*. series). Only one of these patients had neuromyotonia (PNH), but epileptic seizures were common (6 of 7 cases in the Thieben *et al*. series). There was some evidence of improved cognition in these patients on treatment with steroids, plasma exchange and/or intraveneous immunogobulins.

Morvan (1890) described a syndrome of 'fibrillary chorea' that involved severe muscle twitching (myokymia), muscle pain and cramps, excessive sweating and disordered sleep. This syndrome has now been associated with the presence of VGKC antibodies, and the syndrome can now be used to describe a small group of patients with overlapping peripheral, autonomic and CNS involvement. For example, Liguori *et al*. (2001) described a 76-year-old man with peripheral muscle weakness and fasciculation. In the autonomic nervous system, he displayed sweating, itching, cardiac arrhythmias, weight loss, lacrimation, salivation, urinary incontinence and constipation. With respect to the CNS, there was confusion, memory impairment, visual and auditory hallucinations, and insomnia. Potassium channel antibodies were strongly positive. The sleep EEG was dominated by wakefulness, with only short (<1 minute) atypical rapid-eye-movement phases without spindles, K complexes or delta waves. The patient died 26 months after onset. These authors showed that the antibodies bound strongly to neuronal dendrites in rat hippocampus and thalamus. Lee *et al*. (1998) described a similar patient with a much better response to plasmapheresis, immunosuppression and thymectomy. Toosey *et al*. (2005) have recently reported a patient with similar peripheral and autonomic symptoms, but with a different pattern of CNS symptoms. This patient manifested severe frontal behavioural and neuropsychological changes, including confabulation, associated with corresponding hypometabolism on fluorodeoxyglucose-PET in the ventromedial frontal region.

Hypercalcaemia

The clinical manifestations of hypercalcaemia are described in the section on hyperparathyroidism (earlier in chapter). Severe hypercalcaemia is usually caused by malignancy or hyperparathyroidism. Sarcoidosis, adrenal insufficiency, thiazide administration, hyperthyroidism, vitamin D intoxication and milk-alkali syndrome (prolonged ingestion of calcium especially when taken as milk with an antacid) are other rarer causes. Solid tumours, especially squamous cell carcinoma of the lung and carcinomas of the breast and kidney with secondary bone deposits, multiple myeloma and lymphoma are the commonest associated malignancies. Hypercalcaemia associated with malignancy is often due to a combination of increased bone turnover secondary to high levels of tumorally produced parathyroid-related peptide and direct malignant destruction of bone by tumoral invasion (Waxman 1990). Long-term treatment with lithium may very occasionally produce hypercalcaemia by elevating the level of PTH (Christiansen *et al*. 1976).

The severity of symptoms depends on the serum calcium concentration and the associated medical conditions. Changes in mental status commonly occur with serum calcium above 14 mg/dL (3.2 mmol/L). Petersen (1968) reported six examples, mostly due to vitamin D intoxication, with clinical pictures similar to those seen with hyperparathyroidism. Thirst, asthaenia, depression and tension states were the main manifestations, and three showed acute organic psychoses. Weizman *et al.* (1979) reported that 7 of 12 patients with hypercalcaemia of malignancy had prominent psychiatric symptoms. Three showed depression or anxiety, sometimes severe, three developed acute organic reactions and one an acute paranoid psychosis. In all cases the mental symptoms disappeared within 2–6 days of serum calcium being restored to normal. Severe hypercalcaemia with impaired consciousness is more common in malignancy than hyperparathyroidism.

Hypocalcaemia

Hypocalcaemia may result from a deficiency of calcium or vitamin D in the diet, producing rickets in children and osteomalacia in adults. Hypoparathyroidism, acute pancreatitis, rhabdomyolysis and severe liver or renal disease are other possible causes. Anticonvulsant therapy is a cause of hypocalcaemia in patients with epilepsy. Acute severe forms are usually the sequelae of thyroid or parathyroid surgery, or arise as a complication of acute pancreatitis (Riggs 1989).

In children there is a characteristic triad of convulsions, laryngeal stridor and carpopedal spasm (see Hypoparathyroidism, Physical features, earlier). In adults the most important signs are those of neuromuscular irritability: increased deep tendon reflexes and positive Chvostek's and Trousseau's signs. Seizures are the main complication of acute severe hypocalcaemia and are more likely to occur in those with pre-existing epilepsy. Common psychiatric manifestations are described in the section on hypoparathyroidism (see Hypoparathyroidism).

Hypomagnesaemia

Magnesium is predominantly an intracellular ion with less than 10% in the extracellular space, and therefore low serum magnesium usually reflects a severe deficit in whole-body magnesium. Its presence in many foods makes deficiency in normal individuals rare. The most common causes of deficiency are severe protein calorie malnutrition, diabetic ketoacidosis, renal losses secondary to renal tubular necrosis (Hayes *et al.* 1979), sepsis, chronic alcohol dependency, in association with hypocalcaemia, and secondary to the use of drugs such as loop diuretics, aminoglycoside, cisplatin and ciclosporin that lower body stores. The main effects of low magnesium are on cellular membrane function. Calcium, potassium and chloride channel currents are modified and magnesium ions also reversibly occlude the ion channels associated with the excitatory NMDA glutamate receptor. In addition magnesium is involved in many enzyme systems, including those for intermediary metabolism, biosynthesis

of nucleic acids, proteins and lipids, and most systems that require adenosine triphosphate (Pappius 1976).

The clinical picture may be identical to that seen with hypocalcaemia, with hyperexcitability, muscle cramps, carpopedal spasm, tetany with Chvostek's and Trousseau's signs, hyperreflexia and seizures (Vallee *et al.* 1960). Serum calcium may be normal and parenteral magnesium sulphate promptly abolish the symptoms. Other clinical pictures that have been described include convulsions, depression, irritability, vertigo, ataxia and muscle weakness in the absence of tetany (Hanna *et al.* 1960); myoclonic jerks and bizarre multifocal seizures (Fishman 1965); tremors, fasciculation, chorea, athetoid movements, focal signs such as hemiparesis and aphasia, mild confusion and disorientation, delirium of sudden onset and stupor (Flink 1956; Hammarsten & Smith 1957; Randall *et al.* 1959; Hall 1973). All may be reversed by intramuscular or intravenous magnesium sulphate. In one study from the 1960s (Flink 1969) that would struggle to receive ethical committee approval today, volunteers were kept on magnesium-deficient diets for many months. Lethargy, tremors, fasciculations and spontaneous carpopedal spasms developed and all responded to magnesium replacement. However, all symptomatic subjects also developed secondary calcium depletion despite adequate intake and absorption, as well as hypokalaemia, making the specific contribution of magnesium deficiency alone difficult to determine.

Hypermagnesaemia

Clinically significant hypermagnesaemia is rare, mainly occurring as a result of excessive intake in the context of chronic renal failure. Case reports of hypermagnesaemia arising secondary to abuse of laxatives and/or antacids have also been described (Castelbaum *et al.* 1989).

Deep tendon reflexes are lost at lower serum magnesium levels before CNS depression develops, and neuromuscular paralysis may precede the clinical recognition of encephalopathy. Lethargy and confusion are common early manifestations (Alfrey *et al.* 1970) and may progress to areflexia, flaccid neuromuscular paralysis including facially innervated and respiratory muscles, parasympathetic paralysis and coma (Rizzo *et al.* 1993). This may mimic a brainstem stroke and serum magnesium levels should be measured in any patient with renal failure who develops encephalopathy with weakness and areflexia.

Serum magnesium levels have also been investigated in patients with schizophrenia (Kirov *et al.* 1994). Elevated magnesium has often been reported, but also lowered or normal levels, and the literature remains inconsistent (see Alexander & Jackson 1981 for a review).

Hypophosphataemia

Hypophosphataemia is defined as a serum phosphate of less than 0.83 mmol/L and severe hypophosphataemia as a serum phosphate of less than 0.5 mmol/L. Like magnesium and potassium, phosphate is predominantly an intracellular cation, and low serum levels may not necessarily reflect low body stores. Most free phosphate is bound to calcium in bone. Its central role is in cellular energy and enzymatic processes, existing intracellularly predominantly as adenosine monophosphate, diphosphate and triphosphate (AMP, ADP, ATP) or as creatine phosphate. In hypoxia phosphate activates phosphofructokinase, the enzyme that controls glycolysis, and stimulates anaerobic metabolism.

Hypophosphataemia may arise from loss of total body phosphate or more commonly from shifts into the cellular compartment from the serum, a situation encountered in the treatment of diabetic ketoacidosis, when refeeding patients following a period of starvation, and in the management of chronic alcoholics (Territo & Tanaka 1973). In the latter case, hypophosphataemia may be at its worst 10 days after admission and the re-instigation of regular nutrition (Knochel 1977). Hypophosphataemia may affect all levels of the nervous system. The mechanism of CNS dysfunction is uncertain. Tissue hypoxia compounded by reduced cerebral blood flow due to decreased red cell 2,3-diphosphoglycerate may be causal, though in clinical practice coexisting disorders such as alcoholism and hypomagnesaemia make it difficult to determine the main factors involved.

Clinically, patients with hypophosphataemia may present with an acute confusional state with irritability and apprehension or with variable motor abnormalities including ataxia, athetosis, myoclonus, weakness, paralysis with loss of peripheral reflexes or a syndrome resembling Guillain–Barré. Lethargy, distal paraesthesiae, dysarthria and abnormal respiratory patterns may also be early features (Prins *et al.* 1973). A syndrome of impaired eye movements, confusion and ataxia resembling Wernicke's encephalopathy has also been described and hypophosphataemia should be considered in patients presenting with a clinical picture of Wernicke's who fail to respond to thiamine (Vanneste & Hage 1986). Reversible coma with and without seizures and cranial nerve areflexia and a reversible paralysis of movements resembling brain death have also been described (Young *et al.* 1982).

While replacing phosphate orally or if necessary parenterally, parenteral nutrition should be temporarily stopped until CNS symptoms resolve. If supplementation is required, milk that contains high levels of phosphate is advised. Magnesium supplementation should also be considered, as hypomagnesaemia will contribute to high urinary losses.

Low serum zinc

Zinc deficiency is rare but occurs in certain malnourished populations and in countries where bread with a high phytate content is consumed. It can be found with regional enteritis and with malabsorption syndromes. The excretion of zinc is increased in liver disease, diabetes, some renal diseases and with certain drugs (Anon. 1973).

The syndrome most closely tied to low serum zinc is diminished acuity of taste and smell (hyposmia, hypogeusia), first described by Henkin *et al.* (1971) and shown to be responsive to the administration of oral zinc sulphate. Many such patients had developed the hypogeusia soon after a respiratory illness, while in others it appeared spontaneously. The strong perversions of taste and smell that were sometimes present could precipitate emotional disturbance including profound depression.

Henkin *et al.* (1975) monitored the low serum zinc produced by histidine in the treatment of six patients with progressive systemic sclerosis. The authors were able to follow the sequential appearance of anorexia, dysfunction of taste and smell, and ultimately the development of neurological and psychiatric features. The patients became dizzy and unsteady, with cerebellar symptoms in the form of ataxic gait and intention tremor. Several were irritable and easily upset, with depression and periods of weeping. Others showed memory impairments, lethargy, auditory and visual hallucinations and pronounced emotional lability. The disturbances correlated with the degree of lowering of serum zinc and with indicators of total body zinc loss. All were quickly reversed following the administration of zinc sulphate.

Staton *et al.* (1976) described a young male patient presenting with a picture resembling catatonic schizophrenia who responded rapidly to zinc administration after failing to respond to other treatments. He had presented with auditory and visual hallucinations, loose associations, blunted affect and disorientation in time and place. Drooling, negativism and catatonic postures became established. Phenothiazines were ineffective and led to severe extrapyramidal disturbance. After some months electroconvulsive therapy was tried and produced only transient improvement. A low serum zinc and high serum copper were discovered and oral zinc sulphate and pyridoxine were commenced. Thenceforward he made excellent progress and remained well 1 year later.

Acid–base disturbances

Systemic arterial pH is tightly maintained between 7.35 and 7.45 by buffering systems together with respiratory and renal regulatory mechanisms. Common clinical disturbances are simple acid–base disorders due to metabolic or respiratory causes; more rarely mixed pictures may develop.

ketoacids in diabetes mellitus), loss of bicarbonate (as
seen in hyperchloraemic acidosis associated with chronic
diarrhoea) or accumulation of endogenous acids (in renal
failure). Ingestion of exogenous acids (e.g. salicylates) produces a more complex picture associated with increased
lactic acid production. The most prominent result is stimulation of the respiratory centre with deep and rapid respiration. Consciousness is progressively impaired and mental
confusion or delirium is seen in varying degree. The precise
clinical picture in the individual case is largely determined
by the underlying condition and other associated metabolic
derangements.

Respiratory acidosis (hypercapnia) provides a more distinctive clinical picture. Inhalation of 6–7% carbon dioxide
can be shown to impair psychological functioning and lead
to perseverative responses. In chronic respiratory disease
mental dulling and drowsiness are common, and it is well
known that if high-concentration oxygen is given to rapidly
correct hypercapnia, respiratory drive can paradoxically be
reduced further, precipitating mental confusion, irrational
behaviour and impairing consciousness. Oxygen therapy
should therefore be titrated carefully in chronic obstructive
lung disease and chronic carbon dioxide retention.

Clinical features vary according to the severity and duration of the respiratory acidosis, the underlying disease and
whether there is associated hypoxia. Chronic hypercapnia is
associated with sleep disturbance, complaints of memory
impairment, daytime somnolence, personality change,
impairment of coordination, and motor disturbances including tremor, myoclonic jerks and asterixis (Kasper & Harrison
2004). Westlake et al. (1955) reviewed the clinical findings in
carbon dioxide retention due to emphysema. Mental disturbances were usually present when the blood pH was below
7.2 or the $Paco_2$ above 10.6 kPa, and ranged from mild impairment of consciousness, with irritability, disorientation and
confusion, to delirium with auditory and visual hallucinations. Headache, muscle twitching and sweating were
common accompaniments. When the pH fell below 7.1 or the
$Paco_2$ rose above 13.1 kPa, there was increasing lethargy and
drowsiness leading ultimately to coma. Intracranial pressure was often raised, and papilloedema was sometimes
seen. The disturbances were usually transient, because the
pH is ultimately restored by renal activity, but in a minority
of cases the outcome could be fatal.

The mental changes are thought to be due to the direct
action of acidaemia or hypercapnia on the metabolism of
cortical neurones. The rise of intracranial pressure is ascribed
to the accompanying cerebral vasodilatation. The EEG
shows delta waves, sometimes paroxysmal or episodic, at
high arterial levels of carbon dioxide.

Uraemia

Uraemia may result from primary disease of the kidneys or
from extrarenal causes. Any process resulting in prolonged

Alkalosis

Metabolic alkalosis usually results from the loss of acid, most
commonly as HCl due to repeated vomiting, or rarely from
the ingestion of large quantities of sodium bicarbonate given,
for example, in the treatment of peptic ulcer. Central and
peripheral nervous system symptoms and signs such as
apathy, delirium and stupor, a predisposition to seizures,
paraesthesiae, muscular cramping and tetany occur that are
similar to those of hypocalcaemia, because the proportion of
ionised calcium is reduced even though the total serum
calcium is normal.

An important cause of respiratory alkalosis from the psychiatric point of view is overbreathing. Attacks of hyperventilation are common in anxiety disorders especially at times
of stress and in panic disorder. Hyperventilation also follows
the ingestion of large quantities of salicylates.

The effects of respiratory alkalosis vary according to severity and duration but are primarily those of the underlying
disease. Rapid decrease in $Paco_2$ may cause dizziness, mental
confusion and seizures even in the absence of hypoxaemia
(Kasper & Harrison 2004). Experimental studies show that
hyperventilation increases suggestibility and facilitates the
induction of hypnosis. At an early stage perception is
increased, but later dulled. As consciousness becomes
impaired and awareness of the environment diminishes, the
EEG begins to slow and high-voltage delta waves ultimately
appear. Impairment of memory and calculation develop
when the dominant frequency reaches 5 Hz. Psychological
studies show impaired performance on tests of reaction time,
manual coordination and word association, and there is
often subsequent amnesia for events of the period (Wyke
1963).

When hyperventilation accompanies anxiety the emotional arousal is increased, creating a vicious circle. Paraesthesiae, circumoral numbness, chest wall tightness or pain,
dizziness, inability to take an adequate breath and vertigo
may themselves be sufficiently stressful to increase the
patient's concern and reinforce the disorder. Mental confusion may become marked, and myoclonic jerks or epileptic
phenomena may be precipitated. In severe cases the condition may progress to loss of consciousness.

It is uncertain whether these clinical phenomena depend
directly on the lowering of carbon dioxide tension in the
blood or on the rising pH and other metabolic changes in the
neuronal environment. Reduced cerebral blood flow as a
consequence of low $Paco_2$ and vasoconstriction of cerebral
arterioles may make a further contribution. The decrease in
ionised calcium of the blood is almost certainly responsible
for the tetanic phenomena.

Acidosis

Metabolic acidosis may result from an increase in
endogenous acid production (e.g. lactate in lactic acidosis or

and severe reduction of renal blood flow may induce renal failure due to tubular epithelial damage, as may urinary tract obstruction at any point from the pelvic calyces to the urethra. Although the term 'uraemia' was originally adopted to reflect the belief that the syndrome was caused by the accumulation of urea and other end-products of metabolism, the true causes of the syndrome remain unknown. In addition to uraemia and other electrolyte disturbances, renal failure is associated with anaemia, malnutrition, impaired carbohydrate, fat and protein metabolism, and endocrine disturbances.

The severity of symptoms and signs of uraemia vary between individuals, depending on the severity of uraemia and the rapidity with which it has developed. It is typically more severe and progresses more rapidly in patients with acute deterioration in renal function (Locke *et al.* 1961). Early manifestations may be subtle (Stenbäck & Haapanen 1967), including drowsiness, apathy, insomnia and impaired concentration, and do not appear until the glomerular filtration rate has fallen to 20–35% of normal. Mild behavioural changes, impairment of memory and errors in judgement develop later, often in association with signs of neuromuscular irritability, hiccups, cramps and fasciculations and twitching of muscles.

A large series of patients seen in a renal unit reported CNS manifestations in 60%, rising to 75% when blood urea exceeded 18.0 mmol/L, with mental changes as common in patients with acute as well as chronic uraemia (Stenbäck & Haapanen 1967). Patients with uraemia usually present to physicians with physical symptoms, but very occasionally the mental changes can be the most prominent manifestation and lead directly to psychiatric consultation. This is more likely when uraemia has developed slowly. The picture may simulate neurasthaenia with complaints of fatigue after mental effort or body weakness and exhaustion after minimal effort, muscular aches and pains, irritability, sleep disturbance and mood disturbance. Uraemia should always be considered in the differential diagnosis of delirium.

Sluggishness, memory impairment and sleep disturbance are not uncommonly seen in patients treated with renal replacement therapies. Psychometric studies have shown deficits in attention/response speed, learning and memory and perceptual coding in patients on both continuous ambulatory dialysis and haemodialysis.

Uraemic encephalopathy

Uraemic encephalopathy is an organic brain syndrome that occurs in untreated renal failure and in association with renal dialysis. The commonest mental disturbance is progressive torpor and drowsiness with the insidious development of intellectual impairment. The earliest symptoms may be subtle and include feeling generally unwell, fatigue, apathy and impaired concentration (Stenbäck & Haapanen 1967).

Difficulty with concentration is characteristically episodic: a patient may perform well for short periods of time but is unable to sustain mental activity.

With further progression the patient may become depressed or emotionally labile, memory becomes obviously impaired, and episodes of disorientation and confusion appear. Frontal lobe symptoms with impaired abstract thinking, listlessness and apathy prevail but anxious restlessness may also sometimes be seen. *Gegenhalten* (an involuntary, variable resistance to passive movement), grasp, palmomental and other frontal release signs also occur. In the later stages acute confusional states develop in one-third, with visual hallucinations, disorientation and agitation. Both the impairment of consciousness and the changes of mood fluctuate markedly, with lucid periods during which behaviour returns to normal. As in acute confusional states due to other causes the picture changes rapidly and paranoid developments are common.

Eventually more profound impairment of consciousness develops, with increasingly sluggish comprehension and reactions, slurring of speech, incontinence and ultimately coma. Seizures, usually generalised tonic–clonic though focal motor seizures are also common, develop in about one-third of cases. They are more frequent in acute than chronic uraemia and are usually a late feature. Meningism may be found in one-third and fascicular twitching, coarse postural and kinetic tremor, multifocal myoclonus and asterixis (a form of negative myoclonus) characterise later stages of the encephalopathy. Raised limb tone, hyperreflexia, ankle clonus and extensor plantar responses may also be seen in uraemic coma. Hemiparesis may occur in up to 45%, and curiously may exchange sides during the illness (Fraser & Arieff 1988). On recovery there is patchy or complete amnesia for the periods of disorientation and confusion.

Peripheral neurological manifestations

Neuropathy occurs in 70% of patients requiring renal replacement therapy, more commonly in men than women (Schaumburg *et al.* 1992). The neuropathy is distal, sensorimotor and predominantly axonal. Occasionally, intensely painful paraesthesiae may occur, typically in the feet or as band-like sensations (Mawdsley 1972). Weakness of dorsiflexion at the ankle is usually the first motor complaint. Nerve conduction studies may show an axonal pattern of impairment even before clinical signs appear. Isolated mononeuropathies are also common, particularly carpal tunnel syndrome. The most commonly affected cranial nerve is the vestibulocochlear (Burn & Bates 1998). The 'restless legs' syndrome (see Chapter 12) develops in a considerable proportion of patients, with or without overt neuropathy, presenting with unpleasant sensations in the lower limbs, worse in the evenings, which are relieved by movement (Raskin 1989). Renal replacement therapy or transplantation usually improves the neuropathy, with sensory symptoms improving before motor and deep tendon reflexes recovering last. Further neurological manifestations include a myopathy, similar to that seen in hyperparathyroidism. For a comprehensive review, see Burn and Bates (1998).

Investigation of uraemic encephalopathy

Blood urea is raised and electrolyte disturbances including hyponatraemia, hyperphosphataemia, hypocalcaemia and hyperkalaemia are common. Anaemia is often marked in chronic renal failure. If performed, CSF analysis typically shows a mildly raised opening pressure and increased protein, although in aseptic meningitis up to 250 lymphocytes (250 mm^3) and polymorphonucleur leucocytes and protein up to 1 g/L have been described (Madonick et al. 1950).

The EEG is usually most abnormal during the acute onset of encephalopathy (Burn & Bates 1998). There is generalised slowing, most marked frontally with an excess of delta and theta waves. In chronic renal failure the changes are less dramatic. They develop roughly in proportion to the severity of the clinical condition (Tyler 1968), with loss of well-developed alpha activity, progressive slowing, then disorganisation with runs of waves occurring at 5–7 Hz that ultimately replace all other activity. Bilateral spike-and-wave complexes in the absence of clinical seizure activity have been reported in up to 14% with chronic renal failure. On MRI, reversible T1 and T2 changes in the basal ganglia, periventricular white matter and internal capsule that resolve following dialysis have been described (Okada et al. 1991). However, CT or MRI are rarely useful in diagnosis though may help to exclude other causes of confusion such as subdural haematoma or hydrocephalus.

Gross lesions in the CNS are rare in the absence of marked hypertension. The most constant change is scattered neuronal degeneration, with chromatolysis and vacuolisation of nerve cells. In chronic cases this progresses to pyknosis and areas of cell loss.

Aetiology of mental disturbances

Although mental and neurological changes become commoner with increasing elevation of blood urea, it is widely accepted that urea cannot be responsible for all or even the majority of the symptoms. Considerable improvement can follow dialysis when urea is present in the dialysis fluid, and experimentally urea has not been found to have a strong neurotoxic effect. Other abnormalities must therefore play a direct aetiological role, with the level of blood urea serving mainly as an indicator of the severity of overall metabolic disturbance. Nevertheless, estimation of blood urea remains an important clinical indicator for monitoring the progress of the patient's condition.

The calcium content of the cerebral cortex is almost double that seen in normals, a change that may be mediated by increased PTH (Raskin 1989). In animal studies both EEG and brain calcium changes may be prevented by parathyroidectomy and in humans EEG and psychological abnormalities have been shown to improve after parathyroidectomy (Cogan et al. 1978).

In renal impairment the cerebral metabolic rate is reduced, with an associated decrease in cerebral oxygen consumption. These changes, which occur in the presence of normal levels of high-energy phosphates, have been attributed to a reduction in neurotransmission. Studies have suggested a reduction in the activity of the Na^+/K^+-ATPase pump, which is important in the release of neurotransmitters, especially noradrenaline and possibly also dopamine in renal failure (Minkoff et al. 1972; Fraser 1992). Endogenous opiates have also been investigated: circulating levels of β-endorphin are elevated in renal failure and there are reports of naloxone reversing encephalopathy in chronic renal failure (Mattana et al. 1993).

Arterial hypertension also contributes to the clinical picture, as verified by the pathological findings, causing transient neurological disturbances, fits and headache. In many cases a part is played by raised intracranial pressure, altered permeability of small blood vessels and anaemia. Erythropoietin therapy is associated with an improvement in cognitive function, with improvements in the speed and accuracy of information processing and an increase in the event-related P300 (Nissenson 1989).

Other derivatives of protein such as uric acid may play a part, as may other toxins so far unidentified. Electrolyte disturbances are certainly important in many cases. Changes in sodium, potassium, calcium, chloride, phosphate, acid–base balance and osmolality can all be blamed in individual instances. The rapidity of the shifts appears to be the essential factor, whether this is in the direction of normality or abnormality (Tyler 1968).

Drugs have been strongly incriminated as a cause of mental disturbance in patients with chronic renal failure, accounting for over one-third of the episodes in some series (Richet & Vachon 1966; Richet et al. 1970). Sedatives and antibiotics appear to be mainly responsible, either by virtue of accumulation when the drug is excreted by the kidneys or as a result of increased susceptibility of the CNS in the uraemic patient.

Other causes of neuropsychiatric disturbance in patients with chronic renal failure also need to be considered. The risk of intracranial infection is increased in uraemia, especially when immunosuppressive drugs are used after renal transplantation; encephalitis due to herpes simplex or cytomegalovirus may be hard to diagnose in the prodromal stages, leading to behavioural disturbance and change of personality. Low-grade meningitis can lack the typical physical signs and present as depression with chronic headache.

The use of anticoagulants in maintenance haemodialysis may result in a subdural haematoma.

Dialysis-related disturbances

The psychological stresses associated with haemodialysis or transplantation bring a range of problems of their own. Salmons (1980) has reviewed the problems inherent in such management of chronic renal failure, with disruptions in work, daily life and family relationships. Not surprisingly there is a high incidence of depression, anxiety and disturbed sexual functioning among such patients. Short-lived psychotic episodes may be observed, usually in clear consciousness but often marked by 'organic' features such as visual hallucinations or loosely held delusions. Gradual improvement usually follows dialysis, with return of mental clarity a short while after chemical normality has been achieved. Occasionally, however, the time lag may be several days in duration.

Dialysis dysequilibrium syndrome

Dialysis dysequilibrium syndrome was first recognised in the 1960s when patients with uraemia were dialysed over shorter time periods, though with modern dialysis techniques severe forms are extremely rarely seen. It may occur during or after haemodialysis or peritoneal dialysis and is more common at the end of the dialysis session. In its mildest form it consists of restlessness, muscle cramps, nausea, fatigue and headaches. Symptoms generally subside over a few hours. A more severe form is characterised by myoclonus, confusion and seizures, sometimes progressing to coma with signs of brainstem compression (Peterson & Swanson 1964; Mawdsley 1972).

The syndrome is believed to develop because of the osmotic gradient that develops between the plasma and the brain during rapid dialysis. The more rapid clearance of urea and other osmotically active substances from the blood than from the CNS results in intracellular acidosis in the brain in association with an increase in organic acids. This results in an osmotic gradient that draws water into the brain parenchyma, producing encephalopathy, raised intracranial pressure and cerebral oedema. EEG carried out during dialysis shows changes consistent with such a hypothesis, these changes being reversible with hypertonic fructose infusion (Kennedy *et al.* 1963).

Dialysis encephalopathy (dialysis dementia)

Dialysis encephalopathy is seen in patients who have been on haemodialysis for many years and is characterised by a mixed speech dysarthria and dysphasia, myoclonus, dementia and eventually seizures and death. Following its description by Alfrey *et al.* (1972), it became recognised as one of the commonest causes of death in some units (Burks *et al.* 1976).

Fortunately, modifications to the dialysis procedure mean that it is now rarely seen.

A mixed dysarthria and dysphasia with dysgraphia during or immediately following dialysis was reported as the earliest clinical sign in the majority of patients. With time the language dysfunction became permanent and progressively more severe, myoclonic jerks were seen and patients became ataxic and dyspraxic. Paranoia, bizarre behaviour and episodes of delirium were sometimes prominent. Slow worsening of the disorder usually led to dementia, immobility then muteness and death. Treatment was ineffective and progression could continue despite restoration of normal renal function by transplantation.

Most patients developing the disorder had been on haemodialysis for several years. The aluminium content of the brain, especially the grey matter, was increased fourfold in uraemic patients dying from dialysis dementia compared with those dying from other causes (Alfrey *et al.* 1976; McDermott *et al.* 1978). This was at first ascribed to the aluminium in the phosphate-binding gels though it was later discovered that the regional incidence of encephalopathy in various centres correlated with the aluminium content of the water used as dialysate (Parkinson *et al.* 1979). Dialysis dementia should be considered in all patients on dialysis, and all forms of aluminium, especially aluminium containing antacids and dialysate, should be withdrawn on the appearance of the symptoms described above. Desferrioxamine, an aluminium chelator, can safely be given long term and may reverse many of the features (Bolton & Young 1990).

Disturbances associated with renal transplantation

The increasing graft survival of renal transplants has led to a dramatic increase in the number of renal transplants performed, with an estimated 10 000 carried out worldwide each year. Approximately 30% of transplant recipients develop neurological complications, which may result from direct side effects of immunosuppressive agents, rejection encephalopathy, CNS infections and post-transplant lymphoproliferative disorder. Emotional disorders are also frequently seen in this group, who are aware that their ongoing quality of life is determined by the future viability of their grafted kidney.

Acute porphyria

The porphyrias are a heterogeneous group of overproduction diseases resulting from genetically determined partial deficiencies in enzymes involved in haem biosynthesis. Their clinical manifestations are broad, leading Waldenström to describe porphyria as the 'little imitator' in contrast to syphilis 'the big imitator'. Three common subtypes of porphyria give rise to neuropsychiatric disorders. Acute intermittent porphyria is the commonest form in the UK. It is inherited through an autosomal dominant gene on the long arm of chromosome 11, resulting in a 50% reduction of porphobilinogen (PBG) deaminase activity. Variegate porphyria, the other major form, is approximately one-third as common and is inherited through an autosomal dominant gene on the long arm of chromosome 1, resulting in reduction of protoporphyrinogen oxidase activity. It typically presents with light-sensitive erythematous or bullous skin lesions alone and is less commonly the cause of recurrent attacks, though it may also present in a similar manner to acute intermittent porphyria (Elder *et al.* 1997). The third acute form, hereditary coproporphyria, is the rarest and results from a deficit in coproporphyrinogen oxidase activity whose gene lies on chromosome 3. It presents with acute attacks and accompanying blistering skin lesions in approximately one-third. Plumboporphyria has only been described in a few cases but resembles acute intermittent porphyria clinically. Other conditions such as lead poisoning and hereditary tyrosinaemia may produce secondary abnormalities of porphyrin metabolism with similar clinical and biochemical findings.

Biochemical studies of relatives of patients with symptomatic acute intermittent porphyria suggest that at least 90% of individuals with acute intermittent porphyria or variegate porphyria are clinically latent. One study of blood donors showed inherited PBG deaminase deficiency in as many as 1 in 500 (Mustajoki *et al.* 1992). Predicting who will go on to develop clinical features has proven difficult, although women appear to be at greater risk than men (Hindmarsh 1993), with acute attacks approximately five times more common in women. Earlier uncontrolled studies had suggested an increased prevalence of PBG deaminase deficiency in psychiatric inpatients (Tishler *et al.* 1985) associated with agitated psychosis and apathetic or depressed withdrawal without neurological abnormalities. However, subsequent findings of a high prevalence of PBG deaminase deficiency in a non-clinical group suggest that this may be a non-specific finding.

The historical researches of MacAlpine and Hunter (1966, 1969) and MacAlpine *et al.* (1968) suggesting that George III's prolonged and puzzling mental illness may have been associated with acute porphyria drew public attention to these disorders, although considerable doubt has since been cast on some of these conclusions (Warren *et al.* 1996). The acute porphyrias have also been associated with the creative genius of Vincent van Gogh (Loftus & Arnold 1991) and with the obstetric history of Queen Anne (Phillips 1992). Acute porphyrias manifest clinically at any time from puberty onwards, most frequently during the second to fourth decades. As the disease exists so frequently in latent form, a family history may often not be forthcoming. Attacks may

take a myriad of forms that make diagnosis difficult. Failure to consider porphyria in the differential diagnosis may lead to the individual suffering multiple acute episodes before the diagnosis is finally made. Valuable reviews of the clinical features are provided by Crimlisk (1997) and Elder *et al.* (1997). Abdominal pain is almost universal, is severe, can occur in any quadrant and may also involve the back, buttocks and thighs. It is sometimes associated with guarding though not by true peritonism and may require large amounts of opioids for its control. Nausea, vomiting and constipation are common accompaniments. Tachycardia and hypertension are frequently described as features, though pulse and blood pressure may only be moderately raised and are of little diagnostic value. Autonomic neuropathy is responsible for many of the systemic manifestations, including abdominal pain, vomiting, constipation, hypertension and tachycardia. Abnormal cardiac reflexes have also been shown to occur during an attack though regress on remission (Laiwah *et al.* 1985).

Severe attacks can progress to a predominantly motor neuropathy, with weakness typically beginning in the proximal muscles, the arms more than the legs. Reflexes are usually diminished though extensor plantar responses can occur and Guillain–Barré syndrome and lead poisoning are important differential diagnoses. Sensory involvement, often with mild dysaesthesiae, occur in one-third often with bizarre distributions that sometimes raise the suspicion of a conversion disorder. Cranial nerve involvement, especially III, VII and X, may also occur. Seizures are seen in over 20% of cases, and status epilepticus may develop. Hyponatraemia, probably caused by SIADH, is also described (Kappas *et al.* 1989). Variegate porphyria presents with skin lesions alone in 75% in the UK, with the remainder split between mixed and neuropsychiatric features alone. Cutaneous features include photosensitivity, skin fragility, bullous lesions, facial hypertrichosis and hyperpigmentation.

'Mental symptoms' accompany attacks in 25–75% of cases and may dominate the clinical picture, although as many of the series have been undertaken by neurologists or physicians this is likely to be an underestimation (Crimlisk 1997). Emotional disturbances with anxiety, restlessness and depression often occur and may be persisting features (Patience *et al.* 1994; Kappas *et al.* 1995). Detailed psychiatric assessments have been limited to small series or case reports; psychotic features resembling schizophrenia with persecutory delusions, auditory hallucinations, social withdrawal and catatonia have been described (Tishler *et al.* 1985) as have affective symptoms with emotional lability, insomnia and grandiose delusions. Clouding of consciousness and confusion may progress to delirium, with hallucinations, delusions and disturbed behaviour. Coma sometimes develops abruptly. The occurrence of monthly luteal-phase attacks in women may lead to the false diagnosis of an acute polymorphic psychotic reaction or a cycloid psychosis.

Precipitation of attacks

Drugs and the menstrual cycle are the most common precipitants of an acute attack (Kauppinen & Mustajoki 1992), though alcohol excess and inadequate malnutrition are also important precipitants. The current list of agents known to precipitate an acute attack is long and the *British National Formulary* or the Cardiff Porphyria Research Group should be consulted before a drug that is not known to be safe is prescribed. Notorious precipitants include antibiotics such as the sulphonamides and erythromycin; sedatives such as barbiturates, benzodiazepines and sulpiride; hormone products such as the oral contraceptive pill, anabolic steroids, hormone-replacement therapy and tamoxifen; antiepileptics such as phenytoin and carbamazepine; drugs of abuse including cocaine and amphetamines; as well as many commonly prescribed drugs such as antihistamines, diuretics, baclofen, metoclopramide, many of the tricyclic antidepressants and diclofenac. Importantly, many of the drugs that would be considered for use in the mental state disturbances commonly seen in acute porphyric attacks have been associated with their precipitation, necessitating considerable care in the use of the agents. Of the antipsychotics chlorpromazine appears the safest, and there are few data on the atypicals. There are no data on amisulpride though sulpiride is associated with precipitating attacks so it should probably be avoided. There are a few case reports describing the uncomplicated use of olanzapine and cell culture studies have suggested that it may be safe. Mixed reports have been associated with risperidone use and there are currently no data on the use of quetiapine or zotepine; clozapine is believed to be safe. Of the antidepressants, most of the tricyclics should be avoided, but fluoxetine and paroxetine appear to be safe though there are currently too few data to comment on the use of the newer agents, mirtazapine, reboxetine or venlafaxine. The above resources should be consulted before the use of any of these newer agents is contemplated. Other drugs judged safe include aspirin, narcotic analgesics, penicillin, streptomycin, tetracycline, propranolol, paraldehyde and probably clomethiazole (Moore & Disler 1988; Kappas *et al.* 1989; McColl *et al.* 1996).

The importance of nutrition is shown by attacks that occur while on reducing diets, especially when these lead to precipitous loss of weight, and cases have been described of attacks occurring after missing several meals (Kappas *et al.* 1989). The mechanism by which starvation may trigger an attack is uncertain, though a rise in urinary excretion of aminolaevulinic acid (ALA) and PBG has been described with calorie restriction, and is reversed by increased carbohydrate intake (Welland *et al.* 1964). Oestrogen and progesterone aggravate porphyria (Welland *et al.* 1964) and cyclic attacks most commonly occur in the luteal phase, associated with high hormonal levels, and decline after the menopause. Previous claims that stress, surgery and infection are precipitants have not been supported by published data.

Investigations

Most difficulties in the diagnosis of the acute attack occur in patients without a family history of porphyria, especially if the combination of symptoms is atypical. Increased urinary excretion of PBG confirms the diagnosis of an acute attack, which is also associated with increased urinary excretion of ALA. Screening tests using Ehrlich's reagent lack sensitivity and may produce false-positive results; although of use in an emergency situation, they should always be confirmed with quantitative assay. Porphyrins are very light sensitive and break down quickly under normal conditions so urinary samples should be stored in the dark and transported to the laboratory as soon as possible. A negative result does not exclude an acute attack since some patients fail to hyperexcrete. If clinical suspicion persists, quantification of PBG and measurement of faecal and plasma porphyrins is essential. This is especially true in variegate porphyria and hereditary coproporphyria where excretion of PBG may fall below the detection level of most assays very soon after symptom onset. Caution is also required on account of the false-positive results that can occur in the urine with certain febrile illnesses, in lead poisoning and in patients receiving phenothiazine drugs (Reio & Wetterberg 1969).

The EEG often shows abnormalities during acute attacks, with slowing of dominant frequencies and an excess of intermediate slow activity. Sometimes, however, it remains entirely normal. Isolated records are therefore of little help in the diagnosis, but serial recordings can occasionally be useful in confirming the organic origin of symptoms in attacks of uncertain nature. A number of case reports have described MRI and other imaging changes in acute attacks, with multifocal cortical and subcortical lesions that resolve with resolution of the attack (King & Bragdon 1991; Aggarwal *et al.* 1994; Kupferschmidt *et al.* 1995; Utz *et al.* 2001). Some have hypothesised a vascular aetiology for these changes in view of their mild enhancement with contrast, rapid resolution following treatment of the attack and similarity to the lesion distribution seen in hypertensive encephalopathy. A report using conventional angiography has also demonstrated cranial vasospasm. Pathological studies of peripheral nerves show a predominantly motor axonal neuropathy with secondary Schwann cell reactions, findings consistent with PBG-deficient mouse models. These studies have suggested that rather than ALA being directly neurotoxic, the axonopathy is likely to be caused by local deficiency of haem-containing proteins such as the mitochondrial cytochromes (Meyer *et al.* 1998; Lindberg *et al.* 1999).

Differential diagnosis

Porphyria is notorious for leading to mistakes in diagnosis, and patients are sometimes admitted repeatedly to psychiatric units before the condition is discovered. An impression of psychiatric illness is reinforced by the patient's emotional instability during attacks, and the long history of intermittent physical complaints for which no cause has previously emerged. Diagnoses of personality disorder or an anxiety, somatisation or conversion disorder are commonly made when the patient complains of weakness of the limbs and varied aches and pains unbacked by physical signs. Psychotic developments may likewise obscure other aspects of the disorder and lead to a primary diagnosis of depressive illness or acute schizophrenia. Other patients are admitted to general medical wards with suspected appendicitis on account of abdominal pain and vomiting. Intestinal obstruction may be diagnosed when there is severe constipation. Other cases may be mistaken for Guillain–Barré syndrome, or the combination of fits and hypertension may suggest hypertensive encephalopathy.

Treatment and outcome

The chief aim should be prevention of attacks by advising the patient on drugs which must be avoided and about the importance of adequate nutritional intake. Abstention from alcohol should be advised, particularly whisky and red wine, though studies in specialist centres have shown that 87% of patients with inducible porphyria continue to drink alcohol (Thunell *et al.* 1992). It seems prudent to advise early consultation and rapid treatment for concurrent intercurrent infections. On occasion the onset of an attack can be aborted by increasing carbohydrate intake. In women with attacks related to menstruation, suppressing ovulation with a luteinising hormone-releasing hormone anologue has been shown to reduce the number of attacks (Herrick *et al.* 1990).

The symptomatic treatment of the acute attack is described by Thadani *et al.* (2000). For severe pain, opioids are safe and pethidine, morphine or diamorphine may be given. Sympathetic overactivity may be treated with propranolol. Seizures may be related to hyponatraemia so electrolytes should be monitored regularly and fluid restriction used if hyponatraemia develops. If an antiepileptic is required, the newer agents vigabatrin and gabapentin have been shown to be safe. The drugs of choice for emotional disturbance are chlorpromazine, promazine or trifluoperazine. Oral and intravenous glucose to maintain a high-energy intake and intravenous haem arginate are the mainstays of treatment, which by reducing the synthesis of ALA results in biochemical and clinical remission. Recently tin protoporphyrin, an inhibitor of haem oxygenase, has been shown to prolong remission when given with haem arginate (Dover *et al.* 1993), although side effects of cutaneous photosensitivity and potential toxicity currently limit its use.

The duration of attacks varies widely from a few days to several months. The majority subside completely without enduring defects. Some patients, however, are left severely crippled with weakness or muscular wasting, and some remain psychotic for long periods of time. Ultimately there is usually full physical and mental recovery.

Klinefelter's syndrome and other sex chromosome aneuploidies

Klinefelter's syndrome (KS) results from the presence of one or more additional X chromosomes in the nucleus of the male. It is the most common of the sex chromosome aneuploidies with a prevalence of approximately 1 in 800 males (Hook 1992). Diagnosis is often not made until puberty or early adulthood when it often presents with delayed sexual maturation or infertility. As originally described, the typical 47XXY phenotype is characterised by small firm testes, infertility with azoospermia, impaired sexual maturation, gynaecomastia and elevated gonadotrophins (Klinefelter *et al.* 1942). Other clinical manifestations may vary depending on the extent of androgen deficiency and include features of eunuchoidism (long legs and wide span, decreased or absent facial, axillary and pubic hair, gynaecomastia, female fat distribution and small testes and penis). Subsequent reports have expanded the clinical phenotype in recognition of associated cognitive, language and behavioural abnormalities (Simpson *et al.* 2003).

Treatment with testosterone replacement from early puberty has been recommended and shown to improve mood and concentration in addition to its virilising effects (Nielsen *et al.* 1988). A high prevalence of psychiatric disorder in KS and the other sex chromosome aneuploidies (47XXX, 48XXXY, 48XXYY, 49XXXXY) and the growing recognition of focal cognitive deficits have been the twin focuses of psychiatric interest in this condition.

Cognitive and language deficits

Early reports of an excess of KS among patients in hospitals for the learning disabled led to the view that severe impairment of intellect was characteristic. However, subsequent case studies and findings from prospective cohort studies begun in the early 1970s to determine the incidence of sex chromosome aneuploidies have suggested that delayed language development with only mildly reduced full-scale IQ are more characteristic of boys with KS (Leonard *et al.* 1979; Walzer *et al.* 1982; Bender *et al.* 1987). The degree of intellectual impairment is proportional to the number of additional X chromosomes, with an approximately 15-point reduction in IQ with each additional chromosome (Simpson *et al.* 2003). More detailed psychometric studies have shown a differential impairment in cognitive functions, with impaired verbal compared with non-verbal abilities in children with KS. Thus Netley and Rovet (1982) found mean verbal and performance WISC IQs of 85 and 101, respectively, in their sample of 33 children with XXY karyotypes. Though still within the normal range, the verbal IQ was significantly lower than performance IQ and verbal IQ in unaffected sibling controls.

From an early age, boys with KS show language problems reflecting delayed language acquisition (Leonard *et al.* 1979) and poor skills in sentence building, intonation and word naming. At a later age they show poorer articulation and comprehension and difficulties with verbal abstraction, syntax production and word finding (Walzer *et al.* 1982). Graham *et al.* (1988) suggested that these problems reflect a more fundamental impairment with accessing, retrieving and applying linguistic information. Rovet *et al.* (1996) reviewed the literature and hypothesised that KS deficits are primarily language based and may stem from an underlying impairment in auditory temporal processing and working memory. Evidence of frontal executive deficits are conflicting, although Temple and Sanfilippo (2003) have recently suggested a specific impairment in inhibitory skills. Spatial abilities and spatial processing speed appear to be spared (Walzer *et al.* 1978; Bender *et al.* 1986). In many respects this pattern of deficits is the reverse of that found in subjects with Turner's syndrome (see following section).

Considerable debate surrounds the relative influence of genetic and hormonal influences on the cognitive profile seen, although there have been few studies comparing adult with childhood cognitive profiles or even comparing testosterone-treated with untreated boys. Boone *et al.* (2001) have suggested that the characteristic cognitive profile seen in boys with KS changes as they mature, with a reduction in performance IQ and associated increase in verbal IQ occurring after adolescence. They argue for an early left hemisphere dysfunction related to developmental slowing in the rate of cell division prenatally followed by right hemisphere disturbance appearing in a subgroup in young adulthood due to a combination of low testosterone and high oestrogen levels. Imaging studies have recently begun to address this problem. Warwick *et al.* (1999) showed a reduction in whole-brain volume in KS with bilaterally enlarged ventricles, whilst Patwardhan *et al.* (2000) showed a reduction of left temporal lobe grey matter consistent with the observed verbal and language deficits and showed that relative preservation of grey matter in the left temporal region was associated with exogenous testosterone during development. Interestingly, testosterone supplementation was also associated with increased verbal fluency scores in this study. Other brain abnormalities have been described in KS: a high prevalence of EEG abnormalities has been reported, chiefly slowed

alpha but also slow-wave dysrhythmias and paroxysmal features (Hambert & Frey 1964). Epilepsy is also commoner than chance expectation.

Psychiatric features

A high prevalence of psychiatric disorder has emerged in this condition. Personality and behaviour may be abnormal and there is a probable excess of psychotic illness. Some psychiatric features appear to be attributable to the endocrine disorder, others to be more directly related to the chromosomal abnormality.

The personality in patients with KS is sometimes abnormal. A variety of pictures has been described, ranging from markedly antisocial conduct to passivity and social withdrawal. Common descriptions are of patients lacking in drive and initiative, with severe restriction of interests and generally indolent, insecure and dependent. At the same time tolerance of frustration tends to be impaired, with explosive irritability and outbursts of aggression. Poor school and work records, marital instability and impoverished social relationships are said to be common.

Nielsen's (1969) review showed histories of alcoholism in 6% and of criminal behaviour in 12% of patients. A small excess of XXY patients has been reported in surveys of institutions caring for severely disturbed criminals, along with the more usual excess of XYY or XXYY karyotypes (Swanson & Stipes 1969). However, Schiavi *et al.* (1984) failed to support any excess of violent or aggressive behaviour among Klinefelter (or XYY) subjects in their comprehensive survey from Copenhagen. The prevalence of criminal convictions was slightly higher than for XY men, but this difference disappeared on controlling for intelligence and parental socioeconomic status. Moreover, the great majority of the offences committed did not involve personal violence.

The endocrine disorder may play a part in hindering personality maturation and contributing to some aspects of personality difficulties. Thus patients with hypogonadism due to other causes are typically shy, timid and markedly lacking in drive. However, they tend to show more stable histories and temperaments than patients with KS, and lack any excess of criminal behaviours. Wakeling (1972) compared 11 patients with KS and nine other hypogonadal patients seen in a psychiatric hospital; both groups showed insecurity and low tolerance of frustration, but passivity was more marked in the hypogonadal patients and impulsive erratic behaviour in the Klinefelter patients. The latter, moreover, frequently had histories of prepubertal maladjustment, with a higher incidence of unsettled schooling, neurosis and behaviour disorder in childhood. It appears, therefore, that in KS delayed cerebral maturation may make a contribution, over and above the androgen deficiency, in leading to poor social adjustment and disturbed personality functioning.

Sexual problems, as might be expected, are not uncommon. Potency tends to be low and to show an early decline, especially when features of hypogonadism are marked (Pasqualini *et al.* 1957). Androgen treatment can be successful in restoring libido and potency (Beumont *et al.* 1972). Occasional reports have described transvestism, exhibitionism and paedophilia in patients with KS, although there is little to suggest that these are over-represented in the syndrome (Orwin *et al.* 1974). Sexual pathology, when it occurs, probably again reflects the restricted personality development and incapacity for deep interpersonal relationships. The more extreme examples of deviant sexual practice have usually occurred in severely antisocial or psychotic individuals.

Mental hospital surveys, reviewed by Forssman (1970), have indicated a threefold increase in patients with KS compared with the general population. This appears to be due mainly to psychotic illnesses of a schizophrenic nature. Nielsen (1969) found that 6% of patients recorded in the psychiatric literature had been given a diagnosis of schizophrenia, and another 7% had psychoses of an uncertain type but almost all with paranoid delusions. Well-documented examples of schizophrenia in association with KS are provided by Pomeroy (1980) and Roy (1981). The increased risk of mental illness may represent another facet of the increased vulnerability to stress of the patient with KS, or may have more direct genetic determinants.

There is little to suggest an increased incidence of organic psychiatric illness. Jablensky *et al.* (1970) have described a patient who demented rapidly in his early forties, showing diffuse white matter degeneration and adrenal cortical atrophy at autopsy; however, this may well have represented a chance association with KS.

Turner's syndrome

The XO karyotype is characterised by primary amenorrhoea with streak ovaries and consequent sexual infantilism, short stature and multiple congenital abnormalities. Somatic anomalies primarily affect the skeleton and connective tissue and include short stature, webbed neck, low hairline, cubitus valgus–wide carrying angle, oedema of hands and feet, nail dysplasia, and widely spaced nipples with a 'shield'-like chest. Facial appearance is often characteristic, with a small jaw, fish-like mouth and low-set ears. Congenital lymphoedema and poor development of the lymphatic channels is believed to be responsible for many of the characteristic phenotypic changes and may also be responsible for coarctation of the aorta. Other systems commonly involved include the cardiovascular system (bicuspid aortic valve in 50%, coarctation of the aorta in up to 20% and frequent hypertension), the urinary system (horseshoe and other structural abnormalities of the kidneys) and endocrine system (primary hypothyroidism in up to 50% and glucose intolerance is common). The classic 45 XO karyotype is seen in half, with the remainder made up of mosaicism, isochromosomes of X, ring or partial deletions of the X chromosome (Jacobs *et al.* 1990). Treatment is frequently with growth hormone, and with oestrogen from adolescence.

Psychiatric interest in the condition has largely centred on the cognitive functioning of such patients. Money (1963, 1964) drew attention to the common finding of a lower performance than verbal IQ paralleled by inferior scores on tests of perceptual organisation when compared with scores on verbal comprehension, discrepancies that became more marked at the higher intelligence levels. Subsequent investigation has identified specific deficits in visuospatial and visuoperceptual abilities (Pennington *et al.* 1985), motor function, non-verbal memory, executive function and attentional abilities (Ross *et al.* 2002). Finer-grained analysis of the language of women with Turner's syndrome has also led to the identification of subtle speech difficulties, in particular reduced oral fluency and abnormal narrative production (Temple 2002). Calculation difficulties (Bruandet *et al.* 2004) and deficiencies in social cognition hypothesised to correlate with previously identified personality characteristics have also been described (Lawrence *et al.* 2003a).

It remains uncertain how far the specific cognitive deficits and difficulties in social functioning seen in girls with Turner's syndrome reflect the direct effects of genes on cerebral maturation or reflect more indirect consequences of hormonal deficiencies resulting from the genetic defect. Ross *et al.* (2002) assessed the neurocognitive profile of 71 adult women with Turner's syndrome who were treated with oestrogen replacement including 10 who had apparently normal ovarian function. As with girls with Turner's syndrome, the adult women continued to show impairment on visuomotor tasks with a spatial component, tasks involving the manipulation of spatial–relational information, and attention tasks requiring control of impulsivity and self-monitoring. Conversely, motor speed and verbal memory in tasks without heavy spatial loading have previously been shown to be oestrogen responsive (Ross *et al.* 2000). They argue that the lack of responsivity of the core cognitive deficit seen in Turner's syndrome to oestrogen replacement, noted even in the 10 women with apparently normal ovarian function, points towards a genetic aetiology. This would be consistent with Murphy *et al.* (1994) who showed that visuospatial ability was negatively correlated with the percentage of lymphocytes containing the XO karyotype in a subset of patients with XO mosaicism. Whilst there is little direct evidence to suggest that the neurocognitive deficits are due to absence of fetal exposure to sex hormones, the identification of steroid receptors in several areas of the primate brain during prenatal and postnatal development and the correlation between periods of early steroid production and periods of rapid brain growth suggest a role for sex hormones in early brain development (Brinton *et al.* 1997).

Structural and functional imaging studies have identified a number of abnormalities in cortical and subcortical brain regions in women with Turner's syndrome. Murphy *et al.* (1993) showed that patients with Turner's syndrome showed significantly smaller cerebral hemisphere volumes, parieto-occipital brain matter volumes, and smaller hippocampi, lenticular nuclei and thalamic nuclei bilaterally. On many of these measures the mosaic patients occupied an intermediate position. Among the group as a whole there was significant right–left asymmetry in parieto-occipital brain matter volumes, that on the right being reduced. Subsequent studies have replicated the parieto-occipital volumetric reduction and functional studies have shown complementary reduction in metabolic activity (Reiss *et al.* 1995; Murphy *et al.* 1997). This decrease in parietal lobe grey matter is consistent with the broad impairment in visuospatial skills described as the core neuropsychological deficit in Turner's syndrome (Brown *et al.* 2002).

Clinical series have frequently found that girls with Turner's syndrome are more immature and have weaker social relationships, school performance and self-esteem than matched controls (Kihlbom 1969; McCauley *et al.* 1995). These difficulties are common and typically worsen at adolescence but rarely progress to frank psychopathology or developmental delay (McCauley *et al.* 1995). Observations have shown that girls with Turner's syndrome make less eye contact during social interactions and have greater difficulties interpreting non-verbal communication (Lawrence *et al.* 2003b). Using a specially developed social cognition questionnaire sensitive to flexibility and responsiveness in social interactions, Skuse *et al.* (1997) showed that quality of social interaction was dependent on whether the X chromosome was maternally (Xm) or paternally (Xp) inherited. Girls with a paternally inherited Xp chromosome were significantly better adjusted, with superior verbal and higher-order executive function skills that mediate social interactions. The same group has further shown that women with maternally inherited Xm chromosome also have impaired facial recognition and are impaired at recognising emotions, especially fear in the faces of others (Lawrence *et al.* 2003b). Also described are impairments in reading intentions and emotions from the eyes, an important component in the development of social cognition that has been shown to be impaired in individuals with autistic spectrum disorders. Together this evidence suggests a role for X expression in relation to the development of sociocognitive abilities and the possibility of an X-linked locus that underlies the development of sexual dimorphism in social behaviour.

References

Abed, R.T., Clark, J., Elbadawy, M.H. & Cliffe, M.J. (1987) Psychiatric morbidity in acromegaly. *Acta Psychiatrica Scandinavica* **75**, 635–639.

Abend, W.K. & Tyler, H.R. (1989) Thyroid disease and the nervous system. In: Aminoff, M.J. (ed.) *Neurology and General Medicine*, ch. 16. Churchill Livingstone, New York.

Abrams, G.M. & Jay, C. (1998) Neurological disorders of mineral metabolism and parathyroid disease. In: Goetz, C.G. & Aminoff, M.J. (eds) *Handbook of Clinical Neurology*, vol. 26, 111–130. Elsevier, New York.

Adams, R.D. & Kubik, C.S. (1944) Subacute degeneration of the brain in pernicious anaemia. *New England Journal of Medicine* **231**, 1–9.

Addison, T. (1849) Anaemia: disease of the supra-renal capsules. *London Medical Gazette* **43**, 517–518.

Aggarwal, A., Quint, D.J. & Lynch, J.P. (1994) MR imaging of porphyric encephalopathy. *American Journal of Roentgenology* **162**, 1218–1220.

Alarcon, R.D. & Franceschini, J.A. (1984) Hyperparathyroidism and paranoid psychosis: case-report and review of the literature. *British Journal of Psychiatry* **145**, 477–486.

Alarcón, R.D. & Franceschini, J.A. (1984) Hyperparathyroidism and paranoid psychosis. Case report and review of the literature. *British Journal of Psychiatry* **145**, 477–486.

Alexander, P.E. & Jackson, A.H. (1981) Calcium and magnesium: relationship to schizophrenia and neuroleptic-induced extrapyramidal symptoms. In: Alexander, P.E. (ed.) *Electrolytes and Neuropsychiatric Disorders*, ch. 9. MTP Press, Lancaster.

Alfrey, A.C., Terman, D.S., Brettschneider, L., Simpson, K.M. & Ogden, D.A. (1970) Hypermagnesemia after renal homotransplantations. *Annals of Internal Medicine* **73**, 367–371.

Alfrey, A.C., Mishell, J.M., Burks, J. *et al.* (1972) Syndrome of dyspraxia and multifocal seizures associated with chronic hemodialysis. *Transactions of the American Society of Artificial Internal Organs* **18**, 257–261.

Alfrey, A.C., Le Gendre, G.R. & Kaehny, W.D. (1976) The dialysis encephalopathy syndrome. *New England Journal of Medicine* **294**, 184–188.

Alpert, J.E., Mischoulon, D., Nierenberg, A.A. & Fava, M. (2000) Nutrition and depression: focus on folate. *Nutrition, Risk Factors and Disease* **16**, 544–546.

American Diabetes Association (2004) Position statement. *Diabetes Care* **27**, S11–S14.

Anand, M.P. (1964) Iatrogenic megaloblastic anaemia with neurological complications. *Scottish Medical Journal* **9**, 388–390.

Anderson, R.J., Freedland, K.E., Clouse, R.E. & Lustman, P.J. (2001) The prevalence of comorbid depression in adults with diabetes. A meta-analysis. *Diabetes Care* **24**, 1069–1078.

Anon. (1973) Zinc deficiency in man. *Lancet* **i**, 299–300.

Anon. (1978) Factitious hypoglycaemia. *Lancet* **i**, 1293.

Arky, R.A., Veverbrants, E. & Abramson, E.A. (1968) Irreversible hypoglycemia. A complication of alcohol and insulin. *JAMA* **206**, 575–578.

Arlt, W. & Allolio, B. (2003) Adrenal insufficiency. *Lancet* **361**, 1881–1893.

Arlt, W., Callies, F., van Vlijmen, J.C. *et al.* (1999) Dehydroepiandrosterone replacement in women with adrenal insufficiency. *New England Journal of Medicine* **341**, 1013–1020.

Arlt, W., Fremerey, C., Callies, F. *et al.* (2002) Well-being, mood and calcium homeostasis in patients with hypoparathyroidism receiving standard treatment with calcium and vitamin, D. *European Journal of Endocrinology* **146**, 215–222.

Arnaldi, G., Angeli, A., Atkinson, A.B. *et al.* (2003) Diagnosis and complications of Cushing's syndrome: a consensus statement. *Journal of Clinical Endocrinology and Metabolism* **88**, 5593–5602.

Asher, R. (1949) Myxoedematous madness. *British Medical Journal* **2**, 555–562.

Askmark, H., Olsson, Y., & Rossitti, S. (2000) Treatable dropped head syndrome in hypothyroidism. *Neurology* **55**, 896–897.

Ataya, K., Mercado, A., Kartaginer, J., Abbasi, A. & Moghissi, K.S. (1988) Bone density and reproductive hormones in patients with neuroleptic-induced hyperprolactinaemia. *Fertility and Sterility* **50**, 876–881.

Auer, R.N. & Siesjo, B.K. (1993) Hypoglycaemia: brain neurochemistry and neuropathology. *Baillières Clinical Endocrinology and Metabolism* **7**, 611–625.

Austin, E.J. & Deary, I.J. (1999) Effects of repeated hypoglycemia on cognitive function: a psychometrically validated reanalysis of the Diabetes Control and Complications Trial data. *Diabetes Care* **22**, 1273–1277.

Avery, T.L. (1973) A case of acromegaly and gigantism with depression. *British Journal of Psychiatry* **122**, 599–600.

Bale, R.N. (1973) Brain damage in diabetes mellitus. *British Journal of Psychiatry* **122**, 337–341.

Barlow, E.D. & De Wardener, H.E. (1959) Compulsive water drinking. *Quarterly Journal of Medicine* **28**, 235–258.

Barnard, R.V., Campbell, M.J. & McDonald, W.I. (1971) Pathological findings in a case of hypothyroidism with ataxia. *Journal of Neurology, Neurosurgery and Psychiatry* **34**, 755–760.

Bastepe, M. & Juppner, H. (2003) Pseudohypoparathyroidism and mechanisms of resistance toward multiple hormones: molecular evidence to clinical presentation. *Journal of Clinical Endocrinology and Metabolism* **88**, 4055–4058.

Bauer, M., Hellweg, R., Graf, K.J. & Baumgartner, A. (1998) Treatment of refractory depression with high dose thyroxine. *Neuropsychopharmacology* **18**, 444–455.

Baum, H., Ludecke, D.K. & Herrmann, H.D. (1986) Carpal tunnel syndrome and acromegaly. *Acta Neurochirurgica (Wien)* **83**, 54–55.

Bellamy, R.J. & Kendall-Taylor, P. (1995) Unrecognized hypocalcaemia diagnosed 36 years after thyroidectomy. *Journal of the Royal Society of Medicine* **88**, 690–691.

Bender, B.G., Puck, M.H., Saldenblatt, J.A. & Robinson, A. (1986) Dyslexia in 47,XXY boys identified at birth. *Behavior Genetics* **16**, 343–354.

Bender, B.G., Linden, M.G. & Robinson, A. (1987) Environment and developmental risk in children with sex chromosome abnormalities. *Journal of the American Academy of Child and Adolescent Psychiatry* **26**, 499–503.

Bennett, S.T., Lucassen, A.M., Gough, S.C.L. *et al.* (1995) Susceptibility to human type 1 diabetes at *IDDM2* is determined by tandem repeat variation at the insulin gene minisatellite locus. *Nature Genetics* **9**, 284–291.

Beumont, P.J.V., Bancroft, J.H.J., Beardwood, C.J. & Russell, G.F.M. (1972) Behavioural changes after treatment with testosterone: case report. *Psychological Medicine* **2**, 70–72.

Bewsher, P.D., Gardiner, A.Q., Hedley, A.J. & Maclean, H.C.S. (1971) Psychosis after acute alteration of thyroid status. *Psychological Medicine* **1**, 260–262.

Bjelland, I., Tell, G.S., Vollset, S.E., Refsum, H. & Ueland, P.M. (2003) Folate, vitamin B12, homocysteine, and the MTHFR 677C→T polymorphism in anxiety and depression: the Hordaland Homocysteine Study. *Archives of General Psychiatry* **60**, 618–626.

Bjorses, P., Halonen, M., Palvimo, J.J. *et al.* (2000) Mutations in the AIRE gene: effects on subcellular location and transactivation function of the autoimmune polyendocrinopathy–candidiasis–ectodermal dystrophy protein. *American Journal of Human Genetics* **66**, 378–392.

Blau, J.N. & Hinton, J.M. (1960) Hypopituitary coma and psychosis. *Lancet* **i**, 408–409.

Bleuler, M. (1951) The psychopathology of acromegaly. *Journal of Nervous and Mental Disease* **113**, 497–511.

Bleuler, M. (1967) Endocrinological psychiatry and psychology. *Henry Ford Hospital Medical Journal* **15**, 309–317.

Bolton, C.F. & Young, G.B. (1990) *Neurological Complications of Renal Disease.* Butterworth, Boston.

Boone, K.B., Swerdloff, R.S., Miller, B.L. *et al.* (2001) Neuropsychological profiles of adults with Klinefelter syndrome. *Journal of the International Neuropsychological Society* **7**, 446–456.

Boscaro, M., Barzon, L. & Sonino, N. (2000) The diagnosis of Cushing's syndrome. *Archives of Internal Medicine* **160**, 3045–3053.

Boscaro, M., Barzon, L., Fallo, F. & Sonino, N. (2001) Cushing's syndrome. *Lancet* **357**, 783–791.

Botez, M.I & Reynolds, E.H. (eds) (1979) *Folic Acid in Neurology, Psychiatry and Internal Medicine.* Raven, New York.

Bottiglieri, T., Laundy, M., Crellin, R., Toone, B.K., Carney, M.W.P. & Reynolds, E.H. (2000) Homocysteine, folate, methylation, and monoamine metabolism in depression. *Journal of Neurology, Neurosurgery and Psychiatry* **69**, 228–232.

Bourdeau, I., Bard, C., Noël, B. *et al.* (2002) Loss of brain volume in endogenous Cushing's syndrome and its reversibility after correction of hypercortisolism. *Journal of Clinical Endocrinology and Metabolism* **87**, 1949–1954.

Bourdeau, I., Bard, C., Forget, H., Boulanger, Y., Cohen, H. & Lacroix, A. (2005) Cognitive function and cerebral assessment in patients who have Cushing's syndrome. *Endocrinology and Metabolism Clinics of North America* **34**, 357–369.

Boyd, A. (1995) Bromocriptine and psychosis: a literature review. *Psychiatric Quarterly* **66**, 87–95.

Bremner, J.D., Krystal, J.H., Southwick, S.M. & Charney, D.S. (1995) Functional neuroanatomical correlates of the effects of stress on memory. *Journal of Traumatic Stress* **8**, 527–553.

Brewer, C. (1969) Psychosis due to acute hypothyroidism during the administration of carbimazole. *British Journal of Psychiatry* **115**, 1181–1183.

Brierley, J.B. (1981) Brain damage due to hypoglycaemia. In: Marks, V. & Rose, F.C. (eds) *Hypoglycaemia*, 2nd edn, ch. 22. Blackwell Scientific Publications, Oxford.

Brinton, R.D., Tran, J., Proffitt, P. & Montoya, M. (1997) 17-beta-Estradiol enhances the outgrowth and survival of neocortical neurons in culture. *Neurochemical Research* **22**, 1339–1351.

Brown, W.A., Kesler, S.R., Eliez, S. *et al.* (2002) Brain development in Turner syndrome: a magnetic resonance imaging study. *Psychiatry Research* **116**, 187–196.

Brownlie, B.E.W., Rae, A.M., Walshe, J.W.B. & Wells, J.E. (2000) Psychoses associated with thyrotoxicosis: 'thyrotoxic psychosis'. A report of 18 cases, with statistical analysis of incidence. *European Endocrinology* **142**, 438–444.

Brozek, J. & Caster, W.O. (1957) Psychologic effects of thiamine restriction and deprivation in normal young men. *American Journal of Clinical Nutrition* **5**, 109–120.

Bruandet, M., Molko, N., Cohen, L. & Dehaene, S. (2004) A cognitive characterization of dyscalculia in Turner syndrome. *Neuropsychologia* **42**, 288–298.

Bruck, E., Abal, G. & Aceto, T. (1968) Pathogenesis and pathophysiology of hypertonic dehydration with diarrhoea. *American Journal of Diseases of Children* **115**, 122–144.

Buckley, C. (2005). Diseases associated with antibodies to voltage-gated potassium channels. *Advances in Clinical Neuroscience and Rehabilitation* **5**, 11–12.

Buckman, M.T. & Kellner, R. (1985) Reduction of distress in hyperprolactinaemia with bromocriptine. *American Journal of Psychiatry* **142**, 242–244.

Bunevicius, R., Kazanavicius, G., Zalinkevicius, R. & Prange, A.J. (1999) Effects of thyroxine as compared with thyroxine plus triiodothyronine in patients with hypothyroidism. *New England Journal of Medicine* **340**, 424–429.

Burks, J.S., Alfrey, A.C., Huddlestone, J., Novenberg, M.D. & Lewin, E. (1976) A fatal encephalopathy in chronic haemodialysis patients. *Lancet* **i**, 764–768.

Burn, D.J. & Bates, D. (1998) Neurology and the kidney. *Journal of Neurology, Neurosurgery and Psychiatry* **65**, 810–821.

Burney, R.E., Jones, K.R., Christy, B. & Thompson, N.W. (1999) Health status improvement after surgical correction of primary hyperparathyroidism in patients with high and low preoperative calcium levels. *Surgery* **125**, 608–614.

Bursten, B. (1961) Psychoses associated with thyrotoxicosis. *Archives of General Psychiatry* **4**, 267–273.

Cardiff University Porphyria Research Group. Available at http://www.cardiff.ac.uk/medicine/medical_biochem/porphyria/index.htm

Carney, M.W.P. & Sheffield, B.F. (1970) Associations of subnormal serum folate and vitamin B$_{12}$ values and effects of replacement therapy. *Journal of Nervous and Mental Disease* **150**, 404–412.

Carney, M.W.P., Wienbren, I., Jackson, F. & Purnell, G.V. (1971) Multiple adenomatosis presenting with psychiatric manifestations. *Postgraduate Medical Journal* **47**, 242–243.

Carney, M.W.P., Williams, D.G. & Sheffield, B.F. (1979) Thiamine-pyridoxine lack in newly-admitted psychiatric patients. *British Journal of Psychiatry* **135**, 249–254.

Carney, M.W.P., Ravindrau, A., Rinsler, M.G. & Williams, D.G. (1982) Thiamine, riboflavin and pyridoxine deficiency in psychiatric in-patients. *British Journal of Psychiatry* **141**, 271–272.

Carney, M.W.P., Chary, T.K.N., Laundy, M. *et al.* (1990) Red cell folate concentrations in psychiatric patients. *Journal of Affective Disorders* **19**, 207–213.

Carroll, B.J. (1976) Psychoendocrine relationships in affective disorders. In: Hill, O.W. (ed.) *Modern Trends in Psychosomatic Medicine*, vol. 3, ch. 7. Butterworth, London.

Castelbaum, A.R., Donofrio, P.D., Walker, F.O. & Troost, B.T. (1989) Laxative abuse causing hypermagnesemia, quadriparesis and neuromuscular junction defect. *Neurology* **39**, 746–747.

Chaudhuri, K.R. (1997) The neurology of diabetes. *British Journal of Hospital Medicine* **58**, 343–347.

Checkley, S.A. (1978) Thyrotoxicosis and the course of manic depressive illness. *British Journal of Psychiatry* **133**, 219–223.

Chiu, H. (1996) Vitamin B$_{12}$ deficiency and dementia. *International Journal of Geriatric Psychiatry* **11**, 851–858.

Christiansen, C., Baastrup, P.C. & Transö, I. (1976) Lithium, hypercalcaemia, hypermagnesaemia, and hyperparathyroidism. *Lancet* **ii**, 969.

Ciechanowski, P., Katon, W.J. & Russo, J.E. (2000) Depression and diabetes: impact of depressive symptoms on adherence, function and costs. *Archives of Internal Medicine* **1160**, 3278–3285.

Clarfield, A.M. (1988) The reversible dementias: do they reverse? *Annals of Internal Medicine* **109**, 476–486.

Clarke, R., Smith, A.D., Jobst, K.A., Refsum, H., Sutton, L. & Ueland, P.M. (1998) Folate, vitamin B12, and serum total homocysteine levels in confirmed Alzheimer's disease. *Archives of Neurology* **55**, 1449–1455.

Clarke, R., Grimley Evans, J., Schneede, J. *et al.* (2004) Vitamin B12 and folate deficiency ini later life. *Age and Ageing* **33**, 34–41.

Cleghorn, R.A. (1951) Adrenal cortical insufficiency: psychological and neurological observations. *Canadian Medical Association Journal* **65**, 449–454.

Cleghorn, R.A. (1965) Hormones and humors. In: Martini, L. & Pecile, A. (eds) *Hormonal Steroids. Biochemistry, Pharmacology, and Therapeutics*, vol. 2, p. 519. Academic Press, New York.

Clinical Society of London (1888) Report of a committee of the Clinical Society of London. Report on myxoedema. *Transactions of the Clinical Society of London* **21** (suppl.), 18.

Clyde, P.W., Harari, A.E., Getta, E.J. & Shakir, K.M.M. (2003) Combined levothyroxine plus liothyronine compared with levothyroxine alone in primary hypothyroidism. A randomized controlled trial. *JAMA* **290**, 2952–2958.

Cogan, M.G., Covey, C.M., Arieff, A.I. *et al.* (1978) Central nervous system manifestations of hyperparathyroidism. *American Journal of Medicine* **65**, 963–970.

Cohen, K.L. & Swigar, M.E. (1979) Thyroid function screening in psychiatric patients. *JAMA* **242**, 254–257.

Cohen, S.I. (1980) Cushing's syndrome: a psychiatric study of 29 patients. *British Journal of Psychiatry* **36**, 120–124.

Colchester, A., Kingsley, D., Lasserson, D. *et al.* (2001) Structural MRI volumetric analysis in patients with organic amnesia. 1. Methods and comparative findings across diagnostic groups. *Journal of Neurology, Neurosurgery and Psychiatry* **70**, 13–22.

Constant, E.L., De Volder, A.G., Ivanoiu, A. *et al.* (2001) Cerebral blood flow and glucose metabolism in hypothyroidism: a positron emission tomographic study. *Journal of Clinical Endocrinology and Metabolism* **86**, 3864–3870.

Conway, M.J., Seibel, J.A. & Eaton, R.P. (1974) Thyrotoxicosis and periodic paralysis: improvement with beta-blockade. *Annals of Internal Medicine* **81**, 332–336.

Cooper, D.S. (2001) Subclinical hypothyroidism. *New England Journal of Medicine* **345**, 260–265.

Cooper, D.S. (2003a) Combined T4 and T3 therapy: back to the drawing board. *JAMA* **290**, 3002–3004.

Cooper, D.S. (2003b) Hyperthyroidism. *Lancet* **362**, 459–468.

Coppen, A. & Bailey, J. (2000) Enhancement of the antidepressant action of fluoxitine by folic acid: a randomised, placebo controlled trial. *Journal of Affective Disorders* **60**, 121–130.

Coppen, A., Chaudhry, S. & Swade, C. (1986) Folic acid enhances lithium prophylaxis. *Journal of Affective Disorders* **10**, 9–13.

Cravioto, J. & Delicardie, E.R. (1970) Mental performance in school age children. Findings after recovery from early severe malnutrition. *American Journal of Diseases of Children* **120**, 404–410.

Crimlisk, H.L. (1997) The little imitator – porphyria: a neuropsychiatric disorder. *Journal of Neurology, Neurosurgery and Psychiatry* **62**, 319–328.

Davis, P.J., Rappeport, J.R., Lutz, H. & Gregerman, R.I. (1971) Three thyrotoxic criminals. *Annals of Internal Medicine* **74**, 743–745.

de Groot, M., Anderson, R., Freedland, K., Clouse, R. & Lustman, P.J. (2000) Association of diabetes complications and depression in type 1 and type 2 diabetes: a meta-analysis [abstract]. *Diabetes* **49**, A63.

Delong, G.R. (1996) The neuromuscular system and brain in thyrotoxicosis. In: Braverman, L.E. & Utiger, R.D. (eds) *Werner and Ingbar's The Thyroid*, 7th edn, pp. 645–652. Lippincott, Philadelphia.

De Moura, M.C., Correia, J.P. & Madeira, F. (1967) Clinical alcohol hypoglycaemia. *Annals of Internal Medicine* **66**, 893–905.

Denko, J.D. & Kaelbling, R. (1962) The psychiatric aspects of hypoparathyroidism. *Acta Psychiatrica Scandinavica Supplementum* **164**, 1–70.

Diabetes Control and Complications Trial Research Group (1996) Effects of intensive diabetes therapy on neuropsychological function in adults in the Diabetes Control and Complications Trial. *Annals of Internal Medicine* **124**, 379–388.

Diabetes Control and Complications Trial Research Group (1997) Hypoglycaemia in the Diabetes Control and Complications Trial. *Diabetes* **46**, 271–286.

Dobbing, J. (1990) Boyd Orr Memorial Lecture. Early nutrition and later achievement. *Proceedings of the Nutrition Society* **49**, 103–118.

Dover, S.B., Moore, M.R., Fitzsimmons, E.J., Graham, A. & McCall, K.E. (1993) Tin protoporphyria prolongs the biochemical remission produced by heme arginate in acute hepatic porphyria. *Gastroenterology* **105**, 500–506.

Dugbartey, A.T. (1998) Neurocognitive aspects of hypothyroidism. *Archives of Internal Medicine* **158**, 1413–1418.

Dunlap, H.F. & Moersch, F.P. (1935) Psychic manifestations associated with hyperthyroidism. *American Journal of Psychiatry* **91**, 1215–1238.

Duyff, R.F., Van den Bosch, J., Laman, D.M., Van Loon, B.J.P. & Linssen, W.H.J.P. (2000) Neuromuscular findings in thyroid dysfunction: a prospective clinical and electrodiagnostic study. *Journal of Neurology, Neurosurgery and Psychiatry* **68**, 750–755.

Eastley, R., Wilcock, G.K. & Bucks, R.S. (2000) Vitamin B12 deficiency in dementia and cognitive impairment: the effects of treatment on neuropsychological function. *International Journal of Geriatric Psychiatry* **15**, 226–233.

Eaton, W.W., Armenian, H., Gallo, J., Pratt, L. & Ford, D.E. (1996) Depression and risk for onset of type II diabetes. A prospective population-based study. *Diabetes Care* **19**, 1097–1102.

Eayers, J.T. (1968) Developmental relationships between brain and thyroid. In: Michael, R.P. (ed.) *Endocrinology and Human Behaviour*, ch. 14. Oxford University Press, Oxford.

Edeh, J. & Toone, B.K. (1985) Antiepileptic therapy, folate deficiency and psychiatric morbidity: a general practice survey. *Epilepsia* **26**, 434–440.

Elder, G.H., Hift, R.T. & Meissner, P.N. (1997) The acute porphyrias. *Lancet* **349**, 1613–1617.

Emsley, R., Potgieter, A., Taljaard, F., Joubert, G. & Gledhill, R. (1989) Water excretion and plasma vasopressin in psychotic disorders. *American Journal of Psychiatry* **146**, 250–253.

Eriksson, P.S., Perfilieva, E., Bjork-Eriksson, T. *et al.* (1998) Neurogenesis in the adult human hippocampus. *Nature Medicine* **11**, 1313–1317.

Expert Committee on the Diagnosis and Classification of Diabetes Mellitus (2003) Report of the expert committee on the diagnosis and classification of diabetes mellitus. *Diabetes Care* **26**, s5–s20.

Fabrykant, M. (1960) Neuropsychiatric manifestations of somatic disease: a review of nutritional, metabolic and endocrine aspects. *Metabolism* **9**, 413–426.

Fava, G.A., Fava, M., Kellner, R., Serafini E & Mastrogiacomo, I. (1981) Depression, hostility and anxiety in hyperprolactinaemic amenorrhoea. *Psychotherapy and Psychosomatics* **36**, 122–128.

Fava, G.A., Sonino, N. & Morphy, M.A. (1987) Major depression associated with endocrine disease. *Psychiatric Developments* **5**, 321–348.

Fava, M., Fava, G.A., Kellner, R. *et al.* (1983) Psychosomatic aspects of hyperprolactinemia. *Psychotherapy and Psychosomatics* **40**, 257–262.

Fenwick, P. (1990) Automatism, medicine and the law. *Psychological Medicine Monograph Supplement* **17**, 1–27.

Ferguson, S.C., Blane, A., Perros, P. *et al.* (2003) Cognitive ability and brain structure in type 1 diabetes: relation to microangiopathy and preceding severe hypoglycemia. *Diabetes* **52**, 149–156.

Fishman, R.A. (1965) Neurological aspects of magnesium metabolism. *Archives of Neurology* **12**, 562–569.

Flink, E.B. (1956) Magnesium deficiency syndrome in man. *JAMA* **160**, 1406–1409.

Flink, E.B. (1969) Therapy of magnesium deficiency. *Annals of the New York Academy of Sciences* **162**, 901–905.

Folks, D.G. & Petrie, W.M. (1982) Thyrotoxicosis presenting as depression. *British Journal of Psychiatry* **140**, 432.

Fontbonne, Berr, C., Ducimetiere, P. & Alperovitch, A. (2001) Changes in cognitive abilities over a 4-year period are unfavorably affected in elderly diabetic subjects: results of the Epidemiology of Vascular Aging Study. *Diabetes Care* **24**, 366–370.

Forrest, K.Y.Z., Becker, D.J., Kuller, L.H., Wolfson, S.K. & Orchard, T.J. (2000) Are predictors of coronary heart disease and lower extremity arterial disease in type 1 diabetes the same? A prospective study. *Atherosclerosis* **148**, 159–169.

Forrest, R.D., Jackson, C.A. & Yudkin, J.S. (1986) Glucose intolerance and hypertension in North London: the Islington Diabetes Survey. *Diabetic Medicine* **3**, 338–342.

Forssman, H. (1970) The mental implications of sex chromosome aberrations. The Blake Marsh Lecture for 1970. *British Journal of Psychiatry* **117**, 353–363.

Fourman, P., Davis, R.H., Jones, K.H., Morgan, D.B. & Smith, J.W.G. (1963) Parathyroid insufficiency after thyroidectomy: review of 46 patients with a study of the effects of hypocalcaemia on the electro-encephalogram. *British Journal of Surgery* **50**, 608–619.

Fourman, P., Rawnsley, K., Davis, R.H., Jones, K.H. & Morgan, D.B. (1967) Effect of calcium on mental symptoms in partial parathyroid insufficiency. *Lancet* **ii**, 914–915.

Fowler, R.C., Kronfol, Z.A. & Perry, P.J. (1977) Water intoxication, psychosis, and inappropriate secretion of antidiuretic hormone. *Archives of General Psychiatry* **34**, 1097–1099.

Frame, B. & Marel, G.M. (1983) Clinical disorders of bone and mineral metabolism. *Annals of Internal Medicine* **99**, 725–727.

Fraser, C.L. (1992) Neurological manifestations of the uremic state. In: Arieff, A.I. & Griggs, R.C. (eds) *Metabolic Brain Dysfunction in Systemic Disorders*, pp. 139–166. Little Brown, Boston.

Fraser, C.L. & Arieff, A.I. (1988) Nervous system complications in uremia. *Annals of Internal Medicine* **109**, 143–153.

Fredericks, E.J. & Lazor, M.Z. (1963) Recurrent hypoglycaemia associated with acute alcoholism. *Annals of Internal Medicine* **59**, 90–94.

Gama, R. Teale, J.D. & Marks, V. (2003) Clinical and laboratory investigation of adult spontaneous hypoglycaemia. *Journal of Clinical Pathology* **56**, 641–646.

Gavard, J.A., Lustman, P.J. & Clouse, R.E. (1993) Prevalence of depression in adults with diabetes. An epidemiological evaluation. *Diabetes Care* **16**, 1167–1178.

Genter, P. & Ipp, E. (1994) Plasma glucose thresholds for counterregulation after an oral glucose load. *Metabolism* **43**, 98.

Gibberd, F.B. & Simmonds, J.P. (1980) Neurological disease in ex-Far-East prisoners of war. *Lancet* **ii**, 135–137.

Godfrey, P.S.A., Toone, B.K., Carney, M.W.P. *et al.* (1990) Enhancement of recovery from psychiatric illness by methylfolate. *Lancet* **336**, 392–395.

Goldman, M.B., Luchins, D.J. & Robertson, G.L. (1988) Mechanisms of altered water metabolism in psychotic patients with polydipsia and hyponatremia. *New England Journal of Medicine* **318**, 397–403.

Goodwin, J.S., Goodwin, J.M. & Garry, P.J. (1983) Association between nutritional status and cognitive functioning in a healthy elderly population. *JAMA* **249**, 2917–2921.

Graham, J.M., Bashir, A.S., Stark, R.E., Silbert, A. & Walzer, S. (1988) Oral and written language abilities of XXY boys: implications for anticipatory guidance. *Pediatrics* **81**, 795–806.

Grainger, D.N. (1992) Rapid development of hyponatraemic seizures in a psychotic patient. *Psychological Medicine* **22**, 513–517.

Gray, J. & Hoffenberg, R. (1985) Thyrotoxicosis and stress. *Quarterly Journal of Medicine, New Series* **54**, 153–160.

Groote Veldman, R.G. & Meinders, A.E. (1996) On the mechanism of alcohol-induced pseudo-Cushing's syndrome. *Endocrine Reviews* **17**, 262–268.

Guisado, R. & Arieff, A.I. (1975) Neurologic manifestations of diabetic comas: correlation with biochemical alterations in the brain. *Metabolism* **24**, 665–679.

Gurney, C., Hall, R., Harper, M., Owen, S., Roth, M. & Smart, G.A. (1967) A study of the physical and psychiatric characteristics of women attending an out-patient clinic for investigation for thyrotoxicosis. Communication to the Scottish Society for Experimental Medicine, Glasgow, 1967. Quoted in Slater, E. & Roth, M. (1969) *Clinical Psychiatry*, 3rd edn. Baillière, Tindall & Cassell, London.

Haddad, P.M. & Wieck, A. (2004) Antipsychotic-induced hyperprolactinaemia. Mechanisms, clinical features and management. *Drugs* **64**, 2291–2314.

Haggerty, J.J. *et al.* (1990) Subclinical hypothyroidism: a review of neuropsychiatric aspects. *International Journal of Psychiatry in Medicine* **20**, 193.

Halbreich, U., Rojansky, N., Palter, S. *et al.* (1995) Decreased bone mineral density in medicated psychiatric patients. *Psychosomatic Medicine* **57**, 485–491.

Hall, R.C.W. (1973) Hypomagnesemia. Physical and psychiatric symptoms. *JAMA* **224**, 1749–1751.

Hambert, G. & Frey, T.S. (1964) The electroencephalogram in the Klinefelter syndrome. *Acta Psychiatrica Scandinavica* **40**, 28–36.

Hammarsten, J.F. & Smith, W.O. (1957) Symptomatic magnesium deficiency in man. *New England Journal of Medicine* **256**, 897–899.

Hanna, S., Harrison, M., Macintyre, I. & Fraser, R. (1960) The syndrome of magnesium deficiency in man. *Lancet* **ii**, 172–176.

Hart, I.K., Maddison, P., Newsom-Davis, J., Vincent, A. & Mills, K.R. (2002) Phenotypic variants of autoimmune peripheral nerve hyperexcitability. *Brain* **125**, 1887–1895.

Haskett, R.F. (1985) Diagnostic categorisation of psychiatric disturbance in Cushing's syndrome. *American Journal of Psychiatry* **142**, 911–916.

Hauw, J.-J., De Baecque, C., Hausser-Hauw, C. & Serdaru, M. (1988) Chromatolysis in alcoholic encephalopathies. *Brain* **111**, 843–857.

Hayes, F.A., Green, A.A., Senzer, N. & Pratt, C.B. (1979) Tetany: a complication of cis-dichlorodiamineplatinum (11) therapy. *Cancer Treatment Reports* **63**, 547–548.

Hayward, C. (1995) Psychiatric illness and cardiovascular disease risk. *Epidemiologic Reviews* **17**, 129–138.

Healton, E.B., Savage, D.G., Brust, J.C., Garrett, T.J. & Lindenbaum, J. (1991) Neurologic aspects of cobalamin deficiency. *Medicine (Baltimore)* **70**, 229–245.

Heath, H. III (1980) Primary hyperparathyroidism. *Lancet* **ii**, 204.

Helweg-Larsen, P., Hoffmeyer, H., Kieler, J. *et al.* (1952) Famine disease in German concentration camps: complications and sequels. *Acta Psychiatrica et Neurologica Scandinavica Supplementum* **83**, 1–460.

Henkin, R.I., Schechter, P.J., Hoyle, R. & Mattern, C.F.T. (1971) Idiopathic hypogeusia with dysgeusia, hyposmia, and dysosmia. A new syndrome. *JAMA* **217**, 434–440.

Henkin, R.I., Patten, B.M., Re, P.K. & Bronzert, D.A. (1975) A syndrome of acute zinc loss. Cerebellar dysfunction, mental changes, anorexia and taste and smell dysfunction. *Archives of Neurology* **32**, 745–751.

Hepburn, D.A. *et al.* (1991) Symptoms of acute insulin-induced hypoglycaemia in humans with and without IDDM: factor-analysis approach. *Diabetes Care* **14**, 949–957.

Herbert, V. (1961) Experimental nutritional folate defiency in man. *Transactions of the Association of American Physicians* **75**, 307.

Herbert, V. (1988) Don't ignore low serum cobalamin (vitamin B12) levels. *Archives of Internal Medicine* **148**, 1705–1707.

Herman, M. & Rost, H. (1937) Psychoses associated with pernicious anemia. *Archives of Neurology and Psychiatry* **38**, 348–361.

Herrick, A.L., McColl, K.E., Wallace, A.M., Moore, A.M. & Goldberg, A. (1990) LHRH analogue treatment for the prevention of premenstrual attacks of acute porphyria. *Quarterly Journal of Medicine* **75**, 355–363.

Herridge, C.F. & Abey-Wickrama, I. (1969) Acute iatrogenic hypothyroid psychosis. *British Medical Journal* **3**, 154.

Hersov, L.A. & Rodnight, R. (1960) Hartnup disease in psychiatric practice: clinical and biochemical features of three cases. *Journal of Neurology, Neurosurgery and Psychiatry* **23**, 40–45.

Hertz, P.E., Nadas, E. & Wojtkowski, H. (1955) Cushing's syndrome and its management. *American Journal of Psychiatry* **112**, 144–145.

Hickman, J.W., Atkinson, R.P., Flint, L.D. & Hurxthal, L.M. (1961) Transient schizophrenic reaction as a major symptom of Cushing's syndrome. *New England Journal of Medicine* **264**, 797–800.

Hindmarsh JT. (1993) Variable phenotypic expression of genotypic abnormalities in the porphyries. *Clinica Chimica Acta* **217**, 29–38.

Hinkle, L.E. & Wolf, S. (1952a) Importance of life stress in course and management of diabetes mellitus. *JAMA* **148**, 513–520.

Hinkle, L.E. & Wolf, S. (1952b) A summary of experimental evidence relating life stress to diabetes mellitus. *Journal of the Mount Sinai Hospital* **19**, 537–570.

Hollowell, J.G., Staehling, N.W., Flanders, W.D. *et al.* (2002) Serum TSH, T4, and thyroid antibodies in the United States population (1988–1994): National Health and Nutrition Examination Survey (NHANES III). *Journal of Clinical Endocrinology and Metabolism* **87**, 489–499.

Holmes, J.M. (1956) Cerebral manifestations of vitamin B_{12} deficiency. *British Medical Journal* **2**, 1394–1398.

Homocysteine Studies Collaboration (2002) Homocysteine and risk of ischaemic heart disease and stroke: a meta-analysis. *JAMA* **288**, 2015–2022.

Hook, E.B. (1992) Prevalence, risks and recurrence. In: Brock, D.J.H., Rodeck, C. & Ferguson-Smith, M. (eds) *Prenatal Diagnosis and Screening*, pp. 351–392. Churchill Livingstone, London.

Hossain, M. (1970) Neurological and psychiatric manifestations in idiopathic hypoparathyroidism: response to treatment. *Journal of Neurology, Neurosurgery and Psychiatry* **33**, 153–156.

Hunt, P.J., Gurnell, E.M., Huppert, F.A. *et al.* (2000) Improvement in mood and fatigue after dehydroepiandrosterone replacement in Addison's disease in a randomized, double blind trial. *Journal of Clinical Endocrinology and Metabolism* **85**, 4650–4656.

Hutto, B.R. (1997) Folate and cobalamin in psychiatric illness. *Comprehensive Psychiatry* **38**, 305–314.

Illowsky, B.P. & Kirch, D.G. (1988) Polydipsia and hyponatremia in psychiatric patients. *American Journal of Psychiatry* **145**, 675–683.

Illum, F. & Dupont, E. (1985) Prevalences of CT-detected calcification in the basal ganglia in idiopathic hypoparathyroidism and pseudohypoparathyroidism. *Neuroradiology* **27**, 32–37.

Ishii, N. & Nishihara, Y. (1981) Pellagra among chronic alcoholics: clinical and pathological study of 20 necropsy cases. *Journal of Neurology, Neurosurgery and Psychiatry* **44**, 209–215.

Jablensky, A., Janota, I. & Shepherd, M. (1970) Neuropsychiatric illness and neuropathological findings in a case of Klinefelter's syndrome. *Psychological Medicine* **1**, 18–19.

Jacobs, P.A., Betts, P.R. & Cockwell, A.E. (1990) *Annals of Human Genetics* **54**, 209–223.

Jadresic, D.P. (1990) Psychiatric aspects of hyperthyroidism. *Journal of Psychosomatic Research* **34**, 603–615.

Jager, J. & Young, R.T. (1974) Sounding board: non-hypoglycemia is an epidemic condition. *New England Journal of Medicine* **291**, 907.

James, W. (1890) What is an emotion? In: *The Principles of Psychology*, vol. 2, pp. 125–142. Dover, New York. (Reprinted 1984 by Oxford University Press, New York.)

Jana, D.K. & Romano-Jana, L. (1973) Hypernatremic psychosis in the elderly: case reports. *Journal of the American Geriatrics Society* **21**, 473–477.

Jeffcoate, W.J., Silverstone, J.T., Edwards, C.R.W. & Besser, G.M. (1979) Psychiatric manifestations of Cushing's syndrome: response to lowering of plasma cortisol. *Quarterly Journal of Medicine* **191**, 465–472.

Jellinek, E.H. (1962) Fits, faints, coma and dementia in myxoedema. *Lancet* **ii**, 1010–1012.

Jellinek, E.H. & Kelly, R.E. (1960) Cerebellar syndrome in myxoedema. *Lancet* **ii**, 225–227.

Jenkins, P.J., Sohaib, S.A., Akker, S. *et al.* (2000) The pathology of median neuropathy in acromegaly. *Annals of Internal Medicine* **133**, 197–201.

Joborn, C., Hetta, J., Rastad, J., Agren, H., Akerstrom, G. & Ljunghall, S. (1988) Psychiatric symptoms and cerebrospinal fluid monoamine metabolites in primary hyperparathyroidism. *Biological Psychiatry* **23**, 149–158.

Joborn, C., Hetta, J., Lind, L., Rastad, J., Akerstrom, G. & Ljunghall, S. (1989) Self-rated psychiatric symptoms in patients operated on because of primary hyperparathyroidism and in patients with long-standing mild hypercalcemia. *Surgery* **105**, 72–78.

Johannsson, G. *et al.* (2002) Low dose dehydroepiandrosterone affects behavior in hypopituitary androgen-deficient women: a placebo-controlled trial. *Journal of Clinical Endocrinology and Metabolism* **87**, 2046–2052.

Johnson, J. (1975) Schizophrenia and Cushing's syndrome cured by adrenalectomy. *Psychological Medicine* **5**, 165–168.

Johnson, W.O. (1928) Psychosis and hyperthyroidism. *Journal of Nervous and Mental Disease* **67**, 558–566.

Jones, S.J., Yu, Y.L., Rudge, P. *et al.* (1987) Central and peripheral SEP defects in neurologically symptomatic and asymptomatic subjects with low vitamin B12 levels. *Journal of the Neurological Sciences* **82**, 55–65.

Jordan, R.M., Kammer, H. & Riddle, M.R. (1977) Sulfonylurea-induced factitious hypoglycaemia: a growing problem. *Archives of Internal Medicine* **137**, 390–393.

Jose, C.J., Barton, J.L. & Perez-Cruet, J. (1979) Hyponatraemic seizures in psychiatric patients. *Biological Psychiatry* **14**, 839–843.

Josephson, A.M. & Mackenzie, T.B. (1980) Thyroid-induced mania in hypothyroid patients. *British Journal of Psychiatry* **137**, 222–228.

Kaminski, H.J. & Ruff, R.L. (1989) Neurologic complications of endocrine diseases. *Neurologic Clinics* **7**, 489–508.

Kappas, A., Sassa, S., Galbraith, R.A. & Nordmann, Y. (1989) The porphyrias. In: Scriver, C.R., Beaudet, A.L., Sly, W.S. & Valle, D. (eds) *The Metabolic Basis of Inherited Disease*, 6th edn, ch. 52. McGraw-Hill, New York.

Kappas, A., Sassa, S., Galbraith, R.A. & Nordmann, Y. (1995) The porphyrias. In: Scriver, C.S., Beaudet, A.L., Sly, W.S. & Valle, D. (eds) *The Metabolic and Molecular Bases of Inherited Disease*, 7th edn, pp. 2103–2160. McGraw-Hill, New York.

Karnaze, D.S. & Carmel, R. (1990) Neurologic and evoked potential abnormalities in subtle cobalamin deficiency states, including deficiency without anemia and with normal absorption of free cobalamin. *Archives of Neurology* **47**, 1008–1012.

Karp, B.I. & Laureno, R. (1995) Pontine and extra-pontine myelinolysis: a neurologic disorder following rapid correction of hyponatraemia. *Medicine* **72**, 359–371.

Karpati, G. & Frame, B. (1964) Neuropsychiatric disorders in primary hyperparathyroidism. *Archives of Neurology* **10**, 387–397.

Kasper, D.L. & Harrison, T.R. (2004) *Harrison's Principles of Internal Medicine*, 16th edn. McGraw Hill, New York.

Kathol, R.G., Turner, R. & Delahunt, J. (1986) Depression and anxiety associated with hyperthyroidism: response to antithyroid therapy. *Psychosomatics* **27**, 501–505.

Kauppinen, R. & Mustajoki, P. (1992) Prognosis of acute porphyria: occurrence of acute attacks, precipitating factors, and associated diseases. *Medicine* **71**, 1–13.

Kawakami, N., Takatsuka, N., Shimizu, H. & Ishibashi, H. (1999) Depressive symptoms and occurrence of type 2 diabetes among Japanese men. *Diabetes Care* **22**, 1071–1076.

Kealey, S.M. & Provenzale, J.M. (2002) Tensor diffusion imaging in B12 leukoencephalopathy *Journal of Computer Assisted Tomography* **26**, 952–955.

Keller, S.K., Neuhaus-Theil, A. & Quabbe, H.J. (1985) Psychological correlates of prolactin secretion: aggression and depression. *Acta Endocrinologica* **108**, 118–119.

Kelly, W.F. (1996) Psychiatric aspects of Cushing's syndrome. *Quarterly Journal of Medicine* **89**, 543–551.

Kelly, W.F., Checkley, S.A., Bender, D.A. & Mashiter, K. (1983) Cushing's syndrome and depression: a prospective study of 26 patients. *British Journal of Psychiatry* **142**, 16–19.

Kennedy, A.C., Linton, A.L., Luke, R.G. & Renfrew, S. (1963) Electroencephalographic changes during haemodialysis. *Lancet* **i**, 408–411.

Kennedy, G.C., German, M.S. & Rutter, W.J. (1995) The minisatellite in the diabetes susceptibility locus IDDM2 regulates insulin transcription. *Nature Genetics* **9**, 293–298.

Kerr, D.S., Campbell, L.W., Applegate, M.D., Brodish, A. & Landfield, P.W. (1991) Chronic stress induced acceleration of electrophysiologic and morphometric biomarkers of hippocampal ageing. *Journal of Neuroscience* **11**, 1316–1324.

Kertesz, S.G. (2001) Pellagra in two homeless men. *Mayo Clinic Proceedings* **76**, 315–318.

Kessing, L.V., Nilsson, F.M., Siersma, V. & Andersen, P.K. (2003) No increased risk of developing depression in diabetes compared to other chronic illness. *Diabetes Research and Clinical Practice* **62**, 113–121.

Khamnei, A.K. (1984) Psychosis, inappropriate antidiuretic hormone secretion, and water intoxication. *Lancet* **i**, 963.

Kihlbom, M. (1969) Psychopathology of Turner's syndrome. *Acta Paedopsychiatrica* **36**, 75–81.

Kind, H. (1958) Die Psychiatrie der Hypophyseninsuffienz speziell der Simmondsschen Krankheit. *Fortschritte der Neurologie-Psychiatrie* **26**, 501–563.

King, P.H. & Bragdon, A.C. (1991) MRI reveals multiple reversible cerebral lesions in an attack of acute intermittent porphyria. *Neurology* **41**, 1300–1302.

Kirov, G.K., Birch, N.J., Steadman, P. & Ramsey, R.G. (1994) Plasma magnesium levels in a population of psychiatric patients: correlations with symptoms. *Neuropsychobiology* **30**, 73–78.

Kleinfeld, M., Peter, S. & Gilbert, G.M. (1984) Delirium as the predominant manifestation of hyperparathyroidism: reversal after parathyroidectomy. *Journal of the American Geriatrics Society* **32**, 689–690.

Klinefelter, H.F., Reifenstein, E.C., & Albright, F. (1942) Syndrome characterized by gynecomastia, aspermatogenesis without a-Leydigism and increased excretion of follicle stimulation hormone. *Journal of Clinical Endocrinology and Metabolism* **2**, 615–627.

Knochel, J.P. (1977) Pathophysiology and clinical characteristics of severe hypophosphataemia. *Archives of Internal Medicine* **137**, 203–220.

Knopman, D., Boland, L.L., Mosley, T. *et al.* (2001) Cardiovascular risk factors and cognitive decline in middle-aged adults. *Neurology* **56**, 42–48.

Kong, M.F. & Jeffcoate W. (1994) Eighty-six cases of Addison's disease. *Clinical Endocrinology (Oxf)* **41**, 757–761.

Kosfeld, M., Heinrichs, M., Zak, P.J., Fischbacher, U. & Fehr, E. (2005) Oxytocin increases trust in humans. *Nature* **435**, 673–676.

Kowdley, K.V., Coull, B.M. & Orwoll, E.S. (1999) Cognitive impairment and intracranial calcification in chronic hypoparathyroidism. *American Journal of the Medical Sciences* **317**, 273–277.

Kraepelin, E. (1896) *Psychiatrie*, 5th edn. Barth, Leipzig.

Kruse, J., Schmitz, N. & Thefeld, W. (2003) German National Health Interview and Examination Survey. On the association between diabetes and mental disorders in a community sample: results from the German National Health Interview and Examination Survey. *Diabetes Care* **26**, 1841–1846.

Kunze, K. & Leitenmaier, K. (1976) Vitamin B$_{12}$ deficiency and subacute combined degeneration of the spinal cord. In: Vinken, P.J. & Bruyn, G.W. (eds) *Handbook of Clinical Neurology, vol. 28. Metabolic and Deficiency Diseases of the Nervous System*, Part II, ch. 6. North-Holland Publishing Company, Amsterdam.

Kupferschmidt, H., Bont, A., Schnorf, H. *et al.* (1995) Transient cortical blindness and biooccipital brain lesions in two patients with acute intermittent porphyria. *Annals of Internal Medicine* **123**, 598–600.

Lahey, F.H. (1931) Non-activated (apathetic) type of hyperthyroidism. *New England Journal of Medicine* **204**, 747–748.

Laiwah, A.C., MacPhee, G.J., Boyle, P., Moore, M.R. & Goldberg, A. (1985) Autonomic neuropathy in acute intermittent porphyria. *Journal of Neurology, Neurosurgery and Psychiatry* **48**, 1025–1030.

Langan, S.J., Deary, I.J., Hepburn, D.A. & Frier, B.M. (1991) Cumulative cognitive impairment following recurrent severe hypoglycaemia in adult patients with insulin-treated diabetes mellitus. *Diabetalogia* **34**, 337–344.

Langdon, F.W. (1905) Nervous and mental manifestations of pre-pernicious anemia. *JAMA* **45**, 1635–1638.

Larner, A.J. (1995) Neurological presentations of hypothyroidism. *Journal of the Royal Society of Medicine* **88**, 721.

Laurent, J., Debry, G. & Floquet, J. (1971) *Hypoglycaemic Tumours*. Excerpta Medica, Amsterdam.

Lawrence, K., Campbell, R., Swettenham, J. *et al.* (2003a) Interpreting gaze in Turner syndrome: impaired sensitivity to intention and emotion, but preservation of social cueing. *Neuropsychologia* **41**, 894–905.

Lawrence, K., Kuntsi, J., Coleman, M., Campbell, R. & Skuse, D. (2003b) Face and emotion recognition deficits in Turner syndrome: a possible role for X-linked genes in amygdala development. *Neuropsychology* **17**, 39–49.

Ledingham, J.G.G. (1983) Water and sodium homeostasis. In: Weatherall, D.J., Ledingham, J.G.G. & Warrell, D.A. (eds) *Oxford Textbook of Medicine*, vol. 2, pp. 18.19–18.28. Oxford University Press, Oxford.

Lee, E.K., Maselli, R.A., Ellis, W.G. & Agius, M.A. (1998) Morvan's fibrillary chorea: a paraneoplastic manifestation of thymoma. *Journal of Neurology, Neurosurgery and Psychiatry* 65, 857–862.

Lee, S., Chow, C.C., Wing, Y.K., Leung, C.M., Chiu, H. & Chen, C.N. (1991) Mania secondary to thyrotoxicosis. *British Journal of Psychiatry* 159, 712–713.

Le Feuvre, M., Isaacs, A.J. & Frank, O.S. (1982) Bromocriptine induced psychosis in acromegaly. *British Medical Journal* 285, 1315.

Leigh, D. (1952) Pellagra and the nutritional neuropathies: a neuropathological review. *Journal of Mental Science* 98, 130–142.

Leigh, H. & Kramer, S.I. (1984) The psychiatric manifestations of endocrine disease. *Advances in Internal Medicine* 29, 413–445.

Leonard, L.B., Cole, B. & Steckol, K.F. (1979) Lexical usage of retarded children: an examination of informativeness. *American Journal of Mental Deficiency* 84, 49–54.

Levistsky, D.A. & Strupp, B.J. (1995) Malnutrition and the brain: changing concepts, changing concerns. *Journal of Nutrition* 125 (8 suppl.), 2221S–2232S.

Levitt, A.J. & Joffe, R.T. (1988) Vitamin B12 in psychotic depression. *British Journal of Psychiatry* 153, 266–267.

Levitt, A.J. & Joffe, R.T. (1993) Folate, B12 and thyroid function in depression. *Biological Psychiatry* 33, 52–53.

Liguori, R., Vincent, A., Clover, L. *et al.* (2001) Morvan's syndrome: peripheral and central nervous system and cardiac involvement with antibodies to voltage-gated potassium channels. *Brain* 124, 2417–2426.

Lindberg, R.L., Martini, R., Baumgartner, M. *et al.* (1999) Motor neuropathy in porphobilinogen deaminase-deficient mice imitates the peripheral neuropathy of human acute porphyria. *Journal of Clinical Investigation* 103, 1127–1134.

Lindenbaum, J., Healton, E.B., Savage, D.G. *et al.* (1988) Neuropsychiatric disorders caused by cobalamin deficiency in the absence of anemia or macrocytosis. *New England Journal of Medicine* 318, 1720–1728.

Lishman, W.A. (1981) Cerebral disorder in alcoholism: syndromes of impairment. *Brain* 104, 1–20.

Lishman, W.A. (1997) *Organic Psychiatry: The Psychological Consequences of Cerebral Disorder*, 3rd edn. Blackwell Publishing, Oxford.

Locke, S., Merrill, J.P. & Tyler, H.R. (1961) Neurologic complications of acute uremia. *Archives of Internal Medicine* 108, 519–530.

Loftus, L.S. & Arnold, W.N. (1991) Vincent van Gogh's illness: acute intermittent porphyria? *British Medical Journal* 303, 1589–1591.

Logothetis, J. (1961) Neurologic and muscular manifestations of hyperthyroidism. *Archives of Neurology* 5, 533–544.

Loosen, P.T., Chambliss, B., Debold, C.R., Shelton, R. & Orth, D.N. (1992) Psychiatric phenomenology in Cushing's disease. *Pharmacopsychiatry* 25, 192–198.

Lovas, K., Loge, J.H. & Husebye, E.S. (2002) Subjective health status in Norwegian patients with Addison's disease. *Clinical Endocrinology* 56, 581–588.

Lovas, K., Gebre-Medhin, G., Trovik, T.S. *et al.* (2003) Replacement of dehydroepiandrosterone in adrenal failure: no benefit for subjective health status and sexuality in a 9-month, randomised, parallel group clinical trial. *Journal of Clinical Endocrinology and Metabolism* 88, 1112–1118.

Lustman, P.J., Griffith, L.S., Clouse, R.E. *et al.* (1997) Effects of nortriptyline on depression and glycemic control in diabetes. Results of a double-blind, placebo-controlled trial. *Psychosomatic Medicine* 59, 241–250.

Lustman, P.J., Griffith, L.S., Freedland, K.E., Kissel, S.S. & Clouse, R.E. (1998) Cognitive behavior therapy for depression in type 2 diabetes: results of a randomized controlled clinical trial. *Annals of Internal Medicine* 129, 613–621.

Lustman, P.J., Anderson, R.J., Freedland, K.E., De Groot, M., Carney, R.M. & Clouse, R.E. (2000) Depression and poor glycemic control: a meta-analytic review of the literature. *Diabetes Care* 23, 434–442.

Luttrell, C.N. & Finberg, L. (1959) Haemorrhagic encephalopathy caused by hypernatraemia: clinical, laboratory and pathological observations. *Archives of Neurology and Psychiatry* 81, 424–428.

MacAlpine, I. & Hunter, R. (1966) The 'insanity' of King George III: a classic case of porphyria. *British Medical Journal* 1, 65–71.

MacAlpine, I. & Hunter, R. (1969) *George III and the Mad-Business.* Allen Lane, The Penguin Press, London.

MacAlpine, I., Hunter, R. & Rimington, C. (1968) Porphyria in the royal houses of Stuart, Hanover, and Prussia: a follow-up study of George III's illness. *British Medical Journal* 1, 7–18.

McCarthy, M.M. (1994) Molecular aspects of sexual differentiation of the rodent brain. *Psychneuroendocrinology* 19, 415–427.

McCauley, E., Ross, J.L., Kushner, H. & Cutler, G. (1995) Self-esteem and behaviour in girls with Turner's syndrome. *Journal of Developmental and Behavioural Pediatrics* 16, 82–88.

McColl, K.E.L., Dover, S., Fitzsimons, E. & Moore, M.R. (1996) Porphyrin metabolism and the porphyrias. In: Weatherall, D.J., Ledingham, J.G.G. & Warrell, D.A. (eds) *Oxford Textbook of Medicine*, 3rd edn, vol. 2, section 11.5. Oxford University Press, Oxford.

McDermott, J.R., Smith, A.I., Ward, M.K., Parkinson, I.S. & Kerr, D.N.S. (1978) Brain-aluminium concentration in dialysis encephalopathy. *Lancet* i, 901–904.

McEwen, B.S., DeKloet, E.R. & Rostene, W. (1986) Adrenal steroid receptors and actions in the nervous system. *Physiological Reviews* 66, 1121–1188.

McFarland, H.R. (1963) Addison's disease and related psychoses. *Comprehensive Psychiatry* 4, 90–95.

McLarty, D.G., Ratcliffe, W.A., Ratcliffe, J.G., Shimmins, J.G. & Goldberg, A. (1978) A study of thyroid function in psychiatric in-patients. *British Journal of Psychiatry* 133, 211–218.

McLester, J.S. (1943) *Nutrition and Diet in Health and Disease*, 4th edn. W.B. Saunders, Philadelphia.

Mace, C.J. (1987) Brittle diabetes in a drug and alcohol abuser. *British Journal of Addiction* 82, 931–934.

Madonick, M.J., Berke, K. & Schiffer, I. (1950) Pleocytosis and meningeal signs in uremia: report on 62 cases. *Archives of Neurology and Psychiatry* 64, 431–436.

Mampalam, T.J., Tyrrell, J.B. & Wilson, C.B. (1988) Transsphenoidal microsurgery for Cushing's disease: a report of 216 cases. *Annals of Internal Medicine* 109, 487–493.

Manyam, B.V. (2005) What is and what is not 'Fahr's disease'. *Parkinsonism & Related Disorders* **11**, 73–80.

Margo, A. (1981) Acromegaly and depression. *British Journal of Psychiatry* **139**, 467–468.

Markowitz, A.M., Slanetz, C.A. & Frantz, V.K. (1961) Functioning islet cell tumours of the pancreas: twenty-five year follow up. *Annals of Surgery* **154**, 877–844.

Marks, V. (1981a) Symptomatology. In: Marks, V. & Rose, F.C. (eds) *Hypoglycaemia*, 2nd edn, ch. 5. Blackwell Scientific Publications, Oxford.

Marks, V. (1981b) Pancreatic hypoglycaemia (hyperinsulinism). In: Marks, V. & Rose, F.C. (eds) *Hypoglycaemia*, 2nd edn, ch. 7. Blackwell Scientific Publications, Oxford.

Marks, V. & Teale, J.D. (2001) Hypoglycemic disorders. *Clinics in Laboratory Medicine* **21**, 79–97.

Marsden, C.D., Meadows, J.C. & Lange, G.W. (1970) Effect of speed of muscle contraction on physiological tremor in normal subjects and in patients with thyrotoxicosis and myxoedema. *Journal of Neurology, Neurosurgery and Psychiatry* **37**, 776–782.

Marshal, R.S. & Mohr, J.P. (1993) Current management of ischemic stroke. *Journal of Neurology Neurosurgery and Psychiatry* **56**, 6–16.

Matos-Santos, A., Nobre, E.L., Costa, J.G.E. *et al.* (2001) Relationship between the number and impact of stressful life events and the onset of Graves' disease and toxic nodular goitre. *Clinical Endocrinology* **55**, 15–19.

Mattana, J., Ahn, J., Desroches, L., Fitzmaurice, S. & Singhal, P.C. (1993) Naloxone reverses encephalopathy in end-stage renal disease. *American Journal of Kidney Diseases* **21**, 669–672.

Mattson, M.P. & Shea, T.B. (2003) Folate and homocysteine in neural plasticity and neurodegenerative disorders. *Trends in Neurosciences* **26**, 137–146.

Mawdsley, C. (1972) Neurological complications of haemodialysis. *Proceedings of the Royal Society of Medicine* **65**, 871–873.

Melamed, E. (1979) Neurological disorders related to folate deficiency. In: Botez, M.I. & Reynolds, E.H. (eds) *Folic Acid in Neurology, Psychiatry, and Internal Medicine*, ch. 38. Raven Press, New York.

Mercier-Guidez, E. & Loas, G. (2000) Polydipsia and water intoxication in 353 psychiatric inpatients: an epidemiological and psychopathological study. *European Psychiatry* **15**, 306–311.

Meyer, A. (1901) On parenchymatous systemic degenerations mainly in the central nervous system. *Brain* **24**, 47–115.

Meyer, U.A., Schuurmans, M.M. & Lindberg, R.L. (1998) Acute porphyrias: pathogenesis of neurological manifestations. *Seminars in Liver Disease* **18**, 43–52.

Michael, R.P. & Gibbons, J.L. (1963) Interrelationships between the endocrine system and neuropsychiatry. *International Review of Neurobiology* **5**, 243–302.

Minkoff, L., Gaertner, G., Darab, M., Mercier, C. & Levin, M.L. (1972) Inhibition of brain sodium-potassium ATPase in uremic rats. *Journal of Laboratory and Clinical Medicine* **80**, 71–78.

Mitchell, J.R.A., Surridge, D.H.C. & Willison, R.G. (1959) Hypothermia after chlorpromazine in myxoedematous psychosis. *British Medical Journal* **2**, 932–933.

Mitchell, W. & Feldman, F. (1968) Neuropsychiatric aspects of hypokalaemia. *Canadian Medical Association Journal* **98**, 49–51.

Money, J. (1963) Cytogenetic and psychosexual incongruities with a note on space-form blindness. *American Journal of Psychiatry* **119**, 820–827.

Money, J. (1964) Two cytogenetic syndromes: psychologic comparisons. 1. Intelligence and specific-factor quotients. *Journal of Psychiatric Research* **2**, 223–231.

Moore, M.R. & Disler, P.B. (1988) Drug-sensitive diseases. 1. Acute porphyrias. *Adverse Drug Reaction Bulletin* **129**, 484–487.

Morgan, M.Y. (1982) Alcohol and the endocrine system. *British Medical Bulletin* **38**, 35–42.

Morvan, A. M. (1890) De la chorée fibrillaire. *Gazette Hebdomadaire de Medicine et de Chirurgie* **27**, 173–176.

Mukherjee, A.B., Svoronos, S., Ghazanfari, A. *et al.* (1987) Transketolase abnormality in cultured fibroblasts from familial chronic alcoholic men and their male offspring. *Journal of Clinical Investigation* **79**, 1039–1043.

Mundy, D.R., Cove, G.H. & Fisken, R. (1980) Primary hyperparathyroidism: changes in the pattern of clinical presentation. *Lancet* **i**, 1317–1320.

Murphy, D.G.M., Decarli, C., Daly, E. *et al.* (1993) X-chromosome effects on female brain: a magnetic resonance imaging study of Turner's syndrome. *Lancet* **342**, 1197–1200.

Murphy, D.G.M., Allen, G., Haxby, J.V. *et al.* (1994) The effects of sex steroids, and the X chromosome, on female brain function: a study of the neuropsychology of adult Turner syndrome. *Neuropsychologia* **32**, 1309–1323.

Murphy, D.G.M., Mentis, M.J., Pietrini, P. *et al.* (1997) A PET study of Turner's syndrome: effects of sex steroids and the X chromosome on brain. *Biological Psychiatry* **41**, 285–298.

Musselman, D.L., Betan, E., Larsen, H. & Phillips, L.S. (2003) Relationship of depression to diabetes types 1 and 2: epidemiology, biology, and treatment. *Biological Psychiatry* **54**, 317–329.

Mustajoki, P., Kauppinen, R., Lannfelt, L., Lilius, L. & Koistinen, J. (1992) Frequency of low erythrocyte porphobilinogen deaminase activity in Finland. *Journal of Internal Medicine* **231**, 389–395.

Nagamine, K., Peterson, P., Scott, H.S. *et al.* (1997) Positional cloning of the APECED gene. *Nature Genetics* **17**, 393–398.

Netley, C. & Rovet, J. (1982) Verbal deficits in children with 47,XXY and 47,XXX karyotypes: a descriptive and experimental study. *Brain and Language* **17**, 58–72.

Newcomer, J.W., Selke, G., Melson, A.K. *et al.* (1999) Decreased memory performance in heathy humans induced by stress-level cortisol treatment. *Archives of General Psychiatry* **56**, 527–533.

Nielsen, J. (1969) Klinefelter's syndrome and the XYY syndrome. *Acta Psychiatrica Scandinavica Supplementum* **209**, 1–353.

Nielsen, J., Pelsen, B. & Sorensen, K. (1988) Follow-up of 30 Klinefelter males treated with testosterone. *Clinical Genetics* **33**, 262–269.

Nilsson, B., Gustavasson-Kadaka, E., Bengtsson, B.A. & Jonsson, B. (2000) Pituitary adenomas in Sweden between 1958 and 1991: incidence, survival, and mortality. *Journal of Clinical Endocrinology and Metabolism* **85**, 1420–1425.

Nissenson, A.R. (1989) Recombinant human erythropoietin: impact on brain and cognitive function, exercise tolerance, sexual potency, and quality of life. *Seminars in Nephrology* **9**, 25–31.

Numann, P.J., Torppar, A.J. & Blumetti, A.E. (1984) Neuropsychologic deficits associated with primary hyperparathyroidism. *Surgery* **96**, 1119–1123.

O'Brien, M.D. & Harris, P.W.R. (1968) Cerebral-cortex perfusion-rates in myxoedema. *Lancet* **i**, 1170–1172.

O'Connor, T.G., Rutter, M., Beckett, C., Keaveney, L. & Kreppner, J.M. (2000) The effects of global severe privation on cognitive competence: extension and longitudinal follow-up. *Child Development* **71**, 376–390.

Oelkers, W., Diederich, S. & Bahr, V. (1992) Diagnosis and therapy surveillance in Addison's disease: rapid adrenocorticotropin (Acth) test and measurement of plasma Acth, renin activity, and aldosterone. *Journal of Clinical Endocrinology and Metabolism* **75**, 259–264.

Okada, J., Yoshikawa, K., Matsuo, H., Kanno, K. & Oouchi, M. (1991) Reversible MRI and CT findings in uremic encephalopathy. *Neuroradiology* **33**, 524–526.

Orwin, A., James, S.R.N. & Turner, R.K. (1974) Sex chromosome abnormalities, homosexuality and psychological treatment. *British Journal of Psychiatry* **124**, 293–295.

Osterweil, D. *et al.* (1992) Cognitive function in non-demented older adults with hypothyroidism. *Journal of the American Geriatrics Society* **40**, 325–335.

Paisley, A.N. & Trainer, P.J. (2003) Medical treatment in acromegaly. *Current Opinion in Pharmacology* **3**, 672–677.

Pappius, H.M. (1976) Inorganic constituents. In: Vinken, P.J. & Bruyn, G.W. (eds) *Handbook of Clinical Neurology*, pp. 423–441. Elsevier, New York.

Parkinson, I.S., Ward, M.K., Feest, T.G., Fawcett, R.W.P. & Kerr, D.N.S. (1979) Fracturing dialysis osteodystrophy and dialysis encephalopathy. An epidemiological survey. *Lancet* **i**, 406–409.

Pasantes-Morales, H. (1996) Volume regulation in brain cells: cellular and molecular mechanisms. *Metabolic Brain Disease* **11**, 187–204.

Pasqualini, R.Q., Vidal, G. & Bur, G.E. (1957) Psychopathology of Klinefelter's syndrome. Review of thirty-one cases. *Lancet* **ii**, 164–167.

Patience, D.A., Blackwood, D.H., McColl, K.E. & Moore, M.R. (1994) Acute intermittent porphyria and mental illness: a family study. *Acta Psychiatrica Scandinavica* **89**, 262–267.

Patten, B.M. & Pages, M. (1984) Severe neurological disease associated with hyperparathyroidism. *Annals of Neurology* **15**, 453–456.

Patwardhan, A.J., Eliez, S., Bender, B., Linden, M.G. & Reiss, A.L. (2000) Brain morphology in Klinefelter syndrome: extra X chromosome and testosterone supplementation. *Neurology* **54**, 2218–2223.

Pennington, B.F., Heaton, R.K., Karzmark, P. *et al.* (1985) The neuropsychological phenotype in Turner syndrome. *Cortex* **21**, 391–404.

Penninx, B.W., Guralnik, J.M., Ferrucci, L., Fried, L.P., Allen, R.H. & Stabler, S.P. (2000) Vitamin B(12) deficiency and depression in physically disabled older women: epidemiologic evidence from the Women's Health and Aging Study. *American Journal of Psychiatry* **157**, 715–721.

Perks, W.H., Horrocks, P.M., Cooper, R.A. *et al.* (1980) Sleep apnoea in acromegaly. *British Medical Journal* **280**, 894–897.

Petersen, P. (1968) Psychiatric disorders in primary hyperparathyroidism. *Journal of Clinical Endocrinology and Metabolism* **28**, 1491–1495.

Peterson, H. De C. & Swanson, A.G. (1964) Acute encephalopathy occurring during haemodialysis. *Archives of Internal Medicine* **113**, 877–880.

Pfeiffer, J.A.F. (1915) Neuropathological findings in case of pernicious anemia with psychical implications. *Journal of Nervous and Mental Disease* **42**, 75.

Phillips, V. (1992) Queen Anne's 'seventeen disappointments'. *Medical Journal of Australia* **156**, 341–342.

Pollitt, E.J. (2000) Developmental sequel from early nutritional deficiencies: conclusive and probability judgements. *Journal of Nutrition* **130**, 350S–353S.

Pomeroy, J.C. (1980) Klinefelter's syndrome and schizophrenia. *British Journal of Psychiatry* **136**, 597–599.

Powers, H.J. (2003) Riboflavin (vitamin B-2) and health. *American Journal of Clinical Nutrition* **77**, 1352–1360.

Price, B.H. & Mesulam, M.M. (1987) Behavioural manifestations of central pontine myelinolysis. *Archives of Neurology* **44**, 671–673.

Prins, J.G., Schrijve, H. & Staghouw, J.H. (1973) Hyperalimentation, hypophosphataemia and coma. *Lancet* **i**, 1253–1254.

Randall, R.E., Rossmeisl, E.C. & Bleifer, K.H. (1959) Magnesium depletion in man. *Annals of Internal Medicine* **50**, 257–287.

Raskin, N.H. (1989) Neurological aspects of renal failure. In: Aminoff, M.J. (ed.) *Neurology and General Medicine*, ch. 14. Churchill Livingstone, New York.

Read, A.E., Gough, K.R., Pardoe, J.L. & Nicholas, A. (1965) Nutritional studies on the entrants to an old people's home, with particular reference to folic acid deficiency. *British Medical Journal* **2**, 843–848.

Reavley, S., Fisher, A.D., Owen, D., Creed, F.H. & Davis, J.R.E. (1997) Psychological distress in patients with hyperprolactinaemia. *Clinical Endocrinology* **47**, 343–348.

Regland, B. *et al.* (1997) Homozygous thermolabile methylenetetrahydrofolate reductase in schizophrenia-like psychosis. *Journal of Neural Transmission* **104**, 931–941.

Reichard, P., Pihl, M., Rosenqvist, U. & Sule, J. (1996) Complications in IDDM are caused by elevated blood glucose level: The Stockholm Diabetes Intervention Study (SDIS) at 10-year follow up. *Diabetologia* **39**, 1483–1488.

Reichlin, S. (1968) Neuroendocrinology. In: Williams, R.H. (ed.) *Textbook of Endocrinology*, 4th edn, ch. 12. W.B. Saunders, Philadelphia.

Reio, L. & Wetterberg, L. (1969) False porphobilinogen reactions in the urine of mental patients. *JAMA* **207**, 148–150.

Reiss, A.L., Mazzocco, M.M., Greenlaw, R., Freund, L.S. & Ross, J.L. (1995) Neurodevelopmental effects of X monosomy: a volumetric imaging study. *Annals of Neurology* **38**, 731–738.

Reynolds, E.H. (1973) Anticonvulsants, folic acid, and epilepsy. *Lancet* **i**, 1376–1378.

Reynolds, E.H. (1979) Folic acid, vitamin B12, and the nervous system: historical aspects. In: Botez, M.I. & Reynolds, E.H. (eds) *Folic Acid in Neurology, Psychiatry and Internal Medicine*, pp. 1–5. Raven Press, New York.

Reynolds, E.H. (1991) Interictal psychiatric disorders: neurochemical aspects. *Advances in Neurology* **55**, 47–58.

Reynolds, E.H. (2002) Benefits and risks of folic acid to the nervous system. *Journal of Neurology, Neurosurgery and Psychiatry* **72**, 567–571.

Reynolds, E.H., Preece, J.M., Bailey, J. & Coppen, A. (1970) Folate deficiency in depressive illness. *British Journal of Psychiatry* **117**, 287–292.

Reynolds, E.H., Wrighton, R.J., Johnson, A.L., Preece, J. & Chanarin, I. (1971) Interrelations of folic acid and vitamin B$_{12}$ in drug-treated epileptic patients. *Epilepsia* **12**, 165–171.

Reynolds, E.H., Rothfeld, P. & Pincus, J.H. (1973) Neurological disease associated with folate deficiency. *British Medical Journal* **2**, 398–400.

Reynolds, E.H., Carney, M.W.P. & Toone, B.K. (1984) Methylation and mood. *Lancet* **ii**, 196–198.

Richardson, J.C., Chambers, R.A. & Heywood, P.M. (1959) Encephalopathies of anoxia and hypoglycaemia. *Archives of Neurology* **1**, 178–190.

Richet, G. & Vachon, F. (1966) Troubles neuro-psychiques de l'urémie chronique. *Présse Medicale* **74**, 1177–1182.

Richet, G., Lopez De Novales, E. & Verroust, P. (1970) Drug intoxication and neurological episodes in chronic renal failure. *British Medical Journal* **1**, 394–395.

Riedel, M., Wiese, A., Schurmeyer, T.H. & Brabant, G. (1993) Quality-of-life in patients with Addison's disease: effects of different cortisol replacement modes. *Experimental and Clinical Endocrinology* **101**, 106–111.

Riggs, J.E. (1989) Neurologic manifestations of fluid and electrolyte disturbances. *Neurologic Clinics* **7**, 509–523.

Rivoal, O., Brezin, A.P., Feldman-Billard, S. & Luton, J.P. (2000) Goldmann perimetry in acromegaly: a survey of 307 cases from 1951 through 1996. *Ophthalmology* **107**, 991–997.

Rizzo, M.A., Fisher, M. & Lock, J.P. (1993) Hypermagnesemic pseudocoma. *Archives of Internal Medicine* **153**, 1130–1132.

Roberts, C.G.P. & Ladenson, P.W. (2004) Hypothyroidism. *Lancet* **363**, 793–803.

Romano, J. & Coon, G.P. (1942) Physiologic and psychologic studies in spontaneous hypoglycaemia. *Psychosomatic Medicine* **4**, 283–300.

Ross, J.L., Roeltgen, D., Feuillan, P., Kushner, H. & Cutler, G.B. (2000) Use of estrogen in young girls with Turner syndrome: effects on memory. *Neurology* **54**, 164–170.

Ross, J.L., Stefanatos, G.A., Kushner, H., Zinn, A., Bondy, C. & Roeltgen, D. (2002) Persistent cognitive deficits in adult women with Turner syndrome. *Neurology* **58**, 218–225.

Rovet, J., Netley, C., Keenan, M., Bailey, J. & Stewart, D. (1996) The psychoeducational profile of boys with Klinefelter syndrome. *Journal of Learning Disabilities* **29**, 180–196.

Roy, A. (1981) Schizophrenia and Klinefelter's syndrome. *Canadian Journal of Psychiatry* **26**, 262–264.

Ruel, J., Faur, R. & Dussault, J.H. (1985) Regional distribution of nuclear T3 receptors in rat brain and evidence for preferential localisation in neurons. *Journal of Endocrinological Investigation* **8**, 343.

Salmons, P.H. (1980) Psychological aspects of chronic renal failure. *British Journal of Hospital Medicine* **23**, 617–622.

Salvatori, R. & Wand, G.S. (2002) Hypothalamic/pituitary function and dysfunction. In: Asbury, A.K., McKhann, G.M., McDonald, W.I. *et al.* (eds) *Diseases of the Nervous System*, 3rd edn, p. 867. Cambridge, UK: Cambridge University Press.

Sandifer, M.G. (1983) Hyponatraemia due to psychotropic drugs. *Journal of Clinical Psychiatry* **44**, 301–303.

Sapolsky, R.M., Steinbehrens, B.A. & Armanini, M.P. (1990) Long-term adrenalectomy causes loss of dentate and pyramidal neurons in the adult hippocampus. *Experimental Neurology* **114**, 246–249.

Saravanan, P., Chau, W.F., Roberts, N. *et al.* (2002) Psychological well-being in patients on 'adequate' doses of L-thyroxine: results of a large, controlled community-based questionnaire study. *Clinical Endocrinology* **57**, 577–585.

Savage, D.G., Lindenbaum, J., Stabler, S.P. & Allen, R.H. (1994) Sensitivity of serum methylmalonic acid and total homocysteine determinations for diagnosing cobalamin and folate deficiency. *American Journal of Medicine* **96**, 239–246.

Sawka, A.M., Gerstein, H.C., Marriott, M.J., MacQueen, G.M. & Joffe, R.T. (2003) Does a combination regimen of thyroxine (T4) and 3,5,3-triiodothyronine improve depressive symptoms in patients with hypothyroidism? Results of a double blind randomized, controlled trial. *Journal of Clinical Endocrinology and Metabolism* **88**, 4551–4555.

Scarlett, J.A., Mako, M.E., Rubenstein, A.H. *et al.* (1977) Factitious hypoglycemia. Diagnosis by measurement of serum C-peptide immunoreactivity and insulin binding antibodies. *New England Journal of Medicine* **297**, 1029–1032.

Schaumburg, H.H. (1992) Uraemic neuropathy In: *Disorders of Peripheral Nerves*, 2nd edn, pp. 156–163. F.A. Davis, Philadelphia.

Scheinberg, P. (1951) Cerebral blood flow and metabolism in pernicious anaemia. *Blood* **6**, 213–227.

Scheinberg, P., Stead, E.A., Brannon, E.S. & Warren, J.V. (1950) Correlative observations on cerebral metabolism and cardiac output in myxoedema. *Journal of Clinical Investigation* **29**, 1139–1146.

Scherer, K. (2003) Neurologic manifestations of vitamin B12 deficiency. *New England Journal of Medicine* **348**, 2208.

Schiavi, R.C., Theilgaard, A., Owen, D.R. & White, D. (1984) Sex chromosome anomalies, hormones, and aggressivity. *Archives of General Psychiatry* **41**, 93–99.

Scrimshaw, N.S. (1998) Malnutrition, brain development, learning and behaviour. *Nutrition Research* **18**, 351–379.

Seggev, J., Shapiro, M.S., Levin, S. & Schey, G. (1986) Alveolar hypoventilation and daytime hypersomnia in acromegaly. *European Journal of Respiratory Diseases* **68**, 381–383.

Serdaru, M., Hausser-Hauw, C., Laplane, D. *et al.* (1988) The clinical spectrum of alcoholic pellagra encephalopathy. A retrospective analysis of 22 cases studied pathologically. *Brain* **111**, 829–842.

Service, F.J. (1995) Medical progress: hypoglycaemic disorders. *New England Journal of Medicine* **332**, 1144–52.

Service, F.J. (1999) Diagnostic approach to adults with hypoglycaemic disorders. *Endocrinology and Metabolism Clinics of North America* **28**, 519–532.

Service, F.J., McMahon, M.M., O'Brien, P.C. & Ballard, D.J. (1991) Functioning insulinoma: incidence, recurrence, and long-term survival of patients – a 60-year study. *Mayo Clinic Proceedings* **66**, 711–719.

Sheehan, H.L. & Summers, V.K. (1949) The syndrome of hypopituitrism. *Quarterly Journal of Medicine* **18**, 319–378.

Shorvon, S.D., Carney, M.W.P., Chanarin, I. & Reynolds, E.H. (1980) The neuropsychiatry of megaloblastic anaemia. *British Medical Journal* **281**, 1036–1038.

Shulman, R. (1967) Psychiatric aspects of pernicious anaemia: a prospective controlled investigation. *British Medical Journal* **3**, 266–270.

Signoret, J.P. & Balthazart, J. (1994) Preface. Proceedings of the International Conference on Hormones, Brain and Behaviour

(Tours, France, August 24–27, 1993). *Psychoneuroendocrinology* **19**, 403–406.

Silverberg, S.J., Shane, E., Jacobs, T.B. *et al.* (1999) 10-year prospective study of primary hyperparathyroidism with or without parathyroid surgery. *New England Journal of Medicine* **341**, 1249–1255.

Simpson, J.L., de la Cruz, F., Swerdloff, R.S. *et al.* (2003) Klinefelter syndrome: expanding the phenotype and identifying new research directions. *Genetics in Medicine* **5**, 460–468.

Singh, S., Padi, M.H., Bullard, H. & Freeman, H. (1985) Water intoxication in psychiatric patients. *British Journal of Psychiatry* **146**, 127–131.

Sivakumar, K. & Williams, M. (1991) Psychiatric aspects of acromegaly: a review and case report. *Irish Journal of Psychological Medicine* **8**, 55–56.

Skuse, D.H., James, R.S., Bishop, D.V. *et al.* (1997) Evidence from Turner's syndrome of an imprinted X-linked locus affecting cognitive function. *Nature* **387**, 705–708.

Smals, A.G., Kloppenborg, P.W., Njo, K.T., Knoben, J.M. & Rutland, C.M. (1976) Alcohol-induced Cushingoid syndrome. *British Medical Journal* **2**, 1298.

Smith, A.D.M. (1960) Megaloblastic madness. *British Medical Journal* **2**, 1840–1845.

Smith, C.D. & Ain, K.B. (1995) Brain metabolism in hypothyroidism studied with ^{31}P magnetic-resonance spectroscopy. *Lancet* **345**, 619–620.

Smith, D.B. & Obbens, E.A.M.T. (1979) Antifolate–antiepileptic relationships. In: Botez, M.I. & Reynolds, E.H. (eds) *Folic Acid in Neurology, Psychiatry, and Internal Medicine*, ch. 28. Raven Press, New York.

Sobrinho, L.G. (1991) *Ballière's Clinical Endocrinology and Metabolism*, 5, 119–142.

Sokoloff, L., Wechsler, R.L., Mangold, R., Balls, K. & Kety, S.S. (1953) Cerebral blood flow and oxygen consumption in hyperthyroidism before and after treatment. *Journal of Clinical Investigation* **32**, 202–208.

Sonino, N., Fava, G.A. & Boscaro, M. (1993a) A role for stressful life events in the pathogenesis of Cushing's disease. *Clinical Endocrinology* **38**, 261–264.

Sonino, N., Fava, G.A., Belluardo, P., Girelli, M.E. & Boscaro, M. (1993b) Course of depression in Cushing's syndrome: response to tratment and comparison with Graves disease. *Hormone Research* **39**, 202–206.

Sonino, N., Raffi, A.R., Boscaro, M. & Fallo, F. (1998) Clinical correlates of major depression in Cushing's disease. *Psychopathology* **31**, 302–306.

Spence, S. (1995) The psychopathology of acromegaly. *Irish Journal of Psychological Medicine* **12**, 142–144.

Spies, T.D., Aring, C.D., Gelperin, J. & Bean, W.B. (1938) The mental symptoms of pellagra: their relief with nicotinic acid. *American Journal of the Medical Sciences* **196**, 461–475.

Spillane, J.D. (1947) *Nutritional Disorders of the Nervous System*. Livingstone, Edinburgh.

Starkman, M.N., Giordani, B., Berent, S., Schork, M.A. & Schteingart, D.E. (2001) Elevated cortisol levels in Cushing's disease are associated with cognitive decrements. *Psychosomatic Medicine* **63**, 985–993.

Starkman, M.N., Schteingart, D.E. & Schork, M.A. (1981) Depressed mood and other psychiatric manifestations of Cush-

ing's syndrome: relationship to hormone levels. *Psychosomatic Medicine* **43**, 3–18.

Starkman, M.N., Gebarski, S.S., Berent, S. & Schteingart, D.E. (1992) Hippocampal formation volume, memory dysfunction, and cortisone levels in patients with Cushing's syndrome. *Biological Psychiatry* **32**, 756–765.

Starkman, M.N., Giordani, B., Gebarski, S.S., Berent, S., Schork, M.A. & Schteingart, D.E. (1999) Decrease in cortisol reverses human hippocampal atrophy following treatment of Cushing's disease. *Biological Psychiatry* **46**, 1595–1602.

Starkman, M.N., Giordani, B., Gebarski, S.S. & Schteingart, D.E. (2003) Improvement in learning associated with increase in hippocampal formation volume. *Biological Psychiatry* **53**, 233–238.

Staton, M.A., Donald, A.G. & Green, G.B. (1976) Zinc deficiency presenting as schizophrenia. *Current Concepts in Psychiatry* **2**, 11–14.

Stenbäck, A. & Haapanen, E. (1967) Azotaemia and psychosis. *Acta Psychiatrica Scandinavica Supplementum* **197**, 1–65.

Sterner, R.T. & Price, W.R. (1973) Restricted riboflavin: within-subject behavioral effects in humans. *American Journal of Clinical Nutrition* **26**, 150–160.

Sterns, R.H., Riggs, J.E. & Schochet, S.S. (1986) Osmotic demyelination syndrome following correction of hyponatremia. *New England Journal of Medicine* **314**, 1535–1542.

Storm, E.E. & Tecott, L.H. (2005) Social circuits: peptidergic regulation of mammalian social behaviour. *Neuron* **47**, 483–486.

Strachan, M.W.J., Deary, I.J., Ewing, F.M.E. & Frier, B.M. (2000) Recovery of cognitive function and mood after severe hypoglycemia in adults with insulin-treated diabetes. *Diabetes Care* **23**, 305–312.

Strachan, M.W.J., Frier, B.M. & Deary I.J. (2003) Type 2 diabetes and cognitive impairment. *Diabetic Medicine* **20**, 1–2.

Strachan, R.W. & Henderson, J.G. (1967) Dementia and folate deficiency. *Quarterly Journal of Medicine* **36**, 189–204.

Sulway, M.R., Broe, G.A., Creasey, H. *et al.* (1996) Are malnutrition and stress risk factors for accelerated cognitive decline? A prisoner of war study. *Neurology* **46**, 650–655.

Surks, M.I., Ortiz, E., Daniels, G.H. *et al.* (2004) Subclinical thyroid disease. Scientific review and guidelines for diagnosis and management. *JAMA* **291**, 228–238.

Surwit, R.S., Schneider, M.S. & Feinglos, M.N. (1992) Stress and diabetes mellitus. *Diabetes Care* **15**, 1413–1422.

Susser, E., Brown, A.S., Klonowski, E., Allen, R.H. & Lindenbaum, J. (1998) Schizophrenia and impaired homocysteine metabolism: a possible association. *Biological Psychiatry* **44**, 141–143.

Sutker, P.B., Galina, Z.H., West, J.A. & Allain, A.N. (1990) Trauma-induced weight loss and cognitive deficits among former prisoners of war. *Journal of Consulting and Clinical Psychology* **58**, 323–328.

Sutker, P.B., Allain, A.N., Johnson, J.L. & Butters, N.M. (1992) Memory and learning performances in POW survivors with history of malnutrition and combat veteran controls. *Archives of Clinical Neuropsychology* **7**, 431–444.

Sutker, P.B., Allain, A.N. & Winstead, D.K. (1993) Psychopathology and psychiatric diagnoses of World War II Pacific theatre prisoner of war survivors and combat veterans. *American Journal of Psychiatry* **150**, 240–245.

Swanson, D.W. & Stipes, A.H. (1969) Psychiatric aspects of Klinefelter's syndrome. *American Journal of Psychiatry* **126**, 814–822.

Swanson, P.D. (1976) Neurological manifestations of hypernatraemia. In: Vinken, P.J. & Bruyn, G.W. (eds) *Handbook of Clinical Neurology*, vol. 28, pp. 443–461. New Holland Publishing Company, Amsterdam.

Taylor, M.J., Carney, S.M., Geddes, J. & Goodwin, G. (2003) Folate for depressive disorders. *Cochrane Database Systematic Review* 2, CD003390.

Temple, C.M. (2002) Oral fluency and narrative production in children with Turner's syndrome. *Neuropsychologia* **40**, 1419–1427.

Temple, C.M. & Sanfilippo, P.M. (2003) Executive skills in Klinefelter's syndrome. *Neuropsychologia* **41**, 1547–1559.

Territo, M.C. & Tanaka, K.R. (1973) Hypophosphataemia in chronic alcoholism. *Archives of Internal Medicine* **134**, 445–447.

Thadani, H., Deacon, A. & Peters, T. (2000) Diagnosis and management of porphyria. *British Medical Journal* **320**, 1647–1651.

Thieben, M.J., Lennon, V.A., Boeve, B.F., Aksamit, A.J., Keegan, M. & Vernino, S. (2004) Potentially reversible autoimmune limbic encephalitis with neuronal potassium channel antibody. *Neurology* **62**, 1177–1182.

Thomas, F.B., Mazzaferi, E.L. & Skillman, T.G. (1970) Apathetic thyrotoxicosis: a distinctive clinical and laboratory entity. *Annals of Internal Medicine* **72**, 679–685.

Thunell, S., Floderus, Y., Henrichson, A., Moore, M.R. & Sinclair, J. (1992) Alcoholic beverages in acute porphyria. *Journal of Studies on Alcohol* **53**, 272–276.

Thygesen, P., Hermann, K. & Willanger, R. (1970) Concentration camp survivors in Denmark. Persecution, disease, disability, compensation. A 23-year follow-up. A survey of the long-term effects of severe environmental stress. *Danish Medical Bulletin* **17**, 65–108.

Tiemeier, H., van Tuijl, H.R., Hofman, A., Meijer, J., Kiliaan, A.J. & Breteler, M.M. (2002) Vitamin B12, folate and homocysteine in depression: the Rotterdam study. *American Journal of Psychiatry* **159**, 2099–2101.

Tishler, P.V., Woodward, B., O'Connor, J. *et al.* (1985) High prevalence of intermittent acute porphyria in a psychiatric patient population. *American Journal of Psychiatry* **142**, 1430–1436.

Tonks, C.M. (1964) Mental illness in hypothyroid patients. *British Journal of Psychiatry* **110**, 706–710.

Toosy, A.T., Burbridge, S.E., Pitkanen, M. *et al.* (2005) Voltage gated potassium antibody associated syndrome with central and peripheral nervous system involvement: a case of Morvan's syndrome.

Trethowan, W.H. & Cobb, S. (1952) Neuropsychiatric aspects of Cushing's syndrome. *Archives of Neurology and Psychiatry* **67**, 281–309.

Trzepacz, P.T., McCue, M., Klein, I., Greenhouse, J. & Levey, G.S. (1988) Psychiatric and neuropsychological response to propranolol in Graves' disease. *Biological Psychiatry* **23**, 678–688.

Trzepacz, P.T., Klein, I., Roberts, M., Greenhouse, J. & Levey, G.S. (1989) Graves' disease: an analysis of thyroid hormone levels and hyperthyroid signs and symptoms. *American Journal of Medicine* **87**, 558–561.

Tunbridge, W.M.G., Evered, D.C., Hall, R. *et al.* (1977) The spectrum of thyroid disease in the community: the Whickham survey. *Clinical Endocrinology* **7**, 481–493.

Turner, T.H. (1984) Psychotic reactions during treatment of pituitary tumours with dopamine agonists. *British Medical Journal* **289**, 1101–1102.

Tyler, H.R. (1968) Neurologic disorders in renal failure. *American Journal of Medicine* **44**, 734–748.

Usdin, T.B., Gruber, C. & Bonner, T.I. (1995) Identification and functional expression of a receptor selectively recognizing parathyroid hormone, the PTH2 receptor. *Journal of Biological Chemistry* **270**, 15455–15458.

Usdin, T.B., Hoare, S.R., Wang, T., Mezey E & Kowalak, J.A. (1999) TIP39: a new neuropeptide and PTH2-receptor agonist from hypothalamus. *Nature Neuroscience* **2**, 941–943.

Utz, N., Kinkel, B., Hedde, J.P. & Bewermeyer, H. (2001) MR imaging of acute intermittent porphyria mimicking reversible posterior leukoencephalopathy syndrome. *Neuroradiology* **43**, 1059–1062.

Vallee, B.L., Wacker, W.E.C. & Ulmer, D.D. (1960) The magnesium-deficiency tetany syndrome in man. *New England Journal of Medicine* **262**, 155–161.

Vanneste, J. & Hage, J. (1986) Acute severe hypophosphataemia mimicking Wernicke's encephalopathy. *Lancet* **i**, 44.

Victor, M. & Lear, A.A. (1956) Subacute combined degeneration of the spinal cord: current concepts of the disease process; value of serum vitamin B12 determinations in clarifying some of the common clinical problems. *American Journal of Medicine* **20**, 896–911.

Vieweg, W.V.R., David, J.J., Rowe, W.T., Wampler, C.J., Burns, W.J. & Spradlin, W.W. (1985) Death from self-induced water intoxication among patients with schizophrenic disorders. *Journal of Nervous and Mental Disease* **173**, 161–165.

Vincent, A., Buckley, C., Schott, J.M. *et al.* (2004) Potassium channel antibody-associated encephalopathy: a potentially immunotherapy responsive form of limbic encephalitis. *Brain* **127**, 701–712.

Wakeling, A. (1972) Comparative study of psychiatric patients with Klinefelter's syndrome and hypogonadism. *Psychological Medicine* **2**, 139–154.

Walsh, J.P., Shiels, L., Lim, E.M. *et al.* (2003) Combined thyroxine/liothyronine treatment does not improve well-being, quality of life, or cognitive function compared to thyroxine alone: a randomised controlled trial in patients wth primary hypothyroidism. *Journal of Clinical Endocrinology and Metabolism* **88**, 4543–4550.

Walstra, G.J.M., Teunisse, S., Van Gool, W.A. & Van Crevel, H. (1997) Reversible dementia in elderly patients referred to a memory clinic. *Journal of Neurology* **244**, 17–22.

Walton, J.N., Kiloh, L.G., Osselton, J.W. & Farrall, J. (1954) The electroencephalogram in pernicious anaemia and subacute combined degeneration of the cord. *Electroencephalography and Clinical Neurophysiology* **6**, 45–64.

Walzer, S., Wolff, P.H., Bowen, D. *et al.* (1978) A method for the longitudinal study of behavioral development in infants and children: the early development of XXY children. *Journal of Child Psychology and Psychiatry and Allied Disciplines* **19**, 213–229.

Walzer, S., Graham, J.M., Bashir, A.S. & Sibert, A.R. (1982) Preliminary observations on language and learning in XXY boys. *Birth Defects Original Article Series* **18**, 185–192.

Wang, H.-X., Wahlin, A., Basun, H. *et al.* (2001) Vitamin B12 and folate in relation to the development of Alzheimer's disease. *Neurology* **56**, 1188–1194.

Warren, M.J., Jay, M., Hunt, D.M., Elder, G.H. & Rohl, J.C. (1996) The maddening business of King George III and porphyria. *Trends in Biochemical Science* **21**, 229–234.

Warwick, M.M., Doodie, G.A., Lowrie, S.M. *et al.* (1999) Volumetric magnetic resonance imaging study of the brain in subjects with sex chromosome aneuploidies. *Journal of Neurology, Neurosurgery and Psychiatry* **66**, 628–632.

Watson, L. (1968) Clinical aspects of hyperparathyroidism. *Proceedings of the Royal Society of Medicine* **61**, 1123.

Watson, L. (1972) Diseases of the parathyroid glands. *Medicine (monthly add-on series, 1972–3)* **2**, 148–156. Medical Education (International) Ltd, London.

Waxman, J. (1990) Hypercalcaemia: a new mechanism for old observations. *British Journal of Cancer* **61**, 647–648.

Wayne, E.J. (1960) Clinical and metabolic studies in thyroid disease. *British Medical Journal* **1**, 1–11, 78–90.

Weizman, A., Eldar, M., Shoenfeld, Y., Hirshorn, M., Wijsenbeek, W. & Pinkhas, J. (1979) Hypercalcaemia-induced psychopathology in malignant diseases. *British Journal of Psychiatry* **135**, 363–366.

Welland, F.H., Hellman, E.S., Collins, A., Hunter, G.W. & Tschudy, D.P. (1964) Factors affecting the excretion of porphyrin precursors by patients with acute intermittent porphyria II. The effect of ethinyl estradiol. *Metabolism* **13**, 251–258.

Westlake, E.K., Simpson, T. & Kaye, M. (1955) Carbon dioxide narcosis in emphysema. *Quarterly Journal of Medicine* **24**, 155–173.

Whybrow, P.C. & Bauer, M. (2000) Behavioural and psychiatric aspects of hypothyroidism. In: Braverman, L.E. & Utiger, R.D. (eds) *Werner and Ingbar's The Thyroid: A Fundamental and Clinical Text*, 8th edn, pp. 837–842. Lippincott Williams & Wilkins, Philadelphia.

Whybrow, P.C. & Hurwitz, T. (1976) Psychological disturbances associated with endocrine disease and hormone therapy. In: Sachar, E.J. (ed.) *Hormones, Behavior and Psychopathology*, p. 516. Raven Press, New York.

Whybrow, P.C., Prange, A.J. & Treadway, C.R. (1969) Mental changes accompanying thyroid gland dysfunction. *Archives of General Psychiatry* **20**, 48–63.

Wieck, A. & Haddad, P. (2002) Hyperprolactinaemia caused by antipsychotic drugs. *British Medical Journal* **324**, 250–252.

Williams, D., Hilton, S.M. & Moore, J. (2002) Cognitive measures of Vietnam-era prisoners of war. *JAMA* **288**, 574.

Wilson, S.A.K. (1940) *Neurology*. Edward Arnold, London.

Wing, R.R., Epstein, L.H., Blair, E. & Nowalk, M.P. (1985) Psychologic stress and blood-glucose levels in nondiabetic subjects. *Psychosomatic Medicine* **47**, 558–564.

Winqvist, O., Karlsson, F.A. & Kampe, O. (1992) 21-Hydroxylase, a major autoantigen in idiopathic Addison's disease. *Lancet* **339**, 1559–1562.

Woltman H.W. (1924) The mental changes associated with pernicious anemia. *American Journal of Medicine* **80**, 435–449.

Woodbury, M.S. (1918) The psycho-neurotic syndrome of hyperthyroidism. *Journal of Nervous and Mental Disorders* **47**, 401–410.

Wredling, R., Levander, S., Adamson, U. & Lins, P.E. (1990) Permanent neuropsychological impairment after recurrent episodes of severe hypoglycaemia in man. *Diabetologia* **33**, 152–157.

Wyatt, K.M., Dimmock, P.W., Jones, P.W. & O'Brien, P.M.S. (1999) Efficacy of vitamin B-6 in the treatment of premenstrual syndrome: systematic review. *British Medical Journal* **318**, 1375–1381.

Wyke, B. (1963) *Brain Function and Metabolic Disorders*. Butterworth, London.

Young, G.P., Amacher, A.L., Paulseth, J.E., Gilbert, J.J. & Sibbald, W.J. (1982) Hypophosphataemia vs. brain death. *Lancet* **i**, 617.

Yudkin, J.S., Forrest, R.D., Jackson, C.A., Burnett, S.D. & Gould M.M. (1993) The prevalence of diabetes and impaired glucose tolerance in a British population. *Diabetes Care* **16**, 1530.

Zellisen, P.M.J. & Croughs, R.J.M. (1994) Relation of osteopenia to glucocorticoid replacement therapy in Addison disease: reply. *Annals of Internal Medicine* **121**, 236–237.

Zucker, D.K., Livingston, R.L., Nakra, R. & Clayton, P.J. (1981) B_{12} deficiency and psychiatric disorders: case report and literature review. *Biological Psychiatry* **16**, 197–205.

CHAPTER 11

Addictive and Toxic Disorders

Mayur Bodani,[1] **Laurence J. Reed**[2] **and Michael D. Kopelman**[2]

[1] West Kent Neurorehabilitation Unit, Sevenoaks Hospital, Kent
[2] Institute of Psychiatry, King's College, London

This chapter is divided into two parts, the first reflecting nervous system toxicity deriving from intentional exposure to addictive substances with implicit yet unintended toxicity (addictive disorders) and the second relating to those disorders arising from incidental exposure to environmental toxins (toxic disorders).

A variety of lines of evidence from animal behavioural research and functional imaging show that a diverse group of substances share distinct reinforcing or 'rewarding' properties. These substances act to alter the function of a common set of neurobiological substrates to produce the compulsive behaviours characterised as addiction. Following a general consideration of the complex processes underpinning addiction, we consider the disorders specific to alcohol, licit and illicit drugs with psychoactive properties and abuse potential in succession.

Non-addictive drugs, certain metals and chemicals are the exogenous toxins that are considered later in this chapter. The effects of toxins derived from invading microorganisms have been briefly considered in Chapter 7 and the toxic products of disordered metabolism in uraemia and hepatic dysfunction in Chapter 10. Poisoning due to metals and other chemical compounds is largely the province of industrial medicine, but must also be borne in mind in occasional patients who present with psychiatric illness of uncertain aetiology.

ADDICTIVE DISORDERS

Addictive disorders have not been separately addressed in previous editions of this book, perhaps reflecting the difficulties in considering addiction as a 'brain disease', the complexity of the disorder as manifested with respect to the variety of substances with abuse liability and, lastly, the competing view of addiction as a moral disorder. Indeed,

Hyman (2007) in a very recent review points out the considerable difficulties in considering such a common yet remarkable condition as addiction as a 'brain disorder' with all the attendant implications for responsibility, voluntary behaviour and free will. That difficulty aside, the disease model of addiction has considerably advanced our understanding of the condition, factors predisposing to its development and its consequences. The earliest coherent consideration of the disease model of addictive disorders was addressed by Himmelsbach (1943) who expressed the view that the disorder required the presence of a physical abstinence syndrome, and that the state of dependence reflected an acquired abnormal state wherein increasing amounts of the substance were required to maintain physiological equilibrium. Clear difficulties arise with such a definition in that, following a period of physiological dependence, the compulsive behaviours are exacerbated rather than lost, requiring definition of a further term 'psychological dependence' (Eddy et al. 1965), again a label that has proved rather unhelpful. Currently, modern diagnostic thought is concentrating on a more precise definition of addiction for the forthcoming *Diagnostic and Statistical Manual of Mental Disorders* (DSM)-V, focusing on compulsive behaviours and marking a distinction from the DSM-IV criteria for substance dependence *per se* (O'Brien et al. 2006).

Koob and Le Moal (1997) have defined drug addiction as a state characterised by (i) a compulsion to seek and take the drug, (ii) a loss of control in limiting intake and (iii) the emergence of negative emotional states (e.g. dysphoria, anxiety, irritability) when access to the drug is prevented. They proposed that the condition arises from the acquisition of unstable 'allostatic' adaptations to specific stress, emotional and reward pathways – hedonic homeostatic dysregulation. Important competing theories, seeking to provide a more complete inclusion of phenomena observed in addiction,

Lishman's Organic Psychiatry: A Textbook of Neuropsychiatry, 4th edition.
© 2009 Blackwell Publishing.   ISBN 978-1-4051-1860-1

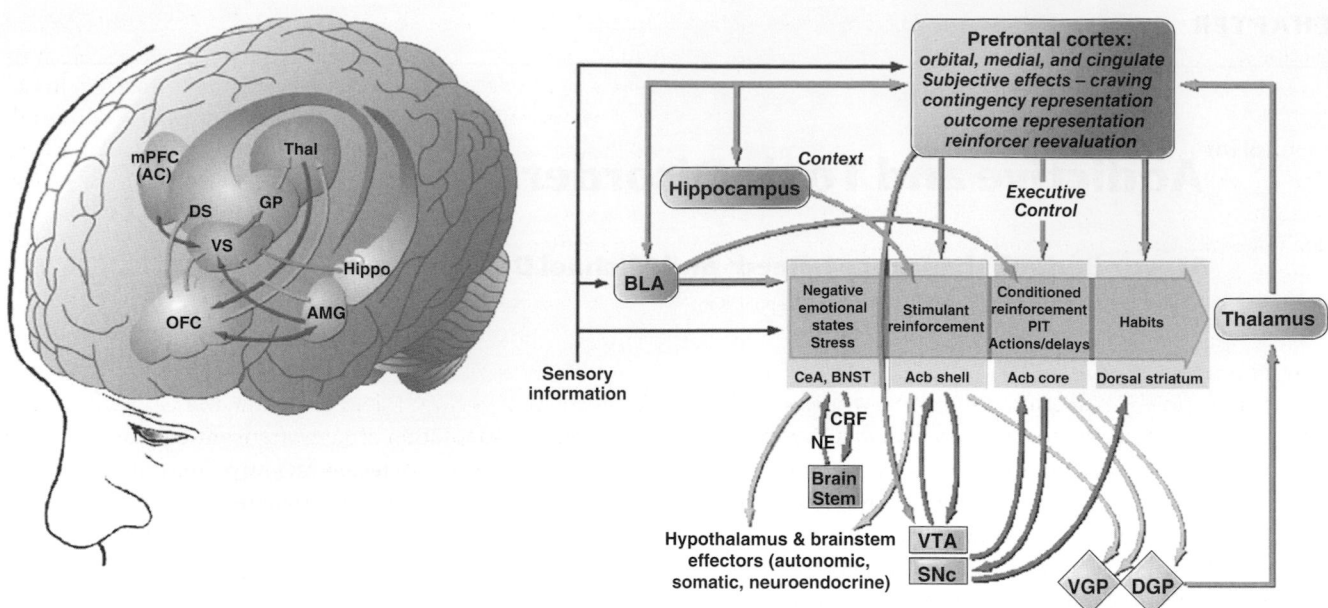

Fig. 11.1 Key elements of the neurocircuitry of addiction (see also Plate 11.1). (From Koob *et al.* 2008 with permission.)

include the incentive–salience model (Robinson & Berridge 1993), wherein neural circuits underpinning the importance or salience of stimuli are sensitised by repeated psychostimulant exposure, leading to compulsive behaviours. This particular theory has the advantage of divorcing the dopaminergic system from function as simple 'reward' system. Everitt and Robbins (2005) have focused on the reinforcement of drug responses related to learning and memory in the transition from episodic 'impulsive' to addictive 'compulsive' drug-taking behaviours. This model emphasises the multiplicity of basic neural systems underpinning addictive behaviours (Fig. 11.1: see also Plate 11.1) (Koob *et al.* 2008). Lastly, a more 'cognitive' view of addictive behaviours has been emphasised by Bechara (2005), positing impairment of prefrontal cortical functions monitoring internal state and guiding future actions as the basis for maladaptive drug-taking. Possibly this works through impaired inhibition of impulsive behaviours, although this latter model may better explain vulnerability to addiction rather than the state itself. Neuroimaging using positron emission tomography (PET) to observe brain metabolic and dopaminergic changes associated with the addicted state has been particularly useful in identifying core networks that may separately or together underpin the compulsive nature of the condition; these include diminished ventral striatal dopamine D_2 receptor availability (Volkow *et al.* 2008a) associated with either impaired reward sensitivity or inhibitory processes (Volkow *et al.* 2008b).

Addictive disorders exhibit common features among the various substances that have abuse liability, involving alterations in a variety of behaviours and implicating a variety of important basic neuronal systems both in the vulnerability to addiction and in attainment of the addicted state. The molecular and genetic basis for adaptation within these networks is now yielding to scrutiny (Nestler 2001). This section considers the neuropsychiatric conditions associated with particular addictive drugs, with regard to the addictive processes themselves and the inadvertent toxicity related to consumption of the drug.

Alcohol

Effects of alcohol on the nervous system

Alcohol is remarkable both for its long history and ubiquity of use (Edwards 2000) and for the diverse range of nervous system disorders that it can produce.

1 Direct effects: alcohol was previously thought to be a simple depressant of CNS functioning, but is highly dose sensitive in its effects.

2 A series of disorders, including fits, hallucinoses and delirium tremens, which are largely due to alcohol withdrawal.

3 Associated nutritional defects leading variously to Wernicke's encephalopathy, Korsakoff's syndrome, peripheral neuropathy and perhaps cerebellar degeneration.

4 Resultant end-stage liver disorder or bone marrow suppression may ensue with their own neuropsychiatric complications.

In addition there is evidence that alcohol and/or its metabolites exert lasting neurotoxic effects, most marked in fetal development but also of relevance in recovery from brain injury. The distinction between these mechanisms cannot be considered absolute for all the syndromes concerned, but in general reaches broad agreement. The direct, nutritional and withdrawal effects of alcohol are considered in the following sections.

Alcohol intoxication

The effects of alcohol consumption are sensitive to dose (measured as blood alcohol level), timing (rising versus declining phase) and social context. Although alcohol is conventionally cited as a central nervous system (CNS) depressant in a manner analogous to that of anaesthetic agents, a specific molecular target has recently been identified on the γ-aminobutyric acid $(GABA)_A$ receptor (Santhakumar *et al.* 2007) leading to augmentation of GABA neurotransmission, although some detailed controversy remains (Lovinger & Homanics 2007). The fact that this has only been discovered recently relates to the relatively high doses of alcohol needed to exert effects, in contrast to high-affinity conventional drug–receptor interactions. The general augmentation of GABA neurotransmission is associated with early net effects on opioidergic and dopaminergic neurotransmission in the ventral striatal 'reward' pathways (Gianoulakis 2001; Barrett *et al.* 2008). These early effects produce stimulation, usually with subjective exhilaration, excitement and loquacity. Personality factors and environmental factors are important at this stage, lively company leading usually to boisterous cheerfulness, whereas alcohol taken alone may intensify feelings of loneliness and depression. Cultural influences are also clearly important in helping to shape the outward evidence of intoxication (Edwards 1974).

At higher doses there are net depressant effects on widespread cortical networks leading to a reduction of psychological efficiency and motor control, which is often at variance with subjective feelings of superiority and skill. Thinking becomes slowed and superficial, with poverty of associations and impaired judgement and reasoning. Learning and retention become faulty, and remote memory unreliable. Acuity of perception is reduced, attention impaired and distractibility increased. Muscular control is impaired at an early stage and reaction times delayed. Later dysarthria, frank incoordination and ataxia appear.

With more severe intoxication there is progressive loss of restraint, self-control becomes undermined and irregularities of behaviour appear. Emotions of hilarity, sadness or self-pity may gain the upper hand, or there may be marked irritability and hostility. With very high blood levels there is increasing drowsiness, leading finally to coma. In alcoholic coma the breathing is slow and stertorous and the temperature subnormal. The pupils may be contracted or widely dilated and the tendon reflexes weak or absent.

A fairly close relationship exists between the intensity of the effects and the level of alcohol in the blood, measured as blood alcohol concentration (BAC), ranging from early euphoria (BAC 0.03–0.12%), lethargy (BAC 0.09–0.25%), confusion (BAC 0.18–0.3%), stupor (BAC 0.25–0.4%), coma

(BAC 0.35–0.5%) and death (BAC > 0.5%). A concentration of 150–250 mg/dL is usually associated with very obvious signs of intoxication. The legal maximum for drivers in the UK is currently set at 80 mg/dL (17.4 mmol/L), although there are arguments for setting this level considerably lower (Fell & Voas 2006). However, the situation is complex, depending on the rate of rise to a given level and also the length of time that alcohol has been in the body, the so-called Mellanby effect. The Mellanby effect refers to the fact that a quick rise will produce effects at a lower level of blood alcohol than a gradual rise, and for a given rate of rise the effects will be less marked if alcohol has been present at a constant level for some time before. Tolerance within the CNS arises both from central adaptation of neurotransmitter signalling and from peripheral metabolic adaptation.

Alcohol and aggression

Alcohol (and other drug) consumption is renowned for its link with the development of violent and aggressive behaviour (Hoaken & Stewart 2003), via a variety of mechanisms including psychostimulant effects, diminished anxiety and pain perception, and impaired inhibition. These factors relating to alchol use *per se* are often confounded by use of additional drugs, and in the case of long-term users by withdrawal effects and cerebral damage.

Against this unequivocal background, the terms 'pathological intoxication' and the DSM-IV term 'alcohol idiosyncratic intoxication' are controversial, referring to occasional examples of irrational combative behaviour that may develop abruptly during the course of alcohol intoxication. This reaction is often apocryphally stated to occur after consumption of relatively small amounts of alcohol, but there is relatively little evidence to support this. In extreme examples the condition is said to present as an outburst of uncontrollable rage and excitement leading to destructive actions against other persons and property. This is the 'pathological reaction to alcohol', 'pathological intoxication', 'acute alcoholic paranoid state' or '*manie à potu*' much discussed in the earlier literature. As typically described, the behaviour is out of character for the individual concerned, the duration is short and there is subsequently amnesia for the entire episode. There have been many critical studies relating to the condition or its antecedents. Coid (1979), in a thorough review, found virtually nothing to support the notion that small amounts of alcohol could trigger such outbursts, and little to suggest that they could develop in persons of stable disposition.

Alcoholic 'blackouts'

Special interest attaches to the abnormalities of memory that may follow a period of severe intoxication. An amnesic gap will of course follow any bout of drinking which is carried to the point of severe impairment of consciousness, but the alcoholic 'blackout' is a phenomenon of a more specific kind. It consists of a dense amnesia for significant events that have occurred during a drinking episode, when at the time outward behaviour perhaps seemed little disordered. Usually the gap extends for a period of several hours, but very occasionally it may cover several days. The subject may have carried on a conversation and gone through quite elaborate activities, for all of which there is no trace of memory next day. On rare occasions grossly abnormal or even criminal conduct may have occurred during the episode, and the amnesic gap can then become a matter of medicolegal importance (Sweeney 1990). The onset, as judged by subjective recall, is usually abrupt, and the end of the amnesic gap may be equally sharp if sleep does not follow directly.

Goodwin *et al.* (1969a,b) presented a detailed description of the nature of blackouts in 64 alcoholic subjects. They confirmed that behaviour during the episode was usually similar to behaviour during any heavy drinking bout, except that some subjects tended to travel long distances as in fugue states. Thus one-quarter of their patients had found themselves in strange places with no recollection of how they got there. The wives of two patients claimed that they could tell when a blackout was in progress on account of a glassy stare, belligerent behaviour or the repetition of questions which showed that experiences were failing to register. En bloc blackouts, as just described, were distinguished from 'fragmentary' losses in which the subject was unaware that events had been forgotten until he was told about them later. Sometimes in this milder variety the memories might return with the passage of time, and sometimes recall was facilitated by further drinking. Thus many subjects had had the experience of hiding money or alcohol when drinking, forgetting it when sober, and later having the memory return in a subsequent drinking bout. The occurrence of blackouts was directly associated with the severity and duration of alcoholism. They appeared only late in the course of the illness, and well after physical dependence and loss of control had become established. Blackouts were very rarely seen unless large amounts of alcohol were being consumed, chiefly in the form of spirits. Goodwin *et al.* also noticed a fairly strong association with a prior history of head injury. Tarter and Schneider (1976) investigated the possibility that alcoholics subject to blackouts might have some enduring impairment of memory when sober, but with negative results. Those with frequent blackouts performed as well as those in whom blackouts were rare on a wide battery of memory measures. The quantity of intake on a given occasion again seemed to be the discriminating factor: the group with many blackouts had a significantly greater tendency to drink to intoxication or until falling asleep, and showed a significantly higher frequency of craving, tolerance and loss of control.

The pathogenesis of these episodes remains uncertain. An interesting suggestion is that they may represent the effects of 'state-dependent learning'. It has been shown that animals trained in a drugged state may 'remember' their training better when retested in a comparable drugged state, indicating that learning depends for its optimum expression on restoration of the original conditions in which the learning was acquired. Goodwin *et al.* (1969c) have demonstrated an analogous situation in volunteers trained and tested under the effects of alcohol. For some tasks, learning transfer proved to be better when the subject was intoxicated in both the first and the second test sessions than when intoxicated in the first but sober in the second. This accords with the observation cited above that events during an alcoholic blackout may sometimes be recalled under subsequent alcoholic intoxication.

Treatment of intoxication

An acute episode of intoxication rarely calls for specific medical treatment, but severely intoxicated persons should be kept under close observation in case alcoholic coma should supervene. Gastric lavage is usually unnecessary since alcohol is rapidly absorbed from the stomach. However, if there is a possibility that drugs have been taken as well, lavage will be indicated. Episodes of paranoid or combative behaviour may, on occasion, require sedation with major tranquillisers, but there are obvious hazards involved in adding one cerebral depressant to another. In actual management the most important factor is usually the handling that the patient receives from those around, who must attempt to react in as good-natured and unprovocative a way as possible. Kelly *et al.* (1971) have shown that intravenous injections of high-potency vitamins B and C can reduce the subjective effects of intoxication and improve performance on reaction time tests, apparently by virtue of a direct effect on the CNS, but this will rarely need to be exploited in practice. Alcoholic coma represents a medical emergency and should be managed in hospital. Care is needed to exclude coincident head injury and its complications, gastrointestinal bleeding, hepatic failure, pneumonia or meningitis. Blood should be taken to confirm the presence of significant amounts of alcohol and to exclude alcoholic hypoglycaemia. A clear airway must be maintained, analeptic drugs may be indicated, and peripheral circulatory failure may require intravenous fluids, vasopressor drugs and steroids. If glucose-containing fluids are transfused, thiamine must always be given in case Wernicke's encephalopathy should be precipitated. Intravenous fructose or even peritoneal dialysis may occasionally be indicated to accelerate the rate of fall in blood alcohol level (O'Neill *et al.* 1984).

Abstinence or withdrawal syndromes

An important group of manifestations occur against a background of severe alcohol abuse but make their appearance usually after a period of complete or relative abstention. It seems therefore that they depend not on the direct toxic effects of alcohol present at the time, but rather on a fall in the level circulating within the body (Victor & Adams 1953; Isbell *et al.* 1955). They include tremulousness, hallucinosis, fits and, most important of all, delirium tremens.

The precise mechanisms underlying these disorders are far from clear. Where hallucinosis and delirium tremens are concerned several complex factors are probably at work. However, all share in common the tendency to occur shortly after drinking has stopped or been abruptly curtailed. Isbell *et al.* (1955) found that the abstinence syndrome, characterised by tremors, weakness, nausea, vomiting, hyperreflexia and fever, was related to the amount of alcohol that had been taken and the duration of consumption. The discovery of the different stages of sleep brought new evidence concerning alcohol withdrawal (Greenberg & Pearlman 1967; Gross & Goodenough 1968). Increasing levels of alcohol suppress the rapid eye movement (REM) phase of sleep (see Chapter 13) and the dreaming associated with it. With continuation of drinking some readjustment occurs, but on withdrawal an abrupt rebound is seen with a great excess of REM sleep. Immediately prior to an attack of delirium tremens, REM sleep may occupy the whole of the sleeping time. It has been suggested that the vivid hallucinations of delirium tremens may represent a 'spilling over' of this active dream material into waking life. The essential mechanisms remain to be clarified, but certainly there appears to be an important relationship between the nature of the sleep disturbances associated with alcohol withdrawal and the clinical manifestations that occur.

Hemmingsen and Kramp (1988) reviewed experimental work indicative of changes in membrane phospholipids and synaptic structure following repeated alcohol withdrawal. They suggested that withdrawal reactions consist essentially of two components: physical signs such as tremor which are determined by the degree of physical dependence developed during the most recent drinking bout; and seizures, hallucinations and delirium that reflect long-term CNS dysfunction accruing over many years of repeated intoxication and withdrawal. A combination of both factors may be operative in some of the withdrawal phenomena encountered.

From clinical evidence it would appear that tremulousness, nausea and transient hallucinations in clear consciousness are among the earliest withdrawal phenomena, occurring often within 3–12 hours of cessation of drinking. Fits occur somewhat later after an interval of 12–48 hours, and the full syndrome of delirium tremens usually only after 3–4 days (Victor & Adams 1953). It is well established that a prolonged period of indulgence is necessary for the more severe effects to occur. With all withdrawal phenomena temporary alleviation follows the taking of alcohol again. All are essentially benign conditions with the exception of delirium tremens.

Alcoholic tremor

This, the commonest withdrawal effect, is usually associated with general weakness, nausea and irritability. In mild form

it can occur after a single night's abstinence and after a period of drinking of only several days. In severe form it usually occurs 12–24 hours after stopping, and only after several weeks of continuous drinking. The patient is alert, startles easily, suffers insomnia and craves the relief which further alcohol will bring. Usually the disorder subsides over several hours or days, but after severe attacks it may be 1 or 2 weeks before the patient is composed and can sleep without sedation.

Hallucinosis

Approximately one-quarter of tremulous patients have disordered sense perception, ranging from transitory misperceptions of familiar objects to illusions and hallucinations (Victor & Adams 1953). Hallucinations usually occur in both the visual and auditory modalities, are generally fleeting, and emerge in clear consciousness. The absence of disorientation, confusion and psychomotor overactivity is important in distinguishing the condition from delirium tremens. It is usually a benign condition, lasting often less than 24 hours and rarely for more than a few days.

Sabot *et al.* (1968) found that the hallucinations are often accompanied by simple auditory and visual sensory disturbances that seem to facilitate their appearance. Tinnitus is common with auditory hallucinations, antedating their appearance and persisting after they have cleared. Visual disturbances in the form of blurring, flashes and spots are usually reported by patients with formed visual hallucinations. The visual hallucinations are mostly of small animals such as rodents and insects, characteristically moving rapidly on the walls, floor or ceiling. Larger animals or human beings may also be seen, or fleeting half-formed images of faces.

As with tremulousness, withdrawal of alcohol appears to be the chief factor leading to transient hallucinations. Occasional patients, however, develop hallucinations while continuing to drink, and in these it has been suggested that thiamine deficiency may be a contributory cause (Morgan 1968). Blackstock *et al.* (1972) followed this possibility further, but were unable to demonstrate a significant difference in indicators of thiamine levels between alcoholics with or without a recent episode of hallucinatory disturbance.

The term *alcoholic hallucinosis* is sometimes used in a more restricted sense to refer to the relatively rare condition in which verbal auditory hallucinations occur alone, again in a setting of clear consciousness. Most examples clear within a few days, but the disorder may sometimes be prolonged. As such the picture may strongly resemble schizophrenia, and a good deal of discussion has centred on its nosological status. The auditory hallucinations often commence as simple sounds such as buzzing, roaring or the ringing of bells. Gradually they take on vocal form, usually the voices of friends or enemies who malign, threaten or reproach the patient. The hallucinations may consist of a single derogatory remark repeated with relentless persistence, or the patient may be assailed by a combination of accusations and admonitions. He may be discovered arguing angrily with his voices, or he may complain to the police about them. Sometimes the voices command the patient to do things against his will, and their compelling quality may be such that he is driven to a suicide attempt or some episode of bizarre behaviour. Usually the voices address the patient directly, but sometimes they converse with one another about him, referring to him in the third person as in schizophrenia. Secondary delusional interpretations follow upon the hallucinatory experiences, and the patient comes to believe firmly that he is watched, hounded or in danger.

The result is an illness which at first sight resembles acute paranoid schizophrenia. However, the delusions will be found to follow only the hallucinatory experiences and not to arise autochthonously. Schizophrenic thought disorder is not seen, nor incongruity of affect, and insight is regained immediately the voices begin to wane. The syndrome must, of course, be viewed separately from the picture seen in established schizophrenic patients who also drink. Such patients may similarly develop abrupt auditory hallucinations when drinking and during withdrawal, since drinking bouts may aggravate the schizophrenic process. The distinction is made on the basis of the preceding history and the features in the mental state as just outlined.

Victor and Hope (1958) reviewed the divergent views about the implications of the illness, ranging from the belief that it represents a form of schizophrenia released by alcohol to the view that it represents an independent psychosis induced by drinking for many years. Of their 76 examples, 90% showed hallucinations that were benign and transient, the great majority clearing within a week. Hallucinations became chronic in only eight patients, persisting then for months or years. In four of the latter the disorder ultimately resolved without the development of more serious psychiatric illness; only in the remaining four was there progression to a true schizophrenia-like illness with ideas of influence, emotional withdrawal and persistent paranoid delusions. Family histories gave no indication of special allegiance with schizophrenia, and the previous personality tended to be cyclothymic rather than schizoid. This applied even in those rare cases which did prove ultimately to develop a schizophrenia-like illness. There is therefore little to suggest that auditory hallucinosis is merely latent schizophrenia made manifest by alcohol. The mechanisms involved remain uncertain, beyond the fact that prolonged indulgence in alcohol is a necessary precursor and that abstinence is frequently observed prior to its onset. Of the 76 cases reported by Victor and Hope (1958), only 15 began while the patient was still drinking, and three of these were reducing their intake substantially at the time. In the remainder the hallucinations began after drinking had stopped entirely, usually setting in 12–48 hours later. The factors that determine the

occasional prolongation of the hallucinosis or transition to a schizophrenia-like illness remain unknown, but there is some indication that repeated attacks may make the patient ultimately more vulnerable to the type of attack which leads on to schizophrenic deterioration. Neuroleptic drugs are usually effective in treatment.

Withdrawal seizures

The consumption of alcohol can precipitate fits in a person suffering from epilepsy, and sometimes this happens after a 'normal' evening's drinking. Commonly the fit then occurs next morning during sobering up. Quite distinct from this are the withdrawal fits that may occur in persons without special epileptic predisposition. These occur only after heavy consumption, and usually within 12–48 hours of the termination of a long-continued bout. They are usually seen only after several years of established alcohol addiction. Very occasionally they occur while consumption continues, presumably as a result of transient falls in the blood alcohol level.

Mostly the fits occur in bouts of two to six at a time, and very occasionally status epilepticus may be precipitated. The fits are usually grand mal in type. If a focal component exists, this is likely to be the result of trauma in addition to alcoholism. In almost 30% of cases the fits are followed by delirium tremens. Conversely, 30% of cases of delirium tremens and 10% of cases of auditory hallucinosis are preceded by fits (Victor & Adams 1953). Electroencephalography (EEG) is abnormal at the time of the fits, but reverts to normal thereafter. It remains normal in the intervals between, thus discrediting the wide belief that they represent a latent epileptic process that has been brought to light (Victor 1966). Furthermore, in epileptic patients seizures may be closely associated with alcohol intake, sometimes repeatedly and in the absence of other predisposing factors (Brennan & Lyttle 1987).

Delirium tremens

Delirium tremens represents by far the most serious of the alcohol withdrawal phenomena, with a mortality of up to 5%. Some large series of cases have been reported to show a lower mortality, but have probably included many partial and incomplete forms.

Definition. The fully developed syndrome consists of vivid hallucinations, delusions, profound confusion, tremor, agitation, sleeplessness and autonomic overactivity. Defined in this way delirium tremens is relatively uncommon, and was found to represent only 5% of a consecutive series of 266 patients admitted to Boston City Hospital with an obvious complication of alcoholism (Victor & Adams 1953). In contrast, in the same series acute tremulousness occurred in 34%, transient hallucinosis with tremor in 11%, auditory hallucinosis in 2%, fits in 12% and Wernicke–Korsakoff syndrome in 3%.

Before diagnosing delirium tremens, McNichol (1970) required the presence of hallucinations along with at least two of the following: confusion and disorientation, tremulousness, increased psychomotor activity, fearfulness and signs of autonomic disturbance. He recognised three grades in the development of the complete syndrome: first, mental sluggishness with tremor and evidence of residual intoxication; later, emotional lability, agitation, fearfulness, increased psychomotor activity, autonomic disturbance, nightmares and disorientation; and finally the onset of definitive delirium tremens with the appearance of hallucinations. The presence of autonomic hyperactivity (tachycardia, sweating, fever) can be of considerable diagnostic importance in pointing to the condition when the cause of a delirious state is not immediately obvious.

Clinical features. Delirium tremens frequently presents in a dramatic manner and appears to have had an explosive onset. However, when opportunities arise for observation during the evolution of the illness, a prodromal phase is commonly seen. The onset is usually at night, with restlessness, insomnia and fear. The patient startles at the least sound, has vivid nightmares and wakes repeatedly in panic. Transient illusions and hallucinations may occur even at this stage, and typically arouse intense anxiety even though insight may still be largely retained.

As the illness becomes more fully declared, the face is anxious or terror stricken. The patient is tremulous, and if out of bed is usually seen to be ataxic. There is evidence of dehydration, with dry lips, a coated tongue and scanty urine. Restlessness is extreme, with agitated activity by day and night, preventing sleep and leading ultimately to dangerous physical exhaustion. Autonomic disturbance shows in perspiration, flushing or pallor, dilated pupils, a weak rapid pulse and mild pyrexia. Epileptic seizures occur in up to one-third of cases, virtually always preceding the delirium (Victor & Adams 1953).

Illusions and hallucinations occur in great profusion, principally in the visual modality but also auditory and haptic. Spots on the counterpane may be mistaken for insects, and cracks on the ceiling for snakes. Visual hallucinations typically consist of fleeting, recurrent and changeable images that compulsively hold the patient's attention. Rats, snakes and other small animals are said to be typical, and can appear in colourful and vivid forms. They are frequently lilliputian in size, and invested with rapid ceaseless activity. The author has observed a patient who followed intently, and with excited comments, a game of football performed continuously for half an hour by two teams of normal-coloured miniature elephants in a corner of his room. Other hallucinations may be normal in size, such as threatening faces or fantastic scenes depicting terrifying situations. Sometimes the hallucinations are amusing or playful in nature, and recapture some of the bonhomie of the patient and his companions

during drinking spells. The patient's occupation and experience may colour the perceptual disorders, the station master seeing trains rapidly approaching him, or the factory worker seeing his bench before him and going through the motions of his work activities.

Auditory hallucinations are commonly of a threatening or persecutory nature. Vestibular disturbances are frequent, and felt by the patient as rotation of the room or movement of the floor. Insects may be felt to be crawling over the skin, perhaps as an elaboration of paraesthesiae.

A marked feature is the intense reality with which the hallucinatory experiences are imbued, and the strong emotional reactions they produce. Apprehension and fear are typical, but amusement and even jocularity may be seen. Sometimes apprehension and amusement are mixed together in a characteristic and paradoxical manner. As with the hallucinations themselves the affective state is often changeable from one moment to another, though fear or even terror is usually uppermost.

The degree of impairment of consciousness varies widely from case to case and in the same patient from one moment to another. It is rarely profound except in the terminal stages, although the true level may be very hard to judge. Diminished awareness of the environment is coupled with overarousal in a characteristic fashion. The patient appears to be alert and over-responsive, but his responsiveness usually proves to be closely tied to his own internal stimuli; he may startle easily but is otherwise largely unaware and indifferent to what proceeds in the real world around him. Disorientation and confusion are very obvious, but the degree of inattention and distractibility may give the impression that consciousness is more severely impaired than is actually the case. When attention can be held fleetingly it is sometimes possible to show that memory and other intellectual functions are intact to a surprising degree.

Speech is usually slurred and with paraphasic errors. In severe examples it may be incoherent and fragmented. Delusions are secondarily elaborated on the faulty perceptual experiences, but are usually fragmented, transitory and as changeable as the hallucinations. Suggestibility is marked and adds to the frequency with which illusions occur; pressing on the eyeballs may cause the patient to see whatever one tells him he sees, and when presented with a blank piece of paper he may proceed to 'read' it on instruction.

EEG typically shows fast activity in delirium tremens. In this it is in marked contrast to the picture seen in most other forms of delirium, where slowing of the dominant rhythms is the characteristic pattern.

Outcome. The disorder is usually short-lived, lasting less than 3 days in the majority of cases. Very rarely recurrent phases may be seen over a longer period of time. Typically it terminates in a prolonged sleep after which the patient feels fully recovered apart from residual weakness and exhaustion. In rare cases a prolonged attack of delirium tremens may clear to reveal an amnesic syndrome, when Wernicke's encephalopathy had been present and unnoticed during the acute stage.

Death when it occurs is usually due to cardiovascular collapse, infection, hyperthermia, or self-injury during the phase of intense restlessness. Any infective process, particularly pneumonia, markedly increases the mortality.

Aetiology. The precise pathophysiology is unknown. Cerebral oedema was formerly thought to be responsible but has not been adequately confirmed. A primary disorder of the reticular formation is strongly suggested by the clinical components of profound inattention coupled with alertness, overactivity and insomnia. The remarkable association with disturbance of REM sleep has already been described.

Cerebral blood flow studies have indicated a state of increased CNS excitability during the course of delirium, in keeping with the characteristic fast frequencies seen on EEG. Hemmingsen *et al.* (1988) performed xenon-labelled single-photon emission computed tomography (SPECT) in patients with actual or impending delirium tremens, with repeat examination on recovery. Increased hemispheric blood flow correlated significantly with the presence of visual hallucinations and psychomotor agitation, and decreased when the acute phase subsided.

Withdrawal of alcohol is the factor most clearly incriminated in the aetiology of the condition, and in the majority of cases can be detected in the antecedent history. Premonitory symptoms often set in within a day or two of cessation of drinking, but the full-blown syndrome usually appears only after 3 or 4 days of abstinence. Refeeding with alcohol has been shown to ameliorate the condition. Nevertheless, some cases undoubtedly begin during a bout of heavy consumption, and reduction of intake below some critical value must then be postulated. It can be shown that trauma or infection are present from the outset in up to half of cases, many others having liver failure, gastrointestinal bleeding or hypoglycaemia. Lundquist (1961) found biochemical evidence of acute liver damage in up to 90% of patients with delirium tremens. A multifactorial aetiology will probably prove to be the complete explanation, involving complex metabolic and neurophysiological pathways.

Treatment
Treatment of minor withdrawal symptoms can often be undertaken on an outpatient basis with the help of sedation from chlordiazepoxide. However, patients with a history of withdrawal seizures, and those with any indication of impending delirium tremens, should be admitted to hospital immediately. Management will in essence consist of close nursing observation at regular intervals, so that the dosage of sedative drugs can be titrated against the symptoms displayed. Edwards (1982) recommends chlordiazepoxide up to 40 mg three or four times daily, starting if necessary with an intramuscular dose of 50–100 mg. Treatment with clomethiazole (chlormethiazole) is an alternative. The drugs are then gradually tailed off over several days at a rate that prevents significant recrudescence of withdrawal symptoms.

With established delirium tremens, treatment must always be in hospital, preferably in a setting where the medical and nursing staff are experienced with the procedures involved. The necessary steps are described by Rix (1978) and Edwards (1982). Fluid replacement and adequate sedation are the first essentials, with careful examination to detect complicating pathologies which aggravate the delirium and greatly worsen prognosis.

Head injury and infection must always be borne in mind. Skull and chest radiography will be required. Coincident intoxication with sedative drugs may lead to particularly severe withdrawal manifestations. Hypoglycaemia, hepatic failure, uraemia and electrolyte imbalance will need to be excluded. Wernicke's encephalopathy must be detected early and treated vigorously. Cardiac failure, gastroduodenal bleeding or bleeding from oesophageal varices may be present. A close watch must be kept at all stages for seizures or circulatory collapse.

The intensity of treatment required will obviously depend on the severity of delirium that has become established. When the syndrome is well developed, half-hourly recordings of temperature, pulse and blood pressure should be made, along with a record of fluid intake and output. At least 6 L of fluid per day will be required, of which 1.5 L should be given as normal saline. If adequate oral intake cannot be ensured, intravenous administration must be started with 5% glucose solution or glucose in saline. Hypokalaemia is a special risk. Hypomagnesaemia may occur.

Adequate sedation is essential, and the dosage should be monitored closely against the patient's clinical state and level of consciousness. Other treatment must always include high-potency vitamin preparations as prophylaxis against Wernicke's encephalopathy or nicotinic acid deficiency encephalopathy. Anticonvulsant medication should be given routinely when there is a past history of withdrawal seizures. Cardiovascular collapse, vomiting or hyperthermia will require appropriate management.

Alcoholic cognitive impairment and cerebral atrophy
The conception of 'alcoholic dementia' has had a chequered history, figuring prominently in early textbooks of psychiatry but later yielding pride of place to Korsakoff's syndrome (Lishman 1981). Nowadays the idea of a genuine dementia caused by alcohol is quite commonly viewed with caution. Many patients labelled as having as alcoholic dementia are indeed suffering from Korsakoff's syndrome (though it seems possible that the reverse also obtains, as described under Korsakoff's sydrome, later in chapter. Others are merely displaying profound social disorganisation in the

context of chronic continuing inebriation. When opportunities arise to assess the latter after a period of total abstinence, intellectual functions may turn out to be substantially intact. Other alcoholics are suffering essentially from a coincident vascular dementia, the effects of multiple head injuries or a dementia of the Alzheimer type.

Nevertheless, clinical experience suggests that the long-continued abuse of alcohol may sometimes lead directly to severe cognitive impairment. Alcohol is suspected of being at least a contributory cause in a substantial number of demented patients seen in hospital, approximately 10% in historical series. Moreover, for every patient who has reached the stage of being investigated for a possible dementia, many others may be suffering from milder, and perhaps protracted, earlier stages of such disorder. Adequate epidemiological studies are not available to clarify the problem directly. Only a proportion of alcoholics come before treatment services, and a comprehensive follow-up of those who do can present formidable problems. Furthermore, it is possible that those who suffer marked cognitive impairment are particularly liable to be lost to view as time goes by. There have been few surveys of 'skid row' alcoholics who may be expected to represent the more deteriorated subjects.

Psychological evidence

Clinical psychologists have presented a now substantial body of evidence which shows that severe alcoholics, even after thorough 'drying out', remain compromised on a broad range of psychological functions. These extend well beyond memory deficits alone to include problems with visuospatial competence, abstracting ability and complex reasoning. Such deficits can be demonstrated even when verbal ability is well preserved, which of course can produce a misleading impression at interview. Again it is noteworthy that they have emerged in subjects presenting themselves for treatment; the cognitive status of those out of contact with medical services has for obvious reasons not been determined.

Psychological assessments during the first few weeks of abstinence show substantial recovery of intellectual and memory functions, so assessment of the stable cognitive state must be deferred for some considerable time. Continuing restitution of function may indeed proceed for a period of several months. Nevertheless, it seems that even after a year of abstinence psychological deficits persist on tests of psychomotor speed, perceptual–motor functioning and visuospatial competence, also measures of abstracting ability and reasoning. Careful tests of memory function can likewise remain impaired, to the extent that a continuum of memory impairment has been postulated, ranging from normality at one extreme to the fully-fledged picture of the Korsakoff amnesic defect at the other (Ryback 1971; Ryan & Butters 1980). New learning capacity has been found to remain impaired after a minimum of 5 years' abstinence, likewise capacity for complex figure–ground analysis

(Brandt *et al.* 1983). Deficits on tests related to frontal lobe function, such as the Wisconsin Card Sorting Test, are particularly noteworthy. Frontal dysfunction could be relevant to aspects of the personality change encountered in alcoholics – the circumstantiality, plausibility and weakness of volition – that may contribute significantly to relapse. A vicious circle may often be established, with worsening cognitive status contributing to the potentiation of the addiction.

Jacobson and Lishman (1987) showed variable degrees of cognitive impairment in Korsakoff and non-Korsakoff alcoholics, and Acker (1985) showed that women were particularly vulnerable to such impairments. More recently, Oscar-Berman and Marinkovic (2003) have documented the cognitive and neurobiological changes in chronic alcoholics, particularly in cognitive functions dependent on the frontal lobes. Sullivan *et al.* (2000a, 2002) have described impairments on tasks such as delayed recall, visuospatial function, and attention; in women, visuospatial function and verbal and nonverbal working memory were particularly affected. This group has also examined changes with abstinence, finding that abstainers improve more than alcoholics who initially abstain but who then return to drinking on aspects of general memory as well as ataxia (Rosenbloom *et al.* 2007). As a heavy drinker gets older, the brain damage occasioned by alcoholism will couple with other pathologies – those of ageing, trauma, vascular changes and hepatic dysfunction – leading to more serious and irreversible change.

Neuropathology

Direct appraisal of cerebral pathology in alcoholics, over and above that concerned with the classic Wernicke lesion, has met with conflicting findings. Cerebral atrophy, mild or moderate in degree, was reported in a high proportion of Courville's (1955) chronic alcoholics at post-mortem, as well as in half of Neuberger's (1957) and all of Lynch's (1960). However, other reports do not find it or do not comment upon it. On microscopy Courville found arachnoidal thickening and cell degeneration and loss, affecting mainly the smaller pyramidal cells of the superficial and intermediate laminae. Disintegration of nerve fibres was also observed. Lynch (1960) described a similar histological picture in 11 chronic alcoholics with adequate nutritional status, when compared with a group of non-alcoholic subjects of the same age and sex. Commenting on the negative reports in the literature, he attributed this to a waning of neuropathological interest in the cortex of alcoholics, with the accent of pathological enquiry centring increasingly on the Wernicke lesion at the base of the brain and on changes in the cerebellum. He also stressed how difficult it is to chart changes, degenerations and loss in such a complex and crowded area as the cortex.

Quantitative studies on brains obtained at post-mortem have confirmed that atrophy or 'shrinkage' is indeed often detectable. Thus in comparison with controls brain weight is slightly but significantly reduced in the alcoholic (Harper & Blumbergs 1982; Torvik *et al.* 1982), and the pericerebral space over the cortex is enlarged (Harper & Kril 1985). This emerges whether or not there is evidence of nutritional brain damage, perhaps pointing to the role of alcohol neurotoxicity. The amount of white matter in the cerebral hemispheres is reduced, and the ventricles enlarged by over one-third, a figure not dissimilar from that found in computed tomography (CT) studies as discussed below (Harper *et al.* 1985; de la Monte 1988). The thickness of the corpus callosum is also significantly reduced by approximately 20% (Harper & Kril 1988).

Lishman (1986, 1990) suggested that the Wernicke–Korsakoff lesion (see below) may sometimes itself be responsible for pictures of dementia by encroaching on key neurochemical nuclei at the base of the brain, with consequent disruption of monoaminergic and cholinergic inputs to the cortex. Pursuing this hypothesis further it is possible to amass evidence that the basal regions of the brain are vulnerable not only to thiamine lack but also to the direct toxic action of alcohol (Lishman 1990). A dual system of this nature could also explain the spectrum of cognitive changes encountered in patients labelled as suffering from Korsakoff's syndrome, ranging from circumscribed memory deficits to more global impairment in a proportion of cases.

Laboratory evidence lends support to the possibility that a direct toxic action of alcohol on the brain may play a considerable role. Leonard (1986) and Charness *et al.* (1989) review its effects on neuronal membranes, cell transport systems and neurotransmitter functions. Studies in mice and rats have shown that brain changes can be induced after a period of several months on a diet supplemented with alcohol (Riley & Walker 1978; Walker *et al.* 1980a,b). Marked alterations in dendritic morphology were found in the hippocampal pyramidal neurones, dentate granular layers and cerebellar vermis, proceeding to cell degeneration and loss. These effects were produced despite the maintenance of good nutrition in all other respects. Detailed cell counts have indicated a 22% reduction in the number of neurones in the superior frontal cortex, along with reduction in the size of neurones in the motor and cingulate cortices (Harper *et al.* 1987; Kril & Harper 1989). Other cortical areas seem not to have been extensively examined. A quantitative study of the extent of dendritic arborisations in layer III pyramidal neurones from the frontal and motor cortex has shown significant reductions in mean dendritic length, number of branches and mean width of basal dendritic fields (Harper & Corbett 1990). Moreover, West *et al.* (1982) showed that alcohol inhibits the reactive sprouting of dendrites in the rat hippocampus that constitutes the normal response to injury. McMullen *et al.* (1984) found that ingestion of alcohol by well-nourished rats leads to reduction of branching in dendritic domains, and a reduction of thickness in corresponding dendritic strata. Abstinence then allows regrowth of dendritic branching and a return to normal thickness of the strata. King *et al.* (1988) have shown similar reversible alterations in the density of dendritic spines in the rat hippocampus. The plasticity inherent in the adult brain with regard to dendritic growth and sprouting (Buell & Coleman 1979, 1981; Flood & Coleman 1986) suggests that continuing growth of the dendritic domains compensates for an age-related decline in neuronal numbers. Dendritic growth may stand to be compromised in the alcoholic subject, with a return to normal levels when prolonged abstinence has been assured. Other factors may also be involved, such as changes in protein or lipid synthesis (Harper 1989; Harper & Kril 1990).

Neuroimaging

Computed tomography and magnetic resonance imaging (MRI) scanning have been conducted on large populations of alcoholics (Ron *et al.* 1982; Lishman *et al.* 1987; Pfefferbaum *et al.* 1995, 2006; Sullivan *et al.* 2000). Compared with normal controls, representative samples of alcoholics have been found commonly to have dilatation of the sulci, fissures and ventricles.

The conclusions to be drawn from these studies are as follows. Some 50–70% of severe chronic alcoholics show indubitable evidence of cortical shrinkage or ventricular dilatation or both. Involvement of the frontal lobes of the brain has sometimes been particularly evident. The changes can be found in quite young alcoholics, appearing well within the first decade of alcohol abuse, although they become more marked in the older age groups studied. Planimetric measures of lateral ventricular size show on average some 50% enlargement compared with age-matched controls. This has emerged even in identical twins discordant for a history of alcoholism (Gurling *et al.* 1984). Atrophy of the cerebellar vermis can also be seen in a high proportion of subjects. However, personal susceptibility to such developments appears to vary widely, in that approximately one-third of subjects continue to show normal scans despite long-continued and severe drinking histories. There are indications that the female brain may be more vulnerable than the male to the development of such CT changes (Jacobson 1986).

MRI has confirmed the ventricular enlargement and the increase in cerebrospinal fluid (CSF) over the cortical surface that is apparent on CT. In Jernigan *et al.*'s (1991a) MRI study, the cortical changes were particularly impressive, and were associated with significant reductions in grey matter in medial temporal, superior frontal and parietal regions. Subcortical grey matter was also reduced, particularly in the caudate nucleus and diencephalon. Sullivan *et al.* (2000a) and Pfefferbaum *et al.* (1995) emphasised the importance of changes in the volume of the third ventricle in non-Korsakoff alcoholics. Jacobson and Lishman (1987) and Oscar-Berman and Marinkovic (2003) have documented the particular vulnerability of the frontal lobes, Sullivan *et al.* (2000b) documented changes in cerebellar volume in relation to ataxia, and Pfefferbaum *et al.* (2006) documented white matter degradation on diffusion tensor imaging.

These cerebral changes clearly antedate clinical evidence of mental impairment, being demonstrable after excluding patients with clinically obvious cognitive deficits. They often appear to set in early during the alcoholic career, and after developing to a certain degree it is possible that they fail to progress further. In seeking clinical associations of the CT findings, few have emerged other than age and duration of abstinence. The duration and severity of alcohol abuse appear to bear little relation to the severity of the cerebral changes once age has been taken into account, although there is some indirect evidence that episodic drinking may be less harmful in this respect than steady continuous drinking.

The most decisive influence, where the drinking history is concerned, has proved to lie with the duration of abstinence. It has been shown that with increasing length of abstinence prior to scanning the CT changes become less pronounced; follow-up over an interval of 1–3 years has confirmed that abstinence in the interim is the factor most closely associated with whether the scans will show improvement (Ron *et al.* 1982; Ron 1983). Even after several years of abstinence, however, as in samples recruited from Alcoholics Anonymous, some degree of persistent ventricular enlargement appears to remain (Jacobson 1986; Lishman *et al.* 1987).

Studies using MRI, which allows more accurate measurement of CSF volumes, have confirmed significant decreases in both ventricular size and subarachnoid spaces during the early weeks of abstinence (Schroth *et al.* 1988). Coincident measurement of T2 values for white matter have served to discount dehydration and rehydration of the brain as the sole explanation; other effects such as increased protein synthesis or increased dendritic growth after withdrawal from alcohol may be more important factors. Pfefferbaum *et al.* (1995, 2006) have also documented changes on MRI following abstinence which suggest that improvement in cortical grey matter, sulcal, and lateral ventricular volumes occurs early in the course of abstinence, with improvement in third ventricular volume appearing later; improvement in white matter microstructural integrity also occurs. This partial reversibility with abstinence is, of course, strong evidence against the possibility that the cerebral changes revealed on the scan may have antedated, and predisposed to, the onset of the alcoholism.

Psychometric testing carried out in conjunction with scanning has indicated, as expected, that a considerable proportion of the alcoholics score poorly on many tests. However, the concordance between measures of functional and structural change has often proved to be low. Bergman *et al.* (1980a,b) found some evidence that impairment of memory and general intelligence was associated with the degree of ventricular enlargement, and that the Halstead Impairment Index was associated with cortical status. However, all such correlations were low. Acker *et al.* (1984) found remarkably few associations on an extensive battery of tests once care had been taken to control for age and estimates of premorbid intellectual competence. However, on CT studies, Acker *et al.* (1987) found that performance on a battery of memory tests was significantly related to the width of the third ventricle in a group of detoxified non-Korsakoff alcoholics. Not dissimilarly, Jacobson and Lishman (1987) divided a sample of non-Korsakoff alcoholics into those with good and poor memory, according to performance on the Logical Memory Test, and compared their scans with those of Korsakoff patients and normal controls. Both the lateral and the third ventricles tended to be larger in alcoholics with poor rather than good memory, the values in the former approaching the values found in Korsakoff patients and the latter the values found in normal controls. The difference in third ventricular size was statistically significant. In general, the findings suggest that cerebral shrinkage *per se* is a poor marker of functional competence, and that only limited reliance can be placed on scan appearances in evaluating the competence of the individual alcoholic patient, but that some more specific correlations between function and focal neuroimaging change can be obtained.

Wernicke's encephalopathy

Wernicke's encephalopathy represents the acute neuropsychiatric reaction to severe thiamine deficiency. It may be defined as a disorder of acute onset characterised by nystagmus, abducens and conjugate gaze palsies, ataxia of gait, and a global confusional state, occurring together or in various combinations (Victor *et al.* 1971). Wernicke first described the condition in 1881 under the title 'polioencephalitis haemorrhagica superior', reporting two cases in chronic alcoholics and one in a patient with persistent vomiting after sulphuric acid poisoning. Initially it was ascribed to an inflammatory process in the CNS, but abundant evidence has since accumulated to show the role of thiamine deficiency. Alexander (1940) was able to demonstrate lesions in the brains of thiamine-deficient pigeons that were similar in distribution and type to those of Wernicke's encephalopathy, and Jolliffe *et al.* (1941) clearly established the efficacy of thiamine in relieving the ophthalmoplegias and in improving clouding of consciousness in human subjects. Nicotinic acid, in contrast, failed to do so.

Wernicke's encephalopathy and alcoholism

Alcoholism is an important but not exclusive cause of the disorder. It leads to thiamine deficiency by several routes: the replacement of vitamin-containing foods by alcohol, impaired absorption of thiamine from the gut, impairment of storage by the liver, decreased phosphorylation to thiamine pyrophosphate (TPP), and excessive requirements for the metabolism of alcohol. Among alcoholics, partial gastrectomy appears to be a significant additional risk factor (Price & Kerr 1985). However, Wernicke's encephalopathy is known to occur in a number of other conditions all closely connected with thiamine deficiency. Campbell and Russell (1941) could find a definite history of alcoholism in only 5 of 21 cases, and Spillane (1947) listed the following additional causes in his review of the literature: carcinoma of the stomach, pregnancy, toxaemia, pernicious anaemia, vomiting, diarrhoea and dietary deficiency. Very occasionally the condition has developed in association with anorexia nervosa (Ebels 1978; Handler & Perkin 1982), and it has been reported after a self-imposed 'hunger strike' in a paranoid patient (Pentland & Mawdsley 1982). Other causes have included prolonged intravenous feeding, renal dialysis, hyperemesis gravidarum (Bergin & Harvey 1992) and severe malnutrition in a chronic schizophrenic patient (Spittle & Parker 1993).

Rimalovski and Aronson (1966) reported a large post-mortem series and found that unequivocal evidence of alcoholism had been recorded in only 50% of patients. In most of the remainder the cause appeared to be carcinoma, especially of the oesophagus, or widespread tuberculosis. Lindboe and Løberg (1989) found that almost one-quarter of their post-mortem cases were non-alcoholics, this rising to 40% in active acute cases. Most of the non-alcoholic patients had suffered from severe cachexia due to a variety of underlying diseases. Nevertheless, in the largest series reported from the USA, Victor et al. (1971) found that all but two of their 245 cases were suffering from established alcoholism. They therefore still regarded Wernicke's encephalopathy as essentially a disease of alcoholics, at least in American urban society.

However, it seems that not all alcoholics are equally at risk. Many neglect their diets severely without developing an overt encephalopathy, whereas others may do so quite early in their alcoholic careers. A young alcoholic reported by Turner et al. (1989) presented with Wernicke's encephalopathy at the age of 18. Even from place to place the prevalence of Wernicke–Korsakoff syndrome appears to be remarkably uneven. First admissions to hospital with the condition have ranged from 65 per million population in Queensland, Australia to 8 per million in New York. At post-mortem it has emerged in 2.8% of persons in Western Australia, 2.2% in Cleveland, Ohio, 1.7% in New York, 0.8% in Oslo and 0.4% in France (Harper et al. 1989, 1995). No obvious correlations can be discerned with the per-capita consumptions of alcohol in these different countries. Numerous factors are likely to be involved: the beverage consumed, its thiamine content, patterns of drinking and patterns of dietary neglect.

However, there may be an important additional factor by way of personal susceptibility. Thiamine is important in relation to several key enzyme systems of the body and brain. It is first phosphorylated to TPP, which acts as a coenzyme, i.e. combines with proteins to form the effective enzyme system. This applies to enzymes such as transketolase, which is essential for the maintenance and synthesis of myelin, and the pyruvate dehydrogenase complex and α-ketoglutarate dehydrogenase complex, both of which play key roles in brain glucose metabolism and energy production (Langlais 1995).

The question therefore arose whether persons vulnerable to thiamine deficiency could have an *inborn abnormality* by way of reduced affinity between TPP and the enzymes with which it must combine. Kaczmarek and Nixon (1983) and Pratt et al. (1985) showed that transketolase is heterogeneous, existing as a number of isoenzyme variants, some differing in their affinity for TPP (Greenwood et al. 1984). Certain variants have seemed to be specific to Korsakoff patients (Blass & Gibson 1977; Nixon 1984). Mukherjee et al. (1987) have presented some preliminary evidence which favours genetic transmission of reduced binding between TPP and transketolase in certain families. Other enzymes that depend on TPP for their proper functioning appear to have been little explored in relation to the syndrome. Pyruvate dehydrogenase and α-ketoglutarate dehydrogenase are just as essential as transketolase to brain cell survival, and all three have been shown to be greatly reduced in samples from the cerebellar vermis in patients with Wernicke–Korsakoff syndrome (Butterworth et al. 1993). Reductions in α-ketoglutarate dehydrogenase were particularly severe, and Butterworth et al. suggest that this could be the trigger for a series of metabolic events that culminate in neuronal death.

Wernicke's encephalopathy and beriberi

The relationship with beriberi proved more of an embarrassment, since the classic neuritic and cardiac forms of the disease seemed rarely to be associated with encephalopathy despite their dependence on thiamine deficiency. During the Second World War, however, experience in prisoner of war camps gave ample opportunity for observing relatively acute deficiency syndromes in large numbers of subjects. In epidemics of beriberi psychological changes were often found to be prominent, with irritability, depression and disturbance of memory (Cruickshank 1961).

More particularly, De Wardener and Lennox (1947) were able to report 52 typical cases of Wernicke's encephalopathy from a prisoner of war camp in Singapore, most of whom at the same time showed neuritic, cardiac or oedematous signs of beriberi. Their classic paper was based on records that spent two years of the war buried in a Siamese cemetery; it was entitled 'Cerebral beriberi (Wernicke's encephalopathy)', and effectively bridged the gap between the two conditions. Response to thiamine was generally excellent in this series. Gross examination of the brains in fatal cases confirmed pathological changes in the distribution typical of Wernicke's encephalopathy. The authors proposed that the encephalopathy appeared when particularly acute and severe thiamine depletion was superimposed on partial deficiency, whereas other forms of beriberi generally resulted from less severe and more prolonged lack of the vitamin. In almost all their cases the encephalopathy had set in when some other factor, such as epidemic diarrhoea, had intensified the vitamin deficiency. The situation was thus analogous to that seen with nicotinic acid, where severe acute depletion produces profound evidence of cerebral dysfunction and more chronic deficiency leads to pellagra.

Clinical features

Victor *et al.*'s (1971, 1989) observations on 245 patients form the basis for much of the description that follows. Wernicke's encephalopathy typically declares itself abruptly, although sometimes it may be several days before the full picture is manifest. The commonest presenting features are mental confusion or staggering gait. The patient may also be aware of ocular abnormalities, with complaints of wavering vision or diplopia on looking to the side. This well-known triad of confusion, ataxia and ophthalmoplegia confers a highly characteristic stamp to the syndrome when it appears in full, but all parts are not always seen together. In an admittedly retrospective analysis of 97 autopsy-proven cases, Harper *et al.* (1986) found that the classic triad had been present in only 16%; 28% had shown two of the signs and 37% only one, but in 19% no feature of the triad was documented. A high index of suspicion is therefore necessary if the condition is not to be missed. Other features include prodromal anorexia, nausea and vomiting. A marked disorder of memory is frequently in evidence and has been insufficiently emphasised in most descriptions. Attention has also been called to lethargy and hypotension which, in the presence of an acute organic mental syndrome, may indicate Wernicke's encephalopathy despite the absence of other definitive signs (Cravioto *et al.* 1961). Rare presentations may be with hypothermia, stupor or coma (Kearsley & Musso 1980).

The age range is evenly distributed throughout adult life, with males affected approximately twice as often as females. This ratio is considerably lower than for alcoholism generally and may be partly a reflection of differences in patterns of drinking. The pattern which leads to Wernicke's encephalopathy appears to be steady drinking extending over months or years and coupled with inadequate intake of food. In Victor *et al.*'s (1971) series, delirium tremens or other withdrawal syndromes had occurred at some time in the past in 40% of cases, withdrawal fits in 10% and liver disease in 10%, indicating the general severity of alcohol abuse.

On examination, Victor *et al.* observed the following signs.

Ocular abnormalities were present in 96% of patients on initial examination. The commonest findings were nystagmus, sixth nerve palsies producing lateral rectus weakness, or some form of conjugate gaze paralysis. The pupils usually showed little more than sluggishness of reactions. Ocular signs can be remarkably evanescent, resolving speedily with treatment or even on feeding thiamine-containing foods. This no doubt accounts for the much lower prevalence of ocular abnormalities reported in cases viewed retrospectively.

Ataxia was observed in 87% of patients who were testable, varying from inability to stand without support to minor difficulties with heel–toe walking. In contrast, intention tremor in the legs or arms was relatively rare.

Peripheral neuropathy was present in 82% of cases, usually confined to the legs. In addition to objective signs there were often subjective complaints of weakness, paraesthesiae and pain.

Serious malnutrition was evident in 84%. Common signs were redness or papillary atrophy of the tongue, cheilosis, angular stomatitis, telangiectases, and dryness and discoloration of the skin. Two-thirds of the patients showed evidence of liver disorder and one-quarter were bedridden when first seen. Overt signs of beriberi were rare but resting tachycardia and dyspnoea on effort were common.

Abstinence syndrome was found at inception in 13%, with epileptic fits, hallucinoses or delirium tremens.

Mental abnormalities were observed in 90% of patients, the rest presenting with ataxia and ophthalmoplegia but remaining lucid throughout. The commonest mental disturbance was a state of quiet global confusion, with disorientation, apathy and derangement of memory. Many were drowsy, sometimes falling asleep in mid-sentence, while others showed marked indifference and inattention to their surroundings. Against the prevailing view, however, almost all were readily rousable and impairment of consciousness was rarely profound or persistent.

In the typical case, spontaneous activity and speech were minimal, and remarks irrational and inconsistent. Grasp, awareness and responsiveness were markedly impaired. Misidentifications were extremely common and made without hesitation. Physical and mental fatiguability was pronounced, and concentration was difficult for the simplest task. In contrast, a small proportion were alert, responsive and voluble, despite obvious confusion and defects of memory.

Evidence of delirium was sometimes seen, with perceptual distortions, vivid hallucinations, insomnia, agitation and autonomic overactivity. In a small number this amounted to frank delirium tremens, but was always evanescent and usually not severe. Hallucinations were rare in the remainder. Loosely knit delusions appeared occasionally and sometimes persisted for weeks after the confusion had cleared.

Assessment of memory was often difficult, but in testable cases a defect of memorising was discovered or else became evident as soon as the major confusion subsided. It was often hard to determine the point at which confusion of thought receded and the memory defect became the most prominent abnormality, since the two usually blended imperceptibly in the course of the illness. In a small number (14%) a typical Korsakoff memory defect was clearly evident from the outset, being the most prominent mental abnormality at the time of initial examination.

Confabulation was common early in the disorder but was not found in every case. In those who showed it, moreover, it could not be elicited on every occasion. The origin could often be traced to confusion of thought or perceptual disorder, and it was sometimes hard to separate confabulations from misidentifications and misinterpretations. As the global confusion receded and memory defects became clearly established, the confabulation subsided and often amounted to translocations in time of genuine past experiences.

Investigations

Diffuse slowing was found on EEG in half of the patients tested by Victor *et al.* (1971). Sometimes, however, the tracings were entirely normal in marked and classic examples of the syndrome. More recent EEG evidence indicates that Wernicke's encephalopathy usually produces prominent generalized asynchronous slow waves and often also causes bisynchronous slow waves and a decrease of the alpha rhythm (Fisch 1999).

The CSF may be abnormal with mild elevation of protein.

In occasional examples, CT has shown symmetrical areas of decreased attenuation in the region of the thalamus (Escobar *et al.* 1983; McDowell & Le Blanc 1984). In the latter study the lesions were observed to improve after several weeks of treatment with thiamine. MRI can show such lesions more clearly, and may also identify atrophy of the mamillary bodies (Charness & DeLaPaz 1987; Bigler *et al.* 1989) or hyperintensities surrounding the third ventricle and aqueduct (Gallucci *et al.* 1990). Meyer *et al.* (1985) demonstrated reductions in both grey and white matter cerebral blood flow, which improves with treatment.

Course and response to treatment

The unique value of Victor *et al.*'s (1971, 1989) series was that a substantial proportion of the patients who survived the acute stage remained under close medical observation for many months or years thereafter. Altogether 17% died during the acute stage, one-quarter were followed for at least 2 months, and more than half were followed for 2–13 years. The long-term outcome with thiamine replacement was accordingly greatly clarified.

Sixth nerve palsies always recovered, often starting to resolve within hours though sometimes taking several days or weeks to disappear completely. Other ocular abnormalities responded similarly, with the exception of horizontal nystagmus which was a permanent residuum in two-thirds of the patients. Ataxia usually began to improve within the first week, but often took a month or two for maximum resolution. In one-quarter of patients the ataxia showed no improvement whatever, and altogether more than half were left with permanent unsteadiness of some degree. Thus residual ataxia and nystagmus can sometimes be useful signs in pointing to the origin of an obscure chronic amnesic syndrome. Polyneuropathy improved only very slowly over several months, and diminution or absence of tendon reflexes was another common permanent sequel.

The global confusion always recovered in survivors, beginning usually within 2–3 weeks and clearing completely within 1–2 months. As the confusion receded the amnesic defects stood out more prominently. Of 186 patients followed for long enough to assess the presence or absence of the Korsakoff state, 84% developed the typical amnesic syndrome. The few who escaped had all shown relatively brief acute illnesses and had lost their confusion within a week. In addition the authors drew attention to the small but important group who presented with the Korsakoff amnesic defect from first contact along with ocular and ataxic signs (some 10% of the total), and their further very small group of nine cases (4%) who had apparently developed the amnesic syndrome without ophthalmoplegia or ataxia at any time (compare Cutting 1978).

Pathology

The pathological changes are remarkable for their predilection for certain circumscribed parts of the brain. Symmetrical lesions are found predominantly in the neighbourhood of the walls of the third ventricle, the periaqueductal region, the floor of the fourth ventricle, certain thalamic nuclei (including especially the paraventricular parts of the medial dorsal nuclei, the anteromedial nuclei and the pulvinar), the mamillary bodies, the terminal portions of the fornices, the brainstem, and the anterior lobe and superior vermis of the cerebellum. In contrast, obvious lesions are rarely seen in the cerebral cortex, corpus striatum, subthalamic and septal regions, cingulate gyri or hippocampal areas. However, Victor *et al.* (1971) found that convolutional atrophy was conspicuous enough to be remarked on in 27% of their cases who came to post-mortem.

Microscopically, the lesions tend to involve all neural elements – neurones, axis cylinders, blood vessels and glia – but with variability from case to case and from one location to another. In general, myelinated fibres tend to be affected more severely than the neurones themselves. Astrocytic and histiocytic proliferation is found in the areas of parenchymal loss. Proliferation of blood vessels and petechial haemorrhages may occur, but the latter may often represent terminal events.

The distribution of lesions is virtually identical in patients dying in the acute stages of Wernicke's encephalopathy and in patients who have shown a chronic Korsakoff syndrome, differing only in the chronicity of the glial and vascular reactions.

In seeking a correlation between symptoms and lesions, Victor *et al.* (1971) suggested that the ophthalmoplegias result from lesions in the third and sixth cranial nerve nuclei and adjacent tegmentum, nystagmus from lesions of the vestibular nuclei, and ataxia from lesions of the vestibular nuclei and the anterior lobes and vermis of the cerebellum. Amnesia in their material appeared to be particularly closely associated with lesions in the medial dorsal nuclei and pulvinar of the thalamus; mammillary lesions, which have traditionally been regarded as crucial for the development of amnesia, were less constant (Victor *et al.* 1971, 1989). More recent studies have disputed this view, arguing that the pathology specifically in the mammillary bodies, the mamillothalamic tract, or the principal anterior nuclei of the thalamus is critical to producing the persistent and severe anterograde memory deficit of the Korsakoff syndrome (Harding *et al.* 2000).

Subclinical Wernicke's encephalopathy

The foregoing description applies to patients who have come dramatically to medical attention on account of an acute disorder. However, it seems probable that milder variants may exist, or indeed that damage may sometimes develop surreptitiously in the Wernicke location without clear clinical indicators of the process (Lishman 1981). The evidence is somewhat indirect but the pointers towards it deserve careful consideration.

Cravioto *et al.* (1961) and Grunnet (1969) found patients with the classic lesion at post-mortem who had died without exhibiting Wernicke's classic signs. Comparison of patients dying in the 1930s and 1960s suggested that the clinical presentations had become less severe, perhaps as a result of the wider availability and prescription of vitamins. The lesions at post-mortem tended to be more circumscribed in the recent cases, and more often subacute or chronic in nature. Most significant of all, the condition could remain undiagnosed prior to death.

This last point has been strongly reinforced by Harper (1979, 1983). Over the course of 9 years in Perth, Australia, 131 cases of Wernicke's encephalopathy were diagnosed at post-mortem, representing almost 3% of all brains examined in the hospital or referred by the city coroner. Only 26 of these 131 cases had been suspected during life, despite the fact that most had been examined in teaching hospitals. The great majority of affected persons were known to be alcoholics, and several had died suddenly and unexpectedly. A considerable range was encountered in the acuteness or chronicity of the lesions, with the not uncommon conjunction of acute histological changes superimposed on chronic pathology within the same brain regions. Two-thirds showed chronic pathological changes alone.

Some alcoholics may therefore harbour covert undiagnosed pathology of the Wernicke type over a considerable period of time. Whether this evolves insidiously or in stepwise fashion is unknown. It may sometimes represent the cumulative effects of repeated minor episodes of Wernicke's encephalopathy that have largely gone unnoticed at the time.

In favour of the idea is the noted resistance to treatment of many alcoholic Korsakoff states, even when thiamine is administered from the earliest stages. This contrasts with the gratifying responses observed, for example, in De Wardener and Lennox's (1947) nutritionally depleted prisoners of war. The alcoholics appear often to have acquired an entrenched structural pathology that may well have been evolving for some time. Those cases in which the Korsakoff syndrome develops insidiously, without an obvious Wernicke episode (see Chapter 2), could equally be explained on such a basis. It could conceivably be the case that covert pathology of this nature makes a contribution to the memory deficits encountered in alcoholics generally.

The issue is of potential therapeutic importance. If a substantial number of alcoholics develop a thiamine-dependent pathology well before it is clinically apparent, high-potency vitamin therapy should find wider prophylactic application. The feasibility and desirability of routinely supplementing alcoholic beverages with thiamine has indeed received consideration (Centerwall & Criqui 1978; Weinstein 1978; Bishai & Bozzetti 1986; Finlay-Jones 1986; Rouse & Armstrong 1988). Price *et al.* (1987) conclude that fortification of flour alone, as practised in the UK and USA, is insufficient for prophylaxis in problem drinkers. Reuler *et al.* (1985) estimate that the supplementation of alcoholic beverages in the USA would merely cost the consumer an additional 0.1 cent per litre of wine. The identification of persons at special genetic risk (see Wernicke's encephalopathy and alcoholism, earlier) could also prove to be important. However, these are matters to be clarified by future research.

Treatment

Wernicke's encephalopathy represents an acute medical emergency and warrants energetic treatment from the moment the diagnosis is made. Doses of thiamine as small as 2–3 mg can modify the ophthalmoplegias, but much larger doses are indicated to minimise the chance of disabling sequelae, particularly since associated hepatic disorder may interfere with utilisation of the vitamin. In view of the possibility of other concurrent vitamin deficiencies, Pabrinex is usually employed intravenously in place of thiamine alone. Intravenous infusion should always be carried out slowly over 10 minutes on account of the risk of anaphylactic reactions. Each injection of Pabrinex contains thiamine hydrochloride 250 mg, nicotinamide 160 mg, riboflavine 4 mg, pyridoxine hydrochloride 50 mg and ascorbic acid 500 mg. The duration of treatment is controversial, but should be for at least 5 days twice daily, followed by high-dose oral thiamine. In the occasional patient who seems refractory to thiamine replacement, determination of the serum magnesium level may be indicated. Traviesa (1974) showed that hypomagnesaemia impaired both the biochemical and clinical response to treatment. The syndrome of nicotinic acid deficiency encephalopathy (see under Wernicke's encephalopathy and beriberi, earlier) must also be kept in mind when response has been lacking or incomplete to the replacement of thiamine alone.

Other aspects of management must include attention to infection, dehydration or electrolyte imbalance as a result of vomiting. Signs of congestive cardiac failure should be treated. Disturbed behaviour, and particularly that due to coincident delirium tremens, will require appropriate sedation.

Oral vitamin supplements are usually continued for several weeks after the acute illness has resolved. In patients with enduring ataxia, polyneuritis or memory disturbance, high-potency vitamin injections should be pursued energetically as long as improvement is occurring.

Korsakoff's syndrome

The relationship between Wernicke's encephalopathy and Korsakoff's syndrome has gradually been clarified. Korsakoff gave the first comprehensive account of the amnesic syndrome that bears his name in 1887, shortly after Wernicke's description of his syndrome, but the close relationship between the two was not appreciated at the time.

All Korsakoff's cases had polyneuritis, which led him to propose the name 'psychosis polyneuritica'. The great majority of cases were reported in alcoholics and the cause was thought to be some toxic effect of alcohol. Shortly thereafter cases were reported without alcoholism or neuropathy in patients suffering from puerperal sepsis, typhoid or intestinal obstruction. By the 1930s other known causes included gastric carcinoma, intractable vomiting and severe dietary deficiency. Thiamine deficiency therefore came under suspicion as the common metabolic link. Bowman *et al.* (1939) tried the effect of parenteral thiamine and reported encouraging results; disorientation and confabulation responded in many cases, but the memory deficits were largely unaltered.

Meanwhile, evidence accumulated to suggest a clinical link between Wernicke's encephalopathy and Korsakoff's syndrome. Features of the two disorders were sometimes seen together, and the former was often noted to lead to the latter. De Wardener and Lennox's (1947) cases were again important here, showing clear evidence of memory deficits in association with ataxia and ophthalmoplegias. The acuteness of their cases also allowed the memory deficits to respond unequivocally to thiamine in many cases. The link between the two conditions was consolidated when the site of the cerebral lesions in Korsakoff's syndrome was clarified. Malamud and Skillicorn (1956) provided clear evidence that in patients dying with Korsakoff's syndrome the location of cerebral pathology appeared to be identical with that seen in Wernicke's encephalopathy, the two merely differing in the acuteness or chronicity of the pathological process.

The amnesic syndrome can, of course, result from a variety of brain lesions that have nothing to do with thiamine deficiency but, where the nutritionally depleted subject is concerned, Wernicke's encephalopathy and Korsakoff's syndrome appear to be different facets of the same pathological process. Confirmation came from the clinicopathological study of Victor *et al.* (1971), published under the composite title *The Wernicke–Korsakoff syndrome*. Of 186 alcoholic patients who survived the acute illness and were observed for long enough to assess the development of amnesia, 84% developed a typical Korsakoff syndrome. Other cerebral pathology may make additional contributions to the fully developed picture, but lesions in the Wernicke distribution appeared to be fundamental to the amnesic deficits displayed.

Follow-up of the Korsakoff patients showed complete recovery in one-quarter, partial recovery in half, and no improvement whatever in the remainder (Victor *et al.* 1971). Complete recovery was observed even in some very severe examples, although detailed follow-up neuropsychological assessment was not presented. The onset of improvement was commonly delayed for several weeks or months, and once started sometimes continued for as long as 2 years.

In the chronic amnesic stage anterograde and retrograde amnesia are the dominant features, but continuing minor impairments of perceptual and cognitive function could usually be discerned by careful examination. The retrograde amnesia is usually of several years' duration, although with islands of preservation and without a sharply demarcated beginning. Confabulation is rarely encountered in the chronic stage (see Chapter 2).

Over recent years, the following have become evident.
1 The classic lesion at the base of the brain is often associated with more widespread cerebral pathology, including cortical shrinkage and ventricular dilatation. The contribution that this may make to certain aspects of the clinical picture warrants careful appraisal.
2 The rarity of fully fledged Korsakoff's syndrome as a residue of thiamine deficiency in non-alcoholics raises the possibility that a direct neurotoxic action of alcohol may play some part in the evolution of the condition.
3 There is evidence that Korsakoff's syndrome may be misdiagnosed to a considerable extent in clinical practice.

Neuroimaging findings and cortical pathology
Cortical pathology was widely described in the earlier literature before the diencephalic basal brain lesion came to be fully appreciated (Lishman 1981). Thereafter interest in cortical aspects showed a pronounced decline. However, neuroimaging studies have re-emphasised that supratentorial changes are common. Jacobson and Lishman (1990) compared 25 Korsakoff patients, gathered from hospitals around

London, with non-Korsakoff alcoholics of similar age. On CT the Korsakoff patients had wider third ventricles, as might have been expected from their diencephalic lesions, but also significantly larger lateral ventricles, sylvian fissures and interhemispheric fissures. The widening of the interhemispheric fissures, measured between the frontal lobes, was particularly marked and showed significant correlations with certain tests of frontal lobe function (Jacobson 1989). Shimamura *et al.* (1988) found atrophy in frontal sulcal and perisylvian areas on CT in comparison with normal controls, the frontal atrophy correlating with impairment on memory and other tests. Jernigan *et al.* (1991b), using MRI, showed greater grey matter losses in the medial temporal and orbitofrontal cortex when Korsakoff patients were compared with non-amnesic alcoholics. However, Colchester *et al.* (2001) showed statistically significant reduction in thalamic volume in 11 Korsakoff patients whereas medial temporal lobe volumes were relatively preserved, in contrast to patients with herpes encephalitis in whom atrophy was the other way around.

Further evidence of cortical involvement has come from functional brain imaging studies. Hunter *et al.* (1989) examined 10 Korsakoff patients with hexamethylpropyleneamine oxine (HMPAO)-SPECT, revealing impaired blood flow in the frontal regions that correlated significantly with deficits on tests of memory and orientation. Kessler *et al.* (1984) showed that glucose metabolism, as measured by FDG-PET, was reduced overall by 20% in Korsakoff patients, with hypometabolism present in numerous cortical areas in addition to the thalamus and basal ganglia. However, Joyce *et al.* (1994) found that FDG-PET showed robust hypometabolism in only three regions, the anterior cingulate, posterior cingulate and precuneate areas, in comparison with normal controls. Reed *et al.* (2003), using quantified FDG-PET, showed significant hypometabolism in the thalamic, ventromedial frontal, and retrosplenial regions only. EEG studies in Korsakoff's syndrome have revealed mild or moderate generalized slow waves with only a few cases showing more prominent generalized slow waves (Fisch 1999).

A substantial cortical component to the pathology could be relevant to the wider cognitive deficits often detected in Korsakoff patients on detailed psychological testing, sometimes exceeding those in matched non-Korsakoff alcoholics (Jacobson *et al.* 1990). Various authors have demonstrated impairments on executive or frontal lobe tests in Korsakoff's patients (Janowsky *et al.* 1989; Joyce & Robbins 1991; Kopelman 1991). These impairments could also explain some of the striking clinical aspects of the syndrome, in particular apathy, lack of initiative and profound lack of insight that the majority of patients display. As discussed in Chapter 2, these are not inevitable concomitants of severe memory disorder, and can be entirely absent in amnesic syndromes of other aetiologies.

Neurotoxic action of alcohol in Korsakoff's syndrome

Thiamine replacement is not regularly effective in reversing the memory difficulties; and as Freund (1973) pointed out there is a remarkable lack of evidence that permanent memory disorder can follow thiamine deficiency unaccompanied by alcohol abuse. There have been occasional reports of a persistent Korsakoff syndrome following severe vomiting, malabsorption or prolonged intravenous feeding, but in a close examination of these Kopelman (1995) concludes that the evidence for a non-alcoholic nutritional cause must still be regarded as equivocal.

The inevitability of the link between an overt episode of Wernicke's encephalopathy and Korsakoff's syndrome may also be challenged on the basis of clinical experience. In many Korsakoff patients there is evidence of a pre-existing Wernicke encephalopathy, as reported by Victor *et al.* (1971), but in others no such history is forthcoming. Some patients appear to develop their amnesic difficulties insidiously (Cutting 1978), in the context of chronic continuing inebriation. Such patients would be under-represented in Victor *et al.*'s sample, since most of their patients were incepted as cases of Wernicke's encephalopathy then followed through to the Korsakovian development.

Thus while the relationship between thiamine deficiency and Wernicke's encephalopathy cannot be doubted, there is less clear-cut evidence to incriminate thiamine exclusively in the chronic Korsakoff state. A combination of alcohol neurotoxicity and avitaminosis may be necessary for the development of the fully fledged syndrome, as discussed in some detail by Lishman (1990). An alternative explanation is that in alcoholics thiamine deficiency may have been operative over a considerable period of time. In other words, alcoholism may tend to be associated with a 'subclinical' Wernicke pathology which, by the time it becomes overt, has led to fixed and irreversible structural changes.

Continuity hypothesis

It is interesting in this connection that certain continuities have been discerned between the memory deficits seen in Korsakoff's syndrome and those found in chronic alcoholics generally (Ryback 1971). Subtle but definite 'subclinical' memory deficits appear to be widespread in the alcoholic population, and these become more pronounced in alcoholics who complain of memory difficulties. In the latter the severity of the deficits can overlap to some degree with those seen in Korsakoff's syndrome. Continuities are also apparent in measures of third ventricular width as detected on CT. Either alcohol neurotoxicity or 'subclinical' thiamine deficiency could be the common link. Bowden (1990) has argued strongly for the latter, suggesting that in neuropsychological research a rigid distinction between Korsakoff and non-Korsakoff alcoholics should no longer be regarded as valid.

Diagnosis

The diagnosis of Korsakoff's syndrome requires clear evidence of a marked memory disorder along with relative preservation of other cognitive functions. Subtle deficits will often be revealed by special testing, as outlined under Psychological evidence, earlier, particularly with regard to visuoperceptive functions and abstracting ability, but performance on standard intelligence tests should be substantially intact. This was well illustrated by Butters and Cermak's (1980) comparison of intelligence test scores (Wechsler Adult Intelligence Scale, WAIS) in a group of Korsakoff patients and a group of intact normal controls. The latter were carefully matched for age, socioeconomic class and educational background. With the sole exception of the digit–symbol subtest, no significant differences could be discerned in any aspect of test performance. In contrast, on measures such as the Wechsler Memory Scale, Butters and Cermak found that Korsakoff patients can generally be expected to score some 20–30 points below the expectation derived from their IQs.

In clinical practice such careful distinctions are not always observed. In a retrospective survey of 63 alcoholic patients admitted to the Maudsley Hospital, Cutting (1978) found 50 who had been labelled as having Korsakoff's syndrome and 13 as having alcoholic dementia. However, the Korsakoff patients proved to be heterogeneous. Those with a relatively acute onset mirrored the classic syndrome, with an isolated memory deficit and a poor prognosis as judged by capacity to resume independent existence. In contrast, 17 of the 50 differed from these acute cases in significant ways. Their symptoms had been several months in evolution, they tended to be older, females predominated over males, and some two-thirds showed improvement on follow-up. Psychological test profiles, where available, showed that the gradual-onset group, like the alcoholic dements, were impaired across a wider range of cognitive functions in addition to their memory problems. This suggested that several patients with more global cognitive impairments had been falsely labelled as suffering from Korsakoff's syndrome.

Jacobson and Lishman (1987) have also provided evidence of heterogeneity within the syndrome. They obtained separate indices of the severity of memory impairment and of 'generalised intellectual decline' in their sample of 38 chronic Korsakoff patients. The former was derived from the discrepancy between the WAIS IQ and the Wechsler Memory Quotient, the latter from the discrepancy between the WAIS IQ and the National Adult Reading Test which yields an approximate estimate of premorbid IQ. When the two indices were plotted against each other a marked scatter was apparent; some two-thirds of patients showed clear memory impairment with little fall from premorbid IQ (i.e. the classic Korsakoff pattern), others showed both mild memory and mild intellectual decline, whereas 10% showed little memory impairment but marked intellectual decline. Thus it appeared that there was an admixture of patients in the sample, with at one extreme a group that might more properly have been labelled as having more generalised cognitive impairment. Females featured disproportionately among those with generalised impairment as was the case in Cutting's survey. Certain relationships could be discerned with CT scan parameters: widening of the third ventricle tended to be associated with more severe memory deficits, and widened interhemispheric fissures with greater fall from premorbid intellectual functioning.

It would seem therefore that patients with Korsakoff's syndrome show a variable degree of generalised impairment, particularly in executive or frontal lobe impairment but other deficits (e.g. in visuospatial function) can also occur. Certainly the label of Korsakoff's syndrome would appear to be more commonly applied in clinical practice than is strictly warranted.

Treatment

In the established chronic Korsakoff state treatment will often prove to be disappointing. Cutting (1978) reviews the differing reports in the literature, some finding no patients whatsoever with a significant response to thiamine and others obtaining improvement in up to 70% (Victor *et al.* 1971). Nevertheless, the possibility of occasional substantial improvement means that high-dose thiamine replacement must always be attempted by the parenteral route, and oral replacement should be pursued over many months if benefit continues to be observed.

Other nutritional disorders associated with alcoholism

Other disorders in alcoholics are suspected of being nutritional in origin, although the evidence is less complete. Of those considered below peripheral neuropathy is almost certainly due in part to vitamin deficiency, but here and in the others a direct toxic effect of alcohol may also be responsible.

Peripheral neuropathy

Alcoholic peripheral neuropathy may sometimes be symptomless and manifest only by loss of the ankle reflexes, but in most cases there are prominent complaints of sensory disturbance. It begins usually in the feet with numbness, pins and needles, burning sensations and pain. Sensory ataxia may be prominent. Weakness may progress ultimately to foot drop with wasting of the leg muscles. Cutaneous sensory loss is most marked peripherally in the hands and feet, and intense hyperaesthesia may be elicited on stroking the skin. The calf muscles are often very tender. Oedema of dependent parts may develop along with dystrophic changes of the skin and nails.

The condition often accompanies Wernicke's encephalopathy or Korsakoff's syndrome, and some 50% of patients with neuropathy show residua of these disorders. It may also present as an isolated abnormality, or in association with delirium tremens. The main cause appears to be deficiency of thiamine, although other deficiencies may be important as well. Pyridoxine and pantothenic acid deficiency can produce neuropathy and are likely to be involved in some alcoholics. A toxic role for alcohol itself, or other toxic substances in alcoholic beverages, has been proposed, but slow recovery is usual with vitamin therapy even though drinking continues.

Cerebellar degeneration

Victor *et al.* (1959) have described a remarkably uniform cerebellar syndrome in alcoholics, with ataxia of stance and gait as the principal abnormalities. The arms are little affected, and nystagmus and dysarthria may be absent. The typical course is gradual evolution over several weeks or months, after which the disorder remains static for many years. More rarely, slow progression occurs over a number of years. The resemblance to cerebellar degeneration seen with bronchial carcinoma can sometimes be close, and chest radiography is obviously important in every case. CT or MRI may reveal cerebellar cortical atrophy. Gilman *et al.* (1990) have shown hypometabolism in the superior cerebellar vermis with FDG-PET.

Pathological changes are largely restricted to the anterior and superior aspects of the vermis and cerebellar hemispheres. The cell loss affects the Purkinje cells especially. Victor *et al.* (1989) suggest that the ataxia of Wernicke's encephalopathy, at least in its chronic form, is based on a similar type of lesion. They therefore favour a nutritional cause rather than a direct toxic effect of alcohol. There is little evidence to favour the latter, Estrin (1987) finding that estimates of annual and lifetime consumption were *lower* in alcoholics with cerebellar degeneration than in those without. Karhunen *et al.* (1994) have shown a small inverse correlation between Purkinje cell counts and size of daily intake in moderate drinkers, but the variation was wide suggesting important differences in individual susceptibility. Sullivan *et al.* (2000b) have documented correlations between cerebellar grey and white matter volumes and ataxia in alcoholic and Korsakoff patients.

Amblyopia

In rare cases retrobulbar neuritis may develop in alcoholics, progressing over 1 or 2 weeks but rarely extending to complete blindness. Dimness of central vision, especially for red and green, is the more common result. An associated peripheral neuropathy is usual. The smoking of strong pipe tobacco is often incriminated in addition to the alcoholism, and deficiencies of both thiamine and vitamin B_{12} appear to be responsible. Acute blindness is more commonly seen as a result of methyl alcohol consumption, and is then attributed to the direct toxic effects of the poison.

Marchiafava–Bignami disease

This rare disorder was formerly thought to be restricted to Italian males but this is now known to be erroneous, likewise the belief that it was especially related to the drinking of wine. It presents with ataxia, dysarthria, epilepsy and severe impairment of consciousness, or in more slowly progressive forms with dementia and spastic paralysis of the limbs. Delmas-Marsalet *et al.* (1967) reviewed the literature and presented cases with full neuropathological examination. Extensive demyelination affects the corpus callosum and adjacent subcortical white matter, the optic tracts and the cerebellar peduncles. The mortality is high, but patients sometimes survive for several years. Recovery is rare. Characteristic findings have been reported in the corpus callosum on CT or MRI (Kawamura *et al.* 1985). A nutritional origin is suggested by the symmetry and constancy of location of the lesions within the CNS, and the frequent history of dietary deprivation. The fact that virtually all cases have occurred in alcoholics suggests that alcohol may also play a part in causation (Victor *et al.* 1989). The precise factors involved remain uncertain.

Central pontine myelinolysis

This is an acute and often fatal complication of alcoholism, presenting with obtundation, bulbar palsy, quadriplegia and loss of pain sensation in the limbs and trunk. Vomiting, confusion, disordered eye movements and coma are common. Some patients show the 'locked in' syndrome with mutism and paralysis but relatively intact sensation and comprehension (Adams & Victor 1993). The lesion lies in the centre of the basis pontis, varying in extent and sometimes involving other neighbouring structures. It consists essentially of a focus of demyelination, usually demonstrable with MRI.

A nutritional origin has again been strongly suspected (Cole *et al.* 1964). Many cases are seen in association with Wernicke's encephalopathy and polyneuropathy. However, it may also occur with liver disease not due to alcohol, with Wilson's disease, and after liver transplantation/haemodialysis (Compston 1993). Other causes include severe burns, hyperemesis gravidarum and diuretic therapy which have led to hyponatraemia. It has emerged that over-rapid correction of low serum sodium is a common cause in such situations, the pons being unusually vulnerable to rapid changes in electrolyte balance due to its close admixture of white matter bundles and richly vascular grey matter (Leslie *et al.* 1980). This has led to the relabelling of the condition as the 'osmotic demyelination syndrome' (Sterns *et al.* 1986).

Barbiturates

The barbiturates are a large class of related compounds based on barbituric acid with sedative hypnotic properties, once widely prescribed for sleep and anxiety disorders, now in greatly restricted use as anticonvulsants (e.g. phenobarbital) and in anaesthesia (e.g. pentobarbital) (Charney *et al.* 2001). A fascinating review of the history of barbiturate use is provided by López-Muñoz *et al.* (2005), detailing the impact of the widespread availability of compounds with effective anaesthetic, anticonvulsant and anxiolytic properties, followed by the later recognition of their addictive and toxic properties, in particular their role in overdose as exemplified by the death of Marylin Monroe. Acute and chronic toxicity associated with barbiturates reached a peak in the 1960s but are now uncommon as a result of more stringent prescribing practices. Barbiturate use is associated with increasing tolerance so that ultimately enormous quantities can be consumed, and barbiturate addiction is still occasionally seen, most often along with addiction to alcohol and other drugs.

Acute barbiturate intoxication

The barbiturates display a very narrow therapeutic window, with early anxiolysis followed by a period of confusion and drowsiness giving way to deepening anaesthesia (Charney *et al.* 2001). The pulse and respiration are slowed, the blood pressure lowered, and the body temperature often reduced. The tendon reflexes are diminished, or absent in deep coma. The plantar responses may be upgoing. Nystagmus is a prominent feature in the earlier stages together with tremors of the tongue and lips. Death may result from respiratory failure or peripheral circulatory collapse.

During recovery signs of cerebellar disturbance are marked, with nystagmus, ataxia, asynergia, dysarthria and hypotonia. A muddled euphoria is often seen while consciousness is returning, and a period of hypomania may persist after all neurological features have cleared.

Estimation of the blood barbiturate level serves to confirm the cause of the acute intoxication or coma. EEG may also be useful in showing generalised fast beta activity during the first 24 hours after overdose, unlike most other severe intoxications which produce slowing of rhythms in parallel with reduction of the level of consciousness.

Treatment of an acute overdose of barbiturates requires immediate admission to hospital, with facilities at hand for mechanical respiration and dialysis if required. Induced vomiting, gastric lavage or activated charcoal treatment must be carried out urgently, and measures may be needed to control peripheral circulatory failure. Deepening or prolonged coma may necessitate artificial respiration and the use of haemodialysis.

Chronic barbiturate intoxication

Chronic barbiturate intoxication produces drowsiness, fluctuating confusion, dysarthria and ataxia that may closely resemble drunkenness due to alcohol. Withdrawal effects are also similar, with epileptic fits and delirium. It is still important to consider barbiturate abuse in patients who present with intermittent confusion of obscure origin, or who develop fits or delirium of uncertain aetiology on admission to hospital.

Little has been discovered about possible long-term effects of barbiturate abuse on the CNS. The question has rarely been addressed directly, no doubt because of difficulties in the systematic follow-up of subjects. Moreover, polydrug abuse has been a common pattern in barbiturate addicts, with a large number of sedative, narcotic and stimulant drugs often featuring in the histories of patients.

EEG during barbiturate coma shows diminished amplitude and burst suppression, providing a reliable guide to central effects (Winer *et al.* 1991). After withdrawal dramatic changes occur, with high-voltage paroxysmal discharges or bursts of high-amplitude waves at 4–6 Hz during the first 12–48 hours, with seizures similar to the grand mal fits of idiopathic epilepsy (Essig 1967).

γ-Hydroxybutyrate

γ-Hydroxybutyrate (GHB), also known as liquid ecstacy, is a recently recognised drug of abuse related to the sedative hypnotics and used for its anxiolytic and euphoriant properties (Gonzalez & Nutt 2005). Initially synthesised in the 1960s, the recent increase in the recreational use of GHB, and its association with 'drug rape', has focused attention on the compound and its effects. In a randomised controlled study comparing the effects of GHB with a barbiturate and a benzodiazepine, GHB showed intermediate properties with initial euphoria and reduced anxiety, with higher doses producing sedation and nausea (Carter *et al.* 2006). There is evidence for distinct GHB receptors in the brain, although it is probable that the main mechanism of action is to promote GABAergic neurotransmission (Crunelli *et al.* 2006). GHB abuse is associated with acute hospital presentation, with sedation and paradoxical agitation being the main features but with few other distinguishing features, rendering diagnosis difficult (Drasbek *et al.* 2006).

Benzodiazepines

Benzodiazepines are in common use as short-term anxiolytics, hypnotics, anticonvulsants and muscle relaxants, as add-on therapy to selective serotonin reuptake inhibitors in the treatment of obsessive–compulsive disorder, and as adjunctive therapy in treating patients with acute mania or agitation (Chouinard 2004). Prevalence rates of benzodiazepine use (depending on the definition of benzodiazepine use and observation period) range from 0.2 to 8.9%, with the ratio of female to male use constant at 2 : 1 and longer-term benzodiazepine users usually older than 45 years (Zandstra *et al.* 2002).

Increased awareness of the risks of tolerance, dependence and cognitive side effects has contributed to the decline in the prescription of benzodiazepines over the last two decades (O'Brien 2005a), as has increased availability of alternative pharmacological and non-pharmacological treatments for anxiety and insomnia (Stewart & Westra 2002). The rapid development of tolerance limits benzodiazepine use to brief periods only, typically 2–4 weeks. Discontinuation following the development of physical dependence can lead to severe withdrawal effects that can mimic the symptoms for which the drugs were initially prescribed, with exacerbation of anxiety and insomnia. Patients prescribed therapeutic doses over long periods may show an admixture of beneficial and withdrawal effects.

There is a variety of compounds in the benzodiazepine class differing in duration of action, potency and primary metabolism (Chouinard 2004). Of those commonly prescribed, nitrazepam, diazepam and flurazepam have longer half-lives compared with lormetazepam, temazepam and oxazepam. Lorazepam is much more potent compared with, for example, diazepam and temazepam. The risk of physical dependence is much greater with shorter-acting compounds. All benzodiazepines are metabolised in the liver through glucuronidation or nitrogen reduction, and eliminated by the kidneys. In patients with impaired liver function (e.g. the elderly, patients with cirrhosis), caution should be used in prescribing, especially those benzodiazepines that undergo liver oxidation, as the oxidative process is more susceptible to liver impairment compared with glucuronidation and nitrogen reduction. Benzodiazepines metabolised by oxidation use the cytochrome P450 3A4 liver enzyme system. Therefore caution is also required in prescribing to patients already receiving medicines utilising this route of metabolism, e.g. ketoconazole, erythromycin, clarithromycin, diltiazem, verapamil, ritonavir (this list not exhaustive).

All forms of benzodiazepines act by enhancing the actions of the inhibitory neurotransmitter GABA by binding to a specific recognition site on $GABA_A$ receptors containing α1–5 subunits. Compounds that bind at this modulatory site and enhance the inhibitory actions of GABA are classified as agonists, those that decrease the actions of GABA are termed inverse agonists, whereas compounds which bind but have no effect on GABA inhibition are termed antagonists. The clinically used benzodiazepines are full agonists. Attempts have been made to develop compounds that are anxioselective in that they retain the anxiolytic properties of the full-agonist benzodiazepines but have reduced sedation and dependence liabilities (Atack 2003). Early data suggest that α1 $GABA_A$ receptors may mediate sedation, anterograde amnesia and seizure protection, whereas α2 $GABA_A$ receptors may mediate anxiolysis (Mohler et al. 2002).

Research suggests that although benzodiazepine prescribing is high among patients with severe mental illness (e.g. schizophrenia and bipolar disorder) and co-occurring substance misuse disorders, abuse potential is high in this group (Brunette et al. 2003) and there is little evidence to support that their use is helpful either for relief of target symptoms of anxiety and depression or for attaining remission from substance use disorder.

Among intentional abusers of benzodiazepines, benzodiazepines are usually a secondary drug of abuse, used mainly to augment the 'high' received from another drug or to offset the adverse effects of other drugs. Few cases of addiction, as opposed to 'normal' physical dependence, arise from legitimate use of benzodiazepines (O'Brien 2005a). The psychiatric complications attending the general use of benzodiazepines are best considered first in terms of their withdrawal phenomena and secondly their sedative actions.

Withdrawal effects

Dependence on benzodiazepines can occur very quickly and within therapeutic dosage. Withdrawal effects can follow dose reduction or discontinuation. Adverse reactions are commoner with abrupt than gradual withdrawal, after high dosage or prolonged use, and with shorter-acting forms of benzodiazepine, although there is much individual variability. The symptoms of withdrawal are highly variable from patient to patient. The usual time course for the development of symptoms is within 3–10 days of stopping treatment. Withdrawal is more rapid with compounds that have a short half-life. Lorazepam has been associated with particularly early and severe withdrawal effects. Withdrawal of regular night sedation can precipitate nightmares, vivid dreams and 'rebound insomnia', accompanied by increased REM sleep for several weeks. Discontinuation of daytime treatment can lead to agitation, dysphoria and perceptual changes. Somatic symptoms of anxiety tend to be accompanied by restlessness, emotional lability, impaired concentration and depersonalisation. Insomnia is often severe. Panic attacks and paranoid feelings occur. Weakness, dizziness, tremor, muscle twitching, palpitations, headaches and sweating are common, likewise gastrointestinal symptoms including nausea, anorexia, abdominal discomfort and diarrhoea. Perceptual disturbances have been described in many modalities and include sensations of movement or tilting in the visual field leading to feelings of unsteadiness ('perceptual ataxia'), also tinnitus and unusual tactile sensations. Blurring of vision, facial burning and hot and cold feelings may be accompanied by muscle pain and aching. Increased sensitivity may be experienced to light, sounds, smells and taste. The more florid manifestations last on average 5–20 days, but anxiety-related symptoms can persist for 6–12 months. Severe and dangerous manifestations can follow abrupt withdrawal from large dosage. Confusion and hallucinations may progress to delirious states closely similar to delirium tremens. A serious complication is grand mal fits, sometimes with status epilepticus.

Management of withdrawal

After careful assessment of the reasons for commencing the medication, and of the possible need for continuing alternative treatment, the dosage of benzodiazepines should be very gradually tapered. When the patient is on a short-acting compound, substitution with diazepam may facilitate withdrawal. Propranolol may help to ameliorate some of the somatic symptoms, and clonidine has been claimed to be useful. Sedative antidepressants may be indicated when depression is severe. Anxiety management techniques have been shown to be valuable, and self-support groups have come to be widely established. A recent Cochrane review of the management of benzodiazepine monodependence (Denis *et al.* 2006) found support for dose-tapering strategies with little current support for substitution of longer-acting agents or adjunctive medications.

Sedative effects

Despite rapid tolerance to benzodiazepines, sedation can continue to occur especially with escalating dosage, leading to slowed cerebration, increased reaction time and decreased vigilance. This can be hazardous in persons using machinery or when driving. When used for night sedation, 'hangover' effects may be troublesome, particularly in older persons, and especially with long-lasting preparations such as nitrazepam. Severe sedation, from cumulative dosage or excessive intake, can result in a picture of intoxication with slurred speech, ataxia, emotional lability and poor memory and concentration. Impairment of judgement may be compounded by a paradoxical increase in hostility and aggression, ranging from excitement to outbursts of anger and antisocial behaviour (Mancuso 2004). Very large doses lead to coma with respiratory depression, although fatalities from overdosage have proved to be rare.

A good deal of interest attaches to the amnesic effects that may be produced, especially with intravenous administration. This has been utilised prior to surgery or uncomfortable investigatory procedures. Wolkowitz *et al.* (1987) gave incremental doses of diazepam intravenously to volunteers, revealing marked effects on attention and word list recognition. At higher dosage the effects could be so profound that the subject could not remember that a word list had been given. In contrast, access to information acquired prior to the injections was totally spared. Lister (1985) and Hartman (1988) review other studies that have shown impaired recall of new material, apparently due to deficient acquisition into long-term memory. The severity and duration of the memory effects vary according to the particular drug used, the dose and the route of administration, but beyond this the pattern appears to be qualitatively the same: impairment of acquisition without effects on retention or retrieval. In some circumstances the drugs may even facilitate retrieval. How far these effects depend on sedation, reflecting attentional processes rather than memory *per se*, remains uncertain.

It is also unclear whether long-continued use can lead to neuropsychological impairment. Observations suggesting that this is so have usually been on patients taking other medications in addition. Lucki *et al.* (1986) studied patients who had taken benzodiazepines continuously for a mean of 5 years, mostly in normal therapeutic dosage. In comparison with matched controls seeking treatment for anxiety-related disorders, there were few demonstrable effects. The free recall of word lists was unaffected, also performance at digit–symbol substitution and letter cancellation tasks.

Impairment was found only on the critical flicker–fusion threshold. Such results would appear to reflect tolerance to the amnesic and other psychological effects of the drugs with long-term use.

Opiates and opioids

The opiates comprise a series of alkaloids derived from the opium poppy *Papaver somniferum*, including morphine, thebaine and codeine, which have a long history of use for relief of pain and diarrhoea, and of abuse for euphoriant effects. Heroin (diamorphine) is prepared from morphine by acetylation and has a particularly marked euphoriant effect. The opioids refer to all drugs with morphine-like action and include synthetic compounds such as fentanyl (and derivatives), methadone, buprenorphine and oxycodone, as well as the endogenous neurotransmitters enkephalin, endorphin and dynorphin. The major and most valuable property of the opioids is pain relief; indeed the opioids are the most powerful and effective drugs for pain relief known, being particularly effective at reducing pain without effects on other sensations. Unfortunately, such a valuable property is also associated with profound abuse liability, and a major source of abused opioids are those diverted from clinical prescription (Cicero *et al.* 2007).

The central actions of opioid drugs have been clarified by the identification of opiate receptors in the brain. These exist as μ (mu), κ (kappa) and δ (delta) subclasses, of which the most important for analgesic and euphoriant effects is the μ receptor found widely throughout the nervous system, particularly in the dorsal root ganglia of the spinal cord, the ventral tegmental area and the ventral striatum. It is now known that endogenous opioids present in the nervous system (enkephalins, endorphins and dynorphin) have important modulating effects on pain perception. There is evidence that repeated administration of exogenous opioid drugs leads to suppression of endogenous opioid activity and also to augmentation of stress systems, which lead to an important role in relapse to opioid dependence (Koob & Kreek 2007).

Acute effects

Opiates are administered by a variety of routes, some such as methadone and codeine being orally bioavailable; however, for maximal euphoriant effects rapid administration is preferred. For example, heroin is administered by intravenous injection, termed 'shooting up', or by inhalation, called 'chasing the dragon'. Administration is followed by a euphoriant 'rush' and a subsequent 'high' comprising a state of mental detachment and feelings of extreme well-being. They also have sedative effects ('nodding' or 'gouching'), leading to difficulty with concentration, drowsiness and sleep. After large doses depression of the respiratory centres can cause respiratory arrest and death. The characteristic sign of pinpoint pupils with respiratory failure is virtually pathognomonic of opioid overdose. Established treatment for opioid overdose is intravenous administration of the potent opioid antagonist naloxone, which rapidly reverses opioid coma 'on the point of the needle'; however, care needs to be taken that opioid effects do not return given the short (20-minute) half-life of naloxone (Clarke *et al*. 2005).

With repeated use tolerance develops rapidly so that dangerously large doses come to be taken. In particular a withdrawal syndrome develops, with marked motivational and physical signs of dependence that may disrupt the addict's life by constant drug-seeking behaviour. Physical dependence becomes apparent when administration is disrupted or curtailed. The early opiate abstinence syndrome consists of craving, anxiety, sweating, restless sleep and running eyes and nose. More severe degrees show as gooseflesh ('cold turkey'), shivering, muscle twitching, dilated pupils and aching in the bones and muscles. Abdominal cramps develop later with vomiting, diarrhoea, increased pulse and blood pressure, severe insomnia and low-grade fever. Consciousness is unimpaired throughout. The physical withdrawal syndrome tends to reach a peak during the third and fourth days, usually subsiding within a week. Although extremely unpleasant, it is rarely life-threatening. However, the motivational aspects of the withdrawal syndrome persist, leading to intense craving and increased risk of relapse under conditions of drug-primed, cue-primed or stressful circumstances (Bossert *et al*. 2005). Opioid replacement therapy with long-acting orally bioavailable opioids such as methadone or buprenorphine is directed towards preventing development of the withdrawal state, with relapse to more harmful use of opioids (see Mattick *et al*. 2008 for a Cochrane review of current practice). Given that opioid replacement therapy needs to be given on a continuous and costly basis, non-opioid pharmacotherapies are under assessment, such as the opioid antagonist naltrexone which shows some evidence for prevention of craving and relapse (O'Brien 2005b).

One very important exception to this picture of relatively mild physical withdrawal effects is seen in the neonatal abstinence syndrome, which is marked by neonatal irritability, seizures, growth retardation, failure to thrive and an increase in sudden infant death syndrome. This important source of mortality and morbidity necessitates vigilant opioid replacement treatment in expectant opioid-dependent women (Minozzi *et al*. 2008).

Psychiatric disorder

The use of opiates *per se* appears to be relatively free from adverse effects on the CNS. The major identified problems associated with opioid abuse stem from the complications of intravenous administration, including injection of impurities and transmission of infections such as hepatitis B and C and HIV. Overdose, deep vein thrombosis and hypoxic brain damage are recognised causes of comorbidity. Neuroimaging studies have identified abnormalities associated with infection, infarction and anoxia in heroin users presenting for treatment, with a relatively rare leucoencephalopathy associated with 'chasing the dragon' (Borne *et al*. 2005). Neuropsychological studies of opioid use, to quote a recent review, 'remains limited' (Gruber *et al*. 2007). They summarise findings suggesting that the use of opiates is associated with multiple deficits in attention, concentration, recall, visuospatial skills and psychomotor speed, with particularly marked effects on executive functions and behavioural inhibition, but these may be premorbid features associated with both inception of heroin use and persistence with heroin use. However, considerable difficulties are encountered in discerning the possible contributions of individual substances when polydrug abuse is so common a pattern. Thus it is hard to make definitive statements on the issue, in contrast to the obvious cerebral toxicity of several other abused substances. This may in itself be a significant observation.

Cannabis and the cannabinoids

Cannabis refers to products of the plant *Cannabis sativa* (and *Cannabis indica*), widespread in tropical and temperate areas. In the form of marijuana and hashish they have a long history of medicinal and ritual use predicated on their psychoactive properties (Clarke & Watson 2002). Cannabis also has practical use in the form of hemp – strong fibres derived from cannabis used in the production of rope and other fabrics – which may have contributed to the widespread availability of this plant and served as a base for later adoption to psychoactive use. The importance of cannabis and the cannabinoids stems from their current status as the most widely abused illicit drugs within Western societies, their potential medicinal use and their relationship to psychiatric disorder, particularly psychosis and schizophrenia. The cannabinoids comprise the 60-plus cannabis-derived compounds, most importantly Δ^9-tetrahydrocannabinol (Δ^9-THC) derived from *Cannabis sativa* and current synthetic variants, which contribute to psychoactive use. Accepted medical uses of cannabinoids (currently Marinol or Dronabinol, an oral preparation of Δ^9-THC) include treatment for refractory nausea and vomiting associated with chemotherapy and for weight loss associated with anorexia in AIDS and HIV infection.

Cannabinoids, particularly Δ^9-THC, have been shown to exhibit reinforcing effects in animal models, including self-administration and conditioned place preference, and to show tolerance and withdrawal following chronic use. These findings should serve to curtail the frequently encountered question about whether such phenomena are true of human use, but rather focus attention on the nature and degree with which they are present. Using such models, it has been possible to identify important contributions of the endogenous dopamine and opioid systems to the behavioural effects of cannabinoids, and to detect endocannabinoids such as anandamide that have neuromodulatory function within reinforcement systems in the brain. Two cannabinoid receptors, CB_1 (central) and CB_2 (peripheral), have been identified, with the CB_1 receptor clearly implicated in the behavioural effects of cannabinoids. In a series of studies of CB_1 receptor knockout models, attenuation of opioid effects was also demonstrated (Martin *et al.* 2000), emphasising that the effects of opioids are contingent on intact cannabinoid signalling and that cross-talk between systems is often important for the net drug effects to a single agent.

Contemporary views on cannabis use have tended to become an emotive and highly politicised topic, specifically with respect to how control is best achieved through regulation and policing and the status of cannabis as a 'gateway' drug to more harmful drug use. While there is still uncertainty about the prevalence of seriously adverse psychological reactions to the drug, and case reporting has perhaps highlighted the rare and exceptional, the current prevalence and early inception of psychoactive use is such that cannabis use must nowadays be increasingly considered in psychiatric differential diagnosis. Both acute and chronic forms of adverse reaction have been described, the main difficulty being how far these reflect special vulnerability in the patient rather than the direct neuroadaptive properties of cannabis on the nervous system. The relationship between cannabis/cannabinoids and psychiatric disorder is considered here with respect to general behavioural properties of psychoactive use, neuropsychological effects and long-term abstinence effects, as well as their putative and controversial relevance to schizophrenia.

Acute effects of cannabis

Cannabis is most often smoked, with effects noted within 10–15 minutes, but can also be ingested with delayed onset of effects and prolonged action. The active ingredient, Δ^9-THC, has high lipophilicity, which contributes to rapid onset of psychoactive effects. The effects of ingesting or smoking marijuana are distinctive and were described in early reports by Bromberg (1934) and Allentuck and Bowman (1942). Since these early reports, multiple studies have been conducted under both naturalistic and controlled conditions examining acute and non-acute (residual) effects on subjective experience and neuropsychological function (reviewed by Gonzalez *et al.* 2002; Gonzalez 2007).

The most common reported effect of cannabis use is one of 'relaxation', although there is considerable variation in effects between both individuals and occasions (Green *et al.* 2003). Other responses include happiness, laughter and increased sensory perceptions. Negative effects are uncommon and include dizziness, drowsiness, paranoia, anxiety and depression, and occasionally depersonalisation

(Gonzalez 2007). Cognitive functions are affected in many subtle ways. The stream of talk tends to be circumstantial and fragmented. There may be difficulty in linking parts to the whole, or sudden interruptions in the stream of thought resembling the blocking of schizophrenia. Time sense is characteristically distorted, often with remarkable subjective lengthening of time spans. Sometimes there is unawareness of the passage of time, or a curious disturbance in which the present does not seem to arise out of the past. Attention, concentration and comprehension are only slightly impaired in the milder stages of intoxication, although retrieval-based memory deficits have been consistently observed (Gonzalez 2007). Effects of Δ^9-THC have been noted with respect to other cognitive functions, including measures of decision-making and inhibition, but these may relate to risk variables rather than the consequences of cannabis use *per se*. Intriguingly, in one laboratory-based controlled study, haloperidol treatment did little to affect the subjective experience of Δ^9-THC and *worsened* neuropsychological performance, indicating that the effects of Δ^9-THC are not substantially mediated via dopaminergic neurotransmission (D'Souza *et al.* 2008a).

Tolerance to cannabis is now well recognised (D'Souza *et al.* 2008b), as is the existence of a cannabis withdrawal syndrome marked by irritability, aggression, decreased appetite and sleep disturbance (Budney *et al.* 2004). Studies of the non-acute (residual) effects of cannabis have been reviewed by Gonzalez *et al.* (2002), who established basic criteria for inclusion of studies into a meta-analysis. Relatively few studies met such criteria, but supported mild residual effects of cannabis on learning and memory performance, which are alleviated by abstinence, with some evidence of diminished decision-making. In the absence of longitudinal studies, these may relate to pre-existing deficits.

Cannabis and psychiatric disorder

The claim that excessive use of cannabis over long periods of time can result in a chronic psychotic illness akin to schizophrenia, or indeed increase the risk of developing schizophrenia *per se*, is currently a subject of intense controversy. While there is an emerging consensus that cannabis use is a risk factor for developing schizophrenia (Arseneault *et al.* 2004; Moore *et al.* 2007; Murray *et al.* 2007), strong evidence about the magnitude of risk from cannabis use has been hard to obtain and the hypothesis needs to be viewed with caution. When chronic psychoses have developed there may have been important predisposing factors or even pre-existing illness; and where social decompensation is concerned much may be due to social or subcultural influences. A historical study by Halikas *et al.* (1972), in which 100 regular cannabis users were interviewed along with 50 non-user friends of the group, showed clearly how it could be erroneous to attribute causal significance to the drug. A high prevalence of psychopathology was found in both samples, approximately half of each fulfilling criteria for some psychiatric diagnosis. Moreover, almost every diagnosed psychiatric illness among the users had begun before the first exposure to cannabis.

Early examples of *prolonged depersonalisation* lasting for months after cannabis use have been cited, sometimes after relatively brief exposures (Keshavan & Lishman 1986). The patients often considered their chronic symptoms to be identical with those experienced during acute intoxication, adding to the suspicion that neurobiological factors could be responsible. Nevertheless, more recent controlled studies found little evidence for a distinct drug-induced depersonalisation syndrome (Medford *et al.* 2003).

With regard to the *chronic psychoses*, it is generally viewed that cannabis use exacerbates symptomatology, likelihood of relapse and the severity of social impairment, although a recent Cohrane review still regarded the evidence as equivocal (Rathbone *et al.* 2008).

Evidence of *cognitive impairment*, especially some time after cannabis exposure, has been hard to demonstrate after controlling for premorbid cognitive function. Iversen (2005) reviewed the evidence for a link with the somewhat surprising conclusion that 'cannabis could be rated to be a relatively safe drug'. Investigation of structural or functional brain changes associated with cannabis use has been the subject of recent review by Quickfall and Crockford (2006) who analysed in excess of 100 studies on this topic. In general, no strong structural abnormalities were associated with cannabis use. Functional impairments were associated with increases during acute use and decreases during abstinent periods, analogous in many respects to use of psychostimulant drugs in general, without particular specificity for cannabis use *per se*.

Psychostimulants

Cocaine, amphetamines and methamphetamine

The psychostimulants cocaine, amphetamine and methamphetamine comprise a group of drugs with analogous effects to adrenaline (epinephrine) and are often referred to as 'sympathomimetic amines'. They stimulate the CNS and also activate the sympathetic nervous system, producing increased activity, excitement and euphoria. They have a long history of use to alleviate fatigue in the form of tonics (perhaps the most famous example being CocaCola) and a correspondingly long history of abuse and behavioural toxicity. Currently, the most prevalent psychostimulant in the UK is cocaine, although worldwide methamphetamine abuse in the form 'crystal meth' is arguably the greater problem (Buxton & Dove 2008). Prior to the escalation in the use of cocaine, amphetamines were the most abused psychostimulant, and abuse is occasionally seen even now. Sloboda (2002) has highlighted the difficulties in assessing the prevalence of psychostimulant (and other illicit drug) abuse, which occurs largely in illicit markets and hence limits the planning of interventions targeted either on supply of the drug or on dealing with the consequences of abuse.

The use of cocaine has a long history. The alkaloid is obtained from the leaves of the coca bush (*Erythroxylum coca*) which is grown extensively in Colombia, Bolivia and Peru. Coca paste, a crude derivative of the leaves, may be chewed or smoked, but most of the crop is converted into cocaine hydrochloride and sold as a powder, often mixed with various adjuvants. This can be inhaled into the nose (sniffing or snorting) or injected intravenously. Freebase forms are derived from the hydrochloride as preparations suitable for smoking, a simple process yielding the form known as 'crack'. Tiny pellets of crack, representing pure crystalline cocaine, are sold remarkably cheaply and rapidly lead to the most severe form of addiction. Animal experiments have shown that cocaine is a powerful primary reinforcer, largely mediated through the dopaminergic system (Thomas *et al.* 2008), leading the animal to work for drug reward to the exclusion of food and often until death.

Medical use of the amphetamines is now largely restricted to the treatment of narcolepsy (dexamfetamine sulphate, racemic amfetamine sulphate, methylphenidate; see Chapter 13) and of children with attention deficit hyperactivity disorder. Ephedrine, the earliest member of the group, is mainly employed as a nasal decongestant, and its derivatives are ingredients of over-the-counter cold cure remedies: pseudoephedrine (Sudafed), phenylpropanolamine (Triogesic) and phenylephrine. Other related compounds have been used for the treatment of obesity though this is now discouraged: phenmetrazine (Preludin), diethylpropion (Apisate), phentermine (Duromine). Many patients have become dependent as a result of careless prescribing, and all drugs in the group may be abused for their stimulant and euphoriant effects. The use of methylamphetamine (Methedrine) by intravenous injection presented particular problems during the 1960s. Stricter prescribing controls are nowadays offset by illegal manufacture.

Physical and psychological effects

In whatever form they are taken the psychostimulants exert powerful stimulant and euphoriant effects, leading to increased energy and wakefulness for a time and feelings of great well-being. Intravenous use produces an intense 'rush' or 'high' almost instantaneously, gradually receding over 20–30 minutes. The smoking of 'crack' cocaine has a similarly rapid effect, peaking after 5 minutes or so then abating quickly leaving the addict craving another dose. Nasal inhalation leads to a more gradual onset of euphoria, since vasoconstriction occurs within the nasal mucosa. The effects then typically wear off over an hour or so. While under the influence of the drug the subject shows enhanced alertness and mental acuity and feels increased confidence in social interchange. Cocaine is often regarded as an aphrodisiac because of the elation and disinhibition experienced, but higher doses lead to impotence and decreased sexual desire.

The stimulant effect on the sympathetic nervous system leads to tachycardia, raised blood pressure, increased temperature and dilated pupils. Important effects are also exerted on the dopaminergic system, especially in mesolimbic and mesocortical areas (Thomas *et al*. 2008). Large doses can result in a dangerous degree of hypertension, cardiac dysrhythmias or grand mal convulsions. Adulterants by way of procaine or lidocaine increase the risk of cardiovascular complications or status epilepticus. Other toxic effects include muscle twitching, nausea and vomiting, irregular respiration and hyperpyrexia.

Sudden fatalities can occur from cardiovascular complications such as myocardial infarction, ventricular fibrillation or cerebral haemorrhage. Other deaths result from CNS depression, with circulatory and respiratory failure, loss of reflexes and delirium. Unexplained deaths are thought to be due to toxic effects on the myocardium. Persons with a congenital deficiency of pseudocholinesterase are at special hazard from even small doses since this enzyme metabolises cocaine.

Severe malnutrition is common in regular abusers who often present with multiple vitamin deficiencies. The powerful local anaesthetic effect of cocaine serves to obscure pain, so that dental neglect can reach extreme degree. Many addicts therefore present in a severely deteriorated state.

It was formerly thought that tolerance did not occur, based on experience of occasional recreational users of the drug. However, it is now clear that users of freebase forms can come to tolerate immense and frequently repeated doses, with adaptation to the convulsant and cardiovascular effects. It is less clear whether tolerance develops to the euphoriant properties though this is likely.

Behavioural toxicity develops rapidly and soon becomes a major problem. Even the casual weekend user is prone to find that little is enjoyable without the drug, and progresses to more frequent and dangerous forms of administration. As the dosage increases dysphoric effects emerge in the wake of elation, with depression, irritability, anxiety and profound insomnia. Severe craving and intense drug-seeking behaviour can then become entrenched. Withdrawal results in a state of depression, apathy and increased appetite, with lethargy and disinterest often persisting for many weeks. Suicidal feelings are not uncommon. Physical aspects of withdrawal include disturbed sleep patterns, tremors and muscle pain, but the major physiological disruptions seen with opiate and sedative withdrawal do not occur.

Psychostimulants and psychiatric disorder

The psychiatric effects of psychostimulants can be considered in four successive stages: acute intoxication, withdrawal depression, addiction and, most dramatically,

hallucinosis and psychosis. The euphoria of acute intoxication, already described above, shows symptoms analogous to mania, with heightened pleasure, hyperactivity and increased speed of intellectual functioning. Disinhibition and impulsive behaviour are common, including a proneness to violence. A second stage, following withdrawal of the psychostimulant, is marked by dysphoria and can resemble major depression, with anxiety, misery, apathy and irritability occurring when psychostimulant levels are falling or in more prolonged abstinence when the addict is craving another dose. Restlessness and hostility can be prominent and alcohol or other drugs may be used to combat such phases. Distinguishing major depression from cocaine (or other psychostimulant) withdrawal can be a difficult diagnostic problem, most readily resolved by brief psychiatric admission. In a recent review of the syndrome, Rubin *et al*. (2007) demonstrated that measures of depressed mood in cocaine withdrawal resolved with brief abstinence, whether or not overt 'major depression' had been evident. Cocaine and psychostimulant addiction have been associated with subtle neuropsychological impairments, particularly affecting executive and attentional processing, with diminished cognitive control leading to impulsivity (Ersche & Sahakian 2007; Garavan & Hester 2007), although these features may be associated with either inception or persistence of psychostimulant use rather than the consequence of use *per se*.

Psychostimulant use is associated with the development of substance-induced psychotic disorder, which is a surprisingly heterogeneous category. The manifestations are probably closely related to elevated dopamine activity in the brain. In a recent review of this disorder, Mathias *et al*. (2008) noted that many of the publications related to single cases with 'a striking paucity of information on the outcome, treatment, and best practice for substance-associated psychotic episodes'.

Amphetamine or cocaine hallucinosis usually begins with visual and auditory misperceptions. Harmless objects and noises appear to be threatening and the person is hypervigilant and increasingly concerned. Halo effects may appear around lights, or sensations of movement at the periphery of the visual field. Hallucinations then emerge in several modalities: lights sparkling at the periphery of vision ('snow lights'), voices calling the user's name, and the classic tactile hallucinations of insects felt crawling under the skin. At this stage partial insight is retained into the unreal nature of the hallucinations and delusions.

Amphetamine or cocaine psychosis represents further progression to extreme paranoia. It is usually preceded by a transitional period of increasing suspiciousness, ideas of reference, dysphoria and compulsive behaviour (Weiss *et al*. 1994). The patient is restless and talkative, and everyday events are misinterpreted in delusional fashion: he believes others are plotting against him or about to attack him, or that he is being followed by the police or drug dealers. He may act on such beliefs with unusual aggressiveness, damaging property or becoming homicidal or suicidal. Insight is lost into the unreal nature of the hallucinatory experiences; he may pick and scratch at his skin in the search for insects or even claim to see them. A further characteristic feature is repetitive stereotyped behaviour, such as dismantling and reassembling a watch or radio over and again, or compulsively arranging and rearranging a set of objects (Ghodse 1995). Consciousness is fully preserved throughout and there is no disorientation.

Neurological complications

Glauser and Queen (2007) review the multiple non-cardiac complications associated with cocaine and psychostimulant abuse and their relationship to method of administration. Headache, convulsions and cerebrovascular accidents following acute psychostimulant administration are well recognised, with rarer complications such as spinal cord thrombosis documented. All such events could occur in new or occasional users as well as in chronic addicts.

Cerebral vasculitis represents another hazard. This was first suspected in intravenous drug users from angiographic findings, with irregular segmental constrictions in intermediate-sized arteries and complete obstruction in smaller vessels (Rojas *et al.* 2005). The picture is complicated by poly-drug abuse and impurities in the injected material, or by sepsis, which could have been chiefly responsible.

Treatment

Treatment of acute toxic reactions may require barbiturates or diazepam to control severe agitation, overstimulation or seizures (Estroff & Gold 1986). Propranolol helps with tachycardia and hypertension, and further drugs may be needed to deal with cardiac dysrhythmias. Impending circulatory and respiratory failure will warrant urgent supportive measures. Respiratory depression may indicate that opiates have been taken as well, requiring the administration of naloxone. Chlorpromazine or haloperidol may be needed for the control of psychotic reactions.

Approaches to treatment of psychostimulant addiction are largely psychosocial (Knapp *et al.* 2007), as psychopharmacological trials with anticonvulsants (Minozzi *et al.* 2008), antipsychotics (Amato *et al.* 2007), dopamine agonists (Soares *et al.* 2003) and antidepressants (Lima *et al.* 2003) have been shown on meta-analysis and review to offer no great promise.

Ecstasy and the substituted amphetamines

The substituted amphetamines are a large series of so-called designer drugs arising from combinatorial chemical substi-

tutions based on the core amphetamine (phenylethylamine) molecule. Ecstasy (3,4-methylene-dioxymethamphetamine, MDMA) is the most widely known of these compounds, on which this section focuses. However, the substituted amphetamines also include 'Eve' (3,4-methylene-dioxyethamphetamine), 'STP' (2,5-dimethoxy-4-methylamphetamine) and 'DOB' (2,5-dimethoxy-4-bromoamphetamine), which are among the most well known of an astonishing number of unfamiliar or less fashionable varieties. The famous (or infamous) book *PiHKAL: Phenethylamines i Have Known And Loved* by the biochemist Alexander Shulgin details the synthesis and subjective effects of over 100 of these compounds: the book is legally available, the compounds are not, despite the fact that it serves as the source of methods for the clandestine synthesis of this group of compounds.

Ecstasy (MDMA) became well known in the UK in the 1980s in the context of 'raves' (parties organised for energetic dancing) as a euphoriant and to promote feelings of closeness to others. Along with mild stimulation it has some hallucinogenic potential. From time to time it attracts widespread publicity from the sudden tragic deaths that occur, occasionally on first contact with the drug. Tolerance occurs gradually with repeated use, some habitués taking as many as 10–20 tablets during the course of a weekend (Winstock 1991). However, it does not appear to cause physical dependence, although a large research effort has been directed towards the identification of long-term neurotoxic effects of use. While less newsworthy currently, epidemiological surveys in Europe and the USA (National Epidemiologic Survey on Alcohol and Related Conditions) indicate stable and substantial prevalence of use (Keyes *et al.* 2008).

Acute and subacute effects

The acute subjective effects of MDMA use have been well studied from the 1980s onwards. In a comprehensive review of 24 such studies, Baylen and Rosenberg (2006) identified the major categories of subjective effects as 'emotional (e.g. anxiety, depression, closeness, fear, euphoria, calmness) or somatic (e.g. nausea/vomiting, bruxism, muscle aches/headache, sweating, numbness, body temperature changes, fatigue, dizziness, dry mouth, increased energy)'. Interestingly, cognitive effects such as confused thought, perceptual effects such as sensory disturbance and sleep effects such as insomnia were not reported in more than five of the 24 studies, indicating that while they do occur, this is not the experience of the majority of users. In their review of placebo-controlled healthy volunteer studies, Dumont and Verkes (2006) noted marked psychostimulant effects (elevation of heart rate and systolic and diastolic blood pressure) at doses of 1 mg/kg and above occurring together with the characteristic subjective effects. MDMA is typically taken a stereotyped fashion in doses of about 150 mg, with onset of action within an hour and typically lasting 8 hours, with notable subacute effects lasting days. In a study focusing on these subacute effects, Verheyden *et al.* (2003) questioned 466 regular users of MDMA and identified the experience of low mood and impaired concentration in about 80%.

MDMA use has been strongly linked to episodic acute toxicity and death, occurring through a variety of mechanisms (Schifano 2004). The more prevalent complication is hyperpyrexia, arising from the psychomotor stimulant effects, compounded by vigorous dancing and environmentally induced overheating, leading to states of collapse due to dehydration and metabolic acidosis. Conversely, attempts to counter such dehydration can lead to water intoxication and inadvertent hyponatraemia. Convulsions, cerebral haemorrhage, rhabdomyolysis, disseminated intravascular coagulation and acute renal failure have all been reported. Such acute adverse reactions can require urgent medical intervention, with active cooling measures, control of seizures, rehydration and other supportive measures. Long-lasting residual sequelae of acute toxicity is often underestimated: Kopelman *et al.* (2001) reported medial temporal, thalamic and retrosplenial hypometabolism on FDG-PET, associated with profound and sustained amnesia, in such a case.

Long-term consequences

Relatively early after MDMA use became prevalent in the 1980s, it was shown to be a selective serotonergic neurotoxin in animal models, producing a rapid and persistent decrease in brain 5-hydroxytryptamine (5HT) and 5-hydroxyindoleacetic acid in experimental animals (McKenna & Peroutka 1990). Of particular note, structural damage was also shown in non-human primates, affecting serotonergic fibres in the cortex and cell bodies in the dorsal raphe nucleus (Ricaurte *et al.* 1988). The mechanisms by which MDMA produces selective serotonergic toxicity comprise a combination of oxidative stress, excititoxicity and mitochondrial dysfunction (Quinton & Yamamoto 2006), leading particularly to depletion of monoamine neurotransmitters including serotonin and dopamine. Such consistent findings have prompted substantial research into potential long-term neuropsychiatric sequelae in human users of ecstasy, leading to currently in excess of several hundred studies. A range of psychiatric and neuropsychological problems have been identified in current regular ecstasy users and ex-users, with low mood, anxiety and subtle attention and memory deficits being the most consistent findings (reviewed by Karlsen *et al.* 2008). However, the overall conclusion of these studies is that it is not possible to dissociate specific effects due to MDMA over and above those associated with premorbid risk factors and polysubstance misuse, a point highlighted by Gouzoulis-Mayfrank and Daumann (2006). A review of structural and functional MRI studies has not identified any consistent findings, although PET ligand studies have identified potential deficits in serotonin transporter densities in line with the animal literature (Cowan 2007). While the unclear picture emerging from neuropsychological and neuroimaging studies has led to questions about the animal data, focusing on interspecies differences and dose-scaling assumptions (Easton & Marsden 2006), there is a pressing need for appropriately designed longitudinal studies of sufficient power to detect potential neurotoxic effects of MDMA in humans.

Hallucinogens

Hallucinogens, also known as psychedelics (from the Greek meaning 'to make visible the psyche'), are psychoactive substances that may dramatically alter visual, auditory, gustatory and tactile perceptions, and associated cognitions and consciousness. They are generally not associated with dependence or addiction, or physiological toxicity, but this must be viewed with caution. The explosion in use of the hallucinogens, particularly lysergic acid diethylamide (LSD), from the 1950s onwards has provided the basis for our current knowledge of their potential toxic effects, although it should be noted that the use of naturally occurring hallucinogens has been an important part of human ritual and search for ecstatic experience from the earliest times. Interestingly, research into the properties of these compounds first focused attention on the importance of the serotonin system in cerebral disorder, particularly in the generation of 'model psychosis' (Nichols 2004). This section focuses on LSD, while a multiplicity of other drugs with similar hallucinogenic properties to LSD are not discussed in detail. Of these latter compounds, one group are derived from plants and enjoy a vogue in certain parts of the world. Mescaline comes from a cactus grown in Mexico and nearby parts of the USA, and psilocybin and psilocin from 'magic mushrooms' found in a variety of regions. Mace, nutmeg and the morning glory plant contain other hallucinogenic substances. Another group comprising a range of synthetic compounds with hallucinogenic and amphetamine-like activity have also been widely abused: dimethyltryptamine, dimethoxyamphetamine and dimethoxymethylamphetamine, all largely based on a phenethylamine structure.

Phenyclidine (PCP, 'angel dust') is related to pethidine and has been widely abused in North America. Its use is particularly hazardous on account of a tendency to precipitate convulsions and coma, and its unpredictable psychological effects including outbursts of violent bizarre behaviour and prolonged psychoses.

Lysergic acid diethylamide

LSD is an indole derivative of ergot and can be manufactured synthetically. It is the most powerful hallucinogen known, doses as small as 25 μg usually having a demonstrable effect on humans. The mode of action on the brain is thought be inhibition of the serotonergic system, via stimulation of presynaptic $5HT_2$ receptors and consequent feedback effects on serotonergic neurones (Kosten 1990). Soon after its discovery it enjoyed a vogue in experimental psychiatry for the study of 'model psychoses' that could be induced in normal subjects. Thereafter it was employed as an adjunct in psychotherapy, for abreaction and to assist in the recall of long-forgotten experiences. As a result the acute effects of its administration were closely studied and formed the basis of a good deal of theoretical speculation. Nowadays administration under medical supervision is almost unknown, but the drug continues to be widely taken on an illicit basis. The benefits claimed by users include augmented aesthetic sensitivity, enhanced creativity, the occurrence of transcendental experiences, the acquisition of new insights, and aphrodisiac effects. None of these has been properly substantiated. It is widely abused by unstable individuals in search of dramatic experiences, and often by those who abuse other drugs as well. As a drug of abuse LSD carries the special hazard that it can easily be administered surreptitiously without the subject's knowledge, resulting in profoundly disturbing effects that may sometimes lead to psychiatric referral. When taken at intervals of more than 1 week the reaction is just as intense with the same repeated dose; there is no evidence that LSD is a drug of addiction in the sense of creating physical dependence, and there are no withdrawal effects on discontinuation. The danger lies rather in psychological dependence on the effects that are produced.

Acute effects of ingestion

The acute effects are well described by Isbell *et al.* (1956) and Freedman (1968). There is some variation in individual susceptibility, but striking psychological changes usually follow doses in the range 20–120 μg. The predominant effects with small doses are autonomic changes and alterations of mood, while larger doses produce perceptual distortions, vivid hallucinations and striking subjective changes in body image. These remarkably intense phenomena are usually not accompanied by clouding of consciousness or demonstrable impairment of intellectual processes; indeed a heightened state of awareness is maintained, and thought processes characteristically remain clear. The subject becomes preoccupied with the phenomena he is witnessing and experiencing, but usually retains insight into the fact that they are due to the drug. In these respects the 'toxic' state resulting from LSD and related hallucinogens is very different from the acute organic reactions induced by most other agents.

The autonomic effects are the first to appear. They include dilatation of the pupils, piloerection and some rise in body temperature. The tendon reflexes are often increased, and muscular tremors and twitching develop in severe reactions. Weakness, somnolence and giddiness may be marked. The earliest mood changes are of euphoria or anxiety. Euphoria is usually the predominant change and may extend to feelings of ecstasy, but this can be followed later by sudden swings to

depression, panic or a profound sense of desolation. Some subjects become active and excited, while others are quiet, passive and withdrawn. Some are overwhelmed with a sense of mystical experience. Others become paranoid and hostile to their surroundings. Much probably depends on the premorbid personality of the subject, his expectations and the setting in which the drug is taken.

Perceptual distortions, illusions and hallucinations are mainly in the visual sphere but can affect all modalities. Vision may be blurred or astonishingly enhanced and vivid. The perception of depth and distance is changed, size and shape distorted, and colour greatly intensified. Hearing may be dulled or hyperacute, clothing may feel like sandpaper, or the body may feel extremely light or heavy. Synaesthesia often occurs and is fascinating to the subject: sensory data are transformed from one modality to another so that sounds or tactile stimuli appear as bursts of light or scintillating moving spectra. Hallucinations are again mainly visual and occur in both unformed and formed varieties: kaleidoscopic patterns of light in intense and changeable colour, or complex visions of animals and people. Tactile paraesthesiae, metallic tastes and strange smells are not uncommon, but auditory hallucinations are rare.

Distortions of body image can figure prominently and take bizarre forms. Customary boundaries become fluid, so that the patient feels he is one with the chair on which he is sitting or merged with the body of another. His own hands and feet may appear to be transformed into claws or the extremities of a dead person. Sometimes intense somatic discomfort is experienced, with feelings of being twisted, crushed or stretched. Depersonalisation and feelings of unreality may extend to the impression of being outside one's own body, difficulty in recognising the self in a mirror, or difficulty in deciding whether a thought refers to a real event or is merely a spontaneous thought.

Despite these experiences the subject is able to respond to questions, and conceptual and abstract thinking can usually be shown to be substantially intact. Except in the most severe reactions a large measure of critical self-judgement is preserved. However, as the effects of the drug increase, external reality becomes progressively less intrusive and self-control may be lessened, occasionally with dangerous results as described below. Frank delusions may occasionally be expressed but an organised delusional system rarely develops.

The effects of the drug are usually apparent within 30 minutes of ingestion, rising to a maximum 1–4 hours thereafter. The reaction subsides gradually over the next 8–16 hours and there is usually no residuum on waking next morning. However, after the vivid effects of the drug experience, the real world often appears to be drab and dull, and natural events lack the urgent and compelling quality of what has gone before. Some degree of depression and disillusionment may thus be an understandable aftermath.

Adverse reactions

Among habitual users the great majority of LSD experiences are apparently without adverse effect. Occasionally, however, profoundly disturbing results accompany the acute effects of the drug, and lead to emergency medical referral or trouble with the police. Adverse effects appear to be commoner in unstable subjects. Certainly a large proportion of those coming before psychiatrists have a history of previous psychiatric care (Ungerleider *et al.* 1966). It has been estimated that less than 0.1% of normal subjects experience seriously adverse reactions when LSD is taken under medical supervision; among patients undergoing psychotherapy the incidence rises to 0.2–1.0%, and among psychotic subjects to 1–3% (Louria 1968). The frequency among illicit users is unknown but is probably higher still. Much may also depend on the circumstances in which the drug is taken, on impurities in the preparations used and on injudicious doses.

The pictures that result have been described by Frosch *et al.* (1965), Ungerleider *et al.* (1966), Bewley (1967) and Freedman (1968). They may be divided into acute emotional disturbances, the acting out of impulses, and acute psychotic reactions.

Acute emotional disturbances are the most common, especially an acute panic reaction in which the subject feels overwhelmed by experiences beyond his control. He may feel that he is going insane or react in terror to homicidal impulses. He may present himself at hospital seeking relief, or be brought by friends who fear he will come to harm. There is no impairment of consciousness, although recollection of the details of the LSD experience may be hazy. Rapid recovery occurs as the drug effects wear off, usually within 8–12 hours, though sometimes 1 or 2 days are required to regain normality. Other acute emotional disturbances include depression, paranoia and outbursts of explosive anger. Profound depression very occasionally leads to attempted or successful suicide. Acute paranoia may cause the subject to flee about the streets in terror or lead to episodes of explosive anger.

The acting out of impulses is facilitated as self-control becomes diminished. The subject may become unmanageable, run amok, attempt to disrobe or make overt homosexual advances. Sociopathic individuals are more prone to commit acts of violence and attempted homicide has been reported. Feelings of invulnerability may lead the patient to take unwarranted risks with danger of bodily harm. Patients who have fallen from windows or roofs have sometimes apparently acted on the belief that they would float down unharmed.

Acute psychotic reactions are commonly longer lasting, and the majority of Ungerleider *et al.*'s (1966) patients remained in hospital for more than a month. Most are schizophrenia-like illnesses, with hallucinations, delusions and overactive

behaviour. Less commonly they take the form of acute organic reactions with confusion, disorientation and marked emotional lability. However, the latter may often be the product of multiple drug abuse.

Hatrick and Dewhurst (1970) reported two interesting examples in which psychotic illnesses followed a latent interval, well after the effects of acute intoxication had subsided. The illnesses were nevertheless coloured by phenomena reminiscent of the acute phase of intoxication. Both patients were said to have been previously stable and well adjusted, and the illnesses followed a single exposure to LSD.

Features that may be of diagnostic significance in LSD-induced psychoses are discussed by Dewhurst and Hatrick (1972). A particularly striking aspect may be the wide variety of schizophreniform, affective and neurotic symptoms present in the same patient. Suggestive symptoms include regression to childhood, loss of time sense, grandiose delusions of a pseudophilosophical nature, and a wealth of visual hallucinations and perceptual disturbances. Visual hallucinations are said to be more intense than in other acute organic reactions and may be specific, transient and recurring. Auditory hallucinations tend to have a more startling, personal and realistic quality than in schizophrenia. The emotional response is usually constantly shifting, with apprehension, panic, elation or depression in rapidly changing sequence. When an LSD-induced psychosis presents as hypomania, euphoria may alternate with panic, which is an unusual combination in primary affective illness. Many patients with suicidal ruminations have irrational compulsive urges to self-destruction, arising suddenly and sometimes unbacked by other depressive symptoms.

Rosenthal (1964) drew attention to a further rare type of prolonged reaction, consisting of visual hallucinosis in clear consciousness. Rosenthal considered this to be specifically related to multiple exposures to LSD over a considerable period of time. The condition is often heralded by a change in the experience produced by the drug, typically a change to unpleasant reactions that may have led to its discontinuation. Spontaneous visual hallucinations then commence and continue for many months. The hallucinations are similar in form and content to those experienced under the drug: droplets of colour, shimmering panels and brightly coloured shape distortions. Cats, crabs, insects and corpses may also be seen. Pleasant hallucinations were often under semi-voluntary control, in that the patient could make them more or less intense by efforts of concentration, but the unpleasant phenomena were intrusive and liable to provoke severe anxiety. The patients continued to recognise the unreality of the hallucinations, and there was no evidence of thought disorder or other schizophrenic phenomena. Occasionally, however, a secondary delusional system was elaborated to explain the hallucinations.

The issue of longer-term neuropsychological deficits associated with long-term hallucinogen use has been addressed in a meta-analysis and review by Halpern and Pope (1999) who conclude that the evidence for any consistent deficits are at present equivocal and are methodologically confounded by polysubstance misuse in this group.

Recurrences of the LSD effect (flashbacks)

Occasionally, there may be a simple prolongation of the LSD state lasting several days, with undulating anxiety and persisting visual aberrations, but Frosch et al. (1965) have described more remarkable phenomena in which the LSD experiences recur for many weeks or months after discontinuation of the drug. Sometimes it is merely bewilderment or fear that recur in milder form, but quite commonly sensory phenomena are involved as well. Two of Frosch et al.'s patients experienced depersonalisation and perceptual distortions 2 months later. Another had many transient episodes of catatonia and visual hallucinations over the course of a year, similar to those that had been induced by LSD.

Horowitz (1969) suggests that perhaps as many as 5% of users experience mild recurrences from time to time, while others have put the estimate much higher. Sensory recurrences have been reported in all modalities, but the visual system is most often involved. Horowitz described three main varieties. The commonest consists of the repeated intrusion into awareness of some image derived from the LSD experience. This arrives unbidden and is outside voluntary control. It may be accompanied by distortion of time sense or reality sense. It is usually the same image that recurs, often of a frightening nature, and considerable psychiatric disturbance can occasionally be provoked. The second variety consists of the spontaneous return of perceptual distortions: halo effects, blurring, shimmering, reduplication, distortion of planes, changes of colour, micropsia or macropsia. In the third variety there may be increased sensitivity to spontaneous imagery for some time after taking LSD. Such imagery is more vivid than usual, less readily suppressed, and occupies a greater proportion of the subject's thought and time than formerly.

Abraham (1983) added additional phenomena, notably geometric pseudohallucinations, false perceptions of movement in the peripheral field, flashes of colour, intensified colours, and 'trailing phenomena' in which after-images remain immediately behind an object as it traverses the visual field. Symptoms were sometimes reported as long as 8 years after the last exposure to LSD. Common precipitants in Abraham's series were emergence into a dark environment, staring at a blank wall or the subsequent use of marijuana. Benzodiazepines were found to be useful in treatment.

Several explanations have been proposed to account for recurrences but none has been substantiated. Brain damage has been blamed, or the release of some stored metabolite, or neurophysiological changes in the mechanisms underlying imagery formation and suppression. Abraham (1982) has obtained evidence that LSD users are impaired on tests of colour discrimination when examined an average of 2 years after their last exposure, and that those experiencing flashbacks are particularly affected. Further visual studies have shown depressed critical flicker frequencies and reduced sensitivity to light during dark adaptation in past users of LSD (Abraham & Wolf 1988). The tendency for recurrences to accompany periods of stress and anxiety has suggested that they may represent a form of conditioned response or learned reaction to anxiety. Psychodynamic theorists have viewed the recurrent imagery as representing screen images to conceal emotional conflict, or as symbolising the breakthrough of repressed ideas.

More recently, hallucinogen persisting perception disorder has been incorporated into the psychiatric diagnostic schedules, characterised by frequent flashbacks involving intense and intrusive visual recollection of prior hallucinations. Halpern and Pope (2003) have reviewed this field and identify the disorder as genuine but highly uncommon.

Solvent abuse

Solvent abuse is defined as the intentional inhalation of volatile substances to achieve an altered mental state. From initial recognition as a problem in the 1970s it continues to be a significant problem worldwide, with a striking variety of distinct solvents and delivery systems being described, according to availability and fashion. An influential classification by Balster (1998) defined three major classes of abused solvents: the volatile solvents, nitrous oxide and the alkyl nitrites. Volatile solvents include glues, thinners, fuels and anaesthetics, with street names such as 'air blast', 'discorama', 'hippie crack' and 'moon gas'. Nitrous oxide, known as laughing gas or 'shoot the breeze', can be obtained from diverted medical anaesthetics, but is also found in whipped-cream dispenser chargers (known as whippets). Volatile alkyl nitrites, known as 'poppers', 'snappers' or 'boppers', are also commercially available as Rush, Bolt, Thrust, Climax, Locker Room and tend to be associated with adult use, particularly in groups where men have sex with men.

Intriguingly, volatile solvent misuse is mainly a problem affecting young adolescents of school age, with a stable rate of 10% of adolescents admitting to having used solvents at some time (Williams & Storck 2007). In the UK it came to widespread recognition in the form of 'glue sniffing', carried out sporadically as a small-group activity, and prompted restrictions on the sale of a variety of previously readily available volatile products in 1999. As with all psychoactive drugs, use may be experimental or episodic. Serious complications are rare, although accidental injury while intoxicated and 'sudden sniffing death syndrome' related to cardiac toxicity are significant problems. Neurotoxic and systemic side effects are strongly associated with regular use over long periods. Detection of solvent misuse is a particular problem as initial effects are short-lived and the intoxicant itself is volatile; however, as it may be exhaled, a characteristic odour may persist and findings such as perioral rashes, glitter or paint stains, and self-neglect provide clues.

Acute effects

Glue is commonly inhaled from a plastic bag ('bagging'), either nasally ('sniffing or snorting') or through the mouth ('huffing'), with depth of inhalation being adjusted for maximal euphoriant effect. Aerosols may be sprayed directly into the mouth or nose, a particularly hazardous procedure: 'dusting' refers to the direct application of computer cleaning products to the nose or mouth through the nozzle provided. Solvents are rapidly absorbed in the lungs, with immediate and brief effects. They act directly on the CNS through a variety of mechanisms identified in the action of alcohol or anaesthetics (Balster 1998), with a number of downsteam effects on neurotransmitter systems, including promotion of GABA and opioid systems and inhibition of N-methyl-D-aspartate (NMDA) neurotransmission (for review see Bowen *et al.* 2006).

The subjective effects are a period of euphoria and exhilaration, known as the 'rush', setting in rapidly and accompanied by giddiness and disorientation. This phase may be prolonged for several hours by repeated inhalation, otherwise effects are brief and there is relatively rapid recovery. Nausea, slurred speech, dizziness, diplopia, ataxic gait and disorientation occur as the inhalant dose increases, and coma can supervene though uncommonly as this prevents the ability to repeat inhalation. Hallucinations may occur, chiefly in the visual modality and often frightening in nature. Spatial distortions, macropsia, micropsia and body image disturbances are commonly experienced. Disinhibition and feelings of omnipotence during the phase of intoxication may lead to risk-taking, accidents and aggressive antisocial behaviour. Amnesia for the events of the episode is common on recovery.

Nitrites differ pharmacologically from other inhalants, primarily causing vascular vasodilatation and smooth muscle relaxation. The sensations are of dizziness, tachycardia, light-headedness and skin warmth occurring within seconds, with effects wearing off in minutes. Nitrites are primarily inhaled to enhance sexual experience, with penile engorgement and anal sphincter relaxation (Romanelli *et al.* 2004).

Adverse consequences

The great majority of solvent misusers do not come before medical attention, and at the level of mild sporadic use appear usually to escape long-term physical damage. Nevertheless, it is a highly dangerous activity with a considerable number of acute deaths reported in occasional users, due to sudden sniffing death syndrome, inhalation of vomit or

suffocation from the plastic bag, aspiration, trauma, drowning or fire. Sudden sniffing death syndrome was described by Bass (1970) and arises from myocardial cell 'stabilisation', which increases the risk of cardiac arrhythmias, especially on sudden stress; this effect can be both acute and delayed, occurring hours after the period of use. Tolerance can develop if regular abuse persists over many months so that very large quantities come to be employed, whereas physical dependence by contrast appears to be uncommon.

The danger lies chiefly for those vulnerable individuals for whom inhalation becomes a regular and entrenched habit. A number of chronic complications, some serious, have now been reported, both with glue sniffing itself and with abuse of other solvents. These include cardiomyopathies, haematological complications such as aplastic anaemia, and renal toxicity. A range of CNS toxicities is seen, including toluene leucoencephalopathy, cerebellar ataxia, cranial neuropathy including optic neuropathy, encephalopathy both acute and chronic, and peripheral neuropathies. Much may depend on individual susceptibility to the chemicals involved.

Toluene leucoencephalopathy has been described since the early 1960s and is now a well-recognised syndrome, characterised by cerebellar ataxia, corticospinal tract dysfunction, brainstem signs and cranial neuropathies (Filley *et al.* 2004). An early example was reported by Grabski (1961) and followed up by Knox and Nelson (1966).

After some years of regular toluene inhalation, a 21-year-old man presented with confusion, inappropriate laughter and long periods of staring into space. He showed the classic titubating gait and intention tremors of cerebellar dysfunction. Over the years he became increasingly slowed and forgetful. On occasions when he stopped inhaling for several days the ataxia would remit considerably. Eight years later he was still abusing toluene and was ataxic, tremulous and emotionally labile.

Following on from these early reports a number of case series and case–control studies confirmed a characteristic neuropsychological syndrome regarded as prototypical of white-matter dementia (Filley *et al.* 2004). Characteristically, the dementia comprises inattention, apathy, memory dysfunction, visuospatial impairment, but with preservation of language. MRI shows, as indicated by the early air encephaolograms, diffuse cerebral and cerebellar atrophy with characteristic white matter hyperintensities that correlate with extent of neuropsychological dysfunction (Yücel *et al.* 2008). Neuropathological examination at post-mortem shows cerebral and cerebellar myelin loss, perivascular macrophages containing debris, and gliosis in agreement with findings in animal models that support astrocyte activation by toluene as the likely pathophysiological mechanism underpinning the white matter encephalopathy (Yamaguchi *et al.* 2002). During pregnancy, toluene abuse at high dose, rather than low-level environmental exposure, causes a constellation of teratogenic features known as fetal solvent syndrome, similar in nature to the fetal alcohol syndrome (Costa *et al.* 2002). Recent advances in MRI neuroimaging techniques, including diffusion tensor imaging, may improve early detection of toxicity and help resolve mechanisms of prognosis and recovery.

Petrol sniffing. In contrast to toluene leucoencephalopathy, less is known about the toxicity associated with petrol sniffing, a form of solvent abuse particularly associated with the most marginalised of groups in society. Intoxication is liable to continue for some hours after exposure, and prolonged or rapid inhalation may lead to a phase of violent excitement followed by coma. Chronic inhalation leads ultimately to loss of appetite and weight, neurasthenic symptoms, and muscular weakness and cramps. A special complication is encephalopathy due to the tetraethyl lead added to petrol, leading to a lead encephalopathy superadded to potential solvent encephalopathy that requires specific hospital management. In a follow-up study of 29 cases of neuropsychological impairment specifically occurring following petrol sniffing, Cairney *et al.* (2005) noted almost complete recovery with only the most severely affected showing residual signs of toxicity. However, given the example provided by toluene leucoencephalopathy, this finding should be regarded as provisional.

TOXIC DISORDERS

Certain metals and chemicals are the exogenous toxins considered in this section. Poisoning due to metals and other chemical compounds is largely the province of industrial medicine, but must also be borne in mind in occasional patients who present with psychiatric illness of uncertain aetiology. This section considers the role of environmental toxins in the development of neurodegenerative disorders *per se*, before considering the specific features of drug-induced toxicity and toxicity induced by lead, mercury, manganese, arsenic, thallium, organophosphorus compounds and carbon disulphide.

Environmental toxins and neurodegenerative disorders

Neurodegenerative disorders such as Alzheimer's disease and Parkinson's disease are increasingly recognised as involving environmental exposure to various toxins, in interaction with age and genotype. The clearest example of this model is provided by the designer drug 1-methyl-4-phenyl-1,2,3,6-tetrahydropyridine (MPTP), which resulted in the development of acute parkinsonism, similar to idiopathic Parkinson's disease, in a group of heroin addicts in California (Langston *et al.* 1983). Since this observation, several epidemiological studies have indicated that different environmental agents, including pesticides, increase the risk of Parkinson's disease (Langston 2002; Steece-Collier *et al.* 2002). With regard to Alzheimer's disease, while the link with aluminium exposure continues to be controversial (Flaten 2001), the link with type 2 diabetes, a condition with substantial environmental determinants, is increasingly accepted (Nicolls 2004).

Toxic effects of other drugs

Many other drugs can produce toxic effects on the CNS and lead to psychiatric disturbance. The number involved is legion, and the variety of their effects too great to be discussed in detail here. Comprehensive reviews of drug toxicity are presented by Dukes (1992), and aspects of particular relevance to psychiatric practice are dealt with by Tornatore *et al.* (1987), Ciraulo *et al.* (1989) and Lipowski (1990). These cover the adverse reactions seen with steroids, insulin, narcotics, analgesics, hypnotics, anticonvulsants, tranquillisers, anticholinergic agents, antiparkinsonian drugs, rauwolfia alkaloids, antihypertensive drugs, digoxin, diuretics, antituberculous drugs, other antibacterial agents, androgens, estrogens and oral contraceptives. Only some of these are considered below. In a critical review of the association of psychoactive medications and delirium in hospitalised inpatients, Gaudreau *et al.* (2005) identified relatively few firm associations, with opioids, benzodiazepines and corticosteroids most robustly implicated.

Sometimes the toxic reaction is an idiosyncratic response to the drug given in normal therapeutic dosage, or to several drugs being prescribed in combination. For this reason it is essential to review the patient's current medication when dealing with psychiatric illnesses of obscure origin, and particularly when these take the form of acute organic reactions. Sometimes the cause is excessive self-medication, either in error or when the patient is addicted. The range of drugs surreptitiously abused tends to increase steadily. As a corollary, inadequate use of analgesic medications with concomitant breakthrough pain may be mistaken for anxiety, depression and addiction, so-called pseudoaddiction, which is now well recognised especially in palliative care settings (Porter-Williamson *et al.* 2003).

The commonest form of disturbance is an acute organic reaction of variable duration, usually with features typical of delirium and often with prominent hallucinations. Neurological and other systemic signs specific for the drug in question may be in evidence. However, some drugs are associated primarily with mood changes or psychotic reactions in clear consciousness, as described below.

The elderly are especially at risk of adverse drug reactions. Concomitant physical illness or incipient dementia will reduce the margins by which delirium is provoked. Common offending drugs include digoxin, minor and major tranquillisers, antihypertensives and diuretics. Hypnotics such as nitrazepam readily accumulate, leading to daytime confusion. Anticholinergic agents (antispasmodics, tricyclic antidepressants, phenothiazines and antiparkinsonian drugs) are particularly liable to induce confusion or memory impairment in the elderly (Potamianos & Kellett 1982). Anticholinergics have also been clearly incriminated as a major factor leading to postoperative delirium (Tune *et al.* 1981).

Antidepressants

Among psychotropic drugs, severe reactions may occasionally be seen with antidepressant medication or combinations of antidepressant drugs. These are reviewed by Connell (1968) and McClelland (1986). Minor degrees of disturbance are probably quite frequent; Davies *et al.* (1971) reported episodes of impaired memory and orientation in 13% of patients taking tricyclic antidepressant drugs, rising to 35% in those over 40 years of age. Withdrawal reactions may occasionally be seen when monoamine oxidase inhibitors, or more rarely tricyclic antidepressants, are stopped abruptly, with nausea, gastrointestinal upset, headache, anxiety and panic (Anon. 1986).

Lithium

Lithium can have serious effects on CNS functioning. A fine tremor, representing exaggeration of normal physiological tremor, must often be accepted, likewise some minor forgetfulness and lethargy. When such symptoms develop in patients on long-term lithium treatment, the possibility of induced hypothyroidism must be borne in mind (see Chapter 10). More marked symptoms – muscle fasciculation, coarse tremor, ataxia, incoordination or extrapyramidal signs – call for abrupt cessation of treatment. The development of confusion or impairment of consciousness constitutes a medical emergency; the severe encephalopathic reactions that then ensue sometimes prove to be irreversible or result in permanent brain damage. Increasing confusion is accompanied by seizures, cerebellar signs, marked generalised tremor or decerebrate rigidity. States of stupor or coma may be prolonged. For reasons that are unclear such reactions may sometimes set in despite normal serum concentrations of lithium (Spiers & Hirsch 1978; Newman & Saunders 1979). On recovery there may be long-lasting cerebellar and extrapyramidal deficits (Sellers *et al.* 1982; Schou 1984). Smith and Kocen (1988) have described two patients in whom the clinical picture closely resembled Creutzfeldt–Jakob disease, with rapid onset of dementia, rigidity and in one case myoclonic jerks. EEG closely supported such a diagnosis. In both cases discontinuation of lithium led to resolution of the symptoms and EEG abnormalities over the course of 2–3 weeks.

The combination of lithium and haloperidol was specially incriminated by Cohen and Cohen (1974) in leading to severe reactions. Two of their patients were left with permanent parkinsonian–cerebellar deficits and dementia, and two with persistent dyskinesias. Loudon and Waring (1976) reported similar though milder reactions of this nature, and Spring (1979) described severe neurotoxic developments with the combination of lithium and thioridazine. Sometimes the same combination of drugs has been given previously without ill effect as in the following example.

> A patient reported by Thomas (1979) had been maintained on lithium within the normal therapeutic range for many years. Haloperidol was then added on account of a hypomanic swing, in a dose of 1.5 mg three times per day. Two days later she developed gross extrapyramidal signs with marked rigidity and orofacial dyskinesia. She became severely confused and disorientated, and EEG showed diffuse slow waves. Both drugs were stopped, with gradual resolution of the extrapyramidal disturbance over the course of the next 3 months. However, she was left with persistent evidence of brain damage by way of disorientation and memory impairment. This patient had experienced the combination of lithium and haloperidol 3 years previously without adverse effect.

Such reports must be viewed in the context of the many patients treated safely on the same combinations of drugs. Nevertheless, close monitoring of the clinical situation and of serum lithium levels would seem essential whenever lithium is coupled with other neuroleptic agents. Episodes of sleep-walking have also been reported after adding neuroleptics to patients established on lithium; Charney *et al.* (1979) reported 10 examples, involving haloperidol, thioridazine, chlorpromazine and other neuroleptics, usually occurring within a few days of starting the second drug. Neurotoxicity has also been reported when lithium is given with carbamazepine, phenytoin or methyldopa (Beeley 1986).

Neuroleptic malignant syndrome

The extrapyramidal disorders associated with the phenothiazines and butyrophenones are described in Chapter 12. The neuroleptic malignant syndrome is a more recently recognised complication of such drugs, seemingly rare but of great importance in that it is not infrequently fatal. Reviews of the condition are provided by Caroff (1980), Cope and Gregg (1983), Addonizio *et al.* (1987) and Kellam (1987). It has been described sporadically since the 1960s but the syndrome still lacks clear definition. Buckley and Hutchinson (1995) review its uncertain nosological status. An excess of cases has sometimes been described in patients below the age of 40 but the age range is wide. Males appear to be affected more commonly than females.

The patient develops severe extrapyramidal rigidity and akinesia, usually setting in abruptly or over the course of several days. Pyrexia is a characteristic accompaniment, along with autonomic disturbances by way of sweating, sialorrhoea, tachycardia, hyperventilation and labile blood pressure. Muscular rigidity is the cardinal feature, but may be accompanied by tremor, oro-bucco-lingual dyskinesias and sometimes dysphagia and dysarthria. Fluctuating impairment of consciousness can lead to confusion, stupor or coma. Agitation is common and may be severe. Dehydration and prostration can become extreme. Common laboratory findings include a leucocytosis, raised creatine phosphokinase activity and abnormal liver function tests, but these are not invariable. EEG sometimes shows diffuse slowing but is usually normal. CT is uninformative. The picture may be mistaken for encephalitis or meningitis, but CSF examination is negative. Catatonia may be diagnosed on account of the stupor, posturing or waxy flexibility. Anticholinergic intoxication should be considered in the differential diagnosis. Death is estimated to occur in up to 20% of cases, usually from cardiorespiratory failure, pneumonia or renal failure secondary to rhabdomyolysis and myoglobinuria.

The syndrome has been reported in association with butyrophenones, phenothiazines and thioxanthines, though perhaps most commonly with haloperidol and depot fluphenazines. It sets in usually within the first 2 weeks of treatment. It may begin shortly after the first dose, though a puzzling feature is its occasional development after many months on the drugs. Earlier courses of the identical drugs may have been given without adverse effect. In a small but important subgroup an identical syndrome has developed in parkinsonian patients when antiparkinsonian medications such as levodopa or amantadine are withdrawn (Kellam 1987). Rare examples have been reported following lithium, metoclopramide, carbamazepine, desipramine, dothiepin, tetrabenazine and other non-neuroleptics (Buckley & Hutchinson 1995).

Medically ill psychiatric patients appear to be at increased risk, many examples developing in patients with dehydration, malnutrition or concomitant neurological disease (Sternberg 1986). Indeed Levinson and Simpson (1986) have questioned the unitary nature of the syndrome, suggesting that a number of examples merely represent extrapyramidal reactions complicated by fever due to remediable medical conditions. Dehydration with electrolyte imbalance and infections such as pneumonia appeared to be the factors most often responsible.

Treatment consists of the withdrawal of all neuroleptic medication immediately the condition is suspected, along with intensive supportive measures to maintain respiratory, renal and cardiovascular function. Dehydration or electrolyte imbalance must be remedied, and a thorough search made for infections and other medical conditions that may be complicating the picture. Active cooling measures may be required. Benefit has been reported from treatment with dantrolene sodium, a peripheral muscle relaxant, and the dopamine agonist bromocriptine (Granato *et al.* 1983; Miyasaki & Lang 1995). Electroconvulsive treatment has sometimes been found to be rapidly beneficial, although obviously this must be undertaken with care (Davis *et al.* 1991). From Davis *et al.*'s review such treatment appears to be safe, with the proviso that neuroleptics are discontinued beforehand.

The disorder usually lasts for 5–10 days after stopping the drugs, or rather longer with depot preparations. Resolution is typically complete in those who recover, although occasional patients are left with neurological residua (Miyasaki & Lang 1995). When treatment of the original psychiatric disorder continues to be necessary, alternative drugs such as carbamazepine or lithium should be tried. If it is essential to reintroduce phenothiazines, those with low potency should be given initially. Careful monitoring of blood pressure and temperature will then be necessary, with vigilance if extrapyramidal rigidity should develop. There are indications that 'rechallenges' with neuroleptics are in fact often safely accomplished, provided a gap of at least 2 weeks is left after resolution of the syndrome (Rosebush *et al.* 1989). Clozapine should be considered when conventional neuroleptics cannot be tolerated (Weller & Kornhuber 1992).

Dopamine receptor blockade in the basal ganglia or hypothalamus has been postulated as the cause, though with little direct supportive evidence. However, significantly decreased levels of homovanillic acid, the major metabolite of dopamine, have been found in the CSF both during active phases and after recovery from the syndrome (Nisijima & Ishiguro 1990). Some evidence also points to serotonergic involvement (Buckley & Hutchinson 1995). At post-mortem, no specific abnormalities have yet been discovered.

Attention has been drawn to certain similarities between the condition and the 'fatal catatonia' of the pre-neuroleptic era (Caroff 1980; Kellam 1987). Some examples of adverse reactions to the combination of lithium and haloperidol may also represent variants of the syndrome, particularly the cases reported by Cohen and Cohen (1974) where extrapyramidal dysfunction was accompanied by fever, leucocytosis and elevated serum enzymes. On present evidence the condition would seem to represent an idiosyncratic reaction to neuroleptic medication, although it remains possible that this may merely have served as a trigger to some largely independent pathogenic process.

Withdrawal effects

Withdrawal effects must be considered where drugs with a depressant action on the CNS are concerned. Drugs other than alcohol or barbiturates can lead to severe withdrawal phenomena including epileptic fits, hallucinations and periods of delirium. Such pictures have been reported for glutethimide (Doriden) and ethchlorvynol (Placidyl) in patients admitted to hospital for investigation of long-standing intermittent confusion (Lloyd & Clark 1959; Hudson & Walker 1961). Similar results may follow withdrawal from paraldehyde, meprobamate, methaqualone (Mandrax) and carbromal (Granville-Grossman 1971). The withdrawal effects that can be seen with benzodiazepines are described earlier under Benzodiazepines/Withdrawal effects.

Analgesics

Chronic analgesic abuse may readily cause diagnostic confusion. Bizarre behaviour and hyperventilation may lead to a mistaken diagnosis of hysteria. When consciousness is severely impaired diabetic coma may be suspected. Greer *et al.* (1965) reported examples of chronic salicylate intoxication producing pictures of confusion, amnesia, agitation, stupor and coma. Some patients were hallucinated, paranoid and combative. Hyperventilation and tinnitus were important signs, also coarse irregular tremors of the hands and ataxia of gait.

Murray *et al.* (1971) drew attention to another possible hazard of chronic analgesic abuse. Of eight patients who had consumed very large doses of compound analgesics containing phenacetin, four showed definite evidence and two possible evidence of dementia. Neuropathological studies of the brains of nine other analgesic abusers showed a surprisingly high frequency of histological changes typical of Alzheimer's disease even though cerebral atrophy was absent. These interesting findings merit further investigation.

Steroid therapy

Mood changes accompanying steroid therapy more often consist of mild elation than depression, and are much commoner than confusion or delirium (Granville-Grossman 1971). The elation and social activation seen while on steroids may be replaced by depression when the drugs are withdrawn (Carpenter & Bunney 1971). More florid reactions have been reported in up to 10% of patients given steroids in large dosage: excited elated behaviour, intense anxiety with panic attacks, severe depression, or transient psychoses with perceptual abnormalities, hallucinations, derealisation and paranoia. Such reactions are often deeply alarming to the patient, but generally subside within a few weeks when the drugs can be withdrawn.

Their determinants will often be complex when the steroids are given for conditions that implicate the CNS. However, Hall *et al.* (1979) restricted attention to the psychoses seen in patients in whom there was no reason to suspect a cerebral lesion. They found that the clinical pictures defied formal classification, often representing a complex admixture of affective, schizophreniform and organic features.

Moreover, a single episode in a given patient could show a great variety of symptoms from one moment to another, and little was characteristic except this changeability. A common constellation of symptoms was emotional lability, anxiety, distractibility, pressured speech, insomnia, perplexity, agitation, hypomania, auditory and visual hallucinations, delusions, intermittent memory impairment, mutism and body image disturbance. The onset was usually within 3 weeks of the start of treatment, mostly within 5 days, and response to phenothiazines was excellent. EEG changes of a non-specific type commonly accompanied the disturbances, reverting to normal on recovery. There was no evidence that a history of previous psychiatric illness was a predisposing factor.

Other drug reactions

An important group of drugs are those which produce mood changes or psychotic reactions without evidence of confusion or impairment of consciousness. With reactions of this type it is less likely that the essentially 'toxic' nature of the disturbance will be appreciated. Rauwolfia alkaloids were an early example, leading to severe depressive mood changes unaccompanied by organic mental symptoms. The rauwolfia reaction may develop only after several weeks or months on the drug, and has been attributed to a fall in cerebral monoamines.

Heavy metals and other chemicals

Heavy metals are chemical elements with a specific gravity at least five times that of water. There are at least 23 such elements. The heavy elements most implicated in human poisoning are lead, mercury, arsenic and cadmium. Some heavy metals such as zinc, copper, iron and manganese are required in the body in small amounts but are toxic in large quantities.

Lead

Lead is found in cosmetics, plastics, batteries, insecticides, pottery glaze, soldered pipes and paint. Modern building specifications prevent a previous major source of lead exposure, namely drinking water from old lead-piped plumbing systems. Older buildings remain a risk. Domestic water supplies remain a risk in areas where the water is soft, and some outbreaks have been traced to beer or cider stored overnight in lead pipes. Industrial causes have been greatly reduced as a result of stringent precautions, but a risk exists in the following occupations: painting, plumbing, ship building, lead smelting and refining, brass founding, pottery glazing, vitreous enamelling; the manufacture of storage batteries, white lead, red lead, rubber, glass and pigments; and among compositors who handle type metal. The list is important because a history of exposure is often the crucial factor in arousing suspicion of the disorder. Overt lead poisoning is now a great deal rarer than during the early part of the twentieth century. 'Subclinical' lead poisoning refers to low-level lead exposure, particularly in children, who are especially vulnerable because they absorb more lead than adults due to their developing nervous system. A blood lead concentration of 10 µg/dL or higher in children is cause for concern. In 1984, the Centers for Disease Control and Prevention estimated that 3–4 million American children had unacceptably high levels of lead in their blood. A recent report evidences a progressive decline in the overall prevalence of a blood lead level of 10 µg/dL or more in US children aged 1–5 years from 8.6% (1988–1991) to 1.4% (1992–2004). The authors found that 55% of children overall have a blood lead level between 1 and <2.5 µg/dL but non-Hispanic black US children remain at highest risk. Risk factors for higher blood lead levels are residing in older housing, poverty, and being a child in a younger age group (Jones *et al.* 2009). A number of behavioural effects are recognised complications of raised lead levels, including impaired cognitive performance.

Needleman *et al.* (1990) found that adolescents who had high dentine lead levels in childhood 10 years earlier had poorer hand–eye coordination, longer reaction times and slower finger-tapping than children who had low dentine lead levels in childhood. Bellinger *et al.*'s (1992) prospective study indicated that higher blood lead levels at age 24 months were significantly predictive of lower global scores on the Wechsler Intelligence Scale for Children (WISC)-R and measures of educational attainment at age 10. Even over the range 0–25 µg/L, a 10-µg increase in blood lead at 24 months was associated with a 5.8-point reduction in WISC IQ at 10. Tong *et al.*'s (1996) follow-up of children from a lead smelting town in Australia has lent strong support to this finding. Seeber *et al.* (2002) detected cognitive deficits with average blood lead levels between 370 and 520 µg/L. The unborn fetus and the elderly are also at risk of neuropsychiatric complications.

The principal manifestations include abdominal colic, 'lead neuropathy' and 'lead encephalopathy'. Lassitude is almost invariably the earliest symptom. Aching in joints and limbs is also common. Gastrointestinal disturbances then appear, with anorexia, constipation and attacks of severe intestinal colic. The child is pale and often irritable. Acute phases of disturbance tend to be precipitated by intercurrent infection or other sources of acidosis which mobilise lead from the bones. 'Peripheral neuropathy' was formerly common in adults but has always been rare in children. It is now very rare in both. It is unique in being a purely motor disturbance, perhaps with the primary effect on the muscles themselves, although ultimately the nerves are involved as well. The muscles chiefly affected are those most used, resulting in the classic picture of wrist drop and paralysis of the long extensors of the fingers. Less commonly there is weakness and wasting of the shoulder girdle muscles or of the dorsiflexors of the foot. Lead encephalopathy is the most serious

manifestation. In adults it may present with episodes of delirium, often in association with fits. During crises the blood pressure is elevated. In chronic encephalopathy the patient is dull, with poor memory, impaired concentration, headache, trembling, deafness or transitory episodes of aphasia and hemianopia (Hunter 1959). However, the most pronounced manifestations are seen in children, and cerebral involvement is reported in about half of those affected. The encephalopathy may sometimes set in very rapidly. The intracranial pressure rises abruptly, with headache, projectile vomiting, visual disturbances and severe impairment of consciousness. Convulsions and muscular twitching are common, and acute delirium may lead on to coma. Ocular and limb pareses may develop. Papilloedema is often seen, and meningeal irritation may cause neck stiffness and head retraction. The CSF is under increased pressure, the protein is raised and a moderate pleocytosis may be found. Death can result from medullary compression.

Diagnosis

In the diagnosis of lead poisoning there is no one sign which is pathognomonic. A lead line on the gums may be produced by subepithelial deposits of lead sulphide, especially when the teeth are carious. However, this is rare in children. Anaemia is always present and usually accompanied by basophilic stippling of the erythrocytes. In young children, radiography of the long bones shows a dense band in the lines of provisional calcification. Repeated examination of the blood and urine may reveal a raised lead content, but single readings can be misleading with falsely high or low results. Coproporphyrins are increased in the urine. Lead encephalopathy should be considered in children who develop fits of obscure origin, and when headache and papilloedema are discovered without obvious cause. Anaemia in association with colic or peripheral neuropathy should similarly raise suspicion. Diseases that may be simulated include encephalitis, cerebral tumour, tuberculous meningitis, uraemia and hypertensive encephalopathy.

Treatment

Most of the lead is held in storage in the bones, and as a temporary measure storage can be promoted by giving calcium lactate and extra milk in the diet. Chelating agents are used to promote the urinary excretion of lead and disodium calcium ethylenediaminetetra-acetate (calcium versenate, EDTA) can be given parenterally. Lead replaces the calcium in the compound and the circulating unionised chelate is excreted by the kidneys. Symptoms are rapidly relieved because the chelate is much less toxic than the ionised metal in body fluids. In consequence, chelating agents have been regarded as life-saving in the management of acute lead encephalopathy. Meso-2,3-dimercaptosuccinic acid ('succimer'), an analogue of dimercaprol, has been employed as an oral chelating agent with low toxicity.

Outcome

The risk of permanent intellectual disablement is considerable among the survivors of lead encephalopathy. Children may be left with mental retardation, cerebral palsy, fits, or blindness due to optic atrophy. Perlstein and Attala (1966) reviewed a large group of 425 children who had suffered lead poisoning, finding permanent sequelae in 39%. This rose to 82% among those who had presented with encephalopathy.

Cerebral pathology

The cerebral manifestations have been attributed to a combination of intense cerebral oedema and vascular changes. There is proliferation of the endothelium of small blood vessels, sometimes with occlusion of the lumen, and the development of perivascular nodules of hypertrophied glial cells. Cerebral ischaemia may result from the acute rise in intracranial pressure and lead to cerebral atrophy. In chronic cases the meninges become fibrosed and hyperplastic, and arachnoiditis obstructs the flow of CSF (Akelatis 1941). Internal hydrocephalus is often marked in patients who show residual cerebral impairment.

Mercury

Mercury is both a unique element that has no essential biological function and a ubiquitous environmental toxin that causes a wide range of adverse health effects in humans. It is liquid at room temperature, is 13.6 times heavier than water, and its vapour pressure at 20°C is 0.16 Pa (Tennent 1971). Mercury and zinc are easily volatile metals compared with, for example, magnesium and iron. Mercury has been used in mercury switches, thermostats, thermometers and other instruments. Its ability to amalgamate with gold and silver has been used in mining these precious metals, and is also used as a dental restorative. Its toxic properties have been exploited for medicines, preservatives, antiseptics and pesticides (Gochfeld 2003). There are three forms of mercury from a toxicological point of view, each with its own profile of toxicity: inorganic mercury salts, organic mercury compounds, and metallic (or elemental) mercury. Inorganic mercury salts are water soluble, irritate the gut and can cause severe kidney damage. Organic mercury compounds are fat soluble, can cross the blood–brain barrier and cause neurological damage. Metallic mercury poses two dangers. It can vaporise at room temperature so that poisoning can occur even if mercury metal is spilled in crevices or cracks in the floorboards. Metallic mercury can be biotransformed into organic mercury by bacteria, for example, in lakes. This can be passed along the food chain and eventually to humans (Langford & Ferner 1999).

Chronic mercury poisoning was commoner in former times as a hazard among workers involved in recovering the metal from the ore and in chemical workers, thermometer makers and photo engravers. Groups of cases were reported among fingerprint experts employing a mercury and chalk mixture (Agate & Buckell 1949) and among repairers of direct current electric meters (Bidstrup *et al.* 1951). Mercury was also extensively employed in the felt hat industry, where the toxic effects no doubt contributed to the epithet 'mad as a hatter' and to Lewis Carroll's choice of the hatter in *Alice in Wonderland*. Warkany and Hubbard (1951) discovered that the mercury contained in teething powders was the common cause of acrodynia (pink disease) in infants and young children.

Lead, mercury and arsenic exposures represent the most common causes of toxic metal poisoning. In 1997, 3596 cases of mercury heavy metal poisoning were reported by the American Association of Poison Control Centers (Patrick 2002). The major forms of exposure are mercury vapour, the elemental mercury content of dental amalgam, and methylmercury compounds. Mercury vapour emitted from both natural and anthropogenic sources is globally distributed in the atmosphere. It is returned as a water-soluble form in precipitation and finds its way into bodies of fresh and ocean water. Land run-off also accounts for further input into lakes and oceans. Inorganic mercury present in water sediments is subject to bacterial conversion to methylmercury compounds, which are bioaccumulated in the aquatic food chain to reach the highest concentration in predatory fish (Clarkson 1997). The general population does not face a significant health risk from methylmercury, although certain groups with high fish consumption may attain blood levels associated with a low risk of neurological damage to adults. Since there is a risk to the fetus in particular, pregnant women are advised to avoid a diet high in the intake of certain fish, such as shark, swordfish and tuna. Fish such as pike, walleye and bass taken from polluted fresh waters should also be avoided (Jaerup 2003). In addition, Salonen *et al.* (1995) reported evidence to suggest that a high intake of mercury from non-fatty freshwater fish was associated with an excess risk of acute myocardial infection and death from coronary heart disease in eastern Finnish men, perhaps due to the promotion of lipid peroxidation by mercury. Several studies since have reported statistical associations between cardiovascular disease and mercury but conclusions about cause and effect lack evidence because of the multiple risk factors for cardiovascular disease (Clarkson *et al.* 2003). The European Environment Agency (EEA) suggests that blood concentrations of mercury below 5.8 ng/ml will avoid adverse effects, but cautions that people who eat fish contaminated by methyl mercury have been found to have levels very close to this at 5.6 ng/ml (2002). The balance of published reports suggests that the CNS and kidneys remain the key targets of mercury toxicity.

Elemental mercury vapour accounts for most occupational and accidental exposures by inhalation. Mercury is readily absorbed after inhalation. Mercury can be an indoor air pollutant as well as an industrial emission with resulting ambient air pollution (Goldman & Shannon 2001). Currently, mercury vapour concentrations greater than 0.01 mg/m^3 are considered unsafe (Moienafshari *et al.* 1999). Fetuses are considered the most sensitive subpopulation because of the vulnerability of the developing nervous system. A level of 0.1 μg/kg body weight per day has been reported as a scientifically justified (safe?) level of methylmercury exposure for maternal–fetal pairs (Mahaffey 2000).

Dental amalgam, which consists of about 50% metallic mercury, has been used for over 150 years in dental practice. Mercury is continuously released from dental amalgam and absorbed by several body tissues (Mutter *et al.* 2004). Whether the amounts released are sufficient to cause significant toxicity is controversial (Null & Feldman 2002). It has been suggested that although the mercury vapour generated during removal of amalgams does cause a transient increase in the patient's mercury levels in tissue fluids, biochemical assays demonstrate that the increase is too small to have an adverse impact on organ systems, true also even when patients have all their amalgams removed in a single session (Osborne & Albino 1999). Patients with so-called 'amalgam illness' are thought to be exhibiting psychogenic disorders in a large number of cases, including a high prevalence of somatisation (Langworth 1997). Dentists occupationally exposed to mercury have not been shown to suffer harmful reproductive or other systemic health effects (but cognitive changes have been seen) provided proper mercury hygiene is used (Wahl 2001).

Mercury's several different forms, and the subtlety of its chemical effects at chronic low-level exposure, make the diagnosis of mercury toxicity difficult to establish. Diagnosis is also made difficult because of the lack of specific signs. A high index of suspicion is necessary when patients present with a combination of behavioural and personality changes, movement disorder, memory problems, unusual rashes or neuropsychological deficits. It is only in cases involving a knowledge of mercury that appropriate historic information is obtained, and clinical suspicions confirmed by establishing toxic levels of mercury in blood and urine (Johnson 2004).

Clinical manifestations

Physical symptoms include stomatitis, spongy bleeding gums and excessive salivation. A coarse tremor may develop in the hands, face and tongue, characteristically interrupted by coarse jerking movements (hatters' shakes). A sensorimotor peripheral neuropathy is common, sometimes with prominent sensory ataxia, also varying degrees of visual field constriction.

Psychological symptoms are often an early manifestation. In particular a constellation of symptoms known as 'erythism' has been repeatedly noted. In this the sufferer is nervous, timid and shy, blushes readily and becomes em-

barrassed in social situations. He objects to being watched and seeks to avoid people. He becomes irritable and quarrelsome, sometimes to the extent that he is obliged to give up work. Such symptoms are usually accompanied by lassitude, tremulousness, ataxia and some degree of impairment of intellectual capacity.

> A detective sergeant of 45 was trained in fingerprint work and sent to a division where he investigated up to 300 crimes per year. During this time he became a 'nervous wreck', could not hold a cup without spilling it, and found court appearances acutely distressing because he could not stand still or answer questions without embarrassment. During the early war years the crime rate declined and his symptoms improved, but they worsened again immediately the crime rate rose in the postwar period. On examination he showed a marked tremor and several teeth were loose.

Bidstrup *et al.* (1951) found definite evidence of erythism in 10 and probable evidence in 8 of 161 men engaged in mending direct current electric meters.

> One employee had noticed tremor of his hands for a year and had become irritable, short-tempered and easily embarrassed. He had developed a stammer for the first time in his life. A few months later he became unsteady on his feet and his whole body developed a tremor. His writing became almost illegible. He was ultimately diagnosed as suffering from multiple sclerosis. At this point he read in the daily paper about the above findings in the Lancashire Constabulary and told his general practitioner that he too handled mercury. Six months after transfer to another job he had recovered completely.

Kark *et al.* (1971) report another example with prominent neurological symptoms.

> A man who had worked for 2 years extracting mercury from batteries showed a gradual decline in memory and loss of interest, becoming less talkative and active. He developed gingivitis, decreased visual acuity and insomnia. Tremor ultimately made eating and drinking impossible, and he was virtually unable to stand on account of titubation and truncal ataxia. On examination he showed dysarthria, constricted visual fields, and diminished acuity of both hearing and vision. There were constant choreiform movements of the face and fingers. EEG showed diffuse theta activity and the air encephalogram revealed cerebral atrophy. He recovered slowly on treatment with chelating agents.

Neuropsychological testing has shown identifiable deficits in persons chronically exposed to mercury, often persisting for many years. For example, Ngim *et al.* (1992) found that dentists with a history of contact with mercury vapour were significantly poorer than controls on tests of motor speed, visual scanning, visuomotor coordination and memory. Performance correlated inversely with the cumulative dose of exposure. None showed overt toxic signs but their blood mercury levels were raised. Hartman (1988) and O'Carroll *et al.* (1995) review studies on mercury miners and plant workers that have shown impairment of motor coordination, reaction time and short-term memory. O'Carroll *et al.*'s own patient suffered exposure while cleaning a tank containing phenylmercury ammonium acetate (which releases inorganic mercury in the body) and was chronically disabled thereafter by muscle spasms, shakiness, anxiety and depression. Psychological testing 3–4 years later showed marked and specific deficits in attention and concentration, with performance well below expectation on verbal fluency, Trail-making and Stroop tests and on the Paced Auditory Serial Addition Test (PASAT). MRI showed no abnormality, but SPECT revealed focal hypermetabolism in the posterior cingulate cortex.

Acrodynia is a serious disease of infants and young children. The hands and feet are reddened with desquamation of the skin, itching, burning and evanescent rashes. In severe cases the hair and even the nails may be lost. The child is restless and miserable, showing periods of apathy alternating with extreme irritability. Anorexia, insomnia and photophobia are prominent. On examination there is hypotonia with diminished tendon reflexes and peripheral sensory loss. There is a tachycardia and the blood pressure is raised. The cause was unknown, although a toxic agent had long been suspected. In 1951, Warkany and Hubbard found mercury in the urine in a large number of cases, and proposed that exposure to mercury in hypersensitive infants was the responsible factor. This has since been well established (Dathan 1954), the source being mainly from teething powders, worming pills, ointments or nappy powders. Fortunately, the condition is now very rare indeed.

Organic mercury compounds

Organic mercury compounds are associated with marked neurological and psychiatric disturbances, especially the ethyl and methyl derivatives, which are used in the manufacture of fungicides. From time to time certain accidents have resulted in large outbreaks of poisoning with a heavy mortality. In the Minamata Bay epidemic in Japan, 83 persons were affected, most patients dying or suffering permanent severe disability (Kurland *et al.* 1960). Inorganic mercury derived from industrial processes had been discharged into rivers, methylated by aquatic microorganisms, and eaten by fish which then became poisonous. More recently, Amazonian riverside communities in Brazil have been

affected as a result of mercury used in the course of gold mining (Anon. 1992). In Iraq several outbreaks resulted from the distribution of grain treated with fungicides, intended for planting but made into bread by mistake. In the 1972 epidemic, 6500 persons were admitted to hospital and there were 459 deaths (Bakir *et al.* 1973).

Sensory disturbances are in the foreground, with numbness of the hands, deafness, blurred vision and narrowing of the visual fields progressing to blindness (Hunter 1978). Ataxia and dysarthria may be severe, often in association with sore gums and salivation. Involuntary movements and convulsions are common. Mental dullness is accompanied by restlessness, progressing over the course of weeks or months to coma. Many cases are fatal. At post-mortem, selective cortical damage is seen in numerous areas, with neurone loss, porosity of the underlying white matter and swelling of oligodendrocytes (Hay *et al.* 1963). Extensive spongiosis of the cortex may occur in childhood cases (Takeuchi *et al.* 1979). Severe destruction may also be seen in the cerebellum, basal ganglia and calcarine region (Feldman 1982).

Manganese

Manganese is an essential trace element, functioning as a cofactor in many enzymatic reactions in both animals and humans, but which, in excess, can cause irreversible nervous system damage. Manganese is supplied to the brain via both the blood–brain and blood–CSF barriers. Transferrin may be involved in manganese transport into the brain. A large portion of manganese is bound to manganese metalloproteins, especially glutamine synthetase in astrocytes. Manganese may be present in synaptic vesicles in glutamatergic neurones, and manganese released into the synaptic cleft may influence synaptic neurotransmission (Takeda 2003).

Manganese is a ubiquitous constituent of the environment, comprising about 0.1% of the earth's crust. For the general population food is the most important source of manganese, with daily intake ranging from 2 to 9 mg. Absorption from the gastrointestinal tract occurs as the divalent and tetravalent forms. Homeostatic mechanisms limit absorption of manganese from the gastrointestinal tract. Elimination of manganese occurs primarily by excretion into bile (Barceloux 1999). The CNS, and the basal ganglia in particular, is an important target in manganese neurotoxicity. Manganese neurotoxicity has been known for more than 150 years since Couper in 1837 described a syndrome in Scottish workers exposed to high levels of dust while grinding black oxide of manganese at a chemical industry. Since then the syndrome has been described in several groups of workers and manganese poisoning remains a predominantly occupational disease.

It occurs in manganese ore workers and those involved in steel manufacture, dry battery manufacture, bleaching and electro-welding. Despite the large number of people at risk, manganese poisoning is relatively rare and it is probable that a large quantity can be absorbed over a long period of time before harmful effects are produced. Individual sensitivity also appears to be important in that some subjects exposed for an equally long period show no ill effects. The chief route of entry is inhalation of the dust, fumes or vapour. Since 1976 the organomanganese compound methylcyclopentadienyl manganese tricarbonyl (MMT) has been used as an anti-knock agent and octane enhancer in unleaded gasoline, increasing the atmospheric emission of MMT combustion products from the tailpipe of vehicles, principally manganese phosphate, manganese sulphate and manganese phosphate/sulphate mixtures. Animal exposure studies (oral administration) indicate that brain manganese concentrations are significantly higher in exposures to manganese phosphate and manganese phosphate/sulphate mixtures, with neurobehavioural consequences (Normandin et al. 2004). There remains uncertainty as to whether the small increase in manganese contamination resulting from use of MMT could have neurotoxic effects in humans as a consequence of inhalation exposure (Normandin et al. 2002).

Manganese contamination also occurs as a consequence of the use of the contrast agent mangafodipir trisodium in nuclear magnetic resonance diagnostic imaging. The manganese released from mangafodipir trisodium is initially sequestered by the liver for first-pass elimination, which allows enhanced contrast. Human manganese deficiency is rare but has been reported in patients on parenteral nutrition and in micronutrient studies (Crossgrove & Zheng 2004). In mammalian cells toxic doses of manganese cause DNA damage and chromosome aberrations. Large amounts of manganese affect fertility in mammals and are toxic to the embryo and fetus. The fungicide MANEB and the contrast agent mangafodipir trisodium can also be embryotoxic, the latter only at doses much higher than those employed clinically (Gerber et al. 2002). Learning difficulties have been tentatively linked to the use of infant feeding formulas with high manganese content (Cawte 1985).

Clinical manifestations
The early manifestations usually develop insidiously with headache, asthenia, torpor and hypersomnia. Impotence is common. Psychological abnormalities then become pronounced and may first draw attention to the disorder. There have been reports of marked emotional disturbances in up to 70% of cases, especially episodes of persistent and uncontrollable laughter and crying (Fairhall & Neal 1943). There may be strong impulsions to run, dance, sing or talk which the patient finds difficult to resist. Impulsive acts and stupid crimes are a special risk in the early phases (Penalver 1955). Other abnormalities include forgetfulness, mental dullness, marked irritability and outbursts of aggression. Neuropsychological assessment in refinery workers has shown constructional apraxia, correlating significantly with levels of

exposure to manganese dust (Brown et al. 1991). Very occasionally an acute psychotic picture is seen, with severe excitement, agitation, hallucinations and delusions (Abd El Naby & Hassanein 1965).

Parkinsonism develops later with typical mask-like facies, slow monotonous speech and slowing of voluntary movements. Nocturnal leg cramps are a prominent feature. Fine tremor or gross rhythmical movements develop in the hands, limbs and trunk. The gait becomes typically parkinsonian with retropulsion and propulsion. A characteristic 'cock-step' gait has been described, a peculiar broad-based slapping walk with the legs held stiffly on tip-toe and wide apart. On examination muscular rigidity is found, with increased reflexes and ankle clonus. Cerebellar deficits may also be present. Sensory disturbances are rare. Chronic headache and severe insomnia may accompany the neurological developments.

Severe examples have been misdiagnosed as paralysis agitans, Wilson's disease, postencephalitic parkinsonism or multiple sclerosis. Wilson's disease may be closely simulated since liver damage may also be present. Manganese preferentially damages areas of the brain different to those affected in Parkinson's disease. In Parkinson's disease the pathology is a result of dopamine neurones in the substantia nigra pars compacta, whereas in manganese-induced parkinsonism the damage is localised to the pallidum and striatum. The positive response to levodopa in patients with Parkinson's disease also distinguishes it from manganese-induced parkinsonism in which the response is poor or nil. MRI abnormalities indicative of degeneration of the striatum predicts the evolution of atypical parkinsonism rather than Parkinson's disease. Striatal fluorodopa uptake on PET is consistently reduced in Parkinson's disease (especially in the posterior putamen) but normal in parkinsonism induced by manganese toxicity. These features all help to distinguish Parkinson's disease from magnesium-induced parkinsonism and permit the correct diagnosis to be established (Olanow 2004).

Removal from exposure at an early stage usually allows considerable recovery to occur. The psychological symptoms resolve quickly but disturbance of speech and gait may persist. In well-established cases the neurological disabilities may prove to be irreversible and patients are left permanently disabled. A considerable number have been observed to worsen neurologically even after removal from exposure (Abd El Naby & Hassanein 1965). Treatment with levodopa may sometimes improve the motor abnormalities (Huang et al. 1989).

At post-mortem, the basal ganglia are found to be mainly affected, with cell loss, gliosis and shrinkage. This is most marked in the globus pallidus. The thalamus may also be involved. Diffuse changes are found elsewhere including the cerebral cortex and brainstem, and slight generalised cortical atrophy may be seen (Canavan et al. 1934). In advanced cases the peripheral nerves and muscles may show degenerative changes (Penalver 1955).

The mechanism of neurotoxicity relates to mitochondrial dysfunction, depletion of levels of peroxidase and catalase, and catecholamine biochemical imbalances following manganese exposure. The site specificity of the pathology (basal ganglia) and the nature of the cellular damage caused by manganese have been attributed to its capacity to produce cytotoxic levels of free radicals. There is recent evidence at a molecular level of an aetiological relationship between oxidative stress and manganese-related neurodegeneration (HaMai & Bondy 2004).

At a cellular level, increasing evidence suggests that astrocytes are a site of early dysfunction and damage; chronic exposure to manganese leads to selective dopaminergic dysfunction, neuronal loss, and gliosis in basal ganglia structures together with characteristic astrocytic changes known as Alzheimer type II astrocytosis. Astrocytes possess a high-affinity high-capacity specific transport system for manganese that facilitates its uptake and sequestration in mitochondria, leading to disruption of oxidative phosphorylation. In addition, manganese causes a number of other functional changes in astrocytes, including impairment of glutamate transport, alterations in the glycolytic enzyme glyceraldehyde 3-phosphate dehydrogenase, and increased densities of binding sites for the peripheral-type benzodiazepine receptor (a class of receptor predominantly localised to mitochondria of astrocytes and involved in oxidative metabolism, mitochondrial proliferation and neurosteroid synthesis). Such effects can lead to compromised energy metabolism, resulting in altered cellular morphology, production of reactive oxygen species and increased extracellular glutamate concentration. These consequences may result in impaired astrocyte–neuronal interactions and play a major role in the pathophysiology of manganese neurotoxicity (Normandin et al. 2002).

Arsenic

Arsenic poisoning is encountered in the ore-refining industry, the fur industry, and in the manufacture of glass, insecticides and herbicides. Acute poisoning results in vomiting, diarrhoea and violent abdominal cramps. Headache, delirium and fits develop, and coma and death may follow within 2 or 3 days.

In chronic arsenic poisoning the picture is different. Early signs include dermatitis, conjunctivitis, lacrimation and coryza. Keratosis and skin pigmentation may be extensive, with characteristic white lines across the nails (Mee's lines). Anorexia and weight loss are common, but the abdominal cramps and diarrhoea of acute poisoning are often absent. Headache and vertigo are accompanied by apathy, drowsiness and impairment of mental acuity. At this stage the mental changes can be the leading clinical manifestations,

sometimes closely simulating neurotic disorder (Ecker & Kernohan 1941). Later restlessness, excitability and confusion become marked. Severe memory disturbance can occasionally produce the picture of Korsakoff's syndrome. Peripheral neuritis is common, with paraesthesiae, burning pain in the limbs and conspicuous sensory signs. Distal leg weakness may develop with loss of the ankle reflexes.

Thallium

As John Emsley (1978) has remarked, 'If ever an element was cursed at birth, that element was thallium'. Thallium is a rare but highly toxic heavy metal giving rise to significant human exposure from environmental, industrial and (historically) medicinal sources (Peter & Viraraghavan 2005). Thallotoxicosis following acute exposure is marked by gastroenteritis, polyneuropathy and alopecia, whereas that by chronic exposure is marked by anorexia, headache, muscle pain, alopecia, blindness and even death (reviewed by Peter & Viraraghavan 2005). White streaks (Mee's lines) may be seen on fingernails and toenails. Specific treatment is with chelating agents such as Prussian blue (Hoffman 2003). Involvement of the nervous system is a significant feature of thallium poisoning. After small doses ataxia and paraesthesiae develop and may progress to frank peripheral neuropathy. Retrobulbar neuritis is often seen. Tremor, chorea, athetosis and myoclonic jerking are also common. Mental abnormalities (encephalopathia thallica) may be pronounced, with lethargy, impairment of consciousness, memory deficits, paranoia, depression and dementia (Prick 1979). After large doses cerebral involvement is severe, with cranial nerve palsies, delirium, hallucinations, fits and coma. Death often follows from respiratory paralysis.

Follow-up by Reed et al. (1963) showed that sequelae were limited to the nervous system, both peripherally and centrally, and occurred in half of the survivors. The enduring deficits consisted of features derived from the acute stage: ataxia, tremor, abnormal motor movements, fits and visual disturbance. A recent neuroimaging study of this rare condition identified abnormalities in the striatum in subjects showing otherwise classical presentation of chronic thallium neurotoxicity (Tsai et al. 2006).

Bismuth

Bismuth preparations continue to be used for gastrointestinal and skin disorders as various prescribed and over-the-counter compounds (bismuth subgallate, bismuth subnitrate, tripotassium dicitratobismuthate, bismuth subcitrate and bismuth subsalicylate). Bismuth therapy in gastrointestinal use has shown major efficacy in the treatment of gastroduodenal ulcers. Colloidal bismuth subcitrate is as effective as the histamine H_2-receptor antagonists in peptic ulcer, with a lower rate of relapse (Caron & Rouveix 1991). Rarely, bismuth is reported as having been used in injection form as a health tonic in developing countries (Addrizzo-Harris *et al*. 1997). Chronic uncontrolled use of bismuth salts is associated with a range of toxic symptoms. Most patients affected have been between 40 and 80 years old, with more women than men affected.

Collignon *et al*. (1979) analysed reports of 99 cases in the literature and describe seven patients of their own. Neurological abnormalities are prominent during the prodromal phase, with disturbances of gait and balance, tremors, myoclonic jerks and other disorders of movement. Headache, insomnia and apathy may be accompanied by difficulties with thinking and memory. Some patients show marked oscillations between depression and euphoria. Buge *et al*. (1981) report occasional patients with visual hallucinations and persecutory delusions. Such prodromata can last for several weeks or months.

The acute encephalopathy then presents with confusion and clouding of consciousness, often accompanied by considerable excitement and agitation. Disturbances of memory and praxis sometimes dominate the picture and myoclonic jerks are almost universal. Up to one-third of patients suffer generalised seizures. Motor neurological abnormalities are marked while blood bismuth levels are high. Von Bose and Zaudig (1991) report a more recent example in which rapidly progressive dementia, intermittent delirium, ataxia and myoclonus led to an initial diagnosis of Creutzfeldt–Jakob disease.

As the acute organic reaction subsides the patient may recover completely, or be left with short-term memory difficulties or more global defects of intellectual function. These can persist for more than a year in certain cases. Collignon *et al*. (1979) stress apraxic and agnosic deficits that may remain along with the memory disorder. The picture may mimic the presenile or senile dementias (Summers 1998) or chronic subdural haematoma, or may suggest the presence of a frontal lobe lesion.

Buge *et al*. (1981) have described characteristic CT appearances during the acute phase, with hyperdensities in the cerebral cortex, cerebellum and basal ganglia due to the presence of bismuth. These disappear slowly over 2–3 months on recovery, although enlargement of the cortical sulci may sometimes persist. A characteristic EEG pattern in patients with encephalopathy has been found to consist of monomorphic waves of 3–5 Hz involving tempororolandic and frontal areas, often spreading occipitally. A diffuse beta rhythm of low voltage is also seen but no spikes or other paroxysmal features. The EEG changes appear consistent even in different patients with markedly different blood bismuth levels, ranging from 150 to 1600 µg/L (normal level is ≤5 µg/L). Blood bismuth levels, however, may not accord with actual brain tissue concentrations (Supino-Viterbo *et al*. 1977).

Organophosphorus compounds

Complex esters of phosphoric acid and its derivatives are widely used in industry, horticulture and agriculture. Prominent among them are pesticides such as parathion and malathion, also diazinon and chlorfenvinphos used in sheep dip. Chemical warfare agents include sarin, tabun and soman. Such compounds are potent inhibitors of acetylcholinesterase, first binding to phosphorylation sites, then altering membrane function in a manner that can lead to delayed neurotoxicity. They also interact with adrenergic, dopaminergic and serotonergic mechanisms (Bradwell 1994).

Acute toxic effects consist of cholinergic crises with miosis, bronchoconstriction, diarrhoea, bradycardia and cardiac dysrhythmias. Many patients show weakness due to depolarisation block of neurotransmission, with areflexia and fasciculations (Donaghy 1993). Tremors, ataxia, confusion and agitation may develop, sometimes with bulbar signs and convulsions. Respiratory failure is the usual mode of death. In less severe cases a progressive sensorimotor polyneuropathy follows the acute symptoms after a delay of 1 or 2 weeks. Severe quadriparesis may result. Cognitive deficits have been identified in several epidemiological studies, often persisting for several years after acute exposure (Steenland 1996).

Less intense and intermittent exposure may lead to chronic complaints of nausea, headache, cramps and dizziness, sometimes with muscle fasciculations and difficulty in focusing the eyes. Tiredness and hypersomnia are prominent. Hartman (1988) and Steenland (1996) review neuropsychological studies that have shown impairments of sustained attention and information processing. Florid psychiatric pictures resulting from chronic exposure have been described by Gershon and Shaw (1961) in 16 patients. Most were farmers or greenhouse workers who had used pesticide sprays without adequate protection. After some years of exposure seven developed depressive illnesses, five schizophrenic reactions and four presented with cognitive difficulties. Most had had episodes of acute poisoning in the past with classic symptoms and signs. Bradwell (1994) has reported a farm worker chronically exposed to weedkillers and pesticides who suffered repeated episodes of acute organic psychosis, also periods of depression and mania over several years, all against a background of chronic anergia and hypersomnia. Recent reviews include Rusyniak and Nanagas (2004), Wesseling and Keifer (2002) and Levin and Rodritzky (1976).

Methyl bromide

Methyl bromide is a monohalogenated methane. It exists as a colourless odourless gas and is naturally produced in oceans. It can be pressurised to a liquid and has sometimes been used as a fire extinguisher and refrigerant but more commonly as a fumigant and insecticide.

Over 300 cases of systemic methyl bromide poisoning have been reported, with around 60 fatalities (Herzstein & Cullen 1990; Deschamps & Turpin 1996). Toxic exposures in humans have been documented from inhalation (Deschamps & Turpin 1996), dermal abrasions (Lifshitz *et al.* 2000) and contact with contaminated plastic sheeting (Herzstein & Cullen 1990) and leaking old fire extinguishers (Hoizey *et al.* 2002).

Severe exposures are fatal, with acute pulmonary oedema, renal failure and convulsions (De Jong 1944). Brief exposures are followed by headache, nausea and vertigo, then a characteristic interval of hours or even days during which the patient is symptom-free. This may be followed by the explosive onset of headache, muscular twitching, convulsions, delirium, visual disturbances and somnolence progressing to coma (Baker & Tichy 1953). Chronic mild exposure may be followed by peripheral neuropathy. Fumigation workers with chronic mild exposure were found to show significantly reduced performance on tests of cognition, manual dexterity and olfaction (Calvert *et al.* 1998).

Indirect measures of exposure are provided by serum bromide levels (Buchwald 2001) as the parent agent is rapidly reduced. Methyl bromide shows both enzymatic and non-enzymatic conjugation with glutathione (via the enzyme erythrocyte glutathione transferase). Methyl bromide is metabolised by glutathione conjugation and excreted as carbon dioxide. Methyl bromide causes carcinoma in animal exposures, but data about its carcinogenicity in humans is lacking (Anon. 1999).

Carbon disulphide

Carbon disulphide is an organic solvent. It is a constituent of lacquers and varnishes, and is used in industry in the manufacture of rubber and plastics, notably rayon. Disorders of the CNS are more common the heavier the exposure to carbon disulphide (Krstev *et al.* 2003).

The commonest toxic effect is peripheral neuritis affecting both motor and sensory nerves and producing aching cramp-like pains in the limbs. Visual changes also occur, with central scotomata and concentric narrowing of the visual fields. Auditory symptoms include tinnitus and deafness, and dizziness may occur. Mental changes may be profound and can be the presenting feature. A variety of subjective symptoms are described (Takebayashi *et al.* 1998). These include a heavy feeling in the head, light-headedness, fainting after suddenly standing up, tremor, dullness, and increased sensitivity of the skin in the extremities. An effect on glucose metabolism, with some heavily exposed workers showing increased concentrations of glycosylated haemoglobin, has also been described. Both insidious changes of personality and acute toxic psychoses have been described (Braceland 1942).

Personality changes consist of mood swings, irritability and outbursts of inexplicable rage. The worker may be exhilarated when breathing the fumes in the factory but depressed when at home. Constant fatigue may progress to a state of profound apathy. Headache, anorexia and insomnia are usually marked, and loss of libido is common. Later there may be difficulties with memory, and auditory and visual hallucinations may occur.

In Braceland's survey the more acute psychoses were usually sudden in onset and sometimes closely resembled episodes of mania. These appear to be uncommon today now that levels of exposure in the workplace have been regulated. Severe confusion was accompanied by noisy aggressive behaviour, delusions and hallucinations. Most cleared rapidly on admission to hospital, but some could last for many weeks or months. Residual memory defects occasionally persisted. Examples of acute schizophrenia-like psychoses were also reported, probably in those who were specially predisposed.

Hartman (1988) reviews the cognitive effects of chronic exposure. Motor speed, reaction time, vigilance and visuoconstructive abilities have proved to be affected, sometimes showing significant correlations with duration of exposure. In Huang's study of 10 workers (1996) in a viscose rayon plant subjected to long-term exposure, who had polyneuropathy and various neuropsychiatric symptoms, EEGs were all normal. Brain CT showed mild cortical atrophy in three workers, and low-density basal ganglia lesions in three others. Brain MRI showed multiple lesions in the basal ganglia and corona radiata, but not in all cases. Carotid duplex sonography revealed mild atherosclerosis with plaques in extracranial vessels in over half.

Carbon disulphide neuropathy may persist for a long time. On MRI, multiple high signal intensities in the basal ganglia and subcortical white matter suggest a vascular process, particularly in the small vessels. Diffuse demyelination in the cerebral hemispheres and diffuse decrease in regional cerebral blood flow suggest a microangiopathic process. Carbon disulphide exposure is a risk factor for stroke and a cause of diffuse leucoencephalopathy. Carbon disulphide may induce parkinsonian features and therefore needs to be differentiated from idiopathic parkinsonism (Huang 2004).

References

Abd El Naby, S. & Hassanein, M. (1965) Neuropsychiatric manifestations of chronic manganese poisoning. *Journal of Neurology, Neurosurgery and Psychiatry* **28**, 282–288.

Abraham, H.D. (1982) A chronic impairment of colour vision in users of LSD. *British Journal of Psychiatry* **140**, 518–520.

Abraham, H.D. (1983) Visual phenomenology of the LSD flashback. *Archives of General Psychiatry* **40**, 884–889.

Abraham, H.D. & Wolf, E. (1988) Visual function in past users of LSD: psychophysical findings. *Journal of Abnormal Psychology* **97**, 443–447.

Acker, C. (1985) Performance of female alcoholics on neuropsychological testing. *Alcohol and Alcoholism* **20**, 379–386.

Acker, C., Acker, W.L. & Shaw, G.K. (1984) Assessment of cognitive function in alcoholics by computer: a control study. *Alcohol and Alcoholism* **19**, 223–233.

Acker, C., Jacobson, R.R. & Lishman, W.A. (1987) Memory and ventricular size in alcoholics. *Psychological Medicine* **17**, 343–348.

Adams, R.D. & Victor, M. (1993) *Principles of Neurology*, 5th edn. McGraw-Hill, New York.

Addonizio, G., Susman, V.L. & Roth, S.D. (1987) Neuroleptic malignant syndrome: review and analysis of 115 cases. *Biological Psychiatry* **22**, 1004–1020.

Addrizzo-Harris, D.J., Churg, A. & Rom, W.N. (1997) Radio-opaque punctate opacities on the chest radiograph following intravenous injection of a bismuth compound. *Thorax* **52**, 303–304.

Agate, J.N. & Buckell, M. (1949) Mercury poisoning from fingerprint photography. *Lancet* **ii**, 451–454.

Akelatis, A.J. (1941) Lead encephalopathy in children and adults: a clinico-pathological study. *Journal of Nervous and Mental Disease* **93**, 313–332.

Alexander, L. (1940) Wernicke's disease; identity of lesions produced experimentally by B1 avitaminosis in pigeons with haemorrhagic polioencephalitis occurring in chronic alcoholism in man. *American Journal of Pathology* **16**, 61–70.

Allentuck, S. & Bowman, K.M. (1942) The psychiatric aspects of marijuana intoxication. *American Journal of Psychiatry* **99**, 248–250.

Amato, L., Minozzi, S., Pani, P.P. & Davoli, M. (2007) Antipsychotic medications for cocaine dependence. *Cochrane Database of Systematic Reviews* 3, CD006306.

Anon. (1986) Problems when withdrawing antidepressives. *Drug and Therapeutics Bulletin* **24**, 29–30.

Anon. (1992) Brazil's mercury poisoning disaster. *British Medical Journal* **304**, 1397.

Anon. (1999) Methyl bromide. *IARC Monographs on the Evaluation of Carcinogenic Risks to Humans* **71**, 721–735.

Arseneault, L., Cannon, M., Witton, J. & Murray, R.M. (2004) Causal association between cannabis and psychosis: examination of the evidence. *British Journal of Psychiatry* **184**, 110–117.

Atack, J.R. (2003) Anxioselective compounds acting at the GABA(A) receptor benzodiazepine binding site. *Current Drug Targets. CNS and Neurological Disorders* **2**, 213–232.

Baker, A.B. & Tichy, F.Y. (1953) The effects of the organic solvents and industrial poisonings on the central nervous system. In: Merritt, H.H., Hare, C.C. (eds) *Metabolic and Toxic Diseases of the Nervous System*, ch. 26. Research Publications of the Association for Research in Nervous and Mental Disease vol. 32. Williams & Wilkins, Baltimore.

Bakir, F., Damluji, S.F., Amin-Zaki, L. *et al.* (1973) Methylmercury poisoning in Iraq. An Inter-University Report. *Science* **181**, 230–240.

Balster, R.L. (1998) Neural basis of inhalant abuse. *Drug and Alcohol Dependence* **51**, 207–214.

Barceloux, D.G. (1999) Manganese. *Journal of Toxicology. Clinical Toxicology* **37**, 293–307.

Barrett, S.P., Pihl, R.O., Benkelfat, C., Brunelle, C., Young, S.N. & Leyton, M. (2008) The role of dopamine in alcohol self-administration in humans: individual differences. *European Neuropsychopharmacology* **18**, 439–447.

Bass, M. (1970) Sudden sniffing death. *Journal of the American Medical Association* **212**, 2075–2079.

Baylen, C.A. & Rosenberg, H. (2006) A review of the acute subjective effects of MDMA/ecstasy. *Addiction* **101**, 933–947.

Bechara, A. (2005) Decision making, impulse control, and loss of willpower to resist drugs: a neurocognitive perspective. *Nature Neuroscience* **8**, 1458–1463.

Beeley, L. (1986) Drug interactions with lithium. *Prescriber's Journal* **26**, 160–163.

Bellinger, D.C., Stiles, K.M. & Needleman, H.L. (1992) Low-level lead exposure, intelligence and academic achievement: a long-term follow-up study. *Pediatrics* **90**, 855–861.

Bergin, P.S. & Harvey, P. (1992) Wernicke's encephalopathy and central pontine myelinolysis associated with hyperemesis gravidarum. *British Medical Journal* **305**, 517–518.

Bergman, H., Borg, S., Hindmarsh, T., Ideström, C.-M. & Mützell, S. (1980a) Computed tomography of the brain and neuropsychological assessment of male alcoholic patients and a random sample from the general male population. *Acta Psychiatrica Scandinavica Supplementum* **286**, 77–88.

Bergman, H., Borg, S., Hindmarsh, T., Ideström, C.-M. & Mützell, S. (1980b) Computed tomography of the brain and neuropsychological assessment of male alcoholic patients. In: Richter, D. (ed.) *Addiction and Brain Damage*, ch. 10. Croom Helm, London.

Bewley, T.H. (1967) Adverse reactions from the illicit use of lysergide. *British Medical Journal* **3**, 28–30.

Bidstrup, P.L., Bonnell, J.A., Harvey, D.G. & Locket, S. (1951) Chronic mercury poisoning in men repairing direct-current meters. *Lancet* **ii**, 856–861.

Bigler, E.D., Nelson, J.E. & Schmidt, R.D. (1989) Mamillary body atrophy identified by MRI in alcohol amnesic (Korsakoff's) syndrome. *Neuropsychiatry, Neuropsychology, and Behavioral Neurology* **2**, 189–201.

Bishai, D.M. & Bozzetti, L.P. (1986) Current progress toward the prevention of the Wernicke–Korsakoff syndrome. *Alcohol and Alcoholism* **21**, 315–323.

Blackstock, E.E., Gath, D.H., Gray, B.C. & Higgins, G. (1972) The role of thiamine deficiency in the aetiology of the hallucinatory states complicating alcoholism. *British Journal of Psychiatry* **121**, 357–364.

Blass, J.P. & Gibson, G.E. (1977) Abnormality of a thiamine-requiring enzyme in patients with Wernicke–Korsakoff syndrome. *New England Journal of Medicine* **297**, 1367–1370.

Borne, J., Riascos, R., Cuellar, H., Vargas, D. & Rojas, R. (2005) Neuroimaging in drug and substance abuse. Part II: opioids and solvents. *Topics in Magnetic Resonance Imaging* **16**, 239–245.

Bossert, J.M., Ghitza, U.E., Lu, L., Epstein, D.H. & Shaham, Y. (2005) Neurobiology of relapse to heroin and cocaine seeking: an update and clinical implications. *European Journal of Pharmacology* **526**, 36–50.

Bowden, S.C. (1990) Separating cognitive impairment in neurologically asymptomatic alcoholism from Wernicke–Korsakoff syndrome: is the neuropsychological distinction justified. *Psychological Bulletin* **107**, 355–366.

Bowen, S.E., Batis, J.C., Paez-Martinez, N. & Cruz, S.L. (2006) The last decade of solvent research in animal models of abuse: mechanistic and behavioral studies. *Neurotoxicology and Teratology* **28**, 636–647.

Bowman, K.M., Goodhart, R. & Jolliffe, N. (1939) Observations on the role of vitamin B1 in the etiology and treatment of Korsakoff psychosis. *Journal of Nervous and Mental Disease* **90**, 569–575.

Braceland, F.J. (1942) Mental symptoms following carbon disulphide absorption and intoxication. *Annals of Internal Medicine* **16**, 246–261.

Bradwell, R.H. (1994) Psychiatric sequelae of organophosphorous poisoning: a case study and review of the literature. *Behavioral Neurology* **7**, 117–122.

Brandt, J., Butters, N., Ryan, C. & Bayog, R. (1983) Cognitive loss and recovery in long-term alcohol abusers. *Archives of General Psychiatry* **40**, 435–442.

Brennan, F.N. & Lyttle, J.A. (1987) Alcohol and seizures: a review. *Journal of the Royal Society of Medicine* **80**, 571–573.

Bromberg, W. (1934) Marihuana intoxication. *American Journal of Psychiatry* **91**, 303–330.

Brown, D.S.O., Wills, C.E., Yousefi, V. & Nell, V. (1991) Neurotoxic effects of chronic exposure to manganese dust. *Neuropsychiatry, Neuropsychology, and Behavioral Neurology* **4**, 238–250.

Brunette, M.F., Noordsy, D.L., Xie, H. & Drake, R.E. (2003) Benzodiazepine use and abuse among patients with severe mental illness and co-occurring substance use disorders. *Psychiatric Services* **54**, 1395–1401 (http://ps.psychiatry_online.org).

Buchwald, A.L. (2001) Late confirmation of acute methyl bromide poisoning using S-methylcysteine adduct testing. *Veterinary and Human Toxicology* **43**, 208–211.

Buckley, P.F. & Hutchinson, M. (1995) Neuroleptic malignant syndrome. *Journal of Neurology, Neurosurgery, and Psychiatry* **58**, 271–273.

Budney, A.J., Hughes, J.R., Moore, B.A. & Vandrey, R. (2004) Review of the validity and significance of cannabis withdrawal syndrome. *American Journal of Psychiatry* **161**, 1967–1977.

Buell, S.J. & Coleman, P.D. (1979) Dendritic growth in the aged human brain and failure of growth in senile dementia. *Science* **206**, 854–856.

Buell, S.J. & Coleman, P.D. (1981) Quantitative evidence for selective dendritic growth in normal human ageing but not in senile dementia. *Brain Research* **214**, 23–41.

Buge, A., Supino-Viterbo, V., Rancurel, G. & Pontes, C. (1981) Epileptic phenomena in bismuth toxic encephalopathy. *Journal of Neurology, Neurosurgery and Psychiatry* **44**, 62–67.

Butters, N. & Cermak, L.S. (1980) *Alcoholic Korsakoff's Syndrome: An Information-processing Approach to Amnesia.* Academic Press, New York.

Butterworth, R.F., Kril, J.J. & Harper, C.G. (1993) Thiamine-dependent enzyme changes in the brains of alcoholics: relationship to the Wernicke–Korsakoff syndrome. *Alcoholism: Clinical and Experimental Research* **17**, 1084–1088.

Buxton, J.A. & Dove, N.A. (2008) The burden and management of crystal meth use. *Canadian Medical Association Journal* **178**, 1537–1539.

Cairney, S., Maruff, P., Burns, C.B., Currie, J. & Currie, B.J. (2005) Neurological and cognitive recovery following abstinence from petrol sniffing. *Neuropsychopharmacology* **30**, 1019–1027.

Cala, L.A., Jones, B., Wiley, B. & Mastaglia, F.L. (1980) A computerised axial tomographic (CAT) study of alcohol induced cerebral atrophy in conjunction with other correlates. *Acta Psychiatrica Scandinavica Supplementum* **286**, 31–40.

Calvert, G.M., Mueller, C.A., Fajen, J.M. *et al.* (1998) Health effects associated with sulfuryl fluoride and methyl bromide exposures among structural fumigation workers. *American Journal of Public Health* **88**, 1774–1780.

Campbell, A.C.P. & Russell, W.R. (1941) Wernicke's encephalopathy: the clinical features and their probable relationship to vitamin B deficiency. *Quarterly Journal of Medicine* **34**, 41–64.

Canavan, M.M., Cobb, S. & Drinker, C.K. (1934) Chronic manganese poisoning. *Archives of Neurology and Psychiatry* **32**, 501–512.

Carlen, P.L., Wilkinson, D.A., Wortzman, G. *et al.* (1981) Cerebral atrophy and functional deficits in alcoholics without clinically apparent liver disease. *Neurology* **31**, 377–385.

Caroff, S.N. (1980) The neuroleptic malignant syndrome. *Journal of Clinical Psychiatry* **41**, 79–83.

Caron, F. & Rouveix, B. (1991) Bismuth revisited in *Helicobacter pylori* gastro-duodenal infection. *Therapie* **46**, 393–398.

Carpenter, W.T. & Bunney, W.E. Jr (1971) Behavioral effects of cortisol in man. *Seminars in Psychiatry* **3**, 421–434.

Carter, L.P., Richards, B.D., Mintzer, M.Z. & Griffiths, R.R. (2006) Relative abuse liability of GHB in humans: a comparison of psychomotor, subjective, and cognitive effects of supratherapeutic doses of triazolam, pentobarbital, and GHB. *Neuropsychopharmacology* **31**, 2537–2551.

Cawte, J. (1985) Psychiatric sequelae of manganese exposure in the adult, foetal and neonatal nervous systems. *Australian and New Zealand Journal of Psychiatry* **19**, 211–217.

Centerwall, B.S. & Criqui, M.H. (1978) Prevention of the Wernicke–Korsakoff syndrome: a cost–benefit analysis. *New England Journal of Medicine* **299**, 285–289.

Charness, M.E. & DeLaPaz, R.L. (1987) Mamillary body atrophy in Wernicke's encephalopathy: antemortem identification using MRI. *Annals of Neurology* **22**, 595–600.

Charness, M.E., Simon, R.P. & Greenberg, D.A. (1989) Ethanol and the nervous system. *New England Journal of Medicine* **321**, 442–454.

Charney, D.S., Kales, A., Soldatos, C.R. & Nelson, J.C. (1979) Somnambulistic-like episodes secondary to combined lithium-neuroleptic treatment. *British Journal of Psychiatry* **135**, 418–424.

Charney, D.S., Mihic, S.J. & Harris, R.A. (2001) Hypnotics and sedatives. In: Hardman, J.G. & Limbird, L.E. (eds) *Goodman and Gilman's The Pharmacological Basis of Therapeutics*, 10th edn, pp. 399–427. McGraw-Hill, New York.

Chouinard, G. (2004) Issues in the clinical use of benzodiazepines: potency, withdrawl, and rebound. *Journal of Clinical Psychiatry* **65** (suppl. 5), 7–12.

Cicero, T.J., Inciardi, J.A. & Surratt, H. (2007) Trends in the use and abuse of branded and generic extended release oxycodone and fentanyl products in the United States. *Drug and Alcohol Dependence* **91**, 115–120.

Ciraulo, D.A., Shader, R.I., Greenblatt, D.J. & Creelman, W. (1989) *Drug Interactions in Psychiatry.* Williams & Wilkins, Baltimore.

Clarke, R.C. & Watson, D.P. (2002) Botany of natural cannabis medicines. In: Grotenhermen, F. & Russo, E. (eds) *Cannabis and*

Cannabinoids: Pharmacology, Toxicology, and Therapeutic Potential, pp. 3–13. Haworth Integrative Healing Press, New York.

Clarke, S.F., Dargan, P.I. & Jones, A.L. (2005) Naloxone in opioid poisoning: walking the tightrope. *Emergency Medicine Journal* **22**, 612–616.

Clarkson, T.W. (1997) The toxicology of mercury. *Critical Reviews in Clinical Laboratory Sciences* **34**, 369–403.

Clarkson, T.W., Loszlo, M. & Myers, G.J. (2003) European Environment Agency, risks to health and the environment related to the use of mercury products, report prepared for and published by the European Commission, London 2002. *New England Journal of Medicine* **349**, 1731–1737.

Cohen, W. & Cohen, N.H. (1974) Lithium carbonate, haloperidol, and irreversible brain damage. *Journal of the American Medical Association* **230**, 1283–1287.

Coid, J. (1979) Mania à potu: a critical review of pathological intoxication. *Pychological Medicine* **9**, 709–719.

Colchester, A., Kingsley, D., Lasserson, D. *et al.* (2001) Structural MRI volumetric analysis in patients with organic amnesia. I. Methods and comparative findings across diagnostic groups. *Journal of Neurology, Neurosurgery and Psychiatry* **71**, 13–22.

Cole, M., Richardson, E.P. & Segerra, J.N. (1964) Central pontine myelinolysis: further evidence relating the lesion to malnutrition. *Neurology* **14**, 165–170.

Collignon, R., Brayer, R., Rectem, D., Indeiceu, P. & Laterre, E.C. (1979) Analyse sémiologique de l'encéphalopathie bismuthique. Confrontation avec sept cas personnels. *Acta Neurologica Belgica* **79**, 73–91.

Compston, A. (1993) Non-infective inflammatory demyelinating, and paraneoplastic diseases of the nervous system. In: Walton, J. (ed.) *Brain's Diseases of the Nervous System*, 10th edn, ch. 10. Oxford University Press, Oxford.

Connell, P.H. (1968) Central nervous system stimulant and antidepressant drugs. In: Meyler, L. & Herxheimer, A. (eds) *Side Effects of Drugs*, ch. 1. Excerpta Medica, Amsterdam.

Cope, R.V. & Gregg, E.M. (1983) Neuroleptic malignant syndrome. *British Medical Journal* **286**, 1938.

Costa, L.G., Guizetti, M., Burr, Y.M. & Oberdoerster, L. (2002) Developmental neurotoxicity: do similar phenotypes indicate a common mode of action? A comparison of fetal alcohol syndrome, toluene embryopathy, and maternal phenylketonuria. *Toxicology Letters* **127**, 197–205.

Courville, C.B. (1955) *The Effects of Alcohol on the Nervous System of Man*. San Lucas Press, Los Angeles.

Cowan, R.L. (2007) Neuroimaging research in human MDMA users: a review. *Psychopharmacology (Berl)* **189**, 539–556.

Cravioto, H., Korein, J. & Silberman, J. (1961) Wernicke's encephalopathy: a clinical and pathological study of 28 autopsied cases. *Archives of Neurology* **4**, 510–519.

Crossgrove, J. & Zheng, W. (2004) Manganese toxicity upon overexposure. *NMR in Biomedicine* **17**, 544–553.

Cruickshank, E.K. (1961) Neuropsychiatric disorders in prisoners-of-war. In: Gruhle, H.W., Jung, R., Mayer-Gross, W. & Muller, M. (eds) *Psychiatrie det Gegenwar*, vol. 3, pp. 807–836. Springer, Berlin.

Crunelli, V., Emri, Z. & Leresche, N. (2006) Unravelling the brain targets of gamma-hydroxybutyric acid. *Current Opinion in Pharmacology* **6**, 44–52.

Cutting, J. (1978) The relationship between Korsakov's syndrome and 'alcoholic dementia'. *British Journal of Psychiatry* **132**, 240–251.

Dathan, J.G. (1954) Acrodynia associated with excessive intake of mercury. *British Medical Journal* **1**, 247–249.

Davies, R.K., Tucker, G.J., Harrow, M. & Detre, T.P. (1971) Confusional episodes and antidepressant medication. *American Journal of Psychiatry* **128**, 95–99.

Davis, J.M., Janicak, P.G., Sakkas, P., Gilmore, C. & Wang, Z. (1991) Electroconvulsive therapy in the treatment of the neuroleptic malignant syndrome. *Convulsive Therapy* **7**, 111–120.

De Jong, R.N. (1944) Methyl bromide poisoning. *Journal of the American Medical Association* **125**(ii), 702–703.

De la Monte, S.M. (1988) Disproportionate atrophy of cerebral white matter in chronic alcoholics. *Archives of Neurology* **45**, 990–992.

Delmas-Marsalet, P., Vital, C., Julien, J., Béraud, C., Bourgeois, M. & Bargues, M. (1967) La maladie de Marchiafava et Bignami. *Journal de Médicine de Bordeaux* **144**, 1627–1646.

Denis, C., Fatséas, M., Lavie, E. & Auriacombe, M. (2006) Pharmacological interventions for benzodiazepine mono-dependence management in outpatient settings. *Cochrane Database of Systematic Reviews* 3, CD005194.

Deschamps, F.J. & Turpin, J.C. (1996) Methyl bromide intoxication during grain store fumigation. *Occupational Medicine (Oxford)* **46**, 89–90.

De Wardener, H.E. & Lennox, B. (1947) Cerebral beri beri (Wernicke's encephalopathy). *Lancet* **i**, 11–17.

Dewhurst, K. & Hatrick, J.A. (1972) Differential diagnosis and treatment of lysergic acid diethylamide induced psychosis. *Practitioner* **209**, 327–332.

Donaghy, M. (1993) Toxic and environmental disorders. In: Walton, J. (ed.) *Brain's Diseases of the Nervous System*, 10th edn, ch. 15. Oxford University Press, Oxford.

Drasbek, K.R., Christensen, J. & Jensen, K. (2006) Gamma-hydroxybutyrate: a drug of abuse. *Acta Neurologica Scandinavica* **114**, 145–156.

D'Souza, D.C., Braley, G., Blaise, R. *et al.* (2008a) Effects of haloperidol on the behavioral, subjective, cognitive, motor, and neuroendocrine effects of Δ-9-tetrahydrocannabinol in humans. *Psychopharmacology (Berl)* **198**, 587–603.

D'Souza, D.C., Ranganathan, M., Braley, G. *et al.* (2008b) Blunted psychotomimetic and amnestic effects of Δ-9-tetrahydrocannabinol in frequent users of cannabis. *Neuropsychopharmacology* **33**, 2505–2516.

Dukes, M.N.G. (1992) *Meyler's Side Effects of Drugs. An Encyclopedia of Adverse Reactions and Interactions*, 12th edn. Elsevier, Amsterdam.

Dumont, G.J. & Verkes, R.J. (2006) A review of acute effects of 3,4-methylenedioxymethamphetamine in healthy volunteers. *Journal of Psychopharmacology* **20**, 176–187.

Easton, N. & Marsden, C.A. (2006) Ecstasy: are animal data consistent between species and can they translate to humans? *Journal of Psychopharmacology* **20**, 194–210.

Ebels, E.J. (1978) How common is Wernicke–Korsakoff syndrome? *Lancet* **ii**, 781–782.

Ecker, A. & Kernohan, J.W. (1941) Arsenic as a possible cause of subacute encephalomyelitis. *Archives of Neurology and Psychiatry* **45**, 24–43.

Eddy, N.B., Halbach, H., Isbell, H. & Seevers, M.H. (1965) Drug dependence: its significance and characteristics. *Bulletin of the World Health Organization* **32**, 721–733.

Edwards, G. (1974) Drugs, drugs dependence and the concept of plasticity. *Quarterly Journal of Studies on Alcohol* **35**, 176–195.

Edwards, G. (1982) *The Treatment of Drinking Problems*. Grant McIntyre, London.

Edwards, G. (2000) *Alcohol: The World's Favorite Drug*. St Martin's Press, New York.

Emsley, J. (1978) The trouble with thallium. *New Scientist* **79** (Aug. 10) August, 392–394.

Ersche, K.D. & Sahakian, B.J. (2007) The neuropsychology of amphetamine and opiate dependence: implications for treatment. *Neuropsychology Review* **17**, 317–336.

Escobar, A., Aruffo, C. & Rodriguez-Carbajal, J. (1983) Wernicke's encephalopathy. A case report with neurophysiologic and CT-scan studies. *Acta Vitaminologica et Enzymologica* **5**, 125–131.

Essig, C.F. (1967) Clinical and experimental aspects of barbiturate withdrawal convulsions. *Epilepsia* **8**, 21–30.

Estrin, W.J. (1987) Alcoholic cerebellar degeneration is not a dose-dependent phenomenon. *Alcoholism: Clinical and Experimental Research* **11**, 372–375.

Estroff, T.W. & Gold, M.S. (1986) Medical and psychiatric complications of cocaine abuse with possible points of pharmacological treatment. *Advances in Alcohol and Substance Abuse* **5**, 61–76.

Everitt, B.J. & Robbins, T.W. (2005) Neural systems of reinforcement for drug addiction: from actions to habits to compulsion. *Nature Neuroscience* **8**, 1481–1489.

Fairhall, L.T. & Neal, P.A. (1943) *Industrial Manganese Poisoning*. National Institutes of Health Bulletin No. 182. United States Government Printing Office, Washington, DC.

Feldman, R.G. (1982) Neurological manifestations of mercury intoxication. *Acta Neurologica Scandinavica Supplementum* **92**, 201–209.

Fell, J.C. & Voas, R.B. (2006) The effectiveness of reducing illegal blood alcohol concentration (BAC) limits for driving: evidence for lowering the limit to .05 BAC. *Journal of Safety Research* **37**, 233–243.

Filley, C.M., Halliday, W. & Kleinschmidt-DeMasters, B.K. (2004) The effects of toluene on the central nervous system. *Journal of Neuropathology and Experimental Neurology* **63**, 1–12.

Finlay-Jones, R. (1986) Should thiamine be added to beer? *Australian and New Zealand Journal of Psychiatry* **20**, 3–6.

Fisch, B. (ed.) (1999) Generalised changes of amplitude: Symmetrically high and low amplitude. In: *Fisch and Spehlmann's EEG Primer*, 3rd edn, p. 413. Elsevier, Amsterdam.

Flaten, T.P. (2001) Aluminium as a risk factor in Alzheimer's disease, with emphasis on drinking water. *Brain Research Bulletin* **55**, 187–196.

Flood, D.G. & Coleman, P.D. (1986) Failed compensatory dendritic growth as a pathophysiological process in Alzheimer's disease. *Canadian Journal of Neurological Science* **13**, 475–479.

Freedman, D.X. (1968) On the use and abuse of LSD. *Archives of General Psychiatry* **18**, 330–347.

Freund, G. (1973) Chronic central nervous system toxicity of alcohol. *Annual Review of Pharmacology* **13**, 217–227.

Frosch, W.A., Robbins, E.S. & Stern, M. (1965) Untoward reactions to lysergic acid diethylamide (LSD) resulting in hospitalisation. *New England Journal of Medicine* **273**, 1235–1239.

Gallucci, M., Bozzao, A., Splendiaini, A., Masciocchi, C. & Passariello, R. (1990) Wernicke encephalopathy: MR findings in five patients. *American Journal of Neuroradiology* **11**, 887–892.

Garavan, H. & Hester, R. (2007) The role of cognitive control in cocaine dependence. *Neuropsychology Review* **17**, 337–345.

Gaudreau, J.D., Gagnon, P., Roy, M.A., Harel, F. & Tremblay, A. (2005) Association between psychoactive medications and delirium in hospitalized patients: a critical review. *Psychosomatics* **46**, 302–316.

Gerber, G.B., Léonard, A. & Hantson, P. (2002) Carcinogenicity, mutagenicity and teratogenicity of manganese compounds. *Critical Reviews in Oncology and Hematology* **42**, 25–34.

Gershon, S. & Shaw, F.H. (1961) Psychiatric sequelae of chronic exposure to organophosphorus insecticides. *Lancet* **i**, 1371–1374.

Ghodse, H. (1995) *Drugs and Addictive Behaviour. A Guide to Treatment*, 2nd edn. Blackwell Science, Oxford.

Gianoulakis, C. (2001) Influence of the endogenous opioid system on high alcohol consumption and genetic predisposition to alcoholism. *Journal of Psychiatry and Neuroscience* **26**, 304–318.

Gilman, S., Adams, K., Koeppe, R.A. *et al.* (1990) Cerebellar and frontal hypometabolism in alcoholic cerebellar degeneration studied with PET. *Annals of Neurology* **28**, 775–785.

Glauser, J. & Queen, J.R. (2007) An overview of non-cardiac cocaine toxicity. *Journal of Emergency Medicine* **32**, 181–186.

Gochfeld, M. (2003) Cases of mercury exposure, bioavailability, and absorption. *Ecotoxicology and Environmental Safety* **56**, 174–179.

Goldman, L.R. & Shannon, M.W. (2001) Technical report: mercury in the environment: implications for pediatricians. American Academy of Pediatrics Committee on Environmental Health. *Pediatrics* **108**, 197–205.

Gonzalez, A. & Nutt, D.J. (2005) Gamma hydroxy butyrate abuse and dependency. *Journal of Psychopharmacology* **19**, 195–204.

Gonzalez, R. (2007) Acute and non-acute effects of cannabis on brain functioning and neuropsychological performance. *Neuropsychology Review* **17**, 347–361.

Gonzalez, R., Carey, C. & Grant, I. (2002) Nonacute (residual) neuropsychological effects of cannabis use: a qualitative analysis and systematic review. *Journal of Clinical Pharmacology* **42**, 48S–57S.

Goodwin, D.W., Crane, J.B. & Guze, S.B. (1969a) Alcoholic blackouts: a review and clinical study of 100 alcoholics. *American Journal of Psychiatry* **126**, 191–198.

Goodwin, D.W., Crane, J.B. & Guze, S.B. (1969b) Phenomenological aspects of the alcoholic 'blackout'. *British Journal of Psychiatry* **115**, 1033–1038.

Goodwin, D.W., Powell, B., Bremer, D., Hoine, H. & Stern, J. (1969c) Alcohol and recall: state-dependent effects in man. *Science* **163**, 1358–1360.

Gouzoulis-Mayfrank, E. & Daumann, J. (2006) The confounding problem of polydrug use in recreational ecstasy/MDMA users: a brief overview. *Journal of Psychopharmacology* **20**, 188–193.

Grabski, D.A. (1961) Toluene sniffing producing cerebellar degeneration. *American Journal of Psychiatry* **118**, 461–462.

Granato, J.E., Stern, B.J., Ringel, A. *et al.* (1983) Neuroleptic malignant syndrome: successful treatment with dantrolene and bromocriptine. *Annals of Neurology* **14**, 89–90.

Granville-Grossman, K. (1971) *Recent Advances in Clinical Psychiatry.* Churchill, London.

Green, B., Kavanagh, D. & Young, R. (2003) Being stoned: a review of self-reported cannabis effects. *Drug and Alcohol Review* **22**, 453–460.

Greenberg, R. & Pearlman, C. (1967) Delirium tremens and dreaming. *American Journal of Psychiatry* **124**, 133–142.

Greenwood, J., Jeyasingham, M., Pratt, O.E., Ryle, P.R., Shaw, G.K. & Thomson, A.D. (1984) Heterogeneity of human erythrocyte transketolase: a preliminary report. *Alcohol and Alcoholism* **19**, 123–129.

Greer, H.D., Ward, H.P. & Corbin, K.B. (1965) Chronic salicylate intoxication in adults. *Journal of the American Medical Association* **193**, 555–558.

Gross, M.M. & Goodenough, D.R. (1968) Sleep disturbances in the acute alcoholic psychoses. *Psychiatric Research Reports of the American Psychiatric Association* **24**, 132–147.

Gruber, S.A., Silveri, M.M. & Yurgelun-Todd, D.A. (2007) Neuropsychological consequences of opiate use. *Neuropsychology Review* **17**, 299–315.

Grunnet, M.L. (1969) Changing incidence, distribution, and histopathology of Wernicke's polioencephalopathy. *Neurology* **19**, 1135–1139.

Gurling, H.M.D., Reveley, M.A. & Murray, R.M. (1984) Increased cerebral ventricular volume in monozygotic twins discordant for alcoholism. *Lancet* **i**, 986–988.

Halikas, J.A., Goodwin, D.W. & Guze, S.B. (1972) Marijuana use and psychiatric illness. *Archives of General Psychiatry* **27**, 162–165.

Hall, C.W., Popkin, M.K., Stickney, S.K. & Gardner, R. (1979) Presentation of the steroid psychoses. *Journal of Nervous and Mental Disease* **167**, 229–236.

Halpern, J.H. & Pope, H.G. Jr (1999) Do hallucinogens cause residual neuropsychological toxicity? *Drug and Alcohol Dependence* **53**, 247–256.

Halpern, J.H. & Pope, H.G. Jr (2003) Hallucinogen persisting perception disorder: what do we know after 50 years? *Drug and Alcohol Dependence* **69**, 109–119.

HaMai, D. & Bondy, S.C. (2004) Oxidative basis of manganese neurotoxicity. *Annals of the New York Academy of Sciences* **1012**, 129–141.

Handler, C.E. & Perkin, G.D. (1982) Anorexia nervosa and Wernicke's encephalopathy: an underdiagnosed association. *Lancet* **ii**, 771–772.

Harding, A., Halliday, G., Caine, D. & Kril, J. (2000) Degeneration of anterior thalamic nuclei differentiates alcoholics with amnesia. *Brain* **123**, 141–154.

Harper, C. (1979) Wernicke's encephalopathy: a more common disease than realised. A neuropathological study of 51 cases. *Journal of Neurology, Neurosurgery and Psychiatry* **42**, 226–231.

Harper, C. (1983) The incidence of Wernicke's encephalopathy in Australia: a neuropathological study of 131 cases. *Journal of Neurology, Neurosurgery and Psychiatry* **46**, 593–598.

Harper, C. (1989) Brain damage and alcohol misuse. *Current Opinion in Psychiatry* **2**, 434–438.

Harper, C.G. & Blumbergs, P.C. (1982) Brain weights in alcoholics. *Journal of Neurology, Neurosurgery and Psychiatry* **45**, 838–840.

Harper, C. & Corbett, D. (1990) Changes in the basal dendrites of cortical pyramidal cells from alcoholic patients: a quantitative Golgi study. *Journal of Neurology, Neurosurgery and Psychiatry* **53**, 856–861.

Harper, C. & Kril, J. (1985) Brain atrophy in chronic alcoholic patients: a quantitative pathological study. *Journal of Neurology, Neurosurgery and Psychiatry* **48**, 211–217.

Harper, C.G. & Kril, J.J. (1988) Corpus callosum thickness in alcoholics. *British Journal of Addiction* **83**, 577–580.

Harper, C.G. & Kril, J.J. (1990) Neuropathology of alcoholism. *Alcohol and Alcoholism* **25**, 207–216.

Harper, C.G., Kril, J.J. & Holloway, R.L. (1985) Brain shrinkage in chronic alcoholics: a pathological study. *British Medical Journal* **290**, 501–504.

Harper, C.G., Giles, M. & Finlay-Jones, R. (1986) Clinical signs in the Wernicke–Korsakoff complex: a retrospective analysis of 131 cases diagnosed at necropsy. *Journal of Neurology, Neurosurgery and Psychiatry* **49**, 341–345.

Harper, C., Kril, J. & Daly, J. (1987) Are we drinking our neurones away? *British Medical Journal* **294**, 534–536.

Harper, C., Gold, J., Rodriguez, M. & Perdices, M. (1989) The prevalence of the Wernicke–Korsakoff syndrome in Sydney, Australia: a prospective necropsy study. *Journal of Neurology, Neurosurgery and Psychiatry* **52**, 282–285.

Harper, C., Fornes, P., Duyckaerts, C., Lecomte, D. & Hauw, J.-J. (1995) An international perspective on the prevalence of the Wernicke–Korsakoff syndrome. *Metabolic Brain Disease* **10**, 17–24.

Hartman, D.E. (1988) *Neuropsychological Toxicology: Identification and Assessment of Human Neurotoxic Syndromes.* Pergamon Press, Oxford.

Hatrick, J.A. & Dewhurst, K. (1970) Delayed psychosis due to LSD. *Lancet* **ii**, 742–744.

Hay, W.J., Rickards, A.G., McMenemy, W.H. & Cumings, J.N. (1963) Organic mercurial encephalopathy. *Journal of Neurology, Neurosurgery and Psychiatry* **26**, 199–202.

Hemmingsen, R. & Kramp, P. (1988) Delirium tremens and related clinical states: psychopathology, cerebral pathophysiology and psychochemistry. A two-component hypothesis concerning etiology and pathogenesis. *Acta Psychiatrica Scandinavica Supplementum* **345**, 94–107.

Hemmingsen, R., Vorstrup, S., Clemmesen, L. *et al.* (1988) Cerebral blood flow during delirium tremens and related clinical states studied with xenon-133 inhalation tomography. *American Journal of Psychiatry* **145**, 1384–1390.

Herzstein, J. & Cullen, M.R. (1990) Methyl bromide intoxication in four field-workers during removal of soil fumigation sheets. *American Journal of Industrial Medicine* **17**, 321–326.

Himmelsbach, C.K. (1943) Can the euphoric, analgetic and physical dependence effects of drugs be separated? IV. With reference to physical dependence. *Federation Proceedings* **2**, 201–203.

Hoaken, P.N. & Stewart, S.H. (2003) Drugs of abuse and the elicitation of human aggressive behavior. *Addictive Behaviors* **28**, 1533–1554.

Hoffman, R.S. (2003) Thallium toxicity and the role of Prussian blue in therapy. *Toxicological Reviews* **22**, 29–40.

Hoizey, G., Souchon, P.F., Trenque, T. *et al.* (2002) An unusual case of methyl bromide poisoning. *Journal of Toxicology. Clinical Toxicology* **40**, 817–821.

Horowitz, M.J. (1969) Flashbacks: recurrent intrusive images after the use of LSD. *American Journal of Psychiatry* **126**, 565–569.

Huang C.-C. (1996) Chronic carbon disulphide encephalopathy. *European Journal of Neurology* **36**, 364–368.

Huang, C.C. (2004) Carbon sulphide neurotoxicity: Taiwan experience. *Acta Neurologica Taiwanica* **13**, 3–9.

Huang, C.-C., Chu, N.-S., Lu, C.-S. *et al.* (1989) Chronic manganese intoxication. *Archives of Neurology* **46**, 1104–1106.

Hudson, H.S. & Walker, H.I. (1961) Withdrawal symptoms following ethchlorvynol (placidyl) dependence. *American Journal of Psychiatry* **118**, 361.

Hunter, D. (1959) *Health in Industry*. Penguin Books, Harmondsworth.

Hunter, D. (1978) *The Diseases of Occupations*, 6th edn. Hodder & Stoughton, London.

Hunter, R., McLuskie, R., Wyper, D. *et al.* (1989) The pattern of function-related regional cerebral blood flow investigated by single photon emission tomography with ^{99m}Tc-HMPAO in patients with presenile Alzheimer's disease and Korsakoff's psychosis. *Psychological Medicine* **19**, 847–855.

Hyman, S.E. (2007) The neurobiology of addiction: implications for voluntary control of behavior. *American Journal of Bioethics* **7**, 8–11.

Isbell, H., Fraser, H.F., Wickler, A., Belleville, R.E. & Eisenman, A.J. (1955) An experimental study of aetiology of 'rum fits' and delirium tremens. *Quarterly Journal of Studies on Alcohol* **16**, 1–33.

Isbell, H., Belleville, R.E., Fraser, H.F., Wikler, A. & Logan, C.R. (1956) Studies on lysergic acid diethylamide (LSD-25): 1. Effects in former morphine addicts and development of tolerance during chronic intoxication. *Archives of Neurology and Psychiatry* **76**, 468–478.

Iversen, L. (2005) Long-term effects of exposure to cannabis. *Current Opinion in Pharmacology* **5**, 69–72.

Jacobson, R.R. (1986) The contribution of sex and drinking history to the CT brain scan changes in alcoholics. *Psychological Medicine* **16**, 547–559.

Jacobson, R.R. (1989) Alcoholism, Korsakoff's syndrome and the frontal lobe. *Behavioral Neurology* **2**, 25–38.

Jacobson, R.R. & Lishman, W.A. (1987) Selective memory loss and global intellectual deficits in alcoholic Korsakoff's syndrome. *Psychological Medicine* **17**, 649–655.

Jacobson, R.R. & Lishman, W.A. (1990) Cortical and diencephalic lesions in Korsakoff's syndrome: a clinical and CT scan study. *Psychological Medicine* **20**, 63–75.

Jacobson, R.R., Acker, C.F. & Lishman, W.A. (1990) Patterns of neuropsychological deficit in alcoholic Korsakoff's syndrome. *Psychological Medicine* **20**, 321–334.

Jaerup, L. (2003) Hazards of heavy metal contamination. *British Medical Bulletin* **68**, 167–182.

Janowsky, J.S., Shimamura, A.P., Kritchevsky, M. & Squire, L.R. (1989) Cognitive impairment following frontal lobe damage and its relevance to human amnesia. *Behavioral Neuroscience* **103**, 548–560.

Jernigan, T.L., Butters, N., Ditraglia, G. *et al.* (1991a) Reduced cerebral grey matter observed in alcoholics using MRI. *Alcoholism: Clinical and Experimental Research* **15**, 418–427.

Jernigan, T.L., Schafer, K., Butters, N. & Cermak, L.S. (1991b) Magnetic resonance imaging of alcoholic Korsakoff patients. *Neuropsychopharmacology* **4**, 175–186.

Johnson, C.L. (2004) Mercury in the environment: sources, toxicities, and prevention of exposure. *Pediatric Annals* **33**, 437–442.

Jolliffe, N., Wortis, H. & Fein, H.D. (1941) The Wernicke syndrome. *Archives of Neurology and Psychiatry* **46**, 569–597.

Jones, R.J., Homa, D.M., Meyer, P.E., *et al.* (2009) Trends in blood lead levels and blood lead testing among US children aged 1 to 5 years, 1988–2004. *Pediatrics* **123**, e376–385.

Joyce, E.M. & Robbins, T.W. (1991) Frontal lobe function in Korsakoff and non-Korsakoff alcoholics: planning and spatial working memory. *Neuropsychologia* **29**, 709–723.

Joyce, E.M., Rio, D.E., Ruttimann, U.E. *et al.* (1994) Decreased cingulate and precuneate glucose utilization in alcoholic Korsakoff's syndrome. *Psychiatry Research* **54**, 225–239.

Kaczmarek, M.J. & Nixon, P.F. (1983) Variants of transketolate from human erythrocytes. *Clinica Chimica Acta* **130**, 349–356.

Karhunen, P.J., Erkinjuntti, T. & Laippala, P. (1994) Moderate alcohol consumption and loss of cerebellar Purkinje cells. *British Medical Journal* **308**, 1663–1667.

Kark, R.A.P., Poskanzer, D.C., Bullock, J.D. & Boylen, G. (1971) Mercury poisoning and its treatment with N-acetyl-D, L-penicillamine. *New England Journal of Medicine* **285**, 10–16.

Karlsen, S.N., Spigset, O. & Slørdal, L. (2008) The dark side of ecstasy: neuropsychiatric symptoms after exposure to 3,4-methylenedioxymethamphetamine. *Basic and Clinical Pharmacology and Toxicology* **102**, 15–24.

Kawamura, M., Shiota, J., Yagishita, T. & Hirayama, K. (1985) Marchiafava–Bignami disease: computed tomographic scan and magnetic resonance imaging. *Annals of Neurology* **18**, 103–104.

Kearsley, J.H. & Musso, A.F. (1980) Hypothermia and coma in the Wernicke–Korsakoff syndrome. *Medical Journal of Australia* **2**, 504–506.

Kellam, A.M.P. (1987) Neuroleptic malignant syndrome, so-called. A survey of the world literature. *British Journal of Psychiatry* **150**, 752–759.

Kelly, M., Myrsten, A.-L. & Goldberg, L. (1971) Intravenous vitamins in acute alcoholic intoxication: effects on physiological and psychological functions. *British Journal of Addiction* **66**, 19–30.

Keshavan, M.S. & Lishman, W.A. (1986) Prolonged depersonalization following cannabis abuse. *British Journal of Addiction* **81**, 140–142.

Kessler, R.M., Parker, E.S., Clark, C.M. *et al.* (1984) Regional cerebral glucose metabolism in patients with alcoholic Korsakoff's syndrome [Abstract]. *Society for Neuroscience* **10**, 541.

Keyes, K.M., Martins, S.S. & Hasin, D.S. (2008) Past 12-month and lifetime comorbidity and poly-drug use of ecstasy users among young adults in the United States: results from the National Epidemiologic Survey on Alcohol and Related Conditions. *Drug and Alcohol Dependence* **97**, 139–149.

King, M.A., Hunter, B.E. & Walker, D.W. (1988) Alterations and recovery of dendritic spine density in rat hippocampus following long-term ethanol ingestion. *Brain Research* **459**, 381–385.

Knapp, W.P., Soares, B.G., Farrel, M. & Lima, M.S. (2007) Psychosocial interventions for cocaine and psychostimulant amphetamines related disorders. *Cochrane Database of Systematic Reviews* **3**, CD003023.

Knox, J.W. & Nelson, J.R. (1966) Permanent encephalopathy from toluene inhalation. *New England Journal of Medicine* **275**, 1494–1496.

Koob, G. & Kreek, M.J. (2007) Stress, dysregulation of drug reward pathways, and the transition to drug dependence. *American Journal of Psychiatry* **164**, 1149–1159.

Koob, G.F. & Le Moal, M. (1997) Drug abuse: hedonic homeostatic dysregulation. *Science* **278**, 52–58.

Koob, G., Everitt, B. & Robbins, T. (2008) Reward, motivation and addiction. In: Squire, L.R., Bloom, F.E. & Spitzer, N.C. (eds) *Fundamental Neuroscience*, 3rd edn Academic Press, Amsterdam.

Kopelman, M.D. (1991) Frontal dysfunction and memory deficits in the alcoholic Korsakoff syndrome and Alzheimer-type dementia. *Brain* **114**, 117–137.

Kopelman, M.D. (1995) The Korsakoff syndrome. *British Journal of Psychiatry* **166**, 154–173.

Kopelman, M.D., Reed, L.J., Marsden, P. *et al.* (2001) Amnesic syndrome and severe ataxia following the recreational use of MDMA ('ecstasy') and other substances. *Neurocase* **7**, 423–432.

Kosten, T.R. (1990) Neurobiology of abused drugs. Opioids and stimulants. *Journal of Nervous and Mental Disease* **178**, 217–227.

Kril, J.J. & Harper, C.G. (1989) Neuronal counts from four cortical regions of alcoholic brains. *Acta Neuropathologica* **79**, 200–204.

Krstev, S., Perunicic, B., Farleic, B. *et al.* (2003) Neuropsychiatric effects in workers with occupational exposure to carbon disulphide. *Journal of Occupational Health* **45**, 81–87.

Kurland, L.T., Faro, S.N. & Siedler, H. (1960) The outbreak of a neurologic disorder in Minamata, Japan, and its relationship to the ingestion of seafood contaminated by mercuric compounds. *World Neurology* **1**, 370–395.

Langford, N. & Ferner, R. (1999) Toxicity of mercury. *Journal of Human Hypertension* **13**, 651–656.

Langlais, P.J. (1995) Alcohol-related thiamine deficiency. Impact on cognitive and memory functioning. *Alcohol Health and Research World* **19**, 113–121.

Langston, J.W. (2002) Parkinson's disease: current and future challenges. *Neurotoxicology* **23**, 443–450.

Langston, J.W., Ballard, P., Tetrud, J.W. & Irwin, I. (1983) Chronic parkinsonism in humans due to a product of mepiridine-analog synthesis. *Science* **219**, 979–980.

Langworth, S. (1997) Experiences from the amalgam unit at Huddinge hospital: somatic and psychosomatic aspects. *Scandavanian Journal of Environment and Health* **23**, 65–67.

Leonard, B.E. (1986) Is ethanol a neurotoxin? The effects of ethanol on neuronal structure and function. *Alcohol and Alcoholism* **21**, 325–338.

Leslie, K.O., Robertson, A.S. & Norenberg, M.D. (1980) Central pontine myelinolysis: an osmotic gradient pathogenesis. *Journal of Neuropathology and Experimental Neurology* **39**, 370.

Levin, H.S. & Rodritzky, R.L. (1976) Behavioral effects of organophosphate in man. *Clinical Toxicology* **9**, 391–403.

Levinson, D.F. & Simpson, G.M. (1986) Neuroleptic-induced extrapyramidal symptoms with fever. *Archives of General Psychiatry* **43**, 839–848.

Lifshitz, M., Gavrilov, V. *et al.* (2000) Central nervous system toxicity and early peripheral neuropathy following dermal exposure to methyl bromide. *Journal of Toxicology. Clinical Toxicology* **38**, 799–801.

Lima, M.S., Reisser, A.A., Soares, B.G. & Farrell, M. (2003) Antidepressants for cocaine dependence. *Cochrane Database of Systematic Reviews* 2, CD002950.

Lindboe, C.F. & Løberg, E.M. (1989) Wernicke's encephalopathy in non-alcoholics. An autopsy study. *Journal of the Neurological Sciences* **90**, 125–129.

Lipowski, Z.J. (1990) *Delirium: Acute Confusional States*, 2nd edn. Oxford University Press, Oxford.

Lishman, W.A. (1981) Cerebral disorder in alcoholism: syndromes of impairment. *Brain* **104**, 1–20.

Lishman, W.A. (1986) Alcoholic dementia: a hypothesis. *Lancet* **i**, 1184–1186.

Lishman, W.A. (1990) Alcohol and the brain. *British Journal of Psychiatry* **156**, 635–644.

Lishman, W.A., Jacobson, R.R. & Acker, C. (1987) Brain damage in alcoholism: current concepts. *Acta Medica Scandinavica Supplementum* **717**, 5–17.

Lister, R.G. (1985) The amnesic action of benzodiazepines in man. *Neuroscience and Biobehavioral Reviews* **9**, 87–94.

Lloyd, E.A. & Clark, L.D. (1959) Convulsions and delirium incident to glutethimide (doriden) withdrawal. *Diseases of the Nervous System* **20**, 524–526.

López-Muñoz, F., Ucha-Udabe, R. & Alamo, C. (2005) The history of barbiturates a century after their clinical introduction. *Neuropsychiatric Disease and Treatment* **1**, 329–343.

Loudon, J.B. & Waring, H. (1976) Toxic reactions to lithium and haloperidol. *Lancet* **ii**, 1088.

Louria, D.B. (1968) Lysergic acid diethylamide. *New England Journal of Medicine* **278**, 435–438.

Lovinger, D.M. & Homanics, G.E. (2007) Tonic for what ails us? High-affinity GABAA receptors and alcohol. *Alcohol* **41**, 139–143.

Lucki, I., Rickels, K. & Geller, A.M. (1986) Chronic use of benzodiazepines and psychomotor and cognitive test performance. *Psychopharmacology* **88**, 426–433.

Lundquist, G. (1961) Delirium tremens: a comparative study of pathogenesis, course, and prognosis with delirium tremens. *Acta Psychiatrica Scandinavica* **36**, 443–466.

Lynch, M.J.G. (1960) Brain lesions in chronic alcoholism. *Archives of Pathology* **69**, 342–353.

McClelland, H.A. (1986) Psychiatric reactions to psychotropic drugs. *Adverse Drug Reaction Bulletin* **119**, 444–447.

McDowell, J.R. & Le Blanc, H.J. (1984) Computed tomographic findings in Wernicke–Korsakoff syndrome. *Archives of Neurology* **41**, 453–454.

McKenna, D.J. & Peroutka, S.J. (1990) Neurochemistry and neurotoxicity of 3,4-methylenedioxymethamphetamine (MDMA, 'ecstasy'). *Journal of Neurochemistry* **54**, 14–22.

McMullen, P.A., Saint-Cyr, J.A. & Carlen, P.L. (1984) Morphological alterations in rat CA1 hippocampal pyramid cell dendrites resulting from chronic ethanol consumption and withdrawal. *Journal of Comparative Neurology* **225**, 111–118.

McNichol, R.W. (1970) *The Treatment of Delirium Tremens and Related States*. Thomas, Springfield, IL.

Mahaffey, K.R. (2000) Recent advances in the recognition of low-level methylmercury poisoning. *Current Opinion in Neurology* **13**, 699–707.

Malamud, N. & Skillicorn, S.A. (1956) Relationship between the Wernicke and the Korsakoff syndrome. *Archives of Neurology and Psychiatry* **76**, 585–596.

Mancuso, C.E. (2004) Paradoxical reactions to benzodiazepines: literature review and treatment options. *Pharmacotherapy* **24**, 1177–1185.

Martin, M., Ledent, C., Parmentier, M., Maldonado, R. & Valverde, O. (2000) Cocaine, but not morphine, induces conditioned place preference and sensitization to locomotor responses in CB1 knockout mice. *European Journal of Neuroscience* **12**, 4038–4046.

Mathias, S., Lubman, D.I. & Hides, L. (2008) Substance-induced psychosis: a diagnostic conundrum. *Journal of Clinical Psychiatry* **69**, 358–367.

Mattick, R.P., Kimber, J., Breen, C. & Davoli, M. (2008) Buprenorphine maintenance versus placebo or methadone maintenance for opioid dependence. *Cochrane Database of Systematic Reviews* 2, CD002207.

Medford, N., Baker, D., Hunter, E. *et al*. (2003) Chronic depersonalization following illicit drug use: a controlled analysis of 40 cases. *Addiction* **98**, 1731–1736.

Meyer, J.S., Tanahashi, N., Ishikawa, Y. *et al*. (1985) Cerebral atrophy and hypoperfusion improve during treatment of Wernicke–Korsakoff syndrome. *Journal of Cerebral Blood Flow and Metabolism* **5**, 376–385.

Minozzi, S., Amato, L., Vecchi, S. & Davoli, M. (2008a) Maintenance agonist treatments for opiate dependent pregnant women. *Cochrane Database of Systematic Reviews* 2, CD006318.

Minozzi, S., Amato, L., Davoli, M. *et al*. (2008b) Anticonvulsants for cocaine dependence. *Cochrane Database of Systematic Reviews* 2, CD006754.

Miyasaki, J.M. & Lang, A.E. (1995) Treatment of drug-induced movement disorders. In: Kurlan, R.J.B. (ed.) *Treatment of Movement Disorders*, ch. 11. Lippincott, Philadelphia.

Mohler, H., Fritschy, J.M. & Rudolph, U. (2002) A new benzodiazepine pharmacology. *Journal of Pharmacology and Experimental Therapeutics* **300**, 2–8.

Moienafshari, R., Bar-Oz, B. & Koren, G. (1999) Occupational exposure to mercury: what is a safe level? *Canadian Family Physician* **45**, 43–45.

Moore, T.H., Zammit, S., Lingford-Hughes, A. *et al*. (2007) Cannabis use and risk of psychotic or affective mental health outcomes: a systematic review. *Lancet* **370**, 319–328.

Morgan, H.G. (1968) Acute neuropsychiatric complications of chronic alcoholism. *British Journal of Psychiatry* **114**, 85–92.

Mukherjee, A.B., Svoronos, S., Ghazanfari, A. *et al*. (1987) Transketolase abnormality in cultured fibroblasts from familial chronic alcoholic men and their male offspring. *Journal of Clinical Investigation* **79**, 1039–1043.

Murray, R.M., Greene, J.G. & Adams, J.H. (1971) Analgesic abuse and dementia. *Lancet* **ii**, 242–245.

Murray, R.M., Morrison, P.D., Henquet, C. & Di Forti, M. (2007) Cannabis, the mind and society: the hash realities. *Nature Reviews of Neuroscience* **8**, 885–895.

Mutter, J., Naumann, J., Sadaghiani, C., Walach, H. & Drasch, G. (2004) Amalgam studies: disregarding basic principles of mercury toxicity. *International Journal of Hygiene and Environmental Health* **207**, 391–397.

Needleman, H.L., Schell, A., Bellinger, D., Leviton, A. & Allred, E. N. (1990) The long-term effects of exposure to low doses of lead in childhood. An 11-year follow-up report. *New England Journal of Medicine* **322**, 83–88.

Nestler, E.J. (2001) Molecular basis of long-term plasticity underlying addiction. *Nature Reviews of Neuroscience* **2**, 119–128.

Neuberger, K.T. (1957) The changing neuropathological picture of chronic alcoholism. *Archives of Pathology* **63**, 1–6.

Newman, P.K. & Saunders, M. (1979) Lithium neurotoxicity. *Postgraduate Medical Journal* **55**, 701–703.

Ngim, C.H., Foo, S.C., Boey, K.W. & Jeyaratnam, J. (1992) Chronic neurobehavioural effects of elemental mercury in dentists. *British Journal of Industrial Medicine* **49**, 782–790.

Nichols, D.E. (2004) Hallucinogens. *Pharmacology and Therapeutics* **101**, 131–181.

Nicolls, M.R. (2004) The clinical and biological relationship between Type II diabetes mellitus and Alzheimer's disease. *Current Alzheimer Research* **1**, 47–54.

Nisijima, K. & Ishiguro, T. (1990) Neuroleptic malignant syndrome: a study of CSF monoamine metabolism. *Biological Psychiatry* **27**, 280–288.

Nixon, P.F. (1984) Is there a genetic component to the pathogenesis of the Wernicke–Korsakoff syndrome? *Alcohol and Alcoholism* **19**, 219–221.

Normandin, L., Panisset, M. & Zayed. J. (2002) Manganese neurotoxicity: behavioural, pathological, and biochemical effects following various routes of exposure. *Reviews on Environmental Health* **17**, 189–217.

Normandin, L. Ann Beaupré, L., Salehi, F. *et al*. (2004) Manganese distribution in the brain and neurobehavioral changes following inhalation exposure of rats to three chemical forms of manganese. *Neurotoxicology* **25**, 433–441.

Null, G. & Feldman, M. (2002) Mercury dental amalgams: the controversy continues. *Journal of Orthomolecular Medicine* **17**, 85–110.

O'Brien, C.P. (2005a) Benzodiazepine use, abuse, and dependence. *Journal of Clinical Psychiatry* **66** (suppl. 2), 28–33.

O'Brien, C.P. (2005b) Anticraving medications for relapse prevention: a possible new class of psychoactive medications. *American Journal of Psychiatry* **162**, 1423–1431.

O'Brien, C.P., Volkow, N. & Li, T.K. (2006) What's in a word? Addiction versus dependence in DSM-V. *American Journal of Psychiatry* **163**, 764–765.

O'Carroll, R.E., Masterton, G., Dougall, N., Ebmeier, K.P. & Goodwin, G.M. (1995) The neuropsychiatric sequelae of mercury posioning. The Mad Hatter's disease revisited. *British Journal of Psychiatry* **167**, 95–98.

Olanow, C.W. (2004) Manganese-induced Parkinsonism and Parkinson's disease. *Annals of the New York Academy of Sciences* **1012**, 209–223.

O'Neill, S., Tipton, K.F., Pritchard, J.S. & Quinlan, A. (1984) Survival after high blood alcohol levels. Association with first-order elimination kinetics. *Archives of Internal Medicine* **144**, 641–642.

Osborne, J.W. & Albino, J.E. (1999) Psychological and medical effects of mercury intake from dental amalgam. A status report for the American Journal of Dentistry. *American Journal of Dentistry* **12**, 151–156.

Oscar-Berman, M. & Marinkovic, K. (2003) Alcoholism and the brain: an overview. *Alcohol Research and Health* **27**, 125–133.

Patrick, L. (2002) Mercury toxicity and antioxidants. Part 1: Role of glutathione and alpha-lipoic acid in the treatment of mercury toxicity. *Alternative Medicine Review* **7**, 456–471.

Penalver, R. (1955) Manganese poisoning. *Industrial Medicine and Surgery* **24**, 1–7.

Pentland, B. & Mawdsley, C. (1982) Wernicke's encephalopathy following hunger strike. *Postgraduate Medical Journal* **58**, 427–428.

Perlstein, M. & Attala, R. (1966) Neurologic sequelae of plumbism in children. *Clinical Pediatrics* **5**, 292–298.

Peter, A.L. & Viraraghavan, T. (2005) Thallium: a review of public health and environmental concerns. *Environment International* **31**, 493–501.

Pfefferbaum, A., Sullivan, E.V., Mathalon, D.H., Shear, P.K., Rosenbloom, M.J. & Lim, K.O. (1995) Longitudinal changes in magnetic resonance imaging brain volumes in abstinent and relapsed alcoholics. *Alcoholism: Clinical and Experimental Research* **19**, 1177–1191.

Pfefferbaum, A., Adalsteinsson, E. & Sullivan, E.V. (2006) Supratentorial profile of white matter microstructural integrity in recovering alcoholic men and women. *Biological Psychiatry* **59**, 364–372.

Porter-Williamson, K., Heffernan, E. & Von Gunten, C.F. (2003) Pseudoaddiction. *Journal of Palliative Medicine* **6**, 937–939.

Potamianos, G. & Kellett, J.M. (1982) Anti-cholinergic drugs and memory: the effects of benzhexol on memory in a group of geriatric patients. *British Journal of Psychiatry* **140**, 470–472.

Pratt, O.E., Jeyasingham, M., Shaw, G.K. & Thomson, A.D. (1985) Transketolase variant enzymes and brain damage. *Alcohol and Alcoholism* **20**, 223–232.

Price, J. & Kerr, R. (1985) Some observations on the Wernicke–Korsakoff syndrome in Australia. *British Journal of Addiction* **80**, 69–76.

Price, J., Kerr, R., Hicks, M. & Nixon, P.F. (1987) The Wernicke–Korsakoff syndrome: a reappraisal in Queensland with special reference to prevention. *Medical Journal of Australia* **147**, 561–565.

Prick, J.J.G. (1979) Thallium poisoning. In: Vinken, D.J. & Bruyn, G.W. (eds) *Intoxication of the Nervous System*, pp. 239–278. Handbook of Clinical Neurology, vol. 36. Elsevier North-Holland Biochemical Press, Amsterdam.

Quickfall, J. & Crockford, D. (2006) Brain neuroimaging in cannabis use: a review. *Journal of Neuropsychiatry and Clinical Neurosciences* **18**, 318–332.

Quinton, M.S. & Yamamoto, B.K. (2006) Causes and consequences of methamphetamine and MDMA toxicity. *AAPS Journal* **8**, E337–E347.

Rathbone, J., Variend, H. & Mehta, H. (2008) Cannabis and schizophrenia. *Cochrane Database of Systematic Reviews* 3, CD004837.

Reed, D., Crawley, J., Faro, S.N., Pieper, S.J. & Kurland, L.T. (1963) Thallotoxicosis. *Journal of the American Medical Association* **183**, 516–522.

Reed, L.J., Stevens, T.G. & Kopelman, M.D. (2003) Neuropsychiatric disorders. In: Warrell, D., Benz, E., Cox, T.M. & Firth, J.D. (eds) *Oxford Textbook of Medicine*, 4th edn, vol. 3, pp. 1273–1282. Oxford University Press, Oxford.

Reuler, J.B., Girard, D.E. & Cooney, T.G. (1985) Medical intelligence: current concepts. Wernicke's encephalopathy. *New England Journal of Medicine* **312**, 1035–1039.

Ricaurte, G.A., Forno, L.S., Wilson, M.A. *et al.* (1988) (±)3,4-Methylenedioxymethamphetamine selectively damages central serotonergic neurons in nonhuman primates. *Journal of the American Medical Association* **260**, 51–55.

Riley, J.N. & Walker, D.W. (1978) Morphological alterations in hippocampus after long-term alcohol consumption in mice. *Science* **201**, 646–648.

Rimalovski, A.B. & Aronson, S.M. (1966) Pathogenic observations in Wernicke–Korsakoff encephalopathy. *Transactions of the American Neurological Association* **91**, 29–31.

Rix, K.J.B. (1978) Alcohol withdrawal states. *Hospital Update* July, 403–407.

Robinson, T.E. & Berridge, K.C. (1993) The neural basis of drug craving: an incentive-sensitization theory of addiction. *Brain Research. Brain Research Reviews* **18**, 247–291.

Rojas, R., Riascos, R., Vargas, D., Cuellar, H. & Borne, J. (2005) Neuroimaging in drug and substance abuse. Part I: cocaine, cannabis, and ecstasy. *Topics in Magnetic Resonance Imaging* **16**, 231–238.

Romanelli, F., Smith, K.M., Thornton, A.C. & Pomeroy, C. (2004) Poppers: epidemiology and clinical management of inhaled nitrite abuse. *Pharmacotherapy* **24**, 69–78.

Ron, M.A. (1983) The alcoholic brain: CT scan and psychological findings. *Psychological Medicine Monograph Supplement* **3**.

Ron, M.A., Acker, W. & Lishman, W.A. (1980) Morphological abnormalities in the brains of chronic alcoholics. A clinical, psychological and computerised axial tomographic study. *Acta Psychiatrica Scandinavica Supplementum* **286**, 41–46.

Ron, M.A., Acker, W., Shaw, G.K. & Lishman, W.A. (1982) Computerised tomography of the brain in chronic alcoholism. A survey and follow-up study. *Brain* **105**, 497–514.

Rosebush, P.I., Stewart, T.D. & Gelenberg, A.J. (1989) Twenty neuroleptic rechallenges after neuroleptic malignant syndrome in 15 patients. *Journal of Clinical Psychiatry* **50**, 295–298.

Rosenbloom, M.J., Rohlfing, T., O'Reilly, A.W., Sassoon, S.A., Pfefferbaum, A. & Sullivan, E.V. (2007) Improvement in memory and static balance with abstinence in alcoholic men and women: selective relations with change in brain structure. *Psychiatry Research* **155**, 91–102.

Rosenthal, S.H. (1964) Persistent hallucinosis following repeated administration of hallucinogenic drugs. *American Journal of Psychiatry* **121**, 238–244.

Rouse, I.L. & Armstrong, B.K. (1988) Thiamin and alcoholic beverages: to add or not to add? *Medical Journal of Australia* **148**, 605–607.

Rubin, E., Aharonovich, E., Bisaga, A., Levin, F.R., Raby, W.N. & Nunes, E.V. (2007) Early abstinence in cocaine dependence: influence of comorbid major depression. *American Journal on Addictions* **16**, 283–290.

Rusyniak, D.E. & Nanagas, K.A. (2004) Organophosphate poisoning. *Seminars in Neurology* **24**, 197–204.

Ryan, C. & Butters, N. (1980) Further evidence for a continuum-of-impairment encompassing male alcoholic Korsakoff patients and chronic alcoholic men. *Alcoholism: Clinical and Experimental Research* **4**, 190–198.

Ryback, R.S. (1971) The continuity and specificity of the effects of alcohol on memory. *Quarterly Journal of Studies on Alcohol* **32**, 995–1016.

Sabot, L.M., Gross, M.M. & Halpert, E. (1968) A study of acute alcoholic psychoses in women. *British Journal of Addiction* **63**, 29–49.

Salonen, J.T., Seppänen, K., Nyyssönen, K. et al. (1995) Intake of mercury from fish, lipid peroxidation, and the risk of myocardial infarction and coronary, cardiovascular, and early death in eastern Finnish men. *Circulation* **91**, 645–655.

Santhakumar, V., Wallner, M. & Otis, T.S. (2007) Ethanol acts directly on extrasynaptic subtypes of GABAA receptors to increase tonic inhibition [Review]. *Alcohol* **41**, 211–221.

Schifano, F. (2004) A bitter pill. Overview of ecstasy (MDMA, MDA) related fatalities. *Psychopharmacology (Berl)* **173**, 242–248.

Schou, M. (1984) Long-lasting neurological sequelae after lithium intoxication. *Acta Psychiatrica Scandinavica* **70**, 594–602.

Schroth, G., Naegele, T., Klose, U., Mann, K. & Peterson, D. (1988) Reversible brain shrinkage in abstinent alcoholics, measured by MRI. *Neuroradiology* **30**, 385–389.

Seeber, A., Meyer-Baron, M. & Schäper, M. (2002) A summary of two meta-analyses on neurobehavioural effects due to occupational lead exposure. *Archives of Toxicology* **76**, 137–145.

Sellers, J., Tyrer, P., Whiteley, A., Banks, D.C. & Barer, D.H. (1982) Neurotoxic effects of lithium with delayed rise in serum lithium levels. *British Journal of Psychiatry* **140**, 623–625.

Shimamura, A.P., Jernigan, T.L. & Squire, L.R. (1988) Korsakoff's syndrome: radiological (CT) findings and neuropsychological correlates. *Journal of Neuroscience* **8**, 4400–4410.

Shulgin, A. & Shulgin, A. (1991) *PiHKAL: Phenethylamines i Have Known And Loved. A Chemical Love Story*. Transform Press, Berkeley, CA.

Sloboda, Z. (2002) Changing patterns of 'drug abuse' in the United States: connecting findings from macro- and microepidemiologic studies. *Substance Use and Misuse* **37**, 1229–1251.

Smith, S.J.M. & Kocen, R.S. (1988) A Creutzfeldt–Jakob like syndrome due to lithium toxicity. *Journal of Neurology, Neurosurgery and Psychiatry* **51**, 120–123.

Soares, B.G., Lima, M.S., Reisser, A.A. & Farrell, M. (2003) Dopamine agonists for cocaine dependence. *Cochrane Database of Systematic Reviews* **2**, CD003352.

Spiers, J. & Hirsch, S.R. (1978) Severe lithium toxicity with 'normal' serum concentrations. *British Medical Journal* **1**, 815–816.

Spillane, J.D. (1947) *Nutritional Disorders of the Nervous System*. Livingstone, Edinburgh.

Spittle, B. & Parker, J. (1993) Wernicke's encephalopathy complicating schizophrenia. *Australia and New Zealand Journal of Psychiatry* **27**, 638–682.

Spring, G.K. (1979) Neurotoxicity with combined use of lithium and thioridazine. *Journal of Clinical Psychiatry* **40**, 135–138.

Steece-Collier, K., Maries, E. & Kordower, J.H. (2002) Etiology of Parkinson's disease: genetics and environment revisited. *Proceedings of the National Academy of Sciences USA* **99**, 13972–13974.

Steenland, K. (1996) Chronic neurological effects of organophosphate pesticides. *British Medical Journal* **312**, 1312–1313.

Sternberg, D.E. (1986) Neuroleptic malignant syndrome: the pendulum swings. *American Journal of Psychiatry* **143**, 1273–1275.

Sterns, R.H., Riggs, J.E. & Schochet, S.S. (1986) Osmotic demyelination syndrome following correction of hyponatremia. *New England Journal of Medicine* **314**, 1535–1542.

Stewart, S.H. & Westra, H.A. (2002) Benzodiazepine side-effects: from the bench to the clinic. *Current Pharmaceutical Design* **8**, 1–3.

Sullivan, E.V., Rosenbloom, M.J. & Lim, K.O. (2000a) Longitudinal changes in cognition, gait, and balance in abstinent and relapsed alcoholic men: relationships to changes in brain structure. *Neuropsychology* **14**, 178–188.

Sullivan, E.V., Deshmukh, A., Desmond, J.E., Lim, K.O. & Pfefferbaum, A. (2000b) Cerebellar volume decline in normal aging, alcoholism, and Korsakoff's syndrome: relation to ataxia. *Neuropsychology* **14**, 341–353.

Sullivan, E.V., Rosenbloom, M.J. & Pfefferbaum, A. (2002) A profile of neuropsychological deficits in alcoholic women. *Neuropsychology* **16**, 74–83.

Summers, W.K. (1998) Bismuth toxicity masquerading as Alzheimer's dementia. *Journal of Alzheimer's Disease* **1**, 57–59.

Supino-Viterbo, V., Sicard, C., Risvegliato, M., Rancurel, G. & Buge, A. (1977) Toxic encephalopathy due to ingestion of bismuth salts: clinical and EEG studies of 45 patients. *Journal of Neurology, Neurosurgery and Psychiatry* **40**, 748–752.

Sweeney, D.F. (1990) Alcoholic blackouts: legal implications. *Journal of Substance Abuse Treatment* **7**, 155–159.

Takebayashi, T., Omae, K., Ishizuka, C. et al. (1998) Cross-sectional observations of the effects of carbon disulphide on the nervous system, endocrine system, and subjective symptoms in rayon manufacturing workers. *Occupational and Environmental Medicine* **55**, 473–479.

Takeda, A. (2003) Manganese action in brain function. *Brain Research. Brain Research Reviews* **41**, 79–87.

Takeuchi, T., Eto, N. & Eto, K. (1979) Neuropathology of childhood cases of methylmercury poisoning (Minamata disease) with prolonged symptoms, with particular reference to the decortication syndrome. *Neurotoxicology* **1**, 1–20.

Tarter, R.E. & Schneider, D.U. (1976) Blackouts: relationship with memory capacity and alcoholism history. *Archives of General Psychiatry* **33**, 1492–1496.

Tennent, R.M. (1971) *Science Data Book*. Oliver and Boyd, Edinburgh.

Thomas, C.J. (1979) Brain damage with lithium/haloperidol. *British Journal of Psychiatry* **134**, 552.

Thomas, M.J., Kalivas, P.W. & Shaham, Y. (2008) Neuroplasticity in the mesolimbic dopamine system and cocaine addiction. *British Journal of Pharmacology* **154**, 327–342.

Tong, S., Baghurst, P., McMichael, A., Sawyer, M. & Mudge, J. (1996) Lifetime exposure to environmental lead and children's intelligence at 11–13 years: the Port Pirie cohort study. *British Medical Journal* **312**, 1569–1575.

Tornatore, F.L., Sramek, J.J., Okeya, B.L. & Pi, E.H. (1987) *Reactions to Psychotropic Medication*. Plenum Medical Book Co., New York.

Torvik, A., Lindboe, C.F. & Rogde, S. (1982) Brain lesions in alcoholics. A neuropathological study with clinical correlations. *Journal of the Neurological Sciences* **56**, 233–248.

Traviesa, D.C. (1974) Magnesium deficiency: a possible cause of thiamine refractoriness in Wernicke–Korsakoff encephalopathy. *Journal of Neurology, Neurosurgery and Psychiatry* **37**, 959–962.

Tsai, Y.T., Huang, C.C., Kuo, H.C. et al. (2006) Central nervous system effects in acute thallium poisoning. *Neurotoxicology* **27**, 291–295.

Tune, L.E., Holland, A., Folstein, M.F., Damlouji, N.F., Gardener, T.J. & Coyle, J.T. (1981) Association of post-operative delirium with raised serum levels of anticholinergic drugs. *Lancet* **ii**, 651–652.

Turner, S., Daniels, L. & Greer, S. (1989) Wernicke's encephalopathy in an 18-year-old woman. *British Journal of Psychiatry* **154**, 261–262.

Ungerleider, J.T., Fisher, D.D. & Fuller, M. (1966) The dangers of LSD. *Journal of the American Medical Association* **197**, 389–392.

Verheyden, S.L., Henry, J.A. & Curran, H.V. (2003) Acute, subacute and long-term subjective consequences of 'ecstasy' (MDMA) consumption in 430 regular users. *Human Psychopharmacology* **18**, 507–517.

Victor, M. (1966) Treatment of alcoholic intoxication and the withdrawal syndrome. *Psychosomatic Medicine* **28**, 636–650.

Victor, M. & Adams, R.D. (1953) The effect of alcohol on the nervous system. In: *Metabolic and Toxic Diseases of the Nervous System*, ch. 28. Research Publications of the Association for Research in Nervous and Mental Disease, vol. 32. Williams & Wilkins, Baltimore.

Victor, M. & Hope, J.M. (1958) The phenomenon of auditory hallucinations in chronic alcoholism. A critical evaluation of the status of alcoholic hallucinosis. *Journal of Nervous and Mental Disease* **126**, 451–481.

Victor, M., Adams, R.D. & Mancall, E.L. (1959) A restricted form of cerebellar cortical degeneration occurring in alcoholic patients. *Archives of Neurology* **1**, 579–688.

Victor, M., Adams, R.D. & Collins, G.H. (1971) *The Wernicke–Korsakoff Syndrome*. Blackwell Scientific Publications, Oxford.

Victor, M., Adams, R.D. & Collins, G.H. (1989) *The Wernicke–Korsakoff Syndrome and Related Neurologic Disorders due to Alcoholism and Malnutrition*, 2nd edn. F.A. Davis, Philadelphia.

Volkow, N.D., Wang, G.J., Fowler, J.S. & Telang, F. (2008a) Overlapping neuronal circuits in addiction and obesity: evidence of systems pathology. *Philosophical Transactions of the Royal Society of London B* **363**, 3191–3200.

Volkow, N.D., Fowler, J.S., Wang, G.J., Baler, R. & Telang, F. (2008b) Imaging dopamine's role in drug abuse and addiction. *Neuropharmacology* **56** (suppl. 1), 3–8.

Von Bose, M.J. & Zaudig, M. (1991) Encephalopathy resembling Creutzfeldt–Jakob disease following oral, prescribed doses of bismuth nitrate. *British Journal of Psychiatry* **158**, 278–280.

Wahl, M.J. (2001) Amalgam-resurrection and redemption. Part 2. The medical mythology of anti-amalgam. *Quintessence International* **32**, 696–710.

Walker, D.W., Barnes, D.E., Riley, J.N., Hunter, B.E. & Zornetzer, S.F. (1980a) Neurotoxicity of chronic alcohol consumption: an animal model. In: Sandler, M. (ed.) *Psychopharmacology of Alcohol*, p. 607. Raven Press, New York.

Walker, D.W., Barnes, D.E., Zornetzer, S.F., Hunter, B.E. & Kubanis, P. (1980b) Neuronal loss in hippocampus induced by prolonged ethanol consumption in rats. *Science* **209**, 711–713.

Warkany, J. & Hubbard, D.M. (1951) Adverse mercurial reactions in the form of acrodynia and related conditions. *American Journal of Diseases of Children* **81**, 335–373.

Weinstein, M.C. (1978) Prevention that pays for itself. *New England Journal of Medicine* **299**, 307–308.

Weiss, R.D., Mirin, S.M. & Bartel, R.L. (1994) *Cocaine*, 2nd edn. American Psychiatric Press, Washington, DC.

Weller, M. & Kornhuber, J. (1992) Clozapine rechallenge after an episode of 'neuroleptic malignant syndrome'. *British Journal of Psychiatry* **161**, 855–856.

Wesseling, C. & Keifer, M. (2002) Long term neurobehavioural effects of mild poisonings with organophosphate and N-methyl carbamate pesticides among banana workers. *International Journal of Occupational and Environmental Health* **8**, 27–34.

West, J.R., Lind, M.D., Demuth, R.M. *et al.* (1982) Lesion-induced sprouting in the rat dentate gyrus is inhibited by repeated ethanol administration. *Science* **218**, 808–810.

Williams, J.F. & Storck, M. (2007) American Academy of Pediatrics Committee on Substance Abuse and American Academy of Pediatrics Committee on Native American Child Health. Inhalant abuse. *Pediatrics* **119**, 1009–1017.

Winer, J.W., Rosenwasser, R.H. & Jimenez, F. (1991) Electroencephalographic activity and serum and cerebrospinal fluid pentobarbital levels in determining the therapeutic end point during barbiturate coma. *Neurosurgery* **29**, 739–741.

Winstock, A.R. (1991) Chronic paranoid psychosis after misuse of MDMA. *British Medical Journal* **302**, 1150–1151.

Wolkowitz, O.M., Weingartner, H., Thompson, K., Pickar, D., Paul, S.M. & Hommer, D.W. (1987) Diazepam-induced amnesia: a neuropharmological model of an 'organic amnesic syndrome'. *American Journal of Psychiatry* **144**, 25–29.

Yamaguchi, H., Kidachi, Y. & Ryoyama, K. (2002) Toluene at environmentally relevant low levels disrupts differentiation of astrocyte precursor cells. *Archives of Environmental Health* **57**, 232–238.

Yücel, M., Takagi, M., Walterfang, M. & Lubman, D.I. (2008) Toluene misuse and long-term harms: a systematic review of the neuropsychological and neuroimaging literature. *Neuroscience and Biobehavioral Reviews* **32**, 910–926.

Zandstra, S.M., Furer, J.W., van de Lisdonk, E.H. *et al.* (2002) Different study criteria affect the prevalence of benzodiazepine use. *Social Psychiatry and Psychiatric Epidemiology* **37**, 139–144.

CHAPTER 12

Movement Disorders

Max Henderson[1] and John D.C. Mellers[2]

[1] Institute of Psychiatry, King's College, London
[2] Maudsley Hospital, London

The movement disorders form a substantial part of neurological practice and have gradually attracted increasing psychiatric interest. This is partly on account of their psychiatric concomitants, for example a high incidence of depression in Parkinson's disease and of behavioural disturbance in the opening stages of hepatolenticular degeneration. Biochemical research, particularly in relation to dopamine metabolism, has revealed analogies between the changes thought to underlie certain movement disorders and those postulated to occur in major psychiatric illnesses. Yet more striking has been the explosion in the use of functional neuroimaging techniques, which have produced a more detailed understanding of both normal and abnormal cerebral activity. An increased awareness of biological substrates for aspects of neurological conditions previously thought to be 'functional' has followed. Ultimately these developments promise new treatment options.

Traditional neuroleptic medications induced a wide range of movement disorders. Both neurologists and psychiatrists were required to be conversant in their management. Whilst this undoubtedly remains the case, the growth in the use of the atypical antipsychotics has resulted in a fall in the incidence of drug-induced motor symptoms. Prescribers now need to be aware of other complications such as obesity and diabetes.

Other movement disorders, such as spasmodic torticollis, blepharospasm and Gilles de la Tourette's syndrome, reflect the striking influence that mental factors may bring to bear on motor dysfunction. So close is this interaction that psychogenic factors may appear to be solely responsible for causing such conditions, yet other evidence suggests that cerebral malfunction may be primarily to blame. Marked psychosensitivity need carry no implications for psychogenesis *per se*, yet attempts to discern the true situation can prove to be difficult. In the discussion of such disorders below, the arguments advanced in both directions will be presented.

Drug-induced disorders

Soon after the introduction of phenothiazines to psychiatric practice it became apparent that extrapyramidal movement disorders ranked high among the unwanted effects of treatment. Until the introduction of clozapine, the successive development of new neuroleptics failed to solve the problem, in that all major tranquillisers appeared to share these side effects in some degree. Indeed, their propensity to disturb extrapyramidal function proved to be roughly proportional to their antipsychotic effect, although earlier ideas that the two were necessarily linked to one another have not been upheld.

Among the phenothiazines, those with a piperazine side chain (e.g. trifluoperazine) show more marked extrapyramidal effects than those with aliphatic or piperidine side chains (e.g. chlorpromazine, thioridazine). The butyrophenones (haloperidol, benperidol, droperidol) are particularly potent in this regard. The thioxanthenes (e.g. flupentixol) may induce the whole range of disorders considered below. The atypical antipsychotics show a much reduced propensity to produce movement disorders but the risk is not eliminated.

Clinical pictures

Four main syndromes have been delineated, namely parkinsonism, akathisia, acute dystonic reactions and the group of disorders at present subsumed under the term 'tardive dyskinesia'. Tardive dystonia and tardive akathisia have been recognised more recently. Precise estimates of the incidence of all such conditions have been hard to obtain, on account of variations in prescribing practice and differences in the populations surveyed. Nevertheless, it is now firmly established that the drugs are to be blamed rather than inherent aspects of the psychiatric disorders themselves. Exactly analogous movement disorders are induced whether the neuroleptics are given for schizophrenia, affective disorder, neurotic disability or for the control of chronic pain. It must be granted, however, that the stereotypies and mannerisms of chronic schizophrenia can at times lead to diagnostic difficulty and even obscure for a while the development of the extrapyramidal symptoms.

The clinical pictures encountered are fully described in comprehensive reviews by Marsden *et al.* (1975), Miyasaki and Lang (1995) and Sachdev (2005) and may be summarised as follows.

Parkinsonism

Parkinsonian features usually develop insidiously, often within a week and almost always within the first month of treatment, often coincident with the onset of antipsychotic activity (Wirshing 2001). The development of parkinsonism is broadly dose dependent, increasing as higher levels of neuroleptics are achieved. However, it emerges in only some 20–40% of persons, individual susceptibility being important. The incidence increases with age, as with idiopathic Parkinson's disease.

All the features of idiopathic Parkinson's disease (see Parkinson's disease and the parkinsonian syndrome, later in the chapter) may be induced. Bradykinesia is the earliest and commonest sign, with muscular rigidity and disturbance of posture and gait developing later. The upper extremities are commonly affected first followed by the jaw and then the lower extremities. The symptoms are usually bilateral (Sachdev 2005) and are more commonly symmetrical than in idiopathic Parkinson's disease (Rodnitzky 2002). Tremor is a good deal less common than with the idiopathic disease, the exception being the occasional appearance late in the course of treatment of fine perioral tremor ('rabbit' syndrome). The latter generally sets in after months or years of therapy as with tardive dyskinesia. Sialorrhoea may occur due to a reduced swallowing rate, in contrast to that associated with clozapine which is caused by increased saliva production (Wirshing 2001).

With continuation of the drugs the parkinsonian features may gradually subside as tolerance develops. Short of this they will usually resolve over the course of several weeks when the drugs are stopped. However, Marsden and Jenner (1980) stress that occasional patients continue to show parkinsonism for as long as 18 months after cessation of therapy. In the rare examples that fail to recover thereafter, one may usually presume that idiopathic Parkinson's disease had already been present.

With the more severe extrapyramidal reactions provoked by potent neuroleptics, the clinical picture may occasionally come to resemble 'catatonia'. Gelenberg and Mandel (1977) described a group of patients showing negativism, withdrawal, posturing and waxy flexibility, of gradual onset usually in the first few weeks of treatment. Incontinence of urine was sometimes observed. Behrman (1972) has described mutism, sometimes progressing to the full syndrome of akinetic mutism. Such developments may easily be confused with worsening of schizophrenic symptomatology, leading to increase in dosage of the offending medication. In contrast, stopping the drugs can lead to slow resolution. The differential diagnosis includes neuroleptic malignant syndrome.

Akathisia

Akathisia consists of motor restlessness accompanied by subjective feelings of inner tension and discomfort referable chiefly to the limbs. It often coexists with parkinsonian features but is possibly even more common: it occurs in up to 90% of young patients but the incidence decrease with age. The symptoms can be considerably distressing and are a frequent cause of poor drug compliance. The patient complains of being driven to move, of pulling sensations in the legs and an inability to keep them still. The disorder usually appears within the first few days of treatment but may only develop as higher dosage is achieved. Both subjective and objective aspects need to be present for the diagnosis and it is now thought that the observable behaviours are a response to these inner feelings of tension (Wirshing 2001). Barnes (1989) has produced a rating scale for assessment of both the observable and subjective components of the syndrome. Sometimes the latter are lacking (pseudoakathisia), chiefly in patients with negative psychotic symptoms (Barnes & Braude 1985).

Braude *et al.* (1983) investigated motor restlessness in detail by ratings of subjective sensations and objective manifestations in a large group of patients on antipsychotic medication. A principal components analysis served to delineate the akathisia syndrome more precisely. Mild examples presented mainly subjectively; inner restlessness was a common and non-specific symptom, but complaints clearly referable to the legs characterised the akathisia group. These leg sensations are deep – paraesthesiae are uncommon. Patients with moderate akathisia showed in addition a tendency to rock from foot to foot or to walk on the spot, along with coarse tremor or myoclonic jerks in the feet. Patients with severe akathisia showed difficulty in maintaining their position, for example shuffling or tramping the feet when sitting, rising repeatedly when seated, or walking or pacing when attempting to stand still. In the most severe forms patients may be unable to tolerate any position, whether sitting, lying or standing, for more than a few minutes.

Continuation of the drugs may allow the symptoms to subside, but this is not invariable. An extrapyramidal origin is postulated, but the evidence for this is mainly inferential.

Akathisia must be distinguished from the restless legs syndrome (Ekbom's syndrome) which may resemble it closely (Trenkwalder *et al.* 2005). This is seen in the absence of neuroleptic medication, usually in patients who are otherwise in normal health. However, associations have been noted with iron-deficiency anaemia, renal failure and pregnancy. Physical examination typically shows no neurological abnormality. The condition is more common than previously thought with a prevalence of 6–9% in community surveys. The majority of patients have mild symptoms with spontaneous remissions and never seek medical attention. It may occur at any age, including childhood, but is more common in older people. There is a female preponderance and a strong genetic predisposition.

Diagnostic criteria for restless leg syndrome have recently been defined (Allen *et al.* 2003). An urge to move the legs is usually accompanied by marked leg discomfort, with creeping sensations, dysaesthesiae or sensations of cold or weakness, usually most pronounced in the calves. The desire to move arises directly from such discomforts, which are temporarily relieved by activity such as stretching or walking. Symptoms characteristically show a marked diurnal variation and occur only, or are worse, in the evening and at night. Insomnia and daytime sleepiness are common and may occaisionally be severe. In part this is attributable to difficulty getting to sleep because of the symptoms. In addition, however, some 80% of patients have periodic limb movements during sleep: frequent, involuntary, repetitive, stereotyped movements of the legs during sleep that can be associated with microarousals and sleep deprivation. Central dopaminergic abnormalities and disturbances of iron metabolism have been implicated in the disorder. All patients should be investigated for iron deficiency and iron supplements given if serum ferritin is low. Dopaminergic agents are recognised as first-line treatment. Alternatives include opioids, gabapentin and other antiepileptic drugs, clonazepam and clonidine. Long-term treatment wth dopaminergic agents may be associated with exacerbation of symptoms, emphasising the importance of treating only significantly disabling symptoms.

Acute dystonia

Acute dystonic reactions are considerably rarer than the above reactions, affecting perhaps some 2% of patients. They develop abruptly and early in the course of treatment, within a few days of oral treatment or within hours of intramuscular injection. The more potent piperazine phenothiazines and the butyrophenones are chiefly responsible. Young adults and children appear to be particularly susceptible, and males have outnumbered females in most surveys. It is more common in those who have previously had a dystonic reaction and in those known to have abused cocaine (Cortese *et al.* 2004; Stubner *et al.* 2004).

The patient is seized with strong sustained or intermittent uncontrolled muscular contractions that are frequently painful and deeply alarming. Deviation of the eyes, blepharospasm, trismus and grimacing are common. Severe examples show tongue protrusion, dysphagia and respiratory stridor. Extension to the neck and trunk can lead to torticollis, retrocollis, writhing and opisthotonos. Continuous slow writhing may affect the limbs, with dystonic postures of hyperpronation and adduction.

Marked examples may be mistaken for status epilepticus or tetanus by the inexperienced observer. Hysteria may be diagnosed when muscular spasms are remittent. The disorder is self-limiting and usually of no more than several hours' duration, although therapeutic intervention will often be indicated for the relief of acute distress.

Tardive dyskinesia

As experience was gained of long-term neuroleptic medication it became apparent that a range of movement disorders make their first appearance only late in the course of treatment. These have attracted considerable attention, on account of their sometimes seriously disabling nature and because in a proportion of patients they can prove to be irreversible. The term 'tardive dyskinesia' is used to refer to such late developments rather than to any phenomenologically distinct dyskinetic picture. Although tardive dystonia and perhaps tardive akathisia are now seen as distinct entities, tardive dyskinesia may include choreiform, myoclonic and athetoid movements.

The commonest site of the abnormal movements is around the mouth and tongue, which become involved in a more or less continuous flow of choreiform activity (orofacial dyskinesia, bucco-linguo-masticatory dyskinesia). The tongue protrudes, twists and curls, along with incessant chewing, pouting and sucking movements of the lips, jaw and cheeks. In severe examples talking and eating can be hampered. The upper face tends typically to be spared, but may show tic-like blinking or blepharospasm. The neck may be affected with twisting dystonic movements.

Involvement of the trunk, arms, hands and legs may also be observed (Kidger *et al.* 1980). The distal extremities show choreiform and athetotic movements, with finger twisting and spreading, tapping of the feet and dorsiflexion of the toes. Abnormalities of gait and posture show as lordosis, rocking and shoulder shrugging. Grunting and disturbance of the respiratory rhythm may be in evidence. Overall, three-quarters of patients have orofacial involvement, half have limb involvement and one-quarter have involvement of the trunk. Factor analysis applied to ratings of involvement of different body regions has suggested that there may be relatively independent subvarieties, affecting respectively the jaws and tongue, the face and lips, and the extremities and trunk (Glazer *et al.* 1988). These may possibly have differing aetiological and prognostic connotations.

Altogether the picture may come to involve a complex admixture of tics, chorea, athetosis, dystonia and myoclonic jerks; however, rhythmic tremor is not seen. It may worsen dramatically with emotional stress and it decreases with drowsiness. Choreiform movements appear to be commoner in the elderly, and dystonic pictures in the young. Age also influences the topography, orolingual movements being especially common in the elderly.

A similar disorder is known to occur spontaneously, especially in the elderly, with up to 6% of those in their seventh decade affected (Klawans 1980). In patients on long-term neuroleptics, however, tardive dyskinesia is far from uncommon. Variable estimates have resulted from different surveys, depending among other factors on readiness to include very minor degrees of movement disorder. The working party appointed by the American Psychiatric Association (Task Force on Late Neurological Effects of

Antipsychotic Drugs 1980) concluded that 10–20% of people given antipsychotic drugs for a year or more could be expected to develop a clinically appreciable tardive dyskinesia, the rate probably being higher in the elderly. A review by Yassa and Jeste (1992) suggested a median figure of 24%. Woerner *et al.* (1998) found a rate of 25% after 1 year's exposure, which increased to 53% after 3 years' exposure. However, disabling degrees are rare. Sachdev (2000) reported that 5–10% of patients will have some degree of functional impairment relating to their tardive dyskinesia. In particular, eating difficulties have led to weight loss. Although cases can follow only 1 month's exposure (Jeste *et al.* 1999), the great majority of patients will have been on neuroleptics for at least 2 years when the disorder makes its first appearance and often for considerably longer. Operational criteria for duration of neuroleptic exposure and chronicity are included in the Diagnostic and Statistical Manual of Mental Disorders (DSM)-IV: 3 months' exposure to neuroleptics is required in the under-60s and 1 month's exposure in the over-60s. The symptoms must last more than 4 weeks. It is labelled 'persistent' if lasting longer than 3 months and 'chronic' if more than 6 months.

Among the predisposing factors highlighted in certain surveys are age, sex and evidence of brain damage. There is a marked increase in incidence after the age of 40, and a female preponderance among the elderly. The influence of pre-existing brain damage has been less uniformly upheld (Sachdev 2005), but associations have been reported with a history of exposure to electroconvulsive therapy (ECT) or leucotomy, likewise evidence of cognitive dysfunction or negative symptoms in schizophrenia (Waddington & Youssef 1986; Barnes 1987). In McClelland *et al.*'s (1991) long-term follow-up of hospitalised patients, the development of facial dyskinesia was significantly associated with ventricular enlargement on computed tomography (CT). More than one study has suggested that patients with a history of acute dyskinesias are at greater risk. Patients with organic psychiatric disorders have shown an especially high prevalence (Yassa *et al.* 1984). An increased risk has been reported in diabetics (Ganzini *et al.* 1991) and van Os *et al.* (1997) reported a threefold increase in risk of tardive dyskinesia in patients who had abused alcohol. A single study has found an association with a variant of the dopamine D_3 receptor gene (Steen *et al.* 1997), and Andreassen *et al.* (1997) reported an increased risk in patients homozygous for mutated alleles of the cytochrome P450 2D6 gene.

The evidence that patients with affective disorders may be more at risk than patients with schizophrenia is reviewed by Barnes (1987), likewise indications that depressive symptomatology in the course of schizophrenia may confer additional risk. There is some evidence that prolonged exposure or exposure to high dosage of neuroleptics may increase the chance of developing the condition, but this is disputed. The Yale study, in which a large cohort of patients was followed

prospectively for evidence of the condition developing, has been exceptional in finding a clear positive relationship to neuroleptic dose (Morganstern & Glazer 1993). It is clear, however, that most patients will have received large total quantities before tardive dyskinesia supervenes. The concomitant administration of anticholinergics appears to increase the severity of the disorder but probably does not alter the risk of its development. Use of atypical antipsychotics carries a significantly lower risk. Jeste *et al.* (1999) reported a 5–10 times lower incidence with risperidone than haloperidol, and Tollefson *et al.* (1997) observed similar results with olanzapine. A noteworthy feature is that the first signs very often make their appearance when the drugs are discontinued or the dosage is lowered. Indeed the previously common practice of 'drug holidays' is associated with an increased risk of tardive dyskinesia (Goldman & Luchins 1984).

A disturbing aspect of the condition is its liability to persist despite stopping the medication. A majority of patients will improve substantially, usually within months but sometimes taking 1 or 2 years for complete resolution. Between one-quarter and half of all patients may be expected to improve markedly within a year (Task Force on Late Neurological Effects of Antipsychotic Drugs 1980). More recent 5-year follow-up data from Bergen *et al.* (1989) showed about half were stable and unchanging, one-quarter showed a fluctuating course, 11% improved and 8% worsened. Between years 5 and 10, half of patients will show a reduction in symptoms of 50%. In children complete recovery can be predicted, but in some 30% of adults the condition seems destined to be permanent, especially in the elderly.

In addition to neuroleptics, the condition may follow the prescription of other medications that also affect dopamine neurotransmission. Examples include oral contraceptives, anticonvulsants, tricyclic antidepressants and dopaminergic drugs which are not antipsychotics such as metoclopramide (Leo 1996). Similar dyskinesias are seen in frank neurological disorders such as Huntington's disease, Sydenham's chorea, Hallervorden–Spatz syndrome and Fahr's disease.

Tardive dystonia

Burke *et al.* (1982) and more recently Rodnitzky (2002) have described a syndrome of 'tardive dystonia' that appears to be attributable to antipsychotic medication. As with tardive dyskinesia it typically follows several years of treatment with the drugs, and once established tends to be persistent. However, the nature of the movement disorder is quite different. The dystonia consists of sustained slow twisting movements affecting the limbs, trunk, neck or face. Unlike tardive dyskinesia, it typically causes severe distress to the patient and can result in significant neurological disability.

The disorder typically begins after 3–7 years of neuroleptic exposure but may occur within the first year (Burke *et al.*

1982; Kang *et al.* 1986, 1988). Males may be affected earlier than females (Kiriakakis *et al.* 1998). Onset in some two-thirds of patients is focal. As the dystonia progresses there is usually spread so that by the time the condition plateaus, usually after several months, over two-thirds of cases have a segmental dystonia, with some 15% having a generalised distribution. Younger patients tend to have a more generalised picture, older patients more focal. Focal cases may present identical pictures to torticollis, blepharospasm or oromandibular dystonia. The presentation in generalised cases may be indistinguishable from idiopathic torsion dystonia, though a family history of such a condition is lacking. Sustained postures are sometimes seen in addition to the slow twisting movements, sometimes relieved by small tactile manoeuvres as in dystonia generally (see under The dystonias, later in chapter). The movements generally abate during sleep. A history of tardive dyskinesia is seen in approximately half of patients, although pharmacologically the two disorders are distinct: anticholinergic agents are sometimes beneficial for the dystonic movements but tend to exacerbate tardive dyskinesia. Withdrawal of neuroleptics is the mainstay of treatment but prognosis is disappointing. Up to half of patients will show some improvement but remission is seen in less than 15%. Exposure to neuroleptics for less than 10 years predicted a favourable outcome in one study (Kiriakakis *et al.* 1998).

Davis *et al.* (1988) extended the spectrum of disorders encountered, reporting three patients with laryngospasm as part of the clinical picture, sometimes developing abruptly and requiring tracheostomy, and two patients with spasmodic dysphonia.

In all cases differentiation must be made from Wilson's disease by appropriate diagnostic studies, also from other symptomatic dystonias when there are abnormal neurological signs. A primary blepharospasm, oromandibular dystonia or torticollis must be considered when there are no dyskinetic movements. The distinction from classic tardive dyskinesia can at times be difficult and both may occur together; the distinction is chiefly important because of the different options presented for treatment (see Management/Tardive dystonia, later in chapter). Finally, it is important to beware of mistaking the picture for a psychogenic disorder, particularly when the movements are bizarre or influenced transiently by emotion, suggestion or an interview after amobarbital administration.

Tardive akathisia

A syndrome of 'tardive' or 'chronic' akathisia has been distinguished from the acute form, usually developing after some years on neuroleptics. It may coexist with features of tardive dyskinesia, including orofacial dyskinesia and choreoathetoid movements of the limbs, and like tardive dyskinesia it may worsen on dose reduction whereas acute akathisia tends to be aggravated by increase in dosage.

Burke *et al.* (1989) have presented the features seen in 52 cases. The condition had developed after a mean of 4.5 years on dopamine antagonists, but in on-third had developed within a year. Complex stereotyped movements consisted of marching on the spot, frequent crossing and uncrossing of the legs, trunk rocking, grunting, moaning and face rubbing or scratching. Half of the patients managed to stop neuroleptics, and the symptoms then persisted for a mean of 2.5 years. The younger patients did better than the old. Attempts at therapy were frequently disappointing (see Management/Tardive akathisia). The condition can be profoundly disabling, leading to inner torment, irritability and inability to concentrate.

Pathophysiology

The pathophysiology of the neuroleptic-induced movement disorders appears to be associated with various aspects of the dopamine–acetylcholine balance within the brain, more particularly within the corpus striatum. However, earlier views have become progressively more complex, with the discovery of both inhibitory and excitatory dopamine receptors in the striatum, and the demonstration of feedback striatonigral pathways that may be mediated in part by cholinergic or γ-aminobutyric acid (GABA)ergic mechanisms. The maintenance of correct dopamine and acetylcholine levels in the striatum is clearly under highly complex control and stands to be disturbed in a multitude of ways. Hence, no doubt, the variety of movement disorders encountered when this balance is altered by drugs. Discussions of the hypotheses put forward in attempts at explanation are provided by Marsden and Jenner (1980), Baldessarini and Tarsy (1980), Miyasaki and Lang (1995) and Casey (2004).

Among their many pharmacological actions, all neuroleptics have powerful effects on cerebral dopamine mechanisms. These correlate highly with their antipsychotic potency. The phenothiazines, butyrophenones and thioxanthenes act specifically to block cerebral dopamine D_2 receptors. Reserpine and tetrabenazine operate differently, interfering with the intraneuronal granular uptake and storage of dopamine. Clozapine differs from the typical antipsychotics in that it has weak effects on striatal dopamine D_2 receptors, high affinity for D_4 and D_1 receptors, and a relatively strong blocking effect on serotonin S_2 receptors (Advokat 2005).

Drug-induced parkinsonism appears to be chemically closely analogous to naturally occurring Parkinson's disease. The blockade of dopamine receptors within the striatum amounts to 'chemical denervation', resulting in relative dopamine deficiency. Anticholinergic drugs can accordingly be of benefit by helping to restore the correct dopamine–acetylcholine balance. More complex theories are now emerging that relate to the speed with which the drug dissociates from the dopamine receptor (Kapur & Seeman 2001). The rapid dissociation hypothesis suggests that atypical antipsychotics bind to D_2 receptors for long enough to be antipsychotic but not long enough to cause parkinsonism.

The genesis of akathisia is little understood, but may rest on dopamine receptor blockade in brain areas other than the striatum. It is interesting that this is the only form of movement disorder which may develop within a few hours of starting treatment, i.e. within the time frame of dopamine receptor blockade with neuroleptics. However, it is clear from pharmacological responses that other neurotransmitters must also be involved, including central adrenergic systems. Separate pathophysiology is thought to be involved in the acute and tardive forms given that acute forms worsen with an increase in neuroleptic dose whereas the tardive form improves.

The mechanisms underlying acute dystonic reactions also remain obscure. Their peak incidence at 24–48 hours from the initiation of therapy is well after the peak onset of dopamine receptor blockade. They may reflect interference with presynaptic dopamine mechanisms, or there may be a mismatch between excess release of dopamine and coincident hypersensitivity of dopamine receptors. Neuroleptics principally occupy D_2 receptors, and the increased dopamine turnover may be expressed through overactivation of unblocked D_1 receptors. Again, however, it is likely that other neurotransmitter systems are also implicated; Jeanjean *et al.* (1997) suggest neuroleptic binding to σ opiate receptors is important.

There is probably not a unitary pathophysiology for tardive dyskinesia; various patterns of movement emerge after varying lengths of treatment and differ in their persistence. It has been especially difficult to explain why drugs which block striatal dopamine receptors should eventually produce forms of dyskinesia known to be associated with dopamine overactivity in the striatum. Thus the choreiform movements of tardive dyskinesia resemble those seen as a complication of levodopa therapy in Parkinson's disease, and the administration of levodopa or anticholinergic drugs exacerbates the condition. The prolonged blockade may have led to this end-result by virtue of increased dopamine turnover coupled with upregulation of receptor numbers, possibly with an imbalance between D_1 and D_2 receptors. Alternatively, hypersensitivity of D_2 receptors may cause them to respond abnormally to the dopamine reaching them (Klawans *et al.* 1980). Hypersensitivity of this nature probably accounts for the worsening of the condition on withdrawal of neuroleptics and the success of their reintroduction in ameliorating the condition. However, attempts to demonstrate dopamine receptor supersensitivity by positron emission tomography (PET) or at autopsy have been relatively unsuccessful.

Animal studies have indicated that over the course of prolonged neuroleptic administration, dopamine receptor blockade may actually slowly disappear, giving way to supersensitivity in its place. Moreover, the latter can be shown to persist for many months after withdrawal, providing an analogy to the possible situation in tardive dyskinesia in humans (Clow *et al.* 1979a,b). It remains difficult, nevertheless, to reconcile the very late appearance of tardive dyskinesia with the supersensitivity known to develop soon after starting neuroleptics, and it is likely that complex interactions with other neurotransmitters are also partly responsible. A role for GABA neurones in the striatum has been suggested (Gerlach & Casey 1988).

No convincing pathology has been described in the brain to account for those tardive dyskinesias that become irreversible. Structural or neurotoxic changes in the neurones, affecting their membranes or the cell respiratory mechanisms, must nevertheless be postulated in such cases. One such theory is suggested by Cadet and Lohr (1989) and Gunne and Andren (1993), who argue that tardive dyskinesia results from neuronal loss especially of GABAergic neurones projecting from the globus pallidus to the thalamus. This may be due to excess free radicals or excitotoxicity, both of which lead to apoptotic cell death. This cell death leads to disinhibition of lateral pallidal neurones, which may be responsible for the hyperkinetic state of tardive dyskinesia. A number of lines of evidence support this hypothesis. Neuroleptics increase catecholamine turnover, which leads to excess free radical production. They also lead to accumulation of iron in the basal ganglia. Some (mixed) reports find a beneficial role for antioxidants in the treatment and prevention of tardive dyskinesia. Finally, it is consistent with age, diabetes, smoking and brain damage being additional risk factors (Sachdev 2000).

Management

The management of movement disorders occurring as side effects of antipsychotic treatment must take into account every effort at prevention. As we have seen, the range of movement disorders encountered is, at the very least, stigmatising and at worst profoundly disabling and tormenting. Most physicians are now reluctant to prescribe neuroleptics as first-line drugs and will instead opt for atypical antipsychotics. If a conventional neuroleptic is to be prescribed, there is no firm evidence that any particular phenothiazine, butyrophenone or thioxanthene is less hazardous than others. Dosage and duration of neuroleptics should be kept to a minimum and long-term maintenance therapy strictly reserved for patients in whom definite benefit can be expected. In practice this usually means patients with chronic schizophrenia of a type liable to manifest ongoing positive symptoms in the absence of medication. Where a movement disorder has developed, clearly drug withdrawal is the first step. In cases where antipsychotic treatment is still required there is obviously an even more compelling argument in favour of switching to an atypical agent.

Parkinsonism

Anticholinergic drugs are of value in controlling drug-induced parkinsonism. It often transpires, however, that once parkinsonian features have come under control, the antiparkinsonian medication can be withdrawn without recrudescence of the motor disorder. It should therefore be tapered off after 3 months for a trial period. Long-continued anticholinergic administration as a routine adjunct to neuroleptic treatment is now considered to be contraindicated. Levodopa should theoretically help drug-induced parkinsonism, but has been little used to date. Some reviewers suggest it is ineffective (Sachdev 2005).

Akathisia

When akathisia is a persisting and disabling complaint the most decisive remedy is reduction of drug dosage (Braude *et al.* 1983). Benzodiazepines may help in some degree as may amantadine or clonidine (Miller & Fleischhacker 2000). Anticholinergics are now rarely used because of a lack of effectiveness and because of the risk of exacerbating tardive dyskinesia. However, the most encouraging results appear to be obtained with beta-blockers such as propranolol, which can reduce both subjective and objective manifestations of the syndrome (Adler *et al.* 1986) possibly by having some cross-affinity with serotonergic receptors.

Acute dystonia

For acute dystonic reactions, anticholinergic drugs are best given parenterally. Benzatropine, diphenhydramine and procyclidine can be administered intravenously and are often dramatically effective. Intravenous diazepam can also help. For milder reactions it is important to remember the efficacy of non-specific calming of the patient, or simple sedation with diazepam. The previous occurrence of dystonic reactions constitutes one of the few indications for the prophylactic prescription of anticholinergic drugs from the start of a course of neuroleptic medication, although care needs to be taken with elderly patients.

Tardive dyskinesia

Once tardive dyskinesia is detected, anticholinergic drugs should be discontinued immediately. The next step is to reduce the dosage of neuroleptics gradually and if possible stop them altogether. This may lead to an initial worsening of the condition, but in favourable cases it will be a temporary exacerbation. Some 30–50% of patients will improve as a result, but this may occur only gradually over a number of months or years. If the mental state does not permit total withdrawal, it may be possible to settle for a lower dose. Current practice often consists of substituting the current medication with another (Taylor *et al.* 2005). Some evidence suggests that clozapine may be an effective treatment for tardive dyskinesia (Casey 1989; Louza & Bassitt 2005). When

the movements persist, other treatments may be tried but the number advocated indicates that none is universally successful. Drugs that deplete striatal dopamine may be used (Teoh 1988). Tetrabenazine is the only licensed treatment in the UK but should be avoided in patients with pre-existing depression. Donepezil has shown benefits in a single study (Caroff *et al.* 2001). Benzodiazepines may be useful by virtue of their sedating effect and are widely used. More recent treatments evaluated by double-blind comparisons include clonazepam (Thaker *et al.* 1990) and vitamin E used as a free-radical scavenging agent (Elkashef *et al.* 1990). Gabapentin appears to be effective, adding weight to the theory that GABAergic mechanisms improve tardive dyskinesia (Hardoy *et al.* 1999). Evidence is also available for melatonin (Shamir *et al.* 2001) and pyridoxine (Lerner *et al.* 2001).

Quite often, however, it will be found that no available therapy ameliorates the condition and one must merely hope for spontaneous resolution. The temptation to control the dyskinesia by reintroducing neuroleptics at increased dosage is strictly to be avoided, except in those rare cases where life is threatened by the severity of the involuntary movements. While it may be highly efficacious in producing short-term relief, this merely postpones the problem by reinstating the original pathogenesis and can be expected to worsen the ultimate disability.

Tardive dystonia

Tardive dystonia presents equally severe management problems and the results of treatment are often disappointing. The first step should be to taper or discontinue the causative drugs or change to alternative therapy. Anticholinergic drugs such as trihexyphenidyl (benzhexol) can help, though at the expense of worsening any coincident tardive dyskinesia. Reserpine or tetrabenazine were associated with improvement in two-thirds of patients (Kang *et al.* 1986). Diazepam, lorazepam or baclofen may also be successful.

Clozapine holds special promise and has been reported to help after fruitless attempts with other drugs, leading to slow improvement over several months (Lamberti & Bellnier 1993). It would certainly appear to be the drug of choice in patients whose psychosis requires the continuation of neuroleptics (Friedman 1994; Van Harten *et al.* 1996; Karp *et al.* 1999). The combination of clozapine and clonazepam has sometimes proved to be particularly effective (Shapleske *et al.* 1996). If the dystonia is localised, for example in the cervical region, botulinum toxin might be used (Brashear *et al.* 1998; Molho *et al.* 1998). There is a single report of bilateral thalamotomy being effective (Yadalam 1990).

Tardive akathisia

Treatment of tardive akathisia can be particularly difficult, not least because discontinuation of neuroleptics may lead to transient worsening. This should nevertheless be attempted, even though few cases will benefit substantially. Burke *et al.* (1989) found that reserpine and tetrabenazine were the most successful drugs, though only one-third of their patients achieved complete resolution of symptoms. Anticholinergics and beta-blockers were without effect, although lorazepam improved occasional patients markedly. Sometimes the reintroduction of neuroleptics at higher dosage may ultimately need to be tried.

Parkinson's disease and the parkinsonian syndrome

The cardinal neurological deficits that comprise the syndrome of parkinsonism are tremor, muscular rigidity, bradykinesia and postural abnormality. A large number of other associated features are also characteristic as described below.

By far the commonest form is idiopathic parkinsonism or paralysis agitans, as described by James Parkinson in 1817. This owes its origin to a specific degeneration of pigmented cells in the brainstem, particularly those of the substantia

nigra. Substantial changes in our understanding of the genetic aspects of the disease have occurred in the last decade. The background lifetime risk of 2% (Elbaz *et al.* 2002) doubles where there is a positive family history (Fahn 2003) and a genetic component is more likely in those whose symptoms start before the age of 50 (Tanner *et al.* 1999).

Since 1997 at least 11 genes or genetic loci have been associated with Parkinson's disease (Dekker *et al.* 2003; Pankratz & Foroud 2004; Hague *et al.* 2005). At present these genes account for only a very small proportion of patients with the disorder and yet these discoveries have led to a better understanding of the pathogenesis of Parkinson's disease and promising directions for developing entirely new approaches to treatment. The genes and loci have been designated *PARK-1, PARK-2,* etc., corresponding approximately to the order in which they were discovered (Table 12.1). In most cases the genes and loci have been identified in very rare families showing a simple mendelian pattern of disease inheritance, but some of these findings are now being

Table 12.1 Genes and loci associated with Parkinson's disease. (Adapted from Dekker *et al.* 2003 and Hague *et al.* 2005.)

Locus	Gene	Chromosomal location	Inheritance	Onset	Clinical features	Estimated attributable risk
PARK-1	α-Synuclein	4q21–q23	AD	Late	Less tremor, rapid progression	Small
PARK-2	Parkin	6q25.2–q27	AR	Early: juvenile	Dyskinesia, dystonia Slow progression	PD overall: 0.4–0.7% Early onset PD: 9–18% Early-onset recessive PD: 49%
PARK-3		2p13	AD	Late	Dementia in some patients	Small
PARK-4	α-Synuclein triplication	4q21–q23	AD	Early	Rapid progression, postural tremor, late dementia	Single report
PARK-5	UCHL-1	4p14	AD	Late	None	Single report
PARK-6	PINK-1	1p35–p36	AR	Early	Slow progression	Early-onset recessive PD: up to 15%
PARK-7	DJ-1	1p36	AR	Early	Slow progression	Locally in Dutch isolate: 33% early-onset PD Generally: unknown
PARK-8	LRRK-2	12p11.2–q13.1	AD	Late	None	1–6% prevalence in familial and sporadic PD
PARK-9		1p36	AR	Juvenile	Kufor–Rakeb syndrome, spasticity, dementia, supranuclear gaze paralysis	Single report
PARK-10		1p32	NM	Late	None	Linkage to age at onset reported in Icelandic study
PARK-11		2q36–q37		Late	None	

AD, autosomal dominant; AR, autosomal recessive; LRRK-2, leucine-rich repeat kinase 2; NM, non-mendelian; PD, Parkinson's disease; UCHL-1, ubiquitin carboxy-terminal hydrolase 1.

extended in order to identify putative genetic vulnerability factors in apparently sporadic (idiopathic) Parkinson's disease. The first gene to be identified was α-synuclein on chromosome 4. Three autosomal dominantly inherited point mutations in this gene have been described, including the original Greek family, other southern Mediterranean families and a single German family. A family with triplication of a large region that included the α-synuclein gene has also been reported. In contrast, many different mutations have been described in the parkin gene on chromosome 6. Parkin mutations may account for up to 50% of early-onset cases showing an autosomal recessive pattern of inheritance, but have also been described in patients with late-onset apparently sporadic Parkinson's disease and have been reported as showing autosomal dominant inheritance. Leucine-rich repeat kinase 2 has been identified as the causative gene at the *PARK-8* locus for an autosomal dominantly inherited disease. More significantly, a mutation in this gene has now been described in up to 6% of patients with apparent sporadic Parkinson's disease.

While the α-synuclein gene has been identified in only a few families, its discovery has been of great importance because it has provided new insights into the pathogenesis of Parkinson's disease. The identification of α-synuclein in particular, but also that of parkin and some of the other genes, have disclosed an important pathogenic role for the ubiquitin–proteosome system, a cytoplasmic complex that breaks down aggregates of misfolded, unassembled or damaged protein. Aggregates of α-synuclein are a substrate for breakdown by the ubiquitin–proteosome system. Mutant α-synuclein protein is associated with excess aggregate formation, as are a variety of environmental factors including oxidative stress, heavy metals and pesticides. Although such aggregation may represent a protective mechanism, it appears that when aggregate formation exceeds the capacity of the proteosome system, it accumulates (as Levy bodies) and is associated with cell death (apoptosis). Genetic mutations in parkin and ubiquitin carboxy-terminal hydrolase 1 (in *PARK-5*) lead to impaired protein degradation by the proteosome. Novel therapeutic possibilities include neuroprotective strategies targeting proteins in the proteosome system, aiming to inhibit aggregate formation or enhance protein degradation. There has been considerable interest in the possibility of genetic testing but because the genes identified so far are relatively rare and in many cases of uncertain penetrance, there is no agreed protocol for genetic testing or counselling. However, the field is developing rapidly.

A parkinsonian picture may be induced by certain medications such as reserpine, phenothiazines, butyrophenones and methyldopa (drug-induced parkinsonism). This tends to remit slowly over several weeks or months when the offending drug is withdrawn. A similar syndrome, postencephalitic parkinsonism, was a common aftermath of the pandemics of encephalitis lethargica that occurred almost 80 years ago (see Course and outcome, later). Cases could appear up to 20 years after the original infection, which was sometimes very mild. An early age of onset suggested the postencephalitic variety, also oculogyric crises, abnormal pupil reactions or continuing marked sleep disturbance.

Many other conditions that affect the basal ganglia may cause akinetic rigid syndromes along with other features resulting from diffuse brain damage, for example repeated head injuries in boxing, cerebral syphilis, anoxia due to cardiac arrest, or poisoning with carbon monoxide or manganese. Such a syndrome may appear as part of other degenerative disorders, such as progressive supranuclear palsy, multiple system atrophy, Alzheimer's disease, Lewy body dementia, Wilson's disease or cerebral arteriosclerosis. The latter, however, is no longer recognised as a cause of Parkinson's disease *per se*, and the category of 'arteriosclerotic parkinsonism' has fallen into disrepute (Eadie & Sutherland 1964; Pallis 1971). Certainly the clinical features that were used to delineate this form of the syndrome were variable from one observer to another. An arteriosclerotic origin tended to be blamed when the onset had been acute or progression had occurred in a step-like manner, when progressive dementia coincided with or preceded the parkinsonism, or when pseudobulbar palsy or pyramidal deficits were present. *Marche à petit pas* seemed also to be characteristic of the variety. However, it is hard to establish a causal relationship to cerebral arterial disease when this exists, and the two disorders may simply occur together by coincidence. In Eadie and Sutherland's (1964) study no more clinical evidence of arterial disease could be found in a large group of parkinsonian patients than among equivalent age-matched controls. Nonetheless, the area remains of interest to a number of investigators. Improvements in clinical diagnosis mean that only 1% of the UK Parkinson's Disease Brain Bank series needed reclassifying to vascular parkinsonism. It has been estimated to account for only 3% of cases of parkinsonism in elderly Europeans (de Rijk *et al.* 1997). Winikates and Jankovic (1999) have devised a rating scale for the diagnosis of vascular parkinsonism.

Clinical features

The idiopathic disease is slightly commoner among men than women. The mean age of onset is 55 years with two-thirds of cases beginning between 50 and 59 (Hoehn & Yahr 1967). Excellent accounts of the clinical features and natural history are given by Selby (1990), Pearce (1992) and Fahn (2003).

Tremor is the presenting feature in about three-quarters of the idiopathic cases and consists of alternating contractions of opposing muscle groups (frequency 4–6 Hz). It is present at rest but ceases during sleep, and may become less marked when the limb is engaged in voluntary movement. It is worsened by excitement, anxiety and fatigue.

Most typically it appears in the hands as flexio-extension movements affecting the metacarpophalangeal joints of the fingers and thumb. It is common also in the jaw and tongue and may come to affect the head or the lower limbs. In some cases it is predominantly or entirely unilateral.

Rigidity affects the large and small muscles of the limbs, trunk and neck, involving agonists and antagonists equally and through the whole range of passive movement. In these respects it is quite unlike the spasticity that results from corticospinal tract damage, and feels to the examining hand to have a 'lead pipe' or 'plastic' quality. When tremor is also present, the rigidity is broken up ('cogwheel' rigidity). Rigidity, like tremor, can be predominantly unilateral. It persists during sleep and is unaffected by emotional factors.

Bradykinesia consists of poverty and slowness of movement. This is not due solely to rigidity since stereotactic surgery can relieve rigidity without improving bradykinesia. Bradykinesia is not always sufficiently emphasised in descriptions of the disorder yet can be the most disabling aspect to the patient. Sometimes it dominates the entire picture. It shows in slowness in the initiation and execution of motor acts, and poverty of automatic and associated movements such as the normal swinging of the arms when walking. Fleminger (1992) has shown that it can be distinguished from the motor retardation of depression by certain dual task performance tests. Bradykinesia probably accounts for many of the classic features of parkinsonism: the mask-like face, infrequent blinking, clumsiness of fine finger movement, crabbed writing and monotonous speech. The striking disorder of prosody evident in the speech of patients with Parkinson's disease has been shown to be related to motor control, not loss of linguistic knowledge or associated depression (Darkins et al. 1988). The gait is affected in many characteristic ways, with slowness, shuffling, difficulty in starting and turning, and impaired equilibrium. It may show an episodic quality, causing periodic freezing of action or episodes of complete immobility. More than any other feature, bradykinesia can be profoundly affected by the patient's mental state. There are numerous reports of severely disabled patients achieving surprising feats of motor behaviour in response to fear, excitement or other environmental stimulation.

Postural changes show as a characteristic flexion of the trunk and neck bringing the chin to the chest, with arms adducted at the shoulders and flexed at elbows, wrists and knuckles. The typical 'festinant' gait appears to be a product of the abnormal posture along with difficulty in controlling the centre of gravity. Postural instability leads to frequent falls.

Other features include oculomotor abnormalities, excessive salivation, seborrhoea, constipation, urinary disturbance, subjective sensory discomfort and marked fatigue. Infrequent blinking is common in all forms of parkinsonism, and paresis of convergence may occur. The latter is par-

ticularly common in postencephalitic parkinsonism, which may also show oculogyric crises. Sialorrhoea is mainly the result of difficulties in coping with normal quantities of saliva on account of dysphagia. Constipation is a major symptom of the disease and a cause of much distress. Urinary frequency and incontinence are frequent complaints. Sensory discomforts include feelings of tightness, pain and cramp in the limbs and back. The fatigue associated with the disorder is often particularly distressing and disabling. It has been found to correlate better with coexistent depression than with the severity of motor symptoms but is often independent of both (Friedman & Friedman 1993).

There has been increased interest in the olfactory dysfunction that is present in 70–100% of patients (Hawkes & Shephard 1998; Katzenschlager et al. 2004). Many patients are unaware of a loss of smell but if they are it can predate the onset of motor disturbance by over a year (Henderson et al. 2003). As such it may be an aid to early diagnosis.

In the detection of early cases the following observations can be useful. The patient shows difficulty when asked to maintain a steady rhythmic movement, as in tapping or making polishing movements. The handwriting often reveals changes at an early stage, as do attempts to draw parallel lines or spirals. The glabellar tap reflex is elicited by tapping over the root of the nose between the eyebrows; parkinsonian patients are said to blink in response to each tap no matter how often or at what frequency, and fail to habituate as normal subjects do. Observation of the gait can also be revealing in early cases when attention is directed at the lack of arm swinging, difficulty in turning sharply or the exacerbation of tremor in the hands.

Course and outcome

Idiopathic parkinsonism is usually a progressive disease. Difficulties with diagnostic certainty mean studies of prognosis and mortality must be viewed cautiously, although improved treatment has had a definite impact on survival. Life expectancy in well-treated idiopathic Parkinson's disease should be nearly normal. Several studies have found a mortality rate of 1.6 compared with control groups. Mean life expectancy from diagnosis is 14 years. A small number, however, show very slow progression and remain without severe disablement after 20 years or more. Factors associated with increased mortality include advanced age, dementia, depression and lack of levodopa responsiveness. There is evidence that smoking is protective. Common causes of death are cardiac and cerebral vascular disease, bronchopneumonia and neoplasia. The prognosis in terms of rate of progression and mortality is better for postencephalitic cases and worse for vascular parkinsonism and those in whom the diagnosis is unsure since a number of these will ultimately be diagnosed with multiple system atrophy or progressive supranuclear palsy.

Pathology and pathophysiology

Parkinson's disease is associated with lesions in component parts of the extrapyramidal nervous system. The most striking finding is degeneration and loss of neurones in the pars compacta of the substantia nigra, seen macroscopically as nigral pallor. The surviving neurones characteristically show Lewy bodies within their cytoplasm, the pathological hallmark of the condition. These are inclusion bodies with characteristic eosinophilic staining surrounded by a clear halo (Fig. 12.1: see also Plate 12.1). Gibb and Lees (1989) were able to demonstrate Lewy bodies in the remaining pigmented nuclei of the substantia nigra in every case that conformed to strict clinicopathological criteria for idiopathic Parkinson's disease. Lewy bodies consist of ubiquitin and α-synuclein. They are found in other brainstem nuclei, especially the locus caeruleus, raphe nuclei and dorsal vagal nucleus, as well as in the hypothalamus and nucleus basalis of Meynert. In up to one-third of cases they are also apparent in the parahippocampus and temporal neocortex (Gibb & Lees 1987). Glial scarring is seen in the brainstem in the islands from which neurones have disappeared. Cellular degeneration is often apparent in the globus pallidus, putamen and caudate, possibly by virtue of trans-synaptic degeneration. Diffuse cortical atrophy has been reported to be common, and possibly greater than would be expected for healthy individuals of equivalent age. Braak *et al.* (2004) have described six stages through which the pathology of Parkinson's disease progresses. Wider cerebral involvement occurs at each stage. Of note is that in the first two stages symptoms are most unlikely. They suggest that symptoms only arise when a critical degree of neuronal loss, about 70%, has occurred.

In postencephalitic parkinsonism the pigmented cells of the substantia nigra and locus caeruleus are similarly lost, but neurofibrillary changes rather than Lewy bodies are seen in those that remain.

The cardinal biochemical feature of parkinsonism is striatal dopamine deficiency caused by loss of dopaminergic fibres in the nigrostriatal tract, which passes from the pars compacta of the substantia nigra to the caudate and putamen. Consequently, dopamine concentrations in these regions may be reduced to 10–20% of normal levels. The net result is increased inhibitory striatal input to the globus pallidus and thence changes in many parts of the extrapyramidal system, which conspire to produce the parkinsonian picture (Stacy & Jankovic 1992).

The connections of the basal ganglia, and the neurotransmitters involved, are complex and as yet incompletely understood (Stacy & Jankovic 1992; Harding 1993). Multiple parallel loops are present in the extrapyramidal system, two of which predominate. The striatum (i.e. caudate nucleus and putamen) receives glutamatergic projections from all parts of the cortex that pass to their small spiny neurones. These neurones use GABA and a variety of peptides as their neurotransmitters. They project to the lateral globus pallidus and from there to the subthalamic nucleus. This in turn sends glutamatergic projections to the internal segment of the globus pallidus, which projects to the ventrolateral nucleus of the thalamus and back to the cortex.

The second major loop involves GABAergic projections from the striatum to the pars reticulata of the substantia nigra, and dopaminergic projections back from the pars compacta of the substantia nigra in the dense nigrostriatal pathway. The striatum also contains large cholinergic interneurones; dopamine and acetylcholine appear to be

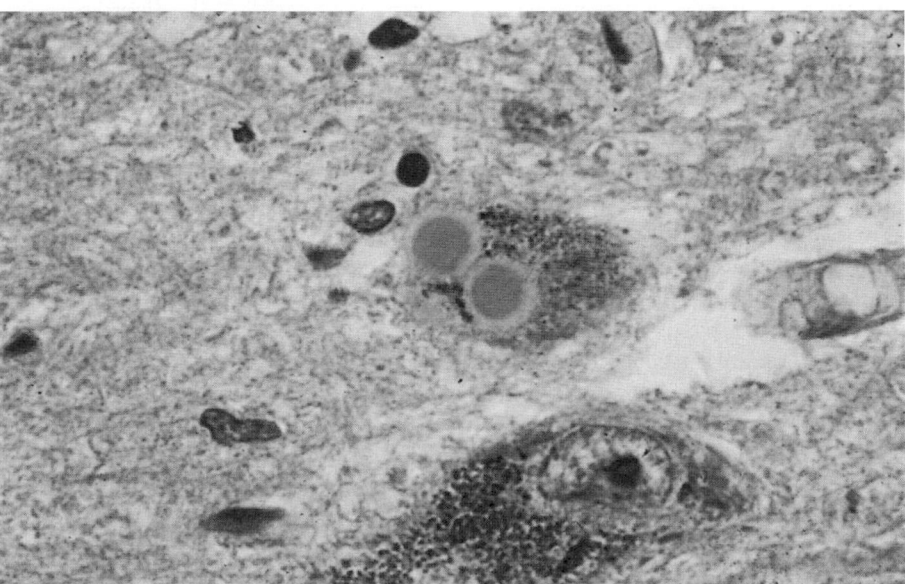

Fig. 12.1 Lewy bodies in the substantia nigra (haematoxylin and eosin). Magnification ×600. (Courtesy of Professor Peter Lantos.) See also Plate 12.1.

antagonistic in their effects in the striatum, and any condition that alters the balance in the direction of marked cholinergic dominance leads to parkinsonism. However, it is clear that dopamine deficiency will also alter the balance of excitatory and inhibitory activity in many parts of the extrapyramidal system, and that the evolution of parkinsonian symptoms will depend on changes in several of its components.

The losses of dopamine in the striatum can be detected by functional neuroimaging. The presynaptic uptake of ^{18}F-labelled dopa by the dopamine transporter is reduced in the caudate and putamen in comparison with age-matched controls, the degree of decline correlating with severity of locomotor disability (Brooks *et al.* 1990). The posterior part of the putamen is most severely affected, with reductions averaging 45% of normal, the anterior putamen and caudate being less markedly involved (62% and 84% of normal levels respectively). This pattern differs from that seen with progressive supranuclear palsy (see Corticobasal degeneration, later in chapter), which shows equally severe reductions in all parts of the putamen and caudate. There is also evidence from studies with ^{11}C-raclopride that the density of D$_2$ binding sites is slightly upregulated in the putamen in untreated Parkinson's disease, but without change in the caudate (Sawle *et al.* 1990). Studies using single photon emission computed tomography (SPECT) have found that postsynaptic D$_2$ receptors are preserved, suggesting that only presynaptic fibres are affected in Parkinson's disease. Studies using ^{18}F-fluorodeoxyglucose PET have shown reduced glucose metabolism in the lentiform nucleus contralateral to the affected limb in early disease; much more widespread dysfunction is seen in advanced disease. Colloby and O'Brien (2004) provide a helpful review. Reductions in presynaptic dopamine transporter are also detectable by both SPECT and PET using a number of tropane-based tracers (Brooks *et al.* 2003). These techniques have a sensitivity of around 90% in distinguishing patients with early symptomatic Parkinson's disease from normals and from those with essential tremor and are increasingly becoming part of clinical practice. However, the extent to which a normal dopamine transporter scan might be relied upon to exclude the diagnosis of Parkinson's disease in the presence of symptoms is still uncertain.

In addition to the nigrostriatal pathway, other dopaminergic neurones in the ventral tegmental area of the brainstem project to the cortex and limbic structures. There is evidence that these 'mesolimbic' and 'mesocortical' pathways are also impaired in Parkinson's disease, which may be relevant to some of the psychiatric complications discussed below.

Interesting evidence has recently been obtained concerning the possible origin of the selective degeneration of dopaminergic neurones in the substantia nigra in the disease. The discovery that 1-methyl-4-phenyl-1,2,3,6-tetrahydropyridine (MPTP) taken by drug addicts could result in parkinsonism (Langston *et al.* 1983) has led to the hypothesis that environmental toxins could conceivably play a part. MPTP induces neuronal death via its metabolite, 1-methyl-4-phenyl-pyridine (MPP), which has been shown to inhibit NADH-CoQ$_1$ reductase (complex I), the first enzyme of the mitochondrial respiratory chain (Nicklas *et al.* 1985). Complex I was then shown to be selectively deficient in the substantia nigra of patients with Parkinson's disease, with normal activities of this and other respiratory chain enzymes in other brain areas (Schapira *et al.* 1989, 1990a,b). No such abnormality was present in patients with multiple system atrophy, which also leads to parkinsonism, suggesting that it may be causally related to Parkinson's disease rather than a consequence of the neuronal degeneration. MPP$^+$ is produced by the action of monoamine oxidase B on MPTP; it is taken up by the presynaptic dopamine transporter and is then actively absorbed and concentrated in mitochondria. Inhibition of complex I of the mitochondrial respiratory chain results in the formation of a highly toxic superoxide anion (Zhang *et al.* 2000). MPTP intoxication is now widely used as a model for studying Parkinson's disease.

Additional evidence comes from the finding of abnormalities in sulphur metabolism and *N*-methylation in the disease (Steventon *et al.* 1989; Green *et al.* 1991). Both reflect deficiencies in the metabolic pathways for removing toxins from the body, suggesting that patients with Parkinson's disease may have been unusually susceptible to environmental toxins with MPP-like activity. Support for such an idea comes from the observation that several environmental toxins can cause parkinsonism, for example carbon monoxide and manganese. Efforts continue to find an environmental toxin that acts in a similar way that might be responsible for sporadic disease. Genetic susceptibility to these or other widespread toxic agents could conceivably play a role in the genesis of the disorder.

There is now increased awareness of the role played by non-dopaminergic neurotransmitter systems in Parkinson's disease. Several strands of evidence point to serotonergic dysfunction. There are reduced serotonergic binding sites in the frontal cortex and basal ganglia (Paulus & Jellinger 1991) and lower levels of the 5-hydroxytryptamine (5HT) metabolite 5-hydroxyindoleacetic acid in the cerebrospinal fluid of patients with Parkinson's disease (Mayeux *et al.* 1988a). Changes in 5HT may be implicated in depression (see Affective disorder, later). Depressed parkinsonian patients have greater neuronal loss from the dorsal raphe, which contains serotonergic neurones, than non-depressed patients (Mayberg *et al.* 2000). Neuronal loss also occurs in the noradrenergic cells of the locus caeruleus (Bertrand *et al.* 1997; Soldani & Fornai 1999). Noradrenergic projections to the frontal cortex are impaired (Everitt *et al.* 1990). These changes would be expected to disrupt attentional processes and Bedard *et al.* (1998) have produced supporting neuropsychological evidence of noradrenergic dysfunction. Improvement in attentional performance followed administration of a noradrenergic agonist. Evidence of a cholinergic deficit comes from a number of areas. Patients with Parkinson's disease show loss of ascending cholinergic projection from the nucleus basalis of Meynert and reductions in neurotransmitter enzymes such as choline acetyltransferase (Perry *et al.* 1985; Rinne *et al.* 1991; Shinotoh *et al.* 1999).

Differential diagnosis

The diagnosis is usually apparent once the disease is reasonably well advanced but mistakes can occur in the early stages, particularly if tremor is absent. In elderly patients the signs may be overlooked and complaints of back or limb pain may lead to a diagnosis of arthritis or osteoporosis. Alternatively, the presentation may be with unexpected falls, which are attributed to vertebrobasilar insufficiency. Strictly unilateral rigidity in the absence of tremor can raise suspicion of a cerebral tumour. Marked bradykinesia may at first raise the question of myxoedema or depressive illness. In patients with evidence of intellectual deterioration the parkinsonian features may be overlooked in favour of a diagnosis of Alzheimer's disease (see Chapter 9).

Rapid fluctuations in the early stages can suggest a psychiatric disorder by way of neurosis, hysteria or even malingering. Such suspicion will be increased if the family reports that the patient can function entirely normally in the face of a stressful situation. In the presence of known psychiatric disorder under treatment with neuroleptic drugs, considerable difficulty may be encountered in distinguishing side effects of therapy from the ingravescent development of idiopathic Parkinson's disease. Here it can be important to remember that the parkinsonian side effects of neuroleptic drugs usually make their appearance early in the course of therapy, then often tend to subside (see first page of chapter). In cases of doubt withdrawal may be necessary for very long periods, sometimes a year or more, before the true situation is clarified.

Benign essential tremor (juvenile, adult or senile: Minor's disease) may lead to difficulties with diagnosis. This can begin at any age, a positive family history is often forthcoming and improvement with alcohol is characteristic. The hands are principally affected, the tremor disappears when the limbs are inactive, and titubation of the head is commoner than in Parkinson's disease. There is no bradykinesia or rigidity and the condition is static or perhaps very slowly progressive over several decades.

Other neurological diseases that must sometimes be considered include Huntington's disease and Wilson's disease. The rigid and akinetic forms of Huntington's disease may at first resemble Parkinson's disease. Wilson's disease must be carefully excluded when parkinsonian symptoms begin in adolescence or early adult life. The rigidity of Wilson's disease is similar to that of parkinsonism, but the involuntary movements are more varied including choreic jerking, athetoid and dystonic movements, or flapping tremor of the outstretched hands. Other degenerative conditions which must be borne in mind include progressive supranuclear palsy, corticobasal degeneration and multiple system atrophy. Diffuse Lewy body disease may sometimes present with parkinsonian features alone. Hughes *et al.* (1992) found that almost one-quarter of patients diagnosed as suffering from Parkinson's disease are wrongly so labelled: of 100 cases coming to autopsy, 24 had been misdiagnosed, showing the pathological features of progressive supranuclear palsy, multiple system atrophy, Alzheimer's disease or basal ganglia vascular disease. Schrag *et al.* (2002) analysed data on 202 patients who had been diagnosed with Parkinson's disease, prescribed antiparkinsonian medication or who presented with tremor. A diagnosis of Parkinson's disease was correct in 83%; additionally, 19% of those given an alternative diagnosis were subsequently found to have the disease.

Treatment (Fig. 12.2)

In historical terms the aim of treatment has been the relief of symptoms. With the passage of time, questions have arisen about the possible impact of treatment on mortality and whether current treatments such as levodopa may actually be harmful in the long run. Much current research is focused on discovering agents that modify the disease process. As things stand a large proportion of patients can obtain a gratifying degree of relief from their more disabling symptoms, certainly during the earlier stages of the disorder. Some severely crippled patients are enabled to lead relatively independent lives. Specific therapies must be accompanied by general measures to keep the patient active for as long as possible, with physiotherapy or the use of simple mechanical aids. Psychosocial aspects often need attention, especially since the degree of physical disability may be considerably worsened by stress or concurrent depression.

Drugs

Anticholinergic drugs are still used alone in mild cases. The best known are trihexyphenidyl, benzatropine (Cogentin®), orphenadrine (Disipal®), procyclidine (Kemadrin®) and biperiden (Akineton). Their effect is variable. Mobility is usually improved, with some decrease in rigidity and tremor. Bradykinesia is usually little affected. Atropine-like side effects limit the dose that can be employed, not least the possibility of revealing or worsening any underlying cognitive impairment. The role of anticholinergic drugs in the management of Parkinson's disease has been the subject of a recent Cochrane Collaboration review (Katzenschlager *et al.* 2003).

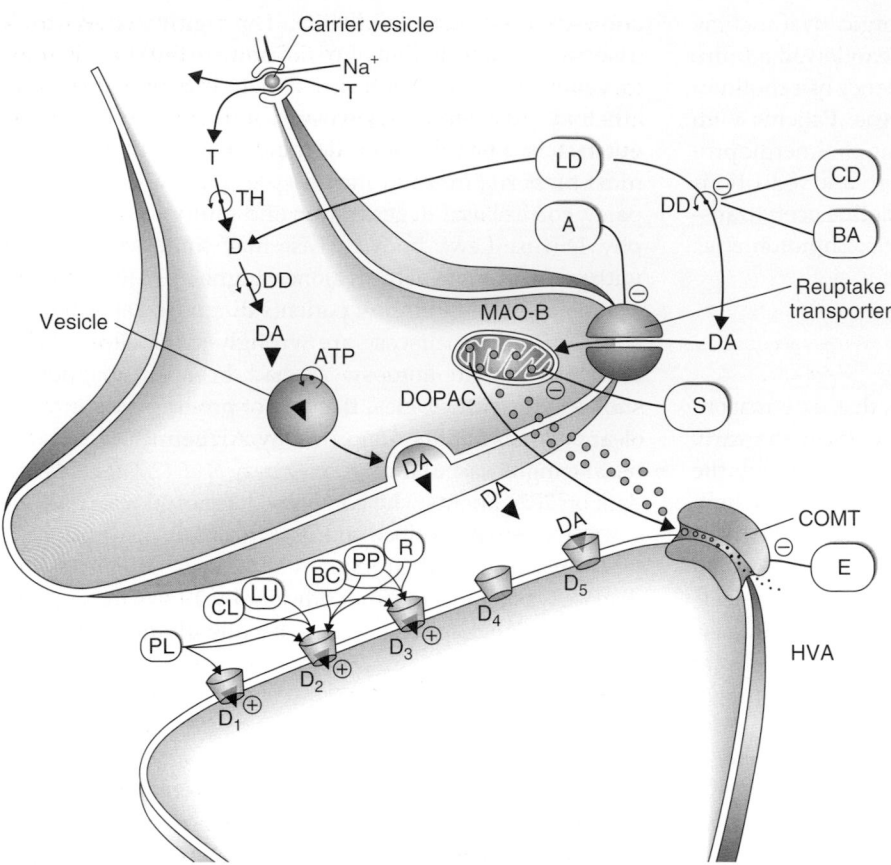

Fig. 12.2 The dopaminergic synapse. A, amantadine; ATP, adenosine triphosphate; BA, benserazide; BC, bromocriptine; CL, cabergoline; CD, carbidopa; COMT, catechol-o-methyl transferase; D, dopa; DA, dopamine; DD, dopa decarboxylase; DOPAC, 3,4-dihydroxyphenulacetic acid; E, entacapone; HVA, homovanillic acic, LD, levodopa; LU, lysuride; MAO, monoamine oxidase; MAO-B, monoamine oxidase type B; PL, pergolide, PP, pramipexole; R, ropinirole; S, selegiline; T, tyrosine; TH, tyrosine hydroxylase.

Amantadine hydrochloride (Symmetrel®) stimulates dopamine release in the central nervous system, and may be indicated if anticholinergic drugs fail and the patient is only mildly disabled. Among the severely disabled it finds application in patients who cannot tolerate levodopa. Amantadine helps with bradykinesia and postural instability in addition to improving rigidity. Mobility may thereby be considerably improved. Hallucinations and confusion are common side effects. In a recent Cochrane Collaboration review (Crosby *et al.* 2003), all six studies showed a positive effect with amantadine but the poor quality of the data was highlighted. It has also been shown to improve levodopa dyskinesia, although the effects were short-lived (Thomas *et al.* 2004).

Selegiline (deprenyl; Eldepryle®) inhibits monoamine oxidase B, one of the enzymes responsible for the breakdown of dopamine in the brain. It has limited antiparkinsonian action, but when used with levodopa can potentiate and prolong its action, sometimes helping with mild dose-related fluctuations of response. It may also allow the dose of levodopa to be reduced. However, it can sometimes worsen dyskinesias and aggravate psychiatric adverse reactions.

Selegiline became widely regarded as the treatment of first choice for newly diagnosed patients because it proved to be 'neuroprotective' in animals, preventing damage to the nigrostriatal system when they were exposed to the toxin MPTP (Heikkila 1984). Evidence was obtained from the DATATOP study that Parkinson's disease progressed more slowly in patients who started on treatment with selegiline, in that the need for levodopa was delayed for almost a year in relation to controls (Parkinson Study Group 1989; Tetrud & Langston 1989). This research has been criticised as the improvements may have been due the symptomatic effects of the drug (Horn & Stern 2004). UK findings (Lees 1995) then suggested that selegiline was associated with an increased mortality when used with levodopa. Subsequent analysis of that data could find no clear reason for the increased mortality and in fact when corrected for baseline covariates the significance became borderline (hazard ratio 0.99–1.72) (Ben-Shlomo *et al.* 1998). A more recent meta-analysis of all selegiline trials in early Parkinson's disease has shown no increased mortality (Ives *et al.* 2004). A new preparation of selegiline, Zydis selegiline, avoids first-pass metabolism, and two studies have shown it can improve 'on' time (Shellenberger *et al.* 2000; Waters *et al.* 2004). An alternative monoamine oxidase B inhibitor, rasagiline, is now available.

Levodopa (L-dopa) is now well established as a highly effective drug with a wide range of activity on different parkinsonian symptoms. It would appear a logical form of treatment, L-dopa being the immediate precursor of dopamine that is known to be deficient in the brain, although the precise mechanism of action remains unknown. Approximately one-third of patients can be expected to obtain marked relief, one-third moderate benefit, and the remainder show a modest or disappointing response. Perhaps some 15% do not respond at all; in such cases the possibility of some alternative diagnosis, such as progressive supranuclear palsy or multiple system atrophy, should be considered.

Levodopa is therefore widely regarded as the treatment of choice in patients who can tolerate it. A synergistic action is seen when given in conjunction with anticholinergic drugs and perhaps with amantadine as well. It may take several months before maximal benefit is obtained, and it cannot be said to have failed until it has been tried for 6 months or preferably a year. The variability of response seen from one individual to another cannot yet be accurately predicted.

Levodopa is now always given in combination with a peripheral dopa decarboxylase inhibitor such as carbidopa (in Sinemet) or benserazide (in Madopar). This prevents its metabolism in the gastrointestinal tract, reducing nausea and vomiting, and allows higher blood levels to be achieved with smaller doses. Moreover, the combined preparations increase the turnover of dopamine in the nigrostriatal system more selectively than does levodopa alone, and maximal benefit is obtained earlier.

Concerns have been expressed that long-term L-dopa may be toxic to dopaminergic neurones. Several studies have demonstrated that L-dopa can be harmful to cultured dopaminergic neurones by stimulating the production of highly reactive oxygen species including free radicals (Mena et al. 1992; Mytilineou et al. 1993). However, the clinical significance of these findings has been questioned. The human brain has high levels of ascorbic acid that acts as an antioxidant. When ascorbic acid is added to culture media, it provides almost complete protection from neurotoxicity (Pardo et al. 1993; Walkinshaw & Waters 1995; Cheng et al. 1996). In vivo animal experiments have largely failed to show L-dopa toxicity. The question was addressed by the ELLDOPA trial in a clinical population (Fahn 2005). No evidence of a detrimental effect from L-dopa was found; in fact there was some evidence that it could be neuroprotective.

Rigidity is helped and tremor also improves but less consistently. Propranolol or some other beta-blocker may further help the latter. Outstanding benefit is seen where bradykinesia and postural instability are concerned, both of which are rarely responsive to anticholinergic drugs. Thus facial mobility is improved, salivation lessened and the voice strengthened. Gait, handwriting and ability to perform fine manipulative tasks all improve. The overall result can be dramatic, with the patient able to do such things as shaving, knitting or getting out of bed unaided when these have not been possible for some considerable time.

Unfortunately, as time goes by the efficacy of levodopa may diminish. In general, over a 5-year period one-third of those who responded initially retain their benefit, one-third lose some and another third lose all their gains becoming worse than they were before (Marsden & Parkes 1977). This is most probably due to progression of the underlying disease. Variations in benefit may emerge for hours or days at a time, or the effects of each dose may become shorter-lasting. The first sign of fluctuation may be early-morning bradykinesia when the effects of the previous day's dose have worn off. End-dose deterioration then appears, with bradykinesia or tremor returning as each dose is due. In time this shows as the 'on–off' effect, with swings from complete relief to total immobility, often occurring with startling rapidity and sometimes many times a day (Marsden & Parkes 1976). By this time, peak-dose dyskinetic movements have also usually developed. In extreme form the patient may be precipitated within minutes, or even seconds, from a state of dyskinetic mobility to one of profound rebound parkinsonism (Quinn 1995).

Tests carried out serially during on and off phases have shown some mild impairment of cognition and adverse swings of affect during the latter phases (Brown et al. 1984). In a detailed study of nine patients experiencing severe on–off phenomena, Nissenbaum et al. (1987) found that four had clear-cut depression and anxiety when 'off', one also showing features of elation and disinhibition when 'on'. In a questionnaire survey, two-thirds of 31 such patients reported some degree of parallel mood change, usually towards depression when akinetic but also with feelings of irritability, aggressiveness and frustration. In rare cases hallucinations and delusions may accompany the transient depressions.

A 69-year-old woman on treatment with Sinemet progressed after 7 years to severe and abrupt changes characteristic of the on–off phenomenon. One year later she began to experience parallel fluctuations in mood. In the 'off' condition she showed depressed mood, agitation, hypochondriacal and nihilistic delusions, and an unshakeable belief that something dreadful was about to happen. She had ideas of guilt, and auditory and visual hallucinations. Although agitated she remained fully orientated and could retain information provided her attention could be sustained. In this condition she was chair-bound. When mobile and 'on' she had a mildly depressed mood, but was not agitated, deluded or hallucinated, and had partial insight into the psychotic phenomena experienced when immobile (Nissenbaum et al. 1987).

A 35-year-old man who had taken Sinemet for 4 years developed manic features during 'on' phases alternating with depression when 'off'. During 'on' phases he showed choreoathetoid movements and became overactive and talkative. He was extremely elated and expressed grandiose ideas that he would marry several women and live for 100 years. On reverting to severe immobility he showed profound depression and nihilistic thought content and expressed the wish to be dead. Between the fluctuations in mood and movement he improved, exhibiting neither mood abnormalities nor dyskinesias. There was no past or family history of affective disorder. His condition was ameliorated by giving smaller doses of medication more frequently (Keshavan *et al.* 1986).

Considerable improvement may be obtained by giving the drug in small divided doses, even every 2 or 3 hours through the day, or by the use of sustained-release preparations. Other approaches are to add selegiline, or to partially substitute an agonist drug such as bromocriptine or pergolide. Apomorphine can find a special place in the treatment of refractory on–off oscillations as described below.

Adverse effects commonly include anorexia, nausea, vomiting and hypotension. These can usually be overcome by starting with low dosage and increasing very gradually. The gastrointestinal effects can be largely avoided by the use of combined preparations of levodopa with a selective extracerebral decarboxylase inhibitor (Sinemet or Madopar). Tremors, tachypnoea, flushing and cardiac dysrhythmias may also be troublesome.

The commonest dose-limiting factor is the appearance of dyskinetic movements. Such dyskinesias can take any form, including orofacial dyskinesia, chorea, dystonia or athetosis of the limbs, analogous in form, and probably in pathophysiology, to the movements seen in tardive dyskinesia (see Drug-induced disorders/Clinical pictures/Akathisia, earlier). Three main varieties are recognised: peak-dose dyskinesia, with choreic or dystonic movements; diphasic dyskinesia, which occurs at the beginning and end of the dose and is often ballistic in character; and 'off-period' dystonia, with fixed, often painful, spasms mainly involving the feet. A compromise quite often has to be sought between the severity of such adventitious movements and the degree of relief of parkinsonian disability. Levodopa produces motor complications at the rate of 10% per year (Quinn *et al.* 1986). Olanow *et al.* (1994) has described how the onset of dyskinesias depends on the state of the nigrostriatal neurones. In MPTP models of the disease, there can be 95% neuronal loss; in this situation, dyskinesias can appear within days. In older patients with advanced disease, dyskinesias appear in months although in general they take many years.

Historically, treatment has started with levodopa and then been adjusted to include dopamine agonists as levo-dopa dyskinesias appear. Recent consideration has been given to delaying the onset of dyskinesias. Two studies have examined the use of slow-release preparations but failed to show any difference (Dupont *et al.* 1996; Block *et al.* 1997). An alternative approach is to start treatment with a dopamine agonist and several randomised controlled trials have examined this issue (Rinne *et al.* 1998; Parkinson Study Group 2000; Rascol *et al.* 2000). Initial treatment with a dopamine agonist was associated with delay in the onset of dyskinesias and other motor complications, although this was to some degree offset by clear evidence that those whose treatment commenced with levodopa had a better clinical response. There remains debate as to the optimal approach (Albin & Frey 2003).

Bromocriptine acts as a direct stimulant of dopamine receptors. Only about one-third of patients obtain a response to bromocriptine alone, but when given with levodopa it allows a smaller dose of the latter to be employed. Some prefer to use it initially on its own in order to defer the introduction of levodopa with its attendant long-term risks of fluctuation in response and dyskinesias. Early combination therapy with levodopa and bromocriptine has some advocates. It finds a special place in the management of patients who experience fluctuations in response to levodopa as described above.

Bromocriptine must be used with caution in the presence of peripheral vascular disease since it is derived from ergot, and it is contraindicated in the presence of ischaemic heart disease. Postural hypotension can be a problem when starting treatment, also nausea and vomiting, which are helped by domperidone. Psychiatric side effects are similar to those seen with levodopa (see Drugs, earlier).

Other dopamine agonists include cabergoline, lisuride, pramipexole, pergolide and ropinirole. Their role in the management of Parkinson's disease has been reviewed by the Movement Disorders Society Task Force (2002). Pergolide, ropinirole and pramipexole have all been studied in early disease. They appear equally effective and are less likely to lead to dyskinesias, although as noted above they do not produce the same clinical improvement as levodopa. They all appear to be effective as adjunctive treatments (Cochrane library issue 2004), reducing 'off' time and improving motor impairments and activities of daily living. Pergolide and cabergoline are ergot-derived drugs and their use is associated with serosal reactions such as retroperitoneal fibrosis. In one study valvular heart disease was demonstrated in one-third of patients taking pergolide (Van Camp *et al.* 2004). There is some evidence that dopamine agonists have a neuroprotective disease-modifying action. The CALM-PD trial studied pramipexole over 4 years and showed significantly reduced decline in striatal neurone loss assessed with SPECT (Parkinson Study Group 2002). The REAL-PET study showed lower decline in ^{18}F-labelled dopa in patients taking ropinirole (Whone *et al.* 2003).

However, the methodologies of both studies have been criticised (Clarke & Guttman 2002; Wooten 2003) and to date neither drug is licensed as 'disease-slowing' in Parkinson's disease.

Apomorphine has a special place in the treatment of late-stage fluctuations in response to levodopa when other approaches have failed, and can on occasion be life-saving (Stibe *et al.* 1988; Hughes *et al.* 1993). It is also a D_1 and D_2 receptor agonist but must be given by subcutaneous injection. Oral domperidone is given concurrently to prevent vomiting. Patients and their relatives can be instructed to inject the drug when 'off' periods occur, relief occurring within 15 minutes and lasting for up to an hour. Continuous daytime infusion can be achieved through a portable pump. Long-term use appears safe and effective (Manson *et al.* 2002; Tyne *et al.* 2004). The injections work with high reliability and tolerance does not develop, but drowsiness and local reactions at injection sites can be troublesome. Intranasal apomorphine is currently being developed as an alternative (Koller *et al.* 1997; Dewey *et al.* 1998).

Catechol *O*-methyltransferase (COMT) is one of the enzymes that metabolise L-dopa and dopamine. Entacapone inhibits COMT peripherally, thus increasing the availability of both dopamine and L-dopa. Another drug, tolcapone, has been withdrawn. Entacapone appears effective as adjunctive therapy, having the advantage over dopamine agonists that it does not need titration (Parkinson Study Group 1997). A new combination drug (containing levodopa, peripheral decarboxylase inhibitor and entacapone) was appreciated by patients and improved compliance (Myllyla *et al.* 2003). A possible additional benefit of the combined use of entacapone and levodopa may be that levodopa pulsatility, believed to contribute to the onset of motor complications, is reduced (Smith *et al.* 2005).

Surgery

There have been considerable developments in the surgical management of Parkinson's disease. The best results are seen in patients with true idiopathic disease who have had dopamine-responsive symptoms (Walter & Vitek 2004). Goals of surgical treatment may be core symptoms of the disease or drug-induced motor complications. Lesions in the ventral intermediate nucleus of the thalamus are effective in relieving tremor, including essential tremor (Walter & Vitek 2004). However, bilateral disease requires bilateral thalamotomies. Alvarez *et al.* (2001) showed a 58% improvement in 'off' medication motor scores 2 years after bilateral thalamotomy. Postoperative chorea was common but short-lived. Bilateral thalamotomies carry the risk of adverse events such as speech problems or gait disturbance (Matsumoto *et al.* 1976; Speelman 1991). Deep brain stimulation is an alternative to lesioning. Again, bilateral stimulation appears more effective than unilateral stimulation (Ondo *et al.* 2001) but dysarthria can be a problem (Walter &

Vitek 2004). One study has compared thalamic lesions to thalamic stimulators (Schuurman *et al.* 2000). Both were equally effective in terms of tremor control but lesions were associated with more adverse events. Matsumoto *et al.* (1984) and Wester and Hauglie-Hanssen (1990) argue that stimulation-related side effects can be reversed, but lack of effect on non-tremor symptoms has limited the use of the thalamic approach (Benazzouz *et al.* 2002).

Two randomised controlled trials confirmed that pallidotomy can improve contralateral tremor, rigidity, bradykinesia and drug-induced dyskinesias (de Bie *et al.* 1999; Vitek *et al.* 2003). In the study by de Bie *et al.* (1999), gait and postural benefits had been lost at 1 year follow-up, although in the study by Vitek *et al.* (2003) significant benefits in ipsilateral rigidity, bradykinesia and drug-induced dyskinesias were still present at 2 years. Surgical complications with bilateral pallidotomy include hypophonia, dysarthria and cognitive problems (Favre *et al.* 2000; Intemann *et al.* 2001; Merello *et al.* 2001; de Bie *et al.* 2002).

Neural transplantation has been shown to be successful in restoring function in primates with lesions of the dopamine pathways, and limited experience has been obtained in patients with Parkinson's disease (Hitchcock 1992; Lindvall 1994; Hauser *et al.* 1995). Despite occasional reports of striking success with autologous transplantation of tissue from the adrenal medulla, this approach has proved disappointing and the use of fetal dopaminergic cells appears to hold more promise. However, this raises considerable ethical problems.

Adrenal medullary transplantation seems commonly to be followed by behavioural complications in the immediate postoperative period, including sleep disturbance, hallucinations, delusions, confusion and mood changes (Stebbins & Tanner 1992). Techniques of this nature may yet find a place in the management of younger patients whose disease is difficult to control by other means, but continuing improvements in drug therapy may overtake their further development.

Psychiatric aspects of parkinsonism

Interest in the psychiatric aspects of parkinsonism has increased as a result of advances in knowledge of the disease. The advent of stereotactic surgery focused renewed attention on the problem of intellectual impairment in the disorder, and the demonstration of disturbance of amine metabolism has brought new interest to its association with depression.

There is a good deal of disagreement in different reports regarding the frequency of mental symptoms, undoubtedly depending on the particular population under scrutiny. Thus behavioural disturbance is likely to be more common when a substantial number of postencephalitic cases are examined, and intellectual impairment will be more frequent when patients with 'arteriosclerotic parkinsonism' are included in the sample. The difficulties of achieving anything like a reliable estimate are increased by the problems inherent in distinguishing these different varieties one from another.

Mjönes (1949) reviewed the earlier work in detail. Three main groups of mental disturbance gradually came to be recognised and were sometimes regarded as an integral part of the pathological picture: a change of personality towards suspicion, irritability and egocentricity; an impairment of memory and intellect; and psychotic developments with depression, paranoia and sometimes visual hallucinations. Some felt that there was a typical paralysis agitans psychopathy, others a characteristic psychosis. Some found a great excess of dementia, others of depression. Mjönes' own investigation of 262 cases of paralysis agitans revealed mental symptoms in approximately 40%. 'Organic' changes predominated over 'reactive' changes, the former consisting of impaired memory and intellect, the latter of depression with irritability, egocentricity and hypochondriasis. Transitional forms were also encountered in which the relative contributions of organic or reactive elements were uncertain.

More recent studies have served to underline the associations with depression and cognitive impairment, the latter chiefly in later-onset Parkinson's disease. It now seems indubitable that the risk of dementia is increased above expectation and several hypotheses have been advanced to account for this. A typical personality change, or a characteristic form of psychotic reaction, are no longer recognised. Those psychoses that do emerge are largely seen in the context of treatment with levodopa and other drugs. These matters are dealt with in detail in the sections that follow.

Cognitive impairment and dementia

The question of cognitive impairment in Parkinson's disease has attracted a great deal of interest, particularly since the advent of treatments that may be effective in prolonging life. There is no doubt that some patients show impairment of cognitive function, sometimes severe and pervasive enough to amount to an easily recognised progressive dementia. Others in contrast remain intellectually intact despite gross physical disablement. The issue which has been hard to resolve is whether, as a group, patients with idiopathic Parkinson's disease are more prone to develop such difficulties than would be expected by virtue of their age alone. The present consensus is that the risk of dementia is definitely increased, perhaps some two- or three-fold. Possible reasons for this have turned out to be complex, and are gradually being disentangled as discussed below.

Brown and Marsden (1984) review the differing estimates of the prevalence of dementia in Parkinson's disease, ranging from 10% to over 80%, and the possible reasons for such wide discrepancies.

Sampling errors are compounded by difficulties in excluding other causes of akinetic–rigid syndromes during life, particularly in separating idiopathic Parkinson's disease from 'arteriosclerotic parkinsonism' (see under Parkinson's disease and the parkinsonian syndrome, earlier). If some examples of parkinsonism merely reflect an accent of diffuse cerebral vascular disease on the basal ganglia, then the cognitive impairments encountered could be due to the widespread cerebral changes in this group. On the other hand, when cognitive impairment is used as a criterion for separating arteriosclerotic from idiopathic parkinsonism, the idiopathic cases will tend to be reported as intact.

Problems with the definition and assessment of dementia are also considerable, and the criteria employed have varied from one study to another. Some have sought to identify the clinical syndrome of dementia, using behavioural criteria and brief mental state tests, whereas others have used batteries of psychological tests to look for specific cognitive deficits. With both approaches the assessment of parkinsonian patients can raise special difficulties. Behavioural criteria must allow for the curtailment of activities occasioned by the disease; psychological testing must take into consideration slowness of response, which may be largely attributable to motor handicap. Care must be taken to allow for what is to be expected in any ageing group of persons, and to differentiate cognitive failure from the depression common with Parkinson's disease. Drugs taken for treatment of the condition may further complicate assessments.

An impressive early survey was carried out by Marttila and Rinne (1976) involving all traceable patients with Parkinson's disease in a defined area of Finland. Of 144 patients, 29% were thought to be demented, 50% of these being mildly, 30% moderately and 20% severely affected. Patients with evidence of arteriosclerosis were more often demented than those without (56% and 18% of cases respectively). There was a clear rise with age, from 20% among those under 70 to 65% among those over 80. The severely physically disabled showed dementia more often than the mildly affected, with increasing severity of rigidity and bradykinesia showing a positive correlation with the degree of intellectual decline. This association pointed to a role for subcortical structures in the pathophysiology of the dementia.

Lieberman *et al.* (1979) found moderate to marked dementia in one-third of 520 patients, this being 10 times the prevalence in spouses used as controls. The demented patients, in addition to a later onset, had become more physically disabled in a shorter time and had responded less well to levodopa. Two distinct forms of Parkinson's disease, with and without dementia, thus seemed a possibility. Lees and Smith (1983) restricted attention to mildly disabled patients, all under the age of 65 and with normal CT scans. Comparisons with age-matched controls showed no impairment on tests of intelligence or memory, but revealed significant deficits on the Wisconsin Card Sorting Test and a verbal fluency test. Frontal cognitive deficits were therefore highlighted.

More recent surveys have attempted to allow for the various sources of artefact outlined above, in particular adopting stringent criteria for the diagnosis of dementia.

The great majority have confirmed an increased prevalence of dementia in the disease. Rajput *et al.* (1984) reviewed the Mayo Clinic records of all parkinsonian patients seen over a 13-year period, charting dementia only when this had been diagnosed on at least two separate occasions. For every patient, two sex- and age-matched controls were selected from residents in the area. Of the 138 new parkinsonian patients seen, 13 (9.4%) were demented compared with 2.9% of controls. When none of the three matched individuals showed dementia at the time the parkinsonism was first recognised, these were followed further and dementia emerged more frequently among the patients than the controls.

Mayeux *et al.* (1988b) performed a similar review of records from a medical centre in New York. Among 339 patients with idiopathic Parkinson's disease, 10.9% were demented according to DSM-III criteria. The demented patients were significantly older than the remainder, had a later age of onset and a more rapid progression of physical disability. When the parkinsonism had begun after the age of 70, dementia was noted almost three times as often as when the onset had been earlier. Among patients over 60 years old the prevalence was judged to be almost four times that expected for a population of equivalent age. Equivalent results were obtained from a register-based survey of patients in the Netherlands, incepted with a hospital discharge diagnosis of Parkinson's disease and followed an average of 8 years later (Breteler *et al.* 1995). In comparison with a reference group of patients with non-cerebral diseases, the risk of developing dementia during this period was increased threefold.

The most clear-cut evidence, however, has come from Mindham's group, who have reported the first truly prospective study of dementia in idiopathic Parkinson's disease (Biggins *et al.* 1992).

Serial assessments were made of cognition, mood and level of disability in a group of 87 patients and 50 healthy matched controls over a 4.5-year period, each subject being examined at 9-month intervals. The mean age of the patients was 64 years. Patients were excluded if they had a history of stroke, hypertension or transient ischaemic attacks, or when there were indications of other neurological disorder. An extensive battery of psychometric tests was administered at each examination, along with rating scales for depression, anxiety and physical disability. The accumulated data sheets were reviewed at the end of the study, blind to whether the subject was a parkinsonian patient or control, and diagnoses of dementia were made according to DSM-III criteria. Judgements were made as to the assessment at which these criteria were first satisfied.

Of the 87 patients, five (6%) were considered to have been demented from the outset of the study, and 10 more became demented during the follow-up period. No control subject did so. After allowing for patients who dropped out during the course of the survey, the cumulative incidence of dementia over this period was 19%. Comparisons between those who demented and those who did not showed that the former were older, older at onset of Parkinson's disease, had a longer duration of illness, and had lower initial performance on certain cognitive tests. This last might indicate that their dementia

had already been present in milder form while not yet meeting DSM-III criteria.

It therefore seems clear that dementia, identifiable clinically, is increased above expectation in Parkinson's disease, even when care has been taken to exclude vascular and other pathologies that might have contributed towards it. Cognitive impairments, insufficient in themselves to lead to such a diagnosis, seem also to be common, though there is insufficient information to judge how often these may be a prelude to dementia.

Psychometric studies show a wide spectrum of deficits among cognitively impaired parkinsonian subjects, as reviewed by Ross *et al.* (1992). In some the picture resembles 'subcortical dementia' (see Chapter 1 under Clinical picture in focal cerebral disorder/Basal ganglia), particularly with respect to memory functioning, and executive function deficits are often prominent suggesting disruption of frontal–subcortical connections. In others, however, there are language and other impairments that point to cortical dysfunction. Sometimes, indeed, the clinical picture appears to overlap with that of Alzheimer's disease. Ross *et al.* conclude that the heterogeneity of the pictures seen suggests that there are multiple dementia syndromes in Parkinson's disease, associated with varying structural and biochemical pathology.

The causation of these deficits remains uncertain and a number of possibilities must be considered. First, they may be due in part to the classic pathology of Parkinson's disease and the dopamine deficiency that ensues. The subcortical nature of the dementia in many examples would fit with such a pathogenesis, especially since mesolimbic and mesocortical projections are known to be involved along with disruption of the nigrostriatal system. Such projections arise from the medial substantia nigra and the ventral tegmental area, and these have been found to be particularly severely affected in parkinsonian patients with dementia (Rinne *et al.* 1989). Neuronal counts and noradrenaline (norepinephrine) levels have also proved to be reduced in the locus caeruleus in the presence of dementia, suggesting that diminished noradrenergic inputs to the cortex may make an additional contribution (Gaspar & Gray 1984; Chui *et al.* 1986; Cash *et al.* 1987). Together these observations support a subcortical origin for the dementia.

To a notable degree, however, dementia is rare in younger patients with Parkinson's disease, even though in all other respects the course and pathology of the disorder appears to be similar whatever the age of onset (Gibb 1989). Dementia has emerged as exceptional with onset below the age of 50, even with disease of long duration, and it becomes commoner with later onset, especially after 70 years. Indeed the factor of age of onset has emerged as one of the firmest risk factors for the development of dementia.

With age there is increasing likelihood of finding Alzheimer-type pathology in the cortex, and certain studies have suggested that this may play a major role in producing the dementia. Alvord *et al.* (1974) and Hakim and Mathieson (1978, 1979) found Alzheimer changes to be commoner in patients with Parkinson's disease than in age-matched controls, and Boller *et al.* (1980) found the prevalence of plaques and tangles in the cortex to rise as the severity of dementia increased. A cortical pathology of Alzheimer type might thus be accelerated in the presence of Parkinson's disease and account for the cognitive deficits seen. However, further detailed studies have given conflicting results and this hypothesis is now regarded as uncertain (Jellinger & Riederer 1984; Gibb 1989).

A third possible explanation involves the nucleus basalis of Meynert. Perry *et al.* (1985) demonstrated marked cholinergic deficits in the cerebral cortex of parkinsonian patients, which in the temporal neocortex correlated with the severity of mental impairment assessed prior to death. The cholinergic deficits were of a similar order to those seen in Alzheimer's disease, despite the dementia being milder, but lacked correlation with the degree of tangle and plaque formation. Rather they correlated with the extent of neuronal loss in the nucleus basalis of Meynert. This was always pronounced, with losses of up to 70% in the presence of parkinsonian dementia. Thus the cortical cholinergic deficits seemed not to be explicable in terms of cortical pathology, but more probably resulted from degeneration of cholinergic axons associated with the loss of cells in the Meynert nucleus. Such loss might itself be due to a pathological process analogous to that inducing changes in the substantia nigra.

This striking set of observations has been both confirmed and refuted in other studies, as reviewed by Ross *et al.* (1992) and Chui and Perlmutter (1992). And it has become apparent that, at least in some cases, dementia can occur in Parkinson's disease in the absence of either Alzheimer-type pathology in the cortex or cell loss in the nucleus basalis of Meynert.

These various possible contributions to dementia are discussed in detail by Dubois and Pillon (1992). It seems probable that many of the cognitive changes are largely due to subcortical pathology, with dopamine deficiency being compounded by loss of inputs from noradrenergic and cholinergic nuclei. In the older patient with Parkinson's disease and severe dementia, concomitant changes of Alzheimer type in the cortex are likely to make an additional contribution.

Structural brain imaging has not contributed substantially to this cortical/subcortical debate. Air encephalography (Selby 1968) and CT (Sroka *et al.* 1981) have shown a high prevalence of cerebral atrophy in patients with Parkinson's disease, and in several studies ventricular enlargement has correlated with the presence of cognitive impairment (Huber & Glatt 1992). Third ventricular width and the intercaudate distance have also shown such associations, whereas the contribution of cortical atrophy usually disappears on controlling for age. To this extent structural imaging supports the relevance

of subcortical pathology. Magnetic resonance imaging has not clarified the situation further (Huber *et al.* 1989).

PET and SPECT have in contrast tended to underline the importance of cortical pathology, showing deficits in metabolism in the frontal and parietal regions that are marked in the presence of dementia. Metter *et al.* (1990), using fluorodeoxyglucose-PET, found essentially the same pattern of hypometabolism in parkinsonian dementia and Alzheimer's disease, with global reductions in brain metabolism and an accent on the parietal regions. These could be observed to progress with worsening of the cognitive impairment. Peppard *et al.* (1992) showed widespread cortical and subcortical reductions in glucose metabolism in non-demented parkinsonian patients, though with significant further reductions in the cortical regions in the presence of dementia. The temporoparietal regions were again particularly affected. It remains unclear, however, whether such patterns reflect intrinsic cortical pathology or the cortical effects of deafferentation from subcortical structures.

Finally, a fourth element has been added now that it is appreciated that Lewy bodies are often found in the cerebral cortex as well as in brainstem nuclei. How far diffuse Lewy body disease may make its own contribution to cognitive failure in patients with Parkinson's disease remains to be determined, but no doubt this may operate as a substantial additional factor.

Affective disorder

An association between parkinsonism and depression is well established. However, debate continues on whether depression is best seen as an understandable response to a debilitating disease or is part of the disease process itself.

Estimates of the prevalence vary widely between 5% and 90% (Hoehn & Yahr 1967; Mindham 1970; Tandberg *et al.* 1996). Early studies have limited validity in light of changes to the diagnostic criteria for both depression and Parkinson's disease. Most notably, early studies tended to use a clinical interview to assess depression rather than a standardised tool. Starkstein *et al.* (1990) assessed 105 patients using the Present State Examination (Wing *et al.* 1974) to produce DSM-III diagnoses; 21 patients had 'major' depression and 20 'minor' depression. Cummings (1992a) suggested a figure of 40%, including both 'major' and 'minor' depression in a single category.

The nature of the population being studied has a great bearing on the findings. Tandberg *et al.* (1996) assessed a large community sample in Norway and found that only 8% had major depression although 45% had depressive symptoms. Studies involving patients who attend specialist clinics identify higher prevalences. Liu *et al.* (1997) found that 17% of patients attending a neurological clinic had major depression, with a further 25% having milder symptoms. Schrag *et al.* (2001) found that 20% of their patients attending a specialist clinic had moderate or severe depression. The precise status of 'mild' or 'sub-syndromal' depression is yet to be determined – the exact point at which a patient can be labelled 'depressed' is of course somewhat arbitrary. However, there is increasing evidence that patients with depressive symptoms who fail to meet current diagnostic criteria for major depressive disorder nonetheless suffer a degree of psychosocial dysfunction as a result of these symptoms, are more likely to have a major depressive episode in the future and can benefit from intervention (Judd *et al.* 2002). Thus, all depressive symptoms warrant careful clinical appraisal.

A number of possible risk factors, such as age, sex, disease duration and duration of levodopa treatment, are not consistently found to predict depression in Parkinson's disease. Fleminger (1991) showed that depression and anxiety were both more common when unilateral Parkinson's disease affected the left rather than the right side of the body, and noted this to be the reverse of what might have been expected if the symptoms were purely a response to functional disability. However, other studies found depression more often in patients with right-sided disease (Starkstein *et al.* 1990; Cole *et al.* 1996). Early disease onset (Kostic *et al.* 1994; Cole *et al.* 1996), a positive family history of depression (Tandberg *et al.* 1997) and atypical parkinsonian signs such as prominent autonomic signs or presence of pyramidal symptoms or rapidly progressive disease (Quinn *et al.* 1986) appear better predictors. Several authors report an association with cognitive impairment (Tandberg *et al.* 1996; Schrag *et al.* 2001; Rojo *et al.* 2003; Lauterbach 2004). Starkstein *et al.* (1989) have suggested that these may cluster together as a subtype of Parkinson's.

A great deal of discussion has surrounded the possible association between disease severity and depression. In individual patients depression can sometimes be clearly reactive in nature, setting in immediately the patient is informed of the nature of the disease, or developing later as an understandable response to the limitations and discomforts imposed by physical disability. Mindham (1974), for example, was able to show a significant correlation between the severity of the leading signs of parkinsonism and the severity of depression in a group of patients attending a neurological clinic. This relationship persisted during treatment with levodopa, those improving physically showing a fall in the severity of affective symptoms. However, the findings of other studies (reviewed by Brown & Jahanshahi 1995) fail to support this simple model.

Starkstein *et al.* (1990) compared rates of depression with stage of disease (as determined by Hoehn and Yahr's method) and found an inverted U-shaped curve, with depression being more common in the early and late stages of the disease. This finding has been replicated by Schrag *et al.* (2001). Hoehn and Yahr stages may be a coarse measure of function and further studies have examined the association of depression with disability and handicap. In this context, impairment relates to the objective disease severity, whilst disability reflects the functional impact of that disease

severity for the individual and handicap describes the broader disadvantages perceived by the individual, for example in being able to fulfil particular roles. Brown *et al.* (1988) demonstrated an association between depression and disability but not simple disease impairment. Schrag *et al.* (2001) found that disease severity accounted for only 28% of the variance in depression but handicap predicted more than 50% of this variance. In other words, depression relates not solely to what an individual patient can or cannot do but more to what such impairments mean for that individual within his own personal social environment.

However, there are also indications that depression may sometimes bear a more integral relationship to the disease process itself, reflecting in some way the causative brain pathology. The high prevalence of depression has impressed many observers and it has seemed to be commoner than in equivalently disabling illnesses (Warburton 1967; Horn 1974; Singer 1974). Robins (1976), for example, supported such an interpretation. In a carefully controlled study, 45 patients with Parkinson's disease were matched for age and sex with chronically disabled people drawn from the same institutions (patients with hemiplegia, paraplegia and arthritis). The groups resembled each other with regard to the frequency of a pre-illness history of depression or of neurotic symptoms. The duration of disablement was similar in both but the degree of handicap greater in the non-parkinsonian group. Nevertheless, the patients with Parkinson's disease were significantly more depressed than the controls as measured by the Hamilton rating scale. In neither group did the severity of disability affect the presence or absence of depression, suggesting that the latter was not solely reactive in nature. However, Gotham *et al.* (1986) found that depression was as common in rheumatoid arthritis as in Parkinson's disease. A growing body of evidence supports the suggestion that at least a proportion of the depression seen in Parkinson's disease is an expression of the disease itself. One piece of this evidence comes from the observation that rather than being a reaction to the disease, depression commonly precedes the emergence of parkinsonian motor symptoms (Santamaria *et al.* 1987; Fukunishi *et al.* 1991). Gonera *et al.* (1997) suggest that depression may be part of a prodromal syndrome occurring 4–6 years ahead of the motor symptoms. Shiba *et al.* (2000) used a medical records linkage system to overcome some of the problems associated with recall bias. In their sample the odds ratio for a preceding diagnosis of depression in parkinsonian patients was 1.9 compared with controls.

Noradrenergic and serotonergic abnormalities are strongly associated with depression in non-parkinsonian patients. Widespread degeneration of monoaminergic neurotransmitter systems are known to occur in Parkinson's disease (Fibiger 1984; Mayeux *et al.* 1984; Lemke *et al.* 2004). Remy *et al.* (2005) showed that depressed patients have reduced catecholaminergic transport in the locus caeruleus, thalamus, striatum and amygdala, and particularly highlighted that loss of noradrenaline and dopamine in the amygdala may contribute to depressive symptomatology. Weintraub *et al.* (2004) used SPECT to show that depressed patients had decreased dopamine transporter availability in the left anterior putamen.

Other studies have focused on the frontal areas of the brain. Taylor *et al.* (1986) showed that depressed parkinsonian patients showed greater impairment on frontal lobe testing than non-depressed patients and suggested that depression was associated with abnormalities in the links between the caudate and the frontal lobe. Mayberg *et al.* (1990) showed reduced glucose metabolism in the orbital and inferior frontal areas of depressed patients, whereas Ring *et al.* (1994) demonstrated reduced regional cerebral blood flow in the anteromedial part of the medial frontal cortex. This area has already been associated with depression in non-parkinsonian patients (Bench *et al.* 1992).

In a large postal survey, Gotham *et al.* (1986) were able to show that depression was related to the degree of impairment in activities of daily living, but even so much of the variability was left unaccounted for. Individual differences in coping style and the availability of social support were probably also influential. The symptom profiles observed included pessimism, hopelessness, decreased motivation and increased concern over health; in contrast, guilt, self-blame and worthlessness were usually absent.

Several studies allude to phenomenological differences between depression in parkinsonian and non-parkinsonian patients. Lemke *et al.* (2004) suggests that parkinsonian depression is characterised by increased levels of dysphoria and irritability and lower levels of guilt and suicidality. In another study, Lemke *et al.* (2005) found marked anhedonia in 80% of depressed parkinsonian patients.

Increased tearfulness has been found to be common in patients with Parkinson's disease, sometimes with 'emotionalism' as indicated by sudden weeping with loss of normal social control (Madeley *et al.* 1992). Almost half of a group of patients with idiopathic Parkinson's disease reported being more tearful since the onset, and 10% showed emotionalism of the type following cerebrovascular accidents (Chapter 8). Such disturbances were sometimes evident in the absence of lowered mood or cognitive impairment.

One obvious problem in the assessment of depression in Parkinson's disease is deciding if 'somatic' features such as slowness and paucity of facial expression are due to the depression or the disease. As a result there has been interest in the use of screening questionnaires. Levin *et al.* (1988) studied the Beck Depression Inventory (Beck *et al.* 1961) using cluster analysis and showed that the somatic questions 'scored true' rather than producing large numbers of false positives. However, Leentjens *et al.* (2000a) has drawn attention to the limitations of the Beck Depression Inventory. In their study, a cut-off of 8/9 gave high sensitivity but

low specificity, i.e. too many false positives. It was not until the cut-off was raised to 16/17 that the specificity was acceptable, but at the expense of the sensitivity, i.e. too many missed cases. Meara *et al.* (1999) have used the Geriatric Depression Scale but found the somatic elements did overscore, producing an excess of false positives. Leentjens *et al.* (2000b) compared the Montgomery–Asberg Depression Rating Scale and the Hamilton Depression Rating Scale, using the Schedule for the Assessment in Neuropsychiatry to provide DSM-IV gold standard diagnoses. The Hamilton Depression Rating Scale appeared to perform better.

Depression impacts substantially on the patient with Parkinson's disease. Physical symptoms progress more quickly in depressed patients (Starkstein *et al.* 1992a); for example, Rochester *et al.* (2004) showed that depression was independently associated with a reduced speed of walking during functional tasks. Brown *et al.* (1988) and Starkstein *et al.* (1992a) reported greater decline in self-care in depressed patients. Starkstein *et al.* (1992a) demonstrated that cognitive function declined more quickly in depressed patients over a year, and that the decline was greatest in the most depressed patients. Previously Starkstein *et al.* (1990) observed that the decline in Mini Mental State Examination scores in patients treated for depression was about half that of untreated controls. Two large studies have examined the factors which contribute to overall health-related quality of life in Parkinson's disease. Kuopio *et al.* (2000) found that patients' Hoehn and Yahr stage accounted for 48% of the variance in their scores on the physical function domain of the SF36, followed by depression. For all of the other seven domains, depression was the strongest predictor. The Global Parkinson's Disease Survey examined patients in seven countries (Global Parkinson's Disease Survey 2002); knowing the disease stage and the medication the patients were taking explained 17% of the variance in quality of life, whereas depression measured on the Beck Depression Inventory accounted for more than 50%.

Patient depression can have an adverse impact on the spouse or carer (Lawton *et al.* 1995). Carers of patients with Parkinson's disease have a heavy burden, performing up to 30 care-related activities per day. Carter *et al.* (1998) and O'Reilly *et al.* (1996) found five times the level of psychiatric illness in spouses who were carers compared with spouses who were not main carers. Meara *et al.* (1999) also reported high levels of depression in carers of parkinsonian patients, the best predictor of which was depression in the patient.

Early research on levodopa's effects examined whether it had an antidepressant effect. Yahr *et al.* (1969) suggested that it improved depression, although Damasio (1970) found it caused depression. More recently, Choi *et al.* (2000) followed up a group of patients starting levodopa for up to 28 months and concluded that long-term levodopa had no impact on depression in Parkinson's disease. Klaassen *et al.* (1995) have reviewed the use of antidepressant medication. Several studies were found that used selegiline as an antidepressant, with mixed results. More recently, Lemke *et al.* (2005) and Reichmann *et al.* (2003) have demonstrated the antidepressant effects of pramipexole in parkinsonian patients.

Tricyclic antidepressants are the most commonly studied drugs, although the methodologies used have been heavily criticised. The Parkinson's disease population is particularly susceptible to many of the adverse effects of tricyclics, such as orthostatic hypotension and confusion secondary to their anticholinergic effects. Additionally, absorption of levodopa can be impaired.

Since Klaassen *et al.*'s review there have been a number of studies investigating the efficacy of selective serotonin reuptake inhibitors (SSRIs) (Ghazi-Noori *et al.* 2003). With fewer noradrenergic and anticholinergic side effects, SSRIs would appear to be better tolerated in a parkinsonian population. Several open-label studies have been reported (Hauser & Zesiewicz 1997; Meara & Hobson 1998; Ceravolo *et al.* 2000; Rampello *et al.* 2002). Dell'Agnello *et al.* (2001) have concluded that SSRIs do not worsen the motor symptoms of the disease despite several case reports that they can produce parkinsonian signs in healthy individuals (Meltzer *et al.* 1979; Bouchard *et al.* 1989). Wermuth *et al.* (1998) have performed the only randomised controlled trial to date and found no benefit from citalopram over placebo.

ECT is not contraindicated, and may result in pronounced motor benefit while alleviating the affective disorder (Lebensohn & Jenkins 1975; Douyon *et al.* 1989). There are numerous reports of ECT successfully treating depression in Parkinson's disease, although no controlled trials have been performed (see Kennedy *et al.* 2003 for a comprehensive review). A large proportion of patients experienced confusion or delirium afterwards, somewhat limiting the usefulness of this approach in all but the most resistant cases.

Psychological therapies for depression, such as cognitive behavioural therapy, are safe, effective and popular with patients and now widely used in the general population. However, almost no work has been done in parkinsonian patients. In a small study Dreisig *et al.* (1999) suggested that younger patients may benefit. Crews and Harrison (1995) have suggested possible adaptations to cognitive behavioural therapy for use in an elderly population. Secker and Brown (2005) suggest that cognitive behavioural therapy may be helpful in the management of carer distress.

Relative to depression, anxiety in Parkinson's disease has received very little attention (Marsh 2000). Anxiety symptoms are common: Marinus *et al.* (2002) used the Hospital Anxiety and Depression Scale (Zigmond & Snaith 1983) to show that 20% of patients had 'probable' anxiety and 29% had 'possible' anxiety. Often the anxiety symptoms are part of a broader depressive syndrome but this is not always the case (Henderson *et al.* 1992). Like depression, anxiety symptoms often precede the onset of motor symptoms (Hender-

son *et al.* 1992). Shiba *et al.* (2000) found that a history of anxiety disorders was more common in patients with Parkinson's disease than in controls (odds ratio 2.2), however far back the history was examined. In a large prospective study of male health-care professionals, Weisskopf *et al.* (2003) identified anxiety as a predictor of subsequent Parkinson's disease even when caffeine intake, smoking and anxiolytic medication had been controlled for. Menza *et al.* (1999) associated anxiety in Parkinson's disease with a functional polymorphism on the serotonin transporter gene. There is no evidence for the treatment of anxiety in Parkinson's disease: SSRIs are probably the best option and benzodiazepines should be used with great caution. Intriguingly, several reports have shown an improvement in anxiety symptoms following pallidal surgery (Troster *et al.* 1997; Scott *et al.* 1998; Junque *et al.* 1999; Higginson *et al.* 2001).

Personality changes

Increasing disability may understandably lead to irritability, as in any disease which results in restriction of activities and dependence on others. Egocentricity, querulousness and an exacting attitude towards those around have often been stressed, likewise a change towards suspiciousness or even frank paranoia. However, the prevalence of such changes is hard to assess. Obsessional traits in the premorbid personality may become exaggerated, and hypochondriasis can be marked. In contrast, euphoria appears to be distinctly rare and when present is probably closely tied to intellectual deterioration.

There does not appear to be any form of personality change specific for parkinsonism. The majority of the features outlined above are generally held to be accountable in terms of individual vulnerability and the psychological and social stresses which operate on the disabled person.

Psychoses

Psychosis in untreated Parkinson's disease is rare. When it does occur it is usually affective in nature. This is almost always depressive, Mindham (1970) finding no examples of mania in a retrospective survey of 89 patients admitted to a psychiatric hospital. Only two had schizophrenic illnesses, one with postencephalitic and one with arteriosclerotic parkinsonism. Davison and Bagley (1969) note that reports of schizophrenia-like psychoses in association with idiopathic Parkinson's disease are rare and review the occasional examples in the literature. Crow *et al.* (1976) report four further cases, two with postencephalitic and two with idiopathic parkinsonism. Today, psychotic symptoms in parkinsonian patients are most often due to medication, as discussed below.

Psychiatric complications of anticholinergic drugs

Anticholinergic drugs may produce an acute organic reaction that sometimes leads to diagnostic difficulty. Porteous and Ross (1956) reported mental disturbance in 20% of patients treated with trihexyphenidyl (Artane), sometimes in response to small doses. Symptoms included confusion, excitement, agitation, paranoid delusions, hallucinations and suicidal intentions, all rapidly disappearing when the drug was withdrawn. The disorder was usually evident soon after starting the drug, for example Minagar *et al.* (1999) report a case that followed the single administration of a sco-polamine patch for travel sickness. Others could sometimes be gradual in evolution, with a risk that the relationship to treatment would be overlooked. Stephens (1967) and Craw-shaw and Mullen (1984) have reported misuse of trihexy-phenidyl in high dosage for its hallucinogenic properties, sometimes with outbursts of severe pathological excitement. Adverse reactions in parkinsonian patients are mostly seen in the elderly. They are also especially common when anti-cholinergics are added to levodopa, even in low dosage (De Smet *et al.* 1982). Anticholinergic psychoses often occur in the context of a delirium, which distinguishes them from other forms of psychosis seen in parkinsonian patients. Hal-lucinations are more often multimodal and are more likely to be perceived as threatening (Saint-Cyr *et al.* 1993).

Amantadine in high dosage may likewise provoke acute organic reactions where hallucinations occur within a delir-ium (Schwab *et al.* 1969; Dallos *et al.* 1970; Postma & Van Tilburg 1975; Timberlake & Vance 1978).

Psychiatric aspects of treatment with levodopa and dopamine agonists

Prior to the advent of dopaminergic medication, psychosis in parkinsonian patients whilst observed was rare. Mjönes (1949) could find no support for the idea of a special paraly-sis agitans psychosis and many of the earlier examples, with florid delusions and auditory and visual hallucinations, were no doubt the product of overmedication with hyos-cine, atropine or other solanaceous drugs. Others probably did not have idiopathic disease; in Mindhams's retrospec-tive study (1970) one psychotic patient had 'arteriosclerotic' Parkinson's disease whilst the other was postencephalitic. Reports of psychosis increased with the availability of levodopa (Cotzias 1969; Celesia & Wanamaker 1972). In an early review, Goodwin (1971) noted that psychiatric symptoms were the third most common group of levo-dopa side effects after dyskinesias and gastrointestinal disturbance.

The definition of psychosis used has a substantial bearing on any estimate of prevalence. Some early reports used a broad definition of psychosis that included confusion and agitation; Sweet *et al.* (1976) found psychosis in 60% of their patients. Tighter definitions yield lower rates. In his review Cummings (1991) suggested a figure of 40%. In a thorough community-based survey using the NeuroPsychiatric Inventory, Aarsland *et al.* (1999a) found hallucinations in 27% and delusions in 16%. Fenelon *et al.* (2000) included

'minor' hallucinatory experiences that may be missed with standardised assessment tools. These include 'presence' hallucinations in which the patient has the sensation of another person in the room, often behind them, and 'passage' hallucinations where the experience is one of a person (or animal) passing briefly by on one side. If these experiences were included, 39.8% of their 216 patients had psychosis.

Visual hallucinations are the most common feature of psychoses emerging with treatment in Parkinson's disease. Typically they occur in a clear sensorium, thus distinguish-ing them from a delirium. They occur with eyes open, often in dim surroundings (Barnes *et al.* 2003), and more fre-quently in the afternoon or evening (Manford & Ander-mann 1998; Barnes *et al.* 2003). They are distinguished from illusions by their complexity and the vivid colours and detail with which they are reported. They are usually brief, lasting seconds or minutes (Barnes *et al.* 2003).

Hallucinations in other modalities are reported much less frequently. Auditory hallucinations occasionally occur in isolation (Moskovitz *et al.* 1978) or alongside visual halluci-nations (Graham *et al.* 1997; Fenelon *et al.* 2000; Factor & Molho 2004; Paleacu *et al.* 2005). They are first- or second-person, non-distinct, like voices in a crowd, and not gener-ally threatening. It is rare for a visual hallucination to be the source of any auditory hallucination (Inzelberg *et al.* 1998). Tactile (Fenelon *et al.* 2002; Paleacu *et al.* 2005), gustatory (Holroyd *et al.* 2001) and olfactory (Tousi & Frankel 2004) hal-lucinations have also been reported. Jimenez-Jimenez *et al.* (1997) reported synaesthetic hallucinations, whilst Factor and Molho (2004) reported a case of Cotard syndrome.

Delusions occur less frequently than hallucinations (Cummings 1992b). They are often persecutory (Naimark *et al.* 1996; Sanchez-Ramos *et al.* 1996). Capgras syndrome has been reported (Lipper 1976). Formal thought disorder is very rare indeed (Cummings 1992b; Fernandez *et al.* 1999). An unexpected increase in sexual drive was noted by several authors soon after the introduction of levodopa (Barbeau 1969; Jenkins & Groh 1970). On occasions this might take the form of paraphilias (Harvey 1988; Cummings 1991; Quinn 1996).

No particular feature of the disease has been shown to be associated with the emergence of psychosis (Friedman 1991). Aarsland *et al.* (1999a) found a trend towards a higher score on the NeuroPsychiatric Inventory in patients with predom-inantly left-sided disease, although Shergill *et al.* (1998) reported more right-sided disease in patients with psychotic symptoms. Several authors have noted that a number of their psychotic patients had a past psychiatric history of both affective and psychotic disorders (Mendis 1996; Sanchez-Ramos *et al.* 1996; Juncos 1999). Increased age and duration of illness are frequently reported to be risks for the development of psychosis in Parkinson's disease (Cummings 1988; Vieregge 1996; Parkinson Study Group 1999; Fenelon *et al.* 2000).

That reports of psychoses became more frequent after the introduction of levodopa has led to a perception that there is a direct relationship between the two, i.e. that these are drug-induced psychoses. Tobias and Merlis (1970) showed that levodopa aggravated the mental status of patients with schizophrenia and several early studies claimed that there was a dose–response relationship between levodopa and psychosis (Cotzias *et al.* 1971; Ryback & Schwab 1971). However, these claims have largely been refuted (Sanchez-Ramos *et al.* 1996; Graham *et al.* 1997; Klein *et al.* 1997; Aarsland *et al.* 1999a) and other evidence points to a more complex relationship between levodopa and psychosis. Most obviously, despite the high prevalence of psychosis, most patients tolerate levodopa for many years without becoming psychotic. Additionally, Goetz *et al.* (1998) gave intravenous levodopa to parkinsonian patients who had already experienced hallucinations and observed no worsening in symptoms.

Psychosis has also been reported to complicate treatment with dopamine agonists, including bromocriptine (Burton *et al.* 1985; Montastruc *et al.* 1989; Cummings 1991), lisuride (Vaamonde *et al.* 1991), pergolide (Jankovic 1985) and apomorphine (Frankel *et al.* 1990). Recent evidence shows that psychosis is two to three times more likely with dopamine agonists than with levodopa (Rinne *et al.* 1998; Parkinson Study Group 2000; Rascol *et al.* 2000); indeed psychiatric side effects are the most common reason for their discontinuation (Montastruc *et al.* 1993). Several authors claim that the psychoses seen with dopamine agonists are more florid and persistent than those seen with levodopa (Lieberman *et al.* 1985; Vaamonde *et al.* 1991). Again, however, a simple relationship is questioned: Turner *et al.* (1984) noted that few patients receiving dopamine agonists for other indications become psychotic.

Aarsland *et al.* (1999a) have reported that approximately one-quarter of parkinsonian patients have vivid dreams and recent research has focused on the association between sleep disturbance and psychosis. High rates of vivid and abnormal dreams are seen in patients who had hallucinations or delusions (Moskovitz *et al.* 1978; Pappert *et al.* 1999). A 'continuum hypothesis' has emerged, suggesting that vivid dreams can be followed by sleep fragmentation and then visual hallucinations emerge in a temporally predictable sequence (Moskovitz *et al.* 1978; de Maindreville *et al.* 2005). This has been questioned (Goetz 2005) and remains unproven. Schenck *et al.* (1987) first reported an association between Parkinson's disease and rapid eye movement (REM) sleep behaviour. Arnulf *et al.* (2002) found that 39% of patients had brief periods of REM sleep during the day. Many of these REM periods corresponded with periods when they complained of hallucinations. Nomura *et al.* (2003) repeated these findings and also discovered that hallucinating patients had higher proportions of stage 1 REM sleep. In contrast, Manni *et al.* (2002) studied hypnopompic

and hypnagogic hallucinations and found that they were embedded in non-REM sleep rather than REM sleep.

Visual hallucinations in Parkinson's disease have been associated with abnormal ocular or visual functioning. Double vision, reduced visual acuity, impaired colour vision, impaired spatial contrast discrimination and impaired facial recognition have all been associated with hallucinations (Diederich *et al.* 1998; Holroyd *et al.* 2001; Crevits 2003; Davidsdottir *et al.* 2005).

One of the strongest predictors of psychosis in Parkinson's disease is cognitive impairment (Aarsland *et al.* 1999a,b; Fenelon *et al.* 2000; Paleacu *et al.* 2005). Papapetropoulos *et al.* (2005) found that prolonged disease, greater disease severity and greater cognitive impairment were each independent predictors of hallucinations. Aarsland *et al.* (2001a) found psychosis with increasing frequency in patients with non-demented Parkinson's disease, demented Parkinson's disease and dementia with Lewy bodies. One conclusion might be that psychotic symptoms are related to the density of cortical Lewy bodies. Barnes *et al.* (2003) suggest that the association between cognitive impairment and hallucinations may represent a final common pathway of general degradation in information processing, a marker of diffuse brain disease or a specific impairment in complex visuospatial functions.

There is evidence for the involvement of the dopamine, serotonin and acetylcholine neurotransmitter systems. Clearly, there is a role for the dopaminergic system, although the simple explanation of receptor hypersensitivity must be questioned. For example, Mellers *et al.* (1995) compared the growth hormone response of both psychotic and non-psychotic patients to apomorphine. No differences were found between the two groups, suggesting equal levels of dopamine sensitivity. Birkmayer *et al.* (1974) found lower levels of tryptophan in the brainstem and increased serotonin in the substantia nigra of psychotic patients. They suggested that hallucinations might arise from an imbalance of serotonin and dopamine. Visual hallucinations also occur with lysergic acid diethylamide (LSD), which acts at the $5HT_2$ receptor (Sadzot *et al.* 1989). The association of cognitive impairment with hallucinations suggests a role for the cholinergic system. Reduced levels of cortical choline acetyltransferase have been found in psychotic patients (Perry *et al.* 1990; Choi *et al.* 2000), and Nakano and Hirano (1984) found atrophy of the nucleus basalis in both Lewy body disease and Alzheimer's disease.

Psychosis impacts on the quality of life of patients and their carers. Initially, many patients retain insight into the nature of their experiences. Graham *et al.* (1997) reported that 70% of their patients had retained insight. Aarsland *et al.* (1999a) found that in 1 week 10% of patients had hallucinations retaining insight, whereas 6% of patients had hallucinations with no insight. Later as the disease progresses, insight is often lost. With advancing disease the burden of caring for the patient increases (Carter *et al.* 1998). Psychosis is the single greatest factor precipitating nursing home placement in parkinsonian patients (Goetz & Stebbins 1993; Aarsland *et al.* 2000). Goetz and Stebbins (1995) showed higher mortality in hallucinating patients, but a more recent study from the same group showed that prognosis has improved (Factor *et al.* 2003).

Dose reduction or drug withdrawal is the initial strategy in the management of psychosis in Parkinson's disease. Any recently added medications should be adjusted first. In patients on stable medication, anticholinergics, followed by dopamine agonists and then COMT inhibitors should be withdrawn if motor symptoms permit (Duncan & Taylor 1996; Fernandez 1999; Juncos 1999).

The introduction of atypical antipsychotic medication brought hope that effective drug treatment would be possible. This has only been partly fulfilled. There were initial positive studies of risperidone (Meco *et al.* 1994; Allen, R.L. *et al.* 1995; Koponen 1997) and olanzapine (Wolters *et al.* 1996; Beasley *et al.* 1997). However, Meco *et al.* (1997) followed up their initial group, finding marked deterioration in motor function, and Graham *et al.* (1998) and Aarsland *et al.* (1999c) have shown that few patients are able to tolerate the sedating effects of olanzapine. More recently, Breier *et al.* (2002) reported that two randomised controlled trials have failed to show a benefit of olanzapine over placebo. Quetiapine has so far been shown to be safe and effective (Fernandez *et al.* 1999; Juncos *et al.* 2004). However, some worsening of motor signs has been reported (Fernandez *et al.* 2000; Friedman & Factor 2000), more often in cognitively impaired patients (Reddy *et al.* 2002).

Perhaps the drug that has been shown to be most effective is clozapine. Despite an early randomised controlled trial showing disappointing results (Wolters *et al.* 1990), many positive studies have been published. The Parkinson Study Group (1999) and the French Clozapine Parkinson Study Group (1999) performed randomised controlled trials which showed that clozapine was safe and effective at doses very much smaller than those used in the treatment of schizophrenia. A follow-up study has shown this remains true after 2 years (Fernandez *et al.* 2004). Fernandez *et al.* (2005) and Pollak *et al.* (2004) both report high rates of psychotic relapse if clozapine is withdrawn. The drawback in using clozapine is the risk of agranulocytosis, necessitating frequent blood tests. There is a single case report of clozapine-induced aplastic anaemia in a psychotic parkinsonian patient (Ziegenbein *et al.* 2003).

An alternative approach is the use of anticholinesterase drugs developed for use in Alzheimer's disease. In a small case series performed by Bergman and Lerner (2002) it appeared safe and effective, although Cummings (2000) has observed worsening of parkinsonian motor signs in dementia with Lewy bodies. Reading *et al.* (2001) found rivastigmine to be effective in improving hallucinations, cognitive

function and carer distress. The drug was relatively well tolerated, although nausea was a dose-limiting side effect. ECT has also been shown to be effective (Hurwitz *et al.* 1988; Friedman & Gordon 1992). A novel and successful approach was reported by Factor *et al.* (1995a) who initially treated two patients with both clozapine and ECT and then used clozapine as maintenance therapy.

Premorbid personality and psychological precipitation of Parkinson's disease

As with certain other neurological diseases, there have been occasional suggestions that the premorbid personality of patients with Parkinson's disease has characteristic features. Closely associated is the proposition that psychological influences may be important in the development of the disorder. None of the observations in this area can be regarded as well founded, but neither can it be said that they have been decisively disproved.

Certain striking qualities in patients with Parkinson's disease have been stressed: their industriousness, rigid moralistic attitudes and habitual suppression of aggression prior to the appearance of the disease. Sands (1942) and Booth (1948) championed the view that persons of a particular psychological make-up were at special risk of developing the disorder. Sands (1942) described what he called the 'masked personality', finding a marked discrepancy between the outward appearance of coping and the turmoil within. Premorbid histories showed the patients to have been exemplary citizens, successful in their undertakings and externally calm, undemonstrative and stable. Close acquaintance, however, revealed a subjective state of tension that was suppressed and concealed from outsiders. With the development of parkinsonism a decompensation could often be observed, exposing the inner turmoil in the form of complaints, demands and self-centred behaviour. Sands suggested that the habitual suppression of emotion, doubtless involving intense physiological activity in many parts of the brain, may have led in some way to the degenerative changes responsible for the disease.

Booth (1948) developed such concepts further in a clinical study of 66 patients supplemented with Rorschach protocols. Some were postencephalitic and some 'senile degenerative' in origin. He concluded that the personality structure had been more decisive for the development of parkinsonism than the immediately obvious pathogenic mechanism; the latter had merely served to precipitate or actualise the disorder. Features stressed by Booth included a habitual impulse to action and a striving for success, independence and authority. Tension was prone to arise between this and the equally strong drive towards social conformity. But such tensions, like other emotions and impulses, were firmly suppressed. Regarding their success in life, he found this to be usually the result neither of great intelligence nor of unusual vitality, but attributable to aggressive perseverance and instinctive social conformity. An externally virtuous and docile disposition concealed hostile and sadistic impulses of unusual strength.

Such a character structure would be vulnerable to frustration in a number of ways. In many examples the first clinical symptoms of parkinsonism were preceded by a situation that had imposed a serious handicap to the execution of self-willed strivings and activities – arthritis, exhaustion, economic losses or professional disappointments. In other patients psychological conflicts could be identified as precipitants. Booth saw the major symptoms of parkinsonism as reflecting the original personality and its conflicts, rigidity for example being the product of a balance between overcoming obstacles and submission to restrictive influences, and the parkinsonian posture being related to unconscious hostility. Psychotherapy, in conjunction with antiparkinsonian medication, was claimed to meet with success in alleviating the symptoms.

There has been little support for these ideas from more recent studies. Diller and Riklan (1956) attempted an objective assessment of personality and background in a large number of patients referred for stereotactic surgery, but found nothing that could be regarded as characteristic for Parkinson's disease. Smythies (1967) compared 40 consecutive patients referred for surgery with control groups on a questionnaire relating to childhood disturbance, premorbid neurotic symptoms and life adjustment. No excess of premorbid emotional disability could be discerned, and no unusual difficulties in life adjustment antedating the illness. However, Pollock and Hornabrook (1966) were impressed with the high proportion of teetotallers among their large unselected series of parkinsonian patients, and found that many lacked hobbies and showed narrow intellectual horizons. Poewe *et al.* (1990) compared groups of patients with Parkinson's disease and benign essential tremor with healthy controls, using Cattell's personality inventory and a structured interview. Both patient groups were significantly more likely to be introverted, rigid, pedantic and self-reproachful than the controls, confirming previous impressions of personality. However, the similarity between the parkinsonian and tremor patients suggested that such traits were merely the product of chronic disability.

More interesting findings have come from comparisons between pairs of monozygotic twins, one of whom had Parkinson's disease while the other did not (Duvoisin *et al.* 1981; Ward *et al.* 1984). The affected members tended to describe themselves as more nervous, quiet, serious and introspective, whereas their co-twins were more outgoing and lighthearted. Moreover, a group of traits showed significant differences before the onset of the Parkinson's disease: the affected twin was less commonly the leader, less aggressive, more self-controlled and less confident. These differences in personality sometimes dated well back into adolescence and early adult life. It seemed possible therefore that neuro-

chemical differences between the twins might have existed from early in their lives, or that there had been some error of fetal development in the member destined for the disease.

Twin studies have also been employed to detect risk factors for the illness. The only possible association that has emerged is that affected twins have smoked less often and less heavily than their co-twins (Ward *et al.* 1984; Bharucha *et al.* 1986), which is interesting in that animal studies have indicated a dopaminergic effect of smoking on the brain. Baron (1986) reviews the epidemiological evidence from many case–control studies which also suggest that smoking may be protective, though with occasional negative reports (Golbe *et al.* 1986). It is possible, however, that differences in smoking habits reflect no more than differences in personality.

Lack of motivation, or apathy, often seen simply as part of a depressive disorder, has now been studied in its own right. Marin (1996) defined apathy as amotivation in affect behaviour and cognition. This was operationalised by Starkstein *et al.* (1992b) as (i) diminished goal-directed behaviour, (ii) diminished goal-directed cognitions and (iii) diminished concomitants of goal-directed behaviour, which (iv) cause distress and (v) are not due to reduced level of consciousness or effects of medication. The prevalence of apathy in Parkinson's disease ranges from 17% (Aarsland *et al.* 1999b) to 42% (Starkstein *et al.* 1992b). Apathy is more common in Parkinson's disease than in control subjects with osteoarthritis matched for disability (Pluck & Brown 2002), suggesting that it may be part of the disease process itself. Levy *et al.* (1998) showed that apathy was a feature of all neurodegenerative diseases. In this study apathy was variably associated with depression in each condition, although many studies confirm that they can be seen as discrete conditions (Starkstein *et al.* 1992b; Aarsland *et al.* 1999b; Shulman 2000; Pluck & Brown 2002). Pluck and Brown (2002) showed that apathy was associated with cognitive impairment. Apathy responds poorly to antidepressants and is not alleviated by levodopa (Pluck & Brown 2002). Chatterjee and Fahn (2002) have reported a case that improved with methylphenidate, whilst Lieberman *et al.* (1997) have suggested that pramipexole can be effective. Ready *et al.* (2004) showed that almost half of their male sample of apathetic patients were testosterone deficient and Okun *et al.* (2002) have suggested testosterone as a treatment.

Dopamine is the 'reward' neurotransmitter and major drugs of addiction stimulate dopamine release in the ventral striatal reward circuit. Although there is functional underactivity of the dopamine system in Parkinson's disease, PET studies show that amphetamine can stimulate prefrontal dopamine release even in advanced disease. It is perhaps unsurprising then that a small subgroup of patients report significant non-motor responses to levodopa. Some patients report that levodopa boosts energy and productivity independently of its effects on the motor system (Priebe 1984) and euphoria can occur during medication peaks (Serrano-

Duenas 2002). Conversely, drug withdrawal can be associated with dysphoria, anhedonia, anxiety and irritability (Serrano-Duenas 2002; Funkiewiez *et al.* 2003).

Giovannoni *et al.* (2000) have suggested criteria for a dopamine dysregulation syndrome.

1 Levodopa-responsive Parkinson's disease.

2 Need for increased doses of dopaminergic drugs.

3 Pattern of pathological use: demands for excessive medication in the presence of dyskinesias, drug-seeking behaviour, unwillingness to reduce dose.

4 Impairment in occupational or social functioning.

5 Development of manic syndrome in relation to dopaminergic medication.

6 Development of withdrawal syndrome in relation to dopaminergic medication.

7 Disturbance lasts at least 6 months.

Pathological use of levodopa has been reported. Evans and Lees (2004) described how patients can become impatient for the next dose and start to make dose increases themselves, whilst Nausieda (1985) described hoarding behaviours and patients seeking clandestine supplies of levodopa. Merims *et al.* (2000) reported the case of a patient who became quadriplegic yet still demanded levodopa. The removal of the drug led to signs of withdrawal that rapidly abated when levodopa was reintroduced. Such behaviours are most commonly reported with levodopa, often short-acting dispersable drugs. Abuse of dopamine agonists does occur though rarely in isolation from levodopa (Lawrence *et al.* 2003). Houeto *et al.* (2002) have reported compulsive use of a subthalamic nucleus stimulator.

Hepatolenticular degeneration (Wilson's disease)

Hepatolenticular degeneration is a rare inherited disorder affecting both the liver and the central nervous system first described by Wilson in 1912. The disease occurs in approximately 1 in 40 000 and is inherited in an autosomal recessive fashion. Over 200 mutations have been identified in the responsible gene, which is located on the long arm of chromosome 13 (Ferenci 2004). The gene encodes a membrane-bound copper-binding protein (ATP7B) expressed primarily in the liver that is responsible for transporting copper into the secretory pathway for incorporation in apocaeruloplasmin and excretion in bile (Bull *et al.* 1993; Yamaguchi *et al.* 1993). Imaired elimination leads to copper accumulation in many organs and tissues, which gives rise to the clinical features of the disease.

Clinical features

The onset is usually in childhood or adolescence, but may be delayed as late as the fifth decade of life. Approximately half of patients are symptomatic by the age of 15. The presentation may be with hepatic disorder, neurological disorder or both. In addition, as discussed below, a considerable proportion present initially with psychiatric disturbance. One-quarter of patients have involvement of more than one organ system at the time of presentation (El-Youssef 2003). Bearn (1957) estimated that some 40% of cases first show hepatic dysfunction, 40% neurological symptoms, and perhaps 20% psychiatric illness or behavioural disorder. There is a marked tendency for the liver disorder to be the first to appear when the onset is in childhood.

Hepatic involvement is almost invariable but may sometimes be found only on liver biopsy or at autopsy. Jaundice or hepatosplenomegaly can be the presenting features. Initial investigation may yield a hepatitic or cirrhotic picture. Fulminant presentations are described with severe liver failure ascites, ankle swelling or haematemesis from rupture of oesophageal varices.

The neurological disorder is confined to the motor system and takes the form of extrapyramidal disturbance with a characteristic accent on the facial and bulbar muscles (Harding 1993). There may be rigidity, tremor, athetoid writhing movements and abnormal dystonic postures of the limbs. In the early stages the disabilities may be transient and sensitive to emotional influences, leading to an erroneous impression of conversion hysteria. A flapping tremor may be seen at the wrists, or characteristic 'wing beating' at the shoulders when the arms are abducted and the elbows flexed. The facial expression is stiff and motionless, often with open mouth and a rigid silent smile. Bulbar symptoms take the form of spastic dysarthria and dysphagia.

Occasional patients develop epileptic seizures, usually of Jacksonian type. Dening *et al.* (1988) found that seizures were 10 times as frequent as in the general population. Hemiplegia is not uncommon. Periods of coma or semicoma may develop, persisting for several weeks but not necessarily heralding a fatal outcome.

Variations in the clinical picture depend to some extent on the age at presentation (Bearn 1957). In young subjects dystonia or spastic rigidity tend to dominate the picture and tremor may be slight. The course is then liable to be acute and rapidly progressive. In adults tremor predominates and rigidity may be unobtrusive, with a milder course and slower progression. A good deal of overlap occurs, however, and mixed pictures are common. In the earlier literature the term 'lenticular degeneration' was used for cases showing spasticity, rigidity and dystonia, and 'pseudosclerosis' for cases with marked tremor and dysarthria. The lenticular presentation is said to occur earlier, with the pseudosclerotic presentation more common in adulthood (El-Youssef 2003).

The Kayser–Fleischer ring is a diagnostic sign of great importance. It is situated at the margin of the cornea, is brown or greyish-green in colour, and is often evident to the naked eye although all patients should be examined with a slit-lamp. It consists of copper deposits in Descemet's membrane in the limbic area of the cornea. Absence of a Kayser–Fleischer ring makes the diagnosis of Wilson's disease improbable in the presence of neuropsychiatric symptoms, but it may be absent in purely hepatic forms of the disease. However, Kayser–Fleischer rings are not pathognomonic; they may also be seen in primary biliary cirrhosis and autoimmune hepatitis. Sunflower cataracts may also be seen in Wilson's disease.

Computed tomography and magnetic resonance imaging (MRI) have been found to show a characteristic picture (Williams & Walshe 1981; Aisen *et al.* 1985). Ventricular dilatation, cortical atrophy and enlargement of the cisterns around the brainstem are common, and may be accompanied by typical hypodense areas in the basal ganglia on CT. This combination is considered to be specific for Wilson's disease. The hypodense areas are most frequent in patients with neurological disability, but can also be seen in those presenting with hepatic disorder or even in presymptomatic cases. MRI characteristically shows symmetrical focal areas of increased signal, especially in the lenticular nuclei (i.e. putamen and globus pallidus) but also in the thalamus, caudate nuclei, dentate nuclei and brainstem (Aisen *et al.* 1985). Focal white matter lesions may be observed in addition to hypointense areas on T2-weighted imaging (King *et al.* 1996). T2-weighted scans may show the 'face of the giant panda' sign, consisting of high signal intensity in the tegmentum except for red nucleus, preservation of signal intensity of the lateral portion of the pars reticulata of the substantia nigra, and hypointensity of the superior colliculus (Hitoshi *et al.* 1991). Rescanning after treatment with chelating agents may show resolution of the changes. PET has shown diffusely reduced brain metabolism, with a particular accent on the lenticular nuclei (Hawkins *et al.* 1987). It is not known why copper has a predilection for accumulating in certain parts of the brain.

Other features include abnormalities of renal function. Azotaemia occurs in 20% of patients and glomerular filtration rate can be lowered by 10%. Copper excess may not be responsible for glomerular dysfunction but is clearly linked to tubular disease. Aminoaciduria is seen in a high proportion of cases. Electrolyte abnormalities may precipitate nephrocalcinosis. Degenerative changes around joints are commonly seen on radiographic examination, even in young persons, and fractures and fragmentations of the bones of the hands and wrists may be detected. Copper deposits in the synovium can cause an arthritis. Cardiomyopathy, heart failure and conduction abnormalities have been described. Episodes of haemolytic anaemia may occur, presumably due to sudden release of copper from the tissues.

Course and outcome

Remissions may be seen in the earlier stages, and even thereafter marked fluctuations in severity can occur. Ultimately,

however, severe crippling results from spasticity and dystonic contractions. Dysphagia is often profound, and intellectual deterioration is common in the later stages. The prognosis is worse the younger the age of onset. Formerly children rarely survived for more than 4 years, whereas adults might survive without severe disablement for 12 years or more. Death usually occurs from liver failure, rupture of oesophageal varices, inhalation or intercurrent infection. With treatment this gloomy outlook has been altered as described below.

Pathology

Smith (1976) describes the pathological findings as follows. The brain is usually normal externally, but on section the corpus striatum is found to be shrunken and brownish or brick-red in colour. The putamen often shows cavitation. Microscopically, neuronal loss is seen in the caudate and putamen, and the latter contains large numbers of astrocytic nuclei, many having a characteristic enlarged and vesicular appearance ('Alzheimer nuclei'). In contrast, the globus pallidus often shows relatively little change. Pericapillary concretions that stain for copper may also be detected. Other abnormal elements include large phagocytic 'Opalski' cells, possibly derived from histiocytes.

The thalamus, subthalamic nuclei and brainstem nuclei may also show Alzheimer nuclei and Opalski cells. Phagocytes containing iron pigment are commonly found in the substantia nigra. Degeneration of the dentate nuclei and superior cerebellar peduncles has occasionally been observed.

Foci of degeneration are not uncommon in the cerebral cortex, especially in the frontal lobes. Diffuse loss of neurones and fibres may occur, or status spongiosus involving both the cortex and the white centres of the convolutions. Astrocytic and oligodendrocytic proliferation may be seen.

The liver may be enlarged in the early stages but is usually smaller than normal at autopsy. It is coarsely cirrhotic, varying in colour from yellow to brown or brick-red depending on the relative amounts of copper storage, fatty degeneration and bile staining. Microscopically, the picture is of multilobular cirrhosis. The spleen is usually enlarged.

Biochemical abnormalities

The liver and brain contain a marked excess of copper, the basal ganglia being particularly heavily affected. The Kayser–Fleischer ring in the cornea is due to deposition of copper there, and levels may be raised in the kidneys and other tissues. The total serum copper is usually low and the excretion of copper in the urine is high (>100 µg in 24 hours).

More than 75% of patients have abnormally low caeruloplasmin. Caeruloplasmin is a globulin synthesised in the liver; 90% of serum copper is normally bound to caeruloplasmin, the remainder being loosely attached to serum albumin. This free copper is the toxic pool, probably representing the part in transition to other body regions, and it is raised in the disease. While important as a screening test, low values of caeruloplasmin are not invariable, some 5% of patients having normal levels and 10–20% of heterozygotes showing a deficiency (Starosta-Rubinstein 1995). Levels may also be reduced in protein-deficiency states and in the presence of liver disease. When the index of suspicion is high and caeruloplasmin is normal, a radioactive ^{64}Cu incorporation test can be valuable, revealing a lack of uptake of orally administered copper into newly synthesised caeruloplasmin. Definitive diagnosis can depend on liver biopsy, which reveals elevated copper levels and the histological changes of nodular cirrhosis.

With the advent of effective treatment, special attention must be directed towards the detection of asymptomatic but vulnerable individuals in the families of patients so that prophylactic treatment can be commenced. Once the disease has been diagnosed all siblings of the patient should be examined: 25% will be at risk and 50% will be heterozygote carriers. Discovery of a low caeruloplasmin should then lead to liver biopsy, which in the heterozygote may show a mild increase in liver copper, though not in the range of Wilson's disease, while liver histology is normal (Harding 1993).

Treatment

The aim of treatment is to eliminate excessive copper from the body and prevent its reaccumulation. Treatment must begin as soon as the diagnosis is made and continue for life. Dimercaprol (BAL) was the first chelating agent to be tried (Denny-Brown & Porter 1951). Results were encouraging but the injections were painful and liable to lead to toxic reactions. Penicillamine was the treatment of choice for many years. However, acute sensitivity reactions were common, sometimes ameliorated by steroids. Moreover, 50% of those presenting neurologically got worse, and half of these did not recover. Late side effects included skin changes, renal damage, systemic lupus erythematosus, myasthenia gravis, optic neuritis, bone marrow suppression and loss of the sense of taste. Low-copper diets no longer have a place in the management of the disease.

Alternatives to penicillamine have been developed. Trientine is considered by many to be the drug of choice as it has a lower incidence of adverse effects than penicillamine. Its exact mechanism of action is unknown. Sideroblastic anaemia is the major side effect. Tetrathiomolybdate, although yet to be licensed, shows considerable promise and is well tolerated. Brewer (2000a) suggests tetrathiomolybdate as the initial chelating agent for those presenting with neurological or psychiatric presentations. It complexes copper with food protein and prevents copper absorption. Zinc is the treatment of choice for lifelong maintenance. It

induces metallothionein in intestinal cells, which then prevents copper absorption, particularly that present in saliva and gastric secretion that would normally be reabsorbed. Zinc is essentially non-toxic, although 10% of patients experience gastric discomfort (Brewer 2000a).

Most patients make an excellent recovery from both hepatic and neurological disorder, although a small proportion fail to respond to medication and follow a steady downhill course to death over several weeks or months (Walshe 1986). Neurological improvement is often more rewarding than hepatic improvement given that almost all patients have a degree of cirrhosis at presentation. However, all aspects of the picture can respond. Tremor, rigidity, dystonia, dysarthria and dysphagia may all gradually resolve and some patients become entirely symptom-free. In general, improvement is more complete the earlier treatment has been commenced. Dramatic results have been reported from states of hopeless incapacity to relative independence, though such cannot always be achieved. Psychiatric symptoms have been found to improve as well, some more impressively than others. This is discussed in the next section.

Occasional patients will warrant liver transplantation, which effectively treats the Wilson's disease as well as the liver failure, restoring copper excretion to normal. Polson *et al.* (1987) have reported its success in reversing severe neurological manifestations, this occurring with unusual rapidity in one of their patients.

A man of 30 had a 14-month history of hepatic and neurological impairment. Despite treatment with penicillamine he developed increasing dysarthria, dysphagia, akinesia and rigidity of the limbs, requiring continuous nursing care. After transplantation liver function became virtually normal from 4 weeks onwards, and neurological recovery began 2–3 months later. By 8 months postoperatively no neurological signs were detectable.

Psychiatric manifestations of Wilson's disease

Psychiatric symptoms can form a prominent part of the clinical picture along with the neurological defects. On this account it is not uncommon for patients to present to psychiatrists before their disease is diagnosed, with a risk that treatment will be dangerously delayed. Dening and Berrios (1989a) recommend that serum caeruloplasmin should be measured in all psychiatric patients who show personality change, especially towards disinhibited, bizarre or reckless behaviour, in those who show neurological signs not accounted for by medication, and in patients with unexplained hepatic disease. Brewer (2000b) believes that all new behavioural abnormalities in patients under 40 should lead to screening for Wilson's disease. Dysarthria and other bulbar symptoms will be a strong indication for investigation in patients below middle age, likewise deterioration in school or work performance in children or young adults. The following case illustrates the diagnostic difficulties that can arise.

A 17-year-old girl developed emotional lability, nervousness, difficulty with handwriting and deterioration in school performance. She was at first thought to be suffering from adolescent adjustment problems. Chlorpromazine was prescribed, leading to increasing tremor, and she became withdrawn. Abnormal liver function tests were noted, likewise mild extrapyramidal dysfunction, but both were ascribed to the drug. She was later hospitalised with a diagnosis of schizoaffective disorder. Finally, she was noted to show excessive drooling, a mask-like face, dysphagia, choreoathetoid movements, dystonia, spasticity, splenomegaly and Kayser–Fleischer rings. A diagnosis of Wilson's disease was confirmed 22 months after the first manifestations. Two years of treatment with penicillamine left her still dysphonic and with severe motor disability (Cartwright 1978).

Wilson (1912) stressed the prominence of psychiatric symptoms in his initial description and believed them to be a fundamental part of the clinical picture. He noted psychotic and hysterical manifestations, later adding affective change and disordered behaviour (Wilson 1940). Impairment of mental function seemed often to be more apparent than real, being to a large extent suggested by the patient's appearance and dysarthria. These various aspects have been reiterated in subsequent case reports and small series.

A more comprehensive picture emerges from a series of publications on the large number of patients referred to Dr John Walshe at Cambridge, this representing the largest series available in the UK (Dening & Berrios 1989a,b, 1990). Akil and Brewer (1995) have described a large series of patients from the USA. The careful documentation employed and the application of operationally defined criteria for the assessment of psychiatric disorder increase the validity of the findings, even though matters of special selection cannot be excluded. The principal conclusions are that personality change and 'incongruous behaviour' are undoubtedly common in Wilson's disease, while psychotic phenomena are rare. Irritability, aggression and depression appear to be frequent, likewise cognitive impairment of mild degree. Many of these psychiatric features appear to have an organic cerebral basis.

Dening and Berrios (1989a) first assessed 195 cases by retrospective case note review. Half were rated as showing some psychiatric disturbance at index admission and 20% had seen a psychiatrist before the disease had been diagnosed. Reasons for referral included deterioration in school or work performance, outbursts of abnormal behaviour and strange disorders of movement.

Personality change, in terms of alterations in lifestyle, relationships or behaviour, was judged as present or possible in one-quarter of patients. A similar proportion showed incongruous behaviour by way of disinhibition, bizarre or reckless behaviour, often leading to forensic problems. Evidence of such behavioural abnormality was significantly associated with high scores on ratings of neurological symptomatology, especially dysarthria. Irritability emerged in 18% and showed similar associations, and aggression was noted in 14%. Cognitive impairment was present or suspected in almost one-quarter, being generally mild, and depression in 21%. Depression showed associations with long duration of admission and the presence of family problems but little relationship to neurological symptoms.

In contrast, delusions and hallucinations occurred in less than 2% of patients, casting doubt on any significant relationship between psychotic illness and Wilson's disease. Disorientation was relatively rare at 7% and closely associated with liver failure.

A more intensive prospective study was made of 31 consecutive attenders at the clinic (Dening & Berrios 1989b). These ranged in severity from patients who had never been symptomatic to patients who were mute and bedridden. More than half were rated as abnormal on the Personality Assessment Schedule, the main factor on factor analysis reflecting traits such as impulsiveness, irresponsibility and aggression. One-third were 'cases' as judged by scores on the General Health Questionnaire. No psychotic symptoms were observed. Only four patients scored below the threshold for cognitive impairment on the Mini Mental State Examination, and in general such impairment was not severe.

Disorders of personality and behaviour were again significantly related to the presence of neurological symptoms, especially dysarthria, bradykinesia and rigidity, strongly suggesting that they had an organic basis. Depressive symptoms were related to hepatic dysfunction. Cognitive impairment, being mild in this sample, showed less marked correlation with neurological disorder than might have been expected; it was evident, moreover, that some patients who seemed superficially to be impaired performed well on psychometric tests.

Finally, an attempt was made to assess the response of neurological and psychiatric symptoms to treatment by retrospective review of 129 patients over a mean period of 10 years (Dening & Berrios 1990). Most gains had occurred during the early years of treatment, with improvement in cognition and 'incongruous behaviour' being significant. In contrast, depression and irritability seemed not to improve. Aspects of neurological disability also decreased significantly, both early and later during treatment, including tremor, rigidity and overall neurological scores. However, dysphagia appeared often to persist and dysarthria to have a poor prognosis.

Other studies also report a high prevalence of depression, 27% in the study by Oder *et al.* (1991). Recent work by Hesse *et al.* (2003) has shown reduced central serotonergic activity and reduction in activity of the presynaptic serotonin transporter, thus calling into question whether the psychiatric features of Wilson's disease are caused directly by copper deposition. Cognitive impairment has been reported by Akil and Brewer (1995) and Rathbun (1996). It is generally mild, although Portala *et al.* (2000) found a range of deficits including concentration problems and lack of appropriate emotion even in treated patients.

Although Dening reported positive response of symptoms to treatment with penicillamine, this drug can also produce adverse neuropsychiatric consequences including seizures and psychosis (McDonald & Lake 1995). This is possible even if the patient were previously psychiatrically asymptomatic (Glass *et al.* 1990). Early reports of the use of tetrathiomolybdate suggest that psychiatric symptoms respond well without adverse effects (Brewer 1995).

Progressive supranuclear palsy (Steele–Richardson–Olszewski syndrome)

Steele *et al.* (1964) described a group of patients with an unusual progressive neurological disorder that manifested as an akinetic–rigid syndrome with ocular and mental features. Outstanding signs include supranuclear paralysis of external ocular movements, particularly in the vertical plane and involving downward gaze. This is sometimes described as a 'Mona Lisa stare'. Dysarthria is common and can be heard as a slurred growl. Pseudobulbar palsy, dystonic rigidity of the trunk and neck, cognitive impairment and signs of pyramidal tract and cerebellar dysfunction may also be seen. A tendency to fall over backwards is characteristic. In the later stages the eyes are fixed centrally, and widespread rigidity reduces the patient to a helpless bedridden state. The estimated prevalence is 5–6 per 100 000 (Schrag *et al.* 1999; Nath *et al.* 2001). The onset is usually in the sixth decade, with death some 5–10 years later. Subsequent reports have confirmed the main features of the syndrome (Steele 1972; Maher & Lees 1986; de Bruin & Lees 1992). Treatment with levodopa may sometimes ameliorate the rigidity and ophthalmoplegia for a time, but treatment response is often disappointing.

The pathology shows cell loss, neurofibrillary tangles, gliosis and demyelination, particularly affecting the basal ganglia, brainstem and cerebellar nuclei. The tangles consist of hyperphosphorylated tau proteins. Under the electron microscope they appear as bundles of straight filaments and do not show the paired helical structure seen in Alzheimer's disease. Tau is also found in glial inclusion bodies. The distribution of changes is remarkably constant and usually there is a surprising lack of cortical involvement. Steele *et al.* (1964) commented on the resemblance of the histological features to those of postencephalitic parkinsonism or the parkinsonism–dementia complex of Guam, although the distribution of changes is different. The aetiology is unknown. Degenerative or viral processes are suspected, but attempts at transmission to primates have been unsuccessful. Rojo *et al.* (1999) believe that familial cases may be more common than previously thought. H1 is one form of the tau gene. Many patients are H1/H1 homozygous, 89% in one study compared with 65% of controls. However, H1 does not seem to influence age of onset or disease severity (Litvan 2001). Tau exists as six different isoforms, three of which have three repeated microtubule-binding domains whereas the remaining three have four repeated microtubule-binding domains. The normal brain has roughly equal amounts of three- and four-repeat tau, whereas Flament *et al.* (1991) have shown that in progressive supranuclear palsy the brain has three to four times more four-repeat than three-repeat tau.

Diagnosis can be difficult and the presentation may be confused with stroke, idiopathic Parkinson's disease, multiple system atrophy and corticobasal degeneration. Litvan *et al.* (1996) have described the clinical diagnostic criteria. Other findings include reduced set-shifting ability and concentration and more apathy and disinhibition in progressive supranuclear palsy than in idiopathic Parkinson's disease (Soliveri *et al.* 2000; Aarsland *et al.* 2001b). Schrag *et al.* (2000) suggested a set of MRI criteria including an axial midbrain diameter of less than 17 mm, signal increase in the midbrain, atrophy or signal increase in the red nucleus, and signal increase in the globus pallidus. Sphincter electromyography can be used to distinguish progressive supranuclear palsy from idiopathic Parkinson's disease but not from multiple system atrophy.

Among the psychiatric manifestations cognitive impairment is very common, affecting over 80% of the patients in de Bruin and Lees' (1992) survey to some degree. Of the 67 patients, five had presented with symptoms leading to an initial diagnosis of Alzheimer's disease, though early aphasia, apraxia and agnosia were never observed. Personality change, abnormal behaviour, emotional lability, depression and social withdrawal were all common.

The most striking cognitive change is bradyphrenia, with slowing of response. Apathy is significantly more common than in idiopathic Parkinson's disease (Aarsland *et al.* 2001b). Judgement is often found to be impaired and abstracting ability may be poor. The question of memory impairment in the disease has been controversial, with differing reports in different series. Here the clearest evidence has come from

Litvan et al.'s (1989) comparison of 12 patients with matched healthy controls. This revealed significant deficits in learning, consolidation and retrieval, also abnormally rapid rates of forgetting. In contrast, 'information scanning', which requires the use of short-term memory processes, remained intact. Verbal fluency tests also showed definite impairment. Both Schrag et al. (2003) and Aarsland et al. (2001b) report that one-third of their patients complained of difficulties with memory and concentration.

The memory disorder may owe much to deafferentation of the subcortical–frontal projections, since the cortical neurones themselves are generally spared. D'Antona et al. (1985) and Brooks (1993) have shown marked prefrontal hypometabolism on PET in comparison with controls of equivalent age. These observations are relevant to the question of 'subcortical dementia' discussed below.

Ovsiew and Schneider (1993) have reported a patient with autopsy confirmation of the disease in whom a schizophrenic psychosis was a central feature and present from the earliest stages. Josephs and Dickson (2003) found that 18% of their patients had a history of psychosis. Schrag et al. (2003) reported findings on 27 patient; using the Quality of Life Assessment Schedule, 54% reported depression and 29% reported anxiety. Depression was strongly linked to overall quality of life. Aarsland et al. (2001b) assessed 61 patients with the NeuroPsychiatric Inventory. Very high levels of apathy and disinhibition were found; depression and anxiety were as common as in the controls with Parkinson's disease.

Subcortical dementia

While the disease itself is rare, certain observations made on the mental state of such patients by Albert et al. (1974) have provoked considerable interest. The pattern of cognitive impairment seen in progressive supranuclear palsy appears to have distinctive features that may reflect the relative confinement of pathology to subcortical structures. Albert et al. termed this picture 'subcortical dementia'. In this they made a valuable contribution, by underlining the fact that cognitive failure does not always imply cortical disease. The cortex depends for its functioning on inputs from the reticular activating systems and other subcortical structures, and when these fail the cortex, though intact, may cease to display its potential.

Albert et al. (1974) contrasted the behaviour pattern in patients with progressive supranuclear palsy with that seen in patients with cortical disease processes. Among five cases seen personally and 42 adequately described in the literature, several key features were evident in the mental state. Though described as 'forgetful' it could frequently be shown that the patient could produce the correct answer if given encouragement and an abnormal amount of time in which to respond. Memory as such appeared not to be truly impaired, but rather the timing mechanism that enables the memory system to function at normal speed. Slowness of thought was similarly prominent; tasks requiring verbal manipulation or perceptual–motor skills were performed incorrectly under normal pressures, but adequately when time was extended. Thus, when the patient was allowed to proceed at his own pace, or when provided with structured situations to elicit responses that did not occur spontaneously, his intellect could prove to be surprisingly intact. Defects of higher cortical function such as dysphasia, agnosia or apraxia were strikingly absent, though calculation or ability to deal with abstract material was sometimes defective. Personality and mood changes fell into two categories: the larger group was indifferent, apathetic and depressed, while the smaller showed progressive irritability and/or euphoria. Brief outbursts of rage were common, and inappropriate forced laughing and crying were often in evidence.

A woman of 65 with the disease showed extrapyramidal rigidity, slowed speech and marked limitation of upward and downward gaze. Her cognitive state was described as follows.

She was alert, attentive and socially appropriate. Immediate recall of digits was seven forward and five backwards. Recent memory was deficient in an unusual way: her first answer to almost every question was 'I don't know'. However, if the examiner encouraged her by saying 'Sure you know; just take your time', she would correctly respond to 95% of the questions. The latency between question and response was often inordinately long, in some cases as long as 4.5 minutes (often taxing the patience of the examiner). Remote memory was intact.

Language functions were as follows: no paraphasias were heard; naming was excellent on confrontation for high and very low frequency words. Although she complained of having difficulty with words, she had no naming defect. She did, however, have a time-related word-finding defect: in 1 minute she was able to find only three words beginning with the letter 'b'. At 5 minutes she had listed 12; at 10 minutes 23; at 15 minutes 33. Tests of repetition, comprehension of spoken and written language, and reading aloud were normal, except for the slow reading rate.

For simple mental calculations her responses were quick and accurate. With more complex arithmetic problems, she was slow but correct. Her proverb interpretations were concrete and she had difficulty finding similarities in two similar objects (Albert et al. 1974).

A 58-year-old woman had dysarthria, a broad-based ataxic gait and striking impairment of upward and downward gaze. Evaluation of mental status revealed an awake, generally placid or apathetic woman who reacted in a seemingly angry manner to the examiner's attempts to question her. Despite her apparent anger, she could nonetheless be coaxed to cooperate. Digit span was six forward. Questions designed to test recent and remote memory led to the following situation: either she refused to answer or she answered incorrectly. However, when the examiner waited, either silently or with attempts to encourage her, for longer than normal waiting periods (even as long as 4–5 minutes for a single question) she then gave the correct answer to 70–80% of the questions. This indicated that her stock of knowledge was not impaired as one might otherwise have concluded. Rather, she was delayed in reaching into the stock for the correct answer. Tests of language and gestures revealed no aphasia or apraxia. No inattention or primary perceptual problems were seen. Proverb interpretations tended to be concrete. Her ability to find the categorical similarities between similar items was impaired. Her calculating ability was poor (Albert *et al.* 1974).

Attention was drawn to rather similar pictures in other diseases with subcortical pathology, and the authors tentatively proposed that the common mechanisms underlying them were those of impaired timing and activation. Impaired functioning of the reticular formation, or disconnection of the reticular-activating systems from thalamic and subthalamic nuclei, might be the cause of slowing of intellectual processes, even though the cortical systems for perceiving, storing and manipulating knowledge remained intact.

The situation in progressive supranuclear palsy, in which the cortex is known to be largely spared, is likely to exist in some other dementing processes also. Parkinson's disease with intellectual impairment is an obvious example; Huntington's chorea is another (see Chapter 9 under Huntington's disease). Normal-pressure hydrocephalus, Wilson's disease and the dementia associated with deep lacunar infarcts (see under Premorbid personality and psychological precipitation of Parkinson's disease, earlier) have also been viewed in this way (Benson 1982; Cummings 1982). It could conceivably be the case that some variants of the dementias of old age may have a subcortical rather than a cortical origin to the cognitive difficulties, or at least a prominent subcortical component in the aetiology of the clinical picture. An interesting possibility is that the 'normal' effects of old age on cognitive functioning may reflect subcortical rather than cortical ageing processes (Albert 1978).

That a subcortical dementia might be both clinically and pathologically distinct from the more classical understanding of dementia as a cortical disease has produced much

research and debate (Pillon *et al.* 1993; Darvesh & Freedman 1996). In subcortcial dementia the disease occurs largely in the basal ganglia, cerebellum and brainstem nuclei (Darvesh & Freedman 1996). Cerebrovascular disease is a common cause as are a number of neurodegenerative conditions. Psychiatric features are common, particularly depression, apathy and personality change. Psychosis is a feature in many presentations. Features such as agnosias, dysphasias and dyspraxias are more indicative of cortical dementias such as Alzheimer's disease.

The idea that dementias are either subcortical or cortical has since been challenged (Turner *et al.* 2002) and it would seem more likely that a spectrum exists between the two. Cortical pathologies do sometimes occur in subclinical diseases, Alzheimer-type pathology in Parkinson's disease for example (Hughes *et al.* 1992), whilst subcortical neuronal loss is seen in Alzheimer's. Moreover, a clinical picture very similar to Alzheimer's disease may be produced by (subcortical) thalamic lesions (Kopelman 1991).

Corticobasal degeneration (cortical–basal ganglionic degeneration)

This rare disorder was first described by Rebeiz *et al.* in 1968. Further series of patients have been reported by Gibb *et al.* (1989) and Riley *et al.* (1990). The condition is reviewed by Watts *et al.* (1994). Corticobasal degeneration consists of degeneration in defined regions of the cerebral cortex coupled with marked pathology in the striatonigral system and other subcortical nuclei. The clinical presentation can resemble progressive supranuclear palsy (see beginning of previous section: Progressive supranuclear palsy), while the pathological changes share features in common with Pick's disease. A clinical hallmark is the asymmetry of the motor manifestations, such that one limb may become completely incapacitated before symptoms develop on the other side.

It presents usually in late middle or early old age, with akinesia, rigidity, limb apraxia and a combination of supranuclear gaze palsy, myoclonus, limb dystonia or cortical sensory loss. Postural instability may be marked. The myoclonus is induced by action, and is often markedly stimulus sensitive. Ataxia, chorea, blepharospasm and pyramidal tract signs may also be seen. Not infrequently the patient develops an 'alien limb', whereby the hand and arm feel 'foreign' to the patient and tend to wander involuntarily and uncontrollably. This feature is discussed by Sawle *et al.* (1991) who ascribe it to damage to the medial frontal cortex and supplementary motor area.

Cognitive disabilities may be notably mild or absent even when severe apraxia hampers the majority of voluntary activity. Other patients, however, develop marked parietal lobe deficits that manifest as dyscalculia, constructional apraxia or visuospatial impairment. Severe generalised dementia supervenes in perhaps one-third of cases. High rates of depression are seen, especially in comparison to progressive supranuclear palsy (Litvan *et al.* 1998), but less apathy and disinhibition. Psychosis appears to be infrequent. Rarely, cases show marked frontal lobe dysfunction, including aggression and even Kluver–Bucy syndrome (Nasreddine *et al.* 1999; Stover & Watts 2001). Onset is typically in the seventh decade (Wenning 1998). Progressive incapacity leads to death after 4–10 years. Treatment with levodopa is often ineffective, though baclofen may help the rigidity and clonazepam may dampen the myoclonus (Thompson & Marsden 1992).

Pathological findings consist of cortical atrophy with cell loss and gliosis, mainly affecting the peri-rolandic frontal and parietal regions in contrast to the frontotemporal atrophy of Pick's disease. Subcortical regions are also markedly affected, especially the globus pallidus, putamen, substantia nigra and lateral thalamus. The subthalamic nucleus, red nucleus and locus caeruleus are also involved. Abnormal neurones show marked resistance to staining methods (achromasia) and a swollen appearance similar to the ballooning of Pick cells. However, classic Pick bodies are not present. Basophilic inclusions are seen, especially in the substantia nigra, also globose neurofibrillary tangles similar to those of progressive supranuclear palsy. The same elevated ratio of four-repeat to three-repeat tau observed in progressive supranuclear palsy is also seen in corticobasal degeneration. As in progressive supranuclear palsy, the H1 allele is very common, 93% in one study (Houlden *et al.* 2001). Lang (2003) suggests this implies that corticobasal degeneration and progressive supranuclear palsy share a common genetic predisposition, although he notes that pathological evidence currently points to them being discrete entities (Ishizawa & Dickson 2001; Dickson *et al.* 2002).

Computed tomography and MRI show ventricular enlargement and cortical atrophy, which may be asymmetrical in distribution. Brain imaging with PET has revealed distinctive features that mirror the pattern of pathological involvement (Eidelberg *et al.* 1991; Sawle *et al.* 1991). Cortical hypometabolism is evident in the superior temporal, inferior parietal, posterior frontal and occipital association cortices, with a markedly asymmetrical pattern that may be of value in differential diagnosis. ^{18}F-fluorodopa uptake is reduced in the caudate and putamen, again in an asymmetrical manner.

Striatonigral degeneration (multiple system atrophy)

Adams *et al.* (1964) drew attention to this rare disorder, closely similar to Parkinson's disease in clinical manifestations but with a distinctive pathological basis. Affected patients show rigidity, akinesia, slowed movements and a flexed posture. At autopsy the striking features are extensive neuronal loss in the zona compacta of the substantia

nigra, but without Lewy bodies, and marked degenerative changes in the putamen and caudate nuclei.

One of Adams *et al.*'s four cases also showed olivopontocerebellar degeneration. Many cases have since been reported with this striking combination, prominent cerebellar ataxia then preceding the parkinsonian symptoms. Moreover, approximately half are handicapped by fainting due to postural hypotension, and other signs of autonomic failure may include impotence and sphincter and deglutition disturbances. Such patients show neuronal loss in the intermediolateral tract of the spinal cord and the dorsal vagal nuclei of the brainstem (Shy–Drager syndrome). Dementia may develop but is uncommon. Gosset *et al.* (1983) reviewed 35 cases with both striatonigral degeneration and olivopontocerebellar degeneration, ranging in age from 30 to 75, half of whom also showed progressive autonomic failure. They termed this combination 'progressive multisystem degeneration'. Several patients also showed pyramidal signs, slight muscle atrophy, intention myoclonus and upward gaze palsy.

Nowadays it is usual to group these various conditions together under the title of multiple system atrophy. The neuropathological picture has now been more completely described. Cell loss and gliosis are widespread throughout the brainstem, cerebellum, basal ganglia and central autonomic nervous system. The hallmark is the diffuse presence of cytoplasmic inclusions that are positive for both α-synuclein and tau (Lantos & Papp 1994; Wenning & Quinn 1997; Dickson *et al.* 1999).

The condition should be suspected when a parkinsonian syndrome coexists with ataxia, vertical gaze palsy, pyramidal signs and evidence of autonomic failure such as postural hypotension. Quinn (1989) considers that it is less rare than commonly supposed, perhaps accounting for up to 10% of patients with parkinsonism, whereas Schrag *et al.* (1999) have estimated the prevalence to be 4.4 per 100 000. The condition starts most commonly in the sixth decade (Wenning & Geser 2003) and is associated with a median time to death of 9 years (Wenning *et al.* 1994). Diagnosis can be difficult, especially as autonomic problems are often missed by both patient and clinican (Colosimo & Pezzella 2002), but consensus criteria now exist (Gilman *et al.* 1998, 1999). The response to levodopa can be variable (Albanese *et al.* 1995; Wenning *et al.* 1995). Although Colosimo *et al.* (1995) reported a response rate of 68%, Quinn and Wenning (1994) have shown that the response to levodopa declines within a few years. Wenning and Quinn (1997) reported high rates of dyskinesias. Dopamine agonists tend to be no more effective than levodopa. Lang (2003) reports disappointing results from stereotactic surgery.

Clincally, there are prominent parkinsonian features in about 80% whilst cerebellar features dominate in the remaining 20% (Gilman *et al.* 1998). Postural or rest tremors may be seen. Dysautonomia is central to both subtypes. This may include postural hypotension (Mathias & Kimber 1999), which is related to loss of preganglionic sympathetic neurones in the inferomedial cell column (Oppenheimer 1980). Bladder dysfunction is very common and results from detrusor hyperreflexia and urethral sphincter weakness (Bonnet *et al.* 1997). This contrasts with the urinary problems seen in Parkinson's disease where incontinence, if seen, is a late sign (Wenning *et al.* 1999). Sexual dysfunction (Wenning *et al.* 1994), constipation (Stocchi *et al.* 2000) and respiratory dysfunction (Wenning *et al.* 1994) are further examples of autonomic difficulties.

Sleep disorders, such as daytime sleepiness, insomnia and REM sleep behaviour disorder, are very common (Wenning *et al.* 1994; Ghorayeb *et al.* 2005). These do not appear to be related to depression, which is also common (Pilo *et al.* 1996; Fetoni *et al.* 1999; Gill *et al.* 1999). Benrud-Larson *et al.* (2005) in a study of 99 patients found that 39% had moderate to severe depression. Depression and, more strongly, autonomic dysfunction contributed substantially to the reported very low levels of life satisfaction. Importantly in contrast to the other parkinsonian syndromes dementia is not a feature, although mild frontal impairment or emotional lability might be seen (Pillon *et al.* 1995; Marti *et al.* 2003).

The dystonias

The dystonias comprise a group of disorders in which sustained muscle spasms invade muscle groups, causing writhing or twisting movements or distorting the body and limbs into characteristic postures. The abnormal movements differ from tics or choreiform movements in being much slower and sustained, and in their tendency to involve the proximal and axial musculature. Dystonias represent the third most common movement disorder after Parkinson's disease and essential tremor (Butler 2002). Reviews of the classification of these disorders and changing conceptions about them are provided by Fahn *et al.* (1998), Cavalho (2002) and Nemeth (2002).

Almost any body part may be involved. Typically at the onset the dystonia occurs only during some specific motor act, affecting a restricted group of muscles (focal dystonia). It may remain localised, or spread to involve contiguous body parts (segmental dystonia) or virtually all of the body (generalised dystonia). Axial dystonia is a focal dystonia affecting the trunk. Hemidystonia affects one half of the body alone, and multifocal dystonia affects several discrete regions. The different syndromes that result are often specially labelled: torticollis in the neck, blepharospasm in the muscles around the eyes, and dystonia musculorum deformans when the disorder is generalised. Focal and segmental dystonias greatly outnumber other forms; in the large series of almost 1000 cases reported from the Dystonia Clinical Research Center in New York these accounted for some

three-quarters of cases, generalised dystonia occurring in less than one-fifth (Fahn *et al.* 1987).

All dystonic movements and postures are worsened by attempts to move. When the spasms are continuous they result in characteristic postures that are maintained except during sleep. When intermittent they cause repetitive, often rhythmic, jerks and spasms, for example in torticollis. The shorter the spasms, the more 'myoclonic' the dystonia. Some patients may show an additional component of tremor. This can produce diagnostic confusion, with dystonias being mistaken for chorea, tremor or myoclonus (Langlois *et al.* 2003).

Some dystonias are symptomatic of structural or metabolic brain disease, following in the wake of perinatal hypoxia or kernicterus (athetoid cerebral palsy) or accompanying Huntington's or Wilson's disease. The basal ganglia, with their high oxidative metabolism, are particularly sensitive to hypoxic damage (Trost 2003). The symptomatic dystonias tend to be asymmetrical or unilateral, and to show other evidence of brain damage by way of seizures, intellectual impairment or pyramidal tract damage. Other dystonias may be induced by drugs such as neuroleptics or levodopa. The range of possible causes is legion, as listed by Marsden and Quinn (1990). In the majority of cases, however, no cause is found and the condition is labelled as a primary or idiopathic dystonia. A pathological cause is identified in some 45% of patients with generalised or multifocal dystonia, but only in 10% of those with focal dystonia. In contrast, hemidystonia is due to a structural cause in over 80% of cases, for example a stroke, head injury or brain tumour. It is essential that Wilson's disease, though rare, is excluded in all patients with onset of dystonia below the age of 50.

Age affects the chances of identifying a cause; in Fahn *et al.*'s (1987) series, 40% of cases were symptomatic when onset was in childhood, 30% when onset was in adolescence and 13% when onset was over the age of 20. Age also has a marked though ill-understood effect on the likelihood of progression to generalised dystonia. This occurred in 60% of Fahn *et al.*'s patients with onset in childhood, in 25% with adolescent onset, but in only 3% of adult-onset cases. The legs are usually affected first in children, less commonly in adolescents, and very rarely in adults.

An interesting small group of patients has been reported by Burke *et al.* (1980) in whom persistent dystonia developed after a considerable delay of 1–14 years following static cerebral insults such as anoxia, trauma or infarction. In the trauma and infarction cases, the body part affected corresponded to the site of the cerebral damage. Schott (1985) has drawn attention to patients who developed segmental dystonias in the wake of quite mild peripheral injuries such as falls, twisting the back or straining the arm or thumb, the movement disorder developing as the symptoms from the injury subsided. The site of the dystonia corresponded closely to that of the initial injury. Such rare examples contribute to the mystery surrounding the genesis of this group of conditions. Dystonias are the most common movement disorders after severe head injury. The mean latency is nearly 2 years. The physiological basis of dystonia post head injury remains unclear, as it may occur when damage is apparently confined to cortical structures and not the basal ganglia (Trost 2003).

The dystonias are of importance to psychiatrists on many counts. Both acute and chronic forms can emerge as side effects of neuroleptic treatment, the latter providing considerable problems of management (see Acute dystonia, under Drug-induced disorders/Clinical pictures, earlier). They are also of interest in that they are markedly 'psychosensitive', being readily aggravated by intercurrent stresses and tensions (Fish *et al.* 1991). This can be so marked that at least in the earlier stages a psychogenic disorder is suspected, this being reinforced when psychological treatment leads to amelioration. Diagnostic mistakes can also arise from the bizarre nature of the movement disorder and the strange postures induced, leading to an impression of simulation, hysteria or catatonic posturing. Strange paradoxes can add to the confusion, as when the patient can run, dance or mount stairs normally while walking provokes considerable difficulty. Some patients can even walk backwards when walking forwards is a problem. Strange tricks or manoeuvres, such as the *geste antagoniste*, may be discovered by the patient to control the movement disorder. Difficulties with diagnosis are increased by the absence of abnormalities on formal neurological examination and investigation in the idiopathic dystonias, where diagnosis depends essentially on familiarity with the clinical pictures produced.

Not surprisingly, in view of the above, differing opinions have been held about the causation of dystonia from time to time. Many examples, and particularly the focal forms, were long considered to be psychogenic in origin, for example torticollis and blepharospasm. However, evidence now increasingly favours the view that both focal and generalised dystonias form part of a spectrum, founded in some subtle disturbance of brain biochemistry and physiology. One model focuses on the role of the basal ganglia in regulating motor activity, suggesting that there is functional impairment in output from the globus pallidus interna and the substantia nigra pars reticulata. This reduced activity leads to disinhibition of the thalamus and the motor cortex, producing abnormal movements (Berardelli *et al.* 1998; Vitek 2002). Vitek (2002) further suggests that dystonias arise from alterations in the rate, pattern, somatosensory responsiveness and synchronisation of neural activity in the pallido-thalamo-cortical circuits. The resurgence of such a view has depended on a number of factors: the demonstration of relationships between the different forms, observation of transitions from one form to another, the similarities in clinical picture between symptomatic and idiopathic cases, and not least the provocation of classic examples by a range of pharmacological agents. Moreover, careful control comparisons have increasingly failed to confirm an excess of personality abnormalities or other psychopathology among the persons affected.

Genetic studies have pointed to an inherited vulnerability to idiopathic dystonia and a common origin for the different subvarieties. Fletcher *et al.* (1990) surveyed 100 British families containing 107 members with generalised, segmental or multifocal dystonia (53 generalised dystonia, 46 segmental, 7 multifocal and 1 hemidystonia). Of the index cases 58 had affected relatives. Altogether 79 secondary cases were discovered, almost half being unaware of their problem (generalised dystonia in 15 cases, segmental in 25, focal in 27, multifocal in 6 and tremor in 6). It was concluded that 85% of the cases were caused by an autosomal dominant gene or genes, with approximately 40% penetrance and highly variable expression. About 14% of singleton cases possibly represented fresh mutations. The estimated risk for siblings or children in familial cases was 21%, and the risk in sporadic cases 8–14%. There was no evidence of increased parental consanguinity. Nemeth (2002) and Cavalho (2002) review the current evidence regarding the genetics of dystonia. At least 10 dystonia genes have now been identified.

A genetic contribution to adult-onset focal dystonia is less clearly established but also seems probable. Waddy *et al.* (1991) examined the relatives of 40 patients with torticollis and orofacial dystonias. Ten of them had relatives with some form of dystonia, segregation analysis again suggesting the presence of an autosomal dominant gene or genes with reduced penetrance.

In a small proportion of cases it is nonetheless still accepted, even by experienced observers, that the dystonia is primarily psychogenic in origin. And of course in many patients there will be a strong interaction between organic predisposition and the modulating influence of emotional and environmental factors.

Dystonia musculorum deformans (generalised torsion dystonia)

Generalised torsion dystonia leads to severe and progressive crippling. A genetic basis is apparent in many cases. It must be distinguished from the symptomatic torsion dystonia that may follow severe perinatal anoxia or kernicterus; a similar picture may also be the presenting feature in Wilson's disease and was occasionally encountered after encephalitis lethargica. Within families who inherit the major disease other members may show formes frustes of the disorder: abnormalities of gait, abnormal arm postures, minor speech defects, or static postural abnormalities such as pes equinovarus or kyphoscoliosis.

Ozelius *et al.* (1997) reported the discovery of the gene *DYT1* on the long arm of chromosome 9, inherited in autosomal dominant fashion with partial penetrance, which is responsible for a form of early-onset dystonia. This form of dystonia has become a model for understanding the disease. The gene produces a mutant form of the protein torsin A, whose precise role awaits clarification. However, it is notable that post-mortem studies have revealed an imbalance of dopamine signalling in the striatum of brains with genetically confirmed DYT1 dystonia (Augood *et al.* 2002). Pathological studies have occasionally reported abnormal findings in the basal ganglia, substantia nigra and elsewhere, but these are regarded as non-specific or even artefactual. However, the evidence points to involvement of the basal ganglia, both by analogy with examples that are symptomatic of known brain lesions and the response that may be observed to stereotactic surgery.

Clinical features

The symptoms usually commence in childhood or early adolescence. The first symptom is commonly a disturbance of gait, with plantar flexion, inversion and adduction of the foot when walking. At first the picture is sometimes bizarre with respect to the precise functions affected, as already mentioned. More rarely the initial disturbance may appear in the upper limbs with abnormal postures or actions. A characteristic dystonic posture consists of extension and hyperpronation of the arms, with flexion of the wrist and extension of the fingers. Occasionally the onset is with involvement of the trunk or with torticollis.

In the early stages the motor abnormalities may become apparent only when activity is attempted and nothing unusual can be found on examination at rest. Remissions lasting for several months at a time may occur, all adding to the erroneous impression that the disorder is psychogenic in origin. Indeed, a hysterical disturbance is not infrequently diagnosed initially, particularly when there are coexistent emotional problems or adverse environmental factors. Thus patients are occasionally encountered who have undergone years of psychotherapy for 'hysterical spasms' before progression of the disorder reveals the true state of affairs. The mistake is easily made in view of the rarity of the disorder and the bizarre nature of the symptoms. Other objective signs of a cerebral lesion are absent, with normal tendon reflexes and unimpaired intelligence. Moreover, the dystonic postures that can occur in conversion hysteria are sometimes indistinguishable from the transient early disturbances of dystonia musculorum deformans.

Later, the muscle spasms occur even when the body is relaxed, producing irregular spontaneous movements or fixed dystonic postures. Muscle groups may hypertrophy. The movements cease during sleep but plague the patient continually while awake. Other parts of the body come to be affected, usually with symmetrical involvement of all four limbs, the trunk and the neck. The proximal muscles tend to be affected more than the distal, and a rotatory element in the axial musculature is typical. The trunk is forced into marked lordosis or scoliosis, and fixed contractures of the limbs lead eventually to severe crippling and permanent deformity. Speech, swallowing and breathing may ultimately be affected. Tendon reflexes become difficult to obtain or may be exaggerated, but the plantar responses

remain down-going. There are no abnormalities of sensation.

Rapid progress and widespread involvement is usual when the onset is in childhood or adolescence. Maximum disability is usually reached within 5–10 years, after which the disease tends to arrest or sometimes may even improve very slightly. In about 5% of patients spontaneous remission occurs, usually lasting for only weeks or months but very occasionally being permanent (Harding 1993).

An important subgroup that must not be overlooked comprises patients with dopa-responsive dystonia or Segawa's disease (Nygaard *et al.* 1988, 1991). This accounts for an estimated 5–10% of patients with onset in childhood or adolescence. The gene responsible for this has been termed *DYT5*. It is found on the long arm of chromosome 14 and inherited in autosomal dominant fashion. The onset is typically with a curious abnormality of gait, for example walking on the toes with a wide base, progressing thereafter to the axial muscles producing lordosis and scoliosis. Parkinsonian features are prone to develop, with bradykinesia, rigidity and tremor, and spasticity with pyramidal signs may be present. Diurnal fluctuations and improvement after sleep have been emphasised, but probably do not discriminate the group from other dystonias. Worsening after exertion is characteristic. In Nygaard *et al.*'s review of 86 cases, 36 were sporadic and the rest had more than one family member affected.

The dramatic response to levodopa sets the group apart. Small doses give immediate benefit, with a return to normal or near normal after several days or months. Minor gait abnormalities may persist, but full functional capacity is usually regained. Doses as small as 100 mg have proved effective, though the average is in the range of 500–1000 mg.

Dyskinesias have not emerged as a problem with long-continued therapy. Patients have responded after remaining untreated for 25–45 years, and the benefit has been sustained in follow-ups of 10–20 years.

Treatment

Treatment of generalised torsion dystonia is often disappointing in the present state of knowledge, but in favourable cases drugs can bring substantial benefit. It is essential that all children and adolescents should have a 3-month trial of levodopa to see if they have the dopa-responsive form, particularly if the dystonia has started in the legs. If this fails the next drug to try is an anticholinergic, which helps about half of cases, sometimes very considerably (Burke *et al.* 1986; Greene *et al.* 1988). A start must be made very gradually, building up to high dosage over several months in order to avoid side effects. In children doses of up to 120 mg daily may prove to be well tolerated. Other drugs that may help if trihexyphenidyl fails include diazepam, clonazepam, baclofen, carbamazepine, tetrabenazine, or neuroleptics such as phenothiazines, haloperidol or pimozide. A combination which can be helpful in very severe dystonia is low-dosage tetrabenazine with pimozide and trihexyphenidyl (Marsden & Quinn 1990). Care needs to be taken with phenothiazenes, which may worsen the dystonia or cause tardive dyskinesia (Adler & Kumar 2000). Stereotactic brain surgery, including the use of deep brain stimulators, has shown positive effects but the optimum site is unclear. Unilateral thalamotomy may be helpful although bilateral procedures can be associated with dysphagia. There are a number of reports suggesting a positive outcome from bilateral pallidotomy (Lozano *et al.* 1997; Lai *et al.* 1999; Vitek 2002). Pallidal stimulation is an alternative (Coubes *et al.* 2000; Volkmann & Benecke 2002).

Increase rates of major depressive disorder are seen in DYT1 dystonia (Pittock *et al.* 2000). In one study patients and neurologically asymptomatic carriers both had four times the rate compared with healthy controls, suggesting that depression was part of the phenotype rather than a result of a debilitating and stigmatising condition (Heiman *et al.* 2004). Whatever their origin, treatment should also be directed towards helping the patient and his family adjust to the profound emotional problems generated by the distressing and long drawn-out illness. Psychotherapy can sometimes be of considerable assistance (Das & Choudhary 2000). Some bring astonishing powers of adaptation to bear in learning to cope with their severe disablement. The Dystonia Society gives valuable support and information.

Spasmodic torticollis (cervical dystonia)

Spasmodic torticollis is characterised by involuntary spasms of the musculature that lead to repeated dystonic movements of the head and neck, or sustained abnormal postures, or both. The element of sustained spasm in the picture serves in the differentiation from a tic. It may at times represent either a focal or a segmental dystonia, the latter when it spreads to involve the upper limbs.

Clinical features

Females are up to twice as likely to develop the condition, with an onset mainly between the ages of 30 and 50 (Epidemiologic Study of Dystonia in Europe Collaborative Group 1999). Two forms are distinguished (Stacy 2000). Primary (or idiopathic) cervical dystonia may be genetic or sporadic. History, examination and investigations reveal no obvious cause, although it may be part of a wider generalised dystonia. Secondary (or symptomatic) dystonia occurs after trauma, dopamine antagonist drugs or degenerative disease that affects the basal ganglia. The movements are typically irregular, forcible and writhing in character, involving several of the neck muscles along with the upper parts of the trapezii. The sternomastoid is usually prominently involved, drawing the head laterally and rotating the chin in a characteristic manner. Less commonly there may be simple lateral flexion, or the head may be pulled directly forwards (antecol-

lis) or backwards (retrocollis). In time the spasms come to be almost continuous and the affected muscle groups may show considerable hypertrophy. Pain is common, occurring in 70–80% of patients (Chan *et al.* 1991; Muller *et al.* 2002), and contributes much to the associated disability (Lobbezoo *et al.* 1996). Other abnormal movements are occasionally detected: facial twitches and grimaces, blinking, shrugging of the shoulders, or twisting athetoid movements of the upper limbs.

Once the condition is well developed, the patient finds himself powerless to relax the offending muscle groups or to resist the abnormal movements except for short periods of time. The movements are noticeably affected by emotional influences, becoming more powerful and frequent under tension, excitement or distress. Any sudden startle or shock is likely to be followed immediately by a spasm. Self-consciousness usually aggravates the condition, likewise walking or engaging in strenuous activity.

The movements subside during sleep, and may temporarily come under a greater measure of control when the patient is engaged in activities such as eating or drinking. An unexplained but striking feature is the ability of some patients to control the spasms by resting a hand or finger lightly against the chin, and not infrequently on the side away from which the turning movements are made (*geste antagoniste*).

The course is usually slow progression over many years but the outcome is extremely variable (Lowenstein & Aminoff 1988). Some patients are only mildly affected and can continue with their usual occupations, while others become permanently and severely incapacitated. A few show arrest or resolution of the disorder, others show spontaneous remissions varying from a few days to several years. This uncertain natural history adds greatly to the difficulties of gauging the effects of treatment. The picture may also modify as to detail over time, quick movements changing to slower spasms, or spasms giving way to sustained postures. Different muscle groups may come to be implicated, subsequent relapses even involving turning to the opposite side.

Among 103 cases, Patterson and Little (1943) found that 13% pursued a static course, 42% were progressive, 40% were recurrent or intermittent, and two patients had complete remissions without treatment. On follow-up 25% were worse, 12% unchanged, 12% slightly improved, 42% much improved and 7% 'cured'; 10% were unable to work, 49% were partially incapacitated for work and 29% were able to work as well as ever.

Meares (1971) found that patients tended in general to deteriorate in the first 5 years and then become static. After the first 10 years slight improvement might be seen (Dauer *et al.* 1998), those who had had the disability for this length of time often showing considerable adaptation to its effects. Remissions may occur, although research in the area is hampered by the lack of a universal definition of remission

(Friedman & Fahn 1986; Lowenstein & Aminoff 1988; Jahanshahi *et al.* 1990). They are often incomplete and short-lived, and most patients have relapsed by 5 years. The only consistent clinical predictor of remission is younger age of onset (Dauer *et al.* 1998).

Aetiology

Hypotheses about aetiology have been widely divergent, ranging from psychodynamic to organic, with many suggestions that both sets of factors may be at work. The condition is now firmly classified among the dystonias, but that does not entirely end the argument. In some cases the torticollis is clearly intimately related to other dystonic manifestations, whereas in others it develops as an isolated manifestation in a setting of emotional trauma. In the latter it can sometimes be hard to escape the conclusion that psychological factors are primarily responsible, albeit operating in an individual who is constitutionally predisposed.

More recent evidence underlines the organic basis of many cases of cervical dystonia. Genetic factors have been shown to play a role in a number of dystonias, as described above. A familial aspect to cervical dystonia has been highlighted by Uitti and Maraganore (1993) and Defazio *et al.* (2004). In the series of Chan *et al.* (1991), 12% of patients had a positive family history. A mutation on chromosome 18 (*DYT7* gene), inherited in an autosomal dominant fashion with incomplete penetrance, has been associated with the development of cervical dystonia in 15 of 18 families in Germany (Leube *et al.* 1997). The discovery of other contributing genes appears highly likely (Jarman & Warner 1998).

Whilst the hypothesis that trauma may be a cause of cervical dystonia is controversial, the prevalence of pain as a symptom has suggested it may contribute to the aetiology (Jankovic 1994). Much of this idea is based on increased recognition of the role played by the basal ganglia in nociception (Jones *et al.* 1991). Evidence of basal ganglia abnormalities has come from functional imaging studies. Galardi *et al.* (1996) have shown that patients with cervical dystonia have greater rates of glucose metabolism in the basal ganglia, thalamus, cerebellum and premotor cortex. Magyar-Lehmann *et al.* (1997) provided supporting evidence with a study showing hypermetabolism in the lentiform nuclei. Naumann *et al.* (1998) showed that patients with cervical dystonia had reduced striatal D_2 dopamine binding compared with healthy controls.

Irrespective of whether psychological factors are causative in cervical dystonia, they are most certainly strongly associated with the disorder. Depression is much more common than in the general population. Nickel *et al.* (1996) found that 24% of their sample were depressed, whilst Muller *et al.* (2002) reported that 15% scored over 18 on the Beck Depression Inventory. Moraru *et al.* (2002) found a similar figure although if milder cases were included the prevalence was 42%. Neck pain (Muller *et al.* 2002) but not duration of disease (Moraru *et al.* 2002) was associated with depression. Anxiety disorders, including social phobia and generalised anxiety disorder, are also common (Gundel *et al.* 2001, 2003; Lauterbach *et al.* 2003). A number of studies highlight that depression and anxiety often predate the dystonic symptoms and as such they are not simply a reaction to a disability (Moraru *et al.* 2002; Gundel *et al.* 2003; Duane & Vermilion 2004; Lauterbach *et al.* 2004). Patients with cervical dystonia have impaired quality of life to which pain and psychological factors contribute significantly (Ben-Shlomo *et al.* 2002; Camfield *et al.* 2002; Muller *et al.* 2002).

Treatment

Physical methods such as massage, traction or immobilisation in collars and braces usually meet with disappointing results. Attempts at immobilisation commonly lead to bruising and chafing, and any benefit is promptly lost on removal of the restraint.

Drug therapy has also proved disappointing (Adler & Kumar 2000). Anticholinergics such as trihexyphenidyl are sometimes helpful but less so than in the dystonias which set in during childhood. Adults are more prone to side effects, and often cannot tolerate the high dosage required for therapeutic response. Benzatropine, diazepam and neuroleptics such as phenothiazines or haloperidol may help a proportion of patients in the early stages, but benefits are often transient. The treatment that has emerged as most useful is injection of botulinum toxin (Botox, Dysport) into the affected muscle groups (Tsui *et al.* 1986; Stell *et al.* 1988; Blackie & Lees 1990). The use of botulinum A and botulinum B has been reviewed by the Cochrane Collaboration (Costa *et al.* 2005a–d). This should be undertaken only in clinics which have special experience of using the technique. It leads to relief from the neck deviations and associated pain in a high proportion of patients.

Careful choice of injection sites is important, the aim being to weaken the most active muscles from among the sternomastoid, splenius capitis and trapezius. Improvement usually follows within a week. Mild neck weakness may be experienced for some days after the injections, also dysphagia that may persist for a week or two and nausea (Jankovic & Schwartz 1991). The beneficial effect typically lasts for 2–4 months, after which repeat injections become necessary. The affected neuromuscular junctions are permanently inactivated, the waning of effect resulting from the establishment of new junctions by a process of sprouting from presynaptic axons. Experience has shown the feasibility of continuing treatments over many years, although antibodies to the toxin may ultimately develop and lead to unresponsiveness. The toxin appears to act by cleaving a membrane-bound protein required for release of acetylcholine. Most treatment is with botulinum type A. Studies have shown that in most cases treatment can be given successfully over many years (Brashear *et al.* 2000; Hsiung *et al.* 2002). Although less than 2% cease treatment due to intolerable side effects, 7.5% can develop a secondary unresponsiveness. Botulinum toxin exists in a number of serotypes: type A and type B both block the action of acetylcholine, but by binding to different receptors. The use of type B appears effective even in patients resistant to type A. The use of type F is currently being explored.

Alternative approaches have included intensive behaviour therapy employing massed practice, aversion techniques or systematic desensitisation to the anxiety induced by the head movements (Agras & Marshall 1965; Brierley 1967; Meares 1973). Biofeedback may meet with substantial success in certain patients, either as an aid to simple relaxation or more directly by electromyographic feedback from the offending muscle groups (Korein & Brudny 1976; Fischer-Williams *et al.* 1981). Psychotherapy directed at the exploration of conflicts, or analysis of the settings in which the movements first appeared, has been reported to produce improvement and even complete relief in occasional patients (Whiles 1940; Paterson 1945). Surgical approaches have included selective division of cervical nerve roots, peripheral denervation, thalamotomy and even sternomastoid myotomy in very disabled patients, but the advent of treatment with botulinum toxin should reduce the need for such invasive procedures.

Blepharospasm and oromandibular dystonia (cranial dystonia, orofacial dystonia)

Blepharospasm consists of an uncontrollable tendency to spontaneous and forcible eye closure. It may begin unilaterally but both eyes are usually soon affected (Malinovsky 1987). Repeated contractions of the orbicularis oculi can progress to almost constant involuntary spasm, sometimes rendering the patient virtually unable to see. Spasms are provoked by bright light, embarrassment, attempts at reading or looking upward. Facial grimacing may be extensive in the effort to keep the eyes open. Some patients find tricks that help: yawning, humming, touching the eyelids or eyebrows, neck extension or forced jaw opening. All spasms disappear during sleep.

It is most common in middle-aged or elderly women, with onset particularly in the sixth decade. Its prevalence is 1.2–5 per 100 000 but there is some evidence of marked geographical differences, for example high rates in northern Italy (Muller *et al.* 2002; Defazio *et al.* 2004). For some considerable time, even years, it may be intermittent, and the aggravation by emotional influences may give a strong impression that psychological factors are operative. A considerable proportion of patients show depression around the time of onset (Marsden 1976a). The affected patients are typically stable, however, and without precipitants that could explain the disorder (Bender 1969).

Oromandibular dystonia has a similar range of onset and also more frequently affects women than men. Prolonged spasms affect the muscles of the mouth, jaw and sometimes the tongue (lingual dystonia). They last for up to a minute and are repetitive but irregular in timing. The lower perioral muscles and the platysma may also be involved. The jaw may be forced open or abruptly closed, the lips purse or retract, and the tongue protrudes or curls within the mouth. Severe grimacing occurs and talking and eating may be rendered difficult. The condition can cause great social embarrassment. Spasmodic dysphonia and dysphagia may also be present.

The picture can at first sight resemble the orofacial dyskinesias seen as a late effect of neuroleptic medication (see Tardive dyskinesia, under Drug-induced disorders/Clinical pictures, earlier) but in essence the movements are different (Marsden 1976a,b). Orofacial dystonia consists of repetitive prolonged spasms rather than the incessant flow of choreiform lip smacking, chewing and tongue rolling movements seen in tardive dyskinesia.

The spasms are typically provoked by embarrassment, fatigue or attempts at speaking, chewing or swallowing. Certain tricks may be learned to abort them, such as grasping the lower jaw firmly or shaking the head. In the early stages the capricious nature of the spasms may produce bizarre results, for example one of Marsden's (1976a) patients could not speak without provoking spasms but could sing normally, and in another where the reverse was obtained.

While each of these two disorders can be seen in isolation, there is a strong tendency for them to be coupled together. Marsden's (1976a) composite material showed blepharospasm alone in 13 cases, oromandibular dystonia alone in 9, and both together in 17. In a later series of 264 patients with blepharospasm, 188 (71%) also showed oromandibular dystonia (Grandas *et al.* 1988). When both are present they usually begin contemporaneously, although sometimes the blepharospasm antedates the oromandibular dystonia by several years. The composite picture has been labelled Meige's syndrome, or Brueghel's syndrome, since both aspects are well depicted in the famous painting. Ben Simon and McCann (2005) suggest that isolated blepharospasm occurs only in a minority of patients. Most have a combination of blepharospasm with oromandibular dystonia or a segmental cranial dystonia. Patients may also exhibit frowning, torticollis titubation, or hyperexcitable trigeminal reflex blinks (Mauriello *et al.* 1996). Spasm are often absent during sleep (Shorr *et al.* 1985).

The course is usually chronic and protracted, but can be intermittent over many years. Blepharospasm remains mild in some 20% of cases, whereas other patients become profoundly disabled (Tolosa & Martí 1988). Grandas *et al.* (1988) found that some 10% of patients with blepharospasm had experienced a partial or complete remission, lasting from months to several years, but with ultimate recurrence in the great majority. Half of Marsden's (1976a) patients with both blepharospasm and oromandibular dystonia progressed to dystonia elsewhere: torticollis, dystonic posturing of the arms, respiratory spasms or flexion spasms of the trunk.

Aetiology

The aetiology of both conditions remains obscure, but they are now firmly included within the dystonia spectrum. Blepharospasm was formerly often considered to be psychological in origin, but its frequent association with oromandibular dystonia has served to dispel this view. An organic basis is supported by its emergence as a side effect of treatment with neuroleptics or levodopa, and its occasional development in Parkinson's disease or as a sequel to encephalitis lethargica. Similar associations apply to oromandibular dystonia, which may also accompany Wilson's disease. In both conditions the nature of the spasms – prolonged, repetitive and irregular in timing – is typical in all respects of other dystonias.

Functional neuroimaging has demonstrated increased metabolism in the thalamus and striatum (Esmaeli-Gutstein *et al.* 1999; Schmidt *et al.* 2003). Baker *et al.* (2003), also using functional MRI, suggest that the cortical and subcortical areas, including the limbic system and the cerebellum, involved in normal blinking may show increased activation. Several authors focus on basal ganglia abnormalities as the cause of blepharospasm (Berardelli *et al.* 1985; Schicatano *et al.* 1997), probably in combination with an alteration in the trigeminal sensorimotor system. The response of one patient to cannabinoids (Gauter *et al.* 2004) suggests a possible role for central GABAergic and glutaminergic systems.

Continuous chronic blepharospasm has also been reported after head injury or subarachnoid haemorrhage, or in association with cerebral tumours, degenerative conditions or cerebral arterial disease. Rostral midbrain lesions appear to be particularly closely related to its development (Poewe *et al.* 1989). In all such settings blepharospasm can sometimes resemble a psychogenic disorder but for the history and abnormal findings on neurological examination. In the large group of patients reported by Grandas *et al.* (1988), dystonia was observed in other parts of the body in 78% of cases: oromandibular dystonia in 71%, torticollis in 23%, laryngeal dystonia in 17%, respiratory dystonia in 15%, arm or hand in 10%, pharyngeal in 7%, trunk in 2% and leg or foot in 2%. A postural tremor was evident in the arms in 12%. A family history suggestive of blepharospasm or dystonia elsewhere was found in almost 10% of cases, suggesting a genetic predisposition. A variety of *gestes antagonistes* appear effective for many patients. These include talking, singing, yawning, whistling, coughing, humming, or placing a finger on the lateral margin of the orbit (Anderson *et al.* 1998).

Although there is now overwhelming evidence of an organic basis for blepharospasm, it is also clear that symptoms may be triggered or exacerbated by psychological factors, and that comorbid psychiatric diagnoses are common. Muller *et al.* (2002) examined 89 consecutive patients attending a specialist clinic and found that 37% were depressed, almost half of these at least moderately. Women were more depressed than men. Wenzel *et al.* (2000) studied a smaller group using the Structured Clinical Interview for DSM-IV and found that 71% had a current or lifetime psychiatric diagnosis; 32% had major depression or recurrent depressive disorder.

Treatment

Treatment can raise very considerable problems as responses to drug treatment are often ill-sustained. With both blepharospasm and oromandibular dystonia there may be a good response to anticholinergic medication provided this can be tolerated in adequate dosage. Levodopa and lisuride helped a proportion of Grandas *et al.*'s patients with blepharospasm. Tetrabenazine, lithium, benzodiazepines or neuroleptics such as haloperidol and pimozide are also often tried. Severe cases of blepharospasm may require section of branches of the facial nerve, or muscle-stripping operations to remove selected parts of the orbicularis oculi muscles.

Injection of botulinum toxin into the orbicularis oculi muscle is now the first-line treatment for blepharospasm. Peak effects occur within 5–7 days. The mean duration of benefit is approximately 3 months but can be as long as 6 months (Dutton & Buckley 1988). There is a suggestion that in the long term drug therapy and even eyelid surgery may augment the effects of botulinum toxin (Mauriello *et al.* 1996). Systemic adverse effects are very rare. Local or regional side effects occur though rarely. These include ptosis, diplopia, perioral asymmetry and dysphagia.

Other dystonias and spasms

Other forms of dystonia rarely present to psychiatrists, although laryngeal dystonia may sometimes suggest a hysterical aphonia. In the adductor type the voice is choked and strangled, whereas with the abductor type it is breathy and effortful with whispered segments. Drugs are of little help, but skilled botulinum injections can again give substantial relief. Pharyngeal dystonia presents with difficulty in swallowing, and respiratory dystonia with difficulty in breathing. For details neurological textbooks should be consulted. Hemifacial spasm consists of twitching, tonic spasm and often synkinesis of the muscles innervated by the facial nerve. Though not a dystonic manifestation, this too can now be treated effectively with botulinum injections to the facial muscles (Brin *et al.* 1995). Other than this, the spasms can be helped in some degree by phenytoin, carbamazepine or clonazepam.

Gilles de la Tourette's syndrome (Tourette's syndrome)

Gilles de la Tourette's syndrome, though relatively rare, has attracted a good deal of attention, chiefly on account of the striking nature of the clinical picture. Multiple tics are accompanied by forced involuntary vocalisations that can sometimes take the form of obscene words or phrases (copro-lalia). One of the chief interests of the condition has centred on this verbal component, which has been interpreted as giving a clue to the underlying psychopathological mecha-nisms. However, our knowledge of the biological basis for this condition is increasing.

Clinical features

Valuable reviews of the clinical picture are presented by Shapiro *et al.* (1978), Lees (1985) and Robertson (1989, 1994). The DSM-IV criteria for diagnosis of the syndrome are as follows:

• presence of both multiple motor and one or more vocal tics at some time during the illness (though not necessarily concurrently);
• such tics occur many times a day, nearly every day or intermittently for more than a year and without a tic-free period exceeding three consecutive months;
• onset before the age of 18 years;
• marked distress or significant impairment in social or occupational functioning occasioned by the disorder;
• absence of general medical conditions or substances such as stimulants that could account for it.

Hanna *et al.* (1999) suggest the prevalence is 0.7%. Patients referred for specialist help can certainly be markedly disa-bled, but it has become increasingly clear that the majority of sufferers are only mildly affected and unknown to health professionals (Robertson & Gourdie 1990). Many of the latter would therefore fail to meet the DSM-IV criteria completely. The failure to identify mild cases thus limits the accuracy of prevalence data. A study of Israeli army recruits found a prevalence of 4.3 per 1000 (Apter *et al.* 1993), but in a study of UK schoolchildren the figure was 1.85% (Hornsey *et al.* 2001).

The condition is a good deal commoner among boys than girls, in a ratio of approximately 3:1 (Spencer *et al.* 1999). Onset is rare after 11, the great majority beginning between the ages of 3 and 8. In these respects the syndrome resembles the generality of tics in childhood. Motor tics tend to begin around the age of 7, vocal tics some 4 years later, and coprola-lia at the time of puberty. Very occasional examples have been reported with onset in adult life (Marneros 1983), though of course these do not conform to the full DSM-IV criteria above.

Tics are simple non-purposeful movements of function-ally related muscle groups. They can be divided into simple and complex tics. Simple tics include (i) clonic tics such as eye-blinking, (ii) tonic tics such as arm-stretching and (iii) dystonic tics such as grimacing. Complex tics tend to appear semi-purposeful, for example touching parts of the body or grooming behaviours. Vocal tics may also be simple, due to contractions of the respiratory, laryngeal, oral or nasal musculature (e.g. sounds and grunts), or complex (e.g words or phrases). Tics may be preceded or accompanied by sensory phenomena such as unusual bodily sensations or an irresistible urge to move. These are relieved by the move-ment of the tic (Kurlan *et al.* 1989; Leckman *et al.* 1993; Marcus & Kurlan 2001; Banaschewski *et al.* 2003; Kwak *et al.* 2003). They are distinct from chorea and other abnormal motor movements in their stereotyped pattern, the same event occurring time and again, and in the ability of the subject to hold the movements in check for a short while at the expense of mounting inner tension.

Simple tics are usually the first manifestation. They usually commence around the eyes or in the face, head and neck, spreading later to the limbs and trunk. Before long there are typically multiple tics, often of great force and severity: blinking, grimacing, jerking of the head, shrug-ging of the shoulders or jerks of the arms and legs. Whole body movements may be involved, leading to bending, jumping, skipping, hopping, stamping or twirling. Com-pulsions to touch or smell objects, smelling the hands, or to hit and strike objects or the subject's own body are often observed. Complex coordinated movements occasionally appear, such as brief slapping of the face or thighs, or wring-ing of the hands. The picture may at times be highly bizarre, and the detailed pattern may change over time.

Vocalisations can occur from the outset but are usually added later. Most begin within 5 years of onset. At first they are often inarticulate sounds – sniffs, grunts, barks, throat clearing, snorting or coughing noises that accompany the motor movements. These may then progress to the enuncia-tion of words, sometimes muttered and barely discernible but sometimes loudly and clearly articulated. The vocal tics commonly occur at the end of sentences or clauses, without impairing the overall speech rhythm.

Common oaths and expletives are frequently involved, or brief obscene phrases of aggressive or sexual content (copro-lalia). The obscenities are often uttered loudly, with an unusual cadence or pitch, and sometimes with imprecise pronunciation of phonemes (Lees 1985). The coprolalia occurs without any appropriate stimulus, and in common with other vocal tics it usually breaks through in the pauses between sentences. Some patients repeatedly utter the same swear word over and over again, or use long strings of elabo-rate obscenities. About one-third of patients also utter emo-tionally charged words of great personal significance, again often spoken oddly with unusual emphasis on particular syllables. One of Lees' patients would occasionally shout the word 'cat', and another 'Elvis'.

The utterance of obscenities commonly sets in at about the time of puberty, but may start as early as 10 or be delayed until well into adult life. It ultimately develops in perhaps one-third of patients reported from clinic samples, though with great variation in different reports. Among sufferers generally it is probably quite rare. Stern *et al.* (2005) suggests a prevalence of only 10%, much less common than echolalia and palilalia. 'Mental coprolalia' in the form of a compul-sion to think obscenities is perhaps commoner than overt coprolalia, and transition from the former to the latter may be observed. Copropraxia is the involuntary and inappropriate making of obscene gestures, the commonest in the UK being the palm-backed 'V' sign. Non-obscene socially inappropriate comments (and behaviours) are now also recognised (Kurlan *et al.* 1996).

It has been shown that when computer programs generate letters or phonemes in a random manner, second- and third-order texts appear increasingly more like English language (Nuwer 1982). There is also an unexpected repeated occurrence of physical obscenities, which by the fourth order of processing have largely disappeared. Similar results are obtained with second-order German. Thus coprolalia in Gilles de la Tourette's syndrome may conceivably result from a 'short-circuiting' in brain function, leading to the production of high probability strings of phonemes out of proportion to other words.

Both the tics and the utterances are affected by emotional stress, becoming more severe with anxiety, excitement, anger, boredom or self-consciousness. The patient may struggle greatly to conceal the coprolalia, disguising or distorting obscene words so that their true nature is not at first detected. Intense efforts at control may succeed for a while, but at the expense of mounting inner tension and ultimately an explosive recrudescence. The coprolalia tends to cease when the patient is alone but the tics do not. Both are often markedly relieved by alcohol. In the past, tics were said to cease or diminish markedly during sleep; however, they can persist during sleep (Rothenberger *et al.* 2001) and have even been observed to increase during REM sleep (Cohrs *et al.* 2001). They disappear during sexual arousal (Shapiro *et al.* 1973). They usually diminish during periods of intense concentration or when the patient is firmly preoccupied with matters that do not arouse anxiety. Jankovic (2001) points out that tics may actually increase with relaxation following a period of stress, for example on coming home after a day at school. He described these as 'releasing tics'.

Echo-phenomena have often been stressed in the literature but occur in less than one-third of cases. There may be compulsive repetition of words spoken by others (echolalia) or compulsive imitation of actions (echopraxia).

The intelligence of affected persons varies widely but in some series a surprising number have shown superior ability. Most studies have shown the distribution of intelligence to be within normal limits (Singer 2005). Robertson (1989) reviews studies that have looked for evidence of specific impairments, noting that language skills appear to be essentially unimpaired whereas visuopractic deficits have emerged with fair consistency. As a result significant discrepancies have often been observed between verbal and performance IQ scores. Attentional deficits have also been highlighted, and may account for Tourette children often falling behind their peers at school despite normal intellectual ability. Channon *et al.* (1992) made comparisons between adult patients with the disorder and matched controls on a

variety of attentional tests, demonstrating significant impairments on serial addition, block span sequence, Trail-making and several vigilance tasks. Impairment was found both in sustaining attention and in focusing and shifting sets between salient stimuli. Such deficits were not explicable in terms of depression, anxiety or obsessionality, and showed no relationship to the dosage of drugs taken. The syndrome is more common in children with autistic spectrum disorder (Baron-Cohen *et al.* 1999), although this is not related to the severity of the autistic symptoms.

Other features that have often been claimed include a high prevalence of childhood neurotic symptoms and disturbed family backgrounds, but proper controlled comparisons are not available. Similar difficulties surround the reports of antisocial behaviour and conduct disorder in a high proportion of patients, including lying, stealing and aggressive behaviour generally. Inappropriate sexual behaviour, including exhibitionism, has also sometimes been stressed.

A high prevalence of self-injurious behaviour has occasionally been reported, including head banging, lip biting and pummelling of the head and chest (Robertson 1992). More serious but rare instances include eye damage and touching hot objects The precise prevalence depends on the definition of the injury caused. Hence in a study of 3500 patients, Freeman *et al.* (2000) found a rate of 14%, whereas Robertson (2000) reports 25%, Stern *et al.* (2005) approximately 33% and Mathews *et al.* (2004) 60%. Self-injurious behaviour is more likely if the patient has an additional psychiatric diagnosis (Freeman *et al.* 2000). Mathews *et al.* (2004) distinguished a 'severe' form, associated with impulse control problems, found in only 4% of cases.

More convincing associations have emerged with behavioural disturbances antedating the appearance of the syndrome, including attention deficit hyperactivity disorder (ADHD). These are often the symptoms for which patients are referred to a physician. In Freeman's cohort of 3500 patients, ADHD occurred in 31–91% (Freeman *et al.* 2000). Occurrence of ADHD is not associated with severity of the tic disorder, although ADHD symptoms are common in severe disease (Robertson & Stern 1998). Knell and Comings (1993) found that ADHD was more common in the siblings of children with Tourette's syndrome and suggested that there may be a common genetic basis for the two conditions. The additional burden of ADHD symptoms impacts substantially on the psychosocial difficulties of Tourette's patients (Bawden *et al.* 1998; Carter *et al.* 2000; Sukhodolsky *et al.* 2003).

Sleep disturbances including nightmares, somnambulism and night terrors have occurred in up to one-third. There is also some evidence that depression and anxiety may be more common in adults with the disorder than in the normal population (Robertson *et al.* 1988, 1993). Freeman *et al.* (2000) reported that 20% had depression and 18% anxiety. There is little to suggest any special relationship with psychotic illness, though not surprisingly there have been occasional reports of patients with bipolar affective disorder or schizophrenia.

Increasingly, however, there is evidence of a close association with obsessive–compulsive disorder, to the extent that this is sometimes regarded as an integral part of the condition, perhaps with a shared genetic predisposition. In addition to ritualistic behaviours and compulsions to touch objects, a high proportion of patients report obsessional thoughts and activities. These sometimes amount to frank obsessive–compulsive illness. Frankel *et al.* (1986) found that half of their patients had significantly elevated scores on a questionnaire for obsessional–compulsive symptoms, many scoring as highly as patients with obsessive–compulsive illness. Robertson *et al.* (1993) similarly showed elevated scores on the Leyton Obsessional Inventory. Obsessional features were observed in two-thirds of the patients reported by Nee *et al.* (1982) and Montgomery *et al.* (1982). The latter study also found a high prevalence of obsessive–compulsive illness among the first-degree relatives of patients. Obsessive compulsive behaviours were present in 32% of Freeman *et al.*'s (2000) cohort, whilst Scahill *et al.* (2003) suggested that up to 89% of patients showed obsessive–compulsive behaviours.

Caine *et al.* (1988) found that almost half of the children in their epidemiological survey had obsessional ideas, often with associated ritualistic motor behaviour. The commonest included 'evening up', whereby a series of rituals ensured that the body was symmetrical and balanced, also counting games and touching rituals to ward off bad omens. Coffey *et al.* (1998) and Cath *et al.* (2000) also report on the need for symmetry and 'doing things right'. Cummings and Frankel (1985) drew attention to certain similarities between the syndrome and obsessive–compulsive disorder, including age of onset, lifelong course with waxing and waning, involuntary intrusive experiences and worsening with depression and anxiety. They advanced the hypothesis that the tics and vocalisations of Gilles de la Tourette's syndrome may be aberrant manifestations of simple motor programmes generated in the basal ganglia, and that obsessions and compulsions represent more complex motor plans initiated by similar anomalous neural activity. Obsessive–compulsive behaviours in adults are associated with ADHD and self-injurious behaviour (Eapen *et al.* 2004), whilst in children they are associated with impulsive and aggressive behaviour (Banaschewski *et al.* 2003).

Course and outcome

Over time the severity of the disorder tends to wax and wane, periods of partial remission alternating with exacerbations. The symptomatology may also change as to detail, new tics developing as old ones disappear. Occasionally there may be periods lasting for days or weeks during which the movements remit completely.

Firm information about the longer-term outcome is hard to obtain since there have been few prolonged follow-up studies. Leckman *et al.* (1998) reviewed a cohort of 36 patients for tic severity in the first two decades. Half the patients were free of tics by the age of 18. It seems that the disorder may ameliorate in early adult life, and coprolalia has been said to remit in about one-tenth of subjects without medication (Shapiro *et al.* 1978). Bruun and Budman (1992) report a rather more encouraging picture. Of 136 patients who were followed for 5–15 years, 59% had been rated as mild to moderate when first encountered, but at follow-up 91% were now in these categories. More than one-quarter had discontinued medication and most others were on lower doses than originally required. Half stated that they had improved spontaneously, most commonly in their late teenage years. A review of several studies suggested that some 30–40% of cases may remit completely by late adolescence, though it cannot be judged whether such remissions are permanent. Symptoms in adulthood appear more stable; 65% of patients studied by de Groot *et al.* (1994) had shown no change in symptoms in the past 5 years. Anecdotal evidence indicates that elderly Tourette patients rarely exhibit severe symptoms, and it is noteworthy that there have been few reports of elderly patients with the disorder.

The social impact of the illness, at least in the early years, is often disastrous. Some patients withdraw to a considerable extent, while others appear to maintain surprisingly good work records and social relationships despite their disability. Some patients remain only mildly affected throughout, clinical impressions of the gravity of the disorder being influenced by those referred for specialist help. Elstner *et al.* (2001) studied 90 adult patients and found that their quality of life was poor overall. Factors associated with this poor quality of life were employment status, tic severity, obsessive–compulsive behaviours, anxiety and depression.

Nosology and aetiology

Different views have been put forward about the nosological status of the condition. Some regard it as a rare and distinct disease entity, while others view it as merely the most severe and persistent presentation of the tic syndrome in childhood.

Gilles de la Tourette (1855) himself allied the condition with certain other rare motor and speech disorders reported from various parts of the world: the 'latah' reaction among Malays, the 'myriachit' of Siberia, and the 'jumping Frenchmen of Maine'. It is now realised, however, that this was erroneous. Latah is manifest as echopraxia, echolalia and coprolalia but tic-like phenomena do not occur. Automatic obedience is a prominent feature. It is essentially a severe startle reaction and does not occur without a provoking stimulus. Yap (1952) regards it as a culturally determined fear response found only in primitive cultures where persons have limited powers of control over the environment. Myriachit is similar. The Jumpers of Maine displayed analogous features as part of a religious ritual.

Psychogenic theories

Psychogenic theories regard emotional traumas and conflicts as fundamental to the genesis of tics. Emotional precipitants can sometimes be discerned at the time of onset, and a high prevalence of psychiatric disturbance has been reported in patients and their families. The tics are seen as the direct or symbolic expression of emotional disturbance, aggression, anxiety or the handling of sexual conflicts.

Psychoanalysts have conceived of tics as the involuntary motor equivalents of emotional activity, allowing repressed impulses, usually of a sexual or sadistic nature, to make their appearance in disguised form (Fenichel 1945). Such impulses have become 'independent of the organised ego', that is to say they lack the normal integration with the totality of the personality. In a similar vein, Mahler and Rangell (1943) regarded the symptoms of Gilles de la Tourette's syndrome as expressing the conflict between erotic and aggressive drives on the one hand and internalised censoring controls on the other.

These psychoanalytic conceptions may not seem particularly convincing when applied to tics generally, but it is interesting that in Gilles de la Tourette's syndrome one may meet with vocal and verbal manifestations that lend some support to such views. The noises can often be construed as aggressive or erotic in character, while coprolalia displays such themes in unmistakable form. Morphew and Sim (1969) argued strongly for a psychogenic aetiology for Gilles de la Tourette's syndrome, noting precipitating factors that were largely psychological in nature, and the improvements that could be seen after psychotherapy, leaving home or admission to hospital. However, susceptibility to psychological influences need not imply that these are causative. It would seem wiser merely to conclude that Gilles de la Tourette's syndrome may reveal psychodynamic factors at work in an unusually clear fashion, rather than to grant them a primary role in the genesis of the disorder. Some observers with wide experience of the condition have been unable to find evidence of inhibition of hostility or other special personality characteristics, and suggest that any observed psychopathology is most likely to be a product of the illness rather than playing a causative role (Shapiro *et al.* 1972).

Learning theory

The learning theory model views tics as conditioned avoidance responses which have originally been evoked in a traumatic situation, then reinforced by the reduction of anxiety that follows (Yates 1958). Because of stimulus generalisation, the anxiety that the tic reduces will eventually be provoked by many more situations so that the tic becomes an increasingly stronger habit. In essence the tic is a simple learned response that has attained maximal habit strength.

Corbett (1971) pointed out that there is a striking similarity between tic movements and the movements seen in the startle response. This applies to both the nature of the movements and their distribution. Thus tics most frequently involve blinking, the face, head and neck, and the limbs, in that order, which parallels the distribution of motor activity during startle. Startle responses, moreover, are sometimes associated with vocalisation, and are easily conditioned to neutral stimuli.

Even if such a model is felt inadequate to explain the origin of the tic, it is easy to see how secondary reinforcing properties may come to attach to it and help to perpetuate the habit. To the extent that problems of aggression and hostility are prominent in patients with Gilles de la Tourette's syndrome, the effects of their behaviour on others may sometimes powerfully gratify the habit. Behavioural treatment based on the learning theory model has met with some success, though apparently less so with Gilles de la Tourette's syndrome than with simple motor tics.

Developmental theories

A developmental defect has been proposed as the basis of tics and derives support from certain indirect evidence. Such a conception presupposes no necessary special nexus of psychological conflict in the patient, nor some covert form of acquired brain damage, but merely that the normal maturational processes of control over motor movements have not been fully achieved. The patient is accordingly vulnerable to faulty conditioning procedures as set out above, or if he is destined for emotional disturbance his neurosis will be liable to choose the form of a tic on account of his motor lability.

Much of the evidence presented by Corbett *et al.* (1969) fits with a conception of developmental defect. The preponderance in boys accords with their proneness to other developmental disorders. The restricted age of onset between 6 and 8 years suggests a developmental defect, similarly the marked tendency for simple tics to remit at adolescence. Corbett *et al.*'s patients showed an excess of other developmental disorders, such as encopresis and speech defects, compared with the clinic population generally.

It is less clear whether developmental failure could account for the genesis of the more florid manifestations of Gilles de la Tourette's syndrome. The frequency of a family history of simple tics argues in favour of some form of constitutional motor lability, but the tendency for the syndrome to persist through adolescence and indeed well into adult life would suggest that more than developmental immaturity is involved.

Organic theories

Organic theories presuppose that some specific brain disorder contributes directly to the development of tics, and various biochemical, neuroimaging and genetic studies contribute to the conclusion that Gilles de la Tourette's syndrome is an inherited developmental disorder of synaptic neurotransmission resulting in disinhibition of the cortical–striatal–thalamic–cortical system. Pasamanick and Kawi (1956) explored the possibility of brain damage resulting from prenatal or perinatal factors by identifying 83 children with tics and tracing the birth records of each. When compared with the next child born, matched for sex, race, maternal age and place of birth, the frequency of complications of pregnancy and parturition was found to have been significantly higher among the children with tics. A number of perinatal factors have now been associated with an increased risk of Tourette's syndrome. These include severe first-trimester nausea, severe maternal stress during pregnancy, maternal use of caffeine, alcohol and tobacco during pregnancy, being an identical twin with a lower birthweight, and transient hypoxia during birth (Leckman 2002).

The success of treatment with dopamine-blocking agents, and the occasional emergence of a not dissimilar syndrome along with tardive dyskinesia after long-term neuroleptic medication (De Veaugh-Geiss 1980; Mueller & Aminoff 1982), point to dopaminergic hypersensitivity as a possible mechanism. The observations that Tourette patients have a higher blink rate at rest and an exaggerated audiogenic startle response also suggest a dopaminergic abnormality (Stell *et al.* 1995; Tulen *et al.* 1999; Gironell *et al.* 2000), although investigations of genetic links to dopamine receptors have repeatedly been negative (Brett *et al.* 1995). Caine (1985) reviews several neurochemical investigations into the disorder, some showing reduced cerebrospinal fluid levels of homovanillic acid, the major metabolite of dopamine, but such findings have been questioned on methodological grounds. More recently, Singer and colleagues have reported increased numbers of presynaptic dopamine carrier sites in the striatum in three Tourette patients studied at autopsy, and also reductions of cyclic AMP in the cerebral cortex (Singer *et al.* 1991; Singer 1992, 2000).

Brain imaging studies support the presence of subtle cerebral defects. Abnormalities in the size of the caudate nucleus and asymmetries in other basal ganglia structures have occasionally been reported (Hyde *et al.* 1995; Peterson *et al.* 2001; Swerdlow & Young 2001). Volumetric MRI studies show changes in the premotor, prefrontal and orbitofrontal areas in boys (Peterson *et al.* 1993). PET and SPECT have indicated hypoperfusion in the basal ganglia, thalamus, frontal and temporal cortex (Braun *et al.* 1995; Crespo-Facorro *et al.* 1999; Stern *et al.* 2000), and possibly decreased availability of striatal D_2 receptors (Chase *et al.* 1986; Riddle *et al.* 1992; Robertson 1994; Moriarty *et al.* 1995). Neurophysiological studies have shown that Tourette patients fail to manifest cortical electrical potentials preceding their simple tics, whereas they have a normal pre-movement negative potential (Bereitschaftspotential) when they voluntarily mimic the same movements (Obeso *et al.* 1981). This suggests that the tics are not generated through the normal cortical motor pathways utilised in willed movement but have a subcorti-

cal origin. Recent work has focused on the neural substrates of habit formation, most notably differential metabolic activity in cortical neurones projecting into the striatum. The area is reviewed by Leckman (2002).

Genetics

Though the disorder is often sporadic, recent studies have increasingly supported a genetic contribution, with links between narrowly defined Gilles de la Tourette's syndrome, chronic multiple tics without vocalisations, and obsessive–compulsive disorder. The precise genetic mechanisms remain unclear, but the presence of a single autosomal gene with varying penetrance has been suggested by some investigators. Polygenic inheritance is another possibility, and X-linked modifying genes may account for the increased prevalence among males.

Price *et al.* (1985) investigated 30 monozygotic and 13 dizygotic pairs of same-sex twins where at least one co-twin had Gilles de la Tourette's syndrome. The concordance rates were 53% in the former and 8% in the latter. When the criteria were broadened to include tics of any sort, the concordances rose to 77% and 23% respectively. The lack of full concordance among monozygotic pairs emphasises the additional role of non-genetic factors, and Leckman *et al.* (1987) were able to show that in non-concordant pairs the unaffected co-twin always had the higher birthweight. This suggests that prenatal events or exposures may have played a part in actualising the disorder.

Large family studies have shown an increased prevalence of Gilles de la Tourette's syndrome and of chronic multiple tics in the relatives of probands, segregation analysis sometimes suggesting the presence of a major autosomal gene with incomplete penetrance (Robertson 1989). Family studies have also indicated that the same gene may be expressed as obsessive–compulsive disorder. Thus many relatives of Tourette patients describe obsessional–compulsive thoughts and actions in the absence of tics or vocalisations (Robertson 1989), and obsessive–compulsive disorder has been found to be especially common among family members where Gilles de la Tourette's syndrome appears to be an inherited disorder (Cummings & Frankel 1985). Family aggregations have been confirmed in two particularly large pedigrees, one of 122 members from six generations in a British family (Curtis *et al.* 1992) and one of 161 members over four generations in the USA (McMahon *et al.* 1992). More recently, studies on a large French-Canadian family showed linkage on the long arm of chromosome 11 (Merette *et al.* 2000). Sib-pair analysis by the Tourette Syndrome Association International Consortium for Genetics (1999) identified two possible locations on chromosomes 4 and 8, whilst a study of a South African family identified possible areas on chromosomes 2 and 8 (Simonic *et al.* 1998, 2001). Thus while the exact mode of inheritance remains to a large extent uncertain, both family and genetic studies combine to suggest that there is a spectrum of disorder, extending from classic examples of the syndrome to other forms of tic and including also obsessive–compulsive disorder.

A new line of investigation has been the possible role of childhood infection (Allen *et al.* 1995; Hallett *et al.* 2000). Elevated titres of antibodies to group A β-haemolytic streptococci have been found in some patients (Swedo *et al.* 1997). Tourette's was one of a number of disorders included wihin the category 'paediatric autoimmune neuropsychiatric disorders associated with streptococcus' (Swedo *et al.* 1998). Church *et al.* (2003) found high levels of anti-basal ganglia antibodies in a group of UK patients, of whom 91% also had raised antistreptolysin O titres. However, there is a growing consensus that a postinfective aetiology accounts for only a small proportion of patients with Tourette's. There appears to be no relationship between the presence of anti-neuronal antibodies and age of onset or severity of tics (Singer *et al.* 1998). Two prospective longitudinal studies have shown no clear link between new group B streptococcal infection and either the development or exacerbation of tic or obsessive–compulsive symptoms (Luo *et al.* 2004; Perrin *et al.* 2004).

Treatment

Until the advent of pharmacotherapy the treatment of Gilles de la Tourette's syndrome was mostly disappointing. Moreover, it was difficult to evaluate the effectiveness of interventions on small numbers of cases because of the tendency of the disorder to show spontaneous fluctuations.

Psychotherapy often met with failure but improvements were sometimes reported, very occasionally with seeming total recovery (Mahler & Luke 1946; Eisenberg *et al.* 1959; Kurland 1965). Nevertheless, supportive psychotherapy and group counselling procedures find an important place in helping patients to cope with their disability. Abreaction has been attempted with a wide range of drugs, and Michael (1957) reported a patient who underwent a striking remission after a series of carbon dioxide inhalations when intensive psychotherapy had met with no response.

The main aim of tic treatment is not to abolish tics entirely, but rather reduce the frequency to the point where normal function is possible. Behavioural therapy can be effective with simple tics, for example 'massed practice', which is based on the theory that voluntary practice of the tics for long periods of time will build up reactive inhibition to their recurrence (Yates 1958). Clark (1966) reported remarkably good results with the technique in two of three cases of Gilles de la Tourette's syndrome. Coprolalia was eliminated by asking the patient to repeat the most frequently used obscenity as often as possible in a large number of treatment sessions. Others, however, have had less success, finding that practice may aggravate the tics by generating increased anxiety (Sand & Carlson 1973). Techniques in which the patient is taught to practise movements incompatible with the tic, or to substitute a neutral word for an obscenity, have also occasionally helped (Friedman 1980). Cohen and Marks (1977) have reported the value of an operant conditioning programme, involving rewards for tic-free periods of increasing length, which can be implemented in the patient's home. Behavioural techniques also find a special place in the management of severe obsessive–compulsive behaviour when this is part of the condition.

Drugs such as diazepam may help temporarily by reducing anxiety, but dopamine receptor antagonists emerged as the first truly valuable medications. Connell *et al.* (1967) convincingly showed the effectiveness of haloperidol in simple tics in a double-blind comparison with diazepam, and Chapel *et al.* (1964) were among the first to report excellent results in Gilles de la Tourette's syndrome. Haloperidol has since received enthusiastic support and remains among the drugs of first choice. Shapiro and Shapiro (1982) conclude that over 80% of patients gain improvement, though some 13% discontinue it because of side effects. Dysphoria and sleepiness can be troublesome and may outweigh the benefits in terms of tic control. A start is usually made with very small dosage, for example 0.25–0.5 mg daily, thereafter building up very gradually to an end-point of maximal improvement with the minimum of side effects. In many patients 2–3 mg daily is adequate for symptom relief, but sometimes much larger doses are required. Dosage can often later be reduced over several months or years without loss of benefit, sometimes to very low levels. Pimozide is effective in many patients and is often less sedating, likewise sulpiride which is less prone to provoke extrapyramidal disturbance. Haloperidol and pimozide are both licensed by the Food and Drug Administration in the USA for the treatment of Tourette's. Sallee *et al.* (1997) suggest that pimozide may be preferable. A number of small studies show promising results for atypical antipsychotic drugs such as ziprasidone (Sallee *et al.* 2000, 2003), olanzapine (Budman *et al.* 2001; Stephens *et al.* 2004) and quetiapine (Mukaddes & Abali 2003). Risperidone was effective in two randomised controlled trials (Dion *et al.* 2002; Gaffney *et al.* 2002), although may be associated with weight gain or dysphoria (Margolese *et al.* 2002). Centrally active α-adrenergic agonists such as clonidine or guanfacine, have also been shown to be effective in several randomised controlled trials (Leckman *et al.* 1991; Tourette's Syndrome Study Group 2002). However, differences in response by individual patients may indicate a trial of several different agents. The anticonvulsant clonazepam and the antidepressant clomipramine have also occasionally shown success, likewise calcium channel blockers such as nifedipine and verapamil. Documented responses have been reported with naloxone, lithium carbonate, tetrabenazine and fluvoxamine (Robertson 1989; Kurlan & Trinidad 1995). Although dopamine receptor antagonists have proven efficacy, dopamine agonists such as pergolide (Gilbert *et al.* 2003) and ropinirole

(Anca *et al.* 2004) also appear beneficial. It is believed that they are acting at presynaptic rather than postsynaptic receptors in the striatum or the cortex. Hoopes (1999) reported the successful use of donepezil, whilst Muller-Vahl (2003) described improvement in a single patient following the administration of Δ^9-tetrahydrocannabinol. Other currently experimental drug regimens are described in the comprehensive review by Jimenez-Jimenez and Garcia-Ruiz (2001).

Leckman (2002) advises treating comorbid obsessive–compulsive symptoms and ADHD prior to treating the tic disorder. Obsessive–compulsive disorders are typically treated with serotonergic drugs such as clomipramine or SSRIs. Scahill *et al.* (1997) reported that tic frequency was not increased with the use of fluoxetine. Management of ADHD is most effective with stimulant drugs such as dexamfetamine or methylphenidate. There is now consistent evidence that the use of stimulants does not worsen tic behaviour (Gadow *et al.* 1999; Tourette's Syndrome Study Group 2002).

Porta *et al.* (2004) treated 30 patients with vocal cord injections of botulinum toxin. They showed that not only could this be effective for vocal tic and coprolalia but reports of the preceding sensory phenomena declined and overall quality of life improved. Operative intervention by way of stereotactic surgery to the dentate nucleus of the cerebellum, or the rostral intralaminar and medial thalamic nuclei, has been found to help occasional patients (Hassler & Dieckmann 1970, 1973; Nadvornik *et al.* 1972). Vandewalle *et al.* (1999) showed that tics could be reduced with high-frequency stimulation of the nucleus ventralis oralis of the internal thalamus. Even in severely affected patients much can often be achieved by careful adjustment of drug regimens and proper attention to psychosocial aspects of management. Valuable support and information can be provided to patients by the Tourette Syndrome Associations in both the UK and the USA.

Psychogenic movement disorder

Approximately one-third of patients referred to a general neurology clinic have symptoms that are at best only partially explained by organic disease (Carson *et al.* 2000). Follow-up studies have demonstrated that less than 5% of these patients will subsequently be found to have an underlying medical condition that was initially missed (Couprie *et al.* 1995; Crimlisk *et al.* 1998; Carson *et al.* 2003). Movement disorder is a relatively unusual presentation in this context, but in specialist movement disorder clinics 5% of patients may be diagnosed as having a disorder that has no basis in medical disease (Factor *et al.* 1995b; Thomas & Jankovic 2004). There is some suggestion in the literature that this figure may be an underestimate: Thomas and Jankovic (2004) present evidence that the rate at which this diagnosis is made is increasing exponentially, a fact they attribute to a

better understanding of the spectrum of organic movement disorders among both general and specialist neurologists. There is also a grey area between syndromes that are demonstrably organic and those regarded as psychogenic, for example the syndrome of fixed dystonia (Schrag *et al.* 2004) (see below) and the closely related problem of post-traumatic dystonia. Without simple diagnostic tests, debate will continue about the nature of such syndromes but it seems likely that in some cases prevailing views about aetiology stand to be revised in favour of the psychogenic.

The neurological literature has retained the term 'psychogenic movement disorders' to describe this group of conditions. In the absence of a clear consensus about suitable alternatives, this term will be adopted here. However, it should be recognised that this term groups together the different categories of psychiatric disorder that may present with somatic symptoms or signs, namely conversion or somatoform disorder and factitious disorder. In clinical practice, having decided that a patient's movement disorder cannot be attributed to organic disease, reaching a psychiatric diagnosis requires judgements to be made in two stages. Firstly, the clinician must decide whether the symptoms are generated unconsciously or consciously. If unconscious, the diagnosis is one of conversion (somatoform) disorder. Secondly, if the symptoms are judged to be wilfully feigned, the clinician must decide why the patient is simulating illness: if the motive is thought to be understandable primarily in terms of psychological needs (to adopt the sick role), the diagnosis is one of factitious disorder; if the motives appear to be purely practical (e.g. to avoid a criminal conviction or for some obvious financial gain), the term 'malingering' (not a medical diagnosis as such) is used. In practice the distinction between factitious disorder and malingering is often difficult to make, let alone the distinction between unconscious and conscious symptom generation, and both dichotomies are undoubtedly better conceived of as dimensions. The area remains controversial and the final diagnosis will be influenced as much by the clinician's opinions about this area in general as by any objective evidence gleaned during clinical assessment.

Clinical features

Using diagnostic criteria proposed by Fahn and Williams (1988) (Table 12.2), several series of patients with psychogenic movement disorder (PMD) have been described (Factor *et al.* 1995b; Williams *et al.* 1995; Feinstein *et al.* 2001). Patients, two-thirds of whom are female, tend to present in their early forties. Tremor is the most common symptom (accounting for around 40% of patients), closely followed by dystonia (in around one-third) (Lang 2006). Gait disorder, myoclonus and psychogenic parkinsonism are less common. No single clinical feature allows the diagnosis to be made with certainty. Rather it is a deviation from the typical clini-

Table 12.2 Diagnostic criteria for psychogenic movement disorder. (From Fahn & Williams 1988)

Degree of diagnostic certainty	Criteria
Documented*	Persistent relief by psychotherapy, suggestion or placebo; or observed without the movement disorder when the patient believed himself to be unobserved
Clinically established*	Incongruent with classical movement disorder or inconsistent over time, plus at least one of the following: other psychogenic signs; multiple somatisations; or an obvious psychiatric disturbance
Probable	Incongruent or inconsistent over time as above, or psychogenic signs or multiple somatisations
Possible	Evidence of emotional disturbance

*The first two categories have subsequently been amalgamated to comprise a clinically definite category (Williams *et al.* 1995).

cal profile of any of the recognised organic syndromes that raises the possibility of PMD (Schrag & Lang 2005). Thus, the diagnosis is best made by a neurologist with experience in movement disorders. The most important features on history that favour a diagnosis of PMD include abrupt onset, rapid progression to maximal severity and inconsistencies over time (in particular a history of variable movement disorders migrating between different parts of the body). A history of previous medically unexplained symptoms is highly suggestive. On examination (Table 12.3), particular attention should be paid to the consistency of abnormal movements, whether the disorder is modified by attention or distraction, and the presence of other non-physiological abnormalities such as functional weakness or sensory complaints.

The 'gold standard' diagnostic criterion for PMD is widely regarded to be the demonstration of persistent relief following psychotherapy, suggestion or placebo. However, organic cases may occasionally demonstrate some of these characteristics (Thomas & Jankovic 2004). Cervical dystonia, for example, may be associated with transient remission in as many as 25% which, if it were to coincide with psychotherapy, could lead to misdiagnosis. Psychogenic disorders may be associated with the secondary physical consequences of prolonged immobility, or the maintenance of abnormal postures. For example, contractures are seen in psychogenic fixed dystonia that can account for persistence of abnormal postures in sleep and under anaesthesia.

An exception to the general rule that variability over time points to a psychogenic aetiology concerns the syndrome of fixed dystonia, which deserves special consideration. Idiopathic or primary dystonia typically displays some variation over time, including being triggered by activity or specific tasks (e.g. writing), and temporary relief by sensory

tricks (*geste antagoniste*). In contrast, fixed dystonia, as its name implies, is relatively constant. In a careful investigation of a series of patients with fixed dystonias, Schrag *et al.* (2004) demonstrated compelling evidence of a psychogenic aetiology in the majority of cases. From a series of 103 patients with fixed dystonia, 41 were investigated prospectively. Detailed neuropsychiatric assessment was conducted in a subgroup of 26 who were compared with a control group of 20 patients with classical dystonia. In the prospective group, 37% met criteria for clinically definite PMD and 29% for somatisation disorder. The authors considered both figures to be underestimates and in the prospectively examined group found only 10% in whom there was no suggestion of a psychogenic disorder. In comparison with the control group patients with fixed dystonia had higher rates of dissociative and affective disorders. The onset of fixed dystonia occurred after a peripheral injury in 68% of cases (compared with 5% in the control group) and 44% of patients had associated features of complex regional pain syndrome (reflex sympathetic dystrophy). The authors conclude that fixed dystonia commonly occurs after peripheral injury and overlaps with complex regional pain syndrome. The study provides compelling evidence that this syndrome has a psychogenic basis in the majority of patients.

The presence of a psychiatric history is often cited as evidence in favour of a psychogenic origin for the presenting movement disorder. However, caution is clearly required as many organic movement disorders are associated with high rates of psychiatric comorbidity and in some, Huntington's disease for example, psychiatric and behavioural problems may develop long before more obvious neurological features. However, patients with PMD do have very high rates of psychiatric disorder. Feinstein *et al.* (2001) have reported the prevalence of psychiatric disorders defined using DSM-

Table 12.3 Examination procedures in psychogenic movement disorders.* (From Stone *et al.* 2005a.)

Disorder	Feature	Examination procedure	Specific caveat
Tremor	Variability	Observe for spontaneous variability in frequency, amplitude or distribution	All movement disorders vary to some degree and will often worsen with anxiety
	Distraction	Observe for improvement while the patient performs a distraction task. Distraction tasks include asking the patient to perform tests of mental concentration (e.g. serial subtraction) or physical tasks with his normal limbs (e.g. rapid alternating hand movements)	Organic disorders may be susceptible to attentional factors to a minor degree
	Entrainment	The patient is asked to make a rhythmical movement with his normal hand or foot. In psychogenic tremor the normal limb either 'entrains' to the same rhythm as the abnormal side, or the requested rhythm becomes irregular or incomplete. A slower (3 Hz) rhythm may be a more sensitive test than faster rhythms	
	Coactivation	A load (weight or pressure) is applied to the affected limb. Organic tremor tends to diminish whereas functional tremor may increase in amplitude. This may be because of coactivation of agonist and antagonist muscle groups. In this situation increased load triggers physiological clonus	
Dystonia	Distraction	As above	
Myoclonus	Variability in stimulus response	Psychogenic myoclonus may be triggered by a variety of stimuli (e.g. noise, light or eliciting tendon reflexes). Observe for variability in the delay between stimulus and jerk. The delay is also usually longer than seen in stimulus-sensitive organic myoclonus	

*In each case a negative test does not exclude a psychogenic basis for the disorder. As with any clinical examination, the usefulness of these tests will depend on the clinician's experience in applying these procedures to patients with both organic and psychogenic disorders.

IV criteria in a series of 42 patients with PMD. The lifetime prevalence rates for the most common comorbid diagnoses were 43% for major depression, 38% for anxiety disorders, and 28.6% for mixed major depression and anxiety. Personality disorders were identified in 45%, and 38% had prominent features of other medically unexplained symptoms.

Investigations

Functional imaging with ^{123}I-2β-carboxymethoxy-3-β-(4-iodophenyl)-tropane and SPECT may be helpful in confirming a diagnosis of Parkinson's disease, with over 90% of patients having abnormal scans early in the course of the disease (Jennings *et al.* 2004). A very high specificity for this technique has also been reported but studies involving substantial numbers of patients with PMD are required before the utility of this procedure can truly be gauged. Almost all reporting of scans is currently based on qualitative assessment and in clinical settings the extent of false negatives and positives will undoubtedly vary between centres.

Electromyography can be used to verify some of the characteristics of psychogenic tremor and myoclonus listed in Table 12.3, including variability in tremor frequency, coactivation, entrainment and prolonged latency (>75 ms) in psychogenic myoclonus (Schrag & Lang 2005). However, the sensitivity and specificity of these techniques has yet to be established. Combined electroencephalographic and electromyographic recordings may be helpful in assessing myoclonus. The demonstration of a prolonged pre-movement Bereitschaftspotential is good evidence of a psychogenic basis but this may be attenuated or even absent in healthy subjects under certain conditions (Terada *et al.* 1995). Furthermore, this technique requires back-averaging of multiple events, which may be impractical if the jerks occur infrequently. A pathological 4–7 Hz drive to peripheral muscles has recently been demonstrated in patients with DYT1 dystonia (Grosse *et al.* 2004). This finding was present in 10 of 12 patients with this disorder but not in healthy controls or patients with PMD. However, the specificity and sensitivity of this abnormality is unknown.

Aetiology

No studies have specifically sought to identify putative aetiological factors in PMD. However, there is considerable overlap between different somatoform presentations (Wessely *et al.* 1999) and it is reasonable to assume that the biological, psychological and social factors that may act to predispose, trigger and maintain other somatoform disorders also operate in PMD (Stone *et al.* 2005b). Onset after minor physical injury is common and much more frequently reported than onset after a psychological trauma (Factor *et al.* 1995b; Feinstein *et al.* 2001; Schrag *et al.* 2004).

The physiological mechanisms by which PMDs might be maintained have received little attention. Raethjen *et al.* (2004) have proposed two alternative mechanisms that might underlie psychogenic tremor. In the first, the movements are essentially construed simply as arising from voluntary-like activity. The second mechanism involves co-contraction of normally opposing agonist/antagonist muscle groups. In this case tremor arises through physiological clonus, as seen in shivering or with prolonged tonic muscular exertion.

Management and prognosis

There have been no controlled treatment trials in PMD and few detailed outcome studies. Factor *et al.* (1995b) reported resolution of symptoms in 35% of 28 patients over a 6-year period. Williams *et al.* (1995) describe outcome in 25 patients who participated in an intensive treatment programme combining psychotherapy in all cases with family sessions (58%), hypnosis (42%) and placebo therapy (13%). Antidepressants were prescribed in 71%. An impressive 52% were felt to have benefited significantly from treatment, with complete resolution of symptoms in 25%; 35% of patients returned to employment. A less optimistic view comes from the most detailed study to date by Feinstein *et al.* (2001). These authors describe outcome in 42 patients (from a series of 88) followed up after a mean interval of 3.2 years from initial assessment. The PMD had remitted in only four patients and in two of these had been replaced by a different mental disorder. Symptoms had improved in one-third of the patients but were the same or worse in over half. Poor outcome was associated with long duration of symptoms at initial presentation, gradual onset and by the presence of psychiatric comorbidity. This was a naturalistic outcome study and treatment given, if any, was not described. These findings are broadly similar to those of recent studies of long-term prognosis in other motor somatoform disorders; if anything, they suggest that PMD may carry a particularly poor prognosis. Thus, Crimlisk *et al.* (1998) report resolution of the presenting symptom in 28% of 64 patients (half of whom had a PMD) followed over 6 years. In a study of functional motor and sensory symptoms in 47 patients, Stone *et al.* (2003) found that 83% reported significant somatic symptoms after a mean follow-up period of 12.5 years. These authors commented on a strong tendency for initial symptoms to be replaced or joined by new ones.

There is little evidence on which to base any specific recommendations for treatment in PMD. Principles and techniques that have proven useful in other somatoform conditions are likely to be of benefit, although many have yet to be fully evaluated. A careful explanation of the diagnosis is of paramount importance (Stone *et al.* 2005b). Psychiatric assessment should include detailed enquiry into the patient's psychosocial background, aiming in particular to identify significant maintaining factors that might otherwise be barriers to recovery. Antidepressant medication may be helpful, even in the absence of significant depression or anxiety (O'Malley *et al.* 1999). Cognitive behavioural therapy is a well-established treatment for a variety of somatoform disorders (Kroenke & Swindle 2000), but other forms of psychotherapy may be preferable for some patients. A multidisciplinary approach combining psychotherapy with physiotherapy and other rehabilitation services has been recommended but again requires evaluation (Schrag *et al.* 2004).

References

Aarsland, D., Larsen, J.P. *et al.* (1999a) Prevalence and clinical correlates of psychotic symptoms in Parkinson disease: a community-based study. *Archives of Neurology* **56**, 595–601.

Aarsland, D., Larsen, J.P. *et al.* (1999b) Range of neuropsychiatric disturbances in patients with Parkinson's disease. *Journal of Neurology, Neurosurgery, and Psychiatry* **67**, 492–496.

Aarsland, D., Larsen, J.P. *et al.* (1999c) Olanzapine for psychosis in patients with Parkinson's disease with and without dementia. *Journal of Neuropsychiatry and Clinical Neuroscience* **11**, 392–394.

Aarsland, D., Larsen, J.P. *et al.* (2000) Predictors of nursing home placement in Parkinson's disease: a population-based, prospective study. *Journal of the American Geriatric Society* **48**, 938–942.

Aarsland, D., Ballard, C. *et al.* (2001a) A comparative study of psychiatric symptoms in dementia with Lewy bodies and Parkinson's disease with and without dementia. *International Journal of Geriatric Psychiatry* **16**, 528–536.

Aarsland, D., Litvan, I. *et al.* (2001b) Neuropsychiatric symptoms of patients with progressive supranuclear palsy and Parkinson's disease. *Journal of Neuropsychiatry and Clinical Neuroscience* **13**, 42–49.

Adams, R.D., Bogaert, L.V. & Eecken, H.V. (1964) Striato-nigral degeneration. *Journal of Neuropathology and Experimental Neurology* **23**, 584–608.

Adler, C.H. & Kumar, R. (2000) Pharmacological and surgical options for the treatment of cervical dystonia. *Neurology* **55** (12 suppl. 5), S9–S14.

Adler, L., Angrist, B., Peselow, E., Corwin, J., Masiansky, R. & Rotrosen, J. (1986) A controlled assessment of propranolol in the treatment of neuroleptic-induced akathisia. *British Journal of Psychiatry* **149**, 42–45.

Advokat, C. (2005) Differential effects of clozapine versus other antipsychotics on clinical outcome and dopamine release in the brain. *Essential Psychopharmacology* **6**, 73–90.

Agras, S. & Marshall, C. (1965) The application of negative practice to spasmodic torticollis. *American Journal of Psychiatry* **122**, 579–582.

Aisen, A.M., Martel, W., Gabrielsen, T.O. *et al.* (1985) Wilson disease of the brain: MR imaging. *Radiology* **157**, 137–141.

Akil, M. & Brewer, G.J. (1995) Psychiatric and behavioral abnormalities in Wilson's disease. *Advances in Neurology* **65**, 171–178.

Albanese, A., Colosimo, C. *et al.* (1995) Multiple system atrophy presenting as parkinsonism: clinical features and diagnostic criteria. *Journal of Neurology, Neurosurgery and Psychiatry* **59**, 144–151.

Albert, M.L. (1978) Subcortical dementia. In: Katzman, R., Terry, R.D. & Bick, K.L. (eds) *Alzheimer's Disease: Senile Dementia and Related Disorders, Aging*, vol. 7, pp. 173–180. Raven Press, New York.

Albert, M.L., Feldman, R.G. & Willis, A.L. (1974) The 'subcortical dementia' of progressive supranuclear palsy. *Journal of Neurology, Neurosurgery and Psychiatry* **37**, 121–130.

Albin, R.L. & Frey, K.A. (2003) Initial agonist treatment of Parkinson disease: a critique. *Neurology* **60**, 390–394.

Allen, A.J., Leonard, H.L. *et al.* (1995) Case study: a new infection triggered, autoimmune subtype of pediatric OCD and Tourette's syndrome. *Journal of the American Academy of Child and Adolescent Psychiatry* **34**, 307–311.

Allen, R.L., Walker, Z. *et al.* (1995) Risperidone for psychotic and behavioural symptoms in Lewy body dementia. *Lancet* **346**, 185.

Allen, R.P., Picchietti, D. *et al.* (2003) Restless legs syndrome: diagnostic criteria, special considerations, and epidemiology. A report from the restless legs syndrome diagnosis and epidemiology workshop at the National Institutes of Health. *Sleep Medicine* **4**, 101–119.

Alvarez, L., Macias, R. *et al.* (2001) Dorsal subthalamotomy for Parkinson's disease. *Movement Disorders* **16**, 72–78.

Alvord, E.C. Jr, Forno, L.S., Kusske, J.A., Kauffman, R.J., Rhodes, J.S. & Goetowseci, C.R. (1974) The pathology of Parkinsonism: a comparison of degenerations in cerebral cortex and brain stem. *Advances in Neurology* **5**, 175–193.

Anca, M.H., Giladi, N. *et al.* (2004) Ropinirole in Gilles de la Tourette syndrome. *Neurology* **62**, 1626–1627.

Anderson, R.L., Patel, B.C. *et al.* (1998) Blepharospasm: past, present, and future. *Ophthalmic Plastic and Reconstructive Surgery* **14**, 305–317.

Andreassen, O.A., MacEwan, T. *et al.* (1997) Non-functional CYP2D6 alleles and risk for neuroleptic-induced movement disorders in schizophrenic patients. *Psychopharmacology* **131**, 174–179.

Apter, A., Pauls, D.L. *et al.* (1993) An epidemiologic study of Gilles de la Tourette's syndrome in Israel. *Archives of General Psychiatry* **50**, 734–738.

Arnulf, I., Konofal, E. *et al.* (2002) Parkinson's disease and sleepiness: an integral part of PD. *Neurology* **58**, 1019–1024.

Augood, S.J., Hollingsworth, Z. *et al.* (2002) Dopamine transmission in DYT1 dystonia: a biochemical and autoradiographical study. *Neurology* **59**, 445–448.

Baker, R.S., Andersen, A.H. *et al.* (2003) A functional magnetic resonance imaging study in patients with benign essential blepharospasm. *Journal of Neuroophthalmology* **23**, 11–15.

Baldessarini, R.J. & Tarsy, D. (1980) The pathophysiologic basis of tardive dyskinesia. In: Fann, W.E., Smith, R.C., Davis, J.M. & Domino, E.F. (eds) *Tardive Dyskinesia: Research and Treatment*, pp. 451–455. MTP Press, Lancaster.

Banaschewski, T., Woerner, W. *et al.* (2003) Premonitory sensory phenomena and suppressibility of tics in Tourette syndrome: developmental aspects in children and adolescents. *Developmental Medicine and Child Neurology* **45**, 700–703.

Barbeau, A. (1969) L-dopa therapy in Parkinson's disease: a critical review of nine years' experience. *Canadian Medical Association Journal* **101**, 59–68.

Barnes, J., Boubert, L. *et al.* (2003) Reality monitoring and visual hallucinations in Parkinson's disease. *Neuropsychologia* **41**, 565–574.

Barnes, T.R.E. (1987) The present status of tardive dyskinesia and akathisia in the treatment of schizophrenia. *Psychiatric Developments* **4**, 301–319.

Barnes, T.R.E. (1989) A rating scale for drug-induced akathisia. *British Journal of Psychiatry* **154**, 672–676.

Barnes, T.R.E. & Braude, W.M. (1985) Akathisia variants and tardive dyskinesia. *Archives of General Psychiatry* **42**, 874–878.

Baron, J.A. (1986) Cigarette smoking and Parkinson's disease. *Neurology* **36**, 1490–1496.

Baron-Cohen, S., Scahill, V.L. *et al.* (1999) The prevalence of Gilles de la Tourette syndrome in children and adolescents with autism: a large scale study. *Psychological Medicine* **29**, 1151–1159.

Bawden, H.N., Stokes, A. *et al.* (1998) Peer relationship problems in children with Tourette's disorder or diabetes mellitus. *Journal of Child Psychology and Psychiatry and Allied Disciplines* **39**, 663–668.

Bearn, A.G. (1957) Wilson's disease: an inborn error of metabolism with multiple manifestations. *American Journal of Medicine* **22**, 747–757.

Beasley, C.M. Jr, Tollefson, G.D. *et al.* (1997) Efficacy of olanzapine: an overview of pivotal clinical trials. *Journal of Clinical Psychiatry* **58** (suppl. 10), 7–12.

Beck, A.T., Ward, C.H. *et al.* (1961) An inventory for measuring depression. *Archives of General Psychiatry* **4**, 561–571.

Bedard, M.A., el Massioui, F. *et al.* (1998) Attentional deficits in Parkinson's disease: partial reversibility with naphtoxazine (SDZ NVI-085), a selective noradrenergic alpha 1 agonist. *Clinical Neuropharmacology* **21**, 108–117.

Behrman, S. (1972) Mutism induced by phenothiazines. *British Journal of Psychiatry* **121**, 599–604.

Benazzouz, A., Breit, S. *et al.* (2002) Intraoperative microrecordings of the subthalamic nucleus in Parkinson's disease. *Movement Disorders* **17** (suppl. 3), S145–S149.

Bench, C.J., Friston, K.J. *et al.* (1992) The anatomy of melancholia: focal abnormalities of cerebral blood flow in major depression. *Psychological Medicine* **22**, 607–615.

Bender, M.B. (1969) Disorders of eye movements. In: Vinken, P.J. & Bruyn, G.W. (eds) *Handbook of Clinical Neurology*, vol. 1, ch. 18. North-Holland Publishing Company, Amsterdam.

Benrud-Larson, L.M., Sandroni, P. *et al.* (2005) Depressive symptoms and life satisfaction in patients with multiple system atrophy. *Movement Disorders* **20**, 951–957.

Ben-Shlomo, Y., Churchyard, A. *et al.* (1998) Investigation by Parkinson's Disease Research Group of United Kingdom into excess mortality seen with combined levodopa and selegiline treatment in patients with early, mild Parkinson's disease: further results of randomised trial and confidential inquiry. *British Medical Journal* **316**, 1191–1196.

Ben-Shlomo, Y., Camfield, L. *et al.* (2002) What are the determinants of quality of life in people with cervical dystonia? *Journal of Neurology, Neurosurgery and Psychiatry* **72**, 608–614.

Ben Simon, G.J. & McCann, J.D. (2005) Benign essential blepharospasm. *International Ophthalmology Clinics* **45**, 49–75.

Benson, D.F. (1982) The treatable dementias. In: Benson, D.F. & Blumer, D. (eds) *Psychiatric Aspects of Neurologic Disease*, ch. 6. Grune & Stratton, New York & London.

Berardelli, A., Rothwell, J.C. *et al.* (1985) Pathophysiology of blepharospasm and oromandibular dystonia. *Brain* **108**, 593–608.

Berardelli, A., Rothwell, J.C. *et al.* (1998) The pathophysiology of primary dystonia. *Brain* **121**, 1195–1212.

Bergen, J.A., Eyland, E.A. *et al.* (1989) The course of tardive dyskinesia in patients on long-term neuroleptics. *British Journal of Psychiatry* **154**, 523–528.

Bergman, J. & Lerner, V. (2002) Successful use of donepezil for the treatment of psychotic symptoms in patients with Parkinson's disease. *Clinical Neuropharmacology* **25**, 107–110.

Bertrand, E., Lechowicz, W. *et al.* (1997) Qualitative and quantitative analysis of locus coeruleus neurons in Parkinson's disease. *Folia Neuropathologica* **35**, 80–86.

Bharucha, N.E., Stokes, L., Schoenberg, B.S. *et al.* (1986) A case–control study of twin pairs discordant for Parkinson's disease: a search for environmental risk factors. *Neurology* **36**, 284–288.

Biggins, C.A., Boyd, J.L., Harrop, F.M. *et al.* (1992) A controlled, longitudinal study of dementia in Parkinson's disease. *Journal of Neurology, Neurosurgery and Psychiatry* **55**, 566–571.

Birkmayer, W., Danielczyk, W. *et al.* (1974) Nucleus ruber and L-dopa psychosis: biochemical post-mortem findings. *Journal of Neural Transmission* **35**, 93–116.

Blackie, J.D. & Lees, A.J. (1990) Botulinum toxin in the treatment of spasmodic torticollis. *Journal of Neurology, Neurosurgery and Psychiatry* **53**, 640–643.

Block, G., Liss, C. *et al.* (1997) Comparison of immediate-release and controlled release carbidopa/levodopa in Parkinson's disease. A multicenter 5-year study. The CR First Study Group. *European Neurology* **37**, 23–27.

Boller, F., Mizutani, T., Roessmann, U. & Gambetti, P. (1980) Parkinson disease, dementia and Alzheimer disease: clinicopathological correlations. *Annals of Neurology* **7**, 329–335.

Bonnet, A.M., Pichon, J. *et al.* (1997) Urinary disturbances in striatonigral degeneration and Parkinson's disease: clinical and urodynamic aspects. *Movement Disorders* **12**, 509–513.

Booth, G. (1948) Psychodynamics in parkinsonism. *Psychosomatic Medicine* **10**, 1–14.

Bouchard, R., Pourcher, E. *et al.* (1989) Fluoxetine and extrapyramidal side effects. *American Journal of Psychiatry* **146**, 1352–1353.

Braak, H., Ghebremedhin, E. *et al.* (2004) Stages in the development of Parkinson's disease-related pathology. *Cell and Tissue Research* **318**, 121–134.

Brashear, A., Ambrosius, W.T. *et al.* (1998) Comparison of treatment of tardive dystonia and idiopathic cervical dystonia with botulinum toxin type A. *Movement Disorders* **13**, 158–161.

Brashear, A., Bergan, K. *et al.* (2000) Patients' perception of stopping or continuing treatment of cervical dystonia with botulinum toxin type A. *Movement Disorders* **15**, 150–153.

Braude, W.M., Barnes, T.R.E. & Gore, S.M. (1983) Clinical characteristics of akathisia: a systematic investigation of acute psychiatric in-patient admissions. *British Journal of Psychiatry* **143**, 139–150.

Braun, A.R., Randolph, C. *et al.* (1995) The functional neuroanatomy of Tourette's syndrome: an FDG-PET Study. II. Relationships between regional cerebral metabolism and associated behavioral and cognitive features of the illness. *Neuropsychopharmacology* **13**, 151–168.

Breier, A., Sutton, V.K. *et al.* (2002) Olanzapine in the treatment of dopamimetic-induced psychosis in patients with Parkinson's disease. *Biological Psychiatry* **52**, 438–445.

Breteler, M.M.B., De Groot, R.R.M., Van Romunde, L.K.J. & Hofman, A. (1995) Risk of dementia in patients with Parkinson's disease, epilepsy and severe head trauma: a register-based follow-up study. *American Journal of Epidemiology* **142**, 1300–1305.

Brett, P.M., Curtis, D. *et al.* (1995) The genetic susceptibility to Gilles de la Tourette syndrome in a large multiple affected British kindred: linkage analysis excludes a role for the genes coding for dopamine D1, D2, D3, D4, D5 receptors, dopamine beta hydroxylase, tyrosinase, and tyrosine hydroxylase. *Biological Psychiatry* **37**, 533–540.

Brewer, G.J. (1995) Practical recommendations and new therapies for Wilson's disease. *Drugs* **50**, 240–249.

Brewer, G.J. (2000a) Recognition, diagnosis, and management of Wilson's disease. *Proceedings of the Society for Experimental Biology and Medicine* **223**, 39–46.

Brewer, G.J. (2000b) Wilson's disease. *Current Treatment Options in Neurology* **2**, 193–204.

Brierley, H. (1967) Treatment of hysterical spasmodic torticollis by behaviour therapy. *Behaviour Research and Therapy* **5**, 139–142.

Brin, M.F., Jankovic, J., Comella, C., Blitzer, A., Tsui, J. & Pullman, S.L. (1995) Treatment of dystonia using botulinum toxin. In: Kurlan, R.J.B. (ed.) *Treatment of Movement Disorders*, ch. 6. Lippincott, Philadelphia.

Brooks, D.J. (1993) Functional imaging in relation to parkinsonian syndromes. *Journal of the Neurological Sciences* **115**, 1–17.

Brooks, D.J., Ibanez, V., Sawle, G.V. *et al.* (1990) Differing patterns of striatal F-dopa uptake in Parkinson's disease, multiple system atrophy and progressive supranuclear palsy. *Annals of Neurology* **28**, 547–555.

Brooks, D.J., Frey, K.A. *et al.* (2003) Assessment of neuroimaging techniques as biomarkers of the progression of Parkinson's disease. *Experimental Neurology* **184** (suppl. 1), S68–S79.

Brown, R. & Jahanshahi, M. (1995) Depression in Parkinson's disease: a psychosocial viewpoint. *Advances in Neurology* **65**, 61–84.

Brown, R.G. & Marsden, C.D. (1984) How common is dementia in Parkinson's disease? *Lancet* **ii**, 1262–1265.

Brown, R.G., Marsden, C.D., Quinn, N. & Wyke, M.A. (1984) Alterations in cognitive performance and affect-arousal state during fluctuations in motor function in Parkinson's disease. *Journal of Neurology, Neurosurgery and Psychiatry* **47**, 454–465.

Brown, R.G., MacCarthy, B. *et al.* (1988) Depression and disability in Parkinson's disease: a follow-up of 132 cases. *Psychological Medicine* **18**, 49–55.

Bruun, R.D. & Budman, C.L. (1992) The natural history of Tourette syndrome. *Advances in Neurology* **58**, 1–6.

Budman, C.L., Gayer, A. *et al*. (2001) An open-label study of the treatment efficacy of olanzapine for Tourette's disorder. *Journal of Clinical Psychiatry* **62**, 290–294.

Bull, P.C., Thomas, G.R. *et al*. (1993) The Wilson disease gene is a putative copper transporting P-type ATPase similar to the Menkes gene. *Nature Genetics* **5**, 327–337.

Burke, R.E., Fahn, S. & Gold, A.P. (1980) Delayed-onset dystonia in patients with 'static' encephalopathy. *Journal of Neurology, Neurosurgery and Psychiatry* **43**, 789–797.

Burke, R.E., Fahn, S. *et al*. (1982) Tardive dystonia: late-onset and persistent dystonia caused by antipsychotic drugs. *Neurology* **32**, 1335–1346.

Burke, R.E., Fahn, S. & Marsden, C.D. (1986) Torsion dystonia: a double-blind, prospective trial of high-dosage trihexyphenidyl. *Neurology* **36**, 160–164.

Burke, R.E., Kang, U.J., Jankovic, J., Miller, L.G. & Fahn, S. (1989) Tardive akathisia: an analysis of clinical features and response to open therapeutic trials. *Movement Disorders* **4**, 157–175.

Burton, K., Larsen, T.A. *et al*. (1985) Parkinson's disease: a comparison of mesulergine and bromocriptine. *Neurology* **35**, 1205–1208.

Butler, A.G., Duffey, P.O., Hawthorne, M.R. & Barnes, M.P. (2004) An epidemiological survey of dystonia within the entire population of North East England over the past 9 years. *Advances in Neurology* **94**, 95–99.

Cadet, J.L. & Lohr, J.B. (1989) Possible involvement of free radicals in neuroleptic-induced movement disorders. Evidence from treatment of tardive dyskinesia with vitamin E. *Annals of the New York Academy of Sciences* **570**, 176–185.

Caine, E.D. (1985) Gilles de la Tourette's syndrome. A review of clinical and research studies and consideration of future directions for investigation. *Archives of Neurology* **42**, 393–397.

Caine, E.D., McBride, M.C., Chiverton, P., Bamford, K.A., Rediess, S. & Shiao, J. (1988) Tourette's syndrome in Monroe County school children. *Neurology* **38**, 472–475.

Camfield, L., Ben-Shlomo, Y. *et al*. (2002) Impact of cervical dystonia on quality of life. *Movement Disorders* **17**, 838–841.

Caroff, S.N., Campbell, E.C. *et al*. (2001) Treatment of tardive dyskinesia with donepezil: a pilot study. *Journal of Clinical Psychiatry* **62**, 772–775.

Carson, A.J., Ringbauer, B. *et al*. (2000) Do medically unexplained symptoms matter? A prospective cohort study of 300 new referrals to neurology outpatient clinics. *Journal of Neurology, Neurosurgery and Psychiatry* **68**, 207–210.

Carson, A.J., Best, S. *et al*. (2003) The outcome of neurology outpatients with medically unexplained symptoms: a prospective cohort study. *Journal of Neurology, Neurosurgery and Psychiatry* **74**, 897–900.

Carter, A.S., O'Donnell, D.A. *et al*. (2000) Social and emotional adjustment in children affected with Gilles de la Tourette's syndrome: associations with ADHD and family functioning. *Journal of Child Psychology and Psychiatry and Allied Disciplines* **41**, 215–223.

Carter, J.H., Stewart, B.J. *et al*. (1998) Living with a person who has Parkinson's disease: the spouse's perspective by stage of disease. *Movement Disorders* **13**, 20–28.

Cartwright, G.E. (1978) Diagnosis of treatable Wilson's disease. *New England Journal of Medicine* **298**, 1347–1350.

Casey, D.E. (1989) Clozapine: neuroleptic-induced EPS and tardive dyskinesia. *Psychopharmacology*, **99**, S47–S53.

Casey, D.E. (2004) Pathophysiology of antipsychotic drug-induced movement disorders. *Journal of Clinical Psychiatry* **65** (suppl. 9), 25–28.

Cash, R., L'Heureux, R., Raisman, R., Javoy-Agid, F. & Scatton, B. (1987) Parkinson's disease and dementia: norepinephrine and dopamine in locus caeruleus. *Neurology* **37**, 42–46.

Cath, D.C., Spinhoven, P. *et al*. (2000) The relationship between types and severity of repetitive behaviors in Gilles de la Tourette's disorder and obsessive-compulsive disorder. *Journal of Clinical Psychiatry* **61**, 505–513.

Cavalho, A. (2002) Classification and genetics of dystonia. *Lancet Neurology* **1**, 316–325.

Celesia, G.G. & Wanamaker, W.M. (1972) Psychiatric disturbances in Parkinson's disease. *Diseases of the Nervous System* **33**, 577–583.

Ceravolo, R., Nuti, A. *et al*. (2000) Paroxetine in Parkinson's disease: effects on motor and depressive symptoms. *Neurology* **55**, 1216–1218.

Chan, J., Brin, M.F. *et al*. (1991) Idiopathic cervical dystonia: clinical characteristics. *Movement Disorders* **6**, 119–126.

Channon, S., Flynn, D. & Robertson, M.M. (1992) Attentional deficits in Gilles de la Tourette syndrome. *Neuropsychiatry, Neuropsychology, and Behavioral Neurology* **5**, 170–177.

Chapel, J.L., Brown, N. & Jenkins, R.L. (1964) Tourette's disease: symptomatic relief with haloperidol. *American Journal of Psychiatry* **120**, 608–610.

Chase, T.N., Geoffrey, V., Gillespie, M. & Burrows, G.H. (1986) Structural and functional studies of Gilles de la Tourette syndrome. *Revue Neurologique (Paris)* **142**, 851–855.

Chatterjee, A. & Fahn, S. (2002) Methylphenidate treats apathy in Parkinson's disease. *Journal of Neuropsychiatry and Clinical Neuroscience* **14**, 461–462.

Cheng, N., Maeda, T. *et al*. (1996) Differential neurotoxicity induced by L-DOPA and dopamine in cultured striatal neurons. *Brain Research* **743**, 278–283.

Choi, C., Sohn, Y.H. *et al*. (2000) The effect of long-term levodopa therapy on depression level in de novo patients with Parkinson's disease. *Journal of the Neurological Sciences* **172**, 12–16.

Chui, H.C. & Perlmutter, L.S. (1992) Pathological correlates of dementia in Parkinson's disease. In: Huber, S.J. & Cummings, J.L. (eds) *Parkinson's Disease: Neurobehavioral Aspects*, ch. 13. Oxford University Press, Oxford.

Chui, H.C., Mortimer, J.A., Slager, U., Zarow, C., Bondareff, W. & Webster, D.D. (1986) Pathologic correlates of dementia in Parkinson's disease. *Archives of Neurology* **43**, 991–995.

Church, A.J., Dale, R.C. *et al*. (2003) Tourette's syndrome: a cross sectional study to examine the PANDAS hypothesis. *Journal of Neurology, Neurosurgery and Psychiatry* **74**, 602–607.

Clarke, C.E. & Guttman, M. (2002) Dopamine agonist monotherapy in Parkinson's disease. *Lancet* **360**, 1767–1769.

Clark, D.F. (1966) Behaviour therapy of Gilles de la Tourette's syndrome. *British Journal of Psychiatry* **112**, 771–778.

Clow, A., Jenner, P. & Marsden, C.D. (1979a) Changes in dopamine mediated behaviour during one year's neuroleptic administration. *European Journal of Pharmacology* **57**, 365–375.

Clow, A., Jenner, P., Theodorou, A. & Marsden, C.D. (1979b) Striatal dopamine receptors become supersensitive while rats are given trifluoperazine for six months. *Nature* **278**, 59–61.

Coffey, B.J., Miguel, E.C. *et al.* (1998) Tourette's disorder with and without obsessive-compulsive disorder in adults: are they different? *Journal of Nervous and Mental Disease* **186**, 201–206.

Cohen, D. & Marks, F.M. (1977) Gilles de la Tourette's syndrome treated by operant conditioning. *British Journal of Psychiatry* **130**, 315.

Cohrs, S., Rasch, T. *et al.* (2001) Decreased sleep quality and increased sleep related movements in patients with Tourette's syndrome. *Journal of Neurology, Neurosurgery and Psychiatry* **70**, 192–197.

Cole, S.A., Woodard, J.L. *et al.* (1996) Depression and disability in Parkinson's disease. *Journal of Neuropsychiatry and Clinical Neuroscience* **8**, 20–25.

Colloby, S. & O'Brien, J. (2004) Functional imaging in Parkinson's disease and dementia with Lewy bodies. *Journal of Geriatric Psychiatry and Neurology* **17**, 158–163.

Colosimo, C. & Pezzella, F.R. (2002) The symptomatic treatment of multiple system atrophy. *European Journal of Neurology* **9**, 195–199.

Colosimo, C., Albanese, A. *et al.* (1995) Some specific clinical features differentiate multiple system atrophy (striatonigral variety) from Parkinson's disease. *Archives of Neurology* **52**, 294–298.

Connell, P.H., Corbett, J.A., Mathews, A.M. & Horne, D.J. (1967) Drug treatment of adolescent ticquers. A double blind trial of diazepam and haloperidol. *British Journal of Psychiatry* **113**, 375–381.

Corbett, J.A. (1971) The nature of tics and Gilles de la Tourette's syndrome. *Journal of Psychosomatic Research* **15**, 403–409.

Corbett, J.A., Mathews, A.M., Connell, P.H. & Shapiro, D.A. (1969) Tics and Gilles de la Tourette's syndrome: a follow-up study and critical review. *British Journal of Psychiatry* **115**, 1229–1241.

Cortese, L., Jog, M. *et al.* (2004) Assessing and monitoring antipsychotic-induced movement disorders in hospitalized patients: a cautionary study. *Canadian Journal of Psychiatry* **49**, 31–36.

Costa, J., Borges, A. *et al.* (2005a) Botulinum toxin type A versus botulinum toxin type B for cervical dystonia. *Cochrane Database of Systematic Reviews* **1**, CD004314.

Costa, J., Espirito-Santo, C. *et al.* (2005b) Botulinum toxin type A therapy for cervical dystonia. *Cochrane Database of Systematic Reviews* **1**, CD003633.

Costa, J., Espirito-Santo, C. *et al.* (2005c) Botulinum toxin type B for cervical dystonia. *Cochrane Database of Systematic Reviews* **1**, CD004315.

Costa, J., Espirito-Santo, C. *et al.* (2005d) Botulinum toxin type A versus anticholinergics for cervical dystonia. *Cochrane Database of Systematic Reviews* **1**, CD004312.

Cotzias, G., Papavasiliou, P. & Gellene, R. (1969) Modification of parkinsonism: chronic treatment with L-dopa. *New England Journal of Medicine* **280**, 337–345.

Cotzias, G.C., Papavasiliou, P.S. *et al.* (1971) Metabolic modification of Parkinson's disease and of chronic manganese poisoning. *Annual Review of Medicine* **22**, 305–326.

Coubes, P., Roubertie, A. *et al.* (2000) Treatment of DYT1-generalised dystonia by stimulation of the internal globus pallidus. *Lancet* **355**, 2220–2221.

Couprie, W., Wijdicks, E.F. *et al.* (1995) Outcome in conversion disorder: a follow up study. *Journal of Neurology, Neurosurgery and Psychiatry* **58**, 750–752.

Crawshaw, J.A. & Mullen, P.E. (1984) A study of benzhexol abuse. *British Journal of Psychiatry* **145**, 300–303.

Crespo-Facorro, B., Cabranes, J. *et al.* (1999) Regional cerebral blood flow in obsessive-compulsive patients with and without a chronic tic disorder. A SPECT study. *European Archives of Psychiatry and Clinical Neurosciences* **249**, 156–161.

Crevits, L. (2003) Abnormal psychophysical visual perception in Parkinson's disease patients. *Acta Neurologica Belgica* **103**, 83–87.

Crews, W.D. Jr & Harrison, D.W. (1995) The neuropsychology of depression and its implications for cognitive therapy. *Neuropsychology Review* **5**, 81–123.

Crimlisk, H.L., Bhatia, K. *et al.* (1998) Slater revisited: 6 year follow up study of patients with medically unexplained motor symptoms. *British Medical Journal* **316**, 582–586.

Crosby, N.J., Deane, K.H. *et al.* (2003) Amantadine for dyskinesia in Parkinson's disease. *Cochrane Database of Systematic Reviews* **2**, CD003467.

Crow, T.J., Johnstone, E.C. & McClelland, H.A. (1976) The coincidence of schizophrenia and parkinsonism: some neurochemical implications. *Pychological Medicine* **6**, 227–233.

Cummings, J.L. (1982) Cortical dementias. In: Benson, D.F. & Blumer, D. (eds) *Psychiatric Aspects of Neurologic Disease*, vol. 2, ch. 5. Grune & Stratton, New York.

Cummings, J.L. (1988) Intellectual impairment in Parkinson's disease: clinical, pathologic, and biochemical correlates. *Journal of Geriatric Psychiatry and Neurology* **1**, 24–36.

Cummings, J.L. (1991) Behavioral complications of drug treatment of Parkinson's disease. *Journal of the American Geriatric Society* **39**, 708–716.

Cummings, J.L. (1992a) Depression and Parkinson's disease: a review. *American Journal of Psychiatry* **149**, 443–454.

Cummings, J.L. (1992b) Neuropsychiatric complications of drug treatment in Parkinson's disease. In: Huber, S. & Cummings, J.L. (eds) *Parkinson's Disease: Neurobehavioral Aspects*, pp. 313–327. Oxford University Press, New York.

Cummings, J.L. (2000) Cholinesterase inhibitors: expanding applications. *Lancet* **356**, 2024–2025.

Cummings, J.L. & Frankel, M. (1985) Gilles de la Tourette syndrome and the neurological basis of obsessions and compulsions. *Biological Psychiatry* **20**, 1117–1126.

Curtis, D., Robertson, M.M. & Gurling, H.M.D. (1992) Autosomal dominant gene transmission in a large kindred with Gilles de la Tourette syndrome. *British Journal of Psychiatry* **160**, 845–849.

Dallos, V., Heathfield, K. *et al.* (1970) Use of amantadine in Parkinson's disease. Results of a double-blind trial. *British Medical Journal* **4**, 24–26.

Damasio, A., Antunes, J. & Macedo, C. (1970) L-Dopa, parkinsonism and depression. *Lancet* **19**, 611–612.

D'Antona, R., Baron, J.C., Samson, Y. *et al.* (1985) Subcortical dementia. Frontal cortex hypometabolism detected by positron tomography in patients with progressive supranuclear palsy. *Brain* **108**, 785–799.

Darkins, A.W., Fromkin, V.A. & Benson, D.F. (1988) A characterization of the prosodic loss in Parkinson's disease. *Brain and Language* **34**, 315–327.

Darvesh, S. & Freedman, M. (1996) Subcortical dementia: a neurobehavioral approach. *Brain and Cognition* **31**, 230–249.

Das, S.K. & Choudhary, S.S. (2000) A spectrum of dystonias: clinical features and update on management. *Journal of the Association of Physicians of India* 48, 622–630.

Dauer, W.T., Burke, R.E. *et al.* (1998) Current concepts on the clinical features, aetiology and management of idiopathic cervical dystonia. *Brain* 121, 547–560.

Davidsdottir, S., A. Cronin-Golomb, *et al.* (2005) Visual and spatial symptoms in Parkinson's disease. *Vision Research* 45, 1285–1296.

Davis, R.J., Cummings, J.L. & Hierholzer, R.W. (1988) Tardive dystonia: clinical spectrum and novel manifestations. *Behavioural Neurology* 1, 41–47.

Davison, K. & Bagley, C.R. (1969) Schizophrenia-like psychoses associated with organic disorders of the central nervous system: a review of the literature. In: Herrington, R.N. (ed.) *Current Problems in Neuropsychiatry*, pp. 113–184. British Journal of Psychiatry Special Publication No. 4. Headley Brothers, Ashford, Kent.

de Bie, R.M., de Haan, R.J. *et al.* (1999) Unilateral pallidotomy in Parkinson's disease: a randomised, single-blind, multicentre trial. *Lancet* 354, 1665–1669.

de Bie, R.M., de Haan, R.J. *et al.* (2002) Morbidity and mortality following pallidotomy in Parkinson's disease: a systematic review. *Neurology* 58, 1008–1012.

De Bruin, V.M.S. & Lees, A.J. (1992) The clinical features of 67 patients with clinically definite Steele–Richardson–Olszewski syndrome. *Behavioural Neurology* 5, 229–232.

Defazio, G., Abbruzzese, G. *et al.* (2004) Epidemiology of primary dystonia. *Lancet Neurology* 3, 673–678.

de Groot, C.M., Bornstein, R.A. *et al.* (1994) The course of tics in Tourette syndrome: a 5-year follow-up study. *Annals of Clinical Psychiatry* 6, 227–233.

Dekker, M.C., Bonifati, V. *et al.* (2003) Parkinson's disease: piecing together a genetic jigsaw. *Brain* 126, 1722–1733.

Dell'Agnello, G., Ceravolo, R. *et al.* (2001) SSRIs do not worsen Parkinson's disease: evidence from an open-label, prospective study. *Clinical Neuropharmacology* 24, 221–227.

de Maindreville, A.D., Fenelon, G. *et al.* (2005) Hallucinations in Parkinson's disease: a follow-up study. *Movement Disorders* 20, 212–217.

Dening, T.R. & Berrios, G.E. (1989a) Wilson's disease. Psychiatric symptoms in 195 cases. *Archives of General Psychiatry* 46, 1126–1134.

Dening, T.R. & Berrios, G.E. (1989b) Wilson's disease: a prospective study of psychopathology in 31 cases. *British Journal of Psychiatry* 155, 206–213.

Dening, T.R. & Berrios, G.E. (1990) Wilson's disease: a longitudinal study of psychiatric symptoms. *Biological Psychiatry* 28, 255–265.

Dening, T.R., Berrios, G.E. & Walshe, J.M. (1988) Wilson's disease and epilepsy. *Brain* 111, 1139–1155.

Denny-Brown, D. & Porter, H. (1951) The effect of BAL (2,3-dimercaptopropanol) on hepatolenticular degeneration (Wilson's disease). *New England Journal of Medicine* 245, 917–925.

de Rijk, M.C., Tzourio, C. *et al.* (1997) Prevalence of parkinsonism and Parkinson's disease in Europe: the EUROPARKINSON Collaborative Study. European Community Concerted Action on the Epidemiology of Parkinson's disease. *Journal of Neurology, Neurosurgery and Psychiatry* 62, 10–15.

De Smet, Y., Ruberg, M., Serdaru, M., Dubois, B., Lhermitte, F. & Agid, Y. (1982) Confusion, dementia and anticholinergics in Parkinson's disease. *Journal of Neurology, Neurosurgery and Psychiatry* 45, 1161–1164.

De Veaugh-Geiss, J. (1980) Tardive Tourette syndrome. *Neurology* 30, 562–563.

Dewey, R.B. Jr, Maraganore, D.M. *et al.* (1998) A double-blind, placebo-controlled study of intranasal apomorphine spray as a rescue agent for off-states in Parkinson's disease. *Movement Disorders* 13, 782–787.

Dickson, D.W., Lin, W. *et al.* (1999) Multiple system atrophy: a sporadic synucleinopathy. *Brain Pathology* 9, 721–732.

Dickson, D.W., Bergeron, C. *et al.* (2002) Office of Rare Diseases neuropathologic criteria for corticobasal degeneration. *Journal of Neuropathology and Experimental Neurology* 61, 935–946.

Diederich, N.J., Goetz, C.G. *et al.* (1998) Poor visual discrimination and visual hallucinations in Parkinson's disease. *Clinical Neuropharmacology* 21, 289–295.

Diller, L. & Riklan, M. (1956) Psychosocial factors in Parkinson's disease. *Journal of the American Geriatric Society* 4, 1291–1300.

Dion, Y., Annable, L. *et al.* (2002) Risperidone in the treatment of Tourette syndrome: a double-blind, placebo-controlled trial. *Journal of Clinical Psychopharmacology* 22, 31–9.

Douyon, R., Serby, M. *et al.* (1989) ECT and Parkinson's disease revisited: a naturalistic study. *American Journal of Psychiatry* 146, 1451–1455.

Dreisig, H., Beckmann, J. *et al.* (1999) Psychological effects of structured cognitive psychotherapy in young patients with Parkinson disease. *Nordic Journal of Psychiatry* 53, 217–221.

Duane, D.D. & Vermilion, K.J. (2004) Cognition and affect in patients with cervical dystonia with and without tremor. *Advances in Neurology* 94, 179–189.

Dubois, B. & Pillon, B. (1992) Biochemical correlates of cognitive changes and dementia in Parkinson's disease. In: Huber, S.J. & Cummings, J.L. (eds) *Parkinsons's Disease: Neurobehavioral Aspects*, ch. 14. Oxford University Press, Oxford.

Duncan, D. & Taylor, D. (1996) Treatment of psychosis in Parkinson's disease. *Psychiatric Bulletin* 20, 157–159.

Dupont, E., Andersen, A. *et al.* (1996) Sustained-release Madopar HBS compared with standard Madopar in the long-term treatment of de novo parkinsonian patients. *Acta Neurologica Scandinavica* 93, 14–20.

Dutton, J.J. & Buckley, E.G. (1988) Long-term results and complications of botulinum A toxin in the treatment of blepharospasm. *Ophthalmology* 95, 1529–1534.

Duvoisin, R.C., Eldridge, R., Williams, A., Nutt, J. & Calne, D. (1981) Twin study of Parkinson disease. *Neurology* 31, 77–80.

Eadie, M.J. & Sutherland, J.M. (1964) Arteriosclerosis in parkinsonism. *Journal of Neurology, Neurosurgery and Psychiatry* 27, 237–240.

Eapen, V., Fox-Hiley, P. *et al.* (2004) Clinical features and associated psychopathology in a Tourette syndrome cohort. *Acta Neurologica Scandinavica* 109, 255–260.

Eidelberg, D., Dhawan, V., Moeller, J.R. *et al.* (1991) The metabolic landscape of cortico-basal ganglionic degeneration: regional asymmetries studied with positron emission tomography. *Journal of Neurology, Neurosurgery and Psychiatry* 54, 856–862.

Eisenberg, L., Ascher, E. & Kanner, L. (1959) A clinical study of Gilles de la Tourette's disease (maladie des tics) in children. *American Journal of Psychiatry* 115, 715–723.

Elbaz, A., Bower, J.H. *et al.* (2002) Risk tables for parkinsonism and Parkinson's disease. *Journal of Clinical Epidemiology* **55**, 25–31.

Elkashef, A.M., Ruskin, P.E., Bacher, N. & Barrett, D. (1990) Vitamin E in the treatment of tardive dyskinesia. *American Journal of Psychiatry* **147**, 505–506.

Elstner, K., Selai, C.E. *et al.* (2001) Quality of Life (QOL) of patients with Gilles de la Tourette's syndrome. *Acta Psychiatrica Scandinavica* **103**, 52–59.

El-Youssef, M. (2003) Wilson disease. *Mayo Clinic Proceedings* **78**, 1126–1136.

Epidemiologic Study of Dystonia in Europe (ESDE) Collaborative Group (1999) Sex-related influences on the frequency and age of onset of primary dystonia. *Neurology* **53**, 1871–1873.

Esmaeli-Gutstein, B., Nahmias, C. *et al.* (1999) Positron emission tomography in patients with benign essential blepharospasm. *Ophthalmic Plastic and Reconstructive Surgery* **15**, 23–27.

Evans, A.H. & Lees, A.J. (2004) Dopamine dysregulation syndrome in Parkinson's disease. *Current Opinion in Neurology* **17**, 393–398.

Everitt, B., Robbins, T. *et al.* (1990) Functions of the locus coeruleus noradrenergic system: a neurobiological and behavioural synthesis. In: Heal, D. & Marsden, C.D. (eds) *The Pharmacology of Noradrenaline in the Central Nervous System*, pp. 349–378. Oxford University Press, New York.

Factor, S.A., Molho, E.S. *et al.* (1995a) Combined clozapine and electroconvulsive therapy for the treatment of drug-induced psychosis in Parkinson's disease. *Journal of Neuropsychiatry and Clinical Neuroscience* **7**, 304–307.

Factor, S.A., Podskalny, G.D. *et al.* (1995b) Psychogenic movement disorders: frequency, clinical profile, and characteristics. *Journal of Neurology, Neurosurgery and Psychiatry* **59**, 406–412.

Factor, S.A., Feustel, P.J. *et al.* (2003) Longitudinal outcome of Parkinson's disease patients with psychosis. *Neurology* **60**, 1756–1761.

Factor, S.A. & Molho, E.S. (2004) Threatening auditory hallucinations and Cotard syndrome in Parkinson disease. *Clinical Neuropharmacology* **27**, 205–207.

Fahn, S. (2003) Description of Parkinson's disease as a clinical syndrome. *Annals of the New York Academy of Sciences* **991**, 1–14.

Fahn, S. (2005) Does levodopa slow or hasten the rate of progression of Parkinson's disease? *Journal of Neurology* **252** (suppl. 4), IV37–IV42.

Fahn, S. & Williams, D.T. (1988) Psychogenic dystonia. *Advances in Neurology* **50**, 431–455.

Fahn, S., Marsden, C.D. & Calne, D.B. (1987) Classification and investigation of dystonia. In: Marsden, C.D. & Fahn, S. (eds) *Movement Disorders*, vol. 2, ch. 17. Butterworth, London.

Fahn, S., Bressman, S.B. *et al.* (1998) Classification of dystonia. *Advances in Neurology* **78**, 1–10.

Favre, J., Burchiel, K.J. *et al.* (2000) Outcome of unilateral and bilateral pallidotomy for Parkinson's disease: patient assessment. *Neurosurgery* **46**, 344–353; discussion 353–355.

Feinstein, A., Stergiopoulos, V. *et al.* (2001) Psychiatric outcome in patients with a psychogenic movement disorder: a prospective study. *Neuropsychiatry, Neuropsychology, and Behavioral Neurology* **14**, 169–176.

Fenelon, G., Mahieux, F. *et al.* (2000) Hallucinations in Parkinson's disease: prevalence, phenomenology and risk factors. *Brain* **123**, 733–745.

Fenelon, G., Thobois, S. *et al.* (2002) Tactile hallucinations in Parkinson's disease. *Journal of Neurology* **249**, 1699–1703.

Fenichel, O. (1945) *The Psychoanalytic Theory of Neurosis*. Norton & Co., New York.

Ferenci, P. (2004) Pathophysiology and clinical features of Wilson disease. *Metabolic Brain Disease* **19**, 229–239.

Fernandez, H.H. (1999) The role of atypical antipsychotics in the treatment of movement disorders. *CNS Drugs* **11**, 467–483.

Fernandez, H.H., Friedman, J.H. *et al.* (1999) Quetiapine for the treatment of drug-induced psychosis in Parkinson's disease. *Movement Disorders* **14**, 484–487.

Fernandez, H.H., Lannon, M.C. *et al.* (2000) Clozapine replacement by quetiapine for the treatment of drug-induced psychosis in Parkinson's disease. *Movement Disorders* **15**, 579–581.

Fernandez, H.H., Donnelly, E.M. *et al.* (2004) Long-term outcome of clozapine use for psychosis in parkinsonian patients. *Movement Disorders* **19**, 831–833.

Fernandez, H.H., Trieschmann, M.E. *et al.* (2005) Rebound psychosis: effect of discontinuation of antipsychotics in Parkinson's disease. *Movement Disorders* **20**, 104–105.

Fetoni, V., Soliveri, P. *et al.* (1999) Affective symptoms in multiple system atrophy and Parkinson's disease: response to levodopa therapy. *Journal of Neurology, Neurosurgery and Psychiatry* **66**, 541–544.

Fibiger, H.C. (1984) The neurobiological substrates of depression in Parkinson's disease: a hypothesis. *Canadian Journal of Neurological Sciences* **11** (1 suppl.), 105–107.

Fischer-Williams, M., Nigl, A.J. & Sovine, D.L. (1981) *A Textbook of Biological Feedback*. Human Sciences Press, New York and London.

Fish, D.R., Sawyers, D. *et al.* (1991) Motor inhibition from the brainstem is normal in torsion dystonia during REM sleep. *Journal of Neurology, Neurosurgery and Psychiatry* **54**, 140–144.

Flament, S., Delacourte, A. *et al.* (1991) Abnormal Tau proteins in progressive supranuclear palsy. Similarities and differences with the neurofibrillary degeneration of the Alzheimer type. *Acta Neuropathologica* **81**, 591–596.

Fleminger, S. (1991) Left-sided Parkinson's disease is associated with greater anxiety and depression. *Psychological Medicine* **21**, 629–638.

Fleminger, S. (1992) Control of simultaneous movements distinguishes depressive motor retardation from Parkinson's disease and neuroleptic parkinsonism. *Brain* **115**, 1459–1480.

Fletcher, N.A., Harding, A.E. & Marsden, C.D. (1990) A genetic study of idiopathic torsion dystonia in the United Kingdom. *Brain* **113**, 379–395.

Frankel, J.P., Lees, A.J. *et al.* (1990) Subcutaneous apomorphine in the treatment of Parkinson's disease. *Journal of Neurology, Neurosurgery and Psychiatry* **53**, 96–101.

Frankel, M., Cummings, J.L., Robertson, M.M., Trimble, M.R., Hill, M.A. & Benson, D.F. (1986) Obsessions and compulsions in Gilles de la Tourette's syndrome. *Neurology* **36**, 378–382.

Freeman, R.D., Fast, D.K. *et al.* (2000) An international perspective on Tourette syndrome: selected findings from 3,500 individuals in 22 countries. *Developmental Medicine and Child Neurology* **42**, 436–447.

French Clozapine Parkinson Study Group (1999) Clozapine in drug-induced psychosis in Parkinson's disease. *Lancet* **353**, 2041–2042.

Friedman, A. & Fahn, S. (1986) Spontaneous remissions in spasmodic torticollis. *Neurology* **36**, 398–400.

Friedman, J. & Gordon, N. (1992) Electroconvulsive therapy in Parkinson's disease: a report on five cases. *Convulsive Therapy* **8**, 204–210.

Friedman, J.H. (1991) The management of the levodopa psychoses. *Clinical Neuropharmacology* **14**, 283–295.

Friedman, J.H. (1994) Clozapine treatment of psychosis in patients with tardive dystonia: report of three cases. *Movement Disorders* **9**, 321–324.

Friedman, J.H. & Factor, S.A. (2000) Atypical antipsychotics in the treatment of drug-induced psychosis in Parkinson's disease. *Movement Disorders* **15**, 201–211.

Friedman, J.H. & Friedman, H. (1993) Fatigue in Parkinson's disease. *Neurology* **43**, A237.

Friedman, S. (1980) Self-control in the treatment of Gilles de la Tourette's syndrome: case study with 18-month follow-up. *Journal of Consulting and Clinical Psychology* **48**, 400–402.

Fukunishi, I., Hosokawa, K. *et al.* (1991) Depression antedating the onset of Parkinson's disease. *Japanese Journal of Psychiatry and Neurology* **45**, 7–11.

Funkiewiez, A., Ardouin, C. *et al.* (2003) Acute psychotropic effects of bilateral subthalamic nucleus stimulation and levodopa in Parkinson's disease. *Movement Disorders* **18**, 524–530.

Gadow, K.D., Sverd, J. *et al.* (1999) Long-term methylphenidate therapy in children with comorbid attention-deficit hyperactivity disorder and chronic multiple tic disorder. *Archives of General Psychiatry* **56**, 330–336.

Gaffney, G.R., Perry, P.J. *et al.* (2002) Risperidone versus clonidine in the treatment of children and adolescents with Tourette's syndrome. *Journal of the American Academy of Child and Adolescent Psychiatry* **41**, 330–336.

Galardi, G., Perani, D. *et al.* (1996) Basal ganglia and thalamocortical hypermetabolism in patients with spasmodic torticollis. *Acta Neurologica Scandinavica* **94**, 172–176.

Ganzini, L., Heintz, R.T. *et al.* (1991) The prevalence of tardive dyskinesia in neuroleptic-treated diabetics. A controlled study. *Archives of General Psychiatry* **48**, 259–263.

Gaspar, P. & Gray, F. (1984) Dementia in idiopathic Parkinson's disease. A neuropathological study of 32 cases. *Acta Neuropathologica* **64**, 43–52.

Gauter, B., Rukwied, R. *et al.* (2004) Cannabinoid agonists in the treatment of blepharospasm: a case report study. *Neuroendocrinology Letters* **25**, 45–48.

Gelenberg, A.J. & Mandel, M.R. (1977) Catatonic reactions to high potency neuroleptic drugs. *Archives of General Psychiatry* **34**, 947–950.

Gerlach, J. & Casey, D.E. (1988) Tardive dyskinesia. *Acta Psychiatrica Scandinavica* **77**, 369–378.

Ghazi-Noori, S., Chung, T. *et al.* (2003) Therapies for depression in Parkinson's disease. *Cochrane Database of Systematic Reviews* **2**, CD003465.

Ghorayeb, I., Bioulac, B. *et al.* (2005) Sleep disorders in multiple system atrophy. *Journal of Neural Transmission* **112**, 1669–1675.

Gibb, W.R.G. (1989) Dementia and Parkinson's disease. *British Journal of Psychiatry* **154**, 596–614.

Gibb, W.R.G. & Lees, A.J. (1987) Dementia in Parkinson's disease. *Lancet* **i**, 861.

Gibb, W.R.G. & Lees, A.J. (1989) The significance of the Lewy body in the diagnosis of idiopathic Parkinson's disease. *Neuropathology and Applied Neurobiology* **15**, 27–44.

Gibb, W.R.G., Luthert, P.J. & Marsden, C.D. (1989) Corticobasal degeneration. *Brain* **112**, 1171–1192.

Gilbert, D.L., Dure, L. *et al.* (2003) Tic reduction with pergolide in a randomized controlled trial in children. *Neurology* **60**, 606–611.

Gill, C.E., Khurana, R.K. *et al.* (1999) Occurrence of depressive symptoms in Shy–Drager syndrome. *Clinical Autonomic Research* **9**, 1–4.

Gilles de la Tourette, G. (1855) Étude sur une affection nerveuse charactérisée par de l'incoordination motrice accampagnée d'écholalie et de coprolalie (jumping, latah, myriachit). *Archives de Neurologie* **9**, 19–42, 158–200.

Gilman, S., Low, P. *et al.* (1998) Consensus statement on the diagnosis of multiple system atrophy. American Autonomic Society and American Academy of Neurology. *Clinical Autonomic Research* **8**, 359–362.

Gilman, S., Low, P.A. *et al.* (1999) Consensus statement on the diagnosis of multiple system atrophy. *Journal of the Neurological Sciences* **163**, 94–98.

Giovannoni, G., O'Sullivan, J.D. *et al.* (2000) Hedonistic homeostatic dysregulation in patients with Parkinson's disease on dopamine replacement therapies. *Journal of Neurology, Neurosurgery and Psychiatry* **68**, 423–428.

Gironell, A., Rodriguez-Fornells, A. *et al.* (2000) Abnormalities of the acoustic startle reflex and reaction time in Gilles de la Tourette syndrome. *Clinical Neurophysiology* **111**, 1366–1371.

Glass, J.D., Reich, S.G. *et al.* (1990) Wilson's disease. Development of neurological disease after beginning penicillamine therapy. *Archives of Neurology* **47**, 595–596.

Glazer, W.M., Morgenstern, H., Niedzwiecki, D. & Hughes, J. (1988) Heterogeneity of tardive dyskinesia. A multivariate analysis. *British Journal of Psychiatry* **152**, 253–259.

Goetz, C.G., Wuu, J., Curgian, L.M. & Leurgans, S. (2005) Hallucinations and sleep disorders in PD: six-year prospective longitudinal study. *Neurology* **64**, 81–86.

Goetz, C.G. & Stebbins, G.T. (1993) Risk factors for nursing home placement in advanced Parkinson's disease. *Neurology* **43**, 2227–2229.

Goetz, C.G. & Stebbins, G.T. (1995) Mortality and hallucinations in nursing home patients with advanced Parkinson's disease. *Neurology* **45**, 669–671.

Goetz, C.G., Vogel, C. *et al.* (1998) Early dopaminergic drug-induced hallucinations in parkinsonian patients. *Neurology* **51**, 811–814.

Golbe, L.I., Cody, R.A. & Duvoisin, R.C. (1986) Smoking and Parkinson's disease. Search for a dose response relationship. *Archives of Neurology* **43**, 774–778.

Goldman, M.B. & Luchins, D.J. (1984) Intermittent neuroleptic therapy and tardive dyskinesia: a literature review. *Hospital and Community Psychiatry* **35**, 1215–1219.

Gonera, E.G., van't Hof, M. *et al.* (1997) Symptoms and duration of the prodromal phase in Parkinson's disease. *Movement Disorders* **12**, 871–876.

Goodwin, F.K. (1971) Behavioural effects of ʟ-dopa in man. *Seminars in Psychiatry* **3**, 477–492.

Gosset, A., Pellissier, J.F., Delpuech, F. & Khalil, R. (1983) Dégénérescence striato-nigrique associée à une atrophie olivo-ponto-cérébelleuse. *Revue Neurologique (Paris)* **139**, 125–139.

Gotham, A.-M., Brown, R.G. & Marsden, C.D. (1986) Depression in Parkinson's disease. A quantitative and qualitative analysis. *Journal of Neurology, Neurosurgery and Psychiatry* **49**, 381–389.

Global Parkinson's Disease Survey (2002) Factors impacting on quality of life in Parkinson's disease: results from an international survey. *Movement Disorders* **17**, 60–67.

Graham, J.M., Grunewald, R.A. *et al.* (1997) Hallucinosis in idiopathic Parkinson's disease. *Journal of Neurology, Neurosurgery and Psychiatry* **63**, 434–440.

Graham, J.M., Sussman, J.D. *et al.* (1998) Olanzapine in the treatment of hallucinosis in idiopathic Parkinson's disease: a cautionary note. *Journal of Neurology, Neurosurgery and Psychiatry* **65**, 774–777.

Grandas, F., Elston, J., Quinn, N. & Marsden, C.D. (1988) Blepharospasm: a review of 264 patients. *Journal of Neurology, Neurosurgery and Psychiatry* **51**, 767–772.

Green, S., Buttrum, S., Molloy, H. *et al.* (1991) N-methylation of pyridines in Parkinson's disease. *Lancet* **338**, 120–121.

Greene, P., Shale, H. *et al.* (1988) Experience with high dosages of anticholinergic and other drugs in the treatment of torsion dystonia. *Advances in Neurology* **50**, 547–556.

Grosse, P., Edwards, M. *et al.* (2004) Patterns of EMG–EMG coherence in limb dystonia. *Movement Disorders* **19**, 758–769.

Gundel, H., Wolf, A. *et al.* (2001) Social phobia in spasmodic torticollis. *Journal of Neurology, Neurosurgery and Psychiatry* **71**, 499–504.

Gundel, H., Wolf, A. *et al.* (2003) High psychiatric comorbidity in spasmodic torticollis: a controlled study. *Journal of Nervous and Mental Disease* **191**, 465–473.

Gunne, L.M. & Andren, P.E. (1993) An animal model for coexisting tardive dyskinesia and tardive parkinsonism: a glutamate hypothesis for tardive dyskinesia. *Clinical Neuropharmacology* **16**, 90–95.

Hague, S.M., Klaffke, S. *et al.* (2005) Neurodegenerative disorders: Parkinson's disease and Huntington's disease. *Journal of Neurology, Neurosurgery and Psychiatry* **76**, 1058–1063.

Hakim, A.M. & Mathieson, G. (1978) Basis of dementia in Parkinson's disease. *Lancet* **ii**, 729.

Hakim, A.M. & Mathieson, G. (1979) Dementia in Parkinson's disease: a neuropathologic study. *Neurology* **29**, 1209–1214.

Hallett, J.J., Harling-Berg, C.J. *et al.* (2000) Anti-striatal antibodies in Tourette syndrome cause neuronal dysfunction. *Journal of Neuroimmunology* **111**, 195–202.

Hanna, P.A., Janjua, F.N. *et al.* (1999) Bilineal transmission in Tourette syndrome. *Neurology* **53**, 813–818.

Harding, A.E. (1993) Movement disorders. In: Walton, J. (ed.) *Brain's Diseases of the Nervous System*, 10th edn, ch. 11. Oxford University Press, Oxford.

Hardoy, M.C., Hardoy, M.J. *et al.* (1999) Gabapentin as a promising treatment for antipsychotic-induced movement disorders in schizoaffective and bipolar patients. *Journal of Affective Disorders* **54**, 315–317.

Harvey, N.S. (1988) Serial cognitive profiles in levodopa-induced hypersexuality. *British Journal of Psychiatry* **153**, 833–836.

Hassler, R. & Dieckmann, G. (1970) Traitement stéréotaxique des tics et cris inarticulés ou coprolaliques considérés comme phénomène d'obsession motrice au cours de la maladie de Gilles de la Tourette. *Revue Neurologique (Paris)* **123**, 89–100.

Hassler, R. & Dieckmann, G. (1973) Relief of obsessive–compulsive disorders, phobias and tics by stereotactic coagulation of the rostral intralaminar and medial-thalamic nuclei. In: Laitinen, L.V. & Livingston, K.E. (eds) *Surgical Approaches in Psychiatry*, ch. 19. Medical and Technical Publishing, Lancaster.

Hauser, R.A. & Zesiewicz, T.A. (1997) Sertraline for the treatment of depression in Parkinson's disease. *Movement Disorders* **12**, 756–759.

Hauser, R.A., Freeman, T.B. & Olanow, C.W. (1995) Surgical therapies for Parkinson's disease. In: Kurlan, R.J.B. (ed.) *Treatment of Motor Disorders*, ch. 2. Lippincott, Philadelphia.

Hawkes, C.H. & Shephard, B.C. (1998) Olfactory evoked responses and identification tests in neurological disease. *Annals of the New York Academy of Sciences* **855**, 608–615.

Hawkins, R.A., Mazziotta, J.C. & Phelps, M.E. (1987) Wilson's disease studied with FDG and positron emission tomography. *Neurology* **37**, 1707–1711.

Heikkila, R.E. (1984) Pharmacological basis of therapeutics: dopamine receptors. *Journal of the Medical Society of New Jersey* **81**, 1084–1086.

Heiman, G.A., Ottman, R. *et al.* (2004) Increased risk for recurrent major depression in DYT1 dystonia mutation carriers. *Neurology* **63**, 631–637.

Henderson, J.M., Lu, Y. *et al.* (2003) Olfactory deficits and sleep disturbances in Parkinson's disease: a case–control survey. *Journal of Neurology, Neurosurgery and Psychiatry* **74**, 956–958.

Henderson, R., Kurlan, R. *et al.* (1992) Preliminary examination of the comorbidity of anxiety and depression in Parkinson's disease. *Journal of Neuropsychiatry and Clinical Neuroscience* **4**, 257–264.

Hesse, S., Barthel, H. *et al.* (2003) Regional serotonin transporter availability and depression are correlated in Wilson's disease. *Journal of Neural Transmission* **110**, 923–933.

Higginson, C.I., Fields, J.A. *et al.* (2001) Which symptoms of anxiety diminish after surgical interventions for Parkinson disease? *Neuropsychiatry, Neuropsychology, and Behavioral Neurology* **14**, 117–121.

Hitchcock, E. (1992) Neural implants and recovery of function: human work. In: Rose, F.D. & Johnson, D.A. (eds) *Recovery from Brain Damage. Reflections and Directions*, pp. 67–78. Plenum Press, New York.

Hitoshi, S., Iwata, M. *et al.* (1991) Mid-brain pathology of Wilson's disease: MRI analysis of three cases. *Journal of Neurology, Neurosurgery and Psychiatry* **54**, 624–626.

Hoehn, M.M. & Yahr, M.D. (1967) Parkinsonism: onset, progression and mortality. *Neurology* **17**, 427–442.

Holroyd, S., Currie, L. *et al.* (2001) Prospective study of hallucinations and delusions in Parkinson's disease. *Journal of Neurology, Neurosurgery and Psychiatry* **70**, 734–738.

Hoopes, S.P. (1999) Donepezil for Tourette's disorder and ADHD. *Journal of Clinical Psychopharmacology* **19**, 381–382.

Horn, S. (1974) Some psychological factors in parkinsonism. *Journal of Neurology, Neurosurgery and Psychiatry* **37**, 27–31.

Horn, S. & Stern, M.B. (2004) The comparative effects of medical therapies for Parkinson's disease. *Neurology* **63** (7 suppl. 2), S7–S12.

Hornsey, H., Banerjee, S. *et al.* (2001) The prevalence of Tourette syndrome in 13–14-year-olds in mainstream schools. *Journal of Child Psychology and Psychiatry and Allied Disciplines* **42**, 1035–1039.

Houeto, J.L., Mesnage, V. *et al.* (2002) Behavioural disorders, Parkinson's disease and subthalamic stimulation. *Journal of Neurology, Neurosurgery and Psychiatry* **72**, 701–707.

Houlden, H., Baker, M. *et al.* (2001) Corticobasal degeneration and progressive supranuclear palsy share a common tau haplotype. *Neurology* **56**, 1702–1706.

Hsiung, G.Y., Das, S.K. *et al.* (2002) Long-term efficacy of botulinum toxin A in treatment of various movement disorders over a 10–year period. *Movement Disorders* **17**, 1288–1293.

Huber, S.J. & Glatt, S.L. (1992) Neuroimaging correlates of dementia in Parkinson's disease. In: Huber, S.J. & Cummings, J.L. (eds) *Parkinson's Disease: Neurobehavioral Aspects*, ch. 12. Oxford University Press, Oxford.

Huber, S.J., Shuttleworth, E.C., Christy, J.A., Chakeres, D.W., Curtin, A. & Paulson, G.W. (1989) Magnetic resonance imaging in dementia of Parkinson's disease. *Journal of Neurology, Neurosurgery and Psychiatry* **52**, 1221–1227.

Hughes, A.J., Daniel, S.E. *et al.* (1992) Accuracy of clinical diagnosis of idiopathic Parkinson's disease: a clinico-pathological study of 100 cases. *Journal of Neurology, Neurosurgery and Psychiatry* **55**, 181–184.

Hughes, A.J., Bishop, S., Kleedorfer, B. *et al.* (1993) Subcutaneous apomorphine in Parkinson's disease: response to chronic administration for up to five years. *Movement Disorders* **8**, 105–170.

Hurwitz, T.A., Calne, D.B. & Waterman, K. (1988) Treatment of dopaminomimetic psychosis in Parkinson's disease with electroconvulsive therapy. *Canadian Journal of Neurological Science* **15**, 32–34.

Hyde, T.M., Stacey, M.E. *et al.* (1995) Cerebral morphometric abnormalities in Tourette's syndrome: a quantitative MRI study of monozygotic twins. *Neurology* **45**, 1176–1182.

Intemann, P.M., Masterman, D. *et al.* (2001) Staged bilateral pallidotomy for treatment of Parkinson disease. *Journal of Neurosurgery* **94**, 437–444.

Inzelberg, R., Kipervasser, S. *et al.* (1998) Auditory hallucinations in Parkinson's disease. *Journal of Neurology, Neurosurgery and Psychiatry* **64**, 533–535.

Ishizawa, K. & Dickson, D.W. (2001) Microglial activation parallels system degeneration in progressive supranuclear palsy and corticobasal degeneration. *Journal of Neuropathology and Experimental Neurology* **60**, 647–657.

Ives, N.J., Stowe, R.L. *et al.* (2004) Monoamine oxidase type B inhibitors in early Parkinson's disease: meta-analysis of 17 randomised trials involving 3525 patients. *British Medical Journal* **329**, 593.

Jahanshahi, M., Marion, M.H. *et al.* (1990) Natural history of adult-onset idiopathic torticollis. *Archives of Neurology* **47**, 548–552.

Jankovic, J. (1985) Long-term study of pergolide in Parkinson's disease. *Neurology* **35**, 296–299.

Jankovic, J. (1994) Post-traumatic movement disorders: central and peripheral mechanisms. *Neurology* **44**, 2006–2014.

Jankovic, J. (2001) Tourette's syndrome. *New England Journal of Medicine* **345**, 1184–1192.

Jankovic, J. & Schwartz, K.S. (1991) Clinical correlates of response to botulinum toxin injections. *Archives of Neurology* **48**, 1253–1256.

Jarman, P.R. & Warner, T.T. (1998) The dystonias. *Journal of Medical Genetics* **35**, 314–318.

Jeanjean, A.P., Laterre, E.C. *et al.* (1997) Neuroleptic binding to sigma receptors: possible involvement in neuroleptic-induced acute dystonia. *Biological Psychiatry* **41**, 1010–1019.

Jellinger, K. & Riederer, P. (1984) Dementia in Parkinson's disease and (pre)senile dementia of Alzheimer type: morphological aspects and changes in the intracerebral MAO activity. *Advances in Neurology* **40**, 199–210.

Jenkins, R.B. & Groh, R.H. (1970) Mental symptoms in Parkinsonian patients treated with L-dopa. *Lancet* **ii**, 177–179.

Jennings, D.L., Seibyl, J.P., Oakes, D., Eberly, S., Murphy, J. & Marek, K. (2004) (^{123}I) β-CIT and single-photon emission computed tomographic imaging vs clinical evaluation in Parkinsonian syndrome: unmasking an early diagnosis. *Archives of Neurology* **61**, 1224–1229.

Jeste, D.V., Lacro, J.P. *et al.* (1999) Lower incidence of tardive dyskinesia with risperidone compared with haloperidol in older patients. *Journal of the American Geriatric Society* **47**, 716–719.

Jimenez-Jimenez, F.J. & Garcia-Ruiz, P.J. (2001) Pharmacological options for the treatment of Tourette's disorder. *Drugs* **61**, 2207–2220.

Jimenez-Jimenez, F.J., Orti Pareja, M. *et al.* (1997) Cenesthetic hallucinations in a patient with Parkinson's disease. *Journal of Neurology, Neurosurgery and Psychiatry* **63**, 120.

Jones, A.K., Brown, W.D. *et al.* (1991) Cortical and subcortical localization of response to pain in man using positron emission tomography. *Proceedings. Biological Sciences/The Royal Society* **244**, 39–44.

Josephs, K.A. & Dickson, D.W. (2003) Diagnostic accuracy of progressive supranuclear palsy in the Society for Progressive Supranuclear Palsy brain bank. *Movement Disorders* **18**, 1018–1026.

Judd, L.L., Schettler, P.J. *et al.* (2002) The prevalence, clinical relevance, and public health significance of subthreshold depressions. *Psychiatric Clinics of North America* **25**, 685–698.

Juncos, J.L. (1999) Management of psychotic aspects of Parkinson's disease. *Journal of Clinical Psychiatry* **60** (suppl. 8), 42–53.

Juncos, J.L., Roberts, V.J. *et al.* (2004) Quetiapine improves psychotic symptoms and cognition in Parkinson's disease. *Movement Disorders* **19**, 29–35.

Junque, C., Alegret, M. *et al.* (1999) Cognitive and behavioral changes after unilateral posteroventral pallidotomy: relationship with lesional data from MRI. *Movement Disorders* **14**, 780–789.

Kang, U.J., Burke, R.E. *et al.* (1986) Natural history and treatment of tardive dystonia. *Movement Disorders* **1**, 193–208.

Kang, U.J., Burke, R.E. *et al.* (1988) Tardive dystonia. *Advances in Neurology* **50**, 415–429.

Kapur, S. & Seeman, P. (2001) Does fast dissociation from the dopamine D(2) receptor explain the action of atypical antipsychotics? A new hypothesis. *American Journal of Psychiatry* **158**, 360–369.

Karp, B.I., Goldstein, S.R. *et al.* (1999) An open trial of clozapine for dystonia. *Movement Disorders* **14**, 652–657.

Katzenschlager, R., Sampaio, C. *et al.* (2003) Anticholinergics for symptomatic management of Parkinson's disease. *Cochrane Database of Systematic Reviews* **2**, CD003735.

Katzenschlager, R., Zijlmans, J. *et al.* (2004) Olfactory function distinguishes vascular parkinsonism from Parkinson's disease. *Journal of Neurology, Neurosurgery and Psychiatry* **75**, 1749–1752.

Kennedy, R., Mittal, D. *et al.* (2003) Electroconvulsive therapy in movement disorders: an update. *Journal of Neuropsychiatry and Clinical Neuroscience* **15**, 407–421.

Keshavan, M.S., David, A.S., Narayanen, H.S. & Satish, P. (1986) 'On–off' phenomena and manic-depressive mood shifts: case report. *Journal of Clinical Psychiatry* **47**, 93–94.

Kidger, T., Barnes, R.E., Trauer, T. & Taylor, P.J. (1980) Sub-syndromes of tardive dyskinesia. *Psychological Medicine* **10**, 513–520.

King, A.D., Walshe, J.M. *et al.* (1996) Cranial MR imaging in Wilson's disease. *AJR American Journal of Roentgenology* **167**, 1579–1584.

Kiriakakis, V., Bhatia, K.P. *et al.* (1998) The natural history of tardive dystonia. A long-term follow-up study of 107 cases. *Brain* **121**, 2053–2066.

Klaassen, T., Verhey, F.R. *et al.* (1995) Treatment of depression in Parkinson's disease: a meta-analysis. *Journal of Neuropsychiatry and Clinical Neuroscience* **7**, 281–286.

Klawans, H.L., Goetz, C.G. *et al.* (1980) Tardive dyskinesia: review and update. *American Journal of Psychiatry* **137**, 900–908.

Klein, C., Kompf, D. *et al.* (1997) A study of visual hallucinations in patients with Parkinson's disease. *Journal of Neurology* **244**, 371–377.

Knell, E.R. & Comings, D.E. (1993) Tourette's syndrome and attention-deficit hyperactivity disorder: evidence for a genetic relationship. *Journal of Clinical Psychiatry* **54**, 331–337.

Koller, W., Pahwa, R. *et al.* (1997) High-frequency unilateral thalamic stimulation in the treatment of essential and parkinsonian tremor. *Annals of Neurology* **42**, 292–299.

Kopelman, M.D. (1991) Frontal dysfunction and memory deficits in the alcoholic Korsakoff syndrome and Alzheimer-type dementia. *Brain* **114**, 117–137.

Koponen, H.J. (1997) Risperidone in the treatment of psychosis and concomitant buccolinguomasticatory dyskinesia in the elderly. *International Journal of Geriatric Psychiatry* **12**, 412–413.

Korein, J. & Brudny, J. (1976) Integrated EMG feedback in the management of spasmodic torticollis and focal dystonia: a prospective study of 80 patients. *Research Publications of the Association for Research in Nervous and Mental Disease* **55**, 385–426.

Kostic, V.S., Filipovic, S.R. *et al.* (1994) Effect of age at onset on frequency of depression in Parkinson's disease. *Journal of Neurology, Neurosurgery and Psychiatry* **57**, 1265–1267.

Kroenke, K. & Swindle, R. (2000) Cognitive-behavioral therapy for somatization and symptom syndromes: a critical review of controlled clinical trials. *Psychotherapy and Psychosomatics* **69**, 205–215.

Kuopio, A.M., Marttila, R.J. *et al.* (2000) The quality of life in Parkinson's disease. *Movement Disorders* **15**, 216–223.

Kurlan, R. & Trinidad, K.S. (1995) Treatment of tics. In: Kurlan, R.J.B. (ed.) *Treatment of Movement Disorders*, ch. 9. Lippincott, Philadelphia.

Kurlan, R., Lichter, D. *et al.* (1989) Sensory tics in Tourette's syndrome. *Neurology* **39**, 731–734.

Kurlan, R., Daragjati, C. *et al.* (1996) Non-obscene complex socially inappropriate behavior in Tourette's syndrome. *Journal of Neuropsychiatry and Clinical Neuroscience* **8**, 311–317.

Kurland, M.L. (1965) Gilles de la Tourette's syndrome: the psychotherapy of two cases. *Comprehensive Psychiatry* **6**, 298–305.

Kwak, C., Dat Vuong, K. *et al.* (2003) Premonitory sensory phenomenon in Tourette's syndrome. *Movement Disorders* **18**, 1530–1533.

Lai, T., Lai, J.M. *et al.* (1999) Functional recovery after bilateral pallidotomy for the treatment of early-onset primary generalized dystonia. *Archives of Physical Medicine and Rehabilitation* **80**, 1340–1342.

Lamberti, J.S. & Bellnier, T. (1993) Clozapine and tardive dystonia. *Journal of Nervous and Mental Disease* **181**, 137–138.

Lang, A. (2003) Corticobasal degeneration: selected developments. *Movement Disorders* **18** (suppl. 6), S51–S56.

Lang, A. (2006) General overview of psychogenic movement disorders: epidemiology, diagnosis and prognosis. In: Hallett, M., Fahn, S., Jankovic J. *et al.* (eds) *Psychogenic Movement Disorders*, pp. 35–41. Lippincott Williams & Wilkins, Philadelphia.

Langlois, M., Richer, F. *et al.* (2003) New perspectives on dystonia. *Canadian Journal of Neurological Sciences* **30** (suppl. 1), S34–S44.

Langston, J.W., Ballard, P., Tetrud, J.W. & Irwin, I. (1983) Chronic parkinsonism in humans due to a product of mepiridine-analog synthesis. *Science* **219**, 979–980.

Lantos, P.L. & Papp, M.I. (1994) Cellular pathology of multiple system atrophy: a review. *Journal of Neurology, Neurosurgery and Psychiatry* **57**, 129–133.

Lauterbach, E.C. (2004) The neuropsychiatry of Parkinson's disease and related disorders. *Psychiatric Clinics of North America* **27**, 801–25.

Lauterbach, E.C., Freeman, A. *et al.* (2003) Correlates of generalized anxiety and panic attacks in dystonia and Parkinson disease. *Cognitive and Behavioral Neurology* **16**, 225–33.

Lauterbach, E.C., Freeman, A. *et al.* (2004) Differential DSM-III psychiatric disorder prevalence profiles in dystonia and Parkinson's disease. *Journal of Neuropsychiatry and Clinical Neuroscience* **16**, 29–36.

Lawrence, A.D., Evans, A.H. *et al.* (2003) Compulsive use of dopamine replacement therapy in Parkinson's disease: reward systems gone awry? *Lancet Neurology* **2**, 595–604.

Lawton, M., Moss, M. *et al.* (1995) The quality of life among elderly care receivers. *Journal of Applied Gerontology* **14**, 150–171.

Lebensohn, Z.M. & Jenkins, R.B. (1975) Improvement in parkinsonism in depressed patients treated with ECT. *American Journal of Psychiatry* **132**, 283–285.

Leckman, J.F. (2002) Tourette's syndrome. *Lancet* **360**, 1577–1586.

Leckman, J.F., Price, R.A., Walkup, J.T., Ort, S., Pauls, D.L. & Cohen, D.J. (1987) Nongenetic factors in Gilles de la Tourette's syndrome. *Archives of General Psychiatry* **44**, 100.

Leckman, J.F., Hardin, M.T. *et al.* (1991) Clonidine treatment of Gilles de la Tourette's syndrome. *Archives of General Psychiatry* **48**, 324–328.

Leckman, J.F., Walker, D.E. *et al.* (1993) Premonitory urges in Tourette's syndrome. *American Journal of Psychiatry* **150**, 98–102.

Leckman, J.F., Zhang, H. *et al.* (1998) Course of tic severity in Tourette syndrome: the first two decades. *Pediatrics* **102**, 14–19.

Leentjens, A.F., Verhey, F.R. *et al.* (2000a) The validity of the Beck Depression Inventory as a screening and diagnostic instrument for depression in patients with Parkinson's disease. *Movement Disorders* **15**, 1221–1224.

Leentjens, A.F., Verhey, F.R. *et al.* (2000b) The validity of the Hamilton and Montgomery–Asberg depression rating scales as screening and diagnostic tools for depression in Parkinson's disease. *International Journal of Geriatric Psychiatry* **15**, 644–649.

Lees, A.J. (1985) *Tics and Related Disorders*. Churchill Livingstone, Edinburgh.

Lees, A.J. (1995) Comparison of therapeutic effects and mortality data of levodopa and levodopa combined with selegiline in patients with early, mild Parkinson's disease. *British Medical Journal* **311**, 1602–1607.

Lees, A.J. & Smith, E. (1983) Cognitive deficits in the early stages of Parkinson's disease. *Brain* **106**, 257–270.

Lemke, M.R., Fuchs, G. *et al.* (2004) Depression and Parkinson's disease. *Journal of Neurology* **251** (suppl. 6), VI/24–27.

Lemke, M.R., Brecht, H.M. *et al.* (2005) Anhedonia, depression, and motor functioning in Parkinson's disease during treatment with pramipexole. *Journal of Neuropsychiatry and Clinical Neuroscience* **17**, 214–220.

Leo, R.J. (1996) Movement disorders associated with the serotonin selective reuptake inhibitors. *Journal of Clinical Psychiatry* **57**, 449–454.

Lerner, V., Miodownik, C. *et al.* (2001) Vitamin B(6) in the treatment of tardive dyskinesia: a double-blind, placebo-controlled, crossover study. *American Journal of Psychiatry* **158**, 1511–1514.

Leube, B., Hendgen, T. *et al.* (1997) Evidence for DYT7 being a common cause of cervical dystonia (torticollis) in Central Europe. *American Journal of Medical Genetics* **74**, 529–532.

Levin, B.E., Llabre, M.M. *et al.* (1988) Parkinson's disease and depression: psychometric properties of the Beck Depression Inventory. *Journal of Neurology, Neurosurgery and Psychiatry* **51**, 1401–1404.

Levy, M.L., Cummings, J.L. *et al.* (1998) Apathy is not depression. *Journal of Neuropsychiatry and Clinical Neuroscience* **10**, 314–319.

Lieberman, A., Dziatolowski, M., Kuperrsmith, M. *et al.* (1979) Dementia in Parkinson disease. *Annals of Neurology* **6**, 355–359.

Lieberman, A., Ranhosky, A. *et al.* (1997) Clinical evaluation of pramipexole in advanced Parkinson's disease: results of a double-blind, placebo-controlled, parallel-group study. *Neurology* **49**, 162–168.

Lieberman, A.N., Leibowitz, M. *et al.* (1985) The use of pergolide and lisuride, two experimental dopamine agonists, in patients with advanced Parkinson disease. *American Journal of the Medical Sciences* **290**, 102–106.

Lindvall, O. (1994) Transplantation: the clinical position. In: Marsden, C.D. & Fahn, S. (eds) *Movement Disorders*, vol. 3, ch. 12. Butterworth-Heinemann, Oxford.

Lipper, S. (1976) Psychosis in patient on bromocriptine and levodopa with carbidopa [letter]. *Lancet* **ii**, 571–572.

Litvan, I. (2001) Diagnosis and management of progressive supranuclear palsy. *Seminars in Neurology* **21**, 41–48.

Litvan, I., Grafman, J. *et al.* (1989) Memory impairment in patients with progressive supranuclear palsy. *Archives of Neurology* **46**, 765–767.

Litvan, I., Agid, Y. *et al.* (1996) Clinical research criteria for the diagnosis of progressive supranuclear palsy (Steele–Richardson–Olszewski syndrome): report of the NINDS-SPSP international workshop. *Neurology* **47**, 1–9.

Litvan, I., Cummings, J.L. *et al.* (1998) Neuropsychiatric features of corticobasal degeneration. *Journal of Neurology, Neurosurgery and Psychiatry* **65**, 717–721.

Liu, C.Y., Wang, S.J. *et al.* (1997) The correlation of depression with functional activity in Parkinson's disease. *Journal of Neurology* **244**, 493–498.

Lobbezoo, F., Thu Thon, M. *et al.* (1996) Relationship between sleep, neck muscle activity, and pain in cervical dystonia. *Canadian Journal of Neurological Sciences* **23**, 285–290.

Louza, M.R. & Bassitt, D.P. (2005) Maintenance treatment of severe tardive dyskinesia with clozapine: 5 years' follow-up. *Journal of Clinical Psychopharmacology* **25**, 180–182.

Lowenstein, D.H. & Aminoff, M.J. (1988) The clinical course of spasmodic torticollis. *Neurology* **38**, 530–532.

Lozano, A.M., Kumar, R. *et al.* (1997) Globus pallidus internus pallidotomy for generalized dystonia. *Movement Disorders* **12**, 865–870.

Luo, F., Leckman, J.F. *et al.* (2004) Prospective longitudinal study of children with tic disorders and/or obsessive-compulsive disorder: relationship of symptom exacerbations to newly acquired streptococcal infections. *Pediatrics* **113**, 578–585.

McClelland, H.A., Metcalfe, A.V., Kerr, T.A., Dutta, D. & Watson, P. (1991) Facial dyskinesia: a 16-year follow-up study. *British Journal of Psychiatry* **158**, 691–696.

McDonald, L.V. & Lake, C.R. (1995) Psychosis in an adolescent patient with Wilson's disease: effects of chelation therapy. *Psychosomatic Medicine* **57**, 202–204.

McMahon, W.M., Leppert, M., Filloux, F., Van De Wetering, J.M. & Hasstedt, S. (1992) Tourette symptoms in 161 related family members. *Advances in Neurology* **58**, 159–165.

Madeley, P., Biggins, C.A., Boyd, J.L., Mindham, R.H.S. & Spokes, E.G.S. (1992) Emotionalism in Parkinson's disease. *Irish Journal of Psychological Medicine* **9**, 24–25.

Magyar-Lehmann, S., Antonini, A. *et al.* (1997) Cerebral glucose metabolism in patients with spasmodic torticollis. *Movement Disorders* **12**, 704–708.

Maher, E.R. & Lees, A.J. (1986) The clinical features and natural history of the Steele–Richardson–Olszewski syndrome (progressive supranuclear palsy). *Neurology* **36**, 1005–1008.

Mahler, M. & Rangell, L. (1943) A psychosomatic study of maladies des tics (Gilles de la Tourette's disease). *Psychiatric Quarterly* **17**, 579–603.

Mahler, M.S. & Luke, J.A. (1946) Outcome of the tic syndrome. *Journal of Nervous and Mental Disease* **103**, 433–445.

Malinovsky, V. (1987) Benign essential blepharospasm. *Journal of the American Optometric Association* **58**, 646–651.

Manford, M. & Andermann, F. (1998) Complex visual hallucinations. Clinical and neurobiological insights. *Brain* **121**, 1819–1840.

Manni, R., Pacchetti, C. *et al.* (2002) Hallucinations and sleep–wake cycle in PD: a 24-hour continuous polysomnographic study. *Neurology* **59**, 1979–1981.

Manson, A.J., Turner, K. *et al.* (2002) Apomorphine mono-therapy in the treatment of refractory motor complications of Parkinson's disease: long-term follow-up study of 64 patients. *Movement Disorders* **17**, 1235–1241.

Marcus, D. & Kurlan, R. (2001) Tics and its disorders. *Neurologic Clinics* **19**, 735–758, viii.

Margolese, H.C., Annable, L. *et al.* (2002) Depression and dysphoria in adult and adolescent patients with Tourette's disorder treated with risperidone. *Journal of Clinical Psychiatry* **63**, 1040–1044.

Marin, R.S. (1996) Apathy: concept, syndrome, neural mechanisms, and treatment. *Seminars in Clinical Neuropsychiatry* **1**, 304–314.

Marinus, J., Leentjens, A.F. *et al.* (2002) Evaluation of the hospital anxiety and depression scale in patients with Parkinson's disease. *Clinical Neuropharmacology* **25**, 318–324.

Marneros, A. (1983) Adult onset of Tourette's syndrome: a case report. *American Journal of Psychiatry* **140**, 924–925.

Marsden, C.D. (1976a) Blepharospasm–oromandibular dystonia syndrome (Brueghel's syndrome). A variant of adult-onset torsion dystonia? *Journal of Neurology, Neurosurgery and Psychiatry* **39**, 1204–1209.

Marsden, C.D. (1976b) The problem of adult-onset idiopathic torsion dystonia and other isolated dyskinesias in adult life (including blepharospasm, oromandibular dystonia, dystonic writer's cramp, and torticollis, or axial dystonia). *Advances in Neurology* **14**, 259–276.

Marsden, C.D. & Jenner, P. (1980) The pathophysiology of extrapyramidal side-effects of neuroleptic drugs. *Psychological Medicine* **10**, 55–72.

Marsden, C.D. & Parkes, J.D. (1976) 'On–off' effects in patients with Parkinson's disease on chronic levodopa therapy. *Lancet* **i**, 292–296.

Marsden, C.D. & Parkes, J.D. (1977) Success and problems of long-term levodopa therapy in Parkinson's disease. *Lancet* **i**, 345–349.

Marsden, C.D. & Quinn, N.P. (1990) The dystonias. Neurological disorders affecting 20,000 people in Britain. *British Medical Journal* **300**, 139–144.

Marsden, C.D., Tarsy, D. & Baldessarini, R.J. (1975) Spontaneous and drug-induced movement disorders in psychotic patients. In: Benson, D.F. & Blumer, D. (eds) *Psychiatric Aspects of Neurologic Disease*, ch. 12. Grune & Stratton, New York.

Marsh, L. (2000) Neuropsychiatric aspects of Parkinson's disease. *Psychosomatics* **41**, 15–23.

Marti, M.J., Tolosa, E. *et al.* (2003) Clinical overview of the synucleinopathies. *Movement Disorders* **18** (suppl. 6), S21–S27.

Marttila, R.J. & Rinne, U.K. (1976) Dementia in Parkinson's disease. *Acta Neurologica Scandinavica* **54**, 431–441.

Mathews, C.A., Waller, J. *et al.* (2004) Self injurious behaviour in Tourette syndrome: correlates with impulsivity and impulse control. *Journal of Neurology, Neurosurgery and Psychiatry* **75**, 1149–1155.

Mathias, C.J. & Kimber, J.R. (1999) Postural hypotension: causes, clinical features, investigation and management. *Annual Review of Medicine* **50**, 317–336.

Matsumoto, K., Asano, T. *et al.* (1976) Long-term follow-up results of bilateral thalamotomy for parkinsonism. *Applied Neurophysiology* **39**, 257–260.

Matsumoto, K., Shichijo, F. *et al.* (1984) Long-term follow-up review of cases of Parkinson's disease after unilateral or bilateral thalamotomy. *Journal of Neurosurgery* **60**, 1033–1044.

Mauriello, J.A. Jr, Dhillon, S. *et al.* (1996) Treatment selections of 239 patients with blepharospasm and Meige syndrome over 11 years. *British Journal of Ophthalmology* **80**, 1073–1076.

Mayberg, H.S., Starkstein, S.E. *et al.* (1990) Selective hypometabolism in the inferior frontal lobe in depressed patients with Parkinson's disease. *Annals of Neurology* **28**, 57–64.

Mayberg, H.S., Brannan, S.K. *et al.* (2000) Regional metabolic effects of fluoxetine in major depression: serial changes and relationship to clinical response. *Biological Psychiatry* **48**, 830–843.

Mayeux, R., Stern, Y., Cote, L. & Williams, J.B.W. (1984) Altered serotonin metabolism in depressed patients with Parkinson's disease. *Neurology* **34**, 642–646.

Mayeux, R., Stern, Y., Sano, M., Williams, J.B.W. & Cote, L.J. (1988a) The relationship of serotonin to depression in Parkinson's disease. *Movement Disorders* **3**, 237–244.

Mayeux, R., Stern, Y., Rosenstein, R. *et al.* (1988b) An estimate of the prevalence of dementia in idiopathic Parkinson's disease. *Archives of Neurology* **45**, 260–262.

Meara, J. & Hobson, P. (1998) Sertraline for the treatment of depression in Parkinson's disease. *Movement Disorders* **13**, 622.

Meara, J., Mitchelmore, E. *et al.* (1999) Use of the GDS-15 geriatric depression scale as a screening instrument for depressive symptomatology in patients with Parkinson's disease and their carers in the community. *Age Ageing* **28**, 35–38.

Meares, R. (1971) Natural history of spasmodic torticollis, and effect of surgery. *Lancet* **ii**, 149–150.

Meares, R. (1973) Spasmodic torticollis. *British Journal of Hospital Medicine* **9**, 235–241.

Meco, G., Alessandria, A. *et al.* (1994) Risperidone for hallucinations in levodopa-treated Parkinson's disease patients. *Lancet* **343**, 1370–1371.

Meco, G., Alessandri, A. *et al.* (1997) Risperidone in levodopa-induced psychosis in advanced Parkinson's disease: an open-label, long-term study. *Movement Disorders* **12**, 610–612.

Mellers, J.D., Quinn, N.P. *et al.* (1995) Psychotic and depressive symptoms in Parkinson's disease. A study of the growth hormone response to apomorphine. *British Journal of Psychiatry* **167**, 522–526.

Meltzer, H.Y., Young, M. *et al.* (1979) Extrapyramidal side effects and increased serum prolactin following fluoxetine, a new antidepressant. *Journal of Neural Transmission* **45**, 165–175.

Mena, M.A., Pardo, B. *et al.* (1992) Neurotoxicity of levodopa on catecholamine-rich neurons. *Movement Disorders* **7**, 23–31.

Mendis, T. (1996) Drug-induced psychosis in Parkinson's disease. *CNS Drugs* **5**, 166–174.

Menza, M.A., Palermo, B. *et al.* (1999) Depression and anxiety in Parkinson's disease: possible effect of genetic variation in the serotonin transporter. *Journal of Geriatric Psychiatry and Neurology* **12**, 49–52.

Merello, M., Starkstein, S. *et al.* (2001) Bilateral pallidotomy for treatment of Parkinson's disease induced corticobulbar syndrome and psychic akinesia avoidable by globus pallidus lesion combined with contralateral stimulation. *Journal of Neurology, Neurosurgery and Psychiatry* **71**, 611–614.

Merette, C., Brassard, A. *et al.* (2000) Significant linkage for Tourette syndrome in a large French Canadian family. *American Journal of Human Genetics* 67, 1008–1013.

Merims, D., Galili-Mosberg, R. *et al.* (2000) Is there addiction to levodopa in patients with Parkinson's disease? *Movement Disorders* 15, 1014–1016.

Metter, E.J., Kuhl, D.E. & Riege, W.H. (1990) Brain glucose metabolism in Parkinson's disease. *Advances in Neurology* 53, 135–139.

Michael, R.P. (1957) Treatment of a case of compulsive swearing. *British Medical Journal* 1, 1506–1508.

Miller, C.H. & Fleischhacker, W.W. (2000) Managing antipsychotic-induced acute and chronic akathisia. *Drug Safety* 22, 73–81.

Minagar, A., Shulman, L.M. *et al.* (1999) Transderm-induced psychosis in Parkinson's disease. *Neurology* 53, 433–434.

Mindham, R.H.S. (1970) Psychiatric symptoms in parkinsonism. *Journal of Neurology, Neurosurgery and Psychiatry* 33, 188–191.

Mindham, R.H.S. (1974) Psychiatric aspects of Parkinson's disease. *British Journal of Hospital Medicine* 11, 411–414.

Miyasaki, J.M. & Lang, A.E. (1995) Treatment of drug-induced movement disorders. In: Kurlan, R.J.B. (ed.) *Treatment of Movement Disorders*, ch. 11. Lippincott, Philadelphia.

Mjönes, H. (1949) Paralysis agitans: a clinical and genetic study. *Acta Psychiatrica et Neurologica Scandinavica Supplementum* 54, 1–195.

Molho, E.S., Feustel, P.J. *et al.* (1998) Clinical comparison of tardive and idiopathic cervical dystonia. *Movement Disorders* 13, 486–489.

Montastruc, J.L., Rascol, O. *et al.* (1989) A randomised controlled study of bromocriptine versus levodopa in previously untreated Parkinsonian patients: a 3 year follow-up. *Journal of Neurology, Neurosurgery and Psychiatry* 52, 773–775.

Montastruc, J.L., Rascol, O. *et al.* (1993) Current status of dopamine agonists in Parkinson's disease management. *Drugs* 46, 384–393.

Montgomery, M.A., Clayton, P.J. & Friedhoff, A.J. (1982) Psychiatric illness in Tourette syndrome patients and first-degree relatives. *Advances in Neurology* 35, 335–339.

Moraru, E., Schnider, P. *et al.* (2002) Relation between depression and anxiety in dystonic patients: implications for clinical management. *Depression and Anxiety* 16, 100–103.

Morganstern, H. & Glazer, W.M. (1993) Identifying risk factors for tardive dyskinesia among long-term outpatients maintained with neuroleptic medications. *Archives of General Psychiatry* 50, 723–733.

Moriarty, J., Campos Costa, D., Schmitz, B., Trimble, M.R., Ell, P.J. & Robertson, M.M. (1995) Brain perfusion abnormalities in Gilles de la Tourette's syndrome. *British Journal of Psychiatry* 167, 249–254.

Morphew, J.A. & Sim, M. (1969) Gilles de la Tourette's syndrome: a clinical and psychopathological study. *British Journal of Medical Psychology* 42, 293–301.

Moskovitz, C., Moses, H. III, *et al.* (1978) Levodopa-induced psychosis: a kindling phenomenon. *American Journal of Psychiatry* 135, 669–675.

Movement Disorders Society Task Force (2002) Management of Parkinson's disease: an evidence-based review. *Movement Disorders* 17 (suppl. 4), S1–S166.

Mueller, J. & Aminoff, M.J. (1982) Tourette-like syndrome after long-term neuroleptic drug treatment. *British Journal of Psychiatry* 141, 191–193.

Mukaddes, N.M. & Abali, O. (2003) Quetiapine treatment of children and adolescents with Tourette's disorder. *Journal of Child and Adolescent Psychopharmacology* 13, 295–299.

Muller, J., Kemmler, G. *et al.* (2002) The impact of blepharospasm and cervical dystonia on health-related quality of life and depression. *Journal of Neurology* 249, 842–846.

Muller-Vahl, K.R. (2003) Cannabinoids reduce symptoms of Tourette's syndrome. *Expert Opinion on Pharmacotherapy* 4, 1717–1725.

Myllyla, A., Miettinen, T. *et al.* (2003) New triple combination of levodopa/carbidopa/entacapone is a preferred treatment in patients with Parkinson's disease. *Neurology* 60 (suppl. 1), A289.

Mytilineou, C., Han, S.K. *et al.* (1993) Toxic and protective effects of L-dopa on mesencephalic cell cultures. *Journal of Neurochemistry* 61, 1470–1478.

Nadvornik, P., Sramka, M., Lisy, L. & Svicka, I. (1972) Experiences with dentatotomy. *Confinia Neurologica* 34, 320–324.

Naimark, D., Jackson, E. *et al.* (1996) Psychotic symptoms in Parkinson's disease patients with dementia. *Journal of the American Geriatric Society* 44, 296–9.

Nakano, I. & Hirano, A. (1984) Parkinson's disease: neuron loss in the nucleus basalis without concomitant Alzheimer's disease. *Annals of Neurology* 15, 415–418.

Nasreddine, Z.S., Loginov, M. *et al.* (1999) From genotype to phenotype: a clinical pathological, and biochemical investigation of frontotemporal dementia and parkinsonism (FTDP-17) caused by the P301L tau mutation. *Annals of Neurology* 45, 704–715.

Nath, U., Ben-Shlomo, Y. *et al.* (2001) The prevalence of progressive supranuclear palsy (Steele–Richardson–Olszewski syndrome) in the UK. *Brain* 124, 1438–1449.

Naumann, M., Pirker, W. *et al.* (1998) Imaging the pre- and postsynaptic side of striatal dopaminergic synapses in idiopathic cervical dystonia: a SPECT study using [123I] epipride and [123I] beta-CIT. *Movement Disorders* 13, 319–323.

Nausieda, P.A. (1985) Sinemet abusers. *Clinical Neuropharmacology* 8, 318–327.

Nee, L.E., Polinsky, R.J. & Ebert, M.H. (1982) Tourette syndrome: clinical and family studies. *Advances in Neurology* 35, 291–295.

Nemeth, A.H. (2002) The genetics of primary dystonias and related disorders. *Brain* 125, 695–721.

Nickel, T., Heinen, F. *et al.* (1996) Spasmodic torticollis: a multicenter study on behavioural aspects. III. Psychosocial changes and coping. *Behavioural Neurology* 9, 25–34.

Nicklas, W.J., Vyas, I. & Heikkila, R.E. (1985) Inhibition of NADH-linked oxidation in brain mitochondria by 1-methyl-4-phenyl-pyridine, a metabolite of the neurotoxin, 1-methyl-4-phenyl-1,2,5,6-tetrahydropyridine. *Life Sciences* 36, 2503–2508.

Nissenbaum, H., Quinn, N.P. *et al.* (1987) Mood swings associated with the 'on–off' phenomenon in Parkinson's disease. *Psychological Medicine* 17, 899–904.

Nomura, T., Inoue, Y. *et al.* (2003) Visual hallucinations as REM sleep behavior disorders in patients with Parkinson's disease. *Movement Disorders* 18, 812–817.

Nuwer, M.R. (1982) Coprolalia as an organic symptom. *Advances in Neurology* 35, 363–368.

Nygaard, T.G., Marsden, C.D. & Duvoisin, R.C. (1988) Dopa-responsive dystonia. *Advances in Neurology* **50**, 377–384.

Nygaard, T.G., Marsden, C.D. & Fahn, S. (1991) Dopa-responsive dystonia: long-term treatment response and prognosis. *Neurology* **41**, 174–181.

Obeso, J.A., Rothwell, J.C. & Marsden, C.D. (1981) Simple tics in Gilles de la Tourette's syndrome are not prefaced by a normal premovement EEG potential. *Journal of Neurology, Neurosurgery and Psychiatry* **44**, 735–738.

Oder, W., Grimm, G. *et al.* (1991) Neurological and neuropsychiatric spectrum of Wilson's disease: a prospective study of 45 cases. *Journal of Neurology* **238**, 281–287.

Okun, M.S., Walter, B.L. *et al.* (2002) Beneficial effects of testosterone replacement for the nonmotor symptoms of Parkinson disease. *Archives of Neurology* **59**, 1750–1753.

Olanow, C.W., Fahn, S. *et al.* (1994) A multicenter double-blind placebo-controlled trial of pergolide as an adjunct to Sinemet in Parkinson's disease. *Movement Disorders* **9**, 40–47.

O'Malley, P.G., Jackson, J.L. *et al.* (1999) Antidepressant therapy for unexplained symptoms and symptom syndromes. *Journal of Family Practice* **48**, 980–990.

Ondo, W., Dat Vuong, K. *et al.* (2001) Thalamic deep brain stimulation: effects on the nontarget limbs. *Movement Disorders* **16**, 1137–1142.

Oppenheimer, D.R. (1980) Lateral horn cells in progressive autonomic failure. *Journal of the Neurological Sciences* **46**, 393–404.

O'Reilly, F., Finnan, F. *et al.* (1996) The effects of caring for a spouse with Parkinson's disease on social, psychological and physical well-being. *British Journal of General Practice* **46**, 507–512.

Ovsiew, F. & Schneider, J. (1993) Schizophrenia and atypical motor features in a case of progressive supranuclear palsy (the Steele–Richardson–Olszewski syndrome). *Behavioural Neurology* **6**, 243–247.

Ozelius, L.J., Hewett, J. *et al.* (1997) Fine localization of the torsion dystonia gene (DYT1) on human chromosome 9q34: YAC map and linkage disequilibrium. *Genome Research* **7**, 483–494.

Paleacu, D., Schechtman, E. *et al.* (2005) Association between family history of dementia and hallucinations in Parkinson disease. *Neurology* **64**, 1712–1715.

Pallis, C.A. (1971) Parkinsonism: natural history and clinical features. *British Medical Journal* **3**, 683–690.

Pankratz, N. & Foroud, T. (2004) Genetics of Parkinson disease. *NeuroRx* **1**, 235–242.

Papapetropoulos, S., Argyriou, A.A. *et al.* (2005) Factors associated with drug-induced visual hallucinations in Parkinson's disease. *Journal of Neurology* **252**, 1223–1228.

Pappert, E.J., Goetz, C.G. *et al.* (1999) Hallucinations, sleep fragmentation, and altered dream phenomena in Parkinson's disease. *Movement Disorders* **14**, 117–121.

Pardo, B., Mena, M.A. *et al.* (1993) Ascorbic acid protects against levodopa-induced neurotoxicity on a catecholamine-rich human neuroblastoma cell line. *Movement Disorders* **8**, 278–284.

Parkinson, J. (1817) *An Essay on the Shaking Palsy.* Sherwood, London.

Parkinson Study Group (1989) Effect of deprenyl on the progression of disability in early Parkinson's disease. *New England Journal of Medicine* **321**, 1364–1371.

Parkinson Study Group (1997) Entacapone improves motor fluctuations in levodopa-treated Parkinson's disease patients. *Annals of Neurology* **42**, 747–755.

Parkinson Study Group (1999) Low-dose clozapine for the treatment of drug-induced psychosis in Parkinson's disease. *New England Journal of Medicine* **340**, 757–763.

Parkinson Study Group (2000) Pramipexole vs levodopa as initial treatment for Parkinson disease: a randomized controlled trial. *JAMA* **284**, 1931–1938.

Parkinson Study Group (2002) Dopamine transporter brain imaging to assess the effects of pramipexole vs levodopa on Parkinson disease progression. *JAMA* **287**, 1653–1661.

Pasamanick, B. & Kawi, A. (1956) A study of the association of prenatal and paranatal factors with the development of tics in children. *Journal of Pediatrics* **48**, 596–601.

Paterson, M.T. (1945) Spasmodic torticollis: results of psychotherapy in twenty-one cases. *Lancet* **ii**, 556–559.

Patterson, R.M. & Little, S.C. (1943) Spasmodic torticollis. *Journal of Nervous and Mental Disease* **98**, 571–599.

Paulus, W. & Jellinger, K. (1991) The neuropathologic basis of different clinical subgroups of Parkinson's disease. *Journal of Neuropathology and Experimental Neurology* **50**, 743–755.

Pearce, J.M.S. (1992) *Parkinson's Disease and its Management.* Oxford University Press, Oxford.

Peppard, R.F., Martin, W.R.W., Carr, G.D. *et al.* (1992) Cerebral glucose metabolism in Parkinson's disease with and without dementia. *Archives of Neurology* **49**, 1262–1268.

Perrin, E.M., Murphy, M.L. *et al.* (2004) Does group A beta-hemolytic streptococcal infection increase risk for behavioral and neuropsychiatric symptoms in children? *Archives of Pediatric and Adolescent Medicine* **158**, 848–856.

Perry, E.K., Curtis, M., Dick, D.J. *et al.* (1985) Cholinergic correlates of cognitive impairment in Parkinson's disease: comparisons with Alzheimer's disease. *Journal of Neurology, Neurosurgery and Psychiatry* **48**, 413–421.

Perry, E.K., Marshall, E. *et al.* (1990) Evidence of a monoaminergic–cholinergic imbalance related to visual hallucinations in Lewy body dementia. *Journal of Neurochemistry* **55**, 1454–1456.

Peterson, B., Riddle, M.A. *et al.* (1993) Reduced basal ganglia volumes in Tourette's syndrome using three-dimensional reconstruction techniques from magnetic resonance images. *Neurology* **43**, 941–949.

Peterson, B.S., Staib, L. *et al.* (2001) Regional brain and ventricular volumes in Tourette syndrome. *Archives of General Psychiatry* **58**, 427–440.

Pillon, B., Deweer, B. *et al.* (1993) Explicit memory in Alzheimer's, Huntington's, and Parkinson's diseases. *Archives of Neurology* **50**, 374–379.

Pillon, B., Blin, J. *et al.* (1995) The neuropsychological pattern of corticobasal degeneration: comparison with progressive supranuclear palsy and Alzheimer's disease. *Neurology* **45**, 1477–1483.

Pilo, L., Ring, H. *et al.* (1996) Depression in multiple system atrophy and in idiopathic Parkinson's disease: a pilot comparative study. *Biological Psychiatry* **39**, 803–807.

Pittock, S.J., Joyce, C. *et al.* (2000) Rapid-onset dystonia–parkinsonism: a clinical and genetic analysis of a new kindred. *Neurology* **55**, 991–995.

Pluck, G.C. & Brown, R.G. (2002) Apathy in Parkinson's disease. *Journal of Neurology, Neurosurgery and Psychiatry* **73**, 636–642.

Poewe, W., Benke, T.H., Felber, S.T. & Aichner, F. (1989) Symptomatic blepharospasm accompanying the paramedian diencephalic syndrome: report of a case. *Behavioural Neurology* **2**, 143–151.

Poewe, W., Karamat, E., Kemmler, G.W. & Gerstenbrand, F. (1990) The premorbid personality of patients with Parkinson's disease: a comparative study with healthy controls and patients with essential tremor. *Advances in Neurology* **53**, 339–342.

Pollak, P., Tison, F. *et al.* (2004) Clozapine in drug induced psychosis in Parkinson's disease: a randomised, placebo controlled study with open follow up. *Journal of Neurology, Neurosurgery and Psychiatry* **75**, 689–695.

Pollock, M. & Hornabrook, R.W. (1966) The prevalence, natural history and dementia of Parkinson's disease. *Brain* **89**, 429–448.

Polson, R.J., Rolles, K., Calne, R.Y., Williams, R. & Marsden, D. (1987) Reversal of severe neurological manifestations of Wilson's disease following orthotopic liver transplantation. *Quarterly Journal of Medicine* **64**, 685–691.

Porta, M., Maggioni, G. *et al.* (2004) Treatment of phonic tics in patients with Tourette's syndrome using botulinum toxin type A. *Neurological Sciences* **24**, 420–423.

Portala, K., Westermark, K. *et al.* (2000) Psychopathology in treated Wilson's disease determined by means of CPRS expert and self-ratings. *Acta Psychiatrica Scandinavica* **101**, 104–109.

Porteous, H.B. & Ross, D.N. (1956) Mental symptoms in parkinsonism following benzhexol hydrochloride therapy. *British Medical Journal* **2**, 138–140.

Postma, J.U. & Van Tilburg, W. (1975) Visual hallucinations and delirium during treatment with amantadine (Symmetrel). *Journal of the American Geriatric Society* **23**, 212–215.

Price, R.A., Kidd, K.K., Cohen, D.J., Pauls, D.L. & Leckman, J.F. (1985) A twin study of Tourette syndrome. *Archives of General Psychiatry* **42**, 815–820.

Priebe, S. (1984) Levodopa dependence: a case report. *Pharmacopsychiatry* **17**, 109–110.

Quinn, N. (1989) Multiple system atrophy: the nature of the beast. *Journal of Neurology, Neurosurgery and Psychiatry* **52** (special supplement), 78–89.

Quinn, N. (1995) Drug treatment of Parkinson's disease. *British Medical Journal* **310**, 575–579.

Quinn, N. (1996) Parkinson's disease. *Journal of Neurosurgery* **85**, 528–529.

Quinn, N. & Wenning, G. (1994) Multiple system atrophy. *British Journal of Hospital Medicine* **51**, 492–494.

Quinn, N., Critchley, P. *et al.* (1986) When should levodopa be started? *Lancet* **ii**, 985–986.

Raethjen, J., Kopper, F. *et al.* (2004) Two different pathogenetic mechanisms in psychogenic tremor. *Neurology* **63**, 812–815.

Rajput, A.H., Offord, K., Beard, C.M. & Kurland, L.T. (1984) Epidemiological survey of dementia in parkinsonism and control population. *Advances in Neurology* **40**, 229–234.

Rampello, L., Chiechio, S. *et al.* (2002) The SSRI, citalopram, improves bradykinesia in patients with Parkinson's disease treated with L-dopa. *Clinical Neuropharmacology* **25**, 21–24.

Rascol, O., Brooks, D.J. *et al.* (2000) A five-year study of the incidence of dyskinesia in patients with early Parkinson's disease who were treated with ropinirole or levodopa. *New England Journal of Medicine* **342**, 1484–1491.

Rathbun, J.K. (1996) Neuropsychological aspects of Wilson's disease. *International Journal of Neuroscience* **85**, 221–229.

Reading, P.J., Luce, A.K. *et al.* (2001) Rivastigmine in the treatment of parkinsonian psychosis and cognitive impairment: preliminary findings from an open trial. *Movement Disorders* **16**, 1171–1174.

Ready, R.E., Friedman, J. *et al.* (2004) Testosterone deficiency and apathy in Parkinson's disease: a pilot study. *Journal of Neurology, Neurosurgery and Psychiatry* **75**, 1323–1326.

Rebeiz, J.J., Kolodny, E.H. & Richardson, E.P. (1968) Corticodentatonigral degeneration with neuronal achromasia. *Archives of Neurology* **18**, 20–33.

Reddy, S., Factor, S.A. *et al.* (2002) The effect of quetiapine on psychosis and motor function in parkinsonian patients with and without dementia. *Movement Disorders* **17**, 676–681.

Reichmann, H., Brecht, M.H. *et al.* (2003) Pramipexole in routine clinical practice: a prospective observational trial in Parkinson's disease. *CNS Drugs* **17**, 965–973.

Remy, P., Doder, M. *et al.* (2005) Depression in Parkinson's disease: loss of dopamine and noradrenaline innervation in the limbic system. *Brain* **128**, 1314–1322.

Riddle, M.A., Rasmusson, A.M., Woods, S.W. & Hoffer, P.B. (1992) SPECT imaging of cerebral blood flow in Tourette syndrome. *Advances in Neurology* **58**, 207–211.

Riley, D.E., Lang, A.E., Lewis, A. *et al.* (1990) Cortical–basal ganglionic degeneration. *Neurology* **40**, 1203–1212.

Ring, H.A., Bench, C.J. *et al.* (1994) Depression in Parkinson's disease. A positron emission study. *British Journal of Psychiatry* **165**, 333–339.

Rinne, J.O., Rummukainen, J., Paljärui, L. & Rinne, U.K. (1989) Dementia in Parkinson's disease is related to neuronal loss in the medial substantia nigra. *Annals of Neurology* **26**, 47–50.

Rinne, J.O., Myllykyla, T. *et al.* (1991) A postmortem study of brain nicotinic receptors in Parkinson's and Alzheimer's disease. *Brain Research* **547**, 167–170.

Rinne, U.K., Bracco, F. *et al.* (1998) Early treatment of Parkinson's disease with cabergoline delays the onset of motor complications. Results of a double-blind levodopa controlled trial. *Drugs* **55** (suppl. 1), 23–30.

Robertson, M.M. (1989) The Gilles de la Tourette syndrome: the current status. *British Journal of Psychiatry* **154**, 147–169.

Robertson, M.M. (1992) Self-injurious behavior and Tourette syndrome. *Advances in Neurology* **58**, 105–114.

Robertson, M.M. (1994) Annotation: Gilles de la Tourette syndrome – an update. *Journal of Child Psychology and Psychiatry* **35**, 597–611.

Robertson, M.M. (2000) Tourette syndrome, associated conditions and the complexities of treatment. *Brain* **123**, 425–462.

Robertson, M.M. & Gourdie, A. (1990) Familial Tourette's syndrome in a large British pedigree. Associated psychopathology severity, and potential for linkage analysis. *British Journal of Psychiatry* **156**, 515–521.

Robertson, M.M. & Stern, J.S. (1998) Tic disorders: new developments in Tourette syndrome and related disorders. *Current Opinion in Neurology* **11**, 373–380.

Robertson, M.M., Trimble, M.R. & Lees, A.J. (1988) The psychopathology of the Gilles de la Tourette syndrome. A phenomenological analysis. *British Journal of Psychiatry* **152**, 383–390.

Robertson, M.M., Channon, S., Baker, J. & Flynn, D. (1993) The psychopathology of Gilles de la Tourette's syndrome. A controlled study. *British Journal of Psychiatry* **162**, 114–117.

Robins, A.H. (1976) Depression in patients with parkinsonism. *British Journal of Psychiatry* **128**, 141–145.

Rochester, L., Hetherington, V. *et al.* (2004) Attending to the task: interference effects of functional tasks on walking in Parkinson's disease and the roles of cognition, depression, fatigue, and balance. *Archives of Physical Medicine and Rehabilitation* **85**, 1578–1585.

Rodnitzky, R.L. (2002) Drug-induced movement disorders. *Clinical Neuropharmacology* **25**, 142–152.

Rojo, A., Pernaute, R.S. *et al.* (1999) Clinical genetics of familial progressive supranuclear palsy. *Brain* **122**, 1233–1245.

Rojo, A., Aguilar, M. *et al.* (2003) Depression in Parkinson's disease: clinical correlates and outcome. *Parkinsonism and Related Disorders* **10**, 23–28.

Ross, G.W., Mahler, M.E. & Cummings, J.L. (1992) The dementia syndromes of Parkinson's disease: cortical and subcortical features. In: Huber, S.J. & Cummings, J.L. (eds) *Parkinson's Disease: Neurobehavioral Aspects*, ch. 11. Oxford University Press, Oxford.

Rothenberger, A., Kostanecka, T. *et al.* (2001) Sleep and Tourette syndrome. *Advances in Neurology* **85**, 245–259.

Ryback, R.S. & Schwab, R.S. (1971) Manic response to levodopa therapy. Report of a case. *New England Journal of Medicine* **285**, 788–789.

Sachdev, P.S. (2000) The current status of tardive dyskinesia. *Australian and New Zealand Journal of Psychiatry* **34**, 355–369.

Sachdev, P.S. (2005) Neuroleptic-induced movement disorders: an overview. *Psychiatric Clinics of North America* **28**, 255–274, x.

Sadzot, B., Baraban, J.M. *et al.* (1989) Hallucinogenic drug interactions at human brain 5-HT2 receptors: implications for treating LSD-induced hallucinogenesis. *Psychopharmacology* **98**, 495–499.

Saint-Cyr, J.A., Taylor, A.E. *et al.* (1993) Neuropsychological and psychiatric side effects in the treatment of Parkinson's disease. *Neurology* **43** (12 suppl. 6), S47–S52.

Sallee, F.R., Nesbitt, L. *et al.* (1997) Relative efficacy of haloperidol and pimozide in children and adolescents with Tourette's disorder. *American Journal of Psychiatry* **154**, 1057–1062.

Sallee, F.R., Kurlan, R. *et al.* (2000) Ziprasidone treatment of children and adolescents with Tourette's syndrome: a pilot study. *Journal of the American Academy of Child and Adolescent Psychiatry* **39**, 292–299.

Sallee, F.R., Gilbert, D.L. *et al.* (2003) Pharmacodynamics of ziprasidone in children and adolescents: impact on dopamine transmission. *Journal of the American Academy of Child and Adolescent Psychiatry* **42**, 902–907.

Sanchez-Ramos, J.R., Ortoll, R. *et al.* (1996) Visual hallucinations associated with Parkinson disease. *Archives of Neurology* **53**, 1265–1268.

Sand, P.L. & Carlson, C. (1973) Failure to establish control over tics in the Gilles de la Tourette syndrome with behaviour therapy techniques. *British Journal of Psychiatry* **122**, 665–670.

Sands, I.R. (1942) The type of personality susceptible to Parkinson disease. *Journal of the Mount Sinai Hospital* **9**, 792–794.

Santamaria, J., Tolosa, E.S. *et al.* (1987) Mental depression in untreated Parkinson's disease of recent onset. *Advances in Neurology* **45**, 443–446.

Sawle, G.V., Brooks, D.J., Ibanez, V. & Frackowiak, R.S.J. (1990) Striatal D2 receptor density is inversely proportional to dopa uptake in untreated hemi-Parkinson's disease: a positron emission tomography study. Proceedings of the Association of British Neurologists, London, 28–30 September 1989. *Journal of Neurology, Neurosurgery and Psychiatry* **53**, 177.

Sawle, G.V., Brooks, D.J., Marsden, C.D. & Frackowiak, R.S.J. (1991) Corticobasal degeneration. A unique pattern of regional cortical oxygen, hypometabolism and striatal fluorodopa uptake demonstrated by positron emission tomography. *Brain* **114**, 541–556.

Scahill, L., Riddle, M.A. *et al.* (1997) Fluoxetine has no marked effect on tic symptoms in patients with Tourette's syndrome: a double-blind placebo-controlled study. *Journal of Child and Adolescent Psychopharmacology* **7**, 75–85.

Scahill, L., Kano, Y. *et al.* (2003) Influence of age and tic disorders on obsessive-compulsive disorder in a pediatric sample. *Journal of Child and Adolescent Psychopharmacology* **13** (suppl. 1), S7–S17.

Schapira, A.H.V., Cooper, J.M., Dexter, D., Jenner, P., Clark, J.B. & Marsden, C.D. (1989) Mitochondrial Complex I deficiency in Parkinson's disease. *Lancet* **i**, 1269.

Schapira, A.H.V., Cooper, J.M., Dexter, D., Clark, J.B., Jenner, P. & Marsden, C.D. (1990a) Mitochondrial Complex I deficiency in Parkinson's disease. *Journal of Neurochemistry* **54**, 823–827.

Schapira, A.H.V., Mann, V.M., Cooper, J.M. *et al.* (1990b) Anatomic and disease specificity of NADH CoQ$_1$ reductase (Complex I) deficiency in Parkinson's disease. *Journal of Neurochemistry* **55**, 2142–2145.

Schenck, C.H., Bundlie, S.R. *et al.* (1987) Rapid eye movement sleep behavior disorder. A treatable parasomnia affecting older adults. *JAMA* **257**, 1786–1789.

Schicatano, E.J., Basso, M.A. *et al.* (1997) Animal model explains the origins of the cranial dystonia benign essential blepharospasm. *Journal of Neurophysiology* **77**, 2842–2846.

Schmidt, K.E., Linden, D.E. *et al.* (2003) Striatal activation during blepharospasm revealed by fMRI. *Neurology* **60**, 1738–1743.

Schott, G.D. (1985) The relationship of peripheral trauma and pain to dystonia. *Journal of Neurology, Neurosurgery and Psychiatry* **48**, 698–701.

Schrag, A. & Lang, A.E. (2005) Psychogenic movement disorders. *Current Opinion in Neurology* **18**, 399–404.

Schrag, A., Ben-Shlomo, Y. *et al.* (1999) Prevalence of progressive supranuclear palsy and multiple system atrophy: a cross-sectional study. *Lancet* **354**, 1771–1775.

Schrag, A., Good, C.D. *et al.* (2000) Differentiation of atypical parkinsonian syndromes with routine MRI. *Neurology* **54**, 697–702.

Schrag, A., Jahanshahi, M. *et al.* (2001) What contributes to depression in Parkinson's disease? *Psychological Medicine* **31**, 65–73.

Schrag, A., Ben-Shlomo, Y. *et al.* (2002) How valid is the clinical diagnosis of Parkinson's disease in the community? *Journal of Neurology, Neurosurgery and Psychiatry* **73**, 529–534.

Schrag, A., Selai, C. *et al.* (2003) Health-related quality of life in patients with progressive supranuclear palsy. *Movement Disorders* **18**, 1464–1469.

Schrag, A., Trimble, M. *et al.* (2004) The syndrome of fixed dystonia: an evaluation of 103 patients. *Brain* **127**, 2360–2372.

Schuurman, P.R., Bosch, D.A. *et al.* (2000) A comparison of continuous thalamic stimulation and thalamotomy for suppression of severe tremor. *New England Journal of Medicine* **342**, 461–468.

Schwab, R.S., England, A.C. Jr., *et al.* (1969) Amantadine in the treatment of Parkinson's disease. *JAMA* **208**, 1168–1170.

Scott, R., Gregory, R. *et al.* (1998) Neuropsychological, neurological and functional outcome following pallidotomy for Parkinson's disease. A consecutive series of eight simultaneous bilateral and twelve unilateral procedures. *Brain* **121**, 659–675.

Secker, D.L. & Brown, R.G. (2005) Cognitive behavioural therapy (CBT) for carers of patients with Parkinson's disease: a preliminary randomised controlled trial. *Journal of Neurology, Neurosurgery and Psychiatry* **76**, 491–497.

Selby, G. (1968) Cerebral atrophy in Parkinsonism. *Journal of the Neurological Sciences* **6**, 517–559.

Selby, G. (1990) Clinical features. In: Stern, G.M. (ed.) *Parkinson's Disease*, ch. 12. Chapman & Hall, London.

Serrano-Duenas, M. (2002) Chronic dopamimetic drug addiction and pathologic gambling in patients with Parkinsons's disease: presentation of four cases. *German Journal of Psychiatry* **5**, 62–66.

Shamir, E., Barak, Y. *et al.* (2001) Melatonin treatment for tardive dyskinesia: a double-blind, placebo-controlled, crossover study. *Archives of General Psychiatry* **58**, 1049–1052.

Shapiro, A.K. & Shapiro, E. (1982) Clinical efficacy of haloperidol, pimozide, penfluridol, and clonidine in the treatment of Tourette syndrome. *Advances in Neurology* **35**, 383–386.

Shapiro, A.K., Shapiro, E., Wayne, H. & Clarkin, J. (1972) The psychopathology of Gilles de la Tourette's syndrome. *American Journal of Psychiatry* **129**, 427–434.

Shapiro, A.K., Shapiro, E., Wayne, H.L., Clarkin, J. & Bruun, R.D. (1973) Tourette's syndrome: summary of data on 34 patients. *Psychosomatic Medicine* **35**, 419–435.

Shapiro, A.K., Shapiro, E.S., Bruun, R.D. & Sweet, R.D. (1978) *Gilles de la Tourette Syndrome*. Raven Press, New York.

Shapleske, J., McKay, A.P. & McKenna, P.J. (1996) Successful treatment of tardive dystonia with clozapine and clonazepam. *British Journal of Psychiatry* **168**, 516–518.

Shellenberger, M., Clarke, A. *et al.* (2000) Zydis selegiline reduces off time and improves symptoms in patients with Parkinson's disease. *Movement Disorders* **15** (suppl. 3), S116–S117.

Shergill, S.S., Walker, Z. *et al.* (1998) A preliminary investigation of laterality in Parkinson's disease and susceptibility to psychosis. *Journal of Neurology, Neurosurgery and Psychiatry* **65**, 610–611.

Shiba, M., Bower, J.H. *et al.* (2000) Anxiety disorders and depressive disorders preceding Parkinson's disease: a case–control study. *Movement Disorders* **15**, 669–677.

Shinotoh, H., Namba, H. *et al.* (1999) Positron emission tomographic measurement of acetylcholinesterase activity reveals differential loss of ascending cholinergic systems in Parkinson's disease and progressive supranuclear palsy. *Annals of Neurology* **46**, 62–69.

Shorr, N., Seiff, S.R. *et al.* (1985) The use of botulinum toxin in blepharospasm. *American Journal of Ophthalmology* **99**, 542–546.

Shulman, L.M. (2000) Apathy in patients with Parkinson's disease. *International Review of Psychiatry* **12**, 298–306.

Simonic, I., Gericke, G.S. *et al.* (1998) Identification of genetic markers associated with Gilles de la Tourette syndrome in an Afrikaner population. *American Journal of Human Genetics* **63**, 839–846.

Simonic, I., Nyholt, D.R. *et al.* (2001) Further evidence for linkage of Gilles de la Tourette syndrome (GTS) susceptibility loci on chromosomes 2p11, 8q22 and 11q23–24 in South African Afrikaners. *American Journal of Medical Genetics* **105**, 163–167.

Singer, E. (1974) The effect of treatment with levodopa on Parkinson patients' social functioning and outlook on life. *Journal of Chronic Diseases* **27**, 581–594.

Singer, H.S. (1992) Neurochemical analysis of postmortem cortical and striatal brain tissue in patients with Tourette syndrome. *Advances in Neurology* **58**, 135–144.

Singer, H.S. (2000) Current issues in Tourette syndrome. *Movement Disorders* **15**, 1051–1063.

Singer, H.S. (2005) Tourette's syndrome: from behaviour to biology. *Lancet Neurology* **4**, 149–159.

Singer, H.S., Hahn, I.-H. & Moran, T.H. (1991) Abnormal dopamine uptake sites in postmortem striatum from patients with Tourette's syndrome. *Annals of Neurology* **30**, 558–562.

Singer, H.S., Giuliano, J.D. *et al.* (1998) Antibodies against human putamen in children with Tourette syndrome. *Neurology* **50**, 1618–1624.

Smith, L.A., Jackson, M.J. *et al.* (2005) Multiple small doses of levodopa plus entacapone produce continuous dopaminergic stimulation and reduce dyskinesia induction in MPTP-treated drug-naive primates. *Movement Disorders* **20**, 306–314.

Smith, W.T. (1976) Intoxications, poisons and related metabolic disorders. In: Blackwood, W. & Corsellis, J.A.N. (eds) *Greenfield's Neuropathology*, 3rd edn, ch. 4. Edward Arnold, London.

Smythies, J.R. (1967) The previous personality in parkinsonism. *Journal of Psychosomatic Research* **11**, 169–171.

Soldani, P. & Fornai, F. (1999) The functional anatomy of noradrenergic neurons in Parkinson's disease. *Functional Neurology* **14**, 97–109.

Soliveri, P., Monza, D. *et al.* (2000) Neuropsychological follow up in patients with Parkinson's disease, striatonigral degeneration-type multisystem atrophy, and progressive supranuclear palsy. *Journal of Neurology, Neurosurgery and Psychiatry* **69**, 313–318.

Speelman, J. (1991) *Parkinson's Disease and Asteroetaxic Surgery*. Elsevier Science Publishers, Amsterdam.

Spencer, T., Biederman, J. *et al.* (1999) Attention-deficit/hyperactivity disorder and comorbidity. *Pediatrics Clinics of North America* **46**, 915–927, vii.

Sroka, H., Elizan, T.S., Yahr, M.D., Burger, A. & Mendoza, M.R. (1981) Organic mental syndrome and confusional states in Parkinson's disease. Relationship to computerised tomographic signs of cerebral atrophy. *Archives of Neurology* **38**, 339–342.

Stacy, M. (2000) Idiopathic cervical dystonia: an overview. *Neurology* **55** (12 suppl. 5), S2–S8.

Stacy, M. & Jankovic, J. (1992) Clinical and neurobiological aspects of Parkinson's disease. In: Huber, S.J. & Cummings, J.L. (eds) *Parkinson's Disease: Neurobehavioral Aspects*, ch. 2. Oxford University Press, New York.

Starkstein, S.E., Preziosi, T.J. *et al.* (1989) Depression and cognitive impairment in Parkinson's disease. *Brain* **112**, 1141–1153.

Starkstein, S.E., Preziosi, T.J. *et al.* (1990) Depression in Parkinson's disease. *Journal of Nervous and Mental Disease* **178**, 27–31.

Starkstein, S.E., Mayberg, H.S. *et al.* (1992a) A prospective longitudinal study of depression, cognitive decline, and physical impairments in patients with Parkinson's disease. *Journal of Neurology, Neurosurgery and Psychiatry* **55**, 377–382.

Starkstein, S.E., Mayberg, H.S. *et al.* (1992b) Reliability, validity, and clinical correlates of apathy in Parkinson's disease. *Journal of Neuropsychiatry and Clinical Neuroscience* **4**, 134–139.

Starosta-Rubinstein, S. (1995) Treatment of Wilson's disease. In: Kurlan, R. (ed.) *Treatment of Movement Disorders*, ch. 4. Lippincott, Philadelphia.

Stebbins, G.T. & Tanner, C.M. (1992) Behavioral effects of intrastriatal adrenal medullary surgery in Parkinson's disease. In: Huber, S.J. & Cummings, J.L. (eds) *Parkinson's Disease: Neurobehavioral Aspects*, ch. 24. Oxford University Press, Oxford.

Steele, J.C. (1972) Progressive supranuclear palsy. *Brain* **95**, 693–704.

Steele, J.C., Richardson, J.C. & Olszewski, J. (1964) Progressive supranuclear palsy. *Archives of Neurology* **10**, 333–359.

Steen, V.M., Lovlie, R. *et al.* (1997) Dopamine D3-receptor gene variant and susceptibility to tardive dyskinesia in schizophrenic patients. *Molecular Psychiatry* **2**, 139–145.

Stell, R., Thompson, P.D. & Marsden, C.D. (1988) Botulinum toxin in spasmodic torticollis. *Journal of Neurology, Neurosurgery and Psychiatry* **51**, 920–923.

Stell, R., Thickbroom, G.W. *et al.* (1995) The audiogenic startle response in Tourette's syndrome. *Movement Disorders* **10**, 723–730.

Stephens, D.A. (1967) Psychotoxic effects of benzhexol hydrochloride (Artane). *British Journal of Psychiatry* **113**, 213–218.

Stephens, R.J., Bassel, C. *et al.* (2004) Olanzapine in the treatment of aggression and tics in children with Tourette's syndrome: a pilot study. *Journal of Child and Adolescent Psychopharmacology* **14**, 255–266.

Stern, E., Silbersweig, D.A. *et al.* (2000) A functional neuroanatomy of tics in Tourette syndrome. *Archives of General Psychiatry* **57**, 741–748.

Stern, J.S., Burza, S. *et al.* (2005) Gilles de la Tourette's syndrome and its impact in the UK. *Postgraduate Medical Journal* **81**, 12–19.

Steventon, G.B., Heafield, M.T.E., Waring, R.H. & Williams, A.C. (1989) Xenobiotic metabolism in Parkinson's disease. *Neurology* **39**, 883–887.

Stibe, C.M.H., Lees, A.J., Kempster, P.A. & Stern, G.M. (1988) Subcutaneous apomorphine in Parkinsonian on–off oscillations. *Lancet* **i**, 403–406.

Stocchi, F., Badiali, D. *et al.* (2000) Anorectal function in multiple system atrophy and Parkinson's disease. *Movement Disorders* **15**, 71–76.

Stone, J., Sharpe, M. *et al.* (2003) The 12 year prognosis of unilateral functional weakness and sensory disturbance. *Journal of Neurology, Neurosurgery and Psychiatry* **74**, 591–596.

Stone, J., Carson, A. & Sharpe, M. (2005a) Functional symptoms and signs in neurology: assessment and diagnosis. *Journal of Neurology, Neurosurgery and Psychiatry* **76** (suppl. 1), i2–i12.

Stone, J., Carson, A. *et al.* (2005b) Functional symptoms in neurology: management. *Journal of Neurology, Neurosurgery and Psychiatry* **76** (suppl. 1), i13–i21.

Stover, N.P. & Watts, R.L. (2001) Corticobasal degeneration. *Seminars in Neurology* **21**, 49–58.

Stowe, R.L., Ives, N.J., Clarke, C. *et al.* (2008) Dopamine agonist therapy in early Parkinson's disease. Cochrane Database of Systematic Reviews, Issue 2.

Stubner, S., Rustenbeck, E. *et al.* (2004) Severe and uncommon involuntary movement disorders due to psychotropic drugs. *Pharmacopsychiatry* **37** (suppl. 1), S54–S64.

Sukhodolsky, D.G., Scahill, L. *et al.* (2003) Disruptive behavior in children with Tourette's syndrome: association with ADHD comorbidity, tic severity, and functional impairment. *Journal of the American Academy of Child and Adolescent Psychiatry* **42**, 98–105.

Swedo, S.E., Leonard, H.L. *et al.* (1997) Identification of children with pediatric autoimmune neuropsychiatric disorders associated with streptococcal infections by a marker associated with rheumatic fever. *American Journal of Psychiatry* **154**, 110–112.

Swedo, S.E., Leonard, H.L. *et al.* (1998) Pediatric autoimmune neuropsychiatric disorders associated with streptococcal infections: clinical description of the first 50 cases. *American Journal of Psychiatry* **155**, 264–271.

Sweet, R.D., McDowell, F.H., Feigenson, J.S., Loranger, A.W. & Good, H. (1976) Mental symptoms in Parkinson's disease during chronic treatment with levodopa. *Neurology* **26**, 305–310.

Swerdlow, N.R. & Young, A.B. (2001) Neuropathology in Tourette syndrome: an update. *Advances in Neurology* **85**, 151–161.

Tandberg, E., Larsen, J.P. *et al.* (1996) The occurrence of depression in Parkinson's disease. A community-based study. *Archives of Neurology* **53**, 175–179.

Tandberg, E., Larsen, J.P. *et al.* (1997) Risk factors for depression in Parkinson disease. *Archives of Neurology* **54**, 625–630.

Tanner, C.M., Ottman, R. *et al.* (1999) Parkinson disease in twins: an etiologic study. *JAMA* **281**, 341–346.

Task Force on Late Neurological Effects of Antipsychotic Drugs (1980) Tardive dyskinesia: summary of a task force report of the American Psychiatric Association. *American Journal of Psychiatry* **137**, 1163–1172.

Taylor, A.E., Saint-Cyr, J.A. *et al.* (1986) Parkinson's disease and depression. A critical re-evaluation. *Brain* **109**, 279–292.

Taylor, D., Kerwin, R. *et al.* (2005) *The Maudsley 2005–2006 Prescribing Guidelines.* Taylor & Francis, London.

Teoh, R. (1988) Tardive dyskinesia. *Adverse Drug Reaction Bulletin* **132** (October), 496–499.

Terada, K., Ikeda, A. *et al.* (1995) Presence of Bereitschaftspotential preceding psychogenic myoclonus: clinical application of jerk-locked back averaging. *Journal of Neurology, Neurosurgery and Psychiatry* **58**, 745–747.

Tetrud, J.W. & Langston, J.W. (1989) The effect of deprenyl (Selegiline) on the natural history of Parkinson's disease. *Science* **245**, 519–522.

Thaker, G.K., Nguyen, J.A. *et al.* (1990) Clonazepam treatment of tardive dyskinesia: a practical GABAmimetic strategy. *American Journal of Psychiatry* **147**, 445–451.

Thomas, A., Iacono, D. *et al.* (2004) Duration of amantadine benefit on dyskinesia of severe Parkinson's disease. *Journal of Neurology, Neurosurgery and Psychiatry* **75**, 141–143.

Thomas, M. & Jankovic, J. (2004) Psychogenic movement disorders: diagnosis and management. *CNS Drugs* **18**, 437–452.

Thompson, P.D. & Marsden, C.D. (1992) Corticobasal degeneration. In: Rossor, M.N. (ed.) *Unusual Dementias*, pp. 677–686. Baillière Tindall, London.

Timberlake, W.H. & Vance, M.A. (1978) Four-year treatment of patients with parkinsonism using amantadine alone or with levodopa. *Annals of Neurology* **3**, 119–128.

Tobias, J.A. & Merlis, S. (1970) Levodopa and schizophrenia. *JAMA* **211**, 1857.

Tollefson, G.D., Beasley, C.M. Jr., *et al.* (1997) Blind, controlled, long-term study of the comparative incidence of treatment-emergent tardive dyskinesia with olanzapine or haloperidol. *American Journal of Psychiatry* **154**, 1248–1254.

Tolosa, E. & Martí, M.J. (1988) Blepharospasm–oromandibular dystonia syndrome (Meige's syndrome): clinical aspects. *Advances in Neurology* **49**, 73–84.

Tourette Syndrome Association International Consortium for Genetics (1999) A complete genome screen in sib-pairs affected with the Gilles de la Tourette syndrome. *American Journal of Human Genetics* **65**, 1428–1436.

Tourette's Syndrome Study Group (2002) Treatment of ADHD in childen with tics: a randomised controlled trial. *Neurology* **58**, 527–536.

Tousi, B. & Frankel, M. (2004) Olfactory and visual hallucinations in Parkinson's disease. *Parkinsonism and Related Disorders* **10**, 253–254.

Trenkwalder, C., Paulus, W. *et al.* (2005) The restless legs syndrome. *Lancet Neurology* **4**, 465–475.

Trost, M. (2003) Dystonia update. *Current Opinion in Neurology* **16**, 495–500.

Troster, A.I., Fields, J.A. *et al.* (1997) Unilateral pallidal stimulation for Parkinson's disease: neurobehavioral functioning before and 3 months after electrode implantation. *Neurology* **49**, 1078–1083.

Tsui, J.K.C., Eisen, A., Stoessl, A.J., Calne, S. & Calne, D.B. (1986) Double-blind study of botulinum toxin in spasmodic torticollis. *Lancet* **ii**, 245–247.

Tulen, J.H., Azzolini, M. *et al.* (1999) Quantitative study of spontaneous eye blinks and eye tics in Gilles de la Tourette's syndrome. *Journal of Neurology, Neurosurgery and Psychiatry* **67**, 800–802.

Turner, M.A., Moran, N.F. *et al.* (2002) Subcortical dementia. *British Journal of Psychiatry* **180**, 148–151.

Turner, T.H., Cookson, J.C. *et al.* (1984) Psychotic reactions during treatment of pituitary tumours with dopamine agonists. *British Medical Journal* **289**, 1101–1103.

Tyne, H.L., Parsons, J. *et al.* (2004) A 10 year retrospective audit of long-term apomorphine use in Parkinson's disease. *Journal of Neurology* **251**, 1370–1374.

Uitti, R.J. & Maraganore, D.M. (1993) Adult onset familial cervical dystonia: report of a family including monozygotic twins. *Movement Disorders* **8**, 489–494.

Vaamonde, J., Luquin, M.R. *et al.* (1991) Subcutaneous lisuride infusion in Parkinson's disease. Response to chronic administration in 34 patients. *Brain* **114**, 601–617.

Van Camp, G., Flamez, A. *et al.* (2004) Treatment of Parkinson's disease with pergolide and relation to restrictive valvular heart disease. *Lancet* **363**, 1179–1183.

Vandewalle, V., van der Linden, C. *et al.* (1999) Stereotactic treatment of Gilles de la Tourette syndrome by high frequency stimulation of thalamus. *Lancet* **353**, 724.

Van Harten, P.N., Kampuis, D.J. *et al.* (1996) Use of clozapine in tardive dystonia. *Progress in Neuropsychopharmacology and Biological Psychiatry* **20**, 263–274.

van Os, J., Fahy, T. *et al.* (1997) Tardive dyskinesia: who is at risk? *Acta Psychiatrica Scandinavica* **96**, 206–216.

Vieregge, P. (1996) Visual hallucinations in Parkinson's disease: a controlled study. *Movement Disorders* **11** (suppl. 1), 158.

Vitek, J.L. (2002) Pathophysiology of dystonia: a neuronal model. *Movement Disorders* **17** (suppl 3), S49–S62.

Vitek, J.L., Bakay, R.A. *et al.* (2003) Randomized trial of pallidotomy versus medical therapy for Parkinson's disease. *Annals of Neurology* **53**, 558–569.

Volkmann, J. & Benecke, R. (2002) Deep brain stimulation for dystonia: patient selection and evaluation. *Movement Disorders* **17** (suppl. 3), S112–S115.

Waddington, J.L. & Youssef, H.A. (1986) An unusual cluster of tardive dyskinesia in schizophrenia: association with cognitive dysfunction and negative symptoms. *American Journal of Psychiatry* **143**, 1162–1165.

Waddy, H.M., Fletcher, N.A., Harding, A.E. & Marsden, C.D. (1991) A genetic study of idiopathic focal dystonias. *Annals of Neurology* **29**, 320–324.

Walkinshaw, G. & Waters, C.M. (1995) Induction of apoptosis in catecholaminergic PC12 cells by L-DOPA. Implications for the treatment of Parkinson's disease. *Journal of Clinical Investigation* **95**, 2458–2464.

Walshe, J.M. (1986) Wilson's disease. In: Vinken, P.J., Bruyn, G.W. & Klawans, H.L. (eds) *Handbook of Clinical Neurology. Vol. 5. Extrapyramidal Disorders*, ch. 12. Elsevier Science Publishers, Amsterdam.

Walter, B.L. & Vitek, J.L. (2004) Surgical treatment for Parkinson's disease. *Lancet Neurology* **3**, 719–728.

Warburton, J.W. (1967) Depressive symptoms in Parkinson patients referred for thalamotomy. *Journal of Neurology, Neurosurgery and Psychiatry* **30**, 368–370.

Ward, C.D., Duvoisin, R.C., Ince, S.E. *et al.* (1984) Parkinson's disease in twins. *Advances in Neurology* **40**, 341–344.

Waters, C.H., Sethi, K.D. *et al.* (2004) Zydis selegiline reduces off time in Parkinson's disease patients with motor fluctuations: a 3-month, randomized, placebo-controlled study. *Movement Disorders* **19**, 426–432.

Watts, R.L., Mirra, S.S. & Richardson, E.P. (1994) Corticobasal ganglionic degeneration. In: Marsden, C.D. & Fahn, S. (eds) *Movement Disorders*, vol. 3, ch. 14. Butterworth-Heinemann, Oxford.

Weintraub, D., Moberg, P.J. *et al.* (2004) Effect of psychiatric and other nonmotor symptoms on disability in Parkinson's disease. *Journal of the American Geriatrics Society* **52**, 784–788.

Weisskopf, M.G., Chen, H. *et al.* (2003) Prospective study of phobic anxiety and risk of Parkinson's disease. *Movement Disorders* **18**, 646–651.

Wenning, G.K. & Geser, F. (2003) Multiple system atrophy. *Revue Neurologique (Paris)* **159**, 3S31–3S38.

Wenning, G.K. & Quinn, N.P. (1997) Parkinsonism. Multiple system atrophy. *Baillières Clinical Neurology* **6**, 187–204.

Wenning, G.K., Ben Shlomo, Y. *et al.* (1994) Clinical features and natural history of multiple system atrophy. An analysis of 100 cases. *Brain* **117**, 835–845.

Wenning, G.K., Ben-Shlomo, Y. *et al.* (1995) Clinicopathological study of 35 cases of multiple system atrophy. *Journal of Neurology, Neurosurgery and Psychiatry* **58**, 160–166.

Wenning, G.K., Litvan, I., Jankovic, J. *et al.* (1998) Natural history and survival of 14 patients with corticobasal degeneration confirmed at postmortem examination. *Journal of Neurology, Neurosurgery and Psychiatry* **64**, 184–189.

Wenning, G.K., Scherfler, C. *et al.* (1999) Time course of symptomatic orthostatic hypotension and urinary incontinence in patients with postmortem confirmed parkinsonian syndromes: a clinicopathological study. *Journal of Neurology, Neurosurgery and Psychiatry* **67**, 620–623.

Wenzel, T., Schnider, P. *et al.* (2000) Psychiatric disorders in patients with blepharospasm: a reactive pattern? *Journal of Psychosomatic Research* **48**, 589–591.

Wermuth, L., Sorensen, P. *et al.* (1998) Depression in idiopathic Parkinson's disease treated with citalopram. A placebo-controlled trial. *Nordic Journal of Psychiatry* **52**, 163–169.

Wessely, S., Nimnuan, C. *et al.* (1999) Functional somatic syndromes: one or many? *Lancet* **354**, 936–939.

Wester, K. & Hauglie-Hanssen, E. (1990) Stereotaxic thalamotomy: experiences from the levodopa era. *Journal of Neurology, Neurosurgery and Psychiatry* **53**, 427–430.

Whiles, W.H. (1940) Treatment of spasmodic torticollis by psychotherapy. *British Medical Journal* **1**, 969–971.

Whone, A.L., Watts, R.L. *et al.* (2003) Slower progression of Parkinson's disease with ropinirole versus levodopa: The REAL-PET study. *Annals of Neurology* **54**, 93–101.

Williams, D.T., Ford, B. *et al.* (1995) Phenomenology and psychopathology related to psychogenic movement disorders. *Advances in Neurology* **65**, 231–257.

Williams, F.J.B. & Walshe, J.M. (1981) Wilson's disease. An analysis of the cranial computerised tomographic appearances found in 60 patients and the changes in response to treatment with chelating agents. *Brain* **104**, 735–752.

Wilson, S.A.K. (1912) Progressive lenticular degeneration: a familial nervous disease associated with cirrhosis of the liver. *Brain* **34**, 295–509.

Wilson, S.A.K. (1940) *Neurology*. Edward Arnold, London.

Wing, J.K., Cooper, J.E. & Sartorius, N. (1974) *The Measurement and Classification of Psychiatric Symptoms. An Instruction Manual for the PSE and Catego Program*. Cambridge University Press, Cambridge.

Winikates, J. & Jankovic, J. (1999) Clinical correlates of vascular parkinsonism. *Archives of Neurology* **56**, 98–102.

Wirshing, W.C. (2001) Movement disorders associated with neuroleptic treatment. *Journal of Clinical Psychiatry* **62** (suppl. 21), 15–18.

Woerner, M.G., Alvir, J.M. *et al.* (1998) Prospective study of tardive dyskinesia in the elderly: rates and risk factors. *American Journal of Psychiatry* **155**, 1521–1528.

Wolters, E.C., Hurwitz, T.A. *et al.* (1990) Clozapine in the treatment of parkinsonian patients with dopaminomimetic psychosis. *Neurology* **40**, 832–834.

Wolters, E.C., Jansen, E.N. *et al.* (1996) Olanzapine in the treatment of dopaminomimetic psychosis in patients with Parkinson's disease. *Neurology* **47**, 1085–1087.

Wooten, G.F. (2003) Agonists vs levodopa in PD: the thrilla of whitha. *Neurology* **60**, 360–362.

Yadalam, K.G., Korn, M.L. & Simpson, G.M. (1990) Tardive dystonia: four case histories. *Journal of Clinical Psychiatry* **51**, 17–20.

Yahr, M.D., Duvoisin, R.C., Schear, M.J., Barrett, R.E. & Hoehn, M.M. (1969) Treatment of parkinsonism with levodopa. *Archives of Neurology* **21**, 343–354.

Yamaguchi, Y., Heiny, M.E. *et al.* (1993) Isolation and characterization of a human liver cDNA as a candidate gene for Wilson disease. *Biochemical and Biophysical Research Communications* **197**, 271–277.

Yap, P.M. (1952) The Latah reaction: its pathodynamics and nosological position. *Journal of Mental Science* **98**, 515–564.

Yassa, R. & Jeste, D.V. (1992) Gender differences in tardive dyskinesia: a critical review of the literature. *Schizophrenia Bulletin* **18**, 701–715.

Yassa, R., Nair, V. & Schwartz, G. (1984) Tardive dyskinesia and the primary psychiatric diagnosis. *Psychosomatics* **25**, 135–138.

Yates, A. (1958) The application of learning theory to the treatment of tics. *Journal of Abnormal and Social Psychology* **56**, 175–182.

Zhang, J., Graham, D.G. *et al.* (2000) Enhanced N-methyl-4-phenyl-1,2,3,6-tetrahydropyridine toxicity in mice deficient in CuZn-superoxide dismutase or glutathione peroxidase. *Journal of Neuropathology and Experimental Neurology* **59**, 53–61.

Ziegenbein, M., Steinbrecher, A. *et al.* (2003) Clozapine-induced aplastic anemia in a patient with Parkinson's disease. *Canadian Journal of Psychiatry* **48**, 352.

Zigmond, A.S. & Snaith, R.P. (1983) The Hospital Anxiety and Depression Scale. *Acta Psychiatrica Scandinavica* **67**, 361–370.

13

Sleep Disorders

Meryl Dahlitz and Michael D. Kopelman

Institute of Psychiatry, King's College, London

Normal sleep

No one knows what sleep is for. However, our waking performance, vigilance and vigour, our health and happiness and the quality of our waking lives are profoundly affected by the way we sleep. Some of these features can be measured but others, such as peace of mind and feeling refreshed, cannot. One of the most important functions of sleep, as shown by the prominence of sleep in the young of all species, may be the promotion of brain development. Sleep and waking occur about the same time every day and an important characteristic of sleep is its strong circadian rhythmicity (Fig. 13.1) (Parkes 1985). Although the body has a capacity to make up recent sleep loss, there appears to be no capacity to recuperate from ancient or chronic sleep deprivation. Despite some recent advances, much of the normal physiology of sleep, its anatomical basis and the neurotransmitters involved remain unexplained.

Many laboratories have demonstrated that sleep is not a passive event but an active physiological process, with clearly defined electrocorticographic and behavioural changes, and which depends on specific neurochemical mechanisms and activity of brainstem nuclei and areas extending from the medulla to the posterior diencephalon. The hypothalamus was recognized as a regulator of sleep and wakefulness with the encephalitis lethargica epidemic of 1917–24, when individuals developed major sleep abnormalities and were found to have hypothalamic lesions at post-mortem (Von Economo 1931). The sleep control systems of the hypothalamus interact with the circadian pacemaker in the suprachiasmatic nucleus as well as interacting with other hypothalamic functions such as the regulation of food intake, metabolism, hormone release and core temperature regulation (Mignot *et al.* 2002a). The finding that hypothalamic pathology is associated with aspects of motor control in narcolepsy has led to the hypothesis that the hypothalamus also plays a role in facilitating motor activity tonically and phasically in association with motivated behaviours (Siegel 2004), as well as in the normal atonia of sleep (see below). Animal models of narcolepsy have demonstrated involvement of the hypothalamic neuropeptide hypocretin (also called orexin) in sleep mechanisms. The hypocretin system encompasses two peptides, hypocretin-1 (orexin A) and hypocretin-2 (orexin B), that are both cleaved from a precursor molecule, preprohypocretin, produced by a small number (about 50 000) of specialised cells located in the lateral and perifornical regions of the hypothalamus. Hypocretin neurones have widespread connections throughout the body. The hypocretin system directly and strongly innervates and potently excites noradrenergic, dopaminergic, serotonergic, histaminergic and cholinergic neurones. Hypocretin also has a major role in modulating the release of glutamate and other amino acid transmitters. There is evidence that the arousal effect of hypocretin-1 depends on the activation of histaminergic neurotransmission mediated by the H_1 histamine receptor (Huang *et al.* 2001). Behavioural investigations in animals have revealed that hypocretin is released at high levels in waking especially during periods of increased motor activity and also in rapid eye movement (REM) sleep and at minimal levels in non-REM (NREM) sleep (Siegel 2004). Hypocretin activity may be critical in opposing sleep propensity during periods of prolonged wakefulness (Yoshida *et al.* 2001). There are two known receptors, hcrtr-1 and hcrtr-2, with differential affinity for the two ligands.

Regular cycles of sleep and wakefulness are determined by external factors (zeitgebers) and internal oscillators or biochemical clocks. When separated from all external time cues most humans have a daily sleep–wake cycle and also a temperature cycle time nearer to 25 than 24 hours. More than 100 biological functions vary between maximum and minimum levels over a 24-hour period. Many different

Lishman's Organic Psychiatry: A Textbook of Neuropsychiatry, 4th edition.
© 2009 Blackwell Publishing.   ISBN 978-1-4051-1860 1

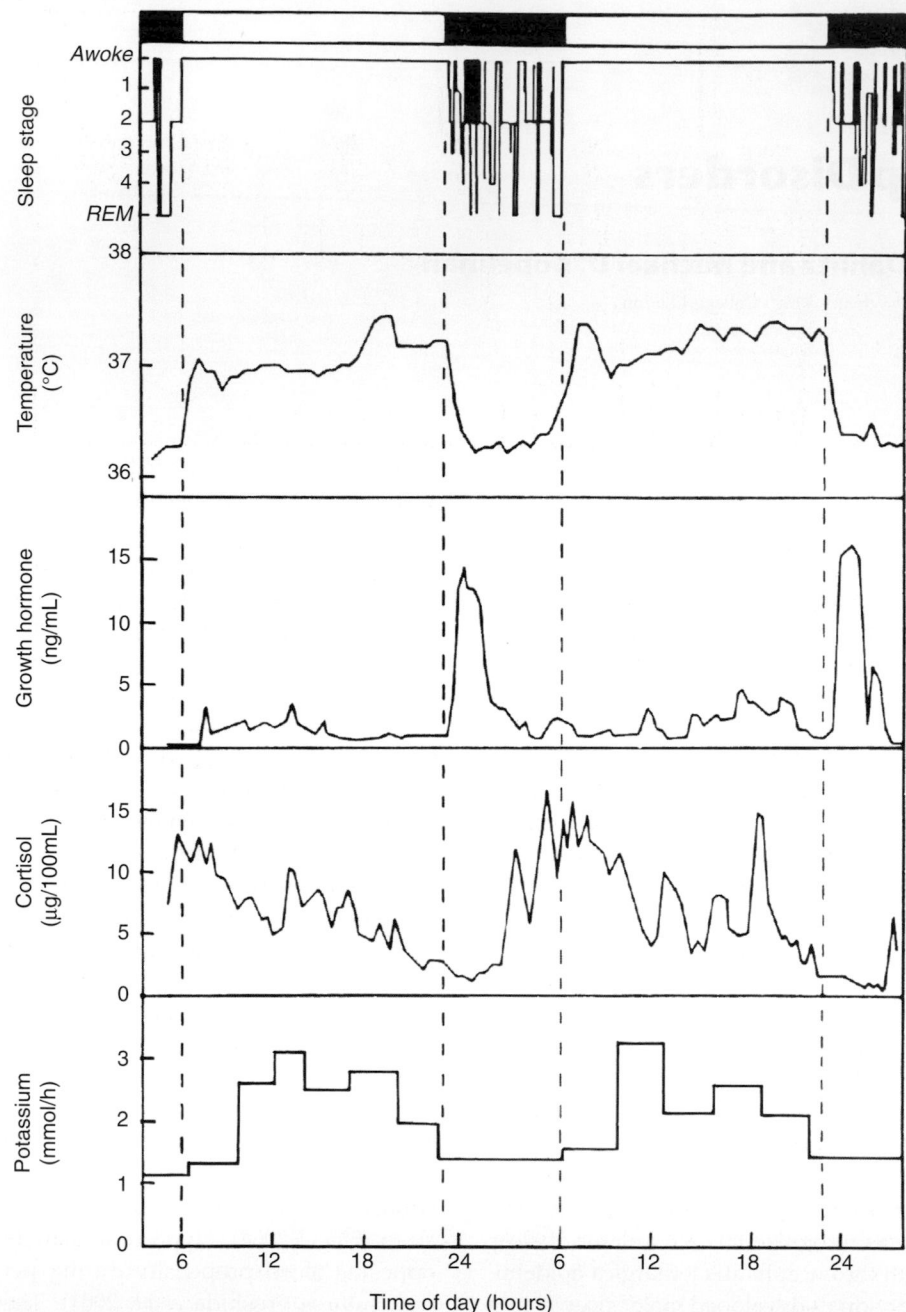

Fig. 13.1 Circadian rhythms in sleep. (Reprinted from Czeisler, C.A. & Richardson, G.S. Circadian timekeeping in health and disease. Part 1. Basic properties of circadian timekeepers. *New England Journal of Medicine* (1983) **309**, 469–476, with permission from Moore-Ede *et al.*)

genetically coded circadian oscillators have been discovered throughout the body but the control of sleep–wake timing appears to be orchestrated by the paired suprachiasmatic nuclei of the hypothalamus. The sensitivity of circadian timekeeping and sleep–wake alternation is exquisite. The phase relationships of oscillatory processes during entrainment to the 24-hour day is timed to facilitate the ability to maintain a consolidated episode of sleep at night (Dijk &

Czeisler 1994). Minor variations in the duration of sleep–wake cycles are corrected within the next and, to a smaller amount, the next but one cycle and a complete phase reversal due to a 12-hour time zone shift can normally be accommodated within a few days. However, adjustment to night shift-work takes longer than recovery from jet-lag and although symptoms usually improve after a week, long-term night-workers often have persistent sleep abnormalities. Although

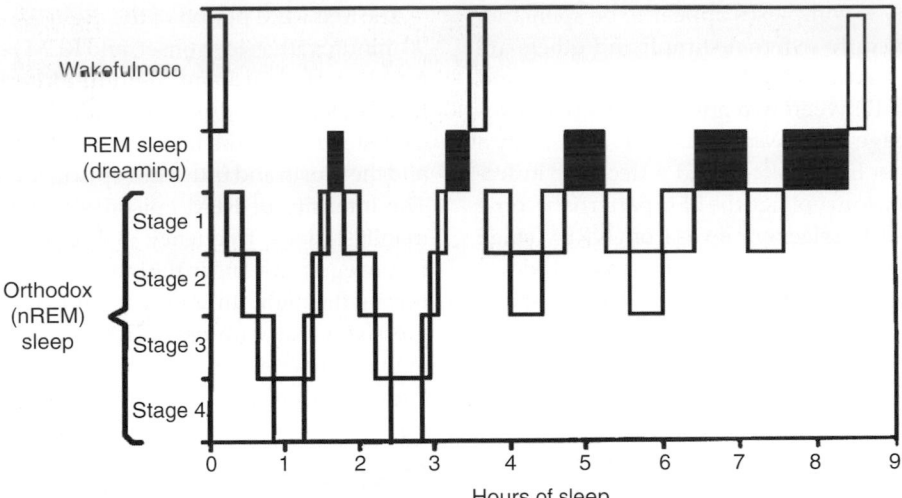

Fig. 13.2 Typical pattern of sleep in a young adult. Sleep stages are shown here during an 8-hour night. The subject enters sleep from wakefulness through Stage 1 and enters progressively deeper sleep stages. The cyclical pattern of progression through sleep stages is evident. REM sleep does not occur until more than 1 hour after sleep onset. REM episodes become more prevalent during the sleep period and are particularly evident in the last third of the night. Brief arousals into wakefulness are common after REM episodes. One is shown here just before the fourth hour of sleep.

adaptation to shiftwork depends on many factors, the most important are the pattern of the shiftwork and the regularity or irregularity of the work schedule. Rotating shiftwork patterns are much more disruptive than fixed shift changes and non-24-hour cycles are particularly difficult. Rotating shifts cause less disturbance to sleep if they progressively phase delay rather than phase advance. There is considerable individual variation in the capacity to synchronise to external time cues (entrain) but generally young people adapt much better than old, with the greatest deterioration in the fourth decade. Normal sleep habits play a large part in determining ability to adapt to shiftwork. People who spontaneously wake early, 'larks' on the Horne and Ostberg (1976) scale, generally have less variable sleep and awakening times and less capacity to adapt to shiftwork than 'owls'.

Different behavioural forms of sleep were described by Macnish (1830) but the concurrent brain electrical changes were not clearly recognised until the development of the electroencephalogram (EEG). Loomis *et al.* (1935) identified five different patterns of electrical activity in the brain that formed the basis for all subsequent classifications of sleep stages. In 1953, Aserinski and Kleitman identified periodic bursts of eye movement during sleep that were different from the slow rolling eye movements that accompany sleep onset. These periodic eye movements were associated with dreaming by Dement and Kleitman (1957). This state of sleep is now commonly known as REM sleep.

Three basic parameters are required to define sleep stage: EEG, electro-oculogram and electromyogram. With regard to EEG, sleep is composed of four NREM stages and one REM stage. The two very different kinds of sleep alternate in regular cycles (Fig. 13.2). In addition to characteristic variations in spontaneous activity of the brain, there are also changes in evoked activity with sensory stimulation. During both wakefulness and sleep, spontaneous EEG activity can be divided into four frequency bands: beta (>12 Hz), alpha (8–12 Hz), theta (4–8 Hz) and delta (1–3 Hz). The amplitude of these waves is generally greater for slow than for fast frequencies, partly because of a filter effect of the skull and scalp. At sleep onset, the alpha rhythm of relaxed wakefulness gradually reduces in frequency, waxing and waning and eventually giving way to a low-voltage irregular pattern characteristic of stage 1 NREM sleep. The rapid eye movements of wakefulness give way to slow rolling or horizontal eye movements.

Stage 1 NREM sleep lasts about 30 seconds to 7 minutes. If aroused, subjects usually report being half-awake. Three characteristic patterns emerge on the EEG of stage 2 NREM sleep: sleep spindles, vertex sharp waves and K potentials. Sleep spindles are so called because the waves at the start and the end of brief bursts of activity of 12–15 Hz are of lower amplitude than the waves in the middle, thereby resembling a spindle shape. Sleep spindles are present in NREM stages 2, 3 and 4. However, since they are superimposed on large-amplitude slow waves in NREM stages 3 and 4, they are difficult to see with the naked eye. About five spindles occur each minute in stage 2 and some are associated with K complexes. K complexes appear to be non-specific evoked potentials characteristic of NREM sleep, and combine a frontal slow wave, a central spindle and a vertex sharp wave. On the EEG, they appear as an initial negative wave followed 0.75 seconds later by a positive wave simultaneously over all areas of the head. Although many K complexes appear to be spontaneous, some are responses to external stimuli and others are provoked by internal autonomic activity such as gut and bladder contractions. Between two and three K complexes occur each minute. Stage 3 NREM sleep is characterised by a continuous increase in EEG voltage and a decrease in frequency. With the increase in voltage the EEG patterns become more synchronised. As the sleeper moves from NREM stage 3 to NREM stage 4 sleep, the EEG becomes increasingly dominated by slow delta waves. Stage 3 sleep is relatively stable across different age groups but the high abundance of slow waves characteristic of stage 4 is typical of sleep in young people. The proportion of stage 4 rapidly diminishes with age so that there is little or none left by the age of 60.

There is a progressive increase in the stimulus threshold necessary to produce arousal through NREM stages 1 to 4. Noise stimuli that are subthreshold for arousal may not cause any alteration in the EEG. NREM stages 3 and 4 occur within 30–45 minutes in healthy young adults and last from a few minutes to an hour. Usually, NREM stage 4 is followed by a brief episode of stage 2 NREM before the first REM period.

The first REM period of the night usually commences 75–90 minutes after sleep onset, and REM periods alternate with NREM periods at about 90-minute intervals during a normal night's sleep. The duration of REM episodes increases with each sleep cycle, the first lasting between 5 and 10 minutes and the fourth and fifth REM episodes lasting 20–60 minutes. The intensity of REM episodes in terms of physiological manifestations, frequency of eye movements and respiratory irregularity, and in the intensity of dreams, also increases during the night. In contrast, NREM stages 3 and 4 are progressively lost, with less NREM stages 3–4 in the second than in the first cycle, and often no NREM stages 3–4 at all in the late cycles (see Fig. 13.3).

Sleep disorders

Sleep disorders are increasingly recognised and are associated with significant morbidity (Kryger *et al.* 2000). There are four main categories of sleep disorder in recent classification: dyssomnias, parasomnias, medical/psychiatric sleep disorders, and proposed sleep disorders. Although the term

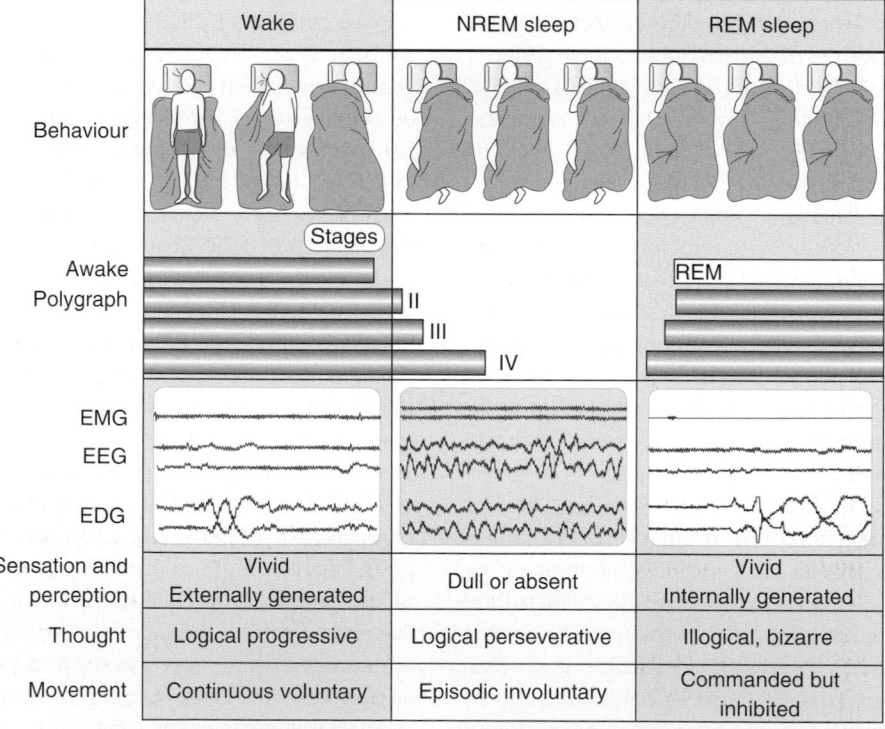

Fig. 13.3 Behavioural states in humans. States of waking, NREM sleep and REM sleep have behavioural, polygraphic and psychological manifestations. In the row labelled behaviour, changes in position (detectable by time-lapse photography or video) can occur during waking and in concert with phase changes of the sleep cycle. Two different mechanisms account for sleep immobility. The first is disfacilitation (during stages I–IV of NREM sleep). The second is inhibition (during REM sleep). During dreams, we imagine that we move, but we do not. Sample tracings of three variables used to distinguish the state are shown: an electromyogram (EMG), an electroencephalogram (EEG) and electro-oculogram (EOG). The EMG tracings are highest during waking, intermediate during NREM sleep and lowest during REM sleep. The EEG and EOG are both activated during waking and inactivated during NREM sleep. Each sample shown is approximately 20 seconds long. The three bottom rows describe other subjective and objective state variables. From J Allan Hobson (2005) Sleep is of the brain, by the brain and for the brain. *Nature* **437**, 1254–1256.

'dyssomnia' was previously applied to any disorder of sleep or wakefulness, it is now confined to the primary sleep disorders. Dyssomnias produce insomnia and/or excessive sleepiness and without these symptoms the dyssomnias would not exist. The dyssomnias are divided into three groups: intrinsic sleep disorders, extrinsic sleep disorders and circadian rhythm disorders.

The international classification of sleep disorders is based on assumptions about the pathophysiology of the disorders and may seem arbitrary at first glance. For example, post-traumatic hypersomnia would not exist without the external event that produced the head injury. However, because the hypersomnia appears to be of central nervous system (CNS) origin and persists after the traumatic event, it is classified as an intrinsic sleep disorder. Similarly, an adjustment sleep disorder is due to psychological factors and so could be considered to be internally generated. However, an external event is the cause and if removed the sleep disorder resolves. Consequently, this is classified as an extrinsic sleep disorder.

Intrinsic dyssomnias: insomnia

Insomnia is a subjective phenomenon of difficulty falling asleep, repeated waking and/or early-morning arousal. Also patients may report not feeling refreshed by sleep. Insomnia is difficult to verify objectively and there is often little correlation between the report of sleeplessness and laboratory recordings of sleep. Psychological factors contribute to insomnia in up to 80% of cases (Nicholson & Marks 1983) Nevertheless, people who do complain of insomnia mostly sleep worse than controls, sleep less, and wake up in the night more often (Frankel et al. 1976). It is unknown whether some people need more sleep, or sleep of a different pattern from that which they habitually obtain. Some subjects, who have very disturbed sleep whilst in the sleep laboratory, do not complain about either sleeping or waking. Sleep laboratory investigations rarely reveal a cause but a diagnosis may be reached by taking a careful clinical history.

The complaint of insomnia is far more common than any other complaint about sleep. Questionnaire surveys show that up to one-third of the general population experiences sleeplessness, although the prevalence varies from country to country. Family practice surveys show that far fewer complain to their doctors about insomnia than experience sleeplessness from time to time. About 3% of the population take hypnotic medication at least occasionally. Overall, women complain twice as often about their sleep as men, and housewives are particularly bad sleepers. Insomnia is frequently associated with depression, mania, anxiety, anorexia nervosa, obsessive–compulsive neurosis and schizophrenia. In normal subjects, insomnia may be caused by stress, such as bereavement, examinations or sickness. Kales and Kales (1983) showed that the complaint of insomnia was most common in subjects from lower socioeconomic groups and of poor education. Unsurprisingly, both heavy drinkers and heavy smokers describe themselves as sleeping less than non-drinkers and non-smokers. Paradoxically, oversleeping for long periods or merely staying in bed can lead to a feeling of poor sleep and sometimes the complaint of insomnia.

The frequency and severity of insomnia increase with age in both sexes. In the normal population, periods of waking during the night become increasingly common with age. Total sleep time decreases from an average of 8 hours daily in young adulthood to about 6 hours daily at age 90. This is accompanied by more nocturnal arousals. These changes begin in early adulthood: 30-year-olds have only half as much stage 4 NREM as 20 year olds and experience twice as much nocturnal wakefulness. In comparison the proportion of REM sleep remains relatively constant, at about 22% of total sleep time, but the preservation of REM sleep in the elderly correlates with the preservation of intelligence. There is much less REM sleep time amongst the elderly demented. The causes of insomnia in the elderly include medical disorders, pain, psychological and social factors, absence of regular activities, minimal exercise, daytime naps, and worries about health, money and/or ultimate destiny. Sleep apnoea and sleep myoclonus, both of which are increasingly prevalent with age, may present as insomnia in some cases. However, the normal deterioration of sleep processes with age may be responsible for much insomnia experienced in the elderly (Regelstein 1980). There is much evidence that the ubiquitous overuse of sedative medication in the elderly is harmful. Daytime sedation, agitation, confusion and disturbed behaviour may disappear when the sedatives are stopped. Sleep apnoea, present in up to 50% of people over 65, is exacerbated by hypnotics (Guilleminault et al. 1978). In patients with dementia, who often experience an exaggeration of the normal age-related changes in sleep and are often confused and restless at night, sedatives can be particularly unhelpful and can cause paroxysmal rage and exacerbate behavioural disturbance.

Common observation shows that the more deeply one sleeps, the more alert one is when awake but this is surprisingly difficult to quantify. Initiation and motivation may suffer after a poor night's sleep, although there may be no deterioration in simple motor or memory tasks. The major effect of insomnia in patients is to cause sleepiness, fatigue, lack of concentration, and sometimes muscle-aching and mild depression, similar to the effects of sleep deprivation experiments in healthy young adults.

In those who regularly sleep for only short periods, the mortality rate is surprisingly high (Kripke et al. 1979; Kripe et al. 1983). Medical conditions inducing insomnia and leading to the taking of sleeping pills would be expected to produce a high death rate. Amongst those who sleep only 6 hours or less, there is a high mortality rate for ischaemic heart disease, stroke and cancer (Wingard 1983). The relative mortality rate of short sleepers was 1.3 times that of normal sleepers when correction was made for age, sex, race, socioeconomic status, physical health, weight, smoking and alcohol consumption.

Much information can be derived from a consideration of the pattern of the insomnia. Difficulty falling asleep, with a sleep latency greater than 30 minutes, is usually related to anxiety, depression, bereavement, accident, environmental stimuli or drugs. The high level of arousal that prevents sleep onset may be associated with high plasma noradrenaline (norepinephrine) levels. High noradrenaline levels may also explain the insomnia of physiological starvation. Sleep maintenance insomnia, with frequent arousals, has many causes. Drugs, particularly alcohol or daytime stimulants, and hypnotic withdrawal should be considered. Medical and psychiatric illness, parasomnias, sleep apnoea, restless legs and sleep myoclonus are also common causes. Frequent arousals at 90-minute intervals are almost always due to REM sleep nightmares. Awakenings from REM sleep are also characteristic of cluster headaches. Random arousals from both REM and NREM sleep are typical of sleep apnoea and anxiety. Early-morning awakening without further sleeping is characteristic of both depression and hypomania, although it may occur with any kind of excitement. Phase-shift disorders can masquerade as insomnia; however, despite unusual sleep onset times, sleep is normal in duration. Cyclical insomnia can be due to recurrent unipolar or bipolar depression, or occasionally menstrual or endocrine disorders.

The history of the insomnia is also helpful diagnostically. Transient insomnia is experienced by everyone several times during their lives and has many causes, including stress, illness, childbirth, drugs, emotional crisis and jet-lag. The patient may experience sleep-onset insomnia, maintenance insomnia or premature awakening. Regardless of form, transient insomnia recovers within 2–4 weeks.

In contrast, chronic insomnia may be lifelong. Idiopathic chronic insomnia accounts for up to one-quarter of all cases of chronic insomnia. It begins early in life with fragmented short sleep episodes and persists as fitful sleep of only 3–4 hours at night in adulthood with early waking and insomnia by day as well as by night. Patients complain of fatigue, irritability and symptoms of somatic depression. It is sometimes familial. Occasionally there are signs of minimal brain damage, dyslexia or hyperkinesis and there may be minor EEG abnormalities during sleep. Clinically, idiopathic insomnia may be impossible to differentiate from chronic psychophysiological insomnia when it presents in adulthood. Both conditions are difficult to treat successfully using drugs, conditioning or biofeedback. Relaxation therapy may be helpful in a proportion of patients.

Most chronic insomnias are secondary to an obvious medical, psychiatric or behavioural problem. Common neurological causes of insomnia include head injury, infection, parkinsonism, encephalitis, psychomotor and general-ised seizures, cortical and subcortical lesions, spinal cord damage, cerebrovascular disease and dementia. Insomnia in neurological disorders may be the result of (i) primary involvement of sleep mechanisms, for example in progressive supranuclear palsy; (ii) abnormal sensory mechanisms, for example in spinal cord lesions; or (iii) stress, discomfort and pain as with nerve or root compression, disc lesions, night cramps or fibrositis. Common medical causes of night waking due to pain include ulcer pain, nocturnal angina, nocturnal asthma and chronic or intermittent airflow obstruction. Metabolic diseases can disturb sleep by affecting sleep mechanisms. Chronic renal insufficiency causes short, fragmented, disorganised sleep. Following dialysis or transplantation, sleep may improve but it rarely becomes normal. Poor sleep in uraemia has been attributed to irreversible neuronal damage but is more likely to be the result of metabolic disturbance. Hyperthyroidism can cause fragmented short sleep with excessive delta activity; hypothyroidism causes excessive sleepiness with lack of delta activity and obstructive sleep apnoea. Following return to the euthyroid condition, sleep can be slow to recover, taking up to 1 year to become normal. Up to one-quarter of acromegalics develop disturbed sleep due to obstructive sleep apnoea. Hypogonadism and menopause can also cause insomnia.

Psychiatric illness frequently causes a greater degree of sleep disturbance than any other cause of insomnia. Severe depression is usually accompanied by difficulty staying asleep and early-morning arousal, but often without delay in sleep onset, whereas in mania the onset of sleep is delayed and sleep is short. Most patients with bipolar illness sleep more when they are depressed and less when they are manic. During the switch from depression to mania, several days may pass without sleep. Sleep is always shortened in mild manic disorder (hypomania) and gravely disturbed in severe mania. There is more variation in the pattern of sleep disturbance in depression; some depressed patients sleep for excessively long not short periods, whilst others have apparently normal sleep. Patients often find that their sleep is unrefreshing. Sleep disturbance is often the first symptom of depression, and restoration of sleep may be the first sign of recovery. The sleep pattern in obsessive–compulsive neurosis is similar to that found in depression, with poor sleep and frequent awakenings, short sleep time, short REM latency and little stage 4 NREM. As in depression, some patients develop hypersomnia.

Anxiety characteristically causes sleep-onset insomnia. Ruminations may maintain a level of arousal that prevents sleep onset. Sleep disturbance as the result of anxiety is more common in young people than in the elderly. Many patients with insomnia dread a further bad night's sleep. This may result in fear and panic, increased arousal and a self-fulfilling prophecy. A phobia of sleepless nights may develop. Relaxation and behaviour therapy may be helpful to these patients. Schizophrenia may be accompanied by severe sleep disturbance, but the sleep pattern in chronic schizophrenia is usually normal and with a normal proportion of REM.

Drugs are a common cause of chronic insomnia. Alcohol can have a profound effect on sleep, and sleep may be totally abolished during heavy binges. More moderate doses of alcohol shorten sleep latency but cause subsequent sleep disruption. Intoxication causes an increase in delta sleep and a decrease with withdrawal. There is a marked but variable decrease in slow-wave sleep following alcohol withdrawal, perhaps related to different levels of tolerance. There is a dose-dependent depression of REM sleep with a compensatory increase on withdrawal. Depending on the alcohol dose, the compensatory REM sleep rebound on withdrawal may occur on the same night or on the following night. Delirium tremens is closely correlated with increased REM time, and some of the agitation in delirium tremens may be caused by REM breakthrough into wakefulness. Chronic alcoholics have fragmented sleep, with little or no delta sleep, decreased REM sleep and many arousals. The sleep–wake cycle becomes disrupted, with excessive daytime sleepiness and frequent naps. Normal motor inhibition of REM sleep may be lost and electromyographic activity during REM is increased not decreased. The sleep of alcoholics can remain disturbed for as long as 2 years after alcohol withdrawal, with difficulty falling asleep, frequent arousals and reduced delta sleep. Sleep changes, particularly loss of REM sleep and alcohol-provoked sleep apnoea, may contribute to memory impairment in chronic alcoholics.

Caffeine, mainly from coffee, tea, cola and chocolate, is another common cause of sleep disruption. The caffeine dose in four cups of coffee at bedtime will cause a marked increase in nocturnal arousals in normal subjects. Caffeine increases arousals even in people who claim to be unaffected by it.

The acute administration of a short half-life hypnotic may cause early-morning rebound insomnia and anxiety, not sedation, the morning after. Withdrawal from chronic use of short-acting hypnotic drugs can lead to a temporary insomnia of profound severity. The severity of rebound insomnia is related to dose, the period of administration and the pharmacokinetics of the drug used, and in some cases the pharmacokinetics of the drug's metabolites. With a short-acting benzodiazepine (e.g. triazolam) the rapid disappearance of the drug from the receptors to which it is bound can result in severe rebound insomnia and anxiety that can last for a few days and nights after a short period of drug administration; after a more prolonged period of use, the rebound insomnia may last as long as 2–3 weeks. Drugs that are more rapidly eliminated give rise to an earlier withdrawal syndrome; withdrawal of drugs with long half-lives may have a latency of several days before rebound symptoms occur. Severe

rebound insomnia is usually more prominent in old rather than young people.

Drugs other than alcohol, caffeine and hypnotics may disrupt sleep. Common culprits include nicotine, beta-blockers, α-methyldopa, phenytoin, bronchodilators, monoamine oxidase inhibitors, amphetamine and other CNS stimulants, anorectic drugs, thiazides and other diuretics.

Patients with acute insomnia may benefit from the short-term use of hypnotics. To obtain maximum benefit, hypnotics should be prescribed at the minimum therapeutic dose and for the briefest period. Tolerance may be minimised by taking a low-dose sedative only intermittently, perhaps every third night. Despite their sedative properties, antidepressants and antihistamines should not be used primarily to treat insomnia due to their long half-lives and their peripheral side effects. The use of two sedatives simultaneously should be avoided as they may potentiate each other and result in dangerous oversedation. Most hypnotics target GABAergic activity globally in the brain. The choice of hypnotic should be informed by a match of pharmacokinetic profiles and the clinical presentation. A rapidly absorbed drug that quickly reaches a peak plasma concentration and has a rapid elimination half-life would be appropriate for a patient with acute sleep-onset insomnia but offers no benefit for an individual with early-morning awakening. Sedation during the following day is a more common effect of drugs with longer elimination half-lives. However, there is considerable variation in the elimination half-life between individuals taking the same drug. Absorption, metabolism and elimination become slower with age. Changes in protein binding, the volume of distribution of the drug as well as changes in tissue sensitivity also occur with advancing years. It is important that the plasma half-life of the drug and its active metabolites is less than 24 hours (or the interdose interval), because the drug may accumulate and cause a confusional state. Hypnotics depress respiration and so should be avoided in patients in whom respiration is already compromised, for example patients with sleep apnoea or chronic airflow obstruction. However, 'pink puffers' may benefit from the use of tranquillisers.

Circadian rhythm disturbances

Circadian disturbance of the sleep–wake rhythm may account for about 10% of insomnia. This may be due to entrainment failure that is sometimes secondary to blindness but may also occur in subjects with normal vision. Weitzman *et al.* (1981) identified a group of insomniacs with a phase-lag syndrome. Patients with the delayed sleep phase syndrome complain of sleep-onset insomnia and difficulty awakening at the desired time. Typically they experience chronic difficulty falling asleep until 2–6 a.m. but do not have difficulty maintaining sleep. There is a severe or, very rarely, absolute inability to advance the sleep phase and enforced wake times result in sleep deprivation. Daytime sleepiness and irritability, particularly in the morning hours, depends largely on the amount of sleep loss that has resulted from the patient's effort to wake up 'on time'. Patients usually score very high as 'owls' on the 'owl–lark' scale (Horne & Ostberg 1976) and feel most alert during the late evening and night hours. When given the opportunity to sleep late, for example on holidays or weekends, waking times are fairly consistently delayed. Hypnotic drugs and alcohol may complicate the presentation and a sleep–wake log may help to demonstrate the pattern of insomnia. Patients often try hypnotics in an effort to advance sleep onset but they are rarely effective in normal doses, although they may aggravate morning sleepiness. The syndrome usually develops in adolescents, although childhood cases have been described. Familial cases have been reported and it appears to be more common in males. Motor activity monitoring and melatonin profiles are normal (Alvarez *et al*. 1992). Sleep hygiene is very important. Depression should be considered if the symptoms are refractory to behavioural intervention in an apparently cooperative patient.

An advanced sleep phase syndrome, with sleep onset at 8–9 p.m. and waking at 3–5 a.m. has been recognised but is much less common than delayed sleep phase syndrome. Recent studies have shown that mutations in the *hPER2* gene are associated with autosomal dominant familial advanced sleep phase syndrome (Taheri & Mignot 2002). Certainly early-onset sleep and waking cause much less social and work disruption than the opposite pattern.

Disturbance of circadian rhythms may be due to damage of the circadian pacemaker in the hypothalamus, perhaps as a result of a tumour. A totally irregular sleep–wake pattern is occasionally seen following head injury.

Narcolepsy

The narcoleptic syndrome is characterised by excessive daytime sleepiness with attacks of daytime somnolence, usually irresistible in intensity and leading to several short episodes of sleep per day ('narcoleptic attacks'). Cataplexy, in which the patient abruptly loses muscle tone in response to some emotionally provoking stimulus, usually laughter, must also be present in order to make a definite diagnosis. Hypnagogic hallucinations and episodes of sleep paralysis are also characteristic of the syndrome in its most complete expression, and considerable disturbance of nocturnal sleep commonly occurs.

Gelineau (1880) gave the first definite description of the disorder, and analysed 14 cases in his monograph (Gelineau 1881). Thereafter, the term 'narcolepsy' came to be applied rather indiscriminately to many varieties of morbid somnolence, some due to structural brain lesions and others associated with psychiatric disorders, resulting in a good deal of nosological confusion and faulty discussion about aetiology.

Gradually the condition was established as a distinct disease entity. Both the strong association with the human leucocyte antigen (HLA) discovered in 1984 (Honda *et al*. 1984; Langdon *et al*. 1984) and low cerebrospinal fluid (CSF) hypocretin levels are most closely associated with cataplexy rather than any of the other features of the syndrome. Association with these biological markers underscores the specificity of cataplexy in clinical diagnosis. The great majority of cases have no gross structural brain pathology but microscopic postmortem studies have found absence of the 50 000 cells that produce preprohypocretin in the lateral hypothalamus. Family members may have narcoleptic symptoms, particularly the relatives of non-HLA-associated cases. Fresh interest has been brought to the syndrome since the finding of a mutation in the gene coding for one of the hypocretin receptors in narcoleptic dogs and the demonstration of a narcolepsy-like state in preprohypocretin knockout mice. However, with one interesting exception, narcoleptic humans do not have mutations of the genes coding for preprohypocretin or either of its known receptors (Mignot 2004).

Clinical features

Detailed accounts of the disorder are to be found in Guilleminault *et al*. (1976) and Parkes (1985). The onset is usually between the ages of 10 and 30 years and is rare after 40. The precise time of onset may be hard to determine, relatives often becoming aware of the problem before the patient himself. Males and females are probably equally liable to the disorder. At least one-quarter of cases have relatives with excessive daytime sleepiness but cataplexy is rare except in the 2% of families where the proband does not carry the HLA type DQB1*0602 usually associated with the syndrome. Of the handful of HLA-typed twins reported in the literature, only the HLA-non-associated cases were concordant for cataplexy.

Approximately three-quarters of cases have at least one of the accessory symptoms in addition to excessive daytime sleepiness and cataplexy: hypnagogic hallucinations in 20–80% and sleep paralysis in 20–60%. The 'tetrad' of all four symptoms occurs in less than 10%. Between 60% and 80% of patients complain of poor nocturnal sleep. Diagnostic uncertainty may arise in the early stages of the disease when narcoleptic attacks antedate the development of cataplexy. In a large series of patients with cataplexy, Yoss and Daly (1960) found that this had set in at the same time as the narcoleptic attacks in 55%, 1–5 years later in 25% and more than 10 years later in 15%. One may therefore encounter patients in whom daytime sleep attacks constitute the sole manifestation for some considerable time. Cataplexy antedating narcolepsy is distinctly uncommon but 'isolated cataplexy', without excessive daytime sleepiness, has been reported. In contrast, sleep paralysis and hypnagogic hallucinations are frequently encountered in the general population. These relatively non-specific symptoms may be precipitated by drugs or changes in sleep habit.

Once it has commenced the disorder appears to persist throughout life. Apparent diminution in severity may be the consequence of deliberate effort to avoid the emotionally provocative stimuli of cataplexy, strategic napping during the day and/or the effect of medication. However, there is no evidence that long-term use of any medications alters the eventual prognosis. Very occasionally remissions and exacerbations have been described, but in most large series this has not been the case. Narcolepsy does not appear to affect lifespan.

Narcoleptic attacks consist of an overwhelming sense of drowsiness, usually leading to a brief period of actual sleep. They are commonly of daily occurrence and with several attacks per day. The period of sleep usually lasts some 10–15 minutes though may be much longer according to circumstances. If the majority of attacks exceed 30 minutes, Roth (1980) classifies the disorder as idiopathic hypersomnia. However, both long and short sleep episodes occur in the daytime in patients with narcoleptic syndrome, as well as in patients with daytime drowsiness from other causes such as sleep apnoea, and the boundary between short sleep attacks and more prolonged daytime sleep episodes is sometimes doubtful (Parkes 1985). The patient may complain either of episodic sleep attacks with reasonable alertness between, or more rarely of fighting a constant battle against drowsiness during the day. Yoss and Daly (1957) divided the syndrome into type I and type II varieties on this basis. Patients with circumscribed sleep attacks will often be found to have episodes of quite profound drowsiness between, although they may not themselves be fully aware of this. Brief 'microsleeps' lasting 10–20 seconds are also common, as shown by electroencephalography (EEG), yet may not be apparent to the patient or observers.

Sleep episodes are commoner in situations normally conducive to drowsiness: after meals, in monotonous, warm surroundings, whilst travelling and as the day progresses. Usually there is a period of a minute or two during which the patient struggles against actual sleep. However, in severe examples attacks can occur in any situation: while talking, eating, working or when engaged in other activities. Attacks while swimming or driving may very occasionally endanger life, though the prodromal drowsiness will almost always serve as a warning. Some patients are extremely irritable when prevented from falling asleep or when suddenly awakened. Typically the patient awakes refreshed, and there is then a refractory period of several hours before the next attack can occur. Some, however, remain drowsy and obtunded on awaking.

Cataplectic attacks consist of sudden immobility or decrease of muscle tone, which may be generalised or limited to certain muscle groups. In severe attacks the patient collapses in a flaccid heap and is totally unable to move or speak. Serious falls and injuries are uncommon because there is usually a brief period of awareness preceding episodes of generalised cataplexy where the subject can assume a protective posture. Tendon reflexes are abolished for a while and extensor plantar reflexes have been observed. However, the patient typically remains fully alert and is aware of what is proceeding around him. Mild episodes may show only as drooping of the jaw, head nodding, or a sense of weakness obliging the patient to sit down or lean against a wall. Objects may be dropped or the knees buckle. Dysarthria, aphonia or ptosis may accompany attacks, and double vision or momentary difficulty with focusing may be the sole manifestation. Facial fasciculation is not uncommon and is the result of oscillating degrees of paresis. Brief partial cataplexy may be so subtle as to pass unnoticed by others. Pallor, pupillary dilation, sweating and an increase in pulse rate are sometimes observed but may be due to the shock that precipitated the attack and not the attack itself. The respiratory muscles are relatively spared and incontinence, when it occurs, is not due to cataplexy but to stress. Very occasionally, consciousness may be briefly clouded during attacks but this should be regarded as exceptional (Roth 1980).

The attacks are of short duration, usually lasting several seconds and rarely more than a minute. Occasionally, the emotional response of the patient, either to the original stimulus or to the cataplexy, may provoke further episodes of cataplexy in succession. This is called status cataplecticus. Alternatively, status cataplecticus may occur spontaneously without any apparent trigger. Status cataplecticus is confined to patients with severe cataplexy and may last minutes, hours or days. It is most likely to occur at the onset of the illness or during tricyclic drug withdrawal. The frequency and severity of cataplexy varies from several episodes per day to a single attack in many years. Episodes are more likely to occur when background vigilance is low, particularly after sleep deprivation or the use of sedative drugs (Parkes 1985).

Over 95% of cataplexy attacks are the result of sudden increases in emotional arousal. The typical triggering stimuli are so specific that cataplexy can almost always be diagnosed with confidence. Precipitation by emotional stimuli is usually strikingly evident in the history, in particular precipitation by laughter. Cataplexy is also likely to occur when the subject feels a combination of excitement, anticipation and the need for a motor response, for example during sport, sexual intercourse, being tickled, hunting, attempts at repartee, showing off or joke telling, but any strong emotion may bring on an attack: surprise, fear, outbursts of anger or feelings of exaltation. Cataplexy may very occasionally be precipitated by sneezing, coughing or nose blowing. Many patients learn to avoid provoking situations, and to check any inclination to laugh in order to avoid attacks. Sometimes, however, they can occur without any discernible affective stimulus.

Cataplexy may occur with no hint of excessive sleepiness. One possibility is that isolated cataplexy is an unusual manifestation of the narcoleptic syndrome in which the other symptoms have not yet made their appearance. In individual cases presenting with cataplexy it is not possible to predict whether they will develop additional symptoms of the narcoleptic syndrome (Roth 1980). Bogaert (1936) first described its familial occurrence. Geladi and Brown (1967) reported a rare example of a family in which typical laughter-induced cataplexy appeared to be transmitted as an autosomal dominant trait. Eleven members were affected from childhood onwards, with no hint of narcoleptic attacks in eight. Sleep paralysis was an occasional accompaniment. Roth (1980) reported families with cataplexy only and no other symptoms of the narcoleptic syndrome. HLA typing has not been reported in these families.

Hypnagogic hallucinations are vivid perceptual experiences occurring at sleep onset, often with the realistic awareness of the presence of someone or something. Up to 50% of narcoleptic individuals have frequent hypnagogic hallucinations but some are anxious about disclosing their experiences because they erroneously fear a psychiatric aetiology. Hypnagogic episodes in normal subjects occur in stage 1 NREM sleep, whilst those of narcoleptics are often accompanied by REM sleep and so should more accurately be termed 'pre-sleep dreams' (Parkes 1986). In the narcoleptic syndrome, pre-sleep dreams most commonly occur in multiple modalities, usually auditory, visual and/or tactile. They are experienced during the transition from wakefulness to sleep, or rather less commonly during the phase of recovery from sleep (hypnopompic dreams). Not uncommonly they occur simultaneously with episodes of sleep paralysis. They may be experienced in the middle of the night when the patient has roused for a while, and they sometimes accompany daytime narcoleptic attacks. Typically, pre-sleep dreams are intensely vivid and seem to be real at the time. The patient may react momentarily in accordance with what he is experiencing. Later, however, when fully awake, he almost always recognises their alien character. Lively accompanying affects, especially of terror, are widely reported as characteristic. Roth and Bruhova (1969) stressed the kaleidoscopic nature and bizarre character of the visions. (Zarcone 1973) suggested that the pre-sleep experiences of narcoleptics differ from those of normals in their complex dream-like quality and the intensity of the accompanying emotion, whereas non-narcoleptics usually experience a mere word or image with little affective meaning.

Sleep paralysis consists of attacks of transient inability to move that emerge in the stage between wakefulness and sleep. In narcoleptics they typically occur while falling asleep, both at night and with daytime sleep attacks. Usually they are infrequent, rarely occurring more than once or twice per week.

The onset is abrupt, with the patient suddenly aware that he can neither speak nor move. The paralysis is flaccid and usually complete, though some patients can open their eyes or even cry out briefly. As with cataplectic attacks the episodes are brief, lasting several seconds and rarely more than a minute. Unlike cataplexy, the episode is usually dispelled abruptly if the patient's name is called or if he is touched or shaken. Otherwise it resolves spontaneously. Intense alarm is usually provoked. Dream mentation sometimes accompanies the attack and may lead the patient to fear that he is to be harmed or attacked.

Sleep paralysis is not specific to the narcoleptic syndrome and may occur in up to 62% of the normal population (Dahlitz & Parkes 1993). It is more likely at times of sleep disruption, for example with jet-lag or the use of sedative hypnotic medication. Frequent sleep paralysis without other symptoms is very rare but may be strongly familial (Roth & Bruhova 1969).

Disturbed nocturnal sleep is also characteristic of narcoleptics, occurring in 60–80% of patients. They fall asleep promptly but thereafter are restless, wake again often and may speak, shout or even walk about the room. Sleep myoclonus occurs in up to half of patients. The lost nocturnal sleep is made up during the daytime, so overall the total sleep time per 24 hours is normal. Vivid and terrifying dreams are common, occurring in some 60% of patients with the narcoleptic syndrome and some 20% of those with excessive daytime sleepiness alone (Roth & Bruhova 1969). Themes of murder or of being pursued are said to be common.

Other symptoms. A variety of other symptoms are reported from time to time. Somnambulism is occasionally a pronounced feature. A rapid weight gain at onset may be observed, and libido or potency may become impaired. Hypogenitality, a feminine hair distribution, polyuria and polydipsia are very occasionally present. Bouts of amnesia can occur as an occasional complication; the patient suddenly realises he has no knowledge of the past few minutes and has to check what has been done, usually discovering that he has continued to function normally during most of the time. Roth (1980) and Parkes (1986) also report that automatic behaviour may feature in narcolepsy. The patient tries to overcome his sleepiness and carry on activities but loses awareness of what transpires; he may continue talking without making sense, his handwriting may suddenly change to meaningless scribble, or he may continue walking and wake in fresh surroundings. Such episodes are prone to occur in one-third of patients, sometimes closely resembling episodes of transient global amnesia.

Differential diagnosis

Sometimes the patient's symptoms have long been attributed by relatives or employers to laziness, irresponsibility or emotional instability. There are no abnormalities on physical examination or routine laboratory tests, and the diagnosis rests essentially on a careful history. REM episodes at sleep onset may be discovered with polysomnography, and although they may support a diagnostic suspicion the clinical history has proved the most robust basis for diagnosis in genetic studies. HLA typing may be useful in confirming the diagnosis, since if the patient is negative for the HLA antigen in question (DQB1*0602) the diagnosis of narcolepsy must be considered very unlikely (Parkes 1986).

In mild cases of excessive daytime sleepiness it may be impossible to draw a definite distinction from normal drowsiness. In the absence of the classic accessory symptoms it can be important to note that attacks of drowsiness are irresistible despite the absence of fatigue, or that attacks occur in inappropriate circumstances. The Epworth Sleepiness Scale (Box 13.1) (Johns 1991) is a clinically useful self-rating scale of excessive daytime sleepiness. Epworth Sleepiness Scale scores correlate well with far more expensive and time-consuming sleep laboratory investigations.

Box 13.1 The Epworth Sleepiness Scale. (Reprinted with permission from M. Johns.)

Name: _____

Today's date: _____ Your age (year): __ _____

Your sex (male = M; female = F): _____

How likely are you to doze off or fall asleep in the following situation, in contrast to feeling just tired? This refers to your usual way of life in recent times. Even if you have not done some of these things recently try to work out how they would have affected you. Use the following scale to choose the most *appropriate number* for each situation:

> 0 = would *never* doze
> 1 = *slight* chance of dozing
> 2 = *moderate* chance of dozing
> 3 = *high* chance of dozing

Situation	Chance of dozing
Sitting and reading	_____
Watching TV	_____
Sitting, inactive in a public place (e.g. a theatre or a meeting)	_____
As a passenger in a car for an hour without a break	_____
Lying down to rest in the afternoon when circumstances permit	_____
Sitting and talking to someone	
Sitting quietly after a lunch without alcohol	
In a car, while stopped for a few minutes in traffic	_____

Thank you for your cooperation

Fatigue based on anxiety or depression is a common misdiagnosis, especially if the patient presents his complaint as a feeling of tiredness instead of describing periods of excessive sleepiness. Neurosis is liable to be suspected when emotional complications have arisen from disrupted social or economic circumstances. However, narcoleptics rarely complain of muscular and physical exhaustion as do patients with fatigue of emotional origin, and they often awake from naps refreshed whereas the neurotic patient does not. The depressed and anxious patient will rarely complain of drowsiness as such, nor of recurring periods of uncontrollable sleep.

Hysterical dissociation may occasionally take the form of sleep, but this typically follows well-defined precipitants. The hysterical 'sleep' represents an active withdrawal, is usually prolonged, and the patient resists being woken. The question of hysteria or of schizophrenia may be raised when hypnagogic phenomena are particularly vivid or fantastic. Daniels (1934) described such a patient who saw forms appearing at the windows and entering the room, and felt as if snakes, birds and other creatures were moving about in her abdomen and emerging from her mouth. All such symptoms disappeared with ephedrine.

Hypothyroidism may be the initial diagnosis when the patient complains of dullness and fatigue, or hypoglycaemia when he describes dizziness or light-headedness as part of the attacks. Epilepsy will be suspected when the episodes are described as 'black-outs', but a careful history will reveal drowsiness before the loss of consciousness and full alertness on recovery. Witnesses will describe an episode of normal sleep from which the patient can be woken and the absence of convulsions. Cataplectic attacks may be mistaken for petit mal akinetic seizures. Precipitation by emotion and the preservation of full alertness are important distinguishing features.

Some patients first seek help on account of diplopia due to latent ocular imbalance brought about by episodes of drowsiness: multiple sclerosis or myasthenia gravis may then be suspected. Attacks of diplopia or ptosis may also be the principal manifestations of the patient's cataplexy. In older patients cataplexy may be mistaken for drop attacks due to vertebrobasilar insufficiency. Early symptoms of dementia may occasionally be attributed to narcolepsy.

The history will usually distinguish narcolepsy from other hypersomnias, such as idiopathic hypersomnia, Kleine–Levin syndrome or sleep apnoea syndrome. The presence of obesity may cause confusion with the latter. Hypersomnia due to structural brain lesions is likely to be long-lasting and with other ancillary evidence by way of neurological abnormalities.

Aetiology

The precise cause of narcolepsy remains elusive. The extremely close association between narcolepsy and HLA class II antigens in linkage disequilibrium with DQB1*0602 raises the possibility of an immunological basis, especially since these antigens are widely distributed in the brain, but this remains to be clarified. Administration of IgG and corticosteroids to a case of developing narcolepsy was not sufficient to abort disease development and no discernible benefit was derived from the administration of IgG in two established cases.

In Labrador and Doberman dogs, narcolepsy is caused by a mutation in the hcrtr-2 receptor gene. There is evidence that absence of hcrtr-2 receptors eliminates hypocretin-evoked excitation of histaminergic neurones in the hypothalamus, which gate NREM sleep onset in mice (Willie *et al.* 2003). Preprohypocretin gene knockout mice and a mouse model with ataxin-3 driven hypocretin cell loss have abnormal wake–REM transitions, behavioural arrests possibly analogous to cataplexy and increased sleep during the active period (Mignot *et al.* 2002a). These findings have led to the conclusion that narcolepsy is caused by deficient hypocretin neurotransmission in these animals. Administration of hypocretin can reverse symptoms of narcolepsy in animals (Siegel 2004).

In humans, CSF hypocretin levels are abnormally low in many subjects with the narcoleptic syndrome, although low CSF hypocretin-1 levels may also be low in some subjects with excessive daytime sleepiness and hypersomnia (Krahn *et al.* 2002; Mignot *et al.* 2002b; Ebrahim *et al.* 2003; Martinez-Rodriguez *et al.* 2003). At post-mortem the number of preprohypocretin cells in the lateral hypothalamus of narcoleptic subjects has been found to be significantly lower than in controls. Some authors have suggested that the absence of preprohypocretin cells with increased gliosis in the region but preservation of the intermingled cells is evidence of specific, possibly immune mediated, destruction of the preprohypocretin cells. A single case has been reported of a mutation in the human preprohypocretin gene which resulted in unusually severe symptoms that developed in early childhood. However, unlike dogs most human narcoleptics do not have mutations in any of the hypocretin genes. This also applies to the rare HLA-DQB1*0602-negative subjects, who appear to have more affected relatives than HLA-DQB1*0602-positive subjects. Although the cause is still unknown in humans, depletion of hypocretin in both animals and humans is associated with the development of narcoleptic symptoms. However, many narcoleptic subjects who are clinically indistinguishable from those with low CSF hypocretin have normal hypocretin levels. The role of the hypocretins in relation to the critical balance between catecholamines, serotonin and acetylcholine in the pons is unknown and the disease pathway in narcolepsy has yet to be explained.

In very occasional patients narcolepsy has been reported in the presence of structural brain pathology (secondary narcolepsy) but the authenticity of most of these cases is doubtful (Parkes 1985). Indeed the rarity of clear-cut examples would suggest that coincidence has often been responsible. Thus narcolepsy has been described with tumours of the hypothalamus and third ventricle, also with general paresis, cerebral arteriosclerosis and multiple sclerosis. Occasionally it has followed encephalitis or head injury, sometimes after a considerable interval.

Most cases with cerebral pathology are atypical, and are probably more accurately regarded as hypersomnias than narcolepsy, having sleep of long duration or sustained severe drowsiness. Cataplexy has been extremely rare in such examples. The exception appears to be encephalitis lethargica, which has occasionally been followed by cataplexy as well as narcolepsy (Adie 1926; Sours 1963), but again these cases have usually been atypical in that they tend to recover and show pupillary abnormalities and personality changes. When narcolepsy and cataplexy are found together, it is unusual to find any evidence of structural brain disease.

It has been established that routine EEG shows no abnormalities in narcolepsy, beyond the expected changes when the subject is drowsy and the normal sleep changes while asleep. During cataplectic attacks and episodes of sleep paralysis, the EEG remains unchanged. However, more discriminating assessment of the stages of sleep shows interesting differences from normals. Rechtschaffen *et al.* (1963) discovered a distinctive feature in the nocturnal sleep of narcoleptics, namely that a REM period occurred at the onset, or shortly after the onset, instead of after the usual period of 90 minutes or so. Daytime sleep attacks have also been shown to consist of REM-type sleep, most often when the patient suffers from cataplexy as well as excessive daytime sleepiness (Dement *et al.* 1964, 1966; Hishikawa & Kaneko 1965; Hishikawa *et al.* 1968). In patients with excessive daytime sleepiness alone, however, the early REM phase may not be seen, and daytime attacks may be accompanied by NREM slow-wave sleep. Pre-sleep dreams and sleep paralysis have proved to occur exclusively in the sleep-onset REM periods, and where recordings could be obtained during cataplectic attacks the REM picture was again obtained. Night-time sleep is also generally deranged. In addition to direct or early onset into REM there are often marked phasic REM bursts, poorly regulated sleep cycles, many shifts of phase and frequent awakenings. Altogether, sleep-onset REM may help to confirm a diagnosis of narcolepsy, emerging in over 95% of cases if daytime naps are studied as well as sleep recordings (Parkes 1985). However, false diagnoses may occur if patients have not adhered to the strict recording requirements, particularly relating to the use of sedative and stimulant drugs and sleep episodes during the period immediately prior to the study. Moreover, the cost of sleep studies may restrict their widespread use.

Thus it seems that the pathogenesis of the narcolepsy syndrome lies in an abnormality of REM sleep timing and the dissociation of different aspects of REM (the dream mentation and the motor inhibition) which then appear when the patient is conscious. It is likely that the NREM system is abnormal as well, as witnessed by the frequent periods of drowsiness that occur apart from attacks of sleep, also the frequent failure of nocturnal NREM sleep to reach the normal depth (Roth & Bruhova 1969).

Genetic factors have emerged as significant in the narcoleptic syndrome. Many authors have found a family history of excessive daytime sleepiness in approximately one-third of narcoleptic probands. It is very rare for multiple cases of cataplexy to occur in a family unless they do not carry the HLA-DQB1*0602 haplotype associated with the disease. Although there are very few case reports, affected subjects in HLA-DQB1*0602-negative families sometimes do not carry the same HLA type. In these cases the disease may be caused by genes remote from the HLA system, but no mutations have yet been found in the preprohypocretin gene or either of the hypocretin receptor genes in HLA-DQB1*0602 familial cases. Environmental factors may contribute to familial clustering. However, HLA-DQB1*0602-negative half-sisters who were reared apart from birth both developed the narcoleptic syndrome in adulthood, suggesting that if common environmental factors were important here, the effect occurs very early in life. One study shows that more narcoleptic individuals are born in March and fewest in September. This suggests that environmental factors during the fetal or perinatal period may be important (Dauvilliers *et al.* 2003). Twin studies of the narcoleptic syndrome are too few to allow an estimate of the relative concordance between monozygotic and dizygotic pairs. Of more than a dozen reported monozygotic twin pairs, only two have been reported to be concordant. This may appear to implicate environmental factors, but could be an artefact of reporting bias.

Treatment

The treatment of narcolepsy is outlined by Parkes (1985) and Cooper (1994). Analeptic drugs are the mainstay of treatment for daytime sleep attacks, though their use is unsatisfactory in a number of ways. High dosage of amphetamines may be required to control attacks, resulting in side effects of insomnia, anorexia, irritability, tremor, hypertension and, on rare occasions, acute paranoid psychoses. Moreover, when pushed to high dosage nocturnal insomnia may lead to an increase in daytime drowsiness and sleep attacks. Addiction is an additional risk, though this appears to be rare among narcoleptics.

In practice it is best to try the effect of one of the less potent stimulant drugs, such as mazindol or modafanil, and reserve dexamfetamine sulphate (Dexedrine) or methylphenidate (Ritalin) for those whose symptoms are not adequately controlled. Alternative preparations can be tried when difficulties arise. High doses may produce unwanted effects, such as sweating and irritability, and may have the paradoxical effect of increasing rather than reducing daytime drowsiness. In

many patients tolerance can be controlled by using low doses of short acting stimulants only as required. Stimulants suppress the REM stage of sleep, and this may contribute to the therapeutic effect in narcolepsy. However, these drugs do not improve cataplexy and usually have little effect on the other symptoms.

Cataplexy is helped by tricyclic antidepressants such as imipramine and desipramine and particularly by clomipramine (Anafranil). The latter has been shown to be effective in a dosage considerably lower than is required for an antidepressant effect, the cataplexy often lessening within 24 hours of starting treatment. Sleep paralysis and hypnagogic hallucinations are also reduced. Tricyclic antidepressants have no direct effect on narcoleptic sleep attacks, but when employed with amphetamines they may allow the dosage of these to be reduced. In theory the combination could be dangerous, with risk of hypertensive crises, but Zarcone (1973) employed imipramine with methylphenidate in 45 cases with no apparent harm. Selective serotonin reuptake inhibitors and the serotonin and noradrenaline (norepinephrine) reuptake inhibitor venlafaxine may control cataplexy with fewer side effects than the tricyclics. Most narcoleptics avoid alcohol because of its sedative effects and consume caffeine only in the mornings to avoid sleepless nights.

Counselling has an important part to play, with advice about acquiring a regular pattern of sleep and daytime activities, and perhaps establishing schedules for daytime naps to ward off spontaneous attacks. Shiftwork must be avoided, or work where drowsiness or falls could be a hazard. In general, untreated subjects should not drive and patients must inform their car insurance company of their diagnosis to ensure that they will be covered in case of a driving accident. Psychotherapy may help where social and personal adjustments must be made to the disability.

The impact of the disorder on patients' lives was illustrated in a questionnaire study by Broughton and Ghanem (1976). Many reported recurrent depression, often severe, and almost half described subjective worsening of memory since the onset of the disease. Employment difficulties were common, both on account of sleep attacks and personality difficulties. A surprising number had suffered accidents, either while driving or while engaged in household activities. Recreational pursuits were commonly hampered to a distressing degree.

Roth (1980) reviewed evidence of a special association between narcolepsy and depression, which appeared to be commoner than in the general population. The sleep attacks tended to become more pronounced during phases when the patient was depressed.

Other sleep disorders

Other syndromes of sleep disturbance have come to be recognised, including idiopathic hypersomnia, hypersomnia with 'sleep drunkenness', the sleep apnoea syndromes and Kleine–Levin syndrome. In addition there are hypersomnias based on identifiable cerebral disease and metabolic dysfunction, and others which appear to be based on psychological factors alone. Brief mention will also be made of the parasomnias, including somnambulism and 'night terrors', which very occasionally come to medical attention in adult patients. REM sleep behaviour disorder arises in older adults and must be distinguished from epilepsy.

Surveys show enormous variation in referral rates of these various conditions to specialist sleep clinics depending on the local availability and subspecialisation of sleep services. Coleman *et al.* (1982) surveyed almost 4000 patients attending sleep disorder clinics in the USA. Half suffered from some form of hypersomnia, one-third from insomnia and 15% from a parasomnia. Of the hypersomnias, 43% represented sleep apnoea syndromes, 25% narcolepsy, 9% idiopathic hypersomnia, and 5% other hypersomnias including sleep drunkenness and Kleine–Levin syndrome; 4% appeared to be due to psychiatric disorder, mainly depression, 3% to medical or toxic conditions and 2% to drugs or alcohol.

Idiopathic hypersomnia

Under this title Roth (1980) delineated a sizeable group of patients rarely mentioned in the literature but considered by him to represent an independent nosological entity. Among patients referred to Roth's clinic in Prague, this group came second only to narcolepsy in frequency. Others, however, have found it less frequently, and in particular much less commonly than the sleep apnoea syndrome as shown in Coleman *et al.*'s survey above.

The chief difference from narcolepsy lies in the longer duration of the daytime sleeps, which typically last from half an hour to several hours at a time. Cataplexy and the other classic accessory symptoms of narcolepsy are absent. The periods of daytime somnolence lack the irresistible quality of narcolepsy but the patient is nevertheless obliged to fight against sleepiness for a large part of the day. The daytime naps are not refreshing and are typically preceded by long periods of drowsiness (Guilleminault & Faull 1982). 'Microsleep' episodes may be detected by continuous recordings, especially when trying to read or watch television, but also at times during conversation. At night the patient falls asleep quickly and sleeps deeply, often with difficulty waking in the morning. Sleep drunkenness (see below) may be a feature on rising. Prolongation of nocturnal sleep may be present, as well as daytime somnolence. At weekends some patients sleep more or less continuously while undisturbed. Sleep-onset REM is not detected, and daytime sleep is of the NREM type (Cooper 1994).

Idiopathic hypersomnia is suspected clinically when daytime somnolence is the sole symptom, i.e. in the absence of the accessory symptoms of narcolepsy, of snoring at night or of nocturnal sleep disturbance. Polysomnography confirms the lack of nocturnal apnoeic periods or hypoventilation. A significantly increased amount of stage 2 NREM sleep may be detected along with a decrease in stages 3 and 4 (Guilleminault & Faull 1982).

The condition sets in usually between the ages of 10 and 20, developing over the course of several months and then tending to remain stable as a source of lifelong disability. Occasionally the onset may be later, even well into middle age. Males are affected slightly more commonly than females. In some 30% of cases it occurs familially. In all these respects the resemblance to narcolepsy is obvious.

Among Roth's 167 cases, almost half showed psychological difficulties (neurotic problems, personality disturbances and depression). During phases of depression the periods of sleepiness were usually increased. Sexual problems occurred in 16%, with lack of libido or potency in the men and menstrual disturbances in the women. As with narcolepsy, problems with education, jobs and recreation were frequent, and often even more severe on account of the long duration of daytime sleeps.

The cause is unknown but presumably rests on biochemical disturbances of the neural mechanisms underlying sleeping and waking. Roth discounted psychogenic factors, likewise any known brain pathology, by his criteria for accumulating the sample. EEG and polygraphic records showed NREM patterns to be prominent during diurnal sleeps, often proceeding to stages 3 and 4. All-night records revealed normal sleep organisation except for its long duration. Treatment consists of the administration of central stimulant drugs, as in narcolepsy, but response is often poor.

Hypersomnia with sleep drunkenness

Roth *et al.* (1972) initially reported this as an independent clinical syndrome, representing 30% of the patients in Prague who were referred for investigation of sleep disturbances. Now, however, it is viewed essentially as a variant or complication of idiopathic hypersomnia (Roth 1980).

Sleep drunkenness consists of difficulty in achieving complete wakefulness, accompanied by confusion, disorientation, poor motor coordination, slowness and repeated returns to sleep. A large group of patients showed this as a chronic symptom, occurring with almost every awakening and typically persisting as a lifelong tendency (Roth *et al.* 1972). In the great majority daytime hypersomnia was present as well. The patients were rarely capable of waking spontaneously but needed vigorous and persistent stimulation. Even when so awakened they were confused, disorientated and ataxic in a manner resembling drunkenness for between 15 minutes and 1 hour or longer. Many showed impaired efficiency for up to 4 hours.

The majority reported extremely deep and prolonged nocturnal sleep, often failing to wake spontaneously for 16–17 hours. At night they fell asleep rapidly within seconds of retiring. Associated symptoms consisted of headache, recurrent depression, difficulty with concentration or emotional lability. Eight patients had severe personality disorders or showed psychotic features. However, there was no characteristic personality type or psychopathology, and psychiatric symptoms were not invariable accompaniments.

The course appeared to be stationary in the absence of treatment: once declared, the disability could last until advanced age. Most patients responded well to analeptic drugs taken by day and immediately before retiring. Alternatively, they could be administered immediately after the initial awakening, the patient being allowed thereafter to sleep for half an hour more, after which he would either wake spontaneously or could be easily roused.

In 52 of the 58 examples there was no apparent cause. Six were possibly symptomatic of brain disorder, setting in shortly after severe head injury, encephalitis or a cerebrovascular accident. In the idiopathic cases the pathophysiology remained obscure. Essentially, the disorder appeared to represent an extension and intensification of the normal processes of sleep.

Apart from the chronic syndrome described above, sleep drunkenness can also occur as an occasional symptom in healthy persons if, for example, they are suddenly awakened after too little sleep. It is facilitated by fatigue or the consumption of alcohol or hypnotics before retiring. It has also been described in persons of irritable disposition and in people subject to frequent terrifying dreams. Roth et al. (1972) refer to such examples in the older psychiatric and criminological literature, including persons who have become aggressive or even homicidal while in a state of sleep drunkenness.

Sleep apnoea syndromes

The importance of hypersomnias accompanied by alveolar hypoventilation has been increasingly recognised. Best known is the Pickwickian syndrome, so-called by Burwell et al. (1956) after the fat boy of *Pickwick Papers*. However, this is merely a special instance of a general class of problems. The topic is comprehensively reviewed by Parkes (1985), Whyte et al. (1989) and Douglas (1994).

A division is traditionally made into apnoeas of obstructive or central origin, but this is now regarded as being to some extent artificial. The great majority, over 90%, are associated with airway obstruction and it is this that must be detected if treatment is to be successful. The rarer 'central' forms include those associated with lesions of the medulla due to a variety of congenital or acquired pathologies, and 'Ondine's curse', seen mainly in infants, in which abnormalities of the respiratory centres are manifest as loss of automaticity of breathing while asleep (Severinghaus & Mitchell 1962). Rare familial forms are probably due to inherited insensitivity of the respiratory centres to hypercapnia. An element of obstructive apnoea usually accompanies these central cases because the pharyngeal and

diaphragmatic muscles are responsive to chemical respiratory stimuli.

Obstructive sleep apnoea is usually due to occlusion or narrowing of the upper airway behind the tongue or palate. Fibreoptic endoscopy shows that the lateral walls of the oropharynx oppose during episodes of apnoea, commencing with constriction in the upper oropharynx (Parkes 1985). During inspiration the pressure within the upper airway is always subatmospheric, and the patency of the airway depends on the bracing effect of the surrounding musculature. Since muscle tone drops during sleep, there is an enhanced tendency towards narrowing at this time, being greatest when lung volume is minimal at the onset of respiration (Bradley et al. 1986). Snoring can result from the turbulent flows engendered, or periods of apnoea when occlusion is complete. Once apnoea has occurred, normal breathing is only restored following arousal for a few seconds, resulting chiefly from the negative intrapleural pressure as the patient struggles to breathe (Douglas 1994). The cycle of recurrent apnoeas and arousals may occur up to 100 times per hour, leading to great disruption of normal sleep patterns.

Many of the sufferers from sleep apnoea are obese but this is not invariable. Fat deposition in the submucous tissues around the nasopharynx then contributes to the obstruction. Others may have grossly enlarged tonsils or small mandibular size, the latter often being associated with palatal, tongue or pharyngeal deformity. Rarer causes are hypothyroidism, acromegaly, failure of the laryngeal abductors (as in Shy–Drager syndrome) or myotonic dystrophy, which leads to respiratory muscle stiffness and weakness.

Most cases of obstructive sleep apnoea commence over the age of 40, with a steady increase in prevalence thereafter. Males outnumber females by 10:1. In contrast, the rare central forms can affect all age groups and without definite sex distribution.

The usual presentation is with excessive daytime sleepiness occasioned by the disrupted nocturnal sleep. A hallmark of the condition is loud snoring or honking at night as reported by sleeping partners, but the absence of snoring does not exclude the condition. Obesity is common, being found in perhaps 50% of subjects, often with a characteristic facial appearance caused by a short thick neck and heavy jowls. The phases of daytime sleepiness are usually profound and often compelling, leading to a significant increase in accidents including road traffic accidents (George et al. 1987). Among 80 patients, Whyte et al. (1989) reported that five had fallen asleep while driving cars, four while driving heavy goods vehicles and one while flying his private plane. The daytime naps are typically of brief duration and are frequent throughout the day. Hypnagogic hallucinations and periods of automatic behaviour may occur.

During sleep, by day and by night, respiratory disturbances give a characteristic stamp to the picture. The breathing becomes periodic, with apnoeic intervals lasting 10–20 seconds during which the level of sleep steadily deepens. Resumption of breathing is accompanied by deep sighing and guttural snoring. While the subject is apnoeic, blood oxygen falls and blood carbon dioxide rises. Muscular twitching may be marked. Nocturnal sleep is characterised by restlessness, frequent changes of posture, flailing arm movements and repeated awakenings. Nocturia or enuresis may occur. While awake, respiratory function studies typically show normal results or there may be persistent alveolar hypoventilation.

Reported complications include pulmonary hypertension resulting from the increase in pulmonary blood pressure during apnoeic periods, and cor pulmonale with right heart failure. Systemic hypertension may develop, likewise cyanosis and polycythaemia. The classic Pickwickian syndrome consists of somnolence with obesity, cor pulmonale and secondary polycythaemia, coupled with daytime hypoxia and carbon dioxide retention. Cardiac dysrhythmias, myocardial infarction and cerebrovascular accidents may contribute further to mortality in marked examples of the syndrome. Not surprisingly, a high incidence of unexpected deaths has been reported (MacGregor *et al.* 1970).

These varied adverse effects on health have been widely discussed in the literature, but it can be difficult to apportion the blame between sleep apnoea *per se* and the confounding effects of such variables as obesity and age. In a systematic review of the evidence, Wright *et al.* (1997) conclude that a causal association between sleep apnoea and a range of poor health outcomes has not been firmly established, except with regard to daytime sleepiness and possibly vehicle accidents.

In severe examples mental features can figure prominently. Many patients find morning arousal difficult, with sleep drunkenness, disorientation, headache and motor incoordination (Parkes 1985). Such difficulties may persist during the day with poor memory and concentration. Sackner *et al.* (1975) found a high prevalence of personality disturbance with paranoia, hostility and sometimes agitated depression. Millman *et al.* (1989) reported that almost half of their patients scored highly on the Zung Depression Scale, with sustained improvement once the sleep apnoea had been relieved. Sudden outbursts of violent behaviour and marked anxiety have also been attributed to the condition, likewise sexual problems including impotence.

Greenberg *et al.* (1987) have documented impairments in neuropsychological functioning in patients with sleep apnoea, more pervasive and severe than in controls suffering from other causes of daytime somnolence. Tests of attention and motor efficiency were particularly affected. The severity and duration of hypoxaemic episodes correlated significantly with measures of perceptual organisation (Block Design Test) and manual motor speed. Children with sleep apnoea may show a deterioration in school performance and failure to thrive. Guilleminault and Anders (1976) reported

that one-third of children showed borderline mental retardation when first seen. Such features, and the daytime drowsiness, appear to exceed what might be expected from insomnia and hypoxia alone, and probably owe much to the frequent shifts of sleep phase that occur throughout the night and the loss of deep slow-wave NREM sleep.

In the investigation of suspected examples it can be invaluable to obtain a history from the patient's sleeping partner. The patient himself is often unaware of his snoring and frequent brief arousals. Short of this, direct observation of the patient while asleep can be informative. Useful screening tests include lateral computed tomography of the neck to gauge any generalised airway narrowing, a 24-hour ECG to detect the bradycardia accompanying apnoeas and the rebound tachycardias that follow, or oximetry to monitor the repeated cycles of desaturation. Rauscher *et al.* (1993) have reported the value of pulse oximetry, coupled with indices of weight, height, sex, witnessed episodes of apnoea and reports of falling asleep when reading, in leading to a correct diagnosis of snorers referred to a sleep laboratory.

However, polysomnography provides the definitive diagnosis when facilities are available and permits assessment of the severity of the condition. Overnight recordings allow continuous monitoring of the EEG, the respiratory movements and airflow during sleep. Apnoeas should occur during both REM and NREM phases to be certain of the diagnosis, but are usually of greater frequency during REM sleep. Hence they are typically more severe during the second half of the night. In practice, sleep is sometimes so disrupted that little REM sleep is achieved, and little or no stage 3 or 4 NREM sleep. Concurrent oximetry allows the severity as well as the frequency of desaturations to be measured.

Treatment should first involve loss of weight when this is indicated, and the strict avoidance of alcohol in the evenings or the use of sedatives or hypnotics. Otolaryngological investigation will often be indicated to explore possibilities of remediable airway obstruction. Contributory factors such as hypothyroidism, acromegaly or retrognathia should receive attention. No truly effective drug treatment has been achieved.

Patients who fail to respond to simpler measures may, if the condition is severe, be considered for continuous positive airway pressure (CPAP) treatment each night. A pressure of 4–10 cmH$_2$O is applied continuously through a mask fitted over the nose and mouth to prevent the recurrent collapse of the upper airways during sleep. Many patients find that they can adjust to this satisfactorily, with consequent improvement in daytime somnolence and both physical and mental symptoms. Surgical procedures to the upper airway have sometimes been performed but their place in treatment is controversial. Nevertheless, tracheostomy still finds a place in severely compromised patients when CPAP is unsuccessful, or as an emergency when some other operative procedure must be undertaken. Occasional patients with true central apnoeas may require intermittent positive pressure respiration while asleep.

Kleine–Levin syndrome of recurrent hypersomnia

Levin (1936) drew attention to a rare syndrome of periodic somnolence, often lasting for days or weeks at a time and associated with intense hunger. Irritability, excitement and motor unrest also characterised the somnolent phases. Kleine (1925) had earlier reported several examples. Critchley (1962) carried out a detailed analysis of the 15 cases in the literature at that time and added 11 of his own. Kleine–Levin syndrome is a long-cycle hypersomnia, the episodes being separated by months or even years of normal health.

The majority of reported cases have been in young men (68%) and with onset in early adolescence. In a review by Annulf *et al.* (2005) 186 patients were identified from 139 articles, of which there were 168 primary cases of Kleine–Levin syndrome. In this series the median age of onset was 13 years (range 4–82 years), 81% during the second decade. The median duration of the syndrome was 8 years with seven episodes of 10 days recurring every 3.5 months. The disease lasted longer in women and in patients with less frequent episodes during the first year. They found that it was precipitated most frequently by infections (38.2%). Other factors including head injury, alcohol consumption, exposure to sunlight, sea sickness or a period of physical stress have anteceded the first attack (Billiard 1981; Will *et al.* 1988).

Common symptoms were hypersomnia (100%), cognitive changes (96%, including a specific feeling of derealization), eating disturbances (80%), hypersexuality (43%), compulsions (29%) and depressed mood (48%) (Annulf *et al.* 2005).

The somnolence may set in abruptly or follow gradually after several days of mounting malaise and tiredness. The patient sleeps excessively by day and night, rousing only to eat or empty bladder and bowels. Incontinence does not occur. External stimuli will wake the patient as from natural sleep, but rousing usually results in intense irritability and truculence. The most common eating disturbance is a dramatic increase in the consumption of food. Critchley (1962) preferred the term 'megaphagia' to 'morbid hunger': compulsive eating in a wolfish and greedy manner is a conspicuous feature. The patient does not complain of hunger itself and rarely demands food when this is not in sight, although any food in the immediate vicinity will be devoured. Hypersexuality may be observed in one-quarter of subjects both during and after attacks (Parkes 1986). Occasionally, sexual behaviour may be disinhibited.

Throughout the attack there are few if any abnormal physical signs. Unexplained mild fever is sometimes reported, also pupillary changes, nystagmus or an extensor plantar response. Laboratory investigations are usually entirely normal, including examination of the CSF, though reduced growth hormone secretion has been reported (Chesson *et al.* 1991). CSF white cell counts and protein levels were normal

on all patients, ruling out infectious meningitis (Annulf *et al.* 2005). CSF levels of hypocretin-1 were normal in five patients but slightly decreased in two patients during an episode (Katz & Ropper 2002; Migrot *et al.* 2002; Dauvilliers *et al.* 2003). The EEG shows the usual changes of drowsiness or sleep, but sleep studies may show an increase in total sleep time to 12–14 hours, reduced sleep latency and REM latency, and a reduction in stages 3 and 4 of NREM sleep (Pike & Strores 1994). Elian and Bornstein (1969) reported a patient who showed paroxysmal delta and diffuse theta activity during attacks, but this is distinctly unusual. Each episode ends spontaneously, typically in a gradual manner but sometimes abruptly.

Mental abnormalities during attacks have attracted much attention.

Irritability is typically marked, extending at times to severe aggression when the patient is disturbed. Uninhibited insolent behaviour may emerge, or fidgety behaviour, agitation and tearing at the bed clothes. The bizarreness of behaviour can be an alerting sign; the patient described by Pike and Stores (1994), for example, chased a friend with a carving knife, stole a cucumber, hit a woman in the street with a bag, and repeatedly changed the position of ornaments in the home. Confusion of thought is usually evident too, with disorientation, forgetfulness, depersonalisation and muddled speech. Vivid imagery may be prominent, with waking fantasies that are difficult to disentangle from vivid dreams. Visual and auditory hallucinations may occur. One of Critchley's patients felt responsible for all the events of which he was aware, and believed he could stop a clock with his thoughts and control his own hearing and vision.

Usually the mental abnormalities subside as the period of somnolence ends, but sometimes they persist for days, weeks or a few months thereafter. Half of patients experience depressed mood during episodes. In two of Gallinek's (1954) patients, severe depression persisted for several weeks after every attack, with suicidal tendencies, retardation and pathological guilt. A period of elation lasting several weeks has occasionally been reported (Gilbert 1964), also a phase of sexual hyperactivity when the sleep is over (Passouant *et al.* 1967). Quite often anorexia, headache and malaise follow the attack before the patient feels fully refreshed and regains normal clarity of thought. Thereafter, however, the normal personality is resumed, usually with partial or total amnesia for what has occurred.

The rarity of the syndrome can lead to diagnostic difficulties. It may not be recognised until several attacks have occurred, especially since the overeating is often not apparent to the patient. Other causes of morbid somnolence are likely to be diagnosed and a primary emotional disturbance may easily be suspected. Disturbed behaviour may dominate the picture, suggesting that the essential problem is a personality disorder or even schizophrenia. When circumstances prevent the patient from taking to bed he may become slovenly, unkempt and very erratic in conduct, as in the following case reported by Robinson and McQuillan (1951).

> An army officer cadet of 19 came to the notice of the army doctors in an abnormal mental state. He was unkempt, offhand, casual and disinterested, answering vaguely and smiling fatuously. Affect was shallow and inappropriate and he experienced auditory hallucinations. He was clearly confused, cerebration was slow and there was evidence of thought blocking. In hospital he was hostile and insolent. Behaviour was often bizarre and he masturbated openly, grinning broadly. He slept a great deal and his appetite could not be satisfied. After 4 days in hospital the disturbance cleared abruptly, and he again became smart, respectful and well mannered. He was amnesic for the events of the previous days, though he realised that he had behaved badly and had been unable to control himself.
>
> A history was then obtained of previous attacks, 2 years and 3 years earlier, each lasting several days and accompanied by somnolence and excessive hunger. In the first he had become strange and distant, avoiding company and seeming unaware of what was said to him. On two successive nights he had micturated into a pair of gumboots. He had sold a bicycle for 25 shillings and spent the money on preserved fruits which he consumed at one sitting. In the second attack he again became drowsy and with an insatiable appetite, and created much disturbance with laughing and shouting. After each attack he had returned abruptly to his normal personality.

Follow-up suggests that in the majority of cases attacks gradually lessen in duration, frequency and severity over several years and ultimately cease. The median duration of the disease in Annulf *et al*'s series (2005) was 4–8 years. However, most case reports do not fit the classic description and in some cases the diagnosis is not justified. It is unknown how many chronic cases are incorrectly diagnosed.

Amphetamines have been claimed to reduce the frequency and severity of the attacks (Gallinek 1962). Lithium proved remarkably effective in preventing attacks in a typical example of the syndrome, with recurrence immediately when the drug was withdrawn (Ogura *et al.* 1976). Similar success with lithium has also been reported in periodic hypersomnia unaccompanied by appetite changes (Abe 1977; Goldberg 1983). Annulf *et al.* (2005) found a 41% response rate for stopping relapses compared with medical abstention (1%). Neither, Carbamazepine nor other antiepileptics are effective.

Patients with secondary Kleine–Levin syndrome are older and experience more frequent and longer episodes, but have clinical symptoms and treatment responses similar to primary cases. The disease usually lasts longer in female patients, with less frequent episodes during the first year (Annulf *et al.* 2005).

The cause is not known. Physical and mental health are usually normal between attacks, and few patients have shown evidence of significant maladjustment. Discernible precipitants can rarely be discovered for individual attacks. The similarity between one case and another and the uniform course pursued both suggest an organic basis. Diencephalic dysfunction is suggested by the combination of sleep and appetite disturbance. There has been only one possible familial case report: a pair of siblings who experienced uncharacteristically prolonged episodes of sleep and who also coincidentally shared HLA-DQB1*0602, the haplotype usually associated with the narcoleptic syndrome. However, CSF orexin (hypocretin) was normal when tested during an attack in one of the siblings (Katz & Ropper 2002).

Movement disorders during sleep

Hypnic jerks at sleep onset are a normal phenomenon and occur only during the early stages of sleep. A hypnic jerk is usually a single asymmetric body twitch, sometimes accompanied by a perception of falling, a vivid dream or hallucination, a sharp cry or a sensory flash. Oswald (1959) considered that hypnic jerks were part of an arousal response to minimal stimuli. They are increased by prior physical work, emotional stress and caffeine and reduced by alcohol and hypnotics. Their apparent association with anxiety may be due to heightened recall and difficulty falling asleep when anxious. Hypnic jerks are not related to other forms of myoclonus or epilepsy and no EEG or clinical abnormality has been associated with them.

The waking involuntary movements of extrapyramidal disease may be modified by sleep. During sleep the reduction in awareness, the loss of voluntary motor control and the diminution of muscle tone result in a reduction or abolition of the spasticity and ridgidity of pyramidal and extrapyramidal disease. In Parkinson's disease, tremor may persist but only during stages 1 and 2 of NREM sleep and gross body movements are reduced by sleep. The non-rhythmic involuntary movements and abnormal postures of choreoathetosis and dystonia may partly disappear during deep sleep but return during REM. The multiple tics of Gilles de la Tourette's syndrome occur throughout sleep in all stages, including REM as well as NREM sleep. Epileptic discharge rates may be constant across all sleep stages, although the convulsive movements may diminish in intensity with the atonia of NREM and REM sleep. Different forms of myoclonus show varied changes during sleep.

Restless legs syndrome and periodic limb movement syndrome

Restless legs syndrome was clearly defined by Ekbom (1945) but had been described much earlier and was probably known in ancient times. It usually presents as a sensory complaint, with deep, creeping, unpleasant or unbearable dysaesthesiae, sensations of cold, discomfort or weakness, usually most pronounced in the calves. It is accompanied by the irresistible desire to move the legs and the inability to keep them still. The restlessness is most common in the evening and is most severe before sleep onset and may persist into light sleep. The restless legs syndrome has close similarity to the whole body restlessness induced by neuroleptic drugs. However, sensory discomfort and motor 'impatience' are prominent in restless legs syndrome but not in akathisia. Whilst the legs and less commonly the arms are affected in restless legs syndrome, the whole body is usually involved in akathisia.

Rapid exercise, walking, leg rubbing or kicking may bring temporary relief Curiously, symptoms may be abolished with fever. Severity usually increases with age, sleep deprivation and mental stress. It may commence or be exacerbated by pregnancy, CNS stimulants including caffeine, alcohol or antidepressant medication. It usually results in sleep-onset insomnia and consequently daytime sleepiness. The discomfort may be extreme and cause severe emotional disturbance. In addition, bed partners are at risk of being kicked or struck.

Many medical conditions have been associated with restless legs syndrome, including motor neurone disease, acute poliomyelitis, subclinical sensory neuropathy, amyloidosis, diabetes, anaemia, uraemia, malnutrition and various deficiency states. The age of onset varies, but it usually commences during the second decade. The course may be slowly progressive with wide fluctuations in severity. CSF hypocretin-1 levels were increased in subjects with restless legs syndrome, and were particularly high in subjects with early onset of the condition (Allen *et al.* 2002). There is a family history in up to 60% of cases and it may be transmitted as an autosomal dominant trait. Both familial and nonfamilial forms are very strongly associated with nocturnal myoclonus or periodic limb movement syndrome.

Periodic limb movement syndrome of sudden stereotyped limb movements throughout sleep is about three times more common than restless legs syndrome. The rhythmic repetitive movements are brief (0.5–5 seconds) and occur at regular 20–40 second intervals throughout the night. The repetitive muscle contractions last several minutes to an hour or more. The frequency and severity vary on different nights and physical and emotional stress make the condition worse. The jerking does not occur at sleep onset and is confined to NREM sleep. The movements are independent of other body movements during sleep and do not occur during waking. It affects 2% of the elderly population but up to 15% of patients investigated for insomnia. Although patients may be unaware of arousals caused by sleep myoclonus, sleep disturbance is common, with increased awakenings, decreased stage 4 NREM and complaints of both insomnia and excessive daytime sleepiness. Onset is

rarely before middle age and the prevalence increases with age.

Jerking must be differentiated from myoclonus with epilepsy as well as jerking and restlessness in sleep apnoea. Electromyographic monitoring may help to confirm the diagnosis. Good sleep hygiene is important. A warm bath at bedtime, gentle stretches of the leg muscles and relaxation tapes before sleep onset may be helpful. Some patients obtain benefit from the use of dopaminergic drugs.

Hypersomnias due to identifiable organic disease

The hypersomnias seen with overt cerebral or metabolic disease differ from the syndromes described above in many respects. They are rarely episodic and lack the transient and overwhelming nature of the narcoleptic attack. Sustained drowsiness is characteristic, or periods of sleep greatly in excess of normal requirements. Sometimes sleep inversion is seen with agitated delirium at night. In contrast to many cases of narcolepsy, the sleep of such hypersomnias does not refresh. Depending on the responsible pathology the patient may be roused with ease or difficulty, and to varying levels of alertness. The sleep is usually undisturbed and vivid dreams are rare.

Lesions involving the midbrain tegmentum or posterior hypothalamus are a common cause. The responsible pathology may be a tumour, vascular lesion or degenerative process. Excessive hunger and weight gain may be seen with the somnolence of hypothalamic lesions, likewise polyuria and polydipsia. Prolonged hypersomnia may follow encephalitis lethargica, general paresis or cerebral oedema from any cause. After head injury a variety of sleep disturbances can be seen, including excessive daytime somnolence and sleep apnoea syndromes (Guilleminault *et al.* 1983). These may cause significant disability and raise medicolegal problems. Infective processes such as encephalitis, typhoid, trypanosomiasis or tuberculous meningitis are regularly accompanied by somnolence. Guilleminault and Mondini (1986) have reported patients with prolonged and disabling daytime sleepiness following infectious mononucleosis.

Metabolic disorders such as uraemia occasionally present with somnolence, similarly the encephalopathies associated with anoxia, chronic respiratory insufficiency or hepatic disorder. Endocrine causes include hypothyroidism, Cushing's and Addison's diseases, diabetes mellitus and hyperinsulinism. Rarer causes are industrial toxins and lead encephalopathy. Abed and Bhalla (1991) have reported cases of prolonged hypersomnia following the administration of combined oral and depot neuroleptics, persisting for several months after discontinuation.

Sometimes organic hypersomnias are accompanied by psychiatric symptomatology, chiefly neurasthenic or depressive pictures. A patient described by Roth (1980) showed periodic hypersomnia and manic–depressive psychosis following a head injury, the hypersomnia phases accompanying the depression; while depressed he slept for 20 hours per day, while hypomanic for 3 or 4 hours per day.

The EEG in such conditions generally shows the picture of sleep together with various anomalies in the form of diffuse slow components or bursts of bifrontal or generalised slow waves. The cyclic organisation of REM and NREM sleep is often modified or disrupted.

Insomnia due to organic disease

Insomnia following cerebral lesions has very occasionally been described. Bricolo (1967) reported a patient who developed total insomnia for 96 hours following bilateral stereotactic thalamotomy for Parkinson's disease. Thereafter he showed inversion of the sleep–wake rhythm which very gradually became more regular.

A remarkable post-traumatic example was described by Webb and Kirker (1981). A 33-year-old woman still showed severe insomnia 2.5 years after a relatively mild head injury. On some nights she claimed she did not sleep at all, while on others she slept for about an hour. In the evenings she felt exhausted but not somnolent. EEG and polygraph recordings on four consecutive nights supported her story, showing brief light sleep for less than an hour and no REM sleep. Hypnotics and sedatives were ineffective in doses that left her alert the following day. Nevertheless, four consecutive nightly doses of L-5-hydroxytryptophan, the precursor of serotonin, were dramatically effective, restoring normal sleep that persisted during several months' follow-up. In the absence of further examples it is hard to interpret such a response, though it remains possible that the drug served to trigger normal sleep mechanisms in the presence of some discrete brainstem lesion.

Fatal familial insomnia is an extremely rare disorder, consisting of progressively worsening insomnia with impairment of autonomic and endocrine functions, and motor signs including dysarthria, ataxia, myoclonus and pyramidal disturbance (Lugaresi *et al.* 1986; Medori *et al.* 1992a). It is inherited as an autosomal dominant with onset in middle age. The sleep disorder is characterised by reduction or loss of both slow-wave and REM phases of sleep. Over several months confusion and complex hallucinations ('enacted dreams') give way to progressive memory loss and impairment of consciousness. Death follows a period of coma 6 months to 3 years from the onset. Neuronal degeneration and astrocytosis are most pronounced in the anterior ventral and dorsomedial nuclei of the thalamus, but can extend to other thalamic nuclei, the olives, and the cerebral and cerebellar cortex. Spongiosis is occasionally observed and DNA analysis has shown mutations in the prion protein gene (Medori *et al.* 1992a,b).

Hypersomnias associated with psychiatric disorder

Most studies of patients with hypersomnia reveal cases in which psychological factors are clearly of aetiological impor-

tance. However, the proportion varies according to the orientation of the observer. Roth (1980) points out that during the nineteenth century most hypersomnias were thought to be emotional in origin, but then organic causes and clear-cut syndromes such as narcolepsy came gradually to be delineated. It still remains uncertain what proportion of cases have a definite psychological causation, as opposed to prominent psychological accompaniments to some other definable cause. Mixed patterns can present especial difficulties, since many of the recognised syndromes described above are strongly influenced by prevailing mood and environmental factors.

The nosology as well as the prevalence of psychogenic hypersomnias remains unclear. In the course of accumulating 88 narcoleptics, Sours (1963) found seven patients with hypersomnia that was symptomatic of organic conditions and 20 with hypersomnia attributable to psychiatric disorder; of the latter, nine were regarded as neurotic in origin, two as depressive reactions, two as hysterical and seven as schizophrenic. Smith (1958) suggested that most reported cases of psychogenic hypersomnia would be labelled more accurately as hysterical trances or psychotic stupors.

All agree that hysterical dissociation and depression are the major factors in well-marked examples, with a frequent theme of withdrawal from conflict-laden situations. The somnolence may set in abruptly after traumatic events or emotional upheavals, persisting thereafter for hours or days, or the condition may present recurrently over many months or years.

The following examples almost certainly reflect hysterical mechanisms at work.

One remarkable report concerned a patient who slept for 32 years, but during that time she cried when hearing bad news, would allow only certain persons to attend her, and was heard occasionally to speak (Froderstrom 1912).

A woman of 49 had a history of sleeping attacks for a year, sometimes lasting 36 hours at a time. Hysterical conversion features were present and became intensified during somnolent phases. When confronted with painful topics from her past life, drowsy attacks could be precipitated, but if caught in time and persuaded to expose the conflict-laden material she would return to normal alertness within minutes. She had had an incestuous relationship with her father and had also had a lover throughout her married life. 'Confessional catharsis' led to a great lessening of attacks in the years that followed (Spiegel & Obernborf 1946).

Depressive rather than hysterical mechanisms may have been operative in the following patient.

A 31-year-old teacher had suffered meningoencephalitis at 3 and was widowed at 22. From the age of 30 she frequently felt ill and suffered from headaches and giddiness when upset. After a 10-year relationship she broke off her engagement saying that her fiancé was not sufficiently well educated. After this she claimed to have slept for a whole week. Since then she had often fallen asleep, sometimes against her will and usually for a whole day. This always occurred after an emotionally upsetting experience. She ultimately improved with psychotherapy and light sedation (Roth 1980).

Hysterical states of somnolence will usually differ in several respects from true sleep. The patient may be unrousable even to painful stimuli, or show gross hysterical stigmata. The prolonged maintenance of certain postures, eyelid tremor, increased muscle tension or contraction of the masseters may be in evidence. EEG recordings made during such states may show wakefulness, perhaps even greater desynchronisation than usual, with a preponderance of fast activity and a good deal of muscle artefact.

Depressive hypersomnias, in contrast, may consist of long periods of genuine sleep; hence the difficulties that may be encountered in reaching a firm diagnosis. It is well recognised that hypersomnia may accompany depression or be the presenting feature (Detre *et al.* 1972; Kupfer *et al.* 1972; O'Regan 1974). In depressive hypersomnias attacks will rarely extend beyond 24 hours at a time, the posture during sleep will be normal and rousing will usually be possible. However, many so-called depressive hypersomnias may represent examples of Roth's 'idiopathic hypersomnia' accompanied by depression.

Patients who display negativism, flexibilitas cerea or other catatonic phenomena in the absence of extrapyramidal disease will be suspected of psychotic illness, either affective or schizophrenic in nature.

Unfortunately, few modern laboratory studies appear to have been carried out on patients with psychogenic hypersomnia. These would seem essential in working towards adequate differentiation between cases that rest on organic or pathophysiological factors and those which are primarily due to psychological causes. In the mean time, it is necessary to evaluate each patient as fully as possible for neurological and psychiatric disorder. It can be helpful to consider the following aspects individually (Roth 1980):

• determination from clinical observation of whether or not the attacks represent genuine sleep;
• evaluation of the course, whether static over years or intermittent, and the effect of external factors upon it;
• exclusion of any possible organic cause;
• assessment of the personality for evidence of pre-existent abnormalities;

• the mounting of combined EEG and polygraphic studies, wherever possible during attacks.

Where psychiatric factors appear to be causative, their alleviation may be decisive in clarifying the diagnosis. Treatment with stimulant drugs carries obvious hazards in any patient whose hypersomnia is due to psychological disturbance.

Somnambulism

Sleep-walking occurs predominantly in males. There is frequently a family history of the disorder and an association with enuresis. The great majority of cases occur in children, and the rare examples coming to attention in adult life are often among servicemen or men under indictment for an offence carried out during an alleged sleep-walking spell. Some 15% of children are alleged to have at least one sleep-walking episode, compared with 2–5% of the adult population (Kales *et al.* 1987).

Behaviour during the somnambulistic episode may sometimes consist of no more than sitting up in bed and making banal repeated movements for a minute or two. More prolonged examples consist of walking aimlessly about, or more rarely running, jumping or searching for something. In the main the behaviour is simple and stereotyped. The subject has a blank expression and movements tend to be repetitive and purposeless, though investigatory eye movements may be apparent and dangerous obstacles are usually avoided. Self-injury is rare but serious examples have been reported. Typically the subject behaves as though indifferent to the environment, with low levels of awareness and reactivity. However, if spoken to he may answer monosyllabically. Some are suggestible during the episode and carry out simple commands.

There is disagreement about the level of motor performance and dexterity that can be observed. Fenwick (1990), for example, states that acts can appear to be purposeful, directed and coordinated. The subject may dress or partially undress, open and shut doors and put himself seriously at risk. Cases have been reported in which patients have walked onto fire escapes or allegedly driven cars in a somnambulistic state. The question of violence during sleep-walking is considered further below.

Most attacks last for less than 10 minutes though some may last for half an hour or more. Spontaneous awakening sometimes occurs, but usually the subject returns to bed and continues normal sleep. Attempts at arousal result in gradual return to full awareness, often with marked disorientation and sleep drunkenness. Dream recall is not reported, and there is usually complete amnesia for what has transpired.

In children, sleep-walking is usually a benign condition, outgrown in later childhood, suggesting that it rests on delayed cerebral maturation. In a retrospective analysis, Kales *et al.* (1980) showed that when the onset was before the age of 10 years it was usually outgrown by 15. However, the cases which come to attention in adult life appear frequently to be associated with severe psychopathology. Sours (1963) studied 14 patients aged between 17 and 27 referred from US Air Force bases. In most the disorder had begun at the time of puberty, and persisted thereafter with attacks every 1–4 months. Traumatic psychological events had seemed to precipitate the onset in many cases: parental death or divorce, a change of school or the birth of a sibling. In some patients each episode was precipitated by interpersonal tensions or other emotional problems. There was strong evidence of disturbed family backgrounds and difficult relationships with the parents. The majority had a past history of acting out behaviour, delinquency and thefts, and many showed evidence of anxiety, depression or depersonalisation. Hysterical conversion symptoms were common. Of the 14 patients, five were diagnosed as schizophrenic and four others were markedly schizoid in personality. The remainder were regarded as having character disorders.

Kales *et al.* (1980) similarly found that 29 adults with a present history of sleep-walking showed high levels of psychopathology on the Minnesota Multiphasic Personality Inventory (MMPI), whereas 21 who had outgrown it had essentially normal patterns. In the former, the sleep-walking had begun later, was more frequent and had more intense manifestations. However, it is difficult to know how typical these results may be of adult sleep-walkers generally.

The cause of somnambulism remains unclear. An explanation in psychodynamic terms was previously favoured, especially where episodes had an apparent purpose and the content was explicable in terms of current conflicts. The sleep-walking was then viewed as a dissociative state, similar to the hysterical fugue. It is now apparent, however, that sleep-walking rests on an abnormality of the sleep mechanisms of the brain and represents partial arousal out of the deep NREM stages of sleep. It occurs most often during the first third of the night when stages 3 and 4 predominate, stages during which dreaming is least likely to occur. Kales and Kales (1974) review laboratory studies confirming this in children, and running counter to the popular notion that sleep-walking represents the acting out of a dream. Episodes could sometimes be induced by lifting somnambulists to their feet during NREM sleep, whereas this did not provoke attacks in children not subject to the disorder.

An organic basis for sleep-walking has been established by the demonstration of a genetic association of the condition with HLA-DQB1 genes. A significant excess in transmission was observed in familial cases of somnambulism for the DQB1*05 and DQB1*04 haplotypes. This suggests that a DQB1 polymorphic amino acid might be more tightly associated than any single allele. This recent finding may implicate the HLA-DQB1 genes in disorders of motor control during sleep generally since specific DQB1 genes are also associated

with narcolepsy and REM behaviour disorder (Lecendreux *et al.* 2003).

Conditions that predispose to higher levels of slow-wave sleep, such as sleep deprivation, shiftwork or alcohol consumption, can be expected to increase the frequency of sleep-walking (Driver & Shapiro 1993). It may be commoner during periods of stress and anxiety. Attention has also been drawn to the liability of certain drugs, taken at bedtime, to induce somnambulism in susceptible individuals (Huapaya 1979; Nadel 1981). Hypnotics, neuroleptics, antidepressants, tranquillisers, stimulants and antihistamines have been incriminated, often in combination and sometimes when taken with alcohol. Luchins *et al.* (1978) reported an example, apparently induced by thioridazine and a derivative of chloral hydrate, during which a 44-year-old psychotic woman stabbed her daughter to death. Sleep laboratory studies confirmed the liability of thioridazine to lead to sleep-walking in this patient, which occurred repeatedly out of stage 4 NREM sleep.

The question of violence towards others during sleep-walking can raise important medicolegal issues and such a defence not uncommonly comes before the courts. Simple aggression usually results from the terror and disorientation of partial arousal from deep slow-wave sleep (Parkes 1985). More difficulty is encountered when weapons have been employed or purposeful coordinated behaviour has been implicit in the act. Oswald and Evans (1985) described a 14-year-old boy who stabbed and severely injured his 5-year-old cousin with a knife, and Fenwick (1987, 1990) reviews other examples from the literature where violence has occurred. Sleep-walking may also be put forward as a defence against sexual assault.

In appraising such cases, Fenwick (1987, 1990) points out that a family history and childhood history of sleep-walking greatly increase the chance that the episode in question is genuine. A first episode occurring in adulthood should be viewed with suspicion. Consequently, it is vital to establish the authenticity of an apparent history of childhood sleep-walking. Genuine sleep-walking is most likely to occur within 2 hours of sleep onset; any witnesses are likely to report inappropriate automatic behaviour, usually with an element of confusion, and there will be substantial amnesia for what transpired. Trigger factors such as drugs, alcohol, excessive fatigue and stress will often feature in the episode. Attempts to conceal the crime will be unusual, the natural response on waking being to summon help immediately. It is helpful if the offence can be shown to be motiveless and out of character for the individual. When there is a sexual element in the offence, careful enquiry should be made for sexual arousal with penile tumescence, since its presence would make a sleep automatism highly unlikely.

In the past sleep-walking has been regarded by the law in England and Wales as a 'sane automatism', leading to acquittal when successfully raised as a defence. However, in the case of *R. v. Burgess* (1991), it was agreed that since somnambulism has a genetic cause and arises from internal factors (i.e. a specific stage of sleep) it should be regarded as an 'insane automatism' and likely to recur (Fenwick 1990). Previously, a verdict of insane automatism inevitably led to detention in a psychiatric hospital. However, since the Criminal Procedure (Insanity and Unfitness to Plead) Act 1991 discretion may be exercised by the court as to the appropriate disposal. This may take the form of a supervision and treatment order. Somnambulism is still regarded as a sane automatism in some jurisdictions.

With regard to treatment, the most important factor is protection from injury. Doors and windows should be locked and dangerous objects removed. Patients should be advised to avoid situations leading to sleep deprivation and to avoid taking alcohol before going to bed. Psychiatric treatment is rarely indicated in children, since most outgrow the disorder and in any case are not markedly disturbed. In adults, however, full psychiatric evaluation and treatment may be required. In persistent cases drugs such as diazepam or flurazepam, which suppress stages 3 and 4 of NREM sleep, may warrant a trial (Kales *et al.* 1987). Their effectiveness has been more convincingly shown with night terrors, discussed immediately below.

Night terrors

Night terrors also arise out of stages 3 and 4 of NREM sleep, differing sharply in this respect from nightmares which occur during phases of REM sleep (Rechtschaffen *et al.* 1963; Kales & Kales 1974). Night terrors and sleep-walking often occur in the same individual and a family history of both is common. Kales *et al.* (1980) suggest that the two form a continuum, with sleep-walking the mild end and night terrors the more extreme end of a spectrum. The usual time of occurrence is within an hour or so of going to sleep. Episodes are rare after the middle of the night, because stages 3 and 4 of NREM sleep become shorter later on.

The episode is accompanied by intense anxiety, autonomic discharge, vocalisations by way of screams, moans and gasps, a racing heart and panting respiration. It typically lasts for only a few minutes and the patient is usually amnesic for the event thereafter. If any content is recalled, this is usually limited to a single frightening image of being attacked, choked or crushed (Oswald & Evans 1985). Occasionally, destructive acts may be carried out such as slashing at objects or hitting other persons (Fenwick 1987).

Follow-up studies show that most children outgrow the disorder in later childhood. As with somnambulism, psychological disturbance is common in affected adults but not in children. Daytime anxiety is also high in adults with the disorder. Diazepam and flurazepam are effective in diminishing night terrors, both in children and in adults. Propranolol can also be markedly beneficial (P. Fenwick, personal communication).

REM sleep behaviour disorder

Schenck *et al.* (1986) and Schenck and Bundlie (1987) have identified a form of acute behavioural disturbance occurring during sleep which, unlike somnambulism or night terrors, emerges during the REM phases and represents the acting out of altered dreams. This has been confirmed by polysomnographic studies. It seems that in these patients the normal inhibitory outflow from pontine centres to the spinal motor neurones during REM sleep is diminished, allowing motor behaviours to emerge (see Fig. 13.4).

Typically the patient develops a progressive sleep disorder, with the abnormal behaviours appearing during the middle or final third of the night and almost always more than 60–90 minutes after sleep onset. The episodes characteristically occur during nightmares of being chased or attacked. Concurrently there has usually been a change in the nature of the dreams experienced, which come to involve motor overactivity and violent confrontations with dream characters. The patient talks, shouts or jumps out of bed during sleep, often injuring himself or grabbing at others in a frenzied or aggressive manner. Such behaviours often clearly represent the attempted enactment of dream material.

A 52-year-old salesman of placid temperament began to talk, yell and sit up during sleep. After 2 years be began to punch, kick and jump out of bed between one and seven nights weekly, often striking and bruising his wife and once punching through a wall. These episodes, Which always occurred at least 2 hours after sleep onset, were often the enactment of dreams that had become more vivid, action-filled and violent. 'Usually something is scaring me or is going to hurt my family and I try to protect them. Then I get most violent.'

A 67-year-old man developed a progressive sleep disorder in conjunction with a dementing illness. Limb jerking, moaning and talking appeared every night, with episodes of punching, kicking and running into furniture. On one occasion his wife saw him throw punches while he dreamed he was fighting squirrels in an attic. Both he and his wife had received numerous injuries during sleep (Schenck & Bundlie 1987).

Schenck and Mahowald (1990) have reported 70 consecutive cases with a marked predominance among older males. The mean age at onset was 53, with a range from 9 to 73 years. Many had initially been suspected of nocturnal epilepsy, obstructive sleep apnoea or various psychiatric conditions. The majority were otherwise healthy, but one-third showed

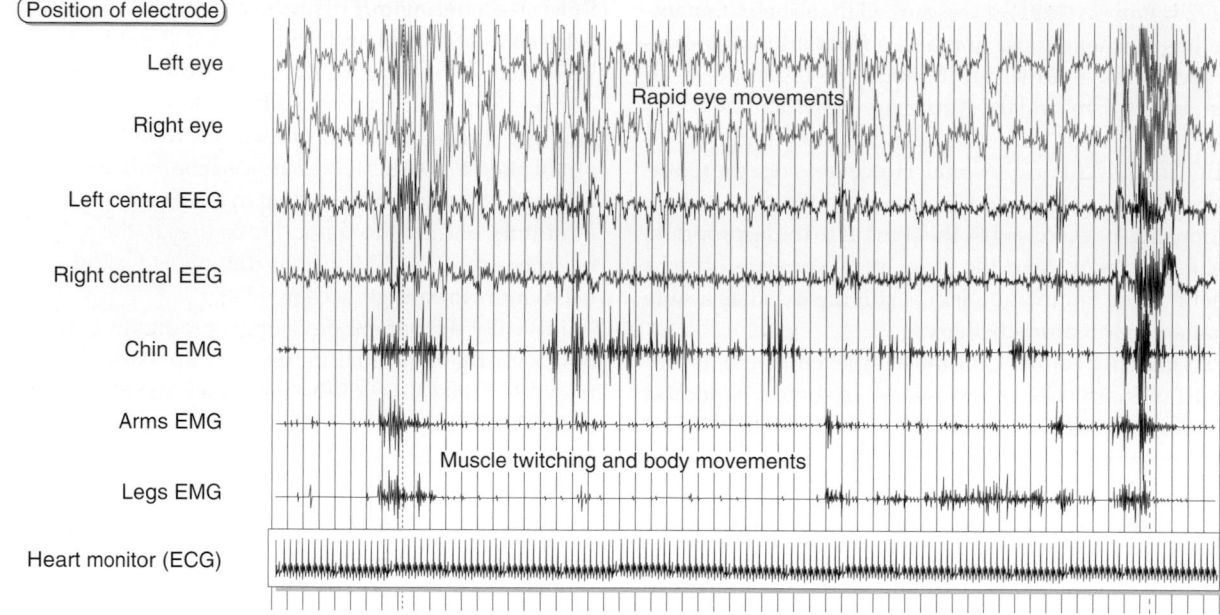

Fig. 13.4 REM sleep without atonia in a patient with REM sleep behaviour disorder. Note the prominent muscle activity and body movements during REM sleep, which is normally accompanied by active muscle paralysis. EEG, electroencephalogram; EMG, electromyogram. From Mark W. Mahowald and Carlos H. Schenck (2005) Insights from studying human sleep disorders. *Nature* **437**, 1279–1285.

evidence of a causal association with CNS disorders such as dementia, Parkinson's disease, narcolepsy, or occasionally vascular or other brainstem lesions. In some cases there was an apparent association with drug or alcohol withdrawal, or the condition set in after major stressors. In most cases the disorder proved to be gradually or rapidly progressive up to the time of treatment. Three-quarters of the subjects had sustained repeated injuries, mostly bruises or lacerations but extending occasionally to fractures or dislocations.

Schenck and Mahowald (1992) have reported additional cases in narcoleptic patients, these appearing to represent almost 12% of the narcoleptics undergoing polysomnographic studies in their clinic. Treatment with stimulants or tricyclic antidepressants had sometimes induced or exacerbated the condition. Curiously, REM behaviour disorder is associated with HLA-DQw1, a supratype of DQB1*0602 associated with the narcoleptic syndrome (Schenck *et al.* 1996).

Polysomnographic studies show preservation of the usual distribution and cycling of sleep stages, though sometimes with reduced REM latency, increased REM density and increased stage 3 or 4 sleep. Periodic and aperiodic limb twitching is common during NREM sleep. The defining characteristic, however, is intermittent loss of the normal electromyographic atonia during REM phases. Seizure activity was never detected in Schenck and Mahowald's cases.

Treatment with clonazepam was rapidly effective in controlling both the disturbing dreams and the problematic sleep behaviours, with only infrequent and minor lapses thereafter. Previous treatments with a variety of sedative–hypnotic drugs had not been helpful. Alternative treatments include desipramine, carbidopa and clonidine, and these can be of value in patients with sleep apnoea where clonazepam may be contraindicated.

References

Abe, K. (1977) Lithium prophylaxis of periodic hypersomnia. *British Journal of Psychiatry* **130**, 312–313.

Abed, R.T. & Bhalla, D. (1991) Persistent neuroleptic-related hypersomnia: two case reports. *Irish Journal of Psychological Medicine* **8**, 130–132.

Adie, W.J. (1926) Idiopathic narcolepsy: a disease sui generis; with remarks on the mechanism of sleep. *Brain* **49**, 257–306.

Allen, R.P., Mignot, E., Ripley, B., Nishino, S. & Earley, C.J. (2002) Increased CSF hypocretin-1 (orexin-A) in restless legs syndrome. *Neurology* **59**, 639–641.

Alvarez, B., Dahlitz, M.J., Vignau, J. & Parkes, J.D. (1992) The delayed sleep phase syndrome: clinical and investigative findings in 14 subjects. *Journal of Neurology, Neurosurgery and Psychiatry* **55**, 665–670.

Aserinski, E. & N. Kleitman (1953) Regularly occurring periods of eye motility and concomitant phenomena during sleep. *Science* **118**, 273–274.

Billiard, M. (1981) The Kleine–Levin syndrome. In: Koella, W.P. (ed.) *Sleep 1980*, pp. 124–127. Basel, Karger.

Billiard, M. & Carlander, B. (1998) [Wake disorders. I. Primary wake disorders]. *Revue Neurologique (Paris)* **154**, 111–129.

Bogaert, L. v. (1936) Les aspects familiaux des paroxysmes reflexes du tonus. *Annales Medico-Psychologiques (Paris)* **94**, 1–4.

Bradley, T.D., Brown, I.G., Grossman, R.F., Zamel, N., Martinez, D., Phillipson, E.A. & Hoffstein, V. (1986) Pharyngeal size in snorers, nonsnorers and patients with obstructive sleep apnoea. *New England Journal of Medicine* **315**, 1327–1331.

Bricolo, A. (1967) Insomnia after bilateral stereotactic thalamotomy in man. *Journal of Neurology, Neurosurgery and Psychiatry* **30**, 154–158.

Broughton, R. & Ghanem, Q. (1976) *The Impact of Compound Narcolepsy on the Life of the Patient*. Spectrum Publications, New York.

Burwell, C.S., Robin, E.D. & Whalley, R.D. (1956) Extreme obesity associated with alveolar hypoventilation: a Pickwickian syndrome. *American Journal of Medicine* **21**, 811–818.

Chesson, A.L., Levine, S.M., Long, L.S. & Lee, S.C. (1991) Neuroendocrine evaluation in Kleine–Levin syndrome: evidence of reduced dopaminergic tone during periods of hypersomnolence. *Sleep* **14**, 226–232.

Coleman, R.M., Roffwarg, H.P. & Kennedy, S. (1982) Sleep–wake disorders based on a polysomnographic diagnosis. A National Cooperative Survey. *Journal of the American Medical Association* **247**, 997–1003.

Cooper, R. (1994) *Normal Sleep*. Chapman & Hall, London.

Critchley, M. (1962) Periodic hypersomnia and megaphagia in adolescent males. *Brain* **85**, 627–656.

Dahlitz, M. & Parkes, J.D. (1993) Sleep paralysis. *Lancet* **341**, 406–407.

Daniels, L.W. (1934) Narcolepsy. *Medicine* **13**, 1–122.

Dauvilliers, Y., Baumann, C.R. & Carlander, B. (2003) CSF hypocretin-1 levels in narcolepsy, Kleine–Levin syndrome, and other hypersomnias and neurological conditions. *Journal of Neurology, Neurosurgery and Psychiatry* **74**, 1667–1673.

Dement, W.C. & Kleitman, N. (1957) The relation of eye movements during sleep to dream activity: an objective method for the study of dreaming. *Journal of Experimental Psychology* **53**, 339–346.

Dement, W.C., Rechtschaffen, A.R. & Gulevitch, G. (1964) A polygraphic study of the narcoleptic sleep attack. *Electroencephalography and Clinical Neurophysiology* **17**, 608–609.

Dement, W.C., Rechtschaffen, A.R. & Gulevitch, G. (1966) The nature of the narcoleptic sleep attack. *Neurology* **16**, 18–33.

Detre, T., Himmelhoch, J., Swartzburg, M., Anderson, C.M., Byck, R. & Kupfer, D.J. (1972) Hypersomnia and manic depressive disease. *American Journal of Psychiatry* **128**, 1303–1305.

Dijk, D.J. & Czeisler, C.A. (1994) Paradoxical timing of the circadian rhythm of sleep propensity serves to consolidate sleep and wakefulness in humans. *Neuroscience Letters* **166**, 63–68.

Douglas, N.J. (1994) *The Sleep Apnoea/Hypopnoea Syndrome*. Chapman & Hall, London.

Driver, H.S. & Shapiro, C.M. (1993) Parasomnias. *British Medical Journal* **306**, 921–924.

Ebrahim, I.O., Sharief, M.K., de Lacy, S. *et al.* (2003) Hypocretin (orexin) deficiency in narcolepsy and primary hypersomnia. *Journal of Neurology, Neurosurgery and Psychiatry* **74**, 127–130.

Ekbom, K. (1945) Restless legs. *Acta Medica Scandinavica Supplementum* **158**, 4–122.

Elian, M. & Bornstein, B. (1969) The Kleine–Levin syndrome with intermittent abnormality in the EEG. *Electroencephalography and Clinical Neurophysiology* **27**, 601–604.

Fenwick, P. (1987) Somnambulism and the law: a review. *Behavioural Sciences and the Law* **5**, 343–357.

Fenwick, P. (1990) Automatism, medicine and the law. *Psychological Medicine Monograph Supplement* **17**.

Frankel, B.L., Coursey, R.D., Buchbinder, R. & Snyder, F. (1976) Recorded and reported sleep in chronic primary insomnia. *Archives of General Psychiatry* **33**, 615–623.

Froderstrom, H. (1912) La dormeuse d'Okno: 32 ans de stupeur: guerison complete. *Nouvelle Iconographie de la Salpetriere* **25**, 267–279.

Gallinek, A. (1954) Syndrome of episodes of hypersomnia, bulimia and abnormal mental states. *Journal of the American Medical Association* **154**, 1081–1083.

Gallinek, A. (1962) The Klein–Levin syndrome: hypersomnia, bulimia and abnormal mental states. *World Neurology* **3**, 235–243.

Geladi, J.M. & Brown, J.W. (1967) Hereditary cataplexy. *Journal of Neurology, Neurosurgery and Psychiatry* **30**, 455–457.

Gelineau, J.B. (1880) De la narcolepsie. *Gazette Hopital* **53**, 626–628, 635–637.

Gelineau, J.B. (1881) *De la Narcolepsie*. Imprimerie du Surgeries, Paris.

George, C.F., Nickerson, P.W., Hanly, P.J., Millet, T.W. & Kryger, M.H. (1987) Sleep apnoea patients have more automobile accidents. *Lancet* **ii**, 447.

Gilbert, G.J. (1964) Periodic hypersomnia and bulimia: the Klein–Levin syndrome. *Neurology* **14**, 844–850.

Goldberg, M.A. (1983) The treatment of Klein–Levin syndrome with lithium. *Canadian Journal of Psychiatry* **28**, 491–493.

Greenberg, G.D., Watson, R.K. & Deptula, D. (1987) Neuropsychological dysfunction in sleep apnoea. *Sleep* **10**, 254–262.

Guilleminault, C. & Anders, T.F. (1976) Sleep disorders in children. *Advances in Pediatrics* **22**, 151–174.

Guilleminault, C. & Faull, K.F. (1982) Sleepiness in non-narcoleptic, non-sleep apneic EDS patients: the idiopathic CNS hypersomnolence. *Sleep* **5**, S175–S181.

Guilleminault, C. & Mondini, S. (1986) Mononucleosis and chronic daytime sleepiness. A long-term follow up study. *Archives of Internal Medicine* **146**, 1333–1335.

Guilleminault, C., Dement, W.C. & Passouant, P. (eds) (1976) *Narcolepsy: Proceedings of the First International Symposium on Narcolepsy*. Advances in Sleep Research, vol. 111. Spectrum Publications, New York.

Guilleminault, C., Faull, K.F., Miles, L. & Van der Hoed, J. (1983) Post traumatic excessive daytime sleepiness: a review of 20 patients. *Neurology* **33**, 1584–1589.

Guilleminault, C., Tilkian, A.T. & Dement, W.C. (eds) (1978) *Sleep Apnoea Syndrome*. New York: Alan R. Liss, pp. 1–12.

Hishikawa, Y. & Kaneko, Z. (1965) Electroencephalographic study on narcolepsy. *Electroencephalography and Clinical Neurophysiology* **18**, 249–259.

Hishikawa, Y., Nan'no, H., Tashibana, M., Furuya, E., Koida, M. & Kaneko, Z. (1968) The nature of sleep attack and other symptoms of narcolepsy. *Electroencephalography and Clinical Neurophysiology* **24**, 1–10.

Honda, Y., Doi, Y., Juji, T. & Sataki, M. (1984) Narcolepsy and HLA: positive DR2 as a prerequisite for the development of narcolepsy. *Folia Psychiatrica et Neurologica Japonica* **38**, 360.

Horne, J.A. & Ostberg, O. (1976) A self assessment questionnaire to determine morningness–eveningness in human circadian rhythm. *International Journal of Chronobiology* **4**, 97–110.

Huang, Z.L., Qu, W.M., Li, W.D. *et al.* (2001) Arousal effect of orexin A depends on activation of the histaminergic system. *Proceedings of the National Academy of Sciences USA* **98**, 9965–9970.

Huapaya, L. (1979) Seven cases of somnambulism induced by drugs. *American Journal of Psychiatry* **136**, 985–986.

Johns, M.W. (1991) A new method of measuring daytime sleepiness. The Epworth Sleepiness Scale. *Sleep* **14**, 540–545.

Kales, A. & Kales, J.D. (1974) Sleep disorders: recent findings in the diagnosis and treatment of disturbed sleep. *New England Journal of Medicine* **290**, 487–499.

Kales, A. & Kales, J.D. (1983) Sleep laboratory studies of hypnotic drugs: efficacy and withdrawal effects. *Journal of Clinical Psychopharmacology* **3**, 140–150.

Kales, A., Soldatos, C.R., Caldwell, A.B. *et al.* (1980) Somnambulism: clinical characteristics and personality patterns. *Archives of General Psychiatry* **37**, 1406–1410.

Kales, A., Soldatos, C.R. & Kales, J.D. (1987) Sleep disorders: insomnia, sleepwalking, night terrors, nightmares, and enuresis. *Annals of Internal Medicine* **106**, 582–592.

Katz, J.D. & Ropper, A.H. (2002) Familial Kleine–Levin syndrome: two siblings with unusually long hypersomnic spells. *Archives of Neurology* **59**, 1959–1961.

Kleine, W. (1925) Periodische Schlafsucht. *Monatsschrift fur Psychiatrie und Neurologie* **57**, 285–320.

Krahn, L.E., Pankratz, V.S., Oliver, L., Boeve, S.E. & Siber, M.H. (2002) Hypocretin (orexin) levels in cerebrospinal fluid of patients with narcolepsy: relationship to cataplexy and HLA DQB1*0602 status. *Sleep* **25**, 733–736.

Kripke, D.F., Simons, R.N., Garfinkel, L. & Hammond, E.C. (1979) Short and long sleep and sleeping pills. *Archives of General Psychiatry* **36**, 103–116.

Kripke, D.F., Ancoli-Israel, S., Mason, M. & Messin, S. (1983) Sleep related mortality and morbidity in the aged. In: XXX *Sleep Disorders: Basic and Clinical Research*, pp. 415–444. Spectrum Publications, New York.

Kryger, M., Roth, T. & Dement, W.C. (2000) *Principles and Practice of Sleep Medicine*. W.B. Saunders, New York.

Kupfer, D.J., Himmelhoch, J.M., Swartzburg, M., Anderson, C., Byck, R. & Detre, T.P. (1972) Hypersomnia in manic-depressive disease (a preliminary report). *Diseases of the Nervous System* **33**, 720–724.

Langdon, N., Welsh, K., Van Dam, M., Vaughan, R.W. & Parkes, J.D. (1984) Genetic markers in narcolepsy. *Lancet* **ii**, 1178–1180.

Lecendreux, M., Bassetti, C., Dau, E. *et al.* (2003) HLA and genetic susceptibility to sleepwalking. *Molecular Psychiatry* **8**, 114–117.

Levin, M. (1936) Periodic somnolence and morbid hunger: a new syndrome. *Brain* **59**, 494–504.

Loomis, A.L., Harvey, E.N. & Hobart, G.A. (1935) Potential rhythms of the cerebral cortex during sleep. *Science* **81**, 597–598.

Luchins, D.J., Sherwood, P.M., Gillin, J.C., Mendelson, W. & Wyatt, J. (1978) Filicide during psychotropic-induced somnambulism: a case report. *American Journal of Psychiatry* **135**, 1404–1405.

Lugaresi, E., Medori, R., Montagna, P. *et al.* (1986) Fatal familial insomnia and dysautonomia with selective degeneration of thalamic nuclei. *New England Journal of Medicine* **315**, 997–1003.

MacGregor, M.I., Block, A.J. & Ball, W.C. (1970) Serious complications and sudden death in the Pickwickian syndrome. *Johns Hopkins Medical Journal* **126**, 279–295.

Macnish, R. (1830) *The Philosophy of Sleep*. E. McPhun, Glasgow.

Martinez-Rodriguez, J.E., Lin, L., Iranzo, A. *et al.* (2003) Decreased hypocretin-1 (orexin-A) levels in the cerebrospinal fluid of patients with myotonic dystrophy and excessive daytime sleepiness. *Sleep* **26**, 287–290.

Medori, R., Montagna, P., Tritschler, H.J. *et al.* (1992a) Fatal familial insomnia: a second kindred with mutation of prion protein gene at codon 178. *Neurology* **42**, 669–670.

Medori, R., Tritschler, H.J., Le Blanc, A. *et al.* (1992b) Fatal familial insomnia: a prison disease with a mutation at codon 178 of the prion protein gene. *New England Journal of Medicine* **326**, 444–449.

Mignot, E. (2004) Sleep, sleep disorders and hypocretin (orexin). *Sleep Medicine* **5** (suppl. 1), S2–S8.

Mignot, E., Taheri, S. & Nishino, S. *et al.* (2002a) Sleeping with the hypothalamus: emerging therapeutic targets for sleep disorders. *Nature Neuroscience* **5** (suppl.), 1071–1075.

Mignot, E., Lammers, G.J., Ripley, B. *et al.* (2002b) The role of cerebrospinal fluid hypocretin measurement in the diagnosis of narcolepsy and other hypersomnias. *Archives of Neurology* **59**, 1553–1562.

Millman, P.P., Fogel, B.S., McNamara, M.E. & Carlisle, C.C. (1989) Depression as a manifestation of obstructive sleep apnoea: reversal with nasal continuous positive airway pressure. *Journal of Clinical Psychiatry* **50**, 348–351.

Nadel, C. (1981) Somnambulism, bed-time medication and overeating. *British Journal of Psychiatry* **139**, 79.

Nicholson, A. & Marks, J. (1983) *Insomnia. A Guide for Medical Practitioners*. MTP Press, Lancaster.

Ogura, C., Okuma, T., Nakazawa, K. & Kishimoto, A. (1976) Treatment of periodic somnolesence with lithium carbonate. *Archives of Neurology* **33**, 143.

O'Regan, J.B. (1974) Hypersomnia and MAOI antidepressants. *Canadian Medical Association Journal* **111**, 213.

Oswald, I. (1959) Sudden bodily jerks on falling asleep. *Brain* **82**, 92–103.

Oswald, I. & Evans, J. (1985) On serious violence during sleepwalking. *British Journal of Psychiatry* **147**, 688–691.

Parkes, J.D. (1985) *Sleep and its Disorders*. W.B. Saunders, London.

Parkes, J.D. (1986) Sleep disorders. *Progress in Clinical Neurosciences* **2**, 1–22.

Passouant, P., Cadilhac, J. & Baldy-Moulinier, M. (1967) Physiopathologie des hypersomnies. *Revue Neurologique (Paris)* **116**, 585–629.

Pike, M. & Strores, G. (1994) Kleine–Levin syndrome: a cause of diagnostic confusion. *Archives of Disease in Childhood* **71**, 355–357.

Rauscher, H., Popp, W. & Zwick, H. (1993) Model for investigating snorers with suspected sleep apnoea. *Thorax* **48**, 275–279.

Rechtschaffen, A.R., Wolpert, E.A., Dement, W., Mitchell, S.A. & Fisher, C. (1963) Nocturnal sleep of narcoleptics. *Electroencephalography and Clinical Neurophysiology* **15**, 599–609.

Regelstein, Q.R. (1980) Insomnia and sleep disturbances in the aged. Sleep and insomnia in the elderly. *Journal of Geriatric Psychiatry* **13**, 153–171.

Robinson, J.T. & McQuillan, J. (1951) Schizophrenic reaction associated with the Klein–Levin syndrome. *Journal of the Royal Army Medical Corps* **96**, 377–381.

Roth, B. (1980) *Narcolepsy and Hypersomnia*. Basel, Karger.

Roth, B. & Bruhova, S. (1969) Dreams in narcolepsy, hypersomnia and dissociated sleep disorders. *Experimental Medicine and Surgery* **27**, 187–209.

Roth, B., Nevsimalova, S. & Rechtschaffen, A. (1972) Hypersomnia with sleep drunkenness. *Archives of General Psychiatry* **26**, 456–462.

Sackner, M.A., Landa, J., Forrest, T. & Greeneltch, D. (1975) Periodic sleep apnoea: chronic sleep deprivation related to intermittent upper airway obstruction and central nervous system disturbance. *Chest* **67**, 164–171.

Schenck, C.H. & Bundlie, S.R. (1987) Rapid eye movement sleep behavior disorder. A treatable parasomnia affecting older adults. *Journal of the American Medical Association* **257**, 1786–1789.

Schenck, C.H. & Mahowald, M.W. (1990) Polysomnographic, neurologic, psychiatric, and clinical outcome report on 70 consecutive cases with REM sleep behavior disorder (RBD): sustained clonazepam efficacy in 89.5% of 57 treated patients. *Cleveland Clinic Journal of Medicine* **57** (suppl.), S9–S23.

Schenck, C.H. & Mahowald, M.W. (1992) Motor dyscontrol in narcolepsy: rapid-eye-movement (REM) sleep without atonia and REM sleep behavior disorder. *Annals of Neurology* **32**, 3–10.

Schenck, C.H., Bundlie, S.R., Mignot, E. & Mahowald, M.W. (1986) Chronic behavioral disorders of human REM sleep: a new category of parasomnia. *Sleep* **9**, 293–308.

Schenck, C.H., Garcia-Rill, E., Segall, M., Noreen, H. & Mahowald, M.W. (1996) HLA class II genes associated with REM sleep behavior disorder. *Annals of Neurology* **39**, 261–263.

Severinghaus, J.W. & Mitchell, R.A. (1962) Ondine's curse: failure of respiratory centre automaticity while awake. *Clinical Research* **10**, 122.

Siegel, J.M. (2004) Hypocretin (orexin): role in normal behavior and neuropathology. *Annual Review of Psychology* **55**, 125–148.

Smith, C.M. (1958) Comments and observations on psychogenic hypersomnia. *Archives of Neurology and Psychiatry* **80**, 619–624.

Sours, J.A. (1963) Narcolepsy and other disturbances in the sleep–waking rhythm: a study of 115 cases with review of the literature. *Journal of Nervous and Mental Disease* **137**, 525–542.

Spiegel, L.A. & Obernborf, C.P. (1946) Narcolepsy as a psychogenic symptom. *Psychosomatic Medicine* **8**, 28–35.

Taheri, S. & Mignot, E. (2002) The genetics of sleep disorders. *Lancet Neurology* **1**, 242–250.

Von Economo, C. (1931) Sleep as a problem of localization. *Journal of Nervous and Mental Disease* **71**, 249–269.

Webb, M. & Kirker, J.G. (1981) Severe post-traumatic insomnia treated with L-5–hydroxytryptophan. *Lancet* **i**, 1365–1366.

Weitzman, E.D., Czeisler, C.A., Coleman, R.M. *et al.* (1981) Delayed sleep phase syndrome, a chronobiological disorder with sleep-onset insomnia. *Archives of General Psychiatry* **38**, 737–746.

Whyte, K.F., Allen, M.B., Jefferey, A.A., Gould, G.A. & Douglas, N.J. (1989) Clinical features of the sleep apnoea/hypopnoea syndrome. *Quarterly Journal of Medicine* **72**, 659–666.

Will, R.G., Young, J.P.R. & Thomas, D.J. (1988) Kleine–Levin syndrome: report of two cases with onset of symptoms precipitated by head trauma. *British Journal of Psychiatry* **152**, 410–412.

Willie, J.T., Chemelli, R.M., Sinton, C.M. *et al.* (2003) Distinct narcolepsy syndromes in orexin receptor-2 and orexin null mice: molecular genetic dissection of non-REM and REM sleep regulatory processes. *Neuron* **38**, 715–730.

Wingard, D.L. & Berkman, L.F. (1983) Mortality risk associated with sleeping pattern among adults. *Sleep* **6**, 102–107.

Wright, J., Johns, R., Watt, I., Melville, A. & Sheldon, T. (1997) Health effects on obstructive sleep apnoea and the effectiveness of continuous positive airways pressure: a systematic review of the research evidence. *British Medical Journal* **314**, 851–860.

Yoshida, Y., Fujiki, N., Nakajima, B., *et al.* (2001) Fluctuation of extracellular hypocretin-1 (orexin A) levels in the rat in relation to the light–dark cycle and sleep–wake activities. *European Journal of Neuroscience* **14**, 1075–1081.

Yoss, R.E. & Daly, D.D. (1957) Criteria for the diagnosis of the narcoleptic syndrome. *Proceedings of the Staff Meetings of the Mayo Clinic* **32**, 320–328.

Yoss, R.E. & Daly, D.D. (1960) Narcolepsy. *Medical Clinics of North America* **44**, 953–968.

Zarcone, V. (1973) Narcolepsy. *England Journal of Medicine* **288**, 1156–1166.

14

Other Disorders of the Nervous System

Simon Lovestone

Institute of Psychiatry, King's College, London

Several disorders of the nervous system not falling within the province of the foregoing chapters remain to be considered. Attention is restricted to those which have attracted some degree of psychiatric interest, either on account of the psychological, cognitive or behavioural symptoms that accompany them or because they can raise problems of differential diagnosis in the overlap between neurology and psychiatry.

Patients with neurological disease sometimes first come before the psychiatrist, usually at an early stage and before there is unequivocal evidence of central nervous system (CNS) pathology. The incidence of erroneous diagnoses is hard to assess but the findings of Tissenbaum *et al.* (1951) may not be unrepresentative even today. On reviewing approximately 400 neurological patients attending a Veterans Administration clinic, they found that 53 (13%) had been considered to suffer from a psychiatric disorder before the neurological diagnosis was established, the commonest psychiatric diagnoses being conversion hysteria, neurosis or affective disorder. The situation was particularly common among patients with Parkinson's disease or multiple sclerosis. In some instances organic disease had been suspected for some time, although the suspicion of non-organic psychiatric disorder persisted until the underlying disease had progressed much further.

In some neurological disorders psychiatric symptoms are an integral part of the disease process, representing the direct effects of CNS involvement on mental functioning. This is most clearly discerned in the numerous disorders that can lead to cognitive impairment, but cerebral pathology may also play a part in determining subtle changes of personality, disorder of affect or even psychotic developments. Where there is evidence on such matters this is discussed. Other psychiatric disturbances in neurological disease have little to do directly with brain pathology, but reflect the reaction of the patient to his disablement. Neurological disability can

pose severe threats to independence and security, or provide obstacles to free communication. Not unnaturally these may tax the individual's capacity for psychological adjustment over time. Emotional symptoms and even frank mental illness may then result, and owe their origin predominantly to the patient's problems and aspects of his social situation. Sometimes, of course, both organic and non-organic factors will be operative together. The correct appreciation of such matters is an essential prelude to planned intervention and help and the neuropsychiatrist and the liaison psychiatrist have an important, and increasingly recognised, role to play in the management of patients with chronic neurological disease and disability.

Some of the disorders considered below are not uncommon. Others are very rare, but can nonetheless be important in the present context if they are liable to have marked psychiatric sequelae.

Multiple sclerosis

Multiple sclerosis (MS) is by far the most frequent of the demyelinating diseases, and indeed is one of the commonest diseases of the nervous system in temperate climates. It is particularly common in the northern hemisphere but rare in tropical and subtropical regions. Although the actual incidence is low, the chronicity of the disorder leads it to rank as a major cause of disability.

The aetiology remains unknown despite a large amount of research and a number of tantalising clues. At various times causative theories have involved vascular, infective, dietary and metabolic mechanisms but none can be considered well established. The present consensus is that the disease results from an interplay between genetic and environmental factors, resulting in an immunologically mediated inflammatory response within the CNS. Two very large studies have shown that the most important genetic susceptibility

Lishman's Organic Psychiatry: A Textbook of Neuropsychiatry, 4th edition.
© 2009 Blackwell Publishing.   ISBN 978-1-4051-1860-1

factors are within the human leucocyte antigen (HLA) class II region of the major histocompatibility complex (MHC) (Lincoln *et al*. 2005; Sawcer *et al*. 2005). Although the data for association with this region are very strong and other regions of the genome are unlikely to play significant effects on aetiopathogenesis, the association is not simple and epistatic effects and interactions with other genes, perhaps with other regions of the MHC, appear to play important roles.

Three sources of evidence point to a strong effect of the environment: twin discordancy, migration studies and gradients in prevalence, especially comparing northern and southern hemispheres. Compston (1993) reviews data from Australia and New Zealand which indicate that living in the southern hemisphere is relatively protective. The environmental effect appears to exert its influence in adolescence, as place-of-birth risk is carried over in adult migrants but is similar to the acquired environment in child migrants. The 'hygiene' hypothesis postulates that the relatively disease-free childhoods of the developed world act to prevent the fullest development of the immune system and the frequent immunological challenges of early life in the less developed world are protective. Giovannoni and Ebers (2007) review recent evidence addressing this attractive hypothesis, including cohort and sibship studies, and find no evidence in favour and much to challenge the hypothesis. On the other hand, the evidence is growing that vitamin D, or exposure to high levels of sunlight associated with vitamin D generation, is protective and vitamin D supplementation may also offer some therapeutic protection against relapse (Brown 2006). Smoking increases risk of MS, with an odds ratio of 1.36 in a meta-analysis (Hawkes 2005). A variety of specific infectious agents have also been proposed as factors that increase risk. Of these the evidence is strongest for Epstein–Barr virus (EBV) (Giovannoni & Ebers 2007) as demonstrated by meta-analyses of case–control and cohort studies of people with EBV exposure, evidence for increased risk for MS in those with anti-EBV antibodies, an association between Hodgkin's lymphoma and MS, and some evidence for EBV activity in people with MS.

Clinical features

The onset is chiefly in young adults between 20 and 40 years of age. In the UK females are affected more often than males. The disorder is protean in its neurological manifestations, traditional diagnostic criteria laying emphasis on both the multifocal and relapsing nature of the symptoms and signs. Typically there is evidence, over time if not at a single examination, of disseminated lesions in the CNS, which at least in the early stages show a tendency to remission and relapse.

Early manifestations frequently include retrobulbar neuritis, disorders of oculomotor function leading to diplopia or nystagmus, or lesions of the long ascending or descending tracts of the cord producing paraesthesiae or spastic paraparesis. Precipitancy of micturition may be an early symptom, likewise ataxia or intention tremor due to cerebellar involvement. Retrobulbar neuritis is particularly common and can occur as a transient disturbance antedating other manifestations by many years.

The initial symptoms tend to settle within weeks or months, sometimes disappearing completely but sometimes leaving residual disability. Further attacks bring new symptoms or an intensification of those already present. The interval between attacks is extremely variable but in exceptional cases remissions may last for 25 years or more. It is 8 years (median value) before patients experience limited walking ability, 20 years before they are able to walk no more than 100 m using unilateral aids, and 30 years before they can walk no further than 10 m (Vukusic & Confavreux 2007). Although these average figures are consistent, there is wide individual variation in natural history and, as yet, no reliable means of predicting prognosis. At presentation most patients show a relapsing–remitting disease course (RRMS) and almost all go on to have secondary progressive disease (SPMS). Some 10% show steady progression of disability from the outset (primary progressive MS). The latter is the usual mode of progression with onset after the age of 50 years. The least common presentation, affecting some 5% of patients, is progressive-relapsing MS (characterised by acute attacks superimposed on progressive decline). Ultimately, almost all patients show downward progression with an accumulation of multiple handicaps. In about one-fifth of cases the disease proves to be relatively benign in that there is minimal disability even several years from the onset. However, there can then be sudden deterioration after a period of remaining symptom-free. The outlook is generally better when purely sensory or visual symptoms have been the chief manifestations since the beginning, whereas disorders of motor coordination or balance confer a poorer prognosis. The most sinister development is the appearance of progressive disease, whether from the outset or after a number of relapses. Younger onset tends to result in a less aggressive form of the disease and the clinical courses, whether relapsing–remitting, primary progressive or progressive, are to a large degree age-related manifestations of the same disease process (Vukusic & Confavreux 2007).

On examination typical early pointers to the diagnosis include pallor of the temporal halves of the optic discs, nystagmus, mild intention tremor, exaggerated tendon reflexes, absent abdominal reflexes, extensor plantar responses, and impaired vibration and joint position sense. During early remissions of the disease, however, there may be little or nothing to detect by way of abnormal signs. Later there is evidence of multiple lesions particularly affecting the optic nerves, cerebellum, brainstem and long tracts of the cord. Eventually the patient is likely to show some combination of ataxia, intention tremor, dysarthria, visual impairment, dissociation of conjugate lateral eye movements, paraparesis, sensory loss in the limbs and urinary incontinence. The psychological manifestations described below will emerge in a large proportion of cases, some being attributable to lesions in the cerebral hemispheres. Epileptic seizures are a rare manifestation, occurring in about 2% of cases.

There are no laboratory findings which are pathognomonic for the disease, but abnormalities occur in the cerebrospinal fluid (CSF) in a high proportion of cases. About half show a slight increase of mononuclear cells in the acute stages or a moderate elevation of protein. The γ-globulins are typically abnormally high, with the relative proportion of IgG selectively raised (Luque & Jaffe 2007). Electrophoresis of the CSF commonly shows the striking appearance of oligoclonal bands within the immunoglobulin fraction. However, false positives may occur with both of these tests. Other proteins have promising characteristics as biomarkers either for diagnosis or for monitoring progression, including neurofilament light chain and antibodies against the heavy chain (Teunissen *et al*. 2005; Luque & Jaffe 2007).

Halliday *et al*. (1973) made an important contribution by demonstrating the diagnostic value of visual-evoked responses in patients suspected of MS. Delayed forms of response from one or both eyes on the presentation of visual patterned stimuli have been shown to correlate highly with the diagnosis, even in patients without a history of optic neuritis and with normal optic discs on ophthalmoscopy. Clearly subclinical lesions of the visual pathways are very common in MS and can be readily detected with such a test. Brainstem auditory-evoked responses are also frequently abnormal. Somatosensory-evoked responses, recorded over the cervical spine while stimulating the median nerve at the wrist, can similarly detect subclinical abnormalities in the somatosensory pathways.

Neuroimaging in multiple sclerosis

Magnetic resonance imaging (MRI) has come to play a major role in the diagnosis of MS and in monitoring disease progression, not least in clinical trials (Arnold 2007). It is now apparent that almost all patients with clinically definite MS will show discrete white matter abnormalities on MRI, mostly periventricular lesions but also lesions in the optic nerve, brainstem and spinal cord. Brain atrophy is also a feature of disease and is most widespread in patients with large numbers of plaques. Grey matter shows more atrophy than white matter. Accumulated experience has shown that normal MRI of the brain all but excludes the diagnosis of MS (Armstrong & Keevil 1991). Conversely, the presence of multifocal circumscribed areas of altered signal with predilection for the periventricular regions will strongly suggest that the disease is present when clinical features are equivo-

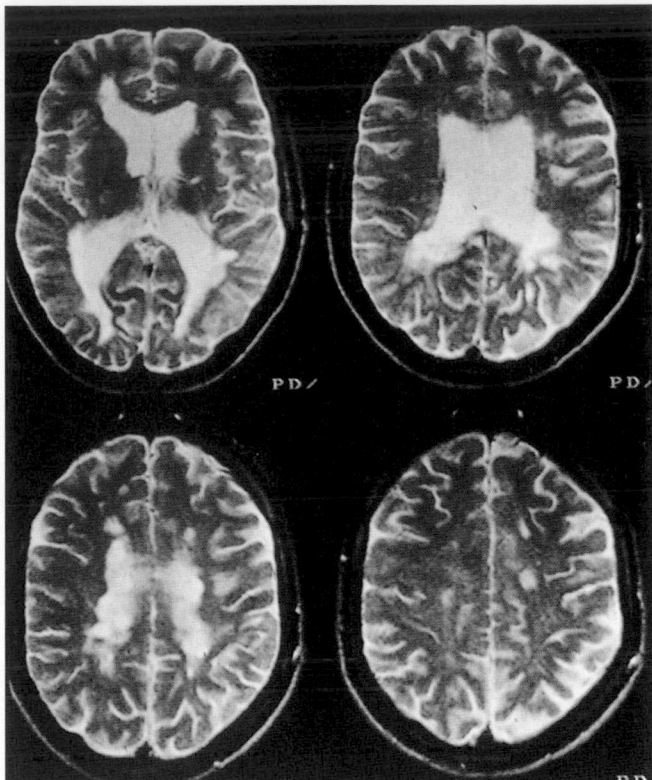

Fig. 14.1 MRI scans showing plaques in the periventricular white matter in a patient with multiple sclerosis. (Reproduced from Hotopf, M.H., Pollock, S. & Lishman, W.A. *Psychological Medicine* (1994), **24**, 525–528, courtesy of Cambridge University Press.)

cal (Fig. 14.1). MS plaques visible on MRI as T2-hyperintense lesions are typically oval in shape, 5 mm or larger in size and are more often to be found in white matter than grey matter (Neema *et al*. 2007). Although some of these lesions resolve over time, most persist. MRI techniques have been developed that are more sensitive than conventional T2-weighted images, including fluid-attenuated inversion recovery (FLAIR) and double inversion recovery (DIR). These approaches are particularly useful in detecting grey matter lesions (Bakshi *et al*. 2001; Pirko *et al*. 2007).

Serial studies in individual patients have shown that the earliest change in an evolving plaque is an increase in permeability of the blood–brain barrier, shown by areas of enhancement with gadolinium-diethylenetriaminepentaacetic acid (DTPA) (Bruck *et al*. 1997). Gadolinium enhancement reflects an early stage in plaque development and can distinguish active lesions from those that have been present for many years.

The criteria for diagnosis of MS include T2-hyperintense lesions and gadolinium-enhancing lesions both for primary diagnosis and for dissemination (Arnold 2007). Thus a change in MRI findings can substitute for clinical symptoms as evidence for dissemination in time as well as dissemination in space (McDonald *et al.* 2001; Polman *et al.* 2005). MRI can be invaluable in making treatment decisions in MS (Arnold 2007).

Proton magnetic resonance spectroscopy (MRS) in MS reveals decreased *N*-acetylaspartate in white matter in the absence of plaques, and elevated choline, myoinositol and lipids (Neema *et al.* 2007). Some evidence suggests stronger correlations between MRS measures and clinical features including both symptoms and prognosis. Other approaches showing promise as MRI-based markers include magnetisation transfer imaging (MTI) and diffusion tensor imaging (DTI), both of which may reveal disease in plaque-free areas and both of which may function as markers of response to putative therapies (Neema *et al.* 2007).

Pathology

The pathological changes within the nervous system consist of scattered sharply circumscribed areas of demyelination and degeneration of long axonal tracts. The blood–brain barrier shows evidence of breakdown and there is widespread evidence of inflammation, gliosis, loss of oligodendrocytes and axonal degeneration. The inflammatory response includes both innate and adaptive immune responses and is directed at both myelin itself and at oligodendrocytes (Dhib-Jalbut 2007; McQualter & Bernard 2007). This autoimmunity probably results from a response of the peripheral immune system being exposed to antigens normally preserved behind the blood–brain barrier but the mechanism for this remains unknown. Moreover, although autoreactive T cells are an invariable component of disease, their induction alone is insufficient to generate a full blown autoimmune disease which must result from other factors combining with autoreactive T-cells and resulting in a complex immune reaction or cascade (McQualter & Bernard 2007).

Macroscopically, the plaques show as greyish translucent areas which may be found in all parts of the neuraxis, chiefly in the white matter but sometimes also in the grey matter of the cortex and spinal cord. Typically, the number of lesions greatly exceeds what would have been expected from the clinical findings. The cerebellum and the periventricular areas of the hemispheres are sites of special predilection.

Microscopically, the acute lesions show degeneration of the myelin sheaths while the axis cylinders remain intact. The perivascular spaces contain lymphocytes and macrophages laden with neutral fats. Later the damaged myelin disappears and astrocytes proliferate to form a glial scar. At this stage axonal destruction is observed within the plaque, although recent evidence demonstrates that axonal degeneration starts early and is a universal and persistent feature of the disease (Dutta & Trapp 2007). Axons may be damaged by

direct imflammatory attack, by the loss of myelin or by other mechanisms and the site of damage is in both grey and white matter (Dutta & Trapp 2007).

Treatment

The arrival of potential disease-modifying treatments for MS brings substantial hope to sufferers. However, the effect of approved therapies on disease progression has been relatively modest, although the effects of some interventions on the frequency of relapse, and on markers of disease, have been confirmed in large trials (Hemmer & Hartung 2007; Kleinschnitz *et al.* 2007). Interferon (IFN)-β delays conversion from a single demyelinating episode to clinically definite MS and is recommended for use early in the disease course in some countries. However, IFN is only partially effective and the majority of patients will still progress to full disease. Glatiramer acetate was approved for use in relapsing–remitting MS, although a large clinical trial found no benefits relative to placebo. Neither IFN-β nor glatiramer acetate are currently recommended for use in the UK by the National Institute for Clinical Excellence (NICE). Modulating the immune system by intravenous immunoglobulins was not supported by large studies, although plasma exchange may be of some benefit in people with particularly aggressive disease. A monoclonal antibody to α4β1 integrin, natalizumab, is approved in the USA and Europe for active relapsing forms of MS and is supported by NICE in the UK. In one trial 96% of patients treated with natalizumab showed absence of new gadolinium-enhancing lesions compared with 68% of placebo-treated patients and in another large randomised controlled trial the addition of natalizumab to IFN-β was shown to be beneficial in relation to both relapse rate and MRI markers of disease (Polman *et al.* 2006; Rudick *et al.* 2006a). Although currently approved, concerns remain about safety following the development of progressive multifocal leucoencephalopathy in two patients receiving both natalizumab and IFN-β (Kleinschnitz *et al.* 2007). Despite this, these two compounds are the first specific, molecularly targeted therapies for MS that have resulted from primary research and many other compounds are in development (Hemmer & Hartung 2007; Kleinschnitz *et al.* 2007).

Recovery from acute exacerbations of the disease is speeded by methylprednisolone, which probably acts by reducing brain oedema in areas of acute inflammation. Prednisolone may be given intravenously or by high-dose oral administration. Immune suppression can stabilise the course in patients with rapidly progressive disease, and a variety of immunosuppressive agents have been tried in attempts to improve the long-term outlook. Azathioprine and mitoxantrone, intravenous immunoglobulins and plasma exchange and short-course high-dose methylprednisolone are all recommended by NICE, albeit under strictly defined circumstances (available at www.nice.org.uk). The NICE guidance also reviews recommendations for a wide variety of treatments for specific sets of symptoms in MS.

Psychiatric aspects

Neuropsychiatric symptoms are a core component of the MS phenotype and include disorders of affect and behaviour and cognitive symptoms. Attention has also been directed to the possibility that psychological factors may be associated with relapses of the disease. The historical development of psychiatric interest in the disorder is traced by Surridge (1969). Early investigators regarded intellectual deficits as the main disturbance, and towards the end of the nineteenth century there were numerous reports of acute psychoses occurring in the disease. However, many of these studies were made before MS could be adequately distinguished from cerebrovascular syphilis. Cottrell and Wilson's (1926) study then had an influential effect. In a consecutive series of 100 outpatients, they found that emotional changes were strikingly common, usually taking the form of increased cheerfulness and optimism. A sense of physical well-being was frequent among the patients despite their severely disabled state. In contrast to these affective changes, intellectual disorders were minimal or negligible. Brain (1930) added hysterical conversion symptoms as a further characteristic of the disease, suggesting that MS might predispose in some way to the mental dissociation responsible for hysteria. From then onward euphoria and hysteria continued to be emphasised in the English literature as typical of MS.

Meanwhile, Ombredane (1929) re-emphasised the occurrence of intellectual deficits. Disturbances of affect were common in the intellectually deteriorated cases, but consisted chiefly of rapid unstable variations in mood rather than constant shifts towards euphoria or depression. Runge (1928) maintained that depression occurred in the early stage but gave way to euphoria as the disease progressed further. Euphoria was seen simply as a concomitant of intellectual deterioration. This view, in sharp contrast to Cottrell and Wilson's findings, became prominent on the European continent thereafter.

More recent investigators have sought to resolve the dilemma by careful surveys of the psychiatric changes in large series of patients. Surridge's (1969) investigation was exceptional for its thoroughness, and in providing a control group suffering from a different progressive disease, namely muscular dystrophy. In this study, 108 patients suffering from MS were visited in their normal places of residence, and separate accounts were obtained from informants to aid in the assessments of mood, intellectual deficits and personality changes. The sample was considered to be representative of patients with MS, except for some possible bias towards more severely disabled cases.

Of the MS patients, 75% were found to suffer some psychiatric abnormality, compared with less than half of the controls. Intellectual deterioration was present in 61%, varying in degree from mild memory loss to profound global dementia. None of the controls showed intellectual impairment. Abnormalities of mood were found in 53% compared with 13% of controls; 27% were depressed, 26% euphoric and 10% showed exaggeration of emotional expression. Euphoria was almost exclusively seen in patients who were intellectually impaired, and a significant correlation emerged between increasing euphoria and increasing intellectual deterioration. Euphoria was also associated with denial of disability which was observed in 11% of the patients. Impaired awareness of disability short of complete denial was found in 31%. Of the MS patients, 40% showed personality change compared with 33% of the controls. This was predominantly a change towards irritability, whereas the muscular dystrophy controls often showed increased patience and tolerance. Psychotic disorders were rare.

These findings effectively set the stage for subsequent studies, which have increasingly used neuropsychological assessments and objective rating procedures for charting the changes observed. Control comparisons have amply confirmed the vulnerability of patients to a range of cognitive and emotional complications, as outlined below. However, considerable difficulties are encountered in reaching firm conclusions about the prevalence of psychiatric disorder in the disease in view of its widely varying manifestations. For example, Dalos et al. (1983) have shown that much depends on whether patients are studied during remissions or relapses; psychiatric symptoms, mainly anxiety and depression, were present in 39% of patients examined during stable periods and in 90% during exacerbations. Certain differences have also emerged between patients with relapsing–remitting and chronic forms of MS, particularly in relation to cognitive deficits (see below).

It can be uncertain how far psychiatric manifestations are attributable to brain pathology rather than representing psychological reactions to the threats and limitations imposed by the physical symptoms. Evidence can sometimes be found for a causal role of brain pathology even where seemingly non-organic symptoms such as depression are concerned, but other influences are also clearly at work. For example, Ron and Logsdail (1989) found that psychiatric morbidity in their sample was strongly related to the degree of social stress perceived by the patient. This suggests an interactional model whereby the vulnerability created by the presence of brain damage enhances the effects of environmental and personal factors in producing psychiatric disorder (Ron & Feinstein 1992). In seeking to define the organic contribution, recent studies have been greatly helped by the availability of sensitive brain-imaging techniques. These have also allowed exploration of the possible contributions of 'covert' brain lesions from early in the disease.

Cognitive impairment

Cognitive impairment occurs in 40–65% of patients with MS (McIntosh-Michaelis *et al.* 1991; Rao *et al.* 1991; Amato *et al.* 2006; Einarsson *et al.* 2006). Much is likely to depend on the stage of the disease at which assessments are made, but even so it is apparent that patients differ markedly in their liability to become impaired. This is perhaps not surprising since the accent of the disease can fall on very different parts of the neuraxis. The severity of impairments also varies widely, from those only detectable on careful testing to pictures of global dementia.

Some studies have found a relationship between cognitive impairment and severity of neurological disability while others have not. Peyser *et al.* (1980a) showed that cognitive deficits could be present or absent in groups with varying levels of disablement. Cognitive impairment may occur early (Ghaffar & Feinstein 2007) and it is clear that psychometric evaluation may reveal deficits that have gone unsuspected on more cursory examination. Peyser *et al.* (1980b) and Heaton *et al.* (1985) found that half of patients judged to be cognitively intact on routine examination were impaired on psychometric testing. In Heaton *et al.*'s study, 46% of relapsing–remitting and 72% of chronic progressive MS patients were found to show cognitive deficits. The progressive group was more severely impaired and on a wider range of functions.

Verbal skills are often relatively well preserved, which may account for other deficits being overlooked. The functions most markedly affected include memory and learning, and capacities to deal with abstract concepts and problem-solving. Attentional processes may be impaired from a very early stage and slowed information processing speed may be the most common cognitive deficit (Benedict & Bobholz 2007).

Memory impairment has been highlighted as one of the commonest deficits encountered, second only to decline in motor skills. Various studies indicate that 40–60% of MS patients perform below expectation on memory tests when compared with control groups (Grafman *et al.* 1991). Again, however, patients vary considerably, some being affected early in the disease while others remain unimpaired. Primary memory as reflected in the digit span appears to remain relatively intact, and rates of forgetting are also largely normal as measured by the Brown–Peterson task. Working, semantic and episodic memories are all affected (Ghaffar & Feinstein 2007). The role of attentional deficits in leading to such problems has not been fully explored, but both depression and psychotropic medication have been exonerated as a complete explanation.

Other cognitive processes emerge as defective in a substantial proportion of patients (Rao 1986; Benedict & Bobholz 2007). Language deficits are rare, except for reductions in verbal fluency. However, marked difficulties may be encountered with psychomotor efficiency and attention and concen-tration. Problems with abstract thinking, conceptualisation and the shifting of sets may resemble those seen with frontal lobe injuries. Perseveration can sometimes be detected. Mahler and Benson (1990) draw an analogy with the pictures seen in 'subcortical dementia'. Such difficulties can emerge in patients who score well on tests of general intelligence, and will then often go unsuspected. In occasional examples the picture amounts to a clinically recognisable dementia.

Thus it is apparent that some patients have not only to adapt to progressive physical disability, but must often do this against a background of diminishing intellect and impaired adaptive capacity. The implications for retraining are obviously important; the presence and severity of impairments such as these may well be crucial in determining the outcome of efforts at rehabilitation.

A consensus conference in 2001 led to the development of a battery of tests designed to detect and assess cognitive impairment in MS: the Minimal Assessment of Cognitive Function in MS (MACFIMS). This battery comprises seven tests covering the cognitive domains known to be affected including processing speed, working memory, episodic memory, verbal memory, executive function and others (Benedict & Bobholz 2007).

The course followed by cognitive impairments may be as variable as the neurological symptoms of the disease. Some patients experience relapses and remissions, while others show steady progression of their cognitive deficits. Attempts to chart the course of decline in patient groups have therefore yielded conflicting results (see Canter 1951; Ivnik 1978). In the first truly prospective study, Filley *et al.* (1990) found remarkably little evidence of progression in a group of 46 patients, only 6 of 36 test measures showing significant deterioration over 1–2 years. On global clinical ratings, however, 7 of 10 patients with chronic progressive disease showed worsening; of the 36 with relapsing–remitting disease, a smaller proportion showed deterioration and this was mainly evident on retesting during a documented relapse. Overall, approximately one-quarter of patients deteriorate, the prevalence of cognitive impairment increasing from 26% to 56% over 10 years and the degree of impairment increasing over this time (Amato *et al.* 1995, 2001).

The high prevalence of cognitive impairment is hardly surprising in view of the finding that plaque formation is widespread. Professor Ron and her colleagues have conducted a series of elegant MRI studies which show that even 'subclinical' brain involvement can lead to detectable cognitive deficits.

Callanan *et al.* (1989) investigated 48 patients with 'clinically isolated lesions' of the type seen in MS. Subtle cognitive deficits were already apparent. On MRI 80% of these showed cerebral abnormalities, by way of increased signal in the periventricular rim or discrete lesions in the brain parenchyma, and the extent of such abnormalities correlated with impairment on tests of abstracting ability and auditory attention.

Feinstein *et al.* (1992a) concentrated on tests of attention and speed of information processing in over 40 patients who had recently suffered a first episode of acute optic neuritis, and who in all other respects were neurologically normal. Approximately half of the sample showed abnormalities on brain MRI, and these were more impaired on the tests than patients without cerebral lesions or normal controls. Thus both studies demonstrated that cognitive deficits can be the only manifestation of otherwise silent brain lesions, emerging as more sensitive indicators of cerebral involvement than neurological symptoms and signs.

The MRI findings mirror clinical findings to the extent that evolution of T2-hyperintense lesions correlates with cognitive decline over a decade or more (Rudick *et al.* 2006b) and grey matter volume loss differentiates those with cognitive impairment from those without (Benedict & Bobholz 2007; Ghaffar & Feinstein 2007). However, there are discrepancies between findings from MRI and from neuropsychology and increasingly studies are turning to functional imaging approaches to explore a putative 'functional reserve' that might explain interindividual variation in cognitive loss (Ghaffar & Feinstein 2007).

Presentation with dementia is occasionally encountered and can raise important problems of differential diagnosis. Koenig (1968) described seven patients in whom dementia was the sole or predominant manifestation of the disease, the MS being of a relatively silent variety neurologically. The onset was usually fairly acute with memory loss, confusion, disorientation or personality change. Some showed slight fluctuations in the level of mental functioning from day to day. Three showed progressive deterioration and only one had a partial remission. Neurological symptoms of brainstem or cord dysfunction had preceded the dementia or accompanied its onset in four cases, but all showed evidence of disseminated CNS disease on careful examination. Koenig suggested that 'silent' or unrecognised MS may be a commoner cause of dementia than is generally recognised. Young *et al.* (1976) reported further examples with intellectual impairment as the presenting symptom or forming a prominent part of the picture from the earliest stages.

Hotopf *et al.* (1994) describe two particularly instructive patients in whom the cognitive changes were at first attributed to psychiatric illness.

A 41-year-old man had a 2-year history of change of personality, becoming quiet, vague and forgetful. He was involved in a series of road traffic accidents and had begun to sleep for long periods. His attitude to his problems was one of bland indifference. There was no family or personal history of psychiatric illness.

On examination he was alert but his affect was strangely inappropriate. He was intermittently disorientated in time and place and there were tendencies to confabulate and perseverate. Concentration, attention and memory were poor, and he had difficulty with verbal fluency and sequential tasks. He made occasional naming errors and paraphasic mistakes when writing. On first contact with the neurological services his mental state had seemed sufficiently bizarre to raise a diagnosis of hysteria, reinforced by his striking lack of concern about his poor performance on tests of cognition.

The only physical signs were an extensor plantar response, which was not present on re-examination, and lack of left arm swinging while walking. Two months later he showed a plantar grasp reflex and a positive glabellar tap. Psychometric testing revealed a verbal IQ of 73 and performance IQ of 63, consistent with moderate to severe decline of intellect. CSF examination showed a raised protein with oligoclonal bands and visual-evoked responses were abnormal. MRI showed periventricular abnormalities and widespread changes in the hemispheres consistent with MS. Screening tests for other causes of dementia were negative. Over the next 8 years he showed steady deterioration to severe global cognitive deficit, with dysphasia, severe ataxia and incontinence of urine.

The second patient presented at the age of 35 with a 3-year history of difficulties with concentration and memory. He had become increasingly withdrawn but showed no concern over his symptoms. When first seen in a neurological clinic a non-organic psychiatric illness was suspected. He had diabetes, and for 6 months there had been an insidious loss of vision. Neurological findings included bilateral optic atrophy and later some evidence of gait disturbance, but there were no other neurological abnormalities. Cognitive examination subsequently showed disorientation, impaired concentration, poor memory, dyscalculia and reduced verbal fluency. Psychometric testing confirmed these deficits and showed a verbal IQ of 73. CSF examination showed oligoclonal bands in the presence of normal total protein, and visual-evoked responses were abnormal. MRI revealed changes consistent with multiple sclerosis (Fig. 14.1). Over the next 18 months he continued to show gradual cognitive decline without any marked physical symptoms or signs.

Sometimes the rate of progression of dementia is astonishingly rapid, as in the patient described by Bergin (1957).

A woman of 30 developed brief retrobulbar neuritis followed 1 year later by diplopia, ataxia and precipitate micturition. Over 3 months she became severely incapacitated, apathetic, retarded and vague. Examination showed a pale left optic disc, fine lateral nystagmus, slight right facial and arm weakness, incoordination of the legs and upgoing plantar responses. The CSF showed 18 lymphocytes/mL and a paretic Lange curve. One week after admission she became confused, uncooperative and disorientated, doubly incontinent and with gross evidence of intellectual impairment. Two weeks later she could not understand even simple sentences. Electroencephalography (EEG) showed random irregular slow waves in all areas and the air encephalogram showed moderate ventricular enlargement. Six weeks after admission she was bedfast, making noises but no recognisable words. The only active limb was her left arm, which was used to strike out at people and tug at her hair. Within 10 weeks she died and post-mortem examination showed well-defined plaques throughout the brain, cerebellum, brainstem and cord.

Abnormalities of mood

Studies from patients in the community or in the clinic show lifetime rates of major depression of up to 50% (Ghaffar & Feinstein 2007). The symptoms are essentially the same as for primary major depressive disorder, although some evidence suggests that irritability is more common than feelings of low esteem. There has been much debate as to the origins of depression in MS. Psychosocial variables are undoubtedly important and increasing attention has turned to psychosocial interventions designed to increase quality of life and reduce mood disturbance with some evidence for efficacy (Malcomson *et al.* 2007). However, there is also evidence from neuroimaging for biological effects of the disease on mood, with some evidence pointing towards left medial inferior prefrontal cortical lesions and dominant anterior temporal atrophy being associated with depression (Feinstein *et al.* 2004). In truth, for most patients it will be a combination of personal circumstances, premorbid predisposing factors and biological effects of disease that give rise to depressive events. Irrespective of its derivation, the degree of depression in MS can be severe, and suicide has been reported in a considerable number of cases.

A variety of other affective changes are common in MS. Euphoria, a bland elevation of mood out of keeping with the patient's physical condition, was once thought to be the usual picture, but it is now clear that depression is at least as common. Much probably depends on the stage at which the patient is examined and whether some degree of intellectual deterioration has occurred. The transition over time from depression to euphoria can sometimes be observed in the individual patient. Frank bipolar affective disorder is twice as common in MS as in the general population (Ghaffar & Feinstein 2007).

Euphoria was defined by Surridge (1969) as a mood of cheerful complacency out of context with the patient's total situation. It differed from the elation of hypomania in not being accompanied by motor restlessness, increased energy or speeding up of thought processes. All but two of the euphoric patients in his series showed intellectual deterioration, and the group as a whole was significantly more disabled than the depressed or normal groups. The phenomenon is possibly related not only to changes of mood but also to denial or impaired awareness of disability. Quite often, however, the initial impression of euphoria proves to be misleading, and the evidence of cheerfulness or complacency subsides as the interview progresses. Indeed Surridge found that 8 of 28 euphoric patients confessed to feeling miserable and depressed despite the strong outward impression that they were unreasonably cheerful. No doubt an element of emotional lability is often associated with euphoria and adds to the difficulty of assessing the patient's true subjective feelings.

Disorders of emotional control include true exaggeration of emotional feeling (lability of affect) or exaggeration of expression that is unbacked by an equivalent degree of feeling (disorder of affective expression). The latter may indeed be incongruous with the underlying mood and is essentially similar to the disorder of emotional expression seen in pseudobulbar palsy. This affective state has been termed 'involuntatry emotional expression disorder' (Cummings *et al.* 2006) and affects up to 10% of people with MS. Antidepressants, levodopa and a dextromethorphan/quinidine combination have all been suggested as possible treatment strategies (Ghaffar & Feinstein 2007).

Psychoses

Psychotic illnesses have been described in the disease, sometimes late in the course but occasionally as a presenting feature. A relatively recent database study suggested rates in MS of more than twice that in the general population (Patten *et al.* 2005). This finding substantiates previous small series or case reports of the co-occurrence of MS and psychosis. With regard to schizophrenia, Davison and Bagley (1969) identified 39 acceptable cases in the literature, 27 with paranoid–hallucinatory and 12 with hebephrenic–catatonic illnesses. The symptomatology did not differ appreciably from that of other schizophrenic psychoses, except that expansive delusional states seemed to be particularly common, and neurological symptoms such as paraesthesiae were sometimes incorporated into paranoid–delusional systems. The psychoses often developed early in the disease, tending to cluster around the time of first appearance of neurological abnormalities.

Feinstein *et al.* (1992b) report an attempt to explore the possible contribution of brain pathology to psychotic illness by comparing groups of 10 patients with and without psychosis. These were well matched for age, disability, duration of disease and disease course. The psychoses were equally divided into two broad categories of schizophrenia and affective psychosis. In all cases the neurological disorder had preceded the onset of psychosis, the mean interval being 8.5 years. On MRI there was a trend for the psychotic group to have a higher total lesion score, particularly in the periventricular regions and in the areas surrounding the temporal horns bilaterally. This reached statistical significance when the left temporal horn and adjacent left trigone areas were combined. Such findings point to a possible aetiological role of brain pathology in contributing to psychotic developments. No differences could be determined in this respect between the schizophrenic and affective psychotic groups.

Presentation with psychosis is rare, but sometimes the neurological abnormalities are so overshadowed by the mental picture that the true diagnosis is missed. Such cases are obviously important. Parker (1956) reported a patient who became apathetic and withdrawn in his early twenties and was diagnosed as suffering from schizophrenia. He showed slight hesitancy of speech and irregular nystagmus but this was ignored at the time. Attempts at treatment and rehabilitation met with no success. A few years later he was fatuous and childish, and by then showed impairment of memory, gross spasticity and pronounced incoordination. He died suddenly and the pathological changes of MS were revealed.

Geocaris (1957) reported four instructive examples of patients admitted with an initial diagnosis of psychosis, three with schizophrenia and one with severe depression, who showed evidence of MS a few weeks or months later. Mur *et al.* (1966) reported three unusual examples in patients over 50 in whom psychotic features dominated the course. One had a paranoid psychosis for 5 years before neurological symptoms appeared in the form of a spastic paresis with dementia; another had a relapsing paranoid syndrome for 11 years accompanied by ataxia of gait and intellectual impairment; and the third had a temporary gait and speech disturbance at the onset of a depressive syndrome that dominated the picture until death. In all three cases the plaques were found to be predominantly in the cerebral hemispheres.

Finally, two patients reported by Matthews (1979) are important in drawing attention to the possibility that acute mental disturbance, remitting completely, may sometimes be the initial manifestation of the disease.

In the first patient, a girl of 19, the presentation was with intermittent confusion and episodes of markedly bizarre behaviour, leading to a diagnosis of probable schizophrenia. No neurological abnormalities were apparent on examination. Epileptic fits developed during a course of electroconvulsive therapy, leading to lumbar puncture which revealed mild pleocytosis in the CSF. EEG was diffusely abnormal, and she was treated with phenytoin. Over the course of the next few weeks she recovered completely, EEG also reverting towards normality. Thereafter she remained well for 3 years. Symptoms typical of MS then made an appearance, the disease following a relapsing and remitting course over the next few years.

The second patient developed depression of acute onset at the age of 24. She became increasingly withdrawn, self-neglectful and intermittently incontinent of urine and faeces. The tendon reflexes were noted to be increased in the lower limbs and the plantar responses were extensor. Examination of the CSF showed abnormalities compatible with MS and EEG showed a marked excess of slow activity bilaterally. Her mental state varied greatly. At times she was almost normally communicative; at others she gave bizarre replies to questions and had outbursts of shouting and kicking. Treatment with prednisolone led to gradual neurological and mental improvement, the patient becoming entirely normal some 3 months from the onset. Several months after recovery she developed unilateral optic neuritis and bilateral abnormalities of visual-evoked responses, clearly indicative of MS.

The question of possible presentations with psychiatric disorder is clearly of great interest, not least in pointing to the need for neurological examination and comprehensive review of the past medical history in psychiatric patients. Particular interest would attach to presentations without organic features in the mental state. In a careful review of 91 patients with MS from a defined region of New Zealand, Skegg (1993) found that 19 had been referred to psychiatrists before the disease was diagnosed, often with non-organic symptomatology. However, only in two cases did a link between such symptoms and developing MS seem plausible. Skegg's review highlights the difficulty of reaching firm conclusions on the issue.

Influence of emotions on the disease

Physical and emotional traumas have often been regarded as precipitants of MS, or as provocative factors that help to determine relapses. Pratt (1951) attempted to examine the situation in detail and found that 38% of MS patients had suffered some emotional stress in the months antedating the onset, compared with 26% of controls suffering from other nervous system disease. The difference fell just short of statistical significance, but in most cases the stresses had not been unduly severe. With regard to later relapses, 25% were preceded by emotional stress, a figure virtually identical with the proportion of controls who had stress antedating their illness. Thus in the group as a whole there was no clear evidence to incriminate emotional factors in causing relapses.

In individual cases, however, a suggestive relationship was sometimes observed. In one patient a relapse occurred within an hour of receiving bad news by letter. In another numbness developed in the legs immediately after a narrow escape from a motor cycle accident, and in another the right arm became useless the morning after breaking off an engagement. Short of major relapses, some patients found that emotional disturbances led to transient exacerbation of the symptoms of a pre-existing lesion. This was significantly commoner than among the controls, and the examples were often clear-cut and impressive, usually occurring within minutes of the emotional upheaval. In different patients, for example, worry led invariably to increased unsteadiness, anger to weakness of a leg, fear or quarrelling to weakness of the legs lasting several hours, self-consciousness to blurring of vision or exacerbation of diplopia.

There is some evidence from animal models of MS that stress might exacerbate the biological process, perhaps by disturbing the hypothalamic–pituitary axis (Bomholt *et al.* 2004; Gold *et al.* 2005; Heesen *et al.* 2007). In addition, recent clinical studies and a meta-analysis have further supported the role of stress (Mohr *et al.* 2004; Mohr & Pelletier 2006). These findings emphasise that ongoing social and psychological support will have an especially important part to play in the management of patients, and may sometimes serve to avert or delay relapses.

Schilder's disease (diffuse cerebral sclerosis, encephalitis periaxialis diffusa, myelinoclastic diffuse sclerosis)

The generic term 'diffuse cerebral sclerosis' has been applied to a variety of conditions in which widespread demyelination and gliosis occur in the white matter of the hemispheres. Histological examination allows a more precise classification, and it seems that reported cases have included examples of familial leucodystrophy and subacute sclerosing leucoencephalitis in addition to cases pathologically related to MS (Greenfield & Norman 1963). Greenfield and Norman suggest that the latter is the most appropriate restricted use for the term 'Schilder's disease'. Nevertheless, some believe that it represents no more than an exceptionally severe variety of MS occurring in early life (Compston 1993). In any case it is rare and most of the evidence comes from case reports (Kotil *et al.* 2002).

Most cases have been reported in children but adults may also be affected (Garell *et al.* 1998). Both sporadic and familial examples are encountered. The varied neurological manifestations include spastic paraparesis, sensory changes and often progressive cerebral blindness. Central deafness may also occur. Mental functions are affected early and severely, dullness and apathy progressing to dementia and stupor. Acute and widespread demyelination may cause cerebral oedema, raised intracranial pressure and papilloedema (Compston 1993). The disease usually runs a rapid course, with death within a few months though some patients survive for 2 or 3 years. Temporary remissions have been described, and very occasionally recovery (Ellison & Barron 1979). A good response to corticosteroids has been reported (Kurul *et al.* 2003). The CSF shows changes resembling those of MS. Brain imaging usually shows a characteristic picture, with symmetrical, sharply defined, low-density lesions in the occipital or frontal regions.

Pathologically, the brain shows large areas of brownish or greyish softening in the white matter, usually maximally involving the occipital lobes and spreading forwards through the hemispheres symmetrically (Greenfield & Norman 1963). Microscopically, they show complete demyelination, and in the older lesions axonal destruction as well. In the smaller lesions the picture is indistinguishable from that of MS.

Psychiatric aspects

A point of psychiatric interest has been the occurrence of pictures indistinguishable from schizophrenia in patients who have later shown Schilder's disease at post-mortem. Several such reports have now accumulated, mostly in patients who had displayed little or nothing by way of neurological disturbance during life. The cerebral pathological findings were in consequence usually unexpected.

Ferraro (1934, 1943) reported two examples in adolescent boys who had been clinically diagnosed as suffering from hebephrenic schizophrenia. In the first, the disorder progressed over 2 or 3 years without neurological abnormalities or features indicative of an organic psychosis at any stage. The second showed fleeting and inconstant neurological abnormalities early in the illness, and obvious intellectual deterioration during the months immediately preceding death 3.5 years later.

Holt and Tedeschi's (1943) patient showed a classic catatonic picture and died within a week. There were no abnormal neurological signs. He had suffered a previous episode of acute catatonic schizophrenia 18 years previously. Roizin *et al.*'s (1945) patient similarly showed a picture of catatonic schizophrenia, with auditory hallucinations and periods of stupor alternating with outbursts of impulsive destructive behaviour. Again, there were no neurological abnormalities and the patient died within a few weeks. Jankowski (1963) described a chronic example in a man of 28 with repeated hospitalisations over 4 years prior to death. Severe affective changes of hebephrenic type developed gradually and without discernible intellectual deterioration. Late in the illness the pupillary reactions to light were lost and he complained of impaired vision, but the CSF remained normal.

Ramani (1981) has reported yet another example, this time diagnosed by computed tomography (CT) during life and subsequently confirmed by biopsy.

> A man of 34 had suffered from chronic schizophrenia, refractory to treatment, for 5 years. It had started with mood swings, leading on to progressive withdrawal, disorganisation of thinking, and paranoid delusions and hallucinations. He showed bizarre posturing at times and echolalia. There was no family history of schizophrenia. On examination the only neurological abnormalities were bilateral extensor plantar responses and a suggestion of a snout reflex. CT showed large, symmetrically situated, low-density areas in the frontal regions.

In most of these examples the accent of the pathological process was on the frontal lobes of the brain, in contrast to the usual predominant involvement of the occipital lobes. This may have accounted for the atypical presentation and development of the disease.

Tuberous sclerosis (tuberose sclerosis, epiloia)

Tuberous sclerosis complex (TSC) is a multisystem disorder most commonly affecting brain, skin, kidneys and heart. It occurs with a birth incidence of 1 in 6000 to 1 in 10000 (Wiederholt *et al.* 1985; Osborne *et al.* 1991) and as might be expected from the systems affected has a complex clinical appearance (Crino *et al.* 2006; Rosser *et al.* 2006). Skin defects include fibromas and hypomelanotic macules seen typically as leaf-shaped dull white patches, particularly over the trunk and buttocks; renal manifestations include cysts and angiomyolipidomas; and cardiac features include rhabdomyomas causing dysrhythmias. However, neurological symptoms are the most common and result in the most impairment. The first clinical manifestations are usually in infancy or childhood although presentation in adulthood can occur, sometimes on account of late-onset epilepsy or sometimes when characteristic skin lesions or neuroimaging signs are discovered. The disorder results from mutations in two genes, *TSC1* (chromosome 9q34) and *TSC2* (16p13.3), which occur spontaneously in approximately two-thirds of cases and are inherited in an autosomal dominant fashion in the remainder (Webb & Osborne 1992).

Neuropsychiatric symptoms

Seizures occur in over 90% of cases at presentation (Rosser *et al.* 2006). All forms of epilepsy, with the probable exception of classic absence seizures, are reported although partial motor and complex partial seizures occur most often. In severe cases the presentation is frequently with infantile spasms. EEG is usually abnormal in patients with severe disease or currently active epilepsy, but can be quite normal in others. No specific pattern is diagnostic. Medical management is the same as for other epilepsies, although severe treatment-resistant seizures are common. Vigabatrin appears to be particularly effective for infantile spasms (Rosser *et al.* 2006) and surgical resection of isolated tubers resulting in epileptic foci can be useful.

Cognitive impairment is common, often profound, but not invariable. In a large study from the UK, the distribution of cognitive ability in TSC was shown to be bimodal as half of the population had a normal IQ and one-third an IQ in the profoundly affected range (Joinson *et al.* 2003). Moderate to severe mental retardation is more common in those with infantile spasms and both epilepsy and cognitive impairment tends to be more severe in those with *TSC2* mutations.

Autistic spectrum disorder is also common in TSC, although prevalence rates vary hugely in different studies probably because of different assessment measures (Rosser *et al.* 2006). Reported rates of autism in TSC range up to 60% but it should be noted that less than 4% of all autism is attributable to TSC.

Psychotic symptoms can occur. Thus Critchley and Earl (1932), reporting institutionalised patients, described the essential psychological feature as a combination of intellectual defect with a 'primitive form of catatonic schizophrenia'. It is now clear that psychotic developments, like the learning disability, are by no means as invariable as these writers believed. Nevertheless, the following case reported by Zlotlow and Kleiner (1965) illustrates the type of schizophrenia-like picture that may be encountered.

> The patient had fits from the age of 4 to 7 years but thereafter excelled at school. Pimples developed on the nose and cheeks from 15 onwards. In adolescence he became shy, solitary and withdrawn, and at 20 a severe mental change occurred: he became nervous and easily upset, with frequent tantrums and childish unreasonable behaviour. Seizures became frequent and he appeared slightly dull mentally. Adenoma sebaceum was by this time well developed, EEG showed abnormalities over the left hemisphere and the air encephalogram showed slight ventricular dilatation.
>
> The mental condition worsened, with fear of leaving the house, feelings that he was losing control of his limbs, and

beliefs that people were laughing and talking about him. In hospital at 23 he was retarded, emotionally dull and spoke slowly in whispers. He denied auditory hallucinations but saw 'moving pictures' before his eyes. The IQ was low (70) with evidence of deterioration. He remained seclusive and withdrawn, with frequent mood swings, irritability and overactivity.

At 34 he was regarded as a chronic schizophrenic, often incontinent, speaking incoherently and with long episodes of mutism. Periods of irritable excitement alternated with catatonic stupor. He remained essentially unchanged over the following years. Skull radiography now showed small calcifications in the pineal region and a number of globular vacuoles in the frontal and temporal bones. EEG showed much disorganised slow activity. He was untestable psychometrically.

Magnetic resonance imaging is used to diagnose TSC and to estimate the extent and document the site of lesions in the brain (Luat *et al.* 2007). Cortical tubers are shown as well-circumscribed lesions on T1-weighted images and as hyper-intensities on T2-weighted sequences. FLAIR and MTI can both add to the sensitivity in detecting cortical tubers. MRS shows decreased *N*-acetylaspartate indicative of neuronal loss. Increasingly, DTI has been used to document tract damage in TSC and may be clinically useful in identifying epileptogenic foci in some studies in combination with various positron emission tomography (PET) imaging techniques (Luat *et al.* 2007).

Pathology

The striking pathological change in the brain consists of pearly white nodules 0.5–3 cm in diameter, situated along the ventricular surfaces and sometimes over the cortical surface as well. The nodules are hard, like rubber or potato (hence 'tuberous'), and may contain minute calcareous fragments. Histologically, they contain dense glial material and curious large cells which are thought to derive from undifferentiated spongioblasts. Frank neoplastic changes may be apparent in the form of glioblastoma multiforme or spongioblastoma. Short of this, the nodular protrusions are occasionally sufficiently large to obstruct the flow of CSF within the ventricles. The intervening brain tissue is often markedly disorganised, with abnormal cytoarchitecture, reduction of neurones and increased gliosis. The cerebellum and cord may be similarly affected.

These changes result from mutations in *TSC1* and *TSC2*, which encode the proteins hamartin and tuberin, respectively. A very large number of mutations in both are noted, many confined to a family or arising spontaneously in an individual. Together these genes account for most of the cases, although there may yet be other *TSC* genes. In a series of over 300 families and patients, approximately one-third had no apparent *TSC1* or *TSC2* mutation (Au *et al.* 2007). The gene products, hamartin and tuberin, interact with each other through coiled-coil domains (van Slegtenhorst *et al.* 1998) and the heterodimer contributes to intracellular signalling in a number of critical pathways. Upstream of *TSC1/TSC2*, these include the mitogen-activated protein kinase, phosphatidylinositol 3-kinase and glycogen synthase kinase-3 pathways. These pathways have been widely implicated in other brain diseases including schizophrenia and Alzheimer's disease (Lovestone *et al.* 2007; Hooper *et al.* 2008) as well as in normal neurodevelopmental processes (Logan & Nusse 2004; Davila *et al.* 2007). Downstream of *TSC1/TSC2*, signalling through mTOR (mammalian target of rapamycin) controls, among other effects, cell growth and differentiation. The mTOR pathway has been clearly shown to be critical to neurodevelopment and to the functioning of the adult nervous system (Swiech *et al.* 2008). It is clear then that the *TSC1/TSC2* genes are at the centre of a network of signalling processes which independently have been shown to be essential to both normal neuronal development and to normal mature neuronal function and are altered in other degenerative and developmental brain diseases. De Vries and Howe (2007) propose that the complex functions as a global regulator and integrator of a range of physiological processes and that the clinical features of the disease can result from disruption of these processes and that tubers and seizures are neither a necessary nor sufficient explanation of the neurocognitive phenotype.

Neurofibromatosis

The neurofibromatoses comprise a number of related conditions characterised by skin pigmentation and tumour formation at a number of sites. Most features arise in tissues of neural crest origin and Schwann cells are the principal components in tumour formation. By far the most common form is von Recklinghausen's disease, now called neurofibromatosis (NF)1, with the characteristic development of peripheral neurofibromas. Prevalence is estimated to be 0.0003 (Littler & Morton 1990). The related disease NF2 can lack distinctive skin manifestations and typically presents with bilateral acoustic neuromas (schwannomas). All other variants are considerably rarer.

Both NF1 and NF2 are inherited as autosomal dominant disorders, although in a very high proportion these represent new mutations. The rate of new mutations of NF1 (1×10^{-4} per gamete per generation) is the highest rate of new mutation in any known human gene and causes half of all cases. Mutations seem to occur most often in paternally inherited chromosomes, suggesting an effect of imprinting (Stephens *et al.* 1992). The *NF1* locus on chromosome 17 encodes the protein neurofibromin (Trovo-Marqui & Tajara 2006). In fact the genetics are complex in a very small minority of cases with mutations in two genes involved in DNA repair (*MLH1* and *MSH2*) that result in somatic mutations in neurofibromin but not germline mutations (Wang *et al.* 2003). The disorder in this case is also called brain tumour-polyposis syndrome 1 or Turcot syndrome. Furthermore, a significant proportion, perhaps as high as 20%, of patients, have deletion of a region containing the *NF1* gene and this causes a more severe form of the disease that includes mental retardation in particular (Dorschner *et al.* 2000; Venturin *et al.* 2004). The neurofibromin protein has complex roles in neurones including regulating the activity of some key protein kinases, modifying microtubule assembly and altering CREB function. All three processes have been implicated in cognitive processes and microtubule function has been shown to be altered in other brain diseases, most notably Alzheimer's disease and some variants of motor neurone disease. The interactions between neurofibromin and the signalling cascades and microtubule function has been reviewed by Weeber and Sweatt (2002).

The *NF2* gene on chromosome 22 encodes the protein neurofibromin-2, also called merlin because it was moesin-, ezrin- and radixin-like. The function of the protein product is not fully understood but it may have tumour-suppressor properties. Most mutations result in a truncation of the gene and result from frameshift or nonsense mutations or splice variants. Genotype–phenotype correlations suggest that splice variants result in markedly different forms of the disorder (Parry *et al.* 1994, 1996).

Clinical manifestations of NF1

The major defining features of von Recklinghausen's disease consist of café-au-lait spots, peripheral neurofibromas and Lish nodules. However, much of the morbidity and mortality in the condition are dictated by additional complications involving many body systems. Diagnostic criteria have been proposed by the National Institutes of Health and can be of particular importance in genetic counselling (NIH Consensus Development Conference 1988).

The café-au-lait spots are brown macules of varying size that appear during childhood, most affected persons having at least six. Those over 0.5 cm in diameter in children and 1.5 cm diameter in adults are of significance. They may be accompanied by freckling in the axillary or inguinal regions. The peripheral neurofibromas usually develop around the time of puberty and gradually increase in size and number with age. They are largely composed of Schwann cells together with perineural fibroblasts and smaller numbers of other cells. Dermal neurofibromas, derived from terminal nerve branches in the skin, appear mainly on the trunk as soft discrete nodules varying in diameter from 1 mm to several centimetres. Nodular neurofibromas are situated on periph-eral nerve trunks and have a firmer consistency. Lish nodules are pigmented hamartomas of the iris, best seen on slit-lamp examination.

Other features of less diagnostic significance include macrocephaly in almost half of patients, and short stature in perhaps one-third (Huson 1994). Campbell de Morgan spots consist of tiny cherry-red skin angiomas. Slight clumsiness and certain aspects of facial appearance also seem to be characteristic. Riccardi (1981) reported that 30–40% of patients showed speech impediments by way of hypernasality, slowing or imprecise pronunciation. Headaches of various types are common.

Several of the complications that develop involve the nervous system. Plexiform neurofibromas consist of large subcutaneous swellings with ill-defined margins, sometimes causing enlargement of part of the face or a limb and often producing marked cosmetic deformity. Those involving peripheral nerve trunks can be painful. They occasionally undergo malignant change to neurofibrosarcoma. Other complications include spinal root and cranial nerve neurofibromas, malignant change in peripheral nerve neurofibromas, and gliomas particularly of the optic nerve and chiasm. Up to one-fifth of children with the disorder develop astrocytomas, often in the optic system resulting in loss of vision (Listernick *et al.* 1994). Aqueduct stenosis may lead to hydrocephalus, and there is a small increased risk of epilepsy. Meningiomas are uncommon except in NF2.

Tumours affecting other parts of the body include rhabdomyosarcoma, phaeochromocytoma and carcinoid tumours of the duodenum. Neurofibromas may be found in the viscera, mediastinum, oral cavity or larynx, sometimes with serious consequences. Skeletal abnormalities include scoliosis, vertebral scalloping, and pseudoarthrosis of the distal long bones. Some 6% of patients develop hypertension.

The clinical course is variable: café-au-lait spots are often recognised in the first year of life, optic gliomas in children between the ages of 3 and 5 years and neurofibromas in adolescence (Zaroff & Isaacs 2005). Prognosis is good even if gliomas develop as they progress slowly and survival rates are greater than 80% at 10 years after onset (Guillamo *et al.* 2003).

Neuropathology

In addition to the pathologies described above, the brain may show subtle abnormalities on detailed examination that reflect cortical dysgenesis (Wiestler & Radner 1994). Disturbances of cytoarchitecture are common, with random orientation of neurones and disarray of cortical lamination. Neuronal heterotopias in the subcortical white matter appear to result from disturbed cell migration during embryogenesis. Gyral abnormalities may be seen such as pachygyria or polymicrogyria.

Focal subependymal glial proliferations may project into the ventricular system or contribute to aqueduct stenosis. Areas of fibrillary gliosis have been described in the cerebellum and adjacent leptomeninges, also scattered micronodular vascular proliferations. Neuropathological features of this nature could be relevant to the mental retardation encountered in a proportion of subjects (see below).

Psychiatric aspects

Intellectual impairment has long been recognised in a proportion of subjects with von Recklinghausen's disease, although severe degrees of handicap are rare. Ferner (1994) concludes that the majority of individuals with NF1 have IQs in the low average range, with about 8–10% scoring below 70. However, some can show superior academic ability. Performance IQs tend to be considerably lower than verbal IQs, and specific learning difficulties appear to be common.

Children with NF1 often show underachievement at school. Language development is sometimes delayed and a high proportion have difficulties with reading and writing. In Huson *et al.*'s (1988) survey in south-east Wales, 10% of 124 patients had attended special schools and a further 17% had required remedial class teaching. Neuropsychological evaluation has shown special problems with language, visuospatial tasks, memory and sustained attention, also difficulties with organisation and planning. Impairments are common with both gross and fine motor coordination in the absence of detectable neurological lesions.

Behavioural disorder has also been stressed in childhood, with hyperactivity and impulsive and aggressive tendencies. Attention deficit hyperactivity disorder type symptoms are present in about one-third of patients (Kayl & Moore 2000). Other problems reported in children include a higher rate of anxiety and depression, social problems and aggression (Johnson *et al.* 1999).

In Rosman and Pearce's (1967) post-mortem study, abnormalities of cerebral architecture and white matter heterotopias were prominent in all patients with intellectual impairment, with less marked changes in those of normal intelligence. However, MRI studies have shown little relationship between intellectual ability and such features as high-intensity lesions on T2-weighted images, suggesting that the cerebral basis of impairment is too subtle to be detected by this means (Ferner 1994).

Other psychiatric disorders have received little attention in neurofibromatosis despite the psychological burden which many subjects must bear. The disfigurement occasioned by the disease can be a grave social handicap, especially when the face is involved. Puzzled or hostile reactions from others are frequently encountered and social ostracism occasionally results. Despite this the majority of patients seem to be reasonably well adjusted and severe psychiatric disturbance appears to be rare. Samuelsson

(1981) reviewed the earlier literature which stressed apathy and depression, also personality disturbance and psychotic states, but these were often in specially selected patients. Samuelsson's own survey involved a thorough psychiatric examination of the 74 cases known to the health services in Gothenburg. Almost one-third were considered to suffer from mental illness in some degree, and 13 had had treatment in psychiatric hospitals. The most common diagnoses were of depression, alcoholism and anxiety. One patient showed social phobia. The patients with mental illness were more often mentally retarded than those without, and showed a significantly increased frequency of neurological abnormalities reflecting CNS involvement. The condition had sometimes had a considerable impact on the patients' lives, including avoidance of sports and other exposures in public, sensitivity about remarks from others, or fear of the nodules becoming malignant. Several patients had decided against procreation.

Samuelsson's study was uncontrolled. Hughes (1994) and Ferner (1994) report an unpublished survey of 103 patients with NF1 which showed that diagnosed psychiatric illness was no more common than in controls matched for age and sex. Moreover, there was no significant increase in anxiety and depression as measured by the Spielberger Anxiety Trait Inventory for Children or the Hospital Anxiety and Depression Scale. One-third of the patients had experienced hostile reactions from strangers because of unsightly neurofibromas. The rates of marriage were similar to those of the control group despite such cosmetic problems.

Riccardi (1981) suggests that the psychological burdens experienced in the disease are among the most important elements for patient care. In particular he stresses that frank discussion of the various features and complications serves to decrease adverse concerns, and provides a realistic context for making future decisions.

Friedreich's ataxia

Friedreich's ataxia is the commonest of the spinocerebellar ataxias and one of the commonest of the hereditary diseases of the nervous system, occurring in approximately 1 in 50 000 white Europeans (Delatycki *et al.* 2000). However, there are variances in this frequency: relatively higher rates have been reported in French Canadians (Barbeau *et al.* 1984) and in southern Italy (Romeo *et al.* 1983) probably due to consanguinity, while relatively lower rates are reported in Finland (Juvonen *et al.* 2002). Clinically, it occurs both sporadically and familially with the pedigrees often having the appearance of autosomal recessive inheritance. However, Friedreich's ataxia is both heterogeneous and, in its main form, a non-mendelian disorder and these combine to give the mixed pedigrees seen in clinical series. The primary locus for the disease (*FRDA1*) is on chromosome 9q in the gene encoding frataxin (FXN). The mutation has been shown to be an expansion in a GAA trinucleotide repeat in exon 1, the normal range of this repeat series being 5–30 and with disease being caused by more than 70 and up to 1000 repeats (Gatchel & Zoghbi 2005; Wells 2008). A second locus for the disease (*FRDA2*) exists in some families on chromosome 9p (Kostrzewa *et al.* 1997).

Clinical features

The onset is typically in the first or second decades of life. Unsteadiness of gait may at first be mistaken for the clumsiness of adolescence. With progression the gait becomes broad-based and lurching, action tremor appears in the arms and titubation may develop in the head. The trunk may eventually be implicated rendering even sitting difficult. Nystagmus is present in one-fifth of cases, and the speech is dysarthric. Cerebellar dysfunction shows also in generalised hypotonia and asynergia of movement. Weakness and wasting sometimes develop distally in the limbs and the tendon reflexes are eventually lost. However, the plantar responses are upgoing, indicating pyramidal tract involvement. Sphincter control is usually unaffected until late in the disease. Posterior column changes are manifest in defective vibration and position sense, although other sensory modalities are usually intact. Rombergism is detectable early on. Characteristic deformities with kyphoscoliosis or pes cavus are found in almost all cases, the latter sometimes long antedating other manifestations. Optic atrophy occurs in about one-quarter of cases and sensorineural deafness in 10%. Myocardial involvement is common and diabetes is prone to develop (Harding 1983; Albin 2003; Bhidayasiri *et al.* 2005).

The disease pursues a slowly progressive course though in occasional cases long stationary periods are encountered. Incomplete and abortive cases also occur in which the condition is static or progresses very slowly indeed. In the typical case severe incapacity with inability to walk is reached within 15 years of onset. Few patients live more than 20 years after the disease is declared, although survival into the sixth or seventh decades is not unknown.

Pathology

The brunt of the pathology falls on the long ascending and descending tracts of the cord. Degeneration is most marked in the posterior columns, spinocerebellar tracts and pyramidal tracts. Fibrous gliosis replaces the atrophied fibres. Atrophy may also be seen in the dorsal roots of the cord and the tracts and nuclei of the lower brainstem. The peripheral nerves show loss of large myelinated fibres and segmental demyelination. Purkinje cell loss has been reported in the cerebellum, also atrophy of the dentate nuclei and superior cerebellar peduncles. It can be hard to distinguish primary degenerative changes from those secondary to circulatory

disturbances arising from the patient's cardiac disease. The myocardium may show hypertrophy of muscle fibres and fibrosis.

The primary genetic defect in Friedreich's ataxia is in the gene encoding frataxin, a mitochondrial protein (Schapira 2006; Wells 2008). As pointed out by Wells (2008), since this discovery Friedreich's ataxia has become one of the most studied neurological disorders at the pathophysiological and molecular level. This work is bearing fruit: the triplet repeat in the gene has been convincingly shown to reduce transcription as it induces the formation of 'sticky' DNA, i.e. the physical association of purine–purine–pyrimidine triplexes in negatively supercoiled plasmids. The relative loss of frataxin results in an imbalance in sulfur–iron metabolism and subsequent hypersensitivity to oxidative stress. This in turn has led to some very clear potential therapeutic strategies which are being intensively investigated (Schols *et al.* 2004; Pandolfo 2008).

Psychiatric aspects

Psychiatric interest in the disorder has centred chiefly on the intellectual impairment noted in some patients (reviewed in Corben *et al.* 2006), and on the severe mental disturbances that occasionally arise.

Intellectual impairment has been reported in some series of patients but not in others. Friedreich himself noted an absence of mental defect in his cases, but later workers suggested that a considerable proportion showed mental deterioration, possibly associated with extension of the pathological process to the cerebral cortex. Bell and Carmichael (1939) reviewed 242 families from the literature and noted that mental impairment had been present in almost one-quarter. This varied in degree, the grade of defect tending to be similar in different affected members of a given family. Severe effects on cognition appeared mainly to be confined to family members afflicted with the neurological disorder, and had usually been conspicuous from the early stages.

More recent studies have shown verbal and visuospatial deficits correlating with cerebellar atrophy (Wollmann *et al.* 2002), slowed reaction times (Hart *et al.* 1986; White *et al.* 2000), and results on neuropsyhchological testing reminiscent of mild frontal lobe disease (Botez-Marquard & Botez 1993).

Psychotic developments have also been recognised in patients with Friedreich's ataxia. Many different forms of abnormal mental state are described, but mostly in isolated cases so that the overall incidence is hard to assess. The form that has attracted most attention is a schizophrenia-like illness characterised by paranoid delusions and outbursts of excitement. Davies (1949) described a patient who illustrates many of the features stressed in the literature: aggressive impulsive behaviour, paranoid beliefs, nocturnal hallucinations and episodes of clouding of consciousness.

A boy of 15 came from a family in which two members showed pes cavus and two others were subject to attacks of depression. He developed scoliosis, ataxia and titubation of the head at 13. At 15 he became stubborn and irritable, started housebreaking and absconded from home. Four months later he tried to poison his father and bought a rope with which to hang his stepmother. Later that month he was found wandering in a state of confusion. He had been observed to behave strangely at school where, following a retrosternal 'feeling of excitement', he would bang desks and shout for several minutes, subsequently having no recollection of this behaviour. In bed he had seen visions before falling asleep, often of a diminutive man in ruffles and buckled shoes who would utter the word 'Transformation'.

On admission to hospital he showed advanced features of Friedreich's ataxia, was unhappy and tearful, and claimed that his father and stepmother were plotting against him. Attention, concentration and memory were unimpaired. During 4 months in hospital he remained paranoid and subject to sudden outbursts of rage. EEG was grossly abnormal, with theta waves predominantly in the right temporo-occipital region. Towards the end of his stay he suddenly became euphoric, denied his hatred of his family and was discharged.

He worked well as a laboratory technician for 6 months then again had a fugue-like episode. One month later he attacked his family, threw vitriol over a neighbour, and was committed to a psychiatric hospital.

Such severe psychotic pictures have sometimes been labelled 'Friedreich's psychosis'. However, it seems unlikely that they are in any way specific for the disease. Some appear to be schizophrenic illnesses, occurring in families already prone to schizophrenia, whereas others may represent the paranoid hallucinatory states of temporal lobe epilepsy.

Motor neurone disease (amyotrophic lateral sclerosis, Lou Gehrig's disease)

Motor neurone disease (MND), or amyotrophic lateral sclerosis (ALS), is a complex disorder with many variants becoming apparent as genes associated with familial forms are discovered. In the sporadic forms it is commoner in males than females and has an onset usually between the ages of 50 and 70 years. Incidence is reported at approximately 2 per 100 000 population (Yoshida *et al.* 1986). The disorder consists of a combination of muscular atrophy of lower motor neurone type together with spasticity due to corticospinal tract damage. Some forms have an accompanying dementia.

The precise clinical picture depends on the relative prominence of symptoms of upper and lower motor neurone lesions.

The onset is insidious, usually with atrophy of the small hand muscles. The thenar and hypothenar eminences are often the first to be affected. Slow progression comes to involve the arms and legs symmetrically, atrophy being accompanied by prominent fascicular twitching. Spasticity is usually most marked in the legs, with hyperactive reflexes and upgoing plantar responses. The combination of upper and lower motor neurone signs is highly characteristic, exaggerated tendon reflexes being found along with considerable muscular atrophy. There are no sensory changes and the sphincters are rarely affected.

Sometimes atrophy is seen alone without spasticity (progressive muscular atrophy). Sometimes the accent is on the bulbar nuclei from the outset (progressive bulbar palsy), with atrophy and fasciculation of the tongue, paralysis of the vocal cords and difficulty with deglutition and articulation. Lesions of the corticospinal tracts above the medulla frequently produce an added element of pseudobulbar palsy, with loss of emotional control, a hyperactive jaw jerk, and spastic dysarthria and dysphagia.

The course is invariably progressive, but the rate varies from case to case. Most patients survive for 2 or 3 years but rarely longer, death resulting from bulbar involvement or weakness of the muscles of respiration. Very occasionally patients are encountered in whom the course is unusually benign.

The pathological changes consist of degeneration of the anterior horn cells and lateral tracts of the cord with secondary gliosis. The motor nuclei of the brainstem and the pyramids in the medulla also show progressive degeneration. The motor neurones of the cord contain filamentous inclusions and dense bodies that stain with anti-ubiquitin antibodies (Leigh *et al.* 1988; Leigh 1994). Affected muscles show denervation atrophy. In the brain there may be loss of Betz cells and degeneration of the pyramidal layers of the precentral cortex. It would appear that in a considerable proportion of patients abnormal gliosis can be detected in the cortex and subcortical nuclear masses, with atrophy sometimes particularly affecting the frontal lobes (Brownell *et al.* 1970; Hudson 1981).

Approximately 10% of cases are familial and the discovery of genes causing disease in some of these families has dramatically altered understanding of this condition. However, only a proportion of familial forms have been explained by gene discoveries. Currently, using genetic linkage studies, 10 forms of MND are recognised: ALS1–ALS8, ALS with frontotemporal dementia (ALS-FTD), and ALS with frontotemporal dementia and Parkinson's disease (ALS-FTDP). ALS2 and ALS5 are transmitted as autosomal recessive and the remainder as autosomal dominant disorders. The first gene to be discovered in an autosomal dominant ALS was *SOD1*, which encodes superoxide dismutase 1, on chromosome 21. This gene is the cause of ALS1 (Rosen *et al.* 1993). Subsequently, mutations were found in the *MAPT* (tau) gene in ALS-FTDP, in the *VAPB* (VAMP-associated protein B) gene in ALS8, in the *DCTN1* (dynactin subunit p150) gene in progressive lower motor neurone disease, in Alsin in ALS2 and in *SETX* (senataxin) in ALS4. Mutations in TDP43 have been identified in familial and sporadic ALS (Sreedharan *et al.* 2008). Gros-Louis *et al.* (2006) review the genetics of ALS and Boillee *et al.* (2006) review the current understanding of the genetics for aetiopathogenesis. As it was the first to be discovered, the largest body of work relates to *SOD1* mutations. Extensive studies in cells and in animal models have led to the conclusion that the mutations result in a gain in toxic function rather than a loss of normal function of the dismutase enzyme. In motor neurones, *SOD1* mutants tend to misfold and to form aggregates. The degree of aggregation is greater in forms that show the most propensity to misfold. It is not known whether the aggregation is itself toxic: it might be a response to some other toxic property of the mutant protein. However, aggregations are a common finding in many neurodegenerative disorders and the argument that this forms a common toxicity pathway is a compelling one (Lovestone & McLoughlin 2002). Whether it is via aggregation or some other toxic property of mutant *SOD1*, ample evidence suggests that the final or proximal cause of motor neurone death is the mitochondrion (Boillee *et al.* 2006).

Another common feature across different neurodegenerative disorders is evidence for loss of neuronal function before neuronal death. MND is no exception and, like Alzheimer's disease, studies in animal models but also in brain from patients suggests axonal damage as a feature of the disease process. Axonal transport is dependent on the axonal cytoskeleton consisting of both microtubules and neurofilaments. In Alzheimer's disease and in forms of MND involving the tau gene (ALS-FTD), microtubules are the site of axonal transport disruption. In most forms of MND, however, the evidence points to neurofilaments. In both animal models and in post-mortem brain there is evidence for neurofilament accumulation, and in animals with mutations in neurofilament genes a phenotype akin to MND is induced (Boillee *et al.* 2006). Some of the other genes associated with MND, particularly the affected dynactin subunit and VAPB, are known to play a role in axonal transport or the axonal cytoskeleton.

Finally, MND is not only a disorder of motor neurones, although it is dysfunction in this cell group that gives rise to the classical symptoms. Microglial cells in particular are activated in MND; likewise, induction of microglial activity in mice exacerbates disease. This has led to trials in mice of agents known to modify microglial activity such as minocycline and cyclooxygenase (COX)-2 inhibitors, with varying degrees of success. Trials in humans are awaited. Many other potential therapeutic avenues are being pursued based on experimental interventions in rodent models including trophic factors and stem cell therapies. However, only one compound, riluzole, has been approved as a disease-modifying therapy.

The treatment of MND is complex and involves a wide range of interventions for the many symptoms that result from motor neurone failure. Radunovic *et al.* (2007) review the range of care required for patients, from diagnosis, through symptomatic treatments to disease-modifying therapies and palliative care. The only specific drug approved, riluzole, increases life expectancy by at least 3 months after 18 months of treatment.

Psychiatric aspects

With the exception of cognitive impairment, the majority of patients appear to show little by way of psychiatric disturbance, except perhaps for understandable depression due to their progressive incapacitation, or emotional lability resulting from pseudobulbar palsy.

Emotional lability and loss of emotional control may be prominent when an element of pseudobulbar palsy is part of the picture. Of 101 cases, Ziegler (1930) reported explosive laughing or crying in 19, all except one of whom had signs of brainstem involvement. Several patients described clearly that their subjective emotional state was at variance with such reactions. One patient, in addition to weeping spasmodically, was prone to violent and uncontrollable outbursts of rage.

Houpt *et al.* (1977) found that one-third of their patients scored as moderately depressed on the Beck Depression Inventory, and more than one-fifth warranted a clinical diagnosis of depression at interview. Hogg *et al.* (1994) have reported the results of a questionnaire survey of 52 patients, finding high scores on the Hospital Anxiety and Depression Scale. Almost half of the sample could be considered depressed, this being significantly related to the severity of physical impairments and dependence on others. Systematic reviews suggest rates of depression of about 50% (McLeod & Clarke 2007), although Wicks *et al.* (2007) note that rates of depression depend on the scale used, finding 44% not depressed with one scale and 75% not depressed with another. Psychosocial factors play a greater role in determining depression and quality of life than physical disability in MND (Goldstein *et al.* 2006; McLeod & Clarke 2007).

Dementia is not a component of most cases of MND. Careful testing may nonetheless reveal deficits in memory and frontal lobe function, even in patients who are superficially intact (David & Gillham 1986; Irwin *et al.* 2007; Phukan *et al.* 2007). In particular, personality change, irritability and executive dysfunction syndromes characterise the deficits and neuropsychological testing suggests frontal lobe dysfunction. This overlap with frontotemporal dementia is marked in some families who present with a full FTD syndrome in addition to MND. These families represent subtypes of the disorder, and in one set of families mutations in the same gene that is associated with FTD (*MAPT*) have been found. Mutations in this gene cause a remarkable range of disorders, from FTD, through FTD-MND variants to corticobasal degeneration and progressive supranuclear palsy. Cortical blood flow and glucose metabolism, especially in frontal areas, have been shown to be reduced on single-photon emission computed tomography and PET (Goulding *et al.* 1990; Ludolph *et al.* 1992). Using PET, Kew *et al.* (1993a,b) have demonstrated abnormal patterns of activation in prefrontal and other brain areas in response to motor tasks, this being especially marked in patients who perform poorly on frontal lobe tests.

Hudson (1981), Ferrer (1992) and Kew and Leigh (1992) review the literature on patients who develop overt dementia and/or parkinsonism along with the disease. The occurrence of dementia has recently gained increased recognition, being mostly of frontal-lobe type. Mental features of behavioural, emotional and memory disorder set in insidiously, usually some 6–12 months before wasting begins. However, the two may evolve concurrently, or the wasting may precede the dementia. The clinical picture is typical of other frontal lobe dementias except for its rapid course. The patient is characteristically euphoric and disinhibited, and restlessness and impulsivity are common. Progressive language difficulties lead to stereotyped phrases, echolalia and ultimately mutism, while perceptual and spatial functions usually remain intact. Some patients develop gluttonous behaviour and hypersexuality (Neary *et al.* 1990). In the presence of cognitive impairment the motor manifestations tend to involve the tongue and proximal upper limb muscles predominantly, while the hands and legs are spared, so that the patient remains mobile until late in the disease. A familial incidence has sometimes been noted.

The pathological changes include spongiform changes in the superficial cortical layers, and it is likely that some cases formerly classified as an amyotrophic variant of Creutzfeldt–Jakob disease were suffering from the present condition. The conjunction between ALS and parkinsonism–dementia in the island of Guam (see below) appears to be different, in particular showing the histopathological hallmark of neurofibrillary tangles.

Amyotrophic lateral sclerosis and the parkinsonism–dementia complex of Guam

Amytrophic lateral sclerosis has been found to occur with extraordinary frequency among the indigenous Chamorro population of the island of Guam in the western Pacific (Kurland & Mulder 1954). Here the prevalence is 100 times greater than in the USA. Cases tend to occur familially but no clear pattern of inheritance has emerged. In the same population a syndrome characterised by parkinsonism and progressive dementia is also found (Lessell *et al.* 1962), and it is now recognised that the two essentially represent different facets of the same disease process. Both also occur in the neighbouring islands of the Mariana group and in the Kii peninsula of Japan.

The ALS is indistinguishable from the classic disease apart from its tendency to be associated with parkinsonism and dementia. The onset also tends to be at a younger age and the course more protracted. The parkinsonism–dementia complex presents with memory deficits and a slowing of mental and motor activity, and progresses to generalised dementia with extrapyramidal rigidity. Some patients develop psychotic disorders in the later stages, with delusions, hallucinations and hostile destructive behaviour.

A re-evaluation of 176 patients from Guam confirmed the close interrelationships between the two disorders (Elizan *et al.* 1966). Of the 104 who presented initially with ALS, five developed parkinsonism–dementia complex on average 5 years later, five developed parkinsonism alone and two an organic mental syndrome without parkinsonism. Of the 72 who presented with parkinsonism–dementia complex, 27 developed ALS on follow-up. In the families concerned, ALS and parkinsonism–dementia complex often occurred indiscriminately and in various combinations, giving further evidence of a close relationship between the two syndromes.

The histological pictures similarly show a good deal of overlap. The parkinsonism–dementia complex shows diffuse cerebral atrophy with widespread neurofibrillary changes in the cortex and subcortical nuclei. Atrophy of the globus pallidus is characteristic, also loss of pigment from the substantia nigra (Hirano *et al.* 1961). The cases with ALS show similar neurofibrillary changes throughout the brain in addition to the classic cord pathology (Hirano *et al.* 1966). Patients who have shown clinical features of only one syndrome are commonly found to show the pathological changes of both.

Myasthenia gravis

Myasthenia gravis is a disorder of the voluntary musculature characterised by abnormal muscle weakness after activity and a marked tendency for recovery of power after a period of rest. It is commoner than chance among patients who have had hyperthyroidism, Hashimoto's thyroiditis or other autoimmune disorders. Thymic abnormalities are usually present in the form of thymus hyperplasia, thymic tumour (thymoma) or more rarely thymus involution. More than two-thirds of cases show characteristic thymic changes, with large germinal centres in the medulla, indicative of B-cell activation and proliferation. There is now abundant evidence that the disease is essentially an autoimmune disorder in which circulating antibodies interfere with motor endplate function. The disorder was first recognised in the seventeenth century, although the first full descriptions of the syndrome were made much later. Hughes (2005) reviews the fascinating history of a remarkable disease.

Clinical features

The disorder can begin at any age, usually appearing in the second or third decades but with evidence for bimodal distribution of onset with peaks before and after the age of 50 years. It is more frequent in females than males (ratio approximately 6 : 4) until late middle age when the sex ratio is reversed. The prevalence in the population is increasing, probably due to increased survival, and is on the order of 80 per million (Phillips 1994; Flachenecker 2006).

The neurological syndrome is extensively described elsewhere. In brief, the first complaint is usually of ready fatiguability of certain muscle groups, or some symptom of cranial nerve involvement such as diplopia, difficulty with chewing or difficulty with swallowing. The onset is sometimes insidious, sometimes sudden, and precipitation by emotional upset or a febrile illness is not uncommon. Ocular muscles are usually involved early leading to ptosis or diplopia. Bulbar symptoms are also common, with difficulty in chewing or swallowing which worsens as the meal progresses, or a characteristic fading and slurring of speech after speaking for several minutes. Facial weakness may produce flattening and loss of wrinkles and the smile may have a characteristic 'snarling' quality. The muscles of the neck are often involved, also the shoulder girdles and flexors of the hip. In general, proximal muscle groups are more severely affected than distal groups, and the arms more than the legs, but the distribution is variable. The respiratory muscles may fatigue easily on laughing or crying, and in crises of the disorder respiration can be dangerously embarrassed.

The muscular weakness is typically variable from day to day and sometimes from hour to hour. It tends to be worse towards the end of the day, but is sometimes paradoxically most marked on waking in the morning. Ultimately, weakness of certain muscle groups may persist even when these have not been exercised for some time. Wasting is occasionally observed. The tendon reflexes almost always remain brisk even when weakness is severe, but may decrease on repeated elicitation. Objective sensory changes are absent but the patient may experience pain in the muscles of the neck and around the eyes, or complain of a feeling of stiffness or paraesthesiae in affected areas.

The course is extremely variable. It is usually slowly progressive but a number of cases prove to be relatively static. Spontaneous remissions and sudden relapses may occur. Diagnosis is by a combination of clinical evaluation and diagnostic tests, including demonstration of autoantibodies to acetylcholine receptors (AChRs) and muscle-specific tyrosine kinase (MuSK) and observation of the response to anticholinesterase drugs. Edrophonium chloride may be injected intravenously, with examination for increased muscle strength during the following 30–60 seconds. Electrophysiological tests include demonstration of an abnormal decrement in compound muscle action potentials on repetitive motor nerve stimulation, or the more sensitive single-fibre electromyography which shows blocking or abnormal 'jitter' (i.e. variations in interpotential intervals).

It is important to perform tomograms of the anterior mediastinum to detect thymic hyperplasia or the presence of a malignant thymoma, also chest radiography to exclude bronchial carcinoma leading to Lambert–Eaton syndrome (see below).

Pathophysiology

Myasthenia gravis has proved to be essentially an autoimmune disorder: antibodies are present at the neuromuscular junction, where the pathology occurs; antibodies from patients and immunisation against the antigen induce disease in experimental animals; and therapies that remove the antibodies are successful in relieving disease (Conti-Fine et al. 2006). The antibodies are of two main types, the most common being against nicotinic AChRs and an MuSK involved in AChR clustering. The biochemical defect at the neuromuscular junction was first thought to be due to competitive blocking by circulating antibodies that impaired the effects of acetylcholine at the motor end-plate. It is now apparent that there is considerable damage to AChRs at the postsynaptic membrane of the neuromuscular junction, brought about by antibodies directed against them (anti-AChRs). This damage is likely induced largely by complement activation, with evidence for a range of complement proteins including the activation fragment of C3 and the membrane attack complex being present in both patients and animal models (Conti-Fine et al. 2006; Vernino 2007). Other mechanisms include cross-linking of the AChR leading to degradation and functional blockade.

Cultures of thymic lymphocytes from myasthenic patients produce anti-AChR antibodies in vitro, particularly those from patients with thymic follicular hyperplasia showing active medullary germinal centres (Ragheb & Lisak 1994). Moreover, certain elements within the thymus share strong structural and antigenic similarities with muscle AChRs. It is therefore possible that an early step in pathogenesis consists of sensitisation of anti-AChR antibodies within the thymus itself. In this way evidence can be assembled to suggest that the thymus is involved not only in perpetuating the disease but perhaps in inducing it as well (De Baets & Kuks 1993). Approximately 10–15% of patients have a thymoma (Tormoehlen & Pascuzzi 2008).

Treatment

Anticholinesterase drugs remain the mainstay of treatment for patients with mild myasthenia or symptoms restricted to a small group of muscles. More recent developments are summarised by Conti-Fine *et al.* (2006). Corticosteroids and other immunosuppressants are essential components of therapy. Plasma exchange (plasmapheresis) and intravenous immunoglobulin are used for severe exacerbations and thymectomy is a therapeutic option, although the evidence base for this is not as strong as it might be. Psychiatric supervision can have an important part to play in patients who develop marked psychological reactions to the disorder. As discussed below the emotional state of the patient may have a considerable influence on clinical progress.

Other myasthenic syndromes

Other myasthenic syndromes may be induced by certain drugs, notably phenytoin, streptomycin and penicillamine. The latter in particular may be associated with a rise in anti-AChR antibodies and does not resolve when the penicillamine is withdrawn. Transient neonatal myasthenia may occur in children born to myasthenic mothers, usually resolving within weeks or months. Congenital myasthenia may be present from birth or become apparent during the first 2 years of life. Juvenile myasthenia can begin at any age from 12 months to 16 years and is generally similar to the adult disease. Lambert–Eaton syndrome is often associated with neoplasia, especially oat-cell carcinoma of the bronchus, sometimes developing several years before the neoplasm is apparent. Perhaps one-third of cases are non-neoplastic. Weakness and wasting, usually insidious, affect the proximal parts of the limbs and trunk, and ptosis and diplopia are not uncommon. Fatiguability is usually less striking than with myasthenia gravis, and autonomic symptoms such as dry mouth are common. Other differences are that the tendon reflexes are diminished or absent but reappear following a sustained muscular contraction, and there may be a 'reversed myasthenic effect' with progressive augmentation of strength during the first few seconds of maximal effort (Erlington & Newsom-Davis 1994). Circulating antibodies to AChRs are absent, but there is evidence of an IgG autoantibody that binds to voltage-regulated calcium channels at neuromuscular junctions. Anticholinesterase drugs lead to little improvement, but guanidine and 3,4-diaminopyridine are of benefit. Prednisone, azathioprine and plasma exchange may be useful in non-neoplastic cases.

Psychiatric aspects

Myasthenia gravis has attracted psychiatric attention on several grounds. Emotional factors have been thought to precipitate onset in some cases and to play a significant role in aggravating the established disease in others. The psychological make-up of myasthenic patients and their responses to the illness have accordingly been studied in some detail. There is also a possibility that memory may be adversely affected in certain patients. Finally, important problems of differential diagnosis not infrequently arise, and can involve psychiatric as well as neurological disorders.

The psychological responses seen in the illness are discussed by MacKenzie *et al.* (1969), Sneddon (1980) and Kulaksizoglu (2007). The patient is faced with the task of adapting to a disease that produces neither physical deformity nor pain and which has ephemeral manifestations. Interpersonal difficulties may be aggravated by the anxiety and uncertainty which the symptoms evoke, and by the tendency for those around to become suspicious of the genuineness of the disorder when there is so little to observe objectively. Patients may be suspected of faking their weakness or of being drunk when the speech is slurred. Meeting strangers can be a source of social embarrassment when facial weakness prevents a smile, likewise eating in public when the jaw must be supported towards the end of a meal.

The individual's reaction to the disease appears to be closely related to his premorbid personality and shows the usual range of responses to physical incapacity (Magni *et al.* 1988). Anxiety can be very marked and the patient's life may come to centre around the schedules of medication. An increase in the dose is regarded as ominous while a decrease leads to fearfulness of symptoms returning. Other patients seek to deny their disability, reducing medication and embarking on too much activity. The dependency induced by the disease often sets in train further psychological reactions. Some patients regress and develop increasing dependence on relatives and doctors. An obsessional attendance on every detail of treatment may result. Others become severely depressed, or hostile and frustrated. Major mental illnesses may occasionally arise with sporadic case reports of co-occurrence of psychosis and myasthenia.

Some, but by no means all, patients report precipitation of crises or exacerbation by emotional stress (Bedlack & Sanders 2000). Specific emotional factors can often be discerned in close relation to the first appearance of symptoms, probably as a result of their aggravating the latent disorder and bringing it to attention. Oosterhuis and Wilde's (1964) study of 150 cases showed that 8% had had some acute emotional disturbance directly preceding the onset. A further one-third had had a fairly long-lasting period of emotional stress coexistent with the onset, such as difficulties at work or marital infidelity. Two-thirds of these patients reported that emotional disturbances worsened their symptoms but one-third were either uncertain or denied an effect of stress or emotion.

Sneddon's patients had often needed to learn techniques for handling anger-provoking situations in order to remain well (Sneddon 1980). For example, half left the room and lay down if they felt themselves becoming angry; others found that crying and swearing relieved the tension and caused less weakness.

Paul *et al.* (2001) reviewed studies of cognition in myasthenia gravis and found none that met at least half of their criteria for study inclusion. However, despite this they conclude that there is some (weak) evidence for mild impairments in learning, although they note that patients frequently complain about cognitive difficulties.

Psychiatric aspects of differential diagnosis

Myasthenia gravis must be distinguished from other neurological disorders including ocular and peripheral neuropathies, brainstem lesions, parkinsonism, MND and carcinomatous myopathy. From the psychiatric point of view mistakes may occur in both directions: patients with weakness and fatigue of neurotic or depressive origin may be suspected of the disease; conversely, patients with myasthenia gravis may initially be diagnosed as suffering from neurosis, conversion hysteria or personality disorder.

Complaints of weakness and excessive fatigue are commonly encountered in routine medical practice and many such patients are mistakenly suspected of myasthenia gravis. Grob (1958) estimated that 20% of patients referred to him as possible myasthenics were in fact suffering from emotional disorders. Schwab and Perlo (1966) in an analysis of 130 patients wrongly diagnosed as having myasthenia gravis, found that by far the greatest proportion (38%) were suffering from a 'chronic fatigue syndrome' attributable to some form of neurosis. Such a mistake is particularly likely to arise when an injection of neostigmine or edrophonium has produced a marked placebo response, and especially if the patient's report of improvement has not been backed by attempts to monitor muscle strength objectively. Sometimes improvement on oral medication alone is accepted as evidence of myasthenia and this can be seriously misleading.

Progressive muscular dystrophies

The progressive muscular dystrophies, or myopathies, comprise a group of genetically determined degenerative diseases primarily affecting the voluntary musculature. Reviewed comprehensively by Emery (2002), one classification system is based on the clinical picture with the distribution of weakness determining the categories of Duchenne and Becker type, Emery–Dreifuss, limb-girdle, facioscapulohumeral, distal and aculopharyngeal.

Clinical features and genetics

The Duchenne, and milder Becker, forms result from mutations in the dystrophin (*DMD*) gene on the X chromosome, most commonly exon deletions. It develops very occasionally in girls when there is a translocation between the short arm of the X chromosome and some other chromosome; a variant resembling limb-girdle dystrophy may also be seen in female carriers when one X chromosome is partially inactivated ('lyonisation'). Female carriers of the disease can be detected by DNA studies, complemented where necessary by serum creatine kinase estimations. Prenatal diagnosis of affected male fetuses is possible (Kemper & Wake 2007). While there are no curative therapies at present, exciting

progress towards molecular interventions are being made (Cossu & Sampaolesi 2007; Wagner *et al.* 2007).

Duchenne dystrophy becomes apparent towards the end of the third year of life with difficulty in walking and climbing stairs, first affecting the pelvic girdles but soon the shoulder girdles as well. Enlargement of the calf muscles is characteristic, also sometimes affecting the quadriceps and deltoids. Most patients are unable to walk by the age of 10 and become confined to a wheelchair. Progressive skeletal deformity tends to develop as a result of atrophy and contractures. Death usually occurs from respiratory infection or cardiac failure; formerly few patients survived the second decade, but with modern supportive care many now live to their late thirties. Myocardial involvement is invariable but may not be detectable in the early stages. Characteristic changes are seen in the ECG in a high proportion of cases.

The Becker form of dystrophy affects muscle groups in a similar distribution but is more benign. Onset is usually between the ages of 5 and 25 years and patients may remain ambulant for two or three decades. Though severely disabled some can survive to a normal age. It is about one-third as common as the Duchenne form in incidence at birth, and is due to different defects in the same gene.

Facioscapulohumeral dystrophy is the third most common dystrophy and occurs equally in males and females, with onset at any time between childhood and late adult life. The facial and scapulohumeral muscles are the first affected, leading to winging of the scapulae and marked facial weakness that gives a characteristic pouting appearance. Muscular hypertrophy is uncommon. Spread may occur elsewhere, particularly to the anterior tibial muscles producing foot drop. Progression is variable, sometimes leading to severe disability after 20–30 years but sometimes following a benign course with periods of apparent arrest. It is inherited as an autosomal dominant disease, with the locus on chromosome 4. Interestingly, the mutation is not in a gene but in a DNA tandem array called D4Z4 where a deletion causes a frameshift disruption in downstream genes (van der Maarel & Frants 2005).

Distal muscular dystrophy is inherited as both an autosomal dominant and a recessive form, with onset usually in middle age. Weakness begins in the small hand muscles and lower legs then gradually spreads proximally. Rates of progression are variable.

Limb-girdle dystrophy affects males and females equally, usually beginning in the second or third decades but sometimes as late as middle age. It is due to an autosomal recessive gene, but sporadic cases are common. Either the shoulder or the pelvic girdles may be affected initially, and enlargement of the calf muscles sometimes occurs. Distinction from the Becker form can be made by muscle biopsy with dystrophin staining. The rate of progression is variable but severe disability is usually present after 20 years.

Oculopharyngeal muscular dystrophy occurs especially in French Canadians and has been traced to immigrants from France in the seventeenth century (Emery 2002). It is due to a GCG expansion in the N-terminal part of the gene for poly(A) binding protein nuclear 1 (PABPN1) at 14q11.2–q13. The Emery–Dreifuss form occurs as autosomal dominant and recessive forms, both being associated with mutations in the gene encoding lamin A/C.

In all varieties the tendon reflexes are diminished or lost in relation to affected muscle groups. All forms of sensation are intact. Histologically, the affected muscles show great variation in the size of individual fibres and a large amount of connective and adipose tissue.

Psychiatric aspects

From the psychiatric point of view the issue that has attracted most attention concerns cognitive function in muscular dystrophy, not least because of interest in the function of some of the dystrophy-associated genes in normal brain (Mehler 2000; D'Angelo & Bresolin 2006). There are obvious difficulties in attempting to assess the intellectual potential of children with severe physical handicaps, and in deciding whether decreased educational performance should be attributed to neurobiological dysfunction or to the psychosocial consequences of physical disablement. Nevertheless, evidence increasingly favours the view that a substantial proportion of patients with the Duchenne form have learning deficits and cognitive dysfunction. There are also indications that this may sometimes reflect cerebral involvement as part of the disease.

In a moderately sized series of patients with facioscapulohumeral dystrophy, clear evidence was found of mild learning difficulties, with severity being associated with the extent of the molecular genetic lesion (Sistiaga *et al.* 2008). A deletion resulting in a fragment size of 24 kb or less gave rise to significantly reduced IQ and visuospatial and other deficits compared with patients with molecularly confirmed but less severe genetic variants. There was no correlation with muscle phenotype. Young children with the Duchenne type show a wide range of, usually, mild cognitive impairments and learning difficulties (Wicksell *et al.* 2004; Cyrulnik *et al.* 2007, 2008; Young *et al.* 2008). Some have attributed these mild changes to cerebellar damage (Cyrulnik & Hinton 2008). However, some patients have severe learning difficulty and there is some evidence for a genotype–phenotype correlation, with severe impairment being related to deletions in the distal part of the gene (Moizard *et al.* 2000; Giliberto *et al.* 2004). Functionally there is evidence for abnormality in the EEG, and in both structural and functional imaging (Rae *et al.* 1998; Mercuri *et al.* 1999; Anderson *et al.* 2002; Quijano-Roy *et al.* 2006; la Coletta *et al.* 2007). Together these data argue for a role, especially for dystrophin, in the normal brain. Animal models with perturbed dystrophin show alteration

in long-term potentiation, the cellular basis of plasticity and perhaps learning and memory, supporting this hypothesis (Anderson *et al.* 2004; Vaillend *et al.* 2004).

Other, non-cognitive symptoms are also found. In a series of patients approximately one-third had a lifetime incidence of psychiatric comorbidity, most often depression or phobias (Kalkman *et al.* 2007). However, there was no phenotype–phenotype correlation either between type of dystrophy or with severity of symptoms. Attention-deficit hyperactivity disorders and other disorders including autism occur more frequently in Duchenne than expected from population rates (Hendriksen & Vles 2008; Young *et al.* 2008).

As adulthood approaches the psychosocial consequences of the disorder increasingly intrude, and the patient's psychological adjustment will often be decisively shaped by the milieu in which he lives. The strain thrown on the families of affected individuals may then be very considerable.

There does not appear to be any special association between non-myotonic forms of muscular dystrophy and psychosis, although occasional families have been reported in which schizophrenia and muscular dystrophy appear to coincide.

Myotonic dystrophies

In the myotonic dystrophies a variable degree of muscle wasting and weakness is combined with the phenomenon of 'myotonia', i.e. delayed relaxation of skeletal muscles after voluntary contraction. The commonest is myotonic dystrophy (dystrophia myotonica, Steinert's disease), in which the myotonia is accompanied by progressive wasting and weakness of selected muscle groups together with other characteristic features such as cataract, hypogonadism and frontal baldness. Myotonia congenita (Thomsen's disease) is a more generalised muscle disorder with myotonia and hypertrophy, setting in very early in life but rarely progressing to serious disablement. Paramyotonia congenita is similar but with the myotonia and weakness appearing only on exposure to cold. Other myotonic disorders include a variant of myotonia congenita with onset later in childhood, and various forms of periodic paralysis which also show myotonic features.

Dystrophia myotonica

The molecular genetics of dystrophia myotonica has revealed a fascinating new molecular pathogenesis of disease, that due to abnormality in RNA resulting from unstable repeat expansion of regions of DNA (Day & Ranum 2005). There are two forms: type 1 (DM1) resulting from an expanded CTG repeat in the 3' non-coding region of the myotonic dystrophy protein kinase (*MDPK*) gene on chromosome 19q35, and type 2 (DM2) resulting from an expanded CCTG repeat in an intron in the zinc finger protein 9 (*ZNF9*) gene on chromosome 3q21. These expansions may be very large indeed, from 37 to thousands in the case of DM1 and from 75 to 11 000 in DM2. Previously, repeat disorders were thought to be only due to triplet repeats, as for Huntington's disease, and were thought to exert their pathogenicity through loss of function of the primary gene or a toxic gain of function due to novel or aberrant protein expression. DM2 demonstrated that the unstable repeat expansions can be tetranucleotide (and indeed pentanucleotide as in the case of spinocerebellar ataxia type 10) and also raised the possibility for the first time of RNA-dominant disease (Osborne & Thornton 2006). All repeat expansion diseases show the phenomenon of anticipation, i.e. increasing severity and earlier onset in successive generations due to germ-cell instability of the expansion resulting in ever larger expansions with each generation. In DM1 this instability is greater in maternal transmission. Transmission patterns are less clear in DM2; although intergenerational expansion is more dramatic than in DM1, the picture is complicated both by somatic mosaicism and by the fact that the effect of expansion size is saturable such that the genotype–phenotype correlation is not as clear-cut as for DM1 (Day & Ranum 2005).

The pathogenetic effects of these two mutations is not fully understood, although much progress has been made. Both expansions are transcribed into RNA but are not translated into protein, ruling out the possibility of a toxic gain of function from a novel protein. Haploinsufficiency of the *MDPK* and *ZNF9* genes themselves was a possibility but the absence of other mutations in these genes and the apparent normality of mice lacking *MDPK* weigh against this potential mechanism (Day & Ranum 2005). Nor do other, nearby, genes in the DM1 or DM2 loci seem to be affected or indeed similar to each other, making a localised effect on gene expression unlikely. Instead, a so-called transdominant effect of RNA seems to be active, the RNA produced regulating other, distant, genes and resulting in the complex clinical picture. The genes affected in DM1 include cardiac troponin T, the insulin receptor, a muscle chloride channel (CLC-1), tau and the *N*-methyl-D-aspartate (NMDA) NR1 receptor, all of which show abnormal splicing in the presence of CUG or CCUG expansion, which in turn alter the regulation of RNA-binding proteins (Day & Ranum 2005; Osborne & Thornton 2006). The alteration in splicing of these genes and the subsequent change in protein expression patterns in both brain and peripheral tissue explains many of the known features of the diseases.

Clinical features

DM1 and DM2 show substantial clinical overlap. The disease is characterised by muscle weakness and myotonia together with multisystem effects in eye, cardiac, central nervous and endocrine systems. Males and females are equally affected. The commonest age of onset is between 20 and 25, and 50% of patients will have developed the disorder by this age.

However, the range covers virtually the whole lifespan as described above. Congenital forms of DM1 are often heralded by pregnancy complications and the children have severe disease accompanied by craniofacial abnormalities. Congenital or juvenile DM2 has not been reported.

The myotonia is usually the first symptom to be declared but is rarely sufficient in itself to lead to medical attention. It chiefly affects the hands, forearms and orbicularis oculi, although the legs may be implicated as well. It is best demonstrated by observing the slowed relaxation of hand grip, or the difficulty in opening the eyes after screwing them up tightly. Delayed relaxation may be noted in the tendon reflexes, or a groove may persist in the tongue after depressing it with a spatula. The smile is sometimes characteristically slow and lingering.

The myotonia is rarely a grave handicap. Involvement of the tongue can cause difficulties with articulation, or sudden falls may result from difficulty in adjusting balance after a trip or stumble. Aggravating factors include exposure to cold or prolonged inactivity. It is characteristically worse on waking and improves as the patient begins to move about. Caughey and Myrianthopoulos (1963) also stress that it is often aggravated by emotional factors such as fright or surprise. One of their patients first noticed the myotonia when his legs seemed to freeze while caught in a burning building, and another when his legs became stiff on the signal to start a race. Fear, anger or sudden joy may temporarily increase the symptoms so that a wave of stiffness is felt to run through the muscles of the body. Another patient was liable to fall rigidly to the ground whenever she was suddenly excited or surprised. Several had become housebound because of fear of falls in the street.

The atrophy and weakness is selective, symmetrically affecting the facial muscles, masticatory muscles, sternomastoids and distal parts of the arms and legs. Hypertrophy can occur in the early stages but atrophy usually prevails. The facial appearance is characteristic, with hollow temples, ptosis, a sad lugubrious expression and a tendency for the mouth to hang partially open. Finger grip is weak and foot drop may occur. The tendon reflexes are normal initially, though diminished or absent as the disease progresses. Sensory changes are rare, but slight sensory disturbances and subjective complaints of pain are occasionally encountered. The pattern of weakness does show some differences between disease types. DM1 cases typically show facial, masticatory and upper limb weakness followed by shoulder and hip girdle involvement, whereas DM2 often presents with hip girdle problems manifested as difficulty in rising or climbing stairs (Day & Ranum 2005).

The progression of the disability is remarkably variable but usually slow. Rare cases may be completely disabled within a year or two, although most patients remain ambulant for 15–20 years or even longer. In general the muscle weakness and wasting will be much less severe in cases of late onset, and the prognosis can then be remarkably good. In the final stages respiration and swallowing may become embarrassed.

On pathological examination the affected muscles show variation of fibre size, fibrosis and fibre degeneration as in other dystrophic processes. A characteristic finding is multiplication of sarcolemmal nuclei, which tend to form long central chains, also sarcolemmal aggregates of mitochondria. Changes have been detected in muscle spindles, with abnormal innervation to the intrafusal fibres and abnormally shaped end-plates.

Associated defects may involve a number of organs and systems of the body. Cataract is one of the commonest additional defects: in some series slit-lamp examination has revealed lens opacities in almost every case. Other ocular abnormalities may include limitation of eye movements, retinal degeneration or partial constriction of the visual fields. Frontal baldness is common in males and occasionally occurs in females. Endocrine abnormalities include testicular atrophy and hypogonadism in the male, and menstrual abnormalities and infertility in the female. Insulin resistance is common and pituitary–adrenal and thyroid abnormalities have occasionally been reported.

Electrocardiographic abnormalities are found in more than half of patients, including varying degrees of heart block and atrial dysrhythmias. Cardiac failure or sudden death due to cardiac arrest may occur. Smooth muscle dysfunction can involve dilatation of the lower oesophagus, peristaltic incompetence of the small intestine, dilatation of the colon, or a flaccid bladder with urinary retention. Anaesthetics present a special risk, particularly of prolonged respiratory arrest following thiopental. Serum immunoglobulins are often abnormally low. Skull radiography may show general thickening of the vault, localised thickening of the frontal bones (hyperostosis frontalis interna), enlarged sinuses or a small sella turcica. Other congenital physical defects include a high narrow palate, hare lip or talipes equinovarus.

Differential diagnosis and treatment
Differentiation from other forms of muscular dystrophy is important on account of the differing prognosis. It can usually be made on the basis of the characteristic distribution of weakness, wasting and myotonia, together with associated abnormalities in other systems as outlined above. The facial appearance may resemble that of facioscapulohumeral dystrophy, although there the limbs are affected proximally rather than distally. Myasthenia gravis may be suspected when ptosis and muscular fatigue are marked. Differentiation from myotonia congenita (see below) can be more difficult when onset is early in life, and indeed the two have sometimes been reported from the same family. Polyneuropathy may be suspected in view of the distal and symmetrical weakness. Peroneal muscular atrophy can usually be distinguished by the associated loss of vibration sense at the ankles.

Psychiatric aspects
Involvement of the CNS is undoubted in the more severe early-onset and congenital cases but likely in adult-onset cases also. In congenital DM1, myotonia and cardiovascular involvement may be absent and cerebral effects predominant or may be the only symptoms. Mental impairment is common: IQ levels are between 40 and 80 in 50–90% of patients (Meola & Sansone 2007). Speech is delayed and a range of behavioural symptoms are reported including hyperactivity, autism and various difficulties in social behaviours (Steyaert *et al.* 1997). In the juvenile form of DM1, CNS effects are predominant and motor signs are typically weak or absent. Learning disabilities and difficulties with relationships with peers occur in school-age children. Attention deficit hyperactivity disorder in preschool children and anxiety disorders in childhood and young adulthood are common (Meola & Sansone 2007).

Adult-onset disease shows more neuropsychological involvement in DM1 than DM2, although in both types cognition, behaviour and personality changes may occur together with fatigue and daytime sleepiness. Meola and Sansone (2007) review the evidence for neuropsychiatric symptoms.

In the absence of frank mental retardation it is uncertain how much global intelligence is affected by DM1 or DM2. A series of studies report low-normal range IQ, although Meola and Sansone (2007) do find abnormally low IQ in those with moderately severe DM1. On the other hand, visuospatial defects undoubtedly do occur in DM1 and may be invariable. Speech is often affected due to motor difficulties but language itself is normal. Malloy *et al.* (1990) carried out a careful study of 20 patients between the ages of 20 and 65, stratified with regard to age and compared with controls matched for age and education. While the sample as a whole showed cognitive deficits, especially on non-verbal spatial tests, there was no evidence of an abnormal age-related decline. In contrast to the motor deficits, which clearly progressed, the cognitive impairments appeared to be relatively stable. Bird *et al.* (1983) could not document definite decline in any of their 29 patients, and there was no deterioration on repeat psychometric testing in five cases after intervals of 11–19 years.

Dysexecutive syndrome, i.e. reduced intitiative and activity, is a feature of DM1 and various studies have shown selective involvement of frontal lobe function. Apathy is common.

Personality abnormalities and *social deterioration* are perhaps even commoner than defective intelligence. However, Bird *et al.* (1983) have warned against stereotyping sufferers from the disease. They examined 29 patients and found that one-third showed prominent personality abnormalities, mainly in the presence of low intellectual ability and advanced physical handicap. However, there was no 'typical' personality type, and the problems that emerged were largely what would be expected in persons with physical and cognitive problems. Subsequently, however, two studies reported avoidant personality traits to be particularly characteristic of DM1 and to be associated with neuroimaging evidence of disease in frontal and parieto-occipital regions (Delaporte 1998; Meola *et al.* 2003).

Somnolence may be a marked feature in the disease, adding to the impression of apathy and perhaps related to diencephalic dysfunction or alveolar hypoventilation. If anything patients tend to minimise the degree of somnolence. True fatigue is also prominent in many cases and goes beyond that expected from the myotonia.

The social decline that can result is usually severe and could be traced in 70% of Thomasen's (1948) patients. Caughey and Myrianthopoulos (1963) encountered several families of distinction where the disease, within two or three generations, had led to a marked deterioration in family fortunes and social status. Perron *et al.* (1989) documented the socioeconomic impact of the disease in the Saguenay–Lac-Saint-Jean region of Quebec where it occurs with remarkable frequency. A representative sample of 218 affected persons over the age of 15 was compared with control data from the same population; only 12% were employed compared with 42% of controls, and the mean income for 1982 was reduced by almost two-thirds. The effect on the families was not surprisingly severe: 43% were living below the poverty line, which was three times as common as in Canadian families generally.

Myotonia congenita

Thomsen (1876) gave a clear account of the disease that bears his name in four generations of his own family. Thomasen (1948) subsequently collected all cases in the literature and described three further families, resulting in a total of 157 families with 470 affected persons. It is nevertheless a rare disease (Colding-Jorgensen 2005; Heatwole & Moxley 2007). The pattern of inheritance is usually autosomal dominant, although an autosomal recessive form has also been described. In both the dominant and the recessive forms mutations in the *CLCN1* gene coding for the skeletal muscle chloride channel CLC-1 have been found (Koch *et al.* 1993), including in Thomasen's own family (Steinmeyer *et al.* 1994). Males and females are affected equally.

Onset is usually from shortly after birth and few cases appear after the age of 12. Myotonia is typically the presenting feature and the sole cause of disability for many years. It presents as a painful stiffness or cramp on attempting voluntary movement, most marked after rest and especially troublesome first thing in the morning. The myotonia is widespread throughout the body muscles, unlike its regional distribution in dystrophia myotonica. Involvement of the tongue and jaw may lead to difficulty with speech, chewing and swallowing. Clumsiness on initial movement may lead to frequent falls. Exposure to cold aggravates it, also excitement, tension or emotional disturbance. Most patients find that with repeated movements the stiffness passes off and learn such manoeuvres as limbering up to run.

Generalised muscular hypertrophy is common and atrophy rare. However, the strength is not proportional to the size of the muscles and patients fatigue easily. The tendon reflexes are usually normal. The associated features seen in dystrophia myotonica are rarely encountered, and when present tend to be minimal. Occasional cases have been reported with cataract, minor lens opacities or endocrine disturbance, but it is hard to be sure that these were not cases of early dystrophia myotonica without atrophy.

The course tends to remain static over the years and progression of myotonia or muscular weakness is rarely observed. The disorder is quite compatible with survival to old age. However, the myotonia is often severe and can require treatment with phenytoin or tocainide.

Psychiatric aspects

Patients with myotonia congenita are usually normal in intelligence and personality. In sharp contrast to dystrophia myotonica, social deterioration was not observed in Thomasen's (1948) large study. Mental changes were conspicuous by their absence. Thomsen (1876) himself drew attention to a hereditary psychosis in several members of his own family, describing it as a 'kind of imbecility, confusion of ideas combined with a tendency for the mind to wander and vacant brooding; it has most in common with a certain kind of mental weakness which occurs in old age'. Since then, however, most investigators have dismissed any association with psychosis as fortuitous, and in fact there are strong indications that the myotonia and the mental disorder were transmitted independently in different branches of Thomsen's family (Caughey & Myrianthopoulos 1963; Johnson 1967). Johnson (1967) has reported a patient with myotonia congenita who developed two acute psychotic episodes of mixed affective and schizophrenic type. Two of the siblings had myotonia congenita, and the father and several other family members had had acute psychoses; but here again the muscle disorder and the psychotic propensity appeared to be transmitted independently in the family, and no direct relationship could be established between the two disorders.

Paramyotonia congenita

Paramyotonia congenita of Eulenburg resembles myotonia congenita except that the myotonia and weakness only appear on exposure to cold. It is transmitted as an autosomal dominant disorder due to mutations in the gene for the α-subunit of the human skeletal muscle sodium channel gene

(*SCN4A*) on chromosome 17 (Ptacek *et al.* 1992). Interestingly, mutations in the same sodium channel gene give rise to other paramyotonias without cold induction (Koch *et al.* 1995) and in a family with hypokalaemic periodic paralysis (Davies *et al.* 2001). Typically, paramyotonia congenita develops early in life, worsens at puberty, then tends to improve or vanish in later decades (Caughey & Myrianthopoulos 1963). It often principally affects the muscles of the face, tongue and hands. Involvement of the legs may cause 'cramps' or inability to rise from a sitting position in the cold. Severe weakness is sometimes induced by cold, with or without myotonia, and lasts on rare occasions for several hours at a time. In severe attacks the patient may be bedridden and unable to turn, leading to a suspicion of hysterical paralysis. There is no hypertrophy of muscles, and power and reflexes are normal between attacks. Psychiatric and social complications appear to be as rare as in myotonia congenita. Associated dystrophic features such as cataracts, testicular atrophy and changes on skull radiography do not occur.

Neuropsychiatric manifestations of carcinoma

Increasing attention is being paid to several neuropsychiatric syndromes that may accompany neoplasia in various parts of the body even when there is no spread of tumour cells to the brain. Thus patients with carcinoma may develop marked nervous system pathology while the tumour remains confined to its original site or when spread is limited to metastases to the regional lymph nodes. Mental symptoms figure prominently in such syndromes as well as neurological defects.

The mechanisms underlying such remote effects remain uncertain. Especially puzzling has been the observation that neuropsychiatric manifestations may precede clinical evidence of the primary tumour by a considerable period of time, sometimes several years. Moreover, the disorders may continue to progress after apparently successful eradication of the neoplasm. Occasionally, they make a first appearance some time after removal of the tumour and without evidence of recurrence of the neoplasm itself.

Before considering these remote effects in detail certain aspects of the orthodox involvement of the nervous system by secondary metastatic deposits are briefly considered.

Metastatic involvement of the CNS

Tumours that commonly metastasise to the brain include those of the lung, breast, alimentary tract, prostate and pancreas. Carcinoma of the lung is undoubtedly the most frequent variety today. Melanomas may similarly metastasise to the CNS. Secondary cerebral deposits are usually multiple and fast-growing, but occasionally a solitary cerebral metastasis may warrant surgical intervention along with treatment

of the primary growth. Not infrequently an intracranial metastasis gives rise to symptoms before the primary lesion, especially when this is in the lung, and sometimes the primary lesion is not discovered until post-mortem.

An 'encephalitic' form of metastatic carcinoma may very occasionally be encountered. Here there is no tumour formation as such within the brain but diffuse infiltration of carcinomatous cells throughout the CNS, i.e. within the brain parenchyma and along the perivascular spaces as well as in the meninges. There is no true inflammatory reaction but the presentation may at first closely simulate an encephalitic process. Carcinomatosis of the meninges may also produce a misleading picture. Secondary deposits invade the leptomeninges diffusely, particularly at the base of the brain, giving rise to an illness which at first resembles meningitis. Pyrexia and neck stiffness may be prominent features. Headache is usually marked and accompanied by cranial nerve palsies and often visual failure. A period of vague ill health has usually preceded more definite manifestations.

Non-metastatic manifestations of neoplasia (paraneoplastic disorders)

The number of non-metastatic syndromes known to be causally related to cancer is now considerable and includes sensory and other peripheral neuropathies, subacute cerebellar degenerations, myelopathies and myopathies (Grant 2002). For some time it was thought that pathological changes were restricted to levels caudal to the basal ganglia, but cerebral involvement is now recognised as well. Severe involvement of the limbic areas on the inferomedial surfaces of the temporal lobes is a well-recognised syndrome, producing an illness with prominent memory disturbances and often some degree of dementia.

Obviously, the clinical pictures that characterise these non-metastatic complications are many and various. Table 14.1 represents an attempt at classification modified from Brain and Adams (1965) and remains useful today with a few additions (Grant 2002). Strict classification is impossible since the various disorders may appear singly or in combination. With the encephalopathies particularly, the pathological evidence suggests that a number of syndromes merge into one another as part of a spectrum. Of the syndromes in the table, only those likely to be of importance to the psychiatrist are considered in detail and these are summarisd in Table 14.2 (Schott 2006).

With regard to prevalence, the non-metastatic complications are relatively uncommon and some varieties exceptionally so. Nevertheless, they constitute an important part of general hospital neurological practice. Among 1476 cases of carcinoma, Croft and Wilkinson (1965) obtained an overall prevalence of 7% with non-metastatic complications. Carcinoma of the lung produced by far the highest frequency at 16%. Hodgkin's disease and lymphoepithelioma of the

Table 14.1 Neuropsychiatric disorders associated with neoplasms. (From Brain & Adams 1965 with permission.)

Encephalopathies
Progressive multifocal leucoencephalopathy
Encephalopathy with subacute cerebellar degeneration
Encephalopathy with brainstem lesions
Diffuse encephalopathies with mental symptoms
Encephalopathies presumed due to metabolic disturbance
Limbic encephalopathy

Myelopathies (including cases resembling motor neurone disease)

Neuropathies
Sensory neuropathy (with degeneration of posterior root ganglia and dorsal columns of cord)
Peripheral sensorimotor neuropathies
Subacute optic nerve or retinal degeneration
Metabolic, endocrine and nutritional neuropathies

Muscle disorders
Polymyopathy (mainly proximal, of limb girdles and trunk)
Myasthenic syndromes including Lambert–Eaton syndrome
Polymyositis
Metabolic myopathies

Table 14.2 Percentage of patients with various clinical features and results of investigations in paraneoplastic limbic encephalitis. (From Schott 2006 with permission.)

Clinical/investigation feature	Gultekin *et al.* (2000)	Lawn *et al.* (2003)
Cognitive impairment	84	92
Psychiatric features	42	50
EEG abnormalities	82	100
CSF abnormalities	80	78
Serum anti-neuronal antibodies	60	64
MRI temporal lobe signal change	57	83
Epileptic seizures	50	58
Primary tumour		
Lung	50	54
Testis	20	8
Breast	8	13

thymus have also been reported in association with such disorders.

Subacute cerebellar degeneration

This was one of the earlier syndromes to gain recognition (Brain *et al.* 1951) and in patients over 50 years old neoplastic origin is the cause of half of all subacute cerebellar degenerations (Bolla & Palmer 1997). The presenting symptom is usually ataxia of gait, spreading later to all four limbs and often to the trunk. Dysarthria is severe but nystagmus often slight or absent. Muscle weakness, dysphagia, diplopia and sensory symptoms may also occur. The CSF is often abnormal with a pleocytosis, elevated immunoglobulins and oligoclonal bands. The diagnosis may sometimes be confirmed by the presence in serum and CSF of antibodies directed against cerebellar Purkinje cells (Clouston *et al.* 1992; Greenlee *et al.* 1992).

Mental symptoms figure prominently in the majority of cases. Most present with dementia but some also with agitation, anxiety and depression. The onset may antedate the appearance of the carcinoma by several months or years, or follow it by a similar interval. Once started the disorder may progress so rapidly that the patient is bedridden within weeks, while in other cases it may take a year to develop fully. Sometimes arrest may be seen after many months of progression, but remission does not occur. The dementia can continue to progress after the cerebellar affliction has stabilised. Treatment of the neoplasm has no demonstrable effect on the progress of the disorder.

The striking pathological change is the disappearance of Purkinje cells from the cerebellum. Diffuse degeneration is seen in other cerebellar neurones, and patchy microglial proliferation in the white matter of the cerebral and cerebellar hemispheres. In contrast, the dentate nuclei are often little affected. Degeneration may occur in the long tracts of the cord, especially the spinocerebellar tracts and posterior columns, and in the oculomotor and lower cranial nerve nuclei. Meningeal and perivascular lymphocytic infiltration is seen in some cases, and inflammatory changes have been observed in the brainstem and subthalamic region.

Rather similar to the above is opsoclonus, consisting of rapid chaotic conjugate eye movements that severely distort ocular fixation and which are often accompanied by ataxia. This can be abrupt in onset, in contrast to subacute cerebellar degeneration, and sometimes progresses to coma and death within several weeks. It may be associated with myoclonus and encephalopathy, but coordination of the individual limbs is preserved. A proportion of cases show a useful clinical response to treatment with corticosteroids, suggesting that the disorder may be due to immune reactions to tumour antigens affecting the brainstem neurones. Pathological changes involve loss of Purkinje cells and neuronal changes in the inferior olives, along with diffuse mononuclear infiltration of the brain parenchyma and leptomeninges. The disorder is characteristically seen with neuroblastoma in childhood, but also with tumours of the lung, breast and ovary in adults.

Encephalopathy with brainstem involvement

This, the so-called 'mixed form of encephalomyelitis' of Brain and Henson (1958), presents with varied neurological signs including cerebellar disorder, bulbar palsy, disordered external ocular movements, wasting and weakness of the limbs, extensor plantar responses, involuntary movements and posterior column sensory disturbance. Mental changes are again prominent in many examples, including dementia. The disorder can follow a prolonged course over 2 years or more. In one case the neurological manifestations had been evident for 2 years before serial radiography revealed carcinoma of the lung.

The pathological changes involve degeneration in the dentate nucleus, superior cerebellar peduncles, brainstem nuclei, motor cells of the cord, and the pyramidal tracts and posterior columns. Inflammatory changes may be conspicuous, with perivascular cuffing and cellular infiltrations of the meninges.

Encephalopathies presumed due to metabolic disturbance

An important but apparently rare group of cases has been described in which marked mental disorders are associated with carcinoma of the lung yet cerebral changes prove to be minimal or absent on detailed pathological examination (Charatan & Brierley 1956). The common feature in such cases was a fluctuating disturbance of consciousness with periods of lucidity, extending over several months prior to death and unaccompanied by neurological abnormalities. Affective disturbances were often prominent in the earlier stages. In all cases the mental disturbance had either preceded or overshadowed the presence of the neoplasm. Here it would seem very likely that metabolic disturbances were fundamental to the development of the mental changes.

The first of Charatan and Brierley's cases was a man of 53 who became depressed and quarrelsome over several months. He later developed paranoid religious delusions and episodes of grossly muddled and odd behaviour. There were no organic features in the mental state and a diagnosis of paranoid schizophrenia was made. After recovering briefly for a week or two he abruptly relapsed, and at this stage carcinoma of the lung was detected. A quick decline led to coma and death.

The second was a man of 43 admitted after wandering from home in a depressed and apathetic state. He had lost his memory but this returned 4 days after admission. The only abnormal sign was some lability of mood. Soon, however, he developed periods of confusion with lucid intervals and deteriorated to death over 4 months. There had been suspicious shadowing of the lung for some months before presentation.

The third was a man of 63 who for 1 year had been slow, lethargic and complaining of feeling tired. Six months before presentation there had been an episode of confused nocturnal rambling, and since then his memory had been failing from time to time. Major epileptic fits had com-

menced at this time and chest radiography had shown shadowing of the lung. Gradual decline was accompanied by lucid intervals lasting a few days at a time. The mental state continued to show marked fluctuation in hospital until he died 2.5 months later.

Electroencephalography had shown little abnormality in the first two cases, and the CSF was normal except in the first. In all three the brain was free from metastases and only a marginal gliosis of the white matter could be detected. However, the livers contained numerous metastases and it was thought possible that liver failure may have contributed to the picture, either with or without other metabolic disturbances occasioned by the neoplasms.

Limbic encephalopathy and 'chemobrain'

Other patients present with mental disturbance in association with pathological changes largely limited to the limbic grey matter of the brain. The carcinoma is often bronchial in origin (small cell), often with metastases in the hilar lymph nodes but without direct spread to the brain, although primaries in testes and lymphomas have been described. In several examples the neoplasm has become evident only at post-mortem examination. Strangely, the primary growth has not always been discovered even then, the only evidence of cancer sometimes being secondary deposits in the mediastinal lymph nodes. Very occasional examples have also been reported with neoplasms of the bladder, mediastinum and thymus (Bakheit et al. 1990; Schott 2006).

This form of encephalopathy was comprehensively described by Corsellis et al. (1968). The outstanding clinical feature is a marked disturbance of memory for recent events, although some degree of generalised intellectual impairment often develops later. Affective disturbance is frequently prominent early in the evolution of the disorder, usually in the form of severe anxiety or depression. Some patients are hallucinated and some have epileptic attacks, but otherwise impairment of consciousness is not observed. Several patients have shown a coincident carcinomatous neuropathy.

The first report of such a picture in association with carcinoma was included among cases reported by Brierley et al. (1960), although the connection was not appreciated at the time. One of their patients with 'subacute encephalitis of later adult life' was a man of 58 who demented over the course of 3 months and died, revealing an intense inflammatory reaction in the brain, most severe in the medial temporal lobe structures. The mediastinal lymph nodes were extensively infiltrated with oat-cell carcinoma though neoplasia had not been suspected during life.

Bakheit et al. (1990) review the more recent literature on the condition. Symptoms had predated the diagnosis of malignancy in almost one-third of cases, and neurological findings were few unless other brain regions were involved. CT was usually unhelpful in diagnosis, and MRI was normal in two of three cases examined and nowadays is often able to detect medial temporal lobe signal change with FLAIR sequences. EEG can also be normal or show non-specific abnormalities over the temporal lobes, in contrast to the distinctive picture seen with herpes encephalitis. The CSF is usually abnormal with a raised lymphocyte count and raised immunoglobulin level. Oligoclonal bands may be detected. The course in various cases has varied widely from a few weeks to up to 5 years.

The pathological picture shows a combination of degenerative and inflammatory changes that are concentrated on the medial temporal lobe structures: the hippocampus, uncus, amygdaloid nucleus, dentate gyrus, hippocampal gyrus, cingulate gyrus, insular cortex and posterior orbital cortex. The changes can sometimes extend throughout the length of the fornices and involve the mamillary bodies. The rest of the hemisphere and the hindbrain are only slightly affected. The changes consist of extensive neuronal loss, marked astrocytic proliferation and fibrous gliosis, and perivascular infiltration with small round cells and the formation of glial nodules. In no cases have tumour cells been identified within the CNS. The severity of the inflammatory component has varied from case to case, but at times has been severe enough to be virtually indistinguishable from viral encephalitis. No inclusion bodies have been seen. Bakheit *et al.* (1990) suggest that immune damage to the limbic neurones is a more plausible explanation than an infective aetiology and this has largely been confirmed (Schott 2006).

The most recent example of this group of disorders is one where antibodies to the NMDA receptor are produced. This has been described in a series of 12 young/middle-aged women who were found to have an ovarian teratoma (Dalmau *et al.* 2007) (Fig. 14.2). Removal of the primary tumour plus immunotherapy usually but not always cured the disorder. Many presented with florid psychopathology including psychotic or catatonic symptoms, 'acute personality change' or panic; most had seizures and generalised slowing on EEG. We have recently seen such a patient, a 21-year-old student with no previous history who became acutely depressed over 24–48 hours. Her overriding mood was of fear. She was mute and perplexed and was admitted initially to a psychiatry ward where her behaviour was extremely disturbed, with incontinence and faecal smearing. As she became more mute and withdrawn, encephalitis was suspected and confirmed by EEG. MRI was normal. Diagnosis was eventually made with the relevant immunological tests, although no underlying malignancy was identified, and the patient was treated with steroids and plasmapheresis. She made a gradual recovery after 2 months.

How commonly mental disturbance in patients with carcinoma may be due to limbic system involvement is hard to assess. As already described some examples are clearly due to more diffuse cerebral pathology or to metabolic disturbances, but where memory failure is a predominant feature the possibility of limbic encephalopathy should be borne in mind.

A wide variety of hypotheses have been proposed to explain the neuropsychiatric, non-metastatic complications of carcinomas. These have included toxins released from the cancer, defective immune system resulting in opportunistic viral infection or a direct effect of perturbation in immune function. Evidence to support an immune aetiology has grown over the last few years.

Also important to patients are the effects of therapy and the impact of disease. An extensive literature points to mild and possibly transient cognitive deficits associated with chemotherapy (Jansen *et al.* 2007; Nelson *et al.* 2007; Taillibert *et al.* 2007). Sometimes called 'chemobrain', a better term has been proposed: 'cancer- or cancer-therapy-associated cognitive change' (Hurria *et al.* 2007; Taillibert *et al.* 2007). Increasing attention is being paid to the long-term consequences as progress in oncology results in more patients living normal lifespans.

Normal-pressure hydrocephalus

Normal-pressure hydrocephalus is a syndrome of gait disturbance, cognitive impairment and urinary incontinence that may be secondary to other diseases such as traumatic brain injury or meningitis or primary, in which case it is known as idiopathic normal-pressure hydrocephalus (INPH) (Gallia *et al.* 2006). It owes its delineation to a group of workers who demonstrated cases in whom marked hydrocephalus was associated with normal or even low intraventricular pressure, sometimes after head injury or subarachnoid haemorrhage but sometimes in patients suspected of a primary dementing illness (Hakim 1964; Adams *et al.* 1965; Hakim & Adams 1965; Adams 1966). Air encephalography showed the absence of any block within the ventricular system, but the air failed to ascend over the surface of the hemispheres betokening obstruction within the basal cisterns or cerebral subarachnoid space. Paradoxically, despite the normal intraventricular pressure, the neurological and mental impairments sometimes proved to be reversible by shunting procedures that reduced the pressure still further.

Clinical features

The incidence of INPH has been estimated to lie between approximately 2 per 100 000 and 2 per 1 million population (Vanneste *et al.* 1992; Krauss & Halve 2004). It is essentially a disorder of the elderly.

The mental changes are a prominent part of the picture throughout. The appearance is of a subcortical dementia type syndrome, with inattention, psychomotor retardation and executive function difficulties (Gallia *et al.* 2006). Aphasias are uncommon. Forgetfulness is usually a prominent early feature, combined with slowing of mental and physical activity, difficulty with thinking and reduced spontaneity, a combination which may lead to a diagnosis of early presenile dementia or depression. Emotional reactions are less vivid

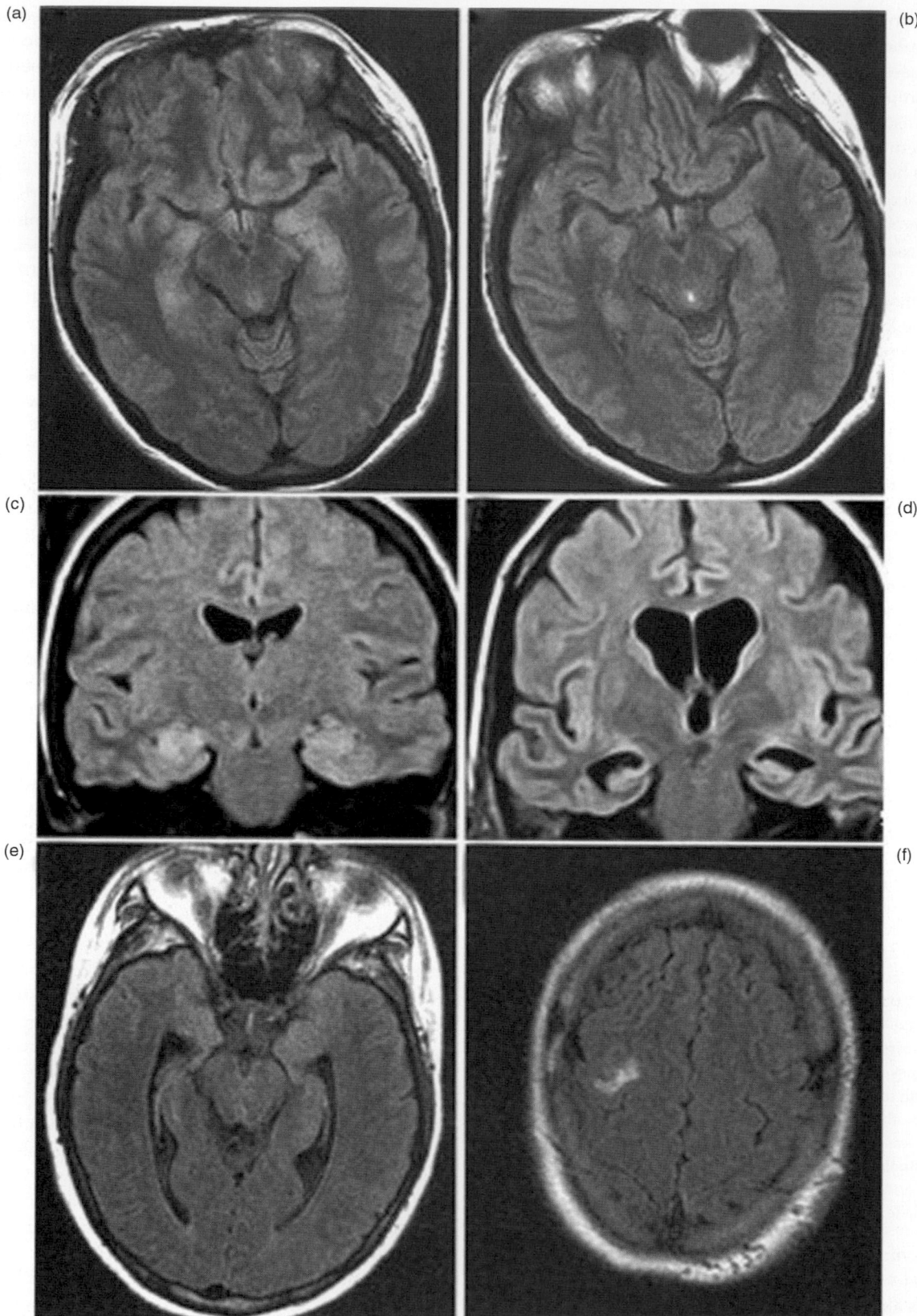

Fig. 14.2 Brain MRI findings in three patients with *N*-methyl-ᴅ-aspartate receptor encephalitis associated with ovarian teratome (Dalmau *et al*. 2007). (a, b) Patient 1 at symptom presentation (a) and after partial clinical improvement and CSF normalisation with immunotherapy (b). (c, d) Patient 2 at symptom presentation (c) and 4 months later (d); this patient developed rapidly progressive neurological deterioration that did not respond to immunotherapy. (e, f) Patient 3 at symptom presentation; note the mild fluid-attenuated inversion recovery hyperintensity in medial temporal lobes and right frontal cortex. After immunotherapy and tumor resection, the MRI was normal (not shown).

and psychic life seems generally impoverished. Insight is limited or absent from an early stage but social comportment is usually well preserved.

Disturbance of gait may be the presenting feature. In mild examples the patient walks slowly on a broad base with a stiff-legged shuffling gait. There is difficulty with turning and often difficulty with initiating movements similar to that seen in parkinsonism. Falls are frequent. The precise nature of the disturbance is hard to characterise but is often described as an uncertainty, unsteadiness or carelessness in walking. The ill-defined term 'gait apraxia' has been applied. When coupled with the mental symptoms, this abnormality of gait is often the feature which leads one to suspect the presence of normal-pressure hydrocephalus. The disturbance may progress eventually to severe difficulty in walking, standing or arising from a seated position, sometimes even to difficulty in turning over in bed. Signs of spastic paraparesis may be evident with hyperactive tendon reflexes and extensor plantar responses. However, even when the disability is pronounced it is rare to find frank ataxia of the limbs, dyssynergia or intention tremor of cerebellar type.

Urinary incontinence usually appears only when other symptoms are evident, but may set in surprisingly early in relation to the degree of mental impairment. Again this may have diagnostic importance in bringing the condition to mind. Bladder hyperactivity can be demonstrated on urodynamic testing (Ahlberg *et al.* 1988). Faecal incontinence is rare and develops only in the most severe examples.

Other features may include slowness of movement in the upper limbs or occasionally some degree of arm tremor or ataxia. Unexplained nystagmus is occasionally present. Late in the course sucking and grasping reflexes may appear. Headache is rare and when present is usually minimal. Papilloedema does not develop. A history of falling spells with brief impairment of consciousness is common, but frank epileptic seizures have not been reported.

The course without treatment is of slow downward progression with increasing neurological and mental disability. Fluctuations from day to day or from week to week are very characteristic. In some of the more prolonged examples a plateau appears to be reached after many months with a relatively fixed pattern of impairments thereafter. Others progress eventually to coma and death.

Investigations

The findings on investigation are characteristic and necessary to confirm the diagnosis (Relkin *et al.* 2005). These include CSF flow analyses and neuroimaging. EEG is frequently abnormal, showing non-specific random theta or delta activity.

Imaging is an essential part of the diagnostic process. Before the advent of CT, air encephalography usually provided the decisive evidence by way of symmetrically enlarged ventricles, often reaching huge proportions, but with little or no air in the cerebral subarachnoid space above the basal cisterns. Following the procedure, however, there was a risk of rapid deterioration, sometimes requiring urgent neurosurgical intervention.

Structural imaging with CT or MRI demonstrates the enlarged ventricles. Other findings may include periventricular hyperintensities, thinning of the corpus callosum and no evidence of obstruction to CSF flow (Relkin *et al.* 2005). MRI finds a special place in the detection of minor obstructive lesions that might otherwise be missed, particularly in the posterior fossa.

Tests of CSF dynamics include the CSF tap test, external CSF drainage and CSF outflow resistance determination. Although there are no definitive diagnostic tests, the judicious use of CSF analyses can increase predictive accuracy to 90% (Marmarou *et al.* 2005). The CSF tap test involves the withdrawal of large volumes (40–50 mL) of CSF and then careful monitoring of symptoms. Improvement suggests, with high accuracy, a good response to intervention is likely but the test has low sensitivity. The test can in effect be extended by external CSF drainage by an indwelling catheter and this gives good sensitivity and specificity but at some cost, as patients must be admitted to hospital and side effects including infection and nerve root irritation are higher than for other investigations. More commonly used is outflow resistance measurement: abnormally high values are associated with an improved response to therapy.

Secondary normal-pressure hydrocephalus

In many examples no antecedent cause can be discovered. In others there is a history of subarachnoid haemorrhage, head injury or meningitis which has presumably led to the organisation of adhesions in the basal cisterns of the brain. After subarachnoid haemorrhage, organisation of exudate within the arachnoid villi at the superior sagittal sinus may contribute further by obstructing the reabsorption of CSF. Very occasionally the typical clinical syndrome may be due to a partially non-communicating hydrocephalus occasioned, for example, by a third ventricular tumour or aqueduct stenosis. A rare cause has been described by Brieg *et al.* (1967) and Ekbom *et al.* (1969): in hypertensive individuals an elongated 'ectatic' basilar artery may indent the floor of the third ventricle and distort the ventricular system upwards and anteriorly, leading to normal-pressure hydrocephalus.

In Ojemann's (1971) material of 50 cases no cause could be found in 18. These 'idiopathic' cases were all in their sixties or seventies. Of the 32 with known causes, 12 followed subarachnoid haemorrhage, 11 head injury and three meningitis. Five were due to tumours or the after-effects of posterior fossa surgery and one was due to aqueduct stenosis. The age range in this group was wider, from 26 to 69 years.

Differential diagnosis

All three core symptoms – urinary incontinence, falls and ataxia and cognitive decline – are common in the elderly. The most important differential diagnosis is from the primary dementias. INPH should be suspected if early in the decline there appears a disorder of gait together with inertia, apathy and psychomotor retardation. Urinary incontinence developing before the mental impairments have proceeded very far should also raise suspicion.

A depressive illness may be simulated early in the course, when physical and mental slowness are prominent and intellectual impairment minimal. Several patients reported by Pujol *et al.* (1989) met *Diagnostic and Statistical Manual of Mental Disorders* (DSM)-III criteria for major depression. Rice and Gendelman (1973) drew attention to other ways in which the patient may first present to a psychiatrist. In five patients behavioural abnormalities were in the forefront of the picture, sometimes tending to obscure the organic features in the mental state. Examples included personality change with paranoid trends or increasing belligerence, acute agitation and paranoia accompanied by visual hallucinations, and marked anxiety and depression accompanying progressive dementia. In each case the hydrocephalus appeared to have aggravated pre-existing emotional difficulties in the patient in addition to producing intellectual impairment.

When the gait disturbance is the presenting feature, differentiation is required from other causes of mild spasticity and ataxia such as cervical spondylosis. Other differential diagnoses for the gait disturbance include arthritis and peripheral neuropathy. Parkinsonism may be suspected initially on account of the pronounced motor slowing. Some of the problems encountered in diagnosis are illustrated in the following cases.

A woman of 66 had had a radical mastectomy for cancer of the breast followed 1 month later by progressive unsteadiness of gait, forgetfulness and intermittent confusion. Within 6 months the memory disorder was pronounced and psychometry showed widespread impairments. There was no evidence of secondary deposits. The CSF was normal but air encephalography showed gross dilatation of the ventricles with no air over the cortical surface. She worsened precipitately after air encephalography and became drowsy, confused and almost mute. She could no longer walk and nystagmus was present in all directions of gaze. The CSF now showed what were thought to be neoplastic cells and a diagnosis of carcinomatous meningeal infiltration was made.

Over the next 15 months she did not deteriorate as expected. She gradually became more alert, though she continued to speak little and took little notice of what went on around her. She lay or sat immobile, idle or watching television. On readmission she was grossly disorientated and with marked memory impairments, and showed no initiative whatsoever. She was incontinent of urine and faeces and could not sit or stand unsupported. The ankle reflexes were brisk and the plantars upgoing but there were no cerebellar signs. The syndrome of normal-pressure hydrocephalus was recognised and a shunt operation performed. Improvement was evident within 3 days and after 7 weeks her mental state had returned to normal. Control of bowel and bladder was regained, and when seen 9 months later she was walking by herself though still with an uncertain gait (Adams *et al.* 1965).

A man of 49 complained of lethargy, easy fatiguability and vague weakness of the legs. For 6 months his family had noted him to be dull and forgetful. He was found to be slow in motor and verbal responses and with a mild impairment of recent memory. The plantar responses were extensor but there were no other abnormal neurological signs. CSF pressure was mildly elevated with a protein of 100 mg/dL. Air encephalography showed symmetrical dilatation of the ventricles with a small amount of air over the surface. A tentative diagnosis of Alzheimer's disease was made. In hospital there was considerable improvement in his apathy and inertia but he relapsed after a few weeks at home. Walking became seriously impaired, with a stiff-legged gait and several falls. On readmission he was now severely amnesic for recent events and disorientated in time and place. He improved again in hospital but the diagnosis of Alzheimer's disease remained.

Over the next 2 months he gradually declined into severe confusion and was readmitted pending transfer to a long-stay psychiatric hospital. He was now unkempt, apathetic and unconcerned, with great slowness on mental tasks. He walked with a wide-based stiff-legged gait and stumbled on turning. Bilateral grasp reflexes were observed, and a prehensile sucking reflex when the lips were touched. The Wechsler Adult Intelligence Scale (WAIS) IQ was 64, whereas 4 months earlier it had been 101. After lumbar puncture he changed remarkably, becoming alert and quick of mind, fully orientated and able to learn new facts, and the WAIS IQ rose to 105. Gait returned to normal but the plantars remained extensor. A shunt operation was performed with excellent results, and a small mass situated on the floor of the third ventricle encroaching on the entrance to the aqueduct was irradiated. Six months later he was back at his usual clerical job (McHugh 1966).

Treatment and response

Treatment involves a shunt operation to lower CSF pressure within the ventricles and maintain it at this low level. An indwelling catheter is inserted into a lateral ventricle, incorporating a low-pressure one-way valve, and opening either into the superior vena cava through the jugular venous system (ventriculocaval shunt) or into the peritoneal cavity (ventriculoperitoneal shunt). The latter are more commonly used. The result, though somewhat unpredictable, is gratifyingly successful in certain cases. Those patients who on intracranial pressure monitoring have shown elevated mean pressures or marked spontaneous pressure waves tend to show the best response (Jeffreys & Wood 1978; Crockard *et al.* 1980).

A wide range of shunts and catheters are available. Adjustable valves with subcutaneous controllers are increasingly used. These can be manipulated by the physician, allowing finer control of CSF pressure and avoiding over- and under-drainage. As the devices are magnetically controlled, this can result in problems for patients near magnetic sources, including MRI scanners (Gallia *et al.* 2006).

Shunt operations, even when dramatically successful initially, are not without their long-term complications (Jeffreys 1993). The catheter may become blocked or infected or shift its position, or the valve may cease to function. Over-drainage can result in headache, lethargy, strabismus, nausea and vomiting, typically relieved by lying down. The 'slit ventricle syndrome', commoner in those who have been shunted since early childhood, presents with a history indicative of intermittent obstruction and is probably also largely a consequence of previous over-drainage (Hendrick 1993).

Among INPH cases, Ojemann (1971) found satisfactory improvement after shunting in all patients where a complete block in the subarachnoid space had been demonstrated. The patients with only partial obstruction showed disappointing results, perhaps because some had a primary dementing illness in addition to their normal-pressure hydrocephalus. Pickard (1982) suggests that complete recovery can be expected in about one-third of patients, with useful improvement in a further 30%.

The improvement is often manifest immediately on recovery from the anaesthetic, with further gains in the days that follow. Sometimes, however, there is little change during the first postoperative week, gradual improvement then taking place over the next several weeks. The neurological deficits are usually the first to resolve, although gait disturbance sometimes responds only gradually. Incontinence typically clears fairly promptly. Intellectual deficits tend to improve more slowly, sometimes with maximal gains after several months. In favourable cases intellectual impairments, aspontaneity and apathy can ultimately clear completely. Follow-up with repeat evaluation of cognitive function has shown gains more obvious at 1 year than at 6 months, and well maintained thereafter (Crockard *et al.* 1980).

In secondary normal-pressure hydrocephalus following subarachnoid haemorrhage, improvement is likely within a few days of shunting but focal neurological deficits related to the local effects of the haemorrhage will often persist unaltered. The response in cases following head injury is governed by the degree and severity of the underlying brain damage. Salmon (1971) reported nine post-traumatic cases, operated at intervals of 6 months to 8 years after injury. Two were 'much improved' and three 'improved', including two patients who showed some evidence of cortical atrophy as well. The improvements often took place slowly over the course of several weeks.

Other forms of hydrocephalus

The best-known form of hydrocephalus is that which declares itself in infancy, resulting from obstruction along the course of the CSF pathways. This is usually due to developmental defects of the brain, haemorrhage following birth trauma, or an attack of meningitis. When the disturbance is manifest before the cranial sutures have closed there is progressive enlargement of the head. Usual accompaniments are varying degrees of spasticity, mental retardation and sometimes blindness, depending on the severity of the obstruction and the presence or absence of associated developmental brain defects. In some patients the hydrocephalus becomes arrested and intellect may occasionally be surprisingly well preserved. In cases due to developmental defects there are often other congenital abnormalities, particularly spina bifida and meningomyelocele. In adults obstructive hydrocephalus is mainly the result of new pathology, such as a tumour strategically situated to impede the CSF circulation within the brain. It commonly presents with symptoms of raised intracranial pressure but sometimes the initial picture can be misleading.

Occasionally, moreover, adult obstructive hydrocephalus is attributable to congenital defects or pathology acquired much earlier in life; a partial balance is then achieved between the production and absorption of CSF. Developmental defects such as aqueduct stenosis or partial obliteration of the foramina of the fourth ventricle can remain latent in this way. Headache is usual but not inevitable, and a spectrum is likely to exist between the cases considered here and those already described under the heading of normal-pressure hydrocephalus. A frequent feature is a history of attacks of abrupt loss of consciousness, lasting a few minutes during which the patient lies motionless and flaccid. Such attacks are often preceded or followed by headache and are presumably due to sudden rises of intracranial pressure. The mental changes, which may or may not accompany the neurological developments, can take the form of listlessness, apathy and inattentiveness, progressing to a picture of dementia and inertia resembling frontal lobe disorder.

Aqueduct stenosis, in particular, may fail to declare itself until adolescence or mid-adulthood. Asymptomatic cases have also been found at post-mortem. The stenosis is usually the result of congenital defect, although some can be traced to an episode of meningitis in childhood and others show gliosis of unknown cause. Sometimes a small mass, such as a periaqueductal glioma, compresses the aqueduct from without. Symptoms of raised intracranial pressure may occur, sometimes following an intermittent crescendo pattern succeeded by periods of unconsciousness, but in others such evidence is completely lacking. Some present with unsteadiness of gait or with epilepsy, usually of psychomotor type. Others show hypothalamic symptoms such as impotence, amenorrhoea or obesity, due to pressure of the distended third ventricle on the pituitary and hypothalamus. Mental symptoms may be the presenting feature, with impairment of memory or generalised dementia. Of the 10 cases reported by Nag and Falconer (1966) only five presented with symptoms indicative of raised intracranial pressure, while memory disorder was the initial manifestation in four. Harrison *et al.* (1974) obtained a history of deterioration of memory and concentration in one-third of their cases. This was usually mild, but in two cases was sufficiently marked to be the feature that brought the patient to medical attention.

A man of 52 showed slow progression of gait disturbance and impotence following the death of his mother to whom he was closely attached. Six years later he was hospitalised and the disorder was ascribed to 'nerves'. Thereafter he developed emotional lability, mild memory impairment and occasional urinary incontinence. One year later mental testing was within normal limits except for moderate slowing of responses, but his gait was strikingly abnormal with tiny shuffling steps and difficulty in initiating movement. The CSF was normal and under normal pressure. Air encephalography showed aqueduct stenosis. Ventriculography showed dilatation of the lateral and third ventricles, and also of the upper 1 cm of the aqueduct. A shunt operation led to excellent resolution of his symptoms. He had had meningitis at the age of 5 and had complained frequently of headache throughout adult life (Wilkinson *et al.* 1966).

An example reported by Ojemann *et al.* (1969) is also instructive:

A woman of 54 had an 18-month history of progressive change of personality and failure of mental functions. She became disinterested in people and activities, and showed inattentiveness and difficulty with calculation. Some months later her gait became unsteady and her left hand tremulous, leading to a diagnosis of parkinsonism. Deterioration progressed relentlessly with marked apathy and incontinence of urine. On examination she showed impairment of memory and other intellectual functions, a slight left hemiparesis and spasticity in the legs. On sitting down she took 30 seconds to complete the last 4 inches, and on approaching a step she raised her foot too early and too high. CSF pressure was normal, and air encephalography showed air in the fourth ventricle but none in the aqueduct. Ventriculography displayed large lateral and third ventricles, with gross dilatation of the rostral part of the aqueduct and a nodular mass projecting from the region of the quadrigeminal plate. A shunt operation produced striking improvement and she was entirely normal 1 year after operation.

An interesting association of aqueduct stenosis has been reported by Reveley and Reveley (1983). In the course of examining the CT scans of schizophrenic patients they found three with aqueduct stenosis. Two were known to be hydrocephalic from shortly after birth, while in the third the condition was entirely unsuspected. The significance of this association remains at present unclear.

The diagnosis rests ultimately on radiographic studies along with CT or MRI. Erosion of the dorsum sellae is shown on plain radiography in the majority, and the lateral and third ventricles are seen to be symmetrically enlarged. The aqueduct is either not displayed or is seen to be very narrow. Intraventricular pressure may be elevated or normal.

Shunt operations can be dramatically successful in relieving the symptoms whether or not the pressure has been raised. However, a considerable failure rate is seen mainly due to obstruction within the subarachnoid space (McMillan & Williams 1977).

Other disorders affecting the CNS

Progressive multifocal leucoencephalopathy

This rare disorder is an uncommon complication of chronic disorders with compromised immune function, most notably HIV/AIDS in recent years (Wyen *et al.* 2005; Berger 2007; Drake *et al.* 2007). Other chronic diseases where progressive multifocal leucoencephalopathy (PML) may be a complication include lymphoma, Hodgkin's disease, leukaemia or sarcoidosis. The disorder results from opportunistic infection of the brain by JC polyomavirus (Khalili & White 2006).

A very few patients receiving natalizumab for MS or Crohn's disease, especially if also being treated with immunosuppressive agents, succumbed to PML (Gold *et al.* 2007). Most affected patients have been between 30 and 60 years of age. Progressive dementia is accompanied by neurological manifestations indicative of focal involvement of the CNS: pareses, ataxia, dysphasia and visual field defects. Rapid mental and neurological deterioration typically leads to death within a few weeks or months, but very occasional cases have shown slow progression over several years. MRI features include hyperintense lesions in periventricular and subcortical white matter most often in parieto-occipital or frontal lobes, but also elsewhere in the brain (Whiteman *et al.* 1993). MRI is more sensitive than CT which shows low-density lesions in the central and convolutional white matter, often with a distinctive 'scalloped' appearance to their lateral borders (Carroll *et al.* 1977). Such lesions do not enhance, and are without mass effect. Despite these changes, diagnosis is complicated and may require biopsy (Pelosini *et al.* 2008), especially since the virus often cannot be detected in CSF in patients treated with antiviral drugs (Koralnik 2004).

At post-mortem, scattered crumbling foci of softening are seen as small round greyish areas throughout the brain. They are situated mainly in the white matter, affecting the cerebral hemispheres, cerebellum and brainstem, and showing a special predilection for the junction of cortex and subcortex. Within such areas there is marked demyelination along with relative preservation of the axis cylinders. Perivascular lymphocytic cuffing is usually well developed. A unique stamp is given by the changes observed in the glial cells. Astrocytes are enormously enlarged, with bizarre distorted nuclei that often show abnormal mitoses. The oligodendroglial nuclei often contain inclusion bodies.

The availaibility of highly active antiretroviral therapy (HAART) has improved the prognosis of PML in HIV/AIDS: 3-month mortality has decreased from 90% to 50% (Koralnik 2004). However, the incidence remains unaffected as does prognosis when PML occurs in the context of other diseases.

Adrenoleucodystrophy

This group of disorders includes neonatal and childhood adrenoleucodystrophy, Zellweger's cerebrohepatorenal syndrome and adult-onset adrenomyeloneuropathy. The biochemical abnormality they share is the accumulation of very-long-chain saturated fatty acids (VLCFA), particularly hexacosanoate, in lipid-containing tissues including the brain. Characteristic lamellar inclusions can be shown in the Schwann cells of the nervous system and the cells of the adrenal cortex. The diagnosis may be made by demonstrating increase in VLCFA (Moser *et al.* 1999) or ultrastructural examination of nerve terminals biopsied from the skin or conjunctiva. The childhood and adult-onset forms are both sex-linked, appearing only in males, and may be found in the same family. MRI lesions are seen in both adult and childhood-onset forms but progress slower in the adult form (Eichler *et al.* 2007). The defect in these X-linked cases is in the *ABCD1* gene, where over 500 separate mutations have been shown to cause disease (Moser *et al.* 2004). The gene encodes a protein that has a role in peroxisomal β-oxidation and hence fatty acid metabolism.

Childhood cerebral adrenoleucodystrophy often presents with inattention, hyperactivity and emotional lability. Visual, auditory and motor symptoms follow and the course of the condition is then very rapid. However, mutations in the *ABCD1* gene in the absence of overt cerebral involvement do not result in an altered IQ (Cox *et al.* 2006). Adrenal insufficiency may not be apparent at the time of presentation but Addison's disease develops eventually. Occasionally this precedes the nervous system involvement.

The neonatal form of infantile adrenoleucodystrophy, Refsum disease and Zellweger's syndrome are all overlapping peroxisome biogenesis disorders caused by mutations in one of the many peroxin genes. As in other adrenoleucodystrophy disorders, VLCFAs accumulate because of the defect in lipid peroxidation. A severe neonatal disorder is the consequence, with facial malformation, renal and hepatic abnormality, death usually before the age of 5 years and histological evidence of leucodystrophic change in the brain.

Adrenomyeloneuropathy presents with spastic paraparesis and sensory loss in the legs due to peripheral nerve involvement, proceeding sometimes to dementia. In rare examples the presentation has been with focal cerebral deficits, Klüver–Bucy syndrome, dementia resembling Alzheimer's disease or spinocerebellar degeneration (Moser *et al.* 1984).

Adrenoleucodystrophy came to the attention of the public with the film *Lorenzo's Oil*. This highly controversial film was reviewed by Moser, a leading clinician and researcher in the field who identified himself as possibly one of the characters in the film (Moser 1993). The film tells the fictional story of a boy affected by the disease and his family's search for a cure. Whether 'Lorenzo's oil' (4:1 glyceryl trioleate-glyceryl trierucate) is efficacious is nearly as controversial as the film. It appears to lower VLCFA and to delay progression of MRI lesions (Moser *et al.* 2005) but clinical benefits have not been demonstrated (Aubourg *et al.* 1993).

Dementia with familial calcification of the basal ganglia (adult-onset bilateral striopallidodentate calcinosis, Fahr's syndrome)

Basal ganglia calcification is, in itself, a benign finding on neuroimaging, with no increase in dementia (Forstl *et al.* 1992). However, in the syndrome of adult-onset bilateral striopallidodentate calcinosis in the absence of calcium or parathyroid hormone imbalance, dementia is a feature. Reports in the literature have included both apparently sporadic cases and those inherited in an autosomal dominant fashion. The largest series comprised 38 patients from five autosomal dominant families and eight isolated individuals (Manyam *et al.* 2001). Cognitive symptoms were the most frequent after motor effects.

Many affected persons are asymptomatic for long periods of time, although it seems likely that most eventually show some form of extrapyramidal dysfunction. Parkinsonism or choreoathetosis usually develop in late middle age, or more rarely cerebellar ataxia or pyramidal deficits. Progressive impairment of memory and intellect frequently accompany the motor manifestations, with slowing of cognitive processes typical of subcortical dementia. Dysphasia and other focal cortical deficits are not observed. In several cases a psychosis indistinguishable from schizophrenia has been reported, often antedating the motor and cognitive manifestations by many years. Francis (1979) and Francis and Freeman (1984) have reported nine patients in four generations of a family in whom a schizophrenia-like psychosis appeared to be the principal accompaniment of the disorder.

Cummings *et al.* (1983) review the literature on the condition, finding indications of two relatively distinct patterns of presentation. Those who present with psychotic episodes tend to do so in their early thirties, those with dementia and motor disorder some 20 years later. Both share the characteristic finding of dense calcification symmetrically involving the basal ganglia and particularly the putamen. The dentate nuclei of the cerebellum and the pulvinar of the thalamus may also be heavily affected.

Other conditions leading to calcification within the basal ganglia must be excluded, the commonest being hypoparathyroidism and pseudohypoparathyroidism. Hyperparathyroidism may occasionally produce a not dissimilar radiological appearance. Investigation of serum calcium and phosphate serves to make the distinction since these have uniformly proved to be normal. Other causes of calcification such as toxoplasmosis, tuberous sclerosis or the sequelae of encephalitis or anoxia will also need consideration when the familial nature of the condition is not apparent.

In a review of the literature, Flint and Goldstein (1992) cast doubt on the syndrome as an independent clinical entity, suggesting that at least some cases are variants of pseudohypoparathyroidism. Some of the associated features of the latter, such as short stature and shortened metacarpals, occurred in their own familial cases and in other reported examples. Flint and Goldstein also conclude that schizophrenia, when carefully delineated, is uncommon and may represent no more than a chance association.

A locus on chromosome 14 was linked to one very large family that had decreasing age of onset in each generation, suggesting the phenomenon of anticipation (Geschwind

et al. 1999). Subsequently some, but not all, families with the condition were shown to have linkage to the same region, demonstrating that this is a heterogeneous condition (Oliveira *et al.* 2004). Interestingly, in one family where probands had basal ganglia calcification, dementia, bipolar affective disorder and parkinsonism, prompting a diagnosis of Fahr's syndrome, the neuropsychiatric symptoms were found to be independent of basal ganglia calcification and linkage to the locus on chromosome 14 was excluded (Brodaty *et al.* 2002).

Neurodegeneration with brain iron accumulation (pantothenate kinase-associated neurodegeneration, Hallervorden–Spatz syndrome)

A heterogeneous group of related disorders result from deposition or accumulation of iron in the basal ganglia. Described first in 1922 by Hallervorden and Spatz in a family with dementia and dysarthria, the condition presents classically in the first decade of life with death before the age of 30 years, although atypical presentations can be later. Dooling *et al.* (1974) describe the typical features of early onset of a motor disorder mainly of extrapyramidal type, the mental changes of dementia, and a relentlessly progressive course leading to death on average 11 years later. Of their 42 examples from the literature, mental changes had been the first manifestations in four. In more than half the onset had been before the age of 10, but one had begun at 30 and two others at 57 and 64 years. The disorder is inherited as an autosomal recessive disease. The late-onset cases were non-familial and died after 5–6 years.

Motor abnormalities consist mainly of rigidity, dystonia and choreoathetoid movements, although spasticity and pyramidal signs may appear. Dysarthria is almost always present and facial grimacing may occur. Myoclonus and tremor are not uncommon. Abnormalities of posture or movement are the usual presenting symptoms, often interfering with walking. Vision may be impaired due to retinopathy or optic atrophy.

A change of personality sometimes sets in early, with depression and outbursts of aggressive behaviour. Intellectual deterioration then gradually develops along with the motor manifestations, often progressing to mutism in the terminal stages.

There are no abnormal findings in the blood or CSF. EEG shows slowing as the disease advances, sometimes with spikes and sharp waves. The CT scan may resemble that seen in Huntington's chorea, with prominent atrophy of the basal ganglia (Dooling *et al.* 1980). Generalised atrophy of the cortex, brainstem and cerebellum may also be apparent. MRI shows destruction of the central part of the globus pallidus, surrounded by dark signal due to iron deposition ("eye of the tiger" sign) (Angelini *et al.* 1992).

At post-mortem the distinctive finding is reddish-brown discoloration of the globus pallidus and pars reticulata of the substantia nigra, due to the accumulation of iron-containing pigment. Microscopy shows loss of neurones in the affected areas with demyelination and gliosis, and numerous oval or rounded structures (spheroids) which are identifiable as axonal swellings. The latter are frequently widely disseminated in the cortex, although this may otherwise show little by way of neuronal loss or gliosis. The Purkinje cells of the cerebellum may be depleted.

Neurodegeneration with brain iron accumulation (NBIA) is found in two variants, type 1 and type 2. NBIA1 is caused by mutations in the *PANK2* gene (Zhou *et al.* 2001) and NBIA2 by mutations in the *PLA2G6* gene. *PANK2* codes for a pantothenate kinase involved in coenzyme synthesis from vitamin B$_5$ (pantothenic acid). Loss of the gene in mouse results in a retinopathy (Kuo *et al.* 2005). A variety of similar syndromes to NBIA1 have been reported. One example, also known as Karak syndrome, was found to have mutations in the *PLA2G6* gene coding for a phospholipase (Mubaidin *et al.* 2003; Morgan *et al.* 2006). The heterogeneity and complexity of these syndromes is illustrated by the fact that a mutation in *PLA2G6* also causes infantile neuroaxonal dystrophy (Khateeb *et al.* 2006) and mutations in *PANK2* also cause the closely related HARP syndrome (hypoprebetalipoproteinaemia, acanthocytosis, retinitis pigmentosa, and pallidal degeneration) (Ching *et al.* 2002).

The names of Julius Hallervorden and Hugo Spatz are notorious as participants in one of medicine's more shameful episodes. Hallervorden, who replaced Max Bielschowsky as head of neuropathology in Berlin when Bielschowsky was dismissed from his post as a Jew, and Spatz, who once worked in Kraepelin's department with Nissl, were Nazi war criminals and the recipients of brain material from the 'euthanasia', or murder, of mentally ill children and adults (http://www.whonamedit.com).

Neuroacanthocytosis (choreoacanthocytosis)

Neuroacanthocytosis is a rare syndrome of progressive neurodegeneration and acanthocytosis most familiar in the autosomal recessive form known as choreoacanthocytosis but also occurring in abetalipoproteinaemia and X-linked McLeod syndrome (Rubio *et al.* 1997). Acanthocytes are abnormal red blood cells, detected in fresh blood films by their spiny protuberances. They must be carefully distinguished from echinocytes, which show a not dissimilar appearance, and from other artefactual changes in red cell morphology (Hardie 1989). Acanthocytes are also found in abetalipoproteinaemia (Bassen–Kornzweig syndrome), a condition usually appearing in the first decade of life and accompanied by fat malabsorption, spinocerebellar ataxia and pigmentary retinopathy. These features are attributed to defective absorption of vitamin E. In neuroacanthocytosis,

however, lipid metabolism is entirely normal. The locus for choreoacanthocytosis has been clearly identified on chromosome 9p21 (Rubio *et al.* 1997) with a novel gene *CHAC* or *VPS13A*, coding for the protein chorein, being the most likely culprit (Rampoldi *et al.* 2001; Dobson-Stone *et al.* 2002; Ruiz-Sandoval *et al.* 2007).

The condition usually comes to attention in early middle age, although the range of onset is wide. Involuntary movements, chiefly choreic, are accompanied by hyporeflexia or areflexia and sometimes by muscle wasting. Seizures occur in perhaps half of cases. Steady and slow progression of deficits is the rule over several decades, though there is much variability. Hardie *et al.* (1991) presented 19 cases with a review of the relevant literature. Movement disorder is virtually universal, with choreiform and dystonic movements affecting the orofacial region and sometimes the limbs. In severe examples there may be biting of the tongue and lips, also pseudobulbar features with difficulty with speech and swallowing. Tongue protrusions and severe grimacing may occur. Tics can also be prominent, along with grunting, sniffing and spitting. Vocalisations sometimes develop, usually of monosyllabic words. A peculiar lurching gait may be seen, with dipping of the knees and foot flap. A minority of cases progress to an akinetic–rigid state. Muscle wasting and weakness can affect distal or proximal groups, hyporeflexia being common even in its absence.

Among psychiatric features depression, anxiety and obsessive–compulsive disorder are not infrequent. Hardie *et al.* (1991) also report a characteristic organic personality change, leading to vagueness, distractibility and neglect of appearance and social skills. In fact the literature is scattered with examples of misdiagnosis emphasising pleiotropy of the condition (Walker *et al.* 2007). Examples of neuroacanthocytosis presenting for example as Huntington's disease (Gold *et al.* 2006), schizophrenia and Tourette's syndrome (Bruneau *et al.* 2003; Muller-Vahl *et al.* 2007) are reported. Dementia has been clinically evident in some half of reported cases, but neuropsychological evaluation may show deficits in many more, particularly on tests of attention and planning indicative of frontal lobe disorder. Investigation in suspected cases must include a careful search for acanthocytes in fresh blood films, repeated if necessary on several occasions since the abnormal cells can be relatively rare in the early stages. The serum creatinine kinase may or may not be elevated. CT often shows caudate atrophy, or generalised cerebral atrophy in the presence of dementia. MRI may show increased T2 signals from the basal ganglia. At post-mortem there is extensive neuronal loss and gliosis in the corpus striatum and globus pallidus, also sometimes in the lateral substantia nigra. The caudate nucleus may be virtually depleted of both large and small neurones. The hemisphere white matter shows mild diffuse gliosis, but the cortex itself is spared.

Differential diagnosis must obviously include Huntington's disease, especially in patients who show a dominant pattern of inheritance. The presence of seizures, muscle wasting, areflexia or evidence of neuropathy should immediately raise suspicion of neuroacanthocytosis, also good preservation of cognitive function late into the disease. Gilles de la Tourette's syndrome may sometimes be closely simulated, likewise tardive dyskinesia if the patient has been on neuroleptic medication. Estimation of serum lipids will reveal those patients whose acanthocytosis is due to abetalipoproteinaemia.

Metachromatic leucodystrophy

This rare cause of dementia and motor disorder is inherited in an autosomal recessive fashion due to mutation in the arylsulphatase A gene (*ARSA*). The two most common mutations in the population occur with a frequency of 13–17% (Barth *et al.* 1994) and have been reported to also occur more often than expected in vascular dementia (Philpot *et al.* 1997). Metachromatic leucodystrophy represents an abnormality of neural lipid metabolism, with accumulation of galactosyl sulphatide in affected tissues. Deposits of the material stain metachromatically. Kihara (1982) describes five allelic variants: late infantile, juvenile, and adult forms, partial cerebroside sulphate deficiency, and pseudoarylsulphatase A deficiency. The infantile form represents the classic disease, setting in before the age of 3 and progressing to severe motor and mental retardation, sometimes with blindness. The juvenile form is less common, presenting with motor and mental dysfunction and sometimes resembling a spinocerebellar disorder.

The adult form is rarest of all. Onset in recorded cases has varied from 19 to 46 years, presenting sometimes with dementia and sometimes with psychotic disorder. Motor dysfunction is less prominent and may develop only later in the disease. In adults the course can be extremely protracted over several decades; mistakes in diagnosis are common and unless a sibling has already been affected, the condition may go unsuspected during life. Common misdiagnoses include early-onset dementia, schizophrenia or multiple sclerosis.

Cummings and Benson (1992) refer to reports of the condition first diagnosed as schizophrenia or presenting with expansive delusions suggestive of mania. When motor abnormalities eventually appear, they take the form of pyramidal and extrapyramidal dysfunction with paresis, dystonic movements, dysarthria and parkinsonism. Ataxia, nystagmus and intention tremor are common. Seizures often occur, and peripheral neuropathy is usually present.

Hyde *et al.* (1992) have drawn attention to the special liability of adolescent and early adult cases to present with psychotic disorder, this appearing to be restricted to such an age of onset. Thus of 129 published case reports, 55 patients had had an onset between the ages of 10 and 30 years, and 29 of these (53%) showed psychotic symptoms. This was the most frequent presenting feature in the age group concerned, and

seemed considerably more common than with other neurological disorders. No such symptoms were apparent in the 74 cases with juvenile or later adult onset. Typical symptoms included auditory hallucinations, sometimes of voices commenting on the patient's behaviour, complex delusions, fragmentation of thinking, inappropriate affect, bizarre behaviour or catatonic posturing. Many of the psychoses appeared at first to be non-organic, and 15 patients had been diagnosed as suffering from schizophrenia. Two showed mania and three personality change. The false diagnoses sometimes persisted for several years before dysarthria, spasticity and hyperreflexia appeared.

Hyde *et al.* (1992) suggest that such psychotic developments may owe much to the disruption of frontal–subcortical connections occasioned by the demyelination. At first this mainly affects the subfrontal and periventricular frontal white matter. As the disease progresses and demyelination spreads more diffusely the psychotic symptoms tend to disappear, being replaced by sensorimotor disturbances and dementia. However, the age of the patient must be an additional determining factor, since a similar distribution of demyelination is seen in the infantile, juvenile and late-onset forms.

A typical diagnostic puzzle is described below.

A woman of 29 was referred for a second opinion, 2.5 years after admission to a psychiatric hospital with a provisional diagnosis of schizophrenia. Certain organic features in her mental state had then given rise to concern. Her birth and early development had been normal, and her early schooling had proceeded smoothly. However, at 11 she changed, becoming increasingly disruptive and attention seeking. At 16 she was found to be of average intelligence but thought to have a personality disorder. On leaving school she held jobs for short periods only, and embarked on the life of a vagrant, obtaining money by petty theft and prostitution. Her behaviour became increasingly erratic and bizarre, and she gave birth to two illegitimate children whom she abandoned. All this was in contrast to her stable family background.

On a number of occasions, while on remand, she was found to be of average intelligence and a label of psychopathic personality was repeatedly applied. At 26 she was found wandering in a dishevelled state which led to her hospitalisation. On examination she was child-like and unable to give an account of herself. She repeated stereotyped phrases such as 'egg but no bacon', smiled fatuously, and would laugh or cry for no reason. She was uncooperative with cognitive testing and the initial diagnosis was of schizophrenia.

Ultimately it was possible to demonstrate grossly impaired short-term memory, poor writing and constructional apraxia. Neurological examination showed primitive reflexes but no other abnormality. However, CT revealed considerable cerebral atrophy and lumbar puncture showed a raised CSF protein. Her WAIS verbal IQ was 59 and performance IQ 40.

On transfer to the Bethlem Royal Hospital she showed right–left disorientation, difficulty in following complex instructions and some nominal dysphasia. However, such features seemed to be in keeping with her level of global intellectual impairment. Neurological signs remained absent, but by now she was occasionally incontinent.

Extensive investigations revealed grossly deficient arylsulphatase A activity in the white blood cells and cultured skin fibroblasts. Metachromatic granules were present in the urine. EEG was normal, but the electromyogram showed slowing of sensory conduction in the lower limbs. A repeat CT scan showed more marked changes than before and MRI showed distinctive hyperintensities in the periventricular white matter (Fig. 14.3) (Fisher *et al.* 1987).

The specific diagnosis depends on showing diminished arylsulphatase A activity in the white blood cells, serum and urine, and demonstration of excessive sulphatide in the urine. Low levels of pseudoarylsulphatase A also occur in the absence of genetic variation in the gene, a condition known as pseudodeficiency. The clinical relevance of this is uncertain, although some studies have reported increased rates of pseudodeficiency in children with neurological signs and syndromes (Sangiorgi *et al.* 1991) not dissimilar to the clinical picture of children with diagnosed leucodystrophy (MacFaul *et al.* 1982) and adults with schizophrenia and other

psychotic disorders (Heavey *et al.* 1990; Mihaljevic-Peles *et al.* 2001).

Metachromatic deposits within Schwann cells may be detected in biopsy specimens from the sural nerve or rectal wall. Peripheral nerve conduction velocity is reduced. The heterozygote state may also be detected by measurement of arylsulphatase in the white blood cells. Waltz *et al.* (1987) emphasise the importance of brain imaging in bringing the disorder to mind, particularly in patients who present with psychiatric disorder. CT usually shows mild atrophy, with symmetrical decrease in white matter attenuation, especially near the frontal and occipital horns. MRI shows such changes more impressively.

At post-mortem severe white matter destruction is seen in the brain, often with cavitation, along with loss of normal myelin sheaths. Accumulations of strikingly metachromatic material appear as spherical granular masses. Similar changes are found in the peripheral nerves and certain visceral organs. The neuronal cell bodies are virtually unaffected, although at the end stage some may show sulphatide accumulations.

Kufs' disease (neuronal ceroid lipofuscinosis, Kufs–Parry disease, Batten–Bielschowsky or Spielmeyer–Vogt–Sjogren disease)

Kufs' disease is the name given to the adult form of cerebral lipidosis in which the abnormal lipopigment deposits consist of a ceroid-like material akin to lipofuscin. It is an example of one of many storage disorders usually evident in infancy and childhood. Interested readers should consult a textbook of paediatric neurology or recent reviews (Goebel & Wisniewski 2004; Rakheja *et al.* 2007) for details.

Symptoms begin in adolescence or adulthood with an insidious dementia accompanied by motor manifestations. Extrapyramidal disturbances and cerebellar disorder appear to be commoner than spasticity in adults. Myoclonic and other forms of seizure are often encountered. In a review of 118 published cases, Berkovic *et al.* (1988) accepted only 50 as true examples of the condition. The remainder showed a variety of atypical features or had evidence of other storage diseases (e.g. Niemann–Pick disease or late-onset gangliosidosis). Two main forms of clinical presentation were apparent: type A with seizures and type B with dementia and motor disturbances, although considerable overlap occurred. The seizures typically took the form of progressive myoclonus epilepsy, often with marked photosensitivity, proceeding ultimately to dementia. Neurological signs developed only late in type A patients and consisted of little more than ataxia and dysarthria. Type B patients usually presented with behavioural change, ranging from disinterest to overt psychosis, the organic nature of the condition becoming obvious when dementia or motor disturbances made an appearance. Cerebellar and extrapyramidal features were

(a) (b)

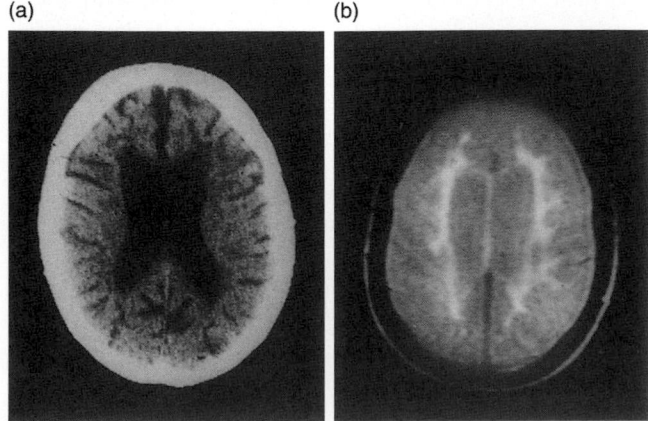

Fig. 14.3 CT and MR scans from a patient with metachromatic leucodystrophy. (Reproduced from Fisher, N.R., Cope, S.J. & Lishman W.A. *Journal of Neurology, Neurosurgery and Psychiatry* (1987), **50**, 488–489, courtesy of BMJ Publishing Group.)

usually prominent, and tic-like facial dyskinesia particularly so. With both varieties the onset tended to be around 30 years of age, although some began in late adolescence. The course of the disease varied considerably, death following a mean of 12 years later.

Recessive inheritance predominates, although families with autosomal dominant inheritance have been described. A number of cases are apparently sporadic. The pathogenetic defect lies in the intracellular processing of lysosomal and perhaps of Golgi membranes. Unlike juvenile forms, there is no pigmentary degeneration of the retina.

Diagnostic classification of neuronal ceroid lipofuscinosis is based on age of onset, although there are other variants. A number of *CLN* genes have been identified (currently eight), mutations in which account for the varying phenotpyes that lead to cellular accumulation of lysosomal storage material which ultrastructurally conforms to fingerprint or curvilinear profiles, or granular osmophilic deposits (Goebel & Wisniewski 2004). The diagnosis of adult neuronal ceroid lipofuscinosis is gained by careful evaluation of skin, rectal or brain biopsies with the electron microscope.

The characteristic finding at post-mortem is striking distension of nerve cells with autofluorescent lipopigment, along with neuronal degeneration and reactive gliosis. Cells in the basal ganglia, brainstem and cerebellum tend to be more heavily involved than those of the cortex (Dekaban & Herman 1974). A variable degree of generalised brain atrophy may accompany such changes.

Whipple's disease

Whipple's disease is a rare multisystem disorder that is infective in origin, the responsible organism being *Tropheryma whippelii* (Mahnel & Marth 2004; Deriban & Marth 2006). An immunological defect in the host is likely to play an important part in causation. It is very much more common in men than women, setting in usually in the sixth decade. The classic presentation is with weight loss, lassitude, chronic diarrhoea and malabsorption, often pursuing a chronic course to extreme emaciation. Multiple arthralgias, serous effusions, uveitis, lymphadenopathy and low-grade pyrexia are other common manifestations.

Involvement of the nervous system occurs sometimes after the systemic disorder is well advanced but occasionally as the dominant feature. Neurological involvement has been reported several times when gastrointestinal and other symptoms are minimal. In very rare examples it has represented the sole clinical or pathological manifestation of the disorder. Louis *et al.* (1996) note that the diagnosis should be considered in any case of systemic illness accompanied by supranuclear vertical gaze palsy, rhythmic myoclonus, dementia with psychiatric symptoms, or hypothalamic manifestations.

The symptoms tend to be non-specific so that diagnosis may be missed or greatly delayed. Pallis and Lewis (1980) describe the common picture as dementia progressing over months or years, external ophthalmoplegias, or myoclonic movements of the head, trunk or limbs. Other patients have presented with focal neurological signs indicative of a space-occupying lesion, or hypothalamic involvement with somnolence, hyperphagia and polydipsia. A slowly progressive dementia has been described in several patients. It may be accompanied by motor disorder, particularly supranuclear gaze palsies or myoclonus, although such are not always in evidence. Lampert *et al.*'s (1962) patient had a 7-year history of progressive mental deterioration leading to an impression of Alzheimer's disease; there was no history of gastrointestinal disturbance though an attack of arthritis had occurred at the onset.

Evidence of malabsorption or anaemia will often be present. The CSF may be normal or show pleocytosis and elevation of protein. The CT scan can be negative, although may show hyperdense regions in the white matter (Ludwig *et al.* 1981). Definitive diagnosis depends on the demonstration of periodic acid–Schiff (PAS)-positive material in macrophages which, in the absence of prior treatment, can almost always be revealed by duodenal biopsy. This must be undertaken whenever the disease is suspected. Lymph node biopsy can be informative too, or the characteristic inclusions may be detected in cells from the CSF. Polymerase chain reaction amplification of the CSF may be performed to detect the DNA sequence specific for *T. whippelii*. Brain biopsy will sometimes be performed (Warren *et al.* 2005), but will stand to be negative in patients with hypothalamic involvement alone.

The findings at post-mortem are distinctive. Tissues involved by the disease show PAS-positive granules within macrophages, representing membrane-like structures derived from bacterial walls (sickle particle-containing cells). The bacilli themselves can sometimes be seen by electron microscopy. CNS involvement shows as collections of PAS-positive cells in the brain and cord, often with widespread perivascular nodules and indolent inflammatory changes.

Treatment with antibiotics usually meets with a good response where gastrointestinal and other systemic manifestations are concerned. In the treatment of neurological complications less success has been reported, although a vigorous attempt should always be pursued. Albers *et al.* (1989) discuss the various treatment regimens employed, emphasising the importance of using antibiotics that cross the blood–brain barrier if neurological involvement is to be controlled.

Mitochondrial myopathy (mitochondrial encephalomyopathy)

The mitochondrial myopathies are a complex group of diseases that share in common a primary dysfunction of mitochondrial metabolism (see De 1993 for a review of these syndromes). Although first described in relation to skeletal muscle, many other organs may be affected, leading sometimes to dysfunction in the liver, heart, kidney, eye or endocrine system (so-called multisystem disease). The CNS is frequently involved and neuropsychiatric disorder can be the predominant manifestation (mitochondrial encephalomyopathy).

The underlying defects in mitochondrial metabolism have been studied in detail, revealing deficiencies in various respiratory chain enzymes, especially complexes I and III. At present, however, the relationship between such defects and the phenotypic manifestations of disease show a good deal of overlap and precise systems of classification have not been achieved. Molecular biological approaches have revealed several point mutations as well as rearrangements of mitochondrial DNA such as partial deletions or duplications (Di Mauro & Moses 1992). However, the nuclear genome also encodes extensively for mitochondrial proteins and may often be involved (Shanske 1992). Mitochondrial myopathies associated with point mutations (e.g. MERRF and MELAS, see below) usually show a maternal pattern of inheritance, whereas large-scale mitochondrial DNA deletions are generally sporadic (Oldfors *et al.* 2006).

A number of clinical syndromes are now well recognised, as reviewed by Lombes *et al.* (1989). Mitochondrial encephalomyopathy, lactic acidosis and stroke-like episodes (MELAS) is the most common maternally inherited mitochondrial disease and may present in children or young adults with stunted growth, seizures and episodic vomiting. Recurrent stroke-like episodes are characteristic with transient hemiplegia, hemianopia or cortical blindness. An A→G mutation in the transfer RNA$^{Leu(UUR)}$ at position 3243 of the mitochondrial DNA accounts for the majority of MELAS cases (Wallace 1992). However, the clinical phenotypes associated with this point mutation are diverse. Chronic progressive external ophthalmoplegia (CPEO) (Mariotti *et al.* 1995) and Leigh syndrome (Makino *et al.* 2000) have also been associated with the A3243G mutation. Kearns–Sayre syndrome is defined by the triad of progressive external ophthalmoplegia, pigmentary retinopathy and cardiac conduction defects, usually with onset before the age of 20 years (Gross-Jendroska *et al.* 1992). The most common molecular defect underlying Kearns–Sayre syndrome is large-scale deletions of mitochondrial DNA (Zeviani *et al.* 1998). Myoclonus epilepsy with ragged red fibres (MERRF) presents with myoclonus, ataxia and muscle weakness and often progresses to generalised seizures and dementia. Onset is again usually before the age of 20. The most common point mutation associated with this condition is at nucleotide 8344 (A8344G) of the tRNA(Lys) gene of mitochondrial DNA (Oldfors *et al.* 1995).

However, the pleomorphic manifestations of mitochondrial disorders do not fit neatly into distinct subsyndromes. Petty *et al.* (1986) reviewed 66 cases. Onset in the majority was before 20 years of age, but presentations occurred up to the age of 68. Relatives were affected in almost one-third of cases. Petty *et al.* made a broad division into three groups. The commonest presentation (55% of cases) was with ptosis, progressive external ophthalmoplegia, and limb weakness induced or increased by exertion. A further 18% presented with limb weakness alone, showing a proximal myopathy with exercise intolerance. These could continue with muscle involvement alone, although a few patients developed neurological manifestations later. The remaining 27% showed predominant involvement of the CNS, with features such as ataxia, deafness, involuntary movements and seizures. Dementia was common in this last group and was severe in many. Whereas overall prognosis was good in patients without CNS involvement the last group fared poorly, half of them becoming dependent on others at a mean of 17 years from onset.

A mitochondrial myopathy will usually be suspected in patients who present with progressive external ophthalmoplegia combined with other symptoms, or when myopathy is accompanied by prominent fatigue. Petty *et al.* suggest that it should also be considered in the absence of such symptoms when there is cerebellar ataxia, deafness or pigmentary retinopathy, and especially when these are combined with involuntary movements or dementia.

Talley and Faber (1989) report a man of 26 suffering from MELAS syndrome who presented with dementia. Admission to hospital was precipitated by failing memory and social withdrawal 1 month after an episode of status epilepticus. He was short in stature and showed a right visual field defect, diminished hearing and neglect of the right upper extremity. Though initially orientated in time and place he was slowed, and his speech was limited to stereotyped phrases. He was unable to read, perform simple calculations or copy geometric figures. His prevailing mood was of apprehension. EEG showed diffuse slowing, and CT revealed calcification in the basal ganglia and right thalamus. Lactic acid levels were raised in the blood and CSF, and muscle biopsy showed diffuse ragged red fibres.

Over the next 3 weeks he became mute, markedly indifferent to what went on around, and with a severe comprehension defect. He developed hemiparesis on the right, and a left visual field defect in addition to the right hemianopia. New findings on CT included lucent areas medially in the left hemisphere. Major seizures developed and he became combative and difficult to manage. Repeated hospitalisations were required on this account over the succeeding 4 years, with periodic stroke-like events, generalised seizures and a fluctuating though declining level of mentation. The patient's mother was of short stature with bilateral sensorineural hearing loss, easy fatiguability and ragged red fibres on muscle biopsy. His half-sister similarly showed indications of MELAS syndrome.

The decisive investigation in mitochondrial myopathies is skeletal muscle biopsy. The appearance of ragged red fibres with the Gomori trichrome stain is almost pathognomonic, representing abnormal accumulations of mitochondria. Histochemical staining techniques such as demonstration of strongly succinate dehydrogenase-reactive blood vessels and electron microscopy provide confirmatory information; subsarcolemmal mitochondria are abnormal in size and morphology as well as increased in numbers. Skeletal muscle tissue obtained by biopsy is also useful for the preparation of intact mitochondria for assaying respiratory enzyme activities, which are frequently abnormal (Thambisetty & Newman 2004).

Other important investigations include raised resting blood lactate levels, or when normal are increased on exercise. Electromyography may show myopathic changes, and CSF protein may be raised. Infarct-like lucencies on CT are a common feature with involvement of the CNS; in MELAS, these hypodensities are transient, correlating with fluctuations in the clinical course. CT or MRI is also likely to show cerebral or cerebellar atrophy with calcification of the basal ganglia also being reported (Thambisetty *et al*. 2002).

Behçet's syndrome

Behçet's syndrome is an uncommon disorder predominantly affecting young males. It is rare in childhood and in persons over 50. It is said to be more common in Mediterranean countries, the Middle East and Japan but occurs worldwide. The classic triple symptom complex consists of oral ulceration, genital ulceration and ocular lesions (uveitis, iridocyclitis, retinal vasculitis), usually occurring in several attacks per year and pursuing a chronic course over many years. Lassitude, malaise and slight pyrexia may accompany attacks but the degree of constitutional disturbance varies. Common additional manifestations include arthritis, thrombophlebitis, erythema nodosum and non-specific skin sensitivity. The overall course is unpredictable, but the illness often abates after one or two decades. Blindness may remain as a permanent sequel.

It is now recognised to be a chronic multisystem disorder with predominant vasculitis (Wechsler & Piette 1992). Diagnostic criteria have been proposed but there is no universally accepted diagnostic test (International Study Group for Behçet's Disease 1990). CNS involvement is recognised as a serious complication, important not for its frequency but on account of its grave prognosis. No part of the nervous system appears to be immune. A great variety of clinical pictures may result from the vasculitis and disseminated encephalomyelitis.

The onset is usually abrupt, coinciding with a relapse of orogenital ulceration or uveitis. Failing this there is almost always a well-established history of the syndrome before nervous system involvement sets in. The patient develops headaches, fever, slight neck stiffness and a variety of neurological signs. Brainstem involvement is particularly common, with giddiness, ataxia, diplopia, cranial nerve palsies or long tract signs. A typical feature is the episodic nature of such defects, the picture seeming to stabilise after several weeks then relapsing with fresh developments. Recurrent attacks of hemiplegia or paraplegia may lead on to pseudobulbar palsy. Periods of remission may result in temporary improvement or in rare cases complete recovery. In general, however, serious neurological defects persist. The course has been likened to that of severe forms of MS and differentiation may occasionally present difficulties (Ashjazadeh *et al*. 2003). Dural venous sinus thrombosis has been found to be common, often presenting with intracranial hypertension (Wechsler *et al*. 1992). The CSF usually shows a slight lymphocytic pleocytosis and increase in protein. When neck stiffness is severe there may be a marked polymorphonuclear response.

Pallis and Fudge (1956) attempted to demarcate three main forms of nervous system involvement: a brainstem form, a meningomyelitic form and a variety with mental symptoms predominating. The last could present either as transient episodes of confusion or in the form of dementia. The patients with dementia usually showed an insidious onset and steady slow progression, sometimes accompanied by features of parkinsonism and sometimes by pseudobulbar palsy. Executive dysfunction and memory impairment occurs even in the absence of overt neurological symptoms and depression (Monastero *et al*. 2004; Erberk-Ozen *et al*. 2006). Depression is common, affecting up to half of all patients, and adversely impacts on quality of life (Taner *et al*. 2007; Uguz *et al*. 2007). Schizoaffective and bipolar symptoms have also been reported, sometimes in multiple members of affected families (Goolamali *et al*. 1976; Berman *et al*. 1979; Alevizos *et al*. 2004).

Involvement of the CNS is usually a serious development. The patient's general condition is often poor, and adverse developments can set in rapidly. However, the course of each episode is unique and unpredictable. Some patients deteriorate after repeated relapses, some remain quiescent for long periods, and others decline steadily and die.

Computed tomography may show single or multiple low-density lesions, principally in the subcortical nuclear masses or brainstem, often with resolution some weeks later. Atrophic changes are also common, with an accent on the posterior fossa cisterns and cerebellar sulci. MRI is more sensitive in revealing focal areas of altered signal intensity (Mizukami *et al*. 1992), and may be especially valuable in showing dural sinus thrombosis. Periventricular lesions similar to those of MS may be seen. Changes at post-mortem include low-grade perivascular inflammation, scattered areas of demyelination and necrosis, and patchy cerebral infarction.

As might be expected in an inflammatory condition, plasma levels of cytokines and also leptin, a proinflammatory mediator, are elevated but are not diagnostic (Evereklioglu *et al.* 2002a,b). The disease tends to aggregate in families but without good evidence for mendelian patterns of inheritance in most cases. The exception are those very rare cases of paediatric onset, which appear to be largely autosomal recessive (Molinari *et al.* 2003). Genetic linkage of Behçet's disease to the HLA-B region has been established (Ohno *et al.* 1982; Ando *et al.* 1997) but the precise genetic variant associated with disease remains to be discovered.

Treatment is entirely symptomatic or palliative (Evereklioglu 2004). Steroids have been claimed to help markedly in some patients, including those with involvement of the CNS, although others have reported no benefit. Immunosuppressive drugs (cyclophosphamide, azathioprine, chlorambucil) may also be of benefit, though side effects limit their usefulness. Other approaches are under investigation including thalidomide and monoclonal antibodies to tumour necrosis factor (TNF)-α and other cytokines (Evereklioglu 2004).

Sarcoidosis

Sarcoidosis is characterised by the development of chronic granulomatous lesions in various parts of the body. The aetiology is unknown, though an immunologically determined alteration in tissue reactivity appears to be fundamental to the disease. It is assumed, but not proven, that this is induced by exposure to some environmental, perhaps infectious, agent. The immunological profile is complex, with an increase in CD4+ helper T cells and yet at the same time a frequent reduction in reaction to immunological challenge; in other words, a combination of activation and suppression profiles. A familial aggregation has long been noted, although this does not appear to fall into any recognised pattern of inheritance (Buck & McKusick 1961). Association with a variety of HLA profiles has been noted (Nowack & Goebel 1987; Rossman *et al.* 2003) and currently the most promising markers of disease are the HLA-DRB1 locus and the *BTNL2* gene, which appears to be an independent susceptibility factor even though it maps close to the HLA-DRB1 locus itself.

The characteristic lesion is the epithelioid cell granuloma or follicle, consisting of a well-demarcated collection of epithelioid cells with occasional giant cells. The centres may show necrosis but the caseation seen with tubercular infection is lacking. The lesions tend to heal spontaneously but provoke surrounding fibrosis. The commonest site is the respiratory system, presenting with hilar lymphadenopathy or reticular shadowing in the lungs. The mildness of symptoms often contrasts with the extent of the lesions, cases sometimes being discovered on routine chest radiography. Erythema nodosum is another characteristic presentation. Ocular manifestations include iridocyclitis and uveitis. The latter

may be accompanied by parotitis (uveoparotid fever). Other parts of the body commonly involved are the superficial lymph nodes, spleen, liver and phalanges of the hands and feet. Overt myopathy is rare but muscle infiltration is often apparent on biopsy.

The onset is usually between the ages of 20 and 40 years. In general sarcoidosis runs an indolent course with relapses and remissions, showing a tendency to subside spontaneously after several years. Individual lesions gradually resolve while others make an appearance, the cycle sometimes being narrowly confined and sometimes widespread in different organs. A minority of patients are left disabled by pulmonary fibrosis or ocular complications. Death, when it occurs, may be due to renal failure or cardiac involvement. Affection of the CNS (see below) can also carry serious hazards. Treatment with steroids is often effective in inducing remission and promoting the healing of lesions, although maintenance therapy must sometimes continue for many years. Immunosuppressive therapy plays a role and newer treatments are emerging (Baughman *et al.* 2003; Grutters & van den Bosch 2006).

A low-grade pyrexia is an inconstant accompaniment. During active phases of the disease there may be a normochromic anaemia, raised erythrocyte sedimentation rate and eosinophilia. Mild leucopenia and thrombocytopenia are sometimes seen. The serum immunoglobulins, especially IgG, are usually elevated and hypercalcaemia of moderate degree is not infrequent. In uncertain cases and with unusual presentations chest radiography may reveal the characteristic picture, likewise radiograph of the phalanges. A raised serum alkaline phosphatase denotes hepatic involvement. Biopsy of skin lesions, lymph nodes or muscle can give confirmatory evidence. The Kveim test consists of an intradermal injection of sarcoid tissue extract; this has fair reliability, yielding a nodule with the histological features of sarcoidosis.

Involvement of the nervous system is estimated to occur in 5% of patients (Vinas & Rengachary 2001; Stern 2004; Joseph & Scolding 2007). Neurological dysfunction may be the presenting feature or indeed the sole clinical manifestation, although cases with lesions entirely confined to the nervous system are very rare (Allen *et al.* 2003). There are no clear demarcations between the various forms of nervous system involvement but certain broad categories can be discerned. The parts most frequently involved are the cranial nerves, meninges, hypothalamus and pituitary.

Lesions of the cranial and peripheral nerves are the commonest neurological feature. The seventh cranial nerve is particularly vulnerable, leading to unilateral or bilateral facial palsies. Involvement of the optic nerves results in blurring of vision, papilloedema, optic atrophy or field defects. The peripheral nerves may be affected singly or in combination. Basal meningitis or brainstem involvement can lead to multiple fluctuating cranial nerve palsies.

Granulomatous meningitis or meningoencephalitis affects mainly the basal brain regions. The meninges become thickened and infiltrated with granulomas and lymphocytes. Lumbar puncture shows elevated protein and a pleocytosis. Chronic headache is accompanied by focal signs as the adjacent chiasm and hypothalamus become infiltrated. An adhesive arachnoiditis can lead to raised intracranial pressure and hydrocephalus. In some cases the meningeal involvement remains entirely subclinical; it was evident in all 14 of Delaney's (1977) post-mortem cases, yet had been suspected during life in only nine.

The brain parenchyma may become involved by contiguous spread or by the formation of tumour-like masses of granulomatous material. Involvement of the hypothalamus and third ventricular region leads to somnolence, obesity, hyperthermia and memory difficulties or change of personality. Pituitary dysfunction may show as diabetes insipidus, menstrual irregularities and other endocrine dysfunctions. Lesions situated within the cerebral hemispheres may be single or multiple. The cerebellum, brainstem or cord may be similarly affected. Solitary deposits have sometimes been mistaken for neoplasms until biopsy is performed. Focal signs may make an abrupt appearance, and seizures can be hard to control.

Mental disturbance will often be prominent when sarcoidosis affects the CNS. Hook (1954) reported patients with a variety of pictures: apathy, lack of judgement and personal neglect progressing over a year to semicoma; acute agitation and hallucinosis leading to residual dementia; profound memory impairment and irritability. Friedman and Gould (2002) similarly report a patient with confusion and psychosis, and others report neurosarcoid presenting as schizophrenia (Duwe & Turetsky 2002; Zielasek *et al.* 2002). Cordingley *et al.*'s (1981) patient presented with progressive dementia, the only abnormal signs being a wide-based gait and incomplete eye abduction together with nystagmus on lateral gaze. Others have described marked changes of character, fluctuating confusion and a variety of psychotic pictures. In some the disturbance will be occasioned by hydrocephalus consequent on basal meningitis or obstruction of CSF flow by granulomatous masses. In others direct brain infiltration will be responsible. In patients with circumscribed failure of memory, as in the following example, localised involvement of the hypothalamus and limbic structures is probably responsible.

A woman developed sarcoidosis at 24, presenting with bilateral hilar lymphadenopathy. Two years later she had a minor seizure and shortly thereafter developed headache, weakness and incoordination. Examination revealed a sensory level at T4 and a myelogram showed obstruction from T4 to T7. CT demonstrated a right frontal granuloma

and basal meningeal involvement with mild ventricular dilatation. Dexamethasone produced marked neurological improvement over the following year which was well maintained.

At 28 she became aware of increasing memory impairment over 3–4 weeks, then abruptly became agitated, deluded and doubly incontinent. She was disorientated in time and place and heard hallucinatory voices at night. The acute organic reaction settled over 6–8 weeks on haloperidol and increased dexamethasone, but her memory remained mildly impaired. Psychometric testing at that time showed a WAIS full scale IQ of 78, with scores of 55% on the Wechsler Logical Memory Test and 45% on the Rey–Osterrieth Test.

Some months later her memory deteriorated further and she developed compulsive eating, weight gain and insomnia. At 30 she was obese, mildly ataxic, and with hyperreflexia in the legs and bilateral extensor plantars. There were no psychotic features but she was disorientated in time and showed a severe defect of short-term memory. She could recall nothing of a name and address or of simple geometrical figures. The WAIS IQ was 82, but the logical memory test now gave a score of only 20% and the Rey–Osterrieth Test 30%. The CT scan was unchanged but pulmonary and hepatic involvement was demonstrated. Steroids were increased to high dosage, with improvement 3 weeks later in orientation and on simple tests of recall. She was discharged to a semi-independent life in her own home which she managed to run with the help of memory aids (Thompson & Checkley 1981).

A further instructive patient was reported by McLoughlin and McKeon (1991), in whom both memory disorder and bipolar affective disorder appeared to be due to involvement of the limbic system.

A 25-year-old mechanic developed hilar lymphadenopathy, and sarcoidosis was confirmed by mediastinoscopy and lymph node biopsy. This resolved with steroids and he remained well for 6 years until sarcoid meningitis appeared. This too resolved with steroids over a number of months and he remained on prednisolone 15 mg daily thereafter. Three years later, at the age of 34, he developed sensorimotor leg neuropathies and bilateral fifth nerve numbness, but CT at this time showed no cerebral abnormalities. Two years later he developed diabetes insipidus and anterior pituitary failure requiring replacement therapy, and the following year was treated with cranial irradiation. CSF analysis showed active CNS sarcoidosis and MRI revealed minimal cortical atrophy.

The following year he became depressed with anorexia, weight loss and marked guilt feelings about his illness. There was no family history of psychiatric disorder. At the same time he noted that his memory was impaired for recent events. Imipramine relieved the depression, but 12 months later he began to experience marked mood swings alternating between episodes of depression and hypomania lasting for a few days at a time. Three months later lithium was added, by which time the mood swings were alternating every 24–28 hours. Neurological examination was normal apart from bilateral facial sensory impairment. CSF analysis showed that the neurosarcoidosis was still active, but repeat MRI showed no change. Psychometric testing confirmed the memory deficit and showed a WAIS-R IQ of 96.

Attempts to stabilise his mood swings with high-dose lithium failed on account of troublesome polyuria, but they nevertheless subsided over several months in hospital. He remained depressed and some months later took an overdose and died. At post-mortem a large granulomatous mass was discovered just anterior to the mamillary bodies at the origin of the pituitary stalk. Histological examination showed that this had infiltrated the dorsomedial nucleus of the thalamus, mamillary bodies, third ventricle, fornices and pituitary stalk. There was patchy basal meningeal fibrosis with isolated meningeal granulomas. The cerebral hemispheres, cerebellum and brainstem were unaffected. Spinal meningeal fibrosis was severe with entrapment of ventral and dorsal roots.

In some cases a combination of structural and metabolic disturbances is likely to shape the psychiatric picture, particularly in the presence of hypercalcaemia or a degree of renal failure. Steroid therapy may make its own contribution to mental disturbances.

In patients with organic psychosyndromes and neurological defects of obscure origin, it is obviously important to bear the possibility of sarcoidosis in mind. Full investigation along the lines described above will almost certainly produce confirmatory evidence of the disorder, even when nervous system involvement has been the presenting manifestation. Neuroimaging may show the intracranial lesions or evidence of basal meningitis, and lumbar puncture may reveal evidence of chronic meningitis.

The prognosis for patients with neuropsychiatric complications is extremely variable, but in general intracranial involvement should be viewed as a grave development. Some show a remittent picture, others slow and incomplete recovery, while others show progressive disability. A few will die of the neurological manifestations. However, the outlook is not uniformly poor. Among the 19 patients followed by Pentland *et al.* (1985), half had had an acute monophasic illness which resolved with steroids, and alto-gether two-thirds showed a surprisingly good outcome 1–16 years later. Those who had shown a relapsing–remitting course had often presented pictures closely simulating MS. Facial nerve palsy is usually transient and shows a good response to steroids. Basal meningitis may slowly ameliorate and subside, although the overall response to treatment is poor. In favourable cases intracerebral granulomas can improve or even resolve with steroid therapy, and surgical removal has occasionally been successful.

Electrical accidents and lightning injuries

Contact with powerful sources of electric current may cause sudden death due to ventricular fibrillation or respiratory arrest, sometimes with severe burns where the current enters and leaves the body. The effects of the shock are strongly influenced by the site of contact as well as the strength of the electrical source. Among survivors transient evidence of neurological dysfunction is not uncommon, although persisting sequelae appear to be rare. The mortality in 60 cases reported by Hammond and Ward (1988) was 3%; neurological complications were noted in one-quarter and psychiatric sequelae in 18%. Psychiatric and neurological sequelae of electrical trauma have been reviewed (Kotagal *et al.* 1982; van Zomeren *et al.* 1998; Duff & McCaffrey 2001; Primeau 2005).

Much of the acute disturbance appears to be due to temporary blockade of neuronal function or vasomotor changes in the brain and cord, although petechial haemorrhages and areas of demyelination and degeneration have been observed. Additional damage may be caused by intense tetanic muscular contractions that sometimes propel the victim for a considerable distance. Acute tetanic spasm of the paraspinus muscles may produce compression fractures of the vertebral bodies. With lightning injuries blast-like lesions may be sustained due to the sudden displacement and return of air in the immediate vicinity of the lightning strike.

A period of unconsciousness may last for hours or days, sometimes being delayed for several moments during which the affected person calls for help. The unconsciousness may be accompanied by epileptic seizures or more commonly myoclonic jerking. Cessation of respiration due to bulbar paralysis can require assisted ventilation for many hours. When consciousness is retained the subject may experience intense pain, tinnitus, deafness or visual disturbance, along with tremors, twitching, local paralysis and sensory changes. Confusion and excitement can then be prominent, with retrograde and post-traumatic amnesia much as with head injury. Severe neurological disturbances such as paraplegia, hemiplegia, mutism and aphonia may resolve over hours or days. Transient unilateral parkinsonism has been attributed to damage to the basal ganglia. Fixed dilated pupils during the acute stage are not necessarily an ominous prognostic sign. All patients should have electrocardiographic monitoring for at least 48 hours to enable detection of cardiac dysrhythmias, and a watch must be kept for acute renal failure due to myoglobin released from injured muscles (Pruitt & Mason 1996).

More prolonged sequelae include cranial nerve damage with loss of taste, facial paresis and auditory and vestibular disturbances. Very occasionally, severe diffuse brain damage may be an enduring aftermath. However, the most common sequelae are peripheral nerve and spinal cord syndromes that are sometimes days or weeks in developing, perhaps as vascular changes progress. Farrell and Starr (1968) stress that a latent period of months may occasionally intervene. The pictures that have been described include delayed atrophy affecting an arm or leg, quadriparesis, or slowly progressive spasticity with sensory changes (so-called spinal atrophic paralysis). The waxing and waning of chronic neurological deficits may sometimes resemble MS. In patients such as these the current may have traversed the spinal cord directly.

Prolonged neuropsychiatric aftermaths include amnesia and impaired cognitive functioning, often compounded by anxiety attaching to the shock and sometimes by compensation issues. Of 60 patients in Hammond and Ward's (1988) series, 11 suffered psychiatric problems similar to those of post-traumatic stress disorder: insomnia, nightmares, anxiety, headache and difficulty in concentration. The following patient illustrates the cognitive and personality changes that may occasionally follow.

A 26-year-old man was rendered unconscious for several hours after sustaining a shock from bare wires which had made contact with his forehead. On recovery he had throbbing headache, was sluggish in cerebration, and complained of feeling depressed and irritable for several weeks thereafter. CT was normal. Two months later he was still vague and forgetful with delayed responses to questions. Five months after the accident he showed significant impairment of memory, lability of mood and psychomotor retardation. His girlfriend described a marked change of personality, with argumentativeness and occasional aggressive behaviour. Cognitive testing showed nominal and expressive dysphasia, impaired right–left discrimination, and difficulty in making simple drawings. He had lost his ability to speak German, which he had learned during the previous 3 years. WAIS scores were well below expectation in view of his educational and occupational history.

Two years later his memory remained impaired and he was still mentally sluggish and rather vacuous in appearance. However, there was no longer evidence of dysphasia or drawing difficulties. Simple arithmetic was poor. His mother confirmed a marked change of personality from a bright extroverted person to one who was slow, sullen and withdrawn. Though no longer depressed he was distractible, and had abandoned his reading and former hobbies.

Brain injury due to diving

Apart from the hazards of anoxia and hypothermia, divers are at risk of two main forms of injury to the nervous system, namely toxicity due to gases breathed under high partial pressure and decompression illness (DCI). These risks increase in relation to the depth and duration of submersion and, perhaps not surprisingly, are increased in younger and less experienced divers (Newton *et al.* 2007). They apply equally to caisson workers who may spend several days at a time working at very considerable depths. When explosives are used divers are also exposed to increased risk of blast injury because of the enhanced transmission of pressure waves in water.

There are also concerns that divers, including sports divers, may sometimes sustain a degree of neurological damage even in the absence of obvious events such as DCI, although the issue remains controversial. Repeated exposures appear to be a special hazard in persons with a patent foramen ovale or other form of right-to-left shunt in the circulation. These matters are considered below, much deriving from accounts by Denison (1996) and Wilmshurst (1997).

Gas toxicity
The gases breathed during submersion must be delivered at the same pressure as the surrounding water. Scuba divers breathe compressed air but are restricted to relatively shallow depths (30–50 m) because of the risk of nitrogen narcosis, which is probably due to the narcotic effects of nitrogen dissolved in nerve membranes impeding neural transmission. The breathing of pure oxygen does not solve the problem, because oxygen is toxic to the lungs when alveolar pressure exceeds 50 kPa (0.5 atmospheres, 5 m of sea water) and to the nervous system when the pressure exceeds 200 kPa (2 atmospheres, 10 m of sea water). Epileptic convulsions are then liable to occur. Deeper dives are accomplished using a mix of oxygen and helium and this has allowed divers to reach astonishing depths (below 600 m). However, deeper than 160 m the risk of high-pressure nervous syndrome increases considerably, resulting in tremor, myoclonic jerks, nausea, vomiting, fatigue, postural instability, somnolence and cognitive dysfunction and other symptoms (Bennett & McLeod 1984).

Decompression illness
During submersion inert gases under pressure become dissolved in body tissues: nitrogen when breathing air, or helium when breathing oxygen–helium mixtures. In the course of the ascent such gases come out of solution as the ambient pressure falls, tending to form bubbles within the tissues and the blood (gas nucleation). Provided the ascent is sufficiently gradual the extra load of gas diffuses into the bloodstream and out of the lungs, but if it is too rapid the bubbles increase in size and number and may come to block blood vessels. This appears to be the principal

cause of DCI or 'bends', which is a risk with any dive below 10 m unless very brief. It is a particular risk after deep 'saturation dives', during which divers are maintained at the pressure of their diving depth for days or weeks on end; chambers are used at the surface for this purpose, to economise the time which would otherwise be needed for repeated very slow ascents.

Two grades of DCI are recognised: type 1 bends, consisting of skin irritation and musculoskeletal pain only; and type 2 bends, with pulmonary and nervous system manifestations and sometimes circulatory collapse. Pulmonary symptoms consist of sudden chest pain, dyspnoea and cough due to bubble formation within the pulmonary circulation. Neurological symptoms, which occur in about half of cases, consist chiefly of spinal cord syndromes, visual disturbances or vertigo, although central focal deficits may occur. Newton *et al.* (2007) review 200 cases of DCI and report that over 85% of these had at least some neurological manifestation. The range of severity is wide, from slight dysaesthesiae, ataxia and ophthalmoplegia to paraparesis, quadriparesis, dysphasia and confusion. Such episodes may be transient or long-lasting and permanent sequelae can result. The episodes are sometimes recurrent, in general resembling thromboembolic cerebrovascular disease except for commonly affecting the cord. The symptoms usually develop some minutes to hours after the dive is over, and must be treated immediately by recompression and the administration of oxygen. The diversity of symptoms associated with DCI may sometimes suggest that psychiatric syndromes occurring in divers might be atypical DCI episodes. Hopkins and Weaver (2001) report two such cases where a psychotic episode occurred in the context of a dive and possible DCI. However, careful consideration of the symptoms, which included muscle pain, weakness and fatigue, made the primary diagnosis of DCI unlikely and treatment with hyperbaric oxygen did not result in a reversal of the psychosis.

Severe examples of DCI may result from a different mechanism, when lung tissue becomes disrupted by the expansion of gases within it (pulmonary barotrauma), allowing gas to enter the pulmonary veins and thus the arterial system. Cerebral gas embolism may then result in severe focal cerebral symptoms. However, the distinction between pulmonary barotrauma and gas nucleation in leading to the various manifestations of DCI is far from established.

Neuropathological effects apparently related to DCI have been described by Palmer *et al.* (1987). In an examination of the spinal cords of 11 divers, mostly dying from diving accidents, they found distended empty blood vessels, sometimes with perivascular haemorrhages, and minor chronic changes with foci of gliosis and hyalinisation of blood vessels. In three cases Marchi staining showed tract degeneration, variously affecting the posterior, lateral or anterior columns of the cord. Examination of the brains of 25 divers, again mostly dying from diving accidents, showed distended empty vessels in two-thirds of subjects, presumably caused by gas bubbles

(Palmer *et al.* 1992). Perivascular lacunae were present in one-third, presumably due to bubble occlusion, along with hyalinisation of blood vessels which may have accrued from periodic rises in luminal pressure. Foci of necrosis were sometimes observed in the cerebral grey matter, and vacuolation in the white matter extending to status spongiosis.

Sequelae of diving

A well-known long-term effect of diving is the presence of aseptic infarcts in the long bones, evident on radiography and presumably due to gas embolism. This is commoner with a history of DCI but is found in many subjects with no such history. The incidence rises with age and diving intensity. Infarcts near the articular surfaces can be severely disabling, and crippling dysbaric osteonecrosis may occasionally ensue.

The neurological disturbances of DCI may fail to resolve completely, and surveys of divers have shown a small but definite prevalence of neurological deficits. Todnem *et al.* (1990) examined 156 commercial divers, aged 21–49 years, along with 100 controls. Half of the divers had experienced frank episodes of DCI. At the time of examination 20% had stopped diving and six had lost their licenses because of neurological problems; 12 (8%) had had problems with vision, vertigo or reduced skin sensitivity in non-diving situations, and six had been referred to neurological clinics on account of seizures, transient cerebral ischaemia or transient amnesia attacks. No controls had such symptoms. The divers complained significantly more often of symptoms referable to the CNS, mainly problems with concentration and memory, and had more peripheral neurological symptoms, chiefly paraesthesiae in the hands and feet. On examination significantly more showed hand tremor, or signs indicative of cord damage such as reduced touch and pain sensation in the feet. Seven had a mild peripheral neuropathy. Scores for neurological symptoms and signs correlated significantly with age, amount of diving exposure, and a history of DCI. In another self-report study, divers with experience of DCI reported considerably more long-term neurological sequelae than other divers (McQueen *et al.* 1994). In a study of construction divers matched to controls, the divers had significantly different error rates in tasks of reference memory and navigation behaviours (Leplow *et al.* 2001). In another investigation of saturation divers, Todnem *et al.* (1991a) found that 18% of divers and 5% of controls had abnormal EEG, with increased temporal slow waves and sharp potentials. Such abnormalities again correlated significantly with diving exposure and a history of DCI but not with neurological symptom scores. Brainstem evoked potential latencies were also increased in the diving group.

Shallow water diving is a variant used professionally for collection of shellfish and recreationally, where instead of using scuba equipment the divers hold their breath. Deep water 'free diving' is a particularly risky and difficult recreational variant of unassisted diving. Neurological sequelae of shallow water diving, including cognitive and motor deficits, result from DCI and from carbon monoxide poisoning (Williamson *et al.* 1987). In a large study of professional abalone divers the incidence of deficits in visual function, psychomotor abilities and recent memory was related to individual characteristics in the divers and attributed to their diving technique (Williamson *et al.* 1989).

A recent cause for concern is the demonstration of hyperintensities on MRI in a proportion of divers and caisson workers, presumably due to microinfarcts in the brain (Warren *et al.* 1988). Reul *et al.* (1995) studied 52 amateur scuba divers (mean age 38 years) and compared them with 50 controls engaged in other sports; 52% of the divers and 20% of the controls showed hyperintensities, principally in the subcortical white matter and basal ganglia. These were significantly larger and more numerous in the divers. Only three had histories pointing to episodes of DCI, suggesting that such lesions may often accrue without clinical indicators of their presence. Others, however, have found no excess of MRI abnormalities in divers compared with controls (Rinck *et al.* 1991; Todnem *et al.* 1991a,b), perhaps due to different selection procedures and imaging protocols. In some studies although no excess of MRI abnormalities was observed in divers, those that were found correlated with faster rate of ascent and other variables suggestive of dive-related events (Tripodi *et al.* 2004). Hyperbaric oxygen exposure in the absence of DCI (in chamber attendants for example) does not appear to be associated with neurological problems or MRI lesions (Ors *et al.* 2006).

Knauth *et al.* (1997) report an investigation of 87 sports divers, none of whom had a history of DCI. Eleven (13%) showed hyperintensities on MRI, but multiple hyperintensities occurred exclusively in three subjects with large right-to-left shunts in the circulation as demonstrated by transcranial Doppler ultrasonography after the venous injection of microbubbles. Ten further subjects with similarly large shunts had normal MRI scans. Nevertheless, the possibility arises that divers with right-to-left shunts may be at particular risk of accumulating microinfarcts in the brain. The great majority of such shunts are likely to reflect a patent foramen ovale, which may well become functional only under the abnormal pressure conditions of diving. Others could be due to small atrial septal defects or pulmonary arteriovenous shunts.

Hyperostosis frontalis interna (hyperostosis cranii, metabolic craniopathy, endocraniosis, Morgagni's syndrome)

Hyperostosis of the frontal region of the skull accompanied by obesity and hypertrichosis (excessive, thick body hair) constitutes this rare syndrome. There are some indications that it may be commoner than chance expectation in patients with organic psychosyndromes.

The radiological picture is of thickening of the inner tables of the frontal bones, with smooth rounded exostoses projecting into the cranial cavity. Part of the problem in discerning any putative clinical associations lies with the frequency of the condition and with the occurrence of minor variations. It may be found at any age from adolescence upwards, increasing markedly from the third or fourth decades onwards. Females are affected very much more often than males. While the pattern of inheritance is not understood, it does occur in families and identical twin-pairs have been reported (Koller *et al.* 2005). As the bone abnormalities are so easily identified in skeletal remains, the condition has frequently been diagnosed in ancient populations, medieval and prehistoric (Hershkovitz *et al.* 1999; Glab *et al.* 2006; Mulhern *et al.* 2006; Sikanjic 2006). The pathogenesis is unknown. Two 'syndromes' have been proposed: Morgagni's syndrome, with hyperostosis, obesity and hirsutism; and Stewart–Morel syndrome, in which neuropsychiatric features predominate. Neither, however, has won wide acceptance.

In most reviews the main features have been headache, obesity, hirsutism and menstrual disorders (Capraro *et al.* 1970). Headache was found in 89% of Silinkova-Malkova and Malek's (1965/66) series compared with 37% of controls; hirsutism was present in 37% compared with 14% of controls. Thirst, water retention, sleep disturbances and a variety of rather minor endocrine changes are also described. Among mental features neurotic complaints figure prominently, also disturbances of personality, memory impairment and occasionally dementia. A number of forms of psychosis have been reported. All agree, however, that the condition is very often entirely asymptomatic.

Walinder (1977) compared a group of patients with hyperostosis frontalis interna to a matched control set and found higher rates of psychiatric morbidity in siblings of probands than in siblings of controls, suggesting a shared genetic susceptibility to psychiatric disorder only sometimes manifesting as Morgagni's syndrome.

Agenesis of the corpus callosum

Absence of the corpus callosum, in whole or in part, occurs as a developmental abnormality, perhaps in as many as 1 in 4000 births (Paul *et al.* 2007). In complete agenesis other associated defects may be present: hydrocephalus, microgyria, heterotopias, arachnoid cysts, spina bifida or meningomyelocele. The anterior and hippocampal commissures may be intact even when the corpus callosum is entirely missing. Paul *et al.* (2007) provide a complete review of the known genetic causes and the underlying neurobiology.

Most cases have been reported in children, although the condition can come to light at any age. It usually presents by virtue of symptoms attributable to other cerebral malformations: seizures, mental retardation or hydrocephalus. Occasionally, however, it is discovered only at post-mortem or in the course of neuroradiological investigations carried out for some other purpose. The discovery of asymptomatic cases is likely to increase now that brain imaging is so frequently performed.

David *et al.* (1993) and Dobyns (1996) note that complete agenesis is associated with a wide variety of genetic anomalies, including trisomies of chromosomes 8, 13 and 18. However as noted by Paul *et al.* (2007), in cases of complete, as opposed to partial, agenesis there appears to be a genetic cause in only 10–15% of cases. It appears sometimes to be the result of intrauterine metabolic disturbances such as hyperglycinaemia, or intrauterine exposure to infections and toxins. Epilepsy, spasticity and other motor defects are common, likewise varying grades of mental subnormality especially in cases of partial agenesis and when associated with other conditions. However, when patients with other malformations are excluded, intelligence is usually in the normal range.

There has been a renewal of interest in the psychological status of such patients in view of the abnormal functioning known to follow surgical section of the commissures and the interest in disconnection syndromes (reviewed by David *et al.* 1993; Paul *et al.* 2007). Various cognitive deficits have been demonstrated, in particular on tests of bimanual coordination and in crossed-responding to visual stimuli and in the matching of visual patterns between left and right visual fields. However, all such deficits are variable, and other tests of interhemispheric transfer appear often to be well performed. Compensatory mechanisms must clearly be at work, by way of bilateral speech representation, increased use of ipsilateral inflow pathways, or utilisation of such other commissural pathways as are intact. Milner (1983) provides a valuable review of neuropsychological studies in such patients, concluding that while it is likely that both cognitive and skilled performances can suffer, there are clearly great individual differences from one case to another. In particular, there is no good evidence that acallosal brains are less laterally specialised than normal brains, despite conflicting findings on the issue.

David *et al.* (1993) and Paul *et al.* (2007) have reviewed the association between developmental defects of the corpus callosum and major psychiatric disturbances. These have included schizophrenia, depression and behavioural disorders of childhood including overlap with autism spectrum disorders. Of the seven new cases presented by David *et al.*, four had clear psychotic symptoms, two of these being schizophrenic and one manic–depressive, one had features of Asperger's syndrome, one a personality disorder with depression and conversion symptoms, and one was an adolescent with behavioural problems. No conclusions could be drawn concerning the relevance of the callosal abnormalities to these clinical manifestations, not least because the prevalence of callosal anomalies in the general population is uncertain.

The radiological diagnosis based on the air encephalogram was first described by Bull (1967). Marked separation is seen between the lateral ventricles; they show angular dorsal margins, concave medial borders and dilatation of the caudal portions. The third ventricle is widened with a large dorsal extension. Equivalent features can be detected on CT or MRI. Characteristic findings are seen in relation to the pericallosal arteries and other vessels on angiography.

Acknowledgements

The editor is grateful to Dr Madhav Thambisetty for his invaluable contributions to this chapter.

References

Adams, R.D. (1966) Further observations on normal pressure hydrocephalus. *Proceedings of the Royal Society of Medicine* **59**, 1135–1140.

Adams, R.D., Fisher, C.M., Hakim, S., Ojemann, R.G. & Sweet, W.H. (1965) Symptomatic occult hydrocephalus with 'normal' cerebrospinal fluid pressure: a treatable syndrome. *New England Journal of Medicine* **273**, 117–126.

Ahlberg, J., Norlen, L., Blomstrand, C. & Wikkelso, C. (1988) Outcome of shunt operation on urinary incontinence in normal pressure hydrocephalus predicted by lumbar puncture. *Journal of Neurology, Neurosurgery and Psychiatry* **51**, 105–108.

Albers, J.W., Nostrant, T.T. & Riggs, J.E. (1989) Neurologic manifestations of gastrointestinal disease. *Neurologic Clinics* **7**, 525–548.

Albin, R.L. (2003) Dominant ataxias and Friedreich ataxia: an update. *Current Opinion in Neurology* **16**, 507–514.

Alevizos, B., Anagnostara, C. & Christodoulou, G.N. (2004) Resistant bipolar disorder precipitated by Behcet's syndrome. *Bipolar Disorders* **6**, 260–263.

Allen, R.K., Sellars, R.E. & Sandstrom, P.A. (2003) A prospective study of 32 patients with neurosarcoidosis. *Sarcoidosis, Vasculitis and Diffuse Lung Diseases* **20**, 118–125.

Amato, M.P., Ponziani, G., Pracucci, G., Bracco, L., Siracusa, G. & Amaducci, L. (1995) Cognitive impairment in early-onset multiple sclerosis. Pattern, predictors, and impact on everyday life in a 4-year follow-up. *Archives of Neurology* **52**, 168–172.

Amato, M.P., Ponziani, G., Siracusa, G. & Sorbi, S. (2001) Cognitive dysfunction in early-onset multiple sclerosis: a reappraisal after 10 years. *Archives of Neurology* **58**, 1602–1606.

Amato, M.P., Zipoli, V. & Portaccio, E. (2006) Multiple sclerosis-related cognitive changes: a review of cross-sectional and longitudinal studies. *Journal of the Neurological Sciences* **245**, 41–46.

Anderson, J.L., Head, S.I., Rae, C. & Morley, J.W. (2002) Brain function in Duchenne muscular dystrophy. *Brain* **125**, 4–13.

Anderson, J.L., Head, S.I. & Morley, J.W. (2004) Long-term depression is reduced in cerebellar Purkinje cells of dystrophin-deficient mdx mice. *Brain Research* **1019**, 289–292.

Ando, H., Mizuki, N., Ohno, S. *et al.* (1997) Identification of a novel HLA-B allele (B*4202) in a Saudi Arabian family with Behcet's disease. *Tissue Antigens* **49**, 526–528.

Angelini, L., Nardocci, N., Rumi, V., Zorzi, C., Strada, L. & Savoiardo, M. (1992) Hallervorden–Spatz disease: clinical and MRI study of 11 cases diagnosed in life. *Journal of Neurology* **239**, 417–425.

Armstrong, P. & Keevil, S.F. (1991) Magnetic resonance imaging 2: clinical uses. *British Medical Journal* **303**, 105–109.

Arnold, D.L. (2007) The place of MRI in monitoring the individual MS patient. *Journal of the Neurological Sciences* **259**, 123–127.

Ashjazadeh, N., Borhani, H.A., Samangooie, S. & Moosavi, H. (2003) Neuro-Behcet's disease: a masquerader of multiple sclerosis. A prospective study of neurologic manifestations of Behcet's disease in 96 Iranian patients. *Experimental and Molecular Pathology* **74**, 17–22.

Au, K.S., Williams, A.T., Roach, E.S. *et al.* (2007) Genotype/phenotype correlation in 325 individuals referred for a diagnosis of tuberous sclerosis complex in the United States. *Genetics in Medicine* **9**, 88–100.

Aubourg, P., Adamsbaum, C., Lavallard-Rousseau, M.C. *et al.* (1993) A two-year trial of oleic and erucic acids ('Lorenzo's oil') as treatment for adrenomyeloneuropathy. *New England Journal of Medicine* **329**, 745–752.

Bakheit, A.M., Kennedy, P.G. & Behan, P.O. (1990) Paraneoplastic limbic encephalitis: clinico-pathological correlations. *Journal of Neurology, Neurosurgery and Psychiatry* **53**, 1084–1088.

Bakshi, R., Ariyaratana, S., Benedict, R.H. & Jacobs, L. (2001) Fluid-attenuated inversion recovery magnetic resonance imaging detects cortical and juxtacortical multiple sclerosis lesions. *Archives of Neurology* **58**, 742–748.

Barbeau, A., Roy, M., Sadibelouiz, M. & Wilensky, M.A. (1984) Recessive ataxia in Acadians and 'Cajuns'. *Canadian Journal of Neurological Sciences* **11**, 526–533.

Barth, M.L., Ward, C., Harris, A., Saad, A. & Fensom, A. (1994) Frequency of arylsulphatase A pseudodeficiency associated mutations in a healthy population. *Journal of Medical Genetics* **31**, 667–671.

Baughman, R.P., Lower, E.E. & Du Bois, R.M. (2003) Sarcoidosis. *Lancet* **361**, 1111–1118.

Bedlack, R.S. & Sanders, D.B. (2000) How to handle myasthenic crisis. Essential steps in patient care. *Postgraduate Medicine* **107**, 211–212.

Bell, J. & Carmichael, E.A. (1939) On hereditary ataxia and spastic paraplegia. *The Treasury of Human Inheritance* **4**, 141–281.

Benedict, R.H. & Bobholz, J.H. (2007) Multiple sclerosis. *Seminars in Neurology* **27**, 78–85.

Bennett, P.B. & McLeod, M. (1984) Probing the limits of human deep diving. *Philosophical Transactions of the Royal Society of London B* **304**, 105–117.

Berger, J.R. (2007) Progressive multifocal leukoencephalopathy. *Current Neurology and Neuroscience Reports* **7**, 461–469.

Bergin, J.D. (1957) Rapidly progressing dementia in disseminated sclerosis. *Journal of Neurology, Neurosurgery and Psychiatry* **20**, 285–292.

Berkovic, S.F., Carpenter, S., Andermann, F., Andermann, E. & Wolfe, L.S. (1988) Kuf's disease: a critical reappraisal. *Brain* **111**, 27–62.

Berman, L., Trappler, B. & Jenkins, T. (1979) Behcet's syndrome: a family study and the elucidation of a genetic role. *Annals of the Rheumatic Diseases* **38**, 118–121.

Bhidayasiri, R., Perlman, S.L., Pulst, S.M. & Geschwind, D.H. (2005) Late-onset Friedreich ataxia: phenotypic analysis, magnetic resonance imaging findings, and review of the literature. *Archives of Neurology* **62**, 1865–1869.

Bird, T.D., Follett, C. & Griep, E. (1983) Cognitive and personality function in myotonic muscular dystrophy. *Journal of Neurology, Neurosurgery and Psychiatry* **46**, 971–980.

Boillee, S., Vande, V.C. & Cleveland, D.W. (2006) ALS: a disease of motor neurons and their nonneuronal neighbors. *Neuron* **52**, 39–59.

Bolla, L. & Palmer, R.M. (1997) Paraneoplastic cerebellar degeneration. Case report and literature review. *Archives of Internal Medicine* **157**, 1258–1262.

Bomholt, S.F., Harbuz, M.S., Blackburn-Munro, G. & Blackburn-Munro, R.E. (2004) Involvement and role of the hypothalamo-pituitary-adrenal (HPA) stress axis in animal models of chronic pain and inflammation. *Stress* **7**, 1–14.

Botez-Marquard, T. & Botez, M.I. (1993) Cognitive behavior in heredodegenerative ataxias. *European Neurology* **33**, 351–357.

Brain, W.R. (1930) Critical review: disseminated sclerosis. *Quarterly Journal of Medicine* **23**, 343–391.

Brain, W.R. & Adams, R.D. (1965) Epilogue: a guide to the classification and investigation of neurological disorders associated with neoplasms. In: Brain, W.R. & Norris, E.H. (eds) *The Remote Effects of Cancer on the Nervous System*, ch. 21. Contemporary Neurology Symposia, vol. 1. Grune & Stratton, New York.

Brain, W.R. & Henson, R.A. (1958) Neurological syndromes associated with carcinoma: the carcinomatous neuromyopathies. *Lancet* **ii**, 971–975.

Brain, W.R., Daniel, P.M. & Greenfield, J.G. (1951) Subacute cortical cerebellar degeneration and its relation to carcinoma. *Journal of Neurology, Neurosurgery and Psychiatry* **14**, 59–75.

Brieg, A., Ekbom, K., Greitz, T. & Kugelberg, E. (1967) Hydrocephalus due to elongated basilar artery: a new clinicoradiological syndrome. *Lancet* **i**, 874–875.

Brierley, J.B., Corsellis, J.A.N., Hierons, R. & Nevin, S. (1960) Subacute encephalitis of later adult life: mainly affecting the limbic areas. *Brain* **83**, 357–368.

Brodaty, H., Mitchell, P., Luscombe, G. *et al.* (2002) Familial idiopathic basal ganglia calcification (Fahr's disease) without neurological, cognitive and psychiatric symptoms is not linked to the IBGC1 locus on chromosome 14q. *Human Genetics* **110**, 8–14.

Brown, S.J. (2006) The role of vitamin D in multiple sclerosis. *Annals of Pharmacotherapy* **40**, 1158–1161.

Brownell, B., Oppenheimer, D.R. & Hughes, J.T. (1970) The central nervous system in motor neurone disease. *Journal of Neurology, Neurosurgery and Psychiatry* **33**, 338–357.

Bruck, W., Bitsch, A., Kolenda, H., Bruck, Y., Stiefel, M. & Lassmann, H. (1997) Inflammatory central nervous system demyelination: correlation of magnetic resonance imaging findings with lesion pathology. *Annals of Neurology* **42**, 783–793.

Bruneau, M.A., Lesperance, P. & Chouinard, S. (2003) Schizophrenia-like presentation of neuroacanthocytosis. *Journal of Neuropsychiatry and Clinical Neuroscience* **15**, 378–380.

Buck, A.A. & McKusick, V.A. (1961) Epidemiologic investigations of sarcoidosis. III. Serum proteins; syphilis; association with tuberculosis: familial aggregation. *American Journal of Hygiene* **74**, 174–188.

Bull, J. (1967) The corpus callosum. *Clinical Radiology* **18**, 2–18.

Callanan, M.M., Logsdail, S.J., Ron, M.A. & Warrington, E.K. (1989) Cognitive impairment in patients with clinically isolated lesions of the type seen in multiple sclerosis. A psychometric and MRI study. *Brain* **112**, 361–374.

Canter, A.H. (1951) Direct and indirect measures of psychological deficit in multiple sclerosis. *Journal of General Psychology* **44**, 3–35 and 27–50.

Capraro, V.J., Dillon, W.P. & Calabrese, J.S. (1970) Morgagni's syndrome: metabolic craniopathy. *Obstetrics and Gynecology* **35**, 565–569.

Carroll, B.A., Lane, B., Norman, D. & Enzmann, D. (1977) Diagnosis of progressive multifocal leukoencephalopathy by computed tomography. *Radiology* **122**, 137–141.

Caughey, J.E. & Myrianthopoulos, N.C. (1963) *Dystrophia Myotonica and Related Disorders*. Thomas, Springfield, IL.

Charatan, F.B. & Brierley, J.B. (1956) Mental disorder associated with primary lung carcinoma. *British Medical Journal* **1**, 765–768.

Ching, K.H., Westaway, S.K., Gitschier, J., Higgins, J.J. & Hayflick, S.J. (2002) HARP syndrome is allelic with pantothenate kinase-associated neurodegeneration. *Neurology* **58**, 1673–1674.

Clouston, P.D., Saper, C.B., Arbizu, T. *et al.* (1992) Paraneoplastic cerebellar degeneration. III. Cerebellar degeneration, cancer, and the Lambert–Eaton myasthenic syndrome. *Neurology* **42**, 1944–1950.

Colding-Jorgensen, E. (2005) Phenotypic variability in myotonia congenita. *Muscle and Nerve* **32**, 19–34.

Compston, A. (1993) Non-infective inflammatory demyelinating, and paraneoplastic diseases of the nervous system. In: Walton, J. (ed.) *Brain's Diseases of the Nervous System*, 10th edn, ch. 10. Oxford University Press, Oxford.

Conti-Fine, B.M., Milani, M. & Kaminski, H.J. (2006) Myasthenia gravis: past, present, and future. *Journal of Clinical Investigation* **116**, 2843–2854.

Corben, L.A., Georgiou-Karistianis, N., Fahey, M.C. *et al.* (2006) Towards an understanding of cognitive function in Friedreich ataxia. *Brain Research Bulletin* **70**, 197–202.

Cordingley, G., Navarro, C., Brust, J.C. & Healton, E.B. (1981) Sarcoidosis presenting as senile dementia. *Neurology* **31**, 1148–1151.

Corsellis, J.A.N., Goldberg, G.J. & Norton, A.R. (1968) 'Limbic encephalitis' and its associations with carcinoma. *Brain* **91**, 481–496.

Cossu, G. & Sampaolesi, M. (2007) New therapies for Duchenne muscular dystrophy: challenges, prospects and clinical trials. *Trends in Molecular Medicine* **13**, 520–526.

Cottrell, S.S. & Wilson, S.A.K. (1926) The affective symptomatology of disseminated sclerosis: a study of 100 cases. *Journal of Neurology and Psychopathology* **7**, 1–30.

Cox, C.S., Dubey, P., Raymond, G.V., Mahmood, A., Moser, A.B. & Moser, H.W. (2006) Cognitive evaluation of neurologically asymptomatic boys with X-linked adrenoleukodystrophy. *Archives of Neurology* **63**, 69–73.

Crino, P.B., Nathanson, K.L. & Henske, E.P. (2006) The tuberous sclerosis complex. *New England Journal of Medicine* **355**, 1345–1356.

Critchley, M. & Earl, C.J.C. (1932) Tuberose sclerosis and allied conditions. *Brain* **55**, 311–346.

Crockard, A., McKee, H., Joshi, K. & Allen, I. (1980) ICP, CAT scans and psychometric assessment in dementia: a prospective analysis. In: Shulman, K., Mannsrou, A., Miller, J.D., Becker, D.P., Hochwald, G.M. & Brock, M. (eds) *Intracranial Pressure IV*, pp. 501–504. Springer-Verlag, Berlin.

Croft, P.B. & Wilkinson, M. (1965) The incidence of carcinomatous neuromyopathy with special reference to carcinoma of the lung and breast. In: Brain, W.R. & Norris, F.H. (eds) *The Remote Effects of Cancer on the Nervous System*, ch. 6. Contemporary Neurology Symposia, vol. 1. Grune & Stratton, New York.

Cummings, J.L. & Benson, D.F. (1992) *Dementia: A Clinical Approach*, 2nd edn. Butterworth-Heinemann, Boston & London.

Cummings, J.L., Gosenfeld, L.F., Houlihan, J.P. & McCaffrey, T. (1983) Neuropsychiatric disturbances associated with idiopathic calcification of the basal ganglia. *Biological Psychiatry* **18**, 591–601.

Cummings, J.L., Arciniegas, D.B., Brooks, B.R. *et al.* (2006) Defining and diagnosing involuntary emotional expression disorder. *CNS Spectrums* **11**, 1–7.

Cyrulnik, S.E. & Hinton, V.J. (2008) Duchenne muscular dystrophy: a cerebellar disorder? *Neuroscience and Biobehavioral Reviews* **32**, 486–496.

Cyrulnik, S.E., Fee, R.J., De, V., Goldstein, E. & Hinton, V.J. (2007) Delayed developmental language milestones in children with Duchenne's muscular dystrophy. *Journal of Pediatrics* **150**, 474–478.

Cyrulnik, S.E., Fee, R.J., Batchelder, A., Kiefel, J., Goldstein, E. & Hinton, V.J. (2008) Cognitive and adaptive deficits in young children with Duchenne muscular dystrophy (DMD). *Journal of the International Neuropsychological Society* **14**, 853–861.

Dalmau, J., Tuzun, E., Wu, H.Y. *et al.* (2007) Paraneoplastic anti-N-methyl-D-aspartate receptor encephalitis associated with ovarian teratoma. *Annals of Neurology* **61**, 25–36.

Dalos, N.P., Rabins, P.V., Brooks, B.R. & O'Donnell, P. (1983) Disease activity and emotional state in multiple sclerosis. *Annals of Neurology* **13**, 573–577.

D'Angelo, M.G. & Bresolin, N. (2006) Cognitive impairment in neuromuscular disorders. *Muscle and Nerve* **34**, 16–33.

David, A.S. & Gillham, R.A. (1986) Neuropsychological study of motor neurone disease. *Psychosomatics* **27**, 441–445.

David, A.S., Wacharasindhu, A. & Lishman, W.A. (1993) Severe psychiatric disturbance and abnormalities of the corpus callosum: review and case series. *Journal of Neurology, Neurosurgery and Psychiatry* **56**, 85–93.

Davies, D.L. (1949) Psychiatric changes associated with Friedreich's ataxia. *Journal of Neurology, Neurosurgery and Psychiatry* **12**, 246–250.

Davies, N.P., Eunson, L.H., Samuel, M. & Hanna, M.G. (2001) Sodium channel gene mutations in hypokalemic periodic paralysis: an uncommon cause in the UK. *Neurology* **57**, 1323–1325.

Davila, D., Piriz, J., Trejo, J.L., Nunez, A. & Torres-Aleman, I. (2007) Insulin and insulin-like growth factor I signalling in neurons. *Frontiers in Bioscience* **12**, 3194–3202.

Davison, K. & Bagley, C.R. (1969) Schizophrenia-like psychoses associated with organic disorders of the central nervous system: a review of the literature. In: Herrington, R.N. (ed.) *Current Problems in Neuropsychiatry*, pp. 84, 190, 191, 225, 230, 234, 282, 284, 354, 387, 657, 665, 697, 706, 708, 716, 728. British Journal of Psychiatry Special Publication No. 4. Headley Brothers, Ashford, Kent.

Day, J.W. & Ranum, L.P. (2005) Genetics and molecular pathogenesis of the myotonic dystrophies. *Current Neurology and Neuroscience Reports* **5**, 55–59.

De, V. (1993) The expanding clinical spectrum of mitochondrial diseases. *Brain and Development* **15**, 1–22.

De Baets, M.H. & Kuks, J.J.M. (1993) Immunopathology of myasthenia gravis. In: De Baets, M.H. & Oosterhuis, H.J.G.H. (eds) *Myasthenia Gravis*, ch. 5. CRC Press, Boca Raton, FL.

Dekaban, R.S. & Herman, M.M. (1974) Childhood, juvenile, and adult cerebral lipidoses. *Archives of Pathology* **97**, 65–73.

Delaney, P. (1977) Neurologic manifestations in sarcoidosis: review of the literature, with a report of 23 cases. *Annals of Internal Medicine* **87**, 336–345.

Delaporte, C. (1998) Personality patterns in patients with myotonic dystrophy. *Archives of Neurology* **55**, 635–640.

Delatycki, M.B., Williamson, R. & Forrest, S.M. (2000) Friedreich ataxia: an overview. *Journal of Medical Genetics* **37**, 1–8.

Denison, D.M. (1996) Diving medicine. In: Weatherall, D.J., Ledingham, J.G.G. & Warrell, D.A. (eds) *Oxford Textbook of Medicine*, 3rd edn, Section 8.5.5(f). Oxford University Press, Oxford.

Deriban, G. & Marth, T. (2006) Current concepts of immunopathogenesis, diagnosis and therapy in Whipple's disease. *Current Medicinal Chemistry* **13**, 2921–2926.

De Vries, P.J. & Howe, C.J. (2007) The tuberous sclerosis complex proteins: a GRIPP on cognition and neurodevelopment. *Trends in Molecular Medicine* **13**, 319–326.

Dhib-Jalbut, S. (2007) Pathogenesis of myelin/oligodendrocyte damage in multiple sclerosis. *Neurology* **68** (22 suppl. 3), S13–S21.

Di Mauro, S. & Moses, L.G. (1992) Mitochondrial encephalomyopathies. *Brain Pathology* **2**, 111–112.

Dobson-Stone, C., Danek, A., Rampoldi, L. *et al.* (2002) Mutational spectrum of the CHAC gene in patients with chorea-acanthocytosis. *European Journal of Human Genetics* **10**, 773–781.

Dobyns, W.B. (1996) Absence makes the search grow longer. *American Journal of Human Genetics* **58**, 7–16.

Dooling, E.C., Schoene, W.C. & Richardson, E.P. Jr (1974) Hallervorden–Spatz syndrome. *Archives of Neurology* **30**, 70–83.

Dooling, E.C., Richardson, E.P. Jr & Davis, K.R. (1980) Computed tomography in Hallervorden–Spatz disease. *Neurology* **30**, 1128–1130.

Dorschner, M.O., Sybert, V.P., Weaver, M., Pletcher, B.A. & Stephens, K. (2000) NF1 microdeletion breakpoints are clustered at flanking repetitive sequences. *Human Molecular Genetics* **9**, 35–46.

Drake, A.K., Loy, C.T., Brew, B.J. *et al.* (2007) Human immunodeficiency virus-associated progressive multifocal leucoencephalopathy: epidemiology and predictive factors for prolonged survival. *European Journal of Neurology* **14**, 418–423.

Duff, K. & McCaffrey, R.J. (2001) Electrical injury and lightning injury: a review of their mechanisms and neuropsychological, psychiatric, and neurological sequelae. *Neuropsychology Review* **11**, 101–116.

Dutta, R. & Trapp, B.D. (2007) Pathogenesis of axonal and neuronal damage in multiple sclerosis. *Neurology* **68** (22 suppl. 3), S22–S31.

Duwe, B.V. & Turetsky, B.I. (2002) Misdiagnosis of schizophrenia in a patient with psychotic symptoms. *Neuropsychiatry, Neuropsychology, and Behavioral Neurology* **15**, 252–260.

Eichler, F., Mahmood, A., Loes, D. *et al.* (2007) Magnetic resonance imaging detection of lesion progression in adult patients with X-linked adrenoleukodystrophy. *Archives of Neurology* **64**, 659–664.

Einarsson, U., Gottberg, K., Von, K.L. *et al.* (2006) Cognitive and motor function in people with multiple sclerosis in Stockholm County. *Multiple Sclerosis* **12**, 340–353.

Ekbom, K., Greitz, T. & Kugelberg, E. (1969) Hydrocephalus due to ectasia of the basilar artery. *Journal of the Neurological Sciences* **8**, 465–477.

Elizan, T.S., Hirano, A., Abrams, B.M., Need, R.L., Van Nuis, C. & Kurland, L.T. (1966) Amyotrophic lateral sclerosis and parkinsonism–dementia complex of Guam. Neurological re-evaluation. *Archives of Neurology* **14**, 356–368.

Ellison, P.H. & Barron, K.D. (1979) Clinical recovery from Schilder disease. *Neurology* **29**, 244–251.

Emery, A.E. (2002) The muscular dystrophies. *Lancet* **359**, 687–695.

Erberk-Ozen, N., Birol, A., Boratav, C. & Kocak, M. (2006) Executive dysfunctions and depression in Behcet's disease without explicit neurological involvement. *Psychiatry and Clinical Neurosciences* **60**, 465–472.

Erlington, G. & Newsom-Davis, J. (1994) Clinical presentation and current immunology of the Lambert–Eaton myasthenic syndrome. In: Lisak, R.P. (ed.) *Handbook of Myasthenia Gravis and Myasthenic Syndromes*, ch. 5. Marcel Dekker, New York.

Evereklioglu, C. (2004) Managing the symptoms of Behcet's disease. *Expert Opinion on Pharmacotherapy* **5**, 317–328.

Evereklioglu, C., Er, H., Turkoz, Y. & Cekmen, M. (2002a) Serum levels of TNF-alpha, sIL-2R, IL-6, and IL-8 are increased and associated with elevated lipid peroxidation in patients with Behcet's disease. *Mediators of Inflammation* **11**, 87–93.

Evereklioglu, C., Inaloz, H.S., Kirtak, N. *et al.* (2002b) Serum leptin concentration is increased in patients with Behcet's syndrome and is correlated with disease activity. *British Journal of Dermatology* **147**, 331–336.

Farrell, D.F. & Starr, A. (1968) Delayed neurological sequelae of electrical injuries. *Neurology* **18**, 601–606.

Feinstein, A., Kartsounis, L.D., Miller, D.H., Youl, B.D. & Ron, M.A. (1992a) Clinically isolated lesions of the type seen in multiple sclerosis: a cognitive, psychiatric, and MRI follow up study. *Journal of Neurology, Neurosurgery and Psychiatry* **55**, 869–876.

Feinstein, A., Du, B.G. & Ron, M.A. (1992b) Psychotic illness in multiple sclerosis. A clinical and magnetic resonance imaging study. *British Journal of Psychiatry* **161**, 680–685.

Feinstein, A., Roy, P., Lobaugh, N., Feinstein, K., O'Connor, P. & Black, S. (2004) Structural brain abnormalities in multiple sclerosis patients with major depression. *Neurology* **62**, 586–590.

Ferner, R.E. (1994) Intellect in neurofibromatosis 1. In: Huson, S.M. & Hughes, R.A.C. (eds) *The Neurofibromatoses*, ch. 9. Chapman & Hall, London.

Ferraro, A. (1934) Histopathological findings in two cases clinically diagnosed dementia praecox. *American Journal of Psychiatry* **90**, 883–903.

Ferraro, A. (1943) Pathological changes in the brain of a case clinically diagnosed dementia praecox. *Journal of Neuropathology and Experimental Neuroloy* **2**, 84–94.

Ferrer, I. (1992) Dementia of frontal lobe type and amyotrophy. *Behavioral Neurology* **5**, 87–96.

Filley, C.M., Heaton, R.K., Thompson, L.L., Nelson, L.M. & Franklin, G.M. (1990) Effects of disease course on neuropsychological functioning. In: Rao, S.M. (ed.) *Neurobehavioral Aspects of Multiple Sclerosis*, ch. 8. Oxford University Press, Oxford.

Fisher, N.R., Cope, S.J. & Lishman, W.A. (1987) Metachromatic leukodystrophy: conduct disorder progressing to dementia. *Journal of Neurology, Neurosurgery and Psychiatry* **50**, 488–489.

Flachenecker, P. (2006) Epidemiology of neuroimmunological diseases. *Journal of Neurology* **253** (suppl. 5), V2–V8.

Flint, J. & Goldstein, L.H. (1992) Familial calcification of the basal ganglia: a case report and review of the literature. *Psychological Medicine* **22**, 581–595.

Forstl, H., Krumm, B., Eden, S. & Kohlmeyer, K. (1992) Neurological disorders in 166 patients with basal ganglia calcification: a statistical evaluation. *Journal of Neurology* **239**, 36–38.

Francis, A.F. (1979) Familial basal ganglia calcification and schizophreniform psychosis. *British Journal of Psychiatry* **135**, 360–362.

Francis, A. & Freeman, H. (1984) Psychiatric abnormality and brain calcification over four generations. *Journal of Nervous and Mental Disease* **172**, 166–170.

Friedman, S.H. & Gould, D.J. (2002) Neurosarcoidosis presenting as psychosis and dementia: a case report. *International Journal of Psychiatry in Medicine* **32**, 401–403.

Gallia, G.L., Rigamonti, D. & Williams, M.A. (2006) The diagnosis and treatment of idiopathic normal pressure hydrocephalus. *Nature Clinical Practice Neurology* **2**, 375–381.

Garell, P.C., Menezes, A.H., Baumbach, G. *et al.* (1998) Presentation, management and follow-up of Schilder's disease. *Pediatric Neurosurgery* **29**, 86–91.

Gatchel, J.R. & Zoghbi, H.Y. (2005) Diseases of unstable repeat expansion: mechanisms and common principles. *Nature Reviews of Genetics* **6**, 743–755.

Geocaris, K. (1957) Psychotic episodes heralding the diagnosis of multiple sclerosis. *Bulletin of the Menninger Clinic* **21**, 107–116.

Geschwind, D.H., Loginov, M. & Stern, J.M. (1999) Identification of a locus on chromosome 14q for idiopathic basal ganglia calcification (Fahr disease). *American Journal of Human Genetics* **65**, 764–772.

Ghaffar, O. & Feinstein, A. (2007) The neuropsychiatry of multiple sclerosis: a review of recent developments. *Current Opinion in Psychiatry* **20**, 278–285.

Giliberto, F., Ferreiro, V., Dalamon, V. & Szijan, I. (2004) Dystrophin deletions and cognitive impairment in Duchenne/Becker muscular dystrophy. *Neurological Research* **26**, 83–87.

Giovannoni, G. & Ebers, G. (2007) Multiple sclerosis: the environment and causation. *Curr Opin Neurol* **20**, 261–268.

Glab, H., Szostek, K. & Kaczanowski, K. (2006) Hyperostosis frontalis interna, a genetic disease? Two medieval cases from Southern Poland. *Homo* **57**, 19–27.

Goebel, H.H. & Wisniewski, K.E. (2004) Current state of clinical and morphological features in human NCL. *Brain Pathology* **14**, 61–69.

Gold, M.M., Shifteh, K., Bello, J.A., Lipton, M., Kaufman, D.M. & Brown, A.D. (2006) Chorea-acanthocytosis: a mimicker of Huntington disease. Case report and review of the literature. *Neurologist* **12**, 327–329.

Gold, R., Jawad, A., Miller, D.H. *et al.* (2007) Expert opinion: guidelines for the use of natalizumab in multiple sclerosis patients previously treated with immunomodulating therapies. *Journal of Neuroimmunology* **187**, 156–158.

Gold, S.M., Mohr, D.C., Huitinga, I., Flachenecker, P., Sternberg, E.M. & Heesen, C. (2005) The role of stress-response systems for the pathogenesis and progression of MS. *Trends in Immunology* **26**, 644–652.

Goldstein, L.H., Atkins, L., Landau, S., Brown, R. & Leigh, P.N. (2006) Predictors of psychological distress in carers of people with amyotrophic lateral sclerosis: a longitudinal study. *Psychological Medicine* **36**, 865–875.

Goolamali, S.K., Comaish, J.S., Hassanyeh, F. & Stephens, A. (1976) Familial Behcet's syndrome. *British Journal of Dermatology* **95**, 637–642.

Goulding, P., Burjan, A., Smith, R. *et al.* (1990) Semi-automatic quantification of regional cerebral perfusion in primary degenerative dementia using 99m technetium-hexamethylpropylene amino oxime and single photon emission tomography. *European Journal of Nuclear Medicine* **17**, 77–82.

Grafman, J., Rao, S., Bernardin, L. & Leo, G.J. (1991) Automatic memory processes in patients with multiple sclerosis. *Archives of Neurology* **48**, 1072–1075.

Grant, R. (2002) What the general neurologist needs to know about the paraneoplastic syndromes. *Practical Neurology* **2**, 318–327.

Greenfield, J.G. & Norman, R.M. (1963) Demyelinating diseases. In: Blackwood, W., McMenemey, W.H., Meyer, A., Norman, R. M. & Russell, D.S. (eds) *Greenfield's Neuropathology*, 2nd edn, ch. 8. Edward Arnold, London.

Greenlee, J.E., Brashear, H.R., Jaeckle, K.A., Geleris, A. & Jordan, K. (1992) Pursuing an occult carcinoma in a patient with subacute cerebellar degeneration and anticerebellar antibodies. Need for vigorous follow-up. *Western Journal of Medicine* **156**, 199–202.

Grob, D. (1958) Myasthenia gravis: current status of psychogenesis, clinical manifestations and management. *Journal of Chronic Diseases* **8**, 536–566.

Gros-Louis, F., Gaspar, C. & Rouleau, G.A. (2006) Genetics of familial and sporadic amyotrophic lateral sclerosis. *Biochimica et Biophysica Acta* **1762**, 956–972.

Gross-Jendroska, M., Schatz, H., McDonald, H.R. & Johnson, R.N. (1992) Kearns–Sayre syndrome: a case report and review. *European Journal of Ophthalmology* **2**, 15–20.

Grutters, J.C. & van den Bosch, J.M. (2006) Corticosteroid treatment in sarcoidosis. *European Respiratory Journal* **28**, 627–636.

Guillamo, J.S., Creange, A., Kalifa, C. *et al.* (2003) Prognostic factors of CNS tumours in neurofibromatosis 1 (NF1): a retrospective study of 104 patients. *Brain* **126**, 152–160.

Gultekin, S.H., Rosenfeld, M.R., Voltz, R., Eichen, J., Posner, J.B. & Dalmau, J. (2000) Paraneoplastic limbic encephalitis: neurological symptoms, immunological findings and tumour association in 50 patients. *Brain* **123**, 1481–1494.

Hakim, S. (1964) *Algunas observaciones sobra la pression del L.C.R. sindrome hidrocefalico en al adulto con 'pression normal' del L.C.R.* Tesis de grado, Universidad Javeriana, Bogota, Colombia. Quoted by Ojemann, R.G. *et al.* (1969) *Journal of Neurosurgery* **31**, 279–294.

Hakim, S. & Adams, R.D. (1965) The special clinical problem of symptomatic hydrocephalus with normal cerebrospinal fluid pressure: observations on cerebrospinal fluid hydrodynamics. *Journal of the Neurological Sciences* **2**, 307–327.

Halliday, A.M., McDonald, W.I. & Mushin, J. (1973) Visual evoked response in diagnosis of multiple sclerosis. *British Medical Journal* **4**, 661–664.

Hammond, J.S. & Ward, C.G. (1988) High-voltage electrical injuries: management and outcome of 60 cases. *Southern Medical Journal* **81**, 1351–1352.

Hardie, R.J. (1989) Acanthocytosis and neurological impairment: a review. *Quarterly Journal of Medicine* **71**, 291–306.

Hardie, R.J., Pullon, H.W., Harding, A.E. *et al.* (1991) Neuroacanthocytosis. A clinical, haematological and pathological study of 19 cases. *Brain* **114**, 13–49.

Harding, A.E. (1983) Classification of the hereditary ataxias and paraplegias, *Lancet* **i**, 1151–1155.

Harrison, M.J.G., Robert, C.M. & Uttley, D. (1974) Benign aqueduct stenosis in adults. *Journal of Neurology, Neurosurgery and Psychiatry* **37**, 1322–1328.

Hart, R.P., Henry, G.K., Kwentus, J.A. & Leshner, R.T. (1986) Information processing speed of children with Friedreich's ataxia. *Developmental Medicine and Child Neurology* **28**, 310–313.

Hawkes, C.H. (2005) Are multiple sclerosis patients risk-takers? *Quarterly Journal of Medicine* **98**, 895–911.

Heaton, R.K., Nelson, L.M., Thompson, D.S., Burks, J.S. & Franklin, G.M. (1985) Neuropsychological findings in relapsing-remitting and chronic-progressive multiple sclerosis. *Journal of Consulting and Clinical Psychology* **53**, 103–110.

Heatwole, C.R. & Moxley, R.T. III (2007) The nondystrophic myotonias. *Neurotherapeutics* **4**, 238–251.

Heavey, A.M., Philpot, M.P., Fensom, A.H., Jackson, M. & Crammer, J.L. (1990) Leucocyte arylsulphatase A activity and subtypes of chronic schizophrenia. *Acta Psychiatrica Scandinavica* **82**, 55–59.

Heesen, C., Gold, S.M., Huitinga, I. & Reul, J.M. (2007) Stress and hypothalamic–pituitary–adrenal axis function in experimental autoimmune encephalomyelitis and multiple sclerosis: a review. *Psychoneuroendocrinology* **32**, 604–618.

Hemmer, B. & Hartung, H.P. (2007) Toward the development of rational therapies in multiple sclerosis: what is on the horizon? *Annals of Neurology* **62**, 314–326.

Hendrick, E.B. (1993) Results of treatment in infants and children. In: Schurr, P.H. & Polkey, C.E. (eds) *Hydrocephalus*, ch. 7. Oxford University Press, Oxford.

Hendriksen, J.G. & Vles, J.S. (2008) Neuropsychiatric disorders in males with Duchenne muscular dystrophy: frequency rate of attention-deficit hyperactivity disorder (ADHD), autism spectrum disorder, and obsessive–compulsive disorder. *Journal of Child Neurology* **23**, 477–481.

Hershkovitz, I., Greenwald, C., Rothschild, B.M. *et al.* (1999) Hyperostosis frontalis interna: an anthropological perspective. *American Journal of Physical Anthropology* **109**, 303–325.

Hirano, A., Malamud, N. & Kurland, L.T. (1961) Parkinsonism–dementia complex, an endemic disease on the island of Guam. II. Pathological features. *Brain* **84**, 662–679.

Hirano, A., Malamud, N., Elizan, T.S. & Kurland, L.T. (1966) Amyotrophic lateral sclerosis and parkinsonism–dementia complex on Guam: further pathologic studies. *Archives of Neurology* **15**, 35–51.

Hogg, K.E., Goldstein, L.H. & Leigh, P.N. (1994) The psychological impact of motor neurone disease. *Psychological Medicine* **24**, 625–632.

Holt, E.K. & Tedeschi, C. (1943) Cerebral patchy demyelination. *Journal of Neuropathology and Experimental Neurology* **2**, 306–314.

Hook, O. (1954) Sarcoidosis with involvement of the nervous system: report of nine cases. *AMA Archives of Neurology and Psychiatry* **71**, 554–575.

Hooper, C., Killick, R. & Lovestone, S. (2008) The GSK3 hypothesis of Alzheimer's disease. *Journal of Neurochemistry* **104**, 1433–1439.

Hopkins, R.O. & Weaver, L.K. (2001) Acute psychosis associated with diving. *Undersea and Hyperbaric Medicine* **28**, 145–148.

Hotopf, M.H., Pollock, S. & Lishman, W.A. (1994) An unusual presentation of multiple sclerosis. *Psychological Medicine* **24**, 525–528.

Houpt, J.L., Gould, B.S. & Norris, F.H. (1977) Psychological characteristics of patients with amyotrophic lateral sclerosis (ALS). *Psychosomatic Medicine* **39**, 299–303.

Hudson, A.J. (1981) Amyotrophic lateral sclerosis and its association with dementia, parkinsonism and neurological disorders: a review. *Brain* **104**, 217–247.

Hughes, R.A.C. (1994) Neurological complications of neurofibromatosis 1. In: Huson, S.M. & Hughes, R.A.C. (eds) *The Neurofibromatoses*, ch. 8. Chapman & Hall, London.

Hughes, T. (2005) The early history of myasthenia gravis. *Neuromuscular Disorders* **15**, 878–886.

Hurria, A., Somlo, G. & Ahles, T. (2007) Renaming 'chemobrain'. *Cancer Investigation* **25**, 373–377.

Huson, S.M. (1994) Neurofibromatosis 1: a clinical and genetic overview. In: Huson, S.M. & Hughes, R.A.C. (eds) *The Neurofibromatoses*, ch. 7. Chapman & Hall, London.

Huson, S.M., Harper, P.S. & Compston, D.A.S. (1988) Von Recklinghausen neurofibromatosis. A clinical and population study in south-east Wales. *Brain* **111**, 1355–1381.

Hyde, T.M., Ziegler, J.C. & Weinberger, D.R. (1992) Psychiatric disturbances in metachromatic leukodystrophy. Insights into the neurobiology of psychosis. *Archives of Neurology* **49**, 401–406.

International Study Group for Behçet's Disease (1990) Criteria for diagnosis of Behçet's disease. *Lancet* **335**, 1078–1080.

Irwin, D., Lippa, C.F. & Swearer, J.M. (2007) Cognition and amyotrophic lateral sclerosis (ALS). *American Journal of Alzheimer's Disease and Other Dementias* **22**, 300–312.

Ivnik, R.J. (1978) Neuropsychological stability in multiple sclerosis. *Journal of Consulting and Clinical Psychology* **46**, 913–923.

Jankowski, K. (1963) A case of Schilder's diffuse sclerosis diagnosed clinically as schizophrenia. *Acta Neuropathologica* **2**, 302–305.

Jansen, C.E., Miaskowski, C.A., Dodd, M.J. & Dowling, G.A. (2007) A meta-analysis of the sensitivity of various neuropsychological tests used to detect chemotherapy-induced cognitive impairment in patients with breast cancer. *Oncology Nursing Forum* **34**, 997–1005.

Jeffreys, R.V. (1993) Investigation and management of hydrocephalus in adults. In: Schurr, P.H. & Polkey, C.E. (eds) *Hydrocephalus*, ch. 8. Oxford University Press, Oxford.

Jeffreys, R.V. & Wood, M.M. (1978) Adult non-tumourous dementia and hydrocephalus. *Acta Neurochirurgica* **45**, 103–114.

Johnson, J. (1967) Myotonia congenita (Thomsen's disease) and hereditary psychosis. *British Journal of Psychiatry* **113**, 1025–1030.

Johnson, N.S., Saal, H.M., Lovell, A.M. & Schorry, E.K. (1999) Social and emotional problems in children with neurofibromatosis type 1: evidence and proposed interventions. *Journal of Pediatrics* **134**, 767–772.

Joinson, C., O'Callaghan, F.J., Osborne, J.P., Martyn, C., Harris, T. & Bolton, P.F. (2003) Learning disability and epilepsy in an epidemiological sample of individuals with tuberous sclerosis complex. *Psychological Medicine* **33**, 335–344.

Joseph, F.G. & Scolding, N.J. (2007) Sarcoidosis of the nervous system. *Practical Neurology* **7**, 234–244.

Juvonen, V., Kulmala, S.M., Ignatius, J., Penttinen, M. & Savontaus, M.L. (2002) Dissecting the epidemiology of a trinucleotide repeat disease: example of FRDA in Finland. *Human Genetics* **110**, 36–40.

Kalkman, J.S., Schillings, M.L., Zwarts, M.J., Van Engelen, B.G. & Bleijenberg, G. (2007) Psychiatric disorders appear equally in patients with myotonic dystrophy, facioscapulohumeral dystrophy, and hereditary motor and sensory neuropathy type I. *Acta Neurologica Scandinavica* **115**, 265–270.

Kayl, A.E. & Moore, B.D. III (2000) Behavioral phenotype of neurofibromatosis type 1. *Mental Retardation and Developmental Disabilities Research Reviews* **6**, 117–124.

Kemper, A.R. & Wake, M.A. (2007) Duchenne muscular dystrophy: issues in expanding newborn screening. *Current Opinion in Pediatrics* **19**, 700–704.

Kew, J.J.M. & Leigh, P.N. (1992) Dementia with motor neurone disease. In: Rossor, M.N. (ed.) *Unusual Dementias*, ch. 7. Baillière Tindall, London.

Kew, J.J.M., Goldstein, L.H., Leigh, P.N. *et al.* (1993a) The relationship between abnormalities of cognitive function and cerebral activation in amyotrophic lateral sclerosis. A neuropsychological and positron emission tomographic study. *Brain* **116**, 1399–1423.

Kew, J.J.M., Leigh, P.N., Playford, E.D. *et al.* (1993b) Cortical function in amyotrophic lateral sclerosis. A positron emission tomographic study. *Brain* **116**, 655–680.

Khalili, K. & White, M.K. (2006) Human demyelinating disease and the polyomavirus JCV. *Multiple Sclerosis* **12**, 133–142.

Khateeb, S., Flusser, H., Ofir, R. *et al.* (2006) PLA2G6 mutation underlies infantile neuroaxonal dystrophy. *American Journal of Human Genetics* **79**, 942–948.

Kihara, H. (1982) Genetic heterogeneity in metachromatic leukodystrophy. *American Journal of Human Genetics* **34**, 171–181.

Kleinschnitz, C., Meuth, S.G., Stuve, O., Kieseier, B. & Wiendl, H. (2007) Multiple sclerosis therapy: an update on recently finished trials. *Journal of Neurology* **254**, 1473–1490.

Knauth, M., Ries, S., Pohimann, S. *et al.* (1997) Cohort study of multiple brain lesions in sport divers: role of a patent foramen ovale. *British Medical Journal* **314**, 701–705.

Koch, M.C., Ricker, K., Otto, M. *et al.* (1993) Evidence for genetic homogeneity in autosomal recessive generalised myotonia (Becker). *Journal of Medical Genetics* **30**, 914–917.

Koch, M.C., Baumbach, K., George, A.L. & Ricker, K. (1995) Paramyotonia congenita without paralysis on exposure to cold: a novel mutation in the SCN4A gene (Val1293Ile). *Neuroreport* **6**, 2001–2004.

Koenig, H. (1968) Dementia associated with the benign form of multiple sclerosis. *Transactions of the American Neurological Association* **93**, 227–228.

Koller, M.F., Papassotiropoulos, A., Henke, K. *et al.* (2005) Evidence of a genetic basis of Morgagni–Stewart–Morel syndrome. A case report of identical twins. *Neurodegenerative Diseases* **2**, 56–60.

Koralnik, I.J. (2004) New insights into progressive multifocal leukoencephalopathy. *Current Opinion in Neurology* **17**, 365–370.

Kostrzewa, M., Klockgether, T., Damian, M.S. & Muller, U. (1997) Locus heterogeneity in Friedreich ataxia. *Neurogenetics* **1**, 43–47.

Kotagal, S., Rawlings, C.A., Chen, S.C., Burris, G. & Npuriouri, S. (1982) Neurologic, psychiatric, and cardiovascular complications in children struck by lightning. *Pediatrics* **70**, 190–192.

Kotil, K., Kalayci, M., Koseoglu, T. & Tugrul, A. (2002) Myelinoclastic diffuse sclerosis (Schilder's disease): report of a case and review of the literature. *British Journal of Neurosurgery* **16**, 516–519.

Krauss, J.K. & Halve, B. (2004) Normal pressure hydrocephalus: survey on contemporary diagnostic algorithms and therapeutic decision-making in clinical practice. *Acta Neurochirurgica* **146**, 379–388.

Kulaksizoglu, I.B. (2007) Mood and anxiety disorders in patients with myasthenia gravis: aetiology, diagnosis and treatment. *CNS Drugs* **21**, 473–481.

Kuo, Y.M., Duncan, J.L., Westaway, S.K. *et al.* (2005) Deficiency of pantothenate kinase 2 (Pank2) in mice leads to retinal degeneration and azoospermia. *Human Molecular Genetics* **14**, 49–57.

Kurland, L.T. & Mulder, D.W. (1954) Epidemiologic investigations of amyotrophic lateral sclerosis. *Neurology* **4**, 355–378 and 438–448.

Kurul, S., Cakmakci, H., Dirik, E. & Kovanlikaya, A. (2003) Schilder's disease: case study with serial neuroimaging. *Journal of Child Neurology* **18**, 58–61.

La Coletta, M.V., Scola, R.H., Wiemes, G.R. *et al.* (2007) Event-related potentials (P300) and neuropsychological assessment in boys exhibiting Duchenne muscular dystrophy. *Arquivos de Neuropsiquiatria* **65**, 59–62.

Lampert, P., Tom, M.I. & Cumings, J.N. (1962) Encephalopathy in Whipple's disease. A histochemical study. *Neurology* **12**, 65–71.

Lawn, N.D., Westmoreland, B.F., Kiely, M.J., Lennon, V.A. & Vernino, S. (2003) Clinical, magnetic resonance imaging, and electroencephalographic findings in paraneoplastic limbic encephalitis. *Mayo Clinic Proceedings* **78**, 1363–1368.

Leigh, P.N. (1994) Ubiquitin. In: Williams, A.C. (ed.) *Motor Neurone Disease*, ch. 16. Chapman & Hall, London.

Leigh, P.N., Anderton, B.H., Dodson, A., Gallo, J.-M., Swash, M. & Power, D.M. (1988) Ubiquitin deposits in anterior horn cells in motor neurone disease. *Neuroscience Letters* **93**, 197–203.

Leplow, B., Tetzlaff, K., Holl, D., Zeng, L. & Reuter, M. (2001) Spatial orientation in construction divers: are there associations with diving experience? *International Archives of Occupational and Environmental Health* **74**, 189–198.

Lessell, S., Hirano, A., Torres, J. & Kurland, L.T. (1962) Parkinsonism–dementia complex. *Archives of Neurology* **7**, 377–385.

Lincoln, M.R., Montpetit, A., Cader, M.Z. *et al.* (2005) A predominant role for the HLA class II region in the association of the MHC region with multiple sclerosis. *Nature Genetics* **37**, 1108–1112.

Listernick, R., Charrow, J., Greenwald, M. & Mets, M. (1994) Natural history of optic pathway tumors in children with neurofibromatosis type 1: a longitudinal study. *Journal of Pediatrics* **125**, 63–66.

Littler, M. & Morton, N.E. (1990) Segregation analysis of peripheral neurofibromatosis (NF1). *Journal of Medical Genetics* **27**, 307–310.

Logan, C.Y. & Nusse, R. (2004) The Wnt signaling pathway in development and disease. *Annual Review of Cell and Developmental Biology* **20**, 781–810.

Lombes, A., Bonilla, E. & Di Mauro, S. (1989) Mitochondrial encephalomyopathies. *Revue Neurologique* **145**, 671–689.

Louis, E.D., Lynch, T., Kaufmann, P., Fahn, S. & Odel, J. (1996) Diagnostic guidelines in central nervous system Whipple's disease. *Annals of Neurology* **40**, 561–568.

Lovestone, S. & McLoughlin, D.M. (2002) Protein aggregates and dementia: is there a common toxicity? *Journal of Neurology, Neurosurgery and Psychiatry* **72**, 152–161.

Lovestone, S., Killick, R., Di Forti, M. & Murray, R. (2007) Schizophrenia as a GSK-3 dysregulation disorder. *Trends in Neurosciences* **30**, 142–149.

Luat, A.F., Makki, M. & Chugani, H.T. (2007) Neuroimaging in tuberous sclerosis complex. *Current Opinion in Neurology* **20**, 142–150.

Ludolph, A.C., Langen, K.J., Regard, M. *et al.* (1992) Frontal lobe function in amyotrophic lateral sclerosis: a neuropsychologic and positron emission tomography study. *Acta Neurologica Scandinavica* **85**, 81–89.

Ludwig, B., Bohl, J. & Haferkamp, G. (1981) Central nervous system involvement in Whipple's disease. *Neuroradiology* **21**, 289–293.

Luque, F.A. & Jaffe, S.L. (2007) Cerebrospinal fluid analysis in multiple sclerosis. *International Review of Neurobiology* **79**, 341–356.

McDonald, W.I., Compston, A., Edan, G. *et al.* (2001) Recommended diagnostic criteria for multiple sclerosis: guidelines from the International Panel on the diagnosis of multiple sclerosis. *Annals of Neurology* **50**, 121–127.

MacFaul, R., Cavanagh, N., Lake, B.D., Stephens, R. & Whitfield, A.E. (1982) Metachromatic leucodystrophy: review of 38 cases. *Archives of Disease in Childhood* **57**, 168–175.

McHugh, P.R. (1966) Hydrocephalic dementia. *Bulletin of the New York Academy of Medicine* **42**, 907–917.

McIntosh-Michaelis, S.A., Roberts, M.H., Wilkinson, S.M. *et al.* (1991) The prevalence of cognitive impairment in a community survey of multiple sclerosis. *British Journal of Clinical Psychology* **30**, 333–348.

MacKenzie, K.R., Martin, M.J. & Howard, F.M. Jr (1969) Myasthenia gravis: psychiatric concomitants. *Canadain Medical Association Journal* **100**, 988–991.

McLeod, J.E. & Clarke, D.M. (2007) A review of psychosocial aspects of motor neurone disease. *Journal of the Neurological Sciences* **258**, 4–10.

McLoughlin, D. & McKeon, P. (1991) Bipolar disorder and cerebral sarcoidosis. *British Journal of Psychiatry* **158**, 410–413.

McMillan, J.J. & Williams, B. (1977) Aqueduct stenosis. *Journal of Neurology, Neurosurgery and Psychiatry* **40**, 521–532.

McQualter, J.L. & Bernard, C.C. (2007) Multiple sclerosis: a battle between destruction and repair. *Journal of Neurochemistry* **100**, 295–306.

McQueen, D., Kent, G. & Murrison, A. (1994) Self-reported long-term effects of diving and decompression illness in recreational scuba divers. *British Journal of Sports Medicine* **28**, 101–104.

Magni, G., Micaglio, G.F., Lalli, R. *et al.* (1988) Psychiatric disturbances associated with myasthenia gravis. *Acta Psychiatrica Scandinavica* **77**, 443–445.

Mahler, M.E. & Benson, D.F. (1990) Cognitive dysfunction in multiple sclerosis: a subcortical dementia? In: Rao, S.M. (ed.) *Neurobehavioral Aspects of Multiple Sclerosis*, ch. 5. Oxford University Press, Oxford.

Mahnel, R. & Marth, T. (2004) Progress, problems, and perspectives in diagnosis and treatment of Whipple's disease. *Clinical and Experimental Medicine* **4**, 39–43.

Makino, M., Horai, S., Goto, Y. & Nonaka, I. (2000) Mitochondrial DNA mutations in Leigh syndrome and their phylogenetic implications. *Journal of Human Genetics* **45**, 69–75.

Malcomson, K.S., Dunwoody, L. & Lowe-Strong, A.S. (2007) Psychosocial interventions in people with multiple sclerosis: a review. *Journal of Neurology* **254**, 1–13.

Malloy, P., Mishra, S.K. & Adler, S.H. (1990) Neuropsychological deficits in myotonic muscular dystrophy. *Journal of Neurology, Neurosurgery and Psychiatry* **53**, 1011–1013.

Manyam, B.V., Walters, A.S. & Narla, K.R. (2001) Bilateral striopallidodentate calcinosis: clinical characteristics of patients seen in a registry. *Movement Disorders* **16**, 258–264.

Mariotti, C., Savarese, N., Suomalainen, A. *et al.* (1995) Genotype to phenotype correlations in mitochondrial encephalomyopathies associated with the A3243G mutation of mitochondrial DNA. *Journal of Neurology* **242**, 304–312.

Marmarou, A., Bergsneider, M., Klinge, P., Relkin, N. & Black, P.M. (2005) The value of supplemental prognostic tests for the preoperative assessment of idiopathic normal-pressure hydrocephalus. *Neurosurgery* **57** (3 suppl.), S17–S28.

Matthews, W.B. (1979) Multiple sclerosis presenting with acute remitting psychiatric symptoms. *Journal of Neurology, Neurosurgery and Psychiatry* **42**, 859–863.

Mehler, M.F. (2000) Brain dystrophin, neurogenetics and mental retardation. *Brain Research. Brain Research Reviews* **32**, 277–307.

Meola, G. & Sansone, V. (2007) Cerebral involvement in myotonic dystrophies. *Muscle and Nerve* **36**, 294–306.

Meola, G., Sansone, V., Perani, D. *et al.* (2003) Executive dysfunction and avoidant personality trait in myotonic dystrophy type 1 (DM-1) and in proximal myotonic myopathy (PROMM/DM-2). *Neuromuscular Disorders* **13**, 813–821.

Mercuri, E., Gruter-Andrew, J., Philpot, J. *et al.* (1999) Cognitive abilities in children with congenital muscular dystrophy: correlation with brain MRI and merosin status. *Neuromuscular Disorders* **9**, 383–387.

Mihaljevic-Peles, A., Jakovljevic, M., Milicevic, Z. & Kracun, I. (2001) Low arylsulphatase A activity in the development of psychiatric disorders. *Neuropsychobiology* **43**, 75–78.

Milner, D. (1983) Neuropsychological studies of callosal agenesis. *Psychological Medicine* **13**, 721–725.

Mizukami, K., Shiraishi, H., Tanaka, Y. *et al.* (1992) CNS changes in neuro-Behcet's disease: CT, MR, and SPECT findings. *Computerized Medical Imaging and Graphics* **16**, 401–406.

Mohr, D.C. & Pelletier, D. (2006) A temporal framework for understanding the effects of stressful life events on inflammation in patients with multiple sclerosis. *Brain, Behavior and Immunity* **20**, 27–36.

Mohr, D.C., Hart, S.L., Julian, L., Cox, D. & Pelletier, D. (2004) Association between stressful life events and exacerbation in multiple sclerosis: a meta-analysis. *British Medical Journal* **328**, 731.

Moizard, M.P., Toutain, A., Fournier, D. *et al.* (2000) Severe cognitive impairment in DMD: obvious clinical indication for Dp71 isoform point mutation screening. *European Journal of Human Genetics* **8**, 552–556.

Molinari, N., Kone, P.I., Manna, R., Demaille, J., Daures, J.P. & Touitou, I. (2003) Identification of an autosomal recessive mode of inheritance in paediatric Behcet's families by segregation analysis. *American Journal of Medical Genetics* **122A**, 115–118.

Monastero, R., Camarda, C., Pipia, C. *et al.* (2004) Cognitive impairment in Behcet's disease patients without overt neurological involvement. *Journal of the Neurological Sciences* **220**, 99–104.

Morgan, N.V., Westaway, S.K., Morton, J.E. *et al.* (2006) PLA2G6, encoding a phospholipase A2, is mutated in neurodegenerative disorders with high brain iron. *Nature Genetics* **38**, 752–754.

Moser, A.B., Kreiter, N., Bezman, L. *et al.* (1999) Plasma very long chain fatty acids in 3,000 peroxisome disease patients and 29,000 controls. *Annals of Neurology* **45**, 100–110.

Moser, H.W. (1993) Lorenzo's oil. *Lancet* **341**, 544.

Moser, H.W., Moser, A.E., Singh, I. & O'Neill, B.P. (1984) Adrenoleukodystrophy: survey of 303 cases: biochemistry, diagnosis, and therapy. *Annals of Neurology* **16**, 628–641.

Moser, H.W., Dubey, P. & Fatemi, A. (2004) Progress in X-linked adrenoleukodystrophy. *Current Opinion in Neurology* **17**, 263–269.

Moser, H.W., Raymond, G.V., Lu, S.E. *et al.* (2005) Follow-up of 89 asymptomatic patients with adrenoleukodystrophy treated with Lorenzo's oil. *Archives of Neurology* **62**, 1073–1080.

Mubaidin, A., Roberts, E., Hampshire, D. *et al.* (2003) Karak syndrome: a novel degenerative disorder of the basal ganglia and cerebellum. *Journal of Medical Genetics* **40**, 543–546.

Mulhern, D.M., Wilczak, C.A. & Dudar, J.C. (2006) Unusual finding at Pueblo Bonito: multiple cases of hyperostosis frontalis interna. *American Journal of Physical Anthropology* **130**, 480–484.

Muller-Vahl, K.R., Berding, G., Emrich, H.M. & Peschel, T. (2007) Chorea-acanthocytosis in monozygotic twins: clinical findings and neuropathological changes as detected by diffusion tensor imaging, FDG-PET and (123)I-beta-CIT-SPECT. *Journal of Neurology* **254**, 1081–1088.

Mur, J., Kümpel, G. & Dostal, S. (1966) An anergic phase of disseminated sclerosis with psychotic course. *Confinia Neurologica* **28**, 37–49.

Nag, T.K. & Falconer, M.A. (1966) Non-tumoral stenosis of the aqueduct in adults. *British Medical Journal* **2**, 1168–1170.

Neary, D., Snowden, J.S., Mann, D.M.A., Northen, B., Goulding, P.J. & MacDermott, N. (1990) Frontal lobe dementia and motor neurone disease. *Journal of Neurology, Neurosurgery and Psychiatry* **53**, 23–32.

Neema, M., Stankiewicz, J., Arora, A., Guss, Z.D. & Bakshi, R. (2007) MRI in multiple sclerosis: what's inside the toolbox? *Neurotherapeutics* **4**, 602–617.

Nelson, C.J., Nandy, N. & Roth, A.J. (2007) Chemotherapy and cognitive deficits: mechanisms, findings, and potential interventions. *Palliative and Supportive Care* **5**, 273–280.

Newton, H.B., Padilla, W., Burkart, J. & Pearl, D.K. (2007) Neurological manifestations of decompression illness in recreational divers: the Cozumel experience. *Undersea and Hyperbaric Medicine* **34**, 349–357.

NIH Consensus Development Conference (1988) Neurofibromatosis. Conference statement. *Archives of Neurology* **45**, 575–578.

Nowack, D. & Goebel, K.M. (1987) Genetic aspects of sarcoidosis. Class II histocompatibility antigens and a family study. *Archives of Internal Medicine* **147**, 481–483.

Ohno, S., Ohguchi, M., Hirose, S., Matsuda, H., Wakisaka, A. & Aizawa, M. (1982) Close association of HLA-Bw51 with Behcet's disease. *Archives of Ophthalmology* **100**, 1455–1458.

Ojemann, R.G. (1971) Normal pressure hydrocephalus. In: *Clinical Neurosurgery*, ch. 16, pp. 745, 746, 748, 749. Proceedings of the Congress of Neurological Surgeons, vol. 18. Williams & Wilkins, Baltimore.

Ojemann, R.G., Fisher, C.M., Adams, R.D., Sweet, W.H. & New, P.J.F. (1969) Further experience with the syndrome of 'normal' pressure hydrocephalus. *Journal of Neurosurgery* **31**, 279–294.

Oldfors, A., Holme, E., Tulinius, M. & Larsson, N.G. (1995) Tissue distribution and disease manifestations of the tRNA(Lys) A→ G(8344) mitochondrial DNA mutation in a case of myoclonus epilepsy and ragged red fibres. *Acta Neuropathologica* **90**, 328–333.

Oldfors, A., Moslemi, A.R., Jonasson, L., Ohlsson, M., Kollberg, G. & Lindberg, C. (2006) Mitochondrial abnormalities in inclusion-body myositis. *Neurology* **66**, 549–555.

Oliveira, J.R., Spiteri, E., Sobrido, M.J. *et al.* (2004) Genetic heterogeneity in familial idiopathic basal ganglia calcification (Fahr disease). *Neurology* **63**, 2165–2167.

Ombredane, A. (1929) *Sur les troubles mentaux de la sclérose en plaques*. Thèse de Paris. Quoted by Surridge, D. (1969) *British Journal of Psychiatry* **115**, 749–764.

Oosterhuis, H.J. & Wilde, G.J. (1964) Psychiatric aspects of myasthenia gravis. *Psychiatria, Neurologia, Neurochirurgica* **67**, 484–496.

Ors, F., Sonmez, G., Yildiz, S. *et al.* (2006) Incidence of ischemic brain lesions in hyperbaric chamber inside attendants. *Advances in Therapy* **23**, 1009–1015.

Osborne, J.P., Fryer, A. & Webb, D. (1991) Epidemiology of tuberous sclerosis. *Annals of the New York Academy of Sciences* **615**, 125–127.

Osborne, R.J. & Thornton, C.A. (2006) RNA-dominant diseases. *Human Molecular Genetics* **15** (special no. 2), R162–R169.

Pallis, C.A. & Fudge, B.J. (1956) The neurological complications of Behcet's syndrome. *AMA Archives of Neurology and Psychiatry* **75**, 1–14.

Pallis, C. & Lewis, P.D. (1980) Neurology of gastrointestinal disease. In: Vinken, P.J. & Bruyn, C.W. (eds) *Neurological Manifestations of Systemic Diseases*, Part II, ch. 21. Handbook of Clinical Neurology, vol. 39. North-Holland Publishing Co., Amsterdam.

Palmer, A.C., Calder, I.M. & Hughes, J.T. (1987) Spinal cord degeneration in divers. *Lancet* **ii**, 1365–1366.

Palmer, A.C., Calder, I.M. & Yates, P.O. (1992) Cerebral vasculopathy in divers. *Neuropathology and Applied Neurobiology* **18**, 113–124.

Pandolfo, M. (2008) Drug Insight: antioxidant therapy in inherited ataxias. *Nature Clinical Practice Neurology* **4**, 86–96.

Parker, N. (1956) Disseminated sclerosis presenting as schizophrenia. *Medical Journal of Australia* **1**, 405–407.

Parry, D.M., Eldridge, R., Kaiser-Kupfer, M.I., Bouzas, E.A., Pikus, A. & Patronas, N. (1994) Neurofibromatosis 2 (NF2): clinical characteristics of 63 affected individuals and clinical evidence for heterogeneity. *American Journal of Medical Genetics* **52**, 450–461.

Parry, D.M., MacCollin, M.M., Kaiser-Kupfer, M.I. *et al.* (1996) Germ-line mutations in the neurofibromatosis 2 gene: correlations with disease severity and retinal abnormalities. *American Journal of Human Genetics* **59**, 529–539.

Patten, S.B., Svenson, L.W. & Metz, L.M. (2005) Psychotic disorders in MS: population-based evidence of an association. *Neurology* **65**, 1123–1125.

Paul, L.K., Brown, W.S., Adolphs, R. *et al.* (2007) Agenesis of the corpus callosum: genetic, developmental and functional aspects of connectivity. *Nature Reviews of Neuroscience* **8**, 287–299.

Paul, R.H., Cohen, R.A., Zawacki, T., Gilchrist, J.M. & Aloia, M.S. (2001) What have we learned about cognition in myasthenia gravis? A review of methods and results. *Neuroscience and Biobehavioral Reviews* **25**, 75–81.

Pelosini, M., Focosi, D., Rita, F. *et al.* (2008) Progressive multifocal leukoencephalopathy: report of three cases in HIV-negative hematological patients and review of literature. *Annals of Hematology* **87**, 405–412.

Pentland, B., Mitchell, J.D., Cull, R.E. & Ford, M.J. (1985) Central nervous system sarcoidosis. *Quarterly Journal of Medicine* **56**, 457–465.

Perron, M., Veillette, S. & Mathieu, J. (1989) Myotonic dystrophy: I. Socioeconomic and residential characteristics of the patients. *Canadian Journal of Neurological Sciences* **16**, 109–113.

Petty, R.K.H., Harding, A.E. & Morgan-Hughes, J.A. (1986) The clinical features of mitochondrial myopathy. *Brain* **109**, 915–938.

Peyser, J.M., Edwards, K.R. & Poser, C.M. (1980a) Psychological profiles in patients with multiple sclerosis. A preliminary investigation. *Archives of Neurology* **37**, 437–440.

Peyser, J.M., Edwards, K.R., Poser, C.M. & Filskov, S.B. (1980b) Cognitive function in patients with multiple sclerosis. *Archives of Neurology* **37**, 577–579.

Phillips, L.H. (1994) The epidemiology of myasthenia gravis. *Neurologic Clinics* **12**, 263–271.

Philpot, M., Lewis, K., Pereria, M.L. *et al.* (1997) Arylsulphatase A pseudodeficiency in vascular dementia and Alzheimer's disease. *Neuroreport* **8**, 2613–2616.

Phukan, J., Pender, N.P. & Hardiman, O. (2007) Cognitive impairment in amyotrophic lateral sclerosis. *Lancet Neurology* **6**, 994–1003.

Pickard, J.D. (1982) Adult communicating hydrocephalus. *British Journal of Hospital Medicine* **27**, 35–44.

Pirko, I., Lucchinetti, C.F., Sriram, S. & Bakshi, R. (2007) Gray matter involvement in multiple sclerosis. *Neurology* **68**, 634–642.

Polman, C.H., Reingold, S.C., Edan, G. *et al.* (2005) Diagnostic criteria for multiple sclerosis: 2005 revisions to the 'McDonald Criteria'. *Annals of Neurology* **58**, 840–846.

Polman, C.H., O'Connor, P.W., Havrdova, E. *et al.* (2006) A randomized, placebo-controlled trial of natalizumab for relapsing multiple sclerosis. *New England Journal of Medicine* **354**, 899–910.

Pratt, R.T.C. (1951) An investigation of the psychiatric aspects of disseminated sclerosis. *Journal of Neurology, Neurosurgery and Psychiatry* **14**, 326–335.

Primeau, M. (2005) Neurorehabilitation of behavioral disorders following lightning and electrical trauma. *NeuroRehabilitation* **20**, 25–33.

Pruitt, B.A. & Mason, A.D. (1996) Lightning and electric shock. In: Weatherall, D.J., Ledingham, J.G.G. & Warrell, D.A. (eds) *Oxford Textbook of Medicine*, 3rd edn, Section 8.5.5(g). Oxford University Press, Oxford.

Ptacek, L.J., George, A.L. Jr, Barchi, R.L. *et al.* (1992) Mutations in an S4 segment of the adult skeletal muscle sodium channel cause paramyotonia congenita. *Neuron* **8**, 891–897.

Pujol, J., Leal, S., Fluvia, X. & Conde, C. (1989) Psychiatric aspects of normal pressure hydrocephalus. A report of five cases. *British Journal of Psychiatry* **154** (suppl. 4), 77–80.

Quijano-Roy, S., Marti-Carrera, I., Makri, S. *et al.* (2006) Brain MRI abnormalities in muscular dystrophy due to FKRP mutations. *Brain and Development* **28**, 232–242.

Radunovic, A., Mitsumoto, H. & Leigh, P.N. (2007) Clinical care of patients with amyotrophic lateral sclerosis. *Lancet Neurology* **6**, 913–925.

Rae, C., Scott, R.B., Thompson, C.H. *et al.* (1998) Brain biochemistry in Duchenne muscular dystrophy: a ^{1}H magnetic resonance and neuropsychological study. *Journal of the Neurological Sciences* **160**, 148–157.

Ragheb, S. & Lisak, R.P. (1994) The immunopathogenesis of acquired (autoimmune) myasthenia gravis. In: Lisak, R.P. (ed.) *Handbook of Myasthenia Gravis and Myasthenic Syndromes*, ch. 12. Marcel Dekker, New York.

Rakheja, D., Narayan, S.B. & Bennett, M.J. (2007) Juvenile neuronal ceroid-lipofuscinosis (Batten disease): a brief review and update. *Current Molecular Medicine* **7**, 603–608.

Ramani, S.V. (1981) Psychosis associated with frontal lobe lesions in Schilder's cerebral sclerosis. *Journal of Clinical Psychiatry* **42**, 250–252.

Rampoldi, L., Dobson-Stone, C., Rubio, J.P. *et al.* (2001) A conserved sorting-associated protein is mutant in chorea-acanthocytosis. *Nature Genetics* **28**, 119–120.

Rao, S.M. (1986) Neuropsychology of multiple sclerosis: a critical review. *Journal of Clinical and Experimental Neuropsychology* **8**, 503–542.

Rao, S.M., Leo, G.J., Bernardin, L. & Unverzagt, F. (1991) Cognitive dysfunction in multiple sclerosis. I. Frequency, patterns, and prediction. *Neurology* **41**, 685–691.

Relkin, N., Marmarou, A., Klinge, P., Bergsneider, M. & Black, P.M. (2005) Diagnosing idiopathic normal-pressure hydrocephalus. *Neurosurgery* **57** (3 suppl.), S4–S16.

Reul, J., Weis, J., Jung, A., Willmes, K. & Thron, A. (1995) Central nervous system lesions and cervical disc herniations in amateur divers. *Lancet* **345**, 1403–1405.

Reveley, A.M. & Reveley, M.A. (1983) Aqueduct stenosis and schizophrenia. *Journal of Neurology, Neurosurgery and Psychiatry* **46**, 18–22.

Riccardi, V.M. (1981) Von Recklinghausen neurofibromatosis. *New England Journal of Medicine* **305**, 1617–1627.

Rice, E. & Gendelman, S. (1973) Psychiatric aspects of normal pressure hydrocephalus. *Journal of the American Medical Association* **223**, 409–412.

Rinck, P.A., Svihus, R. & de Francisco, P. (1991) MR imaging of the central nervous system in divers. *Journal of Magnetic Resonance Imaging* **1**, 293–299.

Roizin, L., Moriarty, J.D. & Weil, A.A. (1945) Schizophrenic reaction syndrome in course of acute demyelination of central nervous system: clinicopathological report of a case, with brief review of the literature. *Archives of Neurology and Psychiatry* **54**, 202–211.

Romeo, G., Menozzi, P., Ferlini, A. *et al.* (1983) Incidence of Friedreich ataxia in Italy estimated from consanguineous marriages. *American Journal of Human Genetics* **35**, 523–529.

Ron, M.A. & Feinstein, A. (1992) Multiple sclerosis and the mind. *Journal of Neurology, Neurosurgery and Psychiatry* **55**, 1–3.

Ron, M.A. & Logsdail, S.J. (1989) Psychiatric morbidity in multiple sclerosis: a clinical and MRI study. *Psychological Medicine* **19**, 887–895.

Rosen, D.R., Siddique, T., Patterson, D. *et al.* (1993) Mutations in Cu/Zn superoxide dismutase gene are associated with familial amyotrophic lateral sclerosis. *Nature* **362**, 59–62.

Rosman, N.P. & Pearce, J. (1967) The brain in multiple neurofibromatosis (von Recklinghausen's disease): a suggested neuropathological basis for the associated mental defect. *Brain* **90**, 829–838.

Rosser, T., Panigrahy, A. & McClintock, W. (2006) The diverse clinical manifestations of tuberous sclerosis complex: a review. *Seminars in Pediatric Neurology* **13**, 27–36.

Rossman, M.D., Thompson, B., Frederick, M. *et al.* (2003) HLA-DRB1*1101: a significant risk factor for sarcoidosis in blacks and whites. *American Journal of Human Genetics* **73**, 720–735.

Rubio, J.P., Danek, A., Stone, C. *et al.* (1997) Chorea-acanthocytosis: genetic linkage to chromosome 9q21. *American Journal of Human Genetics* **61**, 899–908.

Rudick, R.A., Stuart, W.H., Calabresi, P.A. *et al.* (2006a) Natalizumab plus interferon beta-1a for relapsing multiple sclerosis. *New England Journal of Medicine* **354**, 911–923.

Rudick, R.A., Lee, J.C., Simon, J. & Fisher, E. (2006b) Significance of T2 lesions in multiple sclerosis: a 13-year longitudinal study. *Annals of Neurology* **60**, 236–242.

Ruiz-Sandoval, J.L., Garcia-Navarro, V., Chiquete, E. *et al.* (2007) Choreoacanthocytosis in a Mexican family. *Archives of Neurology* **64**, 1661–1664.

Runge, W. (1928) Psychische Störungen bei multipler Sklerose. In: Bumke, O. (ed.) *Handbuch der Geisteskrankheiten*, vol. 7, Special Part 3. Springer, Berlin.

Salmon, J.H. (1971) Surgical treatment of severe post-traumatic encephalopathy. *Surgery, Gynecology and Obstetrics* **133**, 634–636.

Samuelsson, B. (1981) *Neurofibromatosis (v. Recklinghausen's Disease). A clinical–psychiatric and genetic study*. Thesis, translated by A. Jacobs, Psychiatric Department, University of Göteborg, Sweden.

Sangiorgi, S., Ferlini, A., Zanetti, A. & Mochi, M. (1991) Reduced activity of arylsulfatase A and predisposition to neurological disorders: analysis of 140 pediatric patients. *American Journal of Medical Genetics* **40**, 365–369.

Sawcer, S., Ban, M., Maranian, M. *et al.* (2005) A high-density screen for linkage in multiple sclerosis. *American Journal of Human Genetics* **77**, 454–467.

Schapira, A.H. (2006) Mitochondrial disease. *Lancet* **368**, 70–82.

Schols, L., Meyer, C., Schmid, G., Wilhelms, I. & Przuntek, H. (2004) Therapeutic strategies in Friedreich's ataxia. *Journal of Neural Transmission Supplementum* **68**, 135–145.

Schott, J.M. (2006) Limbic encephalitis: a clinician's guide. *Practical Neurology* **6**, 143–153.

Schwab, R.S. & Perlo, V.P. (1966) Syndromes simulating myasthenia gravis. *Annals of the New York Academy of Sciences* **135**, 350–366.

Shanske, S. (1992) Mitochondrial encephalomyopathies: defects of nuclear DNA. *Brain Pathology* **2**, 159–162.

Sikanjic, P.R. (2006) Analysis of human skeletal remains from Nadin iron age burial mound. *Collegium Antropologicum* **30**, 795–799.

Silinkova-Malkova, E. & Malek, J. (1965/66) Endocraniosis. *Neuroendrocrinology* **1**, 68–82.

Sistiaga, A., Camano, P., Otaegui, D. *et al.* (2009) Cognitive function in facioscapulohumeral dystrophy correlates with the molecular defect. *Genes, Brain and Behavior* **8**, 53–59.

Skegg, K. (1993) Multiple sclerosis presenting as a pure psychiatric disorder. *Psychological Medicine* **23**, 909–914.

Sneddon, J. (1980) Myasthenia gravis: a study of social, medical, and emotional problems in 26 patients. *Lancet* **i**, 526–528.

Sreedharan, J., Blair, J.P., Tripathi, V.B. *et al.* (2008) TDP-43 mutations in familial and sporadic amyotrophic lateral sclerosis. *Science* **319**, 1668–1672.

Steinmeyer, K., Lorenz, C., Pusch, M., Koch, M.C. & Jentsch, T.J. (1994) Multimeric structure of ClC-1 chloride channel revealed by mutations in dominant myotonia congenita (Thomsen). *EMBO Journal* **13**, 737–743.

Stephens, K., Kayes, L., Riccardi, V.M., Rising, M., Sybert, V.P. & Pagon, R.A. (1992) Preferential mutation of the neurofibromatosis type 1 gene in paternally derived chromosomes. *Human Genetics* **88**, 279–282.

Stern, B.J. (2004) Neurological complications of sarcoidosis. *Current Opinion in Neurology* **17**, 311–316.

Steyaert, J., Umans, S., Willekens, D. *et al.* (1997) A study of the cognitive and psychological profile in 16 children with congenital or juvenile myotonic dystrophy. *Clinical Genetics* **52**, 135–141.

Surridge, D. (1969) An investigation into some psychiatric aspects of multiple sclerosis. *British Journal of Psychiatry* **115**, 749–764.

Swiech, L., Perycz, M., Malik, A. & Jaworski, J. (2008) Role of mTOR in physiology and pathology of the nervous system. *Biochimica et Biophysica Acta* **1784**, 116–132.

Taillibert, S., Voillery, D. & Bernard-Marty, C. (2007) Chemobrain: is systemic chemotherapy neurotoxic? *Current Opinion in Oncology* **19**, 623–627.

Talley, B.J. & Faber, R. (1989) Mitochondrial encephalomyopathic dementia in a young adult. *Neuropsychiatry, Neuropsychology and Behavioral Neurology* **2**, 49–60.

Taner, E., Cosar, B., Burhanoglu, S., Calikoglu, E., Onder, M. & Arikan, Z. (2007) Depression and anxiety in patients with Behcet's disease compared with that in patients with psoriasis. *International Journal of Dermatology* **46**, 1118–1124.

Teunissen, C.E., Dijkstra, C. & Polman, C. (2005) Biological markers in CSF and blood for axonal degeneration in multiple sclerosis. *Lancet Neurology* **4**, 32–41.

Thambisetty, M. & Newman, N.J. (2004) Diagnosis and management of MELAS. *Expert Review of Molecular Diagnostics* **4**, 631–644.

Thambisetty, M., Newman, N.J., Glass, J.D. & Frankel, M.R. (2002) A practical approach to the diagnosis and management of MELAS: case report and review. *Neurologist* **8**, 302–312.

Thomasen, E. (1948) *Myotonia: Thomsen's Disease (Myotonia Congenita), Paramyotonia, and Dystrophia Myotonica.* Universitetsforlaget, Aarhus.

Thompson, C. & Checkley, S. (1981) Short term memory deficit in a patient with cerebral sarcoidosis. *British Journal of Psychiatry* **139**, 160–161.

Thomsen, J. (1876) Tonische Krämpfe in willkürlich beweglichen Muskeln in Folge von ererbter psychischer Disposition. *Arkiv für Psychiatrie und Nervenkrankheiten* **6**, 702–718. Quoted by Johnson, J. (1967) *British Journal of Psychiatry* **113**, 1025–1030.

Tissenbaum, M.J., Harter, H.M. & Friedman, A.P. (1951) Organic neurological syndromes diagnosed as functional disorders. *Journal of the American Medical Association* **147**, 1519–1521.

Todnem, K., Nyland, H., Riise, T. *et al.* (1990) Analysis of neurologic symptoms in deep diving: implications for selection of divers. *Undersea Biomedical Research* **17**, 95–107.

Todnem, K., Skeidsvoll, H., Svihus, R. *et al.* (1991a) Electroencephalography, evoked potentials and MRI brain scans in saturation divers. An epidemiological study. *Electroencephalography and Clinical Neurophysiology* **79**, 322–329.

Todnem, K., Vaernes, R. & Kambestad, B.K. (1991b) Visual evoked and brain stem auditory evoked potentials in divers. *Aviation, Space and Environmental Medicine* **62**, 982–985.

Tormoehlen, L.M. & Pascuzzi, R.M. (2008) Thymoma, myasthenia gravis, and other paraneoplastic syndromes. *Hematology/Oncology Clinics of North America* **22**, 509–526.

Tripodi, D., Dupas, B., Potiron, M., Louvet, S. & Geraut, C. (2004) Brain magnetic resonance imaging, aerobic power, and metabolic parameters among 30 asymptomatic scuba divers. *International Journal of Sports Medicine* **25**, 575–581.

Trovo-Marqui, A.B. & Tajara, E.H. (2006) Neurofibromin: a general outlook. *Clinical Genetics* **70**, 1–13.

Uguz, F., Dursun, R., Kaya, N. & Cilli, A.S. (2007) Quality of life in patients with Behcet's disease: the impact of major depression. *General Hospital Psychiatry* **29**, 21–24.

Vaillend, C., Billard, J.M. & Laroche, S. (2004) Impaired long-term spatial and recognition memory and enhanced CA1 hippocampal LTP in the dystrophin-deficient Dmd(mdx) mouse. *Neurobiology of Disease* **17**, 10–20.

Van der Maarel, S.M. & Frants, R.R. (2005) The D4Z4 repeat-mediated pathogenesis of facioscapulohumeral muscular dystrophy. *American Journal of Human Genetics* **76**, 375–386.

Vanneste, J., Augustijn, P., Dirven, C., Tan, W.F. & Goedhart, Z.D. (1992) Shunting normal-pressure hydrocephalus: do the benefits outweigh the risks? A multicenter study and literature review. *Neurology* **42**, 54–59.

Van Slegtenhorst, M., Nellist, M., Nagelkerken, B. *et al.* (1998) Interaction between hamartin and tuberin, the TSC1 and TSC2 gene products. *Human Molecular Genetics* **7**, 1053–1057.

Van Zomeren, A.H., Ten Duis, H.J., Minderhoud, J.M. & Sipma, M. (1998) Lightning strike and neuropsychological impairment: cases and questions. *Journal of Neurology, Neurosurgery and Psychiatry* **64**, 763–769.

Venturin, M., Guarnieri, P., Natacci, F. *et al.* (2004) Mental retardation and cardiovascular malformations in NF1 microdeleted patients point to candidate genes in 17q11.2. *Journal of Medical Genetics* **41**, 35–41.

Vernino, S. (2007) Autoimmune and paraneoplastic channelopathies. *Neurotherapeutics* **4**, 305–314.

Vinas, F.C. & Rengachary, S. (2001) Diagnosis and management of neurosarcoidosis. *Journal of Clinical Neuroscience* **8**, 505–513.

Vukusic, S. & Confavreux, C. (2007) Natural history of multiple sclerosis: risk factors and prognostic indicators. *Current Opinion in Neurology* **20**, 269–274.

Wagner, K.R., Lechtzin, N. & Judge, D.P. (2007) Current treatment of adult Duchenne muscular dystrophy. *Biochimica et Biophysica Acta* **1772**, 229–237.

Walinder, J. (1977) Hyperostosis frontalis interna and mental morbidity. *British Journal of Psychiatry* **131**, 155–159.

Walker, R.H., Jung, H.H., Dobson-Stone, C. *et al.* (2007) Neurologic phenotypes associated with acanthocytosis. *Neurology* **68**, 92–98.

Wallace, D.C. (1992) Diseases of the mitochondrial DNA. *Annual Review of Biochemistry* **61**, 1175–1212.

Waltz, G., Harik, S.I. & Kaufman, B. (1987) Adult metachromatic leukodystrophy. Value of computed tomographic scanning and magnetic resonance imaging of the brain. *Archives of Neurology* **44**, 225–227.

Wang, Q., Montmain, G., Ruano, E. *et al.* (2003) Neurofibromatosis type 1 gene as a mutational target in a mismatch repair-deficient cell type. *Human Genetics* **112**, 117–123.

Warren, J.D., Schott, J.M., Fox, N.C. *et al.* (2005) Brain biopsy in dementia. *Brain* **128**, 2016–2025.

Warren, L.P. Jr, Djang, W.T., Moon, R.E. *et al.* (1988) Neuroimaging of scuba diving injuries to the CNS. *American Journal of Roentgenology* **151**, 1003–1008.

Webb, D.W. & Osborne, J.P. (1992) New research in tuberous sclerosis. *British Medical Journal* **304**, 1647–1648.

Wechsler, B. & Piette, J.C. (1992) Behcet's disease. *British Medical Journal* **304**, 1199–1200.

Wechsler, B., Vidailhet, M., Piette, J.C. *et al.* (1992) Cerebral venous thrombosis in Behcet's disease: clinical study and long-term follow-up of 25 cases. *Neurology* **42**, 614–618.

Weeber, E.J. & Sweatt, J.D. (2002) Molecular neurobiology of human cognition. *Neuron* **33**, 845–848.

Wells, R.D. (2008) DNA triplexes and Friedreich ataxia. *FASEB Journal* **22**, 1625–1634.

White, M., Lalonde, R. & Botez-Marquard, T. (2000) Neuropsychologic and neuropsychiatric characteristics of patients with Friedreich's ataxia. *Acta Neurologica Scandinavica* **102**, 222–226.

Whiteman, M.L., Post, M.J., Berger, J.R., Tate, L.G., Bell, M.D. & Limonte, L.P. (1993) Progressive multifocal leukoencephalopathy in 47 HIV-seropositive patients: neuroimaging with clinical and pathologic correlation. *Radiology* **187**, 233–240.

Wicks, P., Abrahams, S., Masi, D., Hejda-Forde, S., Leigh, P.N. & Goldstein, L.H. (2007) Prevalence of depression in a 12-month consecutive sample of patients with ALS. *European Journal of Neurology* **14**, 993–1001.

Wicksell, R.K., Kihlgren, M., Melin, L. & Eeg-Olofsson, O. (2004) Specific cognitive deficits are common in children with Duchenne muscular dystrophy. *Developmental Medicine and Child Neurology* **46**, 154–159.

Wiederholt, W.C., Gomez, M.R. & Kurland, L.T. (1985) Incidence and prevalence of tuberous sclerosis in Rochester, Minnesota, 1950 through 1982. *Neurology* **35**, 600–603.

Wiestler, O.D. & Radner, H. (1994) Pathology of neurofibromatosis 1 and 2. In: Huson, S.M. & Hughes, R.A.C. (eds) *The Neurofibromatoses*, ch. 6. Chapman & Hall, London.

Wilkinson, H.A., Lemay, M. & Drew, J.H. (1966) Adult aqueductal stenosis. *Archives of Neurology* **15**, 643–648.

Williamson, A.M., Clarke, B. & Edmonds, C. (1987) Neurobehavioural effects of professional abalone diving. *British Journal of Industrial Medicine* **44**, 459–466.

Williamson, A.M., Clarke, B. & Edmonds, C.W. (1989) The influence of diving variables on perceptual and cognitive functions in professional shallow-water (abalone) divers. *Environmental Research* **50**, 93–102.

Wilmshurst, P. (1997) Brain damage in divers. Diving itself may cause brain damage: but we need more evidence. *British Medical Journal* **314**, 689–690.

Wollmann, T., Barroso, J., Monton, F. & Nieto, A. (2002) Neuropsychological test performance of patients with Friedreich's ataxia. *Journal of Clinical and Experimental Neuropsychology* **24**, 677–686.

Wyen, C., Lehmann, C., Fatkenheuer, G. & Hoffmann, C. (2005) AIDS-related progressive multifocal leukoencephalopathy in the era of HAART: report of two cases and review of the literature. *AIDS Patient Care and STDs* **19**, 486–494.

Yoshida, S., Mulder, D.W., Kurland, L.T., Chu, C.P. & Okazaki, H. (1986) Follow-up study on amyotrophic lateral sclerosis in Rochester, Minn., 1925 through 1984. *Neuroepidemiology* **5**, 61–70.

Young, A.C., Saunders, J. & Ponsford, J.R. (1976) Mental change as an early feature of multiple sclerosis. *Journal of Neurology, Neurosurgery and Psychiatry* **39**, 1008–1013.

Young, H.K., Barton, B.A., Waisbren, S. *et al.* (2008) Cognitive and psychological profile of males with Becker muscular dystrophy. *Journal of Child Neurology* **23**, 155–162.

Zaroff, C.M. & Isaacs, K. (2005) Neurocutaneous syndromes: behavioral features. *Epilepsy and Behavior* **7**, 133–142.

Zeviani, M., Moraes, C.T., DiMauro, S. *et al.* (1998) Deletions of mitochondrial DNA in Kearns–Sayre syndrome. *Neurology* **51**, 1525–1533.

Zhou, B., Westaway, S.K., Levinson, B., Johnson, M.A., Gitschier, J. & Hayflick, S.J. (2001) A novel pantothenate kinase gene (PANK2) is defective in Hallervorden–Spatz syndrome. *Nature Genetics* **28**, 345–349.

Ziegler, L.H. (1930) Psychotic and emotional phenomena associated with amyotrophic lateral sclerosis. *Archives of Neurology and Psychiatry* **24**, 930–936.

Zielasek, J., Bender, G., Schlesinger, S. *et al.* (2002) A woman who gained weight and became schizophrenic. *Lancet* **360**, 1392.

Zlotlow, M. & Kleiner, S. (1965) Catatonic schizophrenia associated with tuberose sclerosis. *Psychiatric Quarterly* **39**, 466–475.

Index

Note: page numbers in *italics* refer to figures, those in **bold** refer to tables and boxes

A

abscess, cerebral 452–3
absence seizures 312
  antiepileptics **367**
  atypical 312
  childhood 315–16
  continuous (absence status) 338–9
    therapy 375
  infants 318
  juvenile 316, 348–9
  myoclonic 318
acalculia, nominal aphasia 53
N-acetylaspartic acid (NAA) in MRS
  Alzheimer's disease 553
  SLE 520
acetylcholine and head injury 174
acetylcholinesterase inhibitors 595
achromatopsia 66
acid–base disturbances 665–6
acidosis 666
acquired epileptic opercular syndrome 318
acquired immune deficiency syndrome *see*
    AIDS–dementia complex; AIDS–
    related complex; HIV/AIDS
acrodynia, mercury toxicity 728
acromegaly 643–4
action/action disorders
  convergent route model 63
  neuropsychology 62–3
acute brain syndrome 9–13
acute confusional state 9–13
acyclovir 435–6
Addenbrooke's Cognitive Examination
    (ACE) 111
addictive disorders 689–721
  barbiturates 707–8
  benzodiazepines 708–10
  cannabis 711–13
  hallucinogens 716–19
  γ-hydroxybutyrate 708
  neurocircuitry 690, Plate 11.1
  neuroimaging 690
  opiates 710–11
  psychostimulants 713–16
  solvent abuse 719–21
  see also alcohol/alcohol abuse/alcoholism

Addison's disease 649–51
  investigations 650–1
  outcome 651
  psychiatric features 650
  treatment 651
adenoma, pituitary 295
adenovirus encephalitis 442
adolescents *see* juvenile *entries*
adrenal crisis 650
adrenal insufficiency 650–1
adrenal medullary transplantation,
    Parkinson's disease 761
adrenal steroid deficiency 649, 650
adrenocorticotropic hormone (ACTH)
  Addison's disease 650
  Cushing's syndrome 646
adrenoleucodystrophy 877
adrenomyeloneuropathy 877
Adult Memory and Information Processing
    Battery 151
affective disorders *see* mood disorders
affective experiences, temporal lobe
    epilepsy 320–1
Africa, viral encephalitides **432**
age/ageing
  Alzheimer's disease differential diagnosis
    551–2
  antiepileptic drug use 368–9
  epilepsy/epilepsy syndrome onset **314**
  head injury 194
  memory impairment 43
  of onset of epilepsy/epilepsy syndromes
    344
AGECAT 156
aggression
  affective 78
  alcohol abuse 691
  cerebral tumours 78
  disordered control 77–80
  epilepsy 78, 350–1
  frontal lobe dysfunction 80
  head injury 209–11
  hypothalamic tumours 295
  neural substrate for responses 78
  pharmacotherapy 251
  psychosurgery 79

  somnambulism 838
  see also violence
aggressive offenders, habitual 79–80
agitation, post-traumatic 182–3, 251
agnosia
  Alzheimer's disease 547–8
  apperceptive 64
  assessment 114–16
  auditory 68–9, 116
  colour 65–6, 116
  finger 69–70, 118
  focal cerebral disorders 23
  neuropsychology 63–9
  occipital lobe lesions 19
  tactile 69, 116
  unilateral spatial 67–8
  verbal auditory 52
  visual object 63–4, 67, 116
  visuospatial 66–7, 114–15
agoraphobia, head injury 220
agrammatism 48
agraphia 53
AIDS–dementia complex 406, 408–14,
    Plate 7.1, Plate 7.2
  MRS 140
AIDS-related complex 401
  see also HIV/AIDS
air encephalography 146
akathisia
  drug-induced 745, 746–7
    management 749, 751
    pathophysiology 750
  tardive 745, 749
    management 751–2
akinetic mutism
  diencephalic lesions 19
  diencephalic tumours 293
akinetic rigid syndromes 753
Albright's hereditary osteodystrophy
    637–8
alcohol abstinence syndrome 692–6, 699
  Wernicke's encephalopathy 701
alcohol/alcohol abuse/alcoholism
  aggression 691
  amblyopia 707
  blackouts 691–2

blood concentrations 691
central pontine myelinolysis 707
cerebellar degeneration 707
cerebral atrophy 134, 696–9
cognitive impairment 696–9
  HIV disease 414
dementia 590
epilepsy 331–2
head injury 199–200
  imaging 176
high-potency vitamin therapy 703
hypoglycaemia 623
insomnia 822
intoxication 691–2
Klinefelter's syndrome 673
Marchiafava–Bignami disease 707
nervous system effects 690–9
neuroimaging 698–9
neuropathology 697–8
neurosyphilis differential diagnosis 429
nicotinic acid deficiency 655
peripheral neuropathy 706–7
porphyria attacks 671
psychological deficits 697
psychometric testing 699
somnambulism 837–8
subdural haematoma differential
    diagnosis 513
tolerance 691
toxic action on brain 698, 704, 705, 706–7
tumour misdiagnosis 300
Wernicke's encephalopathy 699–700
withdrawal syndromes 692–6
see also delirium tremens; Korsakoff's
    syndrome; Wernicke's
    encephalopathy
alcoholic hallucinosis 693–4
alcoholic tremor 693
alcoholics
  Cushing's syndrome 648
  hypoglycaemia **621**
  hypopituitarism 641
  memory disorders/impairment 699
  multiple sclerosis 848
  progressive supranuclear palsy 776–7
  sarcoidosis 886
Alexander, G.E. 31
alexia
  acquired 55–6
  agnosic 52
  with agraphia 54–5
  occipital 52
  parietotemporal 54–5
  without agraphia 52
alkalosis 666
alkyl nitrites 719, 720
aluminium
  Alzheimer's disease 565
  dialysis encephalopathy 669
Alzheimer type II astrocytosis 729–30
Alzheimer's disease 43, 543, 544–65
  axonal damage 859
  clinical features 546–7
  course and outcome 554–5

diagnostic criteria 554
disease-modifying therapy 544, 559–60
early-onset 544, 560, 561
  autosomal dominant 560
  difference from late-onset 546–7
  familial 558
EEG use 128–9
environmental toxin exposure 721
epilepsy 331
familial 546
  early-onset 558
folate deficiency 660
frontotemporal dementia differential
    diagnosis 576
genetic factors 544, 558, 560–2
  genotype–phenotype correlations
    561–2
  plus psychosis 550
head injury 173, 191, 562
  boxing 239
investigation 552–3
late-onset 544, 546, 548
  brain changes 551–2
  differences from early-onset 546–7
management 544, 559–60, 595
MRI 137, Plate 3.2
MRS 140
neurochemistry 556–7
neuropathology 555–6
  Lewy bodies with/without 573
normal ageing differential diagnosis
    551
Parkinson's disease/parkinsonian
    syndrome 763–4
PET 142–3, Plate 3.4
poststroke 482
prevalence and incidence 545–6
SPECT 145
subacute encephalitis differential
    diagnosis 441
supportive organisations 593
symptoms 547–51
tumour misdiagnosis 300
vascular dementia relationship 570
very late-onset 544, 561
amantadine hydrochloride 758, 768
ambidexterity 46, 47
amblyopia, alcoholism 707
Americas, viral encephalitides **432**
γ-aminobutyric acid (GABA)
  Huntington's disease 583, 584
  Parkinson's disease/parkinsonian
    syndrome 755–6
  signalling in schizophrenia 87
γ-aminobutyric acid (GABA) receptor,
    alcohol effects 691
γ-aminobutyric acid$_A$ (GABA$_A$) receptors,
    benzodiazepine actions 709
aminolaevulinic acid (ALA) 671, 672
Ammon's horn sclerosis 319–20, 332
amnesia
  acute organic reactions 12
  alcoholic blackouts 691–2
  anterograde 32–3, 109

aseptic meningitis 451–2
brain tumours 284
  diencephalic 292
  temporal lobe 290
clinical picture 37–8
consolidation theory 40
contextual information acquisition 39
definition 36–7
dementia 590
  Alzheimer's disease 547
  Huntington's disease 579
denial 73
diencephalic 33–4
  lesions 19
diffuse cerebral disease 42–4
emotional reactions 37
epileptic
  temporal lobe 321
  transient 325
event ordering 38
focal disorders 22–3
hippocampal 34–5, 39
migraine 509
multiple trace theory 40–1
neuropsychological deficits 36–41
parahippocampal 39
personality disturbance 38
post-traumatic (PTA) 183–5, 204
  age at time of injury and 194
  children 241–2
  duration indicating outcome 188–9
  duration indicating severity of injury
    186–8
  pharmacotherapy 250
  rehabilitation 248
  selective 204–5
psychogenic 44–5
retrieval deficit 39
retrograde 38
  assessment 109
  disproportionate 41
  focal 41
  hemispheric differences 40
  lengthy 39–41
  temporal gradient 39–40
semanticisation hypothesis 40
storage deficit 39
stroke 490
subarachnoid haemorrhage 494–6
temporal lobe lesions 18
  medial 34–5
thinking process 38
time sense disturbance 38
transient 33
  epileptic 33, 325
  global 33, 362
amnesic syndrome 38–9
  chronic 6–7
  focal retrograde 44
amphetamines 713–15
  dopamine release stimulation 771
  hallucinosis 714
  Kleine–Levin syndrome of recurrent
    hypersomnia 833

narcolepsy treatment 828
psychosis 714–15
substituted 715–16
amusia 69
amygdala 30
amygdalectomy 79
amyloid angiopathies, cerebral 569–70
haemosiderin deposits 139
amyloid-β peptide/protein
Alzheimer's disease
cascade hypothesis 558–9
formation 557–8
deposition in head injury 173, 562
boxers 239
amyloid-β precursor protein (βAPP)
Alzheimer's disease 557–8
mutations 558, 560
NSAID actions 563
head injury 171
hereditary cerebral haemorrhage with
amyloidosis (Dutch-type) 569
amyotrophic lateral sclerosis 860
anaemia
megaloblastic 658
sideroblastic 774
see also pernicious anaemia
analgesic abuse 724
anaplastic astrocytoma **299**
anarthria, apraxic 52–3
aneurysms, intracranial/cerebral 492
acute clinical picture and management
493, 494
clipping 493, 494–5
giant 499
psychiatric sequelae 494, 495, 496, 497
angel dust 716
angiitis
granulomatous 407
see also vasculitis
angiography
cerebral 146
CT of tumours 299
angular gyrus syndrome 590
ankle reflex, hypothyroidism 629
anomia, colour 66
anorexia, hypopituitarism differential
diagnosis 642
anosognosia 72–4, 119
cerebral lateralisation 73–4
anoxia, cerebral in head injury 170
anterior circulation infarcts 475–6
anti-AChR antibodies 861
antibiotics
Lyme disease 454
syphilis 430
antibodies
autoimmune
antiphospholipid syndrome 521
SLE 513, 514–15, 521
small vessel vasculitides 525–6
see also serological tests
anticholinergic drugs
blepharospasm 786
oromandibular dystonia 786

Parkinson's disease/parkinsonian
syndrome 757
psychiatric complications 767–8
anticholinesterases
Alzheimer's disease 595
head injury 250–1
myasthenia gravis 861–2
Parkinson's disease 770
anticonvulsants 366–73
adverse effects/toxicity 367–8, 369, 370,
371, 377–8
cognitive problems 354
sexual dysfunction 349
brain tumour management 301
in clinical practice 371
drug interactions 368
antidepressants 378–9
antipsychotics 379
failed monotherapy 371–2
first line **367**, 371
GABAergic **372**
head injury 251, 253
hypocalcaemia induction 664
individual agents 369–71
modes of action **372**
newer 371
patient characteristics 368–9
in remission 372–3
second line/alternative **367**, 370, 371, 379
seizure type/syndrome 367
antidepressants
dementia 594–5
epilepsy 378–9
head injury-associated problems
aggression 251
mood disorders 250, 251–2
PTSD 250
HIV patients 420
stroke 486, 487
toxic effects 722–3
antidiuretic hormone (ADH)
deficiency 661
diabetes insipidus 644
antiepileptics see anticonvulsants
antifungal drugs in AIDS patients
candidiasis 420
cryptococcosis 421
anti-inflammatory drug protective effects,
Alzheimer's disease 563
antiphospholipid syndrome 517–18
aetiopathogenesis of neuropsychiatric
problems 520–1
overlap with SLE 517–18
antipsychotics
atypical in Parkinson's disease 770
dementia 595
diabetes mellitus risk 618
epilepsy 379
head injury 251, 252
HIV patients 420
hyperprolactinaemia induction 643
movement disorders 745–52
neurosyphilis 430
parkinsonism 746, 753

PET 143
stroke patients 489
tardive akathisia 749
tardive dyskinesia 747–8
antiretroviral drug therapy 421
depression 416
HAART 877
neuropsychiatric manifestations 401, 402
antiviral drugs, HSV 435–6
anxiety/anxiety disorders
acute organic reaction 13
brain tumours 285, 302
Cushing's syndrome 647
diabetes mellitus 619
epilepsy
ictal 335–6
interictal 342–3
treatment 378
fatigue 826
fear in temporal lobe epilepsy 320–1
generalised
head injury 218–19
stroke 487
head injury 218–23
depression 218
pharmacotherapy 251–2
HIV subjects 415
hyperthyroidism differential diagnosis
634
insomnia 822
insulinoma differential diagnosis 625
migraine 504–6
night terrors 838
Parkinson's disease/parkinsonian
syndrome 767
SLE 515, 517
stroke 487
subarachnoid haemorrhage 496–7
apathy, Parkinson's disease 771
aphasia
Alzheimer's disease 547
amnesic 53
anomic 53
Broca's 48, 49, 50–1, 56
classification 48–9
conduction 53, 56
cortical motor 50–1
dementia with Lewy bodies 574
dynamic 57
expressive 50–1
fluent 112
intelligence 54
jargon 56, 112
neuropsychology 45–58
nominal 53, 113
non-fluent 112
primary motor 50–1, 56
primary sensory 51–2, 56
psychiatric disturbance 56
receptive 51–2
striatal 54
subcortical 54
auditory/visual 52
thalamic 54

transcortical motor/sensory 54
Wernicke's 49, 51–2, 56
aphemia 52–3
aphonia 58
apolipoprotein E
Alzheimer's disease 544, 561
head injury 173, 191
apomorphine 761
apoptosis in head injury 172
apparent diffusion coefficient (ADC)
head injury 177
SLE 519
apraxia
Alzheimer's disease 547
constructional 62, 66–7
corpus callosum lesions 19
for dressing 62
focal cerebral disorders 23
ideational 62
ideomotor 61
limb kinetic 61
neuropsychology 60–2
aprosodias 48
aptitude tests **124**, 157
aqueduct stenosis 876
arboviruses **432**, 433
Argyll Robertson pupil, syphilis 424, 426
Army General Classification Test 190
arousal disorders, non-REM 361
arrhythmia-associated syncope 358, 365
arsenic poisoning 730
arteriosclerosis *see* atherosclerosis
arteriovenous malformations, epilepsy
331
arteritis
giant cell/temporal 526–7
Takayasu's 527
arthropod-borne viruses **432**, 433
arylsulphatase A activity 880, 881
aseptic meningitis *see* meningitis
Asia, viral encephalitides **432**
asomatognosia 72
Asperger's syndrome, facial expression
meaning 65
astatic seizures, myoclonic 318
astheno–emotional disorder, subarachnoid
haemorrhage 497
astrocytoma
case studies 288, 291, 300, 301
imaging *295*, **299**
pilocytic *295*, **299**
posterior fossa 296
temporal lobe *290*
astrocytosis, manganese toxicity 729–30
asymbolia, visual 54–5
ataxias
cerebellar 630
periodic 361
Wernicke's encephalopathy 701, 702
see also Friedreich's ataxia
atherosclerosis
large-artery 474, 475
multi-infarct dementia 566, 567
SLE-related risk 515

athetosis, hyperthyroidism 633
athletes *see* sport
atonic seizures 313
attention
assessment 109, 119
shift 119
tests **124**, 155
attention deficit hyperactivity disorder
(ADHD)
amphetamine therapy 713
paediatric head injury 241, 242, 252
Tourette's syndrome 788, 793
treatment 252, 793
attention disorders
consciousness impairment 9–10
deficit in stroke 490
frontal lobe lesions 17
multiple sclerosis 848
attribution bias, head injury 195–8, 243
auditory association cortex 47
Wernicke's aphasia 52
auditory perceptual defects 68–9
aura
cephalic 310
dysmnestic 321
epigastric 310, 320
epileptic 310, **320**, 335–6
frontal lobe **320**
temporal lobe epilepsy 320, 321–2
migraine with 360, 501, 502, 503, 504, 505,
506, 507
migraine without 501, 502, 503, 505, 506
Australasia, viral encephalitides **432**
autism
facial expression meaning 65
tuberous sclerosis 853
autoantibodies *see* antibodies
Autobiographical Memory Interview 151
autoimmune polyglandular syndrome
type 1 637, 649
type 2 649–50
automatisms 311, 336–7
absence with 312
frontal lobe epilepsy 323
temporal lobe epilepsy 322
autonomic dysfunction, diabetes mellitus
622
autonomic epilepsy 325
autopagnosia 118
autophagy, Huntington's disease 584
autoscopy 75
autosomal dominant arteriopathy with
subcortical infarcts and
leucoencephalopathy, cerebral
(CADASIL) 502, 558, 569
autosomal dominant nocturnal frontal lobe
epilepsy 322, 326
autosomal dominant temporal lobe epilepsy
326
autotopagnosia 74
awakening, generalised tonic–clonic
seizures 316
axonal injury 859
see also diffuse axonal injury

B
BACE (β-amyloid-cleaving peptide) 557,
558, 560, 563
inhibitors 559
bacterial infections
abscess due to 452–3
see also meningitis
Balint's syndrome 66
barbiturates 370, 707–8
intoxication 708
overdose 708
psychostimulant toxic reaction treatment
715
status epilepticus 375
tolerance 708
barotrauma, pulmonary 889
basal areas of brain
amnesia in subarachnoid haemorrhage-
related damage 495–6
personality changes in traumatic damage
206–7
basal cell carcinoma syndrome, naevoid
281
basal ganglia
calcification 877–8
disorders 20
basilar artery
aneurysms 499
migraine related to 501
occlusion 477–8
Batten–Bielschowsky disease *see* Kufs'
disease
B-cell lymphoma, AIDS 404–5
Becker muscular dystrophy 863–4
behaviour
clinical assessment 107
frontal lobe function 116, 118
Behavioural Assessment of Dysexecutive
Syndrome 153
behavioural disturbances
Alzheimer's disease 549
brain tumours 287
chronic organic reaction 15
EEG abnormalities 126
executive syndromes 58–9
head injury
children 242–3
pharmacotherapy 251
rehabilitation 247–8
Huntington's disease 580
neurofibromatosis 856
risk-taking behaviour and anterior
communicating artery aneurysms
496
thalamic infarcts 478
Turner's syndrome 675
Behavioural Inattention Test 147–8
behavioural therapy, Tourette's syndrome
792
Behçet's syndrome 884–5
Bender–Gestalt Test 147
bends 889
benign partial epilepsy of childhood 314
Benton Visual Retention Test 150

benzodiazepines 708–10
  abuse 709
  dependence 708, 709
  GABA$_A$ receptor actions 709
  head injury 251
  metabolism 709
  sedative effects 710
  seizures 370
    status epilepticus 375
  tolerance 708
  withdrawal 709–10
bereavement reactions and AIDS 418
beriberi 652
  Wernicke's encephalopathy 700–1
beta-blockers, head injury 251
bicycle helmets 239–40
Binswanger's disease 569
biofeedback treatment, epilepsy 374–5
biomechanics, head injury 168
biopsy, cortical in primary angiitis 524
bipolar disorder
  insulinoma differential diagnosis 625
  interictal 341
  poststroke 487
  post-traumatic 215–16
birth injury, epilepsy due to 328–9
bismuth poisoning 730–1
bizarre disorientation, basilar artery
    occlusion 478
bleeding, intracranial 474
  traumatic 170
  see also intracerebral haemorrhage,
    subarachnoid haemorrhage
blepharospasm 785–6
Blessed's Dementia Scale 156
blindness, denial 73
blood alcohol concentration (BAC) 691
blood oxygenation-level-dependent
    (BOLD) contrast imaging 140
blood–brain barrier
  glucose transport 623
  HIV infection 405
  multiple sclerosis 846
body awareness disturbances in stroke 490
body image disturbances
  assessment 118–19
  depression 76
  epilepsy 76
  focal cerebral disorders 23
  LSD effects 717
  migraine 509–10
  neuropsychology 71–7
  non-organic psychiatric illness 76–7
  parietal lobe lesions 18
  schizophrenia 76, 77
  unilateral unawareness/neglect 71
border-zone infarcts 476
Borrelia burgdorferi 453–4
Boston Naming Test 148
botulinum toxin
  blepharospasm 786
  spasmodic torticollis 784–5
  Tourette's syndrome 793
boxing 237–9

bradycardia, ictal 358, 365
bradykinesia
  parkinsonism 746
  Parkinson's disease/parkinsonian
    syndrome 754
bradyphrenia, progressive supranuclear
    palsy 776–7
brain, regional dysfunction 77–89
brain electrical activity mapping (BEAM)
    130
brain imaging see named modalities
brain injury
  children 240–3
    mild multiple 227
    non-accidental 170
    pharmacotherapy 252
  diving injuries 888–90
  see also head injury (traumatic brain
    injury)
brain metabolism, regional 141
brain systems 30–1
brain tumour polyposis syndrome 1 855
brain tumours see tumours
brainstem lesions 19–20
Brixton Test 153
Broca, Paul 30, 31
bromocriptine
  head injury 209
  Parkinson's disease/parkinsonian
    syndrome 760
Bruce, D. 31
Brueghel's syndrome 785
buspirone 512
butyrophenones 723

C
CADASIL (cerebral autosomal dominant
    arteriopathy with subcortical infarcts
    and leucoencephalopathy) 502, 558,
    569
  haemosiderin deposits 139
caeruloplasmin 773–4
café au lait spots 855
caffeine, insomnia 822
CAG repeat, Huntington's disease 577
calcification
  hypoparathyroidism 639, **640**, 641
  intracranial 132
  MELAS 641
calcitonin gene-related peptide (CGRP)
  antagonists 511
calcium channel blockade by antiepileptics
  372
calcium level disorders 663–4
  uraemia 668
California Verbal Learning Test 150
callosotomy 374
Cambridge Examination for Mental
    Disorders of the Elderly (CAMDEX)
    156–7
Cambridge Neuropsychological Test
    Automated Battery (CANTAB) 155
candidiasis, AIDS 404, 420
cannabinoid receptors 712

cannabinoids 711–12
cannabis 711–13
  acute effects 712
  depersonalisation 712, 713
  psychiatric disorder 712–13
  tolerance 712
Capgras syndrome/delusion 65
  migraine 509
  stroke 488
carbamazepine 367, 369
  head injury 251
carbidopa 839
carbon disulphide poisoning 732
carcinoma, neuropsychiatric manifestations
    868–71, 872
cardiac causes of syncope 365
  epilepsy differential diagnosis **358**, 358–9
cardiac embolism 475
cardiolipin antibodies 518
cardiological investigations in suspected
    epilepsy 365
cardiovascular risk factors, Alzheimer's
    disease 562–3
caregiver burden
  dementia 594
  stroke 484
  see also family/relatives
carotid artery, internal
  aneurysm 499
  occlusion 476
    transient ischaemic attacks 479
carpal tunnel syndrome
  acromegaly 644
  uraemia 667
carpopedal spasm 638
caspases and head injury 172
catamenial seizures 333
cataplexy
  epilepsy differential diagnosis 361
  narcolepsy 823, 824–5, 827–8
  treatment 828–9
catastrophic reaction 107, 119
  chronic organic reactions 16
catatonia
  encephalitis lethargica 444, 448
  fatal 723
catechol O-methyltransferase (COMT) 761
catecholamine antagonists 250
cavernous haemangiomas 331
cavum septum pellucidum 239
CD4 (helper) T cells in HIV disease
  counts 400, 409
  receptor 399
cell damage markers in head injury 174
cell death
  apoptosis in head injury 172
  see also neuronal loss/death
central nervous system (CNS)
  depressant effects of alcohol 691
  excitability in delirium tremens 696
  metastatic involvement 868
central pontine myelinolysis 707
centrotemporal spikes, benign childhood
    epilepsy 314

cephalic aura 310
cerebellar ataxia, hypothyroidism 630
cerebellar degeneration
  alcoholism 707
  subacute 869
cerebellar tumours 296–7
cerebral abscess 452–3
cerebral amyloid angiopathies 139, 569–70
cerebral angiography 146
cerebral anoxia, head injury 170
cerebral artery aneurysms, middle 493
cerebral artery occlusion
  anterior 476, 477
  imaging 480
  middle 475, 477
  posterior 477
cerebral atrophy
  alcohol abuse/alcoholism 134, 696–9
  CT 133–4
  Cushing's syndrome 649
  dementia 133
  dentatorubral-pallidoluysian **327**, 328
  head injury
    boxers 239
    imaging 175–6
  HIV-associated 407–8
  schizophrenia 133–4
cerebral autosomal dominant arteriopathy
    with subcortical infarcts and
    leucoencephalopathy (CADASIL)
    502, 558, 569
  haemosiderin deposits 139
cerebral blood flow
  Alzheimer's disease 553
  delirium tremens 696
  head injury 178–9
  SLE 520
cerebral disease, diffuse 42–4
cerebral disorders
  acute 4
  chronic 4
  focal 5, 17–20
    diffuse lesion differentiation 22–3
  generalised (diffuse) 5
    focal lesion differentiation 22–3
  regional 29–30
  Tourette's syndrome 791
  see also organic reaction
cerebral dominance for language 46–8
cerebral dysfunction, memory failure 110
cerebral function lateralisation 31
cerebral gas embolism 889
cerebral haemorrhage see intracerebral
    haemorrhage
cerebral hemispheres, traumatic damage
    200, **201**
cerebral infarction, EEG use 127
cerebral ischaemia
  lead toxicity 726
  subarachnoid haemorrhage 493
  see also ischaemic stroke; multi-infarct
    dementia; transient ischaemic attacks
cerebral lesions
  insomnia 835
  schizophrenia association 85–6, 89

cerebral localisation 30–1
cerebral malaria 454
cerebral metabolism
  Alzheimer's disease 553
  head injury 172, 178–9, 232–3
    post-concussion syndrome 232–3
cerebral oedema
  head injury 170
  tumours 285
cerebral sclerosis, diffuse 852–3
cerebral tumours see tumours
cerebral vasculature see cerebrovascular
    disease
cerebral vasculitis 715
  HIV disease 407
cerebrospinal fluid (CSF)
  alcohol effects 698
  multiple sclerosis 845
  Wernicke's encephalopathy 702
cerebrospinal fluid (CSF), assessment/
    examination/tests 131–2
  dementia 592
  HIV-associated dementia 410–11
  meningitis
    aseptic 450, 451
    bacterial 449
  protein content 131–2
  syphilis 423, 427–8
    treatment monitoring and relapse
    430–1
cerebrovascular accidents
  hypothyroidism 630
  medial temporal amnesia 34
  psychostimulants 715
  see also stroke
cerebrovascular disease 473–552
  epilepsy in 331
  tumour misdiagnosis 300
cerebrovascular pathology/lesions
  epilepsy 331
  head injury 169–70
  syphilis 423
CGRP antagonists, migraine 511
channelopathies, epilepsy syndromes **327**,
  372
chemobrain 871
chemotherapy
  brain tumours 302
  cognitive change 871
chickenpox see varicella-zoster virus
children
  adrenoleucodystrophy 877
  agenesis of the corpus callosum 890–1
  brain/head injury 240–3
    mild multiple, and outcome 227
    non-accidental 170
    pharmacotherapy 252
  epilepsy
    antiepileptics 368–9
    cognitive and psychosocial impact 353,
    354
    idiopathic 314–15
    self-induced 317
    situation-related 319
    symptomatic or cryptogenic 315

general paresis in syphilis 426
HIV-associated progressive
    encephalopathy 412–13
Huntington's disease 581–2, 583
hyperekplexia 360–1
hypocalcaemia 664
infections and Tourette's syndrome 792
Kufs' disease 881
lead toxicity 725–6
malnutrition 651–2
mercury toxicity 728
neurofibromatosis 856
posterior fossa tumours 296–7, 303
somnambulism 837
see also infancy
chlordiazepoxide 696
chlorpromazine
  EEG abnormalities 126
  psychostimulant toxic reaction treatment
  715
cholesterol and Alzheimer's disease 565
cholinergic crises 731
cholinergic system
  Alzheimer's disease 556
  head injury 174
    therapeutic targeting 250–1
  Huntington's disease 583
cholinesterase inhibitors
  Alzheimer's disease 595
  head injury 250–1
chorea
  Huntington's disease 578
  hyperthyroidism 633
choreoacanthocytosis 879–80
choreoathetosis 361
chronic fatigue syndrome 863
chronic progressive external
    ophthalmoplegia (CPEO) 883
Churg–Strauss syndrome 525, 526
Chvostek's sign 638, 664
circle of Willis aneurysm 499
cistern enlargement, Wilson's disease 773
citalopram, head injury 252
clinical assessment 103–57
  air encephalography 146
  ancillary investigations 123–46
  appearance 107
  behaviour 107
  cerebral angiography 146
  cognitive state 108–16, **117–18**, 118–19
  CT 132–4
  electroencephalography 124–30
  emotional reactions 107
  encephalography 146
  functional MRI 140–1, Plate 3.3
  history-taking 103–4
  isotope cisternography 146
  lumbar puncture 131–2
  magnetic resonance spectroscopy 139–40
  magnetoencephalography 130–1
  memory 109, 110, 114
  mental state 105, 107–16, **117–18**, 118–19
  mood 107
  MRI 134–5, *136*, 137–9, Plate 3.1, Plate 3.2
  neurotransmitter imaging 145–6

PET 141–4, Plate 3.4
physical examination 104–5, **106**
psychometric 119–23
radioisotope scans 146
skull radiography 132
special investigations 123–47
SPECT 144–5, Plate 3.6
clobazam 370
clomipramine 793
clonazepam
　REM sleep behaviour disorder 839
　seizures 370
clonic seizures 312
　frontal lobe epilepsy 323
clonidine 792, 839
CLOX clock drawing 115
clozapine 770
　EEG abnormalities 126
cluster headache 501
CMV see cytomegalovirus encephalitis
cocaine 713–15
　hallucinosis 714
　psychosis 714–15
coccidioidomycosis 404
cognitive affective syndrome, cerebellar
　296, 297
cognitive and mental impairment
　age-related decline in schizophrenia 81
　alcoholic/alcoholism 696–9
　Alzheimer's disease 547, 551
　anosognosia 73
　aseptic 451
　benzodiazepines 708
　brain tumours 283–4
　　adverse effects of treatment 284, 302,
　　　303
　　corpus callosum 289
　　frontal lobe 286–7
　　management 302
　　parietal lobe 291–2
　　posterior fossa 296, 303
　　prevalence **283**
　　temporal lobe 289–90
　cannabis-induced 713
　cerebral venous sinus thrombosis 528
　chronic organic reaction 15
　Creutzfeldt–Jakob disease 587
　Cushing's syndrome 648
　dementia 133
　　global 9
　　with Lewy bodies 571, 572
　dystrophia myotonica 866
　epilepsy 351–4
　　in epilepsy syndromes 318, 321, 324,
　　　325
　　simple partial seizures 310–11
　Friedreich's ataxia 857
　head injury 198–9, 202–5
　　boxers 238
　　children 241
　　and depression 217–18
　　mild traumatic brain injury 225–6
　　personality change 207–8
　　pharmacotherapy 250–1
　　rehabilitation 246–7

HIV-associated 408–14
HSV-associated 436
Huntington's disease 579–80
hyperthyroidism 633
hypoglycaemia 620–1
hypoparathyroidism 639
hypothyroidism 628
Klinefelter's syndrome 672–3
lead toxicity 725–6
meningitis 449–50
migraine 510
mild 565–6
multiple sclerosis 847, 848–9, **850**
neurofibromatosis 856
Parkinson's disease/parkinsonian
　syndrome 762–4, 769
progressive supranuclear palsy 776
SLE 515–17
stroke 478, 482–3
　rehabilitation 490–1
subarachnoid haemorrhage 494–6
symptom-related in schizophrenia 81–2
tuberous sclerosis 853
Turner's syndrome 674
vascular 566–71
Wernicke's encephalopathy 701–2
Wilson's disease 776
see also mental state examinations
cognitive–behavioural therapy
　PTSD in head injury 250
　seizure patients
　　dissociative 380
　　epileptic 375, 379
Cognitive Estimates Test 116, 152
cognitive impairment, transient in poorly-
　controlled epilepsy 353–4
cognitive state
　assessment 108–16, **117–18**, 118–19
　　initial **111**
　extended examination 110–16, **117–18**,
　　118–19
　routine examination 108–10
coilings, aneurysms 493, 494–5
cold preference, hyperthyroidism 634
colloid cyst 292
coma 5–6
　acute organic reactions 9
　alcoholic 691
　　treatment 692
　diabetic 621–2
　EEG use 128
　head injury 171, 180–1
　hypernatraemia 661
　hyperosmolar non-ketotic 621–2
　see also Glasgow Coma Scale
coma vigil see akinetic mutism
commissures, surgical section 891
communicating artery aneurysms
　anterior (ACoA) 492, 494, 495, 496
　posterior (PCoA) 493
communication problems, post-traumatic
　204
community care, dementia 594
community rehabilitation, head injury
　249

compensation
　head injury 195–8, 233, 243, 244, 245
　whiplash injury 235, 236
comprehension assessment 112–13
Comprehensive Assessment and Referral
　Evaluation Schedule (CARE) 156
compulsions
　encephalitis lethargica 446
　see also obsessive–compulsive disorder
computed tomography (CT) 132–4
　angiography 146
　cerebral atrophy 133–4
　cerebral venous sinus thrombosis 528
　dementia 592
　　Alzheimer's disease 552
　　Huntington's disease 580, 581
　epilepsy 364
　head injury 175
　　assessing severity 185
　　boxers 238
　　MRI advantages 135
　schizophrenia 83
　stroke 480
　subdural haematoma 513
　tumours 297–8
computed tomography angiography,
　tumours 299
computerised psychological tests 155
concentration
　assessment 109
　Cushing's syndrome 648
　frontal lobe lesions 17
　impaired 10
　　hyperthyroidism 633
　　multiple sclerosis 848
concussion 180
　athlete 237
　biomechanics 168
　children 243
　definition 180
　momentary 'concussion' in whiplash
　　injury 235
　multiple 227–8
　symptoms 228, 230
　see also post-concussion syndrome
confabulation 41–2
　assessment 109
　diencephalic tumours 292
　Korsakoff's syndrome 34
　post-traumatic 181, 184
　　pharmacotherapy 252
　provoked 41–2
　source memory deficits 42
　spontaneous 42
　subarachnoid haemorrhage 495
　Wernicke's encephalopathy 702
confidentiality, HIV testing 419
confusion 5
confusional state
　acute 9–13
　migraine 508–9, 509, 511
　post-traumatic 181–2
congenital malformations
　antiepileptic drug-related 368
　epilepsy due to 328–9

conscious awareness level **111**, 112
consciousness, impairment and loss 4
  acute organic reactions 9–11
  attention disorders 9–10
  brain tumours 284
  clouding 5
  EEG use 128
  head injury 168, 171, 180–1
    duration indicating severity 186
    as outcome predictor 188, 227
  in migraine 508, 511
  transient 357
  uraemic encaphalopathy 667
  see also syncope
consent, HIV tests 419
consolidation theory 40
constructional difficulties, assessment 114–15
contingent negative variation (CNV) 129–30
continuous positive airway pressure (CPAP), sleep apnoea syndrome 831
continuous spike–waves in slow-wave sleep, epilepsy with 318–19
contusions, brain 168
conversion disorders 21, 57–8
  head injury 221
  tumour misdiagnosis with 301
convulsions, psychostimulants 715
cooperation level **111**
coordination abnormalities, neurosyphilis 427
corpus callosum
  agenesis 890–1
  developmental defects 890–1
  language 47
  lesions 19
  resection in epilepsy 374
  tumours 289
cortical abnormalities, Turner's syndrome 675
cortical atrophy, Wilson's disease 773
cortical biopsy in primary angiitis 524
cortical border-zone infarcts 476
cortical dysplasia, focal 329
cortical spreading depression and migraine 503
cortical–striatal–thalamic–cortical system, Tourette's syndrome 791
corticobasal degeneration 575, 778–9
corticosteroids *see* steroids
counselling
  pretest for HIV 418–19
  see also genetic counselling
coxsackieviruses 437
cranial (giant cell) arteritis 526–7
cranial fossa tumours, posterior 295–7
cranial nerve palsies
  HIV-associated 413
  SLE 518
cranial nerves
  electrical accidents 888
  sarcoidosis 885
craniopharyngiomas 295–6, **299**, 304

C-reactive protein and SLE 514
creatine signal in MRS 520
Creutzfeldt–Jakob disease (CJD) 584, 585–8
  clinical features 586–7
  EEG use 129
  epidemiology 586
  familial 588
  familial forms 588
  MRI 135, *136*
  pathology 587–8
  variant 585, 586, 587
criminality
  epilepsy 349–51
  Klinefelter's syndrome 673
crowding of thoughts 311
crush closed head injuries, biomechanics 168
crying (pathological) in head injury 218, 252
cryptococcosis, AIDS 404, 421
cryptogenic epilepsy syndromes **314**, 315
cryptotrauma, concept 195
cursive seizures 311
Cushing's syndrome 646–9
  aetiology of mental disturbances 648–9
  outcome 649
  physical features 646–7
  psychiatric features 647–8
Cyclists' helmets 239–40
cyclophosphamide 521
cyst
  colloid 292
  epidermal third ventricle 293
cysticercosis 454–5
cytomegalovirus encephalitis
  HIV disease 403–4, 421
  HIV-associated dementia differential diagnosis 411

D
D₂ receptors
  blocking by antipsychotics 643
  PET 143
Dax, Marc 30
day patient rehabilitation, head injury 248–9
deafness, denial 73
death in epilepsy
  rate 366
  sudden 375–6
decompression illness 888–9
deep vein thrombosis, tumour-related 301
degenerative disorders, epilepsy 331
dehydroepiandrosterone (DHEA) 650, 651
déjà vu 310
  temporal lobe epilepsy 321
delirium 7–8, 10
  aseptic meningitis 451
  clinical features 9–13
  dementia differential diagnosis **23**
  hypernatraemia 661
  occupational 11
  postictal 339
  post-traumatic 181–2
  psychomotor behaviour 11

SLE 515
  Wernicke's encephalopathy 701
delirium tremens 7, 693, 694–6
  aetiology 696
  clinical features 695
  hallucinations 13
  outcome 695–6
  psychomotor behaviour 11
  sedation 696
  treatment 696
delusion(s) 5
  acute organic reactions 11
  Alzheimer's disease 549–50
  brain tumours 285
  chronic organic reactions 15
  schizophrenic symptoms 21–2
  stroke 488
delusional misidentification, post-traumatic 181, 211
dementia 8–9, 543–615
  assessment and differential diagnosis 588–93
  cerebral atrophy 133
  classification **8**, 543–4
  clinical picture 544
  cognitive impairment 133
  cortical **20**
  delirium differential diagnosis **23**
  dialysis 669
  diet 565, 590
  EEG use 128–9
  with familial calcification of basal ganglia 877–8
  folate deficiency 659–60
  frontal lobe 145
  history-taking 589–90
  HIV-associated 406, 408–14
    imaging 410
  imaging 592
    Alzheimer's disease 552–3
    Creutzfeldt–Jakob disease 587
    Huntington's disease 580–1
  insulinoma differential diagnosis 625
  with Lewy bodies, imaging 574
  management 593–5
  motor neurone disease 859–60
  multi-infarct 566
    imaging 567
    SPECT 145
  multiple sclerosis 849, **850**
  neurological examination 105, **106**, 591
  normal-pressure hydrocephalus 871, 874
  P300 response 130
  paralytic (*see* general paresis)
  Parkinson's disease/parkinsonian syndrome 762–4
  personality change 6
  poststroke 482–3, 569
  post-traumatic 191
  presenile 128–9
  pugilistica 238
  questionnaires **124**, 156–7
  rating scales **124**, 156–7
  REM sleep behaviour disorder 839

reversible 656–7
sarcoidosis 886
semantic 43, 574
senile 128–9
speech abnormalities 16
subacute cerebellar degeneration 869
tumour misdiagnosis 300
tumours causing
  diencephalic 293, 294
  frontal lobe 286, 287
vitamin B$_{12}$ deficiency 656–7
see also Alzheimer's disease;
    frontotemporal dementia; multi-
    infarct dementia; subcortical
    dementia; vascular dementia
demyelinating polyneuropathies, HIV-
    associated inflammatory 413
dendrites
  alcohol effects 698
  HIV-related dysmorphology 407–8
dental amalgam 726–7
dentatorubral-pallidoluysian atrophy **327**,
    328
dependence
  benzodiazepines 708, 709
  opioids 710
depersonalisation 72
  acute organic reactions 12
  cannabis 712, 713
depression
  acromegaly 643
  acute organic reaction 13
  Addison's disease 650
  Alzheimer's disease
    as aetiological factor 565
    comorbid 550–1
  bacterial meningitis 450
  body image disturbances 76
  brain tumours 284, 302
  counter-regulatory hormones 620
  Cushing's syndrome 647, 648
  dementia 550–1, 565, 594–5
    Huntington's disease 580
  diabetes mellitus 618, 619–20
  diabetic control 620
  dystonia musculorum deformans 783
  fatigue 826
  folate deficiency 659
  HIV subjects 415–16, 420
  hyperparathyroidism 636
  hypersomnia 835, 836
  hyperthyroidism 633, 635
  hypopituitarism 641
  hypothyroidism 628, 629
  interictal 340–2
  memory impairment 45
  metabolic pathways 620
  migraine 504–6
  motor neurone disease 859
  narcolepsy association 829
  neurosyphilis 426
  normal-pressure hydrocephalus 874
  Parkinson's disease/parkinsonian
    syndrome 764–7

post-traumatic 216–18
  pharmacotherapy 251–2
primary motor aphasia 56
sarcoidosis **886**
SLE 515, 517
stress response 620
stroke 484–7
stupor 25
subarachnoid haemorrhage 496–7
symptoms 22
Wilson's disease 776
see also antidepressants
derealisation
  acute organic reactions 12
  post-traumatic 211
desipramine 839
desmopressin 644
developmental defects
  Gilles de la Tourette syndrome 790
  see also congenital malformations
dexamfetamine
  ADHD treatment 793
  narcolepsy treatment 828
diabetes insipidus 644–5
  primary polydipsia differential diagnosis
    645–6
diabetes mellitus 618–22
  aetiology 618
  Alzheimer's disease 563–4
  brain damage 620–1
  depression 619–20
  diagnosis 618
  dietary restrictions 618–19
  genetic factors 618
  neurological complications 622
diabetic coma 621–2
diabetic ketoacidosis 621
Diagnostic and Statistical Manual of Mental
    Disorders (4th. edition)
  delirium **7**, 8
  dementia **8**
  Structured Clinical Interview in head
    injury 202
dialysis encephalopathy 669
dialysis equilibrium syndrome 669
diazepam
  psychostimulant toxic reaction treatment
    715
  Tourette's syndrome 792
diencephalic epilepsy 325
diencephalic tumours 292–5
diencephalon
  anterograde amnesia 32–3
  lesions 19–20
  see also amnesia, diencephalic
diet, dementia and 590
  Alzheimer's disease 565
diffuse axonal injury 168–9, 171–2
  mild brain injury 224
diffuse poliodystrophy, HIV disease 407
diffusion-weighted imaging 134
  head injury 177
  SLE 518, 519
  stroke 480

Diogenes syndrome 592
diplopia, narcolepsy differential diagnosis
    827
disability/disablement
  head injury (legal issues) 243–5
  WHO definition 247
disconnection syndromes 891
disgust recognition 65
disinhibition
  assessment 119
  brain tumours 288
  frontal lobe lesions 17
  sexual 209, 253, 351
disorganisation 82
disorganisation syndrome 82–3
disorientation, bizarre in basilar artery
    occlusion 478
displacement, illusions 74–6
dispositional changes, frontal lobe tumours
    287
dissociative disorders, tumour misdiagnosis
    301
dissociative seizures 354–5, 359–62, 379–80
  treatment 379–80
distal muscular dystrophy 863
distractibility, Huntington's disease 579
diuretics, thiazide 644–5
diving, brain injuries 888–90
  decompression illness 888–9
  gas toxicity 888
  sequelae 889–90
  shallow water 889–90
dizziness, post-traumatic 234–5
  see also vertigo
donepezil
  dementia 595
  head injury 250–1
  subarachnoid haemorrhage 496
dopamine
  deficiency in Parkinson's disease 755–6
  head injury 174
dopamine agonists
  head injury 209
  Parkinson's disease/parkinsonian
    syndrome 759–61
  psychiatric aspects of treatment 768–70
dopamine dysregulation syndrome 772
dopamine receptor blockade 723
dopamine transporter (DAT)
  ligands 143–4
  Parkinson's disease 143–4, Plate 3.5
dopamine-blocking agents, Tourette's
    syndrome 791
dopaminergic system
  Huntington's disease 583–4
  neuroleptic actions 749–50
  neurotransmitter imaging 145–6
  Parkinson's disease/parkinsonian
    syndrome 755–6
  PET 143
  schizophrenia 87
  synapse 758
doppelgänger phenomenon 75
Dravet's syndrome 318

dreams, pre-sleep 825
dressing
  apraxia 62
  dyspraxia 116
driving and epilepsy 377
drug-induced seizures 332–3
drug interactions, antiepileptics 368
  with antidepressants 378–9
  with antipsychotics 379
drug misuse (illicit substances)
  epilepsy 332
  head injury 199–200
    imaging 176
  HIV patients
    cognitive impairment 414
    psychological morbidity 418
  vasculitis associated with 523
drug therapy
  brain tumours
    cytotoxic agents 302
    medical management 301, 302
    novel agents 304
  dementia 594–5
    Alzheimer's disease 544, 559–60, 595
  diabetes mellitus risk 618
  EEG abnormalities 126
  head injury 174, 250–4
  HIV disease
    opportunistic infection prophylaxis
      419–20
    psychiatric disorders 420
  insomnia 822
  migraine 511–12
  myasthenic syndrome induction 862
  PET examination of influx into brain
    143
  porphyria attack precipitation 671
  SLE 521
  stroke 479
  toxic effects 721–4
  uraemia 668
  withdrawal effects 723–4
  see also named drugs and groups of dugs
DSM-IV Structured Clinical Interview, head
  injury 202
duality, physical 510
dual-task processing impairment, post-
  traumatic 202, 203–4
Duchenne muscular dystrophy 863–4
Dutch-type hereditary cerebral
  haemorrhage with amyloidosis 569
dysarthria 112
  neurosyphilis 427
  progressive supranuclear palsy 776
dyscalculia 70
dysembryoblastic neuroepithelial tumours
  329
dysgraphia, psychogenic 58
dyskinesia
  levodopa side effects 760
  paroxysmal 361
dyslexia
  developmental 55–6
  neuroimaging 55–6

  phonological 55
  psychogenic 58
dysmnestic aura 321
dysphagia, Wilson's disease 773
dysphasia
  central 53
  corpus callosum lesions 19
  fluent 112
  language function assessment **114**
  nominal 53
  non-fluent 112
  parietal lobe lesions 18
  syntactical 53
dyspraxia 114–16
  assessment 116
  constructional 114–15
dysprosody 112
dyssomnias, intrinsic 820–3
dystonias 780–6
  causation 781
  cervical 783–5
  cranial 785–6
  dopa-responsive 782
  DYT1 781–2, 783, 795
  fixed 794
  focal 781
  generalised torsion 781–3
  genetic factors 781–2
  idiopathic 781
  laryngeal 786
  musculorum deformans 781–3
  oromandibular 785–6
  treatment 782–3
  Wilson's disease 772
dystonic reactions, acute
  drug-induced 745, 747, 750
    management 751
  pathophysiology 750
dystrophia myotonica 864–7
  clinical features 865–6
  differential diagnosis 866
  genetic factors 864–5
  psychiatric aspects 866–7
  treatment 866
dystrophin gene 864
DYT1 gene 781–2

E
EBV *see* Epstein–Barr virus
echo-phenomena, Tourette's syndrome 788
echoplanar imaging (EPI) 140
echoviruses 437
ecstasy 715–16
education, protective effects in Alzheimer's
  disease 564
education
  and information, patient/relatives
  dementia 593
  epilepsy 376–7
  post-concussion syndrome 249
EEG *see* electroencephalography (EEG)
elderly patients
  antiepileptics 369
  drug therapy toxic effects 722

  hypernatraemia 661
  stroke rehabilitation 491
electrical accidents 887–8
electrical stimulation of vagus nerve,
    epilepsy 374
electroconvulsive therapy (ECT)
  EEG interpretation 126
  general paresis 430
  Parkinson's disease/parkinsonian
    syndrome 767
electroencephalography (EEG) 124–30
  abnormalities 125, 126
  characteristics 124–5
  dementia 592
    Alzheimer's disease 553
    Creutzfeldt–Jakob disease 587
    Huntington's disease 580
  epilepsy 126–7
  head injury 174–5
  HIV-associated dementia 410
  hypoglycaemia 626
  limitations 125–6
  seizures 362–4
  subacute sclerosing panencephalitis 440
  tumours 297
  uses 126–9
  Wernicke's encephalopathy 702
electrolyte disturbances 660–5
electromyography (EMG) 146–7
electrophysiogical studies, mild traumatic
    brain injury 225
  post-concussion syndrome 233
embolism, cardiac 475
emotional decision-making tests 155
emotional disorders
  Addison's disease 650
  diabetes mellitus 618
  hyperthyroidism 632
  lability/incontinence
    assessment 119
    diencephalic lesions 19
    head injury 218, 252
  LSD 718
  motor neurone disease 859
  multiple sclerosis 850, 851–2
  myasthenia gravis 862
  Parkinson's disease/parkinsonian
    syndrome 766
  porphyrias 670
emotional–motivational blunting disorder
  497
emotional precipitation
  migraine 507
  subarachnoid haemorrhage 498–9
emotional reactions
  acute organic reactions 13
  amnesia 37
  assessment 119
  chronic organic reactions 16
  clinical assessment 107
  glucose blood levels 620
  head injury 195
    affecting recovery 230
  hypoparathyroidism 639

ketone bodies 620
stroke 486–7
employment *see* occupation
encephalitis (non-viral)
 EEG use 127
 limbic paraneoplastic **299**
 periaxalis diffusa 852–3
 Rasmussen's 315
encephalitis (viral) 431–9
 adenovirus 442
 AIDS-related 403–4, Plate 7.1, Plate 7.2
 causes **432**, 433–49
  geographically-restricted **432**, 433–4
  HIV 406, 408–14
  non-geographically-restricted **432**,
   434–8
 clinical presentation 432–3
 cytomegalovirus
  in HIV disease 403–4, 421
  HIV-associated dementia differential
   diagnosis 411
 EEG use 127, *128*
 influenza 442–3, 448
 Japanese B 433
 mumps 438
 see also herpes simplex virus encephalitis;
  postencephalitic disorders
encephalitis lethargica 443–9
 hyperkinetic-type 444, 447
 parkinsonian-type 444
 postencephalitic parkinsonism 753
encephalography 146
encephalomyelitis, mixed form 869–70
encephalomyopathy, mitochondrial 882–4
encephalopathy
 acute nicotinic acid deficiency 654–5
 Binswanger's 569
 bismuth poisoning 730–1
 brainstem involvement 869–70
 dialysis 669
 HIV-associated 406, 408–14
  progressive of childhood 412–13
 hypertensive 499
 lead 725
 limbic 870–1, *872*
 metabolic disturbance 870
 radiation 303–4
 tetraethyl lead 721
 transmissible spongiform 584–8
 uraemic 667, 668
 see also MELAS (mitochondrial
  encephalopathy with lactic acidosis
  and stroke-like episodes)
endocraniosis 890
endocrine deficits/disorders 617–51
 acromegaly 643–4
 Addison's disease 649–51
 brain tumours 301
 Cushing's syndrome 646–9
 diabetes insipidus 644–6
 hyperprolactinaemia 642–3
 hyperthyroidism 632–5
 hypopituitarism 641–2
 hypothyroidism 628–32

Klinefelter's syndrome 672–4
 paroxysmal events 362
enterovirus encephalitis 437
environmental risk factors, Alzheimer's
  disease 562–5
environmental toxins 721
ependymoma **299**
epidermal cyst, third ventricle 293
epigastric aura 310
 temporal lobe epilepsy 320
epilepsia partialis continua of childhood
  315
epilepsy/epilepsy syndromes 309–95, 660
 acute symptomatic 332–3
 aetiology 325–9, 330–5
  SLE and antiphospholipid syndrome
   518
  stroke 482
 aggravating and precipitating factors 333
 aggression 78
 anatomically-localised 315, 319–24
 autonomic 325
 autosomal dominant
  nocturnal frontal lobe 322, 326
  temporal lobe 326
 body image disturbances 76
 cardiological investigations 365
 classification 309–25
  epilepsy syndromes 313–25
  seizures 309–13
 clinical assessment 357–8
 cryptogenic **314**, 315
 definition of seizure 309
 diencephalic 325
 differential diagnosis 356, 358–62
 EEG use 126–7
 frontal lobe 322–3
  auras **320**
 genetic factors 322, 325–8
 hypoparathyroidism differential
   diagnosis 640
 idiopathic 314–15
  cognitive outcome 352
  generalised **314**, 315–18
  localisation-related **314**, 314–15
  tumours misdiagnosis 300
 imaging 364–5
 insulinoma differential diagnosis 625
 investigation 362–5
 migraine and
  comorbid 502–3
  distinction 511
 misdiagnosis 356–7
 movement during sleep 834
 MRI 135, *136*
 narcolepsy differential diagnosis 827
 postinfective 330–1
 post-traumatic in head injury 198, 329–30
  legal aspects 244
  pharmacotherapy 253
 prevalence 325
 psychiatric disability 333–56, 377–80
 sudden death 375–6
 treatment 365–80

tumours causing 329, 331
  management 301
  temporal lobe 289, 291
 Wilson's disease 772
 see also anticonvulsants; generalised
   epilepsy/seizures; myoclonic
   epilepsy/seizures; seizures; status
   epilepticus; temporal lobe epilepsy
   (TLE)
epileptic opercular syndrome, acquired 318
epiloia 853–4
episodic dyscontrol 80
Epstein–Barr virus (EBV) 436–7
 AIDS-related lymphomas and 405
 SLE and 514
Epworth Sleepiness Scale 826
erythism 727
erythropoietin therapy, uraemia 668
ethchlorvynol, withdrawal effects 724
ethnicity (race)
 AIDS 398
 Alzheimer's disease 564
ethosuximide 369
euphoria 119
 multiple sclerosis 850
Europe
 Alzheimer's disease 545
 viral encephalitides **432**
event-related (evoked) potentials
 EEG use 129–30
 mild traumatic brain injury 225
  post-concussion syndrome 233
exanthemata, acute 438
executive disorder 58–60
 Alzheimer's disease 548
 post-traumatic 202, 203–4
 subarachnoid haemorrhage 494, 495
executive function
 neuropsychology 59–60
 tests **124**, 151–4
  working memory and planning 155
exercise, physical
 dementia 594
 SLE 521
exogenous psychoses 4
expansive form of general paresis 425–6
explosive personality disorder 79–80
 intermittent 80
extinction, parietal lobe lesions 18
extrapyramidal symptoms
 dementia with Lewy bodies 572
 sleep 834
eye (ocular/ophthalmological) disorders/
   abnormalities
 aneurysms 493
 diplopia 827
 dystrophia myotonica 865
 encephalitis lethargica 444, 446
 progressive supranuclear palsy 776
 subacute cerebellar degeneration 869
 syphilis 424, 426
 Wernicke's encephalopathy 701
 see also visual *entries*
eyelid myoclonus 316

Eysenck Personality Inventory, migraine 507

F
fabricated AIDS 418
face identity processing 64
facial affect perception 65
facial expressions 65
factitious conditions
  AIDS 418
  hypoglycaemia 624
false memory
  assessment 109
  post-traumatic 184
familial Alzheimer's disease 546
  early-onset 558
familial Creutzfeldt–Jakob disease (CJD) 588
familial hemiplegic migraine 501
familial insomnia, fatal (FFI) 584, 585, 588, 835
family history, dementias 589
family/relatives
  dementia
    burden 594
    support 593
  head injury 254, 254
  stroke rehabilitation 491
  subarachnoid haemorrhage support 493
  see also caregiver burden; education and information, patient/relatives
facioscapulohumeral dystrophy 865
fast low-angle short (FLASH) 140
fatal catatonia 723
fatal familial insomnia (FFI) 584, 585, 588, 835
fatigue
  anxiety/depression 826
  EBV 437
fear
  ictal in temporal lobe epilepsy 320–1
  see also anxiety/anxiety disorders; phobias
febrile seizures/convulsions 319, 332
febrile seizures plus, generalised epilepsy with 326
finger tapping (speed) test 239
FLAIR sequences 134, 135, 175–7, Plate 3.1
fluorescent treponemal antibody absorption (FTA-ABS) test 424, 427
focal cortical dysplasia 329
focal deficits
  brain tumours 283
  head injury
    children 242
    cognitive 204–5
  Huntington's disease 579
focal seizures see partial (focal/localisation-related) seizures
folate (folic acid) deficiency 658–60
  dementia 659–60
  depression 659
  epilepsy 660
  schizophrenia 660
  treatment 660
footballers, head injury 237

forced thinking 310–11
forebrain damage in subarachnoid haemorrhage 495–6
fornix bundles 35
fortification spectra 501
fossa (cranial), tumours of posterior 295–7
frataxin 856–7
FRDA1 gene 856–7
free diving 889–90
Friedreich's ataxia 856–8
  clinical features 857
  genetic factors 856–7
  pathology 857
  psychiatric aspects 857–8
Frontal Assessment Battery 116, **117–18**
frontal lobe
  dementias 145
  dysfunction
    aggression 80
    confabulation 42
  epilepsy 322–3
    auras **320**
  function 59–60
    tests 116, **117–18**, 118
  lesions 17, 22
  memory 35
  tests **124**, 151–4
  traumatic damage 200–1, 203
    children 242
    personality changes 206, 208
  tumours 286–8
frontal lobe syndrome 19, 58–60
  grasp reflex in young adult 105
frontal poles 60
frontotemporal dementia 43, 573–6
  motor neurone disease association 859–60
  MRI 135, 137
  PET 143
  temporal variant 574
fructose, intravenous 692
frustration, primary motor aphasia 56
functional impairment in Alzheimer's disease 548–9
functional neuroimaging
  Alzheimer's disease 553
  epilepsy 364–5
  head injury 178–9
    post-concussion syndrome 232–3
  Huntington's disease 580–1
  see also magnetic resonance imaging, functional (fMRI)
functional seizures 355
fungal infections, AIDS 404, 420
fusiform gyrus, face identity processing 64
fusion inhibitors (anti-HIV) 421

G
GABA see γ-aminobutyric acid (GABA)
GABAergic antiepileptics **372**
gabapentin 370
gait
  Huntington's disease 578
  normal-pressure hydrocephalus 873, 874, **876**

galanthamine 595
Gall, Franz Joseph 30
gamma knife 304
Ganser syndrome, head injury 221
gas embolism, cerebral 889
gas toxicity 888
gaze
  progressive supranuclear palsy 776
  voluntary shift difficulties 66
gelastic seizures 311, 324–5
gender and Alzheimer's disease 564
gene therapy, brain tumours 304
General Memory Index (GMI) 123
general paresis, juvenile 426
general paresis of the insane 444–7
  differential diagnosis 429–30
  grandiose form 425–6
  treatment 430
generalised anxiety disorders
  head injury 218–19
  stroke 487
generalised epilepsy/seizures 309, **310**, 315–18
  antiepileptics **367**
  epilepsy syndromes with **314**
  with febrile seizures plus 326
  secondary 311–13
    partial seizures with 311
genetic counselling
  early-onset autosomal dominant Alzheimer's disease 560
  Huntington's disease 577–8
geographically-restricted causes of viral encephalitis 432
Geriatric Mental State 156
Gerstmann's syndrome
  neuropsychology 69–70
  nominal aphasia 53
Gerstmann–Sträussler–Scheinker (GSS) disease 584, 585
Geschwind syndrome 347–8
giant cell arteritis 526–7
giant cells, multinucleated HIV-related 405, 406, Plate 7.2
giant cerebral aneurysms 499
Gilles de la Tourette syndrome 786–93
  aetiology 789–90
  clinical features 786–9
  course 789
  development theories 790
  genetics 791–2
  learning theory 790
  movement during sleep 834
  nosology 789–90
  organic theories 790–1
  outcome 789
  psychogenic theories 790
  treatment 792–3
Glasgow Coma Scale (GCS) 6
  head injury 185–6, 187, 188
    mild injury 223–4
    as outcome predictor 188
    plus substance abuse 176
  impaired consciousness assessment 112
  subarachnoid haemorrhage 491

Glasgow Outcome Scale, subarachnoid
    haemorrhage 498
glatiramer 846
glioblastoma
    imaging **299**
    symptoms 286
glioma, memory impairment 284
gliomatosis cerebri 289
glucocorticoid deficiency 649, 650
glucose blood levels, emotional stress
    620
glucose transport 623
glue sniffing 719–20
glutamatergic deficits, Alzheimer's disease
    557
glutethimide, withdrawal effects 724
glycaemic control in diabetes mellitus 619
Goldstein–Scheerer tests 154
Gorlin's syndrome 281
Graded Naming Test 148
grand mal *see* tonic–clonic seizures
granulomatosis, Wegener's 525, 526
granulomatous angiitis 523
    HIV disease 407, 407
grasp reflex, young adult 105
Graves' disease 632
growth hormone, acromegaly 643, 644
guanfacine 792
Guillain–Barré syndrome
    HIV-associated 413
    protein content of CSF 132
gustatory hallucinations 321

H
Hachinski index 567
haemangiomas, cavernous 331
haematoma, subdural 512–13
haemodialysis *see* renal replacement
    therapy
Haemophilus influenzae 449
haemorrhage, intracranial 474
    traumatic 170
    see also intracerebral haemorrhage,
        subarachnoid haemorrhage
haemosiderin 139
Hallervorden–Spatz syndrome 878–9
hallucinations 5
    acute organic reactions 12–13
    autoscopic 75
    brain tumours 285
        temporal lobe 291
    chronic organic reactions 16–17
    delirium tremens 13, 694, 695
    dementia
        Alzheimer's disease 550
        with Lewy bodies 572
    dopamine agonist therapy 768
    epilepsy **320**
        occipital lobe 324
        temporal lobe 321
    gustatory 321
    hypnagogic 825
    LSD 717, 718
    migraine 509
    Parkinson's disease 768, 769

post-traumatic 182
    see also visual hallucinations
hallucinogen persisting perception disorder
    719
hallucinogens 716–19
hallucinosis
    alcohol withdrawal 693–4
    amphetamine 714
    cocaine 714
    organic 7
    peduncular 478
    stroke 478, 489
haloperidol 792
    lithium combination 722
    psychostimulant toxic reaction treatment
        715
Halstead Impairment Index 699
Halstead–Reitan Battery 154–5
hamartomas, hypothalamic 293–4
Hamilton Anxiety Rating Scale 517
Hamilton Depression Rating Scale 517
handedness 46–7
handicap, WHO definition 247
Hartnup disease 654
Hayling Test 153
head injury (traumatic brain injury) 167–
        279, 562
    acute effects 180–5
    biochemical changes 171–4
    biomechanics 168
    chronic sequelae 189–201
    crush closed 168
    damage location **201**, 206, 330
    EEG 127, 174–5
    epidemiology 167
    focal 29
    imaging 175–80
        assessing severity 175
        boxers 238
        evidence of permanent damage in mild
            brain injury 224
        post-concussion syndrome 232–3
    management 174, 246–54
    mild 223–35
        definitions 185, 223–4
        evidence for permanent brain damage
            224–5
        multiple 227–8
    open vs. closed 168
    outcome (long-term) 189–91
        predictors 173, 188–9, 227
    pathology 168–70
    pathophysiology 171–4
    penetrating **201**, 206, 330
    personality change 206
    recovery of symptoms 189–91
        after mild injury 228–34
    rehabilitation 246–50
    schizophrenia association 85, 86
    severity, measurement and classification
        185–9
    subarachnoid haemorrhage-related
        disturbances 497
    tau pathology 562
    see also brain injury; concussion

headache
    cluster 501
    migraine 511
        features 500–1
    post-traumatic 234
        therapy 250, 252
    psychostimulants 715
    SLE 517
    subarachnoid haemorrhage 492
headgear 239–40
heart
    cardiological investigations in suspected
        epilepsy 365
    see also cardiac causes of syncope
heat sensitivity, hyperthyroidism 634
heavy metals, toxic effects 724–32
Hebb, D.O. 31
helmets 239–40
helminths 454–5
helper T cells *see* CD4 (helper) T cells in HIV
    disease
hemianopia 67
    see also homonymous hemianopia
hemidepersonalisation 72
hemiparesis, parietal lobe lesions 18
hemiplegia, anosognosia 73
hemiplegic migraine, familial 501
hemisomatognosia 72, 119
Henry and Woodruff sign 360
hepatocellular degeneration *see* Wilson's
    disease
heroin 710, 711
    epilepsy 332
herpes simplex virus encephalitis 434–6
    in AIDS 404, 421
    differential diagnosis 435
        subacute encephalitis 442
    EEG use 127, *128*
    type B/monkey form 346
herpes zoster *see* varicella-zoster virus
heterotopia, periventricular/subcortical
    band 329
highly active antiretroviral therapy
    (HAART) 877
hippocampal amnesia 34–5, 39
hippocampal atrophy, Cushing's syndrome
    649
hippocampal sclerosis 319–20, 332
hippocampal volume in Alzheimer's
    disease 552–3
hirsutism 890
HIV/AIDS 397–421
    AIDS-defining illnesses 400
    antifungal drugs 420, 421
    asymptomatic subjects 399–400
        impairments in 414
    biology of virus 398–9
    case definition of AIDS 401
    classification of disorders 400
    epidemiology and risk groups 397–8
    fabricated/factitious 418
    homosexuals 398, 418
    investigation 418–19
    management/treatment 419–21
    MRI 135

natural history and clinical signs of infection 399–400
neuropsychiatric manifestations 401–2, 408–14, Plate 7.1
primary HIV infection of CNS 405–8
syphilis coinfection 404, 427–8
'worried well' and fear of 415, 417–18
HIV-associated dementia 406, 408–14
genetic factors in susceptibility 409
imaging 410
HMAO-SPECT 145, Plate 3.6
schizophrenia 88
hockey-stick sign 135
homocysteinaemia 562–3
homonymous hemianopia
colour agnosia 65
pure word-blindness 52
homosexuals, HIV disease/AIDS
bereavement and stressful life events 418
transmission 398
Hospital Anxiety and Depression Scale (HADS)
stroke 483
subarachnoid haemorrhage 497
HSV *see* herpes simplex virus encephalitis
human immunodeficiency virus *see* HIV/AIDS
Huntington's disease 576–84
aetiology 577
basal ganglia disorders 20
biochemical studies 583–4
childhood 581–2, 583
clinical features 578–80
course and outcome 581
diagnostic mistakes 582–3
EEG use 129
genetic counselling and presymptomatic testing 577–8
investigations 580–1
juvenile 582
MRI 137, *138*
Parkinson's disease differential diagnosis 757
pathology 583–4
PET 143
SPECT 145
treatment 595
Westphal variant 579
hydrocephalus
adult obstructive 875–6
head injury 177–8
infancy 875
lead toxicity 726
normal pressure 871, 873–6
differential diagnosis 874
response 875
secondary 873, 875
treatment 875
posterior fossa tumours 296
shunts 875, **876**
subarachnoid haemorrhage 493
γ-hydroxybutyrate (GHB) 708
hydroxytryptamine (serotonin) receptor agonists in migraine

5-HT$_{1A}$ 512
5-HT$_{1B/1D}$ 511
see also selective serotonin reuptake inhibitors
hypercalcaemia 663–4
hyperekplexia 360–1
hyperkalaemia 662
hyperkinesis, paediatric head injury 242–3
hyperkinetic-type encephalitis lethargica 444, 447
hypermagnesaemia 664
hypermotor seizures 323
hypernatraemia 661
hyperostosis frontalis interna 890
hyperparathyroidism 635–7
differential diagnosis 637
investigations 636–7
mental disturbance 637
hyperprolactinaemia 642–3
hypersomnia
assessment 119
associated with psychiatric disorder 835–6
diencephalic tumours 292–3
idiopathic 829–30
organic disease 834–5
recurrent in Kleine–Levin syndrome 832–4
with sleep drunkenness 830
hypertension
Alzheimer's disease 562
uraemia 668
hypertensive encephalopathy 499
hyperthyroidism 632–5
apathetic 635
differential diagnosis 634–5
investigations 634
mental disturbances 633, 634, 635
neurological manifestations 633–4
psychological accompaniments 633
hypnagogic hallucinations 825
hypnotic drugs, insomnia 822–3
hypocalcaemia 663–4
hypocretin receptor genes 828
hypocretin system 817
narcolepsy 827, 828
hypoglycaemia
alcohol-induced 623
associated disorders 623
cerebral pathology 626, 628
cognitive deficit 620–1
diabetes mellitus 619
disorders 622–6, **627**, 628
factitious 624
fasting test 625–6, **627**
investigation 625–6
meal-induced 623–4
memory impairment **621**
neurological deficit 620–1
outcome 626
spontaneous 625
treatment 626
hypokalaemia 662
hypomagnesaemia 664

hyponatraemia 661–2
Addison's disease 650
psychotropic medication-induced 645
hypoparathyroidism 637–40, *641*
dementia with familial calcification of basal ganglia differential diagnosis 878
differential diagnosis 639–40, 878
intracranial calcification 639, **640**, *641*
investigations 639
outcome 640
physical features 638
psychiatric features 638–9
hypoperfused zones of ischaemic infarct 480
hypophosphataemia 664–5
hypopituitarism 641–2
hypothalamic function, diencephalic lesions 20
hypothalamic tumours 293–4, 295
endocrine deficits 301
hypothalamotomy, aggression control 79
hypothalamus
amnesia 34
lesion-associated hypersomnia 835
hypothyroidism 628–32
affective psychoses 629
classification 628
differential diagnosis 631
investigations 630
mental disturbance
aetiology 631
outcome 631–2
mild 629
narcolepsy differential diagnosis 827
neurocognitive deficits **630**
neurological features 629–30
neuropsychiatric features 628–9
physical features 628
schizophrenia 629
treatment 631, 632
hysteria
acute dystonia differential diagnosis 747
belle indifférence 21
hysterical dissociation 827, 836
hysterical symptoms, head injury 221

I
ICD-10 *see* International Classification of Disease (ICD-10)
ictal phase
bradycardia 358, 365
EEG 363
psychiatric disorders **335**, 335–9
semiology of temporal lobe epilepsy 322
idiopathic epilepsy/epilepsy syndromes 314–15
cognitive outcome 352
generalised **314**, 315–18
localisation-related **314**, 314–15
tumours misdiagnosed as 300
idiopathic normal pressure hydrocephalus (INPH) 871, 873–6
idiosyncratic reactions, antiepileptics 367–8

illicit substance misuse *see* drug misuse
illusions *see* hallucinations
imaging *see named modalities*
Immediate Memory Index (IMI) 123
immune response, multiple sclerosis 846
immunisation approach, Alzheimer's
    disease 560
immunological markers
  SLE and antiphospholipid syndrome 521
  see also antibodies
immunosuppressive drugs
  primary angiitis of CNS 524
  SLE 521
immunotherapy, brain tumours 304
impairment, WHO definition 247
implicit memory 37
  Huntington's disease 579
impulsiveness 119
  LSD 718
inattention
  parietal lobe lesions 18
  see also attention deficit; attention deficit
    hyperactivity disorder
inborn errors of metabolism 140
incontinence, urinary 288
incoordination in neurosyphilis 427
indolaxine 486
infancy
  agenesis of the corpus callosum 890–1
  hydrocephalus 875
  Kufs' disease 881
  malnutrition 651–2
  mercury toxicity 728
  Ondine's curse 830
  severe myoclonic epilepsy 318
  spasms 317
infarction *see* CADASIL; ischaemic stroke
infections
  intracranial 397–472
    epilepsy following 330–1
  opportunistic in HIV disease/AIDS 400,
    403–4
    prophylaxis 419–20
    treatment 420–1
  parasitic 403, 454–5
  protozoan 403, 454
  see also encephalitis; meningitis
inflammatory polyneuropathies, HIV-
    associated 413
inflammatory process in Alzheimer's
    disease 563
influenza encephalitis 442–3, 448
information, patient *see* education and
    information, patient/relatives
information processing disability, post-
    traumatic 202–3
injury (traumatic)
  birth 328–9
  whiplash 235–7
  see also head injury (traumatic brain
    injury)
in-patient rehabilitation, head injury 248–9
insomnia 820–3
  fatal familial 584, 585, 588, 835

head injury 252–3
  non-REM sleep 821
  organic disease 835
  REM sleep 821
institutional (nursing/residential) care
  dementia 594
  stroke 491
insulin
  factitious hypoglycaemia 624
  signalling and Alzheimer's disease 563–4
insulin gene 618
insulin-like growth factor 1 (IGF-1),
    acromegaly 643, 644
insulinoma 624–5
intellectual impairment *see* cognitive and
    mental impairment
intelligence
  aphasia 54
  assessment 110
  standardised tests 121–3
  see also IQ (intelligence quotient)
intensity-modulated radiation therapy 304
interferon β (IFN-β), multiple sclerosis
    treatment 846
interictal period
  EEG 362, 363
  psychiatric disorders **335**, 340–56
internal border-zone infarcts 476
International Classification of Disease
    (ICD-10)
  delirium **7**, 8
  dementia **8**
  head injury 202
International Classification of Impairments,
    Disabilities and Handicaps (WHO)
    247
International Headache Society
    classification 500
International League Against Epilepsy
    classification system 309–10
  epilepsy syndromes 313, **314**, 315, 316
intoxication, insulinoma differential
    diagnosis 625
intracerebral haemorrhage 474
  stroke due to 473, 474
    Dutch-type hereditary cerebral
      haemorrhage with amyloidosis 569
    imaging 480
    medical management 481
    prognosis 482
intracranial haemorrhage/haematoma,
    traumatic 170
intracranial infections *see* infections
intracranial pressure, raised
  diencephalic lesions 19
  tumours 285
intracranial tumours *see* tumours
ion channels in epilepsy
  antiepileptic drug actions on 372
  genetic mutations **327**
ion channels in migraine 503
IQ (intelligence quotient)
  head injury 204
  Klinefelter's syndrome 673

malnutrition 652
  schizophrenia 81–2
irritability
  acute organic reaction 13
  post-traumatic 218
ischaemic stroke 473, 474–5
  classifications of infarcts 474, 475
  imaging 480
  migraine-related risk 502
  see also multi-infarct dementia; transient
    ischaemic attacks
isolated speech area syndromes 53–4
isotope cisternography 146

J
Jackson, John Hughlings 30
Jacksonian march 310
Jacksonian motor seizures 310
jamais vu 310
  temporal lobe epilepsy 321
Japanese B encephalitis 433
JC virus and AIDS 404
judgement impairment in chronic organic
    reactions 15
juvenile absence epilepsy 316, 348–9
juvenile general paresis 426
juvenile Huntington's disease 582
juvenile myoclonic epilepsy 316

K
Kaposi's sarcoma 401, 420
katastrophenreaktion see catastrophic reaction
Kayser–Fleischer ring, Wilson's disease
    772–3
Kearns–Sayre syndrome 883
ketone bodies, emotional stress 620
kinesogenic dyskinesia, paroxysmal 361
Kleine–Levin syndrome of recurrent
    hypersomnia 832–4
Klinefelter's syndrome 617, 672–4
  cognitive defects 672–3
  language disorders 673
  psychiatric features 673–4
  treatment 672
Klüver–Bucy syndrome
  features
    Alzheimer's disease 458
    frontotemporal dementia 576
  radiotherapy for craniopharyngioma 304
Kojewnikoff's syndrome 315
Korsakoff's syndrome (amnestic disorder)
    34, 696, 704–6
  alcohol neurotoxicity 705
  alcoholic peripheral neuropathy 706
  amnesic symptoms 33–4
  chronic amnesic syndrome 7
  cognitive impairment 697
  confabulation 34, 41
  continuity hypothesis 705–6
  cortical pathology 704–5
  diagnosis 706
  diencephalic lesions 19
  event ordering 38
  heterogeneity 706

memory function 37
memory impairment 45
misdiagnosis 704
neuroimaging 704–5
personality disturbance 38
subarachnoid haemorrhage 495, 497
superadded frontal lobe damage 35
time sense disturbance 38
treatment 706
    resistance 703
Wernicke's encephalopathy relationship
        704, 705
Kufs' disease **327**, 328, 593, 881–2
kuru 584

L
lacunar infarcts 475, 478
Lafora body disease **327**, 328
lamotrigine 369, 370
Landau–Kleffner syndrome 318–19
language
    activities triggering epilepsy 315
    affective components 48
    cerebral dominance 46–8
    function assessment **111**, 112–13, **114**
    laterality 46
    left hemisphere 31
    localisation of functions 48–9
    neuroimaging 49–50, Plate 2.1
    non-dominant hemisphere 47, **47–8**
    tests **124**, 148–9
language disorders
    Alzheimer's disease-related deficits 547
    clinical syndromes 50–8
    Klinefelter's syndrome 673
    neuropsychology 45–58
    parietal lobe lesions 17
    post-traumatic deficits 204
    schizophrenia 56–7
    temporal lobe lesions 18
    Wernicke–Lichtheim model 49
    see also aphasia
large-artery atherosclerosis 474, 475
Lashley, Karl 30, 31
laterality, schizophrenia 46–7, 88
laughing (pathological)
    head injury 218
        pharmacotherapy 252
    seizures with (gelastic) 311, 324–5
lead toxicity 724–6
learning theory, Gilles de la Tourette
        syndrome 790
left-handedness 46, 47
legal issues *see* criminality; medicolegal
        issues
Lennox–Gastaut syndrome 317–18
leucoariosis 475, 567
leucodystrophy, metachromatic 880–1
leucoencephalopathy
    HIV 406–7
    opiates 711
    progressive multifocal 404, 876–7
    subcortical (Binswanger's disease) 569
    toluene 720–1
    see also white matter lesions

levetiracetam 370
levodopa 758–60
    depression effects 766–7
    dopa-responsive dystonias 782
    non-motor responses 771–2
    pathological use 772
    psychiatric aspects of treatment 768–70
    psychosis induction 768–70
Lewy bodies
    dementia with (DLB) 543, 571–3
        management 595
    Parkinson's disease 755, Plate 12.1
Lewy body disease, diffuse 757
Li–Fraumeni syndrome 281
ligand-gated channelopathies, epilepsy
        syndromes **327**
lightning injuries 887–8
limb-girdle dystrophy 863
limbic encephalitis, paraneoplastic **299**
limbic system 30–1
    aggression control 79
    encephalopathy 870–1, *872*
linear accelerator-based radiosurgery
        (LINAC) 304
lipofuscinosis, neuronal ceroid **327**, 328
Lisch nodules 855
list learning tests 150
lithium
    haloperidol combination 722
    toxic effects 722
litigation
    head injury 195–8, 226, 236, 244, 245
    whiplash injury 235, 236
liver disease, Wilson's disease 772
liver transplantation, Wilson's disease 774
localisation-related seizures *see* partial
        (focal/localisation-related) seizures
locked-in syndrome 204
locus coeruleus in Alzheimer's disease
        550
logoclonia 112
long-term potentiation (LTP) 32
lorazepam 375
Lou Gehrig's disease 858–60
louping ill 433
LSD *see* lysergic acid diethylamide (LSD)
lumbar puncture 131–2
    dementia 592–3
lupus erythematosus *see* systemic lupus
        erythematosus
Lyme disease 453–4
lymphadenopathy, persistent generalised
        (PGL) 400–1
lymphocytic meningitis *see* meningitis
lymphoma
    B-cell in AIDS 404–5
    primary CNS
        AIDS-related 404–5
        imaging **299**
        memory impairment 284
lysergic acid diethylamide (LSD) 716–19
    acute effects 717
    adverse reactions 718–19
    flashbacks 719
    recurrence of effect 719

M
macrosomatognosia 74–5, 77
magnesium level disorders 664
magnetic resonance imaging (MRI)
    advantages over CT 135
    brain abnormalities in schizophrenia 86
    cerebral venous sinus thrombosis 528
    coronal *134*, Plate 3.1
    dementia 592
        Alzheimer's disease 552, 553
        Creutzfeldt–Jakob disease 587
        Huntington's disease 580
    diffusion tensor imaging 134–5
    diffusion-weighted imaging 134
        head injury 177
        SLE 518, 519
        stroke 480
    dyslexia 55
    epilepsy 364, 365
    FLAIR 134, *135*, 175–7, Plate 3.1
    head injury 175–7, 178, 179
        boxers 238
        functional MRI 179
    HIV-associated dementia 410
    hypertensive encephalopathy 499
    magnetisation transfer 135
    migraine 502
    safety 137
    schizophrenia 83–4, Plate 2.2
    sequences 134–5, Plate 3.1
    SLE 518–20
    stroke 480
    subdural haematoma 513
    tumours 297–8, *298*, **299**
    whiplash injury 236
    white matter hyperintensities 137–9
magnetic resonance imaging, functional
        (fMRI) 140–1, Plate 3.3
    language 49
    schizophrenia 87–8
magnetic resonance spectroscopy (MRS)
        139–40
    dementia
        Alzheimer's disease 553
        HIV-associated 410
    head injury 180
    SLE 520
    stroke 480
magnetisation transfer imaging (MTI)
    head injury 177
    SLE 519–20
magnetoencephalography (MEG) 130–1
malaria, cerebral 454
malingering, head injury 196–7
malnutrition 651–60
    brain damage 651–2
    chronic severe 651
    infants 651–2
    porphyria attacks 671
    protein–energy 651–2
    psychostimulant use 714
    Wernicke's encephalopathy 701
    young children 651–2
manganese toxicity 728–30
    clinical manifestations 729–30

mania
  HIV-associated 417, 420
  post-traumatic 215–16
    therapy 252
  stroke 487
  stupor 25
manic stupor 25
manic–depressive disorder *see* bipolar
    disorder
Marchiafava–Bignami disease 707
Marie's Three Paper Test 113
mazindol 828
measles virus 439
medical management
  dementia 594–5
  stroke 481
  tumours 301–2
medicolegal issues
  competency in aphasia 54
  head injury 195–8, 243–5
  violence during somnambulism 838
  whiplash injury 235, 236
  see also criminality
medulloblastoma **299**
Mcige's syndrome 785
MELAS (mitochondrial encephalopathy
    with lactic acidosis and stroke-like
    episodes) 328, 883, 884
  basal ganglia calcification *641*
Mellanby effect 691
memantine 595
memory
  assessment 109, 110, 114
  circuitry disruption 35
  declarative 37
  episodic 36–7
    psychoses 45
  explicit 37
  frontal lobe 35
  function assessment **111**
  functional imaging 35–6
  hypothyroidism 628
  immediate 36
  implicit 37
    Huntington's disease 579
  long-term 109–10
  panoramic in simple partial seizures 310
  primary 36
  priming 37
  procedural 37
    Huntington's disease 579
    psychoses 45
  remote 36
  secondary 36
  semantic 36–7
  short-term 36
  tests **124**, 149–51
    standardised 123
  theories 32
  working 36
memory disorders/impairment
  acute organic reactions 12
  alcoholic blackouts 691–2
  Alzheimer's dementia 43
  brain systems 33–6

chronic organic reactions 16
  depression 45
  fornix 35
  hyperparathyroidism 636
  neuropsychology 32–45
  normal ageing 43
  panoramic in simple partial seizures 310
  psychoses 45
  schizophrenia 45
  selective impairment 109
  source 42
  topographical loss 67
  Wernicke's encephalopathy 701–2
  see also amnesia; dementia; false memory
meningiomas
  case studies 287–8
  misdiagnosis 298–300
meningitis 449–52
  aseptic/lymphocytic 450
    HIV-associated 407, 413
  bacterial 449–50
    syphilis 422
    tuberculosis 451–2
  CSF composition 132
  granulomatous 886
meningococcus (*Neisseria meningitidis*) 449,
    450
meningoencephalitis 431
  granulomatous 886
meningovascular syphilis 422, 423
  general paresis differential diagnosis 430
menstrual cycle
  porphyria attack precipitation 671
  seizures related to 333
mental constitution, head injury 192–4
mental impairment *see* cognitive and mental
    impairment
mental state examinations 105, 107–16, **117–**
    18, 118–19
  dementia 591
    Alzheimer's disease 547, 548, 555
mercury toxicity 726–8
  clinical manifestations 727–8
  dental amalgam 726–7
  organic compounds 728
  vapour inhalation 726
MERFF (myoclonic epilepsy with ragged
    red fibres) **327**, 328, 883
mescaline 716
mesencephalic region *see* midbrain
    (mesencephalic) region
mesial temporal lobe
  sclerosis 319–20, 332
  surgery 374
metabolic acidosis 666
metabolic alkalosis 666
metabolic craniopathy 890
metabolic crisis, hypopituitarism 641
metabolic disorders 617–28, 651–75
  acid–base disturbances 665–6
  causing paroxysmal events 362
  EEG use 127–8
  electrolyte disturbances 660–5
  encephalopathies 870
  inborn errors of metabolism 140

malnutrition 651–60
  porphyria 669–72
  uraemia 666–9
  see also diabetes mellitus
metabolic pathways, depression 620
metachromatic leucodystrophy 880–1
metastases
  CNS involvement 868
  neuroimaging **299**
methamphetamine 713–15
methionine 658
methyl bromide poisoning 731
1-methyl-4-phenyl-1,2,3,6-
    tetrahydropyridine (MPTP) 721
  parkinsonism 756
methylcyclopentadienyl manganese
    tricarbonyl (MMT) 728–9
3,4-methylene-dioxymethamphetamine
    (MDMA) 715–16
methylphenidate
  ADHD treatment 793
  brain tumours 302
  head injury 250
  narcolepsy treatment 828
microangiopathy, haemosiderin 139
microscopic polyangiitis 525, 526
microsomatognosia 74–5, 77
midazolam 375
midbrain (mesencephalic) region
  haemorrhage 491
  lesion-associated hypersomnia 835
Middle East, viral encephalitides **432**
Middlesex Elderly Assessment of Mental
    State (MEAMS) 156
migraine 499–512
  with aura 360, 501, 502, 503, 504, 505, 506,
    507
  without aura 501, 502, 503, 505,
    506
  chronic 510–11
  clinical features 500–2
  course and outcome 502–3
  diagnosis and classification 500
  differential diagnosis 511
  genetic factors 503
  hemiplegic familial 501
  imaging 502
  pathophysiology 503–4
  psychiatric aspects 504–6, 508–10
  retinal 501–2
  in SLE 517
  transformed 510–11
  treatment 511–12
Minimal Assessment of Cognitive Function
    in MS (MACFIMS) 848
Mini-Mental State Examination (MMSE)
    110, 111
  Alzheimer's disease 547, 548
    annual changes 555
  frontal lobe function 116, **118**
Minnesota Multiphasic Personality
    Inventory, migraine 506
mirror movements 105
mirror sign 65
mirtazapine 486

misidentification syndromes
  Alzheimer's disease 550
  delusional post-traumatic 181, 211
misoplegia 72
mitochondrial abnormalities, Huntington's
    disease 584
mitochondrial encephalopathy with lactic
    acidosis and stroke-like episodes *see*
    MELAS
mitochondrial myopathy 882–4
modafanil 828
monoclonal antibody therapy
  brain tumours 304
  SLE 521
mood, clinical assessment 107
mood disorders
  Alzheimer's disease 550–1
  antipsychotic-induced tardive dyskinesia
      748
  brain tumours 284
    frontal lobe 287
    temporal lobe 290
  chronic organic reactions 16
  diabetes mellitus 618
  diencephalic lesions 19
  frontal lobe lesions 17
  head injury 215–18
    pharmacotherapy 250, 251–2
    rehabilitation 250
  Huntington's disease 580
  hyperthyroidism 633
  lability 119
  multiple sclerosis 850
  Parkinson's disease/parkinsonian
      syndrome 764–7
  stroke 484–8
  twilight states 5
  vitamin B$_{12}$ deficiency 656
mood stabilisers, HIV patients 420
Morgagni's syndrome 890
mortality, epilepsy 366
motivation
  stroke rehabilitation 491
  see also emotional–motivational blunting
      disorder
motor dysfunction/abnormalities
  Alzheimer's disease 547
  encephalitis lethargica 446
  HIV-associated 408, 409, 410
    minor 411–12
  Huntington's disease 578–9
  mild traumatic brain injury 225
  ritualistic behaviour in Tourette's
      syndrome 789
  Wilson's disease 772
motor dysphasia, subcortical 52–3
motor neurone disease 858–60
  clinical features 858
  genetic factors 858–9
  pathology 858, 860
  psychiatric aspects 859–60
  treatment 859
motor restlessness, drug-induced
    746

motor seizures, partial/focal 310
  frontal lobe epilepsy 323
movement disorders/abnormalities 745–96
  corticobasal degeneration 778–9
  drug-induced 745–52
    clinical picture 745–9
    drug withdrawal 750–1
    management 750–2
    pathophysiology 749–50
  dystonias 780–6
  encephalitis lethargica 445–6
  Gilles de la Tourette syndrome 786–93
  Parkinson's disease/parkinsonian
      syndrome 752–72
  progressive supranuclear palsy 776–8
  psychogenic 793–6
  during sleep 834
  striatonigral degeneration 779–80
  willed movement disturbance in
      encephalitis lethargica 445–6
  Wilson's disease 772–6
movement schemata 61
MR1 mutation 361
multi-infarct dementia 566, 567
  SPECT 145
multinucleated giant cells, HIV-related 405,
    406, 406, Plate 7.2
multiple endocrine neoplasia (MEN)
  hyperparathyroidism 635
  insulinoma 624
Multiple Errands Test 153
  head injury 203
multiple sclerosis 843–52
  clinical features 844–5
  CSF abnormalities 845
  diagnosis 844–5, 845–6
  environmental factors 844
  epilepsy 332
  genetic factors 843–4
  hygiene hypothesis 844
  neuroimaging 845–6
  pathology 846
  psychiatric aspects 847–52
  subacute encephalitis differential
      diagnosis 441–2
  treatment 846–7
  visual evoked responses 845
  vitamin D 844
multiple system atrophy *see* striatonigral
    degeneration
multiple trace theory 40–1
mumps encephalitis 438
Münchausen syndrome, AIDS fabrication
    418
muscle disorders
  HIV-associated 414
  rigidity
    akinetic rigid syndromes 753
    Parkinson's disease/parkinsonian
        syndrome 753, 754, 759
    progressive supranuclear palsy 776
    Wilson's disease 772
  see also dystonias; muscular dystrophy;
      myopathies; myotonic dystrophies

muscle weakness
  hyperthyroidism 634
  hypothyroidism 630
muscular dystrophy
  progressive 863–4
  psychiatric aspects 864
music perception 68
mutism 58
  assessment 119
  catatonic signs 26
  causes 26
  subcortical aphasia 54
  tumours causing
    diencephalic 293
    posterior fossa 296–7
  see also akinetic mutism
myasthenia gravis 860–3
  clinical features 861
  differential diagnosis 863
  hyperthyroidism 634
  pathophysiology 861
  psychiatric aspects 862–3
  treatment 861–2
Mycobacterium tuberculosis 404, 451–2
mycophenolate mofetil 521
myelin pallor, HIV-related 406–7
myelinoclastic diffuse sclerosis 852–3
myelopathy, vacuolar in HIV disease 407,
    412, 413
myoclonic absences 318
myoclonic epilepsy/seizures 312–13
  astatic 318
  eyelid and perioral 316
  infant severe 318
  juvenile 316
  progressive **327**, 327–8
  with ragged red fibres **327**, 328, 883
myoclonus
  with epilepsy 834
  perioral 316
  sleep 826
myofibrillogenesis regulator 1 gene
    mutation 361
myopathies
  acromegaly 644
  HIV-associated 414
  mitochondrial 882–4
myotonia 865
  congenita 867
myotonic dystrophies 864–8
myxoedema 628

N
naevoid basal cell carcinoma syndrome 281
naloxone 711
  psychostimulant toxic reaction treatment
      715
narcolepsy 823–9
  aetiology 827–8
  amphetamine therapy 713
  cataplectic attacks 824–5
  clinical features 824–6
  counselling 829
  differential diagnosis 361, 826–7

disturbed nocturnal sleep 826
epilepsy differential diagnosis 361
genetic factors 827, 828
narcoleptic attacks 824
pre-sleep dreams 825
REM sleep 828
REM sleep behaviour disorder 839
sleep paralysis 825–6
treatment 828–9
natalizumab 846, 877
National Adult Reading Test (NART)
122–3
National Institute for Clinical Excellence
(NICE), multiple sclerosis treatment
guidance 846–7
National Institute of Neurological and
Communicative Disorders and
Stroke and the Alzheimer's Disease
and Related Disorders Association
(NINCDS-ADRDA) criteria
Alzheimer's disease 554
vascular dementia 567, 568
neck
whiplash injuries 235–7
see also torticollis, spasmodic
necrotic cell death, head injury 172
neglect
unilateral 71, 118
visual 67–8
Neisseria meningitidis (meningococcus) 449,
450
neocortical resection in epilepsy 374
neonates, adrenoleucodystrophy 877
neoplasms see tumours
nerve conduction studies 146–7
neural transplantation, Parkinson's disease
761
neurasthenia, hypersomnia 835
neurasthenic symptoms, subarachnoid
haemorrhage 497
neuritic plaques 551–2, 555–6, Plate 9.1
neuroacanthocytosis 593, 879–80
neurodegeneration with brain iron
accumulation 878–9
neurodegenerative disorders
epilepsy 331
Hallervorden–Spatz syndrome 878–9
neuroacanthocytosis 879–80
neuroepithelial tumours, dysembryoblastic
329
neurofibrillary tangles 552, 556, 558, Plate
9.1
progressive supranuclear palsy
776
neurofibromatoses 281, 854–6
clinical manifestations 855
genetic factors 854–5
neuropathology 855–6
psychiatric aspects 856
neurofibromin 855
neuroglycopenia
acute 622–3
chronic 623
subacute 622–3

neuroimaging
language 49–50, Plate 2.1
see also functional neuroimaging; named
modalities
neuroleptic malignant syndrome 722–3
neuroleptics see antipsychotics
neurological examination 104–5
dementia 105, **106**, 591
soft signs 105
neuronal ceroid lipofuscinosis see Kufs'
disease
neuronal degeneration, alcohol-induced
697, 698
neuronal loss/death
Alzheimer's disease 550–1
head injury 172
HIV-associated 407–8
Huntington's disease 583
neuronal plasticity in head injury 173–4
neuronal regeneration and plasticity in head
injury 173–4
neuropathies
carbon disulphide poisoning 732
HIV-associated 407, 413
lead 725
porphyrias 670
in primary angiitis 525
uraemia 667–8
see also peripheral neuropathy
neuropeptides and migraine 503
neuroprotective agents, head injury
174
neuropsychiatry, definition 3–4
neuropsychological tests see psychometric/
psychological/neuropsychological
testing and assessment
neuropsychology 29–89
action disorders 62–3
agnosias 63–9
aphasias 45–58
apraxias 60–2
body image disturbances 71–7
executive function 59–60
Gerstmann's syndrome 69–70
history 29–32
language disorders 45–58
memory disorders 32–45
modern 31–2
non-cognitive disturbances 77–89
perception disorders 63–9
regional brain dysfunction 77–89
schizophrenia 80–9
neurosyphilis see syphilis (neurosyphilis;
T. pallidum)
neurotic disorder 21
neuroticism and migraine 507
neurotoxicity
antiepileptic drugs 354, 377–8
brain tumour treatment 284
chemotherapy/radiotherapy 302
neurotransmitters
Alzheimer's disease 556–7
head injury 174
Huntington's disease 583–4

imaging 145–6
serotonergic in Parkinson's disease
756–7
neutrophil cytoplasmic antibodies (ANCAs)
in small-vessel vasculitides 525–6
nicotinic acid (niacin) deficiency 653, 654
acute encephalopathy 654–5, 704
alcoholism 655
night terrors 838
nigrostriatal tract, Parkinson's disease/
parkinsonian syndrome 755
NINCDS-ADRDA criteria see National
Institute of Neurological and
Communicative Disorders and
Stroke and the Alzheimer's Disease
and Related Disorders Association
criteria
Nipah virus 434
nitrites 719, 720
nitrous oxide abuse 719
N-methyl-d-aspartate (NMDA) receptors
32
Huntington's disease 584
schizophrenia 87
SLE 521
nocturnal frontal lobe epilepsy, autosomal
dominant 322, 326
non-accidental brain injury, children 170
non-cognitive disturbances,
neuropsychology 77–89
non-Hodgkin's lymphoma, AIDS 404–5
non-kinesogenic dyskinesia, paroxysmal
361
non-nucleoside analogue reverse
transcriptase inhibitors 421
non-REM arousal disorders 361
non-steroidal anti-inflammatory drugs
(NSAIDs) 563
noradrenergic system, Alzheimer's disease
556
NOTCH gene/notch proteins 558, 569
nucleoside/nucleotide analogue reverse
transcriptase inhibitors 421
nucleus basalis of Meynert, dementia in
Parkinson's disease/parkinsonian
syndrome 764
number function, assessment 113
nursing care see institutional (nursing/
residential) care

O
obesity
hyperostosis frontalis interna 890
sleep apnoea 830, 831
Object Learning Test 149–50
obscenities, Tourette's syndrome 787–8
obsessive–compulsive disorder
AIDS 416
brain tumours 285
post-traumatic 221–2
Tourette's syndrome 789, 791
treatment 793
see also compulsions
obstructive sleep apnoea 830–1

occipital lobe
  epilepsy 324
    auras **320**
  lesions 19
  traumatic damage 200, **201**
  tumours 292
occipital paroxysms, childhood epilepsy
      314–15
occupation
  carbon disulphide poisoning 732
  delirium 11
  epilepsy impact 377
  head injury rehabilitation 248, 249–50
  manganese toxicity 728
  mercury toxicity 726, 727
  methyl bromide poisoning 731
  organophosphorus compound poisoning
      731
  shiftwork 818–19, 837
ocular disorders/abnormalities *see* eye
oculopharyngeal muscular dystrophy 864
oestrogen and Alzheimer's disease 564
older patients *see* elderly patients
olfactory hallucinations, temporal lobe
      epilepsy 321
oligaemia, ischaemic infarct 480
oligoclonal banding 132
oligodendroglioma **299**
oncogene activation 281–2
Ondine's curse 830
one-carbon metabolism 658
oneiroid states 5
opercular syndrome, acquired epileptic 318
ophthalmological disorders/abnormalities
      see eye
opiates 710–11
  abstinence syndrome 711
  acute effects 710–11
  psychiatric disorder 711
  tolerance 711
opioids 710–11
  dependence 710
  overdose 711
  replacement therapy 711
opsoclonus, subacute cerebellar
      degeneration 869
orbitofrontal cortex traumatic damage,
      personality changes 206
  and cognitive deficits 208–9
orexin *see* hypocretin system
organic personality change 6
organic reaction
  acute 4
    causes **10**, 23–4
    clinical features 9–13
    combination with chronic 17
    differentiation from chronic 22
    hyperthyroidism 633
    hypopituitarism 642
  bismuth poisoning 731
  chronic 4
    causes **14**, 23–4
    clinical features 13–17
    combination with acute 17

differentiation from acute 22
    presentation 13–15
  differential diagnosis 20–6
  drug therapy toxic effects 721
  hypersomnia 834–5
  hypoparathyroidism 638
  non-organic condition differentiation
      20–2
  stupor 25
organic stupor 25
organophosphorus compound toxicity 731
orientation
  assessment 108–9, **111**, 118
  right–left 118
orthostatic syncope 358
osmotic demyelination syndrome 707
out-of-body experience 75
oxcarbazepine 371
oxidative stress and Huntington's disease
      584

P
P50 response 130
P300 response 130
Paced Auditory Serial Addition Task
      (PASAT) 154
  head injury 179, 202, 226
paediatrics *see* children
pain *see* headache; migraine
paired associate learning test 149
palliative care, brain tumours 302
pallido-thalamo-cortical circuits, dystonias
      781
pallidotomy 761
pallilalia 112
panencephalitis
  progressive rubella 440
  subacute 438–42
panic disorders
  ictal anxiety differential diagnosis 336
  LSD 718
panoramic memory in simple partial
      seizures 310
pantothenate kinase-associated
      neurodegeneration 878–9
pantothenic acid deficiency 653
  alcoholism 706
Papez, J.W. 30–1
parahippocampal amnesia 39
paralytic dementia *see* general paresis
paramnesia, post-traumatic reduplicative
      181
paramyotonia congenita 867–8
paraneoplastic disorders 868–71
paraneoplastic limbic encephalitis **299**
paranoid psychosis 583
paraphasic errors 112
parasitic infections 454–5
  AIDS 403
parathyroid hormone (PTH) 636
  see also hyperparathyroidism;
      hypoparathyroidism
parathyroidectomy 637
parietal lobe

epilepsy 323–4
  auras **320**
  lesions 17–18
  traumatic damage 200, **201**
  tumours 291–2
PARK genes 752, 753
parkinsonian syndrome
  clinical features 753–4
  course 754
  differential diagnosis 757
  drug-induced 753
  movement disorder 752–72
  outcome 754
  pathology/pathophysiology 755–7
  premorbid personality 770–2
  psychiatric aspects 761–72
  striatonigral degeneration 779
  treatment 757–61
parkinsonian-type encephalitis lethargica
      444
parkinsonism
  dementia with Lewy bodies 572
  drug-induced 745, 746, 753
    management 751
    pathophysiology 749–50
  idiopathic 754
  manganese toxicity 729
  postencephalitic 437, 445–6, 753
parkinsonism–dementia complex of Guam
      860
Parkinson's disease
  basal ganglia disorders 20
  clinical features 753–4
  course 754
  differential diagnosis 757
  environmental toxin exposure 721
  genetic factors 752–3
  movement disorder 752–72
  movement during sleep 834
  outcome 754
  pathology/pathophysiology 755–7
  PET 143–4, Plate 3.5
  premorbid personality 770–2
  psychiatric aspects 761–72
  REM sleep behaviour disorder 839
  surgery 761
  treatment 757–61
  twin studies 771
paroxysm(s)
  non-epileptic neurological disorders
      causing 360–2
  occipital 314–15
partial anterior circulation infarcts 475, 476
partial (focal/localisation-related) seizures
      309, 310–11
  antiepileptics 367
  cognitive impact 353
  complex 311
  continuous 337–8
  epilepsy syndromes with 313–15, 319–21
  personality 349
  simple 310–11
  surgery 373–4
peduncular hallucinosis 478

pellagra 653–4
penetrating head injury, damage location
  personality change 206
  symptoms **201**
    epilepsy 330
penicillamine 774, 776
  myasthenic syndrome induction 862
penicillin
  Lyme disease 454
  syphilis 430
penumbra of ischaemic infarct 480
perception/perception disorders 63–9
  acute organic reactions 12–13
  auditory defects 68–9
  facial affect 65
  hypothyroidism 628
  LSD effects 717
  self-face 65
  tactile defects 69
  tests **124**, 147–8
perceptual experiences, temporal lobe
    epilepsy 321
perimesencephalic haemorrhage 491
periodic ataxias 361
periodic limb movement syndrome 834
periodic paralysis 361
perioral myoclonus 316
peripheral nerve hyperexcitability (PNH)
    663
peripheral neuropathy 622
  alcoholic 706–7
  HIV-associated 407, 413
  Wernicke's encephalopathy 701, 702
peritoneal dialysis 692
periventricular heterotopia 329
periventricular hyperintensities 138–9
pernicious anaemia 655–8
  investigations 657
  neurological signs 657
  pathology 657
  psychiatric disorders 656–7
  screening 657–8
  treatment 658
peroxisome biogenesis disorders 877
perseveration 10, 107–8
persistent generalised lymphadenopathy
    (PGL) 400–1
persistent vegetative state 204
personality, premorbid
  head injury and influence of 192–4
  Parkinson's disease/parkinsonian
    syndrome 770–2
personality change/difficulties/disorders
    22
  amnesia 38
  brain tumours
    corpus callosum 289
    diencephalic 293
    frontal lobe 288
    temporal lobe 290
  dystrophia myotonica 866–7
  EEG abnormalities 126
  epilepsy 347–9
  explosive disorder 79–80

insulinoma differential diagnosis 625
  migraine 506–7
  organic 6
  Parkinson's disease/parkinsonian
    syndrome 767
  postencephalitic 446–7
  post-traumatic 205–11
    boxers 238
  stroke 483
  subarachnoid haemorrhage 496
  temporal lobe lesions 18–19
  Wilson's disease 775
personification 72
petit mal see absence seizures
petrol sniffing 721
phantom limbs 75–6
pharmacotherapy see drug therapy
phenobarbital 370
  status epilepticus 375
phenothiazines, neuroleptic malignant
    syndrome 723
phencyclidine (PCP) 716
phenytoin 369–70
  myasthenic syndrome induction 862
  status epilepticus 375
phobias
  AIDS in 'worried well' 415, 417–18
  head injury 219–20
  seizure 343, 379
phosphate level disorders 664–5
phospholipid autoantibodies see
    antiphospholipid syndrome
physical aggression see violence
physical duality, migraine 510
physical examination, dementia 591
physical exercise 521, 594
physical illness, psychiatric patients 104, **105**
physostigmine, head injury 250
Pick's disease 575, 576, 588
Pickwickian syndrome 830
pilocytic astrocytoma 295, **299**
pimozide 792
pituitary adenoma
  acromegaly 643, 644
  Cushing's syndrome 646
pituitary tumours 295
  endocrine deficits 301
plasticity, neuronal in head injury 173–4
pleocytosis 131
pneumoencephalography 146
poliodystrophy, diffuse in HIV disease 407
polyangiitis, microscopic 525, 526
polyarteritis nodosa 524–5
polycythaemia rubra vera 527–8
polydipsia, primary 645–6
polymerase chain reaction (PCR)
  HIV 419
  HSV 435
polymicrogyria 329
polyneuritis, Korsakoff's syndrome 704
polyneuropathies
  central pontine myelinolysis 707
  HIV-associated 407, 413
  somatic 622

porphyria
  acute 669–72
    intermittent 670
  attack precipitation 671
  differential diagnosis 672
  iatrogenic 671
  investigations 671–2
  outcome 672
  treatment 672
  variegate 670
positron emission tomography (PET) 141–4
  cerebral activation 142–3, Plate 3.4
  dementia 592
    Alzheimer's disease 553
    Huntington's disease 581
  dyslexia 55
  epilepsy 364–5
  head injury 179
    post-concussion syndrome 232–3
  HIV-associated dementia 410
  language 49–50
  Parkinson's disease 143–4, Plate 3.5
  psychopharmacology 143
  radioligands 143
  schizophrenia 87
  stroke 480–1
  tumours 298
  whiplash injury 236
post-concussion syndrome 193, 218, 221,
    232–3, 246–7
  case studies 231
  children 243
  prevention 246
  rehabilitation 249–50
postencephalitic disorders
  epilepsy 330–1
  parkinsonism 437, 445–6
  personality change 446–7
  psychoses 447
posterior circulation infarcts 475, 477–8
posterior fossa tumours 295–7
postictal disorders 339–40
postinfective epilepsy 330–1
poststroke dementia 482–3, 569
post-traumatic stress disorder (PTSD)
    220–1
  head injury 211, 220–1
    therapy 250
  subarachnoid haemorrhage 497
potassium channel antibody disorders 663
potassium level disorders 662
POUNDing criteria 500
prefrontal cortex, anterior 60
pregabalin 371
pregnancy, antiepileptic use 368
pre-ictal psychiatric disorders 335
presence, feeling of 75
presenilin 1 mutations 560
presyncope 358
primidone 370
prion diseases 584–8
prisoners, epilepsy 350
procedural memory, Huntington's disease
    579

programmed cell death, head injury 172
progressive encephalopathy of childhood,
   HIV-associated 412–13
progressive multifocal
   leucoencephalopathy 876–7
   in AIDS 404, 876, 877
progressive myoclonic epilepsy **327**, 327–8
progressive rubella panencephalitis 440
progressive supranuclear palsy 575, 776–8
   subcortical dementia 777–8
prolactin
   pituitary adenoma secreting 295
   seizures and serum levels of 365
prolactinoma, hyperparathyroidism 635
prolactin-secreting adenoma 642
propranolol, psychostimulant toxic reaction
   treatment 715
prosencephalon (forebrain) damage in
   subarachnoid haemorrhage 495–6
prosopagnosia 64–5
protease inhibitors (anti-HIV) 421
proton magnetic resonance spectroscopy,
   Alzheimer's disease 553
protozoan infections 454
   AIDS 403
PSEN1 mutations 560
pseudo-AIDS 415, 417–18
pseudobulbar palsy 776
pseudocoma, EEG use 128
pseudodementia 566
   Alzheimer's disease differential diagnosis
   550
pseudohypoparathyroidism (PHP) 638
   dementia with familial calcification of
      basal ganglia differential diagnosis
      878
pseudoneurosis, hypoparathyroidism 639
psilocin 716
psilocybin 716
psychogenic attacks/non-epileptic seizures
   356, 362, 365
psychogenic factors
   amnesia 44–5
   whiplash injury 236
psychogenic movement disorder 793–6
   aetiology 796
   clinical features 793–5
   diagnostic criteria 794
   examination 794, *795*
   investigations 795
   management 796
   prognosis 796
Psycholinguistic Assessments of Language
   Processing in Aphasia (PALPA) 149
psychological disturbance 3–4
psychological reactions
   epilepsy related to 333
   HIV disease
      acute 415
      life events 418
      management 420
   migraine 506–7
   as precipitants
      migraine 507–8

subarachnoid haemorrhage 408–9
   see also caregiver burden; post-traumatic
      stress disorder; stress
psychological tests, computerised 155
psychological treatments
   HIV disease 420
   seizure patients
      dissociative 380
      epileptic 374–5, 379
   stroke 486–7, 487
psychometric/psychological/
   neuropsychological testing and
   assessment 119–23, **124**
   advantages 120
   alcoholics 699
   applications 121
   attention 120
   dementia 591
      Huntington's disease 580
   dissociative seizures 355–6
   evidential status 121
   head injury 189, 190
      boxers 238–9
      medicolegal dimensions 197
   limitations 120–1
   motivation 120
   predictive value 120
   sensitivity 120
   specificity 120
   untestable patients 121
psychomotor behaviour
   acute organic reactions 11
   hypothyroidism 628
   multiple sclerosis 848
psychomotor poverty 82
psychopaths, aggressive 79–80
psychoses
   affective in hypothyroidism 629
   Alzheimer's disease 549–50
   amphetamines 714–15
   brain tumours 285
      posterior fossa 297
      temporal lobe 290
   cannabis-induced 713
   chronic organic reactions 16
   Cushing's syndrome 647, 648
   dopamine agonist therapy 768–70
   encephalitis lethargica 444–5, 447
   epilepsy
      interictal 343–7
      postictal 339–40
      treatment 379
   exogenous 4
   Friedreich's ataxia 857
   HIV-associated 415, 416–17
      treatment 420
   Huntington's disease 580
      misdiagnosis 583
   hyperparathyroidism 636
   hyperthyroidism 633, 634, 635
   hypothyroidism 629
   Klinefelter's syndrome 674
   LSD 718
   lupus psychosis 515

memory disorders 45
   multiple sclerosis 850–1
   neurosyphilis differential diagnosis 429
   nicotinic acid response 654
   paranoid 583
   Parkinson's disease/parkinsonian
      syndrome 767
   post-traumatic 182, 211–15
      and mood disorder 215
      pharmacotherapy 252
   progressive supranuclear palsy 777
   psychostimulants 714–15
   SLE 515
   stroke 488–9
   subarachnoid haemorrhage 497
   tuberous sclerosis 853, **853–4**
   vitamin B$_{12}$ deficiency 656
psychosocial dimensions
   childhood epilepsy 354
   subarachnoid haemorrhage 498
psychostimulants 713–16
   neurological complications 715
   physical effects 713–14
   psychiatric disorder 714–15
   psychological effects 713–14
   psychoses 714–15
   tolerance 714
   withdrawal 714
psychosurgery for aggression 79
psychotropic medication
   dementia 594–5
   epilepsy 378
   hyponatraemia 645
   SIADH 645
pulmonary barotrauma 889
pulmonary embolism, tumour-related 301
pulseless disease 527
pulvinar sign 135, *136*
pupils, syphilis 424, 426
Purkinje cells, subacute cerebellar
   degeneration 869
pyramidal signs, asymmetrical in corpus
   callosum lesions 19
pyridoxine deficiency 653
   alcoholism 706

R
rabies 433–4
racial issues
   AIDS 398
   Alzheimer's disease 564
radiography, skull 132
radioisotope scans 146
radiotherapy, brain tumours 303–4
ragged red fibres 883, 884
   see also MERFF (myoclonic epilepsy with
      ragged red fibres)
Rasmussen's encephalitis 315
rauwolfia alkaloid reaction 724
reading
   assessment 113
   Wernicke's aphasia 51–2
   see also dyslexia
reading epilepsy 315

reality distortion 82
reality distortion syndrome 83
reasoning, acute organic reactions 11–12
recognition memory tests 150
reduplication, illusions 75, 76
reduplicative paramnesia, post-traumatic 181
reference, ideas of 11
reflex abnormalities in neurosyphilis 427
reflex seizures 316–17
Refsum disease 877
regeneration, neuronal in head injury 173–4
rehabilitation
    head injury 246–50
        in-patient 248–9
    stroke 473, 489–91
relatives see family/relatives
REM sleep behaviour disorder 361, 838–9
renal disorders
    uraemia 667
    Wilson's disease 773
renal failure
    hyperkalaemia 662
    neuropsychiatric disturbance 668–9
    uraemia 667, 668
renal replacement therapy 669
    uraemia 667–8
renal transplantation 669
    disturbances 669
    uraemia 667–8
reperfusion in stroke recovery 481
repetition defect 53
residential care see institutional (nursing/residential) care
respiratory acidosis 666
respiratory alkalosis 666
restless legs syndrome 834
    akathisia differential diagnosis 746
    diagnostic criteria 747
    uraemia 667–8
Ret proto-oncogene 635
retinal migraine 501–2
retinocochleocerebral vasculopathy 527
retrobulbar neuritis 707
retrograde amnesia
    aseptic meningitis 451–2
    Huntington's disease 579
    post-traumatic 184–5
retroviruses 399
reverse transcriptase of HIV 399
    inhibitors 421
Rey Auditory Verbal Learning Test 150
Rey–Osterrieth Test 150–1
riboflavin deficiency 653
Rickettsia 454
right hemisphere
    language affective components 48
    music perception 68
right–left disorientation 70
risk-taking behaviour and anterior communicating artery aneurysms 496
risperidone 770
rituximab 521

rivastigmine
    dementia 595
    head injury 250–1
Rivermead Behavioural Memory Test 151
RNA, HIV 399
Ro autoantibodies 514
rolandic epilepsy, benign 314
rubella panencephalitis, progressive 440
rugby football helmets 240

S
S-100B in head injury 174
sarcoidosis 885–7
sarcoma, Kaposi's 401, 420
Schilder's disease 852–3
schizophrenia/schizophrenia-like disorders
    Addison's disease 650
    age-related decline 81
    alcoholic hallucinosis relationship 694
    aqueduct stenosis 876
    body image disturbances 76, 77
    cerebral atrophy 133–4
    cerebral lesions 85–6, 89
    chronic 81
    chronic organic reactions 16
    clusters 82–3
    cognitive deficits 81–2
    EEG abnormalities 126
    folate deficiency 660
    functional brain imaging 87–8
    handedness 46–7, 88
    hemispheric differences 88
    Huntington's disease 580
        misdiagnosis 583
    hyperthyroidism 633, 635
    hypothyroidism 629
    insulinoma differential diagnosis 625
    intelligence quotient (IQ) 81–2
    interictal 343–7
    Klinefelter's syndrome 674
    language 56–7, 88
    laterality 46–7, 88
    memory impairment 45
    metachromatic leucodystrophy
        differential diagnosis 880–1, 881
    MRS 140
    neurodevelopmental models 88–9
    neuroleptic therapy 143
    neuropathology 86–7
    neuropsychological impairment 81
    neuropsychology 80–9
    P300 response 130
    postencephalitic 447
    post-traumatic 213–14, 215
    premorbid signs 81–2
    profile 82
    regional brain pathology associations 84–6
    Schilder's disease 852–3
    sex differences 89
    social cognitive deficits 83
    structural brain imaging 83–4, 86
    stupor 25
    susceptibility genes 87

    symptoms 21–2
    temporal lobe tumours 290
    thoughts/thinking disorders 83
    tuberous sclerosis 853, **853–4**
schizophrenic stupor 25
scrapie 588
scuba diving 888, 890
second impact syndrome 237
secondary gain, head injury 195–8, 243
secretases in Alzheimer's disease 557–8
sedation, benzodiazepines 710
Segawa's disease 782
seizures
    acute symptomatic 332–3
    alcohol withdrawal 694
    atonic 313
    clonic 312, 323
    cursive 311
    dissociative 354–5, 359–62, 379–80
    drug-induced 332–3
    febrile 319, 326, 332
    functional 355
    gelastic 311, 324–5
    hypermotor 323
    hypernatraemia 661
    hyperthyroidism 634
    hypocalcaemia 664
    hypothyroidism 630
    motor 310
        frontal lobe epilepsy 323
    myoclonic astatic 318
    non-epileptic 354–5, 359–62
        distinguishing epileptic seizures from 357–8
    reflex 316–17
    self-induced 317
    situation-related **314**, 319
    tonic 312
    tonic–clonic 312, 316, **367**
    tuberous sclerosis 853
    see also absence seizures; epilepsy/epileptic syndromes; generalised epilepsy/seizures; partial (focal/localisation-related) seizures
selective serotonin reuptake inhibitors (SSRIs)
    dementia 594–5
    head injury 251–2
    obsessive–compulsive disorder treatment 793
    Parkinson's disease/parkinsonian syndrome 767
    stroke 487
selegiline 758
self-induced seizures 317
self-injury, Tourette's syndrome 788
self-neglect, senile 592
self-recognition, impaired 65
semantic dementia 43, 574
semantic memory tests 155
semanticisation hypothesis 40
semicoma 6
    assessment 119
senile (neuritic) plaques 551–2, 555–6

senile squalor and self-neglect 592
sensory disorders
  stroke rehabilitation 490
  tabetic syphilis 424
sensory polyneuropathy, distal 407, 413
sensory symptoms
  non-convulsive status epilepticus 338
  simple partial seizures 310
septum pellucidum perforation, boxers 239
seroconversion illness, HIV 399
serological tests
  HIV 418–19
  syphilis 424, 428–9
serotonergic neurotransmitters, Parkinson's
  disease 756–7
serotonin 511, 512
  see also selective serotonin reuptake
    inhibitors (SSRIs)
sertraline
  head injury 252
  stroke 486
sex chromosome aneuploidies 672–5
sexual dysfunction
  epilepsy 349
  head injury
    disinhibition 209, 251, 253
    therapy 253–4
  Klinefelter's syndrome 674
sexual orientation, AIDS and disclosure to
  family 418
sexual transmission, HIV 398
shingles *see* varicella-zoster virus
shopping performance, post-traumatic 203
sialidoses, epilepsy **327**, 328
signal transduction inhibitors, brain
  tumours 304
simian immunodeficiency viruses 398–9
simultanagnosia 66, 116
single-fibre electromyography (SFEMG)
  147
single-photon emission computed
  tomography (SPECT) 144–5, Plate
  3.6
  dementia 592
    HIV-associated 410
    Huntington's disease 581
    with Lewy bodies 574
  epilepsy 364
  head injury 178–9
    boxers 238
    post-concussion syndrome 232
  SLE 520
  stroke 480–1
  tumours 298
  whiplash injury 236
situation-related seizures **314**, 319
SIV 398–9
skull radiography 132
sleep
  behavioural forms 819
  circadian rhythms 817–19
    disturbances 823
  cycles 817–19
  deep 6

extrapyramidal symptoms 834
  hypnic jerks 834
  non-REM 817, 819–20
    insomnia 821
  REM 817, 820
    insomnia 821
  slow-wave, epilepsy with continuous
    spike–waves 318–19
  stages 819–20
sleep apnoea syndromes 830–2
  neuropsychological impairment 831
sleep disorders 817–39
  alcohol intoxication 693
  benzodiazepine withdrawal 709–10
  circadian rhythm disturbances 823
  delirium tremens 694
  deprivation 823, 837
  diencephalic tumours 292–3
  disturbed nocturnal 826
  epilepsy vs. 361–2
  head injury therapy 252–3
  hypersomnia
    associated with psychiatric disorder
     835–6
    due to organic disease 834–5
    idiopathic 829–30
    with sleep drunkenness 830
  hysterical 827
  insomnia 820–3
    due to organic disease 835
  intrinsic dyssomnias 820–3
  Kleine–Levin syndrome of recurrent
    hypersomnia 832–4
  movement disorders 834
  narcolepsy 823–9
  night terrors 838
  Parkinson's disease 769
  periodic limb movement syndrome 834
  pre-sleep dreams 825
  psychiatric illness 822
  REM sleep behaviour disorder 361, 838–9
  restless legs syndrome 834
  SLE 515
  sleep apnoea syndromes 830–2
  somnambulism 826, 836–8
  striatonigral degeneration 780
  Tourette's syndrome 788–9
sleep paralysis 825–6
sleep phase syndromes 823
sleepiness, daytime 823, 831
sleeping sickness 454
sleep-walking *see* somnambulism
slit ventricle syndrome 875
slow-wave sleep, epilepsy with continuous
  spike–waves 318–19
small-vessel disease 474–5
  dementia associated with 567–9
  vasculitis 522, 525–6
smell, hallucinations in temporal lobe
  epilepsy 321
soccer players, head injury 237
social awareness, executive syndromes
  58–9
social decline, dystrophia myotonica 867

social problems in head injury 253–4
sodium ion channels
  blockade by antiepileptics **372**
  migraine 503
sodium ion/potassium (Na$^+$/K$^+$) pump and
  migraine 503
sodium levels *see* hypernatraemia;
  hyponatraemia
sodium valproate *see* valproate
solvent abuse 719–21
somatic polyneuropathy 622
somnambulism 826, 836–8
  aggression 838
  genetic factors 837
somnolence
  diencephalic tumours 292
  dystrophia myotonica 867
  hysterical states 836
somnolent–ophthalmoplegic-type
  encephalitis lethargica 444
space-occupying lesions
  EEG use 127, 128
  insulinoma differential diagnosis 625
spasms, infantile 317
spastic paresis, frontal lobe lesions 17
spatial orientation, focal cerebral disorders
  23
speech
  comprehension 112–13
  motor aspect assessment 112
  repetition 113
  see also verbal *entries*
speech area, isolated, syndromes 53–4
speech disorders
  chronic organic reactions 15–16
  corpus callosum lesions 19
  delirium tremens 695
  dementia 16
  hypothyroidism 628
  hysterical 57–8
  neurosyphilis 427
  poverty 57
  Wernicke's encephalopathy 701
  see also aphasia
speech therapy 489, 490
Speed and Capacity of Language Processing
  Test 149
Spielmeyer–Vogt–Sjögren disease *see* Kufs'
  disease
spinal cord, vacuolar myelopathy in HIV
  disease 407, 412
spinocerebellar ataxias 856
spongiform encephalopathies, transmissible
  584–8
sport and athletes
  epilepsy and risks for 377
  traumatic brain injury due to 237–9
    mild 226–7, 228
SQUID (superconducting quantum
  interference device) 131
startle disease 360–1
startle-induced epilepsy 361
statins, Alzheimer's disease 565
status epilepticus 337–9

acute dystonia differential diagnosis 747
alcohol withdrawal 694
childhood 315
non-convulsive 337–9
therapy 375
Steele–Richardson–Olszewski syndrome *see*
progressive supranuclear palsy
stem cell therapy, brain tumours 304
stereotactic surgery 304
steroids
abuse 724
Alzheimer's disease protective effects 563
brain tumour management 301, 301
SLE 521
Stewart–Morel syndrome 890
strategy application tests 152–3
streptococci, group A β-haemolytic 792
Streptococcus pneumoniae 449, 450
streptomycin, myasthenic syndrome
induction 862
stress
hyperthyroidism 632
multiple sclerosis 852
response in depression 620
see also post-traumatic stress disorder
(PTSD); psychological reactions
striatonigral degeneration 779–80
stroke 473–91
causes 473
migraine 502
definitions and classification 473–9
diagnostic criteria 473, 474
imaging 479–81, 479–81
medical management 481
rehabilitation 473, 489–91
sequelae 481–9, 569
subdural haematoma differential
diagnosis 513
see also intracerebral haemorrhage;
ischaemic stroke
Stroop tests 152
Structured Clinical Interview for DSM-IV
Diagnoses, head injury 202
stupor 6
assessment 119
causes 24–6
types 25
subacute panencephalitides 438–42
subarachnoid haemorrhage 491–9
acute clinical picture and management
492–4
blood in CSF 131
emotional precipitation 498–9
normal-pressure hydrocephalus 873, 875
psychiatric sequelae 494–8
subcortical abnormalities, Turner's
syndrome 675
subcortical band heterotopia 329
subcortical dementia **20**, 777–8
normal-pressure hydrocephalus 871
subcortical leucoencephalopathy 569
subcortical pathology
Huntington's disease 579–80
white matter in SLE 519

subdural haematoma 512–13
subpial transection, multiple 374
substance misuse *see* alcohol/alcohol
abuse/alcoholism; drug misuse
substantia nigra
Parkinson's disease 755, Plate 12.1
striatonigral degeneration 779
sudden death epilepsy 375–6
suicide
AIDS 416
epilepsy 343
head injury 222–3
sulphonylureas, factitious hypoglycaemia
624
sumatriptan 511
supervisory attentional system model 60
supranuclear palsy, progressive 575, 776–8
surgery
brain tumour 302–3
posterior fossa in children 296–7, 302–3
epilepsy 372, 373–4
subarachnoid haemorrhage 493–4, 494–5
subdural haematoma 513
Susac's syndrome 527
symptomatic seizures and epilepsy
syndromes **314**, 315
synaptic loss in Alzheimer's disease 556
syncope 358, 365
cardiac causes 365
epilepsy differential diagnosis **358**,
358–9
causes 358
epilepsy differential diagnosis 356, **358**,
358–9, 365
migraine 508, 511
orthostatic 358
syndrome of inappropriate antidiuretic
hormone secretion (SIADH) 645
α-synuclein
gene 753
Lewy bodies 573
syphilis (neurosyphilis; *T. pallidum*) 421–30
atypical present-day forms 427
diagnostic criteria 427, 428
differential diagnosis 429–30
early asymptomatic 422
HIV 404, 427–8
investigations 428
meningovascular 422, 423, 430
treatment 430–1
systemic lupus erythematosus (SLE) 513–22
clinical features 514–15
genetic factors 514
imaging 518–20
pathogenesis 513–14
psychiatric problems 515–18, 521–2
aetiopathogenesis 520–1
treatment 521–3
systemic vasculitis 522

T
T cells *see* CD4 (helper) T cells in HIV disease
tabes dorsalis 423–4
general paresis and 426

tactile perceptual defects 69
Taenia solium 454
Takayasu's arteritis 527
talk content 107–8
tamoxifen 304
tapeworm, cysticercus stage 454–5
tardive dyskinesia, drug-induced 745,
747–8
irreversible 750
management 751
pathophysiology 750
tardive dystonia, drug-induced 745, 748–9,
751
taste, hallucinations in temporal lobe
epilepsy 321
tau
Alzheimer's disease 556, 558, 559, 560,
561, 562, 563, 564
mutations 560
frontotemporal dementia 575, 576
head injury and 562
progressive supranuclear palsy 776
temper outbursts *see* aggression
Temperament and Character Inventory,
migraine 506
temporal arteritis 526–7
temporal lobe
abscess 453
atrophy 137, Plate 3.2
lesions 18–19
medial
amnesia 34–5
anterograde amnesia 32–3
mesial
sclerosis 319–20, 332
surgery 374
music perception 68
traumatic damage 200, **201**
tumours 289–91
temporal lobe epilepsy (TLE) 319–22, 332
causes 332
genetic/autosomal dominant 326
tumours 289, 291
cognitive impact 352, 353
depression 341
personality traits and 348
surgery 373–4
teratogenicity, antiepileptics 368
teratoma, third ventricle 293
terminology 4–9
Test of Everyday Attention 148
testosterone replacement therapy,
Klinefelter's syndrome 672
tetanus, acute dystonia differential
diagnosis 747
tetraethyl lead 721
Δ^9-tetrahydrocannabinol 711, 712
thalamic infarcts 478
bipolar affective disorder 487–8
dementia 483
thalamic tumours 293
thallium poisoning/thallotoxicosis 730
thiamine
Korsakoff's syndrome treatment 706

metabolism 700
Wernicke's encephalopathy treatment 703–4
thiamine deficiency 34, 652–3, 654
  alcoholic peripheral neuropathy 706
  Korsakoff's syndrome 704, 705
  susceptibility 700
  see also Wernicke's encephalopathy
thiamine pyrophosphate 699, 700
thiazide diuretics 644–5
thinking *see* thoughts/thinking
thioridazine toxic effects 722
thioxanthines 723
thoughts/thinking, content 107–8
thoughts/thinking disorders 56–7
  acute organic reactions 11–12
  amnesia 38
  chronic organic reactions 15
  crowding 311
  epilepsy 310–11
    temporal lobe 321
  forced 310–11
  poverty 57
  schizophrenia 83
thromboangiitis obliterans 527
thromboembolism, tumour-related 301
thrombolytics, stroke 481
thrombosis
  cerebral arterial 474, 475
  cerebral venous sinus 528–9
thyroid crisis 633
thyroid-stimulating hormone (TSH) 628, 629
  hyperthyroidism 634
thyroxine 632
  excess 632, 635
  hyperthyroidism 632, 634, 635
  therapy for hypothyroidism 631, 632
tiagabine 371
tick bite, Lyme disease 453
tics, Tourette's syndrome 786–8, 792
tin protoporphyrin 672
tissue plasminogen activator, recombinant (rt-PA) 481
Todd's paresis 310
Token Test 148–9
tolerance
  barbiturates 708
  benzodiazepines 708
  cannabis 712
  opiates 711
  psychostimulants 714
toluene 720–1
tonic–clonic seizures 312
  antiepileptics **367**
  on awakening 316
tonic seizures 312
'top of the basilar' syndrome 478
topiramate 370
topographical disorientation 67, 118
topographical sense 118
torticollis, spasmodic 783–5
  aetiology 784
  clinical features 783–4
  treatment 784–5

total anterior circulation infarcts (TACI) 475–6
Tourette's syndrome *see* Gilles de la Tourette syndrome
Tower of London Test 153–4
toxic disorders 721–32
  drug therapy toxic effects 721–4
  environmental toxins 721
  epilepsy 331–2
  heavy metals 724–32
  toxic confusional state 5
  see also drug misuse; neurotoxicity
toxoplasmosis, AIDS 403, 420–1
Trail Making Test 154
transformation, illusions 74–6
transient epileptic amnesia 33, 325
transient global amnesia 33, 362
transient ischaemic attacks 478–9
  differential diagnosis 479
    epilepsy 360
transient loss of consciousness 357
transmissible spongiform encephalopathies 584–8
trauma *see* injury
travel phobia, head injury 219
tremor
  alcoholic 693
  benign essential 757
  hyperthyroidism 633
  neurosyphilis 426
  pallidotomy 761
  Parkinson's disease/parkinsonian syndrome 753–4, 757
  see also delirium tremens
Treponema pallidum see syphilis (neurosyphilis; *T. pallidum*)
treponemal tests 424, 428
  see also syphilis
tricyclic antidepressants
  cataplexy treatment 828–9
  epilepsy 378
  Parkinson's disease/parkinsonian syndrome 767
trihexyphenidyl 768
tri-iodothyronine (T_3)
  excess 632
  hyperthyroidism 632, 634
  hypothyroidism treatment 632
triplet repeat disorders 577
triptans 511
'Trojan horse' hypothesis of HIV infection of CNS 405
Tropheryma whippelii (Whipple's disease) 881
Trousseau's sign 664
trypanosomiasis 454
TSC1 and *TSC2* genes 854
tuberculosis (*M. tuberculosis*)
  HIV and 404
  meningeal 451–2
tuberous sclerosis 853–4
tumour suppressor gene mutations 281
tumours 281–308, 329
  aggression 78
  AIDS-related 400, 404–5, 420

cerebellar 296–7
diagnostic errors 298–301
epidemiology and aetiology 281–2
epilepsy 329, 331
  management 301
  temporal lobe 289, 291
general paresis differential diagnosis 429–30
genetic factors 281–2
histological types *282*
imaging 297–8, **299**
investigations 297–8
location/distribution **282**, 286–97
management/treatment 301–4
neuropsychiatric manifestations 868–71, *872*
neuropsychiatric symptoms
  factors governing formation 285–97
  general characteristics 282–5
  management 302
neurotoxicity of treatment 284
  chemotherapy/radiotherapy 302
subdural haematoma differential diagnosis 513
thalamic 293
thromboembolism 301
urinary symptoms 288
Turcot's syndrome 281, 855
Turner's syndrome 617, 674–5
twilight states 5
typhus 454

U
ubiquitin
  frontotemporal dementia 576
  Huntington's disease 584
ultrasonography of tumours 297
unawareness, unilateral 71, 118
unconsciousness *see* consciousness, impairment and loss
Unverricht–Lundborg disease **327**, 328
uraemia 666–9
  hypersomnia 835
  mental disturbances 668–9
  vestibulocochlear nerve 667
uraemic encephalopathy 667, 668
Urbach–Weithe disease 65
utilisation behaviour 59

V
vacuolar myelopathy, HIV-associated 407, 412, 413
vagal nerve stimulation, epilepsy 374
valproate (sodium valproate) 367, 369
  head injury 251
varicella-zoster virus 437–8
  AIDS 404
vascular dementia 128, 562, 566–71
  Alzheimer's disease 570
  epidemiology 571
  management 594, 595
  neuropathology 570–1
  poststroke 482
vascular risk factors, Alzheimer's disease 562–3

vascular syndromes, genetic factors 569–70
vasculitis 522–7
  cerebral 715
    HIV disease 407
  primary 522, 523–4
  systemic 522
vasopressin *see* antidiuretic hormone (ADH)
vasovagal syncope 358, 365
Venereal Disease Research Laboratory
        (VDRL) test 424, 428
venous thrombosis
  cerebral 528–9
  deep tumour-related 301
ventricular dilatation
  alcoholics 698, 699
  Wilson's disease 773
ventriculomegaly, head injury 172, 177–8
verbal aggression in head injury 209
verbal fluency
  assessment 113
  tests 151
verbal memory tests 155
vertebral artery
  aneurysms 499
  occlusion 477–8
vertigo
  epilepsy differential diagnosis 360
  post-traumatic 234–5
very-long-chain saturated fatty acids
        (VLCFA) 877
vestibulocochlear nerve 667
vigabatrin 371
vigilance tests **124**, 154
Vineland Social Maturity Scale 157
violence
  alcohol abuse 691
  epilepsy 350–1
  head injury 209, 210
    caused by emotional reaction 195
  somnambulism 838
  see also aggression
viral infection
  vasculitis secondary to 523
  see also encephalitis; meningitis
visual disorientation 67
visual disturbances
  giant cell arteritis 526–7
  internal carotid artery occlusion 476
  migraine 501
visual evoked responses, multiple sclerosis
        845
visual field defects
  acromegaly 644
  diencephalic lesions 19–20
  occipital lobe lesions 19
  temporal lobe lesions 19
visual hallucinations
  dementia with Lewy bodies 572
  LSD 718
  occipital lobe epilepsy 324
  temporal lobe epilepsy 321
visual memory tests 155
visual neglect 67–8
visual object and Space Perception Battery
        147

visuospatial ability assessment **111**, 114–15
visuospatial difficulties 66–8
  Balint's syndrome 66
  parietal lobe lesions 18
vitamin B
  alcoholic intoxication treatment 692
  deficiency 652–60
vitamin B$_1$ deficiency *see* thiamine
        deficiency
vitamin B$_2$ deficiency 653
vitamin B$_6$ deficiency 653
vitamin B$_{12}$ deficiency 655–8
  dementia 590, 656–7
  mood disorders 656
  one-carbon metabolism 658
  psychosis 656
vitamin C, alcoholic intoxication treatment
        692
vitamin D
  deficiency 664
  intoxication 664
  multiple sclerosis 844
vitamin deficiencies 652–60
  psychostimulant use 714
vitamin therapy, high-potency 703, 704
VLSM maps 50, Plate 2.1
vocalisations, Tourette's syndrome 787–8
vocation *see* occupation
volatile solvents 719–20
volitional movement assessment **111**
voltage-gated ion channels in epilepsy
  antiepileptic drug actions on **372**
  genetic mutations **327**
voltage-gated potassium channel (VGKC)
        antibodies 663
von Economo's disease *see* encephalitis
        lethargica
von Recklinghausen's disease 854–6, 855
voxel-based morphometry, schizophrenia
        83–4, Plate 2.2
VZV *see* varicella-zoster virus

W

Warrington, Elizabeth 31
water intoxication 645
watershed infarcts 476
Wechsler Adult Intelligence Scale (WAIS)
        121–2
Wechsler Memory Scale (WMS) 123
Wegener's granulomatosis 525, 526
Wernicke–Lichtheim model 49
Wernicke's area 47
Wernicke's encephalopathy 34, 699–704
  alcohol/alcohol abuse/alcoholism 34,
        655, 699–700, 706
  alcoholic peripheral neuropathy 706
  beriberi 700–1
  central pontine myelinolysis 707
  chronic amnesic syndrome 7
  clinical features 701–2
  confabulation 41
  course 702
  high-potency vitamin therapy 703
  hypophosphataemia differential
        diagnosis 665

  investigations 702
  Korsakoff's syndrome relationship 704,
        705
  pathology 702–3
  response to treatment 702
  subclinical 703
  susceptibility 700
  thiamine deficiency 653
  treatment 703–4
West Nile virus 432, 433
West syndrome 317
Westphal-variant Huntington's disease 579
whiplash injury 235–7
Whipple's disease 881
white matter hyperintensities 137–9
white matter lesions
  small-vessel disease 567–8
  subcortical in SLE 519
WHO *see* World Health Organization
        (WHO)
willed movement disturbance, encephalitis
        lethargica 445–6
Wilson's disease 593, 772–6
  biochemical abnormalities 773–4
  clinical features 772–3
  course 773
  manganese toxicity 729
  outcome 773
  Parkinson's disease differential diagnosis
        757
  pathology 773
  psychiatric manifestations 774–6
  treatment 774
Wisconsin Card Sorting Test 151–2
word finding 113
word-blindness, pure 52
word-deafness, pure 52
word-dumbness, pure 52–3
work *see* occupation
World Federation of Neurosurgical Societies
        (WFNS) scale for subarachnoid
        haemorrhage 491
World Health Organization (WHO)
  head injury severity scoring 185–6
  HIV clinical staging and case definition
        401
  International Classification of
        Impairments, Disabilities and
        Handicaps 247
writing
  assessment 113
  Wernicke's aphasia 51–2

X
xanthochromia 131

Z
Zellweger's disease 877
zinc
  deficiency 665
  Wilson's disease therapy 774
Zollinger–Ellison syndrome 635
zonisamide 371